The Genetic Basis
of Human Cancer

The Genetic Basis of Human Cancer

Second Edition

EDITORS

Bert Vogelstein, M.D.
Investigator, Howard Hughes Medical Institute
Clayton Professor of Oncology and Pathology
The Johns Hopkins University School of Medicine
Baltimore, Maryland

Kenneth W. Kinzler, Ph.D.
Professor of Oncology
The Johns Hopkins University School of Medicine
Baltimore, Maryland

McGraw-Hill
Medical Publishing Division

New York   Chicago   San Francisco   Lisbon   London   Madrid   Mexico City   Milan   New Delhi
San Juan   Seoul   Singapore   Sydney   Toronto

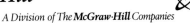

McGraw-Hill

A Division of The McGraw·Hill Companies

1234567890 PBTPBT 098765432

ISBN 0-07-137050-1
This book was set in Times Roman by Progressive Information Technologies, Inc.
The editors were Andrea Seils, Susan R. Noujaim, and Peter J. Boyle; the production supervisor was Phil Galea; the text designer was José R. Fonfrias; the cover designer was Elizabeth Schmitz; Kathrin Unger prepared the index.
Phoenix Book Technology was printer and binder.
This book is printed on acid-free paper.

Acknowledgments
Chapters 1–7, 9–34, and 39–50 were adapted from Scriver CR, Beaudet AL, Sly WS, Valle D (eds.): *The Metabolic & Molecular Bases of Inherited Disease*, 8th edition, copyright © 2001 by The McGraw-Hill Companies, Inc.

Library of Congress Cataloging-in-Publication Data

The genetic basis of cancer / editors, Bert Vogelstein, Kenneth W. Kinzler. – 2nd ed.
    p.; cm.
  Includes bibliographical references and index.
  ISBN 0-07-137050-1
  1. Cancer – Genetic aspects. I. Vogelstein, Bert. II. Kinzler, Kenneth W.
  [DNLM: 1. Neoplasms – genetics. 2. Cell Transformation, Neoplastic – genetics. 3. Gene Expression – genetics. 4. Mutagenesis – genetics. QZ 202 G3297 2002]
  RC268.4.G445 2002
  616.99′4042 – dc21

                                       2001044560

We would like to thank the young investigators
(postdoctoral fellows and students) whose contributions
often go unrecognized but who are largely responsible for the revolution
in cancer research that has occurred over the last two decades.

CONTENTS

PART 4
CANCER BY SITE

Lauri A. Aaltonen, MD, PhD
Senior Fellow, Academy of Finland
Dept. of Medical Genetics
University of Helsinki
Helsinki, Finland
lauri.aaltonen@helsinki.fi
Chapter 20

Naji Al-Dosari, MD
Duke University
Durham, North Carolina
naji@acpub.duke.edu
Chapter 47

Stylianos E. Antonarakis, MD
Professor and Director, Div. of Medical Genetics
University of Geneva Medical School
Geneva, Switzerland
stylianos.antonarakis@medicine.unige.ch
Chapter 2

Arleen D. Auerbach, PhD
Associate Professor, Human Genetics and Hematology
The Rockefeller University
New York, New York
auerbac@rockvax.rockefeller.edu
Chapter 17

Craig T. Basson, MD, PhD
Director, Molecular Cardiology Laboratory
Cardiology Division, Dept. of Medicine
Weill Medical College of Cornell University
New York, New York
ctbasson@med.cornell.edu
Chapter 38

Stephen B. Baylin, MD
Professor of Oncology and Medicine
Associate Director for Research
Dept. of Medicine
The Johns Hopkins Oncology Center
Baltimore, Maryland
Chapter 48

Graham R. Bignell, PhD
Cancer Genome Project, Sanger Centre
Wellcome Trust Genome Campus
Cambridge, England, United Kingdom
grb@sanger.ac.uk
Chapter 37

Sandra H. Bigner, MD
Professor of Pathology
Dept. of Pathology
Duke University Medical Center
Durham, North Carolina
bigne002@mc.duke.edu
Chapter 47

C. Richard Boland, MD
Chief, Division of Gastroenterology
University of California at San Diego
La Jolla, California
crboland@ucsd.edu
Chapter 18

Dirk Bootsma, MD
Dept. of Cell Biology and Genetics
Erasmus University
Rotterdam, the Netherlands
bootsma@gen.fgg.eur.nl
Chapter 14

G. Steven Bova, MD
Assistant Professor, Dept. of Pathology
The Johns Hopkins Hospital
Baltimore, Maryland
gbov@jhmi.edu
Chapter 46

Garrett M. Brodeur, MD
Chief, Division of Oncology
Children's Hospital of Philadelphia
Philadelphia, Pennsylvania
brodeur@email.chop.edu
Chapters 6, 50

Manuel Buchwald, OC, PhD, FRSC
Professor, Molecular and Medical Genetics
Dept. of Genetics
University of Toronto
Chief of Research and Director, Research Institute
Hospital for Sick Children
Toronto, Ontario, Canada
manuel.buchwald@sickkids.on.ca
Chapter 17

Daniel P. Cahill, MD, PhD
Dept. of Medicine
The Johns Hopkins Oncology Center
Baltimore, Maryland
Chapter 7

Paul Cairns, MD
Fox Chase Cancer Center
Philadelphia, Pennsylvania
Chapter 44

Webster Cavenee, MD
Director, Ludwig Institute for Cancer Research
University of California, San Diego
La Jolla, California
Chapter 22

Edward F. Chan, MD
Dept. of Dermatology
University of Pennsylvania Medical Center
Philadelphia, Pennsylvania
Chapter 35

Kathleen R. Cho, MD
Associate Professor, Dept. of Pathology
University of Michigan Medical School
Ann Arbor, Michigan
kathcho@umich.edu
Chapter 43

James E. Cleaver, MD
Dept. of Dermatology
University of California at San Francisco Cancer Center
San Francisco, California
jcleaver@cc.ucsf.edu
Chapter 14

Bruce E. Clurman, MD
Assistant Professor, Div. of Basic Sciences
Fred Hutchinson Cancer Research Center
Seattle, Washington
bclurman@fhcrc.org
Chapter 9

Anne-Marie Codori, PhD
Dept. of Psychiatry and Behavioral Sciences
The Johns Hopkins University School of Medicine
Baltimore, Maryland
Chapter 39

Francis S. Collins, MD
National Center for Human Genome Research
Bethesda, Maryland
fc23@nih.gov
Chapter 25

David N. Cooper, MD
Professor of Human Molecular Genetics
Institute of Medical Genetics
University of Wales College of Medicine
Cardiff, Wales, United Kingdom
cooperdn@cardiff.ac.uk
Chapter 2

Cees J. Cornelisse, PhD
Professor, Dept. of Pathology
Leiden University Medical Center
Leiden, the Netherlands
c.j.cornelisse@lumc.nl
Chapter 36

Fergus J. Couch, MD
Breast Cancer Program
University of Pennsylvania Medical School
Philadelphia, Pennsylvania
Chapter 33

Ramanuj Dasgupta, MD
Dept. of Molecular Genetics and Cell Biology
Howard Hughes Medical Insititute
The University of Chicago
Chicago, Illinois
Chapter 35

Peter Devilee, PhD
Dept. of Human Genetics
Leiden University Medical Center
Leiden, the Netherlands
p.devilee@lumc.nl
Chapter 36

Louis Dubeau, MD, PhD
Professor, Dept. of Pathology
Keck School of Medicine
University of Southern California
Los Angeles, California
ldubeau@hsc.usc.edu
Chapter 41

Lora Hedrick Ellenson, MD
Director, Division of Gynecologic Pathology
Medical College of Cornell University
New York, New York
lhellens@med.cornell.edu
Chapter 42

Nathan A. Ellis, MD
Associate Member, Dept. of Human Genetics
Memorial Sloan-Kettering Cancer Center
New York, New York
n-ellis@ski.mskcc.org
Chapter 16

Lynne W. Elmore, PhD
Dept. of Pathology
The Medical College of Virginia
Richmond, Virginia
Chapter 49

Charis Eng, MD, PhD
Associate Professor and Director
Clinical Cancer Genetics Program
Comprehensive Cancer Center
Ohio State University
Columbus, Ohio
ceng@bcm.tmc.edu
Chapter 31

Eric R. Fearon, MD, PhD
Div. of Molecular Medicine and Genetics
University of Michigan Medical Center
Ann Arbor, Michigan
fearon@umich.edu
Chapter 12

Andrew P. Feinberg, MD
Professor, Dept. of Medicine and Molecular Biology
The Johns Hopkins University
Baltimore, Maryland
Chapter 3

Elaine Fuchs, MD
Amgen Professor of Basic Sciences
Dept. of Molecular Genetics and Cell Biology
Howard Hughes Medical Institute
University of Chicago
Chicago, Illinois
lain@midway.uchicago.edu
Chapter 35

Uri Gat, MD
Silverman Life Sciences Institute
Hebrew University
Jerusalem, Israel
Chapter 35

Richard A. Gatti, MD
Professor, Dept. of Pathology
School of Medicine
University of California, Los Angeles
Los Angeles, California
rgatti@mednet.ucla.edu
Chapter 15

James L. German, III, MD
Professor, Dept. of Pediatrics
Weill Medical College
Cornell University
New York, New York
jlg2003@mail.med.cornell.edu
Chapter 16

James F. Gusella, PhD
Molecular Neurogenetics Unit
Massachussets General Hospital
Charlestown, Maryland
Chapter 26

David H. Gutmann, MD, PhD
Dept. of Neurology
Washington University School of Medicine
St. Louis, Missouri
Chapter 25

Daniel A. Haber, MD
Associate Professor of Medicine
Harvard Medical School
Director, Center for Cancer Risk Analysis
Massachusetts General Hospital Cancer Center
Laboratory of Molecular Genetics
Charlestown, Massachusetts
haber@helix.mgh.harvard.edu
Chapter 24

Theodora Hadjistilianou, MD
Associate Professor, Dept. of Ophthalmology
University of Siena School of Medicine
Siena, Tuscany, Italy
Chapter 22

Curtis C. Harris, MD
Chief, Laboratory of Human Carcinogenesis
National Cancer Institute
Bethesda, Maryland
Chapter 49

Meenhard Herlyn, PhD
Professor, The Wistar Institute
Philadelphia, Pennsylvania
herlynm@wistar.upenn.edu
Chapter 30

Jan H.J. Hoeijmakers, MD
Dept. of Cell Biology and Genetics
Erasmus University
Rotterdam, the Netherlands
hoeijmakers@sgen.fgg.eur.nl
Chapter 14

Michael D. Hogarty, MD
Clinical Associate, Division of Oncology
Children's Hospital of Philadelphia
Philadelphia, Pennsylvania
hogartym@email.chop.edu
Chapter 6

James R. Howe, MD
Assistant Professor of Surgery
University of Iowa College of Medicine
Iowa City, Iowa
james_howe@uiowa.edu
Chapter 21

Ralph H. Hruban, MD
Professor, Dept. of Oncology and Pathology
The Johns Hopkins University School of Medicine
Baltimore, Maryland
Chapter 40

William B. Isaacs, PhD
Professor of Urology and Oncology
Dept. of Urology
The Johns Hopkins Hospital
Baltimore, Maryland
wissacs@mail.jhmi.edu
Chapter 46

Hans Joenje, PhD
Senior Scientist, Dept. of Clinical and Human Genetics
Free University Medical Center
Amsterdam, the Netherlands
h.joenje.humgen@med.vu.nl
Chapter 17

Anne Kallioniemi, MD
Cancer Genetics Branch
National Human Genome Research Institute
Bethesda, Maryland
Chapter 5

Alexander Kamb, PhD
President and Chief Executive Officer
Arcaris, Inc.
Salt Lake City, Utah
kamb@arcaris.com
Chapter 30

Scott E. Kern, MD
Associate Professor
Dept. of Oncology and Pathology
The Johns Hopkins University
Baltimore, Maryland
sk@jhmi.edu
Chapter 40

Kenneth W. Kinzler, PhD
Professor of Oncology
The Johns Hopkins University School of Medicine
Baltimore, Maryland
kinzlke@jhmi.edu
Chapters 1, 13, 34

Richard D. Klausner, MD
National Cancer Institute
Bethesda, Maryland
Chapter 27

Kenneth H. Kraemer, MD
Principal Investigator
Laboratory of Molecular Carcinogenesis
National Cancer Institute
Bethesda, Maryland
kraemer@nih.gov
Chapter 14

Michael Krawczak, MD
Professor, Institute of Medical Genetics
University of Wales College of Medicine
Cardiff, Wales, United Kingdom
krawczak@cardiff.ac.uk
Chapter 2

Christoph Lengauer, MD
The Johns Hopkins Oncology Center
Baltimore, Maryland
Chapter 7

W. Marston Linehan, MD
Chief, Urologic Oncology Branch
National Cancer Institute
Bethesda, Maryland
wml@nih.gov
Chapter 27

Dan L. Longo, MD
Scientific Director
National Institute on Aging
Baltimore and Bethesda, Maryland
longod@grc.nia.nih.gov
Chapter 52

A. Thomas Look, MD
Dana-Farber Cancer Institute
Boston, Massachusetts
thomas_look@dfci.harvard.edu
Chapter 4

Mack Mabry, MD
Medical Director
Matrix Pharmaceutical Inc.
Fremont, California
Chapter 48

Mia MacCollin, MD
Molecular Neurogenetics Lab
Massachusetts General Hospital East
Charlestown, Massachusetts
maccollin@helix.mgh.harvard.edu
Chapter 26

David Malkin, MD
Associate Professor, Dept. of Pediatrics
Hospital for Sick Children
Toronto, Ontario, Canada
david.malkin@sickkids.on.ca
Chapter 23

Stephen J. Marx, MD
Chief, Genetics and Endocrine Sect.
National Institute of Diabetes, Digestive, and Kidney Diseases
Bethesda, Maryland
stephenm@intra.niddk.nih.gov
Chapter 28

Roger E. McLendon, MD
Associate Professor, Dept. of Pathology
Duke University Medical Center
Durham, North Carolina
Chapter 47

Paul S. Meltzer, MD, PhD
Sect. of Molecular Cytogenetics
Laboratory of Cancer Genetics
National Institutes of Health
Bethesda, Maryland
Chapter 5

Tetsuro Miki, MD, PhD
Professor, Dept. of Geriatric Medicine
School of Medicine, Ehime University
Ehime, Japan
miki@m.ehime-u.ac.jp
Chapter 19

Patrice J. Morin, PhD
Investigator
Laboratory of Biological Chemistry
National Institute on Aging
Associate Professor of Pathology
The Johns Hopkins University
Baltimore, Maryland
morinp@grc.nia.nih.gov
Chapter 8

Jun Nakura, MD, PhD
Research Associate, Dept. of Geriatric Medicine
School of Medicine, Ehime University
Ehime, Japan
nakura@m.ehime-u.ac.jp
Chapter 19

Barry D. Nelkin, MD
Associate Professor of Oncology
The Johns Hopkins Oncology Center
Baltimore, Maryland
Chapter 48

Irene F. Newsham, PhD
David and Doreen Hermelin Scholar
Laboratory of Molecular Oncogenetics
Dept. of Neurosurgery and Hermelin Brain Tumor Institute

Henry Ford Hospital
Detroit, Michigan
irene@bogler.net
Chapter 22

Morag Park, MD
Associate Professor
Molecular Oncology Group
Royal Victoria Hospital, McGill University
Montreal, Quebec, Canada
morag@lan1.molonc.mcgill.ca
Chapter 11

Ramon Parsons, MD, PhD
Assistant Professor, Dept. of Pathology
Columbia University Cancer Center
New York, New York
rep15@columbia.edu
Chapter 31

Gloria M. Petersen, PhD
Professor of Clinical Epidemiology
Mayo Foundation
Rochester, Minnesota
peterg@mayo.edu
Chapter 39

B.A.J. Ponder, PhD, FRCP
Professor, CRC Dept. of Oncology
Cambridge Institute for Medical Research
Cambridge, England, United Kingdom
bajp@mole.bio.cam.ac.uk
Chapter 29

Steven M. Powell, MD
Assistant Professor, Div. of Gastroenterology
University of Virginia Health Sciences Center
Charlottesville, Virginia
smp8n@virginia.edu
Chapter 45

Ahmed Rasheed, MD
Research Assistant Professor
Duke University Medical Center
Durham, North Carolina
a.rasheed@duke.edu
Chapter 47

Jonathan L. Rees, MBBS, FRCP
Professor and Chairman, Dept. of Dermatology
The University of Edinburgh
Edinburgh, Scotland, United Kingdom
jonathan.rees@ed.ac.uk
Chapter 32

Gregory J. Riggins, MD, PhD
Assistant Professor of Pathology and Genetics
Duke Univ. Medical Center
Durham, North Carolina
riggi003@mc.duke.edu
Chapter 8

James M. Roberts, MD
Division of Basic Sciences
Fred Hutchinson Cancer Research Center
Seattle, Washington
Chapter 9

Charles M. Rudin, MD
Assistant Professor of Medicine
Howard Hughes Medical Institute, Research Labs
University of Chicago Medical Center
Chicago, Illinois
crudin@medicine.bsd.uchicago.edu
Chapter 10

Gerard D. Schellenberg, PhD
Veterans Affairs Medical Center
Seattle, Washington
zachdad@u.washington.edu
Chapter 19

David Sidransky, MD
Division of Head and Neck Cancer Research
The Johns Hopkins University
Baltimore, Maryland
dsidrans@jhmi.edu
Chapter 44

Michael R. Stratton, MD, PhD
Cancer Genome Project, Sanger Centre
Wellcome Trust Genome Campus
Cambridge, England, United Kingdom
mrs@sanger.ac.uk
Chapter 37

Craig B. Thompson, MD
Howard Hughes Medical Institute
Research Laboratories
University of Chicago
Chicago, Illinois
Chapter 10

Jeffrey M. Trent, MD, PhD
Chief, Laboratory of Cancer Genetics
National Center for Human Genome Research
Bethesda, Maryland
Chapter 5

Andel G.L. van der Mey, MD, PhD
Dept. of Otolaryngology
Leiden University Medical Center
Leiden, the Netherlands
a.g.l.van_der_mey@lumc.nl
Chapter 36

Carl J. Vaughn, MD
Cardiology Div., Dept. of Medicine
Dept. of Cell Biology
Weill Medical College of Cornell University
The New York Presbyterian Hospital
New York, New York
Chapter 38

Mark Veugelers, PhD
Cardiology Div., Dept. of Medicine
Dept. of Cell Biology

Weill Medical College of Cornell University
The New York Presbyterian Hospital
New York, New York
mav2015@med.cornell.edu
Chapter 38

Bert Vogelstein, MD
Investigator
Howard Hughes Medical Institute
Clayton Professor of Oncology and Pathology
The Johns Hopkins University School of Medicine
Baltimore, Maryland
vogelbe@welch.jhu.edu
Chapters 1, 13, 34

Saman Warnakulasuriya, BDS, PhD
Professor in Oral Medicine and Experimental Oral Pathology
Dept. of Oral Medicine and Pathology
WHO Collaborating Center for Oral Cancer and Precancer
Guy's, King's and St Thomas' School of Dentistry
King's College London
London, England, United Kingdom
Chapter 51

Barbara L. Weber, MD
Director, Breast Cancer Program
University of Pennsylvania Medical School
Philadelphia, Pennsylvania
Chapter 33

Charles J. Yeo, MD
Dept. of Surgery and Oncology
The Johns Hopkins Hospital
Baltimore, Maryland
Chapter 40

Chang-En Yu, MD, PhD
Veterans Affairs Puget Sound Health Care System
Dept. of Medicine
University of Washington
Seattle, Washington
changeyu@uwashington.edu
Chapter 19

Berton Zbar, MD
Chief, Laboratory of Immunobiology
Basic Sciences Division, National Cancer Institute
Frederick Cancer Research and Development Center
Frederick, Maryland
zbar@ncifcrf.gov
Chapter 27

PART
1

BASIC CONCEPTS IN CANCER GENETICS

CHAPTER 1

Introduction

Kenneth W. Kinzler ■ *Bert Vogelstein*

As late as the 1970s, human cancers remained a black box. Theories were abundant: Cancer was hypothesized to result from defective immunity, viruses, dysregulated differentiation, mutations. . . . In the absence of hard evidence to confirm or refute any of these theories, it was difficult to be optimistic that cancer would soon be understood, or that there was much hope for patients afflicted with disease.

This has changed dramatically as a result of the revolution in cancer research that has occurred in the last decade. If this revolution were to be summarized in a single sentence, that sentence would be: "Cancer is, in essence, a genetic disease." Although cancer is complex, and environmental and other nongenetic factors clearly play a role in many stages of the neoplastic process, the tremendous progress made in understanding tumorigenesis in large part is owing to the discovery of the genes that, when mutated, lead to cancer. This book pays tribute to this revolution by assembling what is known about the genetic basis of human cancer in a single text, with chapters written by scientists who have made seminal contributions to this knowledge.

The book began as an addition to the classic textbook, *The Metabolic and Molecular Bases of Inherited Disease*. It was soon realized that there was so much information about the genetic basis of human cancer that a separate, more focused book was warranted. It is important to note at the outset that our purpose was not to record everything that is known about cancer; excellent textbooks on the clinical aspects of cancer, on biochemical issues related to cancer, on environmental aspects related to cancer, already exist. Our purpose was to focus on the genes that cause cancer, and to attempt to answer the following questions whenever possible: What fraction of a specific cancer type is associated with a clear genetic component? What are the genes involved? What is the nature of the mutations in these genes? How do these genes work? What are the implications of knowledge about genes for diagnosis and future treatment?

In these introductory comments, we attempt to address some very basic questions about genes and cancer that hopefully will help put the book in perspective and explain its organization.

HOW IS CANCER DIFFERENT FROM OTHER GENETIC DISEASES?

The simplest genetic diseases (e.g., Duchenne muscular dystrophy) are caused by inherited mutations in a single gene that are necessary and sufficient to determine the phenotype (Fig. 1-1). This phenotype generally can be predicted from knowledge of the precise mutation, and modifying genes or environmental influences often play little role. More complex are certain diseases in which single defective genes can predispose patients to pathologic conditions, but the defective gene itself is not sufficient to guarantee the onset of clinically manifest disease. For example, patients who inherit defective low density lipoprotein receptor encoding genes are prone to atherosclerosis, but environmental influences, particularly dietary lipids, play a large role in determining the severity of disease.

Certain cancers display an obvious hereditary influence, but like atherosclerosis, the defective inherited gene is itself not sufficient for the development of cancer. Cancers only become manifest following accumulation of additional somatic mutations. These occur either as a result of the imperfection of the DNA copying apparatus ($\sim 10^{-10}$ mutations per base pair per somatic cell generation) or through DNA damage caused by environmental mutagens.

DO CANCERS OCCUR ONLY IN PATIENTS WHO INHERIT A DEFECTIVE CANCER GENE?

It is estimated that only a small fraction (0.1 to 10 percent, depending on the cancer type) of the total cancers in the Western world occur in patients with a hereditary mutation. However, one of the cardinal principles of modern cancer research is that the same genes cause both inherited and sporadic (noninherited) forms of the same tumor type (Fig. 1-2). This principle, first enunciated by Knudson, is well illustrated by retinoblastomas in children (see Chap. 22) and kidney cancers (see Chap. 27) and colorectal tumors in adults (see Chap. 34). For example, approximately 0.5 percent of colorectal cancer patients inherit a defective *APC* gene from one of their parents. This inherited mutation is not sufficient to initiate tumorigenesis. However, every cell of the colon from such patients is "at risk" for acquiring a second mutation, and two mutations of the right type are believed to be sufficient for initiation. The great majority of colorectal cancer patients (> 99 percent of the total) do not inherit a mutant *APC* gene. However, these sporadic cases also require *APC* mutations to begin the tumorigenic process. In these sporadic cases, the *APC* mutations occur somatically in isolated colorectal epithelial cells. The number of colorectal epithelial cells with *APC* mutations is therefore several orders of magnitude less in the sporadic cases than in the inherited cases, in which every cell has an *APC* mutation. Accordingly, patients with the hereditary mutations often develop multiple tumors instead of single, isolated tumors, and patients with the familial form of the disease develop tumors at an earlier age than the sporadic patients.

What is the "second mutation," alluded to above, that initiates clinically apparent neoplasia in both the hereditary and sporadic types of tumors? In most known examples, the second mutation is believed to result in inactivation of the wild-type allele inherited from the unaffected parent. As described below, genes that, when mutated, lead to cancer predisposition normally suppress tumorigenesis. If one allele of such a gene (e.g., *APC*) is mutated in the germ line, then the cell still has the product of the wild-type allele as a backup. If a somatic mutation of the wild-type allele occurs, however, then the resulting cell will have no functional suppressor gene product remaining and will begin to proliferate abnormally (*clonal expansion*). One of the cells in the proliferating clone is then likely to accumulate another mutation, resulting in further loss of growth control. Through gradual clonal expansion, a tumor will evolve, with each successive mutation providing a further growth advantage, allowing its progeny to continue to replicate in microenvironments inhibitory to the growth of cells with fewer mutations.

A list of standard abbreviations is located immediately preceding the index. Nonstandard abbreviations used in this chapter include: LOH = loss of heterozygosity.

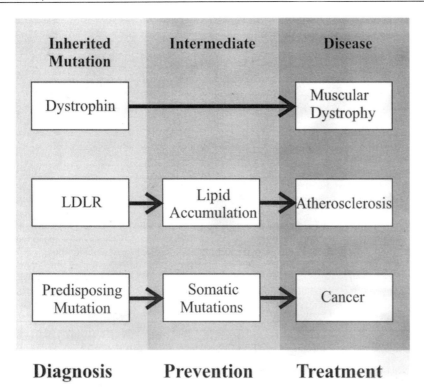

Fig. 1-1 Comparison of genetic diseases. Three types of genetic diseases, of increasing complexity, are illustrated (*Reprinted by permission from Kinzler KW and Vogelstein B: Lessons from hereditary colon cancer Cell 87:161, 1996; copyright 1996 by Cell Press.*)

ARE THE DNA ALTERATIONS IN CANCER DIFFERENT FROM THOSE IN OTHER GENETICALLY DETERMINED DISEASES?

Five different types of genetic alterations have been observed in tumor cells:

1. *Subtle alterations.* Small deletions, insertions, and single base-pair substitutions occur in cancers just as they do in other hereditary diseases (see Chap. 2).

2. *Chromosome number changes.* Somatic losses or gains of chromosomes are often observed in cancers. Although such aneuploidy is occasionally a cause of other inherited diseases (e.g., Down syndrome), the degree of aneuploidy is much more extensive in cancers than ever observed in the phenotypically normal cells of mammals. Most cancers are aneuploid, with chromosome numbers ranging from subdiploid to supratetraploid. Molecular studies have shown that the aneuploidy observed in karyotypic studies actually underestimates the extent of gross chromosomal changes in cancer cells. Even

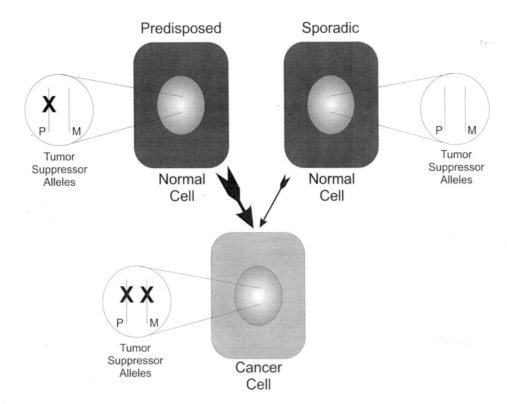

Fig. 1-2 Tumor suppressor gene inactivation. Tumor suppressor gene mutations are thought to initiate many forms of cancer. Both alleles of the tumor suppressor gene must be inactivated for a tumor to form. In familial cancer predisposition syndromes, a mutant allele of a suppressor gene is inherited and is present in every cell. However, tumors are not initiated until the second allele (inherited from the unaffected parent) is inactivated in a somatic cell. In nonfamilial cases, the inactivation of both alleles occurs through somatic mutations. The end result is the same: no functional suppressor gene, leading to tumor initiation.

when cancer cells appear to have two normal copies of a chromosome by karyotype, molecular analyses reveal that both chromosomes often are from the same parent. Thus, instead of one maternal and one paternal chromosome 17 per cell, the cancer cell may have no maternal chromosome 17 and two paternal chromosomes 17. This *loss of heterozygosity* (LOH) often affects more than half the chromosomes in an individual cancer cell. LOH provides an efficient way for the cell to inactivate genes. For example, consider a cell containing two copies of chromosome 5, one with a mutation of a chromosome 5 tumor suppressor gene and the other with a wild-type allele of this gene. The wild-type copy of the gene often will prevent the cell from abnormal proliferation. If the chromosome containing this wild-type allele is lost, then the cell will be left with only the mutant copy of the suppressor gene, and a selective growth advantage will accrue. Such LOH events occur at much higher rates (10^{-5} per generation) than subtle mutations ($\sim 10^{-7}$ per gene per generation), affording the cancer cell a powerful means of ridding itself of wild-type growth-constraining genes. LOH generally occurs through loss of an entire chromosome or through mitotic recombination. Whole chromosome losses are often associated with a duplication of the remaining chromosome, thus making this event invisible by karyotypic methods but detectable by molecular analyses using DNA polymorphisms as probes. Mitotic recombinations generally can be observed only through molecular analyses.

3. *Chromosome translocations.* Balanced and unbalanced translocations are observed frequently in cancers, where they occur by somatic rather than germ-line mutation. In common cancers of epithelial origin (e.g., breast, colon, prostate, stomach), the translocations appear to be random, with no specific breakpoints at the chromosomal or molecular levels. In contrast, leukemias and lymphomas generally contain characteristic translocations that appear to determine many of the biological properties of the neoplasms. For example, acute promyelocytic leukemias virtually always contain a t(15;17) translocation resulting in the fusion of a *Retinoic Acid Receptor* gene on chromosome 17 with the *PML* gene on chromosome 15, and chronic myelogenous leukemias always contain a t(9;22) translocation resulting in fusion of the *abl* oncogene on chromosome 9 with the *BCR* gene on chromosome 22 (see Chap. 4 and 11).

4. *Amplifications.* These alterations are only observed in neoplastic cells in humans and are defined by a five- to hundredfold multiplication of a small region of the chromosome (0.3 to 10 Mb). Gene amplifications generally are observed only in advanced neoplasms. The "amplicons" contain one or more genes whose expression can endow the cell with enhanced proliferative activity, and the higher expression of these genes through an increased copy number is obviously advantageous for the cancer cell (see Chap. 6).

5. *Exogenous sequences.* Certain human cancers are associated with tumor viruses, which contribute genes that result in abnormal cell growth. Representative examples are cervical cancers (see Chap. 43), Burkitt's lymphomas (see Chap. 4), hepatocellular carcinomas (see Chap. 49), and T-cell leukemias (associated with retroviruses). These exogenously introduced genes can best be considered as another class of mutations that contributes to oncogenesis. Like the other mutations described earlier, no exogenous viral gene is sufficient for tumorigenesis. Such viral oncogenes often initiate the tumorigenic process, however, just as defective tumor suppressor genes initiate the process in the many tumors not associated with viral infection.

WHAT GENES ARE MUTATED IN CANCERS?

Two classes of genes are involved in cancer formation. The first class, comprised of oncogenes and tumor suppressor genes, directly controls cellular proliferation. These genes do this by controlling either the rate of cell birth (see Chap. 9) or the rate of cell death (see Chap. 10). Although tumorigenesis largely has been thought of as caused by increases in the rate of cell birth, it is now recognized that tumor expansion represents an imbalance between cell birth and cell death. In normal tissues, cell birth precisely equals cell death, resulting in homeostasis. Defects in either of these processes can result in net growth, perceived as tumorigenesis.

Oncogenes are like the accelerator of an automobile; they normally result in increased cell birth or decreased cell death when expressed (see Chap. 11). A mutation in an oncogene is tantamount to having the cell's "accelerator" pinned to the floor: Cell proliferation continues even when the cell's surrounding environment is giving it clear signals to stop. Mutations in oncogenes include subtle mutations, which change their structure and make them constitutively active, or mutations that increase their expression to levels higher than observed in normal cells.

Continuing with this analogy, tumor suppressor genes are the "brakes" of the cell, normally functioning to inhibit cell growth (see Chap. 12). Just as do automobiles, each cell type has more than one "brake," each of which can be activated under appropriate microenvironmental stimuli. It is only when several of the cell's "brakes" and "accelerators" are rendered dysfunctional through mutation that the cell spins entirely out of control, and cancer ensues.

The second class of genes (caretaker genes) does not control cell growth directly but instead controls the rate of mutation. Cells with defective caretaker genes acquire mutations in all genes, including oncogenes and tumor suppressor genes, at an elevated rate. This higher rate leads to accelerated tumorigenesis. The fact that patients (and cells) with defective caretaker genes are cancer-prone provides one of the most cogent pieces of evidence that mutations in DNA lie at the heart of the neoplastic process.

IS CANCER A SINGLE DISEASE?

Tumors can best be defined as diseases in which a single cell acquires the ability to proliferate abnormally, resulting in an accumulation of progeny. *Cancers* are those tumors which have acquired the ability to invade through surrounding normal tissues. The most advanced form of this invasive process is metastasis, a state in which cancer cells escape from their original location, travel by hematogenous or lymphogenous channels, and take up residence in distant sites. The only difference between a malignant tumor (a.k.a. cancer) and a benign tumor is the capacity of the former to invade. Both benign and malignant tumors can achieve large sizes, but benign tumors are circumscribed and therefore generally can be removed surgically. Malignant tumors often have invaded surrounding or distant tissues prior to their detection, precluding surgical excision of the entire tumor cell population. It is the ability of cancers to destroy other tissues through invasion that makes them lethal.

There are as many tumor types as there are cell types in the human body. Cancers thus represent not a single disease but a group of heterogeneous diseases that share certain biological properties (in particular, clonal cell growth and invasive ability). Cancers can be classified in various ways. Most common cancers of adults are carcinomas, representing cancers derived from epithelial cells. Leukemias and lymphomas are derived from blood-forming cells and lymphoid cells, respectively. Sarcomas are derived from mesenchymal tissues. Melanomas are derived from melanocytes, and retinoblastomas, neuroblastomas, and glioblastomas are derived from stem cells of the retina, neurons, and glia, respectively.

Twenty years ago it could not have been predicted that all these different cancers share common molecular pathogeneses in addition to common biological properties. The cancer research revolution has demonstrated that they do: All result from defects in oncogenes and tumor suppressor genes. Each specific cancer arises through characteristic mutations in specific genes. Although dozens of human oncogenes and tumor suppressor genes have

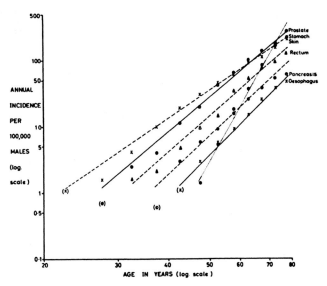

Fig. 1-3 Cancer incidence versus age. The log of the incidence rate and the log of age have a linear relationship, with the incidence increasing dramatically (103- to 107-fold) with age (*Reprinted by permission from Miller DG: On the nature of susceptibility to cancer. The presidential address. Cancer 46:1307,1980; copyright 1980 by the American Cancer Society.*)

been described in the literature, these genes' products appear to converge on a relatively small number of growth-controlling pathways. In some cases, the same gene is involved in multiple cancers. For example, *p53* mutations commonly occur in cancers of the brain, colon, breast, stomach, bladder, and pancreas. In other cases, a defective gene appears to be associated with a single tumor type, such as the *WT1* gene in childhood kidney cancers (see Chap. 24).

HOW MANY MUTATIONS ARE REQUIRED FOR CANCER FORMATION?

Epidemiologic investigations long ago revealed that the incidence of cancer increased exponentially with age (Fig. 1-3). Detailed analysis of age versus incidence curves is consistent with the idea that three to seven mutations are required for full development of cancers. This estimate is consistent with molecular analyses of cancers, in which it is not unusual to observe mutations of four or five different genes. It is generally thought that benign tumors, the precursors of cancers, require fewer mutations (perhaps just two mutations to initiate a small neoplasm). As tumor cells accumulate additional mutations, the resulting clonal expansion causes tumor progression, with progressively larger and more dangerous neoplasms evolving. *Solid tumors* (i.e., those of solid organs such as the colon, bladder, brain, and breast) appear to require a greater number of mutations for their development than *liquid tumors* (i.e., leukemias and lymphomas). The smaller number of mutations required for leukemias may explain the shorter lag time following an initial mutagenic insult. For example, following explosion of the atomic bombs in Japan, leukemias began to appear within a few years, whereas an increased incidence of solid tumors was not evident until at least a decade later.

ORGANIZATION OF THE CANCER CHAPTERS IN THIS BOOK

It is obvious from the preceding that there are numerous interconnections between the principles underlying cancer genetics and that any organization of chapters on cancer is arbitrary. For didactic purposes, however, the chapters are organized into four categories:

The first set of chapters (Chaps. 1–8) focuses on basic concepts in cancer genetics.

The second set of chapters (Chaps. 9–12) is concerned with control of the cell cycle

The third set of chapters (Chaps. 13–39) is devoted to cancers in which heritable mutations of predisposing genes have been identified. These have been divided (see Chap. 13 for additional detail) into those syndromes in which the responsible gene leads to increased mutation rates (caretaker genes) and those in which the responsible gene directly controls cell birth or cell death (gatekeeper genes). Chapter 39 considers the clinical ramifications of inherited predispositions.

The fourth set (Chaps. 40–52) includes chapters on cancers in which heritable predisposing mutations leading to well-defined predisposition syndromes have not been identified. The chapters in this section largely emphasize somatic mutations.

Although this organization necessitates a bit of redundancy, it is hoped that the organization will satisfy those who are searching for information on specific tumor types, those who are interested primarily in specific genes, and those who are interested in acquiring a basic general knowledge of cancer genetics.

The Nature and Mechanisms of Human Gene Mutation

Stylianos E. Antonarakis ■ *Michael Krawczak* ■ *David N. Cooper*

1. There are a variety of different types of mutations in the human genome and many diverse mechanisms for their generation.
2. Single-base-pair substitutions account for the majority of gene defects. Among them, the hypermutability of CpG dinucleotides represents the most important and frequent cause of mutation in humans.
3. Point mutations may affect transcription and translation, as well as mRNA splicing and processing. Mutations in regulatory elements are of particular significance, since they often reveal the existence of DNA domains that are bound by regulatory proteins. Similarly, mutations that affect mRNA splicing can contribute to our understanding of the splicing mechanism.
4. We describe mechanisms of gene deletion and the DNA sequences that may predispose to such lesions, as well as potential mechanisms underlying insertions, duplications, or inversions, with representative examples.
5. Retrotransposition is a rare but biologically fascinating phenomenon that can lead to abnormal phenotypes if the double-stranded DNA is inserted in functionally important regions of a gene. Long interspersed repeat elements (LINEs) and *Alu* repetitive elements and pseudogenes have been shown to function as retrotransposons, and their *de novo* insertion in the genome can produce disease.
6. The expansion of trinucleotide repeats represents a relatively novel category of mutations in humans. There is a growing list of disorders that result from an abnormal copy number of trinucleotides within the 5′ or 3′ untranslated regions, coding sequences, and introns of genes. The pathophysiologic effects of the expansion of the trinucleotide repeat are unknown. Additionally, at least one disorder is caused by expansion of a 12mer repeat (progressive myoclonus epilepsy).
7. The study of mutations in human genes is of paramount importance in understanding the pathophysiology of hereditary disorders, in providing improved diagnostic tests, and in designing appropriate therapeutic approaches.

The study of naturally occurring gene mutations is important for a number of reasons, not the least being that the process of mutational change is fundamental to an understanding of the origins of genetic variation and the mechanisms of evolution. Knowledge of the nature, relative frequency, and DNA sequence context of different gene lesions improves our understanding of the underlying mutational mechanisms and provides valuable insights into the intricacies of DNA replication and repair. It also contributes to the elucidation of the function of proteins and the importance of their structural motifs. Finally, the understanding of the ground rules for assessing and predicting the relative frequencies and locations of specific types of gene lesions may contribute to improvements in the design and efficacy of mutation search strategies. Over the past 20 years, the application of novel DNA technologies has enabled remarkable progress in the analysis and diagnosis of human inherited disease by the characterization of the underlying gene lesions. Many different types of mutation (single-base-pair substitutions, deletions, insertions, duplications, inversions, and repeat expansions) have been detected and characterized in a large number of different human genes. The incidence/prevalence of human genetic diseases is variable; therefore, it is not surprising that the nature, frequency, and location of pathologic gene lesions in the human genome are highly specific. This specificity is largely sequence dependent; thus, some DNA sequences are not only more mutable than others, but they also mutate in characteristic ways. In this chapter, the various types of human gene mutations and their underlying mechanisms are discussed in the order presented in Table 2-1.

NOMENCLATURE OF HUMAN GENE MUTATIONS

Recommendations for the nomenclature of human gene mutations have been published[1] by the Nomenclature Working Group sponsored by the Human Genome Organization (HUGO). These recommendations were the result of a consensus reached after a series of meetings and revisions of the final document, and approved during the 1997 meeting of the American Society of Human Genetics in Baltimore.

It is obvious that the most unambiguous nomenclature system is that based on genomic DNA. Even in that case, however, length polymorphisms can create a problem in the numbering of nucleotides and therefore a standard reference sequence ought to be established, preferably by experts for each gene. Unfortunately, the entire genomic sequence is known for only a minority of human genes. For the vast majority, only the cDNA sequence is available. The existence of more than one transcription start site, alternative splicing, and the utilization of alternative exons and variable number of repeats complicate the nucleotide numbering. Thus, here too, a reference sequence needs to be established. The nomenclature, at least in the present state of the human genome project, needs to be accurate and unambiguous, but flexible. The nucleotide change must always be included in the original report; however, other terms may be used (for example, specifying the amino acid change). The recommendations of the working group are as follows:

- For genomic DNA and cDNA, the A of the ATG of the initiator Met codon is denoted nucleotide +1. There is no

---

A list of standard abbreviations is located immediately preceding the index. Additional abbreviations used in this chapter include: ARE = androgen-response element; C1I = complement component-1 inhibitor; CV = consensus value; CVA = activated cryptic splice site; CVN = consensus value for normal, wild-type splice site; DHFR = dihydrofolate reductase; DMD = Duchenne muscular dystrophy; EBP = enhancer-binding protein; GBA = glucocerebrosidase; GH, growth hormone; HGMD, Human Gene Mutation Database; hnRNP = heterogeneous nuclear ribonucleoprotein; HPFH = hereditary persistence of fetal hemoglobin; HUGO = Human Genome Organization; LCR = locus control region; LINEs = long interspersed repeat elements; OAT = ornithine-δ -aminotransferase; ORF = open reading frame; ss = splice site; STS = steroid sulfatase; TPI1, triosephosphate isomerase I.

Table 2-1 Different Categories of Human Mutations Discussed in This Chapter

Single-base-pair substitutions
   Types of nucleotide substitutions and hypermutable nucleotides
   mRNA splice-junction mutations
   mRNA processing (other than splicing) and translation mutations
   Regulatory mutations
Deletions
Insertions
Duplications
Inversions
Expansion of unstable repeat sequences

nucleotide zero (0). The nucleotide 5′ to +1 is numbered −1. If there is more than one potential ATG, a reference consensus may be used. The numbering of nucleotides in the reference sequence in the databases should not be changed and remains associated with the same (original) accession number.

- The use of lowercase g (for genomic) or c (for cDNA) in front of the nucleotide number is recommended. To avoid confusion, a dot should separate these from the nucleotide number (g. or c. for genomic or cDNA, respectively). The accession number in primary sequence databases (GenBank, EMBL, and DDJB) should also be included in the original publication/database submission of mutations.

- Nucleotide changes start with the nucleotide number, and the change follows this number. 1997G > T denotes that at nucleotide 1997 of the reference sequence, G, is replaced by T.

- Deletions are designated by del after the nucleotide number: 1997delT denotes the deletion of T at nucleotide (nt) 1997, and 1997–1999del denotes the deletion of 3 nts. Alternatively, this mutation can be denoted as 1997–1999delTTC. For deletions in short tandem repeats, the most 3′ position is arbitrarily assigned; e.g., a TG deletion in the sequence AATGTGTGCC is designated 1997–1998delTG or 1997–1998del (where 1997 is the first T before C).

- Insertions are designated by ins after the nucleotide interval number. 1997–1998insT denotes that T was inserted in the interval between nts 1997 and 1998. For insertions in short repeats, the most 3′ nt interval is arbitrarily assigned; e.g., a TG insertion in the sequence AATGTGTGCC is designated 1997–1998insTG (where 1997 is the last G of the short TG repeat).

- Variability of short sequence repeats is designated as $1997(GT)_{6-22}$. In this case, 1997 is the first nucleotide of the dinucleotide GT, which is repeated 6 to 22 times in the population.

- A unique identifier for each mutation should be obtained. The Online Mendelian Inheritance in Man (OMIM) (http://www.ncbi.nlm.nih.gov/Omim/) unique identifier can be used, or database curators may assign such unique identifiers. Other existing databases such as the Human Gene Mutation Database (HGMD; http://www.uwcm.ac.uk/uwcm/mg/hgmd0.html), for example, could also be used as a reference source for cataloged mutations.

- When the full genomic sequence is not known, intron mutations can be designated by the intron intervening sequence (IVS) number, positive numbers starting from the G of the donor site invariant GT, negative numbers starting from the G of the acceptor site invariant AG. IVS4+1G > T denotes the G-to-T substitution at nt +1 of intron 4. IVS4−2A > C denotes the A-to-C substitution at nt −2 of intron 4. Alternatively, the cDNA nucleotide numbering may be used to designate the location of the mutation in the adjacent intron. For example, c.1997+1G > T denotes the G-to-T substitution at nt +1 after nucleotide 1997 of the cDNA. Similarly, c.1997−2A > C denotes the A-to-C substitution at nt −2 upstream of nucleotide 1997 of the cDNA. When the full-length genomic sequence is known, the mutation can be designated by the nt number of the reference sequence.

- Two mutations in the same allele can be listed within brackets as follows: [1997G > T;2001A > C]. This will also enable (1) the designation of mutations that are only deleterious when they occur in the same allele with additional nucleotide substitutions, and (2) the designation of haplotypes of different alleles.

- For amino-acid-based systems, the codon for the initiator *methionine* is codon 1.

- The single-letter amino acid code is recommended, but the three-letter code is also acceptable.

- For the amino-acid-based nomenclature, the format is Y97S (*tyrosine* at codon 97 substituted by *serine*). The *wild-type* amino acid is given before and the mutant amino acid after the codon number. Therefore, there is no confusion as to the significance of G, C, T, and A.

- Stop codons are designated by X, e.g., R97X (*arginine* codon 96 substituted by a termination codon).

- Deletions of amino acids are designated as: T97del denotes that the codon 97 for *threonine* is deleted.

- Insertions of amino acids are designated as: T97–98ins denotes that a codon for *threonine* is inserted at the interval between codons 97 and 98 of the reference amino acid sequence.

- The first report of a mutation in the literature should contain both a nucleotide-based and amino-acid-based name, when appropriate.

No recommendations have yet been made for complex mutations. Detailed description of such mutations and nomenclature proposals can usually be found in the original report or by the unique identifier. A second phase of recommendations will deal with such issues in the future. A discussion paper with further recommendations has recently been published.[2] In addition, the consequences of a mutation (frameshift, particular splicing abnormality, exon skipping, etc.) are not addressed in this nomenclature. However, investigators who maintain mutation databases are encouraged to include a field of mutation consequences or mechanisms (if known) in their databases.

The foregoing recommendations did not always represent a full consensus of the scientific community or the investigators involved in the discussions. Among the numerous other proposals/criticisms, it is worth mentioning the following:

- The "^" sign may be used to determine the interval of an insertion rather than the "−" sign. For example, 1997^1998insG instead of 1997–1998insG.

- The designation of both deleterious mutations in the two alleles of a homozygote for a recessive disorder may be designated as [1997G > T+2001A > G] to indicate the substitution in nt 1997 of one allele and in nt 2001 of the other allele of the same gene.

- Analogous to g. or c. for the genomic or cDNA numbering system, p. may be used to distinguish the protein-based nomenclature clearly.

- X may not be the best symbol for a termination codon.

SINGLE-BASE-PAIR SUBSTITUTIONS

Types of Nucleotide Substitutions

A database containing reports of mutations in the coding regions of human genes causing genetic disease, mainly characterized by DNA sequencing, has been maintained by two authors of this chapter (D.N.C. and M.K.). As of April 15, 2000, this database includes 21,591 entries in 1039 genes (this database is referred to as the Human Gene Mutation Database (HGMD[3]) throughout this chapter; http://www.uwcm.ac.uk/uwcm/mg/hgmd0.html). Earlier versions of the HGMD have been published.[4,5] Only one example of each mutation is recorded, owing to the difficulty in determining whether repeated mutations are identical by descent or truly recurrent. Fig. 2-1 illustrates the spectrum of mutations logged in the database. Missense nucleotide substitutions represent the most common type of mutations, accounting for 50 percent of the total entries. Regarding missense mutations,

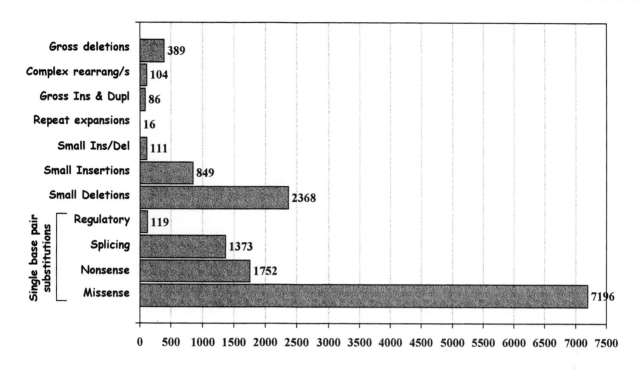

14363 mutations in 783 genes (as of 13sep98)

Fig. 2-1. Spectrum of different types of human gene mutations logged in Human Gene Mutation Database as of September 13, 1998 (*http://www.uwcm.ac.uk/uwcm/mg/hgmd0.html*).

evidence for causality comes from one or more of the following sources:

1. Occurrence of the mutation in a region of known structure or function
2. Occurrence of the lesion in an evolutionarily conserved residue
3. Previous independent occurrence of the mutation in an unrelated patient
4. Failure to observe the mutation in a large sample of normal controls
5. Novel appearance and subsequent cosegregation of the gene lesion and disease phenotype through a family pedigree
6. Demonstration that a mutant protein produced *in vitro* possesses the same biochemical properties and characteristics as its *in vivo* counterpart
7. Reversal of the pathological phenotype in the patient/cultured cells by replacement of the mutant gene/protein with its wild-type counterpart.

The spectrum of single-base-pair substitutions logged in the HGMD by November 1997 (the time it was last subjected to an extensive meta-analysis[6]) is summarized in Table 2-2. Mutations occurring in CpG dinucleotides account for 2133 (29.3 percent) of the total. Therefore, they represent a major cause of human genetic disorders (see below). If only CG-to-TG and CG-to-CA transitions (i.e., consistent with methylation-mediated deamination) are considered, this figure falls to 1675 (23 percent). Breakdown of the data by chromosomal location revealed that the proportion of CG-to-TG or CG-to-CA substitutions was significantly higher for autosomal genes (1325/5296 = 25.0 percent) than for X-chromosomal genes (350/1975 = 17.7 percent; $\chi^2 = 43.21$, 1 *df*, $P < 10^{-5}$). In part, this disparity can be explained by a generally more pronounced CpG suppression observed in X-linked genes: the average CpG content was 3.67 percent for the 401 autosomal cDNA sequences provided by the HGMD, and 2.86 percent for the 45 X-chromosomal cDNAs (Student's $t = 2.35$, 444 *df*, $P < 0.01$). Analysis of Table 13-2 yields transversion (T to A or G, A to T or C, G to C or T, C to G or A) and transition (T to C, C to T, G to A, A to G) frequencies of 37.5 percent and 62.5 percent, respectively. There is therefore a highly significant excess of transitions as compared with the expected frequency (33 percent). Most but not

Table 2-2 Spectrum of Single-Base-Pair Substitutions, in the Human Gene Mutation Database

Initial Nucleotide	Nucleotide Resulting from Single-Base-Pair Change				
	T	C	A	G	Total
T		654	271	312	1237
C	**1632** (940)		371	340	2343
A	201	163		538	902
G	619	453	**1717** (735)		2789
Total	2452	1270	2359	1190	7271

NOTE: A, adenine; C, cytosine; G, guanine; T, thymidine. **Bold** denotes transitions. Figures in brackets refer to transitions that are CG > TG or CG > CA, respectively. These data were based on 7271 single-base-pair substitutions logged on November 1997.[5]

Table 2-3 Relative Single-Base-Pair Substitution Rates in Human Nuclear Genes Causing Inherited Disease

Original Nucleotide	Substituting Nucleotide			
	T	C	A	G
T	—	1.525	0.374	0.410
C	2.702	—	0.541	0.505
A	0.187	0.268	—	1.127
G	0.521	0.712	3.128	—

NOTE: Relative substitution rates are based on data from the Human Gene Mutation Database and have been corrected for confounding effects as described by Krawczak et al.[5] The estimates are unitless and have been scaled so that the average equals unity.

all of this excess can be attributed to the hypermutability of the CpG dinucleotide. However, even when CpG mutations are removed (36.9 percent of all transitions and 16.8 percent of all transversions) from the analysis, the excess of transitions is still significant (55.8 percent vs 33 percent expected). It is important to point out that mutation frequencies observed in the context of human inherited disease are unlikely to reflect the true underlying rates of mutation occurrence. Since different amino acid substitutions have different effects upon protein structure and function, they have necessarily come to clinical attention (and thus entered the HGMD) with different probabilities. Moreover, codon frequencies differ from one another, implying that different amino acid residues are involved in a mutational event with different prior probabilities. Relative single-base-pair substitution rates corrected for these two confounding factors[6] are presented in Table 2-3. The data in this table confirm the existence of a high rate of C-to-T and G-to-A substitutions (48 percent of total).

DNA Polymerase Fidelity and Single-Nucleotide Substitutions. DNA replication occurs as a result of an accurate, yet error-prone, multistep process. The final accuracy depends on the initial fidelity of the replicative step and the efficiency of subsequent error-correction mechanisms.[7] Since DNA polymerases are involved in replication, recombination, and repair processes (Table 2-4),[8] their base incorporation fidelity is probably a critical factor in determining mutation rates in the cell. To test the hypothesis that nonrandom base misincorporation during DNA replication is a major contributory factor in human mutations, Cooper and Krawczak[5] compared the base substitution rates from Table 2-3 with the *in vitro* measured base substitution error rates (data from studies by Kunkel and Alexander[9] and others) exhibited by vertebrate DNA polymerases α, β, and δ. A significant correlation between these two sets of values was

observed for polymerase β but not for polymerases α or δ (Spearman rank correlation coefficient, 0.74; $P < 0.005$). In this comparison, any consideration of the efficacy of the different proofreading and postreplicative mismatch-repair mechanisms was excluded. This is because the purified polymerase preparations used *in vitro* lacked the 3' to 5' exonuclease activities thought to be responsible for proofreading *in vivo*. The result obtained for DNA polymerase β is consistent with the postulate that a substantial proportion of the nucleotide substitutions causing human genetic disease are due to misincorporation of bases during DNA replication.

Slipped Mispairing and Single-Nucleotide Substitutions. A mechanistic model for single-base-pair mutagenesis, the slipped-mispairing model,[10] seeks to explain nucleotide misincorporation through transient misalignment of the primer-template caused by looping out of a template base. During replication synthesis, the template strand slips back one base, resulting in the misincorporation of the next nucleotide on the primer strand. After realignment of both primer and template strand, the mismatch may be corrected in favor of the misincorporated base (Fig. 2-2). *Misalignment* or *dislocation* mutagenesis is thought to be mediated by runs of identical bases or by other repetitive DNA sequences in the vicinity. If misincorporation mediated by one-base-pair (1-bp) slippage is important, then a substantial proportion of point mutations should exhibit identity of the newly introduced base to one of the bases flanking the mutation site. Comparison in the HGMD of the observed and expected frequency of this type of mutation revealed that this is indeed the case, but only at certain codon positions.[6] Mutation toward the 5' flanking nucleotide occurred significantly more often than expected at the second position (642 observed vs 558 expected) but not at the first position (565 observed vs 568 expected) or last position of a codon (167 observed vs 170 expected); mutation toward the 3' flanking base was significantly favored at the first position (490 observed vs 390 expected) but disfavored at the second position (592 observed vs 659 expected) of a codon. These findings suggest a mechanism of mutation at either position 1 or 2 in the codon (both critical in specifying the encoded amino acid residue) that is biased toward the nucleotide at the other position. Inspection of the genetic code reveals that such a bias invariably serves to avoid the *de novo* introduction of termination codons.

CpG Dinucleotides as Hotspots for Nucleotide Substitutions (Methylation-Mediated Deamination of 5-Methylcytosine)

CpG Distribution in the Vertebrate Genome and Its Origins. In eukaryotic genomes, 5-methylcytosine (5mC) occurs predominantly in CpG dinucleotides, the majority of which appear to be methylated.[11,12] Methylation of cytosine results in a high level of

Table 2-4 Eukaryotic DNA Polymerases

	α	β	γ	δ	ε
Catalytic polypeptide	165 kDa	40 kDa	140 kDa	125 kDa	255 kDa
Associated subunits	70, 58, 48 kDa	None	Unknown	48 kDa	Unknown
Cellular localization	Nuclear	Nuclear	Mitochondrial	Nuclear	Nuclear
Associated activities					
3' → 5' Exonuclease	None	None	Yes	Yes	Yes
Primase	Yes	None	None	None	None
Properties					
Processivity	Medium	Low	High	Low	High
Fidelity	High	Low	High	High	High
Major characteristics	Principal replicative DNA polymerase, lagging strand DNA synthesis	Short-patch DNA repair	Mitochondrial DNA polymerase	Leading-strand DNA synthesis	UV-induced repair synthesis

SOURCE: Modified from Wang.[7]

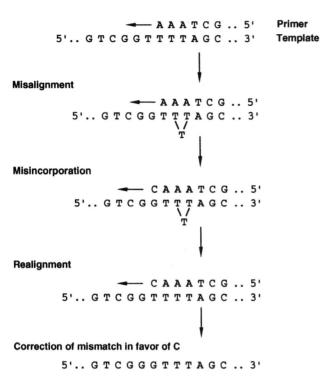

←— A A A T C G .. 5'   **Primer**
5'.. G T C G G T T T T A G C .. 3'   **Template**

Misalignment

←— A A A T C G .. 5'
5'.. G T C G G T T T A G C .. 3'
                    \ /
                     T

Misincorporation

←— C A A A T C G .. 5'
5'.. G T C G G T T T A G C .. 3'
                    \ /
                     T

Realignment

←— C A A A T C G .. 5'
5'.. G T C G G T T T T A G C .. 3'

Correction of mismatch in favor of C

5'.. G T C G G G T T T A G C .. 3'

Fig. 2-2. Schematic representation of the slipped-mispairing model for single nucleotide substitutions.

mutation due to the propensity of 5mC to undergo deamination to form thymine (Fig. 2-3). Deamination of 5mC probably occurs with the same frequency as either cytosine or uracil. However, whereas uracil DNA glycosylase activity in eukaryotic cells can recognize and excise uracil, thymine—being a normal DNA base—is thought to be less readily detectable and hence removable by cellular DNA repair mechanisms. One consequence of the hypermutability of 5mC is the paucity of CpG in the genomes of many eukaryotes, the heavily methylated vertebrate genomes exhibiting the most extreme *CpG suppression*.[12] In vertebrate genomes, the frequency of CpG dinucleotides is between 20 and 25 percent of the frequency predicted from observed mononucleotide frequencies.[13,14] The distribution of CpG in the genome is also nonrandom: About 1 percent of the vertebrate genome consists of a fraction that is rich in CpG and that accounts for about 15 percent of all CpG dinucleotides (reviewed by Bird[15]). In contrast to most of the scattered CpG dinucleotides, these *CpG islands* represent unmethylated domains and in many cases appear to coincide with transcribed regions. The evolution of the heavily methylated vertebrate genome has been

accompanied by a progressive loss of CpG dinucleotides as a direct consequence of their methylation in the germ line.

The CpG Dinucleotide and Human Genetic Disease. An excess of C-to-T transitions was first reported by Vogel and Röhrborn[16] in a study of the mutations responsible for hemoglobin variants in humans. Further studies confirmed the existence of this phenomenon.[17] Many additional studies in eukaryotes (reviewed by Cooper and Krawczak[5]) have now shown that the CpG dinucleotide is specifically associated with a high frequency of C-to-T and G-to-A transitions. The G-to-A transitions arise as a result of a 5mC-to-T transition on the antisense DNA strand, followed by miscorrection of G to A on the sense strand. A high frequency of polymorphism has also been detected in the human genome by restriction enzymes containing CpG in their recognition sequences.[18] CpG was found by molecular analysis to be a hotspot for mutation first in the factor VIII (F8C) gene[19,20] and subsequently in a wide range of different human genes.[21,22] From the relative dinucleotide mutabilities as estimated by Cooper and Krawczak[5,6] (see below for a description), it follows that the CG-to-TG or CG-to-CA substitutions are approximately 13 times more likely than any other substitution in the CG dinucleotide. This is perhaps an underestimate, since in the HGMD each nucleotide substitution has been logged only once, resulting in the systematic exclusion of multiple independent *de novo* mutations. It has been repeatedly noted in various genes that specific CG-to-TG or CG-to-CA mutations recur independently. For example, the number of CG-to-TG or CG-to-CA mutations in the factor VIII (F8C) gene causing hemophilia A is 25 percent of all different single-nucleotide substitutions, but 48 percent if recurrent mutations are considered (based on 586 F8C point mutations; see Kaufman and Antonarakis[23] and should be http://europium.csc.mrc.ac.uk). The observed frequency of CG-to-TG and CG-to-CA mutation varies between human genes; for example, it is less than 10 percent in the β-globin (HBB) and HPRT genes, but it is greater than 50 percent in the ADA gene. In two studies of the coagulation F8C and F9 genes in which almost all mutations in a given set of patients have been identified, approximately 35 percent of nucleotide substitutions were CG to TG or CG to CA.[24–26] The distribution of CpG mutations within a given gene may also be uniform. For example, 9 of 122 single-base-pair substitutions in exon 7 of the protein C (PROC) gene occur in a CpG; by contrast, none of 13 point mutations reported in exons 5 and 6 are in CpG dinucleotides,[27] although these exons contain a larger number of CpGs. In the assumed absence of a detection bias (see below), variation in CpG mutability is due either to differences in germ-line DNA methylation and/or relative intragenic CpG frequency. Indeed, CpG hypermutability in inherited disease implies that the affected sites are methylated in the germ line and thereby rendered prone to 5mC deamination. That 5mC deamination is directly responsible for mutational events has been evidenced by the fact that several cytosine residues known to have undergone a germ-line mutation

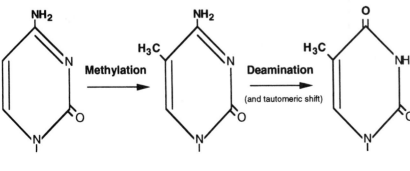

Fig. 2-3. Schematic representation of the molecules for cytosine, 5-methylcytosine, and thymine and the chemical events for the transformation of cytosine to thymine.

Table 2-5 Germ-Line Origin of Mutations in the Clotting Factor IX Gene

	Male	Female	M/F Ratio	p Value
All base substitutions	20	16	2.5	4.99×10^{-3}
All deletions	3	11	0.55	NS
Transitions				
At CpG	10	3	6.7	1.65×10^{-3}
Non-CpG	5	4	2.5	NS
Transversions	5	9	1.1	NS
Deletions				
Small (< 50 bp)	1	8	0.25	NS
Large (> 50 bp)	2	3	1.3	NS
Insertions	1	1		
Total	24	28		

NOTE: Modified from Ketterling *et al.*,[30] with the addition of the Kling *et al.*[31] cases. The observed M/F ratio was corrected for the expected 1:2 (the expected ratio is $z : 1 + z$, where z denotes the probability of an X-linked recessive mutation to have at least one affected male descendant. Since $z \leq 1$, the ratio of 1:2 is a conservative estimate).

in the low-density-lipoprotein receptor gene (LDLR; hypercholesterolemia) and the tumor protein 53 (TP53) gene (various types of tumor) are indeed methylated in sperm DNA.[28]

The frequency of CG-to-TG or CG-to-CA mutations may differ between male and female germ lines because there is a profound difference in DNA methylation in the germ cells of the two sexes: the oocyte is markedly undermethylated, whereas sperm is heavily methylated.[29,30] Thus, it may be that CG-to-TG or CG-to-CA mutations occur more commonly in male germ cells. Table 2-5

shows the germ-line origin of mutations in the F9 gene. In this data set, there is a sevenfold male excess of transitions at CpG dinucleotides.[31] Pattinson et al[32] have noted differences between ethnic groups in the mutation frequency at specific CpG sites within the F8C gene in a small sample. By contrast, the pattern of germ-line CpG mutation in the F9 gene appeared to be indistinguishable between Asians, mostly of Korean origin, and Caucasians.[33] This finding argues for the absence of population-specific methylation patterns and is consistent with no differences in methylation between individuals from different ethnic backgrounds.[34] In somatic tissues, 5mC deamination also appears to be an important mechanism of single-base-pair substitution.[35,36] Indeed, the relative rate of mitotic cancer-associated CG-to-TG or CG-to-CA transitions observed in the TP53 gene, the most widely mutated gene in human tumorigenesis, is very similar to the overall germ-line rate observed in other human genes.[37] Fig. 2-4 depicts the codon usage in human genes (data from 6,130,940 human codons from GenBank release 107 recorded in http://www.dna.affrc.go.jp/nakamura-bin/showcodon.cgi?species = Homo+sapiens+[gbpri]), together with the relative frequency at which codons are affected by any of the 8604 missense/nonsense recorded in the HGMD on July 14, 1998; http://www.uwcm.ac.uk/uwcm/mg/haha1.html). It is obvious from Fig. 2-4 that codons for Arg and Gly underwent more mutations than expected from codon usage alone in human genes. Although four codons for Arg contain CG dinucleotides, it is less clear why the codons for Gly are hypermutable. They all start with G and could therefore be part of a CG dinucleotide. In addition, they all are GGN, and a nearest neighbor analysis of single-base substitutions (Table 2-6) indicated that a mutated G is often flanked by another G at its 5' side. To overcome the bias of counting independent mutations only once, we also compared, in Fig. 2-5, the number of recurrent

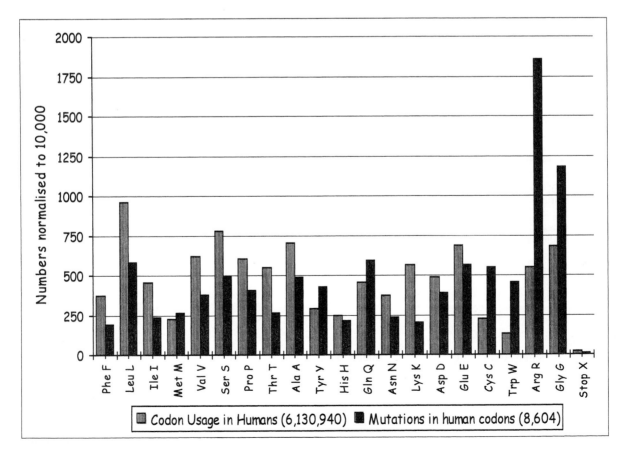

Fig. 2-4. Histogram of codon usage in human genes and mutations found in codons for the various amino acids. The codon usage data are from http://www.dna.affrc.go.jp/nakamura-bin/ showcodon.cgi?species=Homo+sapiens+[gbpri] and the mutation data are from http://www.uwcm.ac.uk/uwcm/mg/haha1.html. The values on the *x*-axis were normalized for 10,000.

Table 2-6 Nucleotide Frequencies at the 3′ and 5′ Sides of Point Mutations Causing Human Genetic Disease

(a) Mutated Base	3′ Neighboring Base				
	T	C	A	G	Total
T	202	240	164	631	1237
C	235	354	619	1135 (195)	2343 (1403)
A	311	218	209	164	902
G	493 (374)	613 (457)	732 (547)	951 (676)	2789 (2054)
Total	1241 (1122)	1425 (1269)	1724 (1539)	2881 (1666)	7271 (5596)

(b) 5′ Neighboring Base	Mutated Base				
	T	C	A	G	Total
T	182	509 (314)	161	669	1521 (1326)
C	438	716 (350)	295	998 (263)	2447 (1346)
A	347	519 (355)	173	345	1384 (1220)
G	270	599 (384)	273	777	1919 (1704)
Total	1237	2343 (1403)	902	2789 (2054)	7271 (5596)

NOTE: Figures in parentheses denote observed nearest-neighbor frequencies when CG-to-TG (**a**) and CG-to-CA (**b**) transitions are excluded.

mutations found in different codons of five X-linked genes (F8C, F9, L1CAM, OTC, and BTK) with the codon usage in these five genes. The information included was extracted from the following locus-specific databases: for BTK, http://www.uta.fi/laitokset/imt/bioinfo/BTKbase/ for F8C, http://europium.csc.mrc.ac.uk for F9, http://www.umds.ac.uk/molgen/haemBdatabase.htm; for L1CAM, http://dnalab-www.uia.ac.be/dnalab/l1/#L1CAM mutations; and, for OTC, http://www.peds.umn.edu/otc/. It is again apparent from Fig. 13-5 that codons for Arg are more vulnerable to point mutations, emphasizing the hypermutability of the CG dinucleotide.

Are other mechanisms also responsible for CpG deamination? The suggestion that CpG deamination may result from endogenous

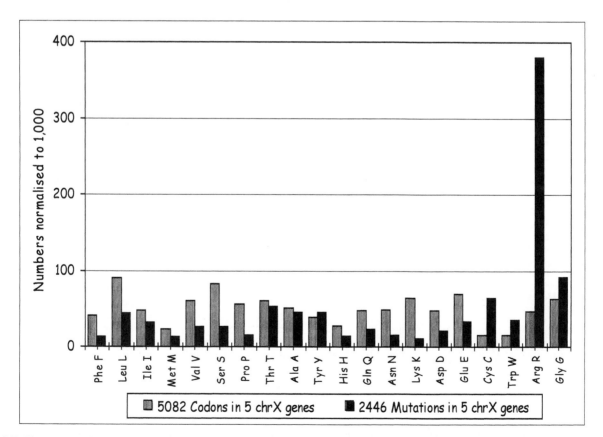

Fig. 2-5. Histogram of the independent recurrent mutations found in codons of five X-linked genes and the occurrence of these codons in these five genes. The genes were F8C, F9, L1CAM, OTC, and BTK. The information for the independent mutations was extracted from the following locus specific databases: for BTK, http://www.helsinki.fi/science/signal/btkbase.html; for F8C, http://146.179.66.63/usr/WWW/WebPages/main.dir/main.htm; for F9, WebPages/database.dir/titlepage.htm; http://dnalab-www.uia.ac.be/dnalab/l1/#L1CAM mutations for L1CAM; and, for OTC, http://www.peds.umn.edu/otc/.

enzymatic activity has been mooted by Steinberg and Gorman,[38] who found that some 70 percent of their (independent) mouse lymphoma cell mutants possessed a specific CGG-to-TGG substitution converting Arg 334 to Trp in the gene-encoding protein-kinase regulatory subunit. In 5 percent of these mutants, a second mutation (CGT to TGT) was found converting Arg 332 to Cys. The co-occurrence of these two mutations at such a high frequency argues for some type of enzymatic mechanism and against two independent methylation-mediated deamination events. Such a mechanism could involve a deaminase, although no such activity has yet been purified. The relevance of the observation to human gene mutation is doubtful, since (1) there are no known examples, including CpG dinucleotides, of pathologic base changes that occur with such a high proportional frequency in humans, and (2) although a very few isolated examples of double mutation have been reported as causes of human genetic disease, these do not involve CpG dinucleotides. Shen et al[39] have reported that DNA methyltransferase is capable of including C-to-T transitions directly in prokaryotes, and the mutation frequency was sensitive to the concentration of the methyl donor, S-adenosylmethionine. The importance of this putative deamination mechanism in eukaryotes is at present unclear.

Non-CpG Point-Mutation Hotspots

In an early and not updated analysis, among the 879 point mutations in HGMD not readily explicable by methylation-mediated deamination, a total of 30 codons in 16 different genes were identified as potential *hotspots* for single-base-pair substitutions. These residues were characterized either by a single base being affected by at least two nonidentical substitutions or by mutations affecting two or three nucleotides within that codon. Some trinucleotide and tetranucleotide motifs are significantly overrepresented within 10 bp on either side of the mutation hotspots. These motifs are TTT (17 observed vs 8 expected), CTT (18 vs 8), TGA (23 vs 11), TTG (20 vs 8), CTTT (8 vs 2), TCTT (8 vs 2), and TTTG (11 vs 2). In addition, Cooper and Krawczak[5] screened a region of 10 bp around 219 non-CpG base substitution sites for triplets and quadruplets that occurred at significantly increased frequencies. Only one trinucleotide was found again to occur at a frequency significantly higher than expected: CTT, the topoisomerase-I cleavage site consensus sequence.[40] CTT was observed 36 times in the vicinity of a point mutation, whereas the expected frequency was 20. By contrast, two tetranucleotides were significantly overrepresented at the screened positions. TCGA was observed 17 times (7 expected; this was probably because *Taq*I restriction enzyme was used for detection of the mutations), whereas TGGA was observed 25 times (12 expected). The latter motif fits perfectly with the deletion hotspot consensus sequence drawn up previously for human genes,[41] which, in turn, resembles the putative arrest site for DNA polymerase α.[42] Thus, it may be that the arrest or pausing of the polymerase at the replication fork disposes the replication complex to misincorporation of nucleotides as well as deletions.

A Nearest-Neighbor Analysis of Single-Base-Pair Substitutions

Methylation-mediated deamination as a primary cause of point mutation is characterized by an increased rate of CG-to-TG and CG-to-CA transitions. However, the relative likelihoods of point mutations at other dinucleotides may also vary, as is suggested by the nearest-neighbor frequencies observed in the HGMD (Table 2-6). (Note that each point mutation can be regarded as occurring within two distinct dinucleotides, depending on whether one considers the 5′ or the 3′ neighboring base.) In Table 2-6, considerable differences are apparent with respect to nucleotides occurring adjacent to sites of point mutation. For example, G residues are clearly overrepresented as 3′ flanking nucleotides when T is mutated, and a mutated G is often flanked by another G residue on the 5′ side.

Differences in the phenotypic consequences of specific point mutations, and thus in the likelihood of their coming to clinical attention, introduce a serious bias to the observed spectrum of mutations underlying human disease. In-depth studies of the phenotypic effect of large numbers of different missense mutations in a specific gene are few. One such study for missense mutations in the F9 gene[43] showed that mutations at *generic* residues (amino acid residues conserved in F9 of other mammalian species and in three related serine proteases) would invariably cause disease. Mutations at F9-specific residues (residues conserved in the factor IX of other mammalian species but not in three related serine proteases) were some sixfold less likely to cause disease, whereas mutations at nonconserved residues were 33 times less likely to result in a hemophilia-B phenotype. Bottema et al[43] estimated that 40 percent of all possible missense changes would cause hemophilia B, implying that 60 percent of residues serve merely as *spacers* to maintain the relative position of critical amino acid residues and probably do not fulfill any specific (known) function. Thus, detectable mutations, identified by virtue of their effect on protein structure and function and subsequently on clinical phenotype, appear to be a subset of a rather larger number of mutations, many of which have no clinical effect, at least in the case of hemophilia B. To what extent this finding in hemophilia B (in which < 5 percent normal F9 activity must be present to generate a clinically abnormal phenotype) can be extrapolated to other genetic disorders is, however, unclear. Nevertheless, it would seem reasonable to suppose that the phenotypic consequences of a given point mutation are determined by the magnitude of the amino acid exchange as assessed by the resulting structural perturbation of the protein. Thus, specific amino acid substitutions might come to clinical attention more readily, depending on the severity of the resulting phenotype. Several methods have been reported for assessing the relative net effect of a specific amino acid exchange.[44,45] Perhaps the best comparative measure of amino acid relatedness available is that devised by Grantham,[45] who combined the three interdependent properties of composition, polarity, and molecular volume to assign each amino acid pair a mean chemical difference. Krawczak et al[6] devised an iterative multivariate procedure that takes into account the phenotypic consequences of a mutation, measured by means of Grantham's chemical difference between the wild type and mutant amino acid. Over and above the hypermutability of CpG dinucleotides, only a subtle and locally confined influence of the surrounding DNA sequence upon relative single-base-pair substitution rates was observed which extended no further than 2 bp from the substitution site.[6] Maximum-likelihood estimates of relative substitution rates taking the immediate 5′ and 3′ flanking nucleotides into account are summarized in Table 2-7. A steady increase in clinical observation likelihood with increasing chemical difference was also noted. Furthermore, nonsense mutations were found to be more than twice as likely to come to clinical attention as the most extreme missense mutations and three times more likely than the average amino acid change. However, the phenotypic consequences of a given mutation must depend not only on the nature of the amino acid substitution, but also on the location of the substitution within the protein. In general, and with the exception of charged residues, most amino acids that make critical interactions (e.g., disulfide bonds, hydrophobic forces, and hydrogen bonds) are rigid or buried within the protein structure, and their mutational substitution will be profoundly destabilizing.

Strand Difference in Base Substitution Rates

A noteworthy feature of Table 2-7 is that it reveals some asymmetry, suggesting a strand difference for single-base-pair substitutions. For example, the relative rates of CT to CC and AG to GG differ by more than twofold. Since the latter transition is complementary to the former, these two figures should coincide if point mutagenesis were acting similarly on both DNA strands. Estimation of relative substitution rates conditional on both the 5′

Table 2-7 Relative Dinucleotide Mutabilities

d	Newly Introduced 5'				Newly Introduced 3' Base			
	T	C	A	G	T	C	A	G
TT	—	1.17	0.31	0.36	—	0.71	0.20	0.28
CT	1.17	—	0.31	0.41	—	1.57	0.27	0.43
AT	0.44	0.20	—	2.06	—	1.53	0.40	0.34
GT	0.86	0.71	3.13	—	—	1.17	0.39	0.30
TC	—	0.93	0.37	0.19	2.06	—	0.37	0.56
CC	1.16	—	0.49	0.32	2.54	—	0.39	0.40
AC	0.23	0.37	—	0.95	2.27	—	0.48	0.44
GC	0.48	0.71	2.68	—	2.06	—	0.51	0.32
TA	—	1.19	0.32	0.34	0.16	0.24	—	1.36
CA	1.28	—	0.43	0.42	0.12	0.43	—	1.23
AA	0.14	0.22	—	0.87	0.12	0.16	—	0.92
GA	0.45	0.60	2.82	—	0.24	0.15	—	0.63
TG	—	1.86	0.37	0.52	0.42	0.62	1.84	—
CG	**9.01**	—	0.88	0.90	0.90	1.17	**12.17**	—
AG	0.10	0.19	—	0.60	0.30	0.46	1.38	—
GG	0.46	0.69	3.09	—	0.49	0.54	1.76	—

NOTE: d, Original dinucleotide. Relative substitution rates are unitless and have been scaled so that the average in each half of the table equals unity.

Table 2-8 A Strand Difference in Relative Single-Base-Pair Substitution Rates

Original Substitution	Relative Rate	Watson-Crick Homologue	Relative Rate
GGT > GTT	1.16 ± 0.16	ACC > AAC	0.51 ± 0.08
TGG > TAG	1.64 ± 0.13	CCA > CTA	0.99 ± 0.09
CGG > CAG	13.01 ± 0.88	CCG > CTG	8.35 ± 0.47
CTT > CCT	1.14 ± 0.20	AAG > AGG	0.35 ± 0.10
CTC > CCC	1.20 ± 0.17	GAG > GGG	0.32 ± 0.07
TGC > TCC	0.76 ± 0.13	GCA > GGA	0.19 ± 0.06
CTG > CCG	1.87 ± 0.15	CAG > CGG	0.81 ± 0.13
GGT > GAT	1.79 ± 0.21	ACC > ATC	0.68 ± 0.14
CTG > CAG	0.22 ± 0.04	CAG > CTG	0.03 ± 0.02
CTT > CGT	0.47 ± 0.11	AAG > ACG	0.12 ± 0.04

NOTE: Relative substitution rates (± SD) are unitless and were scaled so that their average, taken over all 192 possible substitution types, is unity. Estimation of standard deviation and significance assessment was by bootstrapping. Only pairs of substitutions are included for which one relative rate estimate was consistently larger than its counterpart in more than 9995 to 10,000 replications of the estimate procedure.

and 3' flanking nucleotides served to identify 10 pairs of substitutions, complementary to each other, that exhibit the same feature.[6] These are listed in Table 2-8. A strand difference in mutation rates has already been described by Wu and Maeda.[46] By comparison of nonfunctional sequences near the β-globin genes of six primate species, they demonstrated that purine-to-pyrimidine (R-to-Y) transversions occurred approximately 1.5 times more frequently than their pyrimidine-to-purine counterparts. However, complementary transitions were found to occur at equal frequencies. These findings are compatible with the mutational spectrum from the HGMD: R to Y was observed 11 percent more frequently than Y to R, and both T-to-C and A-to-G transitions account for some 10 percent of the mutations in Table 2-2. A slightly different result was obtained for G-to-A transitions, which are 1.4 times more frequent than C-to-T transitions. Nevertheless, Table 2-7 reveals that strand differences in mutation rates depend on the nucleotides flanking the site of mutation. For example, whereas CT to CC is more than 2.5 times more likely than AG to GG, TA is 15 percent more likely to mutate to TG than to CA. A disparity between the likelihoods of CG-to-TG and CG-to-CA transitions is also evident from inspection of Tables 2-7 and 2-8. This observation strongly suggests that, at least within gene coding regions, the two strands are differentially methylated and/or differentially repaired. Holmes et al[47] have demonstrated *in vitro* the existence of a strand-specific correction process in human and *Drosophilia* cells whose efficiency depends on the nature of the mispair. Such differential repair could also account for the observed strand differences in mutation frequency.

Single-Base-Pair Substitutions in Human mRNA Splice Junctions

Single-base-pair substitutions (point mutations) affecting mRNA splicing are nonrandomly distributed, and this nonrandomness can be related to the phenotypic consequences of mutation.[48] Naturally occurring point mutations that affect mRNA splicing fall into four main categories: (1) Mutations within 5' or 3' consensus splice sites. Such lesions usually reduce the amount of correctly spliced mature mRNA and/or lead to the utilization of alternative splice sites in the vicinity. This results in the production of mRNAs that either lack a portion of the coding sequence (*exon skipping*) or contain additional sequence of intronic origin (*cryptic splice-site utilization*). (2) Mutations within an intron or exon that may serve

to activate cryptic splice sites and lead to the production of aberrant mRNA species. (3) Mutations within a branch-point sequence. (4) Mutations in the introns that may regulate the efficiency of splicing, balance of alternative transcripts, and spliceosome assembly. Our understanding of the mechanism of these latter mutations is poor.

Splice-Junction Mutations Causing Human Genetic Disease

Splicing defects are not an uncommon cause of human genetic disease. The vast majority of known gene lesions that affect splicing are point mutations within 5' and 3' splice sites (ss). As shown in Fig. 2-1, the 1373 splicing mutations account for 9.6 percent of the 14363 mutations recorded in the HGMD (as of September 13, 1998). Krawczak et al[48] first collected from the literature (until mid-1991) a total of 101 different examples of point mutation in the vicinity of exon-intron splice junctions of human genes that altered the accuracy or efficiency of mRNA splicing and were responsible for a specific disease phenotype. Since then, the accelerated pace of gene and mutation discovery has greatly enriched our understanding of the importance of different splice signal sequences. Of 1373 different splice-site mutations, 797 (58 percent) affected the 5' ss (donor splice site), 464 (34 percent) were located in 3' ss (acceptor splice site), and most of the remaining 112 resulted in the creation of novel splice sites. Fig. 2-6 shows the consensus splice-site sequences of mammalian genes. For both the wild-type and mutated splice sites, *consensus values* (CVs[49]) can be calculated that reflect the similarity of any one splice site to the consensus sequence. A splice site containing the least frequent bases at each position would yield a CV of 0, whereas splice sites containing only the most frequent bases would have a CV of 1. CV for the wild-type splice sites (consensus value for normal [CVN] splice sites) studied were from 0.7 to 1, with a mean of about 0.83 for the 5' and 3' ss. Sequences with either extremely small or extremely high CVN were lacking. This finding suggested that splice sites that are less than optimal in terms of their similarity to the consensus sequence are especially prone to the deleterious effects of mutation. Splice sites with an already extremely low degree of similarity would not be further functionally impaired by single-base changes. An analysis was also conducted for the CV of mutated splice sites (CVM[48]). These CVMs were from 0.48 to 0.74 for the 3' ss and from 0.5 to 0.84 for the 5' ss. This clearly indicated that mutations at splice-site junctions serve to reduce the similarity to the consensus.

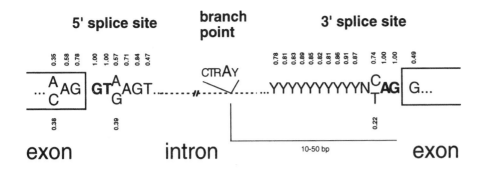

Fig. 2-6. Consensus sequences for the 5′ splice site (ss) (donor site), 3′ ss (acceptor site), and the branch point. Numbers corresponding to the nucleotides represent frequencies of each given nucleotide in the collections of Padget et al[50] and Shapiro and Senapathy.[49]

Location and Spectrum of Splice-Site Mutations

Comparison of the number of mutations in the HGMD reported at particular splice-site positions with their corresponding expectations, based on substitution rates from human gene-coding regions, indicates that point mutations are significantly overrepresented at the invariant positions +1 (observed, 414; expected, 189.5) and +2 (observed, 89; expected, 51.0) of the 5′ ss, and positions −1 (observed, 192; expected, 62.8) and −2 (observed, 168; expected, 23.3) of the 3′ ss. Mutations at all other positions within splice sites were underrepresented. Table 2-9 summarizes the observed and expected frequencies of point mutations at different positions in 5′ ss and 3′ ss. Of the 1373 splicing mutations in the HGMD, 414 (30.1 percent) occur at the 5′-ss position +1 and 89 (6.5 percent) at position +2 (http://www.uwcm.ac.uk/uwcm/mg/haha2.html). The majority (58 percent) of the G+1 mutations were to A, and the majority of the T+2 mutations were to C. In the 3′ ss, there are 168 mutations (12 percent) in the invariant A−2, and 192 (14 percent) in the invariant G−1. The majority (53 percent) of the G−1 mutations were to A, and the majority (69 percent) of the A−2 mutations were to G. Therefore, the four invariant nucleotides (of the 24 involved in the splice-site consensus sequences) in the 5′ ss and the 3′ ss represent a total of 863, i.e., 62.8 percent of the splicing mutations. Fig. 2-7 depicts the distribution of mutations within the consensus 5′ ss and 3′ ss logged in the HGMD. It is of interest that a considerable number of mutations have been found in nucleotides +5 and −1 of the consensus 5′ ss, although these positions are not invariant. At position +5 of the 5′ ss, a total of 103 mutations have been reported, whilst, at position −1, a total of 100 mutations have been found (as of September 13, 1998). Table 2-9, however, shows that these numbers are not higher than expected under a model of random mutations.

It appears very likely that the observed nonrandomness of mutation within splice sites is a reflection of relative phenotypic severity (and hence detection bias) rather than any intrinsic difference in the underlying frequency of mutation. The replacement of G residues at positions +1 and +5 of 5′ ss would be predicted to reduce significantly the stability of base pairing of the splice site with the complementary region of U1 small nuclear RNA (snRNA). Binding to U1 snRNA is essential for the pre-mRNA to be folded correctly before cleavage and ligation can occur within the spliceosome. The same argument holds true for the mutations observed at position −1.[51] Only 42 examples of mutations at the +3 and 20 at the +4 positions of 5′ ss, respectively, were noted; the corresponding residues in U1 snRNA are pseudouridines rather than a cytosine. Thus, the spectrum of 5′-ss mutations observed *in vivo* suggests an important role for U1 snRNA binding.

Mutations Creating Novel Splice Sites

A different category of mutation affecting mRNA splicing is provided by single-base-pair substitutions outside actual splice sites that create novel splice sites that substitute for the wild-type sites. This category may contain more mutations than currently appreciated, because very few sequence data exist for introns as compared with coding regions. A total of 13 mutations creating novel splice sites (13 percent of the 101 splice mutations) were collected in a survey by Krawczak et al;[48] in all but one case, the novel splice site was situated upstream of the original wild-type site. One intriguing finding for mutations creating novel 3′ acceptor splice sites should be noted: All six mutations introduced an A at −2, but never a G at −1. CVs for the activated cryptic splice sites (CVAs) were calculated when possible; in 8 of 12 cases, the CVA was as high as or higher than the wild-type CVN, suggesting that the novel splice sites successfully compete with the wild-type sites for splicing factors. For mutations in the vicinity of 3′ ss, the relative proportion of cryptic splice-site-utilizing mRNA appeared to correlate positively with the CVA/CVN ratio, whereas, at 5′ ss, the distance to the wild-type site may have also played an important role. The current version of the HGMD contains 112 mutations outside the consensus splice sites, and most of them create novel splice sites.

Phenotypic Consequences of Splice-Site Mutation *in Vivo*

The phenotypic consequences of naturally occurring point mutations in the 5′ ss of seven human genes were studied by Talerico and Berget,[52] who observed exon skipping in six cases as compared with only one case (β-globin gene) of cryptic splice-site usage. These initial results suggested that exon skipping might be the preferred *in vivo* phenotype, an assertion confirmed by many subsequent reports. One major mRNA species was usually observed, and this invariably lacked either the exon upstream of the mutated 5′ ss or downstream of the mutated 3′ ss. A detection bias is nevertheless possible, since a single exon-skipped transcript might be easier to detect/identify than a number of less frequent transcripts each resulting from the use of a different cryptic splice site. Several instances of the detection of small amounts of residual

Table 2-9 Observed and Expected Frequencies of Point Mutations at Different Positions in 5′ and 3′ Splice Sites (from the Human Gene Mutation Database, September 13, 1998)

5′ Splice Sites			3′ Splice Sites		
Pos	Obs	Exp	Pos	Obs	Exp
−2	15	84	−6	11	47
−1	100	154	−5	5	57
+1	**414**	**189**	−4	5	48
+2	**89**	**51**	−3	26	45
+3	42	73	−2	**168**	**23**
+4	20	57	−1	**192**	**63**
+5	103	119	−1	4	72
+6	14	68	−2	4	61

NOTE: Pos, position; Obs, observed frequency; Exp, expected frequency.

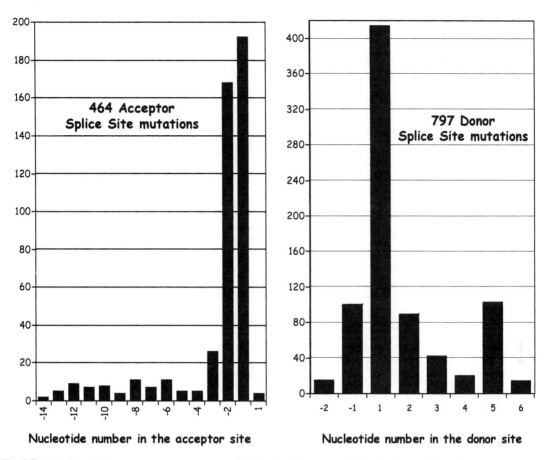

Fig. 2-7. Mutations in the consensus sequences of splice junctions recorded in the Human Gene Mutation Database.

wild-type mRNA from the cells of patients with a 5'-ss defect have also been reported. All these involve the mutation of bases outside the invariant GT dinucleotide, suggesting that normal splicing is still possible in such cases, albeit at greatly reduced efficiency. The choice between exon skipping and cryptic splice-site usage may be visualized merely as a decision about whether to utilize the next available legitimate splice site or the next best, albeit illegitimate, sequence in the immediate vicinity. This choice may be made on the basis of the presence/absence of sites capable of competing with the mutated splice site for splicing factors. Krawczak et al[48] studied the regions both upstream and downstream of their collection of mutations in an attempt to correlate sequence properties with the observed phenotypic consequences of mutation. They presented evidence that, at least for 5'-ss mutations, cryptic splice-site usage is favored under conditions in which a number of such sites are present in the immediate vicinity and exhibit sufficient homology to the splice-site consensus sequence for them to compete successfully with the mutated splice site. Fig. 2-8 schematically represents the consequences of splice mutations with reference to representative examples. In this chapter, exon skipping as a consequence of nonsense mutations in the skipped exon[63,67] is discussed under nonsense mutations.

Mutations within the Pyrimidine Tract

The HGMD contains 69 mutations in the pyrimidine tract of the 3' ss. Some examples include the steroid 21-hydroxylase B (CYP21B) and HBB genes causing adrenal hyperplasia and β thalassemia, respectively.[68-70] It is not clear how and why these mutations at polypyrimidine tracts exert a pathologic influence on efficient mRNA splicing. It may be that some 3' ss are more

susceptible to the effects of pyrimidine loss than are others by virtue of the relative length of the pyrimidine tract.

Mutations at the Branch Point

An intermediate stage in eukaryotic RNA splicing is the formation of a lariat structure utilizing an A (adenosine) residue approximately 10 to 50 nucleotides from the 3' ss. A weak consensus sequence, CTRAY, for this branch point has been observed in mammalian genes. After lariat structure formation, the first downstream AG dinucleotide is usually chosen as the acceptor splice site.[71] In a family with X-linked hydrocephalus, an A-to-C mutation 19 nucleotides upstream from a normal splice acceptor site of exon Q of the L1CAM gene on Xq28 segregated with the disease phenotype.[72] The mutation resulted in several RNA species exhibiting exon-Q skipping, insertion of 69 bp due to utilization of a cryptic splice site, or normal splicing. Another example of such mutation was reported in the COL5A1 gene causing Ehlers-Danlos syndrome type II. Affected members from two British families were heterozygous for a T-to-C point mutation in intron 32 (IVS32, −25T > G), causing loss of the 45-bp exon 33 from the mRNA in 60 percent of transcripts of the mutant gene.[73] The mutation lies only 2 bp upstream of a highly conserved adenosine in the consensus branch-site sequence that is required for lariat formation. A similar branch-site point mutation (IVS4, −22T > C) in the LCAT was observed in a family with fish eye disease, a condition characterized by corneal opacities and low plasma high-density-lipoprotein (HDL) cholesterol. The mutation caused intron retention rather than exon skipping.[74] In a patient with erythropoietic protoporphyria, a C-to-T mutation in intron 2 (IVS2, −23C > T) of the ferrochelatase (FECH) gene was found.[75] This mutation was associated with skipping of exon 2.

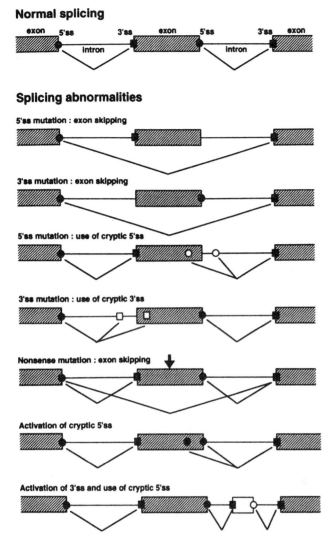

Fig. 2-8. Examples of exon skipping and utilization of cryptic splice sites as a result of mutations in splice sites. *Solid square* and *circle* denote normal or activated 3' ss and 5' ss, respectively. *Open square* and *circle* represent cryptic 3' ss and 5' ss, respectively. The *arrow* denotes a nonsense mutation. Examples of exon skipping due to 5' ss mutations are reported in Weil et al,[53,54] Grandchamp et al,[55] Carstens et al,[56] and Wen et al;[57] exon skipping due to 3' ss mutations is reported in Tromp and Prockop[58] and Dunn et al[59]; use of cryptic 5' ss due to 5' ss mutations is reported in Treistman et al[60] and Atweh et al[61]; use of cryptic 3' ss due to 3' ss mutations is reported in Carstens et al[56] and Su and Lin[62]; exon skipping due to nonsense mutations is reported in Dietz et al[63]; and activation of cryptic 5' ss and 3' ss is reported in Orkin et al,[64] Nakano et al,[65] and Mitchell et al[66]

Mutations in *Alu* Sequences and Creation of a New 5' Splice Site

The creation of 3' ss consequent to a point mutation in a member of the *Alu* family of human repetitive elements was noted by Mitchell *et al.*[76] Analysis of the ornithine aminotransferase mRNA of a patient with gyrate atrophy revealed a 142-nucleotide insertion at the junction of exons 3 and 4. The patient possessed a much reduced level (5 percent) of abnormal mRNA in his fibroblasts and an even smaller amount of normal-sized mRNA. An *Alu* sequence is normally present in intron 3 of the ornithine δ-aminotransferase (OAT) gene, 150 bp downstream of exon 3. The patient was homozygous for a C-to-G transversion in the right arm of this *Alu* repeat, which served to create a new 5' ss. This mutation activated an upstream cryptic 3' ss (the polyT comple-

ment of the *Alu* polyA tail followed by an AG dinucleotide) and a new "exon," containing the majority of the right arm of the *Alu* sequence, was recognized by the splicing apparatus and incorporated into the mRNA. The *splice-mediated insertion* of an *Alu* sequence in reverse orientation may yet prove to be no unusual mechanism of insertional mutagenesis, since *Alu* sequences are interspersed through many coding sequences, the sequence requirements for a functional 3' ss are far from stringent, and the reverse complement of a consensus *Alu* repeat contains at least two cryptic 3' ss and several potential 5' ss.

Other Splicing Mutations

There are certainly several intron sequence motifs, not yet fully recognized, that contribute to the regulation of the splicing mechanism. Mutations for example were detected in IVS3 of the human growth hormone (GH1) gene that affect a novel putative, consensus sequence which also perturb splicing, resulting in exon skipping.[77] These mutations did not occur within the 5' and 3' ss or branch consensus sites. The first was a G to A at nt +28 of the second deleted 18 bp (del+28−45) of IVS3 of the human GH1 gene. These mutations segregated with autosomal dominant GH deficiency in both kindreds, and no other allelic GH1 gene changes were detected. Reverse transcriptase-polymerase chain reaction (RT-PCR) amplification showed a >10-fold preferred use of alternative splicing. Both mutations were located 28 bp downstream from the 5' ss, and both perturbed an intronic XGGG repeat similar to that found to regulate mRNA splicing in chicken β-tropomyosin. Binding of heterogeneous nuclear ribonucleoprotein (hnRNP) to these sequences in pre-mRNA transcripts is thought to play an important role in pre-mRNA packaging and transport as well as 5'-ss selection in pre-mRNAs that contain multiple 5' ss.[77]

In patients with frontotemporal dementia with parkinsonism, three heterozygous mutations in a cluster of 4 nts +13 to +16 of exon 10 of the tau (MAPT) gene were found.[78] All of these mutations destabilized a potential stem-loop structure that is probably involved in regulating the alternative splicing of exon 10. This caused more frequent use of the 5' ss and an increased proportion of tau transcripts that include exon 10. The increase in exon 10+ mRNA was expected to increase the proportion of tau protein containing four microtubule-binding repeats, which is consistent with the neuropathology described in families with this type of frontotemporal dementia. Mutations in intron regions that regulate the proportion of alternatively spliced exons may therefore be an important mechanism for late-onset phenotypes.

mRNA Processing (Other Than Splicing) and Translation Mutations

Mutations affecting mRNA processing and translation may exert their pathologic effects at any one of the various stages between transcriptional initiation and translation. Mutations other than those affecting mRNA splicing are now described and their phenotypic consequences assessed.

Cap-Site Mutants. The transcription of an mRNA is initiated at the cap site (+1), so named because of the posttranscriptional addition of 7-methylguanine at this position to protect the transcript from exonucleolytic degradation. Wong *et al*[79] described an A-to-C transversion at the cap site in the HBB gene of an Indian patient with β thalassemia. Kozak[80] collated known eukaryotic mRNA sequence data and showed that the cap site is an adenine in 76 percent of cases. A cytosine residue at position 1 was noted in only 6 percent of cases. It is not clear, however, whether it is transcription of the β-globin gene that is severely reduced in the above patient or whether transcriptional initiation occurs efficiently but at a different, incorrect site. In the latter case, the resulting transcript could be either incomplete or unstable.

Mutations in Initiation Codons. There are 59 mutations recorded in the HGMD affecting Met (ATG) translational initiation codons, with a preponderance of M-to-V substitutions.

The consequences for mRNA transcription and translation have not been well studied. It is particularly useful to compare and contrast the two ATG mutations reported in the α_1- and α_2-globin genes, respectively. The α_1-globin gene mutation was associated with a reduction in the steady-state α_1-globin mRNA level to one-fourth normal.[81] The corresponding α_2-globin mRNA level consequent to the α_2-globin gene lesion was similarly reduced to one-third normal.[82] The α_2-globin gene mutation results in a greater reduction in α-globin synthesis and a more severe α-thalassemia phenotype than its α_1-globin counterpart. This is presumably because, in normal individuals, the ratio of α_2 to α_1 mRNA produced from the two genes is 2.6, reflecting the relative importance of the α_2-globin gene in α-globin synthesis. The observed reductions in steady-state mRNA levels are reminiscent of the consequences of nonsense mutations (see below). Mitchell et al[66] reported a normal amount of OAT mRNA in Lebanese patients with gyrate atrophy who were homozygous for an initiation codon mutation.

Is the mutant mRNA translated? The answer is likely to be determined by a complex interplay of the different structural features of an mRNA that serve to modulate its translation (reviewed by Kozak[83]). Until fairly recently, it was thought that an AUG codon was an absolute requirement for translational initiation in mammals. However, some exceptions are now known — for example, ACG and CUG (reviewed by Kozak[83]) — indicating that some mutations might be tolerated more than others. The scanning model of translational initiation predicts that the 40S ribosomal subunit initiates at the first AUG codon to be encountered within an acceptable sequence context (GCC A/G CCAUGG is believed to be optimal[83]). Ribosomes may be capable of utilizing mutated AUG codons, albeit with reduced efficiency, or they may be able to initiate translation at the next best available site downstream.[84] The phenotypic consequences of a given ATG mutation are thus likely to depend on the nature of the mutational lesion, the tolerance of the ribosome with respect to translational initiation codon recognition, the presence of alternative downstream ATG codons with flanking translational initiation site consensus sequence, and the functional importance of the absent N-terminal end of the protein.

Creation of a New Initiation Codon. Another type of mutation that interferes with correct initiation is the creation of a cryptic ATG codon (in the context of a favorable Kozak consensus sequence) in the vicinity of the one normally used. An example of this type of lesion is provided by the G-to-A transition at position 122 (relative to the cap site) of the β-globin gene causing β-thalassemia intermedia.[85] This cryptic initiation codon is 26 bp 5' to the normal ATG codon, and its use would lead to a frameshift and premature termination 36 bp downstream. Although the relative extent of utilization of the two ATG codons in this patient is not known, the comparatively mild clinical phenotype suggests that at least some β-globin is correctly initiated and translated. There are 208 cases in the HGMD for the creation of an ATG (Met) codon, but it is unclear how many of these are then used as aberrant initiation codons.

Mutation in Termination Codons

The first reported example of a mutation in a termination codon was that in the α_2-globin (HBA2) gene causing Hemoglobin Constant Spring (Hb$_{constant\ spring}$), an abnormal hemoglobin that occurs frequently in Southeast Asia.[86,87] The associated α-globin chain is 172 amino acids long, rather than the normal 141 amino acids, as a result of a TAA-to-CAA transition in the termination codon. In this patient, translation extends into the 3' noncoding region of the α_2-globin mRNA. The resulting mRNA is highly unstable, resulting in low production of hemoglobin in the red cells of heterozygous carriers.[88] Several other mutations are known to occur in the α_2-globin termination codon, and a similar phenotype to Hb$_{constant\ spring}$ is observed.[89] A total of 15 point mutations in the termination codon have been included in the HGMD. Nine of

these occur in the TGA, five in the TAA, and one in the TAG termination codons, respectively, of the APRT, ARSB, ATM, CTSK, FGFR3, HBA2, IDUA, PROS1, and AIRE1 genes (see the HGMD). With regard to the distribution of termination codons in mammalian genes, TGA is found in 52 percent, TAA in 27 percent, and TAG in 21 percent of these genes. Elongated proteins may also be generated by a second mechanism — a frameshift mutation close to the natural termination codon that results in the extension of translation until the next available downstream termination codon. A number of examples of this type of lesion are known to cause β thalassemia.[69,90–94] All give rise to an imbalance in α- and β-globin chain synthesis and inclusion-body (containing precipitated α and β chains) formation and are associated with the dominant form of the disease.

Polyadenylation/Cleavage Signal Mutations

All polyadenylated mRNA in higher eukaryotes possess the sequence AAUAAA, or a close homologue, 10 to 30 nucleotides upstream of the polyadenylation site. This motif is thought to play a role in 3'-end formation through endonucleolytic cleavage and polyadenylation of the mRNA transcript. Several single-base-pair substitutions are now known in the cleavage/polyadenylation signal sequences of the α_2- and β-globin genes, and all of these cause a relatively mild form of thalassemia due to the reduction of HbA$_2$ synthesis to 3 to 5 percent of the normal level. In the β-globin gene mutants, cleavage and polyadenylation at the normal site are markedly reduced but do still occur at < 10 percent of the normal level as judged by both in vivo and in vitro assays.[95,96] These mutants are characterized by a novel species of β-globin mRNA 1500 nucleotides long and 900 nucleotides larger than the wild-type transcript. This results from the use of an alternative cleavage/polyadenylation site (AATAAAA) 900 bp 3' to the mutated site; polyadenylation occurs within 15 nucleotides of this cryptic site. This abnormal mRNA may be highly unstable, since it was extremely difficult to isolate. Several other polyadenylated mRNA species up to 2900 bp in length have been reported in an Israeli patient with a polyadenylation site mutation;[97] the β+-thalassemia phenotype exhibited by this patient was consistent with the translation of these extended mRNA species. Outside of the globin genes, a polyadenylation mutation has been described (AATAAC to AGTAAC) in the ARSA gene and causes arylsulfatase pseudodeficiency.[98] An unusual T-to-C substitution causing β-globin gene, 12 bp upstream of the AATAAA polyadenylation signal, has been described in an Irish family.[85] It is thought that this lesion may serve to destabilize the β-globin mRNA.

Nonsense Mutations and Their Effect on mRNA Levels

Nonsense mutations obviously cause premature termination of translation and truncated polypeptides, but these lesions may also exert their effects at the transcriptional level. Benz et al[99] first noticed that some patients with β thalassemia who had nonsense codons in the β-globin gene exhibited very low levels (< 1 percent) of β-globin mRNA in erythrocytes. Subsequently, a considerable number of nonsense or frameshift mutations from a variety of different genes have been shown to be associated with dramatic reductions in the steady-state level of cytoplasmic mRNA. However, this rule is not completely inviolable; a few nonsense mutations are associated with normal levels of cytoplasmic mRNA that appears to be efficiently translated to generate a truncated protein (e.g., low-density lipoprotein receptor [LDLR],[100] apolipoprotein C-II [apo C-II]),[101] and β-globin[102]). Moreover, considerable variation in mRNA levels is apparent between different instances of introduced nonsense codons within the same gene: Thus, measured reticulocyte β-globin mRNA varied from < 1 percent normal in a patient with β thalassemia who had a 1-bp frameshift deletion at codon 44 (Kinniburgh et al[103]) to 15 percent in a patient with a nonsense mutation in codon 17 (Chang and Kan[104]). Brody et al[105] observed that mutations that cause premature termination in the terminal exon of the OAT gene have no effect on mRNA level, but termination in the penultimate exon or earlier is associated with markedly reduced levels of mRNA. Decreased *in vitro* accumulation of cytoplasmic mRNA has been reported to be associated with several nonsense mutations in the β-globin gene but not with missense mutations.[106–110] One potential explanation for the observed effect of nonsense mutations on mRNA metabolism is that mRNA which is incompletely translated is not protected properly from RNase digestion on the ribosome and is therefore likely to exhibit an increased turnover rate. Consistent with this postulate, the β-globin mRNA bearing the codon-44 mutation appears to be highly unstable.[111] Moreover, Daar and Maquat[112] reported that all triosephosphate isomerase I (TPI1) gene nonsense and frameshift mutations tested *in vitro* exhibited a reduced mRNA stability but did not alter the rate of transcription. At least for the β-globin codon 39 mutation, however, the decreased steady-state levels of both nuclear and cytoplasmic mRNA have been shown not to be due to increased mRNA instability in the cytoplasm.[106,107,109]

The mechanism by which an in-frame termination codon results in a decrease in concentration of steady-state cytoplasmic mRNA is not understood. One or more parameters could be affected—the transcription rate, the efficiency of mRNA processing or transport to the cytoplasm, or mRNA stability.[113] Urlaub et al[114] showed that whereas nonsense mutations in the dihydrofolate reductase (DHFR) gene located prior to the final exon resulted in drastically reduced (10- to 20-fold) mRNA levels, nonsense mutations in the last exon of the gene yielded normal levels of DHFR mRNA. Nuclear run-on studies and experiments with the transcriptional inhibitor actinomycin demonstrated that the low mRNA levels resulted neither from a reduced rate of transcription nor from decreased mRNA stability. Similar results were obtained for nonsense mutations artificially introduced into the TPI1 gene and expressed *in vitro*.[115] Urlaub *et al.*[114] proposed two explanatory models that imply some form of coupling between processing and/or transport of the mRNA and translation: (1) Translational translocation model: This model proposes that translation of the mRNA on the ribosome would begin as soon as the mRNA emerged from the nuclear pore and would serve to pull the pre-mRNA physically through the splicing apparatus and through the pores in the nuclear membrane. Nonsense mutations would halt the pulling process, leaving the RNA molecule vulnerable to RNase digestion. However, nonsense mutations occurring in the last exon would not be recognized until the translocation of the mRNA from the nucleus was virtually complete. (2) Nuclear scanning of translation frames model: In this model, pre-mRNA are scanned within the nucleus for nonsense mutations prior to their translocation through the nuclear membrane. Detection of an in-frame termination codon would then result in a slowing of mRNA splicing/translocation. Such a mechanism might be an intrinsic part of the mRNA-splicing process since open-reading-frame recognition could be important for exon definition. The translational translocation model would predict a probability gradient from 5' to 3', with a gradually increasing likelihood that an mRNA containing a termination codon would be successfully transported across the nuclear membrane. In support of this hypothesis are the several examples of normal levels of mRNA transcripts derived from genes bearing termination codons in their 3'-most exons (see the OAT example[105]) and the TPI1 and DHFR examples that may imply links between pre-mRNA splicing, mRNA transport, and translation. However, counterexamples, such as the β-globin gene codon-17 and codon-44 nonsense codons quoted above, argue against its validity in all cases, since they are inconsistent with a perfect linear relationship between the relative position of the nonsense mutation and the level of mRNA produced by the mutant allele. The problem with invoking any one model alone is that it cannot adequately explain the inconsistencies observed between studies regarding the possible position effect associated with nonsense

mutations *in vivo* and the role of changes in mRNA stability if they occur. In practical terms, the common finding of greatly reduced or absent cytoplasmic mRNA associated with nonsense mutations has important implications for mutation screening. Attempts to obtain mRNA for RT-PCR amplification and DNA sequencing[116,117] may be thwarted in patients with nonsense mutations by a cellular mechanism that links mRNA processing/transport to translation.

Nonsense Mutations and Exon Skipping

Dietz et al[63] and Naylor et al[67] have reported exon skipping in exons that contain nonsense mutations. In a patient with Marfan syndrome, exon B of the fibrillin gene FBN1 that contained a TAT-to-TAG nonsense mutation was completely skipped.[63] The exon skipping was discovered by RT-PCR analysis of fibroblast mRNA. Two additional examples of this phenomenon have been reported by the same authors in the OAT transcripts of patients with gyrate atrophy: exon 6 was skipped when a Trp 178 to Stop mutation was present in this exon; similarly, exon 8 with a Trp 275 to Stop mutation was skipped. The skipping of the exons with nonsense codons in the OAT cases was partial, that is, there were RNA species that contained the nonsense-mutation-containing exons. The authors proposed a mechanism of *reading* pre-mRNA exon sequences in frame either by direct coupling between translation and RNA processing or by a scanning function of ribosome-like molecules in the nucleus. Naylor et al[67] reported similar observations associated with two different nonsense mutations in exons 19 and 22 in the F8C gene in patients with hemophilia A. Partial skipping has been observed with the exon-19 nonsense mutation whereas, in the case of the exon-22 nonsense codon, only PCR products lacking exon 22 were observed. The exon skipping associated with nonsense mutations has been observed in more than 10 disease-related genes in humans. The mechanism that accounts for these observations is unknown.

Dietz and Kendzior,[118] using chimeric constructs in a model *in vivo* expression system, identified premature termination codons as determinants of splice-site selection. Nonsense codon recognition prior to RNA splicing necessitates the ability to read the frame of precursor mRNA in the nucleus. They proposed that maintenance of an open reading frame can serve as an additional level of scrutiny during exon definition.

Regulatory Mutations

Most mutations causing human genetic disease occur in transcribed regions. A different class of molecular lesion is that represented by regulatory mutations. These lesions disrupt the normal processes of gene activation and transcriptional initiation and serve either to increase or decrease the level of mRNA/gene product synthesized rather than altering its nature. The vast majority of regulatory mutations so far described are found in gene promoter regions—the 5' flanking sequences that contain constitutive promoter elements, enhancers, repressors, the determinants of tissue-specific gene expression, and other regulatory elements. Mutations in the regulatory elements may have several consequences, such as alteration of the amount of mRNA transcript and/or alteration of the developmental expression of a gene. In the majority of regulatory mutations, the mRNA produced is qualitatively normal, and therefore mutation detection methods based on RT-PCR will fail to recognize these lesions. On the other hand, the detection of mutations in potential unknown regulatory elements may predict the existence of such elements. A total of 119 regulatory mutations have been cataloged in the HGMD. Some representative examples of mutations in regulatory elements in the human genome are discussed below.

Mutations in DNA Motifs in the Immediate 5' Flanking Sequences. Single-base-pair substitutions that occur in the promoter region 5' to the β-globin (HBB) gene causing β thalassemia give rise to a moderate reduction in globin synthesis. The known naturally occurring mutations are highly clustered around two regions that have been implicated in the regulation of the human β-globin (HBB) gene. One is a CACCC motif located between −91 and −86 relative to the transcriptional initiation site and the other is the TATA box found at about −30. Mutations have been described in the CACCC motif at positions −92, −90, −88, −87, and −86, and the TATA motif at positions −31, −30, −29, and −28, of the β-globin gene.[60,119–127] Almost all of these mutations are associated with a mild clinical phenotype. The CACCC box binds one or more erythroid-specific nuclear factors involved in the developmental activation of β-globin gene transcription. A −101 mutation occurs in the second upstream CACCC motif between −105 and −101 of the β-globin gene.[128] Matsuda et al[129] have reported a T-to-C transition at position −77 of the δ-globin (HBD) gene in Japanese patients with δ thalassemia. This lesion occurs at the second position of an inverted binding motif (TTATCT) for the DNA-binding protein GATA1. Gel retardation and CAT expression assays demonstrated that this mutation appears to impair δ-globin gene expression by abolishing GATA1 binding to its recognition sequence.

Mutations in *cis*-acting regulatory elements can also increase gene expression. The best examples of such mutations have been observed in hereditary persistence of fetal hemoglobin (HPFH), which is usually a heterozygous condition in which inherited gene lesions cause a marked but variable increase in HbF (α_2 and γ_2) synthesis above the normal adult level of < 1 percent. The molecular analysis of HPFH has revealed both deletion and nondeletion forms. The nondeletion form of HPFH is caused by point mutations within the highly homologous promoter regions of the γ-globin genes. There are three examples of mutation at homologous positions in the Aγ- and Gγ-globin genes at positions −114, −175, and −202.[130–135] The −202 mutation occurs within a GGGGCCCC motif reminiscent of the GC box (GGGCGG) that serves as a binding site for the transcription factor Sp1. The T-to-C mutations at −175 occur within an ATGCAAAT motif (−182 to −175) known as the octamer, found in the promoters of genes encoding immunoglobulins, histones, and snRNA. The −175 lesion has been shown to increase promoter activity between 3- and 20-fold in erythroid cells.[136–140] This lesion appears to reduce or abolish the ability of the ubiquitous octamer-binding protein (OTF-1, which is thought to be a repressor of γ-globin gene transcription) to bind at this site[140–143] and alters the binding of GATA1.[136,139–141] Using gel-retardation assays, Fucharoen et al[132] demonstrated that the −114 mutation abolishes the binding of CP1 to the distal CCAAT motif of the Gγ-globin gene, although the lesion does not affect the binding of erythroid-specific factors.

Hemophilia B$_{leyden}$ is an F9 variant characterized by severe childhood hemophilia ameliorated at puberty, probably under the influence of testosterone,[144] and is an example of developmental specificity of regulatory mutations. The amelioration in clinical phenotype is foreshadowed by an increase in plasma F9 activity/antigen values from < 1 percent to between 30 and 60 percent normal. Several mutations have been found in positions −20, −6, +6, +8, and +13 relative to the transcriptional initiation site in such patients.[145–153] Reitsma et al[146] noted that the region from −5 to +23 possesses significant homology with the region immediately upstream, from −31 to −6. All mutated sites occur within the region of homology. Crossley and Brownlee[154] demonstrated that the +13 mutation lies within a binding site (+1 to +18) for the CCAAT/enhancer-binding protein (C/EBP) and serves to abolish binding of C/EBP to this site. Other transcription factors have been shown to bind in the −32 to +23 region.[155] Hirosawa et al[149] demonstrated that mutations at −20 and −6 were associated with lowered expression of the F9 gene and that restoration of expression in a concentration-dependent fashion was observed on treatment of the cultured cells with androgen. Crossley et al[155] found that an AGCTCAGCTTGTACT motif between −36 and −22, with strong homology to the androgen-response element (ARE) consensus sequence, is functional. It would appear that, before puberty, several transcription

factors (including C/EBP, LF-A1/HNF4, and a further protein that binds to the −6 site) are involved in potentiating the expression of the F9 gene. Since mutations interfering with the binding of any of these factors lead to the abolition of F9 gene transcription, these proteins probably act in concert. It is assumed that at puberty, when a testosterone-dependent mechanism mediated by the ARE comes into play, the binding of all three transcription factors ceases to be an absolute requirement for transcription to occur.

Mutations Outside the Immediate 5′ Flanking Sequences. In addition to known mutations in the remote promoter element known as the *locus control region* (LCR; see below), Berg et al[156] have reported a +ATA/−T mutation at −530 upstream the HBB gene that is associated with reduced β-globin synthesis. This lesion reportedly results in a ninefold increase in the binding capacity of BP1, a protein that may therefore possess the properties of a repressor. In two families with X-linked dominant Charcot-Marie-Tooth neuropathy, a T-to-G transversion at position −528 and a C-to-T transition at position −458 to the ATG start codon of the connexin 32 gene (GJB1) have been found.[157] The first mutation is located in the nerve-specific GJB1 promoter just upstream of the transcription start site, whereas the second is located in the 5′ untranslated region (UTR) of the mRNA.

Regulatory mutations have also been reported in the 3′ flanking sequences of genes. A G-to-A transition 69 bp 3′ to the polyadenylation site appears to be responsible for drastically reducing the expression of the δ-globin gene, causing δ thalassemia.[158] The lesion occurs within a motif homologous to the consensus recognition sequence for the erythroid-specific DNA-binding protein GATA1. Gel-retardation assays have shown that the G-to-A transition resulted in an increased binding affinity for GATA1.[158]

Mutation in Remote Promoter Elements. The first indication that mutations at a considerable distance 5′ to the transcriptional initiation site could affect the expression of a downstream gene came from van der Ploeg et al:[159] A > 40-kb deletion of the Gγ-, Aγ-, and δ-globin genes was found in a Dutch case of γδβ thalassemia, but this deletion had left the β-globin gene intact, together with at least a 2.5-kb 5′ flanking sequence (Fig. 13-9). The implication was that the removal of sequences far upstream of the β-globin gene had resulted in suppression of its transcriptional activity. Kioussis et al[160] then showed that although the β-globin gene in this patient was identical in sequence to that of the wild type, the surrounding chromatin appeared to be in an inactive conformation as judged by DNase-1 sensitivity and methylation analysis. Curtin et al[161] reported a 90-kb deletion of the β-globin gene cluster in an English patient with γδβ thalassemia; the ε-globin gene and part of the Gγ-globin gene were deleted, but Aγ-, ψβ-, δ-, and β-globin genes were intact. A deletion more than 25 kb upstream of the β-globin gene therefore served to abolish its expression. Driscoll et al[162] described an important 25-kb deletion in a Hispanic patient with γδβ thalassemia; the deletion was located between 9.5 and 39 kb upstream of the ε-globin gene and included three of the four erythroid cell-specific DNase-1 hypersensitive sites 5′ to the ε-globin gene. All of the globin genes, including the ε-globin gene, remained intact; the β-globin gene, some 60 kb downstream from the 3′ deletion breakpoint, was nevertheless nonfunctional. Grosveld et al[163] showed that DNA containing the four erythroid-specific hypersensitive sites was capable of directing a high level of position-independent β-globin gene expression *in vitro*. The LCR 5′ to the ε-globin gene is thought to organize the β-globin gene cluster into an active chromatin domain and to enhance the transcription of individual globin genes. The Hispanic γδβ thalassemia deletion results in an altered chromatin structure throughout more than 100 kb in the β-globin gene cluster as revealed by a change in the sensitivity to DNase-1 digestion (see

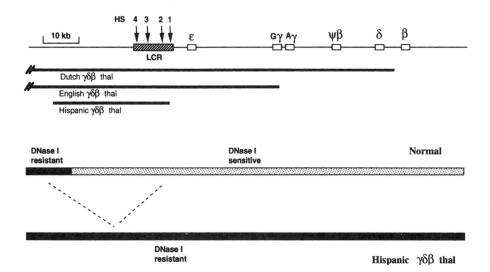

Fig. 2-9. Schematic representation of the deletions in the β-globin gene cluster that eliminate the locus control region (LCR) and result in silencing of the normal β-globin (HBB) gene. The extent of the deletions is shown as thick black line. The LCR and its four DNase hypersensitive sequences (HRS) are depicted. The bottom part of the figure shows the conversion of the entire β-globin gene cluster to a DNase I-resistant state as a result of the Hispanic γδ'-thalassemia deletion.

Fig. 2-9). A similar LCR is also present in the α-globin gene cluster at chromosome 16pter-p13.3.[164] Hatton et al[165] reported a 62-kb deletion causing α thalassemia encompassing the embryonic α-like ζ$_2$-globin gene that left the other genes and pseudogenes of the α-globin gene cluster intact. Though the sequences of the α$_1$- and α$_2$-globin genes were found to be normal, they nevertheless appeared to be transcriptionally inactive. Several other examples of similar deletions 5' to the α-globin gene cluster have now been reported.[166–169] These deletions exhibit an area of overlap between 30 and 50 kb upstream of the α-globin genes. This region contains several DNase-1 hypersensitive sites (two erythroid-specific) and is capable of directing the high-level expression of an α-globin gene both in stably transfected mouse erythroleukemia cells and when integrated into the genomes of transgenic mice.[170,171]

There are also reports of associations of apparently polymorphic variations in the vicinity of certain genes with certain phenotypes. All of these associations require large epidemiologic studies and detailed characterization of the potential regulatory elements to determine whether the polymorphic differences contribute to these phenotypes. For example, there is a G or A polymorphism at position +97 downstream from the termination codon in the 3' UTR of the prothrombin (*F2*) gene. Eighteen percent of patients with a documented familial history of venous thrombophilia had the A at this position as compared with 1 percent of a group of healthy controls.[172] An association was also found between the presence of the A allele and elevated prothrombin levels. This allele could be therefore used as a risk factor for venous thrombophilia. The polymorphism may either be directly responsible for the association or in linkage disequilibrium with another mutation which in turn is responsible for the observed association.

GENE DELETIONS

Gene deletions have so far been found to be responsible for more than 500 different inherited conditions in humans,[4] and these deletions may be broadly categorized on the basis of the length of DNA deleted. Some deletions consist of only one or a few base pairs, whereas others may span several hundred kilobases. By September 1998, the HGMD contained 2739 gross and small deletions.

Gross Gene Deletions

A total of 400 gross gene deletions have been logged in the HGMD. The nonrandomness of these lesions is apparent at two distinct levels. First, in some X-linked recessive conditions of similar incidence, the frequency of gene deletion does not always correlate with the size and complexity of the underlying gene. For example, some 2.5 to 5 percent of patients with hemophilia A have deletions of the F8C gene (26 exons spanning 186 kb of genomic DNA[173,174]), whereas 84 percent of patients with steroid sulfatase (STS) deficiency possess deletions of the STS genes (10 exons spanning 146 kb of genomic DNA[175]). Second, hotspots for deletion breakpoints have been reported within several human genes, including the Duchenne muscular dystrophy (DMD) gene,[176–179] the GH1 gene,[180,181] the LDLR gene,[182] and the α$_1$-globin gene.[183] Two main types of recombination events are thought to cause gross gene deletions—homologous unequal recombination, mediated either by related gene sequences or repetitive sequence elements, and nonhomologous recombination involving DNA with minimal sequence homology. Homologous unequal recombination involves the cleavage and rejoining of nonsister chromatids at homologous but nonallelic DNA sequences and generates fusion genes if the recombination breakpoints are intragenic. By contrast, nonhomologous or illegitimate recombination can occur between two sites that show little or minimal sequence homology.

Homologous Unequal Recombination Between Gene Sequences

Homologous recombination describes recombination occurring at meiosis or mitosis between identical or very similar DNA sequences. Homologous unequal recombination involves the recombination at homologous but nonallelic DNA sequences. This type of homologous recombination is thought to be one cause of deletions of the α-globin genes underlying α thalassemia. The α$_1$- and α$_2$-globin genes have evolved comparatively recently by gene duplication[184] and are thus virtually identical in sequence. These genes also possess flanking regions of homology (see regions *x* and *z* in Fig. 2-10) whose sequence similarity may have been maintained during evolution by gene conversion and unequal crossing-over. These *homology boxes* serve to potentiate homologous unequal recombination through incorrect chromosome alignment at meiosis. Recombinations between homologous *x* boxes, which are 4.2 kb apart (the *leftward crossover*), have been noted to produce chromosomes with a 4.2-kb deletion and only one α-globin gene[185] and chromosomes with three α-globin genes.[186,187] Recombinations between homologous *z* boxes that are 3.7 kb apart (the *rightward crossover*) generate chromosomes with a 3.7-kb deletion as well as the reciprocal product chromosomes carrying three α-globin genes.[186] Such recombination events may be common, since their product chromosomes have been reported in many different ethnic groups.[184] In every case, the breakpoints are located within the *x* or *z* homology boxes.

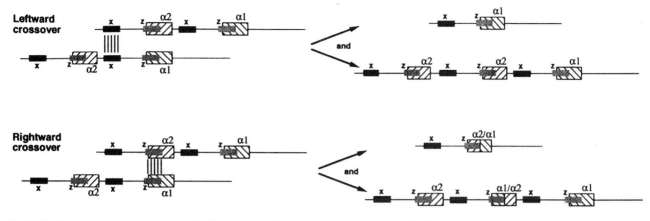

Fig. 2-10. Homologous unequal recombination between the *homology boxes x* and *z* in the human α-globin gene region. The leftward crossover is due to the misalignment of the *x* boxes, whereas the rightward crossover is caused by misalignment of the *z* boxes. The recombination events cause either deletions or duplications as shown.

Homologous Unequal Recombination Between Repetitive Sequence Elements

Recombination with *Alu* Repetitive Elements. Repetitive DNA sequences are thought to cause gene deletions by promoting unequal crossovers. The most abundant repetitive element in the human genome is the *Alu* repeat. There are up to 10^6 copies of *Alu* elements in the human genome, with an average spacing of 4 kb.[188–190] They are about 300 bp long and consist of two similar regions between 120 and 150 bp separated by a short A-rich region. Each *Alu* element is between 70 and 98 percent homologous to the *Alu* consensus sequence. Most of the *Alu* sequences have a polyA tail at their 3′ ends and are flanked by direct repeats (4 to 20 bp). *Alu* sequences are known to contain an internal RNA polymerase-III promoter.[191]

Alu repetitive sequences flanking deletion breakpoints have been noted in many human genetic conditions. *Alu*-sequence-mediated deletions are of essentially three types.

1. Recombination between an *Alu* element and a nonrepetitive DNA sequence that may not possess sequence homology with the *Alu* repeat.
2. Recombination between *Alu* sequences oriented in opposite directions.
3. Recombination between *Alu* sequences oriented in the same direction (Fig. 2-11).

The best examples of the involvement of *Alu* sequences occur in the LDLR and complement component-1 inhibitor (C1I) genes. All but one of the breakpoints associated with five LDLR gene deletions occur within an *Alu* repeat sequence (of which there are a total of 21 within the LDLR gene region). A 5.5-kb deletion[192] involves the formation of a stem-loop structure mediated by inverted repeats on the same DNA strand and derived from oppositely oriented *Alu* sequences in intron 15 and exon 18. A similar mechanism has been postulated for a 5.0-kb LDLR gene deletion[193] but, in this case, while the 3′ breakpoint lies within an *Alu* repeat, the 5′ breakpoint is located in exon 13; two pairs of inverted repeats (10/11 and 7/8 matches) flank the deletion breakpoints and are thought to potentiate the formation of the stem-loop structure. Three other LDLR gene deletions[194–196] are bounded by *Alu* repeats in the same orientation. Here the deletion is proposed to occur by meiotic (or mitotic) recombination between chromosomes misaligned at the highly homologous *Alu* sequences. In the vast majority of cases in which two *Alu* sequences have been implicated in the deletion event, they occur in the same orientation. Therefore, homologous unequal recombination between similarly oriented *Alu* family members, misaligned at meiosis, is probably the most common mechanism of *Alu*-mediated deletion. A clustering of deletion breakpoints within the left arm of *Alu* repeats was first noted by Lehrman et al[197] and has been confirmed on a much larger sample size.[4] However, the reasons for this nonrandomness are less clear. Lehrman et al[197] pointed out that the majority of the left-arm breakpoints lie within the region bounded by the RNA polymerase III promoters A and B and speculated that an open conformation brought about by promoter activity could increase the propensity for recombination to occur. While breakpoints within the right arm of the *Alu* sequence are indeed much less common, Ariga *et al.*[198] have claimed that the breakpoints that do occur within the right arm are invariably located within the region homologous to the sequence between promoters A and B. A similar situation to that found in the LDLR gene pertains in the C1I gene, which possesses a total of 17 *Alu* repeats within a 17-kb region.[199] Deletions and

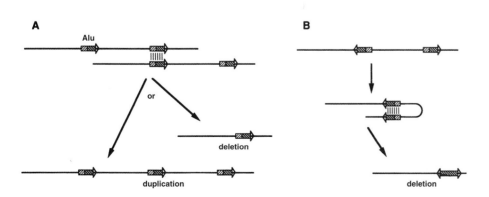

Fig. 2-11. Homologous unequal crossing-over mediated by *Alu* repetitive elements. *Alu*s in the same orientation can mediate unequal crossovers that can cause both deletions and duplications. *Alu*s in the reverse orientation can mediate crossovers via a loop structure that can cause deletions.

partial deletions of the C1I gene appear to account for 15 to 20 percent of the lesions that cause type-1 hereditary angioneurotic edema, and a high proportion of these occur within *Alu* sequences. Clustering of breakpoints is evident; Stoppa-Lyonnet et al[200] have shown that 5/5 deletions/duplications occurred within the first *Alu* sequence element preceding exon 4. However, the breakpoints of these rearrangements were distributed over the entire *Alu* sequence element and were not themselves further clustered.

In contrast to these examples, Henthorn et al[201] collated data on over 30 deletions in the β-globin cluster but noted the presence of *Alu* sequences at only four breakpoints and concluded that the occurrence of deletion breakpoints in *Alu* sequences within the β-globin gene region was not significantly different from that expected by chance alone. However, it could be argued that this was due to the relative paucity of *Alu* sequences (only eight in 60 kb) within the gene cluster. Kornreich et al[202] reached similar conclusions by studying the association between *Alu* sequences and deletion breakpoints in the gene (GLA) encoding α-galactosidase A, a deficiency that causes Fabry disease. Although 12 *Alu* repeats are found in the 12-kb gene region (about 30 percent of the GLA gene comprises *Alu* repeat sequences), deletions were relatively infrequent (only 5 of 130 patients possessed a partial gene deletion); three breakpoints occurred within an *Alu* sequence, and only one resulted from an *Alu-Alu* recombination. Finally, no correlation has been found between the locations of deletion breakpoints and *Alu* sequences in the human HPRT gene.[203] The authors suggested that this might be because the truncated 130- to 210-bp *Alu* repeats in the HPRT gene rarely exhibited more than 30-bp sequence identity, much lower than the 200- to 300-bp sequence identity normally required to promote efficient intrachromosomal recombination in mammalian cells.[204]

Recombination Within Non-*Alu* Repeats. Most gene deletions are not mediated by *Alu* repeat sequences. Indeed, although the 66-kb human growth hormone gene cluster contains some 48 *Alu* sequences, these do not appear to be the cause of the high frequency of clustered GH1 gene deletions causing familial growth hormone deficiency.[180] Vnencak-Jones and Phillips[181] studied 10 such patients and showed that in nine the crossovers had occurred within two 99 percent homologous 594-bp regions flanking the GH1 gene. Other types of repetitive sequence element are also thought to mediate homologous unequal recombination. Approximately 90 percent of individuals with ichthyosis have a deletion at their STS gene.[205] Yen et al[206] reported that 24 of 26 patients with an STS deletion had breakpoints clustered within or around a number of low-copy repetitive sequences flanking the STS gene (called *S232-type repeats*), suggesting that the high frequency of deletion at this locus may be due to recombination between these repetitive sequences. In their study of some 30 deletions of the β-globin gene cluster, Henthorn et al[201] noted breakpoints within five long interspersed repeat elements (LINEs). However, this was no higher than random expectation, and thus it is unnecessary to invoke an important role for LINEs in the causation of deletions at this locus. Sequence analysis of deletion breakpoints located within the intron-43 deletion hotspot in the DMD genes of two unrelated DMD patients has revealed the presence of a transposon-like element belonging to the THE-1 family.[207] Finally, the long terminal repeats of the RTVL-H family have been found to mediate homologous unequal recombinations events.[208]

Gene Fusions Caused by Homologous Unequal Recombination. The classic example of a gene fusion is that of hemoglobin Lepore. First reported by Gerald and Diamond,[209] this hemoglobin, which is synthesized in reduced amounts, is an abnormal molecule, with the first 50 to 80 amino acid residues of δ-globin at its N-terminus and the last 60 to 90 amino acid residues of β-globin at its C-terminus. Three different examples of Hb$_{LEPORE}$ have now been described in which the fusion junction occurs at

different points.[210–217] The recombination of Hb$_{LEPORE/BOSTON}$ genes has occurred within a 59-bp region of DNA (extending from codon 87 to the 11th nucleotide in intron 2) where the δ- and β-globin gene sequences are almost identical, resulting in the deletion of about 7 kb of intervening DNA.[203] Three haplotypes have been reported for Hb$_{LEPORE/BOSTON}$ chromosomes,[218,219] strongly supporting the view that this gene rearrangement has occurred independently on several different occasions. A similar fusion of $^A\gamma$- and β-globin genes due to a 22.5-kb deletion has occurred in Hb$_{KENYA}$.[220–222] These gene fusions appear to have arisen by homologous unequal recombination during meiosis between one globin gene on one chromosome and a misaligned globin gene on the other chromosome. This mechanism would predict the existence of a second abnormal chromosome; an anti-Lepore fusion gene encoding an N-terminal β-globin fused to C-terminal δ-globin. Consistent with this interpretation, several anti-Lepore hemoglobins have been described.[223–226] Another well-characterized example of the creation of fusion genes by homologous unequal recombination is provided by visual dichromacy (red-green color blindness). The genes involved are those encoding the red (RCP) and green (GCP) visual pigments that are highly homologous and linked in tandem on chromosome Xq28.[227] Several other examples of fusion genes generated by unequal recombination between highly homologous, closely linked genes have also been described: between the cytochrome P$_{450}$ genes CYP11B1 and CYP11B2, causing glucocorticoid-suppressible hyperaldosteronism,[228] between the glucocerebrosidase (GBA) gene and a linked GBA pseudogene causing type-1 Gaucher disease[229] and between the α- and β-myosin heavy-chain genes (MYHCA and MYHCB) causing familial hypertrophic cardiomyopathy.[230] Guioli et al[231] have reported a different mechanism for the generation of a fusion gene in a patient with Kallmann syndrome carrying an X;Y translocation. This translocation resulted from recombination between the Kallmann gene (KALX) on chromosome Xp22.3 and its homologue (KALY) on chromosome Yq11.21. The two sequences possess about 92 percent sequence homology, and the breakpoint occurred within an identical 13-bp region. The KALX/Y fusion gene contained the entire KALX gene except the last exon, but no transcription of the novel gene was detectable.

Nonhomologous Recombination. Nonhomologous (illegitimate) recombination occurs between two sites that show minimal sequence homology. This kind of recombination can explain gross DNA rearrangements, sharing only a few nucleotides at the breakpoints, that are also common in mammalian cells. To account for this type of deletion, we postulate that sequences, originally remote from one another, are brought into close proximity through their attachment to chromosome scaffolding. This would serve to explain the observed periodicities in deletions — for example, the similarity in size but not position of some α- and β-globin gene deletions.[183,232] However, Higgs *et al.*[184] found no association between matrix-associated regions and the deletion breakpoints in either globin gene cluster. Several types of junction have been noted in cases of nonhomologous recombination: *flush junctions* resulting from simple breakage and rejoining;[232] *insertional junctions*, which contain novel nucleotides;[233] and *junctions with limited homology*.[234–236] This last category of junction was first noted by Efstratiadis *et al.*[237] in deletions involving the β-globin gene family. These authors proposed that short (2 to 8 bp) direct repeats flanking deletions were involved in their generation. Since these short regions of homology were not long enough to support meiotic recombination between chromosomes, it was postulated that the deletions arose instead by slipped mispairing during DNA replication. Consistent with this postulate, one direct repeat was usually lost in the deletion event. Woods-Samuels *et al.*[238] noted 2- to 3-bp homologies at the breakpoints of three different deletions in the F8C gene and summarized the sequence features identified at 46 rearrangement junctions from large deletions that have been characterized in the human genome: 48 percent shared 2- to 6-bp homology at the breakpoint junction and, in 22 percent, nucleotides were inserted at the junction. In only 17 percent was the deletion due to *Alu-Alu* recombination.

Gene Conversion. *Gene conversion* is the "modification of one of two alleles by the other."[239] The end result is very similar to that consequent to a double unequal crossing-over event. The difference between the two processes is that the modification of one allele (the target) after gene conversion is nonreciprocal, leaving the other allele (the source) unchanged. Gene conversion has been best studied in yeast.[240] In practice, it is usually not possible to distinguish the two mechanisms of interallelic recombination since, in humans, it would be highly unusual to be able to examine both recombination products. Moreover, the haplotypes created by gene conversion and double unequal crossing-over are expected to be identical. The process of gene conversion may involve the whole or only a part of a gene and can occur either between alleles or between highly homologous but nonallelic sequences. Examples of the latter include the $^{A}\gamma$- and $^{G}\gamma$-globin genes[241–243] and the α_1- and α_2-globin genes.[244] The mechanism underlying gene conversion remains elusive but must entail close physical interaction between the homologous DNA sequences. Gene conversion has been invoked in instances in which it is necessary to account for the association of the same disease-causing mutation with two or more different haplotypes—for example, β^E-globin alleles in Southeast Asian populations[245] and the β^S-globin mutation in African populations.[246] In the latter example, the β^S mutation was found on 16 different haplotypes, which could be subdivided into four groups that could not be derived from each other by less than two crossing-over events. Similarly, Kazazian et al[247] and Pirastu et al[248] invoked gene conversion to explain the spread of the nonsense mutation at codon 39 of the β-globin gene to a considerable number of different haplotypes in Mediterranean β-thalassemia patients. Zhang et al[249] described five different β-globin gene mutations causing β thalassemia that occurred on more than one haplotype in the Chinese population. It was considered unlikely that all cases should have occurred either by recurrent mutation on different haplotypes or through multiple recombination events. Matsuno et al[250] reported that a frameshift mutation at codons 41 and 42 in the β-globin gene occurred in association with two different haplotypes in two ethnically distinct groups: Chinese and Southeast Asians. These authors pointed out that six of seven β-thalassemia mutations known to occur on very different haplotypes were located in a 451-bp region between codon 2 and position 16 of intron 2. Similarly, Powers and Smithies[243] have shown that gene conversion events between the $^{G}\gamma$- and $^{A}\gamma$-globin genes usually involve less than 300-bp long. Matsuno et al[250] also noted the existence of a chi sequence (GCTGGTGG) (known to promote recombination in both *Escherichia coli* and in mouse immunoglobulin genes[251]) at the 5′ end of exon 2 near to the site of the proposed gene conversion. Examples of gene conversion involving the steroid 21-hydroxylase (CYP21B) gene and the closely linked and highly homologous (98 percent) pseudogene have been reported by several investigators.[68,252–256] These events often bring in more than one mutation present in the source sequences. Amor et al[253] noted the presence of six chi-like sequences (GCTGGGG) in the region of the CYP21B gene and pseudogene, which they speculated might play a role in the gene conversion events. Other examples of gene conversion events causing human inherited disorders are that of polycystic kidney disease (PKD1[257]), neutrophil cytosolic factor p47-phox (NCF1, chronic granulomatous disease[258]), immunoglobulin λ-like polypeptide 1 (IGLL1, agammaglobulinemia[259]), GBA (Gaucher disease[260]), von Willebrand factor (VWF[261]), and phosphomannomutase (PMM2[262]). These gene-pseudogene pairs are all closely linked, with the exception of the VWF gene (12p13) and its pseudogene (22q11-q13) and the PMM2 gene (16p13) and its pseudogene (18p). Together, these two exceptions have established a precedent for gene conversion between unlinked loci in the human genome.

Short Gene Deletions

A total of 2368 independent human gene deletions of 20 bp or less (as of September 13, 1998) have been logged in the HGMD (http://www.uwcm.ac.uk/uwcm/mg/haha4.html), which greatly extends earlier versions of the database.[263] This size range was selected because: (1) deletion end points are close enough to permit the study of putative sequence elements involved in the deletion process, (2) deletions arising by mechanisms other than homologous recombination were thought likely to predominate in this size range, and (3) most known short gene deletions have been discovered during DNA-sequencing studies so that the sample is likely to be unbiased. For every deletion, 10 bp of DNA flanking the deletion breakpoints were also noted so as to enable the analysis of the local DNA sequence environment. Excluded are deletions of the mitochondrial genome, which, by virtue of its rapid replication time and own distinct DNA polymerase, may not be directly comparable to deletions occurring within the nuclear genome. The distribution of deletion lengths is presented in Fig. 2-12. In 46 percent (1095 of 2368), the deletion involved only one nucleotide and, in 37 percent (868 of 2368), two to four nucleotides; the remaining deletions of 5 to 20 bp account for 17 percent of these lesions. Approximately 85 percent of the small deletions result in an alteration of the reading frame. Some of the DNA sequences in the HGMD share specific properties that may predispose them to deletion-type mutation. In a study of 1828 deletions, performed in October 1997, significance of these findings was assessed by comparing observations made in the HGMD to results from simulation studies, using 10,000 DNA sequences generated randomly according to codon usage for human genes by Wada et al[264] and to a random sample of 448 human cDNA sequences.

Local DNA Sequence Environment. Mononucleotide frequencies were found to differ from those derived from codon usage data[264] in that nucleotides T and A were overrepresented, whereas C and G were underrepresented. Nucleotides immediately flanking the deletion breakpoints revealed a significant excess of T and deficiency of C residues. A total of 13 codons were overrepresented in frame within the DNA sequences examined: TTT, CTT, CCT, AGT, GGT, TTA, ATA, GTA, TCA, AAA, GAA, AGA, and TAG. Several 3- and 4-bp motifs were found to be significantly overrepresented in a region of 10 bp both upstream and downstream of the deletions, regardless of frame. The most dramatic examples were: TTT (721 observed vs 496 expected), AAA (1072 observed vs 727 expected), AGA (1124 observed vs 879 expected), AAGA (416 observed vs 249 expected), AAAA (346 observed vs 204 expected), AGAA (396 observed vs 255 expected), TTTT (208 observed vs 117 expected), GTAA (119 observed vs 56 expected), TTCT (237 observed vs 150 expected), and TCTT (206 observed vs 132 expected).

Direct Repeats and the Generation of Short Deletions

A variety of different mechanisms for the generation of gene deletions involving the misalignment of short direct repeats have been proposed. Most replication-based models are essentially adaptations of the slipped-mispairing hypothesis proposed by Streisinger et al[265] The basic mechanism is as follows (Fig. 2-13): Two direct repeats, R1 and R2, occur in close proximity to each other with complementary sequences R1′ and R2′ on the other strand. As replication proceeds, the DNA duplex becomes single stranded at the replication fork, enabling illegitimate pairing between R2 and the complementary R1′ sequence. As a result, a single-stranded loop is formed containing the R1 repeat and sequence lying between R1 and R2. DNA repair enzymes may then excise this loop and rejoin the broken ends of the DNA strand. The next round of replication would then generate one deleted and

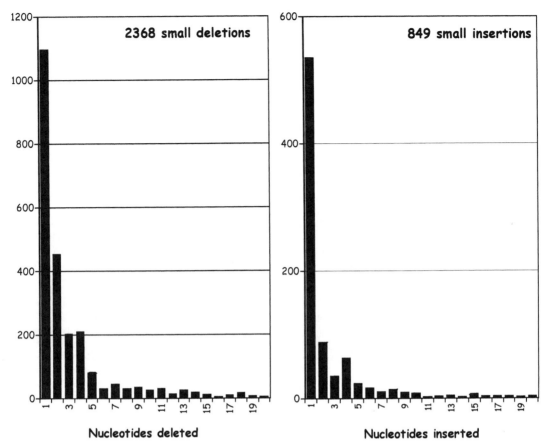

Fig. 2-12. Size distribution of short (< 20 bp) human gene deletions and insertions.

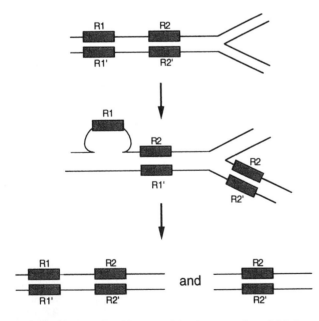

Fig. 2-13. Slipped-mispairing model for the generation of deletions during DNA replication.[237] Top: Double-stranded DNA containing R1 and R2 direct repeats. Middle: Double-stranded DNA becoming single stranded at replication fork and R2 repeat base pairs with complementary R19 repeat producing a single-stranded loop. Bottom: Loop excised and the new double-stranded DNA molecules. One of the two products contains only one of the repeats and lacks the sequences between R1 and R2.

one wild-type duplex. Direct repeats (2 bp or more) could be found flanking and/or overlapping all gene deletions logged in the HGMD. The most frequent length of a direct repeat was 3 bp (793 of 1828; 43.4 percent), while a sizable proportion (869 of 1828; 47.5 percent) were between 4 and 11 bp (Fig. 2-14). The latter occurred more often than expected by chance alone. A strong positive correlation holds between the length of the flanking direct repeats and the amount of DNA deleted, and the likelihood of deletion also appears to increase with the length of the repeat motif. The observations made from the HGMD are thus consistent with the model of slipped mispairing. In accord with the postulate of Efstratiadis et al[237] the deletion of one whole repeat copy plus the sequence between the repeats was observed in 534 (52.7 percent) of 1014 deletions spanning 2 bp or more.

Slipped mispairing can in principle also account for the generation of −1-base frameshift mutations. The production of a frameshift error by these means must involve at least two separate steps: (1) a misalignment occurs within a run of identical bases, followed by (2) further incorporation events that fix the misaligned bases(s). Various lines of evidence from *in vitro* studies now support the validity of this model and demonstrate that deletions/frameshifts can arise during DNA synthesis: (1) Vertebrate polymerases α and β produce many more frameshifts at runs of bases than at nonruns.[9,266] With polβ, hotspots occur predominantly at runs of pyrimidines (particularly TTTT) rather than purines, although this effect is less pronounced with polα. (2) The frequency of frameshift mutations is roughly proportional to the length of the run.[9] (3) The frequency of polβ-dependent frameshift mutation at a run sequence is decreased by experimental interruption of that run.[8] Kunkel and Soni[267] have proposed an alternative mechanism to account for the generation of frameshift

Longest Direct Repeat

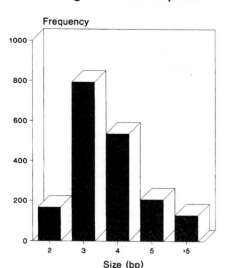

Longest Inverted Repeat

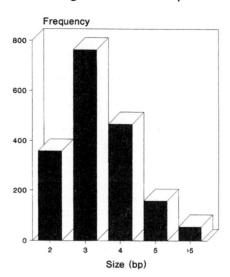

Fig. 2-14. Size distribution of the longest direct (*left*) and inverted (*right*) repeats flanking and/or overlapping short human gene deletions.

mutations at DNA replication: If a misincorporated nucleotide is complementary to the next base 3′, then its translocation to the next position will lead to a frameshift if the misaligned intermediate is rapidly stabilized by further base pairing. Analysis of 814 −1-base frameshifts from the HGMD revealed that the deleted base was identical to one of its neighbors in 500 cases. In addition, 238 deletions overlapped with a run of identical bases of 3 bp or more. Both observations represented a significant excess over expectation. Therefore, a considerable proportion of −1-base frameshift mutations causing human genetic disease may be due to slipped mispairing within runs of identical bases.

Palindromes (Inverted Repeats) and Quasipalindromes in the Vicinity of Short Gene Deletions

Ripley[268] proposed a mechanism of deletion mediated by quasipalindromic (imperfect inverted repeat) sequences. A palindrome possesses self-complementarity within the same DNA strand, which enables this strand to fold back on itself to form a hairpin or cruciform structure. The imperfect self-complementarity of quasipalindromic sequences enables them to form misaligned secondary structures. The nonpalindromic portions of these structures then provide templates for frameshifts and short deletions through the exonucleolytic removal of unpaired bases followed by repair DNA synthesis (Fig. 2-15). This model has been shown to possess predictive value at least in *E. coli.*[269] A search for palindromic sequences that could potentiate the looping out of single-stranded DNA revealed that 1447 of 1828 sequences listed in the HGMD in October 1997 contained at least one pair of

inverted repeats of at least 3 bp; these were found to flank or span the deletion in 1387 cases. There were 128 examples of flanking and/or overlapping inverted repeats of at least 6 bp. A typical case was provided by an 8-bp inverted repeat associated with a lactate dehydrogenase B (LDHB) gene deletion;[270] one repeat was completely removed at the 5′ end of the deletion, whereas the other abutted immediately on the 3′ end of the deletion. In general, however, the exact location of the deleted base(s) was not predictable from the location of inverted repeats. Thus, 421 sequences possessed both direct and inverted repeats of 4 bp or longer flanking and/or overlapping the deletion; the presence of the latter may influence the nature of the deletion regardless of whether it occurs through classic mispairing or via the intrarepeat loop mechanism.

Role for Symmetric Elements?

Sequence motifs that possess an axis of internal symmetry (e.g., CTGAAGTC and GGACAGG) and vary in length between 5 and 18 bp, termed *symmetric elements,*[263] were noted in association with 1527 of the 1828 deletions in the HGMD. Symmetric elements spanning 5 bp or more therefore also appear to be overrepresented in the vicinity of short human gene deletions; their potential significance is unclear, however. An example of the presence of symmetric elements near microdeletions is in the case of the BRCA1 gene where the location of such elements at 5 to 7 bp were shown to be at significantly short distances (0 to 10 bp) from deletion breakpoints.[271]

Deletion Hotspots in Human Genes?

By examining the similarities of DNA sequences among deletions, Krawczak and Cooper[263] previously identified a consensus sequence — TG(A/G)(A/G) (T/T) (A/C) — which appears to be common to deletion *hotspots* found in different human genes. This consensus sequence is similar to the core motifs, TGGGG and TGAGC, found in the tandemly repeated immunoglobulin switch (S μ) regions,[272] and to putative arrest sites for polymerase α, which often contain a GAG motif. Indeed, one arrest site specifically mentioned by Weaver and DePamphilis [(T/A)GGAG[42]] fits perfectly with the deletion hotspot consensus sequence. The arrest of DNA synthesis at the replication fork may increase the probability of either a slipped-mispairing event or the formation of secondary-structure intermediates potentiated by the presence of inverted repeats or symmetric elements. Monnat et al[203] have sought a variety of sequence motifs in their study of 10 somatic deletions of the human HPRT gene causing Werner

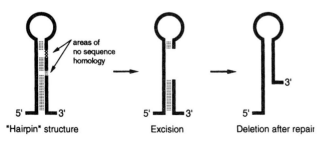

Fig. 2-15. Schematic representation of the excision-repair mechanism for deletions mediated by hairpin structures due to palindrome or quasipalindrome DNA sequences.

syndrome. The same collection of motifs was used for a search of the 1828 deletions and flanking sequences in the HGMD. Only three of these sequence motifs appeared to be overrepresented in the vicinity of short human gene deletions—polypyrimidine runs (C or T) of at least 5 bp, polypurine runs (A or G) of at least 5 bp, and the aforementioned deletion hotspot consensus sequence. Analysis of the precise localization of the deletions logged in the HGMD revealed that 17 codons from seven different genes could be identified as *deletion hotspots* [antithrombin III (AT3) codon 244; cystic fibrosis transmembrane regulator (CFTR) codons 141, 506, 1175, 1200; F8C codon 339; F9 codons 7 and 182; α_2-globin codon 30; β-globin codons 5, 36, 40, 42, 73, 125, and 150; and protein C (PROC) codon 76]. To be classified as a deletion hotspot, the DNA sequence in and around a codon had to be affected by at least two different (and therefore independent) mutations. Either a deletion hotspot consensus-like motif or a run of at least five pyrimidines was found in the vicinity of all these deletion hotspots. That polypyrimidines are significantly associated with deletions is not particularly surprising: Polymerase β-associated deletions occur predominantly in pyrimidine runs and thus, if DNA repair synthesis were a significant cause of frameshift mutation *in vivo*, it would be expected that the mutational spectrum of human gene deletions might show similarities to the polβ-associated mutational spectrum observed *in vitro*. Nevertheless, several differences between these mutational spectra are also apparent. Over 95 percent of polβ-associated frameshift deletions are 1 bp long,[9] whereas only 46.2 percent of the deletions from the HGMD are of this size. Although 988 of the deletions studied in October 1997 included or flanked a pyrimidine run, only 219 (44.9 percent) of these represented losses of a single base pair. This proportion compares with the deletions not associated with pyrimidine runs (595 of 1340; 44.4 percent). Finally, although 76 percent of all nonrun single-base-pair losses *in vitro* involved a G residue, the corresponding figure for human gene mutations was 30.3 percent (i.e., not significantly higher than random expectation).

INSERTIONS

Small Insertions

That insertional mutagenesis might be nonrandom was strongly suggested by the findings of Fearon et al,[273] who reported 10 independent examples of DNA insertion within the same 170-bp intronic region of the *deleted in colorectal carcinoma* (DCC) gene. Currently, 849 small insertions of less than 20 bp are recorded in the HGMD. Figure 13-12 shows the size distribution of these 849 insertions (http://www.uwcm.ac.uk/uwcm/mg/haha5.html). In the majority of cases (63 percent), there is insertion of a single base. Insertions of between 2 and 4 bp represent 22 percent of cases. All other small insertions, i.e., those of 5 to 20 bp, account for 15 percent of such lesions. All mutations interrupt the reading frame of the proteins except for the examples of a three-base insertion in which the novel codons were inserted between existing codons. One of the first such examples was in patients with hereditary elliptocytosis in which the triplet TTG coding for Lys was inserted between codons 147 and 148 in the alpha-spectrin gene (SPTA1)[274] Examples of short insertions leading to human genetic disease have been analyzed previously[41] to determine whether they occur nonrandomly and whether this nonrandomness corresponds to mechanisms of mutagenesis similar to those involved in the generation of short gene deletions.

Insertions due to Slipped Mispairing. In principle, slipped mispairing at the replication fork[237,265] mediated by direct repeats can account for insertion just as for deletion-type mutations: An insertion takes place when the newly synthesized strand disconnects from the primer strand during replication synthesis and slips or folds back so that pairing between different direct-repeat copies becomes possible. If synthesis is resumed so as to stabilize this mispairing, an extra copy plus nucleotide(s) from

between the direct repeats is inserted behind the second repeat. Of the insertions considered by Cooper and Krawczak,[41] at least three occurred within runs of the same base while three were duplications of tandemly repeated sequences. The data were, however, too sparse to confirm any relationship with the DNA sequence environment. Nevertheless, pause sites for DNA polymerase a are known to be hotspots for nucleotide insertion.[275]

Insertions Mediated by Inverted Repeats. Analogous to the process of slipped mispairing between direct repeats, the formation of temporary secondary DNA structures may also be mediated by neighboring inverted repeats. In this situation, the newly synthesized DNA strand, instead of annealing to a direct-repeat copy on the primer strand, snaps back and anneals to itself via the two inverted repeats. If DNA synthesis is then resumed, an insertion would result behind the second palindromic copy. Imperfect self-complementarity can also mediate formation of partially misaligned secondary structures.[268] The nonpalindromic portions of these structures may then provide templates for either deletions (by endonucleolytic removal of bases) or putatively insertions (by gap repair). DNA sequences flanking two insertions considered by Cooper and Krawczak[41] contain such quasipalindromes and would correctly predict the insertion of the appropriate base (thymine) at the appropriate site [Leu 100 of the HBD gene and Cys 1146 of the *type-I* $\alpha 1$-collagen (COL1A1) gene].

Insertions Mediated by Symmetric Elements. Inspection of the insertions collated by Cooper and Krawczak[41] reveals that 8 of 20 of these sequences possess symmetric elements overlapping the site of insertion. With one exception, these insertions all represent inverted duplications of sequence motifs derived from either the 5' or the 3' end of the symmetric element. This finding is suggestive of a common endogenous mechanism of insertional mutagenesis.

Large Insertions — Retrotransposition

The HGMD contains 86 large insertions and duplications (as of September 13, 1998). To date, the largest "foreign" DNA sequence inserted into a gene is 220 kb into the DMD gene.[276] However, neither the inserted sequence nor the breakpoint junctions have been further characterized. One well-characterized insertion is that of the highly repetitive LINEs into the F8C gene, causing severe hemophilia A.[277] LINEs, which belong to the class of autonomous retrotranposons without long terminal repeats, compose approximately 15 percent of the human genome.[278] The insertion of these elements into exon 14 in the F8C genes of two patients involved the duplication of the target sites, a normal occurrence in such cases[279,280] and consistent with a retrotransposition mechanism. Fig. 2-16 is a schematic representation of retrotransposition. Patient JH-27 of reference 277 was shown to possess a 3785-bp truncated LINE complete with 57-bp polyA tract. The insertion produced a target site duplication of 12 to 15 bp. The LINE in patient JH-28 of reference 277 was slightly shorter (2132 bp) but more complex; one portion of LINE sequence (nts 4020 to 5114) was preceded by another (nts 5115 to 6161) in reverse orientation (3' to 5'); there was a polyA tail of 77 residues. Dombroski et al[281] have shown that the LINE found in exon 14 of patient JH-27 is an exact but truncated copy of a full-length LINE with open reading frames (ORFs) found at chromosome 22q11.1-q11.2, which, since it is itself flanked by a target-site duplication, may also be the product of a retrotransposition event. Another patient, JH-25, had an insertion of a truncated LINE in intron 10 of the factor VIII gene.[282] The element, which was 681 bp long, had a 66-bp polyA tail and target-site duplication of 13 to 17 bp, and did not cause any abnormality, since it was found in several members of the patient's family, including his normal maternal grandfather (i.e., the mutation in the F8C gene responsible for hemophilia A in this family was not the insertion of the LINE). The involvement of LINEs in insertional mutagenesis has also been reported in other

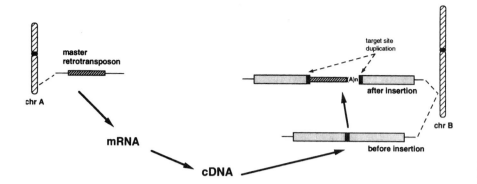

Fig. 2-16. Schematic representation of retrotransposition.

genes causing human disorders such the DMD gene[283] and the adenomatous polyposis of colon (APC) gene in colon carcinoma;[284] in addition, there is an $^A\gamma\delta\beta$ thalassemia due to a large deletion in which insertion of about 50 bp from a LINE has been noted,[285] and breast carcinoma where a LINE element was inserted in the MYC gene.[286] Most of the LINEs found retrotransposition events belong to the Ta subset. It seems likely that only full-length LINEs are the source of active mammalian retrotransposition. There are approximately 3000 to 4000 human full-length LINEs, but most of these are inactive because they contain nonsense and frameshift mutations. However, some elements contain two ORFs: ORF1 and ORF2. The ORF1 encodes an RNA-binding protein that is critical for retrotransposition in HeLa cells[287] and also binds specifically to the ORF2-protein product.[288] The ORF2-protein product contains an N-terminal endonuclease domain[289] and a C-terminal reverse transcriptase domain. The proposed mechanism of LINE retrotransposition is as follows:[278] an active LINE is transcribed in the nucleus and is subsequently transported to and translated in the cytoplasm. The two LINE proteins, ORF1 and ORF2, complex with their encoding LINE transcript in ribonucleoprotein particles. The complex is then transported to recipient DNA sequences where target-primed reverse transcription occurs. The new, integrated LINE copy is usually truncated at its 5' end.

The highly repetitive *Alu*-sequence family has also been shown to be capable of retrotransposition both *in vitro*[290] and *in vivo*. *Alu* elements, which belong to the class of nonautonomous retrotranposons, comprise approximately 10 to 15 percent of the human genome.[278] Insertional inactivation of the NF1 gene by an *Alu* element caused neurofibromatosis type 1, as reported by Wallace *et al.*[291] The insertion, which occurred *de novo*, was localized to intron 5, just 44 bp upstream of exon 33, and resulted in skipping of exon 6. The 320-bp *Alu* repeat was inserted in reverse orientation into a 26-bp stretch of A and T residues. Though the exact mechanism responsible for this interference with splicing is not clear, these findings are consistent with a defect in branch-point recognition. Insertions of *Alu* elements into the human Moloney leukemia virus 12 (MLV 12) oncogene associated with hematopoietic neoplasia B-cell lymphoma,[292] the cholinesterase gene causing acholinesterasemia,[293] the F9 gene causing severe hemophilia B,[294] and the BRCA2 gene in a family with breast cancer[295] have also been reported. The *Alu* element inserted in the MLV12 locus was 308 bp long, contained a polyA tail of 26 residues, and produced an A-rich target-site duplication of 8 bp. The insertion of the 342-bp-long *Alu* element into the cholinesterase gene[293] occurred in an AT-rich region of exon 2. There was a 38-bp-long polyA tail and a target-site duplication of 15 bp. The inserted *Alu* element belonged to the evolutionarily recent subfamily IV. The insertion of the 322-bp-long *Alu* element in the F9 gene[294] occurred in exon 5 and produced a stop codon within the inserted sequence. There was a target-site duplication of 15 bp and a polyA tract of 78 residues. The *de novo* inserted *Alu*

sequences in the NF1 and F9 genes both belong to the same subfamily (*Alu* HS), which is the most recent subfamily in the evolution of *Alu* sequences. The mechanism of retrotransposition of *Alu* sequences is unclear, although the ORF2 protein of LINEs may be involved in this event.[278]

The observation that both *Alu* sequences[295] and LINEs[277] exhibit a preference for integration at AT-rich sequences is reminiscent of the AT-rich insertional target sequences of retroviruses.[296,297] Indeed, the two LINE target sites in the F8C gene[277] are 90 percent homologous to a 10-nucleotide motif (GAAGA-CATAC) present in one of the highly favored retroviral insertion target sequences reported by Shih *et al.*[297]

DUPLICATIONS

The duplication of either whole genes or their constituent exons has played an important role in the evolution of the mammalian genome. However, gene duplication events may also result in disease. The largest duplication reported to date for a single gene is a 400-kb internal duplication of the DMD gene involving exons 13 to 42.[298] Despite this gross alteration in the structure of the gene (and of the resulting protein: about 600 kDa instead of 400 kDa), the patient manifested the relatively mild Becker form of muscular dystrophy. Other gene duplications and partial duplications have been reported, and these vary in size from 45 bp (COL2A1) to 20 kb (HPRT), from a part of an exon (LPL) to an entire gene (HBG2). Usually, the duplicated material exists in tandem with the original sequence, but a particular HPRT gene duplication has been reported by Yang et al[299] that is unusual in that a segment of the gene containing exons 2 and 3 has been placed in the middle of an intron-1 fragment.

One frequent mechanism of gene duplication is homologous unequal recombination. This may take different forms depending on the nature of the DNA sequence at the breakpoints. Thus, homologous unequal recombination in the β-globin gene cluster occurred between the HBG1 and HBG2 genes, whereas in the LDLR gene, it occurred between pairs of *Alu* sequences.[197] In the COL2A1 gene, alignment of two copies of the duplicated exon, in the manner that must have preceded a particular recombination-duplication event, demonstrated 78 percent nucleotide sequence homology around the recombination site.[300] In principle, unequal crossing-over caused by homologous recombination between repetitive sequence elements could lead to either the deletion or the duplication of exons. That the exons found to be duplicated in the C1I[200,301] and COL2A1[300] genes of some patients are deleted in others with deficiencies of these proteins would seem to support this model of mutagenesis. However, other duplication junctions appear to possess little or no homology with each other (e.g., GLA,[202] F8C,[302] and DMD[303,304]). In the lipoprotein lipase (LPL) gene, recombination has occurred between an *Alu* sequence and a region of exon 6, but the sequenced breakpoints exhibited no obvious homology.[305]

One of the best-characterized duplications is in the F8C gene in a family with hemophilia A.[188] The patient had a deletion of 39 kb of exons 23 to 25; however, his normal mother had 23 kb of intron 22 duplicated and reinserted between exons 23 and 24. Since the mother passed on a 39-kb deletion allele to two of her offspring, she must have been a germ-line mosaic for the normal, deletion, and duplication alleles. DNA polymorphism analysis suggested that the deletion and duplication events had occurred on the same chromosome. Gitschier[306] proposed a model in which the duplication had occurred first, either in a grandpaternal gamete or during the mother's early embryogenesis, and the deletion then occurred, probably mediated by the close proximity of the direct repeats, through recombination. The deletion occurred at a pair of CATT sequences normally 39 kb apart in the factor VIII gene. Short repeated sequences are known to mediate recombination events in vertebrate genomes; both $(CAGA)_n$ and $(CAGG)_n$ repeats have been noted in the region of the recombination hotspots found within the murine major histocompatibility gene complex.[307] Several possible topoisomerase-I cleavage sites were noted in the vicinity of the factor VIII gene duplication described by Casula et al[308] Topoisomerase activity has been implicated in several cases of nonhomologous recombination.[40] Other examples of topoisomerase cleavage sites have been reported to be associated with gene duplications;[202,304] potential sites for topoisomerases I and II were found exactly coincident with the breakpoints of a duplication in the dystrophin gene.[304] The significance of these findings remains to be elucidated.

The frequency of gene duplication is difficult to assess on account of the relatively small sample size. As with gene deletions, the frequency of gene duplication is likely to vary dramatically between genes. However, several estimates of the frequency of (partial) gene duplication are available for the dystrophin gene from large studies of patients with Duchenne/Becker muscular dystrophy (DMD/BMD): 6.7 percent,[309] 5.5 percent,[303] and 1.5 percent.[310] Thus, for the DMD gene, a gene for which a disproportionately high rate of large deletions has been reported (>60 percent of total mutations), the duplication frequency is probably 5 to 10 percent of the deletion frequency. A much higher frequency of duplication (uncharacterized and evidenced only by hybridization band intensity) may be found in the CYP21B gene causing 21-hydroxylase deficiency: Haglund-Stengler et al[311] found 11 gene deletions and 9 gene duplications in their study of 43 unrelated patients. However, at other loci, where gene deletions are much less frequent, gene duplications may well be so rare as not to be found. Why are gene duplications usually so much rarer than deletions? One possibility is that deletions are on average more likely to be deleterious and hence more likely to come to clinical attention. This is considered unlikely since with DMD/BMD, for example, it is the maintenance of the reading frame, rather than the nature of the lesion itself, that determines the disease phenotype.[298,303,312,313] A second possibility is that not all mechanisms involved in deletion creation would generate duplications as reciprocal products. Finally, it is possible that duplications are relatively unstable and revert or *decay* to deletions quite rapidly. The F8C partial gene deletion is a case in point. Another example is that of the exon-2+3 duplication in the HPRT gene; cells bearing this gene lesion reverted to wild type in culture through the loss of the duplicated exons.[299,314] Two similar HPRT gene duplications have been reported as spontaneous mutations in the human myeloid leukemia cell line HL60,[314] and these were also found to be highly unstable, exhibiting a reversion rate around 100 times higher than the rate of gene duplication. It would seem therefore that, once duplicated, the enlarged DNA sequence provides the substrate (a premutation) for further rounds of homologous unequal recombination.

Very large duplications also appear to arise from recombination mediated by repeated DNA sequences. Pentao et al[315] have reported that the duplication on chromosome 17p in one patient with Charcot-Marie-Tooth disease type 1A (CMT1A) is a tandem repeat of 1.5 Mb. A repeated element of 17 kb, termed *CMT1A-REP*, flanks the 1.5-Mb CMT1A monomer unit on normal chromosome 17p and was present in an additional copy on the chromosome with the CMT1A duplication. The authors proposed that the CMT1A duplication arose from unequal crossing-over due to misalignment at these CMT1A-REP repeat sequences during meiosis.

INVERSIONS

Inversions appear to be an extremely unusual form of gene mutation. Two examples involving the β-globin gene cluster are presented here: The first is a complex rearrangement of the β-globin gene cluster found in a patient with Indian $^A\gamma\delta\beta$ thalassemia.[316] Two segments—0.83 kb and 7.46 kb, respectively—were deleted, while the intervening segment was inverted and reintroduced between the $^A\gamma$- and δ-gene loci. Jennings et al[316] suggested that this mutation may have been made possible by the chromatin-folding pattern of the cluster region bringing the $^A\gamma$ gene into close proximity with the δ- and β-globin genes. Interestingly, this rearrangement serves to enhance the expression of the upstream fetal $^G\gamma$ gene. A similar example of an inversion has been reported in the APOA1/C3/A4 gene cluster in a patient with premature atherosclerosis and a deficiency of both APOA1 and APOC3.[317] The inversion was 6 kb long, with breakpoints in exon 4 of the APOA1 gene and intron 1 of the APOC3 gene. This inversion resulted in the reciprocal fusion of portions of the two genes and contains exons 1 to 3 of exon 4 from the APOA1 gene plus exons 2 to 4 and intron 1 from the APOC3 gene; the fusion gene is expressed as a stable mRNA. In the process, however, 9 bp from the APOA1 and 21 bp from the APOC3 gene were deleted. Since *Alu* sequences were also noted in the vicinity of the breakpoints of this inversion, Karathanasis et al[317] speculated that the sequences might be involved in the stabilization of a stem-loop structure prior to the inversion event. A final example of an inversion is provided by a Turkish patient with $\delta\beta^0$ thalassemia and a complex rearrangement of the β-globin gene cluster.[318] The rearrangement consists of a deletion of 11.5 kb, including the β- and δ-globin genes, a second 1.6-kb deletion downstream of the first, and a 7.6-kb inversion of the intervening sequence, including the LINE downstream of the β-globin gene.

Perhaps the most important inversion event is that involving the F8C gene causing severe hemophilia A. The high frequency of the inversion (about 40 percent) in these patients provides an explanation for our initial inability to detect the pathologic lesion in about half of all severe hemophilia-A patients[24] and the impossibility of performing PCR amplification across the exon-22/23 boundary by using cDNA derived from these patients.[67] A CpG island, located within intron 22, acts as a bidirectional promoter for two transcribed genes: F8A and F8B. The F8A gene lacks introns and is transcribed in the opposite direction to the factor VIII gene. Two additional homologues of the F8A gene (the A genes), which are also transcribed, exist about 500 kb upstream of the factor VIII gene. These genes are transcribed in the opposite direction to F8A. It is now known that homologous infrachromosomal recombination occurs between one or other of the upstream A genes and the F8A gene, generating an inversion of the intervening factor VIII gene sequence.[319,320] Such inversions result in the separation of exons 1 to 22 from exons 23 to 26 by some 200 to 500 kb. Most inversions (90 percent) involve the distal of the two A genes; this unique mutational mechanism is estimated to occur with a frequency of 7.2×10^{-6} per gene per gamete per generation (D.S. Millar and D.N. Cooper, unpublished results). An international collaborative effort collected data from a total of 2093 patients with severe hemophilia A;[321] of those, 740 (35 percent) had a type-1 (distal) factor VIII inversion, and 140 (7 percent) showed a type-2 (proximal) inversion. Of 532 mothers of patients with inversions, 98 percent were carriers of the abnormal factor VIII gene. When the maternal grandparental origin was examined, the inversions occurred *de novo* in male germ cells in 69 cases and in female germ cells in 1 case.

Molecular Misreading due to Long Runs of Mononucleotides or Dinucleotides

Long runs of adenines (and perhaps other mononucleotides or dinucleotides) promote a phenomenon called *molecular misreading* by which DNA replication/RNA transcription and/or translation result in erroneous products with different numbers of (A)s from the DNA. Linton et al[322] reported a family with hypobetalipoproteinemia in which the deletion of one C in the A_5CA_3 coding sequence of the APOB gene results in a run of $(A)_8$. The patient, however, did not have a severe disease, because there was some ApoB protein made. This was the result of molecular misreading in which approximately 10 percent of the resulting RNAs contained $(A)_9$ instead of the expected $(A)_8$; this partially restored the reading frame and produced low amounts of normal ApoB. Young et al[323] reported a family with mild to moderately severe hemophilia A with a deletion of one T within the coding A_8TA_2 sequence of the F8C gene. The partial "correction" of the phenotype was due to the restoration of the reading frame because of molecular misreading in which approximately 5 percent of the resulting RNAs contained $(A)_{11}$ instead of the expected $(A)_{10}$. In this family, there was also evidence for ribosomal frameshifting during translation of the mutant RNA. Laken et al[324] reported a T-to-A transversion in the coding A_3TA_4 sequence of the APC gene in 6 percent of Ashkenazi Jews and in about 28 percent of Ashkenazim with a family history of colorectal cancer. Rather than altering the function of the encoded protein, this mutation again creates a small hypermutable region, indirectly causing cancer predisposition because there are many somatic cells in which stretches of $(A)_9$ occur instead of the expected $(A)_8$. The $(A)_9$ results in a frameshifting and truncated dysfunctional APC. The mechanisms of transcriptional slippage during elongation at runs of As or Ts has been documented and studied in *E. coli*.[325] Ribosomal frameshifting has also been studied extensively in model organisms.[326]

Van Leeuwen *et al.*[327] found in neurofibrillary tangles, neuritic plaques, and neuropil threads in the cerebral cortex of Alzheimer and Down syndrome abnormal forms of β-amyloid precursor protein and ubiquitin B. These aberrant proteins were produced because of +1 frameshifting that resulted from a deletion of AG in a sequence GAGAG that occurred in the coding regions of both genes. This dinucleotide deletion was again the result of a molecular misreading during transcription or posttranscriptional editing of RNA.

Expansion of Unstable Repeat Sequences

Since the beginning of this decade, a novel mechanism of mutation has been shown to arise through the instability and expansion of certain trinucleotide and other repeat sequences.[328–330] To date, at least a dozen disorders due to trinucleotide repeat, and one due to 12mer-repeat expansion, have been described[331,332] (see Table 2-10 and Fig. 2-17). This mechanism was first reported as a cause of the fragile X syndrome, one of the most frequent causes of inherited mental retardation, which is associated with the presence of a fragile site on Xq27.3. The FMR1 gene underlying the fragile X syndrome[347–350] was found to contain an ~90-bp CGG repeat sequence in the 5′UTR.[350] A length variation of the trinucleotide repeat in the region was noted[348,349] that appeared to correlate with the expression of the fragile X phenotype. Indeed, the $(CGG)_n$ repeat exhibited copy-number variation of between 6 and 52[351] in normal healthy controls although the majority of individuals possessed between 25 and 35 repeat copies.[333] By contrast, phenotypically normal transmitting males exhibited a repeat copy number of between 60 and 200 (the *premutation*), whereas affected males possessed more than 250 and sometimes in excess of 1000 copies (the *full mutation*[333,352–355]). The instability of both the premutation and the full mutation is further exemplified by the existence of somatic mosaicism for different copy-number

alleles in some individuals.[333,356] Alleles with a repeat copy number of <46 exhibit no meiotic instability.[333,352] The premutation represents a small increase in CGG copy number but was not associated with methylation of the gene region or with mental impairment. However, individuals bearing the premutation exhibit a high probability of having either affected children or grandchildren. Expansion of premutations to full mutations only occurs during female meiotic transmission. The probability of repeat expansion correlates with the repeat copy number in the premutation allele.[333] Since the premutation must precede the appearance of the full mutation, all mothers of affected children carried either a full mutation or a premutation; no case of direct conversion of normal copy number to full mutation has been observed.[353] The full mutation was not detected in daughters of normal transmitting males, although small increases in CGG copy number were observed in daughters. All male patients with the fragile X syndrome possessed the full mutation, and all male individuals with the full mutation were mentally retarded. Moreover, 53 percent of females carrying the full mutation also exhibited symptoms of mental retardation. Although the transition from premutation to full mutation was always associated with the expansion of the $(CGG)_n$ repeat, examples of contraction were also observed and were reportedly associated with regression from a full mutation to a premutation.[333,353] Fu et al[333] estimated that about 1 of 500 females in the general population might possess a repeat copy number within the premutation range. In fragile XE mental retardation, the repeat that expands is also a $(CGG)_n$ in the 5′UTR of the FMR2 gene.[334]

The triplet repeats involved in the disorders due to repeat expansions are located in the 5′UTR as in fragile X,[333] the 3′UTR as in myotonic dystrophy,[335] the coding exonic sequences as in Huntington disease,[337] or in an intron as in Friedreich ataxia.[344] The 12mer repeat that is expanded in progressive myoclonus epilepsy type 1 is located in the 5′ flanking region of the CSTB gene.[332] The noncoding repeats could undergo massive expansions to hundreds or thousands copies, which leads to transcriptional suppression. The expansions in coding sequences are less dramatic and result in a gain of function of the abnormal protein that contains longer polyglutamine tracts.

Myotonic dystrophy, which affects approximately 1 in 8000 people, is a progressive disorder of muscle weakness with dominant inheritance and exhibits a unique property termed *anticipation* to denote the earlier onset and increasing severity of the disease in successive generations.[357] It is caused by a $(CTG)_n$ expansion in the 3′UTR of a serine-threonine protein-kinase DMPK.[358–360] The size of the $(CTG)_n$ repeat correlated both with severity and with age of onset; indeed, families in which the severity of the disease had increased in successive generations exhibited a dramatic parallel expansion in repeat copy number. Similarly, infants with severe congenital myotonic dystrophy and their mothers exhibit a greater degree of amplification of CTG repeats than is found in the noncongenital population. In pedigrees exhibiting anticipation, the fragment size increased in successive generations.[335,357,361–363] There are also examples of a contraction rather than an expansion of repeat size,[364] and this may provide an explanation for the incomplete penetrance manifested by myotonic dystrophy. As with the fragile X syndrome, linkage disequilibrium is apparent in heterogeneous populations between myotonic dystrophy and DNA polymorphisms in the vicinity,[359,362] implying either the existence of only one or, at most, a few mutations or that the chromosomal environment predisposes to mutation at the DMPK locus.

In Friedreich ataxia, a recessive disorder, the repeat $(GAA)_n$ is located within an intron of the FRDA1 gene.[344] The age of onset/severity of the phenotype correlates with the size of the repeat.[365] There is a reduction in the amount of frataxin protein (a mitochondrial protein probably involved in cellular iron metabolism) in individuals with abnormal repeat length.[366]

In Huntington disease, spinocerebellar ataxias 1, 2, 3, 6, and 7, dentatorubral-pallidoluysian atrophy, and spinobulbar muscular

Table 2-10 **Various Examples of Disorders of Trinucleotide and Other Repeat Expansion**

	Disorder	Inheritance	Gene	Chr	OMIM no.	Repeat	Normal	Mutant	Repeat Location	Mutation Type	Parental Gender Bias	Ref.
1	Fragile X syndrome	XLD	FMR1	Xq27.3	309550	CGG	6–52	60–200 premut 230–1000 full mut	5′ UTR	LOF, FraX	Maternal	333
2	Fragile E mental retardation	XLD	FMR2	Xq28	309548	GCC	7–35	130–150 premut 230–750 full mut	5′ UTR	LOF, FraX	ND	334
3	Myotonic dystrophy	AD	DMPK	19q13	160900	CTG	5–37	50–3000	3′ UTR	?Dom negative	Maternal	335
4	Spinobulbar muscular atrophy	XLR	AR	Xq13-21	313700	CAG	11–33	38–66	Coding	COF, LOF	ND	336
5	Huntington disease	AD	HD	4p16.3	143100	CAG	6–39	36–121	Coding	GOF	Paternal	337
6	Dentatrubral-pallidoluysian atrophy	AD	DRPLA	12p13.31	125370	CAG	6–35	51–88	Coding	GOF	Paternal	338
7	Spinocerebellar ataxia 1	AD	SCA1/ATX1	6p23	601556	CAG	6–39	41–81	Coding	GOF	Paternal	339
8	Spinocerebellar ataxia 2	AD	SCA2/ATX2	12q24.1	601517	CAG	14–31	35–64	Coding	GOF	Paternal	340
9	Spinocerebellar ataxia 3	AD	SCA3/MJD1	14q32.1	109150	CAG	12–41	40–84	Coding	GOF	Paternal	341
10	Spinocerebellar ataxia 6/Episodic ataxia type 2	AD	CACNA1A	19p13	601011	CAG	7–18	20–23 EA2 21–27 SCA6	Coding	ND	ND	342
11	Spinocerebellar ataxia 7	AD	SCA7	3p12-13	164500	CAG	7–17	38–130	Coding	GOF	Paternal	343
12	Friedreich ataxia	AR	FRDA1	9q13-21.1	229300	GAA	6–34	80 premut 112–1700 full mut	Intron 1	LOF, FraX	Maternal	344
13	Progressive myoclonus epilepsy 1	AR	CSTB	21q22.3	601145	CCCGCCCCGCG	2–3	35–80	5′ Flanking	LOF	Paternal	332
14	Sympolydactyly	AD	HOXD13	2q31-q32	142989	$(GCG)_n(GCT)_n(GCA)_n$	15	22–29	Coding	ND	??	345
15	Oculopharyngeal muscular dystrophy	AD	PABP2	14q11.2-q13	602279	GCG	6	7–13	Coding	ND	??	346

NOTE: Mut, mutation; premut, premutation.

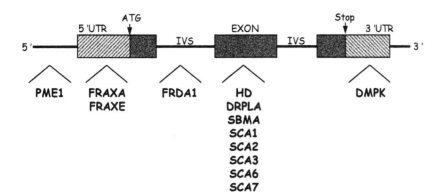

Fig. 2-17. Schematic representation of the location of the different repeat expansions associated with human disorders.

atrophy, the repeat is a (CAG)$_n$ located in the coding regions of the corresponding genes and encodes for polyglutamine.[336,337,339,340-343] The pathophysiology of these neurologic disorders is likely to be due to a gain of function of the abnormal proteins with expanded polyglutamine tracts.[367]

Trinucleotide-repeat expansions are certainly not the only examples of dynamic mutations. Lalioti et al[332] found that the common mutation mechanism in progressive myoclonus epilepsy EPM1 is the expansion of the dodecamer repeat (CCCCGCCCCGCG) in the 5′ flanking region of the CSTB gene. The normal general population contains either two or three copies of this repeat. Alleles with 12 to 17 repeats were also found that were transmitted unstably to offspring. These *premutational* alleles were not connected with a clinical phenotype of EPM1. Abnormal alleles contained between 30 and 75 copies of the 12mer repeat. A marked, cell-specific reduction of CSTB RNA is associated with expanded abnormal alleles. No correlation between number of repeat expansions and age of onset or severity had been found, suggesting a threshold effect of the expansion.[368]

The number of examples of this type of mutation will almost certainly increase and may provide explanations at the molecular level for a variety of intriguing phenomena in human genetics, such as variable expression and multifactorial inheritance.[369]

The following mechanisms could account for repeat instability and expansion: slippage during DNA replication, misalignment with subsequent excision repair, and unequal crossing-over and recombination. The most recently proposed mechanism is that the expansions occur because the triplet repeats form a secondary structure on the 5′ portion of the Okazaki fragments during replication and that may impede the movement of the replication fork. This might in turn result in a double-strand break within the repeat, which could expand during the end joining.[370]

MUTATIONS IN CANCER

A common finding in a diverse array of cancers is genetic instability. Its relationship to tumorigenesis is particularly well understood in hereditary nonpolyposis colon cancer (HNPCC), a syndrome characterized by predisposition to colorectal carcinoma and other cancers of the gastrointestinal and urologic tracts (see Chap. 18). In HNPCC, genetic instability at microsatellite sequences [replication error (RER) positive] has been linked to defects in several mismatch repair (MMR) genes.[371,372] Mutation rates in RER-positive cells are 2 to 3 orders of magnitude higher than in normal RER-negative cells.[371] Multiple mutations are necessary for malignancy, and MMR deficiency greatly speeds the process of accumulating mutations at those loci, which are critical for tumor progression. The target genes of the genome-wide hypermutability evident in MMR-deficient cells are now beginning to be identified. Perhaps the best example is that of the gene encoding the transforming growth factor β (TGFβ) receptor II, which is intimately involved in cellular growth regulation. Colorectal tumors are generally insensitive to the growth-

suppressing hormone TGFβ and, in colorectal tumors manifesting microsatellite instability (MI), this insensitivity is almost invariably due to frameshift mutations within a microsatellite sequence (polyadenine tract) embedded within the TGFβR2 gene.[373-375] Similarly, the target sequence of mutations within the transcription factor E2F-4 gene is a (CAG)$_{13}$ trinucleotide repeat within the putative transactivation domain.[376] Thus, mutation-bearing genes that contribute to the development of colorectal neoplasia may be identified firstly through their involvement in the negative regulation of cell growth and secondly on the basis of their containing repetitive sequences that represent likely targets for mutation in RER-positive cells. Some of the mutated genes are directly involved in growth regulation (e.g., APC,[377] E2F4,[376] and IGF2R[378]) or in promoting apoptosis (e.g., BAX[379]) and are therefore likely to play a role in tumor progression. MMR genes may themselves represent mutational targets[380] ("the mutator that mutates the other mutator"), which increases genomic instability still further. Other genes are not involved in these processes (e.g., HPRT[381]) and their mutation merely represent the consequence of a general genome-wide increase in mutability. It should be noted that the instability resulting from the deficiency of a mismatch-repair enzyme is qualitatively different from the instability associated with the triplet-repeat expansion disorders in which the local DNA structure appears to be critical in promoting expansion.[382]

Mutations may predispose individuals to neoplasia directly, but recent findings show that predisposition may also be indirect. A T-to-A transversion at nucleotide 3920 in the APC gene occurs in about 6 percent of Ashkenazi Jews and about 28 percent of Ashkenazim with a family history of colorectal cancer.[383] This lesion is considered unlikely to predispose individuals to cancer directly by altering the function of the encoded protein. Rather, this transversion generates an (A)$_8$ mononucleotide tract from an existing AAATAAAA sequence motif, thereby creating a hypermutable site within the APC coding sequence. The induced instability of this region manifests itself in terms of a high frequency of frameshift insertions in somatic tissues that have probably arisen through DNA slippage during the replication process.

Krawczak et al[37] demonstrated that the bulk of the spectrum of somatic single-base-pair substitutions in the TP53 gene strongly resembles that of their germ-line counterparts seen in other human genes. The latter set of mutations have, however, arisen in a tissue that is usually well protected against exogenous mutagens and carcinogens: the germ cells. Since spectral similarity is strongly suggestive of the involvement of similar mutational mechanisms, it would appear that many TP53 mutations in the soma have arisen directly or indirectly as a consequence of endogenous cellular mechanisms (DNA repair and replication?) rather than through the action of exogenous mutagens. The similarity noted between the cancer-associated mutational spectrum of TP53 and germ-line gene mutations was consistent with the idea that cancer is a critical mediator of negative selection against excessive germ-line mutation. Sommer[384] has speculated that, for such a mediator function to work, there must be a correlation between germ-line and somatic mutation rates. If specific mutations were to occur that enhanced the rates of both germ-line and somatic mutation, a consequent increase in the incidence of cancer before the end of the normal reproductive period would serve to militate against their survival. It follows that TP53 may act as a critical sensor that is built into the genome's molecular warning system and that, through carcinogenesis, kills the individual and saves the species.[384]

REFERENCES

1. Antonarakis SE, and Members of the Nomenclature Working Group: Recommendations for a nomenclature system for human gene mutations. *Hum Mutat* **11**:1, 1998.
2. Dunnen JT, Antonarakis SE: Mutation nomenclature extensions and suggestions to descrube complex mutations: a discussion. *Hum Mutat* **15**:7–12, 2000.
3. Cooper DN, Ball EV, Krawczak M: The human gene mutation database. *Nucleic Acids Res* **26**:285, 1998.
4. Krawczak M, Cooper DN: The human gene mutation database. *Trends Genet* **13**:121, 1997.
5. Cooper DN, Krawczak M: *Human Gene Mutation.* Oxford, BIOS Scientific, 1993.
6. Krawczak M, Ball EV, Cooper DN: Neighboring nucleotide effects on the rates of germline single base-pair substitution in human genes. *Am J Hum Genet* **63**:474, 1998.
7. Loeb LA, Kunkel TA: Fidelity of DNA synthesis. *Annu Rev Biochem* **52**:429, 1982.
8. Wang TSF: Eukaryotic DNA polymerases. *Annu Rev Biochem* **60**:513, 1991.
9. Kunkel TA, Alexander PS: The base substitution fidelity of eukaryotic DNA polymerases. *J Biol Chem* **261**:160, 1986.
10. Kunkel TA: The mutational specificity of DNA polymerase-β during *in vitro* DNA synthesis. *J Biol Chem* **260**:5787, 1985.
11. Grippo P, Iaccarino M, Parisi E, Scarano E: Methylation of DNA in developing sea urchin embryos. *J Mol Biol* **36**:195, 1968.
12. Cooper DN: Eukaryotic DNA methylation. *Hum Genet* **64**:315, 1983.
13. Bird AP: DNA methylation and the frequency of CpG in animal DNA. *Nucleic Acids Res* **8**:1499, 1980.
14. Nussinov R: Eukaryotic dinucleotide preference rules and their implications for degenerate codon usage. *J Mol Biol* **149**:125, 1981.
15. Bird AP: CpG-rich islands and the function of DNA methylation. *Nature* **321**:209, 1986.
16. Vogel F, Rährborn G: Mutationsvorgänge bei der Entstehung von Hämoglobinvarianten. *Humangenetik* **1**:635, 1965.
17. Vogel F, Kopun M: Higher frequencies of transitions among point mutations. *J Mol Evol* **9**:159, 1977.
18. Barker D, Schäfer M, White R: Restriction sites containing CpG show a higher frequency of polymorphism in human DNA. *Cell* **36**:131, 1984.
19. Youssoufian H, Kazazian HH, Phillips DG, Aronis S, Tsiftis G, Brown VA, Antonarakis SE: Recurrent mutations in hemophilia A give evidence for CpG mutation hotspots. *Nature* **324**:380, 1986.
20. Youssoufian H, Antonarakis SE, Bell W, Griffin AM, Kazazian HH: Nonsense and missense mutations in hemophilia A: Estimate of the relative mutation rate at CG dinucleotides. *Am J Hum Genet* **42**:718, 1988.
21. Green PM, Montandon AJ, Bentley DR, Ljung R, Nilsson IM, Giannelli F: The incidence and distribution of CpG > TpG transitions in the coagulation factor IX gene: A fresh look at CpG mutational hotspots. *Nucleic Acids Res* **18**:3227, 1990.
22. Cooper DN, Krawczak M: Cytosine methylation and the fate of CpG dinucleotides in vertebrate genomes. *Hum Genet* **83**:181, 1989.
23. Kaufman RJ, Antonarakis SE: Structure, biology and genetics of factor VIII, in Hoffman R, Benz EJ, Shattil SJ, Furie B, Cohen HJ, Silberstein LE (eds): *Hematology: Basic Principles and Practice*, 3d ed. New York, Churchill Livingstone, 1999, p 1850.
24. Higuchi M, Kazazian HH, Kasch L, Warran TC, McGinniss MJ, Phillips JA, Kasper C, et al: Molecular characterization of severe hemophilia A suggests that about half the mutations are not within the coding regions and splice junctions of the factor VIII gene. *Proc Natl Acad Sci USA* **88**:7405, 1991.
25. Higuchi M, Antonarakis SE, Kasch L, Oldenburg J, Economou-Petersen E, Olek K, Arai M, et al: Molecular characterization of mild

26. to moderate hemophilia A: Detection of the mutation in 25 of 29 patients by denaturing gradient gel electrophoresis. *Proc Natl Acad Sci USA* **88**:8307, 1991.
26. Koeberl DD, Bottema CDK, Ketterling RP, Lillicrap DP, Sommer SS: Mutations causing hemophilia B: Direct estimate of the underlying rates of spontaneous germ-line transitions, transversions and deletions in a human gene. *Am J Hum Genet* **47**:202, 1990.
27. Reitsma PH, Poort SR, Bernardi F, Gandrille S, Long GL, Sala N, Cooper DN: Protein C deficiency: A database of mutations. *Thromb Haemost* **69**:77, 1993.
28. Rideout WM, Coetzee GA, Olumi AF, Jones PA: 5-Methylcytosine as an endogenous mutagen in the human LDL receptor and p53 genes. *Science* **249**:1288, 1990.
29. Monk M, Boubelik M, Lehnert S: Temporal and regional changes in DNA methylation in the embryonic, extraembryonic and germ lineages during mouse embryo development. *Development* **99**:371, 1987.
30. Driscoll DJ, Migeon BR: Sex differences in methylation of single copy genes in human meiotic germ cells: Implications for X-inactivation, parental imprinting, and origin of CpG mutations. *Somat Cell Mol Genet* **16**:267, 1990.
31. Ketterling RP, Vielhaber E, Bottema CDK, Schaid DJ, Sexauer CL, Sommer SS: Germ-line origin of mutation in families with hemophilia B: The sex ratio varies with the type of mutation. *Am J Hum Genet* **52**:152, 1993.
32. Pattinson JK, Millar DS, Grundy CB, Wieland K, Mibashan RS, Martinowitz U, McVey J, et al: The molecular genetic analysis of hemophilia A: A directed-search strategy for the detection of point mutations in the human factor VIII gene. *Blood* **76**:2242, 1990.
33. Bottema CDK, Ketterling RP, Yoon H-S, Sommer SS: The pattern of factor IX germ-line mutation in Asians is similar to that of Caucasians. *Am J Hum Genet* **47**:835, 1990.
34. Behn-Krappa A, Hölker I, Sandaradura de Silva U, Doerfler W: Patterns of DNA methylation are indistinguishable in different individuals over a wide range of human DNA sequences. *Genomics* **11**:1, 1991.
35. Hollstein M, Sidransky D, Vogelstein B, Harris CC: p53 mutations in human cancer. *Science* **253**:49, 1991.
36. Tornaletti S, Pfeifer GP: Complete and tissue-independent methylation of CpG sites in the p53 gene: Implications for mutations in human cancer. *Oncogene* **10**:1493, 1995.
37. Krawczak M, Smith-Sorensen B, Schmidtke J, Kakkar VV, Cooper DN, Hovig E: The somatic spectrum of cancer-associated single base-pair substitutions in the TP53 gene is determined mainly by endogenous mechanisms of mutation and by selection. *Hum Mutat* **5**:48, 1995.
38. Steinberg RA, Gorman KB: Linked spontaneous CG > TA mutations at CpG sites in the gene for protein kinase regulatory subunit. *Mol Cell Biol* **12**:767, 1992.
39. Shen J-C, Rideout WM, Jones PA: High frequency mutagenesis by a DNA methyltransferase. *Cell* **71**:1073, 1992.
40. Bullock P, Champoux JJ, Botchan M: Association of crossover points with topoisomerase I cleavage sites: A model for non-homologous recombination. *Science* **230**:954, 1985.
41. Cooper DN, Krawczak M: Mechanisms of insertional mutagenesis in human genes causing genetic disease. *Hum Genet* **87**:409, 1991.
42. Weaver DT, DePamphilis ML: Specific sequences in native DNA that arrest synthesis by DNA polymerase α. *J Biol Chem* **257**:2075, 1982.
43. Bottema CDK, Ketterling RP, Li S, Yoon H-P, Phillips JA, Sommer SS: Missense mutations and evolutionary conservation of amino acids: Evidence that many of the amino acids in factor IX function as "spacer" elements. *Am J Hum Genet* **49**:820, 1991.
44. Epstein CJ: Non-randomness of amino-acid changes in the evolution of homologous proteins. *Nature* **215**:355, 1967.
45. Grantham R: Amino acid difference formula to help explain evolution. *Science* **185**:862, 1974.
46. Wu C-I, Maeda N: Inequality in mutation rates of the two strands of DNA. *Nature* **327**:169, 1987.
47. Holmes J, Clark S, Modrich P: Strand-specific mismatch correction in nuclear extracts of human and *Drosophila melanogaster* cell lines. *Proc Natl Acad Sci USA* **87**:5837, 1990.
48. Krawczak M, Reiss J, Cooper DN: The mutational spectrum of single base-pair substitutions in mRNA splice junctions of human genes: Causes and consequences. *Hum Genet* **90**:41, 1992.
49. Shapiro MB, Senapathy P: RNA splice junctions of different classes of eukaryotes: Sequence statistics and functional implications in gene expression. *Nucleic Acids Res* **15**:7155, 1987.

50. Padget RA, Grabowski PJ, Konarska MM, Seiler S, Sharp PA: Splicing of messenger RNA precursors. *Annu Rev Biochem* **55**:1119, 1986.
51. Krainer AR, Maniatis T: Multiple factors including the small nuclear riboproteins U1 and U2 are necessary for the pre-mRNA splicing *in vitro*. *Cell* **42**:725, 1985.
52. Talerico M, Berget SM: Effect of 5′ splice site mutations on splicing of the preceding intron. *Mol Cell Biol* **10**:6299, 1990.
53. Weil D, D'Alessio M, Ramirez F, Eyre DR: Structural and functional characterization of a splicing mutation in the pro-alpha 2(1) collagen gene of an Ehlers-Danlos type VII patient. *J Biol Chem* **265**:16,007, 1990.
54. Weil D, Bernard M, Combates N, Wirtz MK, Hollister DW, Steinmann B, Ramirez F: Identification of a mutation that causes exon skipping during collagen pre-mRNA splicing in an Ehlers-Danlos syndrome variant. *J Biol Chem* **263**:8561, 1988.
55. Grandchamp B, Picat C, de Rooij F, Beaumont C, Wilson P, Deybach JC, Nordmann Y: A point mutation G to A in exon 12 of the PBGD gene results in exon skipping and is responsible for acute intermittent porphyria. *Nucleic Acids Res* **17**:6637, 1989.
56. Carstens RP, Fenton WA, Rosenberg LR: Identification of RNA splicing errors resulting in human ornithine transcarbamylase deficiency. *Am J Hum Genet* **48**:1105, 1991.
57. Wen JK, Osumi T, Hashimoto T, Ogata M: Molecular analysis of human acatalasemia: Identification of a splicing mutation. *J Mol Biol* **211**:383, 1990.
58. Tromp G, Prockop DJ: Single base mutation in the pro-alpha-2(I) collagen gene that causes efficient exon skipping of RNA from exon 27 to exon 29 and synthesis of a shortened but in frame pro-alpha-2(I) chain. *Proc Natl Acad Sci USA* **85**:5254, 1988.
59. Dunn JM, Phillips RA, Zhu X, Becker A, Gallie BL: Mutations in the RB1 gene and their effects on transcription. *Mol Cell Biol* **9**:4596, 1989.
60. Treistman R, Orkin SH, Maniatis T: Specific transcription and RNA splicing defects in five cloned β thalassemia genes. *Nature* **302**:591, 1983.
61. Atweh GF, Wong C, Reed R, Antonarakis SE, Zhu D, Ghosh PK, Maniatis T, et al: A new mutation in IVS1 of the human beta-globin gene causing beta-thalassemia due to abnormal splicing. *Blood* **70**:147, 1987.
62. Su TS, Lin LH: Analysis of a splice acceptor site mutation which produces multiple splicing abnormalities in the human argininosuccinate synthase gene. *J Biol Chem* **265**:19,716, 1990.
63. Dietz HC, Valle D, Francomano CA, Kendzior RJ, Pyeritz RE, Cutting GR: The skipping of consecutive exons *in vivo* induced by nonsense mutations. *Science* **259**:680, 1993.
64. Orkin SH, Kazazian HH, Antonarakis SE, Ostrer H, Goff SC, Sexton JP: Abnormal processing due to the exon mutation of the beta-E-globin gene. *Nature* **300**:768, 1982.
65. Nakano T, Suzuki K: Genetic cause of a juvenile form of Sandhoff disease: Abnormal splicing of beta-hexosaminidase beta chain gene transcript due to a point mutation within intron 12. *J Biol Chem* **264**:5155, 1989.
66. Mitchell GA, Brody LC, Looney J, Steel G, Suchanek M, Dowling C, Kaloustian V der, et al: An initiator codon mutation in ornithine-δ-aminotransferase causing gyrate atrophy of the choroid and retina. *J Clin Invest* **81**:630, 1988.
67. Naylor JA, Green PM, Rizza CR, Giannelli F: Analysis of factor VIII mRNA reveals defects in everyone of 28 hemophilia patients. *Hum Mol Genet* **2**:11, 1993.
68. Higashi Y, Tanae A, Inoue H, Hiromasa T, Fujii-Kariyama Y: Aberrant splicing and missense mutations cause steroid 21-hydroxylase deficiency in humans: Possible gene conversion products. *Proc Natl Acad Sci USA* **85**:7486, 1988.
69. Murru S, Loudianos G, Deiana M, Camaschella C, Sciarratta GV, Agosti S, Parodi MI, et al: Molecular characterization of β-thalassemia intermedia in patients of Italian descent and identification of three novel β-thalassemia mutations. *Blood* **77**:1342, 1991.
70. Beldjord C, Lapoumeroulie C, Pagnier J, Benabadji M, Krishnamoorthy R, Labie D, Bank A: A novel beta-thalassemia gene with a single base mutation in the conversed polypyrimidine sequence at the 3-prime end of IVS2. *Nucleic Acids Res* **16**:4927, 1988.
71. Sharp P: Splicing of messenger RNA precursors. *Science* **235**:767, 1987.
72. Rosenthal A, Jouet M, Kenwrick S: Aberrant splicing of neural cell adhesion molecule L1 mRNA in a family with X-linked hydrocephalus. *Nature Genet* **2**:107, 1992.

73. Burrows NP, Nicholls AC, Richards AJ, Luccarini C, Harrison JB, Yates JR, Pope FM: A point mutation in an intronic branch site results in aberrant splicing of COL5A1 and in Ehlers-Danlos syndrome type II in two British families. *Am J Hum Genet* **63**:390, 1998.
74. Kuivenhoven JA, Weibusch H, Pritchard PH, Funke H, Benne R, Assmann G, Kastelein JJP: An intronic mutation in a lariat branchpoint sequence is a direct cause of an inherited human disorder (fish-eye disease). *J Clin Invest* **98**:358, 1996.
75. Nakahashi Y, Fujita H, Taketani S, Ishida N, Kappas A, Sassa S: The molecular defect of ferrochelatase in a patient with erythropoietic protoporphyria. *Proc Natl Acad Sci USA* **89**:281, 1992.
76. Mitchell GA, Labuda D, Fontaine G, Saudubray JM, Bonnefont JP, Lyonnet S, Brody LC, et al: Splice-mediated insertion of an *Alu* sequence inactivates ornithine δ-aminotransferase: A role for *Alu* elements in human mutation. *Proc Natl Acad Sci USA* **88**:815, 1991.
77. Cogan JD, Prince MA, Lekhakula S, Bundey S, Futrakul A, McCarthy EM, Phillips JA: A novel mechanism of aberrant pre-mRNA splicing in humans. *Hum Mol Genet* **6**:909, 1997.
78. Hutton M, Lendon CL, Rizzu P, Baker M, Froelich S, Houlden H, Pickering-Brown S, et al: Association of missense and 5-prime-splice-site mutations in tau with the inherited dementia FTDP-17. *Nature* **393**:702, 1998.
79. Wong C, Dowling CE, Saiki RK, Higuchi R, Erlich HA, Kazazian HH: Characterization of β-thalassaemia mutations using direct genomic sequencing of amplified single copy DNA. *Nature* **330**:384, 1987.
80. Kozak M: Compilation and analysis of sequences upstream from the translational start site in eukaryotic mRNAs. *Nucleic Acids Res* **12**:857, 1984.
81. Moi P, Cash FE, Liebhaber SA, Cao A, Pirastu M: An initiation codon mutation (AUG to GUG) of the human α1-globin gene. *J Clin Invest* **80**:1416, 1987.
82. Pirastu M, Saglio G, Chang JC, Cao A, Kan YW: Initiation codon mutation as a cause of a thalassemia. *J Biol Chem* **259**:12,315, 1984.
83. Kozak M: Structural features in eukaryotic mRNAs that modulate the initiation of translation. *J Biol Chem* **266**:19,867, 1991.
84. Neote K, Brown CA, Mahuran DJ, Gravel RA: Translation initiation in the HEXB gene encoding the β-subunit of human β-hexosaminidase. *J Biol Chem* **265**:20,799, 1990.
85. Cai S-P, Eng B, Francombe WH, Olivieri NF, Kendall AG, Waye JS, Chui DHK: Two novel β-thalassemia mutations in the 5′ and 3′ noncoding regions of the β-globin gene. *Blood* **79**:1342, 1992.
86. Clegg JB, Weatherall DJ, Milner PG: Haemoglobin Constant Spring: A chain termination mutant? *Nature* **234**:337, 1971.
87. Milner PF, Clegg JB, Weatherall DJ: Haemoglobin H disease due to a unique haemoglobin variant with an elongated a chain. *Lancet* **1**:729, 1971.
88. Hunt DM, Higgs DR, Winichagoon P, Clegg JB, Weatherall DJ: Haemoglobin Constant Spring has an unstable a chain messenger RNA. *Br J Haematol* **51**:405, 1982.
89. Bunn HF: Mutant hemoglobins having elongated chains. *Hemoglobin* **2**:1, 1978.
90. Beris PH, Miesher PA, Diaz-Chico JC, Hans IS, Kutlar A, Hu H, Wilson HB, Huisman TJH: Inclusion body β-thalassaemia trait in a Swiss family is caused by an abnormal hemoglobin (Geneva) with an altered and extended β-chain carboxy terminus due to a modification in codon b114. *Blood* **72**:801, 1988.
91. Ristaldi MS, Pirastu M, Murru S, Casula L, Loudianos G, Cao A, Sciarrata GV, et al: A spontaneous mutation produced a novel elongated β-globin chain structural variant (Hb Agnana) with a thalassemia-like phenotype. *Blood* **75**:1378, 1990.
92. Kazazian HH, Dowling CE, Hurwitz RL, Coleman M, Adams JG: Thalassemia mutations in exon 3 of the β-globin gene often cause a dominant form of thalassemia and show no predilection for malarial-endemic regions of the world. *Am J Hum Genet* **25**(suppl):950, 1989.
93. Fucharoen S, Kobayashi Y, Fucharoen G, Ohba Y, Miyazono K, Fukumaki Y, Takaku F: A single nucleotide deletion in codon 123 of the β-globin gene causes an inclusion body β-thalassaemia trait: A novel elongated globin chain β Makabe. *Br J Haematol* **75**:393, 1990.
94. Thein SL, Hesketh C, Taylor P, Temperley IJ, Hutchinson RM, Old JM, Wood WG, et al: Molecular basis for dominantly inherited inclusion body β-thalassemia. *Proc Natl Acad Sci USA* **87**:3924, 1990.
95. Orkin SH, Cheng T-C, Antonarakis SE, Kazazian HH: Thalassemia due to a mutation in the cleavage-polyadenylation signal of the human β-globin gene. *EMBO J* **4**:453, 1985.
96. Jankovic L, Efremov GD, Petkov G, Kattamis C, George E, Yank K-G, Stoming TA, Huisman THJ: Two novel polyadenylation mutations leading to β⁺-thalassaemia. *Br J Haematol* **75**:122, 1990.

97. Rund D, Dowling C, Najjar K, Rachmilewitz EA, Kazazian HH, Oppenheim A: Two mutations in the β-globin polyadenylation signal reveal extended transcripts and new RNA polyadenylation sites. *Proc Natl Acad Sci USA* **89**:4324, 1992.

98. Gieselmann V, Polten A, Kreysing J, von Figura K: Arylsulfatase A pseudodeficiency: Loss of a polyadenylylation signal and N-glycosylation site. *Proc Natl Acad Sci USA* **86**:9436, 1989.

99. Benz EJ, Forget BG, Hillman DG, Cohen-Solal M, Pritchard J, Cavallesco C, Prensky W, Housman D: Variability in the amount of β-globin mRNA in β⁰-thalassemia. *Cell* **14**:299, 1978.

100. Lehrman MA, Schneider WJ, Brown MS, Davis CG, Elhammer A, Russell DW, Goldstein JL: The Lebanese allele at the low density lipoprotein receptor locus. *J Biol Chem* **262**:401, 1987.

101. Fojo SS, Lohse P, Parrott C, Baggio G, Gabelli C, Thomas F, Hoffman J, Brewer HB: A nonsense mutation in the apolipoprotein C-II Padova gene in a patient with apolipoprotein C-II deficiency. *J Clin Invest* **84**:1215, 1989.

102. Liebhaber SA, Coleman MB, Adams JG, Cash FE, Steinberg MH: Molecular basis for nondeletion α-thalassaemia in American blacks; α₂ 116 GAG > UAG. *J Clin Invest* **80**:154, 1987.

103. Kinniburgh AJ, Maquat LE, Schedl T, Rachmilewitz E, Ross J: mRNA-deficient β⁰-thalassemia results from a single nucleotide deletion. *Nucleic Acids Res* **10**:5421, 1982.

104. Chang JC, Kan YW: β⁰ Thalassemia, a nonsense mutation in man. *Proc Natl Acad Sci USA* **76**:2886, 1979.

105. Brody LC, Mitchell GA, Obie C, Michaud J, Steel G, Fontaine G, Robert MF, et al: Ornithine δ-aminotransferase mutations in gyrate atrophy: Allelic heterogeneity and functional consequences. *J Biol Chem* **267**:3302, 1992.

106. Takeshita K, Forget BG, Scarpa A, Benz EJ: Intranuclear defect in β-globin mRNA accumulation due to a premature translation termination codon. *Blood* **64**:13, 1984.

107. Humphries KR, Ley TJ, Anagnou NP, Baur AW, Nienhuis AW: β⁰⁻³⁹ Thalassemia gene: A premature termination codon causes β-mRNA deficiency without affecting cytoplasmic β-mRNA stability. *Blood* **64**:23, 1984.

108. Baserga SJ, Benz EJ: Nonsense mutations in the human β-globin gene affect mRNA metabolism. *Proc Natl Acad Sci USA* **85**:2056, 1988.

109. Baserga SJ, Benz EJ: β-Globin nonsense mutation: Deficient accumulation of mRNA occurs despite normal cytoplasmic stability. *Proc Natl Acad Sci USA* **89**:2935, 1992.

110. Atweh GF, Brickner HE, Zhu X-X, Kazazian HH, Forget BG: New amber mutation in a β-thalassemic gene with nonmeasurable levels of mutant messenger RNA *in vivo*. *J Clin Invest* **82**:557, 1988.

111. Maquat LE, Kinniburgh AJ, Rachmilewitz EA, Ross J: Unstable β-globin mRNA in mRNA-deficient β⁰-thalassemia. *Cell* **27**:543, 1981.

112. Daar IO, Maquat LE: Premature translation termination mediates triosephosphate isomerase mRNA degradation. *Mol Cell Biol* **8**:802, 1988.

113. Maquat LE: When cells stop making sense: Effects of nonsense codons on RNA metabolism in vertebrate cells. *RNA* **1**:453, 1995.

114. Urlaub G, Mitchell PJ, Ciudad CJ, Chasin LA: Nonsense mutations in the dihydrofolate reductase gene affect RNA processing. *Mol Cell Biol* **9**:2868, 1989.

115. Cheng J, Fogel-Petrovic M, Maquat LE: Translation to near the distal end of the penultimate exon is required for normal levels of spliced triosephosphate isomerase mRNA. *Mol Cell Biol* **10**:5215, 1990.

116. Ploos van Amstel HK, Diepstraten CM, Reitsma PH, Bertina RM: Analysis of platelet protein S mRNA suggests silent alleles as a frequent cause of hereditary protein S deficiency type I. *Thromb Haemost* **65**:808, 1991.

117. Peerlinck K, Eikenboom JCJ, Ploos van Amstel HK, Sangtawesin W, Arnout J, Reitsma PH, Vermylen J, Briet E: A patient with von Willebrand's disease characterized by compound heterozygosity for a substitution of Arg 854 by Gln in the putative factor VIII-binding domain of von Willebrand factor on one allele and very low levels of mRNA from the second allele. *Br J Haematol* **80**:358, 1992.

118. Dietz HC, Kendzior RJ Jr: Maintenance of an open reading frame as an additional level of scrutiny during splice site selection. *Nat Genet* **8**:183, 1994

119. Orkin SH, Antonarakis SE, Kazazian HH: Base substitution at position-88 in a β-thalassemic globin gene: Further evidence for the role of distal promoter element ACACCC. *J Biol Chem* **259**:8679, 1984.

120. Orkin SH, Kazazian HH, Antonarakis SE, Goff SC, Boehm CD, Sexton JP, Waber PG, Giardina PJV: Linkage of β-thalassemia

121. Antonarakis SE, Orkin SH, Cheng TC, Scott AF, Sexton JP, Trusko SP, Charache S, Kazazian HH: β-Thalassemia in American blacks: Novel mutations in the TATA box and an acceptor splice site. *Proc Natl Acad Sci USA* **81**:1154, 1984.

122. Cai SP, Zhang JZ, Doherty M, Kan YW: A new TATA box mutation detected at prenatal diagnosis for β-thalassemia. *Am J Hum Genet* **45**:112, 1989.

123. Takihara Y, Nakamura T, Yamada H, Takagi Y, Fukumaki Y: A novel mutation in the TATA box in a Japanese patient with β⁺ thalassemia. *Blood* **67**:547, 1986.

124. Lin LL, Lin KS, Lin KH, Cheng TY: A novel-34 (C to A) mutant identified in amplified genomic DNA of a Chinese β thalassemia patient. *Am J Hum Genet* **50**:237, 1992.

125. Meloni A, Rosatelli MC, Faa V, Sardu R, Saba L, Murru S, Sciarratta P, et al: Promoter mutations producing mild β-thalassemia in the Italian population. *Br J Haematol* **80**:222, 1992.

126. Faustino P, Osorio-Almeida L, Barbot J, Espirito-Santo D, Goncalves J, Romao L, Martins MC, et al: Novel promoter and splice junction defects add to the genetic, clinical or geographic heterogeneity of β thalassemia in the Portuguese population. *Hum Genet* **89**:573, 1992.

127. Huisman THJ: The β and δ thalassemia repository. *Hemoglobin* **16**:237, 1992.

128. Gonzalez-Rodondo JM, Stoming TA, Kutlar A, Kutlar F, Lanclos KD, Howard EF, Fei YJ, et al: A C to T substitution at nt-101 in a conserved DNA sequence of the promoter region of the β-globin gene is associated with "silent" β thalassemia. *Blood* **73**:1705, 1989.

129. Matsuda M, Sakamoto N, Fukumaki Y: δ-Thalassemia caused by disruption of the site for any erythroid-specific transcription factor, GATA-1, in the δ-globin gene promoter. *Blood* **80**:1347, 1992.

130. Collins FS, Stoeckert CJ, Serjeant GR, Forget BG, Weissman SM: Gγ β⁺ HPFH: Cosmid cloning and identification of a specific mutation 5′ to the Gγ gene. *Proc Natl Acad Sci USA* **81**:4894, 1984.

131. Gilman JG, Mishima N, Wen XJ, Kutlar F, Huisman THJ: Upstream promoter mutation associated with a modest elevation of fetal hemoglobin expression in human adults. *Blood* **72**:78, 1988.

132. Fucharoen S, Shimizu K, Fukumaki Y: A novel C > T transition within the distal CCAAT motif of the G-gamma globin gene in the Japanese HPFH: Implication of factor binding in elevated fetal globin expression. *Nucleic Acids Res* **18**:5245, 1990.

133. Stoming TA, Stoming GS, Lanclos KD, Fei YJ, Kutlar F, Huisman THJ: A A-gamma type of nondeletional hereditary persistence of fetal hemoglobin with a T-C mutation at position −175 to the Cap site of the A-gamma globin gene. *Blood* **73**:329, 1989.

134. Oner R, Kutlar F, Gu LH, Huisman THJ: The Georgia type of nondeletion HPFH has a C to T mutation at nucleotide −114 of the Aγ-globin gene. *Blood* **77**:1124, 1991.

135. Ottolenghi S, Nicolis S, Taramelli R, Malgaretti N, Mantovani R, Comi P, Giglioni B, et al: Sardinian Gγ HPFH: A T to C substitution in a conserved octamer sequence in the Gγ promoter. *Blood* **71**:815, 1988.

136. Martin DIK, Tsai S-F, Orkin SH: Increased gamma-globin expression in a nondeletion HPFH mediated by an erythroid-specific DNA-binding factor. *Nature* **338**:435, 1989.

137. Lloyd JA, Lee RF, Lingrel JB: Mutations in two regions upstream of the A gamma globin gene canonical promoter affect gene expression. *Nucleic Acids Res* **17**:4339, 1989.

138. Gumucio DL, Lockwood WK, Weber JL, Saulino AM, Delgrosso K, Surrey S, Schwartz E, et al: The −175 T > C mutation increases promoter strength in erythroid cells: Correlation with evolutionary conservation of binding sites for two trans-acting factors. *Blood* **75**:756, 1990.

139. McDonagh KT, Lin HJ, Lowrey CH, Bodine DM, Nienhuis AW: The upstream region of the human gamma-globin gene promoter: Identification and functional analysis of nuclear protein binding sites. *J Biol Chem* **266**:11,965, 1991.

140. Nicolis S, Ronchi A, Malgaretti N, Mantovani R, Giglioni B, Ottolenghi S: Increased erythroid-specific expression of a mutated HPFH gamma α-globin promoter requires the erythroid factor NFE-1. *Nucleic Acids Res* **17**:5509, 1989.

141. Mantovani R, Malgaretti N, Nicolis S, Ronchi A, Giglioni B, Ottolenghi S: The effects of HPFH mutations in the human gamma α-globin promoter on binding of ubiquitous and erythroid-specific nuclear factors. *Nucleic Acids Res* **16**:7783, 1988.

142. Gumucio DL, Rood KL, Gray TA, Riordan MF, Sartor CI, Collins FS: Nuclear proteins that bind the human gamma-globin gene promoter: Alterations in binding produced by point mutations associated

with hereditary persistence of fetal hemoglobin. *Mol Cell Biol* **8**:5310, 1988.

143. O'Neil D, Kaysen J, Donovan-Peluso M, Castle M, Bank A: Protein-DNA interactions upstream from the human A gamma globin gene. *Nucleic Acids Res* **18**:1977, 1990.

144. Briet E, Bertina RM, van Tilburg NH, Veltkamp JJ: Haemophilia B Leyden: A sex-linked hereditary disorder that improves after puberty. *N Engl J Med* **306**:788, 1982.

145. Reitsma PH, Bertina RM, Ploos van Amstel JK, Riemans A, Briet E: The putative factor IX gene promoter in hemophilia B Leyden. *Blood* **72**:1074, 1988.

146. Reitsma PH, Mandalaki T, Kasper CK, Bertina RM, Briet E: Two novel point mutations correlate with an altered developmental expression of blood coagulation factor IX (hemophilia B Leyden phenotype). *Blood* **73**:743, 1989.

147. Crossley M, Winship P, Brownlee GG: Functional analysis of the normal and an aberrant factor IX promoter, in *Regulation of Liver Gene Expression.* Cold Spring Harbor, NY, Cold Spring Harbor Laboratory, 1989, p 51.

148. Bottema CDK, Koeberl DD, Sommer SS: Direct carrier testing in 14 families with haemophilia B. *Lancet* **2**:526, 1989.

149. Hirosawa S, Fahner JB, Salier J-P, Wu C-T, Lovrien EW, Kurachi K: Structural and functional basis of the developmental regulation of human coagulation factor IX gene: Factor IX Leyden. *Proc Natl Acad Sci USA* **87**:4421, 1990.

150. Crossley M, Winship PR, Austen DEG, Rizza CR, Brownlee GG: A less severe form of haemophilia B Leyden. *Nucleic Acids Res* **18**:4633, 1990.

151. Gispert S, Vidaud M, Vidaud D, Gazengel C, Boneu B, Goossens M: A promoter defect correlates with an abnormal coagulation factor IX gene expression in a French family (hemophilia B Leyden). *Am J Hum Genet* **45**(suppl):A189, 1989.

152. Reijnen MJ, Sladek FM, Bertina RM, Reitsma PH: Disruption of a binding site for hepatocyte nuclear factor 4 results in hemophilia B Leyden. *Proc Natl Acad Sci USA* **89**:6300, 1992.

153. Freedenberg DL, Black B: Altered developmental control of the factor IX gene: A new T to A mutation at position +6 of the FIX gene resulting in hemophilia B Leyden. *Thromb Haemost* **65**:964, 1991.

154. Crossley M, Brownlee GG: Disruption of a C/EBP binding site in the factor IX promoter is associated with haemophilia B. *Nature* **345**:444, 1990.

155. Crossley M, Ludwig M, Stowell KM, De Vos P, Olek K, Brownlee GG: Recovery from hemophilia B Leyden: An androgen-responsive element in the factor IX promoter. *Science* **257**:377, 1992.

156. Berg PE, Mittelman M, Elion J, Labie D, Schechter AN: Increased protein binding to a −350 mutation of the human β-globin gene associated with decreased β-globin synthesis. *Am J Hematol* **36**:42, 1991.

157. Ionasescu VV, Searby C, Ionasescu R, Neuhaus IM, Werner R: Mutations of the noncoding region of the connexin32 gene in X-linked dominant Charcot-Marie-Tooth neuropathy. *Neurology* **47**:541, 1996.

158. Moi P, Loudianos G, Lavinha J, Murru S, Cossu P, Casu R, Oggiano L, et al: δ-Thalassemia due to a mutation in an erythroid-specific binding protein sequence 3′ to the δ-globin gene. *Blood* **79**:512, 1992.

159. Van der Ploeg LHT, Konings A, Oort M, Roos D, Bernini L, Flavell RA: Gamma-β-thalassaemia studies showing that deletion of the γ- and δ-genes influences β-globin gene expression in man. *Nature* **283**:637, 1980.

160. Kioussis D, Vanin E, de Lange T, Flavell RA, Grosveld FG: β-Globin gene inactivation by DNA translocation in γ-β-thalassaemia. *Nature* **306**:662, 1983.

161. Curtin P, Pirastu M, Kan YW, Gobert-Jones JA, Stephens AD, Lehmann H: A distant gene deletion affects β-globin gene function in an atypical γδβ-thalassaemia. *J Clin Invest* **76**:1554, 1985.

162. Driscoll MC, Dobkin CS, Alter BP: γδβ-Thalassemia due to a de novo mutation deleting the 5′ β-globin gene activation-region hypersensitive sites. *Proc Natl Acad Sci USA* **86**:7470, 1989.

163. Grosveld F, van Assendelft GB, Greaves DR, Kollias G: Position-independent high-level expression of the human β-globin gene in transgenic mice. *Cell* **51**:975, 1989.

164. Jarman AP, Wood WG, Sharpe JA, Gourdon G, Ayyub H, Higgs DR: Characterization of the major regulatory element upstream of the human α-globin gene cluster. *Mol Cell Biol* **11**:4679, 1991.

165. Hatton CSR, Wilkie AOM, Drysdale HC, Wood WG, Vickers MA, Sharpe J, Ayyub H, et al: α-Thalassemia caused by a large (62kb) deletion upstream of the human a globin gene cluster. *Blood* **76**:221, 1990.

166. Wilkie AOM, Lamb J, Harris PC, Finney RD, Higgs DR: A truncated human chromosome 16 associated with α-thalassaemia is stabilized by addition of telomeric repeat (TTAGGG). *Nature* **346**:868, 1990.

167. Romao L, Osorio-Almeida L, Higgs DR, Lavinha J, Liebhaber SA: α-Thalassaemia resulting from deletion of regulatory sequences far upstream of the α-globin structural genes. *Blood* **78**:1589, 1991.

168. Romao L, Cash F, Weiss I, Liebhaber S, Pirastu M, Galanello R, Loi A, et al: Human α-globin gene expression is silenced by terminal truncation of chromosome 16p beginning immediately 3′ of the zeta-globin gene. *Hum Genet* **89**:323, 1992.

169. Liebhaber SA, Griese E-U, Weiss I, Cash FE, Ayyub H, Higgs DR, Horst J: Inactivation of human α-globin gene expression by a de novo deletion located upstream of the α-globin gene cluster. *Proc Natl Acad Sci USA* **87**:9431, 1990.

170. Higgs DR, Wood WG, Jarman AP, Sharpe J, Lida J, Pretorius IM, Ayyub H: A major positive regulatory region located far upstream of the human α-globin gene locus. *Genes Dev* **4**:1588, 1990.

171. Vyas P, Vickers MA, Simmons DL, Ayyub H, Craddock CF, Higgs DR: Cis-acting sequences regulating expression of the human α-globin cluster lie within constitutively open chromatin. *Cell* **69**:781, 1992.

172. Poort SR, Rosendaal FR, Reitsma PH, Bertina RM. A common genetic variation in the 3′-untranslated region of the prothrombin gene is associated with elevated plasma prothrombin levels and an increase in venous thrombosis. *Blood* **88**:3698, 1996.

173. Antonarakis SE, Kazazian HH Jr: The molecular basis of hemophilia A in man. *Trends Genet* **4**:233, 1988.

174. Millar DS, Steinbrecher RA, Wieland K, Grundy CB, Martinowitz U, Krawczak M, Zoll B, et al: The molecular genetic analysis of haemophilia A: Characterization of six partial deletions in the factor VIII gene. *Hum Genet* **86**:219, 1990.

175. Ballabio A, Carrozzo R, Parenti G, Gil A, Zollo M, Persico MG, Gillard E, et al: Molecular heterogeneity of steroid sulfatase deficiency: A multicenter study of 57 unrelated patients at DNA and protein levels. *Genomics* **4**:36, 1989.

176. Forrest SM, Cross GS, Speer A, Gardner-Medwin D, Burn J, Davies KE: Preferential deletion of exons in Duchenne and Becker muscular dystrophies. *Nature* **329**:638, 1987.

177. Forrest SM, Cross GS, Flint T, Speer A, Robson KJH, Davies KE: Further studies of gene deletions that cause Duchenne and Becker muscular dystrophies. *Genomics* **2**:109, 1988.

178. Den Dunnen JT, Bakker E, Klein Breteler EG, Pearson PL, van Ommen GJB: Direct detection of more than 50% of the Duchenne muscular dystrophy mutations by field inversion gels. *Nature* **329**:640, 1987.

179. Wapenaar MC, Kievits T, Hart KA, Abbs S, Blonden LAJ, den Dunnen JT, Grootscholten PM, et al: A deletion hot spot in the Duchenne muscular dystrophy gene. *Genomics* **2**:101, 1988.

180. Vnencak-Jones CL, Phillips JA, Chen EY, Seeburg PH: Molecular basis of human growth hormone deletions. *Proc Natl Acad Sci USA* **85**:5615, 1988.

181. Vnencak-Jones CL, Phillips JA: Hot spots for growth hormone gene deletions in homologous regions outside of *Alu* repeats. *Science* **250**:1745, 1990.

182. Langlois S, Kastelein JJP, Hayden MR: Characterization of six partial deletions in the low density lipoprotein (LDL) receptor gene causing familial hypercholesterolemia (FH). *Am J Hum Genet* **43**:60, 1988.

183. Nicholls RD, Fischel-Ghodsian N, Higgs DR: Recombination at the human α-globin gene cluster: Sequence features and topological constraints. *Cell* **49**:369, 1987.

184. Higgs DR, Vickers MA, Wilkie AOM, Pretorius I-M, Jarman AP, Weatherall DJ: A review of the molecular genetics of the human α-globin gene cluster. *Blood* **73**:1081, 1989.

185. Embury SH, Miller JA, Dozy AM, Kan YW, Chan V, Todd D: Two different molecular organizations account for the single α-globin gene of the α-thalassaemia-2 genotype. *J Clin Invest* **66**:1319, 1980.

186. Trent RJ, Higgs DR, Clegg JB, Weatherall DJ: A new triplicated α-globin gene arrangement in man. *Br J Haematol* **49**:149, 1981.

187. Goossens M, Dozy AM, Embury SH, Zachariades Z, Hadjiminas MG, Stamatoyannopoulos G, Kan YW: Triplicated α-globin loci in humans. *Proc Natl Acad Sci USA* **77**:518, 1980.

188. Hwu HR, Roberts JH, Davidson EH, Britten RJ: Insertion and/or deletion of many repeated DNA sequences in human and higher ape evolution. *Proc Natl Acad Sci USA* **83**:3875, 1986.

189. Moyzis RK, Torney DC, Meyne J, Buckingham JM, Wu JR, Burks C, Sirotkin KM, Goad WG: The distribution of interspersed repetitive DNA sequences in the human genome. *Genomics* **4**:273, 1989.

190. Deininder PL: SINEs: Short interspersed repetitive DNA elements in higher eukaryotes, in Berg DE, Howe MM (eds): *Mobile DNA*. Washington, DC, American Society of Microbiology, 1989, p 619.

191. Jelinek WR, Schmid CW: Repetitive sequences in eukaryotic DNA and their expression. *Annu Rev Biochem* **51**:813, 1982.

192. Lehrman MA, Schneider WJ, Suedhof TF, Brown MS, Goldstein JL, Russell DW: Mutation in LDL receptor: *Alu-Alu* recombination deletes exons encoding transmembrane and cytoplasmic domains. *Science* **227**:140, 1985.

193. Lehrman MA, Russell DW, Goldstein JL, Brown MS: Exon-*Alu* recombination deletes 5 kilobases from the low density lipoprotein receptor gene producing a null phenotype in familial hypercholesterolemia. *Proc Natl Acad Sci USA* **83**:3679, 1986.

194. Hobbs HH, Brown MS, Goldstein JL, Russell DW: Deletion of exon encoding cysteine-rich repeat of low-density lipoprotein receptor alters its binding specificity in a subject with familial hypercholesterolemia. *J Biol Chem* **261**:13,114, 1986.

195. Horsthemke B, Beisiegel U, Dunning A, Havinga JR, Williamson R, Humphries S: Unequal crossing-over between two *Alu*-repetitive DNA sequences in the low-density-lipoprotein-receptor gene. *Eur J Biochem* **164**:77, 1987.

196. Lehrman MA, Russell DW, Goldstein JL, Brown MS: *Alu-Alu* recombination deletes splice acceptor sites and produces secreted low density lipoprotein receptor in a subject with familial hypercholesterolemia. *J Biol Chem* **262**:3354, 1987.

197. Lehrman MA, Goldstein JL, Russell DW, Brown MS: Duplication of seven exons in LDL receptor gene caused by *Alu-Alu* recombination in a subject with familial hypercholesterolemia. *Cell* **48**:827, 1987.

198. Ariga T, Carter PE, Davis AE: Recombinations between *Alu* repeat sequences that result in partial deletions within the C1 inhibitor gene. *Genomics* **8**:607, 1990.

199. Carter PE, Duponchel C, Tosi M, Fothergill JE: Complete nucleotide sequence of the gene for human C1 inhibitor with an unusually high density of *Alu* elements. *Eur J Biochem* **197**:301, 1991.

200. Stoppa-Lyonnet D, Duponchel C, Meo T, Laurent J, Carter PE, Arala-Chaves M, Cohen JHM, et al: Recombination biases in the rearranged C1-inhibitor genes of hereditary angioedema patients. *Am J Hum Genet* **49**:1055, 1991.

201. Henthorn PS, Smithies O, Mager DL: Molecular analysis of deletions in the human β-globin gene cluster: Deletion junctions and locations of breakpoints. *Genomics* **6**:226, 1990.

202. Kornreich R, Bishop DF, Desnick RJ: α-Galactosidase A gene rearrangements causing Fabry disease. *J Biol Chem* **265**:9319, 1990.

203. Monnat RJ, Hackman AFM, Chiaverotti TA: Nucleotide sequence analysis of human hypoxanthine phosphoribosyltransferase (HPRT) gene deletions. *Genomics* **13**:777, 1992.

204. Bollag RJ, Waldman AS, Liskay RM: Homologous recombination in mammalian cells. *Annu Rev Genet* **23**:199, 1989.

205. Shapiro LJ, Yen P, Pomerantz D, Martin E, Rolewic L, Mohandas T: Molecular studies of deletions at the human steroid sulphatase locus. *Proc Natl Acad Sci USA* **86**:8477, 1989.

206. Yen PH, Li X-M, Tsai S-P, Johnson C, Mohandas T, Shapiro LJ: Frequent deletions of the human X chromosome distal short arm result from recombination between low copy repetitive elements. *Cell* **61**:603, 1990.

207. Pizzuti A, Pieretti M, Fenwick RG, Gibbs RA, Caskey CT: A transposon-like element in the deletion-prone region of the dystrophin gene. *Genomics* **13**:594, 1992.

208. Mager DL, Goodchild NL: Homologous recombination between the LTRs of a human retrovirus-like-element causes a 5-kb deletion in two siblings. *Am J Hum Genet* **45**:848, 1989.

209. Gerald PS, Diamond LK: A new hereditary hemoglobinopathy (the Lepore trait) and its interaction with thalassemia trait. *Blood* **13**:835, 1958.

210. Baglioni C: The fusion of two peptide chains in hemoglobin Lepore and its interpretation as a genetic deletion. *Proc Natl Acad Sci USA* **48**:1880, 1962.

211. Barnabus J, Muller CJ: Haemoglobin Lepore Hollandia. *Nature* **194**:931, 1962.

212. Ostertag W, Smith EW: Hemoglobin-Lepore-Baltimore, a third type of a δ, β crossover ($δ^{50}$, $β^{86}$). *Eur J Biochem* **10**:371, 1969.

213. Flavell RA, Kooter JM, DeBoer E, Little PFR, Williamson R: Analysis of δβ-globin gene in normal and Hb Lepore DNA: Direct determination of gene linkage and intergene distance. *Cell* **15**:25, 1978.

214. Baird M, Schreiner H, Driscoll C, Bank A: Localization of the site of recombination in the formation of the Lepore Boston globin gene. *J Clin Invest* **58**:560, 1981.

215. Mavilio F, Giampaolo A, Care A, Sposi NM, Marinucci M: The δβ crossover region in Lepore Boston hemoglobinopathy is restricted to a 59 base pairs region around the 5′ splice junction of a large globin gene intervening sequence. *Blood* **62**:230, 1983.

216. Chebloune Y, Poncet D, Verdier G: S1-nuclease mapping of the genomic Lepore-Boston DNA demonstrates that the entire large intervening sequence of the fusion gene is of β-type. *Biochem Biophys Res Commun* **120**:116, 1984.

217. Metzenberg AB, Wurzer G, Huisman TH, Smithies O: Homology requirements for unequal crossing over in humans. *Genetics* **128**:143, 1991.

218. Lanclos KD, Patterson J, Eframov GD, Wong SC, Villegas A, Ojwang PJ, Wilson JB, et al: Characterization of chromosomes with hybrid genes for Hb Lepore-Washington, Hb Lepore-Baltimore, Hb P-Nilotic, and Hb Kenya. *Hum Genet* **77**:40, 1987.

219. Fioretti G, de Angioletti M, Masciangelo F, Lacerra G, Scarallo A, de Bonis C, Pagano L, et al: Origin heterogeneity of Hb Lepore-Boston gene in Italy. *Am J Hum Genet* **50**:781, 1992.

220. Huisman THJ, Wrightstone RN, Wilson JB, Schroeder WA, Kendall AG: Hemoglobin Kenya, the product of a fusion of gamma and β polypeptide chains. *Arch Biochem Biophys* **153**:850, 1972.

221. Kendall AG, Ojwang PJ, Schroeder WA, Huisman THJ: Hemoglobin Kenya, the product of a γβ fusion gene: Studies of the family. *Am J Hum Genet* **25**:548, 1973.

222. Ojwang PJ, Nakatsuji T, Gardiner MB, Reese AL, Gilman JG, Huisman THJ: Gene deletion as the molecular basis for the Kenya-$^{G}γ$-HPFH condition. *Hemoglobin* **7**:115, 1983.

223. Lehmann H, Charlesworth D: Observations on hemoglobin P (Congo type). *Biochem J* **119**:43, 1970.

224. Badr FM, Lorkin PA, Lehmann H: Haemoglobin P-Nilotic: Containing β-δ chain. *Nature* **242**:107, 1973.

225. Honig GR, Mason RG, Tremaine LM, Vida LN: Unbalanced globin chain synthesis by Hb Lincoln Park (anti-Lepore) reticulocytes. *Am J Hematol* **5**:335, 1978.

226. Honig GR, Shamsuddin M, Mason RG, Vida LN: Hemoglobin Lincoln Park: A βδ fusion (anti-Lepore) variant with an amino acid deletion in the δ chain-derived segment. *Proc Natl Acad Sci USA* **75**:1475, 1978.

227. Nathans J, Piantanida TP, Eddy RL, Shows TB, Hogness DS: Molecular genetics of inherited variation in human color vision. *Science* **232**:203, 1986.

228. Pascoe L, Curnow KM, Slutsker L, Connell JMC, Speiser PW, New MI, White PC: Glucocorticoid-suppressible hyperaldosteronism results from hybrid genes created by unequal crossovers between CYP11B1 and CYP11B2. *Proc Natl Acad Sci USA* **89**:8327, 1992.

229. Zimran A, Sorge J, Gross E, Kubitz M, West C, Beutler E: A glucocerebrosidase fusion gene in Gaucher disease. *J Clin Invest* **85**:219, 1990.

230. Tanigawa G, Jarcho JA, Kass S, Solomon SD, Vosberg H-P, Seidman JG, Seidman CE: A molecular basis for familial hypertrophic cardiomyopathy: An α/β cardiac myosin heavy chain hybrid gene. *Cell* **62**:991, 1990.

231. Guioli S, Incerti B, Zanaria E, Bardoni B, Franco B, Taylor K, Ballabio A, Camerino G: Kallmann syndrome due to a translocation resulting in an X/Y fusion gene. *Nature Genetics* **1**:337, 1992.

232. Vanin EF, Henthorn PS, Kioussis D, Grosveld F, Smithies O: Unexpected relationships between four large deletions in the human β-globin gene cluster. *Cell* **35**:701, 1983.

233. Piccoli SP, Caimi PG, Cole MD: A conserved sequence at c-myc oncogene chromosomal translocation breakpoints in plasmacytomas. *Nature* **310**:327, 1984.

234. Roth DB, Porter TN, Wilson JH: Mechanisms of nonhomologous recombination in mammalian cells. *Mol Cell Biol* **5**:2599, 1985.

235. Roth DB, Wilson JH: Nonhomologous recombination in mammalian cells: Role for short sequence homologies in the joining reaction. *Mol Cell Biol* **6**:4295, 1986.

236. Gilman JG: The 12.6 kilobase DNA deletion in Dutch $β^0$-thalassaemia. *Br J Haematol* **67**:369, 1987.

237. Efstratiadis A, Posakony JW, Maniatis T, Lawn RM, O'Connell C, Spritz RA, DeRiel JK, et al: The structure and evolution of the human β-globin gene family. *Cell* **21**:653, 1980.

238. Woods-Samuels P, Kazazian HH, Antonarakis SE: Nonhomologous recombination on the human genome: Deletions in the human factor VIII gene. *Genomics* **10**:94, 1991.

239. Vogel F, Motulsky AG: *Human Genetics: Problems and Approaches*, 2d ed. Berlin, Springer-Verlag, 1986.

240. Nagylaki T, Petes TD: Intrachromosomal gene conversion and the maintenance of sequence homogeneity among repeated genes. *Genetics* **100**:315, 1982.

241. Shen S, Slightom JL, Smithies O: A history of the human fetal globin gene duplication. *Cell* **26**:191, 1981.

242. Stoeckert CJ, Collins FS, Weissman S: Human fetal globin DNA sequences suggest novel conversion event. *Nucleic Acids Res* **12**:4469, 1984.

243. Powers PA, Smithies O: Short gene conversion in the human fetal globin gene region: A by-product of chromosome pairing during meiosis? *Genetics* **112**:343, 1986.

244. Liebhaber SA, Goossens M, Kan YW: Homology and concerted evolution at the α_1 and α_2 loci of human α-globin. *Nature* **290**:26, 1981.

245. Antonarakis SE, Orkin SH, Kazazian HH, Goff SC, Boehm CD, Waber PG, Sexton JP, et al: Evidence for multiple origins of the β^E-globin gene in Southeast Asia. *Proc Natl Acad Sci USA* **79**:6608, 1982.

246. Antonarakis SE, Boehm CD, Serjeant GR, Theisen CE, Dover GJ, Kazazian HH: Origin of the β^S-globin gene in blacks: The contribution of recurrent mutation or gene conversion or both. *Proc Natl Acad Sci USA* **81**:853, 1984.

247. Kazazian HH, Orkin SH, Markham AF, Chapman CR, Youssoufian H, Waber PG: Quantification of the close association between DNA haplotypes and specific β-thalassaemia mutations in Mediterraneans. *Nature* **310**:152, 1984.

248. Pirastu M, Galanello R, Doherty MA, Tuveri T, Cao A, Kan YW: The same β-globin gene mutation is present on nine different β-thalassaemia chromosomes in a Sardinian population. *Proc Natl Acad Sci USA* **84**:2882, 1987.

249. Zhang J-Z, Cai S-P, He X, Lin H-X, Lin H-J, Huang Z-G, Chebab FF, Kan YW: Molecular basis of β-thalassaemia in South China. *Hum Genet* **78**:37, 1988.

250. Matsuno Y, Yamashiro Y, Yamamoto K, Hattori Y, Yamamoto K, Ohba Y, Miyaji T: A possible example of gene conversion with a common β-thalassaemia mutation and Chi sequence present in the β-globin gene. *Hum Genet* **88**:357, 1992.

251. Smith GR: Chi hotspots of generalized recombination. *Cell* **34**:709, 1983.

252. Harada F, Kimura A, Iwanaga T, Shimozawa K, Yata J, Sasazuki T: Gene conversion-like events cause steroid 21-hydroxylase deficiency in congenital adrenal hyperplasia. *Proc Natl Acad Sci USA* **84**:8091, 1987.

253. Amor M, Parker KL, Gloverman H, New MI, White PC: Mutation in the CYP21B gene (IIe > Asn) causes steroid 21-hydroxylase deficiency. *Proc Natl Acad Sci USA* **85**:1600, 1988.

254. Morel Y, David M, Forest MG, Betuel H, Hauptman G, Andre J, Bertrand J, Miller WL: Gene conversions and rearrangements cause discordance between inheritance of forms of 21-hydroxylase deficiency and HLA types. *J Clin Endocrinol Metab* **68**:592, 1989.

255. Urabe K, Kimura A, Harada F, Iwanaga T, Sasazuki T: Gene conversion in steroid 210-hydroxylase genes. *Am J Hum Genet* **46**:1178, 1990.

256. Tusie-Luna MT, White PC: Gene conversions and unequal crossovers between CYP21 (steroid 21-hydroxylase gene) and CYP21P involve different mechanisms. *Proc Natl Acad Sci USA* **92**:10,796, 1995.

257. Watnick TJ, Gandolph MA, Weber H, Neumann HP, Germino GG: Gene conversion is a likely cause of mutation in PKD1. *Hum Mol Genet* **7**:1239, 1998.

258. Gorlach A, Lee PL, Roesler J, Hopkins PJ, Christensen B, Green ED, Chanock SJ, Curnutte JT: A p47-phox pseudogene carries the most common mutation causing p47-phox-deficient chronic granulomatous disease. *J Clin Invest* **100**:1907, 1997.

259. Minegishi Y, Coustan-Smith E, Wang YH, Cooper MD, Campana D, Conley ME: Mutations in the human lambda5/14.1 gene result in B cell deficiency and agammaglobulinemia. *J Exp Med* **187**:71, 1998.

260. Eyal N, Wilder S, Horowitz M: Prevalent and rare mutations among Gaucher patients. *Gene* **96**:277, 1990.

261. Eikenboom JC, Vink T, Briet E, Sixma JJ, Reitsma PH: Multiple substitutions in the von Willebrand factor gene that mimic the pseudogene sequence. *Proc Natl Acad Sci USA* **91**:2221, 1994.

262. Schollen E, Pardon E, Heykants L, Renard J, Doggett NA, Callen DF, Cassiman JJ, Matthijs G: Comparative analysis of the phosphomannomutase genes PMM1, PMM2 and PMM2psi: The sequence variation in the processed pseudogene is a reflection of the mutations found in the functional gene. *Hum Mol Genet* **7**:157, 1998.

263. Krawczak M, Cooper DN: Gene deletions causing human genetic disease: Mechanisms of mutagenesis and the role of the local DNA sequence environment. *Hum Genet* **86**:425, 1991.

264. Wada K, Wada Y, Doi H, Ishibashi F, Gojobori T, Ikemura T: Codon usage tabulated from the GenBank genetic sequence data. *Nucleic Acids Res* **19**(suppl):1981, 1991.

265. Streisinger G, Okada Y, Emrich J, Newton J, Tsugita A, Terzaghi E, Inouye M: Frameshift mutations and the genetic code. *Cold Spring Harb Symp Quant Biol* **31**:77, 1966.

266. Kunkel TA: The mutational specificity of DNA polymerases α and γ during *in vitro* DNA synthesis. *J Biol Chem* **260**:12,866, 1985.

267. Kunkel TA, Soni A: Mutagenesis by transient misalignment. *J Biol Chem* **263**:14,784, 1988.

268. Ripley LS: Model for the participation of quasi-palindromic DNA sequences in frameshift mutation. *Proc Natl Acad Sci USA* **79**:4128, 1982.

269. DeBoer JG, Ripley LS: Demonstration of the production of frameshift and base-substitution mutations by quasi-palindromic sequences. *Proc Natl Acad Sci USA* **81**:5528, 1984.

270. Maekawa M, Sudo K, Kanno T, Li SS-L: Molecular characterization of genetic mutation in human lactate dehydrogenase A(M) deficiency. *Biochem Biophys Res Commun* **168**:677, 1990.

271. Schmucker B, Krawczak M: Meiotic microdeletion breakpoints in the BRCA1 gene are significantly associated with symmetric DNA-sequence elements. *Am J Hum Genet* **61**:1454, 1997.

272. Gritzmacher CA: Molecular aspects of heavy-chain class switching. *Crit Rev Immunol* **9**:173, 1989.

273. Fearon ER, Cho KR, Nigro JM, Kern SE, Simons JW, Ruppert JM, Hamilton SR, et al: Identification of a chromosome 18q gene that is altered in colorectal cancers. *Science* **247**:49, 1990.

274. Roux AF, Morle F, Guetarni D, Colonna P, Sahr K, Forget BG, Delaunay J, Godet J: Molecular basis of Sp alpha I/65 hereditary elliptocytosis in North Africa: Insertion of a TTG triplet between codons 147 and 149 in the alpha-spectrin gene from five unrelated families. *Blood* **73**:2196, 1989.

275. Fry M, Loeb LA: A DNA polymerase α pause site is a hotspot for nucleotide misinsertion. *Proc Natl Acad Sci USA* **89**:763, 1992.

276. Bettecken T, Müller CR: Identification of a 220 kb insertion into the Duchenne gene in a family with an atypical course of muscular dystrophy. *Genomics* **4**:592, 1989.

277. Kazazian HH, Wong C, Youssoufian H, Scott AF, Phillips DG, Antonarakis SE: Haemophilia A resulting from *de novo* insertion of L1 sequences represents a novel mechanism for mutation in man. *Nature* **332**:164, 1988.

278. Kazazian HH Jr, Moran JV: The impact of L1 retrotransposons on the human genome. *Nat Genet* **19**:19, 1998.

279. Weiner AM, Deininger PL, Efstratiadis A: Nonviral retroposons: Genes, pseudogenes and transposable elements generated by the reverse flow of genetic information. *Annu Rev Biochem* **55**:631, 1986.

280. Fanning TG, Singer MF: LINE-1: A mammalian transposable element. *Biochim Biophys Acta* **910**:203, 1987.

281. Dombroski BA, Mathias SL, Nanthakumar E, Scott AF, Kazazian HH: Isolation of an active human transposable element. *Science* **254**:1805, 1991.

282. Woods-Samuels P, Wong C, Mathias SL, Scott AF, Kazazian HH, Antonarakis SE: Characterization of a non-deleterious L1 insertion in an intron of the human factor VIII gene and evidence for open reading frame in functional L1 elements. *Genomics* **4**:290, 1989.

283. Holmes SE, Dombroski BA, Krebs CM, Boehm CD, Kazazian HH Jr: A new retrotransposable human L1 element from the LRE2 locus on chromosome 1q produces a chimaeric insertion. *Nat Genet* **7**:143, 1994.

284. Miki Y, Nishisho I, Horii A, Miyoshi Y, Utsunomiya J, Kinzler KW, Vogelstein B, Nakamura Y: Disruption of the APC gene by a retrotransposal insertion of L1 sequence in a colon cancer. *Cancer Res* **52**:643, 1992.

285. Mager DL, Henthorn PS, Smithies O: A Chinese $^{G}\gamma + {^{A}\gamma}\delta\beta^{00\text{thalassaemia}}$ deletion: Comparison to other deletions in the human β-globin gene cluster and sequence analysis of the breakpoints. *Nucleic Acids Res* **13**:6559, 1985.

286. Morse J, Rothberg PG, South VJ, Spandorfer JM, Astrin SM: Insertional mutagenesis of the myc locus by a LINE-1 sequence in a human breast carcinoma. *Nature* **333**:87, 1988.

287. Moran JV, Holmes SE, Naas TP, DeBerardinis RJ, Boeke JD, Kazazian HH Jr: High frequency retrotransposition in cultured mammalian cells. *Cell* **87**:917, 1996.

288. Hohjoh H, Singer MF: Cytoplasmic ribonucleoprotein complexes containing human LINE-1 protein and RNA. *EMBO J* **15**:630, 1996.

289. Feng Q, Moran JV, Kazazian HH Jr, Boeke JD: Human L1 retrotransposon encodes a conserved endonuclease required for retrotransposition. *Cell* **87**:905, 1996.

290. Lin CS, Goldthwait DA, Samols D: Identification of *Alu* transposition in human lung carcinoma cells. *Cell* **54**:153, 1988.

291. Wallace MR, Andersen LB, Saulino AM, Gregory PE, Glover TW, Collins FS: A *de novo Alu* insertion results in neurofibromatosis type 1. *Nature* **353**:864, 1991.

292. Economou-Pachnis A, Tsichlis PN: Insertion of an *Alu* SINE in the human homologue of the MIvi-2 locus. *Nucleic Acids Res* **13**:8379, 1985.

293. Muratani K, Hada T, Yamamoto Y, Kaneko T, Shigeto Y, Ohree T, Furuyama J, Higashino K: Inactivation of the cholinesterase gene by *Alu* insertion: Possible mechanism for the human gene transposition. *Proc Natl Acad Sci USA* **88**:11,315, 1991.

294. Vidaud D, Vidaud M, Bahnak BR, Siguret V, Sanchez SG, Laurian Y, Meyer D, et al: Hemophilia B due to a *de novo* insertion of a human-specific *Alu* subfamily member within the coding region of the factor IX gene. *Eur J Hum Genet* **1**:30, 1993.

295. Kariya Y, Kato K, Hayashizaki Y, Himeno S, Tarui S, Matsubara K: Revision of consensus sequence of human *Alu* repeats: A review. *Gene* **53**:1, 1987.

295. Miki Y, Katagiri T, Kasumi F, Yoshimoto T, Nakamura Y: Mutation analysis in the BRCA2 gene in primary breast cancers. *Nat Genet* **13**:245, 1996.

296. Umlauf SW, Cox MM: The functional significance of DNA sequence structure in a site-specific genetic recombination reaction. *EMBO J* **7**:1845, 1988.

297. Shih C-C, Stoye JP, Coffin JM: Highly preferred targets for retrovirus integration. *Cell* **53**:531, 1988.

298. Angelini C, Beggs AH, Hoffman EP, Fanin M, Kunkel LM: Enormous dystrophin in a patient with Becker muscular dystrophy. *Neurology* **40**:808, 1990.

299. Yang TP, Stout JT, Konecki DS, Patel PI, Alford RL, Caskey CT: Spontaneous reversion of novel Lesch-Nyhan mutation by HPRT gene rearrangement. *Somat Cell Mol Genet* **14**:293, 1988.

300. Tiller GE, Rimoin DL, Murray LW, Cohn DH: Tandem duplication within a type II collagen gene (COL2A1) exon in an individual with spondyloepiphyseal dysplasia. *Proc Natl Acad Sci USA* **87**:3889, 1990.

301. Stoppa-Lyonnet D, Carter PE, Meo T, Tosi M: Clusters of intragenic *Alu* repeats predispose the human C1 inhibitor locus to deleterious rearrangements. *Proc Natl Acad Sci USA* **87**:1551, 1990.

302. Murru S, Casula L, Pecorara M, Mori P, Cao A, Pirastu M: Illegitimate recombination produced a duplication within the FVIII gene in a patient with mild hemophilia A. *Genomics* **7**:115, 1990.

303. Hu X, Ray PN, Murphy EG, Thompson MW, Worton RG: Duplicational mutation at the Duchenne muscular dystrophy locus: Its frequency, distribution, origin and phenotype/genotype correlation. *Am J Hum Genet* **46**:682, 1990.

304. Hu X, Ray PN, Worton RG: Mechanisms of tandem duplication in the Duchenne muscular dystrophy gene include both homologous and nonhomologous intrachromosomal recombination. *EMBO J* **10**:2471, 1991.

305. Devlin RH, Deeb S, Brunzell J, Hayden MR: Partial gene duplication involving exon-*Alu* interchange results in lipoprotein lipase deficiency. *Am J Hum Genet* **46**:112, 1990.

306. Gitschier J: Maternal duplication associated with gene deletion in sporadic hemophilia. *Am J Hum Genet* **43**:274, 1988.

307. Steinmetz M, Uematsu Y, Lindahl KF: Hotspots of homologous recombination in mammalian genomes. *Trends Genet* **3**:7, 1987.

308. Casula L, Murru S, Pecorara M, Ristaldi MS, Restagno G, Mancuso G, Morfini M, et al: Recurrent mutations and three novel rearrangements in the factor VIII gene of hemophilia A patients of Italian descent. *Blood* **75**:662, 1990.

309. Den Dunnen JT, Grootscholten PM, Bakker E, Blonden LAJ, Ginjaar HB, Wapenaar MC, van Paassen HMB, et al: Topography of the Duchenne muscular dystrophy (DMD) gene: FIGE and cDNA analysis of 194 cases reveals 115 deletions and 13 duplications. *Am J Hum Genet* **45**:835, 1989.

310. Cooke A, Lanyon WG, Wilcox DE, Dornan ES, Kataki A, Gillard EF, McWhinnie AJM, et al: Analysis of Scottish Duchenne and Becker muscular dystrophy families with dystrophin cDNA probes. *J Med Genet* **27**:292, 1990.

311. Haglund-Stengler R, Ritzen EM, Luthman H: 21-Hydroxy lase deficiency: Disease-causing mutations categorized by densitometry of 21-hydroxylase-specific deoxyribonucleic acid fragments. *J Clin Endocrinol Metab* **70**:43, 1990.

312. Hu X, Worton RG: Partial gene duplication as a cause of human disease. *Hum Mutat* **1**:3, 1992.

313. Roberts RG, Barby TFM, Manners E, Bobrow M, Bentley DR: Direct detection of dystrophin gene rearrangements by analysis of dystrophin mRNA in peripheral blood lymphocytes. *Am J Hum Genet* **49**:298, 1991.

314. Monnat RJ, Chiaverotti TA, Hackmann AFM, Maresh GA: Molecular structure and genetic stability of human hypoxanthine phosphoribosyl-transferase (HPRT) gene duplications. *Genomics* **13**:788, 1992.

315. Pentao L, Wise CA, Chinault AC, Patel PI, Lupski JR: Charcot-Marie-Tooth type 1A duplication appears to arise from recombination at repeat sequences flanking the 1.5 Mb monomer unit. *Nat Genet* **2**:292, 1992.

316. Jennings MW, Jones RW, Wood WG, Weatherall DJ: Analysis of an inversion within the human β-globin gene cluster. *Nucleic Acids Res* **13**:2897, 1985.

317. Karathanasis SK, Ferris E, Haddad IA: DNA inversion within the apolipoproteins AI/CIII/AIV-encoding gene cluster of certain patients with premature atherosclerosis. *Proc Natl Acad Sci USA* **84**:7198, 1987.

318. Kulozik AE, Bellan-Koch A, Kohne E, Kleihauer E: A deletion/inversion rearrangement of the β-globin gene cluster in a Turkish family with δβ-thalassemia intermedia. *Blood* **79**:2455, 1992.

319. Lakich D, Kazazian HH, Antonarakis SE, Gitschier J: Inversions of the factor VIII gene as a common cause of severe hemophilia A. *Nat Genet* **5**:236, 1993.

320. Naylor J, Brinke A, Hassock S, Green PM, Giannelli F: Characteristic mRNA abnormality found in half the patients with severe haemophilia A is due to large DNA inversions. *Hum Mol Genet* **2**:1773, 1993.

321. Antonarakis SE, Rossiter JP, Young M, Horst J, de Moerloose P, Sommer SS, Ketterling RP, et al: Factor VIII gene inversions in severe hemophilia A: Results of an international consortium study. *Blood* **86**:2206, 1995.

322. Linton MF, Pierotti V, Young SG: Reading-frame restoration with an apolipoprotein B gene frameshift mutation. *Proc Natl Acad Sci USA* **89**:11,431, 1992.

323. Young M, Inaba H, Hoyer LW, Higuchi M, Kazazian HH Jr, Antonarakis SE: Partial correction of a severe molecular defect in hemophilia A, because of errors during expression of the factor VIII gene. *Am J Hum Genet* **60**:565, 1997.

324. Laken SJ, Petersen GM, Gruber SB, Oddoux C, Ostrer H, Giardiello FM, Hamilton SR, et al: Familial colorectal cancer in Ashkenazim due to a hypermutable tract in APC. *Nat Genet* **17**:79, 1997.

325. Wagner LA, Weiss RB, Driscoll R, Dunn DS, Gesteland RF: Transcriptional slippage occurs during elongation at runs of adenine or thymine in *Escherichia coli*. *Nucleic Acids Res* **18**:3529, 1990.

326. Jacks T, Varmus HE: Expression of the Rous sarcoma virus pol gene by ribosomal frameshifting. *Science* **230**:1237, 1985.

327. Van Leeuwen FW, de Kleijn DP, van den Hurk HH, Neubauer A, Sonnemans MA, Sluijs JA, Koycu S, et al: Frameshift mutants of beta amyloid precursor protein and ubiquitin-B in Alzheimer's and Down patients. *Science* **279**:242, 1998.

328. Caskey CT, Pizzuti A, Fu Y-H, Fenwick RG, Nelson DL: Triplet repeat mutations in human disease. *Science* **256**:784, 1992.

329. Rousseau F, Heitz D, Mandel J-L: The unstable and methylatable mutations causing the fragile X syndrome. *Hum Mutat* **1**:91, 1992.

330. Mandel J-L: Questions of expansion. *Nat Genet* **4**:8, 1993.

331. Wilmot GR, Warren ST: A new mutational basis for disease, in Wells RD, Warren ST (eds): *Genetic Instabilities and Hereditary Neurological Disorders*. New York, Academic Press, 1998, p 3.

332. Lalioti MD, Scott HS, Buresi C, Rossier C, Bottani A, Morris MA, Malafosse A, Antonarakis SE: Dodecamer repeat expansion in cystatin B gene in progressive myoclonus epilepsy. *Nature* **386**:847, 1997.

333. Fu Y-H, Kuhl DPA, Pizzuti A, Pieretti M, Sutcliffe JS, Richards S, Verkerk AJMH, et al: Variation of the CGG repeat at the fragile X site results in genetic instability: Resolution of Sherman paradox. *Cell* **67**:1047, 1991.

334. Knight SJL, Flannery AV, Hirst MC, Campbell L, Christodoulou Z, Phelps SR, Pointon J, et al: Trinucleotide repeat amplification and hypermethylation of a CpG island in FRAXE mental retardation. *Cell* **74**:127, 1993.

335. Brook JD, McCurrach ME, Harley HG, Buckler AJ, Church D, Aburatani H, Hunter K, et al: Molecular basis of myotonic dystrophy: Expansion of a trinucleotide (CTG) repeat at the 3' end of a transcript encoding a protein kinase family member. *Cell* **68**:799, 1992.

336. La Spada AR, Wilson EM, Lubahn DB, Harding AE, Fischbeck KH: Androgen receptor gene mutations in X-linked spinal muscular atrophy. *Nature* **352**:77, 1991.

337. Huntington's Disease Collaborative Research Group: A novel gene containing a trinucleotide repeat that is expanded and unstable on Huntington's disease chromosomes. *Cell* **72**:971, 1993.

338. Koide R, Ikeuchi T, Onodera O, Tanaka H, Igarashi S, Endo K, Takahashi H, et al: Unstable expansion of CAG repeat in hereditary dentatorubral-pallidoluysian atrophy (DRPLA). *Nat Genet* **6**:9, 1994.

339. Orr HT, Chung MY, Banfi S, Kwiatkowski TJ, Servadio A, Beaudet AL, McCall AE, et al: Expansion of an unstable trinucleotide CAG repeat in spinocerebellar ataxia type 1. *Nat Genet* **4**:221, 1993.

340. Sanpei K, Takano H, Igarashi S, Sato T, Oyake M, Sasaki H, Wakisaka A, et al: Identification of the spinocerebellar ataxia type 2 gene using a direct identification of repeat expansion and cloning technique, DIRECT. *Nat Genet* **14**:277, 1996.

341. Kawaguchi Y, Okamoto T, Taniwaki M, Aizawa M, Inoue M, Katayama S, Kawakami H, et al: CAG expansions in a novel gene for Machado-Joseph disease at chromosome 14q32.1. *Nat Genet* **8**:221, 1994.

342. Zhuchenko O, Bailey J, Bonnen P, Ashizawa T, Stockton DW, Amos C, Dobyns WB, et al: Autosomal dominant cerebellar ataxia (SCA6) associated with small polyglutamine expansions in the alpha(1A)-voltage-dependent calcium channel. *Nat Genet* **15**:62, 1997.

343. David G, Abbas N, Stevanin G, Durr A, Yvert G, Cancel G, Weber C, et al: Cloning of the SCA7 gene reveals a highly unstable CAG repeat expansion. *Nat Genet* **17**:65, 1997.

344. Campuzano V, Montermini L, Molto MD, Pianese L, Cossée M, Cavalcanti F, Monros E, et al: Friedreich's ataxia: Autosomal recessive disease caused by an intronic GAA triplet repeat expansion. *Science* **271**:1423, 1996.

345. Muragaki Y, Mundlos S, Upton J, Olsen BR: Altered growth and branching patterns in synpolydactyly caused by mutations in HOXD13. *Science* **272**:548, 1996.

346. Brais B, Bouchard J-P, Xie Y-G, Rochefort DL, Chretien N, Tome FMS, Lafreniere RG, et al: Short GCG expansions in the PABP2 gene cause oculopharyngeal muscular dystrophy. *Nat Genet* **18**:164, 1998.

347. Pieretti M, Zhang R, Fu Y-H, Warren ST, Oostra BA, Caskey CT, Nelson DL: Absence of expression of the FMR-1 gene in fragile X syndrome. *Cell* **66**:817, 1991.

348. Oberlé I, Rousseau F, Heitz D, Kretz C, Devys D, Hanauer A, Boué J, et al: Instability of a 550 base pair DNA segment and abnormal methylation in fragile X syndrome. *Science* **252**:1097, 1991.

349. Yu S, Pritchard M, Kremer E, Lynch M, Nancarrow J, Baker E, Holman K, et al: Fragile X genotype characterized by an unstable region of DNA. *Science* **252**:1179, 1991.

350. Verkerk AJMH, Pieretti M, Sutcliffe JS, Fu Y-H, Kuhl DPA, Pizzuti A, Reiner O, et al: Identification of a gene (FMR-1) containing a CGG repeat coincident with a breakpoint cluster region exhibiting length variation in fragile X syndrome. *Cell* **65**:905, 1991.

351. Kremer EJ, Pritchard M, Lynch M, Yu S, Holman K, Baker E, Warren ST, et al: Mapping of DNA instability at the fragile X to a trinucleotide repeat sequence p(CCG)n. *Science* **252**:1711, 1991.

352. Rousseau F, Heitz D, Biancalana V, Blumenfeld S, Kretz C, Boué J, Tommerup N, et al: Direct diagnosis by DNA analysis of the fragile X syndrome of mental retardation. *N Engl J Med* **325**:1673, 1991.

353. Hirst M, Knight S, Davies K, Cross G, Ocraft K, Raeburn S, Heeger S, et al: Prenatal diagnosis of fragile X syndrome. *Lancet* **338**:956, 1991.

354. Dobkin CS, Ding X-H, Jenkins EC, Krawczak MS, Brown WT, Goonewardena P, Willner WT, et al: Prenatal diagnosis of fragile X syndrome. *Lancet* **338**:957, 1991.

355. Pergolizzi RG, Erster SH, Goonewardena P, Brown WT: Detection of full fragile X mutation. *Lancet* **339**:271, 1992.

356. Yu S, Mulley J, Loesch D, Turner G, Donnelly A, Gedeon A, Hillen D, et al: Fragile-X syndrome: Unique genetics of the heritable unstable element. *Am J Hum Genet* **50**:968, 1992.

357. Harper PS, Harley HG, Reardon W, Shaw DJ: Anticipation in myotonic dystrophy: New light on an old problem. *Am J Hum Genet* **51**:10, 1992.

358. Harley HG, Brook JD, Rundel SA, Crow S, Reardon W, Buckler AJ, Harper PS, et al: Expansion of an unstable DNA region and phenotypic variation in myotonic dystrophy. *Nature* **355**:545, 1992.

359. Harley HG, Rundle SA, Reardon W, Myring J, Crow S, Brook JD, Harper PS, Shaw DJ: Unstable DNA sequence in myotonic dystrophy. *Lancet* **339**:1125, 1992.

360. Buxton J, Shelbourne P, Davies J, Jones C, van Tongeren T, Aslanidis C, de Jong P, et al: Detection of an unstable fragment of DNA specific to individuals with myotonic dystrophy. *Nature* **355**:547, 1992.

361. Fu Y-H, Pizzuti A, Fenwick RG, King J, Rajnarayan S, Dunne PW, Dubel J, et al: An unstable triplet repeat in a gene related to myotonic muscular dystrophy. *Science* **255**:1256, 1992.

362. Mahadevan M, Tsilfidis C, Sabourin L, Shutler G, Amemiya C, Jansen G, Neville C, et al: Myotonic dystrophy mutation: An unstable CTG repeat in the 3′ untranslated region of the gene. *Science* **255**:1253, 1992.

363. Tsilfidis C, Mackenzie AE, Mrttler G, Barcel3/4 J, Korneluk RG: Correlation between CTG trinucleotide repeat length and frequency of severe congenital myotonic dystrophy. *Nat Genet* **1**:192, 1992.

364. Shelbourne P, Winquist R, Kunert E, Davies J, Leisti J, Thiele H, Bachmann H, et al: Unstable DNA may be responsible for the incomplete penetrance of the myotonic dystrophy phenotype. *Hum Mol Genet* **1**:467, 1992.

365. Filla A, de Michele G, Cavalcanti F, Pianese L, Monticelli A, Campanella G, Cocozza S: The relationship between trinucleotide (GAA) repeat length and clinical features in Friedreich ataxia. *Am J Hum Genet* **59**:554, 1996.

366. Koutnikova H, Campuzano V, Foury F, Dolle P, Cazzalini O, Koenig M: Studies of human, mouse and yeast homologues indicate a mitochondrial function for frataxin. *Nat Genet* **16**:345, 1997.

367. Goldberg YP, Nicholson DW, Rasper DM, Kalchman MA, Koide HB, Graham RK, Bromm M, et al: Cleavage of huntingtin by apopain, a proapoptotic cysteine protease, is modulated by the polyglutamine tract. *Nat Genet* **13**:442, 1996.

368. Lalioti MD, Scott HS, Genton P, Grid D, Ouazzani R, M'Rabet A, Ibrahim S, et al: A PCR amplification method reveals instability of the dodecamer repeat in progressive myoclonus epilepsy (EPM1) and no correlation between the size of the repeat and age at onset. *Am J Hum Genet* **62**:842, 1998.

369. Sutherland GR, Haan EA, Kremer E, Lynch M, Pritchard M, Yu S, Richards RI: Hereditary unstable DNA: A new explanation for some old genetic questions? *Lancet* **338**:289, 1991.

370. Gordenin DA, Kunkel TA, Resnick MA: Repeat expansion: All in a flap? *Nat Genet* **16**:116, 1997.

371. Kinzler KW, Vogelstein B: Lessons from hereditary colorectal cancer. *Cell* **87**:159, 1996.

372. Papadopoulos N, Lindblom A: Molecular basis of HNPCC: Mutations of MMR genes. *Hum Mutat* **10**:89, 1997.

373. Markowitz S, et al: Inactivation of the type II TGF-beta receptor in colon cancer cells with microsatellite instability. *Science* **268**:1336, 1995.

374. Lu S-L, et al: Mutations of the transforming growth factor-beta type II receptor gene and genomic instability in hereditary nonpolyposis colorectal cancer. *Biochem Biophys Res Commun* **216**:452, 1995.

375. Parsons R, et al: Microsatellite instability and mutations of the transforming growth factor beta type II receptor gene in colorectal cancer. *Cancer Res* **55**:5548, 1995.

376. Yoshitaka T, et al: Mutations of E2F-4 trinucleotide repeats in colorectal cancer with microsatellite instability. *Biochem Biophys Res Commun* **227**:553, 1996.

377. Huang J, et al: APC mutations in colorectal tumors with mismatch repair deficiency. *Proc Natl Acad Sci USA* **93**:9049, 1996.

378. Souza RF, et al: Microsatellite instability in the insulin-like growth factor II receptor gene in gastrointestinal tumors. *Nat Genet* **14**:255, 1996.

379. Rampino N, et al: Somatic frameshift mutations in the BAX gene in colon cancers of the microsatellite mutator phenotype. *Science* **275**:967, 1997.

380. Perucho M: Microsatellite instability: The mutator that mutates the other mutator. *Nature Med* **2**:630, 1996.

381. Eshleman JR, et al: Increased mutation rate at the hprt locus accompanies microsatellite instability in colon cancer. *Oncogene* **10**:33, 1995.

382. Goellner GM, et al: Different mechanisms underlie DNA instability in Huntington disease and colorectal cancer. *Am J Hum Genet* **60**:879, 1997.

383. Laken SJ, et al: Familial colorectal cancer in Ashkenazim due to a hypermutable tract in APC. *Nat Genet* **17**:79, 1997.

384. Sommer S: Does cancer kill the individual and save the species? *Hum Mutat* **3**:166, 1994.

Genomic Imprinting and Cancer

Andrew P. Feinberg

1. Genomic imprinting is an epigenetic modification of a specific parental allele of a gene, or the chromosome on which it resides, in the gamete or zygote leading to differential expression of the two alleles of the gene in somatic cells of the offspring.
2. Evidence for genomic imprinting in normal development derives from studies over many years of the whole genome, specific chromosomal regions, and individual imprinted loci. There is now an intense search for an ever-increasing list of imprinted genes that are involved in many different types of cellular processes.
3. Genomic imprinting challenges two assumptions of Mendelian genetics applied to human disease: that the maternal and paternal alleles of a gene are equivalent and that two functional copies of a gene always are associated with health. Imprinted genes probably account for many examples of developmental malformations in humans.
4. Hydatidiform moles and complete ovarian teratomas, the genome of each of which is derived from a single parental origin, show that an imbalance of maternal and paternal genome equivalents leads to neoplastic growth.
5. Several chromosomes show parental origin-specific alterations in cancer, including losses of heterozygosity in Wilms tumor and in acute myelocytic leukemia and gene amplification in neuroblastoma.
6. Beckwith-Wiedemann syndrome, a disorder of prenatal overgrowth and cancer, sometimes involves parental origin-specific germ-line chromosomal rearrangements and uniparental disomy.
7. Loss of imprinting (LOI) is a recently discovered alteration in cancer that involves loss of parental origin-specific gene expression. LOI may include activation of the normally silent copy of growth-promoting genes and/or silencing of the normally transcribed copy of tumor suppressor genes. These changes can involve a switch of a maternal chromosome to a paternal epigenotype.
8. There is a rapidly increasing number of examples of genes and tumors that show LOI. Genes include *IGF2, H19,* and *p57^KIP2*. Tumors include Wilms tumor; hepatoblastoma; rhabdomyosarcoma; Ewing sarcoma; uterine, cervical, esophageal, prostate, lung, and colon cancer; choriocarcinoma; and germ-cell tumors. Thus LOI is one of the most common alterations in human cancer.
9. Normal genomic imprinting is maintained in part by parental origin-specific, tissue-independent DNA methylation of cytosine within CpG islands, regions rich in CpG dinucleotides. Tumors with LOI show abnormal methylation of these CpG islands.
10. Normal genomic imprinting should be viewed as a developmental process rather than as a single event. Thus a combination of both *cis*-acting and *trans*-acting signals is likely to be important in the establishment and maintenance of normal genomic imprinting, and disruption of these same factors can be expected to play a role in LOI in cancer.
11. Since normal imprinting is reversible, LOI also may be reversible and amenable to novel therapeutic approaches, such as modification with 5-aza-2′-deoxycytidine, an inhibitor of DNA methylation.

Genomic imprinting is an epigenetic modification of a specific parental allele of a gene, or the chromosome on which it resides, in the gamete or zygote leading to differential expression of the two alleles of the gene in somatic cells of the offspring. Alterations of genomic imprinting recently have been identified in human cancers. These alterations have generated a great deal of excitement because they appear to occur commonly in both childhood and adult malignancies, lead to altered expression of growth regulatory genes, and represent potentially reversible changes. Thus they may lead to novel forms of therapy for cancer. This chapter presents the experimental foundations on which these recent discoveries have been made, a summary of our current knowledge (which is evolving rapidly), and prospects for future discovery and application.

TYPES OF EPIGENETIC INHERITANCE

Genomic imprinting is a form of epigenetic inheritance, which is a modification of the genome, heritable by cell progeny, that does not involve a change in DNA sequence. Generally, epigenetic inheritance leads to apparently non-Mendelian properties of the gene, such as modification by the other allele or a change from one generation to the next. Examples in *Drosophila* include transvection at the bithorax locus, or pairing-dependent gene expression caused by *trans*-sensing of alleles.[1] The mechanism of transvection is unknown, although interaction between homologous chromosomes appears to influence expression levels from both chromosomes.[2] A second example of epigenetic inheritance is paramutation in plants, a heritable alteration of one allele caused by a second allele of the same gene on the other chromosome.[3]

A third example of epigenetic inheritance is position-effect variegation (PEV) in *Drosophila.* This involves, for example, the spreading of condensed heterochromatin into adjacent euchromatin at sites of chromosomal rearrangement near the white locus;

A list of standard abbreviations is located immediately preceding the index. Nonstandard abbreviations used in this chapter include: PEV = position effect variegation; UPD = uniparental disomy; PWS = Prader-Willi syndrome; AS = Angleman syndrome; LOH = loss of heterozygosity; BWS = Beckwith-Wiedemann syndrome; WT = Wilms tumor; LOI = loss of imprinting.

this leads to variably colored eyes. Two striking features of PEV are the variability of suppression caused by the heterochromatin, leading to very high apparent pseudomutation rates, and the long distances (several megabases) over which PEV can act.[4] Some of the *trans*-acting factors that mediate PEV appear to be involved in the formation or stabilization of heterochromatin.[5,6] Thus their homologues in mammalian cells may be important in understanding genomic imprinting.

An additional example of epigenetic inheritance, similar to PEV but acting over a much shorter distance (several kilobases), is telomere silencing in yeast, caused by the proximity of a gene to telomere sequences. Factors that mediate telomere silencing also are known, and in some cases mammalian homologues have been identified.[7] Two underlying themes of the various forms of epigenetic inheritance are that they appear to involve changes to chromatin and that they act over a distance larger than that of a single gene.

GENOMIC IMPRINTING IN NORMAL DEVELOPMENT

Evidence for genomic imprinting originated from study of the whole genome, then progressed to studies of individual chromosomes and chromosomal regions, and finally led to identification of specific imprinted genes. The definition of genomic imprinting was first introduced by Helen Crouse in 1960 in her studies of the insect *Sciara,* which preferentially sheds paternal chromosomes during development.[8] In the first sentence of this chapter, a modification of Crouse's original definition is used to reflect the modern emphasis on transcriptional regulation. A striking example of possible whole-genome imprinting is the difference between the mule and the hinny. The mule is a cross of a maternal horse and paternal donkey. It is much larger and quite dissimilar to the hinny, which is the reciprocal cross. Of course, there are other alternative explanations for this phenotypic difference, such as mitochondrial inheritance or differing *in utero* environments.

A whole-genome clue to the existence of genomic imprinting in humans derives from the observation of spontaneously aborted triploid human embryos, which show different histopathology depending on whether the excess of chromosomes is paternal or maternal. Embryos with two maternal genome equivalents and one paternal genome equivalent lead to cystic placentas, a large fetus with malformations, and occasionally a term pregnancy. In contrast, embryos with two paternal genome equivalents and one maternal genome equivalent show marked growth retardation and die *in utero.*

Formal proof for imprinting at the level of the genome was offered by Solter and colleagues, who performed pronuclear transplantation experiments in which a maternal pronucleus was replaced with a second paternal pronucleus, or vice versa.[9] *Androgenotes,* defined as containing a normal chromosome number that is entirely of paternal origin, show mainly extraembryonic tissue. In contrast, *gynogenotes,* whose chromosomes are entirely of maternal origin, show mostly embryonic tissue. Thus it appears that the paternal genome equivalent is comparatively more responsible for placental development, and the maternal genome equivalent is comparatively more responsible for embryo development.

Evidence for imprinting of discrete portions of the genome began with studies of X inactivation. This imprinting was first shown by analyzing *PGK* allele expression in mice heterozygous for a polymorphism in the phosphoglycerate kinase gene, detected as an electrophoretic variant in the protein. Although the X chromosome shows random inactivation in embryonic tissues, this is not the case in extraembryonic tissues, which show preferential inactivation of the paternal X chromosome.[10]

The beginning of our understanding of which autosomes undergo genomic imprinting came from studies over many years by Cattanach and colleagues of mice with germ-line chromosomal translocations.[11] When these mice are bred, there is a high frequency of nondisjunction, leading to both paternal and maternal uniparental disomy (UPD) beyond the translocation breakpoint, depending on which parent harbors the translocation. The phenotypes of these animals provide an estimate that 15 percent of the genome is imprinted.[11] Studies of UPD in mice also suggest that when imprinting occurs, an excess of the paternal genome, coupled with maternal loss, leads to prenatal overgrowth, and an excess of the maternal genome leads to decreased growth. Other phenotypes of UPD include embryonic lethality and behavioral disorders.[11] This work provided a critical clue toward identifying imprinted loci in mouse and, by synteny mapping, in humans. UPD studies have shown that imprinting resides at the level of genes and/or chromosomal regions. However, UPD studies have several inherent limitations. The phenotype by which animals are scored is relatively insensitive. The technique used is also relatively nonspecific, in that there may be only a single imprinted gene within the entire chromosomal region that shows UPD.

The first example of a specific imprinted gene was discovered fortuitously by Swain and colleagues, and it did not involve an endogenous gene. It was noted that a C-*myc* transgene fused to an immunoglobulin enhancer was expressed in some tissues only when inherited from the father. When inherited from the mother, the transgene was transcriptionally silent. In addition, the silent maternally inherited copy was methylated.[12] There are now several examples of transgenes that show parental origin-specific methylation, but transcriptional silencing is less common.[13]

The first example of an imprinted endogenous gene also was discovered fortuitously when DeChiara and colleagues disrupted the insulin-like growth factor II (*IGF2*) gene in knockout experiments.[14] When the disrupted allele was inherited from the father, the animals were runted, but there was no phenotype when the disrupted allele was inherited from the mother. When female mice with the disrupted allele themselves had offspring, those animals were of normal size. *In situ* hybridization and RNase protection experiments confirmed that there was no *IGF2*

Table 3-1 Imprinted Genes in Mouse or Humans

Gene	Expression
ASCL2/Mash2	Maternal
GABA receptor	Paternal and Maternal
GNAS Isoforms	Paternal
GRB10	Maternal
Grf1	Paternal
H19	Maternal
IGF2	Paternal
IGF2R	Maternal
Impact	Paternal
INS1	Paternal
Insulin	Paternal
IPW	Paternal
K_VLQT1	Maternal
Mas	Paternal
Necdin	Paternal
P57^{KIP2}	Maternal
PAR-1	Paternal
PAR-5	Paternal
PAR-SN	Paternal
Peg1	Paternal
Peg3	Paternal
SNRPN	Paternal
TSSC3/IPL	Maternal
TSSC5/IMPT1	Maternal
U2afbp-rs	Paternal
UBE3A/E6-AP	Maternal
WT1	Maternal
XIST	Paternal
ZNF127	Paternal

expression in tissues with a disrupted paternal allele. Thus these experiments clearly showed that *IGF2* is imprinted and expressed normally only from the paternal allele.[14] However, *IGF2* is biparentally expressed in two neural tissues, the choroid plexus and the leptomeninges, since animals with a disrupted paternal allele nevertheless expressed the gene in these tissues.[14] These were milestone studies because they showed that genomic imprinting affects normal endogenous genes and also that imprinting is subject to tissue-specific regulation. Recent years have provided more direct approaches to identifying novel imprinted genes.[15] These include positional cloning efforts aimed at identifying imprinted genes near other known imprinted genes, techniques for comparing gene expression in parthenogenetic embryos to that of normal embryos,[16] and restriction landmark genome scanning,[17] which exploits a principle introduced many years ago, to analyze clonality in tumors, and involves a search for DNA methylation near a polymorphic site for which the individual is heterozygous.[18] Approximately 30 imprinted genes have been discovered, although many more are likely to exist. A current inventory (at this writing) of imprinted genes in mouse and humans, which are not necessarily concordant, is provided in Table 3-1. One of the most interesting features of genomic imprinting is that it affects many different cellular processes, including intercellular signaling, RNA processing, and cell cycle control.

GENOMIC IMPRINTING IN HUMAN DISEASE

Two assumptions of Mendelian genetics applied to human disease are that the maternal allele is equivalent to the paternal allele and that two working copies of the gene are associated with normal function. Genomic imprinting challenges the first of these assumptions, since it is a form of epigenetic inheritance that causes parental origin-specific differential gene expression. As will be described later, abnormal imprinting in cancer challenges the second assumption, because loss of imprinting causing biallelic expression of some genes may be a mechanism underlying carcinogenesis.

The literature of the 1970s and 1980s is rich in presumed examples of human genetic disorders that exhibit genomic imprinting. These reports were based primarily on pedigree studies of autosomal dominant disorders that showed parental origin-specific disease penetrance. These disease loci also often show disease anticipation; namely, the phenotype becomes progressively worse from one generation to the next. Although both of these phenomena were ascribed to genomic imprinting,[19] later studies based on molecular cloning of the responsible genes revealed that genomic imprinting often was not the mechanism after all. The classical example is fragile X syndrome, a common cause of mental retardation, which is caused by a trinucleotide repeat expansion.[20,21] This expansion undergoes preferential enlargement in the maternal germ line, accounting for differential disease penetrance as well as anticipation. However, expression is controlled by the length of the repeat and not imprinting per se.[22] Thus parent-of-origin effects may or may not be owing to genomic imprinting. This is not to fault the older studies, since the definition of genomic imprinting itself has evolved somewhat to refer to modification causing parental allele-specific expression rather than any parental allele-specific modification.

Two examples of true imprinted human disease loci are in close proximity on chromosome 15. Their loss causes Prader-Willi syndrome (PWS) or Angelman syndrome (AS). Both involve mental retardation, and PWS also causes obesity, and AS involves gross motor disturbances. Each disorder can be caused by uniparental disomy, PWS by maternal UPD and AS by paternal UPD.[23,24] Similarly, PWS can be caused by intrachromosomal deletions of the paternal chromosome and AS by deletions of the maternal chromosome.[25,26] PWS can be caused by deletions in the small nuclear ribonucleoprotein polypeptide N (*SNRPN*) gene.[27] It has been shown recently that a mutation affecting the splicing of an untranslated upstream exon of *SNRPN* also may lead to AS, as well as abnormal imprinting of other loci.[28] Thus, on chromosome 15, abnormalities of a single gene can affect imprinting of a genomic region and disrupt multiple disease-causing genes, the phenotype depending on the parental origin of the mutated gene. Recently, mutations in *UBE3A,* a ubiquitin protein ligase, also were found in AS patients.[29]

Despite the relative paucity of known human imprinted disease genes, there are probably many more yet to be identified. This seems clear because UPD for specific chromosomes is often associated with multiple congenital anomalies.[30] Chromosomes that likely show this phenomenon include 2, 6, 7, 11, 14, 15, 16, 20, and X.[30] Again, the discovery of these potential imprinted disease-causing regions has been fortuitous, as has much of our knowledge of imprinting. For example, the first such example of UPD pointing the way to an imprinted chromosome was the discovery of a cystic fibrosis patient for whom only the mother was the carrier.[31] Molecular analysis showed that the genotype of the offspring was not owing to gonadal mosaicism but rather to maternal UPD in the offspring. The child also had short stature and possibly Russell-Silver syndrome. This observation indicated that there is at least one imprinted locus on chromosome 7 and that the patient suffered from a deficiency of one or more genes normally expressed only from the paternal allele or duplication of genes normally expressed only from the maternal allele.[31] Not all chromosomes appear to contain disease-related imprinted loci, however, since UPD of chromosomes 4, 5, 9, 10, 13, 21, and 22 has not been associated with birth defects.[30]

INDIRECT EVIDENCE FOR GENOMIC IMPRINTING IN HUMAN CANCER

As in the study of normal genomic imprinting, the idea of a role for genomic imprinting in cancer followed a similar progression of clues regarding whole-genome imprinting, involvement of individual chromosomal regions, and finally imprinting at specific loci. The earliest clues suggesting that genomic imprinting is important in cancer were the whole-genome examples of hydatidiform mole and complete ovarian teratoma. Hydatidiform mole, a malignant tumor of extraembryonic tissue, is caused by an androgenetic embryo arising from two paternal genome equivalents and no maternal genome equivalent.[32] This can be caused by dispermy and loss of the maternal complement or by duplication of the paternal genome and loss of the maternal equivalent. Conversely, complete ovarian teratoma, which is a very curious benign tumor that includes differentiated hair, adipose tissue, and even teeth, arises from a parthenogenetic embryo, with two maternal genome equivalents and no paternal equivalent.[33] Parthenogenesis (literally "virgin birth") is a specialized type of gynogenesis, and it specifically refers to the absence of fertilization and arises within the ovary. These two tumors, although rare, offer two important general lessons for understanding the role of imprinting in cancer. One is that it takes not only 46 chromosomes to create a normal embryo but also a balance of maternal and paternal chromosomes; a relative imbalance of paternal to maternal genetic contributions leads to neoplastic growth. The second lesson is that when there is such an imbalance, the type of neoplasm differs depending on whether there is a maternal or paternal genomic excess.

Another tumor that appears to show imprinting effects is familial paraganglioma, or glomus tumor. In all cases, the transmitting parent is the father.[34] The responsible gene has been localized recently to 11q22.3-q23.[34]

Chromosomal region-specific evidence for a role for imprinting in cancer followed from an observation several years ago involving loss of heterozygosity (LOH) in Wilms tumor. It had been known already that this most common solid tumor of childhood undergoes LOH of chromosome 11 and that the specifically involved region is 11p15.[35] Schroeder and colleagues noted that in each of five nonfamilial cases with LOH, it was always the maternal allele that was lost.[36] In a binomial distribution, five is the minimum number

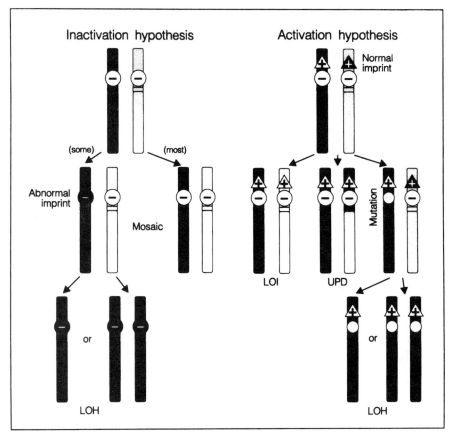

Fig. 3-1 Contrasting hypotheses of genomic imprinting in cancer. The inactivation hypothesis involves loss of expression of a tumor suppressor gene. The paternal allele is inactivated by imprinting, which displays somatic mosaicism (accounting for unilateral tumors), followed by LOH of the maternal allele (arbitrarily shown here affecting the whole chromosome). The activation hypothesis involves normal imprinting of a growth-promoting gene. Overexpression can arise from LOI of the maternal allele or UPD of the paternal allele. LOH of a distinct tumor suppressor gene would be
deleterious to cell growth if it involved the transcriptionally active paternal allele of the growth-promoting gene. Alternatively, both models may be correct, with LOI and LOH leading to epigenetic silencing of a tumor suppressor gene and LOI also leading to abnormal activation of a normally silent growth-promoting gene. Dark shading, paternal chromosome; light shading, maternal chromosome, tumor suppressor gene, growth-promoting gene. (*Reprinted from Feinberg AP: Genomic imprinting and gene activation in cancer. Nature Genet 4:110–113, 1993, with permission.*)

required for statistical significance. Unfortunately, the word *imprinting* did not appear anywhere in this important paper, which stimulated a great deal of speculation and study in the following years.

Sapienza and colleagues confirmed and extended this observation to other so-called embryonal tumors of childhood, all of which involve the development of malignancy within what pathologists believe is fetal tissue that is abnormally residual after birth. Examples include hepatoblastoma and rhabdomyosarcoma.[37] They proposed a model in which imprinting is involved in cancer through epigenetic silencing of a tumor suppressor gene (Fig. 3-1). According to this model, a tumor suppressor gene on 11p15 is imprinted and epigenetically silenced on the paternal allele, accounting for the fact that LOH is seen only on the maternal allele (see Fig. 3-1). After all, LOH of the paternal allele would be inconsequential because the locus is silenced normally.[37]

However, Sapienza and colleagues also pointed out a paradox in this logic. If the locus is normally imprinted and epigenetically silenced, then everyone would have only one functional copy of the gene at birth, and then the locus would behave epidemiologically as if it had undergone a germ-line mutation of a tumor suppressor locus following Knudson's two-hit model of carcinogenesis. According to this model, patients with germ-line mutations show bilateral tumors occurring at an earlier age of onset than patients with sporadically occurring tumors, which require two sequential events to take place within a given somatic cell lineage. Thus, Sapienza and colleagues reasoned, epigenetic

silencing of a tumor suppressor could not be present in all cells of the body because the tumors, such as Wilms tumor (WT), with preferential LOH of the maternal allele are for the most part late-arising unilateral tumors. On the other hand, imprinting must take place no later than the zygote stage while there is still a topologic distinction between the two parental genome equivalents. Therefore, Sapienza and colleagues proposed the following solution to this conundrum: In some individuals during germ-line development or fertilization, aberrant imprinting occurs, preferentially affecting the paternally inherited chromosome. According to this model, imprinting is subsequently erased during development, but not completely, leaving a mosaic pattern of imprinting in various tissues. Thus the imprint would no longer behave as the first hit of a two-hit Knudsonian locus[37,38] (see Fig. 3-1). One puzzle with this model is that it still proposes a relatively large number of cells with this epigenetic alteration, and thus the tumors may appear at an intermediate stage of frequency and age. However, parental origin-specific LOH appears to occur in quite ordinary late-occurring tumors. Furthermore, at least some tumors should not show aberrant imprinting as the first hit, but all tumors show preferential loss of the maternal allele.

There are now several examples of tumor types that show preferential LOH. Most of these involve the maternal chromosome, but not all do. For example, acute myelogenous leukemia (AML) involves preferential loss of the paternal chromosome 7.[39] A summary of chromosome-specific LOH is presented in Table 3-2. However, in the study of human genetic disorders, one must be

Table 3-2 Preferential Chromosomal Alterations in Cancer That Likely Involve Imprinted Genes

Cancer	Chromosome	Alteration	Allele
Wilms tumor	11p	LOH	Maternal
Rhabdomyosarcoma	11p	LOH	Maternal
Osteosarcoma	13q	LOH	Maternal
Acute myelocytic leukemia	7q	LOH	Paternal
Neuroblastoma	1p	LOH	Maternal
Hepatoblastoma	1q	LOH	Paternal
Neuroblastoma	2	Amplification	Paternal

careful not to assume that parent-of-origin effects are owing to genomic imprinting. For example, bilateral retinoblastoma shows preferential loss of the maternal allele. However, this is owing simply to the higher mutation rate of the paternal gamete rather than imprinting, since the *RB* gene is not imprinted.[40]

Preferential involvement of a specific parental chromosome also applies to other types of chromosomal abnormalities in cancer. For example, Haas and colleagues reported preferential involvement of paternal chromosome 9 and maternal chromosome 22 in the Philadelphia chromosome translocation of chronic myelogenous leukemia based on a cytogenetic polymorphism.[41] However, subsequent studies have not shown imprinting of the rearranged *BCR* and *ABL* genes, and molecular studies have not confirmed preferential parental origin of those chromosomes.[42–44]

Other types of parental origin-specific chromosome alterations have withstood the test of time. For example, the N-*myc* gene on chromosome 2 shows preferential amplification of the paternal allele in neuroblastoma.[45] Preferential LOH of the maternal allele of chromosome 1 in neuroblastoma initially was observed by some investigators and not by others.[45,46] However, this controversy was resolved when it was found that advanced tumors, showing N-*myc* amplification, also show preferential LOH of maternal chromosome 1, whereas earlier-stage tumors without N-*myc* amplification do not.[47] Thus genetic disturbances involving imprinted genes in a given type of cancer may involve multiple chromosomes concurrently. This idea of abnormal imprinting affecting multiple chromosomes is a provocative one for which there are other data. For example, Sapienza has found transmission ratio distortion, concordance of 13q loss, and isochromosome 6 of the same parental origin in retinoblastoma, again consistent with a mechanism of generalized disturbance of imprinting in embryogenesis leading to increased cancer risk.[48]

Despite these intriguing observations of diverse tumors, suggesting a role for genomic imprinting in cancer, direct proof for such a role awaited the discovery of specific imprinted human genes and their altered imprinting in cancer. The guidepost toward these genes was the hereditary disorder Beckwith-Wiedemann syndrome.

BECKWITH-WIEDEMANN SYNDROME

Beckwith-Wiedemann syndrome (BWS) is a disorder of prenatal overgrowth and cancer transmitted as an autosomal dominant trait, although most cases arise sporadically. It is reported to affect 1 in 15,000 children, although the frequency may be much higher because close scrutiny of families of BWS patients often shows subtly affected siblings or parents and the phenotype abates with increasing age of the patient.[49,50] Its cardinal features are macroglossia or enlargement of the tongue, macrosomia caused by prenatal overgrowth throughout gestation, abdominal wall defects (including diastasis recti and umbilical hernia), omphalocele, and craniofacial dysmorphism (including facial nevus flameus, ear pits and creases, prominent occiput, maxillary hypoplasia, widened nasal bridge, high arched palate, and

occasionally mild microcephaly). In addition, BWS typically presents with neonatal hypoglycemia, caused in part by overproduction of IGF2.[49,50]

The frequency of embryonal tumors in BWS children is approximately 20 percent, a 1000-fold increase over that of the general population.[51,52] These include WT, hepatoblastoma, rhabdomyosarcoma, and adrenocortical carcinoma.[51,52] In addition, the same organs show dysplastic changes, including adrenal cytomegaly and cysts, nephromegaly with prominent lobulation and nephrogenic rests, hepatomegaly, splenomegaly, and hyperplasia of the islets of Langerhans.[49–52]

A clue to a role for genomic imprinting is increased disease penetrance when BWS is inherited from the mother.[53] As noted earlier, parent-of-origin effects may or may not represent genomic imprinting. However, the tumors these children develop show preferential loss of maternal 11p15, as noted earlier, suggesting that an imprinted locus could cause BWS and also be involved in sporadically occurring tumors.[36,37] Genetic linkage analysis showed that BWS localizes to 11p15, consistent with this idea, and not to 11p13, to which the *WT1* gene had been localized.[54,55]

Further support for the idea that imprinting is involved in BWS came from study of rare chromosomal translocations or inversions affecting approximately 1 percent of BWS patients. About half these rearrangements are balanced, and by analogy with other human genetic disorders, these balanced rearrangements are likely to disrupt the coding sequence of a BWS gene. All the balanced rearrangements have involved the maternally derived chromosome 11.[56,57] The simplest explanation is that the rearrangements are disrupting expression of a maternally expressed gene. Indeed, there are several families in which multiple individuals within the same kindred harbor the same chromosomal rearrangement, but only those inheriting the rearrangement from the mother were affected with BWS.[56,57] The other type of chromosomal rearrangement seen in BWS patients involves unbalanced translocations or duplications. All of these have shown an excess of the paternally derived chromosome.[56] Thus both paternal duplication and maternal rearrangement of chromosome 11 can lead to BWS.

More direct evidence for genomic imprinting of 11p15 in BWS came from studies of Junien and colleagues showing that some patients with BWS have paternal UPD involving a region extending from the β-globin locus to the *ras* gene.[58] This is a very large area of at least 10 Mb and thus does not provide precise localization of an imprinted gene, but it provided an important foundation for later studies of imprinted loci on this chromosome. Curiously, all the patients with UPD are mosaic for this abnormality.[59] Thus it occurs postzygotically and is presumably an early embryonic lethal when present in the zygote.

Paternal UPD causes both duplication of the paternal allele and loss of the maternal allele of the involved genes. Thus UPD by itself is consistent either with loss of function of a gene normally expressed on the maternal chromosome or duplication of a gene normally expressed from the paternal chromosome. The balanced maternal chromosomal rearrangements in other patients could represent loss of function of a maternally expressed gene or, alternatively, disruption of an imprinting control center, a hypothetical *cis*-acting signal that establishes the original imprinting pattern in the germ line. This disruption could lead to abnormal activation of a gene or genes normally silent on the maternal chromosome and thus functional duplication of a gene normally expressed from the paternal chromosome. Evidence for this idea derives from the fact that the balanced chromosomal rearrangements, looked at as a group, span a very large region, > 3 Mb, larger than would be expected for a single locus.[57] However, they are clustered into two distinct regions, each of which could conceivably represent a single large gene.[57] The unbalanced paternal chromosome duplications, however, are difficult to explain other than by a mechanism of increased dosage (doubling) of a gene or genes normally expressed only from the paternal chromosome. Of course, BWS may involve both duplication of paternally expressed genes and loss of maternally expressed genes. The identification of genes involved in BWS followed from the discovery of imprinted genes in human 11p15 and is described in the next section.

IMPRINTED GENES ON 11p15 AND LOSS OF IMPRINTING IN CANCER

The first human gene shown to be imprinted at the molecular level was *IGF2*, which was examined because of its localization to 11p15, for the reasons discussed in the preceding section and because it was known to be imprinted in the mouse. In order to test

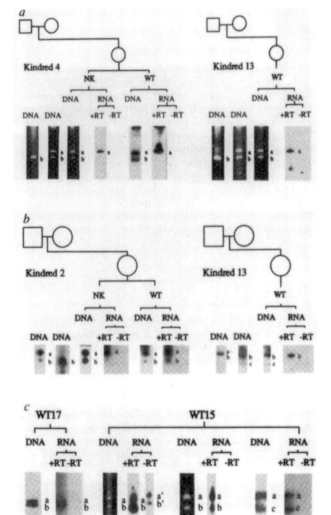

Fig. 3-2 Imprinting of *H19* and *IGF2* genes and loss of imprinting in cancer. *A.* Maternal monoallelic expression of *H19* in normal kidney (NK) and Wilms tumor (WT). Both NK and WT of patient 4 and WT of patient 13 show monoallelic expression of the maternal allele. *B.* Paternal monoallelic expression of *IGF2* in normal kidney. Kindred 2 was analyzed using an ApaI polymorphism and kindred 13 using a dinucleotide repeat (DR) polymorphism. *C.* Biallelic expression of *H19* and *IGF2* in Wilms tumors. WT17 was analyzed using the IGF2/ DR polymorphism and shows biallelic expression. WT15 was informative for all three polymorphisms. Both *H19* and *IGF2* show biallelic expression, as does the WT from patient 2 (see *B*). A single DNA-contaminated RNA sample from patient 15 was deliberately included to illustrate the larger-sized fragments (a′,b′) resulting from amplification of genomic sequences. (*Reprinted from Rainier S, Johnson LA, Dobry CJ, Ping AJ, Grundy PE, Feinberg AP: Relaxation of imprinted genes in human cancer. Nature 362:747–749, 1993, with permission.*)

the hypothesis that *IGF2* is imprinted, it was necessary to reverse transcribe (RT) the gene from RNA in a tissue that expresses it, and then polymerase chain reaction (PCR) amplify the cDNA products. If this RT-PCR is performed on an individual heterozygous for a transcribed polymorphism (i.e., a polymorphic site is present within an exon), then one can determine whether one or both alleles are expressed. If only one allele is expressed, then one can determine if it is maternal or paternal by examining parental genomic DNA samples. In this manner, the *IGF2* gene was found to be normally imprinted, with preferential expression of the paternal allele (Fig. 3-2), as in the mouse.[60–63] In mouse, *H19*, a gene within 100 kb of *IGF2* that encodes an untranslated RNA of unclear function, is oppositely imprinted, with preferential expression of the maternal allele.[64] This gene also was tested for imprinting in humans and was found to be imprinted as well, with preferential expression of the maternal allele.[60,65]

Examination of RNA from WT led to a surprising discovery. Not one, but both *IGF2* alleles were expressed in 70 percent of Wilms tumors.[60,62] In addition, in 30 percent of cases, both alleles of *H19* were expressed[60] (see Fig. 3-2). The term for this novel genetic alteration in cancer is *loss of imprinting* (LOI), which simply means loss of preferential parental origin-specific gene expression and can involve either abnormal expression of the normally silent allele, leading to biallelic expression, or silencing of the normally expressed allele, leading to epigenetic silencing of the locus.[60,66,67] Thus, in addition to the epigenetic silencing suggested earlier by Sapienza and colleagues (see Fig. 3-1), abnormal imprinting in cancer can lead to activation of normally silent alleles of growth-promoting genes[37,38,60,66,67] (see Fig. 3-1).

Subsequently, a large number of additional tumor types have been shown to undergo LOI. At first, LOI was found in other childhood tumors, such as hepatoblastoma, rhabdomyosarcoma, and Ewing sarcoma.[68–71] LOI of *IGF2* and *H19* also have now been found in many adult tumors, including uterine, cervical, esophageal, prostate, lung, and colon cancer, choriocarcinoma, and germ-cell tumors.[72–78] Thus LOI is one of the most common alterations in human cancer. These data are summarized in Table 3-3.

Care must be used in interpreting evidence of biallelic expression of *IGF2* as LOI, since *IGF2* is normally expressed from both alleles of the adult, or P1, promoter.[79] Nevertheless, abnormal imprinting and biallelic expression from the fetal promoters (P2 to P4) has been demonstrated for most of the tumors described earlier.[69,71,72,80] Finally, LOI of *IGF2* has been described in BWS, albeit in a relatively small percentage of patients.[81,82] Additional patients with large stature and WT but not BWS per se also show LOI of *IGF2*.[83]

A third imprinted gene on chromosome 11p15 is *p57^{KIP2}*, encoding a cyclin-dependent kinase (CDK) inhibitor related to p21$^{WAF1/Cip1}$, a target of p53.[84,85] It was mapped to 11p15 and

Table 3-3 Cancers That Show Loss of Imprinting (LOI)

Tumor Type	Gene
Wilms tumor	IGF2, H19, p57^{KIP2}
Rhabdomyosarcoma	IGF2
Hepatoblastoma	IGF2
Bladder	IGF2, H19
Cervical	IGF2, H19
Prostate	IGF2
Testicular	IGF2, H19
Esophageal	H19
Breast	IGF2
Choriocarcinoma	IGF2, H19
Ovarian	IGF2
Colorectal	IGF2

found to be localized within 40 kb of a group of BWS balanced germ-line chromosomal rearrangement breakpoints, in contrast to *IGF2* and *H19,* which are located telomeric to these breakpoints.[57,84] Nevertheless, its chromosomal location suggested that it also may be imprinted and play a role in tumors that show LOH of 11p15. Human *p57^KIP2* was indeed found to be imprinted with preferential expression from the maternal allele.[86] *p57^KIP2* also shows abnormal imprinting and epigenetic silencing in some tumors and in BWS patients.[87] Subsequently, nonsense mutations have been described in BWS, but the frequency is quite low, only 5 percent.[88,89] Interestingly, BWS can arise from *p57^KIP2* mutations transmitted from the father, although with less severity than those transmitted from the mother.[89] Thus the phenotype must in part involve haploinsufficiency of the gene in tissues in which it is not normally imprinted, as well as loss of function in tissues where it is imprinted.[89] This observation is the converse of that made for *UBE3A,* which is mutated at high frequency in AS but is not imprinted in most tissues[29]; yet it must be imprinted in some because it shows UPD effects.

Two additional imprinted 11p15 genes have been identified recently. *TSSC3/IPL* is a maternally expressed homologue of mouse *TDAG51,* which activates Fas and FasL, leading to apoptosis of T lymphocytes.[145,146] TSSC5/IMPT/BWR1C is a putative transmembrane protein that is weakly homologous to bacterial transporter proteins.[147–149] Mutations in *TSSC5* were identified recently in WT and lung cancer[147], suggesting that it may correspond to the long-sought *WT2* gene on 11p15.

A gene spanning a cluster of BWS balanced germ-line chromosomal rearrangement breakpoints has been identified recently as *K_VLQT1*.[131] This gene, which also causes the autosomal dominant cardiac arrhythmia long QT syndrome, spans at least 350 kb and also shows genomic imprinting, with preferential expression of the maternal allele.[131] In addition, the gene undergoes alternative splicing at the 5' end, which involves an untranslated upstream sequence, similar to that observed upstream of the *SNRPN* gene.[131] Thus *K_VLQT1* may be involved in imprint control similar to the function ascribed to *SNRPN* on chromosome 15. Interestingly, *K_VLQT1* is not imprinted in the heart, explaining the lack of parent-of-origin effect in long QT syndrome but marked parent-of-origin effect in translocation-associated BWS.[131]

Finally, a novel antisense transcript, termed LIT1 (Long Intronic Transcript 1), has been identified within *K_VLQT1*.[147] LIT1 is at least 60 kb in size and appears to be unspliced and untranslated. LIT1 is expressed from the paternal allele, in contrast to *K_VLQT1,* which is expressed from the maternal allele.[147] Remarkably, LIT1 undergoes LOI in most patients with BWS.[147]

How can such diverse genetic alterations lead to BWS? One possibility is that some of the genes involved, e.g., *IGF2, p57^KIP2,* and *K_VLQT1,* all are part of the same biochemical pathway. A second possibility is that one or more of these genes may be coordinately regulated as part of a large genomic region of multiple imprinted genes. LIT1 is an intriguing candidate for such a *cis*-acting regulatory role. A summary of genetic alterations in BWS is presented in Table 3-4.

One of the most intriguing recent observations of LOI in cancer was in the normal tissues of colon cancer patients. LOI was found in 12 of 27 informative colorectal cancer patients (44 percent), in the matched normal mucosa of the same patients, and in all four available blood samples from these patients. The colonic mucosa of noncancer patients showed LOI in 2 of 16 informative cases (12 percent) and in 2 of 15 blood samples (13 percent).[150] It is not yet known whether LOI arose in normal tissue before or coincident with LOI in the tumors, but either way, LOI may become a useful new diagnostic or prognostic marker for cancer. In this regard, most patients with microsatellite instability in their tumors showed LOI in the cancer and normal colon, and consistent with this observation, the LOI patients were significantly younger than the non-LOI patients.[150]

THE EFFECTS OF LOI ON GENE EXPRESSION AND TUMOR CELL GROWTH

Since the time of Laennec, it has been known that cancers lose properties of their normal cellular counterparts and gain properties of other types of cells or developmental stages.[90] One of the most intriguing aspects of LOI is that it may help to explain the abnormal gene expression patterns that are responsible for these characteristics.

Quantitative assays of gene expression in WTs with LOI reveal the following: *IGF2* expression is increased approximately twofold, *H19* expression is lost, and *p57^KIP2* expression is lost.[81] This is true even for tumors that show biallelic expression of *H19.*[87] What appears to take place in tumors with LOI is that the maternal chromosome switches to a paternal epigenotype, affecting several genes over a several hundred kilobase domain. Thus the maternal copy of *IGF2* is expressed, hence biallelic expression. Conversely, the maternal alleles of *H19* and *p57^KIP2* are epigenetically silenced as on the paternal chromosome, leading to little or no detectable expression of these genes overall.[81,91]

These observations suggest a unified model of LOI in some cancers, such as WT, which explains epigenetic silencing of tumor suppressor genes as well as activation of normally silent alleles of growth-promoting genes. According to this model, LOI involves a switch in the epigenotype of a chromosomal region in the case of WT from maternal to paternal.[81,91] Thus *IGF2* shows biallelic expression, and *H19* undergoes epigenetic silencing. However, this model is not meant to be universal. For example, not all tumors show a switch in expression of all three genes, *IGF2, H19,* and *p57^KIP2.* Hepatoblastoma shows LOI of *IGF2,* but tumors with biallelic expression of *IGF2* do not necessarily undergo epigenetic silencing of *H19.*[68,69]

What is the biologic effect of these changes in gene expression caused by altered genomic imprinting? IGF2 is an important autocrine and paracrine growth factor.[92–99] Its mitogenic effects are mediated by signaling through the IGF1 receptor.[99] This is clearly an important pathway in cancer because blocking IGF2 at the IGF1 receptor inhibits tumor cell growth and is even the basis of an experimental therapeutic trial.[99–102] In addition, somatic mutations in the *IGF2* receptor gene, which is a metabolic sink for IGF2, have been found in hepatocellular carcinoma, further supporting the idea that signaling by IGF2 is an important mitogenic growth pathway.[103]

Direct evidence for a causative role of insulin-like growth factor II in tumor progression comes from studies of mice harboring an SV40 T-antigen transgene under the control of a rat insulin promoter, known as *RIP-Tag* mice. These animals develop insulinomas at high frequency, and the tumors evolve through sequential stages of tumor progression.[104] When the *RIP-Tag* transgene is bred into a background of mice with homozygously knocked out *IGF2* genes, they still develop tumors, but the tumors

Table 3-4 Genetic Alterations in Beckwith-Wiedemann Syndrome

Genetic Alteration	Allele
Balanced germ-line chromosomal translocations and inversions	Maternal
Unbalanced germ-line chromosomal translocations and duplications	Paternal
Uniparental disomy	Paternal
Loss of imprinting of IGF2	Maternal
Loss of imprinting of p57^KIP2	Maternal
Mutation of p57^KIP2	Maternal
Imprint-specific methylation switch (increased)	Maternal
Gene rearrangement	Maternal
Loss of imprinting of LIT1	Maternal

are arrested at a stage of benign neoplasia.[105] However, when the *RIP-Tag* transgene is bred into a heterozygous *IGF2* knockout background, in which only the paternal allele has been disrupted, the maternal allele undergoes LOI and the tumors progress through malignancy, but the tumors are smaller.[106] Finally, when the maternal allele is knocked out, the tumors still show LOI, in that the neogene is now expressed from the disrupted allele.[106] Thus LOI is a necessary step in tumor progression in this system. This model also provides a clue to one possible effect of LOI. Tumor cells in which *IGF2* has been homozygously knocked out show increased apoptosis, which is overcome by introduction into them of an *IGF2* expression construct.[105] Thus LOI may be one of the factors that allows tumors to escape the apoptosis caused by other carcinogenic mutations.

H19 is an untranslated RNA that accounts for a significant fraction (3 percent) of embryonic mRNA,[107] but significance remains unclear. An *H19* transgene was reported to be an embryonic lethal, but the lethality was caused by a small insertion in the transgene used to mark it.[108,109] An *H19* expression construct caused suppression of growth in soft agar of WT cells into which it was introduced.[110] However, *H19* maps outside the 11p15 region shown to suppress tumor growth in genetic complementation experiments.[111]

The effect of LOI on *p57^{KIP2}* may be as important as that of *IGF2* and *H19*. Most or all WTs tumors undergo epigenetic silencing of *p57^{KIP2}*.[87] In some tumors, this appears to be caused by abnormal imprinting. The same effect is seen in tumors with LOH, since the normally expressed maternal allele is lost.[87] Thus *p57^{KIP2}* may represent an imprinted tumor gene in which epigenetic silencing is the primary carcinogenic event. Indeed, this may turn out to be the first tumor gene in which epigenetic silencing is the only carcinogenic event, if mutations in nonfamilial tumors continue not to be found.

POSSIBLE MECHANISMS OF NORMAL IMPRINTING AND LOSS OF IMPRINTING IN CANCER

DNA Methylation

Cytosine DNA methylation is a covalent modification of DNA in which a methyl group is transferred from *S*-adenosyl methionine to the C-5 position of cytosine by cytosine (DNA-5)-methyltransferase (referred to as *DNA methyltransferase*). DNA methylation occurs almost exclusively at CpG dinucleotides.[112] The pattern of DNA methylation is heritable by somatic cells and maintained after DNA replication by DNA methyltransferase, which has a 100-fold greater affinity for hemimethylated DNA (i.e., parent strand methylated, daughter strand unmethylated) than for unmethylated DNA.[112] However, developing cells in the gamete and embryo undergo dramatic shifts in DNA methylation, which involve both loss of methylation and *de novo* methylation.[112] It is not known what mechanism establishes the original pattern of DNA methylation.

There are two classes of cytosine DNA methylation in the genome. The first occurs throughout the body of genes that show tissue-specific expression, with methylation generally associated with gene silencing. This type of DNA methylation can occur both before and after the changes in gene expression, so they are not necessarily the cause of altered gene expression during development. Rather, they may help to ''lock in'' a given pattern of gene expression.[112,113]

The second class of normal cytosine methylation involves CpG islands, regions rich in CpG dinucleotides. CpG islands are almost always unmethylated in normal cells, and they are usually within the promoter or first exon of housekeeping genes.[114] However, an important exception is CpG islands on the inactive X chromosome, which are methylated. Thus CpG island methylation, unlike non-CpG island methylation, is thought to be involved in epigenetic silencing in general and marking of the inactive X chromosome in particular.[115]

Several recent discoveries suggest a role for DNA methylation in the control of genomic imprinting. First, some imprinted genes in mice, such as *H19,* show parental origin-specific, tissue-independent methylation of CpG islands. For example, the paternal CpG island in *H19* is methylated and the maternal allele unmethylated, in tissues that express the gene as well as those which do not.[116,117] Thus this methylation represents an imprinting mark on the paternal chromosome and is not secondary to changes in gene expression. Second, knockout mice deficient in DNA methyltransferase and exhibiting widespread genome hypomethylation do not show allele-specific methylation of the *H19* CpG island and exhibit biallelic expression of *H19* and loss of expression of *IGF2*.[118] Similar parental origin-specific methylation also has been observed for a CpG island in the first intron of the maternally inherited, expressed allele of the *IGF2* receptor gene (*IGF2R*).[119] Methyltransferase-deficient knockout mice show loss of methylation of *IGF2R* and epigenetic silencing of the gene.[118]

Widespread alterations in DNA methylation in human tumors were discovered 15 years ago.[120] This remains the most commonly found alteration in human cancer, albeit an epigenetic one, and it occurs ubiquitously in both benign and malignant neoplasms.[121] The precise role of these changes has remained unclear, although both decreased and increased methylation has been found at specific sites in tumors, with an overall decrease in quantitative DNA methylation.[122-124]

Recent work using an experimental mouse model system also supports a role for DNA methylation in cancer. "Min" mice carry a mutation for the adenomatous polyposis coli (*APC*) gene and thereby develop colon tumors. When bred to knockout mice deficient in DNA methyltransferase, Min mice are partially protected from the development of tumors, suggesting that cytosine DNA methylation is involved in tumorigenesis.[125] Consistent with this idea, when these mice are treated with 5-azacytidine, a specific inhibitor of DNA methylation, the incidence of tumors is markedly reduced.[125] Of course, in this model system, decreased methylation may simply protect the animals from methylcytosine-to-thymine transition mutations.[125] Decreased methylation also may or may not be linked to genomic imprinting, which has not yet been examined in the Min mouse system, but the studies reinforce the link between altered DNA methylation and cancer.

DNA Methylation and LOI

In humans as in mice, the paternal allele of a CpG island in the *H19* gene and its promoter is normally methylated, and the maternal allele is unmethylated.[81,116,117] Thus CpG island methylation represents an imprint-specific mark on the paternal chromosome. Because tumors with LOI of *IGF2* showed reduced expression of *H19,* and because normal imprinting of *H19* is associated with methylation of the paternal allele, the methylation pattern of *H19* has been examined in tumors with LOI. In all cases showing LOI of *IGF2,* the *H19* promoter exhibits 90 to 100 percent methylation at the sites normally unmethylated on the maternally inherited allele.[81,91] Thus the maternal allele has acquired a paternal pattern of methylation. This is consistent with the fact that the *IGF2* gene on the same (maternally derived) chromosome is expressed in these tumors, as occurs normally only on the paternally derived chromosome. In contrast, tumors without LOI of *IGF2* show no change in the methylation of *H19*, indicating that these changes are related to abnormal imprinting and not malignancy per se.[81,91] The same alterations in methylation of the maternal allele of *H19* are found in BWS patients with LOI of *IGF2,* indicating that LOI can precede the development of malignancy and not arise secondarily.[81,126,127] These observations are consistent with the model presented earlier of a switch in parental epigenotype. According to this model, LOI, at least in WT, involves a switch of the maternal chromosome to a paternal epigenotype, with activation of the maternal *H19* allele, silencing of the maternal *IGF2* allele, silencing of the maternal *p57^{KIP2}* allele, and methylation of the maternal *H19* allele, as on the paternal chromosome.

What is the mechanism of altered DNA methylation in cancer? One mechanism that has been proposed is increased DNA methyltransferase expression itself.[128] Based on a quantitative RT-PCR assay, a 20-fold increase in DNA methyltransferase expression was reported in human colon tumors compared with matched normal mucosa, as well as a 400-fold increase in cancer over the normal mucosa of unaffected patients.[128] However, other RT-PCR experiments showed a more modest change.[129] Furthermore, a sensitive and specific RNase protection assay (RPA) found only a 1.8- to 2.5-fold increase in MTase mRNA.[130] This small difference disappeared entirely when histone H4 was used as an internal control, as a measure of nonspecific tumor cell proliferation. Thus the mechanism of altered methylation and genomic imprinting does not involve the known DNA methyltransferase enzyme itself.[130]

Disruption of an Imprinting Control Center

A second potential mechanism of LOI may involve disruption of an imprinting control center on chromosome 11, similar to that recently described for the PWS/AS region of chromosome 15.[28] A cluster of five BWS balanced germ-line chromosomal rearrangement breakpoints lies between *p57^{KIP2}* on the centromeric side and *IGF2* and *H19* on the telomeric side.[57] Thus disruption of a gene spanning this region could cause abnormal imprinting, as well as BWS and/or cancer, at least when inherited through the germ line. A gene spanning a cluster of BWS-balanced germ-line chromosome rearrangement breakpoints has been identified recently as *K_VLQT1*.[131] This gene spans at least 350 kb, shows genomic imprinting, and undergoes alternative splicing, similar to that observed upstream of the *SNRPN* gene.[130] Thus this gene may be involved in imprint control similar to the function ascribed to *SNRPN* on chromosome 15.

Other Possible Factors Causing LOI

Clues to other potential mechanisms for LOI come from consideration of the factors thought to be important in establishment and maintenance of normal genomic imprinting in mouse and of other forms of epigenetic inheritance in other species, discussed in the opening section of this chapter. One example is the loss of trans-acting factors, which are thought to help maintain a normal pattern of imprinting after it is established in the germ line. *Trans*-acting modifiers of imprinting are likely to exist, since imprinting of transgenes is host strain-dependent.[132] The human homologues of such genes might thus act as tumor suppressor genes.

Another potential mechanism of imprinting that may be disrupted in cancer involves histone deacetylation, which is linked to X inactivation in mammals and to telomere silencing in yeast.[133,134] Trichostatin A, a histone deacetylase inhibitor, may disrupt normal genomic imprinting.[135,136] Genes for both histone acetylase and histone deacetylase have been isolated recently.[137,138] In addition, telomere silencing in yeast also involves the action of specific genes, e.g., *SIR1* to *SIR4*, at least one of which has a homologue in mammals.[7] Similarly, some examples of gene silencing in mammals may resemble position-effect variegation in *Drosophila*, a form of position-dependent epigenetic silencing.[139] Finally, imprinted loci on maternal and paternal chromosomes may interact during DNA replication. Chromosomal regions harboring imprinted genes replicate synchronously.[140] Furthermore, the two parental homologues of some imprinted genes show nonrandom proximity in late S-phase,[141] suggesting some form of chromosomal crosstalk, as has been observed for epigenetic silencing in *Drosophila*.[142] Although the mechanism of imprinting remains unknown, analysis of tumor cells with altered imprinting should provide an additional tool in unraveling this mystery.

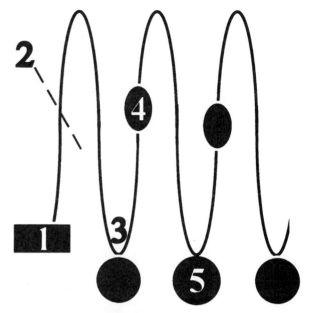

Fig. 3-3 A model of genomic imprinting as a developmental process, at which disturbances of several points may lead to loss of imprinting in cancer. An imprint organizing center (*rectangle*) exerts a long-range *cis*-acting influence on *IGF2* and other imprinted genes (*oval*) via alterations in chromatin structure (represented as DNA loops). This imprint-organizing center establishes the imprinting mark as maternal or paternal. This effect is propagated outward during development similar to the organizing center on the X chromosome. Imprinting is maintained in part by allele-specific methylation of CpG islands, as well as by interactions with *trans*-acting proteins (*circle*). According to this model, loss of imprinting could arise by any of several mechanisms (numbered in the figure): (1) deletion or mutation in the imprint organizing center itself, which would lead to a failure of parental origin-specific switching in the germ line, (2) separation of the imprint-organizing center from the imprinted target genes, as seen in BWS germ-line chromosomal rearrangement cases, (3) abnormal methylation of CpG islands, (4) local mutation of regulatory sequences controlling the target imprinted genes themselves, or (5) loss of or mutations in genes for trans-acting factors that maintain normal imprinting. (*Modified from Feinberg AP, Kalikin LM, Johnson LA, Thompson JS: Loss of imprinting in human cancer.* Cold Spring Harbor Symp Quant Biol *59:357–364, 1994, with permission.*)

In considering these diverse factors that could disrupt imprinting, it is important to view normal genomic imprinting as a developmental process rather than as a single event (Fig. 18-3). In addition to an initial mark on the chromosome, an imprinting signal likely propagates along the chromosome, similar to propagation of a signal along the inactive X chromosome. Furthermore, specific genes show tissue-specific imprinting, and the timing of silencing varies from gene to gene during early embryonic development. Thus a combination of both *cis*-acting and *trans*-acting signals is likely to be important in the establishment and maintenance of normal genomic imprinting, and disruption of these same factors can be expected to play a role in LOI in cancer (see Fig. 3-3). It is also important to note that genomic imprinting normally is erased in primordial germ cells during embryonic development, and thus the aberrant expression in tumors, of factors involved in normal imprint erasure, also could cause loss of imprinting.

IMPLICATIONS FOR CANCER TREATMENT

One of the most exciting aspects of the study of LOI in human cancer is that it is potentially reversible, given that normal imprinting involves epigenetic modifications and that imprinting is normally reversible. A recent experiment suggests that this idea shows some promise.[143] Because tumors with LOI show

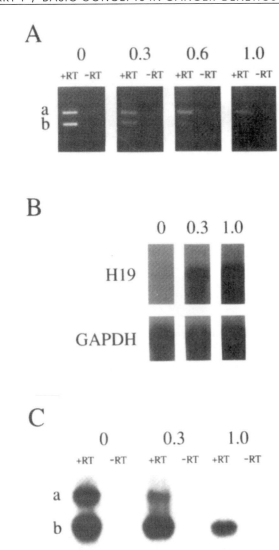

Fig. 3-4 Switch to preferential allelic expression of *IGF2* by 5-aza-2'-deoxycytidine (5-azaCdR) treatment of tumor cells with LOI. RT-PCR was performed on total RNA extracted from JEG-3 choriocarcinoma cells after a single 24-h treatment with 0, 0.3, 0.6, or 1.0 mM 5-azaCdR (indicated). Alternating lanes represent simultaneous experiments with and without reverse transcriptase. PCR products were digested with Apa I. The a and b alleles are 236 and 173 bp, respectively. (*Reprinted from Barletta JM, Rainier S, Feinberg AP: Reversal of loss of imprinting in tumor cells by 5-aza-2'-deoxycytidine. Cancer Res 57:48–50, 1997, with permission.*)

increased methylation of the *H19* CpG island, LOI may be reversed with an inhibitor of DNA methylation, 5-aza-2'-deoxycytidine (5-azaCdR). Two tumor cell lines exhibiting LOI were treated with 5-azaCdR for 24 hours (1 cell division) at concentrations chosen to maximize methylation-related biologic effects. Treatment with increasing doses of 5-azaCdR led to unequal expression of the two *IGF2* alleles in both cell lines (Fig. 3-4). The cells switched from equal expression of the two alleles to predominant expression of the allele represented by the upper uncut band lacking the Apa I polymorphic site, and this effect was nonrandom and specific to one allele. Similarly, 5-azaCdR-treated tumor cells showed a marked increase in *H19* expression similar to that seen in normally imprinted cells. In addition to this reactivation of overall *H19* expression, *H19* also switched from biallelic to monoallelic expression, again consistent with restoration of normal imprinting. Finally, methylation of the imprint-specific CpG island in *H19* switched from virtually complete methylation to the expected pattern of single-allele methylation.[143] In this experiment, since parental DNA was unavailable, the

reestablishment of a normal imprinting pattern could have been due either to a switch of the abnormally imprinted maternal chromosome back to a normal epigenotype. It also could have been due to allele switching, in which the maternal chromosome remained paternally imprinted, but the paternal chromosome switched, to a maternal epigenotype.[143]

Nevertheless, these results are surprising and encouraging because 5-azaCdR may have been expected to show a nonspecific effect on both alleles, similar to that seen in methyltransferase-deficient knockout mice.[118] The fact that 5-azaCdR exerted a specific effect on one chromosome indicates that some imprint-specific information is still retained in tumor cells that show LOI. It further suggests that 5-azaCdR, or drugs with similar effects, may prove useful in the treatment of tumors with LOI, either alone or in conjunction with other agents, and that other strategies for intervention in the pathways regulating genomic imprinting also eventually may be exploited in the design of novel cancer treatments.

ACKNOWLEDGMENT

This work was supported by NIH Grant CA65145.

REFERENCES

1. Tartof KD, Henikoff S: Trans-sensing effects from *Drosophila* to humans. *Cell* **65**:201, 1991.
2. Goldsborough AS, Kornberg TB: Reduction of transcription by homologue asynapsis in *Drosophila* imaginal discs. *Nature* **381**:807, 1996.
3. Patterson GI, Thorpe CJ, Chandler VL: Paramutation, an allelic interaction, is associated with a stable and heritable reduction of transcription of the maze b regulatory gene. *Genetics* **135**:881, 1993.
4. Tartof KD, Bremer M: Mechanisms for the construction and developmental control of heterochromatin formation and imprinted chromosome domains. *Development* (suppl):35, 1990.
5. Tschiersch B, Hofmann A, Krauss V, Dorn R, Korge G, Reuter G: The protein encoded by the *Drosophila* position-effect variegation suppressor gene Su(var)3-9 combines domains of antagonistic regulators of homeotic gene complexes. *EMBO J* **13**:3822, 1994.
6. Gerasimova TI, Gdula DA, Gerasimov DV, Simonova O, Corces VG: A *Drosophila* protein that imparts directionality on a chromatin insulator is an enhancer of position-effect variegation. *Cell* **82**:587, 1995.
7. Brachmann CB, Sherman JM, Devine SE, Cameron EE, Pillus L, Boeke JD: The SIR2 gene family, conserved from bacteria to humans, functions in silencing, cell cycle progression, and chromosome stability. *Genes Dev* **9**:2888, 1995.
8. Crouse H: The controlling element in sex chromosome behavior in Sciara. *Genetics* **45**:1425, 1960.
9. McGrath J, Solter D: Completion of mouse embryogenesis requires both the maternal and paternal genomes. *Cell* **37**:179, 1984.
10. Harper MI, Fosten M, Monk M: Preferential paternal X inactivation in extraembryonic tissues of early mouse embryos. *J Embryol Exp Morphol* **67**:127, 1982.
11. Cattanach BM, Beechey CV: Autosomal and X-chromosome imprinting. *Development* (suppl):63, 1990.
12. Swain JL, Stewart TA, Leder P: Parental legacy determines methylation and expression of an autosomal transgene: A molecular mechanism for parental imprinting. *Cell* **50**:719, 1987.
13. Sapienza C, Paquete J, Tran TH, Peterson A: Epigenetic and genetic factors affect transgene methylation imprinting. *Development* **107**:165, 1989.
14. DeChiara TM, Robertson EJ, Efstratiadis A: Parental imprinting of the mouse insulin-like growth factor-2 gene. *Cell* **64**:849, 1991.
15. Barlow DP, Stoger R, Herrmann BG, Saito K, Schweifer N: The mouse insulin-like growth factor type-2 receptor is imprinted and closely linked to the Tme locus. *Nature* **349**:84, 1991.
16. Kuroiwa Y, Kaneko-Ishino T, Kagitani F, Kohda T, Li L.-L, Tada M, et al: Peg3 imprinted gene on proximal chromosome 7 encodes for a zinc finger protein. *Nature Genet* **12**:186, 1996.
17. Nagai H, Pongliktmongkol M, Kim YS, Yoshikawa H, Matsubara K: Cloning of Not I-cleaved genomic DNA fragments appearing as spots in 2D gel electrophoresis. *Biochem Biophys Res Commun* **213**:258, 1995.

18. Vogelstein B, Fearon ER, Hamilton SR, Feinberg AP: Use of restriction fragment length polymorphisms to determine the clonal origin of human tumors. *Science* **227**:642, 1985.

19. Laird CD: Proposed mechanism of inheritance and expression of the human fragile-X syndrome of mental retardation. *Genetics* **117**:587, 1987.

20. Oberle I, Rousseau F, Heitz D, Kretz C, Devys D, Hanauer A, Boue J, Bertheas MF, Mandel JL: Instability of a 550-base pair DNA segment and abnormal methylation in fragile X syndrome. *Science* **252**:1097, 1991.

21. Fu Y, Kuhl DPA, Pizzuti A, Pieretti M, Sutcliffe JS, Richards S, et al: Variation of the CGG repeat at the fragile X site results in genetic instability: Resolution of the Sherman paradox. *Cell* **67**:1047, 1991.

22. Feng Y, Zhang F, Lokey LK, Chastain JL, Lakkis L, Eberhart D, et al: Translational suppression by trinucleotide repeat expansion at FMR1. *Science* **268**:731, 1995.

23. Nicholls RD, Knoll JHM, Butler MG, Karam S, Lalande M: Genetic imprinting suggested by maternal heterodisomy in nondeletion Prader-Willi syndrome. *Nature* **342**:281, 1989.

24. Knoll JHM, Nicholls RD, Magenis RE, Glatt K, Graham JM Jr, Kaplan L, et al: Angelman syndrome: Three molecular classes identified with chromosome 15q11q13-specific DNA markers. *Am J Hum Genet* **47**:149, 1990.

25. Knoll JH, Nicholls RD, Magenis RE, Graham JM Jr, Lalande M, Latt SA: Angelman and Prader-Willi syndromes share a common chromosome 15 deletion but differ in parental origin of the deletion. *Am J Med Genet* **32**:285, 1989.

26. Mattei MG, Souiah N, Mattei JF: Chromosome 15 anomalies and the Prader-Willi syndrome: Cytogenetic analysis. *Hum Genet* **66**:313, 1984.

27. Nicholls RD: Genomic imprinting and candidate genes in the Prader-Willi and Angelman syndromes. *Curr Opin Genet Dev* **3**:445, 1993.

28. Dittrich B, Buiting K, Korn B, Rickard S, Buxton J, Saitoh S, et al: Imprint switching on human chromosome 15 may involve alternative transcripts of the SNRPN gene. *Nature Genet* **14**:163, 1996.

29. Kishino T, Lalande M, Wagstaff J: UBE3A E6-AP mutations causing Angelman syndrome. *Nature Genet* **15**:70, 1997.

30. Ledbetter DH, Engel E: Uniparental disomy in humans: Development of an imprinting map and its implications for prenatal diagnosis. *Hum Mol Genet* **4**:1757, 1995.

31. Spence JE, Perciaccante RG, Greig GM, Willard HF, Ledbetter DH, Hejtmancik JF, et al: Uniparental disomy as a mechanism for human genetic disease. *Am J Hum Genet* **42**:217, 1988.

32. Kajii T, Ohama K: Androgenetic origin of hydatidiform mole. *Nature* **268**:633, 1977.

33. Linder D, McCaw B, Kaiser X, Hecht F: Parthenogenetic origin of benign ovarian teratomas. *N Engl J Med* **292**:63, 1975.

34. Heutink P, van Schothorst EM, van der Mey AG, Bardoel A, Breedveld G, Pertijs J, et al: Further localization of the gene for hereditary paragangliomas and evidence for linkage in unrelated families. *Eur J Hum Genet* **2**:148, 1994.

35. Reeve AE, Sih SA, Raizis AM, Feinberg AP: Loss of allelic heterozygosity at a second locus on chromosome 11 in sporadic Wilms' tumor cells. *Mol Cell Biol* **9**:1799, 1989.

36. Schroeder W, Chao L, Dao D, Strong L, Pathak S, Riccardi V, et al: Nonrandom loss of maternal chromosome 11 alleles in Wilms tumors. *Am J Hum Genet* **40**:413, 1987.

37. Scrable H, Cavenee W, Ghavimi F, Lovell M, Morgan K, Sapienza C: A model for embryonal rhabdomyosarcoma tumorigenesis that involves genome imprinting. *Proc Natl Acad Sci USA* **86**:7480, 1989.

38. Peterson K, Sapienza C: Imprinting the genome: Imprinted genes, imprinting genes, and a hypothesis for their interaction. *Annu Rev Genet* **27**:7, 1993.

39. Katz F, Webb D, Gibbons B, Reeves B, McMahon C, Chessells J, et al: Possible evidence for genomic imprinting in childhood acute myeloblastic leukaemia associated with monosomy for chromosome 7. *Br J Haematol* **80**:332, 1992.

40. Zhu X, Dunn JM, Phillips RA, Goddard AD, Paton KE, Becker A, et al: Preferential germline mutation of the paternal allele in retinoblastoma. *Nature* **340**:312, 1989.

41. Haas OA, Argyriou-Tirita A, Lion T: Parental origin of chromosomes involved in the translocation t(9;22). *Nature* **359**:414, 1992.

42. Riggins GJ, Zhang F, Warren ST: Lack of imprinting of BCR. *Nature Genet* **6**:226, 1994.

43. Melo JV, Yan XH, Diamond J, Goldman JM: Lack of imprinting of the ABL gene. *Nature Genet* **8**:318, 1994.

44. Melo JV, Yan XH, Diamond J, Goldman JM: Balanced parental contribution to the ABL component of the BCR-ABL gene in chronic myeloid leukemia. *Leukemia* **9**:734, 1995.

45. Cheng JM, Hiemstra JL, Schneider SS, Naumova A, Cheung NV, Cohn SL, et al: Preferential amplification of the paternal allele of the N-myc gene in human neuroblastomas. *Nature Genet* **4**:187, 1993.

46. Caron H, van Sluis P, van Hoeve M, de Kraker J, Bras J, Slater R, et al: Allelic loss of chromosome 1p36 in neuroblastoma is of preferential maternal origin and correlates with N-myc amplification. *Nature Genet* **4**:191, 1993.

47. Caron H, Peter M, van Sluis P, Speleman F, de Kraker J, Laureys G, et al: Evidence for two tumor suppressor loci on chromosomal bands 1p35-36 involved in neuroblastoma: One probably imprinted, another associated with N-myc amplification. *Hum Mol Genet* **4**:535, 1995.

48. Naumova A, Hansen M, Strong L, Jones PA, Hadjistilianou D, Mastrangelo D, et al: Concordance between parental origin of chromosome 13q loss and chromosome 6p duplication in sporadic retinoblastoma. *Am J Hum Genet* **54**:274, 1994.

49. Engstrom W, Lindham S, Schofield P: Wiedemann-Beckwith syndrome. *Eur J Pediatr* **147**:450, 1988.

50. Pettenati MJ, Haines JL, Higgins RR, Wappner RS, Palmer CG, Weaver DD: Wiedemann-Beckwith syndrome: Presentation of clinical and cytogenetic data on 22 new cases and review of the literature. *Hum Genet* **74**:143, 1986.

51. Wiedemann HR: Tumours and hemihypertrophy associated with Wiedemann-Beckwith syndrome. *Eur J Pediatr* **141**:129, 1983.

52. Elias ER, DeBaun MR, Feinberg AP: Beckwith-Wiedemann syndrome, in Jameson JL (ed): *Textbook of Molecular Medicine.* Cambridge, Blackwell Scientific, in press.

53. Viljoen D, Ramesar R: Evidence for paternal imprinting in familial Beckwith-Wiedemann syndrome. *J Med Genet* **29**:221, 1992.

54. Ping AJ, Reeve AE, Law DJ, Young MR, Boehnke M, Feinberg AP: Genetic linkage of Beckwith-Wiedemann syndrome to 11p15. *Am J Hum Genet* **44**:720, 1989.

55. Koufos A, Grundy P, Morgan K, Aleck KA, Hadro T, Lampkin BC, et al: Familial Wiedemann-Beckwith syndrome and a second Wilms tumor locus both map to 11p15. *Am J Hum Genet* **44**:711, 1989.

56. Mannens M, Hoovers JMN, Redeker E, Verjaal M, Feinberg AP, Little P, et al: Parental imprinting of human chromosome region 11p15 involved in the Beckwith-Wiedemann syndrome and various human neoplasia. *Eur J Hum Genet* **2**:3, 1994.

57. Hoovers JMN, Kalikin LM, Johnson LA, Alders M, Redeker B, Law DJ, et al: Multiple genetic loci within 11p15 defined by Beckwith-Wiedemann syndrome: Rearrangement breakpoints and subchromosomal transferable fragments. *Proc Natl Acad Sci USA* **92**:12456, 1995.

58. Henry I, Bonaiti-Pellie C, Chehensse V, Beldjord C, Schwartz C, Utermann G, Junien C: Uniparental paternal disomy in a genetic cancer-predisposing syndrome. *Nature* **351**:609, 1991.

59. Henry I, Peuch A, Riesewijk A, Ahnine L, Mannens M, Beldjord C, et al: Somatic mosaicism for partial paternal isodisomy in Wiedemann-Beckwith syndrome: A post-fertilization event. *Eur J Hum Genet* **1**:19, 1993.

60. Rainier S, Johnson LA, Dobry CJ, Ping AJ, Grundy PE, Feinberg AP: Relaxation of imprinted genes in human cancer. *Nature* **362**:747, 1993.

61. Ohlsson R, Nystrom A, Pfeifer-Ohlsson S, Tohonen V, Hedborg F, Schofield P, et al: IGF2 is parentally imprinted during human embryogenesis and in the Beckwith-Wiedemann syndrome. *Nature Genet* **4**:94, 1993.

62. Ogawa O, Eccles MR, Szeto J, McNoe LA, Yun K, Maw MA, et al: Relaxation of insulin-like growth factor II gene imprinting implicated in Wilms' tumour. *Nature* **362**:749, 1993.

63. Giannoukakis N, Deal C, Paquette J, Goodyer CG, Polychronakos C: Parental genomic imprinting of the human IGF2 gene. *Nature Genet* **4**:98,1993.

64. Bartolomei M, Zemel S, Tilghman SM: Parental imprinting of the mouse H19 gene. *Nature* **351**:153,1991.

65. Zhang Y, Shields T, Crenshaw T, Hao Y, Moulton T, Tycko B: Imprinting of human H19: Allele-specific CpG methylation, loss of the active allele in Wilms tumor, and potential for somatic allele switching. *Am J Hum Genet* **53**:113, 1993.

66. Feinberg AP: Genomic imprinting and gene activation in cancer. *Nature Genet* **4**:110,1993.

67. Feinberg AP, Rainier S, DeBaun MR: Genomic imprinting, DNA methylation, and cancer. *J Natl Cancer Inst Monogr* **17**:21, 1995.

68. Rainier S, Dobry CJ, Feinberg AP: Loss of imprinting in hepatoblastoma. *Cancer Res* **55**:1836, 1995.

69. Li X, Adam G, Cui H, Sandstedt B, Ohlsson R, Ekstrom TJ: Expression, promoter usage and parental imprinting status of insulin-like growth factor II (IGF2) in human hepatoblastoma: Uncoupling of IGF2 and H19 imprinting. *Oncogene* **11**:221, 1995.

70. Zhan SL, Shapiro DN, Helman LJ: Activation of an imprinted allele of the insulin-like growth factor II gene implicated in rhabdomyosarcoma. *J Clin Invest* **94**:445, 1994.

71. Zhan SL, Shapiro DN, Helman LJ: Loss of imprinting of IGF2 in Ewing's sarcoma. *Oncogene* **11**:2503, 1995.

72. Vu TH, Yballe C, Boonyanit S, Hoffman AR: Insulin-like growth factor II in uterine smooth-muscle tumors: Maintenance of genomic imprinting in leiomyomata and loss of imprinting in leiomyosarcomata. *J Clin Endocrinol Metab* **80**:1670, 1995.

73. Doucrasy S, Barrois M, Fogel S, Ahomadegbe JC, Stehelin D, Coll J, et al: High incidence of loss of heterozygosity and abnormal imprinting of H19 and IGF2 genes in invasive cervical carcinomas: Uncoupling of H19 and IGF2 expression and biallelic hypomethylation of H19. *Oncogene* **12**:423, 1996.

74. Hibi K, Nakamura H, Hirai A, Fujikake Y, Kasai Y, Akiyama S, et al: Loss of H19 imprinting in esophageal cancer. *Cancer Res* **56**:480, 1996.

75. Jarrard DF, Bussemakers MJG, Bova GS, Isaacs WB Regional loss of imprinting of the insulin-like growth factor II gene occurs in human prostate tissues. *Clin Cancer Res* **1**:1471, 1995.

76. Kondo M, Suzuki H, Ueda R, Osada H, Takagi K, Takahashi T, et al: Frequent loss of imprinting of the H19 gene is often associated with its overexpression in human lung cancers. *Oncogene* **10**:1193, 1995.

77. Hashomoto K, Azuma C, Koyama M, Ohashi K, Kamiura S, Nobunaga T, et al: Loss of imprinting in choriocarcinoma. *Nature Genet* **9**:109, 1995.

78. Van Gurp RJHLM, Oosterhuis JW, Kalscheuer V, Mariman ECM, Looijenga LHJ: Biallelic expression of the H19 and IGF2 genes in human testicular germ cell tumors. *J Natl Cancer Inst* **86**:1070, 1994.

79. Vu TH, Hoffman AR: Promoter-specific imprinting of the human insulin-like growth factor-II gene. *Nature* **371**:714, 1994.

80. Zhan S, Shapiro D, Zhan S, Zhang L, Hirschfeld S, Elassal J, et al: Concordant loss of imprinting of the human insulin-like growth factor II gene promoters in cancer. *J Biol Chem* **270**:27983, 1995.

81. Steenman MJC, Rainier S, Dobry CJ, Grundy P, Horon IL, Feinberg AP: Loss of imprinting of IGF2 is linked to reduced expression and abnormal methylation of H19 in Wilms' tumor. *Nature Genet* **7**: 433, 1994.

82. Weksberg R, Shen DR, Fei YL, Song QL, Squire J: Disruption of insulin-like growth factor 2 imprinting in Beckwith-Weidemann syndrome. *Nature Genet* **5**:143, 1993.

83. Ogawa O, Becroft DM, Morison IM, Eccles MR, Skeen JE, Mauger DE, et al: Constitutional relaxation of insulin-like growth factor II gene imprinting associated with Wilms' tumour and gigantism. *Nature Genet* **5**:408, 1993.

84. Matsuoka S, Edwards MC, Bai C, Parker S, Zhang P, Baldini A, et al: p57/KIP2, a structurally distinct member of the p21/CIP1 Cdk inhibitor family, is a candidate tumor suppressor gene. *Genes Dev* **9**:650, 1995.

85. Lee M-H, Reynisdottir I, Massague J: Cloning of p57/KIP2, a clini-dependent kinase inhibitor with unique domain structure and tissue distribution. *Genes Dev* **9**:639, 1995.

86. Matsuoka S, Thompson JS, Edwards MC, Barletta JM, Grundy P, Kalikin LM, et al: Imprinting of the gene encoding a human cyclin-dependent kinase inhibitor, p57KIP2, on chromosome 11p15. *Proc Natl Acad Sci USA* **93**:3026, 1996.

87. Thompson JS, Reese KJ, DeBaun MR, Perlman EJ, Feinberg AP: Reduced expression of the cyclin-dependent kinase inhibitor p57KIP2 in Wilms tumor. *Cancer Res* **56**:5723, 1996.

88. Hatada H, Ohashi Y, Fukushima Y, Kaneko M, Inoue Y, Komoto A, et al: An imprinted gene p57KIP2 is mutated in Beckwith-Wiedemann syndrome. *Nature Genet* **14**:171, 1996.

89. Lee MP, DeBaun M, Randhawa G, Reichard BA, Elledge SJ, Feinberg AP: Low frequency of p57KIP2 mutations in Beckwith-Wiedemann syndrome. *Am J Hum Genet* **61**:304, 1997.

90. Pitot HC: Fundamentals of Oncology. New York, Marcel Deckker, 1981.

91. Moulton T, Crenshaw T, Hao Y, Moosikasuwan J, Lin N, Dembitzer F, et al: Epigenetic lesions at the H19 locus in Wilms' tumour patients. *Nature Genet* **7**:440, 1994.

92. Lahm H, Suardet L, Laurent PL, Fischer JR, Ceyhan A, Givel J-C, et al: Growth regulation and co-stimulation of human colorectal cancer cell lines by insulin-like growth factor I, II and transforming growth factor a. *Br J Cancer* **65**:341, 1992.

93. Gelato MC, Vassalotti J: Insulin-like growth factor-II: Possible local growth factor in pheochromocytoma. *J Clin Endocrinol Metab* **71**:1168, 1990.

94. El-Badry OM, Minniti C, Kohn EC, Houghton PJ, Daughaday WH, Helman LJ: Insulin-like growth factor II acts as an autocrine growth and motility factor in human rhabdomyosarcoma tumors. *Cell Growth Diff* **1**:325, 1990.

95. Yee D, Cullen KJ, Paik S, Perdue JF, Hampton B, Schwartz A, et al: Insulin-like growth factor II mRNA expression in human breast cancer. *Cancer Res* **48**:6691, 1988.

96. Lamonerie T, Lavialle C, Haddada H, Brison O: IGF-2 autocrine stimulation in tumorigenic clones of a human colon-carcinoma cell line. *Int J Cancer* **61**:587, 1995.

97. Pommier GJ, Garrouste FL, El Atiq F, Roccabianca M, Marvaldi JL, Remacle-Bonnet MM: Potential autocrine role of insulin-like growth factor II during suramin-induced differentiation of HT29-D4 human colonic adenocarcinoma cell line. *Cancer Res* **52**:3182, 1992.

98. Leventhal PS, Randolph AE, Vesbit TE, Schenone A, Windebank A, Feldman EL: Insulin-like growth factor-II as a paracrine growth factor in human neuroblastoma cells. *Exp Cell Res* **221**:179, 1995.

99. Osborne CK, Coronado EB, Kitten LJ, Arteaga CI, Fuqua SA, Ramasharma K, et al: Insulin-like growth factor-II (IGF-II): A potential autocrine/paracrine growth factor for human breast cancer acting via the IGF-I receptor. *Mol Endocrinol* **3**:1701, 1989.

100. Osborne CK, Clemmons DR, Arteaga CL: Regulation of breast cancer growth by insulin-like growth factors. *J Steroid Biochem Molec Biol* **37**:805, 1990.

101. Vincent TS, Hazen-Martin DJ, Garvin AJ: Inhibition of insulin-like growth factor II autocrine growth of Wilms tumor by suramin in vitro and in vivo. *Cancer Letts* **103**:49, 1996.

102. Miglietta L, Barreca A, Repetto L, Costantini M, Rosso R, Boccardo F: Suramin and serum insulin-like growth factor levels in metastatic cancer patients. *Anticancer Res* **13**:2473, 1993.

103. De Souza AT, Hankins GR, Washington MK, Orton TC, Jirtle RL: M6P/IGF2R gene is mutated in human hepatocellular carcinomas with loss of heterozygosity. *Nature Genet* **11**:447, 1995.

104. Hanahan D: Heritable formation of pancreatic B-cell tumors in transgenic mice expressing recombinant insulin/simian virus 40 oncogenes. *Nature* **315**:115, 1985.

105. Christofori G, Naik P, Hanahan D: A second signal supplied by insulin-like growth factor II in oncogene-induced tumorigenesis. *Nature* **369**:414, 1994.

106. Christofori G, Naik P, Hanahan D: Deregulation of both imprinted and expressed alleles of the insulin-like growth factor 2 gene during B-cell tumorigenesis. *Nature Genet* **10**:196, 1995.

107. Brannan CI, Dees EC, Ingram RS, Tilghman SM: The product of the H19 gene may function as an RNA. *Mol Cell Biol* **10**:28, 1990.

108. Brunkow ME, Tilghman SM: Ectopic expression of the H19 gene in mice causes prenatal lethality. *Genes Dev* **5**:1092, 1991.

109. Pfeifer K, Leighton P, Tilghman SM: The structural H19 gene is required for its own imprinting. *Proc Natl Acad Sci USA* **93**:13876, 1996.

110. Hao Y, Crenshaw T, Moulton T, Newcomb E, Tycko B: Tumor-suppressor activity of H19 RNA. *Nature* **365**:764, 1993.

111. Koi M, Johnson LA, Kalikin LM, Little PFR, Nakamura Y, Feinberg AP: Tumor cell growth arrest caused by subchromosomal transferable DNA fragments from human chromosome 11. *Science* **260**:361, 1993.

112. Cedar H, Razin A: DNA methylation and development. *Biochim Biophys Acta* **1049**:1, 1990.

113. Riggs AD: DNA methylation and cell memory. *Cell Biophys* **15**:1, 1989.

114. Bird AP: CpG-rich islands and the function of DNA methylation. *Nature* **321**:209, 1986.

115. Riggs AD, Pfeifer GP: X-chromosome inactivation and cell memory. *Trends Genet* **8**:169, 1992.

116. Ferguson-Smith AC, Sasaki H, Cattanach BM, Surani MA: Parental-origin-specific epigenetic modification of the mouse H19 gene. *Nature* **362**:751, 1993.

117. Bartolomei M, Webber AL, Brunkow ME, Tilghman SM: Epigenetic mechanisms underlying the imprinting of the mouse H19 gene. *Genes Dev* **7**:1663, 1993.

118. Li E, Beard C, Jaenisch R: Role for DNA methylation in genomic imprinting. *Nature* **366**:362, 1993.

119. Stoger R, Kubicka P, Liu C-G, Kafri T, Razin A, Cedar H, et al: Maternal-specific methylation of the imprinted mouse IGF2 locus identifies the expressed locus as carrying the imprinting signal. *Cell* **73**:61, 1993.

120. Feinberg AP, Vogelstein B: Hypomethylation distinguishes genes of some human cancers from their normal counterparts. *Nature* **301**:89, 1983.

121. Goelz SE, Vogelstein B, Hamilton SR, Feinberg AP: Hypomethylation of DNA from benign and malignant human colon neoplasms. *Science* **228**:187, 1985.

122. Feinberg AP, Gehrke CW, Kuo KC, Ehrlich M: Reduced genomic 5-methylcytosine content in human colonic neoplasia. *Cancer Res* **48**:1159, 1988.

123. Feinberg AP: Alterations in DNA methylation in colorectal polyps and cancer. *Prog Clin Biol Res* **279**:309, 1988.

124. Jones PA, Buckley JD: The role of DNA methylation in cancer. *Adv Cancer Res* **54**:1, 1990.

125. Laird PW, Jackson-Grusby L, Fazeli A, Dickinson SL, Jung WE, Li E, et al: Suppression of intestinal neoplasia by DNA hypomethylation. *Cell* **81**:197, 1995.

126. Reik W, Brown KW, Slatter RE, Sartori P, Elliott M, Maher ER: Allelic methylation of H19 and IGF2 in the Beckwith-Wiedemann syndrome. *Hum Mol Genet* **3**:1297, 1995.

127. Reik W, Brown KW, Schneid H, Bouc YL, Bickmore W, Maher ER: Imprinting mutations in the Beckwith-Wiedemann syndrome suggested by an altered imprinting pattern in the IGF2-H19 domain. *Hum Mol Genet* **4**:2379, 1995.

128. El-Deiry WS, Nelkin BD, Celano P, Yen RC, Falco JP, Hamilton SR, et al: High expression of the DNA methyltransferase gene characterizes human neoplastic cells and progression stages of colon cancer. *Proc Natl Acad Sci USA* **88**:3470, 1991.

129. Schmutte C, Yang AS, Nugyen TT, Beart RB, Jones PA: Mechanisms for the involvement of DNA methylation in colon cancer. *Cancer Res* **56**:2375, 1996.

130. Lee PJ, Washer LL, Law DJ, Boland CR, Horon IL, Feinberg AP: Limited upregulation of DNA methyltransferase in human colon cancer reflecting increased cell proliferation. *Proc Natl Acad Sci USA* **93**:10366, 1996.

131. Lee MP, Hu R-J, Johnson LA, Feinberg AP: Human KVLQT1 gene shows tissue-specific imprinting and encompasses Beckwith-Wiedemann syndrome chromosomal rearrangements. *Nature Genet* **15**:181, 1997.

132. Allen ND, Norris ML, Surani MA: Epigenetic control of transgene expression and imprinting by genotype-specific modifiers. *Cell* **61**:353, 1990.

133. Wolffe AP: Inheritance of chromatin states. *Dev Genet* **15**:463, 1994.

134. Thompson JS, Ling X, Grunstein M: Histone H3 amino terminus is required for telomeric and silent mating. *Nature* **369**:245, 1994.

135. Yoshida M, Kijima M, Akita M, Beppu T: Potent and specific inhibition of mammalian histone deacetylase both in vivo and in vitro by trichostatin A. *J Biol Chem* **265**:17174, 1990.

136. Efstratiadis A: Parental imprinting of autosomal mammalian genes. *Curr Opin Genet Dev* **4**:265, 1994.

137. Brownell JE, Zhou J, Ranalli T, Kobayashi R, Edmondson DG, Roth SY, et al: Tetrahymena histone acetyltransferase A: A homolog to yeast gcn5p linking histone acetylation to gene activation. *Cell* **84**:843, 1996.

138. Taunton J, Hassig CA, Schreiber SL: A mammalian histone deacetylase related to the yeast transcriptional regulator rpd3p. *Science* **272**:408, 1996.

139. Walters MC, Magis W, Fiering S, Eidemiller J, Scalzo D, Groudine M, et al: Transcriptional enhancers act in cis to suppress position-effect variegation. *Genes Dev* **10**:185, 1996.

140. Kitsberg D, Selig S, Brandeis M, Simon I, Keshet I, Driscoll DJ, et al: Allele-specific replication timing of imprinted gene regions. *Nature* **364**:459, 1993.

141. LaSalle JM, Lalande M: Homologous association of oppositely imprinted chromosomal domains. *Science* **272**:725, 1996.

142. Tatof KD, Henikoff S: Trans-sensing effects from *Drosophila* to humans. *Cell* **65**:201, 1991.

143. Barletta JM, Rainier S, Feinberg AP: Reversal of loss of imprinting in tumor cells by 5-aza-2'-deoxycytidine. *Cancer Res* **57**:48, 1997.

144. Feinberg AP, Kalikin LM, Johnson LA, Thompson JS: Loss of imprinting in human cancer. *Cold Spring Harbor Symp Quant Biol* **59**:357, 1994.

145. Lee MP, Feinberg AP: Genomic imprinting of a human apoptosis gene homologue, TSSC3. *Cancer Res* **58**:1052, 1998.

146. Qian N, Frank D, O'Keefe D, Dao D, Zhao L, Yuan L, Wang Q, et al: The IPL gene on chromosome 11p15.5 is imprinted in human and mice and is similar to TDAG51, implicated in Fas expression and apoptosis. *Hum Mol Genet* **6**:2021, 1997.

147. Lee MP, DeBaun MR, Mitsuya K, Galonek HL, Brandenburg S, Oshimura M, Feinberg AP: Loss of imprinting of a paternally expressed transcript, with antisense orientation to K$_V$LQT1, occurs frequently in Beckwith-Wiedemann syndrome and is independent of IGF2 imprinting. *Proc Natl Acad Sci USA* **96**:5203, 1999.

148. Dao D, Frank D, Qian N, O'Keefe D, Vosatka RJ, Walsh CP, Tycko B: IMPT1, an imprinted gene similar to polyspecific transporter and multi-drug resistance genes. *Hum Mol Genet* **7**:597, 1998.

149. Schwienbacher C, Sabbioni S, Campi M, Veronese A, Bernardi G, Menegatti A, Hatada I, et al: Transcriptional map of 170-kb region at chromosome 11p15.5: identification and mutational analysis of the BWR1A gene reveals the presence of mutations in tumor samples. *Proc Natl Acad Sci USA* **95**:3873, 1998.

150. Cui H, Horon IL, Ohlsson R, Hamilton SR, Feinberg AP: Loss of Imprinting in normal tissue of colorectal cancer patients with microsatellite instability. *Nature Med* **4**:1276, 1998.

Genes Altered by Chromosomal Translocations in Leukemias and Lymphomas

A. Thomas Look

1. **Somatically acquired chromosomal translocations activate proto-oncogenes in the hematopoietic cells of both children and adults. This mechanism of gene dysregulation contributes to well over 50 percent of all leukemias that have been characterized cytogenetically and molecularly and to a substantial proportion of lymphomas, notably the Burkitt, large-cell, and follicular types.**

2. **In most instances, chromosomal translocations fuse sequences of a transcription factor or receptor tyrosine kinase gene to those of a normally unrelated gene, resulting in a chimeric protein with oncogenic properties. Repositioning of transcriptional control genes to the vicinity of highly active promoter/enhancer elements, such as those associated with immunoglobulin or T-cell receptor genes, is a second mechanism by which chromosomal translocations induce malignancy.**

3. **The vast majority of translocation-induced leukemias and lymphomas are restricted to cells of a single lineage arrested at a particular stage of development, indicating that the disrupted genes regulate vital processes limited to a subset of committed hematopoietic progenitors. Occasionally, as exemplified by leukemias arising from *MLL* gene abnormalities, more than one lineage or developmental stage is affected, suggesting the involvement of genes active in pluripotent or bipotent stem cells.**

4. **The number of fusion genes with diagnostic and prognostic relevance is increasing rapidly. The hybrid mRNAs produced by these novel structures provide specific molecular probes for identifying affected patients who cannot be diagnosed readily by conventional means or who require chemotherapy tailored to the risk conferred by a particular genetic lesion.**

5. **Studies in murine models, in which specific genes are mutated and homozygously inactivated in "knockout" mice or overexpressed in transgenic mice, have contributed new insights into the essential roles that are played in normal development and oncogenesis by genes discovered because of their proximity to the breakpoints of chromosomal translocations in the human leukemias and lymphomas.**

A list of standard abbreviations is located immediately preceding the index. Nonstandard abbreviations used in this chapter include: bHLH = basic region/helix-loop-helix; bZIP = basic region/leucine zipper; ALL = acute lymphoblastic leukemia; AML = acute myeloid leukemia; DIC = disseminated intravascular coagulation; CMML = chronic myelomonocytic leukemia; APML = acute promyelocytic leukemia; CML = chronic myeloid leukemia; MDS = myelodysplastic syndrome.

The concept that cancer cells contain genetic information not found in normal cells has provided the impetus for molecular approaches to cancer research. A pivotal step in this progress was the realization that gross chromosomal changes—such as translocations, deletions, inversions and amplifications—can perturb genes intimately involved in carcinogenesis.[1-3] Thus a major concern over the past two decades has been the identification of consistent chromosomal abnormalities in specific types of tumor cells, the isolation of genes affected by these changes, and the elucidation of their mechanisms of action and clinical correlations. A surprising dividend of this venture, aided by technology that permits one to create homozygous null animals by inactivating individual genes (e.g., "knockout" mice), has been the discovery of proteins that not only promote cancer but also have essential functions in normal cell development as well.[4]

Specific reciprocal translocations perhaps are the best example of how cytogenetic changes pave the way for cancer induction and spread. These nonheritable abnormalities occur in a high percentage of hematologic cancers—both leukemias and lymphomas—where they disrupt signaling pathways that enhance cell survival.[4-7] Their actions can directly activate occult proto-oncogenes or, more commonly, create cell type-specific fusion proteins that contain elements of one or more transcription factors.[5,8] It is intriguing that many of the genes involved in translocation-mediated fusions have close homologues in genes controlling embryogenesis in *Drosophila* and other invertebrates, underscoring their faithful conservation in nature and their relevance to programs of early cell development.[9-11] Unfortunately, the downstream genetic programs controlled by the various transcription factors affected by chromosomal translocations are largely unknown, so interrelationships between transcription networks and leukemogenesis remain to be assessed.

The medical benefits gained from analysis of chromosomal translocations in the leukemias and lymphomas are still modest. One of the difficulties is that fusion proteins typically are localized to the cell nucleus, making them inaccessible to most available therapies, requiring instead the introduction of therapeutic molecules into the cell. Nonetheless, the chimeric RNA and DNA of these lesions provide highly specific targets for molecular assays that can resolve interpretive ambiguities created by conventional diagnostic or cell classification methods.[12] One emerging application is the use of polymerase chain reaction-(PCR)-based techniques to detect chimeric RNA in residual leukemia cells.[13] Other applications include the detection of specific high-risk genetic lesions, such as the *E2A-PBX1, MLL-AF4,* and *BCR-ABL* fusion genes, to ensure that patients are assigned to sufficiently aggressive treatment programs.[7,14]

This chapter summarizes the molecular consequences of translocations in the human leukemias and lymphomas. Emphasis is placed on disease types with the highest frequencies of productive rearrangements and on those (often rare) types in which study of molecular aberrations has revealed novel principles of pathogenesis.

DYSREGULATION OF TRANSCRIPTIONAL CONTROL GENES

The majority of transcription factors that are altered by chromosomal translocations in the leukemias and lymphomas (Table 4-1) can be classified into four major types on the basis of recurring structural elements within their DNA- and protein-binding domains: basic region/helix-loop-helix (bHLH), basic region/leucine zipper (bZIP), zinc finger, and homeodomain.[6,8,15] Other less common but still functionally significant motifs include A-T hook, Ets-like, Runt homology, and cysteine-rich (LIM). In some cases, a transcription factor gene is rearranged to a site adjacent to a T-cell receptor (*TCR*) or immunoglobulin (*Ig*) locus, resulting in dysregulated expression of the proto-oncogenic sequences. A second, perhaps more common mechanism involves chromosomal rearrangements that fuse transcriptional control genes into functional chimeras. Such fusions are important because they give rise to novel proteins capable of interacting with DNA and other regulatory elements in ways that usurp normal cellular control mechanisms.[6]

The diversity of transcription factor proto-oncogenes implicated in the human leukemias and lymphoma is striking, although increasingly their essential functions can be traced to a fundamental step in cell growth, development, or survival.[8] Currently, more than 10 transcriptional control genes have been shown to play critical roles in normal hematopoiesis (Fig. 4-1). Some of these factors are lineage-specific, whereas others operate early in hematopoietic development, before lineage commitment. Still others are widely expressed but perform unique functions in a limited number of blood cell types, ostensibly by interacting with lineage-restricted proteins.[4] Of major pathobiologic importance, many transcription factors that control blood cell differentiation are targets for productive rearrangement by translocations in the

leukemias and lymphomas, reinforcing their roles as master regulators of hematopoietic cell development. In the following sections I summarize how chromosomal translocations modify transcription factors to generate malignant cells within the hematopoietic system.

Acute Lymphoblastic Leukemias and Non-Hodgkin Lymphomas

The frequency distributions of the various molecular abnormalities mediated by chromosomal translocations are shown diagrammatically in Figs. 4-2 and 4-3, with key associations given in Tables 4-1 and 4-2.

***MYC* Activation in Burkitt Lymphoma and B-Cell Leukemia.** In Burkitt lymphoma and B-cell leukemia, arising in surface Ig-positive "virgin" B lymphoblasts with moderately abundant, vacuolated cytoplasm, the principal genetic change is a juxtapositioning of the *MYC* proto-oncogene next to the *Ig* heavy-chain gene as a result of the t(8;14)(q24;q32).[16-18] *MYC* is a prototypic bHLH/leucine zipper transcription factor whose rearrangement from chromosome 8 to a site near strong *Ig* enhancer elements on chromosome 14 leads to dysregulated expression of the *MYC* oncoprotein. In most instances, the t(8;14) is responsible for inappropriate activation of *MYC*; however, two variants of this rearrangement can produce the same effect, except that they move *Igκ* and *Igλ* light chain genes from chromosome 2 and 22, respectively, to the *MYC* locus on chromosome 8.[19-24] The *MYC* gene often acquires point mutations in its coding or regulatory regions, probably as a result of somatic mutation that occurs after translocation,[25-28] which in some cases encodes proteins that are unable to interact with the *Rb*-related gene *p107*.[29]

A leading question since the discovery of *MYC* activation in Burkitt lymphoma/B-cell leukemia has been: How does the MYC oncoprotein transform B lymphocytes? The answer seems to lie in the effects of *MYC* dysregulation on a transcriptional network comprising at least three other factors, each also harboring bHLH/leucine zipper domains. In this cascade, MYC is able to dimerize with the MAX protein,[30,31] which can bind to DNA, to itself

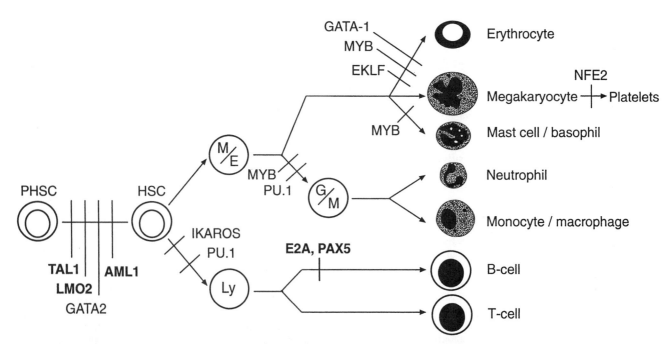

Fig. 4-1 Schematic diagram showing the relative stages at which transcription factors exert their influence on hematopoietic development. Only proteins whose activities have been demonstrated in knockout mice are shown. Factors serving as targets of chromosomal translocations in the leukemias and lymphomas are indicated in boldface type. Note that transcription factor targets can be lineage specific (E2A) or uncommitted to a particular differentiation pathway (AML1). HSC, hematopoietic stem cell; M/E, myeloid/erythroid progenitor; Ly, lymphoid progenitor; G/M, granulocyte/macrophage progenitor. (*Adapted from Shivdasani and Orkin.*[4] Used with permission).

Table 4-1 Transcriptional Control Genes Dysregulated by Chromosomal Translocations that Contribute to Human Leukemias and Lymphomas

Disease	Chromosomal Abnormality	Activated	Mechanism of Activation	Predominate Structural Feature*	Invertebrate Homologue†	References
Lymphoid Leukemia/Lymphoma						
B-cell ALL/Burkitt	t(8;14)(q24;q32)	MYC	Relocation to IgH locus	bHLHzip		16–18
Lymphoma	t(2;8)(p12;q24)	MYC	Relocation to IgL locus	bHLHzip		19, 20, 22, 24
	t(8;22)(q24;q11)	MYC	Relocation to IgL locus	bHLHzip		21, 23
Pre-B-cell All	t(1;19)(q23;p13)	E2A-PBX1	Gene fusion	Homeodomain (PBX1)	exd (D), ceh-20 (C)	130, 131
Pro-B-cell ALL	t(17;19)(q22;p13)	E2A-HLF	Gene fusion	bZIP (HLF)	giant (D), ces-2 (C)	178, 179
Pro-B-cell ALL	t(12;21)(p13;q22)	TEL-AML1	Gene fusion	Runt homology (AML1)	runt (D)	197–201
T-cell ALL	t(8;14)(q24;q11)	MYC	Relocation to TCRα/δ locus	bHLHzip		51–53
	t(7;19)(q35;p13)	LYL1	Relocation to TCRβ locus	HLH		48
	t(1;14)(p32;q11)	TAL1	Relocation to TCRα/δ locus	bHLH		45–47
	t(7;9)(q35;q34)	TAL2	Relocation to TCRβ locus	bHLH		47
	t(11;14)(p15;q11)	LMO1 (RBTN1)	Relocation to TCRα/δ locus	Cysteine-rich		77, 78
	t(11;14)(p13;q11)	LMO2 (RBTN2)	Relocation to TCRα/β locus	Cysteine-rich		79, 80
	t(7;11)(q35;p13)	LMO2 (RBTN2)	Relocation to TCRβ locus	Cysteine-rich		
	t(10;14)(q24;q11)	HOX11	Relocation to TCRα/δ locus	Homeodomain		97–100
	t(7;10)(q35;q24)	HOX11	Relocation to TCRβ locus	Homeodomain		
Diffuse B-cell lymphoma (large cell)	t(3;14)(q27;q32)	BCL6	Relocation to IgH locus	Zinc finger	tramtrack (D)	212–215
	t(3;4)(q27;p11)	BCL6	Relocation to TTF locus	Zinc finger	tramtrack (D)	213, 537
B-CLL	t(14;19)(q32;q13)	BCL3	Relocation to IgH locus	IκB homology		538–540
B-cell lymphoma	t(10;14)(q24;q32)	LYT10	Relocation to IgH locus	Rel homology	dorsal (D)	541
Lymphoplasmacytoid B-cell lymphoma	t(9;14)(p13;q32)	PAX5	Relocation to IgH locus	Paired homeobox	Paired (D)	542
Myeloid Leukemia						
AML (granulocytic)	t(8;21)(q22;q22)	AML1-ETO	Gene fusion	Runt homology (AML1)	runt (D)	226–228, 543
Myelodysplasia	t(3;21)(q26;q22)	AML1-EAP	Gene fusion	Runt homology (AML1)	runt (D)	231
CML (blast crisis)	t(3;21)(q26;q22)	AML1-EVI1	Gene fusion	Runt homology (AML1)	runt (D)	230
AML (undifferentiated)	t(3;v)(q26;v)	EVI1	Aberrant expression	Zinc finger	evil (D)	322, 323
AML (myelomonocytic)	inv(16)(p13;q22)	CBFβ-MYH11	Gene fusion	Complex with AML1 (CBFβ)		251
AML (promyelocytic)	t(15;17)(q21;q21)	PML-RARα	Gene fusion	Zinc finger (RARα)		268–272
AML (promyelocytic)	t(11;17)(q23;q21)	PLZF-RARα	Gene fusion	Zinc finger (RARα)		292
AML (promyelocytic)	t(5;17)(q32;q12)	NPM-RARα	Gene fusion	Zinc finger (RARα)		290
AML (promyelocytic)	t(11;17)(q13;q21)	NₙMA–RARα	Gene fusion	Zinc finger (RARα)		291
AML	t(16;21)(p11;q22)	FUS-ERG	Gene fusion	Ets-like (ERG)		544
AML	t(12;22)(p13;q11)	TEL-MN1	Gene fusion	Ets-like (TEL)		545
Myelodysplasia	t(3;12)(q26;p13)	TEL-EVI1	Gene fusion	Zinc finger (EVI1) / Ets-like (TEL)	evi1 (D)	546
AML (myelomonocytic)	t(8;16)(p11;p13)	MOZ-CBP	Gene fusion	Zinc finger (MOZ) / CREB-binding protein (CBP)	Pointed (D)	547
AML (myelomonocytic)	inv(8)(p11;q13)	MOZ-TIFZ	Gene fusion	Zinc finger (MOZ) / Nuclear receptor coactivator (TIFZ)		548

(Continued on next page)

Table 4-1 (continued)

Disease	Chromosomal Abnormality	Activated	Mechanism of Activation	Predominate Structural Feature*	Invertebrate Homologue[†]	References
Mixed-Lineage Leukemias[‡]						
Pro-B-cell ALL	t(4;11)(q21;q23)	*MLL-AF4*	Gene fusion	A–T hook (MLL)	*trithorax* (D)	342, 344, 345
AML (monocytic)	t(9;11)(q21;q23)	*MLL-AF9*	Gene fusion	A–T hook (MLL)	*trithorax* (D)	363
ALL/AML	t(11;19)(q23;p13.3)	*MLL-ENL*	Gene fusion	A–T hook (MLL)	*trithorax* (D)	341, 355, 363
AML	t(11;19)(q23;p13.1)	*MLL-ELL*	Gene fusion	A–T hook (MLL)	*trithorax* (D)	355, 356
AML	t(1;11)(q21;q23)	*MLL-AF1Q*	Gene fusion	A–T hook (MLL)	*trithorax* (D)	366
AML	t(1;11)(1p32;q23)	*MLL-AF1P*	Gene fusion	A–T hook (MLL)	*trithorax* (D)	549
AML	t(6;11)(q27;q23)	*MLL-AF6*	Gene fusion	A–T hook (MLL)	*trithorax* (D)	389
AML	t(6;11)(q12;q23)	*MLL-AF6QZ1*	Gene fusion	A–T hook (MLL)	*trithorax* (D)	550
AML	t(10;11)(p12;q23)	*MLL-AF10*	Gene fusion	A–T hook (MLL)	*trithorax* (D)	551
AML	t(11;17)(q23;q21)	*MLL-AF17*	Gene fusion	A–T hook (MLL)	*trithorax* (D)	552
AML	t(X;11)(q13;q23)	*MLL-AFX1*	Gene fusion	A–T hook (MLL)	*trithorax* (D)	553
AMML/CMML	t(11;16)(q23;p13)	*MLL-CBP*	Gene fusion	A–T hook (MLL)	*trithorax* (D)	554, 555

Abbreviations: AML, acute myeloid leukemia; ALL, acute lymphoblastic leukemia; CML, chronic myelogenous leukemia; CMML, chronic myelomonocytic leukemia; bHLHzip, basic region/helix-loop-helix/leucine zipper domain; bZIP, basic region/leucine zipper domain.

*Based on analysis of DNA-binding/protein interaction domain. For gene fusions, the partner contributing this structural feature is given in parentheses.

[†]Organism type is shown in parenthesis: D = *Drosophila*; C = *C. Elegans*.

[‡]Only the predominate lineage is given for *MLL* gene rearrangements.

60

Table 4-2 Tyrosine Kinase and Other Genes Dysregulated by Chromosomal Translocations in Human Leukemias and Lymphomas

Disease	Chromosomal Abnormality	Activated Gene	Mechanism of Activation	Predominate Structural Feature*	Invertebrate Homologue†	References
Tyrosine Kinases						
CMML	t(5;12)(q33;p13)	TEL-PDGFRβ	Gene fusion	Tyrosine kinase (PDGFRB)		443
Pre-B-ALL	t(9;12)(p24;p13)	TEL-JAK2	Gene fusion	Tyrosine kinase (JAK2)	Hopscotch (D)	556, 557
T-cell ALL	t(9;12)(p24;p13)	TEL-AK2	Gene fusion	Tyrosine kinase (JAK2)	Hopscotch (D)	
CML (atypical)	t(9;12;14)	TEL-JAK2	Gene fusion	Tyrosine kinase (JAK2)	Hopscotch (D)	
CMML	t(5;7)(q33;q11.2)	HIPI-PDGFβR	Gene fusion	Tyrosine kinase (PDGFβR) Huntington interactin protein (HIP1)		558
AML	t(5;14)(q33;q32)	CEV14-PDGFβR	Gene fusion	Tyrosine kinase (PDGFβR)		559
AML	t(9;12;14)(q34;p13;q22)	TEL-ABL	Gene fusion	Tyrosine kinase (ABL)	abl (D)	203, 442
Anaplastic large-cell lymphoma	t(2;5)(p23;q35)	NPM-ALK	Gene fusion	Tyrosine kinase (ALK)		457
CML	t(9;22)(q34;q11)	BCR-ABL	Gene fusion	Tyrosine kinase (ABL)	abl (D)	407, 413, 416, 417
ALL	t(9;22)(q34;q11)	BCR-ABL	Gene fusion	Tyrosine kinase (ABL)	abl (D)	422–424
T-cell ALL	t(1;7)(p34;q34)	LCK	Relocation to TCRβ locus	Tyrosine kinase		560–562
Other Genes						
Centrocytic B-cell lymphoma	t(11;14)(q13;q32)	Cyclin D1	Relocation to IgH locus	G1 cyclin		493, 494, 499–502
Follicular B cell lymphoma	t(14;18)(q32;q21)	BCL2	Relocation to IgH locus	Antiapoptotic domain	ced-9 (C)	517–520
AML	t(6;9)(p23;q34)	DEK-CAN	Gene fusion	Nucleoporin (CAN)		563
AML	t(9;9)(q34;q34)	SET-CAN	Gene fusion	Nucleoporin (CAN)		528
AML	t(7;11)(p15;p15)	NUP98-HOXA9	Gene fusion	Nucleoporin (NUP98)		529, 530
AML	t(3;5)(q35;q35)	NPM-MLF1	Gene fusion	Nucleolar shuttle protein (NPM)		535
AML	t(10;11)(p13;q14)	CALM-AF10	Gene fusion	Clathrin assembly (CLM)	Cezf (C)	564
T-cell PLL	t(x;14)(q28;q11)	C6.1B	Relocation to TCRα/δ locus	Unknown		565
T-cell ALL	t(7;9)(q34;q34)	TAN1	Relocation to TCRβ locus	EGF cysteine repeats	Notch (D), lin-12 (C)	566
Pre-B-cell ALL	t(5;14)(q31;q32)	IL-3	Relocation to IgH locus	Growth factor		567, 568
T-cell lymphoma	t(4;16)(q26;p13)	IL2-BCM	Gene fusion	Growth factor		569
T-cell PLL	t(14;14)(q11;q32)	TCL1	Relocation to TCRα/δ locus	Unknown		570
	inv(14)(q11;q32)	TCL1	Relocation to TCRα/δ locus	Unknown		
	t(7;14)(q35;q32)	TCL1	Relocation to TCRβ locus	Unknown		
T-cell PLL	t(X;14)(q28;q11)	MTCP1	Relocation to TCRα/δ locus	Unknown		571, 572
B-cell lymphoma	t(11;14)(q23;q32)	RCK	Relocation to IgH locus	Helicase/translation initiation factor		573

Abbreviations: AML, acute myeloid leukemia; ALL, acute lymphoblastic leukemia; CML, chronic myelogenous leukemia; CMML, chronic myelomonocytic leukemia; T-cell PLL, T-cell prolymphocytic leukemia.
*For gene fusions, the partner contributing this structural feature is given in parentheses.
†Organism type is shown in parenthesis: D = *Drosophila*; C = *C. Elegans*.

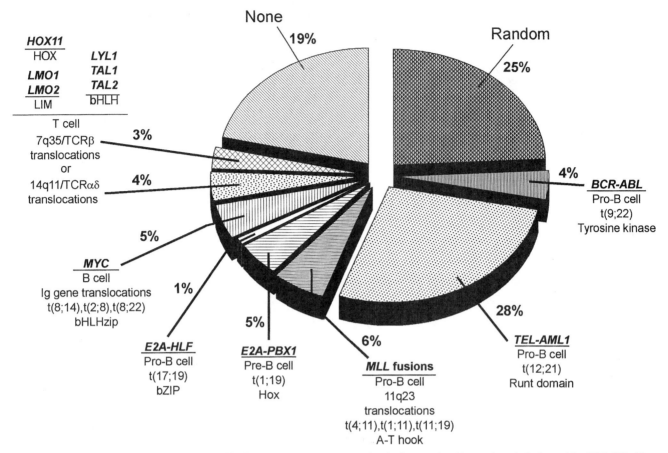

Fig. 4-2 Distribution of translocation-generated fusion genes among the commonly recognized immunologic subtypes of ALL in children and young adults. Key domains for DNA binding and protein-protein interaction of transcription factors are shown in boldface type; an exception is the tyrosine kinase domain indicated for BCR-ABL. The section labeled *random* refers to sporadic rearrangements that have so far been observed only in leukemic cells from single cases. (*Adapted from Look.[211] Used with permission*).

(MAX/MAX homodimers), and to the MAD and MXI-1 family of transcription factors.[32,33] Since MYC/MAX heterodimers activate gene expression,[30,31] whereas MAD/MAX heterodimers act as trans-repressors through an association with a protein called SIN3,[34,35] and since MYC and MAD have equal affinities for MAX,[36,37] increased expression of MYC in B lymphocytes is thought to disrupt the equilibrium of MAX heterodimers, leading to untimely activation of responder genes and ultimately to malignant transformation.[38] Experimental support for this hypothesis comes from the induction of B-cell neoplasms in transgenic mice carrying the *MYC* oncogene driven by an *Ig* gene enhancer.[39,40] An activated *MYC* gene also induces tumorigenic conversion when it is introduced in vitro into B lymphoblasts infected with human Epstein-Barr virus.[41] More recent observations implicate the ornithine decarboxylase gene,[42] the *CDC25* cell-cycle phosphatase gene,[43] and the *ARF* tumor suppressor gene[44] as relevant transcriptional targets of MYC/MAX heterodimers.

***bHLH, LIM,* and *HOX11* Genes.** The role of transcription factors as the preferred targets of chromosomal translocations extends to the T-cell lymphomas and acute leukemias, in which the chromosomal breakpoints consistently appear near enhancers included in the *TCR β* locus on chromosome 7, band q34, or the α/δ locus on chromosome 14, band q11. Highly active in committed T-cell progenitors, these enhancers stimulate the expression of strategically translocated transcription factors that regulate early hematopoietic cell development or the development of other lineages but are not normally expressed in T lymphoid cells (see Table 4-1). Notable examples include the *bHLH* genes, *TAL1/SCL*,[45–47] *TAL2/SCL2*,[47] and *LYL1*,[48] one of which is essential for the development of all blood cell lineages (*TAL1/SCL*).[4,49,50] The more distantly related *MYC* bHLH/ZIP protein is dysregulated in T-cell[51–53] as well as B-cell lymphomas and leukemias.

When rearranged near enhancers within the *TCR β* locus on chromosome 7, band q34, or the α/δ chain locus on chromosome 14, band q11, these regulatory genes become active, and their protein products are thought to bind inappropriately to the promoter/enhancer elements of upstream target genes. The *TAL1* gene, for example, is activated by the t(1;14) or by an intragenic deletion on the 5′ side of the gene that places it under the regulation of the promoter of a gene called *SIL*[54–58]; these rearrangements affect up to one-fourth of all cases of childhood T-cell leukemias and lymphomas.[59,60] Since the TAL1 protein can dimerize with the E2A protein through its bHLH domain to form DNA-binding complexes,[61] and with the LMO2 protein (see below),[61–65] its ectopic expression in T cells bearing the t(1;14) or activating deletions may aberrantly activate specific sets of target genes that are normally quiescent in T-lineage progenitors. It is also possible that TAL1 acts by repressing E2A activity during T-cell development, because E2A/TAL1 heterodimers are inactive as transcriptional trans-activators.[66,67]

Interestingly, TAL1 has emerged as an essential regulator of very early stages of hematopoietic development.[68] Within the hematopoietic system, TAL1 expression is restricted to myeloid and erythroid progenitor cells, megakaryocytes, and mast cells,[69–71] and as noted previously, it is not expressed by normal T lymphocytes or their progenitors.[72] Gene targeting experiments initially showed that mouse embryos lacking a functional *Tal1* gene were devoid of embryonic red blood cells and died at embryonic days 9 to 10.5 of anemia.[49,50] Additional studies of

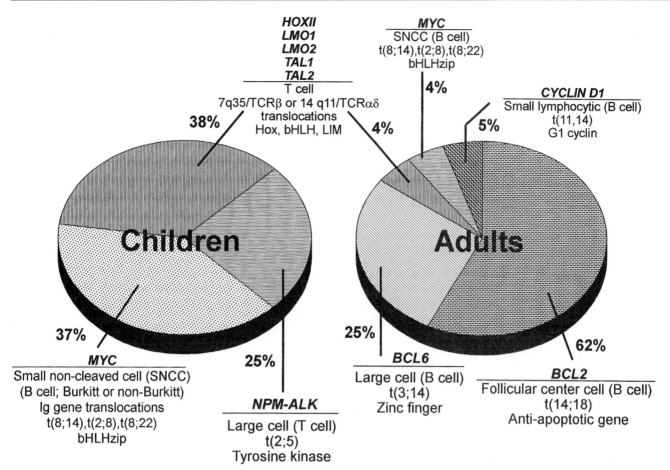

Fig. 4-3 Distribution of histologic subtypes of non-Hodgkin lymphoma in children and adults. Chromosomal translocations and affected genes that occur in a significant fraction (but not all) of the cases within each subtype are shown. (*Adapted from Sandlund, Downing, and Crist.*[574] *Used with permission*).

hematopoietic precursors generated by in vitro differentiation of *Tal* −/− embryonic stem cells, and by assessing the contribution of these cells in vivo to the hematopoietic systems of chimeric mice, have shown that *Tal1* is required for the generation of all hematopoietic cell lineages, including T lymphocytes, suggesting that it plays an essential role in early hematopoietic development, either at the level of mesoderm induction or in maintaining the viability of multipotential hematopoietic progenitors.[68] It would not be surprising if Tal1 were involved in a network of regulatory factors responsible for induction of the hematopoietic lineage, in view of the similar roles of related bHLH proteins as master regulators of mesodermal cell fate, such as those of the MyoD family (MyoD, Myf-5, MRF4, and myogenin),[73,74] which, like the Tal1 protein, form heterocomplexes with the E12/E47 products of the *E2A* gene. An interesting zebrafish mutant cloche affects both blood and endothelial differentiation,[75] and recent microinjection studies suggest that *SCL* acts downstream of cloche to specify hematopoietic and vascular differentiation.[76]

Other types of regulatory genes can be rearranged near *TCR* loci, including those encoding the LMO1 and LMO2 (for cysteine-rich *LIM*-domain *o*nly) proteins (also known as RBTN1/TTG1 and RBTN2/TTG2).[77–80] Although T-cells normally lack expression of either protein, LMO1 is expressed in a segmental and developmentally regulated pattern in the central nervous system,[78] and LMO2 is coexpressed with Tal1 in several lineages, notably in erythroid and other hematopoietic progenitors.[81] Both LMO1 and LMO2 possess zinc finger-like structures in their LIM domains[82] but lack the homeobox DNA-binding domains common to other transcription factors in this family, suggesting that the LIM domain functions in protein-protein rather than protein-DNA

interactions. In fact, LMO2 is coexpressed with TAL1 in several cell lineages, including erythroid progenitors,[81] and these two proteins interact to form a transcriptional complex,[64,83] both in erythroid cells and in human and murine T-cell leukemias induced by these gene products.[64,65,83] The functional relevance of this complex in normal development is exemplified by the fact that gene targeting experiments in mice, in which null mutations were introduced into *Lmo2*, yielded the same phenotype as those described earlier for *Tal1*, indicating that functional complexes are required for normal primitive erythropoiesis and likely the formation of all hematopoietic lineages.[68,81,84,85] Additional studies have expanded this complex to include GATA1,[86] a zinc-finger transcription factor that is also required for erythroid cell development,[87] E2A bHLH proteins, and the newly identified LIM-binding protein Ldb1/NLL, suggesting that oligomeric DNA-binding complexes containing LMO2 play important roles in hematopoiesis.[88] Moreover, both LMO1 and LMO2 induce thymic lymphomas in transgenic mice whose thymocytes express these genes under the control of T-cell-specific or ubiquitously expressed promoters.[89–93] Although it is controversial whether *TAL1* is able to induce T-cell lymphomas in mice on its own,[94,95] it has been shown to shorten the time to development of T-cell lymphomas induced by LMO2 in a double transgenic system, apparently recapitulating the cooperativity that the these two proteins exhibit as components of multimeric transcriptional regulatory complexes in human T-cell tumors.[64,65,96]

HOX11 is an example of a different type of developmental gene that is inappropriately placed under the control of *TCR* loci. Located on chromosome 10, band q24,[97–100] this gene encodes a homeodomain transcription factor that can bind DNA and trans-activate specific target genes.[101] It is most closely related to *Hlx*, a recently described murine homeobox gene expressed in specific hematopoietic cell lineages and during mouse embryogenesis,[102] and is distantly related to the *Antennapedia* homeobox genes of *Drosophila*, which regulate segment-specific gene expression along the anteroposterior axis of the fly embryo.[103] A very specific homeotic role of *Hox11* in mammalian development was demonstrated by homozygous disruption of this gene, which blocked the formation of the spleen in otherwise normal mice.[104] In the mouse, Hox11 is normally expressed in specific regions of the branchial arches and ectoderm of the pharyngeal pouches of the developing hindbrain, as well as from a single site corresponding to the splanchnic mesoderm beginning at embryonic day 11.5.[104] Because the nervous system develops normally in these mice, the roles of Hox11 proteins in branchial arch and hindbrain structures appear to be compensated for by other transcription factors expressed by these cells; however, the role of Hox11 in cellular organization at the site of splenic development is absolutely essential for the genesis of this organ. Further studies have shown that the splenic anlage actually develops normally in *Hox11*−/− mice but that the developing spleen cells undergo apoptosis, suggesting that Hox11 normally acts to promote the survival of splenic precursors during organogenesis.[105] In contrast to *Lmo2* and *Tal1*, which have important roles in hematopoietic cell development, Hox11 proteins are not normally expressed in lymphoid and other types of hematopoietic cells, and hematopoietic cells are not affected by loss-of-function mutations in this gene, except in circulating erythrocytes with asplenia-related Howell-Jolly bodies.

Activation of *HOX11* by chromosomal translocations, either the t(10;14)(q24;q11) or the t(7;10)(q35;q24), in developing T cells is thought to interfere with normal regulatory cascades, thereby promoting malignant transformation. The primary oncogenic importance of aberrant expression of Hox11 in the developing thymus has been demonstrated in transgenic mice, in which this protein was redirected to the thymus, where it was associated with the development of T-cell lymphoma/leukemia at high frequencies.[106] HOX11 has been shown to act as an activator of gene expression, and this activity has been shown to depend on the N-terminal 50 amino acids of the protein.[107] In addition, HOX11 interacts directly with phosphatases that normally regulate a G2-phase cell cycle checkpoint, suggesting that overexpression of this protein in T-cell progenitors may cause accelerated entry into mitosis.[108]

***E2A* Fusion Genes.** The *E2A* gene was cloned by virtue of the fact that it encodes a protein (E12) that binds to the κE2 regulatory site of the *Ig* κ light chain gene promoter.[109] It was subsequently shown to encode three differentially spliced products, E12, E47, and E2-5, each of which belongs to the bHLH family of transcriptional regulatory proteins.[109–113] The bHLH domain is comprised of a basic region responsible for sequence-specific DNA binding followed by a structural domain consisting of two amphipathic helices separated by a loop region of variable length (thus helix-loop-helix), that is responsible for homo- and heterodimerization.[109,110] The bHLH family of proteins includes the *daughterless Drosophila* gene[114,115] and members of the MyoD family of myogenic proteins.[73,74] DNA-binding by E2A is mediated by either homodimers or heterodimers with other bHLH proteins, with the precise binding specificity to variations of the so-called E-box sequence motif determined by the dimerization partners of each complex.[116] Recent structural analysis has supported experimental observations regarding the conformations of homo- and heterodimers formed by the E2A bHLH domains.[117] In addition, the N-terminal sequences of the E2A that are included in leukemogenic fusion proteins (Fig. 4-4) have been shown to contain two discrete transcriptional activation domains, called AD1 and AD2,[112,118,119] the latter of which is also referred to as a *loop-helix (LH) activation domain.*

In most tissues, E2A heterodimerizes with tissue-specific bHLH family members to coordinate gene expression during development.[110,120] These binding partners include TAL/SCL and LYL1 family members, which heterodimerize with E2A[62,121,122] and are themselves dysregulated in T-cell lymphomas/leukemias and aberrantly expressed as a result of translocations involving the *TCR* gene loci.[45–47] In B cells, however, E2A is able to bind E-box sequences as a homodimeric complex,[120,123] apparently due to stabilization of the complex through an intermolecular disulfide bond, which is disrupted in non-B cells.[124] The importance of E2A proteins in B-cell development is indicated by the fact that homozygous mutant mice lacking functional E2A proteins have arrested B-cell development at an early stage.[125,126] Mice deficient in E2A not only lack pro-B cells but also show defects in T-cell development and acquire T-cell malignancies, suggesting that loss of function of E2A may contribute to leukemogenesis in T cells, in addition to its role as a component of heterodimeric complexes with other bHLH proteins.[127,128]

E2A-PBX1. The *E2A* gene participates in two fusion events with major biologic and clinical implications in acute lymphoblastic leukemia (ALL). The first results from the t(1;19)(q23;p13) chromosomal translocation, which rearranges and joins the *E2A* gene within chromosome band 19p13.3 to the *PBX1* gene from chromosome 1, creating an *E2A-PBX1* chimera on the derivative chromosome 19[129–131] (see Fig. 4-2). Because the breakpoints in the *E2A* gene consistently interrupt the ∼3.5-kb intron between exons 13 and 14, the encoded E2A fusion partner invariably consists of the N-terminal two-thirds of the molecule, which includes two transcriptional activation domains (AD1 and AD2), but not the bHLH DNA-binding/protein-interaction domain.[130–132] The PBX1 segment makes up for this deficit by providing a homeodomain motif of ∼60 amino acids that enables the E2A-PBX1 chimera to function as a transcription factor, driven by the potent E2A trans-activating domains.[133–137]

An understanding of the likely oncogenic contribution of the PBX1 fusion partner requires insight into the normal function of PBX proteins. These transcription factors are the mammalian homologues of the *Drosophila* protein extradenticle.[138,139] Mutations in the *exd* gene cause homeotic transformations, changes in which one body segment of the fly is transformed to resemble another segment.[140,141] Thus the extradenticle protein may function as an obligatory cofactor in selector gene activity by forming complexes with major homeotic fly proteins of the Antennapedia and Bithorax clusters, termed *Hom*, which then bind to DNA.[142–145] In view of the close sequence homology shared by extradenticle and PBX proteins, it is perhaps not surprising that the latter interact with specific human homologues of the Hom family, called *HOX proteins*, to determine the target genes recognized by PBX1.[142,144,146,147,147–155]

Given that E2A-PBX1 carries the transcriptional activation domains of E2A and the homeodomain of PBX1, how does the chimera induce malignant transformation? When Kamps and Baltimore[156] infected bone marrow progenitors with retroviruses encoding E2A-PBX1, they reproducibly induced acute myeloid leukemia (AML) in mice repopulated with these progenitors. These myeloid leukemia cells could proliferate for extended periods without maturation so long as they received granulocyte-macrophage colony-stimulating factor (GM-CSF).[157] In the absence of growth factor, the cells died rapidly. These observations are consistent with the block of differentiation characteristic of lymphoid cells carrying the t(1;19) in cases of ALL[158,159] and with arrested T-cell development in lymphomas of *E2A-PBX1* transgenic mice.[160] Thus a major effect of the chimera may be to arrest hematopoietic and lymphoid progenitors at particular stages of development.

Additional studies with cell transformation assays have established the specific E2A-PBX1 domains required for malignant conversion.[161] When either of the two transactivation domains of E2A are abolished, there is a loss or reduction of

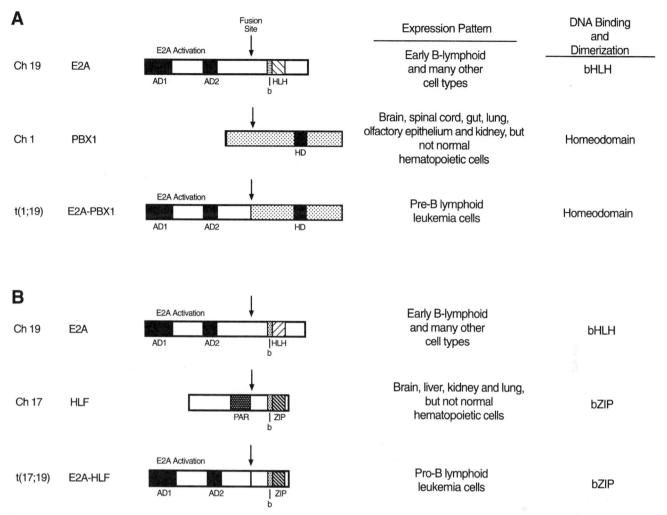

Fig. 4-4 Comparison of the structural features of two major E2A fusion proteins. The E2A portions of the chimeras are identical, retaining both the AD1 and AD2 transcriptional activation domains. The PBX1 fusion partner retains its DNA- and protein-binding domain (homeodomain), as does HLF (bZIP), providing a mechanism for recognition and activation of downstream target genes. Despite the normally wide distribution of E2A and the lack of normal expression of the HLF and PBX1 transcription factors in hematopoietic cells, the two chimeras act specifically on B-cell precursors. HD, homeodomain; bZIP, basic leucine zipper; bHLH, basic helix-loop-helix; Ch, chromosome.

transforming activity. The shortest PBX1 sequence required for oncogenesis includes the homeodomain and its immediately C-terminal 25 amino acids, which also are needed for interaction with specific HOX proteins.[146,162] Unexpectedly, mutant proteins with deletion of the homeodomain and retention of the adjacent flanking region transformed NIH-3T3 cells and induced lymphomas in transgenic mice as efficiently as the full-length chimera.[161,162] Other investigators have confirmed the dispensibility of sequence-specific DNA binding for transformation of fibroblasts while showing that the PBX1 homeodomain is essential for efficient arrest of myeloid cell differentiation.[163] These observations suggest that interaction with members of the HOX family of proteins is sufficient to target the E2A-PBX1 fusion protein to downstream target genes with critical functions in cell transformation but not those which interfere with normal differentiation programs.[161,163] Recent studies have implicated members of related homeodomain families, including Meis1 and pKnox1, as important binding partners and potentially important functional modulators of PBX and HOX proteins.[164–166] Interestingly, these proteins interact through a region of PBX1 that is disrupted in the E2A-PBX1 chimera, suggesting its transforming potential may be augmented by loss of Meis-Knox interactions, which normally may influence target gene recognition, transcriptional properties, or nuclear import of PBX1.[164,165] *E2A-PBX1* is

one of the most common fusion genes in children with ALL, occurring in 20 to 25 percent of cases with a pre-B immunophenotype (defined by cytoplasmic but not surface expression of *Ig* genes).[158,167,168] It is also detected in adults with ALL, as well as occasional cases of pro-B-cell ALL, AML, T-cell ALL, and lymphoma.[14,167–176] Patients with pre-B ALL and the t(1;19) tend to have elevated leukocytes at diagnosis and central nervous system leukemia.[14,167,168] Aside from the adverse impact of these features, the *E2A-PBX1* fusion gene was shown to be independently associated with a poor prognosis,[167] although in recent years intensive chemotherapy has improved clinical outcome significantly in these patients.[168] A prudent clinical management strategy for patients with pre-B ALL is to consider the *E2A-PBX1* fusion gene a high-risk biologic feature that warrants an aggressive approach to therapy. Otherwise, these patients may be undertreated with consequent rapid development of drug-resistant disease.

E2A-HLF. A second *E2A* fusion gene is created by the t(17;19)(q21-q22;13) rearrangement,[177] which joins *E2A* to the *HLF* gene within chromosome band 17q21-22[178,179] (see Fig. 4-2). The breakpoint of this translocation consistently leaves the same portion of *HLF* in the chimeric gene but affects either intron 12 or 13 within *E2A*. The resulting hybrid protein is therefore termed *type I* (intron 13 breakpoint) or *type II* (intron 12 breakpoint),[180] although these structural distinctions do not appear to affect the DNA-binding and transcriptional regulatory properties of E2A-HLF.[181]

The HLF (hepatic leukemia factor) component of the chimera is a novel bZIP transcription factor within the PAR subfamily of proteins (defined by a proline- and acidic amino acid—rich domain).[182–185] HLF recently has been shown to encode two proteins from alternatively spliced transcripts that are regulated by different promoters.[186] One isoform is abundant in brain, liver, and kidney, whereas the other is restricted to hepatocytes; these proteins accumulate with different circadian patterns in the liver and have distinct promoter preferences in trans-activation experiments. Very little is known about the normal function of the PAR proteins, including HLF, but their structural similarity with the CES-2 bZIP protein that orchestrates the death of sertoninergic nerve cells in the developing worm *Caenorhabditis elegans* suggests a regulatory role in cell survival,[187–189] as indicated by the mechanism of E2A-HLF oncogenic activity, described below.

The E2A-HLF fusion product retains the entire DNA-binding/protein-protein interaction domain of HLF, as well as the two N-terminal transactivation domains of E2A.[179,180] In leukemic lymphoblasts, the chimeric protein appears to bind DNA as a homodimer,[190,191] as one might predict given the absence of detectable levels of the known normal PAR proteins in hematopoietic precursors. Like E2A-PBX1, the E2A-HLF oncoprotein can transform NIH-3T3 cells, depending on the integrity of the HLF leucine zipper and the E2A transcriptional activation domains.[192] It also induces lymphoid tumors in transgenic mice.[193] However, E2A-PBX1 induces apoptosis in hematopoietic cells through a p53-independent mechanism that requires the DNA-binding homeodomain of PBX1,[194] which is the direct opposite of the effect of the conditional expression of E2A-HLF.

Analysis of the effects of E2A-HLF on cell survival has provided important insight into how E2A-HLF might take control of immature lymphoid cells. When introduced into leukemic cells carrying the t(17;19), a dominant-negative form of E2A-HLF blocked the usual action of the intact chimera, and as a result, the malignant cells underwent apoptosis.[187] By contrast, the dominant-negative mutant had no effect on apoptotic events in leukemic cells without the t(17;19), suggesting that E2A-HLF may increase the number of developing lymphocytes by preventing their suicide.[187] The homology between HLF and the CES-2 protein of *C. elegans*,[188] which functions early in a genetically controlled cell death pathway, suggests that a comparable pathway operates in human B lymphoblasts and is usurped by E2A-HLF to give rise to ALL.[187] In this model (Fig. 4-5), E2A-HLF activates a downstream target gene that is normally repressed by a CES-2-like protein so that cell survival rather than cell death signals ensue. Thus the leukemogenic activity of E2A-HLF may operate through an evolutionarily conserved pathway that determines the sensitivity of specific lymphoid cells to apoptotic stimuli.

The t(17;19) defines a subset (0.5 to 1 percent) of ALL patients with a pro-B immunophenotype.[177] In several reports this rearrangement was linked to disseminated intravascular coagulation (DIC) and hypercalcemia at initial diagnosis.[177,179,180,195,196] Although the rarity of t(17;19)-positive ALL has hampered efforts to assess its prognostic significance, each of seven patients with molecularly identified *E2A-HLF* fusion died of leukemia despite their enrollment on contemporary treatment protocols.[180,190,195,196] Drug resistance in this type of leukemia may be augmented by the role of E2A-HLF in preventing accelerated apoptosis from therapy-induced DNA damage as well as growth factor deprivation.[187]

TEL-AML1 Fusion Gene. Generally considered a target of chromosomal translocations in myeloid cells, the *AML1* gene is joined to a second transcriptional control gene, called *TEL,* as a result of the t(12;21) in cases of B-lineage ALL.[197–201] Although rarely detected by routine karyotyping (because the telomeric segments of 12p and 21q appear similar in banded metaphase preparations), the t(12;21) rearrangement is apparent by fluorescence in situ hybridization in approximately one-fourth of children with ALL, making *TEL-AML1* the most common genetic abnormality in the lymphoid leukemias.[199] The *TEL-AML1* fusion product consists of the bHLH domain of *TEL* linked to virtually the entire coding region of *AML1,* including the DNA- and protein-binding domain, which bears close amino acid identity to the Runt protein of *Drosophila.* The exact role of the TEL-AML1 oncoprotein in cell transformation remains unclear, but emerging data suggest that the primary effect relates to a compromise of AML1 transcriptional activity,[202] which is required for normal hematopoiesis (see the section in this chapter on the involvement of the AML1-CBFβ complex in the acute myeloid leukemias).

The *TEL* gene is also involved in multiple other fusion genes associated with chronic myelomonocytic leukemia (CMML) (*TEL-PDGFRβ*), AML (*TEL-MN1, TEL-ABL, TEL-EVI1*), and ALL (*TEL-JAK2*) (see Tables 4-1 and 4-2). *TEL* harbors a 65-amino acid helix-loop-helix dimerization motif that is conserved in a subset of the ETS family of proteins, and this region appears to an essential requirement for constitutive tyrosine kinase and transforming activity of the activity of the TEL-PDGFRβ and TEL-ABL fusion proteins.[203–205] TEL-AML1 also appears to dimerize with itself and with normal TEL proteins in the cell, and there is often associated loss of the normal *TEL* allele in leukemias with *TEL-AML1* fusion genes, suggesting that loss of function may contribute to oncogenicity.[204,206] *Tel* has been homozygously disrupted in mice through gene targeting, and interestingly, the *Tel*-deficient mice die at approximately embryonic day 11 with defective yolk sac angiogenesis and intraembryonic apoptosis of mesenchymal and neural cells.[207]

The *TEL-AML1* fusion gene is associated with a superior treatment outcome in patients with B-lineage ALL, and relapse-free survival has approached 90 percent on several different therapeutic regimens.[204,206,208–210] For example, in a recent trial, children with *TEL* gene rearrangements (primarily *TEL-AML1*) had a 5-year event-free survival probability of 91 ± 5 percent (SE) compared with 64 ± 5 percent for those with *TEL* in a germ-line configuration.[208] The prognostic strength of *TEL* rearrangement (usually as a *TEL-AML1* fusion gene) was independent of recognized good-risk features in ALL with B-lineage markers, such as the presenting leukocyte count and hyperdiploidy. Indeed, molecular detection of the *TEL-AML1* fusion gene is the first genetic assay to allow a good-risk subset of patients to be dissected from the otherwise high-risk "pseudodiploid" subset of ALL patients.[211] Thus *TEL-AML1* has been added to the list of genetic abnormalities requiring recognition early in the disease course (Table 4-3).

***BCL6* Activation in Diffuse Large-Cell Lymphoma.** The t(3;14)(q27;q32) and related translocations affect the long arm of chromosome 3 in diffuse large cell lymphomas of the B-cell lineage, leading to the discovery of the *BCL6* proto-oncogene, whose expression is altered in at least 30 percent of these malignancies, the vast majority of which occur in adults.[212–215] *BCL6* encodes a transcription factor containing six zinc-finger DNA-binding motifs near the C-terminus and a POZ regulatory domain near the N-terminus. It is related to the PLZF protein that is fused to RARα as a result of the t(11;17) translocation of acute promyelocytic leukemia. (The postulated developmental roles of highly conserved zinc-finger proteins with POZ domains are discussed in the PLZF section of this chapter.) Like the *AML1-CBFβ* complex in the myeloid cell lineage, but unlike most genes whose expression is altered by translocation to the vicinity of the *Ig* or *TCR* genes, *BCL6* is normally expressed and developmentally regulated in cells of the same lineage in which it is linked to transformation, the B lymphocytes.[216,217] The BCL6 protein is detected in cells of the lymph node germinal center, a region in which antigen-primed B cells normally undergo transformation into either memory B cells or immunoblasts destined to become plasma cells or die as a result of apoptosis.[218] Because BCL6 is

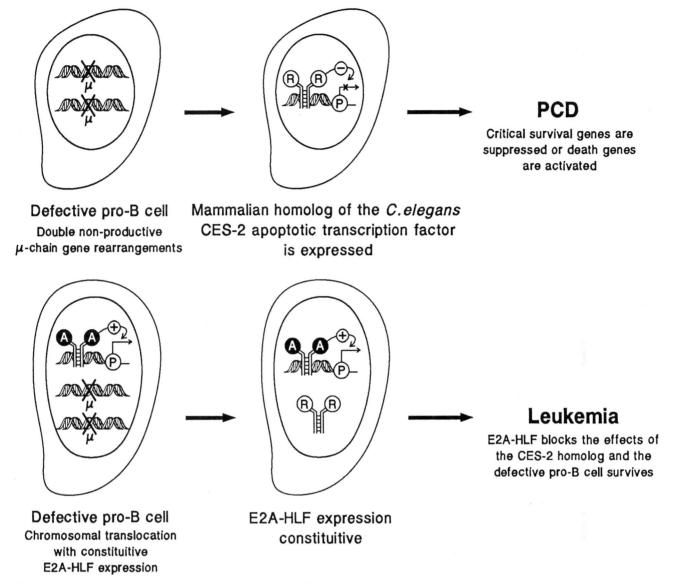

PCD

Critical survival genes are
suppressed or death genes
are activated

Defective pro-B cell

Double non-productive
μ-chain gene rearrangements

Mammalian homolog of the *C.elegans*
CES-2 apoptotic transcription factor
is expressed

Leukemia

E2A-HLF blocks the effects of
the CES-2 homolog and the
defective pro-B cell survives

Defective pro-B cell

Chromosomal translocation
with constituitive
E2A-HLF expression

E2A-HLF expression
constituitive

Fig. 4-5 A proposed model for the anti-apoptotic role of E2A-HLF in leukemogenesis. Leukemic cells with the t(17;19) undergo programmed cell death when E2A-HLF is inhibited through a dominant negative mechanism, suggesting that the primary effect of the hybrid oncoprotein is to prolong cell survival rather than to accelerate cell growth.[187] The close homology of the HLF bZIP domain to that of the CES-2 cell death-specification protein of the nematode *C. elegans*[188] suggests that E2A-HLF may contribute to leukemogenesis by binding to the promoters of target genes normally regulated by a mammalian ortholog of the CES-2 protein, which causes defective pro-B cells to undergo apoptosis. According to this model, E2A-HLF may activate target gene expression in contrast to the proposed repressor effects of CES-2, leading to aberrant survival through an evolutionarily conserved pathway that regulates programmed cell death during B-lymphoid cell development.

Table 4-3 Clinical Risk Assignment in the Childhood Leukemias by Genetic Classification of the Malignant Cells

Abnormality (Risk)	Method of Detection	Treatment
Hyperdiploidy, ≥53 chromosomes (good risk)	DNA flow cytometry	Antimetabolite therapy emphasizing high-dose methotrexate
TEL-AML1 fusion human gene due to t(12;21) (good risk)	RNA PCR to detect *TEL-AML1* fusion transcripts	Antimetabolite therapy emphasizing high-dose methotrexate
E2A-PBX1 fusion gene due to t(1;19) (intermediate risk)	RNA PCR to detect *E2A-PBX1* fusion transcripts	Intensified chemotherapy with alkylating agents and topoisomerase inhibitors
MLL fusion gene due to 11q23 rearrangements and *E2A-HLF* due to t(17;19) (high risk)	RNA PCR to detect *MLL* and *E2A-HLF* fusion transcripts	Experimental forms of intensified chemotherapy or bone marrow transplantation
BCR-ABL fusion gene due to t(9;22), with high leukocyte count (ultra-high risk)	RNA PCR to detect *BCR-ABL* fusion transcripts	Bone marrow transplantation in first remission

normally down-regulated before B cells exit from the germinal center, a reasonable hypothesis is that activated B lymphoblasts constitutively expressing BCL6 are unable to develop normally and instead replicate clonally with the considerable proliferative capacity of a large-cell lymphoma of activated B-lymphocyte origin.[219] This interpretation is supported by the fact that most *BCL6* rearrangements occur within the 5′-noncoding first exon or the first intron of the gene and result in dysregulation of expression of a structurally intact BCL6 protein.[220]

In addition to gene rearrangement mediated by chromosomal translocation, somatic point mutations of the 5′ regulatory regions of the *BCL6* gene have been identified at high frequency in both the diffuse large cell and the follicular lymphomas of B-cell origin, suggesting that dysregulated expression of BCL6 may be linked casually to malignant transformation in high percentages of lymphoid tumors of these pathologic subtypes.[221] Rearrangements of the *BCL6* gene have been shown to have distinct clinicopathologic correlates within the adult diffuse large-cell lymphomas, occurring primarily in extranodal tumors that have not spread to the bone marrow. Importantly, they independently identify a subset of patients with a favorable prognosis.[222]

Acute Myeloid Leukemias

The distribution of gene rearrangements due to chromosomal translocations in AMLs of children and adolescents is shown in Fig. 4-6.

Gene Rearrangements Affecting the *AML1-CBFβ* Complex. The AML1/CBFβ transcription factor complex (Fig. 4-7) is the most frequent target of chromosomal translocations in the human leukemias, in that one of these linked proteins is expressed as an oncogenic chimera in as many as one-third of both ALL and AML patients. This regulatory complex, termed *CBF* because of its identity as a core binding factor (also known as *PEBP2*),[223] consists of a DNA-binding subunit, AML1 (also called *CBFα2* or *PEBP2αB*), and CBFβ (also called *PEBP2β*), a subunit that does not bind DNA independently but rather heterodimerizes with AML1 or one of its closely related family members.[224,225] Chromosomal translocations that modify the AML1/CBFβ complex in myeloid cells include the t(8;21), which generates *AML1-ETO*,[226–229] and the t(3;21), which gives rise to *AML-EVI1, AML-EAP,* or *AML1-MDS1*.[230,231]

The sequence-specific DNA-binding and protein-protein interaction properties of CBF fusion proteins are provided by a large domain within AML1,[232] showing approximately 70 percent homology with the *Drosophila* Runt and Lozenge proteins. The *Drosophila* AML1 homologues participate in several developmental processes, including sex determination, segmentation and neurogenesis (Runt), and determination of photoreceptor identity during eye development (Lozenge). The sequence element recognized by AML1 is TGTGGT,[232] an enhancer core motif that serves as a regulatory element in several viral enhancers, as well as genes whose products are involved in the regulation of hematopoiesis, such as IL-3, GM-CSF, CSF-1, myeloperoxidase, and the TCR receptors.[224,233–240] The binding affinity of AML1 is markedly increased through its heterodimerization with CBFβ, an interaction also mediated through the *runt* homology domain.[232]

The *Aml1* gene was inactivated recently in the germ line of mice by homologous recombination and shown to be essential for definitive hematopoiesis of all lineages.[241,242] Homozygous null

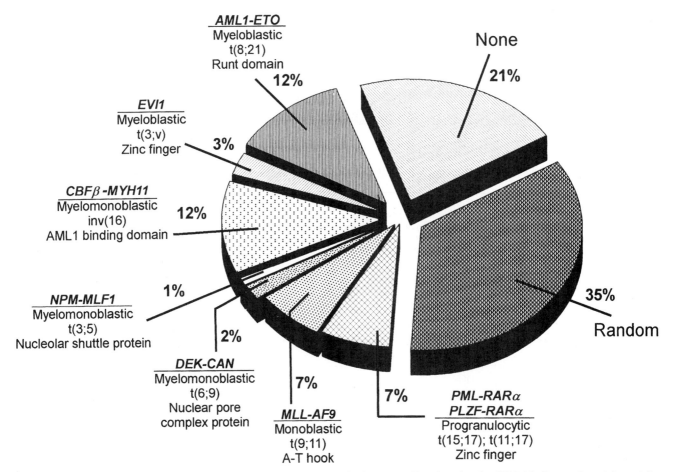

Fig. 4-6 Distribution of translocation-generated fusion genes among the various morphologic subtypes of AML in children and young adults. The section labeled *random* refers to sporadic rearrangements that have so far been observed only in the leukemic cells from single cases. Key domains for DNA binding and protein-protein interaction are given for transcription factors or the type of gene affected for nontranscription factors.

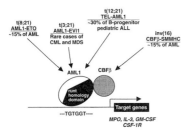

Fig. 4-7 Molecular consequences of chromosomal rearrangements that modify the AML1/CBFβ transcription factor complex, the most frequent target of reciprocal translocations in the human leukemias. In the majority of cases, the structural alteration disrupts the AML1 DNA-binding partner of this complex but not CBFβ, whereas in cases with the inv(16), only the latter protein is affected. The lack of lineage specificity for genetic lesions involving AML1 can be appreciated from the very early site of action of this gene in normal hematopoiesis (see Fig. 19-1), but the molecular basis for the phenotype specificity of each fusion gene in the transformation of myeloid or lymphoid progenitors remains unknown. CML, chronic myeloid leukemia; MDS, myelodysplastic syndrome; AML, acute myeloid leukemia; ALL, acute lymphoblastic leukemia. (*Adapted from Shurtleff et al.*[199] *Used with permission*).

animals display normal morphogenesis and yolk sac-derived erythropoiesis but die between embryonic days 11.5 and 12.5 because of CNS hemorrhage, postulated to be caused by a lack of platelets and possibly potentiated by abnormalities of CNS capillary endothelium.[242] Inactivation of the *Cbfβ* gene in the mouse germ line produced similar effects in homozygous null mice, indicating that CBFβ is required for AML1 function in vivo.[243] From these observations it appears that the AML1/CBFβ complex is an essential regulator of genes required for normal hematopoietic cell development. Hence chromosomal rearrangements that target this complex may interfere with its function in ways that produce arrested differentiation and eventually fully transformed leukemias of specific cell lineages.

The t(8;21), resulting in expression of the AML1-ETO oncoprotein, is the most frequent chromosomal abnormality in the myeloid leukemias of both children and adults; it is found most often in myeloblasts with evidence of granulocytic differentiation (M2 designation by the French-American-British classification system). The fusion protein, which retains the runt homology domain of AML1 and its ability to interact with CBFβ and the core enhancer DNA sequence element, appears to interfere with AML1-mediated transcriptional activation.[232,244] In fact, the C-terminal portion of ETO that is fused in frame with AML1 sequences has been shown to dominantly repress the expression of promoters normally activated by AML1.[240,245,246] The role of ETO in transcriptional repression appears to be directly linked to the ability of sequences included in the fusion protein to recruit the nuclear corepressors N-CoR and mSIN3.[247,248] These proteins assemble in a complex with histone deacetylase, which results in nucleosome assembly and the silencing of gene expression.[249] Thus a biochemical mechanism has been identified that sheds light on the ability of the oncogenic AML1-ETO fusion protein to dominantly oppose the activity of AML1 in the regulation of genes essential for normal myeloid cell development.

The combinatorial versatility of the *AML1* locus is demonstrated by its fusion with sequences from either the *EVI1* gene in t(3;21)-positive chronic myeloid leukemia in blast crisis[230] or to either the *EAP* (Epstein-Barr virus RNA-associated protein) or *MDS1* genes in myelodysplastic syndrome.[231] *EAP* and *MDS1* are located in a region adjacent to *EVI1* on the long arm of chromosome 3 and are often included with *EVI1* in transcripts resulting from these rearrangements.[250] Inclusion of both the Runt-homologous DNA-binding/dimerization domain of AML1 and the zinc-finger DNA-binding domains of EVI1 in the AML1-EVI1 chimeric protein affords ample opportunity for aberrant regulation of target genes.

The CBFβ subunit is involved in another major chromosomal rearrangement in AML, the inversion 16, which affects 15 to 18 percent of AML patients, principally those with myelomonocytic differentiation and increased bone marrow eosinophils (M4-Eo designation in the French-American-British system). This rearrangement joins most of the *CBFβ* gene to the C-terminus of the heavy chain gene of smooth muscle myosin (*MYHII*, also known as *SMMHC*), resulting in formation of a CBFβ-MYH11 protein.[251] Significantly, the fusion protein retains the domain of CBFβ that mediates heterodimerization with AML1.[252,253]

Murine models to study the effects of CBFβ-MYHII on hematopoietic cell development have been produced by inserting the human MYHII cDNA in-frame into the mouse *Cbfb* gene through homologous recombination to "knock in" the fused gene.[254] Similar experiments generated mice in which the *Aml1-ETO* fusion gene has been reconstructed by introducing the appropriate segment of the *ETO* gene into the mouse *Aml1* genomic locus.[255,256] Mouse embryos harboring one allele of *Cbfb-MYHII* or *Aml1-ETO* in the germ line developed CNS hemorrhages at embryologic days 12.5 to 13.5, similar to mice with homozygous loss of *Aml1* or *Cbfb*, indicating that these chimeric proteins dominantly interfere with essential functions of the Aml1/Cbfb complex. Mice expressing Cbfb-MYHII had impairment of primitive as well as definitive hematopoiesis, however, suggesting an additional activity of this fusion protein during hematopoietic cell development.[254] In addition, cells from the fetal livers of embryos expressing the *Aml1-ETO* fusion contained dysplastic multilineage hematopoietic progenitors that had an abnormally high self-renewal capacity and could be established as cell lines in vitro.[255,256] Since both AML1 and CBFβ normally are required for definitive hematopoiesis, the oncogenicity of their respective fusion proteins may stem from disruption of a transcriptional regulatory complex producing arrested myeloid cell differentiation; however, the basis for the phenotypic specificity of leukemias resulting from various types of AML1 and CBFb fusion proteins is unknown (see Fig. 4-7). The available data imply unique activities for each chimeric protein, possibly including gain-of-function as well as loss-of-function effects, as well as global interference with the role of the heterodimeric complex.

Although AML therapy has improved during the past decade, this disease remains extremely difficult to treat with chemotherapy alone, and much of the improvement in survival has arisen from advances in hematopoietic stem cell transplantation. Clinical studies have now demonstrated, however, that the presence of either the *AML1-ETO* or *CBFβ-MYH11* fusion genes in leukemic blast cells at diagnosis will identify patients with a relatively favorable prognosis, especially when treatment consists of intensive chemotherapy including high-dose cytarabine.[12,257–263] The clinical impact of this favorable association with therapeutic outcome is enhanced by the high relative frequency of fusion genes involving the CBF complex in the overall patient population with AML, which approaches approximately one-third of newly diagnosed children and adults with this disease. Molecular analysis of samples taken after the initiation of therapy also has led to the rather surprising finding that both the *AML1-ETO* and the *CBFβ-MYH11* fusion mRNAs can persist in the bone marrow and peripheral blood of AML patients in long-term remission following chemotherapy or bone marrow transplantation.[264–267] These observations illustrate the impact that a more comprehensive understanding of the genetic basis of acute leukemia is having on clinical management and highlight the need for further work to explain the mechanisms that underlie the intriguing correlations that are emerging between molecular findings and therapeutic response.

Retinoic Acid Receptor Rearrangements

PML-RARα. Dysregulated chimeric transcription factors, which induce differentiation arrest at specific stages of development in the myeloid leukemias, offer a new class of intracellular targets for therapeutic attempts to promote differentiation of these leukemias in vivo so that they lose their proliferative capacity. A major example is the fusion product generated by the t(15;17)(q21;q11-22) in acute promyelocytic leukemia (APML), which links critical ligand- and DNA-binding sequences of the retinoic acid receptor-α gene (*RARα*) on chromosome 17 to sequences of the *PML* gene on chromosome 15.[268-273] In its unaltered form, the RARα protein binds to the retinoic acid ligand through a defined ligand-binding domain and to DNA through a separate zinc-finger region as a heterodimer with retinoid X receptor protein.[274] PML proteins, which also possess zinc-finger motifs, are normally located in novel macromolecular nuclear organelles, called *PML oncogenic domains* (PODs), that include at least three other proteins.[275-277] These nuclear bodies are preferential targets of proteins expressed by DNA tumor viruses[278-280] and are up-regulated in activated inflammatory mononuclear cells and by interferon.[281-283] The PML-RARα fusion proteins disrupt these subnuclear structures, causing normal PML, RXR, and other nuclear proteins to disperse in an abnormal microparticulate pattern.[275-277] The fusion proteins interfere with normal myeloid cell development, possibly through adverse effects on assembly of the PODs that contain PML, and dominant inhibitory effects as a homodimeric complex with normal retinoid receptor and peroxisome-proliferator pathways,[284-287] leading to arrested differentiation in the promyelocyte stage. PML-RARα also has been shown to have antiapoptotic activity and to result in cell survival under conditions of growth factor deprivation, which may contribute to its leukemogenic activity.[285,288,289]

PLZF-RARα, NPM-RARα, and NUMA-RARα. Three variant translocations have been identified in AML that unequivocally implicate RARα in leukemias arrested at the promyelocyte stage of differentiation, since both fusion proteins involve the retinoid and DNA-binding domains of this nuclear receptor. Very little is known about the NPM-RARα or NuMA-RARα fusion proteins, which have been identified only in rare patients.[290,291] NPM-RARα links RARα in-frame to N-terminal sequences of nucleophosmin (NPM), a nucleolar shuttle protein that is also involved in NPM-ALK fusion proteins in large-cell lymphoma and NPM-MLF1 in AML, while the NuMA-RARα fusion protein represents a similar in-frame fusion with a protein involved in the nuclear mitotic apparatus.

PLZF-RARα was first recognized several years ago,[292] with subsequent structural and functional studies of PLZF providing intriguing insights into the potential mechanism of action. PLZF is a transcription factor containing nine C-terminal zinc-finger motifs related to those of the Krüppel *Drosophila* segmentation protein and containing an N-terminal POZ (poxvirus and zinc-finger) protein-protein interaction domain.[293] This domain inhibits the binding of transcription factors, including RARα, to DNA when linked in cis, suggesting that PLZF-RARα may act by sequestering RXR or other retinoid receptors within inactive multimeric complexes.[293-296] PLZF is expressed in multiple tissues during development, including elevated expression at Rhombomeric boundaries in the vertebrate hindbrain.[297] It is also expressed by early hematopoietic progenitors with a punctate nuclear distribution and is down-regulated during myeloid cell differentiation.[298] These findings, combined with studies showing heterodimerization of PLZF-RARα with normal PLZF through the POZ domain,[295] suggest that normal PLZF also may play a role in normal hematopoietic cell differentiation, one that is inhibited by the fusion protein. Five additional cases of APML with t(11;17)-mediated expression of PLZF-RARα fusion proteins have been reported,[299] indicating that these patients share a proclivity with PML-RARα patients to develop life-threatening DIC.

The Histone Deacetylase Complex and Its Role in APML. Recent studies have provided an attractive model to explain the mechanism through which the PML-RARα and PLZF-RARα fusion proteins contribute to dysregulated gene expression in

APML. In the absence of ligand, RARs have been shown to repress the expression of target genes. The mechanism involves the recruitment of the NCOR and SMRT corepressors, which in turn mediate the assembly of an histone deacetylase complex that has the ability to silence gene expression.[300-305] The PML-RARα fusion protein retains its ability to interact with the RAR corepressors and block transcription in the absence of ligand. However, unlike normal RAR proteins, which release the repressor complex and function as activators of gene expression in response to physiological concentrations of retinoids, the fusion protein remains in a repressor complex and aberrantly blocks target gene expression.[306-310] Studies in the presence of higher levels of retinoids also have helped explain the responsiveness of APMLs harboring *PML-RARα* fusion genes to ATRA. Pharmacologic dosages of ATRA overcome the association of PML-RARα with the histone deacetylase complex and allow the recruitment of coactivators, resulting in the activation of expression of critical target genes and the induction of growth arrest with granulocytic differentiation within the malignant clone.[311-314] These findings provide a mechanistic rationale for use of ATRA acid in patients with APML, which had been shown already to be effective in empirically initiated trials.[311,313,315-317] In response to pharmacologic doses of this compound, PML and its associated proteins are reorganized into normal-appearing nuclear PODs, with subsequent maturation of the leukemic cells into differentiated myeloid cells with limited life-spans in the circulation. Resistance to ATRA as a single agent generally develops within 3 to 4 months, but its role in the remission induction phase of APML therapy has been established, and clinical trials combining ATRA with cytotoxic chemotherapy have led to improved survival of patients whose promyeloblasts express the PML-RARα fusion protein.[316,317]

Biochemical analysis of the association of histone deacetylase complexes formed with PLZF-RARα fusion proteins also has provided an explanation for the clinical observation that all-trans retinoic acid differentiation therapy is not effective in inducing remissions in patients with this variant RARα fusion protein. The mechanism of transformation appears to be quite similar, in that PLZF-RARα proteins heterodimerize with RXR and form repressor complexes that block target gene expression in a fashion unresponsive to physiological retinoid levels.[300-305] However, the POZ domain of the PLZF portion of the fusion protein independently recruits the SMRT and NCOR nuclear corepressors, in complexes that are not disrupted in the presence of high levels of ATRA. Thus the presence of a second ATRA-unresponsive histone deacetylase complex formed by the PLZF fusion partner provides an explanation for the lack of sensitivity of leukemias harboring this fusion protein to treatment with a ligand that specifically overcomes repression mediated through the RARα moiety of the fusion protein.

Mouse Models of APML. The oncogenic properties of PML-RARα have been studied in transgenic mouse models in which expression of the fusion protein is driven by CD11b or cathepsin G regulatory sequences.[318-320] Mice expressing PML-RARα driven by the cathepsin G promoter develop a myeloproliferative disorder, and 25 to 30 percent of the mice develop AML after a relatively long latency period of 6 to 15 months of age.[307,319,320] By contrast, PLZF-RARα was much more active when its expression was driven by the same promoter, inducing leukemia in all the mice from two lines followed for the same time period, and leukemias in the mice were refractory to pharmacologic dosages of retinoic acid, recapitulating the resistance of human PLZF-RARα leukemias to ATRA therapy.[307] A transformation model, based on retroviral transduction of the *PML-RARα* gene into hematopoietic progenitor cells of chickens also has been used to demonstrate leukemogenicity.[321]

EVI1 Gene Activation. In some cases of AML with high platelet counts, the inv(3)(q21;q26.2) or the t(3;3)(q21;q26.2) moves promoter/enhancer sequences from one site on chromosome 3 into the *EVI1* locus on the same chromosome,[322,323] leading to increased gene expression. The same effect is produced in murine myeloid leukemias by insertional mutagenesis.[324] The EVI1 protein binds to promoter/enhancer sequences containing the GATA sequence motif and may act by interfering with regulatory signals normally mediated by the GATA family of hematopoietic transcriptional regulators.[325–328] The normal function of EVI1 is unknown, although its tissue distribution (oocytes and kidney cells) and its dominant interfering effect on normal myelopoiesis would suggest an important developmental role in regulatory pathways that interface between proliferation and differentiation.

Acute Mixed-Lineage Leukemias: *MLL* Fusion Genes

An extraordinarily diverse group of chromosomal translocations, deletions, and inversions affect chromosome band 11q23. In contrast to the lineage specificity of many other nonrandom rearrangements, these abnormalities occur in both lymphoid and myeloid leukemias (7 to 10 percent of ALL patients, 5 to 6 percent of AML) and in a high percentage of the so-called mixed-lineage leukemias, defined by expression of markers of more than one hematopoietic cell lineage.[329–331] Leukemias with 11q23 translocations also account for a high percentage of acute leukemias in infants less than 1 year of age (80 and 45 percent of infants with ALL and AML, respectively).[332–337] Perhaps the most striking association is the presence of 11q23 translocations in as many as 85 percent of secondary leukemias in patients treated with topoisomerase II inhibitors.[338,339] Taken together, these examples of phenotypic diversity suggest that 11q23 genetic abnormalities mediate the transformation of multipotential hematopoietic stem cells, which give rise to leukemias in which the myeloid or lymphoid progenitors are blocked at various stages of development.

Molecular Biology of *MLL*. Cloning of the gene most often affected by 11q23 abnormalities fulfilled expectations based on phenotypic, cytogenetic, and clinical studies. Many of the breakpoints that occur within the 11q23 locus interrupt the mixed-lineage leukemia gene (*MLL*, also called *HRX*, *ALL-1*, and *HTRX1*), which encodes a large protein of 3968 amino acids with a predicted molecular mass of 431 kDa.[340–345] Most intriguing with regard to function are three regions of homology with the *Drosophila trithorax* (*trx*) gene, two associated with central zinc-finger domains and the third with a 210-amino acid C-terminal region of 61 percent identity called the *SET* (Suvar3-9, Enhancer of zeste, Trithorax) domain.[341,342,346–348] *Trithorax* is a master homeotic gene regulator that positively regulates the actions of a wide spectrum of homeotic (*Hom*) genes in the *Antennapedia* and *Bithorax* complexes of the fly and is required throughout embryogenesis for normal development of the head, thorax, and abdomen.[341–344,349]

The N-terminal region of the MLL protein contains three A-T hook domains, first identified in the so-called HMG (high mobility group) proteins, which are thought to help establish chromatin structure[350] and to bind in the minor groove to DNA segments rich in A and T residues. The intervening region between the A-T hooks and the zinc-finger domains includes a 47-amino acid region of homology with the noncatalytic domains of mammalian DNA methyltransferase (MT), an enzyme that acts on the hemimethylated substrate produced after DNA replication to maintain the methylation pattern of cytosine residues in the genomes of somatic cells.[351] Two additional domains have been defined based on their ability to affect transcriptional control, a trans-repression domain overlapping the MT-homology region and a trans-activation domain in the region C-terminus to the zinc fingers.[352] The SET domain has been shown to mediate interactions with Sbf1, a protein related to dual specificity phosphatases but which lacks a functional catalytic domain.[353] Interestingly, enforced expression of Sbf1 mediates transformation of NIH-3T3 fibroblasts and

primary cultures of B-cell progenitors, suggesting that it functions as a SET domain-dependent positive regulator of growth-inducing kinase signaling pathways.[354]

***MLL* Fusion Genes.** Translocation breakpoints within the *MLL* gene occur exclusively in an 8.5-kb region located between exons 5 and 11 and join *MLL* sequences with genes from numerous other chromosomes to form a large fusion gene (Fig. 4-8). The resulting chimeric proteins, encoded on the derivative 11 chromosome, include the N-terminal half of MLL, with its A-T hook minor groove DNA-binding motifs, the MT-homology domain, and all or part of the associated transcriptional-repression domain.[341,342] Another consistent feature of MLL fusion proteins is the absence of the two zinc-finger regions and the Trithorax homology regions normally located in the C-terminal half of the protein.

In contrast to the similar regions of *MLL* affected by 11q23 rearrangements, an array of structurally diverse protein partners contributes amino acid segments to the MLL fusion proteins found in ALL, AML, and the mixed-lineage leukemias. Twelve of the genes fused to *MLL* by 11q23 translocations have now been cloned and sequenced (see Table 4-1), making it possible to examine their products for functional motifs that might provide clues to the mechanisms leading to the formation of active transforming proteins. At the time of its cloning, each of these fusion partners was a previously unidentified gene with unknown function. The ELL protein (also known as *MEN*) was cloned originally as an MLL fusion partner in translocations involving chromosome subband 19p13.1.[355,356] In an exciting development, the same protein was independently purified as an elongation factor that increases the catalytic rate of RNA polymerase II transcription.[357] This association seems unlikely to be circumstantial, in that ELL has a close functional analogue called *elongin* (SIII), the transcription elongation factor that is also regulated by the von Hippel-Lindau (VHL) tumor suppressor.[358–361] Many questions remain to be answered before the functional significance of the MLL-ELL fusion is known; for example, is the MLL-ELL fusion protein (which contains almost all the ELL coding sequences, fused in-frame to the usual N-terminal segment of MLL) still active as an elongation accelerator? Is ELL subject to regulation by proteins analogous to VHL? If so, does fusion with MLL block this interaction and remove ELL from positive or negative physiological control? And perhaps most important, which genes are controlled in their expression by ELL, and how do they affect cell physiology? Although the full significance of the functional identity of this MLL fusion partner is still unknown, recognition of ELL emphasizes the potentially important roles of such proteins in chimeric constructs, particularly the potential of the chimeras to interfere with the normal roles and regulation of the fusion partner proteins, in addition to their possible inhibitory effects on the normal function of MLL itself.

Another intriguing development in research on *MLL* fusion genes has been the realization that the identity of the fusion partner may determine the phenotypic specificity of the chimera in hematopoietic stem cell transformation. For example, *ENL*, the partner gene on subband 19p13.3, is frequently involved in translocations affecting both ALL (especially in infants and children) and AML,[362] whereas ELL is restricted to *de novo* and therapy-related cases of AML[355] and is rare in children.[362] ENL is one of three related fusion partners, which include *AF-4* on chromosome band 4q21, involved in the frequent 4;11 translocations found in ALL, and *AF-9* on band 9p22, the gene affected by the 9;11 translocation important in both primary and secondary acute monocytic leukemias of children and adults. Each of these proteins appears to contribute domains with similar structural attributes to chimeric proteins,[341,342,345,363–365] in that they contain nuclear localization signals and regions rich in serine and proline that may function as transcriptional trans-activation domains.[363,365] In support of this possibility, ENL was shown to trans-activate reporter gene expression in mammalian cells and

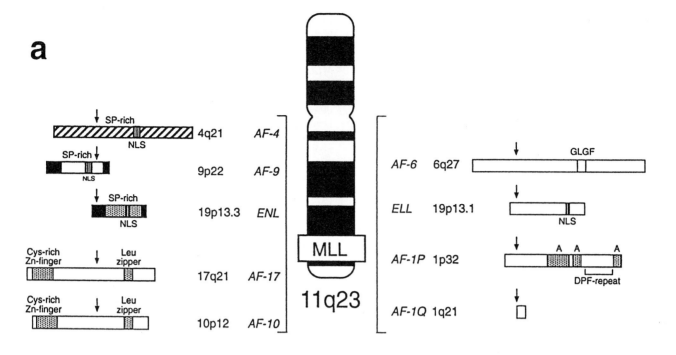

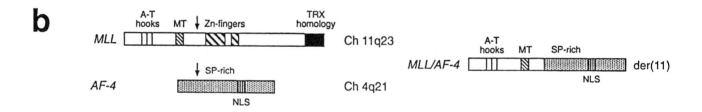

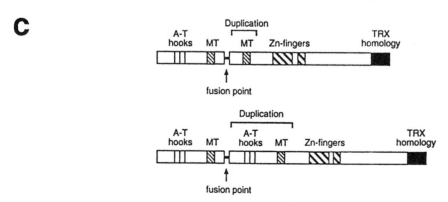

Fig. 4-8 The *MLL* gene and some of its fusion partners. The first three genes shown on the left of the ideogram (*A*) are rich in serine and proline (SP) and contain nuclear localization signals (NLSs), whereas the next two are notable for a cysteine-rich zinc-finger domain and a leucine zipper motif. The AF6 protein contains a novel glycine-leucine-glycine-phenylalanine (GLGF) domain, and AF1P is distinguished by three acidic (A) regions, together with an amino acid repeat motif (aspartic acid-proline-phenylalanine (DPF). AFIQ contributes only a minimal part of its 9-kDa total mass to its fusion with MLL, suggesting that truncation of MLL may itself contribute to leukemogenesis. Regions on the right of the breakpoints (*arrows*) are retained in the fusion product. Of the four major structural elements of *MLL* (*B*), only the A-T hook and mammalian DNA methyltransferase domains are retained in the chimeric proteins. AML cases have been identified recently with "self fusion" rearrangements (*C*), which fuse the same N-terminal *MLL* sequences with duplicated regions of the *MLL* gene. (*Adapted from Downing and Look.*[575] *Used with permission*).

yeast,[365] through the C-terminal serine- and proline-rich region of homology between ENL and AF-9, which is included in the chimeric proteins.

Some *MLL* partner genes appear to contribute functional domains to the chimeric proteins, whereas others truncate *MLL* in ways that may interfere with its normal function. *AF-10* and *AF-17,* potential examples of the first mechanism, are involved in the t(10;11)(p12;q23) and t(11;17)(q23;q21) and contain leucine zipper motifs near their C-termini and cysteine-rich zinc-finger motifs near their N-termini. These structural elements are retained in the oncogenic fusion proteins and may provide dimerization motifs with functional significance. The alternative model is best represented by the *AF1q* gene involved in the t(1;11)(q21;q23). This 9-kDa protein lacks homology to any known protein sequence,[366] and the minimal contribution of its sequences to the uniformly involved MLL N-terminal region implies that loss of MLL function through haploinsufficiency or dominant-negative interference may contribute to leukemogenesis. This interpretation is reinforced by several patients with AML who have lacked 11q23 translocations but have contained partial internal duplications of *MLL* linking the intact gene to a duplication of its N-terminal region.[367,368] In these rearrangements, a region beyond the A-T hook and methyltransferase domains is internally duplicated in-frame with the remainder of the coding sequences (see Fig. 4-4). Thus the partially duplicated *MLL* gene product contains the N-terminal A-T hooks and methyltransferase domains separated from the zinc-finger motifs, indicating that dissociation of N-terminal domains of MLL from regulatory C-terminal regions is a general structural feature of oncogenic MLL fusion proteins.

***Mll, Mll-AF9,* and *MLL-ENL* in Animal Models.** In *Drosophila,* the *MLL* homologue *trx* is a member of a large family of trithorax group proteins that have a positive role in the maintenance of cell-type specific patterns of *HOM-C* gene expression, apparently acting through epigenetic mechanisms that establish and sustain a receptive chromatin configuration.[369] Inactivation of the murine *Mll* gene in the germ line by homologous recombination has suggested that it has a similar function during normal mammalian development.[347,370] Complete loss of *Mll* was lethal during embryogenesis, with the embryos lacking detectable expression of the major *Hox* genes tested, consistent with the requirement for *trx* in maintenance of *HOM-C* gene expression in *Drosophila.* Interestingly, mice lacking function of one *Mll* allele showed a phenotype resulting from haploinsufficiency, with hematopoietic abnormalities that included anemia, thrombopenia and reduced numbers of B cells, bidirectional homeotic transformations of the axial skeleton, and sternal abnormalities. Skeletal abnormalities appeared to be due to shifts in the normal pattern of major *Hox* gene expression, due to inadequate *Mll* gene dosage, so that the hematopoietic cell phenotype may have resulted from a similar mechanism, based on studies that implicate mammalian *Hox* genes in blood cell development.[7,371–376] More recent studies have documented decreased numbers of yolk sac-derived CFU-GEMM, CFU-M, and BFU-E colonies in *Mll*-null embryos.[377] Overall, the results in *Mll*-deficient mice suggest a dual role for 11q23 translocations in human leukemogenesis, including both a gain-of-function effect mediated by the fusion oncogene and simultaneous effects on hematopoietic cell development from haploinsufficiency due to the loss of one normal *MLL* allele.[347]

The leukemogenicity of the *MLL-AF9* fusion gene was demonstrated recently in an animal model by generating this fusion oncogene in embryonic stem (ES) cells and using them to generate chimeric mice.[378] Although ES cells containing the *Mll-AF9* fusion gene gave rise to cells of all lineages in chimeric animals and the cells of numerous tissues expressed the fusion gene, the only tumors to develop in the mice were AMLs, reinforcing the association of this fusion gene with human AML. It also appeared that the fusion genes contributed an early growth advantage to progenitors within the myeloid lineage, because circulating myeloid cells derived from the targeted ES cells were a prominent component of this cell compartment in most of the *Mll-AF9* chimeras from the time of birth. This effect was not observed in mice generated from an ES cell line modified to express a truncated and epitope-tagged *Mll* allele, implying that the disordered growth advantage imparted to myeloid cells did not arise from *Mll* haploinsufficiency but rather from expression of the *Mll-Af9* fusion protein. Although leukemia induction was highly efficient in this model, the latency period ranged from 4 to 12 or more months, implying that additional mutations affecting other oncogenes or tumor suppressors must occur before a fully transformed leukemic clone can emerge.[378]

A retroviral gene transfer assay has been used successfully to document the oncogenic capacity of MLL-ENL (also known as HRX-ENL) by showing its activity in the immortalization and leukemic transformation of myelomonocytic progenitors in mice.[379] Detailed structure-function analysis has indicated that the DNA-binding motifs of MLL are required for the full transforming activity of the fusion protein, including the methyltransferase and A-T hook domains.[380] Within the ENL sequences of the fusion protein, the C-terminal 84 amino acids of ENL, which comprise two helical structures highly conserved with AF9, are both necessary and sufficient for transformation. These structures were shown to function as transcriptional activators, suggesting that the fusion protein acts to dysregulate the expression of target genes that contribute to transformation within the myeloid lineage.

Origins of Therapy-Related AML. *MLL*-associated translocations are a prominent feature of leukemias in patients treated with the epipodophyllotoxins,[338,339,381] but the basis for this association remains uncertain. An intriguing correlation has emerged from analysis of 130 breakpoints by restriction mapping and more than a dozen by genomic DNA sequencing analyses in cases of *de novo* or therapy-related leukemias with 11q23 translocations affecting the *MLL* gene.[382–387] That is, the centromeric portion of the 8.5-kb genomic MLL breakpoint cluster region consistently showed the largest number of breakpoints in cases of *de novo* leukemias, whereas the telomeric portion contained the majority of break-points found in therapy-related cases.[386,387] Scaffold attachment sites have been mapped in the vicinity of these breakpoint regions, as well as high-affinity topoisomerase II cleavage sites, which may influence the distribution of breakpoints.[386]

With regard to the molecular mechanisms involved in the origin of 11q23 translocations in *de novo* and secondary AML, studies to date have focused on (1) recombination within Alu repeats, (2) involvement of V-D-J recombinase enzymes in B-lymphoid progenitors, and (3) the possible role of topoisomerase II inhibitors acting to promote breaks at consensus cleavage sites for this enzyme, which would serve as substrates for recombination events leading to *MLL* translocations in the therapy-related leukemias. The first two possibilities have gained credible support,[368,382,383,385,388] but they do not explain the majority of cases.[382,389]

An intriguing mechanism of genetic recombination involves cleavage by topoisomerase II, as suggested by the frequent identification of *MLL* rearrangements in therapy-related cases of AML of patients treated with agents that inhibit this enzyme.[338,339,381] Antineoplastic drugs with this property include both the epipodophyllotoxin and anthracycline classes of drugs. AML linked to these agents tends to appear as an acute leukemia without a myelodysplastic phase within 6 to 24 months after diagnosis of the primary malignancy, in contrast to the longer latency periods and frequent myelodysplastic prodromes of secondary AML induced by alkylating agents. AML arising after treatment with a topoisomerase inhibitor typically has monoblastic or myelomonoblastic morphology,[338,339,381,390–392] suggesting that the target cell is a myeloid progenitor cell stimulated to enter cell division by chemotherapy-induced neutropenia.

Topoisomerase II catalyzes a two-step reaction involving both double-stranded DNA cleavage and strand relaxation and religation.[393] Both the epipodophyllotoxins and the anthracyclines stabilize the DNA-topoisomerase II complex after cleavage, resulting in the accumulation of double-strand DNA breaks, which are prime substrates for nonhomologous recombination.[394,395] Analysis of several 11q23 translocations has identified topoisomerase II consensus binding sites adjacent to chromosomal breakpoints.[385] Other cases of therapy-related AML lack topoisomerase II-binding sites adjacent to the breakpoints, so additional 11q23 translocation junctions will need to be analyzed before the frequency and importance of this mechanism can be fully assessed.[382,386]

Aside from factors predisposing to nonhomologous recombination, how could topoisomerase inhibitors preferentially induce AML with characteristic MLL fusion proteins? The rapid development of these secondary leukemias suggests a collaborative mechanism in which both the drug and the fusion protein act synergistically to accelerate the multistep process leading to AML. A model incorporating the known effects of the epipodophyllotoxins on G2-phase cell cycle checkpoint control and topoisomerase II activity is shown in Fig. 4-9. These compounds arrest cycling cells in G2 phase, and most committed myeloid progenitors harboring epipodophyllotoxin-induced DNA breaks are likely targeted to undergo apoptosis, based on the degree of neutropenia that accompanies a typical course of therapy with these agents (see Fig. 4-9, top panel). Normal myeloid progenitors arrested in G2 occasionally survive, however, with double-strand DNA breaks at the sites of topoisomerase II integration. As these lesions are repaired, some of the breaks are joined by nonhomologous recombination and result in chromosomal rearrangements. The myeloid progenitors with 11q23 translocations producing in-frame MLL fusion genes begin to proliferate because of a proliferative advantage conferred by the hybrid MLL protein and growth factors produced in response to epipodophyllotoxin-induced neutropenia. According to this model, MLL fusion proteins may exacerbate this process by relaxing

cell cycle checkpoints normally activated by the presence of the integrated topoisomerase II:drug complex, leading to attenuated apoptosis and increased survival of cells with genetic damage at other loci (see Fig. 4-9, bottom panel). In the face of repetitive epipodophyllotoxin treatment, this could lead to the acquisition of additional genetic lesions affecting oncogenes or tumor suppressors in the expanding clone that already expresses an MLL fusion protein, with rapid progression of a multistep process culminating in overt AML.

The exceedingly high frequency of 11q23 translocations associated with infant leukemias suggests a further mechanism that could lead to MLL gene rearrangement and biologically active chimeric proteins. A number of pairs of infant twins have been shown to have identical MLL gene rearrangements.[396,397] In some cases, the leukemias had identical Ig gene rearrangements, consistent with transformation of a common progenitor cell that had completed V-D-J recombination. In other cases the Ig rearrangements differed between twin leukemias, suggesting that transformation occurred before Ig gene recombination and that the leukemic clones had evolved independently. Nonetheless, the identification of identical MLL rearrangements at the DNA sequence level in each twin indicates that the leukemic clone arose in one infant and spread through the placenta to the other sibling. The documentation of MLL rearrangements in utero and the high frequency of 11q23 translocations in infant leukemias (approaching 80 percent of ALL patients and 50 percent of AML patients) suggest that pluripotent progenitor cells with self-renewal capacity are in a proliferative state in the developing bone marrow, rendering them uniquely susceptible to transformation by chimeric MLL oncoproteins. This susceptibility may be related to patterns of gene expression or epigenetic changes in chromatin configuration that are found in subsets of progenitors that are expanding to populate the hematopoietic system during infancy.

Myeloid progenitors similarly susceptible to the transforming effects of chimeric MLL proteins or prone to productive MLL

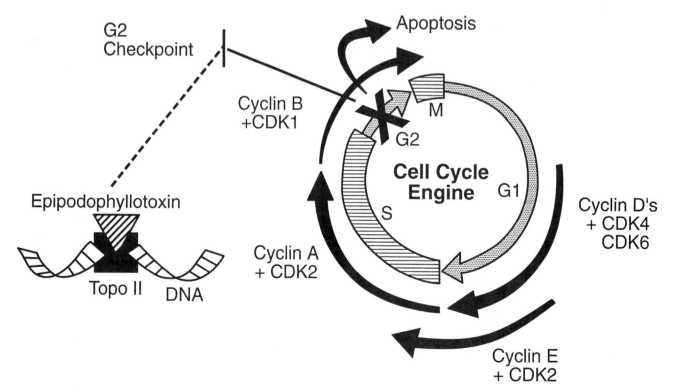

Fig. 4-9 Model accounting for the mechanisms linking epipodophyllotoxin therapy, MLL fusion proteins, cell cycle progression, and the relaxation of cell cycle checkpoints, leading to reduced levels of apoptosis in myeloid progenitor cells after genotoxic chemotherapy (hence increased survival of cells with damaged DNA). The accelerated acquisition of additional genetic lesions in clonogenic preleukemic cells eventually culminates in overt myeloid leukemia. See text for further explanation. (*Adapted from Downing and Look.*[575] *Used with permission*).

rearrangements may be reactivated in patients undergoing therapy with epipodophyllotoxins, accounting for the rapid onset of secondary AML in children and adults treated with these agents. We have recently identified altered transcripts for the p27KIP1 cell cycle kinase inhibitor in leukemias expressing MLL-AF4[398] and have shown that MLL-AF4 induces cell cycle arrest in cell lines when its expression is driven by a conditional promoter,[399] suggesting that hematopoietic stem cells may need to have the capacity to bypass negative cell cycle effects of this fusion protein before they become susceptible to malignant transformation. Moreover, the short latency period between *MLL* rearrangement and overt leukemia following 11q23 translocations in infants and after epipodophyllotoxin therapy suggests that MLL fusion proteins themselves predispose susceptible hematopoietic progenitors to undergo secondary mutations necessary for the development of a fully transformed leukemic clone.

ONCOGENIC ACTIVATION OF TYROSINE KINASES

Cellular tyrosine kinase gene products serve as growth factor receptors or intracellular signal transducers and can be aberrantly activated through a variety of mechanisms, including truncation of the ligand-binding domain of growth factor receptors, loss or replacement of C-terminal regulatory tyrosine residues, and point mutations within intact molecules.[400] In the leukemias and lymphomas, chromosomal translocations produce tyrosine kinase gene fusions that are quite specific for lymphoid progenitor cells of particular lineages and phenotypes. In two instances, the N-terminal sequence of a functionally unrelated protein is fused to a truncated receptor tyrosine kinase. Such kinases normally occupy a proximal position in the transduction of extracellular signals required for cell proliferation, differentiation, and other biologic events that determine cell fate. When activated by growth factors, these transmembrane proteins phosphorylate themselves as well as their substrates, triggering multiple biochemical regulatory cascades. Critical steps in this process are dimerization of two adjacent receptors to initiate signal transduction and phosphorylation of high affinity-binding sites for the SH2 (*Src homology*) domains of GRB2 and other specific cytoplasmic signaling molecules that convert RAS proteins to their GTP-bound forms (reviewed in ref. 401).

The chimeric proteins resulting from receptor tyrosine kinase fusions invariably lack ligand-binding domains and may lack transmembrane domains, yet they clearly function as oncogenic proteins. The mechanism(s) responsible for constitutive activation of a tyrosine kinase in the absence of growth factor binding appear to be related to shuttling of the chimera to a new cellular location[402] and to constitutive activation due to dimerization stimulated by sequences within the nonkinase fusion partner, such as a leucine zipper motif.[403] Thus hybrid proteins with aberrantly activated tyrosine kinase domains represent a novel product of chromosomal rearrangements, further demonstrating the versatility of genetic mechanisms that transform hematopoietic cells.

ABL Fusion Genes in Chronic and Acute Leukemias

The Philadelphia chromosome, produced by a (9;22)(q34;q11) translocation, was first identified in patients with chronic myeloid leukemia (CML) and later shown to occur in 3 to 5 percent of children and 30 to 40 percent of adults with ALL.[404–406] This translocation results in a *BCR-ABL* chimeric tyrosine kinase oncogene, which contains sequences from the *BCR* gene upstream of the second exon of the *ABL* proto-oncogene.[407–412] Thus t(9;22) breakpoints on the distal tip of the long arm of chromosome 9 occur in the first intron of the *ABL* proto-oncogene, which spans a distance of more than 100 kb upstream of sequences encoding the tyrosine kinase domain.[413–415] By contrast, the breakpoints on chromosome 22 are confined to a 5.8-kb region of genomic DNA known as the *major breakpoint cluster region* (M-bcr),[416] which

lies within *BCR*, a gene that encodes a 160-kDa phosphoprotein.[416,417] The 8.5-kb fusion transcript found in CML encodes a 210-kDa hybrid protein that is activated as a tyrosine-specific protein kinase, as is the *v-abl* protein product.[418–421]

Although routine karyotyping does not distinguish between the t(9;22) in CML and ALL, molecular analysis of the *BCR* and *ABL* proto-oncogenes, which are rearranged in both diseases, has revealed differences that apparently mediate the phenotype specificity of these oncogenic fusion kinases.[422–424] In ALL, the rearrangement produces a shorter fusion transcript (6.5 to 7.0 kb) and hybrid protein (185 to 190 kDa) than are generated by the *BCR-ABL* fusion gene in CML[422–424] (Fig. 4-10). The differences are due to unique breakpoints on chromosome 22 in ALL patients that do not lie within the 5.8-kb region of *BCR* that contains the breakpoints in CML. Instead, they are contained within a second minor breakpoint cluster region (M-bcr) located further upstream within the *BCR* gene.[425–427] The ALL fusion protein includes N-terminal *BCR* amino acids but lacks the internal residues that are found in the CML fusion proteins near the *BCR-ABL* junction.

The N-terminal sequences of *ABL* are removed in oncogenic forms of the gene and replaced by the Moloney virus *gag* gene in the case of *v-abl*[428–430] and with *BCR* sequences in the *BCR-ABL* fusion gene of CML and ALL.[418–421] The products of both the *v-abl* and the *BCR-ABL* fusion genes can transform primary hematopoietic cells in vitro, providing a model system for analysis of oncogenic mechanisms.[431]

Both the P185 and P210 BCR-ABL proteins also can induce a CML-like syndrome in vivo in mice when they are expressed in hematopoietic progenitors.[432–435] Mechanistic studies of these fusion proteins have shown that RAS signaling is essential for transformation and that multiple alternative means, including the adapters GRB2, SHC, and CRKL, are used to couple the activated ABL kinase to RAS, resulting in activation of Jun kinase.[436–438] Oncogenic signaling by BCR-ABL also has been shown to involve the cell cycle-regulated genes *MYC* and *cyclin D1*[439,440] and to constitutively activate the transcriptional signal transducer STAT5.[441] The emerging picture is one of multiple signaling pathways that are activated to mediate leukemic transformation by BCR-ABL; hence selective complementation of defective mutant fusion proteins should allow the identification of genetic pathways that are involved in BCR-ABL-mediated hematopoietic cell transformation.[436]

A new mechanism of ABL activation in human leukemia involves a fusion between the Ets transcription factor TEL and the catalytic domain of ABL; the product of this union has been identified in two cases of acute leukemia, one myeloid and the other lymphoid.[203,442] The TEL-ABL fusion kinase resembles the TEL-PDGFβR protein previously described in association with a t(5;12) chromosomal translocation in CML.[443] As with TEL-PDGFβR, the DNA-binding domain of TEL is not incorporated into the chimeric structure. Recently, the TEL-ABL protein was shown to be a constitutively activated kinase located in the cytoskeleton, whose activity depends on oligomerization mediated through a helix-loop-helix domain in the N-terminus of TEL.[203]

Progress also has been made in clarifying the normal role of the ABL kinase. Studies in mice rendered *Abl* deficient by homologous recombination indicate that Abl is not required for embryogenesis; however, mice without this protein develop a wasting syndrome and die shortly after birth.[444,445] In contrast to the BCR-ABL proteins, which are cytoplasmic, normal ABL is a nuclear kinase, whose activity is tightly regulated in vivo.[446] Recent evidence suggests that the kinase is activated by DNA-damaging agents and that it mediates growth arrest in a p53-dependent fashion.[447–450,450,451] Although the precise function of ABL is not known, the available evidence suggests that it regulates pathways that mediate cell cycle arrest after genotoxic damage. It is fascinating that this kinase, which in many ways has functions reminiscent of a tumor suppressor, can be subverted through chromosomal translocation to function in an entirely different

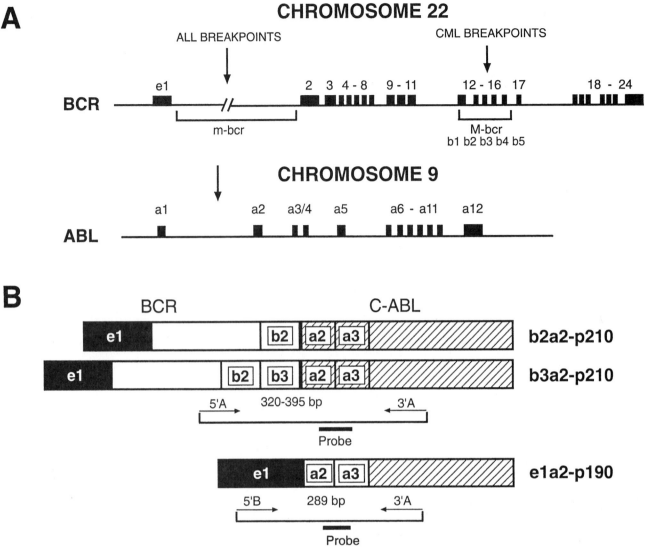

Fig. 4-10 Genomic structure of *BCR* locus on chromosome 22. Breakpoints in chronic myelogenous leukemia (CML) occur primarily in the more 3′ M-bcr region, while those in acute lymphoblastic leukemia (ALL) occur primarily in the m-bcr region. The two common BCR-ABL fusion proteins resulting from M-bcr-type breakpoints are 210 kDa (p210) in size and contain the *BCR* distal exons b1 and b2, with or without b3. By contrast, breakpoints in m-bcr result in a fusion protein of 190 kDa (p190) that contains only the first *BCR* exon, e1. Both the p210 and p190 fusion proteins contain the same portion of ABL. (*Adapted from Okuda, Fisher, and Downing.*[13] *Used with permission*).

cytoplasmic compartment and presumably through different substrates in the malignant transformation of hematopoietic progenitors.

The exceedingly poor prognosis of ALL patients with the Philadelphia chromosome has been attributed to transformation of a primitive hematopoietic stem cell that is inaccessible to most forms of chemotherapy.[406,452–454] Long-term responses (probable cures) have been induced in a subset of children with ALL who have low white blood cell counts at diagnosis, using intensive early-phase chemotherapy, followed by repetitive treatment with pairs of non-cross-resistant drugs.[455] For most patients with BCR-ABL-positive ALL, however, the recommended strategy is allogeneic bone marrow transplantation in first remission, which is also the only known curative approach for CML.[456]

NPM-ALK In Large-Cell Lymphoma

Large-cell lymphomas constitute approximately one-fourth of the non-Hodgkin lymphomas that develop in children and adolescents. In a subset of these tumors, a t(2;5) chromosomal translocation links N-terminal sequences encoded by the ubiquitously expressed nucleophosmin (*NPM*) gene on chromosome 5q35 to the catalytic domain of a previously unidentified tyrosine kinase gene on chromosome 2p23, now termed *ALK* (for *a*naplastic *l*ymphoma *k*inase).[457] The NPM phosphoprotein, which shuttles between the nucleolus and the cytoplasm,[458,459] consists of a putative metal binding site, two acidic amino acid clusters, and two nuclear localization signals.[460] NPM is highly phosphorylated during mitosis and serves as a substrate for CDC2.[461] NPM has been shown to bind to RNA, DNA, the HIV Rev protein, transcription factor YY1, and nucleolar protein p120[461–466] and is thought to play a role in ribosomal assembly, but its specific function remains undefined.

The *ALK* gene product, a tyrosine kinase receptor of 1620 amino acids, shows greatest amino acid identity with members of the insulin receptor subfamily, leukocyte tyrosine kinase in particular (64 percent).[457] Very little is know about the normal function of ALK, with the exception that its murine homologue is exclusively expressed in cells of the central and peripheral nervous systems.[467,468]

The NPM-ALK chimera retains 117 amino acids from NPM and 563 from ALK. In contrast to the cell surface localization of native ALK receptors, immunofluorescence studies with Cos cells have documented both cytoplasmic and nuclear expression of the NPM-ALK chimera.[469,470] The available evidence indicates that the NPM fusion segment contributes an active promoter that drives expression of the ALK kinase domain and a dimerization domain that stimulates its constitutive activation, leading to lymphomagenesis. The transforming potential of NPM-ALK has been demonstrated in NIH-3T3 cells[469,471] and in mice reconstituted with bone marrow cells bearing the chimeric gene.[472] In the latter study, half the animals developed clonal B-lineage large-cell lymphomas that arose in the mesenteric lymph nodes and metastasized to the lungs and kidneys. Experiments with NPM-ALK mutants have established that dimerization mediated by the NPM segment is required to activate the truncated ALK tyrosine kinase for cell transformation and indicate that interactions between ALK and the GRB2 substrate also may be necessary.[469,471]

Discovery of the *NPM-ALK* fusion gene has definite clinical implications. With the availability of ALK-specific antibodies for immunodiagnosis, it is now apparent that a broad morphologic spectrum of large-cell lymphomas expresses the activated chimeric NPM-ALK kinase.[473–476] Other useful assay techniques for this fusion gene include DNA- or RNA-based polymerase chain reaction (PCR) techniques[477,478] and fluorescence *in situ* hybridization assays with interphase cells.[479] Studies to examine the clinical outcome of patients with lymphomas expressing NPM-ALK have demonstrated a favorable prognosis, approaching an 80 percent 5-year survival.[480–482]

In addition to the classic t(2;5), ALK has now been shown to be activated through variant chromosomal rearrangements, including the t(1;2)(q25;p23) and an inv(2)(p23q35), although the presumptive fusion partners remain to be identified.[470,483] In addition, a rare subset of high-risk B-lineage large-cell lymphomas has been described in which the malignant cells express the full-length ALK kinase through an unknown mechanism but clearly lack the t(2;5) chromosomal translocation.[484]

TEL-PDGFRβ in CMML

An attractive hypothesis is that leukemias and lymphomas develop through an accumulation of multiple genetic changes, which eventually give rise to clonal, neoplastic growth. The transition from normal hematopoiesis to myelodysplastic syndrome (MDS) and then to overt AML affords a model in which one might establish the requirement for serial somatic mutations in the genesis of myeloid leukemia.[485] A possible paradigm for the early events in AML pathogenesis was provided by discovery of the t(5;12)(q33;p13) chromosomal translocation in CMML, an MDS subtype characterized by abnormal clonal myeloid cell proliferation and progression to AML.

The t(5;12) produces a fusion transcript in which the tyrosine kinase and transmembrane domains of the platelet-derived growth factor receptor β gene (*PDGFRβ*) on chromosome 5 are linked to a novel *Ets*-like gene (*TEL*) on chromosome 12. The prominent structural features of normal PDGFRβ receptors include five Ig-like extracellular loops and an interrupted intracellular tyrosine kinase domain.[486] This kinase participates in a signal transduction pathway that has a major effect on cell proliferation.[487] Mutated components of the PDGFRβ-related pathway, such as RAS, clearly have transforming potential, as does the PDGFRβ ligand, whose overexpression is associated with a myeloproliferative syndrome in mice.[488]

As emphasized in the preceding section on *AML1* gene fusion, *TEL* is a member of the *Ets* gene family and thus specifies a DNA-binding protein that recognizes the consensus motif C/A GGA A/T.[489] The distinct N-terminal HLH domain of TEL is essential for full transactivating function but probably does not bind DNA directly.[490] By analogy to other transcription factors, such as E2A, MYC, and MYOD, this HLH domain may be involved in protein-protein interactions.[203]

In t(5;12)-induced gene fusion, only the N-terminal HLH domain of *TEL* is incorporated into the chimeric product, which

therefore lacks a legitimate DNA-binding domain. How, then, does the TEL-PDGFRβ protein induce CMML? An obvious model is that the retained TEL HLH domain leads to dimerization (hence activation) of the PDGFRβ kinase. Another possibility, raised by retention of the PDGFRβ transmembrane domain, is that the TEL 5′ region acts as a ligand-binding domain by responding to an unknown cognate binding protein. Finally, PDGFRβ may be moved to a new location in the cell, perhaps the nucleus, through localization signals provided by TEL-binding proteins. Displacement to the nucleus could result in phosphorylation of bound transcription factors with consequent aberrant activation of critical downstream targets. Each of these models has been reviewed in detail.[491]

It therefore appears that *TEL-PDGFRβ* fusion is a pivotal early genetic change in the development of CMML. Patients who progress from this MDS subtype to AML often show numerous additional cytogenetic changes, suggesting that malignant progression results from sequential acquisition of new mutations. Identification of the t(5;12) fusion product thus represents an advance in understanding how one form of MDS predisposes to acute leukemia. A variant t(5;12) translocation, the t(10;12)(q24;p13), also may generate a novel *TEL* fusion gene associated with refractory anemia, eosinophilia in the bone marrow, and increasing monocytosis.[492]

OTHER MECHANISMS OF TRANSFORMATION MEDIATED BY CHROMOSOMAL TRANSLOCATIONS

CYCLIN D1 Activation in Mantle Cell Lymphoma

The t(11;14)(q13;q34) was one of the first chromosomal translocations to be dissected molecularly, based on the realization that the breakpoint on chromosome 14 occurred within the *IgH* gene and use of a probe from this gene to isolate DNA from the so-called *BCL1* region on the long arm of chromosome 11.[493,494] Although additional tumors were identified with breakpoints in this region, it initially proved difficult to identify a proto-oncogene whose expression was altered by the translocation.[495–498] This search has now ended with the identification of the gene encoding cyclin D1 (*CCND1*), located 110 kb distal to the original *BCL1* breakpoint.[499–502] Evidence that *CCND1* is the proto-oncogene targeted by the t(11;14) includes the facts that it is the closest gene to the breakpoint cluster region on chromosome 11 and that the majority of tumors with this translocation aberrantly express this cell cycle regulatory protein (for a recent review, see ref. 503). Cyclin D1 is a member of a family of D-type cyclins that act in concert with their catalytic partners, the cyclin-dependent kinases (CDK4 and CDK6), to initiate the phosphorylation of the retinoblastoma protein, pRB, thus coupling growth factor-induced mitogenic signals to the biochemical machinery of the cell cycle (reviewed in ref. 504). B cells normally express two other cyclin D family members, cyclins D2 and D3, but not cyclin D1, so cyclin D1 expression is abnormally induced in this lineage by the translocation, presumably reflecting the influence of the B-cell-specific *IgH* gene enhancer from chromosome 14. The coding region of cyclin D1 is not altered by these translocations,[501,505,506] the breakpoints of which are often 100 kb or more from the gene itself, implying that uncoupling of cyclin D1 expression from mitogenic signals that would normally regulate the levels of cyclin D2 and D3 provides a constitutive proliferative stimulus.[507] Presumably, small lymphocytes in the mantle zone of the lymph node that harbor this translocation and aberrantly express cyclin D1 are unable to exit the cell cycle on cue and thus are unable to differentiate into Ig-secreting plasma cells.[508]

As molecular probes have become available, first for the *BCL1* locus and more recently to identify expression of the cyclin D1 mRNA and protein, it has been possible to clarify the pathologic diagnosis of B-cell lymphomas harboring the t(11;14). These tumors previously were called *mantle-cell* or *diffuse small cleaved-cell lymphomas,* but the term *mantle-cell lymphoma* now has been uniformly adopted by international agreement.[508–510] Comprising about 5 percent of lymphomas overall, these tumors occur primarily in elderly men, are of intermediate grade, and do not respond well to available therapies. It is now clear that virtually all mantle-cell lymphomas harbor the t(11;14) and express cyclin D1, rendering newly available monoclonal antibodies that recognize this protein especially valuable as immunohistochemical reagents for more accurate diagnosis of this important subset of B-cell malignancies.[511–514]

BCL2 in Follicular Lymphoma

The *BCL2* proto-oncogene was discovered through analysis of genes that are dysregulated by the t(14;18), which is the most common chromosomal translocation among human lymphoid malignancies. The t(14;18) is found in more than 80 percent of follicular center cell lymphomas, a common and generally indolent type of B-cell lymphoma that occurs almost exclusively in adults, and in approximately 20 percent of diffuse adult B-cell lymphomas.[515,516] Molecular analysis of the breakpoints of the 14;18 translocation identified *BCL2* as the gene on chromosome 18 that is overexpressed due to its translocation into the *IgH* locus on chromosome 14.[517–520] Functional studies revealed that BCL2 defines a new class of proto-oncogene products that act to prolong cell survival rather than having more typical effects on cell differentiation or proliferation.[521–523] It has since been learned that BCL2 is a member of a large family of highly conserved proteins that either inhibit or promote apoptosis (reviewed in ref. 524), extending down the phylogenetic tree to the CED-9 protein, which inhibits programmed cell death in *C. elegans.*[525] This interesting family of proteins is discussed further in a separate chapter in this volume (see Chap. 10).

Nuclear Pore Genes in AML

Three translocations in acute myeloid leukemia have been shown to involve nuclear pore genes, the t(6;9) and a cryptic t(9;9) or inv(9) producing the *DEK-CAN* and *SET-CAN* fusion genes[526–528] and the t(7;11) producing a *NUP98-HOXA9* chimera.[529,530] The first of these to be cloned was *DEK-CAN,* which is found in children and young adults with myeloid or myelomonocytic AML (M1, M2, or M4 according to the French-American-British classification). A chimeric DEK-CAN protein is produced, comprising nearly the entire DEK protein fused to the C-terminal two-thirds of the CAN protein.[526,527] A SET-CAN fusion protein was identified subsequently in leukemic cells from a single patient,[528] indicating a central role for CAN amino acids in the transforming capacity of these proteins, since identical portions of CAN were retained in each of the oncogenic hybrids. Insight into the normal role of CAN came when a component of the nuclear pore complex, called *NUP214,* was independently purified and shown to be identical to CAN.[531] CAN was shown to be localized to the nuclear pore by immunofluorescence microscopy; by contrast, DEK-CAN proved to be exclusively nuclear, even though the fusion protein retains the nucleoporin-specific FXFG repeats that are thought to mediate protein-protein interactions important for nuclear transport.[532] The essential role of normal CAN in nuclear transport has been proven through studies of embryos in which the gene was inactivated by homologous recombination,[533] and two cellular proteins have been shown to bind to CAN, of which one, a 112-kDa protein, also interacts with the nucleoporin-specific repeat of DEK-CAN and SET-CAN, suggesting that it might play a role in transformation.[534]

The nucleoporin connection recently has become even more intriguing with the cloning of the t(7;11) fusion gene, which encodes a hybrid protein containing the characteristic FXFG repeat region of another member of the nucleoporin complex, NUP98, fused in-frame to the homeobox domain of the major HOX protein HOXA9.[529,530] A current research focus is to determine whether the nucleoporin repeat regions allow these fusion proteins to interfere with protein or RNA transport across the nuclear membrane, resulting in a novel mechanistic contribution to the transformation of myeloid progenitors.[532–534] Alternatively, the presence of the HOXA9 homeodomain in the more recently identified NUP98-HOXA9 fusion protein raises the possibility that these hybrid proteins could interfere with the transcriptional regulation of genes important for myeloid cell development. According to this scenario, the nucleoporin partner primarily may contribute a protein-protein interaction and effector region to the fusion protein, with domains mediating interaction with DNA prompter/enhancer sequences coming from the other partners in these fusions. This would certainly be a plausible mechanism of transformation for the NUP98-HOXA9 fusion protein, because of the emerging evidence that the major HOX proteins contribute to hematopoietic development,[7,371–376] as already discussed in the section on MLL fusion proteins and the role of mammalian Mll and *Drosophila* trithorax in *HOX* and *Hom* gene regulation.[347]

Nucleolar *NPM-MLF1* Gene in AML

Another translocation specific for hematopoietic neoplasia is the t(3;5)(q25.1;q34), which occurs in a subset of MDSs and AMLs. We recently demonstrated that the t(3;5) interrupts the *NPM* gene, encoding a nucleolar shuttle protein, which is also interrupted by the t(2;5) in large-cell lymphoma and the t(5;17) in APML.[290,528] In the t(3;5), the N-terminal portion of NPM is fused in-frame to sequences of a novel gene on chromosome 3 that we have named *myelodysplasia/myeloid leukemia factor 1.*[535] This *MLF1* gene, which is not expressed by mature blood cells, encodes a cytoplasmic protein containing no identifiable structural motifs. The NPM-MLF1 fusion protein traffics intracellularly under the direction of its NPM amino acid sequences, in that it is predominantly localized within the nucleolus of leukemic cells.[535] These features of MLF1 and NPM-MLF1 suggest that the t(3;5) may contribute to the development of AML through a previously unrecognized mechanism. Current efforts are directed toward the biochemical and biologic characterization of these proteins, as well as that of *MLF2,*[536] an *MLF1*-related gene that we have identified recently.

FUTURE DIRECTIONS

What has been learned about the transforming roles of transcription factors in leukemias and lymphomas? First is the requirement for proto-oncogene activation, usually by chromosomal rearrangement (through reciprocal translocations, inversions, deletions, or tandem duplications), in which the candidate gene comes to lie in the vicinity of a *TCR* or *Ig* gene or is fused with a second gene to form a chimeric protein that may retain many of the key functions of the original factor. Post-activation regulatory events remain largely unknown, although the array of factors so far identified suggests an extraordinarily diverse set of interactions. For example, heterodimerization with other proteins, as in the formation of MYC/MAX, AML1/CBFβ, TAL1/LMO2, or PBX1/HOX complexes, greatly increases the complexity of interactions between oncogenic proteins and transcriptional regulatory networks.

The key to understanding the oncogenic effects of transcription factors lies in the nature of the genes they regulate. Since the majority of these oncoproteins are ectopically expressed, one might predict that they alter the expression of tightly regulated gene programs in normal hematopoietic progenitors. Almost certainly examples will be found in which interaction of these proteins with downstream target genes either activates or represses developmental programs that are normally required only at critical times in the life cycle of the progenitor cell. In some instances, the positive or negative effects of oncogenic transcription factors are probably mediated directly through binding to enhancer sequences in target gene promoters; however, in other cases these proteins may transform cells indirectly, by binding to other transcriptional regulatory proteins and targeting them to nonfunctional or newly functional complexes.

Thus the main challenge for the future is to identify the gene programs controlled by the various transcription factors activated by chromosomal rearrangements. Equally important will be the task of delineating subsequent interactive processes within transcriptional regulatory cascades. This is likely to be even more difficult than deciphering the molecular mechanisms regulating *Drosophila* embryogenesis because of the greater complexity of experimental embryology and genetic analysis in vertebrate model systems. Clues to the normal roles of key gene products will continue to be provided by murine models, in which individual proto-oncogenes are targeted for inactivation by homologous recombination. The oncogenic targets of these proteins in leukemias and lymphomas may still be difficult to decipher because chromosomal translocations often mediate aberrant expression of genes in hematopoietic cells, either as inappropriately expressed intact proteins or as chimeric proteins that contain regulatory subunits from two different proteins.

With increased knowledge of the regulatory networks affected by oncogenic transcription factors, it may be possible to develop new therapeutic strategies for human malignancies, similar to those employing all-*trans*-retinoic acid for the treatment of APML. Indeed, if a fusion protein is crucial to malignant growth, one could alter the disease course by interfering with any of the multiple steps in protein synthesis and action, including oncogene transcription, RNA processing and translation, and DNA or protein-protein interactions. Fused transcription factors would appear ideal for these types of intervention because they represent true chimeras that occur only in rare types of malignant cells. A clear advantage of this approach, which depends on a detailed understanding of the mechanisms underlying each hybrid factor's transforming properties, would be the reduced likelihood of toxicity to normal cells or the development of resistant mutants, by comparison with currently available methods of cancer therapy.

Finally, it is important to realize that aberrant activation of proto-oncogenes by chromosomal translocations is but one event in the multistep process of carcinogenesis. Future molecular research into the leukemias and lymphomas undoubtedly will uncover an array of inactivating mutations affecting tumor suppressors, which act synergistically with proto-oncogenes activated by genetic rearrangement and are required for full expression of malignant phenotypes in hematopoietic cells.

ACKNOWLEDGMENTS

I would like to thank John Gilbert for editorial review and critical comments. This work was supported in part by NIH Grants CA-59571, CA-21765, CA-20180, and CA-71907 and by the American Lebanese Syrian Associated Charities (ALSAC).

REFERENCES

1. Bishop JM: The molecular genetics of cancer. *Science* **235**:305, 1987.
2. Solomon E, Borrow J, Goddard AD: Chromosome aberrations and cancer. *Science* **254**:1153, 1991.
3. Rowley JD: Molecular cytogenetics: Rosetta stone for understanding cancer. Twenty-ninth G. H. A. Clowes Memorial Award Lecture. *Cancer Res* **50**:3816, 1990.
4. Shivdasani RA, Orkin SH: The transcriptional control of hematopoiesis. *Blood* **87**:4025, 1996.
5. Rabbitts TH: Chromosomal translocations in human cancer. *Nature* **372**:143, 1994.
6. Look AT: Oncogenic role of "master" transcription factors in human leukemias and sarcomas: A developmental model, in Vande Woude G (ed): *Advances in Cancer Research.* San Diego, Academic Press, 1995, p. 25.
7. Look AT: Oncogenic transcription factors in the human acute leukemias. *Science* **278**:1059, 1997.
8. Rabbitts TH: Translocations, master genes, and differences between the origins of acute and chronic leukemias. *Cell* **67**:641, 1991.
9. Nusslein-Volhard C, Wieschaus E: Mutations affecting segment number and polarity in *Drosophila*. *Nature* **287**:795, 1980.
10. Nusslein-Volhard C, Frohnhofer HG, Lehmann R: Determination of anteroposterior polarity in *Drosophila*. *Science* **238**:1675, 1987.
11. Levine MS, Harding KW: Drosophila: The zygotic contribution, in Glover DM, Hames BD (eds): *Genes and Embryos*. New York, IRL Press, 1989, p. 39.
12. Rowley JD, Aster JC, Sklar J: The clinical applications of new DNA diagnostic technology on the management of cancer patients. *JAMA* **270**:2331, 1993.
13. Okuda T, Fisher R, Downing JR: Molecular diagnostics in pediatric acute lymphoblastic leukemia. *Mol Diagn* **1**:139, 1996.
14. Pui C-H: Childhood leukemias. *N Engl J Med* **332**:1618, 1995.
15. Papavassiliou AG: Molecular medicine transcription factors. *N Engl J Med* **332**:45, 1995.
16. Dalla-Favera R, Bregni M, Erikson J, Patterson D, Gallo RC, Croce CM: Human c-myc oncogene is located on the region of chromosome 8 that is translocated in Burkitt lymphoma cells. *Proc Natl Acad Sci USA* **79**:7824, 1982.
17. Taub R, Kirsch I, Morton C, Lenoir G, Swan D, Tronick S, Aaronson S, Leder P: Translocation of the C-myc gene into the immunoglobulin heavy chain locus in human Burkitt lymphoma and murine plasmacytoma cell. *Proc Natl Acad Sci USA* **79**:7837, 1982.
18. Adams JM, Gerondakis S, Webb E, et al: Cellular myc oncogene is altered by chromosome translocation to an immunoglobulin locus in murine plasmacytomas and is rearranged similarly in Burkitt lymphomas. *Proc Natl Acad Sci USA* **80**:1982, 1983.
19. Emanuel BS, Selden JR, Chaganti RSK, et al: The 2p breakpoint of a 2;8 translocation in Burkitt lymphoma interrups the V kappa locus. *Proc Natl Acad Sci USA* **81**:2444, 1984.
20. Erikson J, Nishikura K, ar-Rushdi A, et al: Translocation of an immunoglobulin kappa locus to a region 3′ of an unrearranged c-myc oncogene enhances c-myc transcription. *Proc Natl Acad Sci USA* **80**:7581, 1983.
21. Hollis GF, Mitchell KF, Battey J, et al: A variant translocation places the lambda immunoglobulin genes 3′ to the c-myc oncogene in Burkitt's lymphoma. *Nature* **307**:752, 1984.
22. Rappold GA, Hameister H, Cremer T, et al: C-myc and immunoglobulin kappa light chain constant genes are on the 8q+ chromosome of three Burkitt lymphoma lines with t(2;8) translocations. *EMBO J* **3**:2951, 1984.
23. Croce CM, Thierfelder W, Erikson J, Nishikura K, Finan J, Lenoir GM, Nowell PC: Transcriptional activation of an unrearranged and untranslocated c-myc oncogene by translocation of a C lambda locus in Burkitt. *Proc Natl Acad Sci USA* **80**:6922, 1983.
24. Taub R, Kelly K, Battey J, Latt S, Lenoir GM, Tantravahi U, Tu Z, Leder P: A novel alteration in the structure of an activated c-myc gene in a variant t(2;8) Burkitt lymphoma. *Cell* **37**:511, 1984.
25. Rabbitts TH, Hamlyn PH, Baer R: Altered nucleotide sequences of a translocated c-myc gene in Burkitt lymphoma. *Nature* **306**:760, 1983.
26. Pelicci PG, Knowles DM 2, Magrath I, Dalla-Favera R, Knowles DM: Chromosomal breakpoints and structural alterations of the c-myc locus differ in endemic and sporadic forms of Burkitt lymphoma. *Proc Natl Acad Sci USA* **83**:2984, 1986.
27. Taub R, Moulding C, Battey J, Murphy W, Vasicek T, Lenoir GM, Leder P: Activation and somatic mutation of the translocated c-myc gene in burkitt lymphoma cells. *Cell* **36**:339, 1984.
28. Bhatia K, Spangler G, Gaidano G, Hamdy N, Dalla-Favera R, Magrath I: Mutations in the coding region of c-myc occur frequently in acquired immunodeficiency syndrome-associated lymphomas. *Blood* **84**:883, 1994.
29. Gu W, Bhatia K, Magrath IT, Dang CV, Dalla-Favera R: Binding and suppression of the myc transcriptionsl activation domain by p107. *Science* **264**:251, 1994.
30. Blackwood EM, Eisenman RN: Max: A helix-loop-helix zipper protein that forms a sequence- specific DNA-binding complex with Myc. *Science* **251**:1211, 1991.
31. Prendergast GC, Lawe D, Ziff EB: Association of Myn, the murine homolog of Max, with c-Myc stimulates methylation-sensitive DNA binding and Ras cotransformation. *Cell* **65**:395, 1991.
32. Ayer DE, Kretzner L, Eisenman RN: Mad: A heterodimeric partner for Max that antagonizes Myc transcriptional activity. *Cell* **72**:211, 1993.
33. Zervos AS, Gyuris J, Brent R: Mxi1, a protein that specifically interacts with Max to bind Myc-Mas recognition sites. *Cell* **72**:223, 1993.
34. Ayer DE, Lawrence QA, Eisenman RN: Mad-Max transcriptional repression is mediated by ternary complex formation with mammalian homologs of yeast repressor Sin3. *Cell* **80**:767, 1995.

35. Schreiber-Agus N, Chin L, Chen K, Torres R, Rao G, Guida P, Skoultchi AI, DePinho RA: An amino-terminal domain of Mxi1 mediates anti-Myc oncogenic activity and interacts with a homolog of the yeast transcriptional repressor SIN3. *Cell* **80**:777, 1995.

36. Ayer DE, Eisenman RN: A switch from Myc:Max to Mad:Max heterocomplexes accompanies monocyte/macrophage differentiation. *Genes Dev* **7**:2110, 1993.

37. Larsson LG, Pettersson M, Oberg F, Nilsson K, Luscher B: Expression of mad, mxi1, max and c-myc during induced differentiation of hematopoietic cells: Opposite regulation of mad and c-myc. *Oncogene* **9**:1247, 1994.

38. Amati B, Brooks MW, Levy N, Littlewood TD, Evan GI, Land H: Oncogenic activity of the c-Myc protein requires dimerization with Max. *Cell* **72**:233, 1993.

39. Adams JM, Harris AW, Pinkert CA, Corcoran LM, Alexander WS, Cory S, Palmiter RD, Brinster RL: The c-myc oncogene driven by immunoglobulin enhancers induces lymphoid malignancy in transgenic mice. *Nature* **318**:533, 1985.

40. Langdon WY, Harris AW, Cory S, Adams JM: The C-myc oncogene perturbs B lymphocyte development in Emu-myc transgenic mice. *Cell* **47**:11, 1986.

41. Lombardi L, Newcomb EW, Dalla-Favera R: Pathogenesis of Burkitt lymphoma: Expression of an activated c-myc oncogene causes the tumorigenic conversion of EBV-infected human B lymphoblasts. *Cell* **49**:161, 1987.

42. Packham G, Cleveland JL: c-Myc and apoptosis. *Biochim Biophys Acta* **1242**:11, 1995.

43. Galaktionov K, Chen X, Beach D: Cdc25 cell-cycle phosphatase as a target of c-myc. *Nature* **382**:511, 1996.

44. Zindy F, Eischen CM, Randle DH, Kamijo T, Cleveland JL, Sherr CJ, Roussel MF: MYC signaling via the ARF tumor suppressor regulates p53-dependent apoptosis and immortalization. *Genes Dev* **12**:2424, 1998.

45. Begley CG, Aplan PD, Davey MP, Nakahara K, Tchorz K, Kurtzberg J, Hershfield MS, Haynes BF, Cohen DI, Waldmann TA, et al: Chromosomal translocation in a human leukemic stem-cell line disrupts the T-cell antigen receptor delta-chain diversity region and results in a previously unreported fusion transcript. *Proc Natl Acad Sci USA* **86**:2031, 1989.

46. Chen Q, Cheng JT, Tasi LH, Schneider N, Buchanan G, Carroll A, Crist W, Ozanne B, Siciliano MJ, Baer R: The tal gene undergoes chromosome translocation in T cell leukemia and potentially encodes a helix-loop-helix protein. *EMBO J* **9**:415, 1990.

47. Xia Y, Brown L, Yang CY, Tsan JT, Siciliano MJ, Espinosa R, III, Le Beau MM, Baer RJ: TAL2, a helix-loop-helix gene activated by the (7;9)(q34;q32) translocation in human T-cell leukemia. *Proc Natl Acad Sci USA* **88**:11416, 1991.

48. Mellentin JD, Smith SD, Cleary ML: Lyl-l, a novel gene altered by chromosomal translocation in T-cell leukemia, codes for a protein with a helix-loop-helix DNA binding motif. *Cell* **58**:77, 1989.

49. Shivdasani RA, Mayer EL, Orkin SH: Absence of blood formation in mice lacking the T-cell leukaemia oncoprotein tal-1/SCL. *Nature* **373**:432, 1995.

50. Robb L, Lyons I, Li R, Hartley L, Kontgen F, Harvey RP, Metcalf D, Begley CG: Absence of yolk sac hematopoiesis from mice with a targeted disruption of the scl gene. *Proc Natl Acad Sci USA* **92**:7075, 1995.

51. Finger LR, Harvey RC, Moore RC, Showe LC, Croce CM: A common mechanism of chromosomal translocation in T- and B-cell neoplasia. *Science* **234**:982, 1986.

52. McKeithan TW, Shima EA, Le Beau MM, Minowada J, Rowley JD, Diaz MO: Molecular cloning of the breakpoint junction of a human chromosomal 8;14 translocation involving the T-cell receptor alpha-chain gene and sequences on the 3′ side of MYC. *Proc Natl Acad Sci USA* **83**:6636, 1986.

53. Shima EA, Le Beau MM, McKeithan TW, Minowada J, Showe LC, Mak TW, Minden MD, Rowley JD, Diaz MO: Gene encoding the alpha chain of the T-cell receptor is moved immediately downstream of c-myc in a chromosomal 8;14 translocation in a cell line from a human T-cell leukemia. *Proc Natl Acad Sci USA* **83**:3439, 1986.

54. Brown L, Cheng JT, Chen Q, Siciliano MJ, Crist W, Buchanan G, Baer R: Site-specific recombination of the tal-1 gene is a common occurrence in human T cell leukemia. *EMBO J* **9**:3343, 1990.

55. Aplan PD, Lombardi DP, Kirsch IR: Structural characterization of SIL, a gene frequently disrupted in T-cell acute lymphoblastic leukemia. *Mol Cell Biol* **11**:5462, 1991.

56. Aplan PD, Lombardi DP, Reaman GH, Sather HN, Hammond GD, Kirsch IR: Involvement of the putative hematopoietic transcription factor SCL in T-cell acute lymphoblastic leukemia. *Blood* **79**:1327, 1992.

57. Bernard O, Lecointe N, Jonveaux P, Souyri M, Mauchauffe M, Berger R, Larsen CJ, Mathieu-Mahul D: Two site-specific deletions and t(1;14) translocation restricted to human T-cell acute leukemias disrupt the 5′ part of the tal-1 gene. *Oncogene* **6**:1477, 1991.

58. Breit TM, Mol EJ, Wolvers-Tettero IL, Ludwig WD, van Wering ER, van Dongen JJ: Site-specific deletions involving the tal-1 and sil genes are restricted to cells of the T cell receptor alpha/beta lineage: T cell receptor delta gene deletion mechanism affects multiple genes. *J Exp Med* **177**:965, 1993.

59. Baer R: TAL1, TAL2, and LYL1: a family of basic helix-loop-helix proteins implicated in T cell acute leukaemia. *Semin Cancer Biol* **4**:341, 1993.

60. Bash RO, Hall S, Timmons CF, Crist WM, Amylon M, Smith RG, Baer R: Does activation of the TAL1 gene occur in a majority of patients with T-cell acute lymphoblastic leukemia? A pediatric oncology group study. *Blood* **86**:666, 1995.

61. Hsu H-L, Cheng J-T, Chen Q, Baer R: Enhancer-binding activity of the tal-1 oncoprotein in association with the E47/E12 helix-loop-helix proteins. *Mol Cell Biol* **11**:3037, 1991.

62. Hsu HL, Huang L, Tsan JT, Funk W, Wright WE, Hu JS, Kingston RE, Baer R: Preferred sequences for DNA recognition by the TAL1 helix-loop-helix proteins. *Mol Cell Biol* **14**:1256, 1994.

63. Hsu HL, Wadman I, Baer R: Formation of in vivo complexes between the TAL1 and E2A polypeptides of leukemic T cells. *Proc Natl Acad Sci USA* **91**:3181, 1994.

64. Wadman I, Li J, Bash RO, Forster A, Osada H, Rabbitts TH, Baer R: Specific in vivo association between the bHLH and LIM proteins implicated in human T cell leukemia. *EMBO J* **13**:4831, 1994.

65. Larson RC, Lavenir I, Larson TA, Baer R, Warren AJ, Wadman I, Nottage K, Rabbitts TH: Protein dimerization between Lmo2 (Rbtn2) and Tal1 alters thymocyte development and potentiates T cell tumorigenesis in transgenic mice. *EMBO J* **15**:1021, 1996.

66. Voronova AF, Lee F: The E2A and tal-1 helix-loop-helix proteins associate in vivo and are modulated by Id proteins during interleukin 6-induced myeloid differentiation. *Proc Natl Acad Sci USA* **91**:5952, 1994.

67. Hsu HL, Wadman I, Tsan JT, Baer R: Positive and negative transcriptional control by the TAL1 helix-loop-helix protein. *Proc Natl Acad Sci USA* **91**:5947, 1994.

68. Porcher C, Swat W, Rockwell K, Fujiwara Y, Alt FW, Orkin SH: The T cell leukemia oncoprotein SCL/tal-1 is essential for development of all hematopoietic lineages. *Cell* **86**:47, 1996.

69. Green AR, Salvaris E, Begley CG: Erythroid expression of the "helix-loop-helix" gene, SCL. *Oncogene* **6**:475, 1991.

70. Kallianpur AR, Jordan JE, Brandt SJ: The SCL/TAL-1 gene is expressed in progenitors of both the hematopoietic and vascular systems during embryogenesis. *Blood* **83**:1200, 1994.

71. Mouthon MA, Bernard O, Mitjavila MT, Romeo PH, Vainchenker W, Mathieu-Mahul D: Expression of tal-1 and GATA-binding proteins during human hematopoiesis. *Blood* **81**:647, 1993.

72. Visvader J, Begley CG, Adams JM: Differential expression of the LYL, SCL and E2A helix-loop-helix genes within the hemopoietic system. *Oncogene* **6**:187, 1991.

73. Weintraub H: The MyoD family and myogenesis: Redundancy, networks, and thresholds. *Cell* **75**:1241, 1993.

74. Buckingham M: Molecular biology of muscle development. *Cell* **78**:15, 1994.

75. Stainier DY, Weinstein BM, Detrich HW, Zon LI, Fishman MC: Cloche, an early acting zebrafish gene, is required by both the endothelial and hematopoietic lineages. *Development* **121**:3141, 1995.

76. Liao EC, Paw BH, Oates AC, Pratt SJ, Postlethwait JH, Zon LI: SCL/Tal-1 transcription factor acts downstream of cloche to specify hematopoietic and vascular progenitors in zebrafish. *Genes Dev* **12**:621, 1998.

77. McGuire EA, Hockett RD, Pollock KM, Bartholdi MF, O'Brien SJ, Korsmeyer SJ: The t(11;14)(p15;q11) in a T-cell acute lymphoblastic leukemia cell line activates multiple transcripts, including ttg-1, a gene encoding a potential zinc finger protein. *Mol Cell Biol* **9**:2124, 1989.

78. Greenberg JM, Boehm T, Sofroniew MV, Keynes RJ, Barton SC, Norris ML, Surani MA, Spillantini MG, Rabbits TH: Segmental and developmental regulation of a presumptive T-cell oncogene in the central nervous system. *Nature* **344**:158, 1990.

79. Boehm T, Foroni L, Kaneko Y, Perutz MF, Rabbitts TH: The rhombotin family of cysteine-rich LIM-domain oncogenes: distinct members are involved in T-cell translocations to human chromosomes 11p15 and 11p13. *Proc Natl Acad Sci USA* **88**:4367, 1991.

80. Royer-Pokora B, Loos U, Ludwig WD: TTG-2, a new gene encoding a cysteine-rich protein with the LIM motif, is overexpressed in acute T-cell leukaemia with the t(11;14)(p13;q11). *Oncogene* **6**:1887, 1991.

81. Warren AJ, Colledge WH, Carlton MBL, Evans MJ, Smith AJH, Rabbitts TH: The oncogenic cysteine-rich LIM domain protein Rbtn2 is essential for erythroid development. *Cell* **78**:45, 1994.

82. Perez-Alvarado GC, et al: Structure of the carboxy-terminal LIM domain from the cysteine rich protein CRP. *Nature Struct Biol* **1**:388, 1994.

83. Valge-Archer VE, Osada H, Warren AJ, Forster A, Li J, Baer R, Rabbitts TH: The LIM protein RBTN2 and the basic helix-loop-helix protein TAL1 are present in a complex in erythroid cells. *Proc Natl Acad Sci USA* **91**:8617, 1994.

84. Robb L, Elwood NJ, Elefanty AG, Kontgen F, Li R, Barnett LD, Begley CG: The SCL gene product is required for the generation of all hematopoietic lineages in the adult mouse. *EMBO J* **15**:4123, 1996.

85. Yamada Y, Warren AJ, Dobson C, Forster A, Pannell R, Rabbitts TH: The T cell leukaemia LIM protein Lmo2 is necessary for adult mouse hematopoiesis. *Proc Natl Acad Sci USA* **95**:3890, 1998.

86. Osada H, Grutz G, Axelson H, Forster A, Rabbitts TH: Association of erythroid transcription factors: Complexes involving the LIM protein RBTN2 and the zinc-finger protein GATA1. *Proc Natl Acad Sci USA* **92**:9585, 1995.

87. Pevny L, Simon MC, Robertson E, Klein WH, Tsai SF, D'Agati V, Orkin SH, Costantini F: Erythroid differentiation in chimaeric mice blocked by a targeted mutation in the gene for transcription factor GATA-1. *Nature* **349**:257, 1991.

88. Wadman IA, Osada H, Grutz GG, Agulnick AD, Westphal H, Forster A, Rabbitts TH: The LIM-only protein Lmo2 is a bridging molecule assembling an erythroid, DNA-binding complex which includes the TAL1, E47, GATA-1 and Ldb1/NLI proteins. *EMBO J* **16**:3145, 1997.

89. McGuire EA, Rintoul CE, Sclar GM, Korsmeyer SJ: Thymic overexpression of Ttg-1 in transgenic mice results in T-cell acute lymphoblastic leukaemia/lymphoma. *Mol Cell Biol* **12**:4186, 1992.

90. Larson RC, Fisch P, Larson TA, Lavenir I, Langford T, King G, Rabbitts TH: T cell tumours of disparate phenotype in mice transgenic for Rbtn-2. *Oncogene* **9**:3675, 1994.

91. Larson RC, Osada H, Larson TA, Lavenir I, Rabbitts TH: The oncogenic LIM protein Rbtn2 causes thymic developmental aberrations that precede malignancy in transgenic mice. *Oncogene* **11**:853, 1995.

92. Fisch P, Boehm T, Lavenir I, Larson T, Arno J, Forster A, Rabbitts TH: T-cell acute lymphoblastic lymphoma induced in transgenic mice by the RBTN1 and RBTN2 LIM-domain genes. *Oncogene* **7**:2389, 1992.

93. Neale GA, Rehg JE, Goorha RM: Ectopic expression of rhombotin-2 causes selective expansion of CD4-CD8-lymphocytes in the thymus and T-cell tumors in transgenic mice. *Blood* **86**:3060, 1995.

94. Robb L, Rasko JE, Bath ML, Strasser A, Begley CG: Scl, a gene frequently activated in human T cell leukaemia, does not induce lymphomas in transgenic mice. *Oncogene* **10**:205, 1995.

95. Kelliher MA, Seldin DC, Leder P: TAL-1 induces T cell acute lymphoblastic leukemia accelerated by casein kinase IIalpha. *EMBO J* **15**:5160, 1996.

96. Rabbitts TH: LMO T-cell translocation oncogenes typify genes activated by chromosomal translocations that alter transcription and developmental processes. *Genes Dev* **12**:2651, 1998.

97. Hatano M, Roberts CW, Minden M, Crist WM, Korsmeyer SJ: Deregulation of a homeobox gene, HOX11, by the t(10;14) in T cell leukemia. *Science* **253**:79, 1991.

98. Kennedy MA, Gonzalez Sarmiento R, Kees UR, Lampert F, Dear N, Boehm T, Rabbitts TH: HOX11, a homeobox-containing T-cell oncogene on human chromosome 10q24. *Proc Natl Acad Sci USA* **88**:8900, 1991.

99. Lu M, Gong ZY, Shen WF, Ho AD: The tcl-3 proto-oncogene altered by chromosomal translocation in T-cell leukemia codes for a homeobox protein. *EMBO J* **10**:2905, 1991.

100. Dube ID, Kamel Reid S, Yuan CC, Lu M, Wu X, Corpus G, Raimondi SC, Crist WM, Carroll AJ, Minowada J, Baker JB: A novel human homeobox gene lies at the chromosome 10 breakpoint in lymphoid neoplasias with chromosomal translocation t(10;14). *Blood* **78**:2996, 1991.

101. Dear TN, Sanchez Garcia I, Rabbitts TH: The HOX11 gene encodes a DNA-binding nuclear transcription factor belonging to a distinct family of homeobox genes. *Proc Natl Acad Sci USA* **90**:4431, 1993.

102. Allen JD, Lints T, Jenkins NA, Copeland NG, Strasser A, Harvey RP, Adams JM: Novel murine homeobox gene on chromosome 1 expressed in specific hematopoietic lineages and during embryogenesis. *Genes Dev* **5**:509, 1991.

103. McGinnis W, Krumlauf R: Homeobox genes and axial patterning. *Cell* **68**:283, 1992.

104. Roberts CWM, Shutter JR, Korsmeyer SJ: Hox11 controls the genesis of the spleen. *Nature* **368**:747, 1994.

105. Dear TN, Colledge WH, Carlton MB, Lavenir I, Larson T, Smith AJ, Warren AJ, Evans MJ, Sofroniew MV, Rabbitts TH: The Hox11 gene is essential for cell survival during spleen development. *Development* **121**:2909, 1995.

106. Hatano M, Roberts CWM, Kawabe T, Shutter J, Korsmeyer SJ: Cell cycle progression, cell death and T cell lymphoma in HOX11 transgenic mice (abstract). *Blood* **80**:355a, 1992.

107. Masson N, Greene WK, Rabbitts TH: Optimal activation of an endogenous gene by HOX11 requires the NH2-terminal 50 amino acids. *Mol Cell Biol* **18**:3502, 1998.

108. Kawabe T, Muslin AJ, Korsmeyer SJ: HOX11 interacts with protein phosphatases PP2A and PP1 and disrupts a G2/M cell-cycle checkpoint. *Nature* **385**:454, 1997.

109. Murre C, McCaw PS, Baltimore D: A new DNA binding and dimerization motif in immunoglobulin enhancer binding, daughterless, MyoD, and myc proteins. *Cell* **56**:777, 1989.

110. Murre C, McCaw PS, Vaessin H, Caudy M, Jan LY, Cabrera CV, Buskin JN, Hauschka SD, Lassar AB, Weintraub H, Baltimore D: Interactions between heterologous helix-loop-helix proteins generate complexes that bind specifically to a common DNA sequence. *Cell* **58**:537, 1989.

111. Sun XH, Baltimore D: An inhibitory domain of E12 transcription factor prevents DNA binding in E12 homodimers but not in E12 heterodimers. *Cell* **64**:459, 1991.

112. Henthorn P, Kiledjian M, Kadesch T: Two distinct transcription factors that bind the immunoglobulin enhancer E5/E2 motif. *Science* **247**:467, 1990.

113. Henthorn P, McCarrick Walmsley R, Kadesch T: Sequence of the cDNA encoding ITF-1, a positive-acting transcription factor. *Nucleic Acids Res* **18**:677, 1990.

114. Cronmiller C, Schedl P, Cline TY: Molecular characterization of daughterless, a *Drosophila* sex determination gene with multiple roles in development. *Genes Dev* **2**:1666, 1988.

115. Caudy M, Vassin H, Brand M, Tuma R, Jan LY, Jan YN: Daughterless, a *Drosophila* gene essential for both neurogenesis and sex determination, has sequence similarities to myc and the achaete-scute complex. *Cell* **55**:1061, 1988.

116. Blackwell TK, Weintraub H: Differences and similarities in DNA-binding preferences of MyoD and E2A protein complexes revealed by binding site selection. *Science* **250**:1104, 1990.

117. Ellenberger T, Fass D, Arnaud M, Harrison SC: Crystal structure of transcription factor E47: E-box recognition by a basic region helix-loop-helix dimer. *Genes Dev* **8**:970, 1994.

118. Aronheim A, Shiran R, Rosen A, Walker MD: The E2A gene product contains two separable and functionally distinct transcription activation domains. *Proc Natl Acad Sci USA* **90**:8063, 1993.

119. Quong MW, Massari ME, Zwart R, Murre C: A new transcriptional-activation motif restricted to a class of helix-loop-helix proteins is functionally conserved in both yeast and mammalian cells. *Mol Cell Biol* **13**:792, 1993.

120. Lassar AB, Davis RL, Wright WE, Kadesch T, Murre C, Voronova A, Baltimore D, Weintraub H: Functional activity of myogenic HLH proteins requires hetero-oligomerization with E12/E47-like proteins in vivo. *Cell* **66**:305, 1991.

121. Xia Y, Hwang LH, Cobb MH, Baer RJ: Products of the TAL2, oncogene in leukemic T cells: bHLH phosphoproteins with DNA-binding activity. *Oncogene* **9**:1437, 1994.

122. Miyamoto A, Cui X, Naumovski L, Cleary ML: Helix-loop-helix proteins LYL1 and E2a form heterodimeric complexes with distinctive DNA-binding properties in hematolymphoid cells. *Mol Cell Biol* **16**:2394, 1996.

123. Bain G, Gruenwald S, Murre C: E2A and E2-2 are subunits of B-cell-specific E2-box DNA-binding proteins. *Mol Cell Biol* **13**:3522, 1993.

124. Benezra R: An intermolecular disulfide bond stabilizes E2A homo-dimers and is required for DNA binding at physiological temperatures. *Cell* **79**:1057, 1994.

125. Bain G, Robanus Maandag EC, Izon DJ, Amsen D, Kruisbeek AM, Weintraub BC, Krop I, Schlissel MS, Feeney AJ, van Roon M, van der Valk M, te Riele HPJ, Berns A, Murre C: E2A proteins are required for proper B-cell development and initiation of immunoglobulin gene rearrangements. *Cell* **79**:885, 1994.

126. Zhuang Y, Soriano P, Weintraub H: The helix-loop-helix gene E2A is required for B-cell formation. *Cell* **79**:875, 1994.

127. Bain G, Engel I, Maandag EC, te Riele HPJ, Voland JR, Sharp LL, Chun J, Huey B, Pinkel D, Murre C: E2A deficiency leads to abnormalities in αβ T-cell development and to rapid development of T-cell lymphomas. *Mol Cell Biol* **17**:4782, 1997.

128. Yan W, Young AZ, Soares VC, Kelley R, Benezra R, Zhuang Y: High incidence of T-cell tumors in E2A-null mice and E2A/Id1 double-knockout mice. *Mol Cell Biol* **17**:7317, 1997.

129. Mellentin JD, Murre C, Donlon TA, McCaw PS, Smith SD, Carroll AJ, McDonald ME, Baltimore D, Cleary ML: The gene for enhancer binding proteins E12/E47 lies at the t(1;19) breakpoint in acute leukemias. *Science* **246**:379, 1989.

130. Kamps MP, Murre C, Sun XH, Baltimore D: A new homeobox gene contributes the DNA binding domain of the t(1;19) translocation protein in pre-B ALL. *Cell* **60**:547, 1990.

131. Nourse J, Mellentin JD, Galili N, Wilkinson J, Stanbridge E, Smith SD, Cleary ML: Chromosomal translocation t(1;19) results in synthesis of a homeobox fusion mRNA that codes for a potential chimeric transcription factor. *Cell* **60**:535, 1990.

132. Mellentin JD, Nourse J, Hunger SP, Smith SD, Cleary ML: Molecular analysis of the t(1;19) breakpoint cluster region in pre-B cell acute lymphoblastic leukemias. *Genes Chromosomes Cancer* **2**:239, 1990.

133. McGinnis W, Levine MS, Hafen E, Kuroiwa A, Gehring WJ: A conserved DNA sequence in homoeotic genes of the *Drosophila* Antennapedia and Bithorax complexes. *Nature* **308**:428, 1984.

134. Scott MP, Weiner AJ: Structural relationships among genes that control development: sequence homology between the Antennapedia, Ultra-bithorax, and fushi tarazu loci of *Drosophila*. *Proc Natl Acad Sci USA* **81**:4115, 1984.

135. Van Dijk MA, Voorhoeve PM, Murre C: Pbx1 is converted into a transcriptional activator upon acquiring the N-terminal region of E2A in pre-B-cell acute lymphoblastoid leukemia. *Proc Natl Acad Sci USA* **90**:6061, 1993.

136. LeBrun DL, Cleary ML: Fusion with E2A alters the transcriptional properties of the homeodomain protein PBX1 in t(1;19) leukemias. *Oncogene* **9**:1641, 1994.

137. Lu Q, Wright DD, Kamps MP: Fusion with E2A converts the Pbx1 homeodomain protein into a constitutive transcriptional activator in human leukemias carrying the t(1;19) translocation. *Mol Cell Biol* **14**:3938, 1994.

138. Flegel WA, Singson AW, Margolis JS, Bang AG, Posakony JW, Murre C: Dpbx, a new homeobox gene closely related to the human proto-oncogene pbx1 molecular structure and developmental expression. *Mech Dev* **41**:155, 1993.

139. Rauskolb C, Peifer M, Weischaus E: Extradenticle, a regulator of homeotic gene activity, is a homolog of the homeobox-containing human proto-oncogene pbx1. *Cell* **74**:1101, 1993.

140. Weischaus E, Nusslein Volhard C, Jurgens G: Mutations affecting the pattern of the larval cuticle in *Drosophila* melanogaster: III. Zygotic loci on the X chromosome and the fourth chromosome. *Arch Dev Biol* **193**:267, 1984.

141. Peifer M, Wieschaus E: Mutations in the *Drosophila* gene extradenticle affect the way specific homeo domain proteins regulate segmental identity. *Genes Dev* **4**:1209, 1990.

142. Chan S-K, Jaffe L, Capovilla M, Botas J, Mann RS: The DNA binding specificity of ultrabithorax is modulated by cooperative interactions with extradenticle, another homeoprotein. *Cell* **78**:603, 1994.

143. Rauskolb C, Wieschaus E: Coordinate regulation of downstream genes by extradenticle and the homeotic selector proteins. *EMBO J* **13**:3561, 1994.

144. Van Dijk MA, Murre C: Extradenticle raises the DNA binding specificity of homeotic selector gene products. *Cell* **78**:617, 1994.

145. Johnson FB, Parker E, Krasnow MA: Extradenticle protein is a selective cofactor for the *Drosophila* homeotics: Role of the home-odomain and YPWM amino acid motif in the interaction. *Proc Natl Acad Sci USA* **92**:739, 1995.

146. Chang CP, Shen WF, Rozenfeld S, Lawrence HJ, Largman C, Cleary ML: Pbx proteins display hexapeptide-dependent cooperative DNA binding with a subset of Hox proteins. *Genes Dev* **9**:663, 1995.

147. Lu Q, Kamps MP: Structural determinants within Pbx1 that mediate cooperative DNA binding with pentapeptide-containing hox proteins: Proposal for a model of a Pbx1-Hox-DNA complex. *Mol Cell Biol* **16**:1632, 1996.

148. Neuteboom ST, Peltenburg LT, Van Dijk MA, Murre C: The hexapeptide LFPWMR in Hoxb-8 is required for cooperative DNA binding with Pbx1 and Pbx2 proteins. *Proc Natl Acad Sci USA* **92**:9166, 1995.

149. Van Dijk MA, Peltenburg LT, Murre C: Hox gene products modulate the DNA binding activity of Pbx1 and Pbx2. *Mech Dev* **52**:99, 1995.

150. Lu Q, Knoepfler PS, Scheele J, Wright DD, Kamps MP: Both Pbx1 and E2A-Pbx1 bind the DNA motif ATCAATCAA cooperatively with the products of multiple murine Hox genes, some of which are themselves oncogenes. *Mol Cell Biol* **15**:3786, 1995.

151. Knoepfler PS, Kamps MP: The pentapeptide motif of Hox proteins is required for cooperative DNA binding with Pbx1, physically contacts Pbx1, and enhances DNA binding by Pbx1. *Mol Cell Biol* **15**:5811, 1995.

152. Knoepfler PS, Kamps MP: The highest affinity DNA element bound by Pbx complexes in t(1;19) leukemic cells fails to mediate cooperative DNA-binding or cooperative transactivation by E2a-Pbx1 and class I Hox proteins: Evidence for selective targetting of E2a-Pbx1 to a subset of Pbx-recognition elements. *Oncogene* **14**:2521, 1997.

153. Lu Q, Kamps MP: Heterodimerization of Hox proteins with Pbx1 and oncoprotein E2a-Pbx1 generates unique DNA-binding specifities at nucleotides predicted to contact the N-terminal arm of the Hox homeodomain: Demonstration of Hox-dependent targeting of E2a-Pbx1 in vivo. *Oncogene* **14**:75, 1997.

154. Knoepfler PS, Lu Q, Kamps MP: Pbx1-Hox heterodimers bind DNA on inseparable half-sites that permit intrinsic DNA binding specificity of the Hox partner at nucleotides 3′ to a TAAT motif. *Nucleic Acids Res* **24**:2288, 1996.

155. Chang CP, Brocchieri L, Shen WF, Largman C, Cleary ML: Pbx modulation of Hox homeodomain amino-terminal arms establishes different DNA-binding specificities across the Hox locus. *Mol Cell Biol* **16**:1734, 1996.

156. Kamps MP, Baltimore D: E2A-Pbx1, the t(1;19) translocation protein of human pre-B-cell acute lymphocytic leukemia, causes acute myeloid leukemia in mice. *Mol Cell Biol* **13**:351, 1993.

157. Kamps MP, Wright DD: Oncoprotein E2A-Pbx1 immortalizes a myeloid progenitor in primary marrow cultures without abrogating its factor-dependence. *Oncogene* **9**:3159, 1994.

158. Privitera E, Kamps MP, Hayashi Y, Inaba T, Shapiro LH, Raimondi SC, Behm F, Hendershot L, Carroll AJ, Baltimore D, Look AT: Different molecular consequences of the 1;19 chromosomal translocation in childhood B-cell precursor acute lymphoblastic leukemia. *Blood* **79**:1781, 1992.

159. Borowitz MJ, Hunger SP, Carroll AJ, Shuster JJ, Pullen DJ, Steuber PJ, Cleary ML: Predictability of the t(1;19)(q23;p13) from surface antigen phenotype: Implications for screening cases of childhood ALL for molecular analysis. A Pediatric Oncology Group study. *Blood* **82**:1086, 1993.

160. Dedera DA, Waller EK, LeBrun DP, Sen-Majumdar A, Stevens ME, Barsh GS, Cleary ML: Chimeric homeobox gene E2A-PBX1 induces proliferation, apoptosis, and malignant lymphomas in transgenic mice. *Cell* **74**:833, 1993.

161. Monica K, LeBrun DP, Dedera DA, Brown R, Cleary ML: Transformation properties of the E2A-PBX1 chimeric oncoprotein: Fusion with E2A is essential, but the PBX1 homeodomain is dispensable. *Mol Cell Biol* **14**:8304, 1994.

162. Chang CP, de Vivo I, Cleary ML: The Hox cooperativity motif of the chimeric oncoprotein E2a-Pbx1 is necessary and sufficient for oncogenesis. *Mol Cell Biol* **17**:81, 1997.

163. Kamps MP, Wright DD, Lu Q: DNA-binding by oncoprotein E2a-Pbx1 is important for blocking differentiation but dispensable for fibroblast transformation. *Oncogene* **12**:19, 1996.

164. Chang CP, Jacobs Y, Nakamura T, Jenkins NA, Copeland NG, Cleary ML: Meis proteins are major in vivo DNA binding partners for wild-type but not chimeric Pbx proteins. *Mol Cell Biol* **17**:5679, 1997.

165. Knoepfler PS, Calvo KR, Chen H, Antonarakis SE, Kamps MP: Meis1 and pKnox1 bind DNA cooperatively with Pbx1 utilizing an interaction surface disrupted in oncoprotein E2a-Pbx1. *Proc Natl Acad Sci USA* **94**:14553, 1997.

166. Shen WF, Montgomery J, Rozenfeld S, Lawrence HJ, Buchberg A, Largman C: A subset of the Hox homeodomain proteins stabilize Meis protein-DNA binding. *Mol Cell Biol* **17**:6664, 1997.

167. Crist WM, Carroll AJ, Shuster JJ, Behm FG, Whitehead M, Vietti TJ, Look AT, Mahoney D, Ragab A, Pullen DJ, et al: Poor prognosis of children with pre-B acute lymphoblastic leukemia is associated with the t(1;19)(q23;p13). A Pediatric Oncology Group study. *Blood* **76**:117, 1990.

168. Raimondi SC, Behm FG, Roberson PK, Pui C-H, Williams DL, Crist WM, Look AT, Rivera GK: Cytogenetics of pre-B-cell acute lymphoblastic leukemia with emphasis on prognostic implications of the t(1;19). *J Clin Oncol* **8**:1380, 1990.

169. Williams DL, Look AT, Melvin SL, Roberson PK, Dahl G, Flake T, Stass S: New chromosomal translocations correlate with specific immunophenotypes of childhood acute lymphoblastic leukemia. *Cell* **36**:101, 1984.

170. Michael PM, Levin MD, Garson OM: Translocation 1;19: A new cytogenetic abnormality in acute lymphocytic leukemia. *Cancer Genet Cytogenet* **12**:333, 1984.

171. Miyamoto K, Tomita N, Ishii A, Nonaka H, Kondo T, Tanaka T, Kitajima K: Chromosome abnormalities of leukemia cells in adult patients with T-cell leukemia. *J Natl Cancer Inst* **73**:353, 1984.

172. Yamada T, Craig JM, Hawkins JM, Janossy G, Secker-Walker LM: Molecular investigation of 19p13 in standard and variant translocations: The E12 probe recognizes the 19p13 breakpoint in cases with t(1;19) and acute leukemia other than pre-B immunophenotype. *Leukemia* **5**:36, 1991.

173. Secker-Walker LM, Berger R, Fenaux P, Lai JL, Nelken B, Garson M, Michael PM, Hagemeijer A, Harrison CJ, Kaneko Y, Rubin CM: Prognostic significance of the balanced t(1;19) and unbalanced der(19)t(1;19) translocations in acute lymphoblastic leukemia. *Leukemia* **6**:363, 1992.

174. Ohno H, Inoue T, Akasaka T, Okumura A, Miyanishi S, Ohashi I, Kikuchi M, Masuya M, Amano H, Imanaka T, Ohno Y: Acute lymphoblastic leukemia associated with a t(1;19)(q23;p13) in an adult. *Intern Med* **32**:584, 1993.

175. Vagner-Capodano AM, Mozziconacci MJ, Zattara-Cannoni H, Guitard AM, Thuret I, Michel G: t(1;19) in a M4-ANLL. *Cancer Genet Cytogenet* **73**:86, 1994.

176. Wlodarska I, Stul M, DeWolf-Peeters C, Verhoef G, Mecucci C, Cassiman JJ, Van den Berghe H: t(1;19) without detectable E2A rearrangements in two t(14;18)-positive lymphoma/leukemia cases. *Genes Chromosomes Cancer* **10**:171, 1994.

177. Raimondi SC, Privitera E, Williams DL, Look AT, Behm F, Rivera GK, Crist WM, Pui C-H: New recurring chromosomal translocations in childhood acute lymphoblastic leukemia. *Blood* **77**:2016, 1991.

178. Hunger SP, Ohyashiki K, Toyama K, Cleary ML: Hlf, a novel hepatic bZIP protein, shows altered DNA-binding properties following fusion to E2A in t(17;19) acute lymphoblastic leukemia. *Genes Dev* **6**:1608, 1992.

179. Inaba T, Roberts WM, Shapiro LH, Jolly KW, Raimondi SC, Smith SD, Look AT: Fusion of the leucine zipper gene HLF to the E2A gene in human acute B-lineage leukemia. *Science* **257**:531, 1992.

180. Hunger SP, Devaraj PE, Foroni L, Secker-Walker LM, Cleary ML: Two types of genomic rearrangements create alternative E2A-HLF fusion proteins in t(17;19)-ALL. *Blood* **83**:2261, 1994.

181. Hunger SP, Brown R, Cleary ML: DNA-binding and transcriptional regulatory properties of hepatic leukemia factor (HLF) and the t(17;19) acute lymphoblastic leukemia chimera E2A-HLF. *Mol Cell Biol* **14**:5986, 1994.

182. Landschulz WH, Johnson PF, McKnight SL: The leucine zipper: A hypothetical structure common to a new class of DNA binding proteins. *Science* **240**:1559, 1988.

183. O'Shea EK, Klemm JD, Kim PS, Alber T: X-ray structure of the GCN4 leucine zipper, a two-stranded, parallel coiled coil. *Science* **254**:539, 1991.

184. Ellenberger TE, Brandl CJ, Struhl K, Harrison SC: The GCN4 basic region leucine zipper binds DNA as a dimer of uninterrupted alpha helices: Crystal structure of the protein-DNA complex. *Cell* **71**:1223, 1992.

185. Drolet DW, Scully KM, Simmons DM, Wegner M, Chu KT, Swanson LW, Rosenfeld MG: TEF, a transcription factor expressed specifically in the anterior pituitary during embryogenesis, defines a new class of leucine zipper proteins. *Genes Dev* **5**:1739, 1991.

186. Falvey E, Fleury Olela F, Schibler U: The rat hepatic leukemia factor (HLF) gene encodes two transcriptional activators with distinct circadian rhythms, tissue distributions and target preferences. *EMBO J* **14**:4307, 1995.

187. Inaba T, Inukai T, Yoshihara T, Seyschab H, Ashmun RA, Canman CE, Laken SJ, Kastan MB, Look AT: Reversal of apoptosis by the leukaemia-associated E2A-HLF chimaeric transcription factor. *Nature* **382**:541, 1996.

188. Metzstein MM, Hengartner MO, Tsung N, Ellis RE, Horvitz HR: Transcriptional regulator of programmed cell death encoded by *Caenorhabditis elegans* gene ces-2. *Nature* **382**:545, 1996.

189. Thompson CB: A fate worse than death. *Nature* **382**:492, 1996.

190. Inaba T, Shapiro LH, Funabiki T, Sinclair AE, Jones BG, Ashmun RA, Look AT: DNA-binding specificity and trans-activating potential of the leukemia-associated E2A-hepatic leukemia factor fusion protein. *Mol Cell Biol* **14**:3403, 1994.

191. Vinson CR, Hai T, Boyd SM: Dimerization specificity of the leucine zipper-containing bZIP motif on DNA binding: Prediction and rational design. *Genes Dev* **7**:1047, 1993.

192. Yoshihara T, Inaba T, Shapiro LH, Kato J, Look AT: E2A-HLF-mediated cell transformation requires both the trans-activation domain of E2A and the leucine zipper dimerization domain of HLF. *Mol Cell Biol* **15**:3247, 1995.

193. Hunger SP: Chromosomal translocations involving the E2A gene in acute lymphoblastic leukemia: Clinical features and molecular pathogenesis. *Blood* **87**:1211, 1996.

194. Smith KS, Jacobs Y, Chang CP, Cleary ML: Chimeric oncoprotein E2a-Pbx1 induces apoptosis of hematopoietic cells by a p53-independent mechanism that is suppressed by Bcl-2. *Oncogene* **14**:2917, 1997.

195. Devaraj PE, Foroni L, Sekhar M, Butler T, Wright F, Mehta A, Samson D, Prentice HG, Hoffbrand AV, Secker-Walker LM: E2A/HLF fusion cDNAs and the use of RT-PCR for the detection of minimal residual disease in t(17;19)(q22;p13) acute lymphoblastic leukemia. *Leukemia* **8**:1131, 1994.

196. Ohyashiki K, Fujieda H, Miyauchi J, Ohyashiki JH, Tauchi T, Saito M, Nakazawa S, Abe K, Yamamoto K, Clark SC, et al: Establishment of a novel heterotransplantable acute lymphoblastic leukemia cell line with a t(17;19) chromosomal translocation the growth of which is inhibited by interleukin-3. *Leukemia* **5**:322, 1991.

197. Golub TR, Barker GF, Bohlander SK, Hiebert SW, Ward DC, Bray-Ward P, Morgan E, Raimondi SC, Rowley JD, Gilliland DG: Fusion of the TEL gene on 12p13 to the AML1 gene on 21q22 in acute lymphoblastic leukemia. *Proc Natl Acad Sci USA* **92**:4917, 1995.

198. Romana SP, Mauchauffe M, Le Coniat M, Chumakov I, Le Paslier D, Berger R, Bernard OA: The t(12;21) of acute lymphoblastic leukemia results in a tel- AML1 gene fusion. *Blood* **85**:3662, 1995.

199. Shurtleff SA, Buijs A, Behm FG, Rubnitz JE, Raimondi SC, Hancock ML, Chan GC, Pui CH, Grosveld G, Downing JR: TEL/AML1 fusion resulting from a cryptic t(12;21) is the most common genetic lesion in pediatric ALL and defines a subgroup of patients with an excellent prognosis. *Leukemia* **9**:1985, 1995.

200. Romana SP, Poirel H, Leconiat M, Flexor MA, Mauchauffe M, Jonveaux P, Macintyre EA, Berger R, Bernard OA: High frequency of t(12;21) in childhood B-lineage acute lymphoblastic leukemia. *Blood* **86**:4263, 1995.

201. Liang D-C, Chou T-B, Chen J-S, Shurtleff SA, Rubnitz JE, Downing JR, Pui C-H, Shih L-Y: High incidence of TEL/AML1 fusion resulting from a cryptic t(12;21) in childhood B-lineage acute lymphoblastic leukemia in Taiwan. *Leukemia* **10**:991, 1996.

202. Hiebert SW, Sun W, Davis JN, Golub T, Shurtleff S, Buijs A, Downing JR, Grosveld G, Roussel MF, Gilliland DG, Lenny N, Meyers S: The t(12;21) translocation converts AML-1B from an activator to a repressor of transcription. *Mol Cell Biology* **16**:1349, 1996.

203. Golub TR, Goga A, Barker GF, Afar DE, McLaughlin J, Bohlander SK, Rowley JD, Witte ON, Gilliland DG: Oligomerization of the ABL tyrosine kinase by the Ets protein TEL in human leukemia. *Mol Cell Biol* **16**:4107, 1996.

204. Golub TR, Barker GF, Stegmaier K, Gilliland DG: The TEL gene contributes to the pathogenesis of myeloid and lymphoid leukemias by diverse molecular genetic mechanisms. *Curr Top Microbiol Immunol* **220**:67, 1997.

205. Jousset C, Carron C, Boureux A, et al: A domain of TEL conserved in a subset of ETS proteins defines a specific oligomerizaton interface essential to the mitogenic properties of the TEL-PDGFRβ oncoprotein. *EMBO J* **16**:69, 1997.

206. McLean TW, Ringold S, Neuberg D, Stegmaier K, Tantravahi R, Ritz J, Koeffler HP, Takeuchi S, Janssen JW, Seriu T, Bartram CR, Sallan SE, Gilliland DG, Golub TR: TEL/AML-1 dimerizes and is associated with a favorable outcome in childhood acute lymphoblastic leukemia. *Blood* **88**:4252, 1996.

207. Wang LC, Kuo F, Fujiwara Y, Gilliland DG, Golub TR, Orkin SH: Yolk sac angiogenic defect and intra-embryonic apoptosis in mice lacking the Ets-related factor TEL. *EMBO J* **16**:4374, 1997.

208. Rubnitz JE, Downing JR, Pui C-H, Shurtleff SA, Raimondi SC, Evans WE, Head DR, Crist WM, Rivera GK, Hancock ML, Boyett JM, Buijs A, Grosveld G, Behm FG: TEL gene rearrangement in acute lymphoblastic leukemia: A new genetic marker with prognostic significance. *J Clin Oncol* **15**:1150, 1997.

209. Rubnitz JE, Shuster JJ, Land VJ, Link MP, Pullen DJ, Camitta BM, Pui CH, Downing JR, Behm FG: Case-control study suggests a favorable impact of TEL rearrangement in patients with B-lineage acute lymphoblastic leukemia treated with antimetabolite-based therapy. A Pediatric Oncology Group study. *Blood* **89**:1143, 1997.

210. Borkhardt A, Cazzaniga G, Viehmann S, Valsecchi MG, Ludwig WD, Burci L, Mangioni S, Schrappe M, Riehm H, Lampert F, Basso G, Masera G, Harbott J, Biondi A: Incidence and clinical relevance of TEL/AML1 fusion genes in children with acute lymphoblastic leukemia enrolled in the German and Italian multicenter therapy trials. *Blood* **90**:571, 1997.

211. Look AT: Pathobiology of the acute lymphoid leukemia cell, in Hoffman R (ed): *Hematology*, 2d ed. New York, Churchill-Livingstone, 1995, p. 1047.

212. Ye BH, Rao PH, Chaganti RS, Dalla-Favera R: Cloning of bcl-6, the locus involved in chromosome translocations affecting band 3q27 in B-cell lymphoma. *Cancer Res* **53**:2732, 1993.

213. Kerckaert JP, Deweindt C, Tilly H, Quief S, Lecocq G, Bastard C: LAZ-3, a novel zinc-finger encoding gene, is disrupted by recurring chromosome 3q27 translocations in human lymphomas. *Nature Genet* **5**:66, 1993.

214. Miki T, Kawamata N, Hirosawa S, Aoki N: Gene involved in the 3q27 translocation associated with B-cell lymphoma, BCL5, encodes a Kruppel-like zinc-finger protein. *Blood* **83**:26, 1994.

215. Ye BH, Lista F, Lo Coco F, Knowles DM, Offit K, Chaganti RS, Dalla-Favera R: Alterations of a zinc finger-encoding gene, BCL-6, in diffuse large-cell lymphoma. *Science* **262**:747, 1993.

216. Cattoretti G, Chang CC, Cechova K, Zhang J, Ye BH, Falini B, Louie DC, Offit K, Chaganti RS, Dalla-Favera R: BCL-6 protein is expressed in germinal-center B cells. *Blood* **86**:45, 1995.

217. Flenghi L, Ye BH, Fizzotti M, Bigerna B, Cattoretti G, Venturi S, Pacini R, Pileri S, Lo Coco F, Pescarmona E, et al: A specific monoclonal antibody (PG-B6) detects expression of the BCL-6 protein in germinal center B cells. *Am J Pathol* **147**:405, 1995.

218. McLennan ICM: Germinal centers. *Annu Rev Immunol* **12**:117, 1994.

219. Dalla-Favera R, Ye BH, Cattoretti G, Lo Coco F, Chang C-C, Zhang J, Migliazza A, Cechova K, Niu H, Chaganti S, Chen W, Louie DC, Offit K, Chaganti RSK: BCL-6 in diffuse large-cell lymphomas, in De Vita VT, Hellman S, Rosenberg SA (eds): *Important Advances in Oncology*. Philadelphia, Lippincott-Raven, 1996, p. 139.

220. Ye BH, Chaganti S, Chang CC, Niu H, Corradini P, Chaganti RS, Dalla-Favera R: Chromosomal translocations cause deregulated BCL6 expression by promoter substitution in B cell lymphoma. *EMBO J* **14**:6209, 1995.

221. Migliazza A, Martinotti S, Chen W, Fusco C, Ye BH, Knowles DM, Offit K, Chaganti RS, Dalla-Favera R: Frequent somatic hypermutation of the 5′ noncoding region of the BCL6 gene in B-cell lymphoma. *Proc Natl Acad Sci USA* **92**:12520, 1995.

222. Offit K, Lo Coco F, Louie DC, Parsa NZ, Leung D, Portlock C, Ye BH, Lista F, Filippa DA, Rosenbaum A, Ladanyi M, Jhanwar S, Dalla-Favera R, Chaganti RSK: Rearrangement of the BCL-6 gene as a prognostic marker in diffuse large-cell lymphoma. *N Engl J Med* **331**:74, 1994.

223. Speck NA, Stacy T: A new transcription factor family associated with human leukemias. *Crit Rev Eukaryotic Gene Express* **5**:337, 1995.

224. Wang S, Wang Q, Crute BE, Melnikova IN, Keller SR, Speck NA: Cloning and characterization of subunits of the T-cell receptor and murine leukemia virus enhancer core-binding factor. *EMBO J* **13**:3324, 1993.

225. Ogawa E, Inuzuka M, Maruyama M, Satake M, Naito-Fujimoto M, Ito Y, Shigesada K: Molecular cloning and characterization of PEBP2β, the heterodimeric partner of a novel *Drosophila* runt-related DNA binding protein PEBP2α. *Virol* **194**:314, 1993.

226. Miyoshi H, Shimizu K, Kozu T, Maseki N, Kaneko Y, Ohki M: t(8;21) breakpoints on chromosome 21 in acute myeloid leukemia are clustered within a limited region of a single gene, AML1. *Proc Natl Acad Sci USA* **88**:10431, 1991.

227. Gao J, Erickson P, Gardiner K, Le Beau MM, Diaz MO, Patterson D, Rowley JD, Drabkin HA: Isolation of a yeast artificial chromosome spanning the 8;21 translocation breakpoint t(8;21)(q22;q22.3) in acute myelogenous leukemia. *Proc Natl Acad Sci USA* **88**:4882, 1991.

228. Erickson P, Gao J, Chang KS, Look T, Whisenant E, Raimondi S, Lasher R, Trujillo J, Rowley J, Drabkin H: Identification of breakpoints in t(8;21) acute myelogenous leukemia and isolation of a fusion transcript. AML1/ETO, with similarity to *Drosophila* segmentation gene, runt. *Blood* **80**:1825, 1992.

229. Nisson PE, Watkins PC, Sacchi N: Transcriptionally active chimeric gene derived from the fusion of the AML1 gene and a novel gene on chromosome 8 in t(8;21) leukemic cells. *Cancer Genet Cytogenet* **63**:81, 1992.

230. Mitani K, Ogawa S, Tanaka T, Miyoshi H, Kurokawa M, Mano H, Yazaki Y, Ohki M, Hirai H: Generation of the AML1-EVI-1 fusion gene in the t(3;21)(q26;q22) causes blastic crisis in chronic myelocytic leukemia. *EMBO J* **13**:504, 1994.

231. Nucifora G, Begy CR, Erickson P, Drabkin HA, Rowley JD: The 3;21 translocation in myelodysplasia results in a fusion transcript between the AML1 gene and the gene for EAP, a highly conserved protein associated with the Epstein-Barr virus small RNA EBER 1. *Proc Natl Acad Sci USA* **90**:7784, 1993.

232. Meyers S, Downing JR, Hiebert SW: Identification of AML-1 and the (8;21) translocation protein (AML-1/ETO) as sequence specific DNA binding proteins: The runt homology domain is required for DNA binding and protein-protein interactions. *Mol Cell Biol* **13**:6336, 1993.

233. Nuchprayoon I, Meyers S, Scott LM, Suzow J, Hiebert S, Friedman AD: PEBP2/CBF, the murine homolog of the human myeloid AML1 and PEBP2 beta/CBF beta proto-oncoproteins, regulates the murine myeloperoxidase and neutrophil elastase genes in immature myeloid cells. *Mol Cell Biol* **14**:5558, 1994.

234. Takahashi A, Satake M, Yamaguchi-Iwai Y, Bae SC, Lu J, Maruyama M, Zhang YW, Oka H, Arai N, Arai K, et al: Positive and negative regulation of granulocyte-macrophage colony-stimulating factor promoter activity by AML1-related transcription factor, PEBP2. *Blood* **86**:607, 1995.

235. Wotton D, Ghysdael J, Wang S, Speck NA, Owen MJ: Cooperative binding of Ets-1 and core binding factor to DNA. *Mol Cell Biol* **14**:840, 1994.

236. Hernandez-Munain C, Krangel MS: c-Myb and core-binding factor/PEBP2 display functional synergy but bind independently to adjacent sites in the T-cell receptor delta enhancer. *Mol Cell Biol* **15**:3090, 1995.

237. Manley NR, O Connell M, Sun W, Speck NA, Hopkins N: Two factors that bind to highly conserved sequences in mammalian type C retroviral enhancers. *J Virol* **67**:1967, 1993.

238. Sun W, O Connell M, Speck NA: Characterization of a protein that binds multiple sequences in mammalian type C retrovirus enhancers. *J Virol* **67**:1976, 1993.

239. Sun W, Graves BJ, Speck NA: Transactivation of the Moloney murine leukemia virus and T-cell receptor beta-chain enhancers by cbf and ets requires intact binding sites for both proteins. *J Virol* **69**:4941, 1995.

240. Frank R, Zhang J, Uchida H, Meyers S, Hiebert SW, Nimer SD: The AML1/ETO fusion protein blocks transactivation of the GM-CSF promoter by AML1B. *Oncogene* **11**:2667, 1995.

241. Okuda T, van Deursen J, Hiebert SW, Grosveld G, Downing JR: AML1, the target of multiple chromosomal translocations in human leukemia, is essential for normal fetal liver hematopoiesis. *Cell* **84**:321, 1996.

242. Wang Q, Stacy T, Binder M, Marin-Padilla M, Sharpe AH, Speck NA: Disruption of the Cbfa2 gene causes necrosis and hemorrhaging in the central nervous system and blocks definitive hematopoiesis. *Proc Natl Acad Sci USA* **93**:3444, 1996.

243. Wang Q, Stacy T, Miller JD, Lewis AF, Gu T-L, Huang X, Bushweller JH, Bories J-C, Alt FW, Ryan G, Liu PP, Wynshaw-Boris A, Binder M, Marin-Padilla M, Sharpe AH, Speck NA: The CBFβ subunit is essential for CBFα2 (AML1) function in vivo. *Cell* **87**:697, 1996.

244. Meyers S, Lenny N, Hiebert SW: The t(8;21) fusion protein interferes with AML-1B-dependent transcriptional activation. *Mol Cell Biol* **15**:1974, 1995.

245. Meyers S, Lenny N, Hiebert SW: The t(8;21) fusion protein interferes with AML-1B-dependent transcriptional activation. *Mol Cell Biol* **15**:1974, 1995.

246. Westendorf JJ, Yamamoto CM, Lenny N, Downing JR, Selsted ME, Hiebert SW: The t(8;21) fusion product, AML-1-ETO, associates with C/EBP-alpha, inhibits C/EBP-alpha-dependent transcription, and blocks granulocytic differentiation. *Mol Cell Biol* **18**:322, 1998.

247. Wang J, Hoshino TRRL, Kajigaya S, Liu JM: Novel human nuclear receptor co-repressor: cloning and identification as a binding partner for the ETO proto-oncoprotein (abstract). *Blood* **90**:244a, 1998.

248. Lutterbach B, Westendorf JJ, Linggi B, Patten A, Moniwa M, Davie JR, Huynh KD, Bardwell VJ, Lavinsky RM, Rosenfeld MG, Glass C, Seto E, Hiebert SW: ETO, a target of the t(8;21) in acute leukemia, interacts with the N-COR and mSin3 co-repressors. *Mol Cell Biol* (in press).

249. Grunstein M: Histone acetylation in chromatin structure and transcription. *Nature* **389**:349, 1997.

250. Nucifora G, Rowley JD: AML1 and the 8;21 and 3;21 translocations in acute and chronic myeloid leukemia. *Blood* **86**:1, 1995.

251. Liu P, Tarle SA, Hajra A, Claxton DF, Marlton P, Freedman M, Siciliano MJ, Collins FS: Fusion between transcription factor CBFβ/PEBP2β and a myosin heavy chain in acute myeloid leukemia. *Science* **261**:1041, 1993.

252. Shurtleff SA, Meyers S, Hiebert SW, et al: Heterogeneity in CBF beta.MYH11 fusion messages encoded by the inv(16)(p13q22)and the t(16;16)(p13;q22) in acute myelogenous leukemia. *Blood* **85**:3695, 1995.

253. Viswanatha DS, Chen I, Liu PP, Slovak ML, Rankin C, Head DR, Willman CL: Characterization and use of an antibody detecting the CBFβ-SMMHC fusion protein in inv(16)/t(16:16)-associated acute myeloid leukemias. *Blood* **91**:1882, 1998.

254. Castilla LH, Wijmenga C, Wang Q, Stacy T, Speck NA, Eckhaus M, Marin-Padilla M, Collins FS, Wynshaw-Boris A, Liu PP: Failure of embryonic hematopoiesis and lethal hemorrhages in mouse embryos heterozygous for a knocked-in leukemia gene CBFB-MYH11. *Cell* **87**:687, 1996.

255. Yergeau DA, Hetherington CJ, Wang Q, et al: Embryonic lethality and impairment of haematopoiesis in mice heterozygous for an AML-ETO fusion gene. *Nature Genet* **15**:303, 1997.

256. Okuda T, Cai Z, Yang S, et al: Expression of a knocked-in AML1-ETO leukemia gene inhibits the estabalishment of normal definitive hematopoiesis and directly generates dysplastic hematopoietic progenitors. *Blood* **91**:3134, 1998.

257. Martinez-Climent JA, Lane NJ, Rubin CM, Morgan E, Johnstone HS, Mick R, Murphy SB, Vardiman JW, Larson RA, Lebeau MM, Rowley JD: Clinical and prognostic significance of chromosomal abnormalities in childhood acute myeloid leukemia de novo. *Leukemia* **9**:95, 1995.

258. Mrozek K, Heinonen K, de la Chapelle A, Bloomfield CD: Clinical significance of cytogenetics in acute myeloid leukemia. *Semin Oncol* **24**:17, 1997.

259. Berger R, Bernheim A, Ochoa-Noguera ME, Daniel MT, Valensi F, Sigaux F, Flandrin G, Boiron M: Prognostic significance of chromosomal abnormalities in acute nonlymphocytic leukemia: A study of 343 patients. *Cancer Genet Cytogenet* **28**:293, 1987.

260. Samuels BL, Larson RA, Le Beau MM, Daly KM, Bitter MA, Vardiman JW, Barker CM, Rowley JD, Golomb HM: Specific chromosomal abnormalities in acute nonlymphocytic leukemia correlate with drug susceptibility in vivo. *Leukemia* **2**:79, 1988.

261. Keating MJ, Smith TL, Kantarjian H, Cork A, Walters R, Trujillo JM, McCredie KB, Gehan EA, Freireich EJ: Cytogenetic pattern in acute myelogenous leukemia: A major reproducible determinant of outcome. *Leukemia* **2**:403, 1988.

262. Fenaux P, Preudhomme C, Lai JL, Morel P, Beuscart R, Bauters F: Cytogenetics and their prognostic value in de novo acute myeloid leukaemia: A report on 283 cases. *Br J Haematol* **73**:61, 1989.

263. Dastugue N, Payen C, Lafage-Pochitaloff M: Prognostic significance of karyotype in de novo adult acute myeloid leukemia. The BGMT group. *Leukemia* **9**:1491, 1995.

264. Nucifora G, Larson RA, Rowley JD: Persistence of the 8;21 translocation in patients with acute myeloid leukemia type M2 in long-term remission. *Blood* **82**:712, 1993.

265. Miyamoto T, Nagafuji K, Akashi K, Harada M, Kyo T, Akashi T, Takenaka K, Mizuno S, Gondo H, Okamura T, Dohy H, Niho Y: Persistence of multipotent progenitors expressing AML1/ETO transcripts in long-term remission patients with t(8;21) acute myelogenous leukemia. *Blood* **87**:4789, 1996.

266. Tobal K, Johnson PR, Saunders MJ, Yin JA: Detection of CBF/MYH11 transcripts in patients with inversion and other abnormalities of chromosome 16 at presentation and remission. *Br J Haematol* **91**:104, 1995.

267. Jurlander J, Caligiuri MA, Ruutu T, Baer MR, Strout MP, Oberkircher AR, Hoffmann L, Ball ED, Frei-Lahr DA, Christiansen NP, Block AM, Knuutila S, Herzig GP, Bloomfield CD: Persistence of the AML1/ETO fusion transcript in patients treated with allogeneic bone marrow transplantation for t(8;21) leukemia. *Blood* **88**:2183, 1996.

268. de The H, Chomienne C, Lanotte M, Degos L, Dejean A: The t(15;17) translocation of acute promyelocytic leukaemia fuses the retinoic acid receptor alpha gene to a novel transcribed locus. *Nature* **347**:558, 1990.

269. Borrow J, Goddard AD, Sheer D, Solomon E: Molecular analysis of acute promyelocytic leukemia breakpoint cluster region on chromosome 17. *Science* **249**:1577, 1990.

270. Longo L, Pandolfi PP, Biondi A, Rambaldi A, Mencarelli A, Lo Coco F, Diverio D, Pegoraro L, Avanzi G, Tabilio A, et al: Rearrangements and aberrant expression of the retinoic acid receptor alpha gene in acute promyelocytic leukemias. *J Exp Med* **172**:1571, 1990.

271. de The H, Lavau C, Marchio A, Chomienne C, Degos L, Dejean A: The PML-RARα fusion mRNA generated by the t(15;17) translocation in acute promyelocytic leukemia encodes a functionally altered RAR. *Cell* **66**:675, 1991.

272. Kakizuka A, Miller WH Jr, Umesono K, Warrell RP Jr, Frankel SR, Murty VV, Dmitrovsky E, Evans RM: Chromosomal translocation t(15;17) in human acute promyelocytic leukemia fuses RARα with a novel putative transcription factor, PML. *Cell* **66**:663, 1991.

273. Kastner P, Perez A, Lutz Y, Rochette-Egly C, Gaub MP, Durand B, Lanotte M, Berger R, Chambon P: Structure, localization and transcriptional properties of two classes of retinoic acid receptor alpha fusion proteins in acute promyelocytic leukemia (APL): Structural similarities with a new family of oncoproteins. *EMBO J* **11**:629, 1992.

274. Perez A, Kastner P, Sethi S, Lutz Y, Reibel C, Chambon P: PMLRAR homodimers: Distinct DNA binding properties and heteromeric interactions with RXR. *EMBO J* **12**:3171, 1993.

275. Dyck JA, Maul GG, Miller WH Jr, Chen JD, Kakizuka A, Evans RM: A novel macromolecular structure is a target of the promyelocyte-retinoic acid receptor oncoprotein. *Cell* **76**:333, 1994.

276. Weis K, Rambaud S, Lavau C, Jansen J, Carvalho T, Carmo-Fonseca M, Lamond A, Dejean A: Retinoic acid regulates aberrant nuclear localization of PML-RAR alpha in acute promyelocytic leukemia cells. *Cell* **76**:345, 1994.

277. Koken MH, Puvion Dutilleul F, Guillemin MC, Viron A, Linares-Cruz G, Stuurman N, de Jong L, Szostecki C, Calvo F, Chomienne C, Degos L, Puvion E, The HD: The t(15;17) translocation alters a nuclear body in retinoic acid-reversible fashion. *EMBO J* **13**:1073, 1994.

278. Carvalho T, Seeler JS, Ohman K, Jordan P, Pettersson U, Akusjarvi G, Carmo-Fonseca M, Dejean A: Targeting of adenovirus E1A and E4-ORF3 proteins to nuclear matrix-associated PML bodies. *J Cell Biol* **131**:45, 1995.

279. Doucas V, Ishov AM, Romo A, Juguilon H, Weitzman MD, Evans RM, Maul GG: Adenovirus replication is coupled with the dynamic properties of the PML nuclear structure. *Genes Dev* **10**:196, 1996.

280. Everett RD, Maul GG: HSV-1 IE protein Vmw110 causes redistribution of PML. *EMBO J* **13**:5062, 1994.

281. Terris B, Baldin V, Dubois S, Degott C, Flejou JF, Henin D, Dejean A: PML nuclear bodies are general targets for inflammation and cell proliferation. *Cancer Res* **55**:1590, 1995.

282. Lavau C, Marchio A, Fagioli M, Jansen J, Falini B, Lebon P, Grosveld F, Pandolfi PP, Pelicci PG, Dejean A: The acute promyelocytic leukaemia-associated PML gene is induced by interferon. *Oncogene* **11**:871, 1995.

283. Nason-Burchenal K, Gandini D, Botto M, Allopenna J, Seale JR, Cross NC, Goldman JM, Dmitrovsky E, Pandolfi PP: Interferon augments PML and PML/RARalpha expression in normal myeloid and acute promyelocytic cells and cooperates with all-trans-retinoic acid to induce maturation of a retinoid resistant promyelocytic cell line. *Blood* (in press).

284. Jansen JH, Mahfoudi A, Rambaud S, Lavau C, Wahli W, Dejean A: Multimeric complexes of the PML-retinoic acid receptor alpha fusion protein in acute promyelocytic leukemia cells and interference with retinoid and peroxisome-proliferator signaling pathways. *Proc Natl Acad Sci USA* **92**:7401, 1995.

285. Grignani F, Ferrucci PF, Testa U, Talamo G, Fagioli M, Alcalay M, Mencarelli A, Peschle C, Nicoletti I, Pelicci PG: The acute promyelocytic leukemia-specific PML-RARa fusion protein inhibits differentiation and promotes survival of myeloid precursor cells. *Cell* **74**:423, 1993.

286. Grignani F, Testa U, Fagioli M, Barberi T, Masciulli R, Mariani G, Peschle C, Pelicci PG: Promyelocytic leukemia-specific PML-retinoic acid alpha receptor fusion protein interferes with erythroid differentiation of human erythroleukemia K562 cells. *Cancer Res* **55**:440, 1995.

287. Testa U, Grignani F, Barberi T, Fagioli M, Masciulli R, Ferrucci PF, Seripa D, Camagna A, Alcalay M, Pelicci PG, et al: PML/RAR alpha+ U937 mutant and NB4 cell lines: Retinoic acid restores the monocytic differentiation response to vitamin D3. *Cancer Res* **54**:4508, 1994.

288. Fu S, Consoli U, Hanania EG, Zu Z, Claxton DF, Andreeff M, Deisseroth AB: PML/RAα, a fusion protein in acute promyelocytic leukemia, prevents growth factor withdrawal-induced apoptosis in TF-1 cells. *Clin Cancer Res* **1**:583, 1995.

289. Rogaia D, Grignani Fr, Grignani F, Nicoletti I, Pelicci PG: The acute promyelocytic leukemia-specific PML/RARα fusion protein reduces the frequency of commitment to apoptosis upon growth factor deprivation of GM-CSF-dependent myeloid cells. *Leukemia* **9**:1467, 1995.

290. Redner RL, Rush EA, Faas S, Rudert WA, Corey SJ: The t(5;17) variant of acute promyelocytic leukemia expresses a nucleophosmin-retinoic acid receptor fusion. *Blood* **87**:882, 1996.

291. Wells RA, Catzavelos C, Kamel-Reid S: Fusion of retinoic acid receptor α to NuMA, the nuclear mitotic apparatus protein, by a variant translocation in acute promyelocytic leukaemia. *Nature Genet* **17**:109, 1997.

292. Chen Z, Brand N, Chen A, Chen S-J, Tong J-H, Wang Z-Y, Waxman S, Zelent A: Fusion between a novel Krüppel-like zinc finger gene and the retinoic acid receptor-α locus due to a variant t(11;17) translocation associated with acute promyelocytic leukaemia. *EMBO J* **12**:1161, 1993.

293. Bardwell VJ, Treisman R: The POZ domain: A conserved protein-protein interaction motif. *Genes Dev* **8**:1664, 1994.

294. Chen Z, Guidez F, Rousselot P, Agadir A, Chen S-J, Wang Z-Y, Degos L, Zelent A, Waxman S, Chomienne C: PLZF-RARα fusion proteins generated from the variant t(11;17)(q23;q21) translocation in acaute promyelocytic leukemia inhibit ligand-dependent transactivation of wild-type retinoic acid receptors. *Proc Natl Acad Sci USA* **91**:1178, 1994.

295. Dong S, Zhu J, Reid A, Strutt P, Guidez F, Zhong HJ, Wang ZY, Licht J, Waxman S, Chomienne C, Chen Z, Zelent A, Chen SJ: Amino-terminal protein-protein interaction motif (POZ-domain) is responsible for activities of the promyelocytic leukemia zinc finger-retinoic acid receptor-alpha fusion protein. *Proc Natl Acad Sci USA* **93**:3624, 1996.

296. Licht JD, Shaknovich R, English MA, Melnick A, Li JY, Reddy JC, Dong S, Chen SJ, Zelent A, Waxman S: Reduced and altered DNA-binding and transcriptional properties of the PLZF-retinoic acid receptor-alpha chimera generated in t(11;17)-associated acute pro-myelocytic leukemia. *Oncogene* **12**:323, 1996.

297. Cook M, Gould A, Brand N, Davies J, Strutt P, Shaknovich R, Licht J, Waxman S, Chen Z, Gluecksohn-Waelsch S, Krumlauf R, Zelent A: Expression of the zinc-finger gene PLZF at rhombomere boundaries in the vertebrate hindbrain. *Proc Natl Acad Sci USA* **92**:2249, 1995.

298. Reid A, Gould A, Brand N, Cook M, Strutt P, Li J, Licht J, Waxman S, Krumlauf R, Zelent A: Leukemia translocation gene, PLZF, is expressed with a speckled nuclear pattern in early hematopoietic progenitors. *Blood* **86**:4544, 1995.

299. Licht JD, Chomienne C, Goy A, Chen A, Scott AA, Head DR, Michaux JL, Wu Y, DeBlasio A, Miller WH Jr, et al: Clinical and molecular characterization of a rare syndrome of acute promyelocytic leukemia associated with translocation (11;17). *Blood* **85**:1083, 1995.

300. Horlein AJ, Naar AM, Heinzel T, Torchia J, Gloss B, Kurokawa R, Ryan A, Kamei Y, Soderstrom M, Glass CK: Ligand-independent repression by the thyroid hormone receptor mediated by a nuclear receptor co-repressor. *Nature* **377**:397, 1995.

301. Kurokawa R, Soderstrom M, Horlein AJ, Halachmi S, Brown M, Rosenfeld MG, Glass CK: Polarity-specific activities of retinoic acid receptors determined by a co-repressor. *Nature* **377**:451, 1995.

302. Alland L, Muhle R, Hou HJ, Potes J, Chin L, Schreiber-Agus N, DePinho RA: Role for N-CoR and histone deacetylase in Sin3-mediated transcriptional repression. *Nature* **387**:49, 1997.

303. Heinzel T, Lavinsky RM, Mullen TM, Soderstrom M, Laherty CD, Torchia J, Yang WM, Brard G, Ngo SD, Davie JR, Seto E, Eisenman RN, Rose DW, Glass CK, Rosenfeld MG: A complex containing N-CoR, mSin3 and histone deacetylase mediates transcriptional repression. *Nature* **387**:43, 1997.

304. Nagy L, Kao HY, Chakravarti D, Lin RJ, Hassig CA, Ayer DE, Schreiber SL, Evans RM: Nuclear receptor repression mediated by a complex containing SMRT, mSin3A, and histone deacetylase. *Cell* **89**:373, 1997.

305. Chen JD, Evans RM: A transcriptional co-repressor that interacts with nuclear hormone receptors. *Nature* **377**:454, 1995.

306. Lin RJ, Nagy L, Inoue S, Shao W, Miller WHJ, Evans RM: Role of the histone deacetylase complex in acute promyelocytic leukaemia. *Nature* **391**:811, 1998.

307. He LZ, Guidez F, Triboli C, Peruzzi D, Ruthardt M, Zelent A, Pandolfi PP: Distinct interactions of PML-RARα and PLZF-RARα with co-repressors determine differential responses to RA in APL. *Nature Genet* **18**:126, 1998.

308. Grignani F, De Matteis S, Nervi C, Tomassoni L, Gelmetti V, Cioce M, Fanelli M, Ruthardt M, Ferrara FF, Zamir I, Seiser C, Lazar MA, Minucci S, Pelicci PG: Fusion proteins of the retinoic acid receptor-alpha recruit histone deacetylase in promyelocytic leukaemia. *Nature* **391**:815, 1998.

309. Hong S-YDG, Wong C-W, Dejean A, Privalsky ML: SMRT corepressor interacts with PAZF and with the PML-retinoic acid receptor α (RARα) and PLZF-RARα oncoproteins associated with acute promyelocytic leukemia. *Proc Natl Acad Sci USA* **94**:9028, 1997.

310. Guidez F, Ivins S, Zhu J, Soderstrom M, Waxman S, Zelent A: Reduced retinoic acid-sensitivities of nuclear receptor corepressor binding to PML- and PLZF-RARα underlie molecular pathogenesis and treatment of acute promyelocytic leukemia. *Blood* **91**:2634, 1998.

311. Huang ME, Ye YC, Chen SR, Chai JR, Lu JX, Zhoa L, Gu LJ, Wang ZY: Use of all-trans retinoic acid in the treatment of acute promyelocytic leukemia. *Blood* **72**:567, 1988.

312. Castaigne S, Chomienne C, Daniel MT, Ballerini P, Berger R, Fenaux P, Degos L: All-trans retinoic acid as a differentiation therapy for acute promyelocytic leukemia: I. Clinical results. *Blood* **76**:1704, 1990.

313. Warrell RP Jr, Frankel SR, Miller WH Jr, Scheinberg DA, Itri LM, Hittelman WN, Vyas R, Andreeff M, Tafuri A, Jakubowski A, Gabrilove J, Gordon MS, Dimitrovsky E: Differentiation therapy of acute promyelocytic leukemia with tretinoin (all-*trans*-retinoic acid). *N Engl J Med* **324**:1385, 1991.

314. Sun GL, Yang RR, Chen SJ, Gu LJ, Xie WY, Zhang FQ, Li XS, Zhong DH, Cai JR, Chen Z, Wang ZY, Lu JX, Huang LA, Qian ZC, Yu HQ, Wang YL: Treatment of APL with all-trans retinoic acid: A report of five-year experience. *Chin J Cancer* **11**:125, 1993.

315. Chen ZX, Xue YQ, Zhang R, Tao RF, Xia XM, Li C, Wang W, Zu WY, Yao XZ, Ling BJ: A clinical and experimental study on all-*trans* retinoic acid-treated acute promyelocytic leukemia patients. *Blood* **78**:1413, 1991.

316. Warrell RP Jr, Maslak P, Eardley A, Heller G, Miller WH Jr, Frankel SR: Treatment of acute promyelocytic leukemia with all-trans retinoic acid: An update of the New York experience. *Leukemia* **8**:929, 1994.

317. Fenaux P, Chastang C, Chomienne C, Degos L: All transretinoic acid (ATRA) in combination with chemotherapy improves survival in newly diagnosed acute promyelocytic leukemia (APL). *Lancet* **343**:1033, 1994.

318. Early E, Moore MA, Kakizuka A, Nason-Burchenal K, Martin P, Evans RM, Dmitrovsky E: Transgenic expression of PML/RARα impairs myelopoiesis. *Proc Natl Acad Sci USA* **93**:7900, 1996.

319. Grisolano JL, Wesselschmidt RL, Ley TJ: Altered myeloid develop-ment and acute leukemia in transgenic mice expressing PML-RARα under control of cathepsin G regulatory sequences. *Blood* **89**:376, 1997.

320. He LZ, Triboli C, Rivi R, Peruzzi D, Pelicci PG, Soares V, Cattoretti G, Pandolfi PP: Acute leukemia with promyelocytic features in PML/RARα transgenic mice. *Proc Natl Acad Sci USA* **94**:5302, 1997.

321. Altabef M, Garcia M, Lavaue C, Bae S-C, Dejean A, Samarut J: A retrovirus carrying the promyelocyte-retinoic acid receptor PML-RARalpha fusion gene transforms haematopoietic progenitors in vitro and induces acute leukaemias. *EMBO J* **15**:2707, 1996.

322. Morishita K, Parganas E, Bartholomew C, Sacchi N, Valentine MB, Raimondi SC, Le Beau MM, Ihle JN: The human Evi-1 gene is located on chromosome 3q24-q28 but is not rearranged in three cases of acute nonlymphocytic leukemias containing t(3;5)(q25;q34) translocations. *Oncogene Res* **5**:221, 1990.

323. Morishita K, Parganas E, Willman CL, Whittaker MH, Drabkin H, Oval J, Taetle R, Ihle JN: Activation of Evi-1 gene expression in human acute myelogenous leukemias by translocations spanning 300–400 kb on chromosome 3q26. *Proc Natl Acad Sci USA* **89**:3937, 1992.

324. Morishita K, Parker DS, Mucenski ML, Jenkins NA, Copeland NG, Ihle JN: Retroviral activation of a novel gene encoding a zinc finger protein in IL-3-dependent myeloid leukemia cell lines. *Cell* **54**:831, 1988.

325. Delwel R, Funabiki T, Kreider BL, Morishita K, Ihle JN: Four of the seven zinc fingers of the Evi-1 myeloid-transforming gene are required for sequence-specific binding to GA(C/T)AAGA(T/C)AAGATAA. *Mol Cell Biol* **13**:4291, 1993.

326. Perkins AS, Fishel R, Jenkins NA, Copeland NG: Evi-1, a murine zinc finger proto-oncogene, encodes a sequence-specific DNA-binding protein. *Mol Cell Biol* **11**:2665, 1991.

327. Funabiki T, Kreider BL, Ihle JN: The carboxyl domain of zinc fingers of the Evi-1 myeloid transforming gene binds a consensus sequence of GAAGATGAG. *Oncogene* **9**:1575, 1994.

328. Kreider BL, Orkin SH, Ihle JN: Loss of erythropoietin responsiveness in erythroid progenitors due to expression of the Evi-1 myeloid-transforming gene. *Proc Natl Acad Sci USA* **90**:6454, 1993.

329. Mitelman F: *Catalog of Chromosome Aberrations in Cancer.* New York, Wiley-Liss, 1994.

330. Raimondi SC, Kalwinsky DK, Hayashi Y, Behm FG, Mirro J Jr, Williams DL: Cytogenetics of childhood acute nonlymphocytic leukemia. *Cancer Genet Cytogenet* **40**:13, 1989.

331. Raimondi SC: Current status of cytogenetic research in childhood acute lymphoblastic leukemia. *Blood* **81**:2237, 1993.

332. Pui C-H, Frankel LS, Carroll AJ, Raimondi SC, Shuster JJ, Head DR, Crist WM, Land VJ, Pullen DJ, Steuber CP, Behm FG, Borowitz MJ: Clinical characteristics and treatment outcome of childhood acute lymphoblastic leukemia with the t(4;11) (q21;q23): A collaborative study of 40 cases. *Blood* **77**:440, 1991.

333. Kaneko Y, Maseki N, Takasaki M, Sakurai T, Hayashi Y, Nakazawa S, Mori T, Sakurai M, Takeda T, Shikano T, Hiroshi Y: Clinical and hematologic characteristics in acute leukemia with 11q23 translocations. *Blood* **67**:484, 1986.

334. Heerema NA, Arthur DC, Sather H, Albo V, Feusner J, Lange BJ, Steinherz PG, Zeltzer P, Hammond D, Reaman GH: Cytogenetic features of infants less than 12 months of age at diagnosis of acute lymphoblastic leukemia: Impact of the 11q23 breakpoint on outcome. A Report of the Childrens Cancer Group. *Blood* **83**:2274, 1994.

335. Pui CH, Kane JR, Crist WM: Biology and treatment of infant leukemias. *Leukemia* **9**:762, 1995.

336. Chen CS, Sorensen PH, Domer PH, Reaman GH, Korsmeyer SJ, Heerema NA, Hammond GD, Kersey JH: Molecular rearrangements on chromosome 11q23 predominate in infant acute lymphoblastic leukemia and are associated with specific biologic variables and poor outcome. *Blood* **81**:2386, 1993.

337. Chen C-S, Sorensen PHB, Domer PH, Reaman GH, Korsmeyer SJ, Heerema NA, Hammond GD, Kersey JH: Molecular rearrangements on chromosome 11q23 predominate in infant acute lymphoblastic leukemia and are associated with specific biologic variables and poor outcome. *Blood* **81**:2386, 1993.

338. Pui C-H, Behm FG, Raimondi SC, Dodge RK, George SL, Rivera GK, Mirro J, Kalwinsky DK, Dahl GV, Murphy SB, Crist WM, Williams DL: Secondary acute myeloid leukemia in children treated for acute lymphoid leukemia. *N Engl J Med* **321**:136, 1989.

339. DeVore R, Whitlock J, Hainsworth JD, Johnson DH: Therapy-related acute nonlymphocytic leukemia with monocytic features and rearrangement of chromosome 11q. *Ann Intern Med* **110**:740, 1989.

340. Ziemin-van der Poel S, McCabe NR, Gill HJ, Espinosa R, Patel Y, Harden A, Rubinelli P, Smith SD, Lebeau MM, Rowley JD, Diaz MO: Identification of a gene, MLL, that spans the breakpoint in 11q23 translocations associated with human leukemias. *Proc Natl Acad Sci USA* **88**:10735, 1991.

341. Tkachuk DC, Kohler S, Cleary ML: Involvement of a homolog of *Drosophila* trithorax by 11q23 chromosomal translocations in acute leukemias. *Cell* **71**:691, 1992.

342. Gu Y, Nakamura T, Alder H, Prasad R, Canaani O, Cimino G, Croce CM, Cananni E: The t(4;11) chromosome translocation of human acute leukemias fuses the ALL-1 gene, related to *Drosophila* trithorax, to the AF-4 gene. *Cell* **71**:701, 1992.

343. Djabali M, Selleri L, Parry P, Bower M, Young BD, Evans G: A trithorax-like gene is interrupted by chromosome 11q23 translocations in acute leukemias. *Nature Genet* **2**:113, 1992.

344. Domer PH, Fakharzadeh SS, Chen CS, Jockel J, Johansen L, Silverman GA, Kersey JH, Korsmeyer SJ: Acute mixed-lineage leukemia t(4;11)(q21;q23) generates an MLL-AF4 fusion product. *Proc Natl Acad Sci USA* **90**:7884, 1993.

345. Morrissey J, Tkachuk DC, Milatovich A, Francke U, Link M, Cleary ML: A serine/proline-rich protein is fused to HRX in t(4;11) acute leukemias. *Blood* **81**:1124, 1993.

346. Jones RS, Gelbart WM: The *Drosophila* polycomb-group gene enhancer of zeste contains a region with sequence similarity to trithorax. *Mol Cell Biol* **13**:6357, 1993.

347. Yu BD, Hess JL, Horning SE, Brown GA, Korsmeyer SJ: Altered Hox expression and segmental identity in Mll-mutant mice. *Nature* **378**:505, 1995.

348. Simon J: Locking in stable states of gene expression: Transcriptional control during *Drosophila* development. *Curr Opin Cell Biol* **7**:376, 1995.

349. Mazo AM, Huang DH, Mozer BA, Dawid IB: The trithorax gene, a trans-acting regulator of the bithorax-complex in *Drosophila,* encodes a protein with zinc-binding domains. *Proc Natl Acad Sci USA* **87**:2112, 1990.

350. Reeves R, Nissen MS: The A-T-DNA-binding domain of mammalian high mobility group I chromosomal proteins. *J Biol Chem* **265**:8573, 1990.

351. Ma Q, Alder H, Nelson KK, Chatterjee D, Gu Y, Nakamura T, Canaani E, Croce CM, Siracusa LD, Buchberg AM: Analysis of the murine ALL-1 gene reveals conserved domains with human ALL-1 and identified a motif shared with DNA methyltransferases. *Proc Natl Acad Sci USA* **90**:6350, 1993.

352. Zeleznik-Le NJ, Harden AM, Rowley JD: 11q23 translocations split the "AT-hook" cruciform DNA-binding region and the transcriptional repression domain from the activation domain of the mixed-lineage leukemia (MLL) gene. *Proc Natl Acad Sci USA* **91**:10610, 1994.

353. Cui X, de Vivo I, Slany R, Miyamoto A, Firestein R, Cleary ML: Association of SET domain and myotubularin-related proteins modulates growth control. *Nature Genet* **18**:331, 1998.

354. de Vivo I, Cui X, Domen J, Cleary ML: Growth stimulation of primary B cell precursors by the anti-phosphatase Sbf1. *Proc Natl Acad Sci USA* **95**:9471, 1998.

355. Thirman MJ, Levitan DA, Kobayashi H, Simon MC, Rowley JD: Cloning of ELL, a gene that fuses to MLL in a t(11;19)(q23;p13.1) in acute myeloid leukemia. *Proc Natl Acad Sci USA* **91**:12110, 1994.

356. Mitani K, Kanda Y, Ogawa S, Tanaka T, Inazawa J, Yazaki Y, Hirai H: Cloning of several species of MLL/MEN chimeric cDNAs in myeloid leukemia with t(11;19)(q23;p13.1) translocation. *Blood* **85**:2017, 1995.

357. Shilatifard A, Lane WS, Jackson KW, Conaway RC, Conaway JW: An RNA polymerase II elongation factor encoded by the human ELL gene. *Science* **271**:1873, 1996.

358. Duan DR, Humphrey JS, Chen DY, Weng Y, Sukegawa J, Lee S, Gnarra JR, Linehan WM, Klausner RD: Characterization of the VHL tumor suppressor gene product: Localization, complex formation, and the effect of natural inactivating mutations. *Proc Natl Acad Sci USA* **92**:6459, 1995.

359. Duan DR, Pause A, Burgess WH, Aso T, Chen YT, Garrett KP, Conaway RC, Conaway JW, Linehan WM, Klausner RD: Inhibiton of transcription elongation by the VHL tumor suppressor protein. *Science* **269**:1402, 1995.

360. Aso T, Lane WS, Conaway JW, Conaway RC: Elongin (SIII): A multisubunit regulator of elongation by RNA polymerase II. *Science* **269**:1439, 1995.

361. Kibel A, Iliopoulos O, DeCaprio JA, Kaelin WG Jr: Binding of the von Hippel-Lindau tumor suppressor protein to elongin B and C. *Science* **269**:1444, 1995.

362. Rubnitz JE, Behm FG, Curcio-Brint AM, Pinheiro RP, Carroll AJ, Raimondi SC, Shurtleff SA, Downing JR: Molecular analysis of t(11;19) breakpoints in childhood acute leukemias. *Blood* **87**:4804, 1996.

363. Nakamura T, Alder H, Gu Y, Prasad R, Canaani O, Kamada N, Gale RP, Lange B, Crist WM, Nowell PC: Genes on chromosomes 4, 9, and 19 involved in 11q23 abnormalities in acute leukemia share sequence homology and/or common motifs. *Proc Natl Acad Sci USA* **90**:4631, 1993.

364. Chen CS, Hilden JM, Frestedt J, Domer PH, Moore R, Korsmeyer SJ, Kersey JH: The chromosome 4q21 gene (AF-4/FEL) is widely expressed in normal tissues and shows breakpoint diversity in t(4;11)(q21;q23) acute leukemia. *Blood* **82**:1080, 1993.

365. Rubnitz JE, Morrissey J, Savage PA, Cleary ML: ENL, the gene fused with HRX in t(11;19) leukemias, encodes a nuclear protein with transcriptional activation potential in lymphoid and myeloid cells. *Blood* **84**:1747, 1994.

366. Tse W, Zhu W, Chen HS, Cohen A: A novel gene, AF1q, fused to MLL in t(1;11)(q21;q23), is specifically expressed in leukemic and immature hematopoietic cells. *Blood* **85**:650, 1995.

367. Schichman SA, Caligiuri MA, Gu Y, Strout MP, Canaani E, Bloomfield CD, Croce CM: ALL-1 partial duplication in acute leukemia. *Proc Natl Acad Sci USA* **91**:6236, 1994.

368. Schichman SA, Caligiuri MA, Strout MP, Carter SL, Gu Y, Canaani E, Bloomfield CD, Croce CM: ALL-1 tandem duplication in acute myeloid leukemia with a normal karyotype involves homologous recombination between Alu elements. *Cancer Res* **54**:4277, 1994.

369. Schumacher A, Magnuson T: Murine polycomb- and trithorax-group genes regulate homeotic pathways and beyond. *Trends Genet* **13**:167, 1997.

370. Yu BD, Hanson R, Hess JL, Horning SE, Korsmeyer SJ: MLL, a mammalian trithorax-group gene, functions as a transcriptional maintenance factor in morphogenesis. *Proc Natl Acad Sci USA* **95**:1998.

371. Sauvageau G, Lansdorp PM, Eaves CJ, Hogge DE, Dragowska WH, Reid DS, Largman C, Lawrence HJ, Humphries RK: Differential expression of homeobox genes in functionally distinct CD34+ subpopulations of human bone marrow cells. *Proc Natl Acad Sci USA* **91**:12223, 1994.

372. Lawrence HJ, Largman C: Homeobox genes in normal hematopoiesis and leukemia. *Blood* **80**:2445, 1992.

373. Lawrence HJ, Sauvageau G, Ahmadi N, Lopez AR, Lebeau MM, Link M, Humphries K, Largman C: Stage- and lineage-specific expression of the HOXA10 homeobox gene in normal and leukemic hematopoietic cells. *Exp Hematol* **23**:1160, 1995.

374. Sauvageau G, Thorsteinsdottir U, Hough MR, Hugo P, Lawrence HJ, Largman C, Humphries RK: Overexpression of HOXB3 in hematopoietic cells causes defective lymphoid development and progressive myeloproliferation. *Immunity* **6**:13, 1997.

375. Sauvageau G, Thorsteinsdottir U, Eaves CJ, Lawrence HJ, Largman C, Lansdorp PM, Humphries RK: Overexpression of HOXB4 in hematopoietic cells causes the selective expansion of more primitive populations in vitro and in vivo. *Genes Dev* **9**:1753, 1995.

376. Thorsteinsdottir U, Sauvageau G, Hough MR, Dragowska W, Lansdorp PM, Lawrence HJ, Largman C, Humphries RK: Overexpression of HOXA10 in murine hematopoietic cells perturbs both myeloid and lymphoid differentiation and leads to acute myeloid leukemia. *Mol Cell Biol* **17**:495, 1997.

377. Hess JL, Yu BD, Li B, Hanson R, Korsmeyer SJ: Defects in yolk sac hematopoiesis in Mll-null embryos. *Blood* **90**:1799, 1997.

378. Corral J, Lavenir I, Impey H, Warren AJ, Forster A, Larson TA, Bell S, McKenzie AN, King G, Rabbitts TH: An MLL-AF9 fusion gene made by homologous recombination causes acute leukemia in chimeric mice: A method to create fusion oncogenes. *Cell* **85**:853, 1996.

379. Lavau C, Szilvassy SJ, Slany R, Cleary ML: Immortalization and leukemic transformation of a myelomonocytic precursor by retrovirally transduced HRX-ENL. *EMBO J* **16**:4426, 1997.

380. Slany RK, Lavau C, Cleary ML: The oncogenic capacity of HRX-ENL requires the transcriptional transactivation activity of ENL and the DNA binding motifs of HRX. *Mol Cell Biol* **18**:122, 1998.

381. Pui C-H, Ribeiro RC, Hancock ML, Rivera GK, Evans WE, Raimondi SC, Head DR, Behm FG, Mahmoud MH, Sandlund JT, Crist WM: Acute myeloid leukemia in children treated with epipodophyllotoxins for acute lymphoblastic leukemia. *N Engl J Med* **325**:1682, 1991.

382. Gu Y, Alder H, Nakamura T, Schichman SA, Prasad R, Canaani O, Saito H, Croce CM, Canaani E: Sequence analysis of the breakpoint cluster region in the ALL-1 gene involved in acute leukemia. *Cancer Res* **54**:2327, 1994.

383. Gu Y, Cimino G, Alder H, Nakamura T, Prasad R, Canaani O, Moir DT, Jones C, Nowell PC, Croce C M: The t(4;11)(q21;q23) chromosome translocations in acute leukemias involve the VDJ recombinase. *Proc Natl Acad Sci USA* **89**:10464, 1992.

384. Felix CA, Winick NJ, Negrini M, Bowman WP, Croce CM, Lange BJ: Common region of ALL-1 gene disrupted in epipodophyllotoxin-related secondary acute myeloid leukemia. *Cancer Res* **53**:2954, 1993.

385. Negrini M, Felix CA, Martin C, Lange BJ, Nakamura T, Canaani E, Croce CM: Potential topoisomerase II DNA-binding sites at the breakpoints of a t(9;11) chromosome translocation in acute myeloid leukemia. *Cancer Res* **53**:4489, 1993.

386. Strissel Broeker PL, Super HG, Thirman MJ, Pomykala H, Yonebayashi Y, Tanabe S, Zeleznik-Le N, Rowley JD: Distribution of 11q23 breakpoints within the MLL breakpoint cluster region in de novo acute leukemia and in treatment-related acute myeloid leukemia: Correlation with scaffold attachment regions and topoisomerase II consensus binding sites. *Blood* **87**:1912, 1996.

387. Domer PH, Head DR, Renganathan N, Raimondi SC, Yang E, Atlas M: Molecular analysis of 13 cases of MLL/11q23 secondary acute leukemia and identification of topoisomerase II consensus-binding sequences near the chromosomal breakpoint of a secondary leukemia with the t(4;11). *Leukemia* **9**:1305, 1995.

388. Bernard OA, Berger R: Molecular basis of 11q23 rearrangements in hematopoietic malignant proliferations. *Genes Chromosomes Cancer* **13**:75, 1995.

389. Prasad R, Gu Y, Alder H, Nakamura T, Canaani O, Saito H, Huebner K, Gale RP, Nowell PC, Kuriyama K, Miyazaki Y, Croce CM, Canaani E: Cloning of the ALL-1 fusion partner, the AF-6 gene, involved in acute myeloid leukemias with the t(6;11) chromosome translocation. *Cancer Res* **53**:5624, 1993.

390. Super HJG, McCabe NR, Thirman MJ, Larson RA, Lebeau MM, Pedersen-Bjergaard J, Philip P, Diaz MO, Rowley JD: Rearrangements of the MLL gene in therapy-related acute myeloid leukemia in patients previously treated with agents targeting DNA-topoisomerase II. *Blood* **81**:3705, 1993.

391. Hunger SP, Tkachuk DC, Amylon MD, Link MP, Carroll AJ, Welborn JL, Willman CL, Cleary ML: HRX involvement in de novo and secondary leukemias with diverse chromosome 11q23 abnormalities. *Blood* **81**:3197, 1993.

392. Bower M, Parry P, Carter M, Lillington DM, Amess J, Lister TA, Evans G, Young BD: Prevalence and clinical correlations of MLL gene rearrangements in AML-M4/5. *Blood* **84**:3776, 1994.

393. Wang JC: DNA topoisomerases. *Annu Rev Biochem* **54**:665, 1985.

394. Bae YS, Kawasaki I, Ikeda H, Liu LF: Illegitimate recombination mediated by calf thymus DNA topoisomerase II in vitro. *Proc Natl Acad Sci USA* **85**:2076, 1988.

395. Sperry AO, Blasquez VC, Garrard WT: Dysfunction of chromosomal loop attachment sites: Illegitimate recombination linked to matrix association regions and topoisomerase II. *Proc Natl Acad Sci USA* **86**:5497, 1989.

396. Ford AM, Ridge SA, Cabrera ME, Mahmoud H, Steel CM, Chan LC, Greaves M: In utero rearrangements in the trithorax-related oncogene in infant leukaemias. *Nature* **363**:358, 1993.

397. Super HJG, Rothberg PG, Kobayashi H, Freeman AI, Diaz MO, Rowley JD: Clonal, nonconstitutional rearrangements of the MLL gene in infant twins with acute lymphoblastic leukemia: In utero chromosome rearrangement of 11q23. *Blood* **83**:641, 1994.

398. Fujioka K, Caslini C, Jones BG, Komuro H, Naeve CW, Look AT: Aberrant p27Kip1 transcripts identified in human leukemias expressing the MLL-AF4 fusion protein. *Blood* **88**:356a, 1996.

399. Caslini C, Murti KG, Ashmun D, Domer PH, Korsmeyer SJ, Boer JM, Grosveld GC, Look AT: Subcellular localization and cell cycle effects of the MLL-AF4 fusion oncoprotein. *Blood* **88**:557a, 1996.

400. Schlessinger J, Ullrich A: Growth factor signaling by receptor tyrosine kinases. *Neuron* **9**:383, 1992.

401. Schlessinger J: How receptor tyrosine kinases activate Ras. *Trends Biochem Sci* **18**:273, 1993.

402. Greco A, Pierotti MA, Bongarzone I, Pagliardini S, Lanzi C, Della Porta G: TRK-T1 is a novel oncogene formed by the fusion of TPR and TRK genes in human papillary thyroid carcinomas. *Oncogene* **7**:237, 1992.

403. Rodrigues GA, Park M: Dimerization mediated through a leucine zipper activates the oncogenic potential of the met receptor tyrosine kinase. *Mol Cell Biol* **13**:6711, 1993.

404. Anonymous: Chromosomal abnormalities and their clinical significance in acute lymphoblastic leukemia: Third International Workshop on Chromosomes in Leukemia. *Cancer Res* **43**:868, 1983.

405. Rowley JD: Biological implications of consistent chromosome rearrangements in leukemia and lymphoma. *Cancer Res* **44**:3159, 1984.

406. Ribeiro RC, Abromowitch M, Raimondi SC, et al: Clinical and biologic hallmarks of the Philadelphia chromosome in childhood acute lymphoblastic leukemia. *Blood* **70**:948, 1987.

407. Bartram CR, de Klein A, Hagemeijer A, van Agthoven T, Geurts van Kessel A, Bootsma D, Grosveld G, Ferguson-Smith MA, Davies T, Stone M, et al: Translocation of c-abl oncogene correlates with the presence of a Philadelphia chromosome in chronic myelocytic leukaemia. *Nature* **306**:277, 1983.

408. Gale RP, Canaani E: An 8-kilobase abl RNA transcript in chronic myelogenous leukemia. *Proc Natl Acad Sci USA* **81**:5648, 1984.

409. Collins SJ, Kubonishi I, Miyoshi I, Groudine MT: Altered transcription of the c-abl oncogene in K562 and other chronic myelogenous leukemia cells. *Science* **225**:72, 1984.

410. Stam K, Heisterkamp N, Grosveld G, de Klein A, Verna RS, Coleman M, Dosik H, Groffen J: Evidence of a new chimeric bcr/c-abl mRNA in patients with chronic myelocytic leukemia and the Philadelphia chromosome. *N Engl J Med* **313**:1429, 1985.

411. Canaani E, Gale RP, Steiner-Saltz D, et al: Altered transcription of an oncogene in chronic myeloid leukemia. *Lancet* **1**:593, 1984.

412. Shtivelman E, Lifshitz B, Gale RP, Canaani E: Fused transcript of abl and bcr genes in chronic myelogenous leukemia. *Nature* **315**:550, 1985.

413. Heisterkamp N, Stephenson JR, Groffen J, et al: Localization of the c-abl oncogene adjacent to a translocation breakpoint in chronic myelocytic leukaemia. *Nature* **306**:239, 1983.

414. Leibowitz D, Schaefer Rego K, Popenoe DW, et al: Variable breakpoints on the Philadelphia chromosome in chronic myelogenous leukemia. *Blood* **66**:243, 1985.

415. Grosveld G, Verwoerd T, van Agthoven T, de Klein A, Ramachandran KL, Heisterkamp N, Stam K, Groffen J: The chronic myelocytic cell line K562 contains a breakpoint in bcr and produces a chimeric bcr/c-abl transcript. *Mol Cell Biol* **6**:607, 1986.

416. Groffen J, Stephenson JR, Heisterkamp N, et al: Philadelphia chromosomal breakpoints are clustered within a limited region, bcr, on chromosome 22. *Cell* **36**:93, 1984.

417. Heisterkamp N, Stam K, Groffen J, et al: Structural organization of the bcr gene and its role in Ph1 translocation. *Nature* **315**:758, 1985.

418. Kloetzer W, Kurzrock R, Smith L, Talpaz M, Spiller M, Gutterman J, Arlinghaus R: The human cellular abl gene product in the chronic myelogenous leukemia cell line K562 has an associated tyrosine protein kinase activity. *Virology* **140**:230, 1985.

419. Konopka JB, Watanabe SM, Witte ON: An alteration of the human c-abl protein in K562 leukemia cells unmasks associated tyrosine kinase activity. *Cell* **37**:1935, 1984.

420. Konopka JB, Watanabe SM, Singer JW, et al: Cell lines and clinical isolates derived from Ph1-positive chronic myelogenous leukemia patients express c-abl proteins with a common structural alteration. *Proc Natl Acad Sci USA* **82**:1810, 1985.

421. Naldini L, Stacchini A, Cirillo DM, Aglietta M, Gavosto F, Comoglio PM: Phosphotyrosine antibodies identify the p210 c-abl tyrosine kinase and proteins phosphorylated on tyrosine in human chronic myelogenous leukemia cells. *Mol Cell Biol* **6**:1803, 1986.

422. Chan LC, Karhi KK, Rayter SI, et al: A novel abl protein expressed in Philadelphia chromosome-positive acute lymphoblastic leukaemia. *Nature* **325**:635, 1987.

423. Clark SS, McLaughlin J, Crist WM, et al: Unique forms of the abl tyrosine kinase distinguish Ph1-positive CML from Ph1-positive ALL. *Science* **235**:85, 1987.

424. Kurzrock R, Shtalrid M, Romero P, et al: A novel c-abl protein product in Philadelphia-positive acute lymphoblastic leukemia. *Nature* **325**:631, 1987.

425. Hermans A, Heisterkamp N, von Linden M, van Baal S, Meijer D, van der Plas D, Wiedemann LM, Groffen J, Bootsma D, Grosveld G: Unique fusion of bcr and c-abl genes in Philadelphia chromosome positive acute lymphoblastic leukemia. *Cell* **51**:33, 1987.

426. Walker LC, Ganesan TS, Dhut S, Gibbons B, Lister TA, Rothbard J, Young BD: Novel chimaeric protein expressed in Philadelphia positive acute lymphoblastic leukaemia. *Nature* **329**:851, 1987.

427. Fainstein E, Marcelle C, Rosener A, Canaani E, Gale RP, Dreazen O, Smith SD, Croce CM: A new fused transcript in Philadelphia chromosome positive acute lymphocytic leukemia. *Nature* **330**:386, 1987.

428. Witte ON, Ponticelli A, Gifford A, et al: Phosphorylation of the Abelson murine leukemia virus transforming protein. *J Virol* **39**:870, 1981.

429. Reynolds FH Jr, Oroszlan S, Stephenson JR: Abelson urine leukemia virus p120: identification and characterization of tyrosine phosphorylation sites. *J Virol* **44**:1097, 1982.

430. Srinivasan A, Dunn CY, Yuasa Y, Devare SG, Reddy EP, Aaronson SA: Abelson murine leukemia virus: structural requirements for transforming gene function. *Proc Natl Acad Sci USA* **79**:5508, 1982.

431. Daley GQ, McLaughlin J, Witte ON, Baltimore D: The CML-specific P210 bcr/abl protein, unlike v-abl, does not transform NIH/3T3 fibroblasts. *Science* **237**:532, 1987.

432. Daley GQ, Baltimore D: Transformation of an interleukin 3-dependent hematopoietic cell line by the chronic myelogenous leukemia-specific P210bcr/abl protein. *Proc Natl Acad Sci USA* **85**:9312, 1988.

433. Elefanty AG, Hariharan IK, Cory S: bcr-abl, the hallmark of chronic myeloid leukaemia in man, induces multiple haemopoietic neoplasms in mice. *EMBO J* **9**:1069, 1990.

434. Gishizky ML, Johnson White J, Witte ON: Efficient transplantation of BCR-ABL-induced chronic myelogenous leukemia-like syndrome in mice. *Proc Natl Acad Sci USA* **90**:3755, 1993.

435. Kelliher M, Knott A, McLaughlin J, Witte ON, Rosenberg N: Differences in oncogenic potency but not target cell specificity distinguish the two forms of the BCR/ABL oncogene. *Mol Cell Biol* **11**:4710, 1991.

436. Goga A, McLaughlin J, Afar DE, Saffran DC, Witte ON: Alternative signals to RAS for hematopietic transformation by the BCR-ABL oncogene. *Cell* **82**:981, 1995.

437. Senechal K, Halpern J, Sawyers CL: The CRKL adaptor protein transforms fibroblasts and functions in transformation by the BCR-ABL oncogene. *J Biol Chem* (in press).

438. Raitano AB, Halpern JR, Hambuch TM, Sawyers CL: The Bcr-Abl leukemia oncogene activates Jun kinase and requires Jun for transformation. *Proc Natl Acad Sci USA* **92**:11746, 1995.

439. Afar DE, Goga A, McLaughlin J, Witte ON, Sawyers CL: Differential complementation of Bcr-Abl point mutants with c-Myc. *Science* **264**:424, 1994.

440. Afar DE, McLaughlin J, Sherr CJ, Witte ON, Roussel MF: Signaling by ABL oncogenes through cyclin D1. *Proc Natl Acad Sci USA* **92**:9540, 1995.

441. Shuai K, Halpern J, ten Hoeve J, Rao X, Sawyers CL: Constitutive activation of STAT5 by the BCR-ABL oncogene in chronic myelogenous leukemia. *Oncogene* **13**:247, 1996.

442. Papadopoulos P, Ridge SA, Boucher CA, Stocking C, Wiedemann LM: The novel activation of ABL by fusion to an ets-related gene, TEL. *Cancer Res* **55**:34, 1995.

443. Golub TR, Barker GF, Lovett M, Gilliland DG: Fusion of PDGF receptor beta to a novel ets-like gene, tel, in chronic myelomonocytic leukemia with t(5;12) chromosomal translocation. *Cell* **77**:307, 1994.

444. Tybulewicz VL, Crawford CE, Jackson PK, Bronson RT, Mulligan RC: Neonatal lethality and lymphopenia in mice with a homozygous disruption of the c-abl proto-oncogene. *Cell* **65**:1153, 1991.

445. Schwartzberg PL, Stall AM, Hardin JD, Bowdish KS, Humaran T, Boast S, Harbison ML, Robertson EJ, Goff SP: Mice homozygous for the ablm1 mutation show poor viability and depletion of selected B and T cell populations. *Cell* **65**:1165, 1991.

446. Van Etten RA, Jackson P, Baltimore D: The mouse type IV c-abl gene product is a nuclear protein, and activation of transforming ability is associated with cytoplasmic localization. *Cell* **58**:669, 1989.

447. Kharbanda S, Ren R, Pandey P, Shafman TD, Feller SM, Weichselbaum RR, Kufe DW: Activation of the c-Abl tyrosine kinase in the stress response to DNA-damaging agents. *Nature* **376**:785, 1995.

448. Sawyers CL, McLaughlin J, Goga A, Havlik M, Witte O: The nuclear tyrosine kinase c-Abl negatively regulates cell growth. *Cell* **77**:121, 1994.

449. Mattioni T, Jackson PK, Bchini-Hooft van Huijsduijnen O, Picard D: Cell cycle arrest by tyrosine kinase Abl involves altered early mitogenic response. *Oncogene* **10**:1325, 1995.

450. Goga A, Liu X, Hambuch TM, Senechal K, Major E, Berk AJ, Witte ON, Sawyers CL: p53 dependent growth suppression by the c-Abl nuclear tyrosine kinase. *Oncogene* **11**:791, 1995.

451. Yuan Z-M, Huang Y, Whang Y, Sawyers C, Weichselbaum R, Kharbanda S, Kufe D: Role for the c-ABL tyrosine kinase in the growth arrest response to DNA damage. *Nature* **382**:272, 1996.

452. Bloomfield CD, Goldman AL, Berger AR, et al: Chromosomal abnormalities identify high-risk and low-risk patients with acute lymphoblastic leukemia. *Blood* **67**:415, 1986.

453. Jain K, Arlin Z, Mertelsmann R, et al: Philadelphia chromosome and terminal transferase-positive acute leukemia: Similarity of terminal phase of chronic myelogenous leukemia and de novo acute presentation. *J Clin Oncol* **1**:669, 1983.

454. Williams DL, Harber J, Murphy SB, et al: Chromosomal translocation play a unique role in influencing prognosis in childhood acute lymphoblastic leukemia. *Blood* **68**:205, 1986.

455. Roberts WM, Rivera GK, Raimondi SC, Santana VM, Sandlund JT, Crist WM, Pui CH: Intensive chemotherapy for Philadelphia-chromosome-positiveacute lymphoblastic leukemia. *Lancet* **343**:331, 1994.

456. Thomas ED, Clift RA: Indications for marrow transplantation in chronic myelogenous leukemia. *Blood* **73**:861, 1989.

457. Morris SW, Kirstein MN, Valentine MB, Dittmer KG, Shapiro DN, Saltman DL, Look AT: Fusion of a kinase gene, ALK, to a nucleolar protein gene, NPM, in non-Hodgkin's lymphoma. *Science* **263**:1281, 1994.

458. Borer RA, Lehner CF, Eppenberger HM, Nigg EA: Major nucleolar proteins shuttle between nucleus and cytoplasm. *Cell* **56**:379, 1989.

459. Szebeni A, Herrera JE, Olson MO: Interaction of nucleolar protein B23 with peptides related to nuclear localization signals. *Biochemistry* **34**:8037, 1995.

460. Chan W-Y, Liu QR, Borjigin J, Busch H, Rennert OM, Tease LA, Chan P-K: Characterization of the cDNA encoding human nucleophosmin and studies of its role in normal and abnormal growth. *Biochemistry* **28**:1033, 1989.

461. Peter M, Nakagawa J, Doree M, Labbe JC, Nigg EA: Identification of major nucleolar proteins as candidate mitotic substrates of cdc2 kinase. *Cell* **60**:791, 1990.

462. Dumbar TS, Gentry GA, Olson MOJ: Interaction of nucleolar phosphoprotein B23 with nucleic acids. *Biochemistry* **28**:9495, 1989.

463. Fankhauser C, Izaurralde E, Adachi Y, Wingfield P, Laemmli UK: Specific complex of human immunodeficiency virus type 1 rev and

nucleolar B23 proteins: Dissociation by the Rev response element. *Mol Cell Biol* **11**:2567, 1991.

464. Feuerstein N, Mond JJ, Kinchington PR, Hickey R, Karjalainen Lindsberg ML, Hay I, Ruyechan WT: Evidence for DNA binding activity of numatrin (B23), a cell cycle-regulated nuclear matrix protein. *Biochim Biophys Acta* **1087**:127, 1990.

465. Inouye CJ, Seto E: Relief of YY1-induced transcriptional repression by protein-protein interaction with the nucleolar phosphoprotein B23. *J Biol Chem* **269**:6506, 1994.

466. Valdez BC, Perlaky L, Henning D, Saijo Y, Chan PH, Busch H: Identification of the nuclear and nucleolar localization signals of the protein p120. *J Biol Chem* **269**:23776, 1994.

467. Morris SW, Naeve C, Mathew P, James PL, Kirstein MN, Cui X, Witte DP: ALK, the chromosome 2 gene locus altered by the t(2;5) in non-Hodgkin's lymphoma, encodes a neural receptor tyrosine kinase that is highly related to leukocyte tyrosine kinase (LTK). *Oncogene* **14**:2175, 1997.

468. Iwahara T, Fujimoto J, Wen D, Cupples R, Bucay N, Arakawa T, Mori S, Ratzkin B, Yamamoto T: Molecular characterization of ALK, a receptor tyrosine kinase expressed specifically in the nervous system. *Oncogene* **14**:439, 1997.

469. Bischof D, Pulford K, Mason DY, Morris SW: Role of the nucleophosmin (NPM) portion of the non-Hodgkin's lymphoma-associated NPM-anaplastic lymphoma kinase fusion protein in oncogenesis. *Mol Cell Biol* **17**:2312, 1997.

470. Mason DY, Pulford KAF, Bischof D, Kuefer MU, Butler LH, Lamant L, Delsol G, Morris SW: Nucleolar localization of the nucleophosmin-anaplastic lymphoma kinase is not required for malignant transformation. *Cancer Res* **58**:1057, 1998.

471. Fujimoto J, Shiota M, Iwahara T, Seki N, Satoh H, Mori S, Yamamoto T: Characterization of the transforming activity of p80, a hyperphosphorylated protein in a Ki-1 lymphoma cell line with chromosomal translocation t(2;5). *Proc Natl Acad Sci USA* **93**:4181, 1996.

472. Kuefer MU, Look AT, Pulford K, Behm FG, Pattengale PK, Mason DY, Morris SW: Retrovirus-mediated gene transfer of NPM-ALK causes lymphoid malignancy in mice. *Blood* **90**:2901, 1997.

473. Pulford K, Lamant L, Morris SW, Butler LH, Wood KM, Stroud D, Delsol G, Mason DY: Detection of anaplastic lymphoma kinase ALK and nucleolar protein nucleophosmin NPM-ALK proteins in normal and neoplastic cells with the monoclonal antibody ALK1. *Blood* **89**:1394, 1997.

474. Benharroch D, Meguerian Bedoyan Z, Lamant L, Amin C, Brugieres L, Terrier-Lacombe MJ, Haralambieva E, Pulford K, Pileri S, Morris SW, Mason DY, Delsol G: ALK-positive lymphoma: A single disease with a broad spectrum of morphology. *Blood* **91**:2076, 1998.

475. Falini B, Bigerna B, Fizzotti M, Pulford K, Pileri SA, Delsol G, Carbone A, Paulli M, Magrini U, Menestrina F, Giardini R, Pilotti S, Mezzelani A, Ugolini B, Billi M, Pucciarini A, Pacini R, Peliccci P-G, Flenghi L: ALK expression defines a distinct group of T/Null lymphomas ("ALK lymphomas") with a wide morphological spectrum. *Am J Pathol* **153**:875, 1998.

476. Pittaluga S, Wiodarska I, Pulford K, Campo E, Morris SW, Van den Berghe H, De Wolf-Peeters C: The monoclonal antibody ALK1 identifies a distinct morphological subtype of anaplastic large cell lymphoma associated with 2p23/ALK rearrangements. *Am J Pathol* **151**:343, 1997.

477. Sarris AH, Luthra R, Cabanillas F, Morris SW, Pugh WC: Genomic DNA amplification and the detection of t(2;5)(p23;q35) in lymphoid neoplasms. *Leuk Lymphoma* **29**:507, 1998.

478. Downing JR, Shurtleff SA, Zielenska M, Curcio-Brint AM, Behm FG, Head DR, Sandlund JT, Weisenburger DD, Kossakowska AE, Thorner P, Lorenzana A, Ladanyi M, Morris SW: Molecular detection of the (2;5) translocation of non-Hodgkin's lymphoma by reverse transcriptase-polymerase chain reaction. *Blood* **85**:3416, 1995.

479. Mathew P, Sanger WG, Weisenburger DD, Valentine M, Valentine V, Pickering D, Higgins C, Hess M, Cui X, Srivastava DK, Morris SW: Detection of the t(2;5)(p23;q35) and NPM-ALK fusion in non-Hodgkin's lymphoma by two-color fluorescence in situ hybridization. *Blood* **89**:1678, 1996.

480. Shiota M, Nakamura S, Ichinohasama R, Abe M, Akagi T, Takeshita M, Mori N, Fujimoto J, Miyauchi J, Mikata A, Nanba K, Takami T, Yamabe H, Takano Y, Izumo T, Nagatani T, Mohri N, Nasu K, Satoh H, Katano H, Yamamoto T, Mori S: Anaplastic large cell lymphomas expressing the novel chimeric protein p80NPM/ALK: A distinct clinicopathologic entity. *Blood* **86**:1954, 1995.

481. Hutchison RE, Banki K, Shuster JJ, Barrett D, Dieck C, Berard CW, Murphy SB, Link MP, Pick TE, Laver J, Schwenn M, Mathew P,

Morris SW: Use of an anti-ALK antibody in the characterization of anaplastic large-cell lymphoma of childhood. *Ann Oncol* **8(suppl 1)**:37, 1997.

482. Gascoyne RD, Aoun P, Wu D, Chhanabhai M, Skinnider BF, Pulford KAF, Mason DY, Greiner TC, Morris SW, Connors JM, Vose JM, Viswanatha DS, Coldman A, Weisenburger DD: Prognostic significance of ALK protein expression in adults with anaplastic large cell lymphoma. *Blood* (in press).

483. Wlodarska I, De Wolf-Peeters C, Falini B, Verhoef G, Morris SW, Hagemeijer A, Van den Berghe H: The cryptic inv(2)(p23q35) defines a new molecular genetic subtype of ALK-positive ALCL. *Blood* (in press).

484. Delsol G, Lamant L, Mariame B, Pulford K, Dastugue N, Brousset P, Rigal-Huguet F, Saati TA, Cerretti DP, Morris SW, Mason DY: A new subtype of large B-cell lymphoma expressing the ALK kinase and lacking the 2;5 translocation. *Blood* **89**:1483, 1997.

485. Koeffler HP: Myelodysplastic syndromes. *Hematol Oncol Clin North Am* **6**:485, 1992.

486. Yarden Y, Escobedo JA, Kuang WJ, Yang-Feng TL, Daniel TO, Tremble PM, Chen EY, Ando ME, Harkins RN, Francke U, et al: Structure of the receptor for platelet-derived growth factor helps define a family of closely related growth factor receptors. *Nature* **323**:226, 1986.

487. Satoh T, Fantl WJ, Escobedo JA, Williams LT, Kaziro Y: Platelet-derived growth factor receptor mediates activation of ras through different signaling pathways in different cell types. *Mol Cell Biol* **13**:3706, 1993.

488. Yan XQ, Brady G, Iscove NN: Overexpression of PDGF-B in murine hematopoietic cells induces a lethal myeloproliferative syndrome in vivo. *Oncogene* **9**:163, 1994.

489. Nye JA, Petersen JM, Gunther CV, Jonsen MD, Graves BJ: Interaction of murine ets-1 with GGA-binding sites establishes the ETS domain as a new DNA-binding motif. *Genes Dev* **6**:975, 1992.

490. Rao VN, Ohno T, Prasad DD, Bhattacharya G, Reddy ES: Analysis of the DNA-binding and transcriptional activation functions of human Fli-1 protein. *Oncogene* **8**:2167, 1993.

491. Sawyers CL, Denny CT: Chronic myelomonocytic leukemia: Tel-a-kinase what Ets all about. *Cell* **77**:171, 1994.

492. Wlodarska I, Mecucci C, Marynen P, Guo C, Franckx D, La Starza R, Aventin A, Bosly A, Martelli MF, Cassiman JJ, et al: TEL gene is involved in myelodysplastic syndromes with either the typical t(5;12)(q33;p13) translocation or its variant t(10; 12)(q24;p13). *Blood* **85**:2848, 1995.

493. Erikson J, Finan J, Tsujimoto Y, Nowell PC, Croce CM: The chromosome 14 breakpoint in neoplastic B cells with the t(11;14) translocation involves the immunoglobulin heavy chain locus. *Proc Natl Acad Sci USA* **81**:4144, 1984.

494. Tsujimoto Y, Yunis J, Onorato-Showe L, Erikson J, Nowell PC, Croce CM: Molecular cloning of the chromosomal breakpoint of B-cell lymphomas and leukemias with the t(11;14) chromosome translocation. *Science* **224**:1403, 1984.

495. Tsujimoto Y, Jaffe E, Cossman J, Gorham J, Nowell PC, Croce CM: Clustering of breakpoints on chromosome 11 in human B-cell neoplasms with the t(11;14) chromosome translocation. *Nature* **315**:340, 1985.

496. Louie E, Tsujimoto Y, Heubner K, Croce C: *Am J Hum Genet* **41(suppl)**:31, 1987.

497. Rabbitts PH, Douglas J, Fischer P, Nacheva E, Karpas A, Catovsky D, Melo JV, Baer R, Stinson MA, Rabbitts TH: Chromosome abnormalities at 11q13 in B cell tumours. *Oncogene* **3**:99, 1988.

498. Meeker TC, Grimaldi JC, O'Rourke R, Louie E, Juliusson G, Einhorn S: An additional breakpoint region in the BCL-1 locus associated with the t(11;14)(q13;q32) translocation of B-lymphocytic malignancy. *Blood* **74**:1801, 1989.

499. Lammie GA, Fantl V, Smith R, Schuuring E, Brookes S, Michalides R, Dickson C, Arnold A, Peters G: D11S287, a putative oncogene on chromosome 11q13, is amplified and expressed in squamous cell and mammary carcinomas and linked to BCL-1. *Oncogene* **6**:439, 1991.

500. Rosenberg CL, Wong E, Petty EM, Bale AE, Tsujimoto Y, Harris NL, Arnold A: PRAD1, a candidate BCL1 oncogene: Mapping and expression in centrocytic lymphoma. *Proc Natl Acad Sci USA* **88**:9638, 1991.

501. Withers DA, Harvey RC, Faust JB, Melnyk O, Carey K, Meeker TC: Characterization of a candidate bcl-1 gene. *Mol Cell Biol* **11**:4846, 1991.

502. Brookes S, Lammie GA, Schuuring E, Dickson C, Peters G: Linkage map of a region of human chromosome band 11q13 amplified in

breast and squamous cell tumors. *Genes Chromosomes Cancer* **4**:290, 1992.

503. Hall M, Peters G: Genetic alterations of cyclins, cyclin-dependent kinases, and Cdk inhibitors in human cancer, in Vande Woude GF, Klein G (eds): *Advances in Cancer Research*. San Diego, Academic Press, 1996, p. 67.

504. Sherr CJ: Mammalian G1 cyclins. *Cell* **73**:1059, 1993.

505. Rosenberg CL, Motokura T, Kronenberg HM, Arnold A: Coding sequence of the overexpressed transcript of the putative oncogene PRAD1/cyclin D1 in two primary human tumors. *Oncogene* **8**:519, 1993.

506. Rimokh R, Berger F, Bastard C, Klein B, French M, Archimbaud E, Rouault JP, Santa Lucia B, Duret L, Vuillaume M, et al: Rearrangement of CCND1 (BCL1/PRAD1) 3′ untranslated region in mantle-cell lymphomas and t(11q13)-associated leukemias. *Blood* **83**:3689, 1994.

507. Lukas J, Jadayel D, Bartkova J, Nacheva E, Dyer MJ, Strauss M, Bartek J: BCL-1/cyclin D1 oncoprotein oscillates and subverts the G1 phase control in B-cell neoplasms carrying the t(11;14) translocation. *Oncogene* **9**:2159, 1994.

508. Banks PM, Chan J, Cleary ML, Delsol G, De Wolf-Peeters C, Gatter K, Grogan TM, Harris NL, Isaacson PG, Jaffe ES, et al: Mantle cell lymphoma: A proposal for unification of morphologic, immunologic, and molecular data. *Am J Surg Pathol* **16**:637, 1992.

509. Shivdasani RA, Hess JL, Skarin AT, Pinkus GS: Intermediate lymphocytic lymphoma: Clinical and pathologic features of a recently characterized subtype of non-Hodgkin's lymphoma. *J Clin Oncol* **11**:802, 1993.

510. Harris NL, Jaffe ES, Stein H, Banks PM, Chan JKC, Cleary ML, Delsol G, De Wolf-Peeters C, Falini B, Gatter KC, Grogan TM, Isaacson PG, Knowles DM, Mason DY, Muller-Hermelink H-K, Pileri SA, Piris MA, Ralfkiaer E, Warnke RA: A revised European-American classification of lymphoid neoplasms: A proposal from the International Lymphoma Study Group. *Blood* **84**:1361, 1994.

511. Banno S, Yoshikawa K, Nakamura S, Yamamoto K, Seito T, Nitta M, Takahashi T, Ueda R, Seto M: Monoclonal antibody against PRAD1/cyclin D1 stains nuclei of tumor cells with translocation or amplification at BCL-1 locus. *Jpn J Cancer Res* **85**:918, 1994.

512. de Boer CJ, van Krieken JH, Kluin-Nelemans HC, Kluin PM, Schuuring E: Cyclin D1 messenger RNA overexpression as a marker for mantle cell lymphoma. *Oncogene* **10**:1833, 1995.

513. Nakamura S, Seto M, Banno S, Suzuki S, Koshikawa T, Kitoh K, Kagami Y, Ogura M, Yatabe Y, Kojima M, et al: Immunohistochemical analysis of cyclin D1 protein in hematopoietic neoplasms with special reference to mantle cell lymphoma. *Jpn J Cancer Res* **85**:1270, 1994.

514. Yang WI, Zukerberg LR, Motokura T, Arnold A, Harris NL: Cyclin D1 (Bcl-1, PRAD1) protein expression in low-grade B-cell lymphomas and reactive hyperplasia. *Am J Pathol* **145**:86, 1994.

515. Fukuhara S, Rowley JD, Variakojis D, Golomb HM: Chromosome abnormalities in poorly differentiated lymphocytic lymphoma. *Cancer Res* **39**:3119, 1979.

516. Yunis JJ, Frizzera G, Oken MM, McKenna J, Theologides A, Arnesen M: Multiple recurrent genomic defects in follicular lymphoma. A possible model for cancer. *N Engl J Med* **316**:79, 1987.

517. Tsujimoto Y, Gorham J, Cossman J, Jaffe E, Croce CM: The t(14;18) chromosome translocations involved in B-cell neoplasms result from mistakes in VDJ joining. *Science* **229**:1390, 1985.

518. Bakhshi A, Jensen JP, Goldman P, Wright JJ, McBride OW, Epstein AL, Korsmeyer SJ: Cloning the chromosomal breakpoint of t(14;18) human lymphomas: clustering around JH on chromosome 14 and near a transcriptional unit on 18. *Cell* **41**:899, 1985.

519. Cleary ML, Sklar J: Nucleotide sequence of a t(14;18) chromosomal breakpoint in follicular lymphoma and demonstration of a breakpoint-cluster region near a transcriptionally active locus on chromosome 18. *Proc Natl Acad Sci USA* **82**:7439, 1985.

520. Cleary ML, Smith SD, Sklar J: Cloning and structural analysis of cDNAs for bcl-2 and a hybrid bcl-2/immunoglobulin transcript resulting from the t(14;18) translocation. *Cell* **47**:19, 1986.

521. Vaux DL, Cory S, Adams JM: Bcl-2 gene promotes haemopoietic cell survival and cooperates with c-myc to immortalize pre-B cells. *Nature* **335**:440, 1988.

522. Nunez G, London L, Hockenbery D, Alexander M, McKearn JP, Korsmeyer SJ: Deregulated Bcl-2 gene expression selectively prolongs survival of growth factor-deprived hemopoietic cell lines. *J Immunol* **144**:3602, 1990.

523. Korsmeyer SJ: Bcl-2 initiates a new category of oncogenes: Regulators of cell death. *Blood* **80**:879, 1992.

524. Yang E, Korsmeyer SJ: Molecular thanatopsis: A discourse on the BCL2 family and cell death. *Blood* **88**:386, 1996.

525. Hengartner MO, Horvitz HR: *C. elegans* cell survival gene ced-9 encodes a functional homolog of the mammalian proto-oncogene bcl-2. *Cell* **76**:665, 1994.

526. von Lindern M, Poustka A, Lerach H, Grosveld G: The (6;9) chromosome translocation, associated with a specific subtype of acute nonlymphocytic leukemia, leads to aberrant transcription of a target gene on 9q34. *Mol Cell Biol* **10**:4016, 1990.

527. von Lindern M, van Baal S, Wiegant J, Raap A, Hagemeijer A, Grosveld G: Can, a putative oncogene associated with myeloid leukemogenesis, may be activated by fusion of its 3′ half to different genes: characterization of the set gene. *Mol Cell Biol* **12**:3346, 1992.

528. von Lindern M, Breems D, van Baal S, Adriaansen H, Grosveld G: Characterization of the translocation breakpoint sequences of two DEK-CAN fusion genes present in t(6;9) acute myeloid leukemia and a SET-CAN fusion gene in a case of acute undifferentiated leukemia. *Genes Chromosomes Cancer* **5**:227, 1992.

529. Borrow J, Shearman AM, Stanton VP Jr, Becher R, Collins T, Williams AJ, Dube I, Katz F, Kwong YL, Morris C, Ohyashiki K, Toyama K, Rowley J, Housman DE: The t(7;11)(p15;p15) translocation in acute myeloid leukaemia fuses the genes for nucleoporin NUP98 and class I homeoprotein HOXA9. *Nature Genet* **12**:159, 1996.

530. Nakamura T, Largaespada DA, Lee MP, Johnson LA, Ohyashiki K, Toyama K, Chen SJ, Willman CL, Chen IM, Feinberg AP, Jenkins NA, Copeland NG, Shaughnessy JD Jr: Fusion of the nucleoporin gene NUP98 to HOXA9 by the chromosome translocation t(7;11)(p15;p15) in human myeloid leukaemia. *Nature Genet* **12**:154, 1996.

531. Kraemer D, Wozniak RW, Blobel G, Radu A: The human CAN protein, a putative oncogene product associated with myeloid leukemogenesis, is a nuclear pore complex protein that faces the cytoplasm. *Proc Natl Acad Sci USA* **91**:1519, 1994.

532. Fornerod M, Boer J, van Baal S, Jaegle M, von Lindern M, Murti KG, Davis D, Bonten J, Buijs A, Grosveld G: Relocation of the carboxyterminal part of CAN from the nuclear envelope to the nucleus as a result of leukemia-specific chromosome rearrangements. *Oncogene* **10**:1739, 1995.

533. van Deursen J, Boer J, Kasper L, Grosveld G: G2 arrest and impaired nucleocytoplasmic transport in mouse embryos lacking the proto-oncogene CAN/Nup214. *EMBO J* **15**:5574, 1996.

534. Fornerod M, Boer J, van Baal S, Morreau H, Grosveld G: Interaction of cellular proteins with the leukemia specific fusion proteins DEK-CAN amd SET-CAN and their normal counterpart, the nucleoporin CAN. *Oncogene* **13**:1801, 1996.

535. Yoneda-Kato N, Look AT, Kirstein MN, Valentine MB, Raimondi SC, Cohen KJ, Carroll AJ, Morris SW: The t(3;5)(q25.1;q34) of myelodysplastic syndrome and acute myeloid leukemia produces a novel fusion gene, NPM-MLF1. *Oncogene* **12**:265, 1996.

536. Kuefer MU, Look AT, Williams DC, Valentine V, Naeve CW, Behm FG, Mullersman JE, Yoneda-Kato N, Montgomery K, Kucherlapati R, Morris SW: cDNA cloning, tissue distribution, and chromosomal localization of myelodysplasia/myeloid leukemia factor 2 (MLF2). *Genomics* **35**:392, 1996.

537. Dallery E, Galiegue Zouitina S, Collyn-d'Hooghe M, Quief S, Denis C, Hildebrand MP, Lantoine D, Deweindt C, Tilly H, Bastard C, et al: TTF, a gene encoding a novel small G protein, fuses to the lymphoma-associated LAZ3 gene by t(3;4) chromosomal translocation. *Oncogene* **10**:2171, 1995.

538. Ohno H, Takimoto G, McKeithan TW: The candidate proto-oncogene bcl-3 is related to genes implicated in cell lineage determination and cell cycle control. *Cell* **60**:991, 1990.

539. Wulczyn FG, Naumann M, Scheidereit C: Candidate proto-oncogene bcl-3 encodes a subunit-specific inhibitor of transcription factor NF-kappa B. *Nature* **358**:597, 1992.

540. Kerr LD, Duckett CS, Wamsley P, Zhang Q, Chiao P, Nabel G, McKeithan TW, Baeuerle PA, Verma IM: The proto-oncogene bcl-3 encodes an I kappa B protein. *Genes Dev* **6**:2352, 1992.

541. Neri A, Chang CC, Lombardi L, Salina M, Corradini P, Maiolo AT, Chaganti RS, Dalla-Favera R: B cell lymphoma-associated chromosomal translocation involves candidate oncogene lyt-10, homologous to NF-kappa B p50. *Cell* **67**:1075, 1991.

542. Iida S, Rao PH, Nallasivam P, Hibshoosh H, Butler M, Louie DC, Dyomin V, Ohno H, Chaganti RSK, Dalla-Favera R: The t(9;14)(p13;q32) chromosomal translocation associated with lymphoplasmacytoid lymphoma involves the PAX-5 gene. *Blood* **88**:4110, 1996.

543. Shimizu K, Miyoshi H, Kozu T, Nagata J, Enomoto K, Maseki N, Kaneko Y, Ohki M: Consistent disruption of the AML1 gene occurs within a single intron in the t(8;21) chromosomal translocation. *Cancer Res* **52**:6945, 1992.

544. Ichikawa H, Shimizu K, Hayashi Y, Ohki M: An RNA-binding protein gene, TLS/FUS, is fused to ERG in human myeloid leukemia with t(16;21) chromosomal translocation. *Cancer Res* **54**:2865, 1994.

545. Buijs A, Sherr S, van Baal S, van Bezouw S, van der Plas D, Geurts van Kessel A, Riegman P, Lekanne Deprez R, Zwarthoff E, Hagemeijer A, et al: Translocation (12;22) (p13;q11) in myeloproliferative disorders results in fusion of the ETS-like TEL gene on 12p13 to the MN1 gene on 22q11 [published erratum appears in *Oncogene* **11**(4):809, 1995]. *Oncogene* **10**:1511, 1995.

546. Peeters P, Wlodarska I, Baens M, Criel A, Selleslag D, Hagemeier A, Van den Berghe H, Marynen P: Fusion of ETV6 to MDS1/EVI1 as a result of t(3;12)(q26;p13) in myeloproliferative disorders. *Cancer Res* **57**:564, 1997.

547. Borrow J, Stanton VP Jr, Andresen JM, Becher R, Behm FG, Chaganti RS, Civin CI, Disteche C, Dube I, Frischauf AM, Horsman D, Mitelman F, Volinia S, Watmore AE, Housman DE: The translocation t(8;16)(p11;p13) of acute myeloid leukaemia fuses a putative acetyltransferase to the CREB-binding protein. *Nature Genet* **14**:33, 1996.

548. Carapeti M, Aguiar RC, Goldman JM, Cross NC: A novel fusion between MOZ and the nuclear receptor coactivator TIF2 in acute myeloid leukemia. *Blood* **91**:3127, 1998.

549. Bernard OA, Mauchauffe M, Mecucci C, Van den Berghe H, Berger R: A novel gene, AF-1p, fused to HRX in t(1;11)(p32;q23), is not related to AF-4, AF-9 nor ENL. *Oncogene* **9**:1039, 1994.

550. Hillion J, Leconiat M, Jonveaux P, Berger R, Bernard OA: AF6q21, a novel partner of the MLL gene in t(6;11)(q21;q23), defines a forkhead transcriptional factor subfamily. *Blood* **90**:3714, 1997.

551. Chaplin T, Ayton P, Bernard OA, Saha V, Della Valle V, Hillion J, Gregorini A, Lillington D, Berger R, Young BD: A novel class of zinc finger/leucine zipper genes identified from the molecular cloning of the t(10;11) translocation in acute leukemia. *Blood* **85**:1435, 1995.

552. Prasad R, Leshkowitz D, Gu Y, Alder H, Nakamura T, Saito H, Huebner K, Berger R, Croce CM, Canaani E: Leucine-zipper dimerization motif encoded by the AF17 gene fused to ALL-1 (MLL) in acute leukemia. *Proc Natl Acad Sci USA* **91**:8107, 1994.

553. Parry P, Wei Y, Evans G: Cloning and characterization of the t(X;11) breakpoint from a leukemic cell line identify a new member of the forkhead gene family. *Genes Chromosomes Cancer* **11**:79, 1994.

554. Taki T, Sako M, Tsuchida M, Hayashi Y: The t(11;16)(q23;p13) translocation in myelodysplastic syndrome fuses the MLL gene to the CBP gene. *Blood* **89**:3945, 1997.

555. Rowley JD, Reshmi S, Sobulo O, Musvee T, Anastasi J, Raimondi S, Schneider NR, Barredo JC, Cantu ES, Schlegelberger B, Behm F, Doggett NA, Borrow J, Zeleznik-Le N: All patients with the T(11;16)(q23;p13.3) that involves MLL and CBP have treatment-related hematologic disorders. *Blood* **90**:535, 1997.

556. Peeters P, Raynoud SD, Cools J, Wlodarska I, Grosgeorge J, Philip P, Monpoux F, Van Rompay L, Baens M, Van den Berghe H, Marynen P: Fusion of TEL, the ETS variant gene 6 (ETV6) to the receptor-associated kinase JAK2 as a result of t(9;12) in a lymphoid and t(9;15;12) in a myeloid leukemia. *Blood* **90**:2535, 1997.

557. Lachronique V, Boureux A, Della Valle V, Poirel H, Tran Quang C, Mauchauffe M, Berthou C, Lessard M, Berger R, Ghysdael J, Bernard OA: A TEL-JAK2 fusion protein with constitutive kinase activity in human leukemia. *Science* **278**:1309, 1997.

558. Ross TS, Bernard OA, Berger R, Gilliland DG: Fusion of Huntington interacting protein 1 to platelet-derived growth factor β receptor (PDGFβR) in chronic myelomonocytic leukemia with t(5;7)(q33;q11.2). *Blood* **91**:4419, 1998.

559. Abe A, Emi N, Mitsune T, Hiroshi T, Marunouchi T, Hidehiko S: Fusion of the platelet-derived growth factor receptor beta to a novel gene CEV14 in acute myelogenous leukemia after clonal evolution. *Blood* **90**:1997.

560. Tycko B, Smith SD, Sklar J: Chromosomal translocations joining LCK and TCRB loci in human T cell leukemia. *J Exp Med* **174**:867, 1991.

561. Burnett RC, David JC, Harden AM, Le Beau MM, Rowley JD, Diaz MO: The LCK gene is involved in the t(1;7)(p34;q34) in the T-cell acute lymphoblastic leukemia derived cell line, HSB-2. *Genes Chromosomes Cancer* **3**:461, 1991.

562. Wright DD, Sefton BM, Kamps MP: Oncogenic activation of the Lck protein accompanies translocation of the LCK gene in the human HSB2 T-cell leukemia. *Mol Cell Biol* **14**:2429, 1994.

563. von Lindern M, Fornerod M, van Baal S, Jaegle M, de Wit T, Buijs A, Grosveld G: The translocation (6;9), associated with a specific subtype of acute myeloid leukemia, results in the fusion of two genes, dek and can, and the expression of a chimeric, leukemia-specific dek-can mRNA. *Mol Cell Biol* **12**:1687, 1992.

564. Dreyling MH, Martinez Climent JA, Zheng M, Mao J, Rowley JD, Bohlander SK: The t(10;11)(p13;q14) in the U937 cell line results in the fusion of the AF10 gene and CALM, encoding a new member of the AP-3 clathrin assembly protein family. *Proc Natl Acad Sci USA* **93**:4804, 1996.

565. Fisch P, Forster A, Sherrington PD, Dyer MJ, Rabbitts TH: The chromosomal translocation t(X;14)(q28;q11) in T-cell pro-lymphocytic leukaemia breaks within one gene and activates another. *Oncogene* **8**:3271, 1993.

566. Ellisen LW, Bird J, West DC, Soreng AL, Reynolds TC, Smith SD, Sklar J: TAN-1, the human homolog of the *Drosophila* notch gene, is broken by chromosomal translocations in T lymphoblastic neoplasms. *Cell* **66**:649, 1991.

567. Grimaldi JC, Meeker TC: The t(5;14) chromosomal translocation in a case of acute lymphocytic leukemia joins the interleukin-3 gene to the immunoglobulin heavy chain gene. *Blood* **73**:2081, 1989.

568. Meeker TC, Hardy D, Willman C, Hogan T, Abrams J: Activation of the interleukin-3 gene by chromosome translocation in acute lymphocytic leukemia with eosinophilia. *Blood* **76**:285, 1990.

569. Laabi Y, Gras MP, Carbonnel F, Brouet JC, Berger R, Larsen CJ, Tsapis A: A new gene, BCM, on chromosome 16 is fused to the interleukin 2 gene by a t(4;16)(q26;p13) translocation in a malignant T cell lymphoma. *EMBO J* **11**:3897, 1992.

570. Virgilio L, Lazzeri C, Bichi R, Nibu K, Narducci MG, Russo G, Rothstein JL, Croce CM: Deregulated expression of TCL1 causes T cell leukemia in mice. *Proc Natl Acad Sci USA* **95**:3885, 1998.

571. Madani A, Choukroun V, Soulier J, Cacheux V, Claisse JF, Valensi F, Daliphard S, Cazin B, Levy V, Leblond V, Daniel MT, Sigaux F, Stern MH: Expression of p13MTCP1 is restricted to mature T-cell proliferations with t(X;14) translocations. *Blood* **87**:1923, 1996.

572. Gritti C, Choukroun V, Soulier J, Madani A, Dastot H, Leblond V, Radford-Weiss I, Valensi F, Varet B, Sigaux F, Stern MH: Alternative origin of p13MTCP1-encoding transcripts in mature T-cell proliferations with t(X;14) translocations. *Oncogene* **15**:1329, 1997.

573. Seto M, Yamamoto K, Takahashi T, Ueda R: Cloning and expression of a murine cDNA homologous to the human RCK/P54, a lymphoma-linked chromosomal translocation junction gene on 11q23. *Gene* **166**:293, 1995.

574. Sandlund JT, Downing JR, Crist WM: Non-Hodgkins's lymphoma in childhood. *N Engl J Med* **334**:1238, 1996.

575. Downing JR, Look AT: MLL fusion genes in the 11q23 acute leukemias, in Freireich EJ, Kantarjian H (eds): *Leukemia: Advances in Research and Treatment*. Boston, Kluwer Academic Publishers, 1995, p. 73.

CHAPTER 5

Chromosome Alterations in Human Solid Tumors

Paul S. Meltzer ▪ *Anne Kallioniemi* ▪ *Jeffrey M. Trent*

1. Recurring sites of chromosome change represent the byproducts of molecular events that participate in the generation or progression of human cancers. Chromosome abnormalities in patients with hematopoietic cancers have proven to be of diagnostic and prognostic value, and the molecular defects for many have been described (see Chap. 4). Despite solid tumors being exceedingly more common than the blood-borne cancers of man, and their significantly greater contribution to morbidity and mortality relative to hematologic neoplasms, less is known about chromosome changes and their clinical and biologic importance in solid tumors. Nevertheless, significant information is accumulating on recurring chromosome alterations in solid tumors including the molecular dissection of recurring breakpoints in many malignancies.

2. The pattern of chromosome alterations in human solid tumors is decidedly nonrandom. Solid tumors tend to demonstrate multiple clonal structural and numeric chromosome rearrangements and databases are being developed to describe new karyotypic abnormalities in the context of tumor histopathology.

3. General categories of structural chromosome rearrangements in human solid tumors include chromosome translocations, deletions, inversions and changes associated with increases in DNA sequence copy number (double minutes [dmin]; and homogeneously staining regions [HSRs]).

4. Tumor-specific chromosome rearrangements have been identified in human solid tumors. Chromosome alterations in many common cancers are described.

5. Human sarcomas represent a paradigm for molecular dissection of human solid tumors. Tumor-specific chromosome translocations have been described and characterized at the molecular level for several sarcomas including Ewing's sarcoma, alveolar rhabdomyosarcoma, synovial sarcoma, myxoid liposarcoma, and soft tissue clear-cell sarcoma. In general, these translocations juxtapose segments of two genes, which can give rise to a chimeric fusion transcript. Two closely related genes *EWS* (on chromosome 22q12) and *FUS* (on chromosome 16p11) have been demonstrated to participate in tumor-specific translocations in several sarcomas. In each case, *EWS* or *FUS* acquires a DNA-binding domain from the translocation partner chromosome. These tumor-specific chimeric oncoproteins have transcription factor activity, and it appears that they contribute to malignant transformation by leading to dysregulated gene expression.

6. Numerous benign neoplasms, such as lipoma and leiomyoma, exhibit translocations involving members of the HMGI family of DNA-binding proteins. Multiple-partner genes are involved with one of the two HMGI genes in various tumors. The disturbance of HMGI protein function appears to have a profound effect on the proliferation of mesenchymal cells

in multiple lineages, yet these tumors do not become malignant.

7. The clinical value of chromosome rearrangements in the common solid tumors of adults is largely indeterminate. Recent advances and the development of new technical approaches for analysis of complex changes in solid tumors suggest that further insights into chromosome rearrangements (and the genes dysregulated by them) may increase clinical utility.

It is now recognized that most human cancers (including solid tumors) display recurring chromosome abnormalities. However, questions remain in most cases as to their exact biologic significance. How do chromosomal changes relate to changes in expression of important genes (including oncogenes)? What is the significance of a recurring cytogenetic alteration when viewed against a background of other (often multiple) genetic alterations? What clinical significance, if any, do specific cytogenetic abnormalities have for solid tumors? These questions have been the focus of intense study over the past decade and our recognition and recently our molecular understanding of chromosome abnormalities is providing significant insights into neoplasms in general and solid tumors particularly.

Significant progress has been made in tumor cytogenetics in recent years. For example, prior to 1981 there were only 1800 cases of malignancies with abnormal chromosomes reported in all of the world's literature, and < 3 percent were from solid tumors. By the end of 1994, there were > 22,000 published cases of neoplasms with abnormal karyotypes, and 27 percent of those were from solid tumors. Knowledge within this area has continued and through June of 1996, 26,523 cases, including 215 balanced and 1588 unbalanced recurrent aberrations, were identified among 75 different neoplastic disorders. This data is regularly updated by Prof. Felix Mitelman, and is available by CD-ROM,[1] or on the World Wide Web (www.ncbi.nlm.nih.gov/CCAP/NG/).

With this explosion in our knowledge of human chromosome alterations in neoplasia, has come the widespread acceptance of the clinical value of chromosome analysis in studies of human hematologic cancers. Specifically, chromosome analysis of malignant cells from patients with hematopoietic cancers provides diagnostic and equally importantly prognostic information independent of other laboratory and clinical feature of disease (see Chap. 10).[2–4] Despite solid tumors representing almost 95 percent of the cancers of humankind, far less is known about chromosome changes and especially their clinical importance in solid tumors. This chapter focuses on features of solid tumor cytogenetics that can be related to our understanding of the biologic and hopefully clinical utility of this information.

Two excellent books by Heim and Mitelman,[3] and Sandberg,[2] survey the field of cancer cytogenetics and provide in-depth descriptions of chromosome changes by histopathologic subtype. There is also a useful (but didactic) description of all published cytogenetic changes in the reported literature, which may be of interest for those who seek a listings of all chromosome changes, in the *Catalog of Chromosome Aberrations in Cancer.*[1] Finally, Thompson provides a comprehensive manual related to methodology for analysis of solid tumors.[5] The interested reader is referred to these sources for in-depth information on techniques as well as detailed karyotypic information on any given tumor type.

GENERAL ASPECTS OF CHROMOSOME CHANGE IN SOLID TUMORS

The diversity of structural chromosome alterations across the spectrum of human cancers is enormous and increasing rapidly. The central dogma underlying the study of chromosomes in cancer is that karyotypic changes are nonrandom, and thus are distributed erratically throughout the human genome. Specific chromosome bands are preferentially involved in rearrangements in different neoplasms, and increasingly, the underlying molecular defects are being understood. Examination of the nonrandom nature of chromosome alterations has led to the identification of > 200 recurring chromosome changes in > 70 neoplastic disorders (including now many benign proliferations).[1] Every human chromosome, with the exception of the Y chromosome, can be included in some form of neoplasia-associated alteration.

Methodology and Clonality

Technical obstacles are frequently responsible for the relative paucity of cytogenetic information from solid tumor samples. These obstacles include difficulties in sample disaggregation, cell viability due to necrosis of biopsy samples, contamination of samples with normal cells, and the complexity of most tumors (especially carcinomas) that frequently display a heterogeneous pattern of chromosome change. In most solid tumors, the time of clinical manifestation and removal of the tumor mass is thought to occur at a point considerably distant from cellular transformation, resulting in the generation of significant chromosomal rearrangement and imbalances. From a technical point of view, this means that in some solid tumors no two karyotypes from the same specimen may be identical, and that as few as one or as many as 100 chromosome rearrangements may be described within a single karyotype. To confuse matters even more, there is evidence that at least some tumors may arise from multiple stem cells or diverge soon after appearance of an initiating transformation event and then undergo clonal expansion of cell populations with unrelated karyotypes (i.e., they may be "polyclonal" in origin).[6–9] However, even with these complex karyotypes and heterogeneous tumor cell populations it has been possible to describe certain chromosomal abnormalities that are germinal to the development of a given tumor type. *Primary chromosome aberrations* are frequently found as the sole karyotypic abnormality in a neoplastic cell, and reflect their presumed causal role in cellular transformation. *Secondary chromosome aberrations* are thought to be important in tumor progression, do not appear alone, but nevertheless display nonrandom features with distribution patterns that are frequently tumor-type dependent. It is believed that the features of genetic instability, divergence, and heterogeneity observed in most solid tumors, represent significant genetic obstacles to effective patient treatment through "Darwinian" selection of genetically rearranged cells with proliferative (or therapy resistance) advantage.

Despite the difficulty in analyzing solid tumors cytogenetically, there is overwhelming information that most cancers are monoclonal (and thus all cells of a tumor share genetic characteristics of the original transformed cells), and therefore cancer is heritable at the cellular level.[9] This discovery, which was initially based largely on cytogenetic evidence, has been a major factor in reaching the conclusion that changes in DNA sequences of individual cells are responsible for malignant changes in those cells.

Terminology

As described previously, the results of tumor chromosome studies are complex and challenging to summarize. The range of chromosome counts may be quite wide, for example, from hypodiploid (e.g., < 46 chromosomes/cell) to hypertetraploid (> 96 chromosomes), and it is not uncommon to find more than one modal number. It is also generally true that, even when karyotyping cells with the same number of chromosomes, no two karyotypes from the same specimen are completely identical in all numeric as well as structural abnormalities observed. Consequently the field ordinarily describes the *clonal changes* that are evident and that make up a composite karyotype interpretation of the specimen. A numeric abnormality is said to be clonal if a missing chromosome is observed in at least three karyotypes, and an extra chromosome is found in at least two, while a clonal structural abnormality is described if it is found in two or more cells. Karyotypic anomalies, which are found in a majority of cells from a tumor, are said to represent the *stemline* population, while those abnormalities that are found in a small proportion of karyotypes are said to represent a *sideline* population. Multiple sidelines may (and usually do) exist in the same tumor sample. Many of the problems associated with describing complex karyotypes and multiple sidelines have been addressed by international convention according an International System of Cytogenetic Nomenclature (ISCN)[10] and all descriptions of cancer (and constitutional) karyotypic are written in accordance with the ISCN recommendations. Table 5-1 gives representative examples of abbreviations utilized in chromosome nomenclature of solid tumors.

RECURRING CHROMOSOME ALTERATIONS IN HUMAN SOLID TUMORS

General Findings

Although it has been difficult to obtain information on chromosome alterations in solid tumors, nonetheless, many recurring cytogenetic alterations have been described and a summary of nonrandom chromosomal abnormalities is presented in Table 5-2. Representative examples of chromosome rearrangements in human solid tumors are documented in banded cells from two different cancers (Figs. 5-1 and 5-2). Examples of the utility of

Table 5-1 Chromosome Nomenclature

A–G	Chromosome groups
1–22	Autosome numbers
X, Y	Sex chromosomes
/	Diagonal line indicates *mosaicism*, e.g., 46/47 designates a mosaic with 46-chromosome and 47-chromosome cell lines
p	Short arm of chromosome, "petite"
q	Long arm of chromosome
del	Deletion
der	Derivative of chromosome
dup	Duplication
I	Isochromosome
ins	Insertion
inv	Inversion
r	Ring chromosome
t	Translocation
ter	Terminal (may also be written as pter or qter)
+ or −	Placed *before* the chromosome number, these symbols indicate addition (+) or loss (−) of a whole chromosome; e.g., +21 indicates an extra chromosome 21, as in Down syndrome. Placed *after* the chromosome number, these symbols indicate gain or loss of a chromosome part; e.g., 5p − indicates loss of part of the short arm of chromosome 5, as in cri-du-chat syndrome.

From Gelehrter and Collins.[199] Used with permission.

Table 5-2 Recurring Karyotypic Abnormalities in Human Solid Tumors*

Tumor type	Karyotype abnormalities and other findings
Malignant	
Bladder (transitional cell carcinoma)	**+7; del(10)(q22–q24); del(21)(q22)**; del(21)(q22); del and t of 1q21; i(5p); −9; i(11q); del and t of 11p11–q11; del, t, and dup of 13q14
Brain, rhabdoid tumor	−22
Breast (adenocarcinoma)	del(1)p11–p13; del(3)q11–13; del(5q); **−17; i(1q); der(16)t(1;16)(q10;p10); del(1)(q11–q12); del(3)(p12–p13p41–p21); del(6)(q21–q22); +7; +18; +20;** del and t of 1p11–p13; t of 1q21–q23; 3q11–q13, 7q32–q36, and 11q13–q14; dup of 11q13–q14; dmins; hsrs
Colon (adenocarcinoma)	**+7; +20;** i(1q); inv and t of 1p11–q11; i(7q); l(8q); +7; t of 7p11–q11; +8; +12; del of 12q; i(17q); t of 17p11–q11; del of 17p; −18; dmins
Ewing's sarcoma	**t(11;22)(q24;q12)**; t(1;16)(q11;q11.1) +8
Extraskeletal myxoid chondrosarcoma	**−Y; t(9;22)(q22;q12)**
Fibrosarcoma	**−Y**
Giant cell tumors	**+8**; telomeric fusions of 11p15, 13p, 15p, 18p, 19p, 21p; fus(14p;21p); fus(15p;21p)
Glioma†	**+7; −10; −22; −X; +X; −Y;** del(22)(q11–q13); del or t of 9
Hepatoblastoma	gain of 2q
Kidney (renal cell carcinoma)	**del(3)(p14–p21); del(3)(p11–p14); t(3;5)(p13;q22); −3; +7; −8; +10; −Y;** t(3;8)(p14;q24), t(3;11) (p13–p14;p15); i(5p); del(6)(q21–q23)
Kidney (papillary carcinoma)	+7; +17; **t(X;1)(p11;q21)**
Larynx (squamous cell carcinoma)	**−Y**
Liposarcoma (myxoid)	**t(12;16)(q13;p11)**
Lung (adenocarcinoma)	**del(3)(p14p23); +7**
Lung (small cell carcinoma)	**del(3)(p14p23); +7**; del of 5q, 6, 9p, 13q, 17p
Lung (squamous cell carcinoma)	**+7**
Fibrous histiocytoma	**−Y**
Melanoma, cutaneous	t(1;6)(q11–q21; q11–q13); t(1;19)(q11;q13); t of 1q11–q12 that yield 1q gain; del and t of 1p11–q12; i(6p); t of 6p11–q11 that yields 6p gain; other t of 6q11–q13; t of 7q11; +7; del and t 9p
Melanoma, uveal	−3; partial del of 3; +8; i(8q)
Meningioma	**−22; +22; −Y; del(22)(q11–q13)**
Mesothelioma	del, t, dup, or inv of 3p21–p23
Nasopharynx (squamous cell carcinoma)	**−Y**
Neuroblastoma	**del(1)(p32–p36)**; t which yield del of 1p32–p36; der(1)t(1;17)(p36;?); dmins
Ovary (carcinoma)	**+12, +7, +8, −X**; del(6q15–q23), del(3) (p21–p10); +3; +5; loss of 1p; gain of 1q; t(1;17)(p36;?); dmins; hsrs; hsrs of 19q13.1–q13.2, t(6;14)(q21;q24)
Primitive neuroectodermal tumors	i(17q)
Prostate (carcinoma)	**del(10)(q24), +7, −Y**, del(7q)
Retinoblastoma	**i(6p); del(13)(q14.1q14.1)**
Rhabdomyosarcoma (alveolar)	**t(2;13)(q37;q14); t(1;13)(p36;q14)**
Salivary gland (carcinoma)	**del(6)(q22–q25); +8; −Y**
Skin (basal cell carcinoma)	**t(9;16)(q22;p13)**
Oral (squamous cell carcinoma)	**+7**
Synovial sarcoma	**t(X;18)(p11;q11)**
Germ cell tumors (seminoma, teratoma)	i(12p); other structural abnormalities which yield 12p gain
Thyroid (adenocarcinoma)	**inv(10)(q11q21)**
Uterus (adenocarcinoma)	**+10;** i(1q); del or t of 1q21; del(6) (q21)

Table 5-2 (Continued)

Tumor type	Karyotype abnormalities and other findings
Wilms' tumor	**del(11)(p13p13); del(11)(p15p15)**; i(1q); t(1;16)(q10;q10)
Benign	
Barrett's esophagus	**−Y**
Breast fibroadenoma	der(1;16)(q10;p10), del(3p)
Colon (adenoma)	**+7**; **+8**; **+12**; del of 12q, del(1)(p36)
Giant cell tumor	**+8**
Kidney (adenoma)	− Y, +7, +17
Lipoma	**t(1;12)(p33−p34;q13−q15); t(2;12) (p22−p23;q13−q15); t(3;12)(q27−q28;q13−q15); t(5;12)(q33;q13−q15); t(11;12)(q13;q13−q15); del(12)(q13q15); t(12;21)(q13−q15;q21); del(13)(q12−q22)**
Lung (hamartoma)	**t(6;14)(p21;q24)**
Neuorepithelioma	**t(11;12)(q24;q12)**
Neurinoma	**−22; −Y**
Orbital fibroma	**t(X;2)(q26;q33)**
Ovary (adenoma)	**+12**
Ovary (fibroma)	**+12**
Ovary (thecoma)	**+12**
Salivary gland (pleomorphic adenoma)	**t(1;8)(p22;q12); t(3;8)(p21;q12); t(6;8)(p21−p22;q12); t(8;13)(p23;q13−q14); del(8)(q12q21−q22); t(8;9)(q12;p22); t(9;12)(p21−p24;q13−q15); inv(12)(p13q13)**
Thyroid adenoma	**+5, +7, +12, structural abnormalities of 19q**
Uterus (leiomyoma)	**r(1)(p11−p36q11−q14); t(2;12) (q35−q37;q14); del(7)(q21−q22q31−q32); t(12;14)(q14−q15;q23−q24); +12; other translocations of 12q13−q15; structural abnormalities with 1p36 and 6p21 breakpoints**

†Includes glioma, anaplastic glioma, glioblastoma, astrocytoma, oligodendroglioma, and ependymoma. **Primary karyotype changes are in boldface type**, secondary changes are in normal type. Generic structural alterations are given by ISCN abbreviations (e.g., del for deletions; t for translocations; inv for inversions; dup for duplications) to shorten text (see Table 20-1 and Thompson[5]).

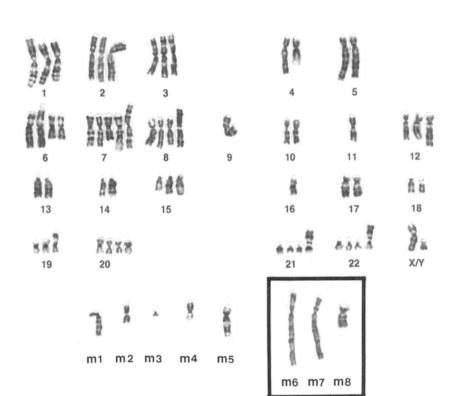

Fig. 5-1 Representative G-banded karyotype from a human malignant melanoma demonstrating numerous structural and numeric alterations. The bottom of the figure illustrates marker (m) chromosomes that represent chromosomes rearranged beyond recognition of their normal component chromosome(s). (*From Kamb A, Gruis NA, Weaver-Feldhaus J, et al.[98] Used by permission of the publisher.*)

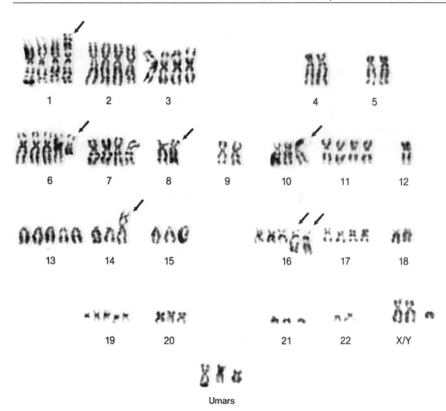

Fig. 5-2 Representative G-banded karyotype from a malignant metastatic colon adenocarcinoma demonstrating numerous structural (arrows) and numeric alterations, as well as unidentifiable marker chromosomes (Umars).

fluorescence *in situ* hybridization (FISH) as a powerful approach to identify either the entire or specific regions of all human chromosomes (Fig. 5-3), and for analysis of complex rearrangements (Fig. 5-4) are provided. More detailed information on these cancers is provided in other chapters. The application of a new technology for independently identifying all chromosomes (termed SKY) has significant potential for elucidating previously unknown chromosomal rearrangements (Fig. 5-3).[11] After a brief discussion of generic classes of chromosome rearrangements, short summaries of recurring chromosome alterations of selected cancers are provided. A detailed description of human sarcomas is presented to highlight the significant and unique (to solid tumors) molecular characterization of these cancers.

Generally, abnormalities of chromosome 1 are nearly universal, and the high frequency of alterations in the majority of solid tumors has led to the suggestion that these changes represent a frequent event in the progression, but not the genesis, of various cancers. In general the reports of clinical relevance have been limited to studies in neuroblastoma where deletion of 1p correlates with specific oncogene (*MYCN*) amplification (see Chap. 50).[12,13] In addition to structural alterations of chromosome 1, gain of chromosome 7 is one of the most common abnormalities in epithelial tumors and has been identified as a primary karyotype abnormality in a number of tumors.[1,14–18]

Cytologic Evidence of Gene Amplification

Another frequent category of chromosome alteration in solid tumors characterizes a clinically important mechanism for activation of oncogene overexpression—DNA sequence amplification (see Chap. 12). This increase in DNA sequence copy number change often results in cytologically recognizable chromosome alterations referred to as either homogeneously staining regions (HSRs), if integrated within chromosomes, or double minutes (dmin), if extrachromosomal in nature (Fig. 5-5). Figures 5-6 and 5-7 illustrate the use of fluorescence in situ hybridization (FISH) technologies and chromosome microdissection combined to identify changes in DNA copy number recognizable within a tumor, as well as

providing specific examples of HSRs and dmin in human breast and ovarian cancer.

Comparative Genomic Hybridization (CGH)

Copy number changes of individual genes and loci, as well as chromosomes and chromosomal subregions, are characteristic of human cancer, especially solid tumors. Conventional cytogenetic studies of solid tumors are sometimes difficult, because metaphases are often impossible to obtain, and genomic instability and clonal heterogeneity make data interpretation difficult. Comparative genomic hybridization (CGH) was developed to allow genome-wide screening of DNA sequence copy number aberrations in cancer (Figs. 5-8 and 5-9).[19,20] Applications of CGH in cancer genetics include characterization of recurrent unbalanced genomic rearrangements, defining novel genes involved in copy number alterations, analysis of progression and clonal evolution of cancer, as well as subclassification and prognostic evaluation of cancer. In this respect, CGH studies have already substantially contributed to our understanding of cancer biology.

CGH has most often been applied to the identification of common clonal chromosomal aberrations in cancer. When CGH data from several studies are combined, consistent patterns of nonrandom genetic aberrations emerge. Some of these changes appear to be common to various kinds of malignant tumors, while others are more tumor-specific. For example, gains of chromosomal regions 1q, 3q, and 8q, as well as losses of 8p, 13q, 16q, and 17p, are common to a number of tumor types, such as breast, ovarian, prostate, renal, and bladder cancer.[21,22] Other alterations, such as 12p and Xp gains in testicular cancer, 13q gain and 9q loss in bladder cancer, 14q loss in renal cancer, and Xp loss in ovarian cancer are more tumor-specific and may reflect the unique pathways of cancer development in different organs.

CGH has also played an important role in pinpointing putative locations of cancer genes, especially at chromosomal sites undergoing DNA amplification. There are several examples of genes whose amplification in cancer were discovered based on leads from CGH analysis. In most cases, the amplification target gene was identified based on candidate genes previously localized

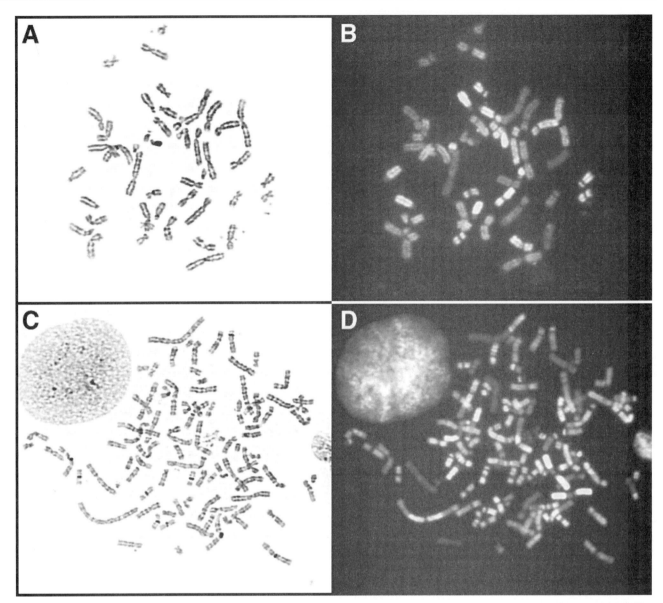

Fig. 5-3 Illustration of a G-banded normal metaphase cell (*A*) and the spectral karyotyping (SKY) of the same cell (*B*) performed following the simultaneous hybridization of 24 combinatorially labeled chromosome painting probes (Schröck et al. Multicolor spectral karyotyping of human chromosomes. *Science* 273:494, 1996). The resulting spectral analysis assigns a unique color to each of the 24 human chromosomes. This is contrasted to the G-banding of a tumor metaphase cell (*C*) and the identical cell following SKY (*D*). In addition to an increase in chromosome number, the combination of colors along the length of a single chromosome in the tumor cell documents extensive interchromosomal rearrangement.

to the region of involvement indicated by CGH. The androgen receptor (AR) (at Xq11-q12) was found to be amplified in recurrent prostate cancer after androgen deprivation therapy.[23] Other CGH studies have implicated amplification of oncogenes whose activation in cancer was previously known to occur by chromosomal translocations only. Such examples include amplification of the REL proto-oncogene (at 2p14-p15) in non-Hodgkin lymphomas,[24,25] BCL2 (at 18q21.3) in recurrent B-cell lymphomas,[26] and PAX7-FKHR fusion gene (fusing 1p36 and 13q14) in alveolar rhabdomyosarcoma.[27] Finally, a common site of amplification in breast and other cancers is at 20q. Several groups have identified novel genes that are involved in this amplification. These include the AIB1 gene, a steroid receptor coactivator,[28] BTAK, a serine/threonine kinase,[29] ZNF217, a transcription factor,[30] and NABC1 gene of unknown function,[30] all of which have been identified as amplified and overexpressed in breast cancers.

Overall, it is likely that many additional examples of novel gene amplifications in cancer are likely to emerge in future studies. The clinical significance of such novel amplified genes needs to be evaluated in large patient materials. The recently developed tissue microarray technology provides a valuable tool for high-throughput molecular profiling of large panels of uncultured tumor specimens.[31,28] This technology can be applied to rapid copy number and expression analyses of several genes in hundreds of tumors in different stages of the disease (Fig. 5-10).

The ability of CGH to evaluate archival tumor tissues makes it especially suitable to the analysis of clonal evolution of cancer progression. Analysis of genetic changes in tumors at different stages, such as premalignant lesions, in situ carcinoma and invasive cancer, may highlight aberrations involved in these specific steps of tumor progression.[32–34] CGH results are particularly informative when clonal relationships between two cancer specimens taken from the same patient are available for analysis.[35] For example, genetic changes that are not found in primary tumors, but do occur in their metastases are informative in

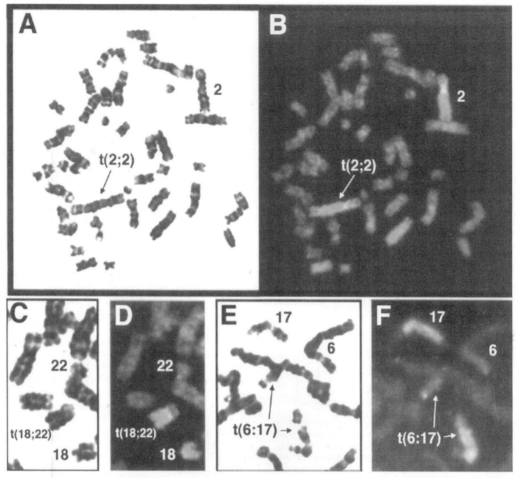

Fig. 5-4 Illustration of the application of fluorescent *in situ* hybridization (FISH) to detect complex chromosome rearrangements in malignancy. In this case, a cancer with three different translocations [t(2;2); t(18;22); and t(6;17)] were studied using probes specific for the long and short arm or each involved chromosome. *A*, G-banded metaphase. *B*, The identical metaphase as *A*, hybridized with fluorescent probes for the long arm and short arm of chromosome 2. A normal copy of chromosome 2 and a rearranged chromosome 2 (arrow) was observed. *C* and *D* represent detection of reciprocal translocations between chromosomes 18 and 22 (C/D) and 6 and 17 (E/F). In both cases, a partial G-banded metaphase is shown on the left, FISH using probes specific for each involved chromosome arm is shown on the right. (*From Guan X-Y, Zhang H, Bittner ML, Jiang Y, Meltzer PS, Trent JM.[117] Used by permission of the publisher.*)

pinpointing genetic changes and genes with important roles in the metastatic progression.

The following sections briefly overview several of the major tumor types for which significant cytogenetic information is available.

Transitional Cell Carcinoma (TCC) of the Bladder. Among the first cytogenetic studies to demonstrate the clinical importance of cytogenetic results in a human solid tumor were reports characterizing the propensity for recurrence of bladder tumors with cytogenetic abnormalities.[36,37] Long-term follow-up demonstrated that patients with abnormal karyotypes had a greater rate of tumor recurrence than patients with normal karyotypes (measured as the presence of detectable gross structural rearrangements). More recent studies corroborate these data and in general patients with diploid tumors appear to have a more favorable outcomes than patients with a mix of diploid and hyperdiploid, or hyperdiploid tumors.[38]

Chromosomes most frequently altered in this tumor type[2,3,39-45] include +7, del(10)(q22–24), and del(21)(q22). Other consistent chromosome alterations are also listed in Table 20-2. Another recurring change characterizing bladder cancers is loss of one copy of chromosome 9 (termed monosomy 9).[44,45] These results have been confirmed by loss of heterozygosity (LOH) studies, and appear to suggest that an

initiating genetic defect in bladder tumors is associated with deletion of 9p.[44,45]

Brain Tumors. In this brief section, we do not attempt to stratify chromosome alterations into the numerous histologic subtypes of brain (and particularly glial) tumors. In general across all subtypes of brain cancer, several examples of recurring chromosome alteration have been observed. These alterations include trisomy 7, monosomy 10, monosomy 22 or del(22)(q11-q13), and loss of one or both sex chromosomes.[2,3,46–49] Cytologic evidence of gene amplification (especially dmin) are found in up to 50 percent of brain tumors[46,47,49] and initial observation of these changes dates back over three decades.[46] Finally, cytogenetic analysis has defined a minimal region of deletion in glial tumors, 10q25, as a likely site of a tumor suppresser gene important to the development of this malignancy.[48]

Breast Carcinoma. Numerous studies defining the chromosome changes in breast carcinoma have been published recently and the interested reader is referred to these for further detailed information.[1–3,50–58] Briefly, among the most frequent changes in breast carcinomas are the loss of chromosome 17 in primary tumors[55] and the amplification in metastatic tumors of the band region on 17 (q13), which encodes the HER-2/neu oncogene.[59,60] More commonly, structural alterations of chromosomes 1, 3, 7,

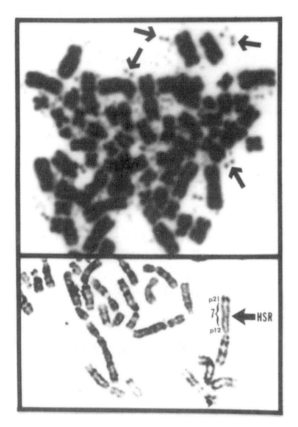

Fig. 5-5 Cytologic evidence of DNA sequence (gene) amplification. Top, example of tumor cell metaphase stained with Giemsa stain and displaying multiple copies of double minutes (dmin) (arrows). Bottom, example of a tumor cell metaphase G-banded and displaying a homogeneously staining region (hsr) involving the short arm of chromosome 7 (arrow).

and 11 are the most frequently structurally altered.[1-3,49-58] As is true for brain cancers, another important feature of breast carcinomas is the common occurrence of gene amplification, most frequently detectable as HSRs in metastatic tumors. As mentioned previously, amplification of the HER-2/*neu* oncogene[59,60] is most characteristic, followed by the recent recognition of amplification of a gene(s) on the long arm of chromosome 20.[50,52,53,61,62]

Karyotypic changes in breast cancer not surprisingly increase in frequency in metastatic tumors in contrast to changes recognized in primary tumors.[50,51,63,64] The most common numeric changes in primary tumors include loss of 17, loss of 19, and gain of chromosome 7, while the chromosomes most frequently structurally altered are chromosomes 1 and 6. Both primary and metastatic lesions often demonstrate overrepresentation of 6p and 1q, frequently with loss of 1p and 6q.[50,51,65] Although common in both primary and metastatic disease, chromosome 1 alterations are even more frequent in metastatic disease. These data have led to the suggestion that a permissive phenotype for generalized genomic instability may be associated with the transition to metastatic disease.[51]

Colon Cancer. Colon cancer is the paradigm in solid tumors demonstrating associated chromosomal (and now defined genetic) changes associated with disease predisposition, initiation, and progression (see Chap. 34).[1-3,66] Initially, cytogenetic studies were particularly useful in defining the association of altered with disease progression; therefore, it is not surprising that the most frequent chromosomal alterations include both the loss of chromosome 5 and structural rearrangements that frequently involve chromosomes 1 and 6 (usually 1p21-q11 and 6q13-q16).

Overall, overrepresentation of 1q, 6p, 8q and chromosomes 7 and 13 is observed while underrepresentation of chromosomes 17, 18, and 15 and 5 are most common.[1-3,67-72] In contrast to breast cancers, studies comparing primary to metastatic samples show a similar overall frequency and distribution of chromosome alterations.

Renal Cell Carcinoma (RCC). Nonpapillary renal cell carcinoma (RCC) is the most common form of adult kidney cancer; and cytogenetic analysis has revealed several recurring sites of chromosome change, including structural alterations of chromosome 3 (particularly 3p11-p14), and the numeric changes +7, − 8, +10, and − Y.[1-3,73-77] The deletion of 3p either as a simple deletion or by translocation has strongly suggested the presence of a predisposing gene to 3p25–36. The autosomal dominant disorder von Hippel-Lindau disease is associated with renal cell carcinoma alone or in combination with other phenotypic abnormalities, and this gene has recently been identified and characterized (see Chap. 27.)

Lung Cancer. The overwhelming number of cytogenetic studies in lung cancer have characterized small cell lung carcinoma (SCLC).[1-3,78-81] The most typical finding is del(3)(p14p23); and LOH and other biologic studies have suggested a gene(s) important in SCLC etiology maps to 3p21-p22. SCLC, as many other solid tumors, is characterized by gain of chromosome 7, which has been reported as a sole or primary change in lung carcinomas, as well as a change frequently observed in adjacent normal lung tissue.[15] Other secondary changes include loss of 5q, 6, 9p, 13q, 17p and 9p.[1-3] As is true of breast and brain tumors, cytologic evidence of gene amplification (principally in the form of dmin) have been observed frequently in SCLC and have been shown most frequently to involve amplification of the MYC and RAS oncogene families (particularly L-MYC) (see Chaps. 6 and 48.)

In non-small cell lung carcinomas, deletions of 3p and 5q are also the most common finding although the frequency of 3 loss is significantly less.[80,82,83] In general, these tumors have complex karyotypes, which show loss of 3p, 5q, 8p, Y, 5p, 10p, and gain of 1q, 3q, and 7q.[1-3,82,83]

Malignant Melanoma. Several recent studies of the chromosomes in malignant melanoma have been reported. Briefly, the chromosomes most often involved in both structural and numeric abnormalities are 1, 6, 7, 9, 10, and 11.[1-3,84-89] Figure 5-11 provides an example of the distribution of breakpoints involved in structural alteration from 158 cases of melanoma.[84] Translocations or deletions of the long arm of chromosome 6 (6p11-q12) are very common in this disorder;[90,91] and recently it was recognized that apparent simple deletions in this disorder in fact represented cryptic translocations where the telomere of another chromosome was "captured" to stabilize the breakage event.[92] Importantly, LOH and biologic evidence also exists to indicate that a gene(s) on chromosome 6 is implicated in the control of tumorigenicity in this disorder.[93-95]

Abnormalities of chromosome 1 are exceedingly frequent, involving most often the pericentromeric region 1p12-q12.[1-3,85] The net effect of these abnormalities is usually loss of 1p segments coupled with overrepresentation of 1q, a finding common in many solid tumors. Finally, several studies have suggested a familial predisposition for a subset of malignant melanomas, with suggested linkage to 1p[96] and, more importantly, the identification of a hereditary melanoma gene on 9p (see Chap. 30).[97-99] Mutations in the *P16/CDCK2N* gene appear responsible for only a subset of patients with familial melanoma (approximately 25 percent). Numerous studies, including work in our laboratory are underway to identify additional genes associated with familial melanoma. Regions of chromosome alteration may help pinpoint the location of genes important in susceptibility to this disease.

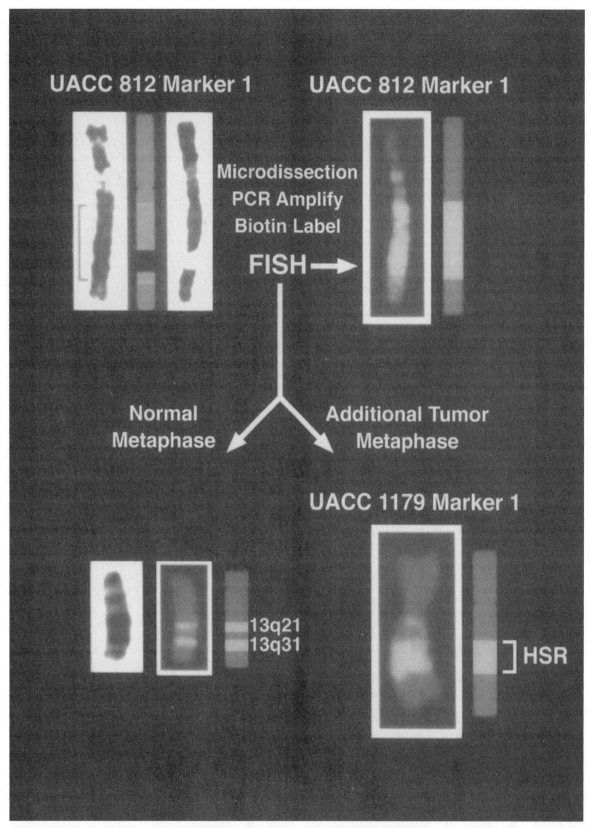

Fig. 5-6 Diagrammatic representation of the detection and characterization of hsrs from human breast cancers by chromosome microdissection (see reference 118). Upper left, G-banded hsr-bearing Marker 1 (left) from case UACC812. Microdissection (right) through the hsr of Marker 1. Upper right, after PCR amplification and biotin labeling of the dissected DNA, the PCR product is purified and hybridized by FISH back to Marker 1 to confirm that the dissection product hybridized to the hsr (bracket). Lower left, the same microdissection probe for the hsr was used to identify the location in the normal cells of the amplified sequences. Results indicated specific hybridization to the two regions of one chromosome (13q21 and 13q31): left, G-banded chromosome 13; right, identical chromosome following hybridization with the hsr probe. Lower right, the same microdissection FISH hsr probe used to hybridize to additional breast tumor cases to determine the commonality of 13q amplification. A representative example of an hsr encoding 13q amplified sequences I presented from case UACC1179 Marker 1. (*From Zhang J, Cui P, Glatfelter AA, Cummings LM, Meltzer PS, Trent JM.*[119] *Used by permission of the publisher.*)

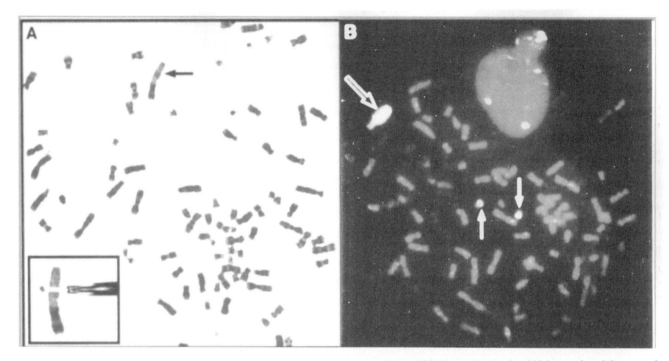

Fig. 5-7 Dissection of a fragment of a homogeneously staining region (hsr) from a human ovarian carcinoma. *A*, G-banded tumor metaphase (insert shows the dissection through the hsr to isolate DNA from the amplified region for use as a FISH probe). *B*, the same case as *A* after FISH illustrating the hsr (thick arrow) and the normal single copy region amplified in this tumor (19q13). (*From Guan X-Y, Cargile CB, Anzick SL, et al.[110] Used by permission of the publisher.*)

Studies from our laboratory have demonstrated that a recurring translocation t(1;6)(q11–21;q11–13) has been observed in a number of melanoma cases,[90] and Fig. 5-12 provides an example of this translocation. This figure also provides an illustration of the dissection of the translocation breakpoint (a starting point for positional cloning studies). Translocation of chromosome 1 segments to chromosomes 19 and 11 have also been reported to occur in a nonrandom fashion.[100,101] Evidence of gene amplification (HSRs) has been identified in melanomas, but the frequency is very low.[102]

Neuroblastoma. Deletion of part of the long arm of chromosome 1 (resulting in net loss of 1p32–p36) is the principal change recognized in this pediatric neoplasm.[1–3,11,12] Loss of this chromosomal segment appears often to be followed by amplification of the oncogene *N-MYC*, which is accompanied by recognition of HSRs or dmin in some clinical samples (see Chap. 6 for additional information).

Ovarian Carcinoma. Descriptive cytogenetics in ovarian carcinoma has been difficult because of the complexity of the clonal

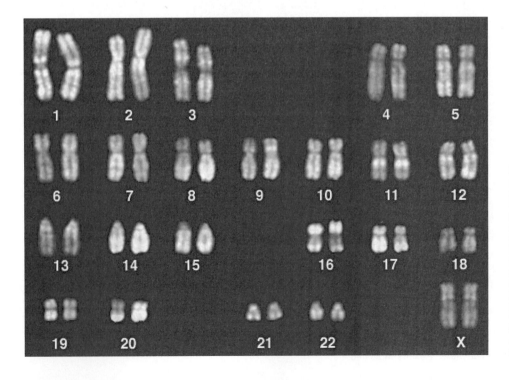

Fig. 5-8 An example of CGH analysis of a breast cancer specimen. Numerous genetic changes in the tumor DNA are visualized as color changes on metaphase chromosomes. Chromosomal regions that appear green reflect DNA gains and amplifications (e.g., 3p14, 8q, 11q13, 12q12–q13, 13q, 17q22–q24, and 20q13) and those that are red, DNA losses and deletions (e.g., 1p21–p31, 4, 8p, 9p, 11p, 11q14-qter, 13q14-qter, 16q12–q21, 18, and X). (*From Heim S, Mitelman F.[3] Used by permission of the publisher.*)

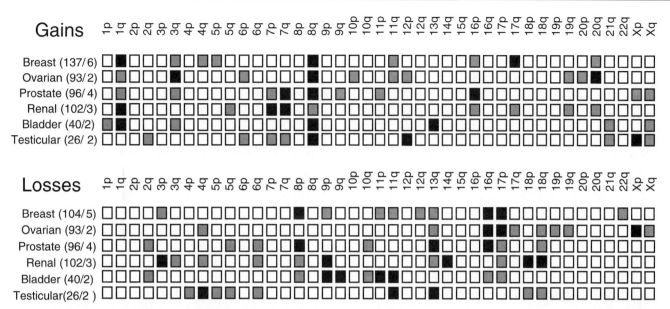

Fig. 5-9 An overview of the most common gains and losses reported in the published CGH studies of selected genital and urological tumors (the references to the original studies can be obtained from www.nhgri.nih.gov/DIR/LCG/CGH). The number of tumors analyzed and the number of studies evaluated for each tumor type are indicated in parenthesis. The black squares (■) indicate the three most-common changes to a particular tumor type, and the gray squares (▦) the next most-common regions of involvement.

Approximately 10 of the most common changes were indicated for each tumor type. The criterion for selecting the most common changes was not only the frequency, but the systematic presence of the change in independent studies. Distinct patterns of losses and gains are seen for each tumor type, whereas some genetic changes are common to several tumor types. (*From Heim S, Mitelman F.[3] Used by permission of the publisher.*)

changes characteristic of this tumor. More so than any other carcinoma, highly fragmented chromosomes, quadriradials, telomeric fusions, and complexly rearranged chromosomes are frequently found.[2,3] Nevertheless, recurring sites of chromosome change have been described, including deletions in the region 6q15–21, and translocation of chromosome 6 with chromosome 14, t(6;14)(q21;q24).[103,104] Although deletion or translocation of chromosome 6 has not been described as the sole primary change, the loss of 6q remains the most frequent abnormality described in this tumor to date. The most frequent chromosome alterations in ovarian cancer are loss of genetic material for several regions including 3p, 6q, 11p, 17q, and 17p13.[1–3,105–107] Cytologic evidence of gene amplification in the forms of HSRs and dmins and molecular evidence for specific amplification (e.g., *KRAS* oncogene) have been seen in several studies.[108–111]

Testicular Germ Cell Tumors. Histopathologic classification of testicular germ cell tumors is based upon the contribution of embryonic (embryonal carcinoma, immature and mature teratomas) or extraembryonic tissues (yolk sac tumors and choriocarcinomas), or combinations of both. Of the published cytogenetic studies of germ cell tumors isochromosomes for 12p, {i(12p)} are the most common and earliest recognizable chromosome change.[1–3,112–114] Structural alterations involving the short arm of chromosome 12 have also been reported but the net change is usually results in an increase relative to the diploid copy number of 12p while decreasing the relative copy number of 12q. This information has been suggested to play a clinically useful role in discriminating patient outcome[115] but the true clinical utility is currently indeterminate.

CHROMOSOME ALTERATIONS AND THE MOLECULAR PATHOGENESIS OF HUMAN SARCOMAS

Although the promise has long been realized, that cytogenetic anomalies might serve as signposts to identify the genes that play critical roles in oncogenesis for numerous leukemias, only recently

have translocations in solid tumors yielded to molecular analysis. The common epithelial malignancies of adults lack recurrent tumor-specific chromosome translocations that have been characterized at the molecular level. However, several tumor-specific translocations of sarcomas have now been analyzed in this fashion Table 5-3). In addition, specific genes are now recognized to be the targets of chromosome change in benign tumors. Certain themes have emerged from the study of these rearrangements, which are well illustrated by the genetic abnormalities present in Ewing's sarcoma and alterations of related genes in other cancers.

Chromosome Translocations in Ewing's Sarcoma

Specific chromosome translocations have been characterized in detail in several sarcomas, including alveolar rhabdomyosarcoma and synovial sarcoma, but Ewing's sarcoma presents the most intriguing example for detailed discussion because of the many ramifications arising from molecular analysis of this cancer.[120–122] Ewing's sarcoma is a rare, highly malignant tumor of children and young adults, which can occur in diverse anatomic sites but most frequently arises in bone. The cell of origin is uncertain, and it can be difficult to distinguish morphologically from other so-called "small round blue cell tumors," which include virtually all the solid tumors of childhood in their undifferentiated form.[123] This difficulty helped to fuel interest in the observation that a reciprocal translocation t(11:22)(q24;q12) is present in most cases of Ewing's sarcoma.[124–125] The existence of a recurrent translocation suggested that this rearrangement probably involved genes that were directly related to the pathogenesis of Ewing's sarcoma. In fact, molecular characterization of the t(11:22) has provided strong support for this proposal. Positional cloning techniques revealed that the t(11:22) results in the juxtaposition of sequences from the *FLI1* gene on chromosome 11 and the *EWS* gene on chromosome 22.[126] Although both the der(22) and der(11) might produce fusion transcripts, loss of the der(11) in some tumors and expression analysis strongly implicate the der(22) as the site of the critical rearrangement. The chromosome breakpoints on chromosomes 11 and 22 occur within introns of these genes, and lead to the generation of a chimeric gene in which the 5′ portion of

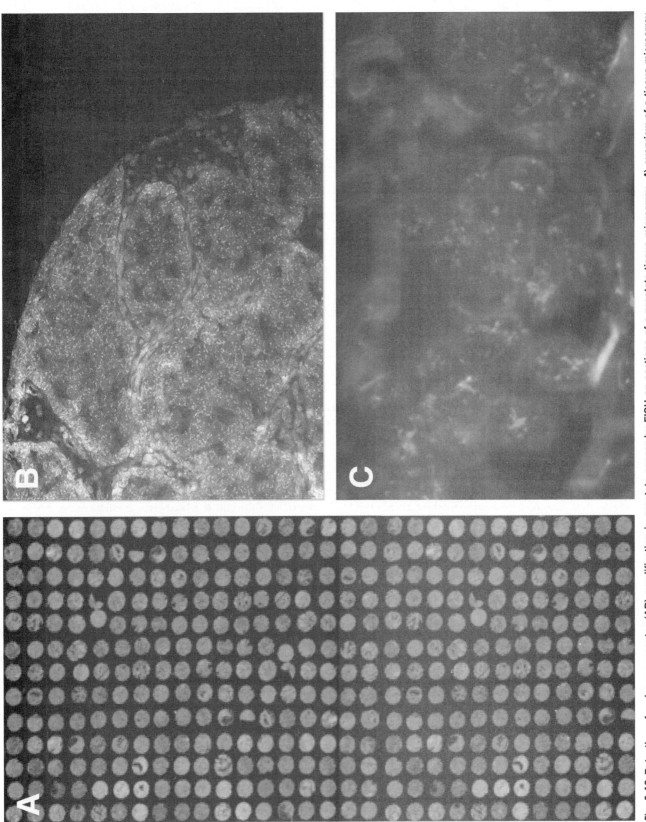

Fig. 5-10 Detection of androgen receptor (AR) amplification in prostate cancer by FISH on sections of a tissue microarray. A) overview of a tissue microarray section containing hundreds of different tumor samples (Ø 0.6 mm, each). ×3. B and C, AR amplification with many clustered AR gene signals and a few centromere X signals. B, ×200; C, ×1000.

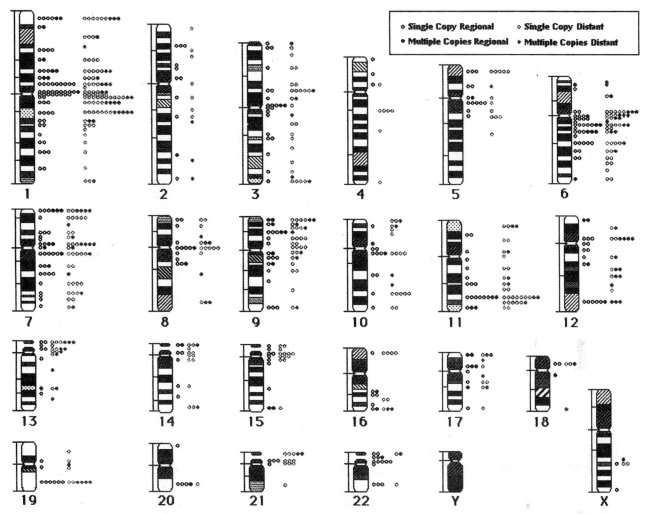

Fig. 5-11 Chromosomal breakpoints identified in clonal structural abnormalities from 158 cases of metastatic melanoma. Dark circles are from cases with tumor limited to the region of surgical dissection, light circles represent cases from patients with disseminated disease at the time of tumor biopsy. (*From Thompson FH, Emerson J, Olson S, et al.*[84] *Used by permission of the publisher.*)

EWS is fused in frame to 3′ sequences from *FLI1* (Figs. 5-13 and 5-14).[127]

Characterization of these genes revealed that *FLI1* has a 97 percent identity with a murine gene (*FLi1* first described as a target of oncogenic retroviral integration on mouse chromosome 9 in a region that is syntenic to human chromosome 11.[128] Sequence analysis demonstrates that *FLI1* is a member of the ETS family of transcription factors that contain a characteristic DNA-binding motif, the ETS domain.[129] The *ETS-1* protooncogene itself was originally defined by the presence of ETS-related sequences in the E26 avian leukosis virus.[130] The 656 amino acid protein encoded by *EWS* was novel but contained a putative RNA-binding domain. Analysis of the genomic structure of *EWS* demonstrated that the gene is composed of 17 exons distributed over approximately 40 kb.[131] The first seven exons encode a repetitive polypeptide with the consensus sequence SYGQQS. This is followed by a hinge region encoded by exons 8 to 10, while the candidate RNA-binding domain is encoded in exons 11 to 13.

The breakpoints in the t(11;22) vary from case to case, but always lead to replacement of the RNA-binding domain of *EWS* by the DNA-binding domain of *FLI1* (Figs. 5-13 and 5-14).[127] The resultant fusion protein would be predicted to have the properties of a transcription factor with a transcriptional activation domain contributed by *EWS* and a DNA-binding domain contributed by *FLI1*. A considerable body of experimental evidence has accumulated to support this interpretation.[134–138]

The EWS/FLI1 fusion protein is localized in the nucleus and retains the DNA-binding specificity of FLI1. Reporter gene assays also demonstrate that it is a potent transcriptional activator, and unlike FLI1 it is able to transform NIH 3T3 cells. The *EWS* sequences clearly confer transcriptional activating function. Because the transforming properties of *EWS* cannot be replaced by other strong transcriptional activation domains, they are likely to provide important protein interaction and regulatory functions.[139]

Important observations have emerged as additional cases of Ewing's sarcoma have been characterized. Although the *EWS* gene is consistently involved in every instance, variant translocation partners for *EWS* have been identified in a subset of cases. The most common alternative to *FLI1* is *ERG*, a gene that maps on chromosome 21q22. ERG is also a member of the ETS family of transcription factors. In a manner quite comparable to the *EWS/FLI1* translocation, the *EWS/ERG* fusion transfers the *ERG* DNA-binding domain to the *EWS* transcriptional activating domain.[127,140] A third variant translocation involves *EWS* with an *ETV1* gene on chromosome 7p22.[141] *ETV1* is yet another member of the ETS family, further emphasizing the importance of the ETS DNA-binding domain contributed to the fusion proteins by each of these three transcription factors. Finally, a fourth variant translocation, t(17;22)(q21;q12) has been described that joins the transactivation domain of *EWS* with a fourth member of the ETS family, the

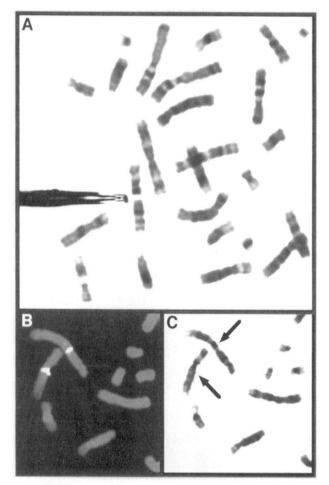

Fig. 5-12 Cytogenetic characterization of a chromosome translocation from a metastatic melanoma. *A,* G-banded tumor metaphase demonstrating a translocation between chromosomes 1 and 6 [t(1;6)(q21;q14)]. Dissection of the chromosomal breakpoint is performed with a glass needle targeted to the translocation breakpoint. *B,* FISH analysis of the dissected material hybridized to a normal human metaphase cell showing chromosome regions involved in the translocation between chromosomes 1 and 6. *C,* the identical cell as *B,* G-banded to confirm the specific chromosomal regions. (*From Zhang J, Cui P, Glatfelter AA, Cummings LM, Meltzer PS, Trent JM.*[119] *Used by permission of the publisher.*)

Table 5-3 Chromosome Translocations in Sarcomas

Tumor	Translocation	Genes
Ewing' sarcoma	t(11;22)(q24;q12)	EWS/FLI-1
	t(21;22)(q22;q12)	EWS/ERG
	t(7;22)(p22;q12)	EWS/ETV1
	t(17;22)(q21;q12)	EWS/ETV4
Malignant melanoma (clear cell sarcoma) of the soft parts	t(12;22)(q13;q12)	EWS/ATF1
Dermatofibrosarcoma protuberans	t(17;22)(q22;q13)	COL1A1/PDGFB
Desmoplastic small round cell tumor	t(11;22)(q13;q12)	EWS/WT1
Extraskeletal myxoid chondrasarcoma	t(9;22)(q22;q12)	EWS/TEC
Infantile fibrosarcoma	t(12;15)(p12;q25)	ETV6/NTRK3
Myxoid liposarcoma	t(12;16)(q13;p11)	FUS/CHOP
	t(12;22)(q13;12)	EWS/CHOP
Alveolar rhabdomyosarcoma	t(2;13)(q35;q14)	PAX3/FKHR
	t(1;13)(p36;q14)	PAX7/FKHR
Synovial sarcoma	t(X;18)(p11;q11)	SYT/SSX

adenovirus E1A enhancer-binding protein (*ETV4*).[142] *ETV4* is known to activate transcription of matrix metalloproteinase genes, thus potentially linking the *EWS/ETV4* fusion protein with the invasive properties of the tumor.

Diagnostic Implications

Ewing's sarcoma can be difficult to distinguish from other cancers that are morphologically similar. This difficulty has led to an examination of the diagnostic importance of the t(11;22). This is well illustrated by consideration of another diagnostic entity, described variously as primitive neuroepithelioma (PN) or peripheral primitive neuroectodermal tumor of childhood (PNET). These tumors are clinically similar to Ewing's sarcoma, though they occur most often in extraosseus sites during adolescence. However, unlike Ewing's sarcoma, PN consistently expresses ultrastructural features of neural differentiation and is therefore felt to be of neural origin. Although PN can be distinguished from Ewing's sarcoma in this basis, it is now recognized that the t(11;22) is also found in PN.[143,144] The presence of the same underlying molecular genetic alteration

suggests that these disorders must be very closely related if not identical. Some pathologists now consider these cancers as part of an as yet incompletely defined Ewing's sarcoma group of peripheral neuroectodermal tumors, all of which are linked by the presence of the t(11;22).[145] In fact, because it is possible to determine the presence of the *EWS/FLI1* fusion gene by either RT-PCR or interphase FISH, it is likely that testing for the presence of this molecular aberration will become part of the routine characterization of these tumors.[146–152] However, the presence of *EWS/FLI1* transcripts in a few tumors with myogenic or biphenotypic features suggests that molecular characterization will supplement, rather than replace, traditional tumor markers.[153] Nonetheless, because of its pathogenic role, the presence of the t(11;22) may ultimately prove more important than markers of cell differentiation, especially if therapies are developed that are directed at the pathways triggered by the *EWS/FLI1* transcription factor.[154] The question also arises as to whether the variant *EWS* translocations within Ewing's sarcoma have different clinical behavior. Currently available data suggest an advantage for patients with *EWS/FLI1* fusions occurring after exon 7 of *EWS* relative to the other variants.[155–157] It will be of interest to define the molecular basis for this effect, which may arise from subtle functional differences in the variant fusion proteins. As illustrated by the following examples, rearrangements involving the *EWS* gene are not confined to Ewing's sarcoma.

***EWS* rearrangements in other sarcomas.** A rare tumor of young adults called malignant melanoma of the soft parts, or clear cell sarcoma, is characterized by a tumor-specific translocation t(12;22)(q13;q12).[158,159] This tumor, which exhibits some neuroectodermal features, most frequently occurs in the tendons and aponeuroses. Molecular characterization of the t(12;22) has revealed that this rearrangement also involves the *EWS* gene, which in this instance gives rise to a chimeric protein carrying sequences from the ATF-1 gene on chromosome 12q13.[160–161] Again in parallel with the t(11;22), ATF-1, a transcription factor in the bZIP family, contributes its DNA-binding domain to the fusion protein.[162,163]

EWS contributes to yet another tumor-specific translocation, the t(11;22)(p13;q12) observed in desmoplastic small round cell tumor.[164,165] This is a tumor that occurs primarily in the abdomen

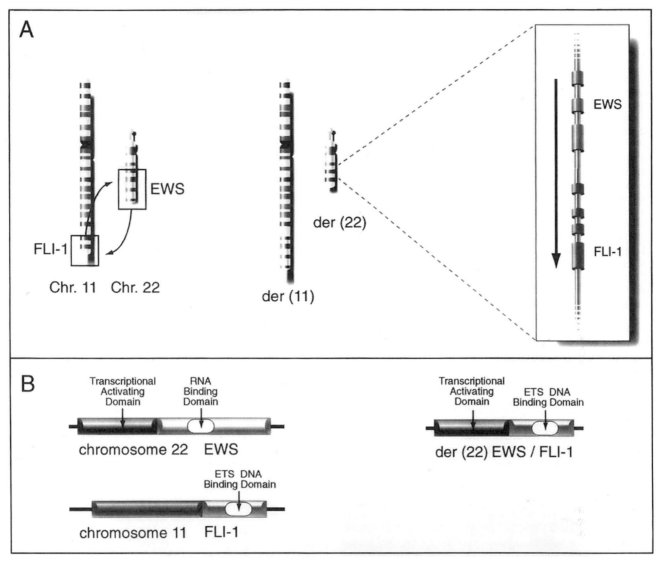

Fig. 5-13 *A*, Translocation of sequences from chromosome 11 to chromosome 22 creates a fusion protein derived from the *EWS* and *FLI1* genes in Ewing's sarcoma. In the diagram on the far right, the arrow indicates the direction of transcription, and exons are represented by enlarged areas. *B*, The fusion protein contains transcriptional activating sequences from the N-terminal portion of *EWS* joined to the ETS DNA-binding domain of *FLI-1*.

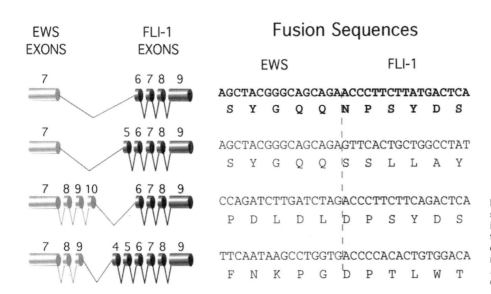

Fig. 5-14 Representative fusion transcripts identified by Zucman et al.[127] illustrating their variability. The most frequent type joins exon 7 of EWS to exon 6 of FLI-1. All of the variants replace the RNA-binding domain of *EWS* with the ETS DNA-binding domain of *FLI-1*.

of adolescent males or in association with other serosal surfaces.[166,167] In this disorder *EWS* forms a chimeric protein with WT-1.[168-171] Remarkably, *WT-1* is the Wilms Tumor gene, which was identified as the target of constitutional deletion in the Wilms tumor-aniridia syndrome.[172] *WT-1*, like the other *EWS* partners is a transcription factor, and the *EWS/WT-1* fusion once again pairs the *EWS* transcriptional activation domain with the zinc finger DNA-binding domain of *WT-1*.

Involvement of *EWS* has been extended to myxoid chondrosarcoma, which exhibits a specific chromosomal translocation t(9;22)(q22–31;q11–12). This rearrangement links *EWS* with almost the entire coding sequence of *CHN*, a member of the steroid hormone receptor superfamily.[173-174] The involvement of *EWS* with multiple partners in so many different sarcomas is remarkable, but even more impressive when one considers *FUS*, a homolog of *EWS*, which is also involved in tumor-specific rearrangements.

An *EWS* homolog also participates in sarcoma translocations. Myxoid liposarcoma (MLPS) is characterized by a t(12;16)(q13;p11).[175] This rearrangement gives rise to a chimeric transcription factor derived from the *CHOP* gene on chromosome 12 and a gene that has been called either *FUS* (for fusion) or *TLS* (for translocated in liposarcoma) on chromosome 16.[176-178] Remarkably, the *FUS/TLS* gene closely resembles the *EWS* gene and contains the same functional domains. *CHOP* is a transcription factor of the C/EBPβ family, and is normally induced in response to starvation or stress stimuli.[179] Heterodimers formed between CHOP and C/EBPβ have reduced DNA-binding activity, and CHOP therefore appears to be a negative regulator.[180-183] However, in the FUS/CHOP chimera the bZIP domain does confer DNA-binding activity. Remarkably, cases of MLPS have now been described that contain *EWS/CHOP* fusions, further emphasizing the functional similarities of *EWS* and *FUS/TLS* as well as the specificity of CHOP for MLPS.[184]

Several conclusions seem inevitable upon consideration of the range of tumors that exhibit rearrangements of either *EWS* or FUS/TLS. These molecular abnormalities appear to be essential to the pathogenesis of the tumors in which they occur. Because all the fusion proteins described above are transcription factors, perturbation of the normal pattern of gene expression must be critical to the malignant transformation of normal precursor cells. Because the occurrence of these translocations is in itself most likely a random event, the emergence of a translocation-bearing tumor clone presumably reflects both the lineage specificity and the oncogenic potency of that specific chimeric transcription factor. The precise reasons for the predominant rearrangement of ETS family genes in Ewing's sarcoma or *CHOP* in myxoid liposarcoma remain to be elucidated, but presumably they relate to the underlying program of gene expression required for the differentiation of the various mesenchymal cell lineages. Elucidation of the detailed downstream biochemical effects of the oncogenic chimeric transcription factors is an important current focus of research. In addition, it should be emphasized that sarcomas bearing chimeric transcription factors are likely to contain additional genetic alterations, such as p53 mutation, which are important to the evolution of the clinically evident malignant tumor.[185,186] However, based on their high incidence in tumors of a given type, it is likely that the translocations that characterize these tumors occur early in their evolution and create a fundamental disturbance of cell function essential to the tumorigenic process.

Rearrangements of the HMGI-C gene in benign tumors. Tumor-specific translocations are not limited to malignant tumors. Benign tumors, notably lipoma and leiomyoma, may be karyotypically abnormal. Rearrangements of chromosome 12q14–q15 have been among the most frequent abnormalities observed in these tumors.[187-189] Diverse partner chromosomes have been observed linked to 12q14–q15 in various tumors.

In addition to lipoma and leiomyoma, rearrangements of the 12q14–q15 region have also been observed in pulmonary chondroid hamartoma, pleomorphic adenomas of the salivary gland, endometrial polyps, and a variety of benign tumors of mesenchymal origin.[190-192] The frequent appearance of the 12q breakpoint strongly suggested that a pathogenically important gene resided at that location, a suspicion borne out when the *HMGI-C* gene was mapped to the site of these breakpoints in both leiomyoma and lipoma.[193,194] *HMGI-C* is the human homolog of the murine pygmy gene and is a member of the HMGI family of small nuclear proteins, including *HMGI-C* and *HMGI(Y)*, which are characterized by the presence of a DNA-binding domain called the AT hook that binds to the minor groove of AT-rich DNA and induces DNA bending.[195] The HMGI-C protein consists of only 109 amino acids encoded by five exons with the three AT hook domains being encoded by the first three exons. The third intron is large (140 kb) and is the site of the translocations that fuse sequences from almost every chromosome to the AT hook domains of *HMGI-C*.[194] HMGI proteins have not been shown to have intrinsic transcription factor activity, but appear to function as accessory factors promoting the binding of other proteins to DNA.[196] In addition, HMGI-C is induced in NIH3T3 cells as a delayed early-response gene suggesting a possible connection between HMGI-C and cell cycle progression. The precise biochemical effects of the fusion proteins have not been established, and the multiple-partner genes have not yet been fully characterized. In one case (a lipoma with a t(3;12)), the partner gene contains two tandem LIM motifs, sequences that are known to function as protein interaction domains.[193,194] The second gene in the HMGI family, HMG-I(Y), maps to chromosome 6p21, and variant translocations in benign tumors may involve this gene instead of HMGI-C.[197,198]

The HMGI family translocations present both parallels and sharp contrasts to those involving the *EWS* gene family. Both categories of translocation involve chimeric DNA-binding proteins that most likely exert their oncogenic effects by perturbing normal gene expression. In both cases, a critical domain is provided by either member of a two-gene family. In the case of HMGI, this is a DNA-binding domain, while in the case of *EWS*, it is the transcriptional activating domain. The benign behavior of tumors with HMGI translocations contrasts with the highly malignant properties of tumors with *EWS* translocations. Benign lipomas and leiomyomas do not appear to evolve into malignant tumors. It is not at all clear how the HMGI-C translocations confer proliferative capacity without a tendency to accumulate further genetic alterations that would promote malignant progression. Comparison of the biochemical consequences of these two categories of translocation is likely to prove important in defining the molecular features that distinguish malignant tumors from their benign counterparts.

CONCLUSION

This brief review of the current progress in identifying recurring sites of chromosome change in human solid tumors, reveals that, despite methodological difficulties, a recurring and decidedly nonrandom pattern of chromosome alterations has clearly emerged. It appears likely that as additional cases of solid tumors are cytogenetically examined, the stratification of some specific histopathologic subtypes will be possible, and this may facilitate diagnostic (and possibly prognostic) analysis.

At present the clinical utility of chromosome analysis in solid tumors is largely indeterminate. However, the pinpointing of regions of the genome that are characteristically altered in solid tumors has been, and will continue to be, of significant benefit in targeting future molecular (and hopefully mechanistic) investigations. Continued study of the basic genetics of solid tumors appears a particularly fruitful avenue to continue, as it assuredly will add to our understanding of the causation, progression, and ultimately the control of these disorders.

ACKNOWLEDGMENT

We want to acknowledge the excellent graphic assistance of Darryl Leja, NHGRI, NIH. Also, we thank Drs. Felix Mitelman and Robert Jenkins for their review of recurring chromosomal alterations.

REFERENCES

1. Mitelman F: *Catalog of Chromosome Aberrations in Cancer, '98: Version 1*. New York, Wiley-Liss, 1998.
2. Sandberg AA: *The Chromosomes in Human Cancer and Leukemia*, 2nd ed. New York, Elsevier Science, 1990.
3. Heim S, Mitelman F: *Cancer Cytogenetics. Chromosomal and Molecular Genetic Aberrations of Tumor Cells*, 2nd ed. New York, Wiley-Liss, 1995.
4. de Klein A, Guerts van Kessel A, Grosveld G, et al.: A cellular oncogene is translocated to the Philadelphia chromosome in chronic myelocytic leukaemia. *Nature* 300:765, 1982.
5. Thompson FH: Cytogenetic methodological approaches and findings in human solid tumors in Barch MJ (ed): *The ACT Cytogenetics Laboratory Manual*, 2nd ed. New York, Raven Press, 1996, p 451.
6. Yang JM, Thompson FH, Knox SM, Dalton WS, Salmon SE, Trent JM: Polyclonal origin of a primary breast carcinoma demonstrated by serial cytogenetic studies of a patient with a history of osteosarcoma [Abstract]. *Cancer Genet Cytogenet* 66:153, 1993.
7. Pandis N, Heim S, Bardi G, Idvall I, Mandahl N, Mitelman F: Chromosome analysis of 20 breast carcinomas: Cytogenetic multiclonality and karyotypic-pathologic correlations. *Genes Chromosomes Cancer* 6:51, 1993.
8. Heim S, Caron M, Jin Y, Mandahl N, Mitelman F: Genetic convergence during serial in vitro passage of a polyclonal squamous cell carcinoma. *Cytogenet Cell Genet* 52:133, 1989.
9. Nowell PC: Tumors as clonal proliferation. *Virchows Arch B Cell Path* 29:145, 1978.
10. Mitelman F (ed): *ISCN (1995): An International System for Human Cytogenetic Nomenclature*. Basel, S. Karger, 1995.
11. Schrock E, du Manoir S, Veldman T, Schoell B, Wienberg J, Ferguson-Smith MA, Ning Y, Ledbetter DH, Bar-Am I, Soenksen D, Garini Y, Ried T: Multicolor spectral karyotyping of human chromosomes. *Science* 273:494, 1996.
12. Christiansen H, Schestag J, Christiansen NM, Grzeschik K-H, Lampert F: Clinical impact of chromosome 1 aberrations in neuroblastoma: A metaphase and interphase cytogenetic study. *Genes Chromosomes Cancer* 5:141, 1992.
13. Caron H, van Sluis P, Van Hoeve M, et al.: Allelic loss of chromosome 1p36 in neuroblastoma is of preferential maternal origin and correlates with N-myc amplification. *Nat Genet* 4:187, 1993.
14. Trent J, Meyskens FL, Salmon SE, et al.: Relation of cytogenetic abnormalities and clinical outcome in metastatic melanoma,. *N Engl J Med* 322:1508, 1990.
15. Korc M, Meltzer P, Trent J: Enhanced expression of epidermal growth factor receptor correlates with alterations of chromosome 7 in human pancreatic cancer. *Proc Natl Acad Sci U S A* 83:5141, 1986.
16. Aly MS, Dal Cin P, Van de Voorde W, et al.: Chromosome abnormalities in benign prostatic hyperplasia. *Genes Chromosomes Cancer* 9:227, 1994.
17. Arps S, Rodewald A, Schmalenberger B, Carl P, Bressel M, Kastendieck H: Cytogenetic survey of 32 cancers of the prostate. *Cancer Genet Cytogenet* 66:93, 1993.
18. Herrmann ME, Lalley PA: Significance of trisomy 7 in thyroid tumors. *Cancer Genet Cytogenet* 62:144, 1992.
19. Kallioniemi A, Kallioniemi O-P, Sudar D, Rutovitz D, Gray JW, Waldman F, Pinkel D: Comparative genomic hybridization: A powerful new method for cytogenetic analysis of solid tumors. *Science* 258:818, 1992.
20. Du Manoir S, Speicher MR, Joos S, Schröck E, Popp S, Dohner H, Kovacs G, Robert-Nicoud M, Lichter P, Cremer T: Detection of complete and partial chromosome gains and losses by comparative genomic hybridization. *Hum Genet* 90:590, 1993.
21. Forozan F, Karhu R, Kononen J, Kallioniemi A, Kallioniemi O-P: Genome screening by comparative genomic hybridization. *TIG* 13:405, 1997.
22. Knuutila S, Björkqvist A-M, Autio K, Tarkkanen M, Wolf M, Monni O, Szymanska J, Larramendy ML, Tapper J, Pere H, El-Rifai W, Hemmer S, Wasenius V-M, Vidgren V, Zhu Y: DNA copy number amplifications in human neoplasms. *Am J Pathol* 152:1107, 1998.
23. Visakorpi T, Kallioniemi A, Syvänen A-C, Hyytinen E, Karhu R, Tammela T, Isola JJ, Kallioniemi O-P: Genetic changes in primary and recurrent prostate cancer by comparative genomic hybridization. *Cancer Res* 55:342, 1995.
24. Houldsworth J, Mathew S, Rao PH, Dyomina K, Louie DC, Parsa N, Offit K, Chaganti RS: REL proto-oncogene is frequently amplified in extranodal diffuse large cell lymphoma. *Blood* 87:25, 1996.
25. Joos S, Otano-Joos MI, Ziegler S, Bruderlein S, du Manoir S, Bentz M, Moller P, Lichter P: Primary mediastinal (thymic) B-cell lymphoma is characterized by gains of chromosomal material including 9p and amplification of the REL gene. *Blood* 87:1571, 1996.
26. Monni O, Joensuu H, Franssila K, Knuutila S: DNA copy number changes in diffuse large B-cell lymphoma—Comparative genomic hybridization study. *Blood* 87:5269, 1996.
27. Weber-Hall S, McManus A, Anderson J, Nojima T, Abe S, Pritchard-Jones K, Shipley J: Novel formation and amplification of the PAX7-FKHR fusion gene in a case of alveolar rhabdomyosarcoma. *Genes Chromosomes Cancer* 17:7, 1996.
28. Anzick SL, Kononen J, Walker RL, Azorsa DO, Tanner MM, Guan XY, Sauter G, Kallioniemi OP, Trent JM, Meltzer PS: AIB1, a steroid receptor coactivator amplified in breast and ovarian cancer. *Science* 277:965, 1997.
29. Sen S, Zhou H, White RA: A putative serine/threonine kinase encoding gene BTAK on chromosome 20q13 is amplified and overexpressed in human breast cancer cell lines. *Oncogene* 14:2195, 1997.
30. Collins C, Rommens JM, Kowbel D, Godfrey T, Tanner M, Hwang SI, Polikoff D, Nonet G, Cochran J, Myambo K, Jay KE, Froula J, Cloutier T, Kuo WL, Yaswen P, Dairkee S, Giovanola J, Hutchinson GB, Isola J, Kallioniemi OP, Palazzolo M, Martin C, Ericsson C, Pinkel D, Gray JW: Positional cloning of ZNF217 and NABC1: Genes amplified at 20q13.2 and overexpressed in breast carcinoma. *Proc Natl Acad Sci U S A* 95:8703, 1998.
31. Kononen J, Bubendorf L, Kallioniemi A, Bärlund M, Schraml P, Leighton S, Torhorst J, Mihatsch MJ, Sauter G, Kallioniemi O-P: Tissue microarrays for high-throughput molecular profiling of tumor specimens. *Nat Med* 4:844, 1998.
32. Bubendorf L, Kononen J, Koivisto P, Schraml P, Moch H, Gasser TC, Willi N, Mihatsch MJ, Sauter G, Kallioniemi OP: Survey of gene amplifications during prostate cancer progression by high-throughput fluorescence in situ hybridization on tissue microarrays. *Cancer Res* 59(4):803, 1999.
33. Heselmeyer K, Schröck E, du Manoir S, Blegen H, Shah K, Steinbeck R, Auer G, Ried T: Gain of chromosome 3q defines the transition from severe dysplasia to invasive carcinoma of the uterine cervix. *Proc Natl Acad Sci U S A* 93:479, 1996.
34. Kuukasjärvi T, Karhu R, Tanner M, Kähkönen M, Schaffer A, Nupponen N, Pennanen S, Kallioniemi A, Kallioniemi OP, Isola J: Genetic heterogeneity and clonal evolution underlying development of asynchronous metastasis in human breast cancer. *Cancer Res* 57:1597, 1997.
35. Gronwald J, Storkel S, Holtgreve-Grez H, Hadaczek P, Brinkschmidt C, Jauch A, Lubinski J, Cremer T: Comparison of DNA gains and losses in primary renal clear cell carcinomas and metastatic sties: Importance of 1q and 3p copy number changes in metastatic events. *Cancer Res* 57:481, 1997.
36. Falor WH: Chromosomes in noninvasive papillary carcinoma of the bladder. *JAMA* 216:791, 1971.
37. Falor WH, Ward RM: Prognosis in early carcinoma of the bladder based on chromosomal analysis. *J Urol* 199:44, 1978.
38. Schapers RFM, Smeets AWGB, Pauwels RPE, Van Den Brandt PA, Bosman FT: Cytogenetic analysis in transitional cell carcinoma of the bladder. *Br J Urol* 72:887, 1993.
39. Wang M-R, Perissel B, Taillandier J, et al.: Nonrandom changes of chromosome 10 in bladder cancer—Detection by FISH to interphase nuclei. *Cancer Genet Cytogenet* 73:8, 1994.
40. Atkin NB, Baker MC: Cytogenetic study of ten carcinomas of the bladder: Involvement of chromosomes 1 and 11. *Cancer Genet Cytogenet* 15:253, 1985.
41. Gibas Z, Prout GR, Connolly JG, Pontes JE, Sandberg AA: Nonrandom chromosomal changes in transitional cell carcinoma of the bladder. *Cancer Res* 44:1257, 1984.
42. Gibas Z, Prout GR, Pontes JE, Connolly JG, Sandberg AA: A possible specific chromosome change in transitional cell carcinoma of the bladder. *Cancer Genet Cytogenet* 19:229, 1986.

43. Poddighe PJ, Ramaekers FCS, Smeets AWGB, Vooijs GP, Hopman AHN: Structural chromosome 1 aberrations in transitional cell carcinoma of the bladder: Interphase cytogenetics combining a centromeric, telomeric, and library DNA probe. *Cancer Res* **52**:4929, 1992.

44. Cairns P, Shaw ME, Knowles MA: Initiation of bladder cancer may involve deletion of a tumour-suppressor gene on chromosome 9. *Oncogene* **8**:1083, 1993

45. Miyao N, Tsai YC, Lerner SP, et al.: Role of chromosome 9 in human bladder cancer. *Cancer Res* **53**:4066, 1993.

46. Lubs HA, Salmon JH: The chromosomal complement of human solid tumors, II. Karyotypes of glial tumors. *J Neurosurg* **22**:160, 1965.

47. Magnani I, Guerneri S, Pollo B, et al.: Increasing complexity of the karyotype in 50 human gliomas. *Cancer Genet Cytogenet* **75**:77, 1994.

48. Rasheed BKA, McLendon RE, Friedman HS, et al.: Chromosome 10 deletion mapping in human gliomas: A common deletion region in10q25. *Oncogene* **10**:2243, 1995.

49. Reifenberger G, Reifenberger J, Ichimura K, Meltzer PS, Collins PV: Amplification of multiple genes from chromosomal region 12q13-14 in human malignant gliomas: Preliminary mapping of the amplicons shows preferential involvement of CDK4, SAS, and MDM2. *Cancer Res* **54**:4299, 1994.

50. Thompson F, Emerson J, Dalton WS, et al.: Clonal chromosome abnormalities in human breast carcinomas I: 28 cases with primary disease. *Genes Chromosomes Cancer* **7**:185, 1993.

51. Trent J, Yang J-M, Emerson J, et al.: Clonal chromosome abnormalities in human breast carcinomas II: 34 cases with metastatic disease. *Genes Chromosomes Cancer* **7**:194, 1993.

52. Tanner MM, Tirkkonen M, Kallioniemi A, et al.: Increased copy number at 20q13 in breast cancer: Defining the critical region and exclusion of candidate genes. *Cancer Res* **54**:4257, 1994.

53. Adelaide J, Penault-Llorca F, Dib A, Yarden Y, Jacquemier J, Birnbaum D: The heregulin gene can be included in the 8p12 amplification unit in human breast cancer. *Genes Chromosomes Cancer* **11**:66, 1994.

54. Almeida A, Muleris M, Dutrillaux B, Malfoy B: The insulin-like growth factor I receptor gene is the target for the 15q26 amplicon in breast cancer. *Genes Chromosomes Cancer* **11**:63, 1994.

55. Nagai MA, Yamamoto L, Salaorni S, et al.: Detailed deletion mapping of chromosome segment 17q12-21 in sporadic breast tumours. *Genes Chromosomes Cancer* **11**:58, 1994.

56. Bieche I, Champeme M-H, Lidereau R: Loss and gain of distinct regions of chromosome 1q in primary breast cancer. *Clin Cancer Res* **1**:123, 1995.

57. Pandis N, Jin Y, Gorunova L, et al.: Chromosome analysis of 97 primary breast carcinomas: Identification of eight karyotypic subgroups. *Genes Chromosomes Cancer* **12**:173, 1995.

58. Hoggard N, Brintnell B, Howell A, Weissenbach J, Varley J: Allelic imbalance on chromosome 1 in human breast cancer. II. Microsatellite repeat analysis. *Genes Chromosomes Cancer* **12**:24, 1995.

59. Slamon DJ, Clark GM, Wong SG, Levin WJ, Ullrich A, McGuire WL: Human breast cancer: Correlation of relapse and survival with amplification of the HER-2/neu oncogene. *Science* **235**:177, 1987.

60. Slamon DJ, Godolphin W, Jones LA, et al.: Studies of the HER-2/neu proto-oncogene in human breast and ovarian cancer. *Science* **244**:707, 1989.

61. Tanner MM, Tirkkonen M, Kallioniemi A, Isola J, Kuukasjärvi T, Collins C, Kowbel D, Guan X-Y, Trent J, Gray JW, Meltzer P, Kallioniemi O-P: Independent amplification and frequent co-amplification of three nonsyntenic regions on the long arm of chromosome 20 in human breast cancer. *Cancer Res* **56**:3441, 1996.

62. Guan X-Y, Xu J, Anzick SL, Zhang H, Trent JM, Meltzer PS: Hybrid selection of transcribed sequences from microdissected DNA: Isolation of genes within an amplified region at 20q11–q13.2 in breast cancer. *Cancer Res* **56**:3446, 1996.

63. Trent J: Cytogenetic and molecular biologic alterations in human breast cancer: A review. *Breast Cancer Res Treat* **5**:221, 1985.

64. Trent JM, Yang J-M, Thompson FH, Leibovitz A, Villar H, Dalton WS: Chromosome alterations in human breast cancer, in: Sluyser M (ed): *Oncogenes and Hormones in Breast Cancer.* Chichester, Ellis Horwood, 1987, p 142.

65. Devilee P, van Vliet M, van Sloun P, et al.: Allotype of human breast carcinoma. A second major site for loss of heterozygosity is on chromosome 6. *Oncogene* **6**:1705, 1991.

66. Vogelstein B, Fearon ER, Hamilton SR, et al.: Genetic alterations during colorectal-tumor development. *N Engl J Med* **319**:525, 1988.

67. Muleris M, Zafrani B, Validire P, Girodet J, Salmon R-J, Dutrillaux B: Cytogenetic study of 30 colorectal adenomas. *Cancer Genet Cytogenet* **74**:104, 1994.

68. Muleris M, Salmon RJ, Zafrani B, Girodet J, Dutrillaux B: Consistent deficiencies of chromosome 18 and of the short arm of chromosome 17 in eleven cases of human large bowel cancer: A possible recessive determinism. *Ann Genet* **28**:206, 1985.

69. Muleris M, Salmon R-J, Dutrillaux B: Chromosome study demonstrating the clonal evolution and metastatic origin of a metachronous colorectal carcinoma. *Int J Cancer* **38**:167, 1986.

70. Thompson FH, Liu Y, Alberts D, Taetle R, Trent JM: Cytogenetic findings in 51 colorectal carcinomas: correlations with sample site [Abstract]. *Am J Hum Genet* **53**:376, 1993.

71. Muleris M, Salmon R-J, Dutrillaux A-M, et al.: Characteristic chromosomal imbalances in 18 near-diploid colorectal tumors. *Cancer Genet Cytogenet* **29**:298, 1987.

72. Bomme L, Bardi G, Pandis N, Fenger C, Kronborg O, Heim S: Clonal karyotypic abnormalities in colorectal adenomas: Clues to the early genetic events in the adenoma-carcinoma sequence. *Genes Chromosomes Cancer* **10**:190, 1994.

73. Berger CS, Sandberg AA, Todd IAD, et al.: Chromosome in kidney, ureter, and bladder cancer. *Cancer Genet Cytogenet* **23**:1, 1986.

74. Kovacs G, Szucs S, De Reise W, Baumbartel H: Specific chromosome aberration in human renal cell carcinoma. *Int J Cancer* **40**:171, 1987.

75. Pathak S, Strong LC, Ferrell RE, Trindade A: Familial renal cell carcinoma with a 3;11 chromosome translocation limited to tumor cells. *Science* **217**:939, 1982.

76. Yoshida MA, Ohyashiki K, Ochi H, et al.: Rearrangement of chromosome 3 in renal cell carcinoma. *Cancer Genet Cytogenet* **19**:351, 1986.

77. Henn W, Zwergel T, Wullich B, Thonnes M, Zang KD, Seitz G: Bilateral multicentric papillary renal tumors with heteroclonal origin based on tissue-specific karyotype instability. *Cancer* **72**:1315, 1993.

78. Rey JA, Bello MJ, de Campos JM, Kusak ME, Moreno S, Benitez J: Deletion 3p in two lung adenocarcinomas metastatic to the brain. *Cancer Genet Cytogenet* **25**:355, 1987.

79. Levin NA, Brzoska P, Gupta N, Gray JW, Christman MF: Identification of frequent novel genetic alterations in small cell lung carcinoma. *Cancer Res* **54**:5086, 1994.

80. Hosoe S, Ueno K, Shigedo Y, et al.: A frequent deletion of chromosome 5q21 in advanced small cell and non-small cell carcinoma of the lung. *Cancer Res* **54**:1787, 1994.

81. Johansson M, Karauzum SB, Dietrich C, et al.: Karyotypic abnormalities in adenocarcinomas of the lung. *Int J Oncol* **5**:17, 1994.

82. Siegfried JM, Hunt JD, Zhou J-Y, Keller SM, Testa JR: Cytogenetic abnormalities in non-small cell lung carcinoma: Similarity of findings in conventional and feeder cell layer cultures. *Genes Chromosomes Cancer* **6**:30, 1993.

83. Siegfried JM, Ellison DJ, Resau JH, Miura I, Testa JR: Correlation of modal chromosome number of cultured non-small cell lung carcinomas with DNA index of solid tumor tissue. *Cancer Res* **51**:3267, 1991.

84. Thompson FH, Emerson J, Olson S, et al.: Cytogenetics in 158 patients with regional or disseminated melanoma: Subset analysis of near diploid and simple karyotypes. *Cancer Genet Cytogenet* **83**:93, 1995.

85. Morse HG, Moore GE, Ortiz LM, Gonzalez R, Robinson WA: Malignant melanoma: From subcutaneous nodule to brain metastasis. *Cancer Genet Cytogenet* **72**:16, 1994.

86. Morse HG, Moore GE: Cytogenetic homogeneity in eight independent sites in a case of malignant melanoma. *Cancer Genet Cytogenet* **69**:108, 1993.

87. Parmiter AH, Nowell PC: Cytogenetics of melanocytic tumors. *J Invest Dermatol* **100**:254S, 1993.

88. Grammatico P, Catricala C, Potenza C, et al.: Cytogenetic findings in 20 melanomas. *Melanoma Res* **3**:169, 1993.

89. Ozisik YY, Meloni AM, Altungoz O, et al.: Cytogenetic findings in 21 malignant melanomas. *Cancer Genet Cytogenet* **77**:69, 1994.

90. Trent JM, Thompson FH, Meyskens FL: Identification of a recurring translocation site involving chromosome 6 in human malignant melanoma. *Cancer Res* **49**:420, 1989.

91. Guan X-Y, Cao J, Meltzer PS, Trent J: Rapid generation of region-specific genomic clones by chromosome microdissection: Isolation of DNA from a region frequently deleted in malignant melanoma. *Genomics* **14**:680, 1992.

92. Meltzer PS, Guan X-Y, Trent JM: Telomere capture stabilizes chromosome breakage. *Nat Genet* **4**:252, 1993.

93. Millikin D, Meese E, Vogelstein B, Trent J: Loss of heterozygosity for loci on the long arm of chromosome 6 in human malignant melanoma. *Cancer Res* **51**:5449, 1991.

94. Trent JM, Stanbridge EJ, McBride HL, et al.: Tumorigenicity in human melanoma cell lines controlled by introduction of human chromosome 6. *Science* **247**:568, 1990.

95. Su YA, Ray ME, Lin T, Seidel NE, Bodine DM, Meltzer PS, Trent JM: Reversion of Monochromosome-mediated suppression of tumorigenicity in malignant melanoma by retroviral transduction. *Cancer Res* **56**:3186, 1996.

96. Goldstein AM, Dracopoli NC, Ho EC, et al.: Further evidence for a locus for cutaneous malignant melanoma-dysplastic nevus (CMM/ DN) on chromosome 1p, and evidence for genetic heterogeneity. *Am J Hum Genet* **52**:537, 1993.

97. Cannon-Albright LA, Goldgar DE, Meyer LJ, et al.: Assignment of a locus for familial melanoma, MLM, to chromosome 9p13-p22. *Science* **258**:1148, 1992.

98. Kamb A, Gruis NA, Weaver-Feldhaus J, et al.: A cell-cycle regulator potentially involved in genesis of many tumor types. *Science* **264**:436, 1994.

99. Goldstein AM, Dracopoli NC, Engelstein M, Fraser MC, Clark WH Jr, Tucker MA: Linkage of cutaneous malignant melanoma/dysplastic nevi to chromosome 9p, and evidence for genetic heterogeneity. *Am J Hum Genet* **54**:489, 1994.

100. Morse HG, Gonzalez R, Moore GE, Robinson WA: Preferential chromosome 11q and/or 17q aberrations in short-term cultures of metastatic melanoma in resections from human brain. *Cancer Genet Cytogenet* **64**:118, 1992.

101. Parmiter AH, Balaban G, Herlyn M, Clark WH, Nowell PC: A t(1;19) chromosome translocation in three cases of human malignant melanoma. *Cancer Res* **46**:1526, 1986.

102. Zhang J, Trent JM, Meltzer PS: Rapid isolation and characterization of amplified DNA by chromosome microdissection: Identification of IGF1R amplification in malignant melanoma. *Oncogene* **8**:2827, 1993.

103. Wake N, Hreshchyshyn MM, Piver SM, Matsui S, Sandberg AA: Specific cytogenetic changes in ovarian cancer involving chromosomes 6 and 14. *Cancer Res* **40**:4512, 1980.

104. Trent JM: Prevalence and Clinical Significance of Cytogenetic Abnormalities in Human Ovarian Cancer. Boston, MA, Nijhoff, 1985.

105. Lee JH, Kavanagh JJ, Wildrick DM, Wharton JT, Blick M: Frequent loss of heterozygosity on chromosome 6q, 11, and 17 in human ovarian carcinomas. *Cancer Res* **50**:2724, 1990.

106. Thompson FH, Emerson J, Alberts D, et al.: Clonal chromosome abnormalities in 54 cases of ovarian carcinoma. *Cancer Genet Cytogenet* **73**:33, 1994.

107. Taetle R, Aickin M, Panda L, Emerson J, Roe D, Thompson F, Davis J, Trent J, Alberts D: Chromosome abnormalities in ovarian adenocarcinoma I. Non-random chromosome abnormalities from 244 cases. *Genes Chromosomes Cancer* (**25**:46, 1999.

108. Guan X-Y, Alberts D, Burgess AC, Thompson FH, Trent JM: Chromosomal analysis of 90 cases of ovarian carcinomas [Abstract]. *Cancer Genet Cytogenet* **41**:291, 1989.

109. Filmus J, Trent JM, Pullano R, Buick RN: A cell line from a human ovarian carcinoma with amplification of the K-ras gene. *Cancer Res* **46**:5179, 1986.

110. Guan X-Y, Cargile CB, Anzick SL, et al.: Chromosome microdissection identifies cryptic sites of DNA sequence amplification in human ovarian carcinoma. *Cancer Res* 1995(**55**:3380, 1999.

111. Sasano H, Garrett CT, Wilkinson DS, Silverberg S, Comerford J, Hyde J: Proto-oncogene amplification in human ovarian neoplasms. *Hum Pathol* **21**:382, 1990.

112. Gibas Z, Prout GR, Pontes JE, Sandberg AA: Chromosome changes in germ cell tumors of the testis. *Cancer Genet Cytogenet* **19**:245, 1986.

113. Oosterhuis JW, de Jong B, Cornelisse CJ, et al.: Karyotyping and DNA flow cytometry of mature residual teratoma after intensive chemotherapy of disseminated nonseminomatous germ cell tumor of the testis: A report of two cases. *Cancer Genet Cytogenet* **22**:149, 1986.

114. Speicher MR, Jauch A, Walt H, et al.: Correlation of microscopic phenotype with genotype in a formalin-fixed, paraffin-embedded testicular germ cell tumor with universal DNA amplification, comparative genomic hybridization, and interphase cytogenetics. *Am J Pathol* **146**:1332, 1995.

115. Bosl GJ, Dmitrovsky E, Reuter VE, et al.: Isochromosome of chromosome 12: Clinically useful marker for male germ cell tumors. *J Natl Cancer Inst* **81**:1874, 1989.

116. Bani MR, Rak J, Adachi D, Wiltshire R, Trent JM, Kerbel RS, Ben-David Y: Multiple features of advanced melanoma recapitulated in tumorigenic variants of early stage (radial growth phase) human melanoma cell lines: Evidence for a dominant phenotype. *J Can Res* **56**:3075, 1996.

117. Guan X-Y, Zhang H, Bittner ML, Jiang Y, Meltzer PS, Trent JM: Rapid generation of human chromosome arm painting probes (CAPs) by chromosome microdissection. *Nat Genet* **12**:10, 1996.

118. Guan, X-Y, Meltzer PS, Dalton WS, Trent JM: Identification of cryptic sites of DNA sequence amplification in human breast cancer by chromosome microdissection. *Nat Genet* **8**:155, 1994.

119. Zhang J, Cui P, Glatfelter AA, Cummings LM, Meltzer PS, Trent JM: Microdissection based cloning of a translocation breakpoint in a human malignant melanoma. *Cancer Res* **55**:4640, 1995.

120. Clark J, Rocques PJ, Crew AJ, Gill S, Shipley J, Chan AM, Gusterson BA, Cooper CS: Identification of novel genes, SYT and SSX, involved in the t(X;18)(p11.2;q11.2) translocation found in human synovial sarcoma. *Nat Genet* **7**:502, 1994.

121. Shapiro DN, Sublett JE, Li B, Downing JR, Naeve CW: Fusion of PAX3 to a member of the forkhead family of transcription factors in human alveolar rhabdomyosarcoma. *Cancer Res* **53**:5108, 1993.

122. Barr FG, Galili N, Holick J, Biegel JA, Rovera G, Emanuel BS: Rearrangement of the PAX3 paired box gene in the paediatric solid tumour alveolar rhabdomyosarcoma. *Nat Genet* **3**:113, 1993.

123. Horowitz ME, Malaner MM, Woo SY, Hicks MJ: Ewing's Sarcoma family of tumors, in Pizzo PA, Poplack DG (eds): *Principles and Practice of Pediatric Oncology*. Philadelphia, JB Lippincott, 1997, 831.

124. Turc-Carel C, Philip I, Berger MP, Philip T, Lenoir GM: Chromosome study of Ewing's sarcoma (ES) cell lines. Consistency of a reciprocal translocation t(11;22)(q24;q12). *Cancer Genet Cytogenet* **12**:1, 1984.

125. Turc-Carel C, Aurias A, Mugneret F, Lizard S, Sidaner I, Volk C, Thiery JP, Olschwang S, Philip I, Berger MP, et al.: Chromosomes in Ewing's sarcoma. I. An evaluation of 85 cases of remarkable consistency of t(11;22)(q24;q12). *Cancer Genet Cytogenet* **32**:229, 1988.

126. Delattre O, Zucman J, Plougastel B, Desmaze C, Melot T, Peter M, Kovar H, Joubert I, de Jong P, Rouleau G, et al.: Gene fusion with an ETS DNA-binding domain caused by chromosome translocation in human tumours. *Nature* **359**:162, 1992.

127. Zucman J, Melot T, Desmaze C, Ghysdael J, Plougastel B, Peter M, Zucker JM, Triche TJ, Sheer D, Turc CC, et al.: Combinatorial generation of variable fusion proteins in the Ewing family of tumours. *Embo J* **12**:4481, 1993.

128. Ben-David Y, Giddens EB, Letwin K, Bernstein A: Erythroleukemia induction by Friend murine leukemia virus: Insertional activation of a new member of the ets gene family, Fli-1, closely linked to c-ets-1. *Genes Dev* **5**:908, 1991.

129. Seth A, Ascione R, Fisher RJ, Mavrothalassitis GJ, Bhat NK, Papas TS: The ets gene family. *Cell Growth Diff* **3**:327, 1992.

130. Watson DK, McWilliams-Smith MJ, Nunn MF, Duesberg PH, O'Brien SJ, Papas TS: The ets sequence from the transforming gene of avian erythroblastosis virus, E26, has unique domains on human chromosomes 11 and 21: both loci are transcriptionally active. *Proc Nat Acad Sci U S A* **82**:7294, 1985.

131. Plougastel B, Zucman J, Peter M, Thomas G, Delattre O: Genomic structure of the EWS gene and its relationship to EWSR1, a site of tumor-associated chromosome translocation. *Genomics* **18**:609, 1993.

132. Ohno T, Rao VN, Reddy ES: EWS/Fli-1 chimeric protein is a transcriptional activator. *Cancer Res* **53**:5859, 1993.

133. Rao VN, Ohno T, Prasad DD, Bhattacharya G, Reddy ES: Analysis of the DNA-binding and transcriptional activation functions of human Fli-1 protein. *Oncogene* **8**:2167, 1993.

134. Mao X, Miesfeldt S, Yang H, Leiden JM, Thompson CB: The FLI-1 and chimeric EWS-FLI-1 oncoproteins display similar DNA binding specificities. *J Biol Chem* **269**:18216, 1994.

135. Lessnick SL, Braun BS, Denny CT, May WA: Multiple domains mediate transformation by the Ewing's sarcoma EWS/FLI-1 fusion gene. *Oncogene* **10**:423, 1995.

136. Bailly RA, Bosselut R, Zucman J, Cormier F, Delattre O, Roussel M, Thomas G, Ghysdael J: DNA-binding and transcriptional activation properties of the EWS-FLI-1 fusion protein resulting from the t(11;22) translocation in Ewing sarcoma. *Mol Cell Biol* **14**:3230, 1994.

137. Magnaghi-Jaulin L, Masutani H, Robin P, Lipinski M, Harel-Bellan A: SRE elements are binding sites for the fusion protein EWS-FLI-1. *Nucleic Acids Res* **24**:1052, 1996.

138. Braun BS, Frieden R, Lessnick SL, May WA, Denny CT: Identification of target genes for the Ewing's sarcoma EWS/FLI fusion protein by representational difference analysis. *Mol Cell Biol* **15**:4623, 1995.

139. Zinszner H, Albalat R, Ron D: A novel effector domain from the RNA-binding protein TLS or EWS is required for oncogenic transformation by CHOP. *Genes Dev* **8**:2513, 1994.

140. Sorensen PH, Lessnick SL, Lopez-Terrada D, Liu XF, Triche TJ, Denny CT: A second Ewing's sarcoma translocation, t(21;22), fuses the EWS gene to another ETS-family transcription factor, ERG. *Nat Genet* **6**:146, 1994.

141. Jeon IS, Davis JN, Braun BS, Sublett JE, Roussel MF, Denny CT, Shapiro DN: A variant Ewing's sarcoma translocation (7;22) fuses the EWS gene to the ETS gene ETV1. *Oncogene* **10**:1229, 1995.

142. Urano F, Umezawa A, Hong W, Kikuchi H, Hata J: A novel chimera gene between EWS and E1A-F, encoding the adenovirus E1A enhancer-binding protein, in extraosseous Ewing's sarcoma. *Biochem Biophys Res Commun* **219**:608, 1996.

143. Stephenson CF, Bridge JA, Sandberg AA: Cytogenetic and pathologic aspects of Ewing's sarcoma and neuroectodermal tumors. *Hum Pathol* **23**:1270, 1992.

144. Giovannini M, Biegel JA, Serra M, Wang JY, Wei YH, Nycum L, Emanuel BS, Evans GA: EWS-erg and EWS-Fli1 fusion transcripts in Ewing's sarcoma and primitive neuroectodermal tumors with variant translocations. *J Clin Invest* **94**:489, 1994.

145. Delattre O, Zucman J, Melot T, Garau XS, Zucker JM, Lenoir GM, Ambros PF, Sheer D, Turc-Carel C, Triche TJ, et al.: The Ewing family of tumors — A subgroup of small-round-cell tumors defined by specific chimeric transcripts. *N Engl J Med* **331**:294, 1994.

146. Desmaze C, Zucman J, Delattre O, Melot T, Thomas G, Aurias A: Interphase molecular cytogenetics of Ewing's sarcoma and peripheral neuroepithelioma t(11;22) with flanking and overlapping cosmid probes. *Cancer Genet Cytogenet* **74**:13, 1994.

147. Selleri L, Giovannini M, Romo A, Zucman J, Delattre O, Thomas G, Evans GA: Cloning of the entire FLI1 gene, disrupted by the Ewing's sarcoma translocation breakpoint on 11q24, in a yeast artificial chromosome. *Cytogenet Cell Genet* **67**:129, 1994.

148. Sorensen PH, Liu XF, Delattre O, Rowland JM, Biggs CA, Thomas G, Triche TJ: Reverse transcriptase PCR amplification of EWS/FLI-1 fusion transcripts as a diagnostic test for peripheral primitive neuroectodermal tumors of childhood. *Diagn Mol Pathol* **2**:147, 1993.

149. Ladanyi M, Lewis R, Garin-Chesa P, Rettig WJ, Huvos AG, Healey JH, Jhanwar SC: EWS rearrangement in Ewing's sarcoma and peripheral neuroectodermal tumor. Molecular detection and correlation with cytogenetic analysis and MIC2 expression. *Diagn Mol Pathol* **2**:141, 1993.

150. Ida K, Kobayashi S, Taki T, Hanada R, Bessho F, Yamamori S, Sugimoto T, Ohki M, Hayashi Y: EWS-FLI-1 and EWS-ERG chimeric mRNAs in Ewing's sarcoma and primitive neuroectodermal tumor. *Int J Cancer* **63**:500, 1995.

151. Scotlandi K, Serra M, Manara MC, Benini S, Sarti M, Maurici D, Lollini PL, Picci P, Bertoni F, Baldini N: Immunostaining of the p30/32MIC2 antigen and molecular detection of EWS rearrangements for the diagnosis of Ewing's sarcoma and peripheral neuroectodermal tumor. *Hum Pathol* **27**:408, 1996.

152. Downing JR, Head DR, Parham DM, Douglass EC, Hulshof MG, Link MP, Motroni TA, Grier HE, Curcio BA, Shapiro DN: Detection of the (11;22)(q24;q12) translocation of Ewing's sarcoma and peripheral neuroectodermal tumor by reverse transcription polymerase chain reaction. *Am J Pathol* **143**:1294, 1993.

153. Sorensen PH, Shimada H, Liu XF, Lim JF, Thomas G, Triche TJ: Biphenotypic sarcomas with myogenic and neural differentiation express the Ewing's sarcoma EWS/FLI1 fusion gene. *Cancer Res* **55**:1385, 1995.

154. Ouchida M, Ohno T, Fujimura Y, Rao VN, Reddy ES: Loss of tumorigenicity of Ewing's sarcoma cells expressing antisense RNA to EWS-fusion transcripts. *Oncogene* **11**:1049, 1995.

155. Zoubek A, Pfleiderer C, Salzer-Kuntschik M, Amann G, Windhager R, Fink FM, Koscielniak E, Delattre O, Strehl S, Ambros PF, et al.: Variability of EWS chimaeric transcripts in Ewing tumours: A comparison of clinical and molecular data. *Br J Cancer* **70**:908, 1994.

156. Zoubek A, Dockhorn-Dworniczak B, Delattre O, Christiansen H, Niggli F, Gatterer-Menz I, Smith TL, Jurgens H, Gadner H, Kovar H: Does expression of different EWS chimeric transcripts define clinically distinct risk groups of Ewing tumor patients? *J Clin Oncol* **14**:1245, 1996.

157. de Alava E, Kawai A, Healey JH, Fligman I, Meyers PA, Huvos AG, Gerald WL, Jhanwar SC, Argani P, Antonescu CR, et al.: EWS-FLI1 fusion transcript structure is an independent determinant of prognosis in Ewing's sarcoma. *J Clin Oncol* **16**:2895, 1998.

158. Stenman G, Kindblom LG, Angervall L: Reciprocal translocation t(12;22)(q13;q13) in clear-cell sarcoma of tendons and aponeuroses. *Genes Chromosomes Cancer* **4**:122, 1992.

159. Mrozek K, Karakousis CP, Perez MC, Bloomfield CD: Translocation t(12;22)(q13;q12.2–12.3) in a clear cell sarcoma of tendons and aponeuroses. *Genes Chromosomes Cancer* **6**:249, 1993.

160. Zucman J, Delattre O, Desmaze C, Epstein AL, Stenman G, Speleman F, Fletchers CD, Aurias A, Thomas G: EWS and ATF-1 gene fusion induced by t(12;22) translocation in malignant melanoma of soft parts. *Nat Genet* **4**:341, 1993.

161. Fujimura Y, Ohno T, Siddique H, Lee L, Rao VN, Reddy ES: The EWS-ATF-1 gene involved in malignant melanoma of soft parts with t(12;22) chromosome translocation, encodes a constitutive transcriptional activator. *Oncogene* **12**:159, 1996.

162. Vallejo M, Ron D, Miller CP, Habener JF: C/ATF, a member of the activating transcription factor family of DNA-binding proteins, dimerizes with CAAT/enhancer-binding proteins and directs their binding to cAMP response elements. *Proc Natl Acad Sci U S A* **90**:4679, 1993.

163. Brown AD, Lopez-Terrada D, Denny C, Lee KA: Promoters containing ATF-binding sites are de-regulated in cells that express the EWS/ATF1 oncogene. *Oncogene* **10**:1749, 1995.

164. Rodriguez E, Sreekantaiah C, Gerald W, Reuter VE, Motzer RJ, Chaganti RS: A recurring translocation, t(11;22)(p13;q11.2), characterizes intra-abdominal desmoplastic small round-cell tumors. *Cancer Genet Cytogenet* **69**:17, 1993.

165. Biegel JA, Conard K, Brooks JJ: Translocation (11;22)(p13;q12): Primary change in intra-abdominal desmoplastic small round cell tumor. *Genes Chromosomes Cancer* **7**:119, 1993.

166. Wills EJ: Peritoneal desmoplastic small round cell tumors with divergent differentiation: A review. *Ultrastruct Pathol* **17**:295, 1993.

167. Parkash V, Gerald WL, Parma A, Miettinen M, Rosai J: Desmoplastic small round cell tumor of the pleura. *Am J Surg Pathol* **19**:659, 1995.

168. Ladanyi M, Gerald W: Fusion of the EWS and WT1 genes in the desmoplastic small round cell tumor. *Cancer Res* **54**:2837, 1994.

169. Brodie SG, Stocker SJ, Wardlaw JC, Duncan MH, McConnell TS, Feddersen RM, Williams TM: EWS and WT-1 gene fusion in desmoplastic small round cell tumor of the abdomen. *Hum Pathol* **26**:1370, 1995.

170. Gerald WL, Rosai J, Ladanyi M: Characterization of the genomic breakpoint and chimeric transcripts in the EWS-WT1 gene fusion of desmoplastic small round cell tumor. *Proc Natl Acad Sci U S A* **92**:1028, 1995.

171. de Alava E, Ladanyi M, Rosai J, Gerald WL: Detection of chimeric transcripts in desmoplastic small round cell tumor and related developmental tumors by reverse transcriptase polymerase chain reaction. A specific diagnostic assay. *Am J Pathol* **147**:1584, 1995.

172. Call KM, Glaser T, Ito CY, Buckler AJ, Pelletier J, Haber DA, Rose EA, Kral A, Yeger H, Lewis WH, Jones C, Housman DE: Isolation and characterization of a zinc finger polypeptide gene at the human chromosome 11 Wilms' tumor locus. *Cell* **60**:509, 1990.

173. Clark J, Benjamin H, Gill S, Sidhar S, Goodwin G, Crew J, Gusterson BA, Shipley J, Cooper CS: Fusion of the EWS gene to CHN, a member of the steroid/thyroid receptor gene superfamily, in a human myxoid chondrosarcoma. *Oncogene* **12**:229, 1996.

174. Gill S, McManus AP, Crew AJ, Benjamin H, Sheer D, Gusterson BA, Pinkerton CR, Patel K, Cooper CS, Shipley JM: Fusion of the EWS gene to a DNA segment from 9q22–31 in a human myxoid chondrosarcoma. *Genes Chromosomes Cancer* **12**:307, 1995.

175. Limon J, Turc-Carel C, Dal Cin P, Rao U, Sandberg AA: Recurrent chromosome translocations in liposarcoma. *Cancer Genet Cytogenet* **22**:93, 1986.

176. Aman P, Ron D, Mandahl N, Fioretos T, Heim S, Arheden K, Willen H, Rydholm A, Mitelman F: Rearrangement of the transcription factor gene CHOP in myxoid liposarcomas with t(12;16)(q13;p11). *Genes Chromosom Cancer* **5**:278, 1992.

177. Crozat A, Aman P, Mandahl N, Ron D: Fusion of CHOP to a novel RNA-binding protein in human myxoid liposarcoma. *Nature* **363**:640, 1993.

178. Rabbitts TH, Forster A, Larson R, Nathan P: Fusion of the dominant negative transcription regulator CHOP with a novel gene FUS by translocation t(12;16) in malignant liposarcoma. *Nat Genet* **4**:175, 1993.

179. Ron D, Habener JF: CHOP, a novel developmentally regulated nuclear protein that dimerizes with transcription factors C/EBP and LAP and functions as a dominant-negative inhibitor of gene transcription. *Genes Dev* **6**:439, 1992.

180. Batchvarova N, Wang XZ, Ron D: Inhibition of adipogenesis by the stress-induced protein CHOP (Gadd153). *Embo J* **14**:4654, 1995.

181. Ubeda M, Wang XZ, Zinszner H, Wu I, Habener JF, Ron D: Stress-induced binding of the transcriptional factor CHOP to a novel DNA control element. *Mol Cell Biol* **16**:1479, 1996.

182. Wang XZ, Ron D: Stress-induced phosphorylation and activation of the transcription factor CHOP (GADD153) by p38 MAP Kinase. *Science* **272**:1347, 1996.

183. Barone MV, Crozat A, Tabaee A, Philipson L, Ron D: CHOP (GADD153) and its oncogenic variant, TLS-CHOP, have opposing effects on the induction of G1/S arrest. *Genes Dev* **8**:453, 1994.

184. Panagopoulos I, Hoglund M, Mertens F, Mandahl N, Mitelman F, Aman P: Fusion of the EWS and CHOP genes in myxoid liposarcoma. *Oncogene* **12**:489, 1996.

185. Komuro H, Hayashi Y, Kawamura M, Hayashi K, Kaneko Y, Kamoshita S, Hanada R, Yamamoto K, Hongo T, Yamada M, et al.: Mutations of the p53 gene are involved in Ewing's sarcomas but not in neuroblastomas. *Cancer Res* **53**:5284, 1993.

186. Hamelin R, Zucman J, Melot T, Delattre O, Thomas G: p53 mutations in human tumors with chimeric EWS/FLI-1 genes. *Int J Cancer* **57**:336, 1994.

187. Sreekantaiah C, Leong SP, Karakousis CP, McGee DL, Rappaport WD, Villar HV, Neal D, Fleming S, Wankel A, Herrington PN, et al.: Cytogenetic profile of 109 lipomas. *Cancer Res* **51**:422, 1991.

188. Mrozek K, Karakousis CP, Bloomfield CD: Chromosome 12 breakpoints are cytogenetically different in benign and malignant lipogenic tumors: localization of breakpoints in lipoma to 12q15 and in myxoid liposarcoma to 12q13.3. *Cancer Res* **53**:1670, 1993.

189. Heim S, Mandahl N, Kristoffersson U, Mitelman F, Rooser B, Rydholm A, Willen H: Reciprocal translocation t(3;12)(q27;q13) in lipoma. *Cancer Genet Cytogenet* **23**:301, 1986.

190. Sreekantaiah C, Sandberg AA: Clustering of aberrations to specific chromosome regions in benign neoplasms. *Int J Cancer* **48**:194, 1991.

191. Kazmierczak B, Rosigkeit J, Wanschura S, Meyer-Bolte K, Van de Ven WJ, Kayser K, Krieghoff B, Kastendiek H, Bartnitzke S, Bullerdiek J: HMGI-C rearrangements as the molecular basis for the majority of pulmonary chondroid hamartomas: a survey of 30 tumors. *Oncogene* **12**:515, 1996.

192. Wanschura S, Kazmierczak B, Pohnke Y, Meyer-Bolte K, Bartnitzke S, Van de Ven WJ, Bullerdiek J: Transcriptional activation of HMGI-C in three pulmonary hamartomas each with a der(14)t(12;14) as the sole cytogenetic abnormality. *Cancer Lett* **102**:17, 1996.

193. Ashar HR, Fejzo MS, Tkachenko A, Zhou X, Fletcher JA, Weremowicz S, Morton CC, Chada K: Disruption of the architectural factor HMGI-C: DNA-binding AT hook motifs fused in lipomas to distinct transcriptional regulatory domains. *Cell* **82**:57, 1995.

194. Schoenmakers EF, Wanschura S, Mols R, Bullerdiek J, Van den Berghe H, Van de Ven WJ: Recurrent rearrangements in the high mobility group protein gene, HMGI-C, in benign mesenchymal tumours. *Nat Genet* **10**:436, 1995.

195. Zhou X, Benson KF, Ashar HR, Chada K: Mutation responsible for the mouse pygmy phenotype in the developmentally regulated factor HMGI-C. *Nature* **376**:771, 1995

196. Chau KY, Patel UA, Lee KL, Lam HY, Crane-Robinson C: The gene for the human architectural transcription factor HMGI-C consists of five exons each coding for a distinct functional element. *Nucleic Acids Res* **23**:4262, 1995.

197. Friedmann M, Holth LT, Zoghbi HY, Reeves R: Organization, inducible-expression and chromosome localization of the human HMG-I(Y) nonhistone protein gene. *Nucleic Acids Res* **21**:4259, 1993.

198. Xiao S, Lux ML, Reeves R, Hidson TJ, Fletcher JA: HMGI(Y) activation by chromosome 6p21 rearrangements in multilineage mesenchymal cells from pulmonary hamartoma. *Am J Pathol* **150**:901, 1997.

199. Gelehrter TD, Collins FS: *Principles of Medical Genetics.* Baltimore, MD, Williams & Wilkins, 1990..

CHAPTER 6

Gene Amplification in Human Cancers: Biological and Clinical Significance

Michael D. Hogarty ■ *Garrett M. Brodeur*

1. Gene amplification is a frequent genetic abnormality in human cancer cells and consists of multiple extra copies of a subchromosomal region of DNA (amplicon). Amplification can be manifested cytogenetically as extrachromosomal double-minute chromosomes (dmins) or as chromosomally integrated homogeneously staining regions (HSRs).

2. Several mechanisms have been proposed to explain the development of gene amplification. These have been based primarily on *in vitro* systems in which there is selection for drug resistance, so the mechanisms involved in *de novo* oncogene amplification may be different. Nevertheless, for gene amplification to occur, it may be necessary to have loss of cell cycle control, DNA damage or instability, and a stimulus to progress through the cell cycle.

3. The size of the amplicon can vary from several hundred to several thousand kilobases. The amplified DNA appears to be in a head-to-tail conformation, and the germ line configuration is largely retained, with relatively few genetic rearrangements. In most cases, only a single expressed gene is consistently amplified, but in other cases, two or more genes from a given chromosomal region may confer a selective advantage, either individually or in concert.

4. Amplification of the *MYCN* oncogene occurs in 20 to 25 percent of all neuroblastomas. *MYCN* amplification is strongly associated with advanced stages of disease and a poor outcome. Currently, the presence of *MYCN* amplification is used to identify patients at high risk who need the most intensive treatment.

5. Amplification of several different genetic regions, especially 11q13 or 12q14, is found in many common types of cancer, including carcinomas of the breast, ovary, lung, head and neck, and gastrointestinal tract. The clinical significance of these findings is somewhat controversial, but in some patients, gene amplification may be associated with a more aggressive tumor behavior and a worse outcome.

6. The most common types of genes amplified are oncogenes and drug-resistance genes. Oncogenes, however, account for the vast majority of genes amplified in human cancers. The most common oncogenes amplified are members of the *MYC* family, the *RAS* family, the *EGFR* family, the *FGF* family, and genes involved in cell cycle regulation (*CCND1, CCNE, MDM2, CDK4*).

7. The mechanisms whereby oncogene amplification confers a selective advantage vary depending on the gene, but include overexpression of (a) a transcription factor (*MYC* family) favoring continued proliferation; (b) a signal transduction molecule (*RAS* family), growth factor, or receptor (*EGFR, FGF* families), that mimicks constitutive growth factor stimulation; or (c) cell-cycle regulatory genes (*CCND1,* *CCNE, MDM2, CDK4*) that lead to loss of cell-cycle control.

8. There are several methods of detecting gene amplification that vary in their difficulty or the need to know the gene (or genes) likely to be amplified. These methods include (a) conventional cytogenetics; (b) Southern blotting; (c) quantitative PCR; (d) fluorescence *in situ* hybridization (FISH); (e) comparative genomic hybridization (CGH); and (f) microarray technology.

INTRODUCTION

Cytogenetically visible rearrangements in human cancer cells fall into three general categories: (a) deletions with a net loss of genetic material; (b) translocations with transposition of genetic material, but no net loss or gain; and (c) gene amplification with a net gain of a specific chromosomal region. Deletions are thought to represent loss of a suppressor gene, whereas translocations and gene amplification generally represent activation of a proto-oncogene. Translocations could result in inactivation of a suppressor gene, but this appears to be a rare event. Gene amplification also can involve drug-resistance genes or other genes that confer a selective advantage when overexpressed. For the purposes of this chapter, gene amplification refers to an increase in copy number (more than six copies per diploid genome) of a specific, subchromosomal region (generally 1 to 2 mb or less). It is not used to refer to numerical gain (generally three to four copies per diploid genome) of whole chromosomes, chromosome arms, or very large chromosomal regions.

Gene amplification usually is apparent cytogenetically, either as extrachromosomal double-minute chromatin bodies, or as chromosomally integrated, homogeneously staining regions. If the copy number is low (e.g., 5 to 10 copies per cell), if the size of the amplified unit (amplicon) is small, or if the karyotype is extremely complex, gene amplification may not be evident by conventional cytogenetics. However, several different molecular approaches have been developed that allow reliable detection of gene amplification in interphase nuclei or from small amounts of tumor DNA (see below). In general, the latter techniques presuppose that the gene (or genes) that might be amplified is known.

Gene amplification almost always results in the overexpression of one or more genes contained in the amplicon. Usually there is a single gene that appears to be the "target" of the gene amplification, but some amplified units may contain two or more genes that could theoretically confer a selective advantage. Furthermore, in some cancers, two or more discrete regions may be amplified. However, in the majority of cases, only a single genetic region is amplified in a given tumor.

Theoretically, the amplification and consequent overexpression of a number of genes could confer a selective advantage on a cancer cell. In practice, the majority of examples that have been studied involve oncogenes or drug-resistance genes. This chapter concentrates on genes that are amplified in a substantial percentage (at least 10 percent) of primary tumors that have been extensively studied (at least 50 cases examined). We discuss *MYCN* amplification in neuroblastomas in detail to illustrate certain points, because it is the most consistent and most extensively studied example of oncogene amplification in a human tumor. However, amplification of the regions 11q13 and 12q14 are also discussed. For the sake of completeness, we discuss amplification of drug-resistance genes in human cancers, but they do not fulfill the criteria for inclusion discussed above.

AMPLIFICATION OF DRUG-RESISTANCE GENES

Culturing mammalian cells under conditions of incrementally increasing concentrations of a cytotoxic drug can lead to amplification of the gene encoding the protein which is the target of that drug.[1] This has suggested the possibility that human cancer cells may become resistant to chemotherapy by amplifying certain genes,[2] such as the dihydrofolate reductase (*DHFR*) gene in methotrexate-resistance, or the multidrug-resistance genes (*MDR1, MRP*) in tumors simultaneously resistant to multiple unrelated chemotherapeutic agents.[3-6] Indeed, there are several reports of human tumor cells that amplified the *DHFR* gene and became resistant to methotrexate.[7-10] However, this occurred in only a few cases, and only after prolonged clinical treatment, so the frequency with which it occurs does not meet our criteria for inclusion in this review. Furthermore, no reports of *MDR1* or *MRP* amplification have been reported in human tumors *in vivo*.[11] Thus, gene amplification appears to be a fairly rare mechanism for the development of drug resistance in humans.

AMPLIFICATION OF ONCOGENES

There are an increasing number of reports of human tumors and cell lines demonstrating amplification of proto-oncogenes. A cataloging of every reported tumor or cell line that has been shown to amplify an oncogene or related genes is beyond the scope of this chapter. Rather, we focus on examples of gene amplification in primary tumors that occur with substantial prevalence (more than 10 percent). The inclusion of cell-line studies would bias these data, because established cell lines in many systems show a higher prevalence of gene amplification than their primary tumor counterparts. For instance, amplification of *MYCN* and *ERBB1* (*EGFR*) are found in ~80 percent of cell lines established from neuroblastomas and head and neck squamous cell carcinomas respectively, whereas they are amplified in ~25 percent and in 10 percent of primary tumor specimens.[12-14]

Many different malignancies have been demonstrated to amplify a variety of oncogenes. These include neuroblastoma, breast and ovarian carcinoma, small cell lung carcinoma (SCLC), and head and neck squamous-cell carcinoma (HNSCC). In these malignancies, the prevalence of gene amplification ranges from 20 to 50 percent (see Table 6-1), often with amplification correlating with an aggressive phenotype (such as with advanced stage or decreased overall survival). In additional malignancies, such as sarcomas, hepatocellular carcinomas, malignant gliomas, and cervical, endometrial, and gastrointestinal cancers, data are accumulating that implicate gene amplification in their pathogenesis or progression as well (Table 6-1).

Genes amplified in human cancers are thought to confer a growth advantage to a clone, analogous to amplification *in vitro* of drug-resistance genes under certain selective external pressures. Genes frequently amplified in cancer tissues include members of the *MYC* (*MYC, MYCN, MYCL*) and *RAS* (*HRAS, KRAS, NRAS*) families of proto-oncogenes, growth factor receptors (*ERBB*-1 and -2, *FGFR*-1 and -2, *MET*), and genes that are involved in cell-cycle regulation (*CCND1, CCNE, MDM2, CDK4*), in addition to other miscellaneous genes (*AKT2, MYB*) (Table 6-2).

Activation of oncogenes is a common mechanism of tumorigenesis, and may occur by point mutation, translocation,

Table 6-1 Recurrent Oncogene Amplification in Human Cancers

Tumor Type	Gene Amplified	Frequency (%)	References
Breast cancer	MYC	20	18, 19, 22, 146
	ERBB2 (EGFR2)	20	18, 19, 22
	CCND1 (Cyclin D1)	15–20	19, 21, 22
	FGFR1	12	22, 24, 56
	FGFR2	12	56
Cervical cancer	MYC	25–50	147
	ERBB2	20	148
Colorectal cancer	HRAS	29	69
	KRAS	22	69
	MYB	15–20	70
Esophageal cancer	MYC	38	149
	CCND1 (Cyclin D1)	25	102
	MDM2	13	150
Gastric cancer	CCNE (Cyclin E)	15	21, 66
	KRAS	10	67
	MET	10	68
Glioblastoma	ERBB1 (EGFR)	33–50	151, 152
	CDK4	15	153
Head and neck cancer	CCND1 (Cyclin D1)	50	14, 72
	ERBB1 (EGFR)	10	14
	MYC	7–10	14, 109
Hepatocellular cancer	CCND1 (Cyclin D1)	13	103, 104
Neuroblastoma	MYCN	20–25	12, 13
Ovarian cancer	MYC	20–30	154, 155
	ERBB2 (EGFR2)	15–30	58, 59
	AKT2	12	60
Sarcoma	MDM2	10–30	110, 111, 150
	CDK4	11	109
Small cell lung cancer	MYC	15–20	62, 63

Table 6-2 Oncogenes Amplified in Human Cancers

Gene Amplified	Locus	Tumors
AKT2	19q13.2	Ovarian cancer
CCND1 (Cyclin D1)	11q13.3	HNSCC, esophageal, breast, HCC
CCNE (Cyclin E)	19q12	Gastric cancer
CDK4	12q14	Sarcoma, glioblastoma
ERBB1 (EGFR)	7p12	Glioblastoma, HNSCC
ERBB2 (EGFR2)	17q11.2-q12	Breast, ovarian, cervical cancer
FGFR1	8p11.1-p11.2	Breast cancer
FGFR2	10q25.3-q26	Breast cancer
HRAS	11p15.5	Colorectal cancer
KRAS	12p13	Colorectal, gastric cancer
MDM2	12q14	Soft tissue sarcomas, osteosarcoma, esophageal cancer
MET	7q31	Gastric cancer
MYB	6q23.3-q24	Colorectal cancer
MYC	8q24.12-q24.13	Ovarian, breast, SCLC, HNSCC, esophageal, cervical cancer
MYCN	2p24.3	Neuroblastoma

or amplification. In many of the malignancies studied to date, amplification of an oncogene is strongly associated with advanced stages of disease and with a poor outcome. In neuroblastoma, for example, *MYCN* amplification is associated with rapid disease progression independent of patient age and stage.[15–17] In other malignancies, however, the presence of amplification does not maintain significance as an independent variable for outcome when stage and histology are considered. In breast cancer, many studies have correlated the presence of ERBB2 (HER-2/*neu*) amplification with clinical parameters such as high stage and grade, lymph node involvement, large tumor size, and steroid hormone-receptor absence.[18,19] In multivariate analysis controlling for the above clinical data, the presence of ERBB2 amplification does not always predict a poor outcome. It remains to be determined, in this instance, whether oncogene amplification is a consequence of aggressive, deregulated cell proliferation and the resulting genomic instability, or if it is an early cellular event that is causative of the more aggressive clinical phenotype.

An amplicon may harbor multiple candidate genes and it may be difficult to determine a putative oncogene target among these. In fact, several genes may act in concert to determine the phenotype arising as a consequence of the amplification event. One widely studied region of amplification is the 11q13 region, amplified in breast and other carcinomas. This amplicon may contain *CCND1* (*Cyclin D1*), *FGF3* (*INT2*), *FGF4* (*HST*), *EMS1*, *GARP*, or a subset of these genes. Though investigators have implicated *CCND1* based on amplification prevalence and expression patterns in the amplified tumors,[20,21] it now appears likely that multiple genes from this region may be the targets of amplification events, as no single gene is invariably present on all amplicons.[22] Other examples include the 12q14 amplicon in the region of *MDM2*, *GLI*, *SAS*, *CDK4*, and 8p11 with *FGFR1*, *PLAT*, and others.[23,24] Likewise, it is possible to exploit the presence of amplified domains to discover potential oncogenes. Amplified DNA fragments can be cloned and mapped within the genome. From the amplified domain, new genes may be sought to explain the biologic significance of the amplification, as well as to elucidate their function in normal cells.[20,25] An example is the recently cloned and characterized AIB1 at 20q13, a steroid receptor co-activator which is amplified in ~6 to 10 percent of primary breast cancers.[26]

The prevalence of gene amplification in different tumors, as well as the biologic and clinical significance of amplifying particular genes, is discussed below, with particular emphasis on the role of *MYCN* amplification in neuroblastoma. Tumors that are presented in detail elsewhere in this volume are discussed briefly.

MYCN Amplification in Neuroblastomas

Neuroblastomas are tumors of the peripheral nervous system that are found almost exclusively in children. The peak age at diagnosis is 22 months, and it is rare after 10 years of age. Neuroblastomas often are localized and have a less aggressive behavior in infants, but they are frequently metastatic and have a poor prognosis in older children. The reason for this apparent discrepancy was unclear initially. However, cytogenetic and molecular analysis of these tumors has identified characteristic differences that allow these tumors to be subclassified into three groups that are distinct in terms of biologic features and clinical behavior (see Chap. 50). The feature that characterizes the most aggressive subset of neuroblastomas is amplification of the *MYCN* oncogene.

Cytogenetic examination of neuroblastomas reveals that a substantial number have either dmins, or HSRs, or both in subpopulations of cells. These two abnormalities are cytogenetic manifestations of gene amplification. Dmins are the predominant form of amplified DNA in primary tumors, but dmins and HSRs are found with about equal frequency in neuroblastoma cell lines.[12,13] Indeed, dmins and/or HSRs occur in about 90 percent of neuroblastoma cell lines, but in only 25 percent of primary tumors. Evidence suggests that this represents selection *in vitro* for cell lines derived from tumors that have pre-existing dmins or HSRs, and there is no evidence to date that these abnormalities develop with time in culture, at least in neuroblastomas. It is unclear why HSRs are a more common form of amplified DNA in established cell lines than in primary tumors.

Although cytogenetic analysis of human neuroblastomas frequently has revealed dmins or HSRs in primary tumors and cell lines,[12,13] the nature of the amplified sequences was not known initially. Evidence for amplification of genes associated with drug resistance was sought, but none was found. However, a study was undertaken to determine if a proto-oncogene was amplified in a panel of neuroblastoma cell lines. An oncogene related to the viral oncogene v-*myc*, but distinct from *MYC*, was amplified in the majority of neuroblastoma cell lines tested.[27] The amplified *MYCN* sequence was mapped to the HSRs on different chromosomes in neuroblastoma cell lines, but the normal single-copy locus was mapped to the distal short arm of chromosome 2.[28] Thus, the *MYCN* locus was amplified in neuroblastomas regardless of whether they had dmins or an HSR, and regardless of the chromosomal location of the HSR.

In collaboration with others, we studied primary tumors from untreated patients to determine if *MYCN* amplification occurred. In the initial analysis of 63 primary tumors, amplification ranging from 3- to 300-fold per haploid genome was found in 24 tumors (38 percent).[15] All cases with *MYCN* amplification in this initial study came from patients with advanced stages of disease. The progression-free survival of these patients was analyzed according to the stage of disease and *MYCN* copy number.[17] *MYCN* amplification clearly was associated with rapid tumor progression and a poor outcome, independent of the stage of the tumor.

Table 6-3 Correlation of *MYCN* Copy Number with Stage and Survival in 3,000 Neuroblastomas

Stage at Diagnosis	*MYCN* Amplification	3-yr. Survival (%)
Benign ganglioneuromas	0/64 (0%)	100
Low stages (1, 2)	31/772 (4%)	90
Stage 4-S	15/190 (8%)	80
Advanced stages (3, 4)	612/1974 (31%)	30
TOTAL	658/3000 (22%)	50

These studies have been extended to over 3000 patients with neuroblastoma enrolled in protocols of the Children's Cancer Group (CCG) and the Pediatric Oncology Group (POG) (Table 21-3).[13,16] It is now clear that among patients with less advanced stages of disease, which is traditionally associated with a good prognosis, a minority (5 to 10 percent) have tumors with *MYCN* amplification.[13,16] Our data indicate that virtually all of these patients are destined to have rapid tumor progression and a poor outcome, similar to their counterparts with advanced stages of disease. Over 30 percent of patients with more advanced tumor stages had *MYCN* amplification, and they also had an expectedly poor outcome. Our finding that *MYCN* amplification is associated with poor outcome regardless of the clinical stage of tumor is supported by independent studies from Japan and Europe.[29–35]

We analyzed the *MYCN* copy number in multiple simultaneous or consecutive samples of neuroblastoma tissue from 60 patients[36] to determine whether the presence or absence of *MYCN* was consistent in different tumor samples from a given patient, or if single-copy tumors ever developed amplification at the time of recurrence. Interestingly, we found a consistent pattern of *MYCN* copy number (either amplified or unamplified) in different tumor samples taken from an individual patient, either simultaneously or consecutively.[36] These studies have been extended to over 150 patients with similar results.[37] This suggests that *MYCN* amplification is an intrinsic biologic property of a subset of neuroblastomas. Tumors that develop *MYCN* amplification generally do so by the time of diagnosis, and cases of neuroblastoma with a single copy (per haploid genome) of *MYCN* at diagnosis rarely develop amplification subsequently.

Twenty-five to 30 percent of the children with neuroblastoma have *MYCN* amplification in their tumors, and virtually all of these children have rapidly progressive and fatal disease. However, there is controversy as to whether high levels of *MYCN* expression in single-copy tumors identify a subset with a particularly poor outcome.[38–43] Differences may depend on whether mRNA or protein expression was measured, as well as other details of the population studied or methods of analysis. Thus, it is still possible that activation of *MYCN* by mechanisms other than amplification or overexpression may play an important role. In addition, it is likely that activation of other oncogenes, deletion of specific suppressor genes, or other genetic lesions may contribute to the poor clinical outcome in these patients.

We sought evidence for amplification of other oncogenes, including *MYC, RAS, HRAS, KRAS, EGFR1, EGFR2, SIS, SRC, MYB, FOS,* and *ETS* in neuroblastomas, but found none.[13] However, there are at least six examples of neuroblastoma cell lines or primary tumors that amplify regions that are remote from the *MYCN* locus at 2p24. These include amplification of genes from 2p22 and 2p13 in the IMR-32 cell line,[44] as well as co-amplification of *MYCN* and *MDM2* (from 12q13) in the NGP, TR-14, and LS cell lines.[23,45,46] Finally, there is one report of co-amplification of *MYCN* and *MYCL* in a neuroblastoma cell line,[47] and this has been seen in at least one primary tumor as well (GM Brodeur, unpublished observations, 1988). These findings indicate that more than one locus can be amplified, but no neuroblastoma has been shown to amplify another gene that did not also amplify *MYCN.*

The presence of *MYCN* amplification in human neuroblastomas has been shown to correlate strongly with advanced clinical stage and poor prognosis.[13,15,17,31,38,41–43] Our recent studies[48] showed that 1p LOH is very common in tumors with *MYCN* amplification (p < 0.001).[12,13] Both *MYCN* amplification and deletion of 1p (as detected by cytogenetic or molecular analysis) appear strongly correlated with a poor clinical outcome and with each other, but it is not yet clear if they are independent prognostic variables.[49–55] Nevertheless, they appear to characterize a genetically distinct subset of very aggressive neuroblastomas.

Our data, which shows the consistency of *MYCN* copy number over time,[36] suggests that *MYCN* amplification is an intrinsic biologic property of a subset of tumors, so it must occur relatively early in these cases. Because patients with *MYCN* amplification represent a subset of patients with 1p deletion, we suspect that the 1p deletion may precede the development of amplification. Both of these genetic findings are uncommon in the tumors of infants less than 1 year of age, a group in which the overall prognosis of neuroblastoma is much better than their older counterparts. These results suggest at least two possibilities: either all neuroblastomas begin as tumors with a more favorable genotype and phenotype, and some evolve into more aggressive tumors with adverse genetic features over time, or there are at least two different subsets of neuroblastoma, and the more aggressive tumors generally occur in children over 1 year of age. Our data and that of other investigators are more consistent with the latter explanation.[13,16,48,51]

Oncogene Amplification in Other Cancers

Breast cancer. Breast cancer is the single most common cancer occurring in women, and represents a genetically heterogeneous disease with frequent amplification of oncogenes and allelic deletions.[18] *MYC, ERBB2,* and *CCND1* (Cyclin D1) are the most frequently amplified genes in breast cancer, each occurring in 10 to 20 percent of cases. Genes of the fibroblast growth factor receptor family (*FGFR1* and *FGFR2*) are also amplified in another 12 percent of cases each, although it is not clear that their expression is increased above baseline (see Table 6-1).[24,56] Many studies have attempted to correlate the presence of a particular amplified gene with outcome or other clinical prognostic factors with contradictory results. Although there is support for the notion that amplification is a late event in the multistep pathogenesis of breast cancer,[18,57] a more recent study has correlated amplification of certain genes or chromosomal regions with distinct breast cancer phenotypes.[22] Amplification of 12q13-q15 (containing *MDM2, CDK4, SAS,* and/or *GLI*) and 20q13 (containing the recently cloned *AIB1*) each occur in fewer than 10 percent of primary tumors.[22,26]

Ovarian cancer. In ovarian cancer, amplification of *ERBB2* and *MYC* are found in 15 to 30 percent of samples.[58,59] *ERBB2* or *MYC* amplification tends to occur in advanced stages of disease and is seen infrequently in early invasive or borderline ovarian epithelial tumors,[58] again implying that these are late genetic events. *AKT2* is a protein serine/threonine kinase with homology to v-*akt,* a viral oncogene that can cause lymphomas in mice. *AKT2* is amplified independently of *MYC* or *ERBB2* in ~12 percent of ovarian cancers and also correlates with invasiveness.[60] Though amplification of *NRAS* and *KRAS* are seen infrequently in ovarian cancers, there is some evidence that these events occur earlier based on their prevalence in low-stage disease, but this remains speculative.[61]

Lung cancer. Lung cancer is one of the most common fatal malignancies and its incidence is increasing in both men and women. Small cell lung carcinoma makes up ~25% of cases and has a distinct clinical course with a propensity for early metastasis. The *MYC* proto-oncogenes are the only genes amplified in a significant number of small cell lung carcinomas (15 to 20 percent of cases), although cell lines derived from SCLC specimens more frequently have gene amplification.[14,62,63] The majority of these cases involve *MYC,* with amplification of *MYCN* and *MYCL* also occurring.[62,63] However, to date, co-amplification of multiple *MYC* family genes has not been described in SCLC specimens. It is possible that the propensity of SCLC cell lines to amplify *MYC in vitro* illustrates this cancer's underlying genetic instability and virulent phenotype.

Although no genes that are frequently amplified in non-SCLC have been identified, a region of amplification at 3q26 has been demonstrated by CGH and reverse chromosome painting in ~40 percent of specimens evaluated.[64,65] The gene target(s) of this amplification remain unknown.

Gastrointestinal cancers. A diverse group of genetic alterations occur in gastrointestinal cancers, involving mutation or deletion of tumor-suppressor genes and DNA repair genes, in addition to amplification of oncogenes. Amplification of *MYC, MDM2,* and *CCND1* occur frequently in esophageal squamous cell carcinoma, the latter being almost uniformly amplified in metastatic disease and correlating with clinical and pathologic staging.[66] In contrast, a plethora of genetic alterations occur in gastric cancer, many presumed to induce cell proliferation via induction of growth factor production or increased growth factor receptor expression, but amplification does not occur commonly. These genetic alterations differ in poorly differentiated and well-differentiated gastric cancers, and *KRAS* or *CCNE* are each amplified in 10 to 15 percent of cases.[21,66,67] Though *MET* is amplified in >10 percent of cases in some series, it is generally not amplified to high copy number.[68]

In colorectal cancers, cytogenetic evidence for gene amplification has long existed in the form of dmins, but with no clear candidate genes. In some series, *MYB, HRAS,* and *KRAS* amplification has been found, but in the majority of colorectal cancers, none of the known oncogenes have been amplified in a significant proportion of cases.[69,70] *MYC* may be amplified in up to 10 percent of tumors, however the level of amplification is often low (two- to five-fold) and the gene is more often overexpressed in the absence of gene amplification, possibly through alterations in *APC*-mediated repression.[71]

HNSCC, other cancers. In HNSCCs, amplification of the 11q13 locus with *CCND1* occurs frequently, while *MYC* and *ERBB1* amplification are also seen.[14,72] These findings are particularly germane in that current clinical prognostic factors are poor for HNSCC and molecular data may in the future become of significant predictive importance. In still other malignancies, gene amplification has been shown to be a prominent feature. In glioblastoma, hepatocellular carcinoma, cervical cancer, and soft tissue sarcomas, the role of oncogene amplification is being elucidated as advanced molecular analyses of these malignancies become more prevalent (see Table 6-1).

MECHANISMS OF GENE AMPLIFICATION

The precise mechanism by which gene amplification occurs in human cancers is not known with certainty.[73] Some information can be obtained by studying amplification of drug-resistance genes in cells grown *in vitro* under selective pressure. However, these systems generally involve the rapid selection for resistance to an antimetabolite or other toxic compound, so it is not clear that these model systems will provide relevant information. It is more likely that the selective pressures that lead to amplification of a gene that provides a growth advantage *in vivo* are not as profound, so the mechanisms leading to gene amplification may be quite different.

Experimentally, it appears that several types of genetic abnormality are required to allow gene amplification to take place. First, there must be loss of cell-cycle control. This occurs frequently by mutation or inactivation of p53 in human tumors,[74,75] but other mechanisms must also be possible, such as overexpression of cyclin D1 (*CCND1*),[76,77] in cells that lack p53 abnormalities. Second, DNA damage or instability must be present. This can be a result of DNA-damaging agents, or due to

mutations in genes such as p53 that affect DNA stability and repair.[78,79] Finally, there needs to be some stimulus to progress through the cell cycle. This can occur as a result of oncogene activation, such as *MYC* overexpression, growth factor/receptor activation, or other mechanisms.[80] The order in which these occur may not be important, but the result is that cells progress through the cell cycle with damaged DNA and are unable to pause for proper repair. The consequence is that gross rearrangements can occur, leading to amplification, deletion, or translocation of genes, with resultant oncogene activation or suppressor gene loss (Fig. 6-1).

Unfortunately, no model system exists for selection of oncogene activation in human tumors. This makes it difficult to draw firm conclusions about early events in the amplification process, so only the end-point of gene amplification can be studied. Some information can be obtained by structural analysis of the amplified unit, as well as by analysis of the genomic configuration of the locus that was amplified. In the majority of cases, the initial form of amplified DNA seen in human cancers is the extrachromosomal dmins. These structures lack centromeres or kinetochores, and they apparently segregate randomly in the two daughter cells after cell division. To remain stable, it is likely that dmins are closed circular molecules. Experimental data supporting this hypothesis have come from the study of amplified units involving the *MYCN* gene in human neuroblastomas, as well as other systems.

Several models have been proposed to explain the development of genomic amplification of specific chromosomal regions. These include the overreplication (onionskin) model, the chromosomal breakage/deletion plus episome formation model, and the duplication and crossing-over model. These models were based on the analysis of genomic rearrangements that followed the rapid, stepwise selection of resistance to a particular drug. None of these models are perfectly consistent with what is known about the structure of DNA in tumors with spontaneous amplification of regions containing oncogenes, such as the *MYCN* oncogene in human neuroblastomas, but some insights can be gained.

Amler and colleagues[81,82] used pulsed-field gel electrophoresis (PFGE) to study the restriction pattern of *MYCN* amplicons, using infrequently cutting enzymes and probes around the *MYCN* gene. These studies led to the conclusion that the amplicons were arranged in tandem, head-to-tail arrays in the HSRs, and that most of the amplicons had a consistent restriction pattern (there was relatively little rearrangement). These conclusions were supported by Schneider and colleagues[83] who cloned a representative amplified domain into yeast artificial chromosomes (YACs) from a cell line with 300 copies of *MYCN* per cell as dmins. They showed that the amplicons in dmins were organized in a head-to-tail, apparently circular, arrangement. Structural rearrangements relative to the normal locus were consistently identified, but there was general preservation of the germ line genomic structure. Finally, Corvi and coworkers[84] showed that the germ line copy of *MYCN* was apparently intact on both homologs of chromosome 2, so that models based on deletion of this locus would not explain the process.

Based on the overreplication model, the resolution of this complex structure would result in considerable rearrangement of the amplified sequences relative to the germ line configuration. There should be a mixture of head-to-head, tail-to-tail, and head-to-tail configurations of the DNA in different or adjacent amplicons. Also, a gradient of amplification would be seen, with the highest level of amplification near the gene that is the presumed target of amplification, with decreasing amplification further away from the amplification epicenter. However, the PFGE data by Amler[81] and YAC-cloning data by Schneider[83] are inconsistent with this model, even though some variation from the germ line pattern was detected by both approaches.

The duplication plus crossing over model would suggest that relatively intact copies of the amplicon would occur *in situ* on a given chromosome, leading to an HSR at the site of the normal

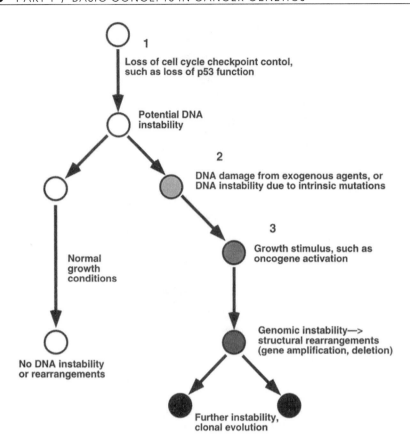

Fig. 6-1 Hypothetical process of gene amplification in mammalian cells. It appears that several types of genetic abnormality are required to allow gene amplification to take place. First, there needs to be loss of cell cycle control. Second, some mechanism of DNA damage or instability must occur. Finally, there needs to be some stimulus to progress through the cell cycle. The events do not need to occur in this order, but the result is that cells progress through the cell cycle with damaged DNA are unable to pause for proper repair. The net result is that gross genetic rearrangements can occur, leading to amplification or other genetic rearrangements.

gene. However, the most common form of amplified DNA is the extrachromosomal dmins, and the chromosomal locations of HSRs representing amplification of *MYCN* in neuroblastomas occur almost everywhere except at the normal chromosomal location of *MYCN* at 2p24.[85] Thus, this model does not seem applicable to what happens when *MYCN* becomes amplified in human neuroblastomas, or perhaps to amplification of oncogenes in general.

However, duplication of the *MYCN* locus has been observed in a few neuroblastoma cell lines that lack true amplification.[86] This may either represent a precursor to amplification of this locus, or an alternate mechanism of *MYCN* activation. Furthermore, amplification of the *MDM2* locus has been seen in a few neuroblastoma cell lines in conjunction with *MYCN* amplification.[23,45,46] In most of these cases, the amplified DNA is in the form of an HSR located at the normal site of *MDM2*. Thus, amplification of this locus may occur by a different mechanism than that involved in *MYCN* amplification.

Finally, the chromosomal breakage/deletion plus episome formation model suggests that one germ line copy of the amplified region is deleted, but this was not detected in the five cell lines studied by Corvi[84] or the cell line studied by Kanda[87] and Shiloh.[44,88] One study by Hunt and Tereba[89] did suggest that one germ line copy of *MYCN* was deleted from a homolog in one cell line by segregating the homologs into separate somatic cell hybrids, but this is inconsistent with data from at least six other cell lines studied by FISH. This suggests that the apparent deletion may have occurred during the formation of the somatic cell hybrids, or that there may be different mechanisms by which *MYCN* amplification can occur.

In summary, none of these models, which are derived primarily from the study of amplification of drug-resistance genes, fully explains the *de novo* amplification of oncogenes in human tumors *in vivo*. It seems likely that a variation of the DNA breakage plus episome formation model without deletion of the normal locus is applicable. Given the apparent retention of the normal parental

copies of the amplified region, it is likely that duplication of the amplified region occurs, followed by excision and circularization to form a dmin. Then the copy number increases by unequal segregation of the replicated minutes, providing a selective advantage to the daughter cell with the largest number of dmins, until maximal advantage is achieved. The *in situ* duplication of this locus identified by Corvi and colleagues[86] may represent an initial step in this process. Also, this mechanism may explain the apparent *in situ* amplification of the *MDM2* locus seen in a few neuroblastoma cell lines with HSRs at 12q14.

Further study will be required to elucidate the precise mechanisms involved, but this will be difficult until a model system for *de novo* oncogene amplification can be found. Nevertheless, the study of drug resistance in mammalian cells suggests that several discrete steps are likely to be involved in the process, including loss of cell-cycle control, DNA instability, and a growth-promoting stimulus. Given the infrequency of p53 mutations in neuroblastomas, some alternative mechanism for loss of cell cycle control and DNA instability must be involved.

STRUCTURAL ANALYSIS OF AMPLICONS

Amplification of the *MYCN* Locus at 2p24

Estimates of the size of the amplified domain around the *MYCN* proto-oncogene in neuroblastomas have ranged from 300 kb to 3000 kb, based on physical, chemical, and electrophoretic measurements of the amplified DNA.[85] However, most approaches to map the size of the amplified domain have been indirect. An attempt was made to clone and map the amplified domain around *MYCN* in a representative neuroblastoma cell line NGP using cosmid and lambda vectors.[90,91] Only 140 kb of contiguous DNA around the *MYCN* locus could be mapped, but a number of additional amplified clones were identified that were not contained in the 140 kb contiguous region. The entire 140 kb contiguous locus was amplified in a panel of 12 primary neuroblastomas with *MYCN* amplification, whereas the non-contiguous fragments were amplified in subsets of them.[91] These data indicate that, although each tumor had a relatively unique pattern of amplified DNA fragments, there was a core region that was consistently amplified in different tumors.

Amler and Schwab[81] have analyzed the amplified domain of a series of neuroblastoma cell lines with *MYCN* amplification, most in the form of chromosomally integrated HSRs. They analyzed the amplified domain by pulsed-field gel electrophoresis and hybridization with DNA probes that represent the 5′ and 3′ ends of the *MYCN* gene. They confirmed the heterogeneity of size of the amplified domain seen in different neuroblastomas demonstrated by earlier studies.[44,88,90,91] They also concluded that most amplified regions of DNA consisted of multiple tandem arrays of DNA segments that were several hundred kilobases in size, and that *MYCN* was at or near the center of the amplified units. Rearrangements were more commonly found in the cell lines with HSRs and with higher *MYCN* copy number (greater than 50 to 100 copies/haploid genome).

To determine the size and structural organization of this region in different tumors and cell lines, as well as the core region that is consistently amplified, we analyzed the amplified domain in human neuroblastomas. Because of the large size of the domain, we used the YAC-cloning vector system.[92] Twenty YACs that contained segments of the amplified domain from a representative neuroblastoma cell line were identified, which could be arranged in a contiguous linear map of ~1.2 Mb.[83,93] In general, the YAC clones were consistent with the germ line configuration of the region, but some rearrangements were identified. Our data also indicated that the core of the domain amplified in different tumors was no more than 130 kb, and that the amplicons of one tumor deleted about half of this core.[94] Although it remains possible that there may be other genes near *MYCN* whose expression is important in mediating the aggressive phenotype associated with *MYCN* amplification, our data suggest that *MYCN* is the primary target of amplification in neuroblastomas (Fig. 6-2).

The closest expressed sequence mapping near *MYCN* is the *DDX1* gene. This gene is an RNA helicase that may play a role in mRNA processing or stability. The *DDX1* gene was found because of its co-amplification with *MYCN* in a retinoblastoma cell line.[95] It also appears to be co-amplified in 50 to 60 percent of neuroblastomas, but it does not appear to be amplified independent of the *MYCN* locus.[96–100] The *DDX1* gene has been mapped about 300 kb 5′ and telomeric of *MYCN*, but in the same transcriptional orientation (Fig. 6-2).[97,98,100] Recent evidence suggests that tumors that co-amplify *MYCN* and *DDX1* may be more aggressive than those amplifying *MYCN* alone.[99] Also, transfection of the NIH3T3 mouse fibroblast line with *DDX1* appears to confer properties of transformation, suggesting that amplification and overexpression of *DDX1* may contribute to a more aggressive phenotype.[101]

Amplification of the 11q13 Locus

The 11q13 region contains a number of genes that are potential targets of the amplification that occurs in HNSCCs, breast carcinomas, hepatocellular carcinomas, and selected other tumors.[14,19,21,22,72,102–104] The genes in this region and representative amplicons are shown in Fig. 6-3. The majority of amplicons involve the *CCND1*, *FGF3* (INT2), and *FGF4* (HST) genes. However, some involve only regions proximal or distal to this, without involving *CCND1*, *FGF3*, or *FGF4*, so there may be multiple targets of amplification in this region. However, it is likely that amplification of *CCDN1* is the most important contributor to the malignant phenotypes, because *FGF3* and *FGF4* expression is generally low or absent.[105]

Amplification of the 12q14 Locus

The 12q14 region also contains a number of genes that are potential targets of the amplification seen in bone and soft tissue sarcomas, glioblastoma, esophageal cancer, and selected other tumors.[22,106–111] The genes in this region and representative amplicons are shown in Fig. 6-4. The majority of amplicons involve *SAS*, *CDK4*, and *MDM2*. However, some involve only *SAS* and *CDK4*, whereas others involve only *MDM2*, so there may be at least two target regions of amplification. Interestingly, for sarcomas, the amplification of one or the other region appears to correlate with particular histologic subtypes.[112]

Patterns of *MYCN* Amplification at 2p24

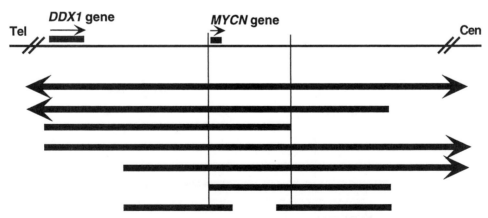

Fig. 6-2 Patterns of *MYCN* amplification at 2p24. Shown at the top is the region of 2p24 containing the *MYCN* and *DDX1* genes. *DDX1* is about 300 kb telomeric of *MYCN,* but both are in the same transcriptional orientation. *MYCN* is amplified in about 22 percent of neuroblastomas, as well as a minority of retinoblastomas, medulloblastomas, small cell lung cancers, and selected other tumors. Shown below are broad lines indicating the extent of amplicons in different tumors. The patterns shown are representative of those seen in human neuroblastomas.[94] Some extend for over a megabase, but all involve the *MYCN* proto-oncogene. About 50 to 60 percent also include the *DDX1* gene, which is overexpressed in these cases, but no tumors amplify *DDX1* unless *MYCN* is also amplified. The core domain that is consistently amplified in all neuroblastomas with *MYCN* amplification is about 130 kb in length. However, one tumor deletes about half of this region, while retaining the *MYCN* gene. Thus, it appears that *MYCN* is the major focus of amplification of this region in neuroblastomas. Nevertheless, recent evidence suggests that overexpression of *DDX1* also has transforming effects, so that co-amplification of both genes may lead to more aggressive tumors than amplification of *MYCN* alone.

Patterns of 11q13 Amplification

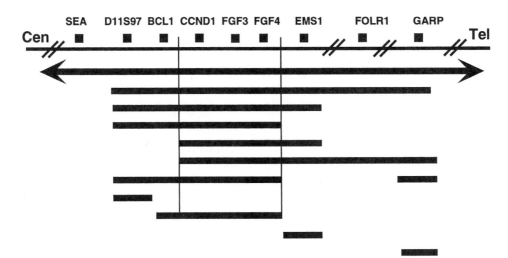

Fig. 6-3 Patterns of 11q13 amplification. Shown at the top is the region of 11q13, which contains a number of genes that are potential targets of the amplification. This region is amplified in head and neck squamous cell carcinomas, breast carcinomas, hepatocellular carcinomas, and selected other tumors. Shown below are broad lines indicating the extent of amplicons in different tumors. The patterns shown are representative of different patterns described in human breast cancers.[22] Some extend over the entire region, but no single gene is consistently amplified in all cases. The majority of amplicons include the *CCND1, FGF3* (INT2), and *FGF4* (HST) genes. However, some include only regions proximal or distal to this, without involving *CCND1, FGF3,* or *FGF4,* so there may be multiple targets of amplification in this region. Furthermore, it is unclear if amplification of *CCDN1, FGF3, FGF4,* or some combination thereof is essential to confer a selective advantage.

BIOLOGICAL SIGNIFICANCE OF GENE AMPLIFICATION

Presumably, the mechanism by which gene amplification confers a selective advantage on the cancer cells is by overexpression of the gene or genes contained within the amplicon. In general, this overexpression is proportional to the increase in copy number, but there is not an absolute correlation. The overexpression of the gene or genes may cause malignant transformation or may alter the cell phenotype by conferring some advantage in cell proliferation or survival. We review briefly what is known about the likely consequences of overexpressing the most frequently amplified genes in human cancers: the *MYC* family, the *RAS* family, the *ERBB* and *FGFR* families, and the cell-cycle control genes, including the cyclins and *MDM2*.

MYC Family Amplification

The structure of the Myc family proteins consists of a transactivating domain at the N-terminal third of the protein, followed by a basic region, helix-loop-helix, and leucine zipper domain (B-HLH-Zip). These proteins are thought to activate transcription by binding to a hexanucleotide motif CACGTG known as an E-box. However, they do not bind well as monomers or as homodimers, but rather as heterodimers with another B-HLH-Zip protein known as Max.[113] This protein lacks a

Patterns of 12q14 Amplification

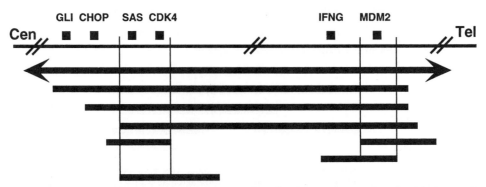

Fig. 6-4 Patterns of 12q14 amplification. Shown at the top is the region of 12q14, which contains a number of genes that are potential targets of the amplification. This region is amplified in bone and soft tissue sarcomas, glioblastoma, esophageal cancer, and selected other tumors. Shown below are broad lines indicating the extent of amplicons in different tumors. The patterns shown are representa- tive of different patterns described in human breast cancers and sarcomas.[22,106–108] Some extend over the entire region, but no single gene is consistently amplified in all cases. The majority of amplicons involve *SAS, CDK4,* and *MDM2*. However, some involve only *SAS* and *CDK4,* whereas others involve only *MDM2,* so there may be at least two target regions of amplification.

transcriptional activation domain, and it can form homodimers that are thought to be transcriptionally repressive.[114–118] Thus, in a state of Max excess, Max homodimers predominate, and transcription is repressed. Conversely, when Myc (or MycN) are expressed at higher levels, Myc-Max heterodimers predominate, resulting in transcriptional activation of Myc target genes, which, to date, remain poorly characterized.[119] Nevertheless, the consequence is progression through the cell cycle and proliferation of the cell population.

Myc oncoproteins have a short half-life (20 to 30 min), so once transcription and translation cease, the levels of Myc fall rapidly, and Max-Max transcriptional repression predominates. However, in tumors that amplify *MYC, MYCN* or *MYCL,* the level of amplification is usually ten- to one hundredfold (or more), with corresponding overexpression of the oncoprotein.[38,41–43,63] This leads to very high steady-state levels of Myc, even when it is not being actively transcribed. This, in turn, presumably favors a state of proliferation, with less likelihood that the cell will enter G0 and become quiescent. This is presumably the selective advantage conferred by overexpressing this family of genes.

RAS Family Amplification

RAS genes encode proteins known as G proteins, which participate in the signaling cascade initiated by the activation of tyrosine kinase receptors or other signaling intermediates. *RAS* activation by specific base-pair mutations or overexpression by amplification leads to enhanced signal transduction through the RAF-1 serine-threonine kinase, the early response kinases (ERK1 and ERK2), and the subsequent induction of transcription of immediate-early genes (e.g., FOS, JUN).[120–122]

The amplification and overexpression of *RAS* genes leads to constitutive signal transduction, mimicking the effects of continual activation of a growth factor receptor, such as EGFR or PDGFR.[120–125] This, in turn, leads to continuous cell proliferation. However, the cellular background is very important, because in certain cellular milieus (such as neural cells), the predominant receptor tyrosine kinase may be signaling differentiation and not proliferation. Activation or overexpression of *RAS* in this context would lead to differentiation of the cell, which would not promote the proliferation of tumor cells.[120–122,125] This may explain why RAS activation is rare in neural tumors, whereas it is one of the most common types of oncogene activation in many other tumor types.[123–125]

Amplification of the *ERBB* and *FGFR* Family

Amplification and overexpression of genes for growth factors or their receptors, such as those of the *EGF/EGFR (ERBB)* and *FGF/FGFR* families, occur in a number of human cancers.[24,56,58] The ERBB and FGF receptors are transmembrane tyrosine kinases, which are involved in cell proliferation. After specific ligand binding, signal transduction occurs through phosphorylation of the SH2 domains of cytoplasmic proteins associated with the receptor. Activation of the Ras-GTP pathway frequently occurs. Kinase activation also leads to PKC phosphorylation, serine/threonine phosphorylations, and changes in phosphatidyl inositol metabolism, with the end result being modulation of specific genes necessary for proliferation.[126,127]

Gastric cancer expresses a number of growth factors and receptors including EGF, TGF-α, ERBB2 and FGFR2.[66,128] EGF is synthesized as a transmembrane precursor, and a secreted protein is released by proteolytic cleavage. It has been shown to enhance growth of cells from most epithelial tumors,[129] and in gastric cancer, EGF expression is associated with poor outcome.[128] Human gastric cancers that possess both EGF and EGFR (or ERBB2) simultaneously have a greater degree of local invasion and lymph node metastasis, further suggesting autocrine stimulation. Additionally, high levels of expression of growth factor receptor alone may result in autophosphorylation and signaling, even in the absence of ligand. Constitutive activation of these growth factor-signaling pathways are a common motif in oncogenesis.[126,127] Amplification and overexpression of either ligand or receptor may cause growth stimulation in an autocrine or paracrine fashion in the appropriate cellular setting and contribute to malignant behavior.

Amplification of the Genes Encoding Regulators of the Cell Cycle

Cells of most higher organisms maintain a stringent "checkpoint control" over progression from G1 into S phase and subsequent cell division. Early in G1, cells are dependent on mitogenic stimuli, but at a certain point a switch to intrinsic cell-cycle machinery occurs with a reduced requirement for growth factor stimuli, apparently ensuring an ordered completion of the cell division cycle. This switch-point is mediated in part by the D-type cyclins, although many proteins may also play important roles as both positive and negative regulators. These proteins include (but are not limited to) other cyclins, cyclin-dependent kinases (cdk), and their inhibitors (cdki). Activation of G1-S cyclins (*CCND1* and *CCNE*) occurs via growth factor signals that induce Cyclin D1 phosphorylation. Activated Cyclins D and E, in association with their predominant cyclin-dependent kinases CDK4 and CDK2, then sequentially phosphorylate the RB protein. This causes the release of E2F from pRB, which activates transcription of genes involved in cell proliferation.[130,131]

Overexpression of *CCND1, CCNE,* or *CDK4* presumably results in a growth advantage for cells by tipping the balance in favor of G1-S transition rather than quiescence. Likewise, overexpression of *MDM2* could have similar effects. MDM2 protein binds p53, a potent cell-cycle inhibitor. By blocking p53-mediated transcriptional activation of cyclin-dependent kinase inhibitors such as p21, cells are more likely to enter S phase.[130,131] This loss of checkpoint control fails to allow time for repair of DNA damage caused by a multitude of insults, such as ionizing radiation, drugs, and cellular toxins, or mutations in DNA repair genes.

METHODS OF DETECTING GENE AMPLIFICATION

A variety of techniques may be used to detect gene amplification.[132] Each technique has its advantages and disadvantages in terms of the amount of tumor tissue or DNA needed, the ease of performing the technique; its sensitivity in detecting low levels of amplification; the size of the amplified unit; and whether the locus (or loci) are known that are likely to be amplified in a given tumor type. The techniques include conventional cytogenetics; Southern analysis; fluorescence *in situ* hybridization (FISH); semiquantitative PCR; comparative genomic hybridization (CGH); and microarray analysis.

Cytogenetic Analysis

Cytogenetic analysis is a labor-intensive technique that is dependent on analyzing dividing cells in the tumor tissue or during adaptation to growth in short-term culture. As a result, it is unsuccessful in the majority of solid tumors and a substantial number of leukemias. The detection of HSRs or dmins provides evidence for gene amplification in the culture, although small HSRs or dmins may escape detection. Also, it is impossible to know with certainty which gene or chromosomal region is amplified. This is a useful technique when investigating a new tumor type, but is not the most efficient or sensitive approach once it is known which gene or genes are likely to be amplified.

Southern Analysis

Southern analysis is the gold standard against which other techniques are compared. This technique relies on the preparation of DNA from tumor tissue that is relatively free of contaminating normal tissue. The DNA is digested with a restriction enzyme, electrophoresed on an agarose gel, blotted to a membrane, and hybridized with a radioactive probe corresponding to the gene or genomic region thought to be amplified.[15,36] This technique is rather labor intensive, and it generally requires 5 to 10 µg of DNA. Frequently, an internal control gene is also hybridized so the intensity of the band of interest can be normalized by quantitative densitometry. However, this technique can miss a small percentage of amplified cells in an unamplified population (such as the bone marrow or a lymph node). Slot blotting is a variation on this technique that requires no digestion, only 1 µg of DNA, and it is easily subjected to densitometric analysis, but low levels of amplification also can be missed.

Fluorescence *In Situ* Hybridization (FISH)

The FISH technique is probably the most efficient and popular technique for the detection of DNA amplification if the gene (or genes) of interest are known.[133,134] It requires only a small amount of tumor tissue, usually a "touch prep" or "cytospin" of several thousand cells on a slide. It can even be done on paraffin-embedded tissue.[134] Hybridization to interphase nuclei takes place overnight under a coverslip, and the results can be interpreted within 24 to 48 h. This technique can also distinguish a small percentage of amplified tumor cells in a population of normal or nonamplified tumor cells, if a counterstain to visualize the "positive" cells is implemented. It may be necessary to utilize a control probe for the centromere or opposite arm of the same chromosome, in order to distinguish between low-level amplification and polysomy for the particular chromosome. However, because this approach requires a fluorescence microscope and sophisticated imaging equipment, and because the probes may be expensive to purchase commercially, FISH is not the ideal approach for all laboratories.

An interesting variation on this technique has been developed whereby amplicons are microdissected and used as FISH hybridization probes to determine the chromosomal origin.[135] This "micro-FISH" approach allows the chromosomal origin of dmins or HSRs to be determined in a single hybridization without knowing a priori the genetic region that is amplified. Indeed, this approach can also identify amplification of previously unsuspected chromosomal regions. However, in addition to the technical demands of FISH, this approach also requires both successful metaphase preparation, with identification of dmins or HSRs, and the ability to perform microdissection and preparation of a microclone library. Therefore, this method is primarily suited for research laboratories.

Semiquantitative PCR

The PCR technique has advantages that might be applied to the detection of genomic amplification in small amounts of tumor DNA.[136–139] As long as the number of cycles of amplification is carefully controlled, and an internal control gene is used for normalization, it is possible to semiquantitatively amplify a given gene or DNA sequence and distinguish the normal copy number from multiple extra copies. Although some claim to detect as low as twofold amplification, generally five- to tenfold amplification is the limit of detection of this technique on primary tumor samples.[136–139]

Comparative Genomic Hybridization (CGH)

This is one of the newest of the approaches to the detection of genomic amplification.[140–142] This approach has the advantage of conventional cytogenetics in that the whole genome is surveyed, not just one or a few specific genomic regions that are known or suspected to be amplified in a given tumor type. Also, because the chromosomal location of the amplified region is known, the likely gene amplified is frequently apparent from past experience. Tumor metaphases are not needed, and only a small amount of DNA is required. However, this approach requires a sophisticated fluorescence microscope and image-capturing capability, as well as software to analyze the data obtained. Furthermore, very small amplicons or low levels of amplification may be missed, and it cannot detect translocations.

Microarray Analysis

DNA microarray technology relies on hybridization just as Southern blotting, FISH, and CGH do. Using this approach, multiple cDNAs, or genomic regions, are "spotted" on a solid-phase support, which may be a glass slide or microchip. Probing with a labeled DNA mixture obtained from tumor samples allows for detection of amplified genomic regions.[143] Comparing data obtained using microarrays and quantitative hybridization has yielded a very good correlation. This technique has the capability to allow high-throughput, although at a substantial cost. The information content requires significant image processing and may not be available in most centers. Commercial development of microarrays containing genomic regions of interest (i.e., those regions with amplification in a particular tumor system) may allow this technology to supplant CGH as the next-generation method of high-resolution genome scanning. Other applications of microarray technology are for analysis of patterns of gene expression,[144] or even analysis of complex genes for mutations.[145]

SUMMARY AND CONCLUSIONS

Gene amplification in human cells is a phenomenon that appears to be restricted to tumor cells. In the majority of cases in which the amplified genomic region has been identified, the target of the amplification appears to be an oncogene, usually of the *MYC, RAS*, or *ERBB* family. A variety of other genes have been shown to be amplified in small numbers of cases, or in tumor-derived cell lines, but the above-mentioned families are found the most consistently. Examples of amplification of genes conferring drug resistance have been found in certain cancers at relapse, but this does not appear to be a common mechanism by which cancer cells become drug resistant *in vivo*.

The mechanism by which amplification of oncogenes in humans occurs is unknown, and it may be different for individual loci. In the majority of cases, however, it probably involves the duplication of a large chromosomal region, followed by deletion and circularization to form an extrachromosomal dmin. Then there is accumulation of these dmins by uneven segregation into the daughter cells during mitosis, until maximal advantage is achieved. This is presumably a consequence of the overexpression of a gene (or genes) on the amplicon that confers the selective advantage. The region amplified may be quite large, from 100 kb to several megabases. However, the region that is consistently amplified may contain little more than the single gene suspected of providing a growth or survival advantage.

The identification of oncogene amplification in certain human cancers provides some insight into the pathogenesis of these diseases. Indeed, in some tumor systems, oncogene amplification had been associated with a greater likelihood of invasion, metastasis, and a poor outcome. Thus, the identification of oncogene amplification in human cancers may have some prognostic value. Ultimately, it may be possible to develop novel therapeutic approaches that target the amplified oncogene or the overexpressed oncoprotein. This approach may be particularly attractive if the amplified gene is mutated or chimeric, allowing the development of selective biological reagents or targeted gene therapy approaches.

ACKNOWLEDGMENTS

This work was supported in part by National Institutes of Health grant RO1-CA-39771.

REFERENCES

1. Schimke RT: Gene amplification in cultured cells. *J Biol Chem* **263**:5989, 1988.
2. Sobrero A, Bertino JR: Clinical aspects of drug resistance. *Cancer Surv* **5**:93, 1986.

3. Pastan I, Gottesman M: Multiple-drug resistance in human cancer. *N Engl J Med* **316**:1388, 1987.

4. Chin JE, Soffir R, Noonan KE, Choi K, Roninson IB: Structure and expression of the human MDR (P-glycoprotein) gene family. *Mol Cell Biol* **9**:3808, 1989.

5. Ling V: P-glycoprotein and resistance to anticancer drugs. *Cancer* **69**:2603, 1992.

6. Grant CE, Valdimarsson G, Hipfner DR, Almquist KC, Cole SPC, Deeley RG: Overexpression of multidrug resistance-associated protein (MRP) increases resistance to natural product drugs. *Cancer Res* **54**:357, 1994.

7. Curt GA, Carney DN, Cowan K, Jolivet J, Bailey BD, Drake JC, Kao-Shan CS, Minna JD, Chabner BA: Unstable methotrexate resistance in human small-cell carcinoma associated with double minute chromosomes. *N Engl J Med* **308**:199, 1983.

8. Horns RCJ, Dower WJ, Schimke RT: Gene amplification in a leukemic patient treated with methotrexate. *J Clin Oncol* **2**:2, 1984.

9. Trent JM, Buick RN, Olson S, Horns RCJ, Schimke RT: Cytologic evidence for gene amplification in methotrexate-resistant cells obtained from a patient with ovarian adenocarcinoma. *J Clin Oncol* **2**:8, 1984.

10. Carman MD, Schornagel JH, Rivest RS, Srimatkandada S, Portlock CS, Duffy T, Bertino JR: Resistance to methotrexate due to gene amplification in a patient with acute leukemia. *J Clin Oncol* **2**:16, 1984.

11. Merkel DE, Fuqua SAW, Tandon AK, Hill SM, Buzdar AU, McGuire WL: Electrophoretic analysis of 248 clinical breast cancer specimens for P-glycoprotein overexpression or gene amplification. *J Clin Oncol* **7**:1129, 1989.

12. Brodeur GM, Green AA, Hayes FA, Williams KJ, Williams DL, Tsiatis AA: Cytogenetic features of human neuroblastomas and cell lines. *Cancer Res* **41**:4678, 1981.

13. Brodeur GM, Fong CT: Molecular biology and genetics of human neuroblastoma. *Cancer Genet Cytogenet* **41**:153, 1989.

14. Leonard JH, Kearsley JH, Chenevix-Trench G, Hayward NK: Analysis of gene amplification in head-and-neck squamous-cell carcinomas. *Int J Cancer* **48**:511, 1991.

15. Brodeur GM, Seeger RC, Schwab M, Varmus HE, Bishop JM: Amplification of N-myc in untreated human neuroblastomas correlates with advanced disease stage. *Science* **224**:1121, 1984.

16. Brodeur GM: Neuroblastoma — Clinical applications of molecular parameters. *Brain Pathol* **1**:47, 1990.

17. Seeger RC, Brodeur GM, Sather H, Dalton A, Siegel SE, Wong KY, Hammond D: Association of multiple copies of the N-myc oncogene with rapid progression of neuroblastomas. *N Engl J Med* **313**:1111, 1985.

18. Garcia I, Dietrich PY, Aapro M, Vauthier G, Vadas L, Engel E: Genetic alterations of c-myc, c-erbB-2, and c-HA-ras proto-oncogenes and clinical associations in human breast carcinomas. *Cancer Res* **49**:6675, 1989.

19. Berns EM, Klijn JG, van Staveren IL, Portengen H, Noordegraaf E, Foekens JA: Prevalence of amplification of the oncogenes c-myc, HER2/neu, and int-2 in one thousand human breast tumours: Correlation with steroid receptors. *Eur J Cancer* **28**:697, 1992.

20. Schuuring E: The involvement of the chromosome 11q13 region in human malignancies: *Cyclin D1* and *EMS1* are two new candidate oncogenes — A review. *Gene* **159**:83, 1995.

21. Karlseder J, Zeillinger R, Schneeberger C, Czerwenka K, Speiser P, Kubista E, Birnbaum D, Gaudray P, Theillet C: Patterns of DNA amplification at band q13 of chromosome 11 in human breast cancer. *Genes Chromosom Cancer* **9**:42, 1994.

22. Courjal F, Cuny M, Simony-Lafontaine J, Louason G, Speiser P, Zeillinger R, Rodriguez C, Theillet C: Mapping of DNA amplifications at 15 chromosomal localizations in 1857 breast tumors: Definition of phenotypic groups. *Cancer Res* **57**:4360, 1997.

23. Van Roy N, Forus A, Myklebost O, Cheng NC, Versteeg R, Speleman F: Identification of two distinct chromosome 12-derived amplification units in neuroblastoma cell line NGP. *Cancer Genet Cytogenet* **82**:151, 1995.

24. Theillet C, Adelaide J, Louason G, Bonnet-Dorion F, Jacquemier J, Adnane J, Longy M, Katsaros D, Sismondi P, Gaudray P, Birnbaum D: FGFRI and PLAT genes and DNA amplification at 8p12 in breast and ovarian cancers. *Genes Chromosom Cancer* **7**:219, 1993.

25. Shiloh Y, Mor O, Manor A, Bar-Am I, Rotman G, Eubanks J, Gutman M, Ranzani GN, Houldsworth J, Evans G, Aviv L: DNA sequences amplified in cancer cells: An interface between tumor biology and human genome analysis. *Mutat Res* **276**:329, 1992.

26. Anzick SL, Kononen J, Walker RL, Azorsa DO, Tanner MM, Guan XY, Sauter G, Kallioniemi OP, Trent JM, Meltzer PS: AIB1, a steroid receptor coactivator amplified in breast and ovarian cancer. *Science* **277**:965, 1997.

27. Schwab M, Alitalo K, Klempnauer KH, Varmus HE, Bishop JM, Gilbert F, Brodeur G, Goldstein M, Trent JM: Amplified DNA with limited homology to myc cellular oncogene is shared by human neuroblastoma cell lines and a neuroblastoma tumour. *Nature* **305**:245, 1983.

28. Schwab M, Varmus HE, Bishop JM, Grzeschik KH, Naylor SL, Sakaguchi AY, Brodeur G, Trent J: Chromosome localization in normal human cells and neuroblastomas of a gene related to c-myc. *Nature* **308**:288, 1984.

29. Tsuda T, Obara M, Hirano H, Gotoh S, Kubomura S, Higashi K, Kuroiwa A, Nakagawara A, Nagahara N, Shimizu K: Analysis of N-myc amplification in relation to disease stage and histologic types in human neuroblastomas. *Cancer* **60**:820, 1987.

30. Rubie H, Hartmann O, Michon J, Frappaz D, Coze C, Chastagner P, Baranzelli MC, Plantaz D, Avet-Loiseau H, Benard J, Delattre O, Favrot M, Peyroulet MC, Thyss A, Perel Y, Bergeron C, Coubon-Collet B, Vannier J-P, Lemerle J, Sommelet D: N-Myc gene amplification is a major prognostic factor in localized neuroblastoma: Results of the French NBL 90 study. *J Clin Oncol* **15**:1171, 1997.

31. Nakagawara A, Ikeda K, Tsuda T, Higashi K, Okabe T: Amplification of N-myc oncogene in stage II and IVS neuroblastomas may be a prognostic indicator. *J Pediatr Surg* **22**:415, 1987.

32. Tonini GP, Boni L, Pession A, Rogers D, Iolascon A, Basso G, Cordero di Montezemolo L, Casale F, De Bernardi B: MYCN oncogene amplification in neuroblastoma is associated with worse prognosis, except in stage 4s: The Italian experience with 295 children. *J Clin Oncol* **15**:85, 1997.

33. Matthay KK, Perez C, Seeger RC, Brodeur GM, Shimada H, Atkinson JB, Black CT, Gerbing R, Haase GM, Stram DO, Swift P, Lukens JN: Successful treatment of stage III neuroblastoma based on prospective biologic staging: A Children's Cancer Group study. *J Clin Oncol* **16**:1256, 1998.

34. Katzenstein HM, Bowman LC, Brodeur GM, Thorner PS, Joshi VV, Smith EI, Look AT, Rowe ST, Nash MB, Holbrook T, Alvarado C, Rao PV, Castleberry RP, Cohn SL: Prognostic significance of age, MYCN oncogene amplification, tumor cell ploidy, and histology in 110 infants with stage D(s) neuroblastoma: The Pediatric Oncology Group experience — A Pediatric Oncology Group study. *J Clin Oncol* **16**:2007, 1998.

35. Kaneko M, Nishihira H, Mugishima H, Ohnuma N, Nakada K, Kawa K, Fukuzawa M, Suita S, Seray Y, Tsuchida Y: Stratification of treatment of stage 4 neuroblastoma patients based on N-myc amplification status. Study Group of Japan for treatment of advanced neuroblastoma, Tokyo, Japan. *Med Pediatr Oncol* **31**:1, 1998.

36. Brodeur GM, Hayes FA, Green AA, Casper JT, Wasson J, Wallach S, Seeger RC: Consistent N-myc copy number in simultaneous or consecutive neuroblastoma samples from sixty individual patients. *Cancer Res* **47**:4248, 1987.

37. Brodeur GM, Maris JM, Yamashiro DJ, Hogarty MD, White PS: Biology and genetics of human neuroblastomas. *J Pediatr Hematol Oncol* **19**:93, 1997.

38. Bartram CR, Berthold F: Amplification and expression of the N-myc gene in neuroblastoma. *Eur J Pediatr* **146**:162, 1987.

39. Bordow SB, Norris MD, Haber PS, Marshall GM, Haber M: Prognostic significance of MYCN oncogene expression in childhood neuroblastoma. *J Clin Oncol* **16**:3286, 1998.

40. Chan H, Gallic B, DeBoer G, Haddad G, Dimitroulakos J, Ikegaki N, Yeger H, Ling V: MYCN protein as a predictor of neuroblastoma prognosis. Annual Meeting of the American Society of Clinical Oncology **16**:513a, 1997.

41. Nisen PD, Waber PG, Rich MA, Pierce S, Garvin JRJ, Gilbert F, Lanzkowsky P: N-myc oncogene RNA expression in neuroblastoma. *J Natl Cancer Inst* **80**:1633, 1988.

42. Seeger RC, Wada R, Brodeur GM, Moss TJ, Bjork RL, Sousa L, Slamon DJ: Expression of N-myc by neuroblastomas with one or multiple copies of the oncogene. *Progr Clin Biol Res* **271**:41, 1988.

43. Slavc I, Ellenbogen R, Jung W-H, Vawter GF, Kretschmar C, Grier H, Korf BR: myc gene amplification and expression in primary human neuroblastoma. *Cancer Res* **50**:1459, 1990.

44. Shiloh Y, Shipley J, Brodeur GM, Bruns G, Korf B, Donlon T, Schreck RR, Seeger R, Sakai K, Latt SA: Differential amplification, assembly and relocation of multiple DNA sequences in human neuroblastomas and neuroblastoma cell lines. *Proc Natl Acad Sci USA* **82**:3761, 1985.

45. Corvi R, Savelyeva L, Breit S, Wenzel A, Handgretinger R, Barak J, Oren M, Amler L, Schwab M: Non-syntenic amplification of MDM2 and MYCN in human neuroblastoma. *Oncogene* **10**:1081, 1995.

46. Corvi R, Savelyeva L, Amler L, Handgetinger R, Schwab M: Cytogenetic evolution of MYCN and MDM2 amplification in the neuroblastoma LS tumor and its cell line. *Eur J Cancer* **31A**:520, 1995.

47. Jinbo T, Iwamura Y, Kaneko M, Sawaguchi S: Coamplification of the L-myc and N-myc oncogenes in a neuroblastoma cell line. *Jpn J Cancer Res* **80**:299, 1989.

48. Fong CT, Dracopoli NC, White PS, Merrill PT, Griffith RC, Housman DE, Brodeur GM: Loss of heterozygosity for chromosome 1p in human neuroblastomas: Correlation with N-myc amplification. *Proc Natl Acad Sci USA* **86**:3753, 1989.

49. Kaneko Y, Kanda N, Maseki N, Sakurai M, Tsuchida Y, Takeda T, Okabe I, Sakurai M: Different karyotypic patterns in early and advanced stage neuroblastomas. *Cancer Res* **47**:311, 1987.

50. Christiansen H, Lampert F: Tumour karyotype discriminates between good and bad prognostic outcome in neuroblastoma. *Br J Cancer* **57**:121, 1988.

51. Hayashi Y, Kanda N, Inaba T, Hanada R, Nagahara N, Muchi H, Yamamoto K: Cytogenetic findings and prognosis in neuroblastoma with emphasis on marker chromosome 1. *Cancer* **63**:126, 1989.

52. Maris JM, White PS, Beltinger CP, Sulman EP, Castleberry RP, Shuster JJ, Look AT, Brodeur GM: Significance of chromosome 1p loss of heterozygosity in neuroblastomas. *Cancer Res* **55**:4664, 1995.

53. Martinsson T, Shoberg P-M, Hedberg F, Kogner P: Deletion of chromosome 1p loci and microsatellite instability in neuroblastomas analyzed with short-tandem repeat polymorphisms. *Cancer Res* **55**:5681, 1995.

54. Gehring M, Berthold F, Edler L, Schwab M, Amler LC: The 1p deletion is not a reliable marker for the prognosis of patients with neuroblastoma. *Cancer Res* **55**:5366, 1995.

55. Caron H, van Sluis P, de Kraker J, Bokkerink J, Egeler M, Laureys G, Slater R, Westerveld A, Voute PA, Versteeg R: Allelic loss of chromosome 1p as a predictor of unfavorable outcome in patients with neuroblastoma. *N Engl J Med* **334**:225, 1996.

56. Adnane J, Gaudray P, Dionne CA, Crumley G, Jaye M, Schlessinger J, Jeanteur P, Birnbaum D, Theillet C: BEK and FLG, two receptors to members of the FGF family, are amplified in subsets of human breast cancers. *Oncogene* **6**:659, 1991.

57. Brison O: Gene amplification and tumor progression. *Biochim Biophys Acta* **1155**:25, 1993.

58. Fajac A, Benard J, Lhomme C, Rey A, Duvillard P, Rochard F, Bernaudin JF, Riou G: c-erbB2 gene amplification and protein expression in ovarian epithelial tumors: Evaluation of their respective prognostic significance by multivariate analysis. *Int J Cancer* **64**:146, 1995.

59. Zhang GL, Zu KL, Yu SY: Amplification of C-erB2 gene in ovarian cancer. *Chung Hua Fu Chan Ko Tsa Chih* **29**:401, 1994.

60. Bellacosa A, de Feo D, Godwin AK, Bell DW, Cheng JQ, Altomare DA, Wan M, Dubeau L, Scambia G, Masciullo V, Ferrandina G, Bennedetti Panici P, Mancuso S, Neri G, Testa JR: Molecular alterations of the AKT2 oncogene in ovarian and breast carcinomas. *Int J Cancer* **64**:280, 1995.

61. Bian M, Fan Q, Huang S: Amplification of proto-oncogenes C-myc, C-N-ras, C-Ki-ras, C-erbB2 in ovarian carcinoma [abstract]. *Chung Hua Fu Chan Ko Tsa Chih* **30**:406, 1995.

62. Chiba W, Sawai S, Hanawa T, Ishida H, Matsui T, Kosaba S, Watanabe S, Hatakenaka R, Matsubara Y, Funatsu T, et al: Correlation between DNA content and amplification of oncogenes (c-myc, L-myc, c-erbB-2) and correlation with prognosis in 143 cases of resected lung cancer. *Gan To Kagaku Ryoho* **20**:824, 1993.

63. Brennan J, O'Connor T, Makuch RW, Simmons AM, Russell E, Linnoila RI, Phelps RM, Gazdar AF, Ihde DC, Johnson BE: myc family DNA amplification in 107 tumors and tumor cell lines from patients with small cell lung cancer treated with different combination chemotherapy regimens. *Cancer Res* **51**:1708, 1991.

64. Brass N, Racz A, Heckel D, Remberger K, Sybrecht GW, Meese EU: Amplification of the genes BCHE and SLC2A2 in 40% of squamous cell carcinoma of the lung. *Cancer Res* **57**:2290, 1997.

65. Balsara BR, Sonoda G, du Manoir S, Siegfried JM, Gabrielson E, Testa JR: Comparative genomic hybridization analysis detects frequent, often high-level, overrepresentation of DNA sequences at 3q, 5p, 7p, and 8q in human non-small cell lung carcinomas. *Cancer Res* **57**:2116, 1997.

66. Tahara E: Genetic alterations in human gastrointestinal cancers, the application to molecular diagnosis. *Cancer* **75**:1410, 1994.

67. Ranzani GN, Pellegata NS, Previdere C, Saragoni A, Vio A, Maltoni M, Amadori D: Heterogeneous proto-oncogene amplification correlates with tumor progression and presence of metastases in gastric cancer patients. *Cancer Res* **50**:7811, 1990.

68. Tsugawa K, Yonemura Y, Hirono Y, Fushida S, Kaji M, Miwa K, Miyazaki I, Yamamoto H: Amplification of the c-met, c-erbB-2 and epidermal growth factor receptor gene in human gastric cancers: Correlation to clinical features. *Oncology* **55**:475, 1998.

69. Salhab N, Jones DJ, Bos JL, Kinsella A, Schofield PF: Detection of ras gene alterations and ras proteins in colorectal cancer. *Dis Colon Rectum* **32**:659, 1989.

70. Greco C, Gandolfo GM, Mattei F, Gradilone A, Alvino S, Pastore LI, Casale V, Casole P, Grassi A, Cianciulli AM: Detection of C-myb genetic alterations and mutant p53 serum protein in patients with benign and malignant colon lesions. *Anticancer Res* **14**:1433, 1994.

71. Tong-Chuan H, Sparks AB, Rago C, Hermeking H, Zawel L, da Costa LT, Morin PJ, Vogelstein B, Kinzler KW: Identification of c-*MYC* as a target of the APC pathway. *Science* **281**:1509, 1998.

72. Merritt WD, Weissler MC, Turk BF, Gilmer TM: Oncogene amplification in squamous cell carcinoma of the head and neck. *Arch Otolaryngol Head Neck Surg* **116**:1394, 1990.

73. Kellems RE (ed): *Gene Amplification in Mammalian Cells*. New York: Marcel Dekker, Inc., 1993.

74. Livingstone LR, White A, Sprouse J, Livanos E, Jacks T, Tlsty TD: Altered cell cycle arrest and gene amplification potential accompany loss of wild-type p53. *Cell* **70**:923, 1992.

75. Yin Y, Tainsky MA, Bischoff FZ, Strong LC, Wahl GM: Wild-type p53 restores cell cycle control and inhibits gene amplification in cells with mutant p53 alleles. *Cell* **70**:937, 1992.

76. Asano K, Sakamoto H, Sasaki H, Ochiya T, Yoshida T, Ohishi Y, Machida T, Kakizoe T, Sugimura T, Terada M: Tumorigenicity and gene amplification potentials of cyclin D1-overexpressing NIH3T3 cells. *Biochem Biophys Res Commun* **217**:1169, 1995.

77. Zhou P, Jiang W, Weghorst CM, Weinstein IB: Overexpression of Cyclin D1 enhances gene amplification. *Cancer Res* **56**:36, 1996.

78. Tlsty TD: Genomic instability and its role in neoplasia. *Curr Top Microbiol Immunol* **221**:37, 1997.

79. Wahl GM, Linke SP, Paulson TG, Huang LC: Maintaining genetic stability through TP53 mediated checkpoint control. *Cancer Surv* **29**:183, 1997.

80. Paulson TG, Almasan A, Brody LL, Wahl GM: Gene amplification in a p53-deficient cell line requires cell cycle progression under conditions that generate DNA breakage. *Mol Cell Biol* **18**:3089, 1998.

81. Amler LC, Schwab M: Amplified N-myc in human neuroblastoma cells is often arranged as clustered tandem repeats of differently recombined DNA. *Mol Cell Biol* **9**:4903, 1989.

82. Amler LC, Schwab M: Multiple amplicons of discrete sizes encompassing N-myc in neuroblastoma cells evolve through differential recombination from a large precursor DNA. *Oncogene* **7**:807, 1992.

83. Schneider SS, Hiemstra JL, Zehnbauer BA, Taillon-Miller P, Le Paslier D, Vogelstein B, Brodeur GM: Isolation and structural analysis of a 1.2-megabase N-myc amplicon from a human neuroblastoma. *Mol Cell Biol* **12**:5563, 1992.

84. Corvi R, Amler LC, Savelyeva L, Gehring M, Schwab M: MYCN is retained in single copy at chromosome 2 band p23-24 during amplification in human neuroblastoma cells. *Proc Natl Acad Sci USA* **91**:5523, 1994.

85. Brodeur GM, Seeger RC: Gene amplification in human neuroblastomas: Basic mechanisms and clinical implications. *Cancer Genet Cytogenet* **19**:101, 1986.

86. Corvi R, Savelyeva L, Schwab M: Duplication of N-MYC at its resident site 2p24 may be a mechanism of activation alternative to amplification in human neuroblastoma cells. *Cancer Res* **55**:3471, 1995.

87. Kanda N, Schreck R, Alt F, Bruns G, Baltimore D, Latt S: Isolation of amplified DNA sequences from IMR-32 human neuroblastoma cells: Facilitation by fluorescence-activated flow sorting of metaphase chromosomes. *Proc Natl Acad Sci USA* **80**:4069, 1983.

88. Shiloh Y, Korf B, Kohl NE, Sakai K, Brodeur GM, Harris P, Kanda N, Seeger RC, Alt F, Latt SA: Amplification and rearrangement of DNA sequences from the chromosomal region 2p24 in human neuroblastomas. *Cancer Res* **46**:5297, 1986.

89. Hunt JD, Valentine M, Tereba A: Excision of N-myc from chromosome 2 in human neuroblastoma cells containing amplified N-myc sequences. *Mol Cell Biol* **10**:823, 1990.

90. Kinzler KW, Zehnbauer BA, Brodeur GM, Seeger RC, Trent JM, Meltzer PS, Vogelstein B: Amplification units containing human N-myc and c-myc genes. *Proc Natl Acad Sci USA* **83**:1031, 1986.

91. Zehnbauer BA, Small D, Brodeur GM, Seeger R, Vogelstein B: Characterization of N-myc amplification units in human neuroblastoma cells. *Mol Cell Biol* **8**:522, 1988.

92. Schneider SS, Zehnbauer BA, Vogelstein B, Brodeur GM: Yeast artificial chromosome (YAC) vector cloning of the *MYCN* amplified domain in human neuroblastomas. *Progr Clin Biol Res* **366**:71, 1991.

93. Reiter JL, Kuroda H, White PS, Schneider-Thabet SS, Taillon-Miller P, Brodeur GM: Physical mapping of the normal and amplified *MYCN* locus. *Genomics*, Submitted, 1999.

94. Reiter JL, Brodeur GM: High-resolution mapping of a 130-kb core region of the MYCN amplicon in neuroblastomas. *Genomics* **32**:97, 1996.

95. Godbout R, Squire J: Amplification of a DEAD box protein in retinoblastoma cell lines. *Proc Natl Acad Sci USA* **90**:7578, 1993.

96. Squire JA, Thorner PS, Weitzman S, Maggi JD, Dirks P, Doyle J, Hale M, Godbout R: Co-amplification of *MYCN* and a DEAD box gene (*DDX1*) in primary neuroblastoma. *Oncogene* **10**:1417, 1995.

97. Noguchi T, Akiyama K, Yokoyama M, Kanda N, Matsunaga T, Nishi Y: Amplification of a DEAD box gene (*DDX1*) with the *MYCN* gene in neuroblastomas as a result of cosegregation of sequences flanking the *MYCN* locus. *Genes Chrom Cancer* **15**:129, 1996.

98. Amler LC, Shurmann J, Schwab M: The DDX1 gene maps within 400 kbp 5' to MYCN and is frequently coamplified in human neuroblastoma. *Genes Chrom Cancer* **15**:134, 1996.

99. George RE, Kenyon RM, McGuckin AG, Malcolm AJ, Pearson AD, Lunec J: Investigation of co-amplification of the candidate genes ornithine decarboxylase, ribonucleotide reductase, syndecan-1 and a DEAD box gene, DDX1, with N-myc in neuroblastoma. United Kingdom Children's Cancer Study Group. *Oncogene* **12**:1583, 1996.

100. Kuroda H, White PS, Sulman EP, Manohar CF, Reiter JL, Cohn SL, Brodeur GM: Physical mapping of the DDX1 gene 340 kb 5' of MYCN. *Oncogene* **13**:156, 1996.

101. George RE, Thomas H, McGuckin AG, Angus B, Pearson AD, Lunec J: The DDX1 gene which is frequently co-amplified with MYCN in neuroblastoma is itself oncogenic. *Med Pediatr Oncol* (In press), 2000.

102. Jiang W, Kahn SM, Tomita N, Zhang YL, Lu SH, Weinstein IB: Amplification and expression of the human cyclin D gene in esophageal cancer. *Cancer Res* **52**:2980, 1992.

103. Nishida N, Fukuda Y, Komeda T, Kita R, Sando T, Furukawa M, Amenomori M, Shibagaki I, Nakao K, Ikenaga M: Amplification and overexpression of the cyclin D1 gene in aggressive human hepatocellular carcinoma. *Cancer Res* **54**:3107, 1994.

104. Zhang YJ, Jiang W, Chen CJ, Lee CS, Kahn SM, Santella RM, Weinstein IB: Amplification and overexpression of cyclin D1 in human hepatocellular carcinoma. *Biochem Biophys Res Commun* **196**:1010, 1993.

105. Gaudray P, Szepetowski P, Escot C, Birnbaum D, Theillet C: DNA amplification at 11q13 in human cancer: From complexity to perplexity. *Mutat Res* **276**:317, 1992.

106. Berner J-M, Forus A, Elkahloun A, Meltzer PS, Fodstad Ø, Myklebost O: Separate amplified regions encompassing CDK4 and MDM2 in human sarcomas. *Genes Chrom Cancer* **17**:254, 1996.

107. Elkahloun AG, Bittner M, Hoskins K, Gemmill R, Meltzer PS: Molecular cytogenetic characterization and physical mapping of 12q13-15 amplification in human cancers. *Genes Chrom Cancer* **17**:205, 1996.

108. Reifenberger G, Ichimura K, Reifenberger J, Elkahloun AG, Meltzer PS, Collins VP: Refined mapping of 12q13-15 amplicons in human malignant gliomas suggests CDK4/SAS an MDM2 as independent amplification targets. *Cancer Res* **56**:5141, 1996.

109. Maelandsmo GM, Berner JM, Florenes VA, Forus A, Hovig E, Fodstad Ø, Myklebost O: Homozygous deletion frequency and expression levels of the CDKN2 gene in human sarcomas—relationship to amplification and mRNA levels of CDK4 and CCND1. *Br J Cancer* **72**:393, 1995.

110. Leach FS, Tokino T, Meltzer P, Burrell M, Oliner JD, Smith S, Hill DE, Sidransky D, Kinzler KW, Vogelstein B: p53 mutation and MDM2 amplification in human soft tissue sarcomas. *Cancer Res* **53**:2231, 1993.

111. Florenes VA, Maelandsmo GM, Forus A, Andreassen A, Myklebost O, Fodstad Ø: MDM2 gene amplification and transcript levels in human sarcomas: relationship to TP53 gene status [see comments]. *J Natl Cancer Inst* **86**:1297, 1994.

112. Kanoe H, Nakayama T, Murakami H, Hosaka T, Yamamoto H, Nakashima Y, Tsuboyama T, Nakamura T, Sasaki MS, Toguchida J: Amplification of the CDK4 gene in sarcomas: Tumor specificity and relationship with the RB gene mutation. *Anticancer Res* **18**:2317, 1998.

113. Blackwood EM, Eisenman RN: Max: a helix-loop-helix zipper protein that forms a sequence-specific DNA-binding complex with Myc. *Science* **251**:1211, 1991.

114. Makela TP, Koskinen P, Vastrik I, Alitalo K: Alternative forms of Max as enhancers or suppressors of Myc-Ras cotransformation. *Science* **256**:373, 1992.

115. Reddy CD, Dasgupta P, Saikumar P, Dudek H, Rauscher FJ III, Reddy EP: Mutational analysis of Max: Role of basic, helix-loop-helix/leucine zipper domains in DNA binding, dimerization and regulation of Myc-mediated transcriptional activation. *Oncogene* **7**:2085, 1992.

116. Kretzner L, Blackwood EM, Eisenman RN: Myc and Max proteins possess distinct transcriptional activities. *Nature* **359**:426, 1992.

117. Amati B, Dalton S, Brooks MW, Littlewood TD, Evan GI, Land H: Transcriptional activation by the human c-Myc oncoprotein in yeast requires interaction with Max. *Nature* **359**:423, 1992.

118. Amati B, Brooks MW, Levy N, Littlewood TD, Evan GI, Land H: Oncogenic activity of the c-Myc protein requires dimerization with Max. *Cell* **72**:233, 1993.

119. Grandori C, Eisenman RN: Myc target genes. *Trends Biochem Sci* **22**:177, 1997.

120. Bar-Sagi D: Ras proteins: Biological effects and biochemical targets [review]. *Anticancer Res* **9**:1427, 1989.

121. Hall A: The cellular functions of small GTP-binding proteins. *Science* **249**:635, 1990.

122. Medema RH, Boss JL: The role of p21ras in receptor tyrosine kinase signaling. *Crit Rev Oncogenes* **4**:615, 1993.

123. Marshall CJ: The ras oncogenes. *J Cell Sci (Suppl)* **10**:157, 1988.

124. Field JK, Spandidos DA: The role of ras and myc oncogenes in human solid tumours and their relevance in diagnosis and prognosis [review]. *Anticancer Res* **10**:1, 1990.

125. Bos JL: Ras oncogenes in human cancer: A review. *Cancer Res* **49**:4682, 1989.

126. Bishop JM: Molecular themes in oncogenesis. *Cell* **64**:235, 1991.

127. Ullrich A, Schlessinger J: Signal transduction by receptors with tyrosine kinase activity. *Cell* **61**:203, 1990.

128. Tokunaga A, Masahiko O, Okuda T, Teramoto T, Fujita I, Mizutani T, Keyama T, Yoshiyuki T, Nishi K, Matsukura N: Clinical significance of epidermal growth factor (EGF), EGF receptor, and c-erbB-2 in human gastric cancer. *Cancer (Suppl)* **75**:1418, 1995.

129. Hamburger AW, White CP, Brown RW: Effect of epidermal growth factor on proliferation of human tumor cells in soft agar. *J Natl Cancer Inst* **67**:825, 1981.

130. Hartwell L: Defects in a cell cycle checkpoint may be responsible for the genomic instability of cancer cells. *Cell* **71**:543, 1992.

131. Sherr CJ: Mammalian G1 cyclins. *Cell* **73**:1059, 1993.

132. Wasson JC, Brodeur GM: Molecular analysis of gene amplification in tumors, in NC Dracopoli, JL Haines, BR Korf, DT Moir, CC Morton, CE Seidman, JG Seidman, DR Smith (eds): *Current Protocols in Human Genetics*. New York: Greene Publishing and John Wiley & Sons, 1994, p. 10.5.1.

133. Shapiro DN, Valentine MB, Rowe ST, Sinclair AE, Sublett JE, Roberts WM, Look AT: Detection of N-myc gene amplification by fluorescence in situ hybridization. Diagnostic utility for neuroblastoma. *Am J Pathol* **142**:1339, 1993.

134. Misra DN, Dickman PS, Yunis EJ: Fluorescence in situ hybridization (FISH) detection of MYCN oncogene amplification in neuroblastoma using paraffin-embedded tissues. *Diag Mol Pathol* **4**:128, 1995.

135. Guan X-Y, Meltzer PS, Dalton WS, Trent JM: Identification of cryptic sites of DNA sequence amplification in human breast cancer by chromosome microdissection. *Nature Genet* **8**:155, 1994.

136. Crabbe DC, Peters J, Seeger RC: Rapid detection of MYCN gene amplification in neuroblastomas using the polymerase chain reaction. *Diag Mol Pathol* **1**:229, 1992.

137. Gilbert J, Norris MD, Haber M, Kavallaris M, Marshall GM, Stewart BW: Determination of N-myc gene amplification in neuroblastoma by differential polymerase chain reaction. *Mol Cell Probes* **7**:227, 1993.

138. Huddart SN, Mann JR, McGukin AG, Corbett R: MYCN amplification by differential PCR. *Pediatr Hematol Oncol* **10**:31, 1993.

139. Boerner S, Squire J, Thorner P, McKenna G, Zielenska M: Assessment of MYCN amplification in neuroblastoma biopsies by differential polymerase chain reaction. *Pediatr Pathol* **14**:823, 1994.

140. Kallioniemi A, Kallioniemi O-P, Sudar D, Rutovitz D, Gray JW, Waldman F, Pinkel D: Comparative genomic hybridization for molecular cytogenetic analysis of solid tumors. *Science* **258**:818, 1992.

141. Kallioniemi A, Kallioniemi O-P, Piper J, Tanner M, Stokke T, Chen L, Smith HS, Pinkel D, Gray JW, Waldman FM: Detection and mapping of amplified DNA sequences in breast cancer by comparative genomic hybridization. *Proc Natl Acad Sci USA* **91**:2156, 1994.

142. Ried T, Peterson I, Holtgreve-Grez H, Speicher MR, Schrock E, du Manoir S, Cremer T: Mapping of multiple DNA gains and losses in primary small cell lung carcinomas by comparative genomic hybridization. *Cancer Res* **54**:1801, 1994.

143. Shalon D, Smith SJ, Brown PO: DNA microarray system for analyzing complex DNA samples using two-color fluorescent probe hybridization. *Genome Res* **6**:639, 1996.

144. DeRisi J, Penland L, Brown PO, Bittner ML, Meltzer PS, Ray M, Chen Y, Su YA, Trent JM: Use of a cDNA microarray to analyse gene expression patterns in human cancer. *Nature Genet* **14**:457, 1996.

145. Hacia JG, Brody LC, Chee MS, Fodor SPA, Collins FS: Detection of heterozygous mutations in BRCA1 using high-density oligonucleotide arrays and two-colour fluorescence analysis. *Nature Genet* **14**:441, 1996.

146. Bieche I, Champeme MH, Lidereau R: A tumor suppressor gene on chromosome 1p32-pter controls the amplification of MYC family genes in breast cancer. *Cancer Res* **54**:4274, 1994.

147. Ocadiz R, Sauceda R, Cruz M, Graef AM, Gariglio P: High correlation between molecular alterations of the c-myc oncogene and carcinoma of the uterine cervix. *Cancer Res* **47**:4173, 1987.

148. Mitra AB, Murty VV, Pratap M, Sodhani P, Chaganti RS: ERBB2 (HER2/neu) oncogene is frequently amplified in squamous cell carcinoma of the uterine cervix. *Cancer Res* **54**:637, 1994.

149. He J, Zhang RG, Zhu D: Clinical significance of c-myc gene in esophageal squamous cell carcinoma. *Chung Hua I Hsueh Tsa Chih* **75**:94, 1995.

150. Momand J, Jung D, Wilczynski S, Niland J: The MDM2 gene amplification database. *Nucleic Acids Res* **26**:3453, 1998.

151. Torp SH, Helseth E, Ryan L, Stolan S, Dalen A, Unsgaard G: Amplification of the epidermal growth factor receptor gene in human gliomas. *Anticancer Res* **11**:2095, 1991.

152. Bigner SH, Wong AJ, Mark J, Muhlbaier LH, Kinzler KW, Vogelstein B, Bigner DD: Relationship between gene amplification and chromosomal deviations in malignant human gliomas. *Cancer Genet Cytogenet* **29**:165, 1987.

153. Galanis E, Buckner J, Kimmel D, Jenkins R, Alderete B, O'Fallon J, Wang CH, Scheithauer BW, James CD: Gene amplification as a prognostic factor in primary and secondary high-grade malignant gliomas. *Int J Oncol* **13**:717, 1998.

154. Baker VV, Borst MP, Dixon D, Hatch KD, Shingleton HM, Miller D: c-myc amplification in ovarian cancer. *Gynecol Oncol* **38**:340, 1990.

155. Bast RCJ, Boyer CM, Jacobs I, Xu FJ, Wu S, Wiener J, Kohler M, Berchuck A: Cell growth regulation in epithelial ovarian cancer. *Cancer* **71**:1597, 1993.

Tumor Genome Instability

Daniel P. Cahill ■ *Christoph Lengauer*

Genetic instability has long been recognized as a cardinal feature of neoplasia.[1,2] However, the causal role of genetic instability in the formation of cancer has only more recently been studied. Accumulating evidence has strengthened the proposal that genetic instability is required early during tumor progression. Instability drives mutations in oncogenes and tumor suppressor genes, providing the tumor cell with a selective growth advantage.[3] While numerous oncogenes and tumor suppressor genes have been identified in the last 20 years, the molecular details underlying genetic instability are just now being revealed.

The clearest molecular evidence for the genetic instability hypothesis comes from the elucidation of the genes causing hereditary nonpolyposis colon cancer (HNPCC). Patients with HNPCC have an increased risk of tumor development over the course of their lifetime but do not display the widespread changes in the at-risk tissue cellular architecture characteristic of other inherited tumor syndromes, for instance, the thousands of polyps in familial adenomatous polyposis (FAP). Instead, they typically develop a single advanced primary tumor at an atypically young age (see Chap. 18 on HNPCC).

Indeed, the tissue specificity is even more of a mystery upon consideration of the underlying genetic defect in these patients. They inherit a mutation in one of the mismatch repair (MMR) genes, such as *MSH2, MLH1, PMS1, PMS2,* or *GTBP(MSH6).*[4–11] Unlike classical tumor suppressor genes such as *p53* or *Rb*, the MMR genes do not directly affect the growth or death of a tumor cell.[12] Experimentally, this distinction can be seen upon reintroduction of a MMR gene into a tumor cell that has two mutant copies. In contrast to reintroduction of a classical tumor suppressor, there is no effect on the tumor cell growth or death.[13]

Instead, the loss of MMR genes imbues these tumors with an elevated nucleotide mutation rate — 2 to 3 orders of magnitude higher than normal cells or MMR-proficient cancers of the same cell type[14–16]. Thus, there is an increased rate of mutation at oncogene and tumor suppressor loci throughout the tumor cell genome. This link between isolated cellular genetic instability and organism-wide tumorigenesis is strong evidence for the genetic instability hypothesis, as sequence instability alone is able to drive the autosomal dominant inheritance of colorectal neoplasia in these families (Fig. 7-1).

Defects of another major DNA repair system have been documented in tumors as well. Nucleotide-excision repair (NER) is responsible for repairing damage caused by many exogenous mutagens.[17] Mutations in one of several different NER genes result in xeroderma pigmentosum and related disorders. Patients with these autosomal recessive, inherited diseases develop numerous skin tumors in sun-exposed areas (see also Chap. 14 on xeroderma pigmentosum).[18,19] Surprisingly, skin tumors represent the major tumor type to which patients with NER defects are susceptible, and the incidence of internal cancers in these patients is not raised to the same degree[20–22]. The simplest

explanation for these results is that ultraviolet light is the major mutagen that results in NER-correctable DNA damage to which humans are exposed (Fig. 7-1).[20–22]

However, there is a more pervasive genomic abnormality of sporadic tumors. Virtually all epithelial solid tumors have structural and numeric chromosome variation — they are aneuploid.[23] The only exceptions are, strikingly, the MMR deficient tumors, which remain diploid throughout tumor progression. Such observations have led to the suggestion that cancers require instability either at the sequence level or at the chromosomal level, but not generally at both levels.[24] This logic would posit that one form of instability is sufficient to drive tumorigenesis. Consistent with this hypothesis, aneuploidy can be found in the earliest neoplastic lesions, such as benign adenomas of the colon, and the accumulation of aneuploid cells is a classic finding in advanced stages of tumorigenesis.[25–28]

Recent analysis has shown that cancer cell aneuploidy is a reflection of an underlying chromosomal instability (CIN).[29] Quantitative studies of aneuploid tumor cell divisions have demonstrated that the chromosomal abnormalities in these cells are the result of an intrinsic segregation instability.[30] This observation gave rise to the proposal that CIN could be considered the primary class of instability required for neoplastic progression in the majority of tumors.

The causes of CIN underlying the widespread aneuploid phenotype are just beginning to be investigated. One theory posits that karyotypic instability in cancer is a truism; it is a natural side effect of the malignant transformation process, driven by the preceding mutations in growth-controlling oncogenes and tumor suppressor genes such as *ras* or *p53*.

However, the existence of karyotypically stable MMR-deficient tumors argues against a causal role for classical oncogenes and tumor suppressors in the CIN phenotype. These tumors have mutations in the same oncogenes and tumor suppressor genes as CIN tumors, and have similar stage-specific growth and progression characteristics, but are not aneuploid. These cases prove that the mutant genes driving advanced neoplastic progression do not inevitability generate or require aneuploidy.

At the other end of the spectrum, a different theory proposes that aneuploidy is not caused by specific genetic alterations but instead results from the altered cellular architecture that ensues whenever an abnormal chromosome complement is present within cells. Thus, a chance abnormal division in an otherwise normal cell gives rise to a karyotypically abnormal daughter cell with a selective growth advantage compared to its neighbors. The abnormal number of chromosomes in this cell destabilizes the segregation machinery, auto-catalyzing chromosome missegregation and further aneuploidy. Aneuploidy begets aneuploidy.[31]

There is some recent evidence to support an alternative to these hypotheses. Perhaps aneuploid tumors sustain an early mutational event in a chromosome stability gene that drives chromosomal instability (Fig. 7-1). In some tumors, CIN has been proposed to be driven by mutations in mitotic checkpoint genes.[30,32,33] For the

Pathways to Genetic Instability

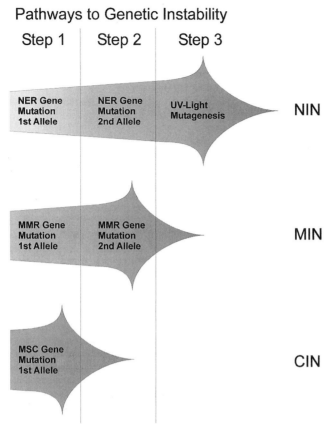

Fig. 7-1 Pathways to genetic instability. Different types of genetic instability require a different number of mutational "hits" in order to engender the respective instability phenotype. In a heterozygote with one defective nucleotide excision repair (NER) allele (step 1), inactivation of the normal allele (step 2) does not immediately lead to mutations. It additionally requires exposure to an environmental agent (i.e., ultraviolet light) (step 3) to create large numbers of mutations (NER-related instability; NIN). In contrast, in a heterozygote with one defective mismatch repair (MMR) allele (step 1), all that is required to begin to develop mutations at a high rate (microsatellite instability; MIN) is the inactivation of the normal allele inherited from the unaffected parent (step 2). Cell fusion and other experiments suggest that chromosomal instability (CIN) can have a dominant quality.[29] One example of a gene that can be mutated in a dominant negative manner to cause CIN is *hBub1*, a component of the mitotic spindle checkpoint (MSC).[30] It apparently requires only a single mutational "hit" of such a gene to engender the CIN phenotype.

majority of tumors, however, the molecular basis of CIN is not known yet. This is an area of active investigation. Many of the known inherited tumor suppressor genes seem to play an important role in genome stability but their mechanistic relationship to genome instability is poorly understood (see chapters 15, 16, 33 and 23 on *ATM, BLM, BRCA1/BRCA2* and *p53*, respectively). It will be interesting to see how many instability genes can be shown to be altered in sporadic cancers.

REFERENCES

1. Loeb LA: Mutator phenotype may be required for multistage carcinogenesis. *Cancer Res* **51**:3075, 1991.
2. Hartwell L: Defects in a cell cycle checkpoint may be responsible for the genomic instability of cancer cells. *Cell* **71**:543, 1992.
3. Lengauer C, Kinzler KW, Vogelstein B: Genetic instabilities in human cancers. *Nature* **396**:643, 1998.
4. Modrich P: Mismatch repair, genetic stability and tumour avoidance. *Philos Trans R Soc Lond B Biol Sci* **347**:89, 1995.
5. Kunkel TA: DNA-mismatch repair. The intricacies of eukaryotic spell-checking. *Curr Biol* **5**:1091, 1995.
6. Peltomaki P, de la Chapelle A: Mutations predisposing to hereditary nonpolyposis colorectal cancer. *Adv Cancer Res* **71**:93, 1997.
7. Sia EA, Jinks-Robertson S, Petes TD: Genetic control of microsatellite stability. *Mutat Res* **383**:61, 1997.
8. Fishel R, Lescoe MK, Rao MR, et al.: The human mutator gene homolog MSH2 and its association with hereditary nonpolyposis colon cancer. *Cell* **75**:1027, 1993.
9. Leach FS, Nicolaides NC, Papadopoulos N, et al.: Mutations of a mutS homolog in hereditary nonpolyposis colorectal cancer. *Cell* **75**:1215, 1993.
10. Bronner CE, Baker SM, Morrison PT, et al.: Mutation in the DNA mismatch repair gene homologue hMLH1 is associated with hereditary non-polyposis colon cancer. *Nature* **368**:258, 1994.
11. Papadopoulos N, Nicolaides NC, Wei YF, et al.: Mutation of a mutL homolog in hereditary colon cancer. *Science* **263**:1625, 1994.
12. Kinzler KW, Vogelstein B: Cancer-susceptibility genes. Gatekeepers and caretakers. *Nature* **386**:761, 1997.
13. Koi M, Umar A, Chauhan DP, et al.: Human chromosome 3 corrects mismatch repair deficiency and microsatellite instability and reduces N-methyl-N'-nitro-N-nitrosoguanidine tolerance in colon tumor cells with homozygous hMLH1 mutation. *Cancer Res* **54**:4308, 1994.
14. Parsons R, Li GM, Longley MJ, et al.: Hypermutability and mismatch repair deficiency in RER+ tumor cells. *Cell* **75**:1227, 1993.
15. Bhattacharyya NP, Skandalis A, Ganesh A, Groden J, Meuth M: Mutator phenotypes in human colorectal carcinoma cell lines. *Proc Natl Acad Sci U S A* **91**:6319, 1994.
16. Eshleman JR, Lang EZ, Bowerfind GK, et al.: Increased mutation rate at the hprt locus accompanies microsatellite instability in colon cancer. *Oncogene* **10**:33, 1995.
17. Wood RD: DNA repair in eukaryotes. *Annu Rev Biochem* **65**:135, 1996.
18. De Weerd-Kastelein EA, Keijzer W, Bootsma D: Genetic heterogeneity of xeroderma pigmentosum demonstrated by somatic cell hybridization. *Nat New Biol* **238**:80, 1972.
19. Bootsma D, Kraemer KH, Cleaver JE, Hoeijmakers JHJ: Nucleotide excision repair syndromes: xeroderma pigmentosum, Cockayne syndrome, and trichothiodystrophy, in Kinzler KW, Vogelstein B, (eds): *The Genetic Basis of Human Cancer.* New York, McGraw-Hill, 1998, p 245–274.
20. Cairns J: The origin of human cancers. *Nature* **289**:353, 1981.
21. Feinberg AP, Coffey DS: Organ site specificity for cancer in chromosomal instability disorders. *Cancer Res* **42**:3252, 1982.
22. Kraemer KH, Lee MM, Scotto J: DNA repair protects against cutaneous and internal neoplasia: evidence from xeroderma pigmentosum. *Carcinogenesis* **5**:511, 1984.
23. Mitelman F: *Catalog of Chromosome Aberrations in Cancer.* Wiley-Liss, 1991.
24. Cahill DP, Kinzler KW, Vogelstein B, Lengauer C: Genetic instability and darwinian selection in tumours. *Trends Cell Biol* **9**:M57, 1999.
25. Auer GU, Heselmeyer KM, Steinbeck RG, Munck-Wikland E, Zetterberg AD: The relationship between aneuploidy and p53 overexpression during genesis of colorectal adenocarcinoma. *Virchows Arch* **424**:343, 1994.
26. Bardi G, Parada LA, Bomme L, et al.: Cytogenetic comparisons of synchronous carcinomas and polyps in patients with colorectal cancer. *Br J Cancer* **76**:765, 1997.
27. Silverstein MJ: *Ductal Carcinoma in Situ of the Breast.* Baltimore, Williams & Wilkins, 1997.
28. Bomme L, Bardi G, Pandis N, Fenger C, Kronborg O, Heim S: Cytogenetic analysis of colorectal adenomas: karyotypic comparisons of synchronous tumors. *Cancer Genet Cytogenet* **106**:66, 1998.
29. Lengauer C, Kinzler KW, Vogelstein B: Genetic instability in colorectal cancers. *Nature* **386**:623, 1997.
30. Cahill DP, Lengauer C, Yu J, et al.: Mutations of mitotic checkpoint genes in human cancers. *Nature* **392**:300, 1998.
31. Duesberg P, Rausch C, Rasnick D, Hehlmann R: Genetic instability of cancer cells is proportional to their degree of aneuploidy. *Proc Natl Acad Sci U S A* **95**:13692, 1998.
32. Li Y, Benezra R: Identification of a human mitotic checkpoint gene: hsMAD2. *Science* **274**:246, 1996.
33. Jin DY, Spencer F, Jeang KT: Human T cell leukemia virus type 1 oncoprotein Tax targets the human mitotic checkpoint protein MAD1. *Cell* **93**:81, 1998.

CHAPTER 8

Gene Expression Profiling in Cancer

Gregory J. Riggins ■ *Patrice J. Morin*

1. **Gene expression profiling is a powerful new approach for viewing the expression of many genes simultaneously in different types of malignant or normal cells. Using computational approaches, differentially expressed genes or informative patterns of expressed genes are mined from large data sets produced by new expression profiling technology. This technology yields the opportunity to classify tumors by gene expression and to locate genes of diagnostic or therapeutic importance.**
2. **DNA array technology uses thousands of DNA fragments arrayed on a solid surface in order to probe many messenger ribonucleic acid (mRNA) levels in one experiment. Both oligonucleotides and portions of complementary deoxyribonucleic acid (cDNA) are used as hybridization probes on the arrays. Clustering and other statistical based algorithms are used to locate patterns of gene expression of importance when analyzing large numbers of RNA samples.**
3. **Serial Analysis of Gene Expression (SAGE) is a sequencing based technology that provides an in-depth quantitative assessment of gene expression. SAGE works by counting transcripts and storing digital values electronically, providing absolute gene expression levels that make historical comparisons and databasing facile. It is useful for studying small numbers of tissue or cellular samples derived from well-controlled experiments.**
4. **Gene expression profiling techniques have been used to obtain global gene expression patterns from several common malignancies and corresponding normal tissues. These studies highlight the potential of gene expression profiling in cancer taxonomy, and in the identification of molecular targets for diagnosis and therapy.**
5. **Gene expression profiling has been used in the dissection of specific oncogenic molecular pathways, including the p53 tumor-suppressor pathway, the APC/β-catenin pathway, and numerous *in vitro* and *in vivo* models of angiogenesis and cancer drug resistance.**

The ability to determine gene expression levels from thousands of genes simultaneously has recently transformed many aspects of cancer research. Large-scale gene expression profiling provides a powerful means to create an overall view of how the genome provides instructions to the cell. Ultimately, the genetic background, mutations, environment, and history of the cell all impact on mRNA and subsequent protein expression. Unlike the positional-cloning approaches that during the last decade revealed the genes mutated during oncogenesis, gene expression profiling does not directly reveal cancer-causing genes, but the pattern of genes used by the malignant (or normal) cell. These patterns, and the differentially expressed genes found within these patterns, have a variety of important uses for improved clinical correlation or therapy design. This chapter reviews the major mRNA profiling techniques and how they are applied to the study of cancer.

Technology advances make research advances possible. Just as the invention of the first compound microscope allowed biologists to view cellular patterns in tissues, the recent advent of gene expression technologies allows the biologist to observe molecular patterns in cells. Although protein levels are the ultimate goal for many uses, large numbers of protein levels cannot be assayed as rapidly as RNA, and this chapter is mostly limited to reviewing RNA profiling methods. High-throughput RNA expression-profiling techniques can be broadly divided into two categories: methods that count transcripts using DNA sequencing and methods that are based on DNA hybridization.

Sequencing is used for profiling to count transcripts from a cDNA library. The relative levels of mRNA can be preserved when reverse-transcribed into cDNA and cloned into a collection of plasmids forming a cDNA library. Automated DNA sequencing[1,2] makes it possible to infer RNA levels of many genes by sequencing cDNA molecules, or fragments of cDNAs, in large numbers.

Alternatively, one can discriminate between different mRNA transcripts by hybridization to a nucleic acid probe of known sequence. Hybridization can be used to either detect mRNA levels by arraying the gene-specific probes on a solid surface, or to subtract sequences from a sample followed by detection of the remaining sequence. By containing many probes arrayed into a small area, DNA Arrays[3–5] can be used to detect thousands of genes simultaneously. Advanced computational methods enable biologists to look for genes with significant differences in expression, or those genes that cluster according to a particular feature.

Collectively all of the expressed mRNA transcripts from a cell are known as the "transcriptome." Significant portions of the transcriptome can be assayed for a given cell population, but the large data sets that are produced by these technologies create new challenges. Expression profiling requires the ability to database and effectively interpret this information. Sophisticated computational and statistical approaches, either new or derived from approaches formally applied to the physical sciences, are now required to interpret the datasets. Other bioinformatics approaches are necessary to draw on the vast and growing archive of information available through public databases or the biomedical literature. Correlating expression levels in malignant cells with the information derived from the recently sequenced human genome is a particularly important example. The genome sequence provides a catalyst for "functional genomic" approaches, such as RNA expression profiling.

Although gene expression profiling techniques are far from reaching their full potential, there have already been several important applications of the technology. Expression profiling has been a useful means for finding the cancer-related genes whose expression levels are dependent on a known oncogene or by the loss of a tumor suppressor. RNA profiling has also been successfully applied to locating cell-type specific genes or gene-expression changes that depend on environmental factors, including drug or hormonal exposures. Even without knowing

Table 8-1 Key Features of Common RNA Profiling Techniques

	Differential Display	DNA Arrays	SAGE
Basis of assay	cDNA fragments compared on gel	Hybridization to spotted DNA	Sequence ligated cDNA tags
Detection method	Electrophoresis of labeled fragments	Optical imaging of hybridization signal	Automated sequencer
Gene identification	Excise band and sequence	DNA probes preidentified	Match SAGE tag to database(s)
Transcript quantification	Comparison of band intensities	Analogue fluorescent signal from DNA spot	Digital counts of SAGE tags
Probe requirements	Starting RNA only	Requires set of arrayed DNA probes	Starting RNA only.
Starting amounts of RNA (approx.)	>5 μg of total RNA	>5 μg of total RNA	>1 μg of total RNA
Number of RNA samples that can be processed per month	Few	Many	Few
Number of genes assayed per sample	Few	Equal to the number of genes on the array	Most all genes expressed above the detection limit
Sensitivity of transcript detection	Higher levels easier to detect	~10 mRNA copies/cell	Dependent on number of tags sequenced

the function of the genes detected by profiling, the overall pattern of genes has been used to help classify tumors by malignant potential or response to therapy. Expression profiling holds the promise of revealing a much more complete picture of the molecular pathways within the malignant cell. However, this data is only the first step for better understanding, diagnosis, and treatment of cancer.

TECHNIQUES FOR EXPRESSION PROFILING

Many techniques have been developed to find those transcripts whose expression level changes between two samples. The first techniques to be widely used to find differentially expressed transcripts were subtractive hybridization and differential display methods. Both could identify transcripts but do not have the same capacity to assay multiple samples like DNA arrays, nor do they provide an in-depth transcriptome characterization of sequencing-based techniques. For this reason, DNA arrays and SAGE are currently the most widely used for transcript profiling of malignant cells. This is, however, a rapidly evolving field. The overview of the features of common RNA profiling techniques (Table 8-1) will likely require significant updating in the not so distant future.

Subtraction Methods

Various methods have been derived to find transcripts that are differentially expressed between two different cell populations.[6] Subtractive hybridization is used to produce a cDNA library that has sequences that are present in one sample of RNA, but not another.[7,8] A typical example is to subtract tumor mRNA from normal mRNA (or *vice versa*) to find transcripts that may have been deleted or amplified in the process of tumor formation. The general approach is to hybridize in solution the two samples (normally cDNA) that are to be subtracted. An excess of one sample (the "driver") hybridizes to most all the unwanted common sequences from the other sample (the "tester" or "tracer"). Typically the driver is labeled in such a way that molecules containing one or both strands in common with the driver are removed or otherwise not cloned. The remaining cDNA consisting mostly of tracer can be cloned to form a library for further analysis such as sequencing.

Other subtractive methods used to find differentially expressed genes include suppression subtractive hybridization[9] and representation difference analysis (RDA).[10] These newer techniques incorporate polymerase chain reaction (PCR) amplification steps in order to work from smaller quantities of starting material. RDA is an effective way to compare two sets of DNA by hybridization

and subtraction, frequently either genomic DNA or cDNA. Overall, the subtractive techniques have been used to locate many important cancer-related genes, but these approaches necessitate a pair-wise analysis of samples and a time-consuming cloning step that make them unsuitable for automated high-throughput gene expression profiling.

Differential Display

In 1992, differential display was described as a method to locate differentially expressed transcripts.[11,12] Differential display works by first producing a set of cDNA fragments that have been identically prepared from each RNA sample, usually based on restriction enzyme digestion of the cDNA or by producing PCR products with arbitrary primers. Next, the fragments are resolved on a gel, producing a characteristic pattern of bands for each sample. The bands from each sample are compared to reveal those bands that differ in intensity between lanes. The cDNA fragment within the band can be excised for further analysis.

The advantage of differential display is that it is performed by one person using equipment available in most molecular biology laboratories. The disadvantage of this technique is that in order to identify most genes they must be excised and sequenced—requiring significant labor for the gene identification step. Also, the technique can be prone to false positives that arise from various factors, including PCR-induced amplification biases. Although there are many successful variations of the differential display approach,[13] differential display approaches do not allow for rapid and efficient identification of expression levels *en mass* that makes it suitable as a transcript "profiling" technique. It has, however, been very useful for identifying differentially expressed genes.

DNA Arrays

A method to detect nucleic acids of a specific sequence supported by a solid surface was developed over 25 years ago by Edwin M. Southern.[14] In 1992, cDNA fragments were arrayed on a solid surface in large numbers and used for parallel gene expression profiling.[5] The idea of large-scale transcript profiling captured the imagination of scientists starting in the mid 1990s, when methods were used to miniaturize DNA arrays;[3,4,15] introducing "chip technology" to biological research. DNA arrays have enormous potential and have an implicit promise that a reliable, low-cost, and standardized format for gene expression profiling will eventually be available to cancer and other researchers. By means of introduction, this section describes basic concepts and readers interested in applying chip technology should consult relevant publications[16–22] and Web sites (Table 8-2).

Table 8-2 Human Transcript Profiling Databases and Resources

Web Site	URL	Description
cDNA Library sequencing		
Body Map	bodymap.ims.u-tokyo.ac.jp	Expression resources for normal tissues based on cDNA library sequencing.
CGAP cDNA xProfiler	cgap.nci.nih.gov/CGAP/ Tissue s/xProfiler	Expression between pools of cDNA libraries can be compared based on extensive database.
DNA Arrays		
Affymetrix	www.affymetrix.com	Vendor of expression chips and other products for expression profiling via DNA arrays.
Brown Lab Homepage	cmgm.stanford.edu/pbrown	Contains useful information on custom cDNA arrays.
Developmental Therapeutics	www.dtp.nci.nih.gov	Microarray and drug response data for NCI 60 cell lines.
Genexpress - CNRS	idefix.upr420.vjf.cnrs.fr/EXPR/	Expression profile of 5,058 human genes by cDNA array.
Microarray Project	www.nhgri.nih.gov/DIR/ Microarray/	Protocols, descriptions and resources for cDNA Microarray technology from the NHGRI.
Molecular Oncology and Development	chroma.mbt.washington.edu/ mod_www/	Protocols and links for DNA arrays from Hood lab at University of Washington.
Molecular Pattern Recognition	waldo.wi.mit.edu/MPR	Protocols, links, software and downloads for DNA arrays from Whitehead/MIT.
UCSD Array Science	array.ucsd.edu	Information and Bioinformatics Tools for expression information.
SAGE		
SAGEmap	www.ncbi.nlm.nih.gov/SAGE	Large RNA expression database from CGAP based on SAGE profiles of malignant and normal cells.
SAGEnet (Johns Hopkins)	www.sagenet.org	SAGE database, protocols, references and links.
Genzyme Molecular Oncology	www.genzyme.com/sage/ welcome.htm	SAGE information and applications for commercial users of the technology.
Other		
Cancer Genome Anatomy Project (CGAP)	cgap.nci.nih.gov/	CGAP homepage with links to expression databases and cancer research resources.
Digital Gene Expression Displayer (DGED)	cgap.nci.nih.gov/CGAP/ Tissues/GXS	CGAP tool that compares gene expression between pools of SAGE and/or cDNA libraries.
Gene Expression Omnibus (GEO)	www.ncbi.nlm.nih.gov/geo	NCBI repository and comparison interface for all types of expression data.
Tissue Microarray Project	www.nhgri.nih.gov/ DIR/CGB/TMA	Protocols and information on tissue microarrays from the NHGRI.

cDNA Arrays. There are many variations of DNA arrays, but they can be viewed in two groups: those that array a fragment of cDNA and those that array a shorter synthetic DNA oligonucleotide. Arraying cDNAs on a membrane for hybridization with a labeled sample was the first DNA array approach (filter arrays), and it is still widely used today.[5,23] Typically, hundreds to thousands of cDNA fragments are amplified by PCR and spotted densely onto a membrane. An RNA or cDNA test sample is then radioactively labeled and hybridized to the targets on the membrane. Expression levels are accessed by the signal intensity produced by the amount of radioactivity hybridized to each probe on the membrane. Several molecular biology companies sell membranes to researchers for use in their studies and services for doing the hybridization and/or analyzing the results.

The technology of cDNA arrays took another leap forward when researchers at Stanford University started spotting cDNA onto glass slides at densities much greater than what could be achieved with nylon membranes.[4] The introduction of cDNA "microarrays" has opened the minds of scientists to the possibility that gene expression patterns could be routinely measured.[24] Robotics are employed for making these arrays that can reproducibly spot well over 5000 cDNAs on a single slide.[25] An additional advancement is the use of two-color hybridization (Fig. 8-1). Two different-colored fluorescent probes, typically red and green, are made from the test and control sample and hybridized to the same array. Each spot on the array is measured in terms of the expression ratio between probes, rather than an absolute level of expression. This approach helps to normalize array-to-array variations in hybridization or printing and provides a more accurate means of comparing expression between chips.

However, this approach does result in the loss of the absolute expression levels since a ratio is being measured. A variety of commercial enterprises make and cell cDNA arrays or services. Additionally most universities have, or are, developing some type of service that provides cDNA arrays technology to investigators.

Oligonucleotide Arrays. Oligonucleotides built on a glass support by photolithography and phosphoramidite DNA synthesis chemistry are commonly known as "DNA Chips."[15,26] This process builds a chip for DNA analysis in a method that is analogous to the mass production of semiconductor chips for the electronics industry. DNA Microchip technology has been developed and commercialized primarily by Affymetrix Corporation. Normally about 20 different oligonucleotides of approximately 20 base pairs (bp) in length are used to represent each gene on mRNA expression chips. The oligonucleotide sequences that represent a particular gene are chosen carefully using algorithms that have been designed to minimize cross-hybridization between different genes. After hybridization with a specially prepared and fluorescently labeled cDNA probe, the chip is read using a laser scanner. Currently, Affymetrix has produced a series of chips that will cover up to a total of 12,000 different known genes plus 48,000 sequences derived from expressed sequence tag (EST) clusters. Thus far, oligonucleotide chips have delivered a more standardized product than the cDNA spotted chips, along with a preoptimized and working infrastructure for array analysis, but at a cost. Although costs for chips have declined, they are still considerably more than glass slide systems.

Oligonucleotides for use in DNA arrays are not limited to Affymetrix chips. Longer oligonucleotides, typically more than

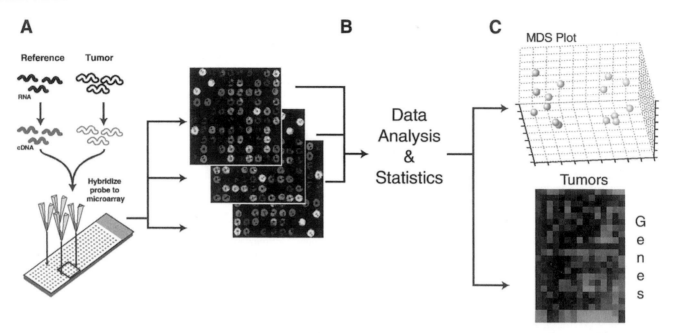

Fig. 8-1 Approach for expression profiling using a two-color cDNA chip. *A.* Two RNA samples are converted to cDNA and are labeled with different florescent dyes; the tumor sample is labeled red and the normal reference is labeled green. The labeled cDNA is hybridized to the DNA on the microarray. *B.* Each DNA spotted on the array is a cDNA fragment that represents a gene. The relative ratio of the gene at each spot is determined by the color after hybridization. Red spots are tumor greater than reference, green spots are tumor less than reference, and yellow spots indicate equal amounts of message. *C.* The signal is scanned in for each array and analyzed. The genes (or RNA samples) can be clustered by expression similarity, and expression can be represented in a multi-dimensional space (MDS) plot. (*Courtesy of Darryl Leja and Ashani Weeraratna from the laboratory of Jeffrey M. Trent, Laboratory of Cancer Genetics, National Human Genome Research Institute.*)

50 bp, can be arrayed by robotic spotting onto glass slides and used in place of PCR fragments amplified from a cDNA template. The choice of arrayed material and support is usually based on what is locally available. It is expected that as the technology continues to evolve, market competition will produce one or more dominant DNA array technologies that will deliver reliability and convenience at a reasonable cost.

cDNA Library Sequencing

Large-scale sequencing of cDNA libraries was first proposed as a rapid means to access transcribed regions from the human genome.[27] Random transcribed sequences generated by cDNA library sequencing are known as expressed sequence tags (ESTs). The Merck/Washington University EST project made one of the first large-scale efforts to disseminate EST sequence data.[28] The Cancer Genome Anatomy Project (CGAP)[29–31] succeeded this effort with its Tumor Gene Index, contributing more than one million ESTs from normal, premalignant, and malignant cells. The data from these projects has greatly reduced the time and effort necessary for many gene-cloning projects, but also serves to reveal which tissues express which transcripts.

Counting transcripts by EST sequencing is a very accurate way of accessing the fractional representation of each transcript, but it is a very expensive and laborious approach. Consequently, expression levels derived from EST data are normally derived from the large public EST sequencing projects. EST-based expression data can be accessed from many of these projects via the World Wide Web as described in the Bioinformatics section below (see Table 8-2 for Web sites). The main advantage of this data is that it is free and easily accessed. The main disadvantages are that the individual experimenter cannot practically generate his own EST data and that the level of detection is low, because often only a few thousand transcripts are assayed for each tissue or cell type, out of the tens of thousands expressed. One must also keep in mind that cDNA libraries used to generate EST data are frequently normalized or subtracted, and that data derived from these libraries can only reveal the presence of a transcript and not quantitative expression levels.

Serial Analysis of Gene Expression

SAGE was first developed in 1995,[32] as a means for efficient counting of mRNA transcripts in large numbers.[33–38] SAGE increases the number of genes that can be counted per sequencing reaction, as compared to cDNA library sequencing, by minimizing the portion of the transcript sequenced. The method (Fig. 8-2) works by cloning and sequencing a 10-bp portion of the cDNA at a defined position near the 3′ end of the transcript. These 10 base pairs, normally next to the last Nla III restriction site, are known as the transcript "tags." The transcript tags from a particular RNA sample are linked together and are cloned into a sequencing vector forming a SAGE library. Automated sequencing then produces tag sequences rapidly in large numbers by the sequencing of many clones simultaneously. Typically, more than 50,000 transcript tags can be counted, with about 2000 sequencing reactions. Although sequencing costs increase proportionally with the number of tags assayed, automated sequencing has increased in efficiency and speed. The SAGE transcript profile from various types of cells can be archived on a computer database and electronically compared to find statistically significant differences in gene expression between cell types. The gene responsible for the differentially expressed tag is identified using informatics or, in rare instances, cloned using the tag sequence. The majority of tags can be matched to a list of possibilities extracted from transcript databases such as the cDNA portion of GenBank,[34] the EST clusters forming the NCBI UniGene database,[39] and coding sequence extracted from the human genome sequence.

Because SAGE counts transcripts by sequencing and avoids the errors inherent in hybridization-based assays, it is often regarded as a very accurate means for expression profiling. SAGE transcript levels are expressed as a fraction of the total transcripts counted, not relative to another experiment or a housekeeping gene, avoiding error-prone normalization between experiments. The absolute nature of SAGE data makes cumulative data sets useful

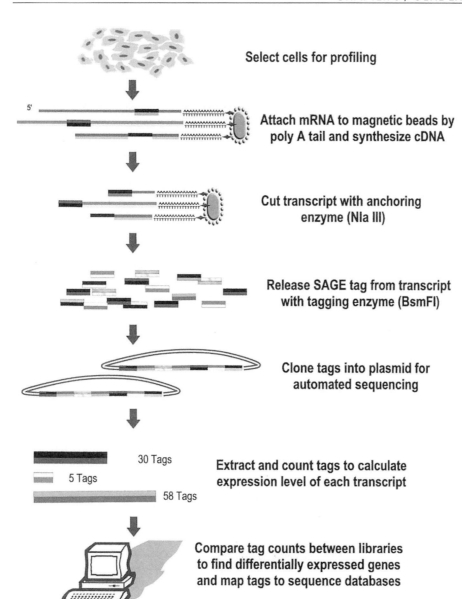

Select cells for profiling

Attach mRNA to magnetic beads by poly A tail and synthesize cDNA

Cut transcript with anchoring enzyme (Nla III)

Release SAGE tag from transcript with tagging enzyme (BsmFI)

Clone tags into plasmid for automated sequencing

30 Tags
5 Tags
58 Tags

Extract and count tags to calculate expression level of each transcript

Compare tag counts between libraries to find differentially expressed genes and map tags to sequence databases

Fig. 8-2 Approach for expression profiling using SAGE. Gene expression is quantified in a population of cells by isolating a transcript tag from the expressed genes. These tags are paired into ditags, ligated to form concatamers, and cloned into a sequencing vector for efficient counting on an automated sequencer. Tag counts from each tissue type are stored electronically and used for comparison to other cell populations. A relative fraction of each transcript can be calculated as well. Informatics are used to match the SAGE tag to a known gene or expressed sequence tag.

and historical comparisons valid.[39,40] An additional strength of SAGE is that it determines expression levels directly from an RNA sample. It is not necessary to have a gene-specific fragment of DNA arrayed to assay each gene. This allows SAGE to identify genes that are not included in an array,[41] and avoids the infrastructure necessary to create and read large DNA arrays. This flexibility has a downside. The number of samples that can be processed using SAGE is small as compared to DNA arrays because it takes 2 weeks or more of skilled labor to construct a SAGE library. The potential to analyze hundreds of samples by SAGE for a single experiment is not a practical option for the technology in its present form. However, when an in-depth and quantitative profile is desired for a small number of samples, the extra work involved in creating a SAGE library can be justified. To date, SAGE has been successful for determining the differentially expressed transcripts in well-controlled experimental systems.[41-48] This type of data generated by SAGE is often complementary to a typical use of DNA arrays in cancer research for a wide survey of many patient tumor samples.

Follow-up Techniques

After a gene expression profile has been obtained on a set of RNA samples, it is desirable to experimentally confirm the expression differences and to extend the analysis to other samples. Normally, a small set of interesting genes is identified by using DNA arrays or SAGE, but several different techniques are more effiicient for assaying this smaller set of interesting genes. In addition, each gene expression technique has inherent errors and an independent method is required for validating the original expression levels.

Northern blotting has been the gold standard for gene expression analysis for many years. Because the transcript being assayed is identified by both molecular weight and by a long hybridization probe, there is normally a low error rate. Although northern blotting is a time-consuming approach, it is still a useful way to confirm profiling data for a limited number of genes.[49] When a good antibody is available for the gene of interest, a western blot or immunohistochemistry are reliable methods for confirming expression changes. This approach is advantageous, particularly when the end point is knowledge of protein levels rather than mRNA levels.

Real-time PCR, sometimes called quantitative or fluorescent PCR, has gained popularity for rapid follow-up and confirmation of profiling data.[50,51] Expression determination by real-time PCR is based on continuous fluorescent monitoring of PCR products[52-54] from a cDNA template. Under the right conditions, the number of cycles required to PCR amplify a product to a certain level is directly proportional to the amount as starting template. Different real-time PCR systems are available from at least four molecular biology vendors. Each of these systems has software for plotting and analyzing fluorescent-labeled PCR products' accumulation for the determination of starting concentration. Normally a serially diluted known sample is used for a standard curve to interpolate concentrations of unknown samples.

There are a variety of methods for detecting the accumulation of PCR products during real-time PCR. A simple method is to incorporate a fluorescent dye directly into the PCR product during amplification. A double-stranded DNA binding dye, SYBR green I (Molecular Probes, Eugene, OR), is effective for this purpose.[52,53] To increase specificity of PCR product detection, additional oligonucleotide can be employed in the assays that hybridize to an internal portion of the PCR product. There are a variety of systems for this purpose marketed by different vendors: TaqMan Assay (PE Biosystems), Hybridization Probes (Roche), and Molecular Beacons (Stratagene). Real-time PCR allows for a quick and low-cost assessment of the expression pattern of several genes in many tumors and can be automated. It is becoming a popular method for the follow-up of profiling data.

To look at protein levels of many samples simultaneously a tissue microarray system has been developed.[55–57] This system allows for up to 1000 small tissue samples, made from a narrow gauge biopsy needle, to be arrayed in a single block of tissue. This block of tissue can then be used to produce hundreds of slides that can be probed by immunohistochemistry or other means. In this way, a standard set of the same samples can be probed for expression levels for many different genes. A digital imaging system is used to record and read the data. Although, robotics are now employed to array the tissues, many good quality samples must be collected and oriented for biopsy in the region of interest oriented by a pathologist. The results must also be scored in some fashion by signal intensity, done manually at this point in the technology's development. Finally, a good antibody is needed for each gene of interest that will work in the normally available formalin-fixed tissue. However, this approach has the potential to make gene expression correlations with a vast archive of preserved tumor material.

BIOINFORMATICS

High-throughput gene expression profiling has produced large data sets that require specialized tools for effective handling and analysis. The earlier RNA expression technologies—subtractive hybridization and differential display—were designed to locate small numbers of differentially expressed genes. With the advent of large-scale gene expression profiling techniques, such as DNA arrays and SAGE, a need has arisen to analyze gene expression level measurements in numbers that are orders of magnitude higher than previous.[58] Although DNA arrays and SAGE have different data formats, there are still elements in common for the data analysis. There is a need to be able to archive and sort through multiple measurements, set statistical confidence levels, recognize patterns within the data, and retrieve information rapidly regarding the detected genes. The large volume of data being generated primarily by DNA arrays has created gene expression informatics challenges that have produced some creative solutions in this rapidly expanding field of research. Perhaps good news for the individual cancer investigator is an increasing amount of publicly available gene expression data. Databases and data-mining approaches are making global expression profiles available to virtually any investigator.

DNA Array Data Analysis

The majority of large-scale gene expression data is currently being generated in the form of images from fluorescent-labeled high-density DNA arrays. While there are many variations particular to each system, there are some features in common. The image from each spotted DNA on the array must be processed to yield a

numeric gene expression level (or ratio between samples). Quality control is key at this step; poorly spotted arrays or other technical artifacts can be excluded at this stage. This initial image analysis step is critical and there are several available options for the signal processing required.[59–61] Most DNA array analysis software has some provision for normalizing the data, based on overall intensity, to account for differences in the probe amount, or other variables altering overall spot detection.

A popular method of analyzing gene expression information from DNA arrays is to cluster the data in a dendogram or "tree" format.[62,63] Clustering programs, now available from commercial sources as well, are based on a variety of statistical algorithms including self-organizing maps and K-means.[64] The genes can be clustered by their expression response to experimental conditions, or the RNA samples used for the array experiment can be clustered by overall similarity of expression patterns. Microarray experiments may address the similarity of expression patterns based on tumor type, response to drugs, response to environmental conditions or a variety of other variables.

SAGE Data Analysis

For handling SAGE data, most investigators rely on the SAGE software generated by the Johns Hopkins SAGE group. This software extracts tag sequences from raw sequence data and tabulates the counts in a database. The software also will make comparisons between libraries of tags and calculate the statistical significance of differences based on Monte-Carlo simulations.[34] Additionally, the software helps create a relational database by extracting tags, gene name and gene information from the sequence database. The program uses this information to match tags to known genes or ESTs. Additional tag-to-gene mapping information can be downloaded from the NCBI from the SAGEmap Web site (Table 8-2). This information that is used by the SAGE software is freely available to noncommercial users of the technology and can be obtained via SAGEnet (Table 8-2).[8]

Databases and Data Mining

Many of the complex expression patterns generated by gene profiling are being deposited on publicly accessible Web sites (Table 8-2) or are commercially available. This data can be very valuable when planning experiments, or for making correlations with potential cancer-related genes.[51,65] It is, therefore, important to access the public expression information for a variety of reasons, but mining the best data and adapting the results for a particular application can be challenging.

To identify genes based on mRNA expression in cDNA libraries, a variety of public databases are available (Table 8-2). These databases range from a display of the number of sequences observed; to more sophisticated statistical approaches that assign confidence levels to differentially expressed genes. The CGAP specializes in creating databases and resources for cancer research,[29–31] and has cDNA-based expression information from malignant, premalignant, and normal cells.

Because SAGE involves digital counts of transcript numbers that are compared electronically, SAGE data naturally lends itself to large-scale collaborative projects and the formation of databases. SAGE libraries constructed at different times or in different laboratories can be accurately compared, resulting in a powerful cumulative database. To complement EST data and to provide a more efficient means for archiving quantitative expression profiles, CGAP adopted SAGE technology starting in 1998, and can be accessed through the SAGEmap Web site.[39,40] From a total of 171,692 sequencing runs, more than 3.4 million valid transcript tags have been processed from 84 different malignant and normal cell types. Online tools built specifically to handle SAGE data[39,40] allow users to make statistical-based comparisons between libraries to find differentially expressed genes by using the xProfiler, or by downloading data for local analysis. SAGE tags can be mapped to UniGene clusters via SAGEmap, making the identification of a gene from a differentially expressed tag easier. The SAGE data generated through this project is also used to create a Digital Northern tool, where the expression level of a particular gene can be determined for each of the tissues used to make SAGE libraries. Expression comparisons based on SAGE have the additional advantage that no normalization to a housekeeping gene or to a reference standard is necessary, because absolute levels of transcripts are compared.

Although there has been significant data generated using DNA arrays, there are challenges in integrating the different expression profiles generated by varying technology platforms. Most DNA array data that is currently publicly available is through laboratory homepages (see Table 8-2 for some links) or as electronic supplements to the journal publications mentioned throughout this chapter.

GENE EXPRESSION PROFILING IN CANCER: DIAGNOSIS AND THERAPY

The expression of the vast majority of the genes remains unchanged during the complex process of tumorigenesis. Indeed, a pioneering study found that the expression of no more than 1–1.5 percent of the genes was significantly altered in colon cancer, as compared to normal colon tissue.[34] Nonetheless, the analysis of human cancer with the techniques described above typically identify hundreds of genes differentially expressed between normal tissues and malignant specimens. Clearly, prioritization rules according to the identity of the genes uncovered or according to specific sets of criteria must be implemented. Efficient techniques for the validation of these genes have been described in the previous section. In addition to the identification of specific differentially expressed genes, global expression profiles can be used for tumor taxonomy. This section will illustrate these principles through the description of some of the most important results of gene profiling obtained in common malignancies.

Colon Cancer

By using SAGE, one study analyzed more than 300,000 transcripts derived from colorectal cancers, pancreatic cancer, and normal colon epithelium. While all the abundant transcripts (more than five copies per cell) represented 75 percent of the mRNA mass, the rare transcripts were responsible for much of the diversity of gene expression: 86 percent of all the different genes were expressed at less than five copies per cell. Interestingly, and perhaps unexpectedly, most of the genes were expressed at similar levels between normal and cancer cells. Indeed, in the case of normal and neoplastic colon, only 548 genes were differentially expressed (less than 1.5 percent of the transcripts present in a given cell). Many genes elevated in cancer represented products known to be involved in growth and proliferation, while genes found in the normal colon were often related to differentiation. Importantly, many of the individual genes found to be differentially regulated may represent targets for mechanism-based therapy or biomarkers for diagnosis. In another study, an Affymetrix oligonucleotide array containing 6500 genes was used to investigate 40 colon tumors and normal colon tissues.[66] Using two-way clustering, clusters of gene with similar patterns of gene expression were identified. Some of these clusters may represent the activation of molecular pathways relevant to colon tumorigenesis.

Breast Cancer

Gene expression in breast cancer has been monitored by using differential display, cDNA arrays, and SAGE in a variety of experimental systems. In a SAGE study of normal and neoplastic breast tissue, at least 50,000 transcripts were analyzed from 4 libraries and highly differentially expressed genes were identified. Small custom arrays were used to validate the genes identified. Claudin-7 was found up-regulated more than a hundredfold in 85 percent and 60 percent of the primary and metastatic tumors, respectively. While differences in gene expression levels can be subtle in other diseases, many genes appear to be vastly differentially regulated in cancer. Similarly, another study used a combination of differential display and cDNA arrays to gain a better understanding of gene expression patterns in breast cancer.[67] This study identified 700 genes differentially expressed between normal and cancer cells, and a cDNA array containing 107 of these genes was constructed. Most of the genes highly expressed in normal cells, and down-regulated in cancer cells, represented genes important for cell adhesion, communication, and maintenance of cell shape. In contrast, most of the genes elevated in cancer were those encoding enzymes involved in metabolism, macromolecular synthesis, and disruption of the extracellular matrix. By using the custom cDNA array, clusters of genes were identified that were associated with relevant clinical parameters, such as estrogen receptor (ER) status, stage, and tumor size. Overall, gene expression patterns allowed the clustering of breast tumors into two major groups that differed in their ER status.

Other studies with large cDNA arrays contributed significantly to our understanding of gene expression in breast cancer.[68,69] Many clusters of genes with related expression patterns were identified. For example, an interferon (IFN)-regulated gene cluster and a proliferation cluster (correlated with mitotic index) were found. Importantly, gene expression clusters corresponding to noncancer tissue such as stroma, lymphocytes, and endothelium were also recognized. These issues are important when primary tumors are analyzed because the gene expression profiles represent a complex environment of interacting tissues. While the large arrays failed to distinguish multiple tumor categories, a smaller, more focused array containing 496 genes clustered the tumors into two groups according to their ER status,[69] in a fashion reminiscent of the differential display study described above.[67] The small array further divided ER-negative breast cancers into two groups. It is unclear whether these two categories may have divergent clinical characteristics, but this experiment emphasizes the power of these techniques in cancer taxonomy. These results suggest the possibility that gene expression patterns may be used effectively for diagnosis and therapeutic decisions in breast cancer. In yet another study, laser capture microdissection, an important validation tool, was used in combination with cDNA arrays for the identification of genes relevant to breast tumorigenesis.[70]

Germ-line mutations in BRCA1 and BRCA2 confer a significant risk of breast and ovarian cancer. Using a large cDNA array, it was recently shown that BRCA1 and BRCA2 tumors could be distinguished from each other and from sporadic breast cancer on the basis of gene expression profiles.[71] Indeed, all the tumors with BRCA1 mutation, and 14 of 15 without the mutation, were appropriately recognized in the BRCA1 classification. Similarly, accurate classification was obtained with BRCA2 tumors. A total of 176 genes were found differentially regulated between BRCA1 and BRCA2 tumors. Interestingly, BRCA1 tumors exhibited increased expression of genes involved in response to cellular stress. A sporadic tumor, which clustered with BRCA1 tumors, proved to exhibit hypermethylation of the BRCA1 promoter. Gene profiling may thus help in the identification of breast cancer genetic status, including the identification of BRCA1 or BRCA2-like phenotype. These different categories may be useful in patient management, as patients with BRCA1-like tumors may require more rigorous follow-up.

Ovarian Cancer

The vast majority of ovarian cancers are diagnosed in late stages and a major emphasis of functional genomics approaches is to identify biomarkers. Schummer et al. constructed a cDNA array consisting of 21,500 randomly selected transcripts from ovarian cDNA libraries.[72] The vast majority of genes were expressed at similar levels in ovarian cancer and ovarian surface epithelium, the presumed normal counterpart of ovarian cancer. However, they were able to identify cDNAs that were expressed more than 2.5-fold in at least 50 percent of the tumors. These clones also had low levels of expression in nonovarian tissues. Many of these cDNAs were novel and corresponded to ESTs, and others had previously been implicated in various cancers. One candidate, HE4, a protease inhibitor, emerged as a promising candidate because it was highly up-regulated in many ovarian tumors and was found at low levels in other tissues. These findings were subsequently confirmed and extended in a SAGE study of ovarian cancer.[73] An analysis was done of 385,000 transcripts from 10 different ovarian libraries, and differentially expressed genes were identified using a strict set of criteria. Selected genes had to be high in all three primary ovarian cancers and low in all three nonmalignant specimens. Twenty-seven genes were identified that met these criteria and that were overexpressed more than tenfold in ovarian tumors. Interestingly, a majority of those genes were predicted to encode membrane or secreted proteins, making them candidates for biomarkers or tumor targeting. Many of these secreted genes encoded protease inhibitors. Another study using a combination of cDNA-RDA and cDNA arrays also found a large number of genes encoding secreted products to be elevated in ovarian cancer.[74]

Prostate Cancer

Prostate cancer originally responds to hormone therapy but typically becomes refractory to this therapy and develops into an androgen-independent tumor.[75] The elucidation of the molecular mechanisms accompanying this phenomenon has begun, but our understanding is still incomplete. To monitor gene expression changes that are associated with hormone-independent growth, the androgen-independent prostate cancer xenograft model CWR22-R and its parental androgen-dependent xenograft CWR22 were analyzed by cDNA microarray.[76,77] Hybridization to a large cDNA array (10,000 clones) revealed that the expression of 160 genes was altered in CWR22 upon androgen removal. The pattern of gene expression changes suggested that the CWR22 cells were undergoing growth arrest upon androgen removal. Interestingly, the majority of these genes were expressed at similar levels between CWR22 and CWR22-R, suggesting that CWR22-R had adapted to growth without androgen and had reentered the cell cycle.[77] Comparison of genes differentially expressed between CWR22 and CWR22-R allow the identification of genes that may be crucial in the progression from androgen dependence to androgen independence.[76,77] Some of these genes were found to be involved in thyroid hormone receptor signaling. IGFBP2 and HSP27 were also found elevated in CWR22-R and were validated through the use of tissue microarrays.[76]

Leukemia

The classification of acute leukemias has long relied on the identity of the precursors. Lymphoid precursors give rise to acute lymphoblastic leukemia (ALL) while myeloid precursor give rise to acute myeloid leukemia (AML). The treatment regimen for these classes is distinct and accurate classification of these tumors can have a significant impact on survival. A cDNA array consisting of 6817 genes was used in order to determine whether global patterns of gene expression could be used to distinguish various classes in leukemias.[78] The original data set, consisting of 38 bone marrow samples (27 ALL, 11 AML), demonstrated that a large number of genes appeared to be correlated with the AML-ALL class distinction. The 50 genes most closely correlated with class distinction were chosen and a class predictor algorithm was developed. In cross-validation analysis by using the original 38 bone marrow samples, 36 of these samples were correctly assigned to the clinical category (AML or ALL). The 50-gene predictor correctly predicted the tumor class in 29 of 34 additional acute leukemias. Interestingly, the number of genes included for prediction was not crucial, as the same results were obtained with predictors containing anywhere from 10 to 200 genes.

An important issue was whether gene expression profiling could be used to determine these classes without a priori knowledge of their existence. This is important because many cancers (prostate, for example) have a variable response to treatment, but cannot readily be divided into classes using current methods. Using self-organizing maps (SOMs), it was possible to identify two categories of acute leukemia that essentially fell along the known ALL-AML classes.[78] Gene profiling could thus identify the two classes of leukemia without previous biological information. Astonishingly, considering the number of clinical specimens studied, SOM could further stratify the acute leukemia classes into four clusters. A first cluster corresponded to AML, a second cluster to T-lineage ALL, and two additional clusters corresponded to B-lineage ALL. The AML, T-cell ALL, and B-cell ALL are the most important clinical distinctions among acute leukemias. These studies demonstrate that gene profiling can accurately identify new classes of cancers (class discovery) and assign tumors to known classes (class prediction). Unfortunately, clinical outcome was not strongly correlated with a particular expression signature. In any event, because leukemic cells can easily be obtained as relatively pure population, these findings may have immediate and important clinical application.

Lymphoma

Diffuse large B-cell lymphoma (DLBCL) is the most common non-Hodgkin lymphoma subtype. DLBCLs are highly heterogeneous, but attempts at further subclassification have failed. A cDNA array containing 17,856 clones was constructed from various lymphoid cell cDNA libraries.[79] DLBCL exhibited a distinct and complex pattern of gene expression and displayed a lymph node signature. Importantly, reclustering the tumors by using genes of the germinal center (GC) B-cell cluster yielded two subtypes: the GC B-like DLBCLs and the activated-B-like DLBCLs. The expression of no single gene correlated well with the new subtypes, but only the analysis of the patterns of a large number of genes could identify these novel groups. Interestingly, these novel subtypes exhibited marked differences in prognosis. Indeed, 76 percent of GC B-like DLBCL patients were alive after 5 years, while only 16 percent of the activated B-like DLBCL patients were still alive after the same period. Gene profiling thus provides a new classification scheme for DLBCL that define prognostic categories. The molecular and clinical differences are significant and suggest that B-like DLBCL and activated B-like DLBCL may represent distinct diseases. Although this last example represents a clear case in which molecular signature involving large number of genes can be of use clinically, there are also examples of gene profiling identifying individual genes for diagnosis. For example, a recent study used Atlas cDNA arrays (Clontech) to identify the gene *clusterin* as a marker for anaplastic large-cell lymphomas.[80]

Melanoma

Thirty-one melanomas and 7 controls were hybridized to a cDNA array that contained probes for nearly 7000 genes.[81] Although no classification schemes for melanoma existed, the gene expression data and hierarchical clustering analysis subdivided the tumors into two groups of 12 and 19. These two groups were analyzed for association with several clinical parameters, such as age and survival, but no associations were found. However, the larger cluster of tumors was predicted, from its expression signature, to consist of tumors with reduced motility and invasiveness. Indeed, these two groups showed differential responses in their ability to migrate into scratch wounds, contract collagen gels, and form tubular networks. Although the analysis did not show association with known clinical parameters, it nonetheless enabled the classification of melanoma into distinct and important classes related to the motility of the tumor cells, and identified genes that may play a role in the invasive ability of this cancer. Further analyses may allow the identification of optimized treatment for each of the classes or other parameters of clinical relevance for melanoma patients.

In another study, melanoma cells were selected for high metastatic potential *in vitro* and analyzed using cDNA arrays.[82]

Several genes involved in extracellular matrix assembly were elevated, including RhoC, which single-handedly enhanced metastasis when overexpressed in melanoma cells. A better understanding of gene expression in highly metastatic cells may lead to improve therapeutic strategies aimed at preventing invasion and metastasis. cDNA arrays and other gene profiling methods will undoubtedly continue to play a major role in this endeavor.

Brain Cancer

Most expression profiling for brain tumors has been applied to glioblastoma multiforme (GBM). DNA arrays,[83–85] SAGE,[40,86] and tissue arrays[55] have all been applied to the study of the genes expressed in GBM and normal neural tissue. Even if the biological implications of the revealed patterns are not yet clear, there are practical uses for this data. One example is the use of large-scale expression data to find potential tumor markers or antigens for GBM.[51] It is also likely that the pattern of expression will be useful for the classification of brain tumors, including the molecularly heterogeneous GBM classification.[87]

Brain tumors other than GBM have been studied by expression profiling. The major malignant pediatric brain tumor, medulloblastoma, has been studied by SAGE.[88] Detailed SAGE expression profiles are also available for medulloblastomas and a variety of gliomas at the CGAP SAGEmap database.[40]

NCI60

A series of 60 cancer cell lines of various histologic origins, known as the NCI60, forms the basis of the National Cancer Institute's cancer drug-screening program.[89] Gene expression in these lines was studied by using a cDNA microarray consisting of approximately 8000 different genes.[90] Except for breast and non–small cell lung carcinoma cell lines, the gene expression patterns clustered the lines according to their presumed histologic origin. The patterns of gene expression in the different tissue were thus sufficiently conserved in the cell lines to be grouped together although it is clear that the establishment of cancer lines is accompanied by changes in gene expression patterns. The clustering of the cell lines depended on the exact genes included in the analysis and other studies have shown that cell lines are significantly different from the tissue of origin in colon[66] and ovarian cancer.[73,74] In any event, analysis of the 60 cell lines allowed the identification of coordinately regulated cluster of genes. The clusters could be labeled according to the genes present in the cluster (proliferation cluster, interferon cluster) or to the patterns of expression of these genes (epithelial cluster, melanoma cluster). Much information might be gained concerning the microenvironment of tumors by comparing expression patterns between primary tumors and their corresponding *in vitro* cultures or cell lines.

The findings with the NCI60 described above validate the use of cell lines for *in vitro* manipulation such as treatment with hormone or chemotherapeutic drugs. Indeed, the same 60 cell lines were clustered according to the growth inhibitory activity (GI_{50}) of 1400 compounds.[91] The cell lines no longer clustered according to their tissue of origin, but according to their drug response. When a subset of these drugs with known mechanisms was used for analysis, several clusters corresponding to mechanisms of action emerged. This could clearly help to identify mechanism of action for unknown drugs. For example, 5-FU appeared with the RNA synthesis inhibitors, suggesting that the main activity of 5-FU may be as an RNA synthesis inhibitor. Further analysis allowed the identification of associations between clusters of genes and clusters of drugs. These relationships may help to identify a genetic basis for certain drug action. For example, an inverse relationship was found between dihydropyrimidine dehydrogenase (DPYD) and 5-FU potency. DPYD is a rate-limiting enzyme in 5-FU degradation. Most cell lines expressing low levels of DPYD were sensitive to 5-FU. DPYD may become useful as a prognosis marker.

Endothelial Cells

Endothelial cells provide the blood supply to solid tumors and are therefore highly relevant to the process of tumorigenesis. A better understanding of angiogenesis may thus provide tools in the fight against cancer. SAGE was used to identify genes differentially expressed *in vivo* between endothelial cells derived from normal and malignant colorectal tissue.[92] The study showed that at least 79 different genes are significantly differentially expressed between these tissues, including 46 that were specifically elevated in tumor-associated endothelial cells. On the basis of these results, it was concluded that neoplastic and normal endothelium are fundamentally different at the molecular level, suggesting that these differences may be clinically relevant. Nine SAGE tags elevated in the tumor corresponded to novel, uncategorized genes. These genes were named tumor endothelial marker (TEM), and designated TEM-1 to TEM-9. Further experiments confirmed the tumor endothelium-specific expression of these genes, not only for colorectal tumors, but also for other major tumor types. These TEMs, or other genes identified in this study, may become targets of antiangiogenic therapies.

Subtractive hybridization techniques and cDNA arrays have also been used for studying the process of angiogenesis.[93,94] Overall, many known and novel genes have been implicated in this process. These candidates await testing as targets for therapeutic interventions.

Gene Profiling Techniques in the Identification of Targets of Specific Oncogenic Molecular Pathways

A main application of techniques such as differential display, SAGE, and cDNA microarrays has been the identification of downstream targets of specific pathways. For example, SAGE was used to identify many genes whose expression is believed to mediate p53-induced apoptosis.[41] Many of these genes were novel and predicted to encode proteins involved in oxidative stress, providing a new paradigm for the mechanism of p53-mediated apoptosis. Similarly, SAGE was used to identify downstream targets of the APC/β-catenin pathway, a pathway activated in the vast majority of colon cancer.[45,46] c-MYC and PPARδ were both identified as direct transcriptional targets of the TCF-β-catenin transcription complex and provided important mechanistic insights into colon tumorigenesis.

cDNA arrays have also been used to identify genes relevant to specific cancer pathways. For example, superoxide dismutase was identified as a target of estrogen derivatives that could kill leukemia cells.[95] In a different approach, ER-responsive breast cancer cells were treated with estrogen and analyzed by SAGE for expression changes leading to the identification of many, possibly useful, estrogen-regulated genes.[48] Differential display was used in the identification of genes involved in Ras transformation.[96,97] Drug resistance has also been studied extensively by gene profiling and genes relevant to cisplatin and taxol resistance have been identified.[98,99] There are no doubts that gene profiling techniques will play a major role in the dissection of the myriad of molecular pathways important in human cancer. The examples above represent a minute fraction of the efforts that have already been dedicated toward this goal.

REFERENCES

1. Smith LM, Fung S, Hunkapiller MW, Hunkapiller TJ, Hood LE: The synthesis of oligonucleotides containing an aliphatic amino group at the 5′ terminus: Synthesis of fluorescent DNA primers for use in DNA sequence analysis. *Nucleic Acids Res* **13**:2399, 1985.
2. Smith LM, Sanders JZ, Kaiser RJ, Hughes P, Dodd C, Connell CR, Heiner C, et al: Fluorescence detection in automated DNA sequence analysis. *Nature* **321**:674, 1986.
3. Lockhart DJ, Dong H, Byrne MC, Follettie MT, Gallo MV, Chee MS, Mittmann M, et al: Expression monitoring by hybridization to high-density oligonucleotide arrays. *Nat Biotechnol* **14**:1675, 1996.

4. Schena M, Shalon D, Davis RW, Brown PO: Quantitative monitoring of gene expression patterns with a complementary DNA microarray. *Science* **270**:467, 1995.

5. Gress TM, Hoheisel JD, Lennon GG, Zehetner G, Lehrach H: Hybridization fingerprinting of high-density cDNA-library arrays with cDNA pools derived from whole tissues. *Mamm Genome* **3**:609, 1992.

6. Carulli JP, Artinger M, Swain PM, Root CD, Chee L, Tulig C, Guerin J, et al: High throughput analysis of differential gene expression. *J Cell Biochem Suppl* **31**:286, 1998.

7. Swendeman SL, La Quaglia MP: cDNA subtraction hybridization: A review and an application to neuroblastoma. *Semin Pediatr Surg* **5**:149, 1996.

8. Sagerstrom CG, Sun BI, Sive HL: Subtractive cloning: past, present, and future. *Annu Rev Biochem* **66**:751, 1997.

9. Diatchenko L, Lau YF, Campbell AP, Chenchik A, Moqadam F, Huang B, Lukyanov S, et al: Suppression subtractive hybridization: A method for generating differentially regulated or tissue-specific cDNA probes and libraries. *Proc Natl Acad Sci U S A* **93**:6025, 1996.

10. Lisitsyn N, Wigler M: Cloning the differences between two complex genomes. *Science* **259**:946, 1993.

11. Liang P, Pardee AB: Differential display of eukaryotic messenger RNA by means of the polymerase chain reaction. *Science* **257**:967, 1992.

12. Welsh J, Chada K, Dalal SS, Cheng R, Ralph D, McClelland M: Arbitrarily primed PCR fingerprinting of RNA. *Nucleic Acids Res* **20**:4965, 1992.

13. Matz MV, Lukyanov SA: Different strategies of differential display: areas of application. *Nucleic Acids Res* **26**:5537, 1998.

14. Southern EM: Detection of specific sequences among DNA fragments separated by gel electrophoresis. *J Mol Biol* **98**:503, 1975.

15. Pease AC, Solas D, Sullivan EJ, Cronin MT, Holmes CP, Fodor SP: Light-generated oligonucleotide arrays for rapid DNA sequence analysis. *Proc Natl Acad Sci U S A* **91**:5022, 1994.

16. Bowtell DD: Options available—from start to finish—for obtaining expression data by microarray. *Nat Genet* **21**:25, 1999.

17. Kurian KM, Watson CJ, Wyllie AH: DNA chip technology. *J Pathol* **187**:267, 1999.

18. Johnston M: Gene chips: Array of hope for understanding gene regulation. *Curr Biol* **8**:R171, 1998.

19. Wilgenbus KK, Lichter P: DNA chip technology ante portas. *J Mol Med* **77**:761, 1999.

20. De Benedetti VM, Biglia N, Sismondi P, De Bortoli M: DNA chips: The future of biomarkers. *Int J Biol Markers* **15**:1, 2000.

21. Wang J: From DNA biosensors to gene chips. *Nucleic Acids Res* **28**:3011, 2000.

22. Lee PS, Lee KH: Genomic analysis. *Curr Opin Biotechnol* **11**:171, 2000.

23. Augenlicht LH, Wahrman MZ, Halsey H, Anderson L, Taylor J, Lipkin M: Expression of cloned sequences in biopsies of human colonic tissue and in colonic carcinoma cells induced to differentiate in vitro. *Cancer Res* **47**:6017, 1987.

24. Brown PO, Botstein D: Exploring the new world of the genome with DNA microarrays. *Nat Genet* **21**:33, 1999.

25. Cheung VG, Morley M, Aguilar F, Massimi A, Kucherlapati R, Childs G: Making and reading microarrays. *Nat Genet* **21**:15, 1999.

26. Lipshutz RJ, Fodor SP, Gingeras TR, Lockhart DJ: High density synthetic oligonucleotide arrays. *Nat Genet* **21**:20, 1999.

27. Adams MD, Soares MB, Kerlavage AR, Fields C, Venter JC: Rapid cDNA sequencing (expressed sequence tags) from a directionally cloned human infant brain cDNA library. *Nat Genet* **4**:373, 1993.

28. Williamson AR: The Merck Gene Index project. *Drug Discov Today* **4**:115, 1999.

29. Strausberg RL, Buetow KH, Emmert-Buck MR, Klausner RD: The cancer genome anatomy project: Building an annotated gene index. *Trends Genet* **16**:103, 2000.

30. Strausberg RL, Dahl CA, Klausner RD: New opportunities for uncovering the molecular basis of cancer. *Nat Genet* **15**:415, 1997.

31. Riggins GJ, Strausberg R: Genome and genetic resources from the Cancer Genome Anatomy Project. *Hum Mol Genet* **10**:663, 2001.

32. Velculescu VE, Zhang L, Vogelstein B, Kinzler KW: Serial analysis of gene expression. *Science* **270**:484, 1995.

33. Velculescu VE, Zhang L, Zhou W, Vogelstein J, Basrai MA, Bassett DE, Jr., Hieter P, et al: Characterization of the yeast transcriptome. *Cell* **88**:243, 1997.

34. Zhang L, Zhou W, Velculescu VE, Kern SE, Hruban RH, Hamilton SR, Vogelstein B, et al: Gene expression profiles in normal and cancer cells. *Science* **276**:1268, 1997.

35. Lal A, Sui I-M, Riggins G: Serial analysis of gene expression: Probing transcriptomes for molecular targets. *Curr Opin Mol Ther* **1**:720, 1999.

36. Powell J: SAGE. The serial analysis of gene expression. *Methods Mol Biol* **99**:297, 2000.

37. Velculescu VE, Vogelstein B, Kinzler KW: Analysing uncharted transcriptomes with SAGE. *Trends Genet* **16**:423, 2000.

38. Madden SL, Wang CJ, Landes G: Serial analysis of gene expression: From gene discovery to target identification. *Drug Discov Today* **5**:415, 2000.

39. Lash AE, Tolstoshev CM, Wagner L, Schuler GD, Strausberg RL, Riggins GJ, Altschul SF: SAGEmap: A public gene expression resource. *Genome Res* **10**:1051, 2000.

40. Lal A, Lash AE, Altschul SF, Velculescu V, Zhang L, McLendon RE, Marra MA, et al: A public database for gene expression in human cancers. *Cancer Res* **59**:5403, 1999.

41. Polyak K, Xia Y, Zweier JL, Kinzler KW, Vogelstein B: A model for p53-induced apoptosis. *Nature* **389**:300, 1997.

42. Madden SL, Galella EA, Zhu J, Bertelsen AH, Beaudry GA: SAGE transcript profiles for p53-dependent growth regulation. *Oncogene* **15**:1079, 1997.

43. Hermeking H, Lengauer C, Polyak K, He TC, Zhang L, Thiagalingam S, Kinzler KW, et al: 14-3-3 sigma is a p53-regulated inhibitor of G2/M progression. *Mol Cell* **1**:3, 1997.

44. Yu J, Zhang L, Hwang PM, Rago C, Kinzler KW, Vogelstein B: Identification and classification of p53-regulated genes. *Proc Natl Acad Sci U S A* **96**:14517, 1999.

45. He TC, Chan TA, Vogelstein B, Kinzler KW: PPARdelta is an APC-regulated target of nonsteroidal anti-inflammatory drugs. *Cell* **99**:335, 1999.

46. He TC SA, Rago C, Hermeking H, Zawel L, da Costa LT, Morin PJ, Vogelstein B, Kinzler KW: Identification of c-MYC as a target of the APC pathway. *Science* **281**:1509, 1998.

47. Inadera H, Hashimoto S, Dong HY, Suzuki T, Nagai S, Yamashita T, Toyoda N, et al: WISP-2 as a novel estrogen-responsive gene in human breast cancer cells. *Biochem Biophys Res Commun* **275**:108, 2000.

48. Charpentier AH, Bednarek AK, Daniel RL, Hawkins KA, Laflin KJ, Gaddis S, MacLeod MC, et al: Effects of estrogen on global gene expression: identification of novel targets of estrogen action. *Cancer Res* **60**:5977, 2000.

49. Taniguchi M, Miura K, Iwao H, Yamanaka S: Quantitative Assessment of DNA microarrays—comparison with northern blot analyses. *Genomics* **71**:34, 2001.

50. Rajeevan MS, Vernon SD, Taysavang N, Unger ER: Validation of array-based gene expression profiles by real-time (kinetic) RT-PCR. *J Mol Diagn* **3**:26, 2001.

51. Loging WT, Lal A, Siu IM, Loney TL, Wikstrand CJ, Marra MA, Prange C, et al: Identifying potential tumor markers and antigens by database mining and rapid expression screening. *Genome Res* **10**:1393, 2000.

52. Wittwer CT, Herrmann MG, Moss AA, Rasmussen RP: Continuous fluorescence monitoring of rapid cycle DNA amplification. *Biotechniques* **22**:130, 1997.

53. Morrison TB, Weis JJ, Wittwer CT: Quantification of low-copy transcripts by continuous SYBR Green I monitoring during amplification. *Biotechniques* **24**:954, 1998.

54. Wittwer CT, Ririe KM, Andrew RV, David DA, Gundry RA, Balis UJ: The LightCycler: A microvolume multisample fluorimeter with rapid temperature control. *Biotechniques* **22**:176, 1997.

55. Kononen J, Bubendorf L, Kallioniemi A, Barlund M, Schraml P, Leighton S, Torhorst J, et al: Tissue microarrays for high-throughput molecular profiling of tumor specimens. *Nat Med* **4**:844, 1998.

56. Moch H, Schraml P, Bubendorf L, Mirlacher M, Kononen J, Gasser T, Mihatsch MJ, et al: High-throughput tissue microarray analysis to evaluate genes uncovered by cDNA microarray screening in renal cell carcinoma. *Am J Pathol* **154**:981, 1999.

57. Schraml P, Kononen J, Bubendorf L, Moch H, Bissig H, Nocito A, Mihatsch MJ, et al: Tissue microarrays for gene amplification surveys in many different tumor types. *Clin Cancer Res* **5**:1966, 1999.

58. Bassett DE, Jr., Eisen MB, Boguski MS: Gene expression informatics—it's all in your mine. *Nat Genet* **21**:51, 1999.

59. Duggan DJ, Bittner M, Chen Y, Meltzer P, Trent JM: Expression profiling using cDNA microarrays. *Nat Genet* **21**:10, 1999.

60. Ermolaeva O, Rastogi M, Pruitt KD, Schuler GD, Bittner ML, Chen Y, Simon R, et al: Data management and analysis for gene expression arrays. *Nat Genet* **20**:19, 1998.

61. Strehlow D: Software for quantitation and visualization of expression array data. *Biotechniques* **29**:118, 2000.

62. Eisen MB, Spellman PT, Brown PO, Botstein D: Cluster analysis and display of genome-wide expression patterns. *Proc Natl Acad Sci U S A* **95**:14863, 1998.

63. Michaels GS, Carr DB, Askenazi M, Fuhrman S, Wen X, Somogyi R: Cluster analysis and data visualization of large-scale gene expression data. *Pac Symp Biocomput* **1**:42, 1998.

64. Sherlock G: Analysis of large-scale gene expression data. *Curr Opin Immunol* **12**:201, 2000.

65. Scheurle D, DeYoung MP, Binninger DM, Page H, Jahanzeb M, Narayanan R: Cancer gene discovery using digital differential display. *Cancer Res* **60**:4037, 2000.

66. Alon U, Barkai N, Notterman DA, Gish K, Ybarra S, Mack D, Levine AJ: Broad patterns of gene expression revealed by clustering analysis of tumor and normal colon tissues probed by oligonucleotide arrays. *Proc Natl Acad Sci U S A* **96**:6745, 1999.

67. Martin KJ, Kritzman BM, Price LM, Koh B, Kwan CP, Zhang X, Mackay A, et al: Linking gene expression patterns to therapeutic groups in breast cancer. *Cancer Res* **60**:2232, 2000.

68. Perou CM, Jeffrey SS, van de Rijn M, Rees CA, Eisen MB, Ross DT, Pergamenschikov A, et al: Distinctive gene expression patterns in human mammary epithelial cells and breast cancers. *Proc Natl Acad Sci U S A* **96**:9212, 1999.

69. Perou CM, Sorlie T, Eisen MB, van de Rijn M, Jeffrey SS, Rees CA, Pollack JR, et al: Molecular portraits of human breast tumours. *Nature* **406**:747, 2000.

70. Sgroi DC, Teng S, Robinson G, LeVangie R, Hudson JR, Elkahloun AG: In vivo gene expression profile analysis of human breast cancer progression. *Cancer Res* **59**:5656, 1999.

71. Hedenfalk I, Duggan D, Chen Y, Radmacher M, Bittner M, Simon R, Meltzer P, et al: Gene-expression profiles in hereditary breast cancer. *N Engl J Med* **344**:539, 2001.

72. Schummer M, Ng WV, Bumgarner RE, Nelson PS, Schummer B, Bednarski DW, Hassell L, et al: Comparative hybridization of an array of 21,500 ovarian cDNAs for the discovery of genes overexpressed in ovarian carcinomas. *Gene* **238**:375, 1999.

73. Hough CD, Sherman-Baust CA, Pizer ES, Montz FJ, Im DD, Rosenshein NB, Cho KR, et al: Large-scale serial analysis of gene expression reveals genes differentially expressed in ovarian cancer. *Cancer Res* **60**:6281, 2000.

74. Ismail RS, Baldwin RL, Fang J, Browning D, Karlan BY, Gasson JC, Chang DD: Differential gene expression between normal and tumor-derived ovarian epithelial cells. *Cancer Res* **60**:6744, 2000.

75. Klotz L: Hormone therapy for patients with prostate carcinoma. *Cancer* **88**:3009, 2000.

76. Bubendorf L, Kolmer M, Kononen J, Koivisto P, Mousses S, Chen Y, Mahlamaki E, et al: Hormone therapy failure in human prostate cancer: Analysis by complementary DNA and tissue microarrays. *J Natl Cancer Inst* **91**:1758, 1999.

77. Amler LC, Agus DB, LeDuc C, Sapinoso ML, Fox WD, Kern S, Lee D, et al: Dysregulated expression of androgen-responsive and nonresponsive genes in the androgen-independent prostate cancer xenograft model CWR22-R1. *Cancer Res* **60**:6134, 2000.

78. Golub TR, Slonim DK, Tamayo P, Huard C, Gaasenbeek M, Mesirov JP, Coller H, et al: Molecular classification of cancer: Class discovery and class prediction by gene expression monitoring. *Science* **286**:531, 1999.

79. Alizadeh AA, Eisen MB, Davis RE, Ma C, Lossos IS, Rosenwald A, Boldrick JC, et al: Distinct types of diffuse large B-cell lymphoma identified by gene expression profiling. *Nature* **403**:503, 2000.

80. Wellmann A, Thieblemont C, Pittaluga S, Sakai A, Jaffe ES, Siebert P, Raffeld M: Detection of differentially expressed genes in lymphomas using cDNA arrays: Identification of clusterin as a new diagnostic marker for anaplastic large-cell lymphomas. *Blood* **96**:398, 2000.

81. Bittner M, Meltzer P, Chen Y, Jiang Y, Seftor E, Hendrix M, Radmacher M, et al: Molecular classification of cutaneous malignant melanoma by gene expression profiling. *Nature* **406**:536, 2000.

82. Clark EA, Golub TR, Lander ES, Hynes RO: Genomic analysis of metastasis reveals an essential role for RhoC. *Nature* **406**:532, 2000.

83. Huang H, Colella S, Kurrer M, Yonekawa Y, Kleihues P, Ohgaki H: Gene expression profiling of low-grade diffuse astrocytomas by cDNA arrays. *Cancer Res* **60**:6868, 2000.

84. Sallinen SL, Sallinen PK, Haapasalo HK, Helin HJ, Helen PT, Schraml P, Kallioniemi OP, et al: Identification of differentially expressed genes in human gliomas by DNA microarray and tissue chip techniques. *Cancer Res* **60**:6617, 2000.

85. Ljubimova JY, Khazenzon NM, Chen Z, Neyman YI, Turner L, Riedinger MS, Black KL: Gene expression abnormalities in human glial tumors identified by gene array. *Int J Oncol* **18**:287, 2001.

86. Gunnersen JM, Spirkoska V, Smith PE, Danks RA, Tan SS: Growth and migration markers of rat C6 glioma cells identified by serial analysis of gene expression. *Glia* **32**:146, 2000.

87. Caskey LS, Fuller GN, Bruner JM, Yung WK, Sawaya RE, Holland EC, Zhang W: Toward a molecular classification of the gliomas: Histopathology, molecular genetics, and gene expression profiling. *Histol Histopathol* **15**:971, 2000.

88. Michiels EMC, Oussoren E, Van Groenigen M, Pauws E, Bossuyt MM, Voûte PA, Baas F: Genes differentially expressed in medulloblastoma and fetal brain. *Physiol Genomics* **1**:83, 1999.

89. Stinson SF, Alley MC, Kopp WC, Fiebig HH, Mullendore LA, Pittman AF, Kenney S, et al: Morphological and immunocytochemical characteristics of human tumor cell lines for use in a disease-oriented anticancer drug screen. *Anticancer Res* **12**:1035, 1992.

90. Ross DT, Scherf U, Eisen MB, Perou CM, Rees C, Spellman P, Iyer V, et al: Systematic variation in gene expression patterns in human cancer cell lines. *Nat Genet* **24**:227, 2000.

91. Scherf U, Ross DT, Waltham M, Smith LH, Lee JK, Tanabe L, Kohn KW, et al: A gene expression database for the molecular pharmacology of cancer. *Nat Genet* **24**:236, 2000.

92. St Croix B, Rago C, Velculescu V, Traverso G, Romans KE, Montgomery E, Lal A, et al: Genes expressed in human tumor endothelium. *Science* **289**:1197, 2000.

93. Kahn J, Mehraban F, Ingle G, Xin X, Bryant JE, Vehar G, Schoenfeld J, et al: Gene expression profiling in an in vitro model of angiogenesis. *Am J Pathol* **156**:1887, 2000.

94. Glienke J, Schmitt AO, Pilarsky C, Hinzmann B, Weiss B, Rosenthal A, Thierauch KH: Differential gene expression by endothelial cells in distinct angiogenic states. *Eur J Biochem* **267**:2820, 2000.

95. Huang P, Feng L, Oldham EA, Keating MJ, Plunkett W: Superoxide dismutase as a target for the selective killing of cancer cells. *Nature* **407**:390, 2000.

96. Ohnami S, Matsumoto N, Nakano M, Aoki K, Nagasaki K, Sugimura T, Terada M, et al: Identification of genes showing differential expression in antisense K- ras-transduced pancreatic cancer cells with suppressed tumorigenicity. *Cancer Res* **59**:5565, 1999.

97. Edamatsu H, Kaziro Y, Itoh H: LUCA15, a putative tumour suppressor gene encoding an RNA-binding nuclear protein, is down-regulated in ras-transformed Rat-1 cells. *Genes Cells* **5**:849, 2000.

98. Johnsson A, Zeelenberg I, Min Y, Hilinski J, Berry C, Howell SB, Los G: Identification of genes differentially expressed in association with acquired cisplatin resistance. *Br J Cancer* **83**:1047, 2000.

99. Duan Z, Feller AJ, Penson RT, Chabner BA, Seiden MV: Discovery of differentially expressed genes associated with paclitaxel resistance using cDNA array technology: Analysis of interleukin (IL) 6, IL-8, and monocyte chemotactic protein 1 in the paclitaxel-resistant phenotype. *Clin Cancer Res* **5**:3445, 1999.

CONTROLS ON CELL CYCLE

Cell Cycle Control: An Overview

Bruce E. Clurman ■ *James M. Roberts*

INTRODUCTION

The process of cell reproduction is known as the cell cycle.[1-3] Usually the cell cycle produces two progeny, or daughter cells, that closely resemble their parent and who are themselves capable of repeating the process. For this to occur, three things are necessary: replication of the genome; a doubling of cell mass (where cell mass refers generally to all cellular components other than chromosomes); and a precise segregation of chromosomes plus a more or less equal distribution of other cell components to the daughter cells. The execution of these events divides the cell cycle into four phases: chromosomes are replicated during S (synthetic) phase; cell constituents are segregated to daughter cells during M (mitotic) phase; and two G (gap) phases intervene between S and M. G1 precedes S phase, and G2 precedes mitosis (Fig. 9-1). Thus, chromosome replication and segregation are confined to discrete intervals of the cell cycle, whereas the third essential component of cell reproduction — growth — occurs continuously in G1, S, G2, and M. It is during G1 and G2 that cells typically respond to the proliferative and antiproliferative signals that determine whether the cell cycle ought to proceed (signals such as growth factors and cytokines). In this way, the cell cycle has the option of stopping within G1 and G2 without interrupting the critical and precarious events of chromosome replication and chromosome segregation.

Faithful reproduction of the cell requires that these events be coordinated with one another. Thus, mitosis ordinarily waits until all chromosomes have been replicated and the cell has doubled in size. However, there are specialized cell cycles where these processes are uncoupled from one another (Fig. 9-2). Repeated S phases with no intervening M phases, known as endocycles, result in the increased chromosome ploidy that is seen in megakaryocytes. Conversely, the basic cell-cycle logic of meiosis is the execution of two sequential M phases without an S phase. A third important variation is seen in the cleavage cycles that occur after fertilization of amphibian eggs. Amphibian eggs are huge cells, which, after fertilization, undergo extremely rapid cell cycles consisting of alternating S and M phases with no cell growth. After approximately 12 cleavage cycles, the embryo consists of 4000 cells, each containing a full complement of genetic material, and each now reduced to the size of a typical somatic cell.[4,5]

These simple examples show that each of the component processes of the cell cycle — growth, chromosome replication, and mitosis — can occur independently of the others. Because cell reproduction could not occur if these processes were executed in random order, there need to be mechanisms for establishing and enforcing the normal sequence of events. This chapter describes the molecules that control progression through the cell cycle, and illustrates how their activities are linked together to orchestrate the orderly process of cell reproduction. Based on these ideas, we suggest that cancer may be a disease of the cell cycle, a hypothesis that is elaborated on in subsequent chapters.

ORIGINS OF MODERN CELL CYCLE BIOLOGY

The current revolution in our understanding of cell-cycle control owes its origins to yeast genetics and amphibian reproductive cell physiology. It was through these seemingly independent lines of investigation that we came to grasp the fundamental logic of the program that controls cell reproduction, identified the genes and molecules responsible for this program, and learned how these molecules are integrated into pathways that have been evolutionarily conserved from yeast to humans.

The yeasts *Saccharomyces cerevisiae* and *Schizosaccharomyces pombe* have been favorites of cell-cycle research since the pioneering studies of Lee Hartwell and Paul Nurse.[6,7] The power of yeast as a model experimental system is in its facile genetics. It is possible to readily isolate mutations that impair the execution of specific biological processes, such as the events of the cell cycle. Identification of the mutated gene provides information about the proteins required for the execution of that biologic pathway. Of special utility are conditional mutations, because they effect the activity of the encoded protein product only under specific restrictive conditions, elevated temperatures for example. Cells harboring conditional mutations can be first collected and propagated by growth under permissive conditions, and the consequences of the mutation then determined by shifting growth to restrictive conditions.

S. cerevisiae is known as budding yeast, because it reproduces by forming a bud that grows to become the daughter cell. The regular pattern of bud development provides convenient morphologic landmarks that can be used to assemble a temporal map of the cell cycle.[8] Thus, an unbudded cell is in G1, a small bud first emerges coincident with initiation of S phase, and a cell with a large bud is in G2/M. Hartwell isolated a large group of genes required for progression through the cell cycle by identifying conditional mutations that caused a cell population to arrest with a uniform morphology (e.g., all unbudded cells). Because the morphology of a yeast cell defines its position within the cell cycle, each mutant presumably had a position-specific defect in the operation of a cell cycle event. He called these cdc mutations (for "cell division cycle").[9] Thus, some cdc mutants were defective in G1-specific events (and arrested as unbudded cells), others in S phase (small-budded cells), and yet others in events that take place in G2/M (large-budded cells). Further analysis of nuclear morphology and the state of the mitotic spindle gave additional information about the specific processes affected by each mutation. In this way, Hartwell successfully identified the vast majority of genes responsible for regulating the eukaryotic cell cycle.[10]

The characterization of cdc mutations revealed a major principle of cell cycle regulation — that the orderly execution of cell cycle events resulted from a series of dependent relationships in which the completion of one event is required for the beginning of the next.[9] For instance, a cell with a mutation in a gene required

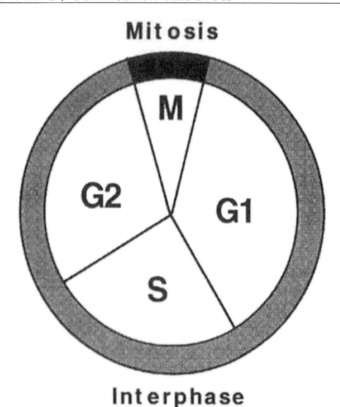

Mitosis

M

G2   G1

S

Interphase

Fig. 9-1 The four phases of the cell cycle. Interphase is composed of S (synthesis) phase, during which time DNA replication occurs, and two G (gap) phases, during which cells respond to various proliferative and antiproliferative stimuli and cell growth occurs. Chromosomes and cellular contents are than distributed to two daughter cells during M (mitosis) phase, and the resulting progeny re-enter the cell cycle in G1.

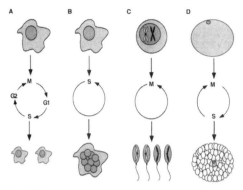

Fig. 9-2 Specialized cell cycles. A, A normal cell cycle is depicted in which a cell gives rise to two identical daughter cells. B, During megakaryopoiesis, promegakaryocytes undergo repeated rounds of DNA replication in the absence of mitosis (endoreduplication), resulting in polyploid megakaryocytes with a DNA content greater than their progenitors. C, In meiosis, two successive cell divisions after DNA replication result in four haploid daughter cells. D, Amphibian eggs undergo 12 rapid cell cycles consisting of alternating S and M phases. No cell growth occurs during these cycles, and the large egg cell is subdivided into approximately 4000 cells, each containing a normal complement of chromosomes.

for DNA replication stops its cell cycle in S phase and does not inappropriately try to begin mitosis (even though it should be capable of doing so). Initially, these dependencies were thought to reflect underlying biochemical pathways in which the product of one event was an essential substrate for the next. Hence, only after an upstream event occurred correctly would the substrates for the next event become available. This is one way to insure that cell cycle events were not executed in random order. The idea that the cell cycle is organized by dependent relationships is still considered one of the most important in cell-cycle biology, but the explanation for dependencies has changed and is discussed shortly.

A particularly important set of dependent pathways is initiated at the transition from G1 into S phase; this is called cell-cycle START.[11] Uniquely at START, the yeast cell senses the external and internal signals that control its proliferation, including mating pheromone, nutrients, and cell size (Fig. 9-3).[12–14] The yeast cell responds by initiating (or failing to initiate) the three parallel pathways required for reproduction of the cell—bud emergence, DNA replication, and spindle pole body duplication (the spindle pole body being the yeast equivalent of the centrosome of the mitotic spindle). The coordinate regulation of these three parallel-reproductive pathways indicates that completion of START represents the commitment of the cell to complete the entire program of events required for cell reproduction. Thus, genes required for START must play pivotal roles in the control of cell proliferation, and among the handful of START-specific genes, the CDC28 gene has gained particular prominence.[6,15,16] Analogous to START, the R POINT (restriction point) in mammalian cells defines a transition within G1 after which completion of the remainder of the cell cycle becomes independent of extracellular mitogens.

In contrast to the budding yeast cell cycle, during which cell growth and cell division are linked in G1 at START, in *S. pombe* (known also as fission yeast), these processes are usually coordinated at the transition between G2 and mitosis.[17] Paul Nurse identified cdc mutants in *S. pombe* that were unable to undergo the G2/M transition and one mutant, called cdc2, received special attention.[18–20] First, CDC2 is required twice during the fission yeast cell cycle, once at the G2/M transition and again at the G1/S transition (where a back-up size control exists). Second, certain dominantly acting mutations of cdc2 caused cells to shorten the length of G2, enter mitosis too quickly, and, consequently, become smaller than normal (known as a "wee" phenotype). This suggests that CDC2 activity is rate limiting for the onset of mitosis. The budding yeast CDC28 gene and the *S. pombe* CDC2 gene are homologs of one another.[17,19] Although CDC28 was first identified through its role at G1/S and cdc2 by its role at G2/M, it is now known that these proteins are required at the G1/S and at G2/M transitions in both types of yeast.[17,21,22] Because of these experiments, CDC2/CDC28 emerged as a key regulator of the cell cycle.

Complementing these genetic analyses of the yeast cell cycle were studies on the meiotic maturation of amphibian eggs. These physiological studies led to the discovery of a natural regulator of cell-cycle progression, an activity named MPF (maturation

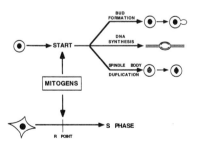

Fig. 9-3 START and the R (restriction) POINT define G1 transitions after which cell cycle progression becomes mitogen independent. At START, budding yeast initiate three independent processes required for cell duplication: bud emergence, DNA synthesis, and spindle-body duplication. A variety of mitogenic and antimitogenic signals determine if cells traverse START, after which cell cycle progression no longer depends upon these stimuli. At the analogous R POINT in mammalian cells, S-phase entry is no longer mitogen dependent. The biochemical bases of START and the R-POINT are discussed in the text.

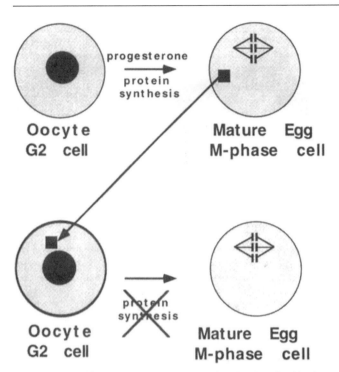

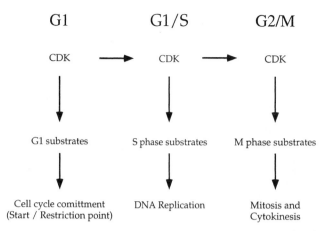

Fig. 9-5 The cdc2 cycle. The enzymatic activity of cdc2 and related kinases (cdks) drives each of the key cell cycle transitions.

Fig. 9-4 MPF stimulates mitosis in G2-oocytes. As described in the text, injection of cytoplasm extract from an M-phase amphibian egg is sufficient to induce maturation of the recipient egg in the absence of progesterone or protein synthesis.

promoting factor).[23-25] Amphibians produce mature eggs in response to the hormone progesterone, which induces immature oocytes to emerge from a prolonged arrest in G2 and resume the meiotic cell cycle. The progesterone-stimulated oocyte completes the reductive meiotic divisions and eventually pauses again in metaphase of meiosis II, but now as a mature egg awaiting fertilization. In other words, oocyte maturation requires cell-cycle progression from G2 of meiosis I to metaphase of meiosis II, and is under the control of MPF. Indeed, injection of MPF isolated from a mature egg into the cytoplasm of an immature oocyte is sufficient to initiate meiotic maturation independently of any hormonal trigger (Fig. 9-4). Furthermore, MPF activity is not restricted to meiosis. MPF activity oscillates during each mitotic cycle, being high in M phase and low in interphase.[24,26,27] This indicates that MPF is a fundamental component of cell-cycle regulation in all cell cycles, mitotic as well as meiotic.

Remarkably, MPF activity will continue to oscillate even in enucleated cells.[28] Because MPF activity can oscillate independently of nuclear events, it has been proposed that the MPF cycle might be an autonomous mitotic clock, and that state of the clock (the "time of day") determines which cell cycle event occurs.[26,28,29] Thus, high MPF activity would permit entry into mitosis, and low MPF activity would permit cells to enter S phase. This model supplanted the earlier idea that the obligate order of cell cycle events might simply be established by substrate-product-type relationships. However, the notion of a mitotic clock would then require the existence of additional feedback controls to keep the clock entrained to actual progress through the cell cycle; the clock must stop if essential cell cycle events do not occur. These feedback controls do exist, and are known as checkpoints.[30]

Perhaps the most far-reaching advance in the cell-cycle field in the last 15 years has been the demonstration that cell-cycle controls are evolutionarily conserved.[31,32] This first became evident when it was discovered that the CDC2 and CDC28 genes in fission and budding yeast encode homologous proteins,[17] now known as the CDC2 protein kinase. Furthermore, gene transfer experiments show that the human CDC2 gene can complement mutations in the yeast CDC2 gene.[33] This was reinforced 6 years

later when MPF was purified (initially from *Xenopus,* and later from other vertebrates), and its catalytic subunit was shown to be a homolog of CDC2.[34-38] These observations set the stage for our current paradigm of eukaryotic cell cycle control, which in its simplest form depicts the cell cycle as a CDC2 cycle (Fig. 9-5).[39] Thus, in organisms ranging from yeast to humans, the catalytic activity of CDC2 and related kinases is required for each of the major transitions within the cell cycle—from G1 into S, and from G2 into M.[40-46]

CDK REGULATION

In budding and fission yeast, the highly regulated action of a single kinase subunit (cdc28 or cdc2, respectively) drives the cell cycle forward.[47] In higher eukaryotes, cell-cycle control is more complex, and several proteins homologous to cdc2 (termed the cyclin-dependent kinases or cdks) have been identified.[48] Cyclin-dependent kinases are protein kinases that vary in size between 30 and 40 kb and share greater than 40 percent sequence identity. In addition to amino acid homology, cdks share many functional and regulatory features with yeast cdc2/28.[49,50] Almost all cdks require association with protein subunits called cyclins to become active kinases. Cdks also contain conserved amino acid residues that modulate kinase activity when phosphorylated or dephosphorylated. Additionally, specific regulatory molecules that bind and inhibit cdk subunits inhibit cdk activity. Each of these regulatory mechanisms is discussed in detail below. Remarkably, while differences among organisms do exist, this multi-tiered regulatory system has been conserved from yeast to humans.

Each phase of the cell cycle is characterized by a unique pattern of cdk activity (Fig. 9-6).[51-53] In mammalian cells, eight cdks have been identified, and most are active (and required) only in specific phases of the cell cycle. Progression through G1 phase depends upon the activities of cdk2, cdk3, cdk4, and cdk6. The recently described cdk8 protein also may function primarily in G1, and may be involved in transcriptional regulation. Cdk2 and cdc2 are active in S-phase, and cdc2 kinase activity also governs mitotic entry and exit. In distinction to its kindred, cdk5 does not appear to be intimately involved in cell-cycle progression, but may, instead, play a role in the developing nervous system, where it associates with the non-cyclin activator p35.[54,55]

Cyclins: Activating Subunits of CDK Enzymes

Monomeric cdk subunits are essentially devoid of enzymatic activity, and kinase activation requires the association of cdks with cyclins.[49] An active cdk is thus a heterodimeric enzyme consisting of regulatory (cyclin) and enzymatic (cdk) subunits. The cyclins are a group of related proteins that contain a conserved region of homology (the cyclin box) and are usually expressed in a cell cycle specific fashion. Cyclin expression is rate-limiting for cdk

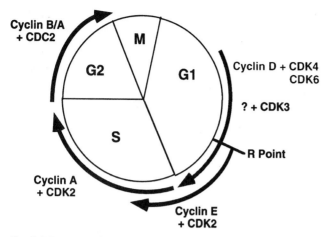

Fig. 9-6 Patterns of cyclin-cdk activity during the mammalian cell cycle. The expression patterns of the key mammalian cyclins is superimposed upon the cell cycle, along with their respective cdk partners. The approximate position of the R POINT is shown (adapted from Sherr[51]).

activation, and control of cyclin expression is a fundamental mechanism underlying cdk periodicity. In general, cyclin levels are determined by both transcriptional control and regulated proteolysis by the ubiquitin-proteosome system.

The recently solved crystal structure of cyclin A bound to cdk2 reveals that cyclins activate cdks in at least two ways. Cyclin binding induces conformational changes in the cdk that first reorients the configuration of the ATP phosphate groups to facilitate phosphotransfer to protein substrates, and second moves the T-loop of the cdk out of a position that would otherwise block entry of protein substrates into the active site (Fig. 9-7).[56,57]

The specificity of cdk action at different times in the cell cycle is in large part determined by its particular cyclin subunit. This functional diversity of cyclins was first established in the yeast *S. cerevisiae* where specific cyclins have been identified that are required for G1, S phase, and mitosis. Budding yeast express three functionally redundant G1 cyclins (cln1, cln2, and cln3), which are required for passage through START.[58–62] While differences between the cln genes have been described, mutant yeast cells with mutated cln alleles can still enter S phase as long as one of these three genes remains functional. Transcription of cln1 and cln2 is controlled by the Swi4/Swi6 transcription factor,[63–65] and cln activity positively reinforces further cln expression.[66–68] Thus, cln1 and cln2 mRNAs rise during G1, reaching peak levels around START.

Once START has been traversed, cln activity is no longer required for subsequent cell-cycle progression. Instead, other cyclins associate with and activate cdc28 during other phases of the cell cycle. Complexes containing cdc28 and the cyclins clb5 and clb6 are required for S phase,[69,70] and the four B-type cyclins, clb1 to clb4 are required for mitosis.[71]

START marks a point of transition in the yeast cell cycle where G1 cyclin expression ends and mitotic cyclin expression begins. This transition comes about because these two classes of cyclin modulate each other's expression. Cln/cdc28 kinase activity directly increases the expression of the clb genes, and conversely clb-cdc28 kinase activity represses cln expression.[72] Not only do G1 cyclins promote the expression of the genes for mitotic cyclins but, as described below, they also increase the stability and functional activity of clb proteins. Furthermore, the cln proteins themselves are rapidly degraded after START. This is discussed below in the section on cell-cycle regulated proteolysis. Together, these controls insure ordered progression through the cell cycle by establishing alternating periods of the cell cycle where either G1 or mitotic cyclins are expressed and functionally active.

Mammalian cyclins C, D1, and E were first identified in a screen for mammalian genes that could complement yeast cyclin

mutations.[73–75] At the same time Cyclin D1 was identified by two other approaches — as a mitogen-responsive gene in a macrophage cell line[76] and as a gene located at a chromosome inversion breakpoint in a parathyroid tumor (and in this guise was originally named PRAD1).[77] A dozen mammalian cyclin genes have been identified that are both structurally and functionally homologous to yeast cyclins.[51,52] Like the yeast cyclins, many of these molecules exhibit cell-cycle-dependent periodicity in their expression and activity (Fig. 9-6).

The primary mammalian G1 cyclins are the D-type cyclins and cyclin E. These cyclins associate with the cdk-4/6, and cdk2 subunits, respectively. There are three D-type cyclins (D1, D2, and D3), which are expressed in a cell-type specific fashion.[51,52,78] The G1 role of the D-type cyclins is revealed by their pattern of expression and by their functional properties. Cyclin D expression begins in early G1 when quiescent cells are stimulated to reenter the cell cycle, and cyclin D expression remains at high levels as long as mitogens are present. In other words, the expression of these labile proteins ($t\frac{1}{2} < 20$ min) is not intrinsically periodic, but instead depends upon the presence of cell-type specific mitogens. Inhibition of cyclin D1 function blocks the cell cycle in G1, demonstrating the necessity of cyclin D for the cell cycle.[79,80] Also, enforced overexpression of cyclin D1 shortens the G1 phase of the cell cycle, and partially diminishes the mitogen requirement for cell proliferation, demonstrating that cyclin D1 levels are limiting for G1 progression.[80,81]

Cyclin E activity is also required in G1, although probably somewhat after cyclin D activity.[81–83] Cyclin E protein expression peaks at the G1-S boundary, and then decays as S-phase progresses.[82,84,85] Determinants of cyclin E periodicity include both transcriptional control by E2F and regulated proteolysis (see below). Overexpression of cyclin E results in G1 contraction and decreased mitogen requirements,[81,86] and cyclin E kinase activity is required for S-phase entry.[82,83] Activation of cyclin D and cyclin E-associated kinases may biochemically constitute the restriction point, the mammalian equivalent of START control in yeast.

Later cell-cycle transitions are governed by the cyclin A and cyclin B proteins. Cyclin A associates with both the cdk2 and cdc2 subunits, and cyclin A kinase activity is required at the start of S phase and at the G2-M transition.[87–89] Cyclin B associates with cdc2 and, like the yeast clb proteins, cyclin B-cdc2 kinase activity regulates both mitotic entry and exit.[90]

The cyclin H protein associates with cdk7, and this heterodimer constitutes the cdk-activating kinase (CAK).[91] CAK is also a component of the human transcription factor TFIIH, and is capable of phosphorylating the carboxy-terminal domain (CTD) of RNA polymerase II. Cyclin C is classed as a G1 cyclin, although its role is not yet defined.[73] Cyclin C has recently been shown to associate with cdk8, and cyclin C-cdk8 complexes also have RNA polymerase II CTD kinase activity, although they do not co-purify with TFIIH.[92] Phosphorylation of the CTD by cyclin-cdk complexes may couple cell-cycle events to the cellular transcriptional machinery.

Comparatively little is known about the remaining cyclins that have been identified to date, including cyclins F, G and I. Cyclin F is the largest cyclin, with a molecular weight of 87, and is most closely related to cyclins A and B. Cyclin F mRNA peaks in G2 and cyclin F protein accumulates in interphase and is destroyed during mitosis.[93] Cyclin G mRNA does not fluctuate in a cell cycle-dependent fashion, but is induced by both the p53 protein and growth stimulation of quiescent cells.[94] The cyclin I protein is expressed most highly in post-mitotic tissues, including muscle and neurons, and may have a unique regulatory role.[95]

CDK Regulation by Phosphorylation and Dephosphorylation

In addition to cyclin binding, phosphorylation and dephosphorylation of conserved cdk residues provides another important level of control over kinase activity.[49] Cdks can be either activated or inactivated by phosphorylation (Fig. 9-8). The site of activating

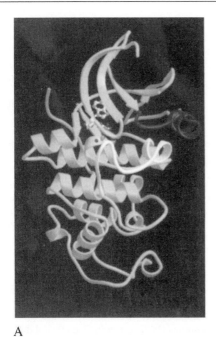

A

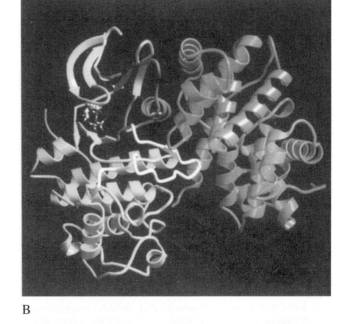

B

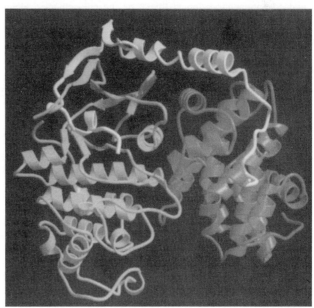

C

D

Fig. 9-7 Crystal structure of cdk2, cyclin A-cdk2, and cyclin A-cdk2-p27 complexes. A, The structure of monomeric cdk2. The T-loop is indicated in yellow, and the PSTAIRE motif in red. An ATP molecule in indicated within the active site. B, The structure of cdk2 bound to an amino-terminal truncated version of cyclin A. Cyclin binding reorients the PSTAIRE helix and moves the T-loop, resulting in the repositioning of ATP-phosphate groups within the complex and allowing substrate accessibility to the active site. C, The structure **of cdk-activating kinase (CAK)-phosphorylated cyclin A bound to cdk2. The yellow ball indicates the position of thr160 within the T-loop. D, The structure of a ternary complex of the amino terminus of p27 bound to cyclin A -cdk2. Separate domains of P27 interact with both cyclin A and cdk2. The structure of this complex reveals that p27 inhibits cdk activity by distorting the structure of the active site, and by binding within the catalytic cleft and preventing ATP binding.**

phosphorylation is a conserved threonine residue in the so-called "T-loop" (e.g., threonine 161 in cdc2, threonine 160 in cdk2).[56] The binding of cyclin to the cdk, and phosphorylation of this residues together move the T-loop away from the catalytic cleft of the enzyme, thereby providing access to protein substrates.[96] Thr160 is phosphorylated by CAK (cyclin H-cdk7), and this phosphorylation is required for cdk activation.[97–100] CAK activity, however, is neither cell-cycle regulated nor limiting, and the major determinant of Thr160 phosphorylation is probably cyclin binding.[91]

Cdks can also be phosphorylated on a specific amino-terminal tyrosine residue (e.g., tyrosine 15 in cdc2 and cdk2). Tyrosine phosphorylated cdk2 is catalytically inactive, even if it is phosphorylated on the activating threonine within the T-loop.[98,100–103] The kinases that phosphorylate tyr15 are evolutionarily conserved and are known as the wee1 and mik1 kinases.[104–107] Conversely, dephosphorylation of tyrosine by the cdc25 phosphatase activates the cdk.[108–112] Regulation of wee1 and cdc25 is complex,[113,114] but the bottom-line is that the relative activities of these enzymes set a threshold for cdk activation and

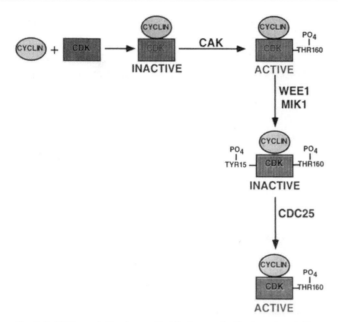

Fig. 9-8 CDK regulation by cyclin binding and cdk phosphorylation. As described in the text, activation of cdks requires cyclin binding and cdk phosphorylation at thr160 by the cdk-activating kinase (CAK). Subsequent phosphorylation of Tyr15 by the wee1 and mik1 kinases and dephosphorylation by cdc25 phosphatases further regulates kinase activity.

determine mitotic entry. Three mammalian cdc25 homologues have been identified (cdc25a, cdc25b, and cdc25c), and each may have a unique cell-cycle role.[115,116] Cdc25a is active in G1 and may be induced by raf-dependent pathways.[117]

CKIs: Inhibitory Subunits of CDK Enzymes

All organisms express proteins that directly bind to and inhibit cdk activity.[118,119] These cdk-inhibitors (CKIs) provide another important strategy by which cdk activity is regulated in response to diverse stimuli. In budding yeast, two kinds of inhibitors have been described. One type is inducible and links the cell cycle to extracellular signals; the other type is an intrinsic component of the mitotic cycle. The best example of the first type of CKI is the FAR1 protein. Mating pheromones induce FAR1, a protein that binds to and inhibits the cln-cdc28 kinase and thereby causes the yeast cell cycle to arrest at START. Another important CDK inhibitor in budding yeast is Sic1, but it is a constitutive element in the mitotic clock and is not known to be induced by extrinsic proliferative signals.[120,121] At the conclusion of each mitosis, Sic1 protein levels rise, inhibiting the clb-cdc28 kinases and facilitating the transition from anaphase to the next G1. Sic1 protein remains at high levels during G1 until activation of the cln-cdc28 kinases at START induce its degradation. This is one mechanism that links activation of the S-phase clb-cdc28 kinases to passage through START.

Mammalian cells express two classes of CKIs that are distinguished by their cdk targets: the Cip/Kip family of CKI's are universal cdk inhibitors, whereas the INK4 proteins are specific cdk4/6 inhibitors (Fig. 9-9).[118] The Cip/Kip family consists of three members: p21, p27, and p57. Overexpression of these molecules causes a G1 arrest in cultured cells, and they are able to inhibit most cyclin-cdk complexes *in vitro*. These molecules bind to assembled cyclin-cdk complexes much more avidly than to monomeric cdk or cyclin subunits. p21 was first identified as a component of cyclin-CDK complexes in proliferating cells[123] and as a protein induced as cells *in vitro* became senescent.[124] Shortly thereafter, it was cloned by a number of independent approaches.[125–128] The p21 protein contains two functional domains, an amino terminal cdk interaction region that is sufficient for cdk inhibition, and a carboxy-terminal region that

binds PCNA, a processivity factor associated with DNA polymerase delta.[129–131]

Two biological roles have been suggested for p21.[118,122] The first is in contributing to the cell-cycle arrest that occurs in cells with damaged DNA.[127] This is discussed in greater detail below. Additionally, p21 has been suggested as a facilitator of withdrawal from the cell cycle in cells undergoing terminal differentiation.[132,133]

The CKI p27Kip1 is structurally related to p21Cip1.[134,135] p21 and p27 share significant amino terminal homology within the cdk inhibitory domain, but p27 does not contain the PCNA interaction region. p27 is not a p53 response gene, but p27 levels respond instead to a variety of extracellular mitogenic and antimitogenic signals.[118] In general, p27 levels are high in nondividing cells and low in proliferating cells. The regulation of p27 is complex, with transcriptional, translational and post-translational mechanisms all implicated in different biological contexts.[136]

The mechanism of cdk inhibition by p27 has been clarified by the crystal structure of p27 bound to cyclin A-cdk2 (Fig. 9-7).[96] In the ternary p27-cyclin A-cdk2 complex, separate domains in p27 interacts with the cyclin and the cdk. Although p27 does not significantly alter the structure of the cyclin, it may bind to a site on the cyclin that the cyclin would ordinarily use for interactions with protein substrates. In this way, p27 might inhibit phosphorylation of physiologically important substrates without inhibiting the catalytic activity of the cdk enzyme. In addition, p27 does have dramatic effects on cdk structure. p27 disrupts the structure of the N-terminal lobe of the cdk, widening and distorting the ATP-binding site. In fact, p27 itself inserts into the catalytic cleft and directly interacts with the amino acids that would bind ATP. This would completely prevent cdk-binding of ATP and completely inhibit catalytic activity.

Less is known about p57, the most recently isolated family member that was cloned by virtue of its homology with p27.[137,138] Both the amino and carboxy-terminal domains of p57 are related to p27. Compared with p27, however, p57 expression is relatively restricted to terminally differentiated tissues.

The INK4 family of CKIs includes four structurally related proteins (p15, p16, p18, p19), each of which contains four ankyrin repeats.[118] The first member of this family to be identified, p16, was found to be associated with cdk4 in transformed cells,[138] and subsequently fingered as a candidate tumor suppressor in familial melanoma.[139,140] INK4 proteins bind to monomeric cdk4/6 subunits, preventing their association with D-type cyclins, and

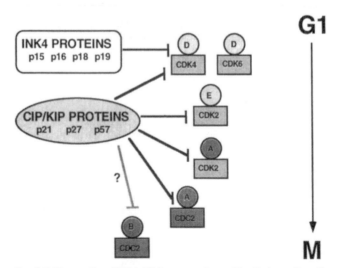

Fig. 9-9 Mammalian CDK-inhibitors are classed by their cyclin-cdk targets. The Cip/Kip proteins (p21, p27, p57) are universal cdk inhibitors that inactivate all cyclin-cdk complexes (with the possible exception of cyclin B-cdc2). In contrast, the INK4 proteins (p15, p16, p18, p19) specifically bind and inhibit only cdk4/6, and cyclin D-cdk4/6 complexes.

INK4 proteins can also inhibit the activity of cyclin D-cdk4/6 complexes. The other INK4 proteins are expressed ubiquitously in mouse tissues and cultured cells, and the expression of p19 does oscillate with the cell cycle.[141,142] While p15 is involved in the anti-proliferative response to TGF-B, the physiological roles of the INK4 protein remain unknown. The frequent deletions of p15 and p16 in primary tumors and the high spontaneous tumor rate in p16-deficient mice indicate that these proteins play a critical role in maintaining normal growth control.[143]

CDK SUBSTRATES

Cdks promote progression through the cell cycle by phosphorylating a group of protein substrates.[53] However, compared with the enormous amount of data concerning cdk regulation, relatively little is known about cdk substrates. The most thoroughly characterized cdk substrates are cell-cycle regulatory proteins themselves. For example, in budding yeast, phosphorylation of p40sic1 by the cln-cdc28 kinase leads to its ubiquitin-mediated proteolysis and progression from G1 to S phase.[120,121] In fact, a yeast strain lacking all cln genes is viable if p40sic1 is also mutated, which suggests that phosphorylation of this CKI is a key function of the cln proteins in promoting cell cycle progression.[144]

A critical regulator of cell-cycle progression in higher eukaryotes, including humans, is the Rb protein. The importance of Rb in cell-cycle control became evident as a result of three separate seminal observations.[145] First, the oncogenic proteins encoded by a variety of DNA tumor viruses (e.g., SV40, adenovirus, and papillomavirus) all bind to the Rb protein.[146–148] Second, the Rb gene is mutated in the germ line in patients suffering hereditary retinoblastoma, and is frequently mutated in tumor cells in patients who develop spontaneous tumors.[149–151] Third, the Rb protein undergoes cell-cycle dependent phosphorylation during G1, and this modifies its interaction with an essential transcription factor known as E2F.[152–156] E2F transcription factors are heterodimeric proteins composed of one E2F subunit and one DP subunit that regulate the transcription of many genes required in S-phase.[157–159] There are five known E2F subunits, which are designated E2F1 to E2F5, and three known DP subunits, which are designated DP1 to DP3. When complexed with Rb, E2F is inactive or it may be a transcriptional repressor, and the cell cycle arrests in the absence of these needed gene products. E2F sequestration is regulated by the phosphorylation state of Rb; unphosphorylated Rb avidly binds E2F while hyperphosphorylated does not. As cells progress through G1, Rb is progressively phosphorylated at multiple sites, ultimately releasing E2F. Viral oncoproteins specifically bind to the unphosphorylated form of Rb, and in doing so automatically release E2F from its Rb-bound inactive state.

The kinases that phosphorylate Rb are the cdks. The pRb protein contains eight consensus cdk-phosphorylation sites, and cyclin D-, E-, and A-cdk complexes have Rb kinase activity *in vitro* and *in vivo*.[160–163] Cyclin D-cdk4 complexes bind stably to Rb, and once Rb is phosphorylated, this complex disassembles.[164] Cyclin D-cdk4/6 and cyclin E-cdk2 complexes probably cooperate to phosphorylate and inactivate Rb during G1. The observation that cyclin D function is dispensable in cells with mutant Rb alleles suggests that pRb phosphorylation is the critical means by which D-type cyclins promote G1 progression.[165–167] Phosphorylation of Rb by cyclin E-cdk2 may also be required prior to S-phase entry, but cyclin E is essential for cell-cycle progression in Rb-mutant cells, demonstrating that other substrates of cyclin E-cdk2 must also exist.[82]

Rb is one member of a family of structurally related "pocket" proteins, which includes p107, p130, and Rb itself.[167] All the pocket proteins bind to members of the E2F family of transcription factors and phosphorylation of these proteins by cyclin-cdk complexes liberates E2F, removing some constraints on cell proliferation. However, neither p107 nor p130 are tumor suppressors, and their function during the cell cycle is poorly understood.

E2F activity is essential for the G1-S transition, but it must also be inactivated for the ensuing S-phase to progress normally.[170,171] E2F/DP heterodimers form stable complexes with cyclin A-cdk2, and phosphorylation of a specific DP residue by cyclin A-cdk2 suppresses E2F DNA-binding. Thus, G1 cyclins activate E2F via Rb phosphorylation, and cyclin A-cdk2 directly inactivates E2F through DP phosphorylation. In this way, sequentially acting cyclin-cdk complexes first initiate and then extinguish E2F activity, causing a pulse of E2F-dependent gene transcription at the G1 to S phase transition.

The elucidation of cdk substrates clearly remains incomplete.[172] For instance, it is thought that proteins directly involved in the initiation of DNA replication will be phosphorylated and activated by cdks at the start of S phase,[173] although not a single such protein has been identified. Almost as short is the list of cdk substrates during mitosis. The first identified mitotic cdk substrates were the nuclear lamins.[174,175] The nuclear lamina is a structure composed of intermediate filament proteins that depolymerizes at the onset of mitosis. The polymerization of lamins is regulated by phosphorylation, and lamins have been shown to be substrates for cyclin B-cdc2. Phosphorylation of lamins promotes their disassembly, and it has been proposed cyclin B-cdc2 lamin kinase activity is responsible for the breakdown of the nuclear lamina at mitosis. Cdc2 kinase activity is also required for assembly of the mitotic spindle.[176] The human Eg5 protein is a kinesin-related motor protein that is needed to build a bipolar spindle. The localization of Eg5 to the spindle apparatus is dependent on phosphorylation at thr927, and this residue is phosphorylated by cyclin B-cdc2. Inhibition of Eg5 function results in a mitotic block, and one mechanism by which cyclin B-cdc2 promotes mitosis is likely to involve Eg5 phosphorylation.

PROTEOLYSIS IN CELL-CYCLE REGULATION

A basic feature of the cell cycle is that its transitions are irreversible. Anaphase cells, for instance, cannot regress to metaphase, nor can S phase cells reverse course and go back to G1. This is accomplished by a cycle of protein destruction that complements the periodic activation of cyclin/cdk complexes. In general, protein destruction eliminates both proteins that have been used in the preceding phase of the cell cycle and proteins that would inhibit progression into the next cell cycle phase.[177] The net effect is to cause the cell cycle to move irreversibly forward.

The paradigm for periodic protein degradation during the cell cycle is the destruction of cyclin B during mitosis (Fig. 9-10).[35,178] The abundance of cyclin B protein oscillates during each cell division cycle, being highest as cells enter mitosis and disappearing after chromosome disjunction has occurred at the metaphase to anaphase transition.[179] This is caused by changes in the rate of its degradation. Many short-lived proteins, including cyclin B, are degraded in the proteosome, a 26S complex that contains multiple proteolytic enzymes and that specifically recognizes and degrades ubiquitinated proteins.[180] Conjugation of a protein to ubiquitin is the signal for its delivery to the proteosome, and this is accomplished in a multistep reaction in which ubiquitin is ultimately transferred through a thiol-ester linkage to lysine side-chains of the target protein.[181,182] Ubiquitin, a 76-amino acid protein, is first attached through its carboxy terminus to an ubiquitin-activating enzyme called E1, in an ATP-dependent reaction. The E1-bound ubiquitin is then transferred to one of a family of carrier proteins called E2, or ubiquitin-conjugating enzymes, which can then transfer ubiquitin to target proteins. Most eukaryotes are thought to have a single E1 gene, but multiple E2 genes (at least 12 in budding yeast). Each of the E2 enzymes recognizes and transfers ubiquitin to only particular proteins, thereby imposing some degree of selectivity on the process of ubiquitin-dependent proteolysis. Further selectivity arises because conjugation of some proteins to ubiquitin requires

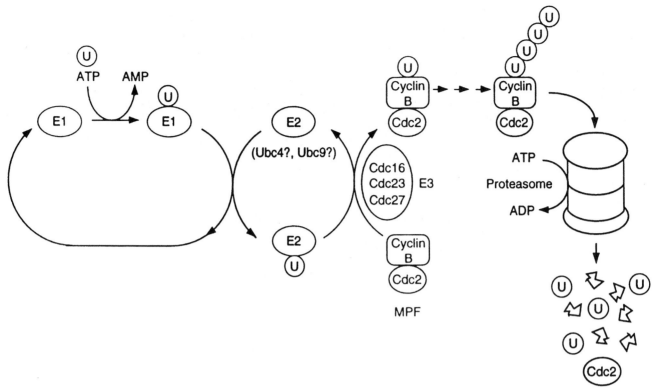

Fig. 9-10 The biochemistry of cyclin destruction. See text for details (reprinted from Murray 1995[190] with permission).

collaboration between an E2 and an E3 enzyme, which is called ubiquitin ligases.

The E2 and E3 enzymes choose proteins for ubiquitination by recognizing specific amino acids motifs.[183] A few types of motifs have been identified, each presumably recognized by certain E2 or E2/E3 combinations. The particular ubiquitination motif within cyclin B is called the cyclin destruction box.[184] A mutant version of cyclin B lacking the destruction box (called cyclin BΔdb) is not conjugated to ubiquitin during mitosis and is not degraded.[185] Consequently, cyclin BΔdb/cdc2 (and its MPF activity) remains active, and the cell cycle becomes blocked in mitosis.[186-188] This important experiment demonstrates that destruction of cyclin B is required for inactivation of cdc2 and MPF activity in anaphase cells, and that inactivation of cdc2 is required for mitosis to be completed. Therefore, just as synthesis of cyclin B is required for a cell to enter mitosis, the destruction of cyclin B is required for a cell to exit mitosis and begin a new cell cycle.[189] Cyclin A also has a destruction box and is degraded in mitosis at about the same time as cyclin B.[190]

The ubiquitination of cyclin B is controlled by an E3-like activity called the anaphase-promoting complex, or APC.[191] As its name implies, the APC is required not only in anaphase for the destruction of cyclin B, but also earlier in mitosis at metaphase to promote the transition into anaphase.[192] It is thought that at the metaphase to anaphase transition the APC is required for the targeted ubiquitination and proteolysis of a protein necessary for cohesion between sister chromatids on the metaphase plate. The APC has been characterized both genetically and biochemically, and shown to be a 20S particle comprising at least three proteins: cdc16, cdc23, and cdc27 (which were originally discovered by Hartwell in the cdc screen described above).[191,193-195]

The activity of the APC is regulated during the cell cycle.[177] The ability of the APC to ubiquitinate B-type cyclins is turned on during mitosis and turned off in G1, leading directly to the periodic accumulation and destruction of these cyclins.[195-197] In this way, the duration of APC activity defines the interval in the cell cycle where the levels of B-type cyclins are kept low; this is a key

element in establishing the G1 phase of the cell cycle. Conversely, inactivation of the APC is required for accumulation of S-phase cyclins, like clb5 and clb6 in yeast, and probably cyclin A in mammalian cells, and is, therefore, a prerequisite for entry into S phase. Thus, cyclin/cdks and the APC are complementary activities that work in parallel to control major transitions within the cell cycle. The mechanisms regulating the APC are incompletely understood, but it seems as though APC activity is directly coupled to cyclin/cdk activity. First, during mitosis it is thought that cyclin B/cdc2 initiates the pathway leading to its own destruction by phosphorylating and activating the APC.[177,196] Second, once activated in mitosis the APC remains active until late in G1, when it is inactivated by G1 cyclin/cdk activity.[196] In yeast, this occurs coincidentally with START, and in mammalian cells, it may be one of the events that leads to cell-cycle commitment at the restriction point.

Protein destruction also controls the abundance of the cyclins and CKIs that regulate entry into S phase. Cyclin E in mammalian cells,[198,199] and the G1 cyclins in yeast (the cln proteins),[200-202] are both degraded by ubiquitin-dependent proteolysis. In both cases, phosphorylation of the cyclin triggers its ubiquitination, which is a common theme in regulated protein turnover.[203-205] Often, phosphorylation of a protein is the end result of a signal transduction pathway, and can be used to allow recognition of proteins by E2 and E3 ubiquitin-conjugating enzymes. In the case of cyclin E and the cln proteins, the cyclins are directly phosphorylated by their associated cdks. Thus, cyclin E/cdk2 activity is inherently self-limited, because cdk2 activity initiates the pathway leading to cyclin E destruction. In essence, this is similar to the control of A and B-type cyclin turnover by the APC, because in each instance cyclin degradation is initiated by cdk activity.

Cdk inhibitor levels are also regulated during G1 by proteolysis. In mammalian cells, the cdk inhibitor p27Kip1 is eliminated from cells after mitogenic stimulation by the ubiquitin-proteosome pathway;[206] in budding yeast, the cdk inhibitor p40Sic1 is regulated in a similar manner.[121,144] In fact, biochemical reconstitution of sic1 turnover *in vitro* has led to the identification of an E3 complex that may rival the importance of the APC in cell-cycle control. The sic1 E3 complex is composed of three proteins, skp1, cdc53, and cdc4.[206a,d–f] The skp1-cdc53-cdc4 complex specifically recognizes and promotes the ubiquitination of phosphorylated sic1 in the presence of cdc34 (an E2) and E1. In addition to sic1, the skp1-cdc53-cdc4 complex also functions as an E3 for the *S. cervesiae* cdk inhibitor far1.[206b]

The components of this E3 complex are members of protein families: cdc4 belongs to a large group of proteins defined by a region of homology called an F-box,[206e,f] and cdc53 belongs to the family of proteins termed cullins.[208] Substitution of different family members within the E3 complex can have dramatic affects on its activity. When other F-box proteins replace cdc4, the substrate specificity of the E3 complex can change. For example, substituting Grr1 for cdc4 confers binding to phosphorylated cln1 and cln2, rather than to sic1, while the met30 F-box protein is involved in repression of genes that regulate methionine synthesis.[206d,e] In recognition of its combinatorial nature, this E3 has been named the SCF complex (Skp-Cullin-F-box). The vast number of SCF complexes that may form through interactions between these protein families may regulate the ubiquitination of a large number of cellular proteins. Numerous human homologs of SCF proteins have been identified, and complexes constraining cyclin A, cul1, and p45skp2 have been observed, which suggests that SCF-like complexes can form.[206c] Thus, this pathway for cell-cycle regulated proteolysis during G1 appears to have been evolutionarily conserved, although E3-like activities of these proteins in mammalian cells has not yet been described.

MOLECULAR BASES OF CELL-CYCLE PHYSIOLOGY

Mitogenic and antimitogenic signals control cell proliferation by starting and stopping the cell cycle, but cells respond differently to these signals at different times in the cell cycle.[209] Immediately after mitosis, cells enter a portion of G1 where the continued presence of mitogenic signals (or the absence of antimitogenic signals) is required for continued progression through the remainder of G1 and into S phase. However, at a fixed point in G1, the cell cycle becomes refractory to these signals, and cell division will be completed even if mitogens are absent or antimitogens are present.[210] The restriction point is defined as the end of the mitogen-responsive portion of G1 (or the moment of transition to mitogen independence), and it reflects the execution of the fundamental proliferative decision made by the cell.[211,212] It has been shown that tumor cells characteristically lose restriction point control over cell-cycle progression (they become constitutively mitogen-independent), highlighting the importance of this pathway in the normal regulation of cell proliferation.[213] The restriction point is physiologically analogous to START in the yeast cell cycle, and shares many of its molecular components. Thus, the requirement for cdc28 at START is paralleled by a requirement for cdks in restriction point control.[214]

Mitogenic and antimitogenic signals control the cell cycle in G1 because they control the activity of the cyclins and cdks that are required for progression through G1. Growth factors and cell-substratum interactions are among the best-studied mitogenic signals, and DNA damage and TGF-β are among the best-studied antimitogenic signals. All of these proliferative signals alter the activity of essential G1 cyclin-cdk complexes and bring about either continued cell-cycle progression or cell-cycle arrest.

Mitogenic growth factors have pleiotropic effects on cell cycle proteins that stimulate progression through G1 and entry into S phase.[213,215,216] They increase expression of G1 cyclins, decrease expression of cdk inhibitors, and promote assembly of G1 cyclin-cdk complexes. Growth factors increase expression of all three cyclins needed for entry into S phase — cyclin D (1, 2, and 3), cyclin E and cyclin A — at least in part by increasing transcription of their respective genes. Cyclin D1 transcription has been shown

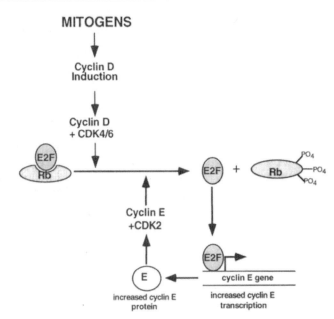

Fig. 9-11 A positive feedback loop reinforces cyclin E transcription. As described in the text, phosphorylation of Rb by cyclin D and cyclin E-associated kinases liberates E2F, which then stimulates cyclin E transcription. Increased cyclin E-cdk2 kinase activity then results in more Rb-phosphorylation, and greater E2F activity. Establishment of this feedback loop renders Rb-phosphorylation mitogen-independent, and may be an important component of the R-point.

to be under the control of at least two growth-factor-modulated signal transduction pathways — the c-myc and ras pathways.[217–219] The biochemical pathways linking c-myc and cyclin D1 transcription are not well defined, but the effects of ras on cyclin D1 transcription appear to be mediated by the MAP kinase pathway.[219] Cyclin D1 transcription begins early in G1, and is followed by an increase in cyclin E gene expression. Cyclin E is one of a large group of genes, which includes DNA polymerase alpha, thymidine kinase, PCNA, dihydrofolate reductase, and many others, that is required for cell proliferation and whose transcription is under control of E2F.[152–159] The induction of cyclin E gene transcription by E2F establishes a positive feedback loop for increasing cyclin E expression (Fig. 9-11).[220] In this pathway, cyclin E-cdk2 phosphorylates Rb, releasing E2F from its Rb-bound inactive state. The free E2F promotes cyclin E gene expression, resulting in increased amounts of cyclin E-cdk2 activity, increasing Rb phosphorylation, and so on. This suggests an interesting and important physiological linkage between cyclin D and cyclin E during the mitogenic response to growth factors. Cyclin D expression is directly elevated by mitogenic growth factors, and this initiates the pathway of Rb phosphorylation and E2F-dependent gene expression. Once initiated, however, Rb phosphorylation can be maintained independently of cyclin D (and, hence, independently of mitogenic growth factors) via the autonomous feedback loop linking Rb to cyclin E. Thus, growth factors are required, through cyclin D, to start the program of E2F-dependent gene expression. These growth factors become dispensable once cyclin E-cdk2 becomes activated and substitutes for cyclin D-cdk4 in phosphorylating Rb. Inherent in this scheme is a transition from a mitogen-dependent to mitogen-independent route for maintaining Rb phosphorylation, and it may be one molecular pathway underlying commitment to cell-cycle progression at the restriction point. Cyclin A transcription also increases in growth factor-stimulated cells just prior to entry into S phase,[51] but the pathways controlling cyclin A transcription are not well understood.

The cdk inhibitor p27Kip1 is another key element in the cell-cycle response to mitogenic growth factors. p27 is required for

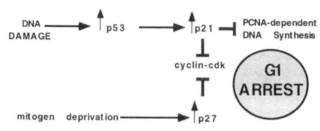

Fig. 9-12 Induction of Cip/Kip proteins by anti-proliferative stimuli imposes a G1 arrest. The p21 and p27 proteins respond to different physiological signals. In the example depicted, DNA damage results in p53 induction and increased p21 transcription, which lead to elevated levels p21 protein and a G1 arrest via cdk inhibition. In addition, p21 inhibits DNA synthesis through the processivity factor PCNA. Similarly, mitogen-deprivation induces p27 expression and cell cycle arrest via cdk inhibition.

cells to stop dividing on schedule when growth factors are withdrawn.[221] p27 is expressed at very low levels in proliferating cells, but its expression greatly increases in cells starved for essential mitogenic growth factors.[222–224] Under these conditions, p27 binds to and inactivates cyclin-cdk complexes and causes the cell cycle to stop (Fig. 9-12). If cells do not make p27, their exit from the cell cycle is delayed, and they will continue to proliferate in the absence of growth factors.[222] Indeed, mice engineered to contain a homozygous deletion of the p27 gene grow twice as fast as control mice, and have increased numbers of cell in all lineages.[225] Conversely, high levels of p27 are sufficient to prevent cell proliferation; therefore, mitogenic stimulation of non-dividing cells requires the elimination of p27.[232] Both control of p27 mRNA translation rate[136] and control of p27 proteolysis by the ubiquitin-proteosome pathway[206] have been implicated in modulating p27 protein levels in response to mitogenic growth factors.

A third mechanism by which growth factors promote cell cycle progression is through assembly of cyclin-cdk complexes. Cyclin D-cdk4 complexes cannot assemble from their individual subunits in growth factor-starved nondividing cells.[226] An assembly factor is induced by growth factors, although its molecular identity is not yet established.

The proliferative response of a cell to environmental signals depends equally on its interactions with soluble extracellular growth factors and on more local interactions with neighboring cells and with the extracellular matrix. Appropriate interactions between specific cell surface receptors (most often the integrin family of proteins) and the extracellular matrix are absolutely required for cell proliferation, a phenomenon known as anchorage-dependence. In fact, loss of anchorage-dependence is the single property of transformed cells that most closely correlates with their ability to form tumors in animals. The effect of cell anchorage on cell-cycle progression, like the effect of growth factors, occurs during G1. Cell anchorage is required for transcription and translation of cyclin D1, for activation of the cyclin E-cdk2 kinase, and for transcription of cyclin A.[227,228] Anchorage regulates cyclin E-cdk2 activity by controlling the levels of the p21 and p27 cdk inhibitors. Therefore, cell anchorage controls the expression and/or activity of all three cyclin/cdk complexes required for the G1/S transition. Cell anchorage and growth factors jointly regulate the cell cycle by modulating the activity of the cyclins and cdks required for G1 and entry into S phase.

The antiproliferative action of agents like TGF-β,[229–234] cyclic-AMP,[235] and DNA damage[125–128,236–238] can also be understood in terms of their effects on cell-cycle proteins. The TGF-β family of cytokines regulates diverse cellular responses, including cell proliferation, cell differentiation, and cell death.[239] The antimitogenic action of TGF-β is a paradigm for the inhibition of cell proliferation by extracellular agents. The active form of TGF-β is a disulfide-linked protein dimer, which, like other members of this cytokine family, signals by bridging together type

I and type II receptor serine/threonine kinases on the cell surface. The signal from the heterodimeric type I and type II receptor complex is transduced to the nucleus by a member of the Smad family of nuclear phosphoproteins. The Smad proteins are thought to be transcription factors that promote expression of genes required for the biologic effects of TGF-β or related cytokines. Mutations in DPC4, a member of the Smad protein family located on chromosome 18q21, have been detected in half of all pancreatic cancers,[240] and this may reflect a role for this protein in transmitting an antimitogenic TGF-β-like signal in pancreatic cells. Ultimately, the TGF-β signal has a plethora of effects on cell-cycle proteins, which together impose a tight blockade on progression through G1. TGF-β blocks the activation of cyclin D-cdk4 complexes by inducing expression of the cdk inhibitor p15[232,241] and by inhibiting translation of cdk4 mRNA.[242] TGF-β also blocks activation of cyclin E-cdk2 in some cases by directly inducing p21 and p27, and in other cases by indirectly by promoting the redistribution of p27 from cyclin D-cdk4 complexes to cyclin E-cdk2.[232,233] The biochemical pathways that link activation of the Smad proteins to these diverse effects on cell-cycle proteins have not been determined.

Normal cells will not replicate a damaged chromosome. Instead, cells pause in G1 to repair the DNA lesion, thereby avoiding duplication of a damaged DNA template and preventing the propagation of genetic misinformation to daughter cells. The p53 tumor-suppressor protein controls this DNA damage response.[243,244] The p53 protein is stabilized in cells containing damaged chromosomal DNA; however, it is not understood how DNA damage is detected by the cell nor how this results in decreased turnover of the p53 protein.[245] p53 is a transcriptional transactivator and up-regulation of p53 leads to increased expression of p53-responsive genes.[246–248] Among these genes is one encoding the cdk inhibitor p21Cip1,[127] and p21 protein levels rise in cells with damaged DNA (Fig. 23-12).[238] Consequently, as p53 levels rise, G1 cyclin-cdk complexes contain elevated amounts of p21 and are inactivated. Additionally, p21 binds to and inactivates the DNA polymerase cofactor PCNA, which contributes to the G1/S phase arrest.[129,130] However, p21 does not inhibit the repair functions of PCNA, which allows DNA repair to continue at the same time DNA replication is blocked.[249] Mice containing an engineered homozygous deletion of the p21 gene are viable, but cells taken from these mice have a defective cell-cycle response to DNA damage.[236,237]

CELL-CYCLE CHECKPOINTS

Cells are usually produced only when a new one is needed.[250] Normal cells are periodically recruited into (or released from) the proliferating state by extracellular signals, and this is mediated by activation (or inactivation) of cell-cycle proteins. Tumor cells, in contrast, proliferate when normal cells would not. Current data show that many, and possibly all, cancer cells contain mutations in cell-cycle regulatory proteins, perhaps partly explaining their unregulated proliferation.[251–256] In particular, one or another element in the Rb regulatory pathway, including p16, cyclin D, cdk4, E2F, or Rb itself, may be mutated in almost 100 percent of human tumors (Fig. 9-13).[251–261] Altered expression of other cell-cycle regulatory proteins is also commonly observed (i.e., cyclin E and p27), but often this occurs by mechanisms other than gene mutation.[262–265]

Although mutations in cell-cycle proteins may directly stimulate proliferation, other considerations suggest that these changes are not sufficient to explain the origin of tumorigenic cells. Epidemiologic, molecular, and genetic evidence all suggest that multiple mutations are required to transform a normal cell into a tumor cell.[266–268] But simple calculations show that at normal mutation rates it is very unlikely for a cell with more than two or three mutations to arise within the lifetime of a typical person. This has suggested that increased genetic mutation rates must be a prerequisite for the evolution of malignant cells, and has given rise

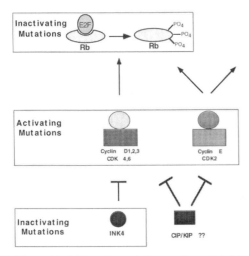

Fig. 9-13 The cyclin D-Rb pathway is frequently mutated in human tumors. Mutations that have been detected in human cancers include both inactivating (recessive) mutations in Rb and the INK4 proteins, and activating (dominant) mutations in the cyclin genes. All result in the deregulation of this pathway.

to the idea that the defining characteristic of a tumor cell may be genetic instability.[269–272] The frequent occurrence in tumor cells of aneuploidy, DNA translocations, DNA deletions, DNA amplifications, and other genetic abnormalities may be a direct manifestation of their genetic instability.

The critical question, therefore, is what controls the genetic stability of a cell? Of course, the accuracy of the enzymes that replicate and segregate chromosomes is largely responsible for the faithful propagation of genetic information. But despite their great fidelity, these enzymes have an intrinsic, spontaneous error rate. Additionally, exogenous agents, such as chemical mutagens, can further elevate the frequency of errors. Therefore, to reduce the accumulation of genetic mistakes normal cells also continually monitor the success of DNA replication and mitosis, and bring the cell cycle to a halt if these do not occur correctly. Once active proliferation is suspended, the cell shifts from duplicating genetic information to repairing it, and only resumes proliferation once the mistakes have been corrected. Checkpoints are the pathways that make progression through the cell cycle dependent on the accurate execution of specific cell-cycle events.[30,269] More specifically, they are the biochemical links between the cyclin-cdk cycle and the macromolecular events of the cell division cycle, such as DNA replication and mitosis.

Checkpoints were first identified experimentally by Weinert and Hartwell in a landmark paper describing the cell-cycle response to DNA damage.[273] DNA damage causes the yeast cell cycle to pause in G2, allowing time for repair enzymes to correct the lesions, thereby preventing the cell from attempting to segregate broken chromosomes during mitosis. It was shown that the RAD9 gene controls this pause in G2, but not because the RAD9 gene was directly involved in the repair process itself. Instead, it was shown that RAD9 is part of a surveillance mechanism, and that activation of the RAD9 pathway by DNA damage prevents cyclin-cdk activity from driving a cell into mitosis.

The molecular mechanism of the DNA damage checkpoint in G2 is beginning to be understood, and it is thought to involve tyrosine phosphorylation and catalytic inactivation of cdc2.[274–278] In cells containing damaged DNA, cdc2 remains inactive because an inhibitory phosphate on tyrosine 15 is not removed.[279–282] The enzyme that ordinarily dephosphorylates tyrosine 15 is the cdc25C phosphatase, but in cells arrested in G2 by the DNA damage checkpoint, this does not happen. The pivotal event in this checkpoint pathway appears to be phosphorylation of cdc25C on

serine 216. When cdc25C is phosphorylated on serine 216, it binds to proteins in the 14-3-3 family, and becomes sequestered in a functionally inactive state. Chk1 is the protein kinase responsible for phosphorylating cdc25C on serine 216, and Chk1 is required for the DNA damage checkpoint.[283–286] It is still not understood how Chk1 is activated by DNA damage, but it is possible that this involves a signal transmitted from damaged DNA to Chk1 by the ATM tumor suppressor protein.[279,287]

Subsequent to the discovery of RAD9 a large number of other genes were identified in yeast that together define an intricate network of pathways that make cell-cycle progression dependent on the faithful duplication of chromosomes during S phase.[288,289] A different, but equally robust, set of pathways checks for the proper attachment of chromosomes to the mitotic spindle, and delays mitosis if this has not occurred correctly.[290,291] This checkpoint is triggered by the absence of spindle-induced tension on kinetochores.[292] Once this checkpoint is triggered, it initiates a MAP kinase-dependent pathway[293] that delays the programmed destruction of mitotic cyclins and prevents the initiation of anaphase. It is likely that this pathway modulates activation of the APC, the mitotic proteolytic machinery. Mutations in these checkpoint genes (the MAD and BUB genes) elevate rates of chromosome nondisjunction. Other less well-defined checkpoint pathways are thought to monitor cell growth, cytokinesis, and centrosome duplication, and to prevent cell-cycle progression should those events be executed incorrectly.

Normal cells use cell-cycle checkpoints as fail-safe mechanisms to avoid the accumulation of genomic errors during cell division. Inactivation of checkpoint pathways is thought to underlie the genetic instability seen in tumor cells. Thus, many tumor suppressor genes might be part of checkpoint pathways, and inactivation of these genes could contribute to the clonal evolution of cancer cells by allowing the accumulation of genomic errors that would normally have resulted in either cycle arrest (and repair) or cell death. Perhaps the best example is the p53 gene, the most commonly mutated gene in human tumors.[245,246,252,255,294] p53 governs the G1 checkpoint in human cells that prevents cells from entering S phase and replicating a damaged chromosome. Also, the gene mutated in the cancer-prone syndrome ataxia-telangiectasia is thought to be required for coordinating cell-cycle progression with the repair of DNA damage during S and G2.[295,296] Human homologs of various yeast checkpoint genes are now being characterized, and their relevance to genetic instability in tumor cells will soon be determined.

In conclusion, the process of tumorigenesis may begin with changes in cell-cycle regulation. Mutations in cell-cycle proteins contribute to tumorigenesis in two ways. The first is to promote cell proliferation directly by allowing the cell to override or bypass controls that ordinarily restrict proliferation. The second is to cause the cell to ignore internal ''alarms'' that signal the presence of errors in the duplication and segregation of genetic information. This results in genetic instability and sets the stage for evolution of malignant cells. For these reasons, cancer can be thought of as a disease of the cell cycle.

REFERENCES

1. Prescott DM: *Reproduction of Eukaryotic Cells.* New York: Academic Press, 1976.
2. Murray A, Hunt T: *The Cell Cycle: An Introduction*, 1st ed. New York: WH Freeman, 1993.
3. Mitchison JM: *The Biology of the Cell Cycle.* London: Cambridge University Press, 1971.
4. Edgar B: Diversification of cell cycle controls in developing embryos. *Curr Opin Cell Biol* **7**:815, 1995.
5. Alberts B, Bray D, Lewis J, Raff M, Roberts K, Watson J: *Molecular Biology of the Cell.* New York: Garland, 1989.
6. Hartwell L: Twenty-five years of cell cycle genetics. *Genetics* **129**:975, 1991.
7. Nurse P: Universal control mechanism regulating onset of M-phase. *Nature* **344**:503, 1990.

8. Hartwell L, Culotti J, Pringle J, Reid B: Genetic control of the cell division cycle in yeast. *Science* **183**:46, 1974.

9. Hartwell L, Mortimer K, Culotti J, Culotti M: Genetic control of the cell division cycle in yeast: V. Genetic analysis of cdc mutants. *Genetics* **74**:267, 1973.

10. Pringle JR, Hartwell LH: The Saccharomyces cerevisiae cell cycle, in Strathern JN, Jones EW, Broach JR (eds): *The Molecular Biology of the Yeast Saccharomyces.* New York: Cold Spring Harbor Laboratory Press, 1981, p. 97.

11. Cross F: Starting the cell cycle: What's the point? *Curr Opin Cell Biol* **7**:790, 1995.

12. Reid B, Hartwell L: Regulation of mating in the cell cycle of Saccharomyces cerevisiae. *J Cell Biol* **75**:355, 1977.

13. Hartwell LH, Unger MW: Unequal division in Saccharomyces cerevisiae and its implications for the control of cell division. *J Cell Biol* **75**:422, 1977.

14. Johnston G, Pringle J, Hartwell L: Coordination of growth with cell division in the yeast S. cerevisiae. *Exp Cell Res* **105**:79, 1977.

15. Nasymth K: Control of the yeast cell cycle by the Cdc28 protein kinase. *Curr Opin Cell Biol* **5**:166, 1993.

16. Lorincz AT, Reed SI: Primary structure homology between the product of the yeast cell cycle control gene CDC28 and vertebrate oncogenes. *Nature* **307**:183, 1984.

17. Nurse P: Genetic control of cell size at cell division in yeast. *Nature* **256**:457, 1975.

18. Hindley J, Phear GA: Sequence of the cell division gene cdc2 from Schizosaccharomyces pombe: Pattern of splicing and homology to protein kinases. *Gene* **31**:129, 1984.

19. Nurse P, Bisset Y: Gene required in G1 for commitment to cell cycle and in G2 for control of mitosis in fission yeast. *Nature* **292**:558, 1981.

20. Beach D, Durkacz B, Nurse P: Functionally homologous cell cycle control genes in fission yeast and budding yeast. *Nature* **300**:706, 1982.

21. Reed SI, Wittenberg C: Mitotic role for the CDC28 protein kinase of S. cerevisae. *Proc Natl Acad Sci U S A* **87**:5697, 1990.

22. Piggot JR, Rai R, Carter BLA: A bifunctional gene product involved in two phases of the yeast cell cycle. *Nature* **298**:391, 1982.

23. Masui H, Markert CL: Cytoplasmic control of nuclear behaviour during meiotic maturation of frog oocytes. *J Exp Zool* **117**:129, 1971.

24. Wasserman WJ, Smith LD: The cyclic behaviour of a cytoplasmic factor controlling nuclear membrane breakdown. *J Cell Biol* **78**:R15, 1978.

25. Reynhout JK, Smith LD: Studies on the appearance and nature of a maturation-inducing factor in the cytoplasm of amphibian oocytes exposed to progesterone. *Dev Biol* **38**:394, 1974.

26. Newport J, Kirschner M: Regulation of the cell cycle during early Xenopus development. *Cell* **37**:731, 1984.

27. Nelkin B, Nichols C, Vogelstein B: Protein factor(s) from mitotic CHO cells induce meiotic maturation in Xenopus Laevis oocytes. *FEBS Lett* **109**:233, 1980.

28. Hara K, Tydeman P, Kirschner M: A cytoplasmic clock with the same period as the division cycle in Xenopus eggs. *Proc Natl Acad Sci U S A* **77**:462, 1980.

29. Murray A, Kirschner MW: Dominoes and clocks: The union of two views of the cell cycle. *Science* **246**:614, 1989.

30. Hartwell L, Weinert T: Checkpoints: Controls that ensure the order of cell cycle events. *Science* **246**:629, 1989.

31. Cross F, Roberts J, Weintraub H: Simple and complex cell cycles. *Ann Rev Cell Biol* **5**:341, 1989.

32. Nurse P: Universal control mechanism regulating onset of M-phase. *Nature* **344**:503, 1990.

33. Lee MG, Nurse P: Complementation used to clone a human homologue of the fission yeast cell cycle control gene cdc2. *Nature* **327**:31, 1987.

34. Gautier J, Norbury C, Lohka M, Nurse P, Maller JL: Purified maturation-promoting factor contains the product of a Xenopus homolog of the fission yeast cell cycle control gene cdc2+. *Cell* **54**:433, 1988.

35. Hunt T: Maturation promoting factor, cyclin and the control of M-phase. *Curr Opin Cell Biol* **1**:268, 1989.

36. Labbe JC, Picard A, Peaucellier G, Cavadore JC, Nurse P, Doree M: Purification of MPF from starfish: Identification as the H1 histone kinase p34 cdc2 and a possible mechanism for its periodic activation. *Cell* **57**:253, 1989.

37. Labbe JC, Lee MG, Nurse P, Picard A, Doree M: Activation at M-phase of a protein kinase encoded by a starfish homologue of the cell cycle gene Cdc2. *Nature* **335**:251, 1988.

38. Dunphy WG, Brizuela L, Beach D, Newport J: The Xenopus cdc2 protein is a component of MPF, a cytoplasmic regulator of mitosis. *Cell* **54**:423, 1988.

39. Murray A: The cell cycle as a cdc2 cycle. *Nature* **342**:14, 1989.

40. Riabowol K, Draetta G, Brizuela L, Vandre D, Beach D: The cdc2 kinase is a nuclear protein that is essential for mitosis in mammalian cells. *Cell* **57**:393, 1989.

41. D'Urso G, Marraccino RL, Marshak DR, Roberts JM: Cell cycle control of DNA replication by a homologue from human cells of the p34-cdc2 protein kinase. *Science* **250**:786, 1990.

42. Th'ng JPH, Wright PS, Hamaguchi J, Lee MG, Norbury CJ, Nurse P, Bradbury EM: The FT210 cell line is a mouse G2 phase mutant with a temperature-sensitive CDC2 gene product. *Cell* **63**:313, 1990.

43. Tsai LE, Lees E, Faha B, Harlow E, Riabowol K: The cdk2 kinase is required for the G1 to S transition in mammalian cells. *Oncogene* **8**:1593, 1993.

44. Fang F, Newport J: Evidence that the G1-S and G2-M transitions are controlled by different cdc2 proteins in higher eukaryotes. *Cell* **66**:731, 1991.

45. Furakawa Y, Piwnica-Worms H, Ernst TJ, Kanakura Y, Griffin JD: Cdc2 gene expression at the to S transition in human T lymphocytes. *Science* **250**:805, 1990.

46. Lamb N, Fernandez A, Watrin A, Labbe J, Cavadore J: Microinjection of the p34cdc2 kinase induces marked changes in cell shape, cytoskeletal organization and chromatin structure in mammalian fibroblasts. *Cell* **60**:151, 1990.

47. Nasymth K: Control of the yeast cell cycle by the Cdc28 protein kinase. *Curr Opin Cell Biol* **5**:166, 1993.

48. Myerson M, Enders GH, Wu C, Su L, Gorka C, Nelson C, Harlow E, Tsai L: The human cdc2 kinase family. *EMBO J* **11**:2909, 1992.

49. Morgan D: Principles of cdk regulation. *Nature* **374**:131, 1995.

50. Lees E: Cyclin-dependent kinase regulation. *Curr Opin Cell Biol* **7**:773, 1995.

51. Sherr C: Mammalian G1 cyclins. *Cell* **73**:1059, 1993.

52. Sherr C: G1 phase progression: Cycling on cue. *Cell* **79**:551, 1994.

53. van den Heuval S, Harlow E: Distinct roles for cyclin-dependent kinases in cell cycle control. *Science* **262**:2050, 1994.

54. Tsai L, Delalle I, Caviness V, Chae T, Harlow E: p35, a neuro-specific regulatory subunit of the cdk5 kinase. *Nature* **371**:419, 1994.

55. Nikoklic M, Dudek H, Kwon Y, Ramos Y, Tsai LH: The cdk5/p35 kinase is essential for neurite outgrowth during neuronal differentiation. *Genes Dev* **8**:816, 1996.

56. De Bondt HL, Rosenblatt J, Jarncarik J, Jones H, Morgan D, Kim S: Crystal structure of the cyclin-dependent kinase 2. *Nature* **363**:595, 1993.

57. Jeffrey PD, Russo AA, Polyak K, Gibbs E, Hurwitz J, Massague J, Paveltich NP: Crystal Structure of a cyclin A-cdk2 complex at 2.3A: Mechanism of cdk activation by cyclins. *Nature* **376**:313, 1995.

58. Cross F: DAF1, a mutant gene affecting size control, pheromone arrest, and cell cycle kinetics of Saccharomyces cerevisiae. *Mol Cell Biol* **8**:4675, 1988.

59. Cross F: Cell cycle arrest caused by CLN gene deficiency in Saccharomyces cerevisiae resembles START-1 arrest and is independent of the mating-pheromone signaling pathway. *Mol Cell Biol* **10**:6482, 1990.

60. Richardson H, Wittenberg C, Cross F, Reed S: An essential G1 function for cyclin-like proteins in yeast. *Cell* **59**:1127, 1989.

61. Hadwiger J, Wittenberg C, Richardson H, Lopes M, Reed S: A family of cyclin homologs that control the G1 phase in yeast. *Proc Natl Acad Sci U S A* **86**:6255, 1989.

62. Wittenberg C, Sugimoto K, Reed SI: G1-specific cyclins of S. cerevisiae: Cell cycle periodicity, regulation by mating pheromone, and association with the p34-CDC28 protein kinase. *Cell* **62**:225, 1990.

63. Koch C, Nasmyth K: Cell cycle regulated transcription in yeast. *Curr Opin Cell Biol* **6**:451, 1994.

64. Koch C, Moll T, Neuberg M, Ahorn H, Nasmyth K: A role for the transcription factors Mbp1 and Swi4 in progression from G1 to S phase. *Science* **261**:1551, 1993.

65. Dirick L, Moll T, Auer H, Nasmyth K: A central role for SWI6 in modulating cell cycle START-specific transcription in yeast. *Nature* **357**:508, 1992.

66. Dirick L, Nasmyth K: Positive feedback in the activation of G1 cyclins in yeast. *Nature* **351**:754, 1991.

67. Cross FR, Tinkelenberg H: A potential positive feedback loop controlling CLN1 and CLN2 gene expression at the start of the yeast cell cycle. *Cell* **65**:875, 1992.

68. Dirick L, Bohm T, Nasmyth K: Roles and regulation of cln-cdc28 kinases at the start of the cell cycle of Saccharomyces cerevisiae. *EMBO J* **14**:4803, 1995.

69. Schwob E, Nasmyth K: CLB5 and CLB6, a new pair of B cyclins involved in S phase and mitotic spindle formation in S. cerevisiae. *Genes Dev* **7**:1160, 1993.

70. Epstein C, Cross F: CLB5: A novel B cyclin from budding yeast with a role in S phase. *Genes Dev* **6**:1695, 1992.

71. Fitch I, Dahmann C, Surana U, Amon A, Nasmyth K, Goetch L, Byers B, Futcher B: Characterization of four B-type cyclin genes of the budding yeast Saccharomyces cerevisiae. *Mol Biol Cell* **3**:805, 1992.

72. Amon A, Tyers M, Futcher B, Nasmyth K: Mechanisms that help the yeast cell cycle clock tick: G2 cyclins transcriptionally activate their own synthesis and repress G1 cyclins. *Cell* **74**:993, 1993.

73. Lew DJ, Dulic V, Reed SI: Isolation of three novel human cyclins by rescue of G1 cyclin (cln) function in yeast. *Cell* **66**:1197, 1991.

74. Koff A, Cross F, Fisher A, Schumacher J, Leguelle K, Philippe M, Roberts JM: Human cyclin E, a new cyclin that interacts with two members of the CDC2 gene family. *Cell* **66**:1217, 1991.

75. Xiong Y, Connolly T, Futcher B, Beach D: Human D-type cyclin. *Cell* **65**:691, 1991.

76. Matsushime H, Roussel M, Ashmun R, Sherr CJ: Colony-stimulating Factor 1 regulates novel cyclins during the G1 phase of the cell cycle. *Cell* **65**:701, 1991.

77. Motokura T, Bloom T, Kim HG, Juppner H, Ruderman JV, Kronenberg HM, Arnold A: A BCL1-linked candidate oncogene which is rearranged in parathyroid tumors encodes a novel cyclin. *Nature* **350**:512, 1991.

78. Sherr C, Kato J, Quell D, Matsuoka M, Roussel M: D-type cyclins and their cyclin-dependent kinases: G1 phase integrators of the mitogenic response. *Cold Spring Harbor Symp Quant Biol* **49**:11, 1994.

79. Baldin V, Lukas J, Marcotte MJ, Pagano M, Draetta G: Cyclin D1 is a nuclear protein required for cell cycle progression in G1. *Genes Dev* **7**:812, 1993.

80. Quelle DE, Ashmun RA, Shurtleff SA, Kato J, Bar-Sagi D, Roussel MF, Sherr CJ: Overexpression of mouse D-type cyclins accelerates G1 phase in rodent fibroblasts. *Genes Dev* **7**:1559, 1993.

81. Resnitzky D, Gossen M, Bujard H, Reed SI: Acceleration of the G1/S phase transition by expression of cyclin D1 and E with an inducible system. *Mol Cell Biol* **14**:1669, 1994.

82. Ohtsubo M, Theodoras AM, Schumacher J, Roberts JM, Pagano M: Human cyclin E: A nuclear protein essential for the G1 to S phase transition. *Mol Cell Biol* **15**:2612, 1995.

83. Knoblich J, Sauer K, Jones L, Richardson H, Saint R, Lehner C: Cyclin E controls S phase progression and its down-regulation during Drosophila embryogenesis is required for the arrest of cell proliferation. *Cell* **77**:107, 1994.

84. Koff A, Giordano A, Desai D, Yamashita K, Harper JW, Elledge S, Nishimoto T, Morgan DO, Franza R, Roberts JM: Formation and activation of a cyclin E/CDK2 complex during the G1 phase of the human cell cycle. *Science* **257**:1689, 1992.

85. Dulic V, Lees E, Reed SI: Association of human cyclin E with a periodic G1-S phase protein kinase. *Science* **257**:1958, 1992.

86. Ohtsubo M, Roberts JM: Cyclin-dependent regulation of G1 in mammalian fibroblasts. *Science* **259**:1908, 1993.

87. Pagano M, Pepperkok P, Verde F, Ansorge W, Draetta G: Cyclin A is required at two points in the human cell cycle. *EMBO J* **11**:961, 1992.

88. Giordano A, Whyte P, Harlow E, Franza BR Jr, Beach D, Draetta G: A 60-kd cdc2-associated polypeptide complexes with the E1A proteins in adenovirus-infected cells. *Cell* **58**:981, 1989.

89. Girard F, Strausfeld U, Fernandez A, Lamb N: Cyclin A is required for the onset of DNA replication in mammalian fibroblasts. *Cell* **67**:1169, 1991.

90. Pines J, Hunter T: Isolation of a human cyclin cDNA: Evidence for cyclin mRNA and protein regulation in the cell cycle and for interaction with p34-cdc2. *Cell* **58**:833, 1989.

91. Nigg E: Cyclin-dependent kinase 7: At the crossroads of transcription, DNA repair and cell cycle control. *Curr Opin Cell Biol* **8**:312, 1996.

92. Tassan JP, Jaquenoud M, Leopold P, Schultz SJ, Nigg EA: Identification of human cyclin-dependent kinase 8, a putative protein kinase partner for cyclin C. *Proc Natl Acad Sci U S A* **92**:8871, 1995.

93. Bai C, Richman R, Elledge SJ: Human cyclin F. *EMBO J* **13**:6087, 1994.

94. Okamoto K, Beach D: Cyclin G is a transcriptional target of the p53 tumor suppressor. *EMBO J* **13**:4816, 1994.

95. Nakamura T, Sanolawa R, Saski Y, Ayusawa D, Oishi M, Mori N: Cyclin I: A new cyclin encoded by a gene isolated from human brain. *Exp Cell Res* **221**:534, 1995.

96. Russo crystal structure.

97. Solomon MJ: The function(s) of CAK, the p34cdc2 activating kinase. *Trends Biochem Sci* **19**:496, 1994.

98. Soloman M, Glotzer M, Lee T, Phillippe M, Kirschner M: Cyclin activation of p34-cdc2. *Cell* **63**:1013, 1990.

99. Solomon MJ, Lee T, Kirschner M: Role of phosphorylation in p34 CDC2 activation: Identification of an activating kinase. *Mol Biol Cell* **3**:13, 1991.

100. Solomon MJ, Harper JW, Shuttleworth J: CAK, the p34 CDC2 activating kinase, contains a protein identical or closely related to p40 MO15. *EMBO J* **12**:3133, 1993.

101. Gould KL, Nurse P: Tyrosine phosphorylation of the fission yeast Cdc2+ protein kinase regulates entry into mitosis. *Nature* **342**:39, 1989.

102. Moreneo S, Hayles J, Nurse P: Regulation of p34-cdc2 protein kinase during mitosis. *Cell* **58**:361, 1989.

103. Simanis V, Nurse P: The cell cycle control gene cdc2+ of fission yeast encodes a protein kinase potentially regulated by phosphorylation. *Cell* **45**:261, 1986.

104. Heald R, McLoughlin M, McKeon F: Human wee1 maintains mitotic timing by protecting the nucleus from cytoplasmically activated Cdc2 kinase. *Cell* **74**:463, 1993.

105. Igarashi M, Nagata A, Jinno S, Suto K, Okayama H: Wee1+-like gene in human cells. *Nature* **353**:80, 1991.

106. Lundgren D, Walworth N, Booher R, Dembski M, Kirschner M, Beach D: mik1 and wee1 cooperate in the inhibitory tyrosine phosphorylation of cdc2. *Cell* **64**:1111, 1991.

107. Russell P, Nurse P: Negative regulation of mitosis by wee1+, a gene encoding a protein kinase homolog. *Cell* **49**:559, 1987.

108. Russell P, Nurse P: cdc25+ functions as an inducer in the mitotic control of fission yeast. *Cell* **45**:145, 1986.

109. Sadhu K, Reed S, Richardson H, Russell P: Human homolog of fission yeast cdc25 mitotic inducer is predominantly expressed in G2. *Proc Natl Acad Sci U S A* **87**:5139, 1990.

110. Kumagai A, Dunphy W: The Cdc25 protein controls tyrosine dephosphorylation of the Cdc2 protein in a cell free system. *Cell* **64**:903, 1991.

111. Sebastian B, Kakizuka A, Hunter T: Cdc25 activation of cyclin-dependent kinase by dephosphorylation of threonine-14 and tyrosine 15. *Proc Natl Acad Sci U S A* **90**:3521, 1993.

112. Strausfield V, Labbe JC, Fesquat O, Cavadore JC, Picard A, Sadhu A, Russell P, Durec M: Dephosphorylation and activation of a p34cdc2/cyclin B complex in vitro by human cdc25 protein. *Nature* **35**:242, 1991.

113. Atherton-Fessler S, Hannig G, Piwnica-Worms H: Reversible tyrosine phosphorylation and cell cycle control. *Semin Cell Biol* **4**:433, 1993.

114. Dunphy W: The decision to enter mitosis. *Trends Cell Biol* **4**:202, 1994.

115. Jinno S, Suto K, Nagata A, Igarashi M, Kanaoka Y, Nojima H, Okayama H: Cdc25A is a novel phosphatase functioning early in the cell cycle. *EMBO J* **13**:1549, 1994.

116. Hoffmann I, Draetta G, Karsenti E: Activation of the phosphatase activity of human cdc25A by a cdk2-cyclin E dependent phosphorylation at the G1/S transition. *EMBO J* **13**:4302, 1994.

117. Galaktionov K, Jessus C, Beach D: Raf1 interaction with Cdc25 phosphatase ties mitogenic signal transduction to cell cycle activation. *Genes Dev* **9**:1046, 1995.

118. Sherr C, Roberts J: Inhibitors of mammalian G1 cyclin-dependent kinases. *Genes Dev* **9**:1149, 1995.

119. Peter M, Herskowitz I: Joining the complex: Cyclin-dependent kinase inhibitory proteins and cell cycle. *Cell* **79**:181, 1994.

120. Mendenhall M: An inhibitor of p34 CDC28 protein kinase activity from Saccharomyces cerevisiae. *Science* **259**:216, 1993.

121. Schwob E, Bohm T, Mendenhall M, Nasmyth K: The B-type cyclins kinase inhibitor p40sic1 controls the G1 to S phase transition in S. cerevisiae. *Cell* **79**:233, 1994.

122. Elledge S, Harper W: Cdk inhibitors: on the threshold of checkpoints and development. *Curr Opin Cell Biol* **6**:847, 1994.

123. Xiong Y, Zhang H, Beach D: Subunit rearrangement of the cyclin-dependent kinases is associated with cellular transformation. *Genes Dev* **7**:1572, 1993.

124. Noda A, Ning Y, Venable S, Pereira-Smith O, Smith J: Cloning of senescent cell-derived inhibitors of DNA synthesis using an expression screen. *Exp Cell Res* **211**:90, 1994.

125. Harper JW, Adami GR, Wei N, Keyomarsi K, Elledge SJ: The p21 cdk-interacting protein cip1 is a potent inhibitor of G1 cyclin-dependent Kinases. *Cell* **75**:805, 1993.

126. Xiong Y, Hannon G, Zhang H, Casso D, Kobayashi R, Beach D: p21 is a universal inhibitor of cyclin kinases. *Nature* **366**:701, 1993.

127. El-Deiry WS, Tokino T, Velculescu VE, Levy DB, Parsons R, Trent JM, Lin D, Mercer WE, Kinzler KW, Vogelstein B: WAF1, a potential mediator of p53 tumor suppression. *Cell* **75**:817, 1993.

128. Gu Y, Turek C, Morgan D: Inhibition of CDK2 activity in vivo by an associated 20K regulatory subunit. *Nature* **366**:707, 1993.

129. Waga S, Hannon G, Beach D, Stillman B: The p21 inhibitor of cyclin-dependent kinases controls DNA replication by interaction with PCNA. *Nature* **369**:574, 1994.

130. Flores-Rozas H, Kelman Z, Dean F, Pan Z, Harper JW, Elledge S, O'Donnell M, Hurwitz J: CDK-interacting protein 1 directly binds with proliferating cell nuclear antigen and inhibits DNA replication catalyzed by the DNA polymerase and holoenzyme. *Proc Natl Acad Sci U S A* **91**:8655, 1994.

131. Luo Y, Hurwitz J, Massague J: Cell-cycle inhibition by independent CDK and CPNA binding domains in p21Cip1. *Nature* **375**:159, 1995.

132. Halevy O, Novitch B, Spicer D, Skapek S, Rhee J, Hannon G, Beach D, Lasser A: Correlation of terminal cell cycle arrest of skeletal muscle with induction of p21 by MyoD. *Science* **267**:1018, 1995.

133. Parker S, Eichele G, Zhang P, Rawls A, Sands A, Bradley A, Olson E, Harper JW, Elledge S: p53-independent expression of p21Cip1 in muscle and other terminally differentiating cells. *Science* **267**:1024, 1995.

134. Polyak K, Lee MH, Erdjument-Bromage H, Koff A, Roberts JM, Tempst P, Massague J: Cloning of p27 kip1 a cyclin-dependent kinase inhibitor and a potential mediator of extracellular antimitogenic signals. *Cell* **78**:59, 1994.

135. Toyoshima H, Hunter T: p27, a novel inhibitor of G1-cyclin-cdk protein kinase activity, is related to p21. *Cell* **78**:67, 1994.

136. Hengst L, Reed SI: Translational control of p27Kip1 accumulation during the cell cycle. *Science* **271**:1861, 1996.

137. Lee M, Reynisdottir I, Massague J: Cloning of p57Kip2, a cyclin-dependent kinase inhibitor with unique domain structure and tissue distribution. *Genes Dev* **9**:639, 1995.

138. Matsuoka S, Edwards M, Bai C, Parker S, Zhang P, Baldini A, Harper JW, Elledge S: p57Kip2, a structurally distinct member of the p21Cip1 cdk inhibitor family, is a candidate tumor suppressor gene. *Genes Dev* **9**:650, 1995.

138a. Serrano M, Hannon GJ, Beach D: A new regulatory motif in cell-cycle control causing specific inhibition of cyclin D-Cdk4. *Nature* **366**:704, 1993.

139. Sheaff R, Roberts J: Lessons in p16 from phylum Falconium. *Curr Biol* **5**:28, 1995.

140. Kamb A: Role of a cell cycle regulator in hereditary and sporadic cancer. *Cold Spring Harbor Symp Quant Biol* **49**:39, 1994.

141. Quelle DE, Ashmun RA, Hannon GJ, Rehberger PA, Trono D, Richter KH, Walker C, Beach D, Sherr CJ, Serrano M: Cloning and characterization of murine p16INK4a and p15INK4b genes. *Oncogene* **11**:635, 1995.

142. Hirai H, Roussel MF, Kato JY, Ashmun RA, Sherr CJ: Novel INK4 proteins, p19 and p18, are specific inhibitors of the cyclin D-dependent kinases CDK4 and CDK6. *Mol Cell Biol* **15**:2672, 1995.

143. Serrano M, Lee H, Chin L, Cordon-Cardo C, Beach D, DePinho RA: Role of the INK4a locus in tumor suppression and cell mortality. *Cell* **85**:27, 1996.

144. Schneider B, Yang Y, Futcher B: Linkage of replication to start by the CDK inhibitor sic1. *Science* **272**:560, 1996.

145. Weinberg RA: The retinoblastoma protein and cell cycle control. *Cell* **81**:323, 1995.

146. Dyson N, Howley PM, Munger K, Harlow E: The human papilloma virus-16 E7 oncoprotein is able to bind to the retinoblastoma gene product. *Science* **243**:934, 1989.

147. Whyte P, Williamson NM, Harlow E: Cellular targets for transformation by the adenovirus E1A proteins. *Cell* **56**:67, 1989.

148. Whyte P, Buchkovich KJ, Horowitz JM, Friend SH, Raybuck M, Weinberg RA, Harlow E: Association between an oncogene and an anti-oncogene: The adenovirus E1A proteins bind to the retinoblastoma gene product. *Nature* **334**:124, 1988.

149. Friend SH, Horowitz JM, Gerber MR, Wang XF, Bogenmann E, Li FP, Weinberg RA: Deletions of a DNA sequence in retinoblastomas and mesenchymal tumors: Organization of the sequence and its encoded protein. *Proc Natl Acad Sci U S A* **84**:9059, 1987.

150. Friend SH, Bernards R, Rogelj S, Weinberg RA, Rapaport JM, Albert DM, Dryja TP: A human DNA segment with properties of the gene that predisposes to retinoblastoma and osteosarcoma. *Nature* **323**:643, 1986.

151. Horowitz JM, Park S, Bogenmann E, Cheng J, Yandell DW, Kaye FJ, Minna JD, Dryja TP, Weinberg RA: Frequent inactivation of the retinoblastoma anti-oncogene is restricted to a subset of human tumor cells. *Proc Natl Acad Sci U S A* **87**:2775, 1990.

152. Buchkovich K, Duffy LA, Harlow E: The retinoblastoma protein is phosphorylated during specific phases of the cell cycle. *Cell* **58**:1097, 1989.

153. Mittnacht S, Lees JA, Desai D, Harlow E, Morgan DO, Weinberg RA: Distinct sub-populations of the retinoblastoma protein show a distinct pattern of phosphorylation. *EMBO J* **13**:118, 1994.

154. Nevins J: E2F: A link between the Rb tumor suppressor protein and viral oncoproteins. *Science* **258**:424, 1992.

155. Sherr CJ: The ins and outs of Rb: Coupling gene expression to the cell cycle clock. *Trends Cell Biol* **4**:15, 1994.

156. Lees JA, Saito M, Vidal M, Valentine M, Look T, Harlow E, Dyson N, Helin K: The retinoblastoma protein binds to a family of E2F transcription factors. *Mol Cell Biol* **13**:7813, 1993.

157. Kaelin WG Jr, Krek W, Sellers WR, DeCaprio JA, Ajchenbaum F, Fuchs CS, Chittenden T, Li Y, Farnham PJ, Blanar MA, Livingston DM, Flemington EK: Expression cloning of a cDNA encoding a retinoblastoma-binding protein with E2F-like properties. *Cell* **70**:351, 1992.

158. Helin K, Lees JA, Vidal M, Dyson N, Harlow E, Fattaey A: A cDNA encoding a pRB-binding protein with properties of the transcription factor E2F. *Cell* **70**:337, 1992.

159. Wu CL, Zukerberg LR, Ngwu C, Harlow E, Lees JA: In vivo association of E2F and DP family proteins. *Mol Cell Biol* **15**:2536, 1995.

160. Lees JA, Buchkovich KJ, Marshak DR, Anderson CW, Harlow E: The retinoblastoma protein is phosphorylated on multiple sites by human cdc2. *EMBO J* **10**:4279, 1991.

161. Dowdy S, Hinds P, Lovic K, Reed S, Arnold A, Weinberg RA: Physical interaction of the retinoblastoma protein with human D cyclins. *Cell* **73**:499, 1993.

162. Ewen M, Sluss K, Sherr CJ, Livingston M, Matsushime H, Kato JY, Livingston DM: Functional interactions of the retinoblastoma protein with mammalian D-type cyclins. *Cell* **73**:487, 1993.

163. Hinds P, Mittnacht S, Dulic V, Arnold A, Reed S, Weinberg R: Regulation of retinoblastoma protein functions by ectopic expression of human cyclins. *Cell* **70**:993, 1992.

164. Kato JY, Matsushime H, Hiebert S, Ewen M, Sherr C: Direct binding of cyclin D to the retinoblastoma gene product and pRb phosphorylation by the cyclin D-dependent kinase, cdk4. *Genes Dev* **7**:331, 1993.

165. Bates S, Parry D, Bonetta L, Vousden K, Dickson C, Peters G: Absence of cyclin D/Cdk complexes in cells lacking functional retinoblastoma protein. *Oncogene* **9**:1633, 1994.

166. Lukas J, Parry D, Aagaard L, Mann DJ, Bartkova J, Strauss M, Peters G, Bartek J: Retinoblastoma-protein-dependent cell-cycle inhibition by the tumour suppressor p16. *Nature* **375**:503, 1995.

167. Lukas J, Bartkova J, Rohde M, Strauss M, Bartek J: Cyclin D1 is dispensable for G1 control in retinoblastoma gene-deficient cells independently of cdk4 activity. *Mol Cell Biol* **15**:2600, 1995.

168. Zhu L, Enders GH, Wu CL, Starz MA, Moberg KH, Lees JA, Dyson N, Harlow E: Growth suppression by members of the retinoblastoma protein family. *Cold Spring Harbor Symp Quantit Biol* **59**:75, 1994.

169. Bandara L, Adamczewski J, Hunt T LaThanghe N: Cyclin A and the retinoblastoma gene product complex with a common transcription factor. *Nature* **352**:249, 1991.

170. Shirodkar S, Ewen M, DeCaprio J, Morgan J, Livingston D, Chittenden T: The transcription factor E2F interacts with the retinoblastoma product and a p107-cyclin A complex in a cell cycle regulated manner. *Cell* **68**:157, 1992.

170a. Dynlacht B, Flores O, Lees J Harlow E: Differential regulation of E2F transactivation by cyclin/cdk2 complexes. *Genes Dev* **8**:1772, 1994.

171. Krek W, Ewen M, Shirodkar S, Arany Z, Kaelin W, Livingston D: Negative regulation of the growth-promoting transcription factor E2F-1 by a stably bound cyclin A-dependent protein kinase. *Cell* **78**:161, 1994.

172. Nigg EA: Targets of cyclin-dependent protein kinases. *Curr Opin Cell Biol* **5**:187, 1993.

173. Heichman K, Roberts JM: Rules to replicate by. *Cell* **79**:1, 1994.

174. Nigg EA: Assembly-disassembly of the nuclear lamina. *Curr Opin Cell Biol* **4**:105, 1992.

175. Heald R, McKeon F: Mutations of phosphorylation sites in lamin A that prevent nuclear lamina disassembly in mitosis. *Cell* **61**:579, 1990.

176. Blangy A, Lane HA, d'Herin P, Harper M, Kress M, Nigg EA: Phosphorylation by p34cdc2 regulates spindle association of human Eg5, a kinesin-related motor essential for bipolar spindle formation in vivo. *Cell* **83**:1159, 1995.

177. Deshaies R: The self-destructive personality of a cell cycle in transition. *Curr Opin Cell Biol* **7**:781, 1995.

178. Maller J: Mitotic control. *Curr Opin Cell Biol* **3**:269, 1991.

179. Evans T, Rosenthal E, Youngblom J, Distel D, Hunt T: Cyclin: A protein specified by maternal mRNA in sea urchin eggs that is destroyed at each cleavage division. *Cell* **33**:389, 1983.

180. Ciechanover A: The ubiquitin-proteosome proteolytic pathway. *Cell* **79**:13, 1994.

181. Hochstrasser M: Ubiquitin, proteosomes, and the regulation of intracellular protein degradation. *Curr Opin Cell Biol* **7**:215, 1995.

182. Jentsch S, Schlenker S: Selective protein degradation: A journey's end within the proteosome. *Cell* **82**:881, 1995.

183. Rogers S, Wells R, Rechsteiner M: Amino acid sequences common to rapidly degraded proteins: The PEST hypothesis. *Science* **234**:364, 1986.

184. Glotzer M, Murray A, Kirschner M: Cyclin is degraded by the ubiquitin pathway. *Nature* **349**:132, 1991.

185. Murray AW, Solomon MJ, Kirschner MW: The role of cyclin synthesis and degradation in the control of maturation promoting factor activity. *Nature* **339**:280, 1989.

186. Ghiara JB, Richardson HE, Sugimoto K, Henze M, Lew DJ, Wittenberg C, Reed SI: A cyclin B homolog in S. cerevisiae: Chronic activation of the CDC28 protein kinase by cyclin prevents exit from mitosis. *Cell* **65**:163, 1991.

187. Surana U, Robitsch H, Price C, Schuster T, Fitch I, Futcher AB, Nasmyth K: The role of CDC28 and cyclins during mitosis in the budding yeast S. cerevisiae. *Cell* **65**:145, 1991.

188. King RW, Jackson P, Kirschner MW: Mitosis in transition. *Cell* **79**:563, 1994.

189. Juca FC, Shibuya EK, Dohrmann EE, Ruderman JV: Both cyclin A∆60 and B∆97 are stable and arrest cells im M phase but only cyclin B∆97 turns on cyclin destruction. *EMBO J* **10**:4311, 1991.

190. Murray AW: Cyclin ubiquitination: The destructive end of mitosis. *Cell* **81**:149, 1995.

191. King R, Peters J, Tugendreich S, Rolfe M, Hieter P, Kirschner M: A 20S complex containing cdc27 and cdc16 catalyzes the mitosis-specific conjugation of ubiquitin to cyclin B. *Cell* **81**:279, 1995.

192. Holloway SL, Glotzer M, King RW, Murray AW: Anaphase is initiated by proteolysis rather than by the inactivation of maturation-promoting factor. *Cell* **73**:1393, 1993.

193. Sudakin V, Ganoth D, Dahan A, Heller H, Hershko J, Luca F, Ruderman J, Hershko A: The cyclosome, a large complex containing cyclin-selective ubiquitin ligase activity, targets cyclins for destruction at the end of mitosis. *Mol Biol Cell* **6**:185, 1995.

194. Irniger S, Piatti S, Michaelis C, Nasmyth K: Genes involved in sister chromatid separation are needed for B-type cyclin proteolysis in budding yeast. *Cell* **81**:269, 1995.

195. Seufert W, Futcher B, Jentsch S: Role of a ubiquitin-conjugating enzyme in degradation of S-phase and M-phase cyclins. *Nature* **373**:78, 1995.

196. Felix M, Labbe J, Doree M, Hunt T, Karsenti E: Triggering of cyclin degradation in interphase extracts of amphibian eggs by cdc2 kinase. *Nature* **346**:379, 1990.

197. Amon A, Irniger S, Nasmyth K: Closing the cell cycle circle in yeast: G2 cyclin proteolysis initiated at mitosis persists until the activation of G1 cyclins in the next cell cycle. *Cell* **77**:1037, 1994.

198. Clurman BE, Sheaff RJ, Thress K, Groudine M, Roberts JM: Turnover of cyclin E by the ubiquitin-proteosome pathway is regulated by CDK2 binding and cyclin phosphorylation. *Genes Dev* **10**:1979, 1996.

199. Won K, Reed S: Activation of cyclin E/CDK2 is coupled to site-specific autophosphorylation and ubiquitin-dependent degradation of cyclin E. *EMBO J* **15**:4182, 1996.

200. Lanker S, Valdivieso M, Wittenberg C: Rapid degradation of the G1 cyclin cln2 induced by CDK-dependent phosphorylation. *Science* **271**:1597, 1996.

201. Tyers M, Tokiwa G, Nash R, Futcher B: The cln2-cdc28 kinase complex of S. cerevisiae is regulated by proteolysis and phosphorylation. *EMBO J* **11**:1773, 1992.

202. Yaglom J, Linskens M, Sadis S, Rubin D, Futcher B, Finley D: p34Cdc28-mediated control of cln3 degradation. *Mol Cell Biol* **15**:731, 1995.

203. Chen Z, Hagler J, Palombella V, Melandri F, Scherer D, Ballard D, Maniatis T: Signal-induced site-specific phosphorylation targets IkBa to the ubiquitin-proteosome pathway. *Genes Dev* **9**:1586, 1995.

204. Treier M, Staszewski L, Bohmann D: Ubiquitin-dependent c-Jun degradation in vivo is mediated by the G domain. *Cell* **78**:787, 1994.

205. Willems AR, Lanker S, Patton EF, Craig KL, Nason TF, Kobayashi R, Wittenberg C, Tyers M: Cdc53 targets phosphorylated G1 cyclins for degradation by the ubiquitin proteolytic pathway. *Cell* **86**:453, 1996.

206. Pagano M, Tam SW, Theodoras A, Beer-Romero P, Del Sal G, Chau V, Yew R, Draetta G, Rolfe M: Role of the ubiquitin proteosome pathway in regulating abundance of the cyclin-dependent kinase inhibitor p27. *Science* **269**:682, 1995.

206a. Feldman RM, Correll CC, Kaplan KB, Deshaies RJ: A complex of Cdc4p, Skp1p, and Cdc53p/cullin catalyzes ubiquitination of the phosphorylated CDK inhibitor Sic1p. *Cell* **91**:221, 1997.

206b. Henchoz S, Chi Y, Catarin B, Herskowitz I, Deshaies RJ, Peter M: Phosphorylation- and ubiquitin-dependent degradation of the cyclin-dependent kinase inhibitor Far1p in budding yeast. *Genes Dev* **11**:3046, 1997.

206c. Lisztwan J, Marti A, Sutterluty H, Gstaiger M, Wirbelauer C, Krek W: Association of human CUL-1 and ubiquitin-conjugating enzyme CDC34 with the F-box protein p45(SKP2): Evidence for evolutionary conservation in the subunit composition of the CDC34-SCF pathway. *EMBO J* **17**:368, 1998.

206d. Patton EE, Willems AR, Sa D, Kuras L, Thomas D, Craig KL, Tyers M: Cdc53 is a scaffold protein for multiple Cdc34/Skp1/F-box protein complexes that regulate cell division and methionine biosynthesis in yeast. *Genes Dev* **12**:692, 1998.

206e. Skowyra D, Craig KL, Tyers M, Elledge SJ, Harper JW: F-box proteins are receptors that recruit phosphorylated substrates to the SCF ubiquitin-ligase complex. *Cell* **91**:209, 1997.

206f. Verma R, Feldman RM, Deshaies RJ: SIC1 is ubiquitinated in vitro by a pathway that requires CDC4, CDC34, and cyclin/CDK activities. *Mol Biol Cell* **8**:1427, 1997.

206g. Bai C, Sen P, Hofmann K, Ma L, Goebl M, Harper JW, Elledge SJ: SKP1 connects cell cycle regulators to the ubiquitin proteolysis machinery through a novel motif, the F-box. *Cell* **86**:263, 1996.

207. Plon S, Leppig KA, Do HN, Groudine M: Cloning of the human homolog of the CDC34 cell cycle gene by complementation in yeast. *Proc Natl Acad Sci U S A* **90**:10484, 1993.

208. Kipreos E, Lander L, Wing J, He WW, Hedgecock E: cul-1 is required for cell cycle exit in C. elegans and identifies a novel gene family. *Cell* **85**:829, 1996.

209. Baserga R: The biology of cell reproduction. Cambridge, MA: Harvard University Press, 1985.

210. Zetterberg A, Larson O: Kinetic analysis of regulatory events in G1 leading to proliferation of quiescence of Swiss 3T3 cells. *Proc Natl Acad Sci U S A* **82**:5365, 1985.

211. Pardee AB: A restriction point for control of normal animal cell proliferation. *Proc Natl Acad Sci U S A* **71**:1286, 1974.

212. Zetterberg A: Control of mammalian cell proliferation. *Curr Opin Cell Biol* **2**:296, 1990.

213. Pardee AB: G1 events and regulation of cell proliferation. *Science* **246**:603, 1989.

214. Zetterberg A, Larsson O, Wiman K: What is the restriction point? *Curr Opin Cell Biol* **7**:835, 1995.

215. Chao M: Growth factor signaling: Where is the specificity? *Cell* **68**:995, 1992.

216. Cantley L, Auger K, Carpenter C, Duckworth B, Graziani A, Kapeller R, Soltoff S: Oncogenes and signal transduction. *Cell* **64**:281, 1991.

217. Winston JT, Pledger WJ: Growth factor regulation of cyclin D1 mRNA expression through protein synthesis-dependent and -independent mechanisms. *Mol Biol Cell* **4**:1133, 1993.

218. Roussel MF, Theodoras AM, Pagano M, Sherr CJ: Rescue of defective mitogenic signaling by D-type cyclins. *Proc Natl Acad Sci U S A* **92**:6837, 1995.

219. Albanese C, Johnson J, Watanabe G, Eklund N, Vu D, Arnold A, Pestell R: Transforming p21ras mutants and c-Ets-2 activate the cyclin D1 promoter through distinguishable regions. *J Biol Chem* **270**:23589, 1995.

220. Hatakeyama M, Herrera R, Makela T, Dowdy S, Jacks T, Weinberg R: The cancer cell and the cell cycle clock. *Cold Spring Harbor Symp Quant Biol* **59**:1, 1994.

221. Roberts JM, Koff A, Polyak K, Firpo E, Collins S, Ohtsubo M, Massague J: Cyclins, cdks, and cyclin kinase inhibitors. *Cold Spring Harbor Symp Quant Biol* **59**:31, 1994.

222. Coats S, Flannagan WM, Nourse J, Roberts J: Requirement of p27Kip1 for restriction point control of the fibroblast cell cycle. *Science* **272**:877, 1996.

223. Nourse J, Firpo E, Flanagan M, Meyerson M, Polyak K, Lee MH, Massague J, Crabtree G, Roberts J: IL-2 mediated elimination of the p27kip1 cyclin-cdk kinase inhibitor prevented by rapamycin. *Nature* **372**:570, 1994.

224. Firpo EJ, Koff A, Solomon M, Roberts J: Inactivation of a cdk2 inhibitor during interleukin-2-induced proliferation of human T lymphocytes. *Mol Cell Biol* **14**:4889, 1994.

225. Fero ML, Rivkin M, Tasch M, Porter P, Carow CE, Firpo E, Polyak K, Tsai L, Broudy V, Perlmutter RM, Kaushansky K, Roberts JM: A syndrome of multi-organ hyperplasia with features of gigantism, tumorigenesis and female sterility in p27 kip1-deficient mice. *Cell* **85**:733, 1996.

226. Matsushime H, Quelle D, Shurtleff S, Shibuya M, Sherr C, Kato JY: D-type cyclin-dependent kinase activity in mammalian cells. *Mol Cell Biol* **14**:2066, 1994.

227. Guadagno T, Ohtsubo M, Roberts J, Assoian R: A link between cyclin A expression and adhesion-dependent cell cycle progression. *Science* **262**:1572, 1993.

228. Zhu X, Ohtsubo M, Bohmer RM, Roberts JM, Assoian R: Adhesion-dependent cell cycle progression linked to the expression of cyclin D1 activation of cyclin E-cdk2 and phosphorylation of the retinoblastoma protein. *J Cell Biol* **133**:391, 1996.

229. Draetta G, Loef E: Transforming growth factor β1 inhibition of p34cdc2 phosphorylation and histone H1 kinase activity is associated with G1/S-phase growth arrest. *Mol Cell Biol* **11**:1185, 1991.

230. Koff A, Ohtsuki M, Polyack K, Roberts J, Massague J: Negative regulation of G1 in mammalian cells: Inhibition of cyclin E-dependent kinase by TGF-beta. *Science* **260**:536, 1993.

231. Laiho M, DeCaprio J, Ludlow J, Livingston D, Massague J: Growth inhibition by TGF-β linked to suppression of retinoblastoma protein phosphorylation. *Cell* **62**:175, 1990.

232. Reynisdottir I, Polyak K, Iavarone A, Massague J: Kip/Cip and INK4 cdk inhibitors cooperate to induce cell cycle arrest in response to TGF-beta. *Genes Dev* **9**:1831, 1995.

233. Slingerland J, Hengst L, Pan C, Alexander D, Stampfer M, Reed S: A novel inhibitor of cyclin-cdk activity detected in transforming growth factor B-arrested epithelial cells. *Mol Cell Biol* **14**:3683, 1994.

234. Polyak K, Kato J, Solomon M, Sherr C, Massaque J, Roberts J, Koff A: p27kip1, a cyclin-cdk inhibitor, links transforming growth factor beta and contact inhibition to cell cycle arrest. *Genes Dev* **8**:9, 1994.

235. Kato JM, Matsuoka M, Polyak K, Massague J, Sherr CJ: Cyclic AMP-induced G1 phase arrest mediated by an inhibitor (p27Kip1) of cyclin-dependent kinase-4 activation. *Cell* **79**:487, 1994.

236. Brugarolas J, Chandrasekaran C, Gordon J, Beach D, Jacks T, Hannon G: Radiation-induced cell cycle arrest compromised by p21 deficiency. *Nature* **377**:552, 1995.

237. Deng C, Zhang P, Harper JW, Elledge S, Leder P: Mice lacking p21Cip1/Waf1 undergo normal development but are defective in G1 checkpoint control. *Cell* **82**:675, 1995.

238. Dulic V, Kaufman W, Wilson S, Tlsty T, Lees E, Harper JW, Elledge S, Reed S: p53-dependent inhibition of cyclin-dependent kinase activities in human fibroblasts during radiation-induced G1 arrest. *Cell* **76**:1013, 1994.

239. Massague J: TGF-beta signaling: Receptors, transducers, and mad proteins. *Cell* **85**:947, 1996.

240. Hahn S, Schutte M, Hoque A, Moskaluk C, da Costa L, Rozenblum E, Weinstein C, Fischer A, Hruban R, Kern S: *Science* **271**:350, 1996.

241. Hannon G, Beach D: p15Ink4b is a potential effector of cell cycle arrest by TGF-beta. *Nature* **371**:257, 1994.

242. Ewen M, Sluss H, Whitehouse L, Livingston D: Cdk4 modulation by TGF-β leads to cell cycle arrest. *Cell* **74**:1009, 1993.

243. Kuerbitz S, Plunkett B, Walsh W, Kastan M: Wild-type p53 is a cell cycle checkpoint determinant following irradiation. *Proc Natl Acad Sci U S A* **82**:7491, 1992.

244. Kastan M, Onyekwere O, Sidransky D, Vogelsein B, Craig R: Participation of p53 protein in the cellular response to DNA damage. *Cancer Res* **51**:6304, 1991.

245. Lane D: p53, guardian of the genome. *Nature* **358**:15, 1992.

246. Vogelstein B, Kinzler K: p53 function and dysfunction. *Cell* **70**:523, 1992.

247. Fields S, Jang S: Presence of a potent transcription activating sequence in the p53 protein. *Science* **249**:1046, 1990.

248. Kern S, Kinzler K, Bruskin A, Jarosz D, Friedman P, Prives C, Vogelstein B: Identification of p53 as a sequence specific DNA binding protein. *Science* **252**:1708, 1992.

249. Li R, Waga S, Hannon G, Beach D, Stillman B: Differential effects by the p21 cdk inhibitor on PCNA dependent DNA replication and DNA repair. *Nature* **371**:534, 1994.

250. Raff M: Size control: The regulation of cell numbers in animal development. *Cell* **86**:173, 1996.

251. Clurman BE, Roberts JM: Cell cycle and cancer. *J Natl Cancer Inst* **87**:1499, 1995.

252. Harlow E: An introduction to the puzzle. *Cold Spring Harbor Symp Quant Biol* **59**:709, 1994.

253. Hunter TJ, Pines J: Cyclins and cancer. *Cell* **66**:1071, 1991.

254. Morgan D: Cell cycle control in neoplastic cells. *Curr Opin Genet Dev* **2**:33, 1992.

255. Hall M, Peters G: Genetic alterations of cyclins, cyclin-dependent kinases and Cdk inhibitor's in human cancer *Adv Cancer Res* **68**:67, 1996.

256. Sherr C: Cancer cell cycles. *Science* **274**:1672, 1996.

257. Jiang WY, Zhang Y, Kahn SM, Hollstein M, Santella M, Lu S, Harris CC, Montesano R, Weinstein IB: Altered expression of the cyclin D1 and retinoblastoma genes in human esophageal cancer. *Proc Natl Acad Sci U S A* **90**:9026, 1993.

258. Lee E, To H, Shew J, Bookstein R, Scully P, Lee WH: Inactivation of the retinoblastoma susceptibility gene in human breast cancers. *Science* **241**:218, 1988.

259. Mori T, Miura K, Aoki T, Nishihira T, Mori S, Nakamura Y: Frequent somatic mutation of the MTS1/CDK4I (multiple tumor suppressor/cyclin-dependent kinase 4 inhibitor) gene in esophageal squamous cell carcinoma. *Cancer Res* **54**:3396, 1994.

260. Kamb A, Gruis NA, Weaver-Feldhaus J, Liu Q, Harshman K, Tavtigian SV, Stockert E, Day III RS, Johnson BE, Skolnick MH: A cell cycle regulator potentially involved in genesis of many tumor types. *Science* **264**:436, 1994.

261. Sheaff R, Roberts J: Lessons in p16 from phylum Falconium. *Curr Biol* **5**:28, 1995.

262. Kawamata N, Morosetti R, Miller S, Park D, Spirin K, Nakamaki T, Takeuchi S, Hatta Y, Simpson J, Wilcyznski S, et al: Molecular analysis of the cyclin dependent kinase inhibitor gene p27/Kip1 in human malignancies. *Cancer Res* **55**:2266, 1995.

263. Keyomarsi K, O'Leary N, Molnar G, Lees E, Fingert H, Pardee A: Cyclin E, a potential prognostic marker for breast cancer. *Cancer Res* **54**:380, 1994.

264. Pietenpol J, Bohlander S, Sato Y, Papadoupolos B, Liu C, Friedman B, Trask B, Roberts J, Kinzler K, Rowley J, Vogelstein B: Assignment of the human p27Kip1 gene to 12p13 and its analysis in leukemias. *Cancer Res* **55**:1206, 1995.

265. Ponce-Castenada M, Lee M, Latres E, Polyak K, Lacombe L, Montgomery K, Mathew S, Krauter K, Sheinfeld J, Massague J, et al: p27Kip1: chromosomal mapping to 12p12-12p13.1 and absence of mutations in human tumors. *Cancer Res* **55**:1211, 1995.

266. Fearon E, Vogelstein B: A genetic model for colorectal tumorigenesis. *Cell* **61**:759, 1990.

267. Loeb L: Mutator phenotype may be required for multistage tumorigenesis. *Cancer Res* **54**:4590, 1990.

268. Knudson AG: Genetics of human cancer. *Annu Rev Genet* **20**:231, 1986.

269. Hartwell L, Weinert T, Kadyk L, Garvik B: Cell cycle checkpoint, genomic integrity, and cancer. *Cold Spring Harbor Symp Quant Biol* **59**:259, 1994.

270. Tlsty T, White A, Livanos E, Sage M, Roelofs H, Briot A, Poulose B: Genomic integrity and the genetics of cancer. *Cold Spring Harbor Symp Quant Biol* **59**:265, 1994.

271. Schimke R, Sherwood S, Hill A, Johnston R: Overreplication and recombination of DNA in higher eukaryotes: Potential consequences and biological implications. *Proc Natl Acad Sci U S A* **83**:2157, 1986.

272. Nowell PC: The clonal evolution of tumor cell populations. *Science* **194**:23, 1976.

273. Weinert T, Hartwell L: The RAD9 gene controls the cell cycle response to DNA damage in Saccharomyces cerevisiae. *Science* **241**:317, 1989.

274. Dasso M, Newport J: Completion of DNA replication is monitored by a feedback system that controls the initiation of mitosis in vitro: Studies in Xenopus. *Cell* **61**:811, 1990.

275. Enoch T, Nurse P: Mutation of fission yeast cell cycle control genes abolishes dependence of mitosis on DNA replication. *Cell* **60**:665, 1990.

276. Rowley R, Hudson J, Young P: The wee1 protein kinase is required for radiation-induced mitotic delay. *Nature* **356**:353, 1992.

277. Smythe C, Newport J: Coupling of mitosis to the completion of S phase in Xenopus occurs via modulation of the tyrosine kinase that phosphorylates p34 CDC2. *Cell* **68**:787, 1992.

278. Walworth N, Davey S, Beach D: Fission yeast chk1 protein kinase links the rad checkpoint pathway to cdc2. *Nature* **363**:368, 1993.

279. Nurse P: Checkpoint pathways come of age. *Cell* **91**:865, 1997.

280. Enoch T, Gould KL, Nurse P: Mitotic checkpoint control in fission yeast. *Cold Spring Harbor Symp Quant Biol* **56**:409, 1991.

281. Rhind N, Furnari B, Russell P: Cdc2 tyrosine phosphorylation is required for the DNA damage checkpoint in fission yeast. *Genes Dev* **11**:504, 1997.

282. Rhind N, Russell P: Tyrosine phosphorylation of cdc2 is required for the replication checkpoint in Schizosaccharomyces pombe. *Mol Cell Biol* **18**:3782, 1998.

283. Hermeking H, Lengauer C, Polyak K, et al: 14-3-3 sigma is a p53-regulated inhibitor of G2/M progression. *Mol Cell* **1**:3, 1997.

284. Sanchez Y, Wong C, Thoma RS, et al: Conservation of the Chk1 checkpoint pathway in mammals: Linkage of DNA damage to cdk regulation through cdc25 [see comments]. *Science* **277**:1497, 1997.

285. Peng CY, Graves PR, Thoma RS, et al: Mitotic and G2 checkpoint control: Regulation of 14-3-3 protein binding by phosphorylation of Cdc25C on serine-216 [see comments]. *Science* **277**:1501, 1997.

286. O'Connell MJ, Raleigh JM, Verkade HM, et al: Chk1 is a wee1 kinase in the G2 DNA damage checkpoint inhibiting cdc2 by Y15 phosphorylation. *EMBO J* **16**:545, 1997.

287. Flaggs G, Plug AW, Dunks KM, et al: Atm-dependent interactions of a mammalian chk1 homolog with meiotic chromosomes. *Curr Biol* **7**:977, 1997.

288. Murray AW: The genetics of cell cycle checkpoints. *Curr Op in Genet Dev* **5**:5, 1995.

289. Sanchez Y, Elledge S: Stopped for repairs. *Bioessays* **17**:545, 1995.

290. Li R, Murray A: Feedback control of mitosis in budding yeast. *Cell* **66**:519, 1991.

291. Hoyt A, Totis L, Roberts BT: S. cerevisiae genes required for cell cycle arrest in response to loss of microtubule function. *Cell* **66**:507, 1991.

292. Murray AW: Tense spindles can relax. *Nature* **373**:560, 1995.

293. Minshull J, Sun H, Tonks N, Murray AW: A MAP kinase-dependent spindle assembly checkpoint in Xenopus egg extracts. *Cell* **79**:475, 1994.

294. Lin J, Wu X, Chen J, Chang A, Levine AJ: Functions of the p53 protein in growth regulation and tumor suppression. *Cold Spring Harbor Symp Quant Biol* **59**:215, 1994.

295. Barlow C, Hirotsune S, Paylor R, Liyanage M, Eckhaus M, Collins F, Shiloh Y, Crawley J, Ried T, Tagle D, Wynshaw-Boris A: Atm-deficient mice: a paradigm of ataxia telangectasia. *Cell* **85**:159, 1996.

296. Meyn MS: Ataxia-telangiectasia and cellular responses to DNA damage. *Cancer Res* **55**:5991, 1995.

Apoptosis and Cancer

Charles M. Rudin ■ *Craig B. Thompson*

1. **Apoptosis is a descriptive term for the phenotype of cells undergoing programmed cell death. Apoptosis is a critical component of development and homeostasis in multicellular eukaryotic organisms. Apoptotic cell death can be distinguished from necrotic cell death by several criteria, including characteristic morphology and a minimal inflammatory reaction.**

2. **The Bcl-2 family of proteins plays a central role in apoptotic control and is conserved evolutionarily. The realization that Bcl-2 functions to prevent apoptosis defined a new category of oncogene: the antiapoptotic gene. Apoptotic regulation is dependent on the relative balance of opposing Bcl-2 family members. Those family members may function by regulating homeostasis between key intracellular organelles and the cytoplasm.**

3. **The caspases are evolutionarily conserved proteases that function as important mediators of apoptosis. Control of caspase activity is dependent on proteolytic processing of cytoplasmic proenzymes. Some of these proteases have autocatalytic potential. The critical downstream targets of caspase family proteolysis have not been fully defined.**

4. **Many cell surface receptors, including the tumor necrosis factor receptor (TNFR) family, have been shown to modify the apoptotic sensitivity of cells. Different members of the TNFR family can promote or inhibit apoptosis. An apoptotic signaling pathway from some of these receptors has been traced by direct protein–protein interaction from receptor engagement to caspase activation.**

5. **Cellular and viral oncogenes that stimulate proliferation are strong inducers of apoptosis. This induction is probably dependent on cell cycle checkpoints (tumor suppressor gene products) that detect abnormally replicating cells and trigger apoptosis. Inhibition of apoptosis therefore is frequently an essential step in the process of oncogenesis.**

6. **Anticancer therapies induce apoptosis in sensitive cells. Inhibition of apoptosis is a major mechanism of chemotherapeutic resistance. Chemotherapy may accelerate the mutagenesis rate and promote aneuploidy of tumors in which apoptosis has been suppressed. New therapies directed at modifying apoptotic signaling pathways may be helpful in circumventing these problems.**

The term *programmed cell death* refers to the induction of cell death by a regulated pathway inherent to the cell. It can be contrasted with necrotic cell death, which is traumatic and depends on factors entirely external to the cell. *Apoptosis* (from the Greek for "falling leaves") is a descriptive term that was used originally to describe the characteristic phenotype of cells that die in the absence of evident trauma. The apoptotic phenotype has been found to be so ubiquitous among cells undergoing programmed cell death that the terms are now used interchangeably. Wyllie and

colleagues in the early 1970s were among the first to observe and record a phenotype of dying cells that appeared to be conserved among widely disparate cell types and was distinct in many respects from necrotic cell death.[1,2] These initial descriptive studies spawned an enormous field of inquiry with direct implications for many problematic areas of medicine, including neurodevelopmental and neurodegenerative diseases, infection, autoimmunity, and cancer.[3-7]

The study of apoptosis has had an important impact on the understanding of organismal growth and differentiation. The characteristic features of the process are conserved widely among multicellular eukaryotes.[8,9] The capacity to initiate an apoptotic pathway appears to be a shared feature of all the cells of the body, including rapidly cycling populations such as leukocytes and long-lived cells such as neurons. Apoptosis plays a crucial role in development, permitting the necessary elimination of surplus cells in the formation of many complex organs, including the brain.[10]

Several morphologic features of apoptotic cells distinguish them from cells that die in response to trauma or hypoxia.[2] Necrotic cell death is characterized by cell swelling and gross disruption of organelles and the cell membrane. Apoptotic cell death is characterized by cell contraction, blebbing of the cytoplasmic membrane, dense condensation of the nucleus, and a pathognomonic autodigestion of the genome into fragments that correspond in size to multiples of the amount of DNA found in individual nucleosomes. If electrophoresed through an agarose gel, DNA from an apoptotic cell therefore can be displayed as a ladder, with rungs corresponding to cleavage between one, two, or multiple nucleosome elements (Fig. 10-1).

Traumatic cell death leads to leakage of intracellular contents and the generation of a potent inflammatory response that depends on multiple cytokines and pyrogens. This response may be critical to confining infection as well as to wound healing and scar formation. In contrast, apoptotic cell death does not lead to uncontrolled cytokine release or the generation of a significant inflammatory response. Apoptotic cell remnants typically are recognized and engulfed by adjacent cells (frequently by cells that are not part of the phagocytic macrophage-monocyte system) prior to breakdown of the cellular membrane and release of intracellular contents.[11-13] The ability to delete cells in an immunologically silent manner may be of central importance in permitting the natural turnover and remodeling of tissues without risking autoimmune disease.

Homeostasis in any cell population requires a balance between the processes of cell proliferation and cell death (Fig. 10-2). Accumulation of abnormal numbers of a clonally related population of cells (i.e., a neoplasm) can result from either uncontrolled proliferation or inhibition of cell death. The regulatory mechanisms that control cell proliferation clearly are extensive and have been the primary focus of research on carcinogenesis for many years. Recently, it has become apparent that the mechanisms of programmed cell death also are tightly regulated, highly responsive to extracellular signals, and similarly integral to the inhibition of carcinogenesis. This chapter outlines the known mechanisms that regulate cell death and some of the implications of dysregulated cell death on carcinogenesis and chemotherapeutic resistance.

A list of standard abbreviations is located immediately preceding the index. Nonstandard abbreviations used in this chapter include: TNFR = tumor necrosis factor receptor; TRAF = TNF receptor-associated factor; IAP = inhibitor of apoptosis.

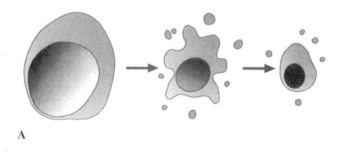

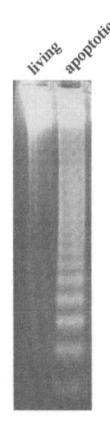

Fig. 10-1 Characteristic cellular changes of apoptosis. *A.* Typical morphologic changes of apoptosis are shown, including blebbing of the cytoplasmic membrane, cell contraction, and marked condensation of the nucleus. Importantly, cytoplasmic contents are not spilled into the extracellular space. *B.* Agarose gel electrophoresis of genomic DNA from apoptotic cells. A pathognomonic laddering of DNA fragments in approximately 200-base pair increments is seen, corresponding to the amount of DNA contained within individual nucleosomes. The cells are murine lymph node cells after 0 h (living) and 48 h (apoptotic) in culture.

BCL-2 AND THE ORIGINS OF THE STUDY OF APOPTOSIS AND CANCER

The *bcl-2* gene (for B-cell lymphoma/leukemia-2) initially was identified as the gene on chromosome 18q21 at the breakpoint of the t(14;18) chromosomal translocation found in the majority of B-cell follicular lymphomas[14-17] (Fig. 10-3). This genomic rearrangement juxtaposes the *bcl-2* gene with the immunoglobulin heavy chain gene enhancer, leading to marked up-regulation and constitutive expression of Bcl-2 in lymphoid cells. The Bcl-2 coding sequence is not altered by this translocation.

The role of Bcl-2 in oncogenesis remained obscure for several years after its discovery. Unlike all previously identified oncogenes, overexpression of the *bcl-2* gene did not increase the proliferative potential of cells in any of the commonly used assays for oncogenic transformation, which depend on a modulation of

the growth rate of the transfected cell. The failure to induce rampant growth correlates with the phenotype of most follicular lymphomas, which have an indolent, slowly progressive natural history, have low proliferative indices, and retain many of the phenotypic characteristics of nontransformed lymphocytes.[18]

The first association between Bcl-2 and inhibition of cell death was made in 1988.[19] Stable *bcl-2* transformants of a cell line dependent on the growth factor interleukin-3 (IL-3) were found to survive for prolonged periods after withdrawal of IL-3, much longer than the parental cell line lacking the upregulated *bcl-2* gene. In addition, Bcl-2 was shown to cooperate with a more traditional oncoprotein, c-myc, to immortalize pre-B cells (see below). Bcl-2 subsequently has been found to be a potent inhibitor of apoptosis in a wide variety of experimental systems.[20]

The discovery of the function of Bcl-2 challenged the prevailing view of carcinogenesis and defined a new category of oncogene.[21] Research on oncogenesis had focused largely on the mechanisms regulating cell proliferation: Cancer was thought to arise from the products of abnormally expressed genes driving cell replication (oncogenes) or failing to inhibit cell replication (tumor suppressor genes). Bcl-2, which is overexpressed by the most common chromosomal rearrangement in lymphoid malignancy, was found to have no direct effect on replication but caused a failure to die. This realization implied for the first time that alteration of either side of the homeostatic balance could contribute not only to cell accumulation but also to carcinogenesis. Subsequent work by many groups has confirmed the carcinogenic potential of antiapoptotic gene dysregulation and has led to a broader view of the types of genetic alterations that contribute to cancer.

To place the effects of apoptotic dysregulation in cancer cells in context, the next section summarizes the current understanding of the mechanisms that regulate apoptosis in normal cells.

THE CENTRAL APOPTOTIC PATHWAY

C. elegans and the Evolutionary Conservation of Apoptotic Regulators

The striking morphologic similarity between disparate cell types undergoing apoptosis suggests that the underlying molecular processes may be similar.[22] Many of the features of this central apoptotic control system have been defined, and the outline of this pathway provides insight into potential mechanisms for viral and cellular oncogenic transformation.

Many of the critical factors involved in the control of apoptosis were first defined in the nematode *Caenorhabditis elegans*. Every cell division and cell death event in the normal pathway of *C. elegans* development is known, and this developmental pathway follows a determined, predictable program.[23] All 131 programmed cell death events in the developing worm depend on the normal function of three proteins: CED-3, CED-4, and CED-9. Loss of CED-3 or CED-4 function or a gain-of-function mutation of the CED-9 protein will lead to complete abrogation of cell death in *C. elegans* development.[24,25] Loss of CED-9 function leads to increased apoptotic cell death.[25] CED-9 appears to function by

Table 10-1 Mammalian Bcl-2-Related Proteins

Antiapoptotic	Proapoptotic	BH-3 Proteins (Inhibit Antiapoptotic Function)
Bcl-2	Bcl-x$_S$	Bad
Bcl-x$_L$	Bax	Bid
Mcl-1	Bak	Bik
Bcl-w	Mtd/Bok	Hrk
A-1		Bim
		Blk

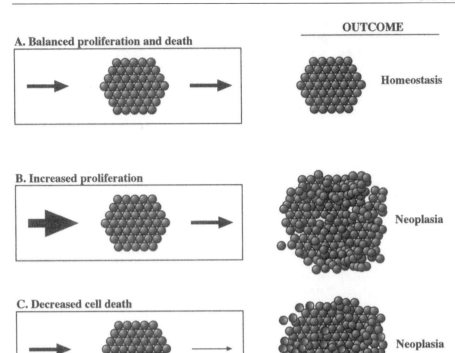

OUTCOME

A. Balanced proliferation and death

Homeostasis

B. Increased proliferation

Neoplasia

C. Decreased cell death

Neoplasia

Fig. 10-2 Dysregulation of either side of the homeostatic balance can lead to neoplasia. *A.* A population of cells in homeostatic balance replicates and dies at equal rates. Mutations that result in either an increase in the proliferative rate (*B*) or a decrease in the death rate (*C*) can lead to the accumulation of clonally related cells.

suppressing inappropriate activity of CED-3 and CED-4.[26] CED-4 interacts with CED-3 to facilitate its activation to a protease capable of generating an apoptotic phenotype.[27–31]

Strong evolutionary pressures would be expected to preserve the mechanisms involved in a process as fundamental to the organism as the control of cell death. Many of the proteins central to apoptotic control indeed have been highly conserved, from the roundworm to the human (Fig. 10-4). CED-9 is highly homologous to mammalian Bcl-2.[32,33] Bcl-2 expression in *C. elegans* mimics a CED-9 gain of function and can partially revert a CED-9 loss-of-function mutant. A mammalian homologue of CED-4, Apaf-1, recently was identified and appears to function as a signal transducer between Bcl-2 family members and CED-3-related molecules.[34] CED-3 was found by database searching to be

related to the mammalian interleukin-1β converting enzyme, now known as *caspase 1*.[35] As discussed below, caspases have been found to play a central role in the effector phase of apoptosis.

The Bcl-2 Family

Bcl-2 overexpression is capable of inhibiting cell death in response to many disparate apoptotic signals, suggesting that it acts at the convergence of many apoptotic pathways. Bcl-2 has been found to be one of a family of related proteins, several members of which appear to play important positive and negative roles in the control of apoptosis (Table 10-1). Antiapoptotic factors including Bcl-2, Bcl-x_L, and Mcl-1 have been found to be overexpressed in several tumor types. Members of the Bcl-2 family have been found to form both homo- and heterodimers, and the relative balance of

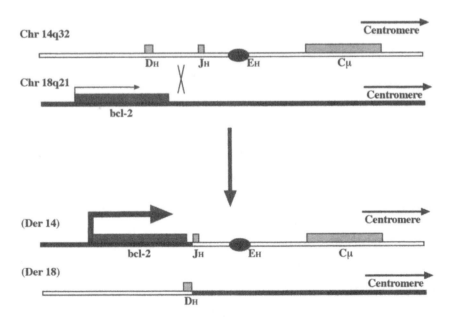

Chr 14q32

Centromere

D_H J_H E_H $C\mu$

Chr 18q21

Centromere

bcl-2

(Der 14)

Centromere

bcl-2 J_H E_H $C\mu$

(Der 18)

Centromere

D_H

Fig. 10-3 The t(14;18) translocation characteristic of follicular lymphomas. Exons of the immunoglobulin heavy chain gene are represented by light boxes, the *bcl-2* gene by a dark box, and the heavy chain enhancer by a black oval. The translocation involves sites in the immunoglobulin heavy chain locus that normally are involved in the rearrangements necessary to generate a functional heavy chain gene and probably occurs in the pre-B-cell stage. The breakpoint in the *bcl-2* gene frequently is in the 3' untranslated region and thus does not affect the coding sequence.

C. elegans:

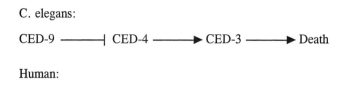

Human:

Fig. 10-4 Critical components of apoptotic regulation have been evolutionarily conserved.

antiapoptotic and proapoptotic members in these complexes may be a critical determinant of apoptotic sensitivity.[43]

Bcl-2 family members can be divided into three categories: antiapoptotic factors such as Bcl-2 that inhibit cell death, proapoptotic factors that when overexpressed trigger cell death, and factors that while not intrinsically proapoptotic nevertheless can bind to and inhibit the function of antiapoptotic factors. Members of the third category typically share only a limited homology with the other family members, in a domain known as BH-3.[44]

The mechanism of action of Bcl-2 family members has not been determined, although several important insights have been established. The structure of $Bcl-x_L$ has been determined by x-ray crystallography and nuclear magnetic resonance (NMR) spectroscopy.[45] The molecular structure of $Bcl-x_L$ surprisingly was found to be similar to that of members of the colicin family of bacterial proteins. Colicins are proteins secreted by bacteria that form pores in the surface membranes of other bacterial strains, causing cell death.[46] The relevance of this unexpected structural link between families of proteins involved in mammalian and bacterial cell death is currently unclear.

Bcl-2 appears to be localized to the nuclear endoplasmic reticular and outer mitochondrial membranes.[47-49] Commitment to apoptotic cell death has been associated with loss of mitochondrial membrane potential, and this membrane potential gradient can be maintained by Bcl-2 overexpression.[50-54] Many of the characteristic nuclear changes of apoptosis can be induced by the addition of dATP and cytochrome c to cytoplasmic extracts in vitro.[55] Since cytochrome c normally is tightly sequestered within mitochondria, Bcl-2 family members may function by directly controlling mitochondrial membrane permeability.[56] Indeed, recent observations indicate that Bcl-2 and $Bcl-x_L$ inhibit, whereas the proapoptotic family member Bax promotes, cytochrome c release from the mitochondrial intermembrane space.[56-59]

Antiapoptotic family members also may function by complexing with and inactivating factors that would otherwise trigger caspase activation. As described earlier, in *C. elegans* CED-9 has been found to interact directly with CED-4; this interaction in turn prevents CED-4 from activating the cysteine protease CED-3.[27,28] $Bcl-x_L$ similarly can interact with the mammalian CED-4 homologue Apaf-1, and this interaction may play a role in the inhibition of Apaf-1 activation of downstream caspases.[34,62,63]

The Caspase Family

Another group of proteins that has been implicated strongly in the central apoptotic pathway are the caspases (*c*ysteine proteases with *asp*artic acid specificity).[64,65] Unlike the Bcl-2 family, which appears to modulate apoptotic threshold without participating directly involved in cellular autodigestion, caspase activity has been associated closely with the apoptotic morphology of the dying cell. The family has at least 13 members, which can be subgrouped on the basis of similarity and target specificity[65-69] (Table 10-2). Overexpression of most caspases has been shown to trigger apoptosis in cell lines, although not all appear to be involved in physiological apoptosis. A central role for this family of proteases in the process of apoptosis in mammalian cells has been suggested by studies showing that specific inhibitors of caspases can prevent cell death, or at least an apoptotic

morphology, in response to many of the known triggers of programmed cell death.[70,71] These inhibitors include viral products such as p35 and crmA (see below) as well as synthetic oligopeptides that occupy and block the protease activity site.

Regulation of caspase activity may occur on several levels. All the caspases are synthesized as larger inactive proenzymes that must undergo proteolytic processing to the active enzymatic forms.[72] The cleavage sites in these proenzymes are consistent with processing by caspases themselves. High local concentrations of some caspases may be sufficient to permit autocatalysis and activation.[73] The processing sites of some family members appear more likely to be target sites for other caspases, suggesting a sequential cascade of protease activation. Initial activation of a caspase may generate a rapidly and irreversibly amplified signal by initiating autocatalysis as well as triggering activation of downstream proteases. An additional layer of regulation may derive from alternate mRNA splicing. At least four of the caspase genes encode truncated forms as well as full-length proteases.[74-77] These truncated proteins may down-regulate protease activity by directly inhibiting the active proteases or by binding and stabilizing the proenzyme forms.

Among the caspase family, caspase 9 has been most clearly implicated in the central pathway of apoptotic induction (Fig. 10-5). Caspase 9, along with cytochrome c and Apaf-1, was identified as a factor required for induction of apoptotic events in a cell-free system.[55,61] Apaf-1 interacts with and activates caspase 9, which can then process other caspases, including caspase 3.[61] Caspase 3, in turn, has been found to be integrally involved in the generation of apoptotic nuclear morphology (condensation and DNA degradation).[78]

Many potential downstream targets with caspase cleavage sites have been identified and together may elucidate some of the mechanisms underlying apoptotic physiology. Among the defined caspase substrates are proteins involved in nuclear and cytoplasmic structure (e.g., nuclear lamins, actin), signal transduction (e.g., c-Abl, Raf-1, NF-κB p65 and p50), cell cycle control (e.g., MDM-2, Rb), genomic repair and integrity (e.g., poly-ADP ribose polymerase (PARP), DNA-dependent protein kinase), and apoptotic regulation ($Bcl-x_L$, Bcl-2).[79-93] Nevertheless, clear definition of the roles and relative importance of the various caspases and their downstream targets has been difficult. For example, PARP can be processed by caspase 3, 8, or 9 and has been used as a marker for the nuclear changes associated with apoptosis.[77,92,93] However, PARP cleavage is neither necessary nor sufficient for apoptosis.[94,95]

CELL SURFACE SIGNALS AFFECTING APOPTOSIS

Survival of most cells in the body is highly dependent on their environment. Cells removed from their in vivo context frequently undergo rapid apoptotic cell death. This suggests that in their natural context many cells continuously receive extracellular signals that result in increased apoptotic resistance.[9] These survival signals may be generated by direct cell–cell contact or by locally diffused soluble factors. Externally derived factors that may increase or decrease apoptotic sensitivity include growth factors, cytokines, interleukins, glucocorticoids, androgens, estrogens, and neurotransmitters. The cell membrane receptors that affect apoptotic sensitivity and the resulting intracellular signaling pathways initiated by engagement of these receptors are being studied intensively.

One critical family of cell surface receptors that affect apoptotic sensitivity is composed of proteins related to the tumor necrosis factor receptors (TNFRs).[96] The family includes the two receptors for TNF (TNFR1 and TNFR2) and at least 10 other related receptors. All TNFR family members have related cysteine-rich extracellular domains, each of which interacts with one of a family of TNF-related signaling proteins. The intracellular domains of these receptors differ widely, suggesting that different signaling pathways may be initiated by engagement

Table 10-2 Mammalian Caspase Subfamilies Grouped by Substrate Specificity

Group 1	Group 2	Group 3
Caspase 1 (ICE)	Caspase 2 (ICH-1/NEDD-2)	Caspase 6 (Mch2)
Caspase 4 (ICE rel II/ICH-2/TX)	Caspase 3 (CPP32/Yama/Apopain)	Caspase 8 (FLICE/MACH/Mch5)
Caspase 5 (ICE rel III/TY)	Caspase 7 (ICE-LAP3/Mch3/CMH-1)	Caspase 9 (ICE-LAP6/Mch6)
Caspase 11 (ICH-3)		Caspase 10 (FLICE2/Mch4)
Caspase 12		
Caspase 13 (ERICE)		

of each receptor. Different family members are capable of producing opposing signals, and in fact, engagement of a single receptor may have different effects in different contexts. In many experimental systems, engagement of some family members (e.g., Fas, TNFR1) promotes apoptosis, whereas engagement of others (e.g., CD30, CD40, TNFR2) promotes survival (Fig. 10-6).

Proapoptotic Signaling

The proapoptotic receptors Fas and TNFR1 share a related sequence in their C-terminal cytoplasmic tails known as the *death domain.* Three cytoplasmic proteins have been isolated on the basis of their ability to associate with these receptors.[97–99] These proteins-RIP, TRADD, and FADD—all contain death domains responsible for association with the receptor tails. RIP and FADD associate most strongly with Fas, and TRADD binds to TNFR1. Overexpression of any of these proteins can initiate apoptosis.

FADD contains a unique N-terminal effector domain that is required for apoptotic induction. In contrast, apoptotic signaling by RIP and TRADD depends only on the death domains, suggesting that these proteins may function primarily by recruitment of FADD or similar effector proteins to an activated receptor. TRADD serves as a link between TNFR1 engagement and multiple downstream signaling pathways.[99–101] The TNFR1-TRADD complex engages TRAF2 (see below), leading to NF-κB and c-Jun N-terminal kinase (JNK) activation, and also recruits

FADD through association of death domains. Mutation of the FADD effector domain blocks TNFR1-mediated apoptosis; although the association between FADD and TNFR1 may be predominantly indirect (i.e., through TRADD), FADD is integral to apoptotic signaling from TNFR1.

FADD has been shown to recruit the unprocessed precursor of caspase 8 to the activated Fas receptor.[102,103] Caspase 8 binds FADD through a portion of the prodomain homologous to the effector domain of FADD. Mutation within the protease domain of caspase 8 blocks apoptosis in response to engagement of either Fas or TNFR1, suggesting that caspase 8 may be a component of both receptor complexes.[73] Procaspase 8 recruitment to such complexes leads to proteolytic processing; activated caspase 8 may then initiate a cascade of caspase activation, leading to apoptosis. This recruitment of a caspase directly to the receptor complex may explain why apoptotic induction by engagement of Fas is, in some contexts, relatively resistant to modulation by Bcl-2.

Antiapoptotic Signaling

Other members of the TNFR family of cell surface receptors mediate signals that increase the apoptotic threshold of a cell. These receptors, including TNFR2, CD30, and CD40, interact with a family of related intracellular proteins known as *TNF receptor-associated factors* (TRAFs). TRAF2, TRAF3, and TRAF5 have similar binding specificities for sites in the

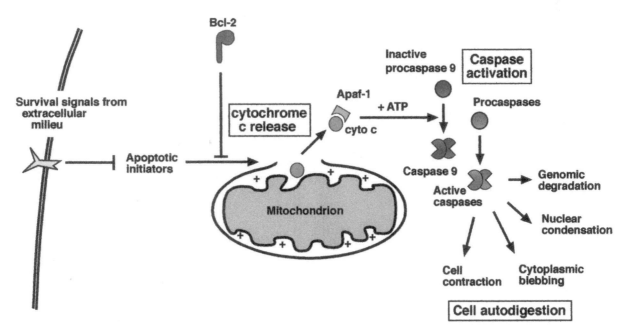

Fig. 10-5 A hypothetical model of the central apoptotic pathway. Initiation of apoptosis is held in check by survival signals received by cell surface receptors. Removal of the cell from its in vivo context or blockade of these survival signals allows induction of the apoptotic pathway, resulting in loss of mitochondrial outer membrane integrity and cytochrome c release. Cytosolic cytochrome c interacts with Apaf-1, which in the presence of ATP leads to caspase 9 processing and activation. This initiates a cascade of caspase activation, and ultimately in the characteristic morphologic changes of apoptosis. Bcl-2 and Bcl-x$_L$ reside in the mitochondrial outer membrane and can inhibit cytochrome c release. Other important apoptotic initiators include cell surface receptor-mediated cell death signals, DNA damage, cell cycle dysregulation, and metabolic alterations.

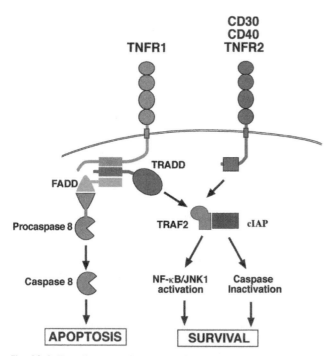

Fig. 10-6 Signaling complexes associated with representatives of the TNFR family. Receptor engagement by extracellular ligand promotes receptor multimerization and initiates formation of the schematically depicted complexes. The cytoplasmic tail of TNFR1 contains a region known as the death domain that interacts with a related domain of TRADD. TRADD serves as a signaling intermediary for both pro- and antiapoptotic pathways through recruitment of additional signaling molecules as shown. The phenotypic result of TNFR1 engagement therefore may be dependent on the relative availability of various second messengers. Signaling through engagement of TNFR2, CD30, or CD40 is also context-dependent. A common pathway for these three receptors is shown: TRAF2 engagement promotes survival through induction of both NF-κB and JNK1 activity and by interaction with the cIAP proteins may lead to inhibition of caspase activity.

cytoplasmic domains of the TNFR2, CD30, and CD40 receptors.[104–111] TRAF1 has been shown to bind directly only to CD30 but forms indirect associations with other receptors through heterodimerization with TRAF2.[104,110] TRAF6 was defined initially as a factor involved in IL-1 receptor signaling but also associates with the cytoplasmic tail of CD40 at a site distinct from the other TRAFs.[112,113]

TRAF proteins associate with multiple sites in the TNFR family cytoplasmic tails and, despite similar binding specificities, may result in distinct biologic responses. NF-κB activation has been associated with increased resistance to apoptosis in several cellular contexts. TRAF2 has been shown to activate NF-κB, whereas TRAF3 may suppress NF-κB activity either directly or by inhibition of TRAF2 function.[114]

The association between TRAF binding and antiapoptotic signaling by these receptors is primarily correlative. The intracellular domains of the TNFR family of proteins are remarkably dissimilar, suggesting that proteins other than the TRAFs are involved in the signaling complexes. The effects of ligand binding to these receptors probably depend on many variables, including the relative numbers of (potentially competing) receptors, the particular set of intracellular second messengers available to associate with these receptors, and the downstream targets present in a given cell.

The TRAF4 protein is unique among the TRAFs in that it has not been reported in association with any cell surface receptors but rather appears to be localized to the nucleus.[115] This factor was identified initially in a screen for proteins overexpressed in

metastatic breast cancer, and high-level expression has been reported subsequently in several breast cancer cell lines.[116] The function of this factor is unknown.

VIRAL MIMICRY AND APOPTOTIC INHIBITION

Apoptosis is an important defense against many types of viral infection. Cell suicide in response to viral infection may both inhibit successful viral replication in lytic infections and defend against viral transformation. Viruses have adapted methods to suppress apoptosis in the host that provide insight into the critical components of apoptotic regulation. Several viral proteins that regulate TNF-related signal transduction, inhibit caspase activity, or mimic Bcl-2 activity have been identified. The fact that viruses specifically target these pathways to prevent host cell death underscores their central importance in the regulation of cell survival.

Recently, a family of four mammalian proteins related to the baculovirus inhibitor of apoptosis (IAP) was identified.[117–122] Baculoviruses are small DNA viruses that infect insect cells. Baculoviral IAP inhibits apoptosis in mammalian as well as in insect cells, again demonstrating the evolutionary conservation of apoptotic pathways. Two IAP-related mammalian proteins, cIAP-1 and cIAP-2, were identified as proteins associating with the TNFR2-TRAF2-TRAF1 complex. A third IAP-related protein, ILP, has been shown to be a potent inhibitor of apoptosis when it is overexpressed in mammalian cells, whereas mutations in the fourth, NAIP, have been implicated in the pathogenesis of the neurodegenerative disorder spinal muscular atrophy. The binding properties of the various IAP-related proteins are distinct, and their relative roles in signaling pathways inhibiting apoptosis have not been fully characterized. They may constitute an important link between TNFR family member ligand binding and antiapoptotic effect.

Baculovirus encodes another potent inhibitor of apoptosis, p35, that functions as a specific inhibitor of caspases.[117] The cowpox crmA protein, although unrelated, has a similar function.[123] Mammalian proteins related to these potent and specific inhibitors have not been identified.

A number of viruses encode Bcl-2 homologues, including Epstein-Barr virus (EBV), African swine fever virus, and adenovirus.[124–126] The adenovirus homologue E1B 19kDa has low sequence similarity to Bcl-2 but was used as a probe to identify three novel proteins that also interact with Bcl-2.[124] These proteins may play important roles in the regulation and/or function of Bcl-2, and the low sequence conservation may help define functional domains of Bcl-2.

EBV has been linked causally to infectious mononucleosis, Burkitt lymphoma, nasopharyngeal carcinoma, AIDS-related lymphomas, and posttransplant lymphoproliferative disorder.[127] One of the necessary components of EBV transformation is the latent membrane protein LMP1. LMP1 is a transmembrane protein that may function in part by mimicking an occupied TNFR-related antiapoptotic receptor.[105] LMP-1 has been found to interact with TRAF proteins and to activate NF-κB; this pathway has been implicated in the pathogenesis of some EBV-positive lymphomas.[128] LMP-1 also has been reported to up-regulate endogenous Bcl-2.[129] BHRF1, an EBV-encoded Bcl-2 homologue, is not expressed in viral latency and therefore is unlikely to play a role in viral transformation; however, this protein may be critical in preventing premature host cell death in the lytic cycle of the virus.

ONCOGENES AND APOPTOTIC INDUCTION

A cell may acquire mutations in any of a variety of known oncogenes that in theory would confer a growth advantage to that cell. To prevent the development of neoplasia, the body must have potent mechanisms by which to inactivate such cells. Immune surveillance may play a role in detecting such transformants, but recent evidence suggests that apoptosis plays a much more critical role: the outgrowth of such potential tumor cells may be prevented by the induction of a suicide response within a premalignant cell. The isolated up-regulation of many oncogenes has been demonstrated to result in host cell apoptosis. Overexpression of Bcl-2 or Bcl-x$_L$ has been found to accelerate carcinogenesis, perhaps by facilitating the acquisition of mutations leading to overexpression of dominant oncogenes.[130]

Cellular Oncogenes

The proto-oncogene that has been most clearly associated with apoptotic induction is c-*myc*. The c-*myc* gene encodes a transcription factor that is up-regulated in many transformed cells and induces rapid cell proliferation.[131] However, isolated c-*myc* overexpression results in apoptosis.[19,132–134] Concomitant overexpression of the *bcl-2* gene prevents apoptosis, resulting in an immortalized, transformed phenotype.[19,134] Overexpression of both c-*myc* and *bcl-2* in lymphocytes of transgenic mice results in synergistic tumorigenesis, generating lymphoid tumors much more rapidly than either transgene alone. c-*myc*-induced apoptosis in fibroblasts can be prevented by cytokines such as insulin-like growth factor I and by high-serum growth conditions.[135]

Two models of c-*myc* function have been proposed to explain these findings[135] (Fig. 10-7). The *conflict model* proposes that c-*myc* generates a purely growth-promoting signal. Under favorable conditions, this leads to cell proliferation, but under adverse conditions, a conflict between proliferative and inhibitory signals is generated, resulting in the triggering of apoptosis. The *dual-signal model* proposes that c-*myc* concurrently generates both proliferative and apoptotic signals. Proliferation then requires the suppression of apoptosis either by cytokine signaling or by expression of antiapoptotic genes such as *bcl-2*.

The t(1;19) chromosomal translocation associated with childhood pre-B-cell leukemia generates a chimeric E2A-PBX1 transcription factor. Transgenic mice with this fusion gene under

A. CONFLICT MODEL

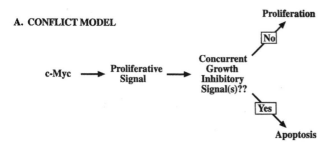

B. DUAL SIGNAL MODEL

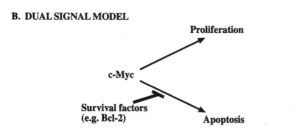

Fig. 10-7 Two models of the signaling pathways of c-*myc*. *A.* The conflict model proposes that c-*myc* generates a purely proliferative signal. Under unfavorable growth conditions, the cell produces inhibitory factors to prevent proliferation. This conflict of opposing signals affecting cell cycle progression results in an apoptotic response. Under favorable growth conditions, no conflict arises, and the cell proliferates. *B.* The dual signal model proposes that c-*myc* generates two signals, one proliferative and the other apoptotic. Proliferation in response to c-*myc* expression depends on suppression of the apoptotic response by survival signals. These signals may be generated by growth factors or antiapoptotic gene up-regulation.

lymphocyte-specific expression demonstrate increased numbers of cycling lymphocyte precursors but also widespread apoptosis in the same populations, resulting in greatly diminished numbers of lymphocytes.[136] All animals died of malignant leukemia/lymphoma within 5 months, presumably because of the outgrowth of cells that acquire secondary mutation(s) that prevent apoptosis.

Viral Oncogenes

Several viral oncogenes also provide insight into the association of oncogene expression with apoptosis. Human papillomavirus has been implicated as a causative agent in cervical carcinoma and other anogenital cancers. Oncogenic papillomaviruses encode a protein, E7, that inactivates the retinoblastoma gene product and is a potent stimulant of cell cycle progression.[137] E7 expression alone causes rapid induction of the cellular *p53* gene (which is involved in cell cycle regulation and apoptotic induction; see below), resulting in apoptotic cell death. These viruses encode a second protein, E6, which binds to and inactivates p53, preventing cell death and thus permitting oncogenic transformation. E7 also induces apoptosis by a p53-independent pathway that is poorly understood; E6 has been shown to be similarly effective in circumventing this p53-independent apoptosis in p53-negative cells.[138]

Adenovirus E1A is another oncogenic protein that induces rapid cell proliferation in transfected cells. Like papillomavirus E7 protein, the adenovirus E1A protein alone is not transforming, because it strongly triggers apoptosis.[139] Viral oncogenes depend on the concurrent expression of the *E1B* gene, which encodes two factors that may both help circumvent apoptosis. E1B 19kDa encodes a Bcl-2 homologue, and E1B 55kDa binds to and inactivates p53.[124,140]

Tumor Suppressor Genes

Tumor suppressor gene function has been found to be much more strongly linked to apoptosis than had been imagined initially. Tumor suppressors, such as p53 and the retinoblastoma gene product pRb, participate in cell cycle regulation and can inhibit proliferation by causing stage-specific cell cycle arrests. These cell cycle arrests are known as *checkpoints*.[141] In yeast, cell cycle checkpoints are thought to function to permit the repair of DNA damage and to ensure integrity of the genome before cell cycle progression. In mammalian cells, in addition to inhibiting the cell cycle progression of abnormal cells, a more important function of checkpoints may be to trigger apoptosis to delete potentially abnormal cells from the body.

p53 is the most commonly mutated gene in human malignancy, and germ-line heterozygous mutation (the Li-Fraumeni syndrome) is associated with high rates of tumorigenesis in many tissues.[142] The p53 protein is a sequence-specific transcription factor that normally is present at very low levels but is up-regulated rapidly by DNA damage or viral infection. p53 induction in response to DNA damage causes a G1-specific cell cycle arrest.[143]

The association between p53 and apoptosis has been demonstrated in vivo and in vitro. Transfection of wild-type p53 into p53-negative tumors results in apoptosis in both solid tumors and hematologic malignancies.[144,145] Loss of p53 in the evolution of experimentally induced tumors of the choroid plexus correlates directly with loss of apoptosis in vivo.[146] Thymocytes from mice with homozygous p53 inactivation demonstrate greatly increased resistance to apoptosis in response to gamma radiation and chemotherapeutic agents.[147,148]

How p53 activation triggers apoptosis is unknown. p53 has been shown to directly up-regulate the transcription of *bax,* a proapoptotic member of the *bcl-2* gene family.[149] However, Bax-deficient mice carry out p53-dependent apoptosis normally, implying that Bax regulation cannot be the primary mechanism of p53-dependent apoptotic signaling.[150] The mechanism of apoptosis induction by p53 may be indirect; strong inhibition of cell cycle progression in a cell primed for proliferation may generate a dichotomy of signals, resulting in activation of a default suicide pathway as proposed in the conflict model for c-*myc* (see Fig. 10-6).

The retinoblastoma gene product pRb also functions as a cell cycle regulator and is inactivated in many human tumors.[151] The pRb protein interacts with at least three members of the E2F family of transcription factors, inhibiting E2F activity and preventing entry into S phase of the cell cycle. Phosphorylation of pRb by cyclin-dependent kinases 4 and 6 releases the E2F factors, permitting E2F-mediated transcriptional regulation and S-phase entry.

Mutation of one *Rb* allele in mice or humans increases the likelihood of tumorigenesis in many tissues. Homozygous inactivation of the *Rb* gene in mice is embryonic lethal, causing massive apoptosis in the brain.[152,153] Again in analogy to c-*myc*, dysregulation of the controls on cell cycle progression by *Rb* inactivation generates not only rapid proliferation but also concurrent apoptotic induction.

The Link Between Proliferative Signals and Apoptosis

In the examples of cellular and viral oncogenes discussed earlier, a surprisingly tight association was found between oncogenic proliferative signals and the triggering of apoptosis. Studies of c-*myc* variants have been unsuccessful in separating the proliferative and apoptotic signals generated by this protein.[132,154] The same regions of c-*myc* that are essential for proliferation are essential for apoptosis. Incremental increases in c-*myc* expression cause parallel increases in both proliferative and apoptotic signals. Both signals are equally dependent on c-*myc* binding to its partner, Max. This unanticipated feature of oncogene activation suggests a fundamental mechanism for avoiding malignant transformation. Gene expression that generates potent proliferative signals may coordinately increase the apoptotic susceptibility of the cell, resulting in cell death unless strong antiapoptotic signals are present. A major function of cell cycle regulatory pathways may be to inextricably link proliferative induction to increased apoptotic sensitivity.

APOPTOSIS AND THE MULTIHIT MODEL OF ONCOGENESIS

The *multihit model* of oncogenesis holds that multiple genetic mutations must occur within a single cell to produce fully malignant transformation. The fact that many potentially oncogenic mutations trigger apoptosis suggests that mutations that inhibit apoptotic control are necessary for tumor cells to grow to sufficient mass to cause problems for the host. In order for the c-*myc* gene to be transforming, a prior event must have occurred to prevent apoptotic induction. *Rb* inactivation alone may promote p53-dependent cell death rather than tumorigenesis unless apoptosis in inhibited. Activation of oncogenes and inactivation of tumor suppressor genes may be insufficient to promote significant expansion of tumor cells without the tumor cell also acquiring defects in its ability to undergo apoptosis. Mutations in genes that affect apoptosis also may be central to the ability of tumor cells to metastasize. Metastatic cells must survive in the absence of many of the survival signals their normal counterparts receive from the extracellular milieu (see Fig. 10-4).

Mutation of apoptotic control genes without secondary mutations in growth regulatory genes similarly is insufficient for tumorigenesis. The characteristic t(14;18) translocation of the *bcl-2* gene has been detected at a low frequency in normal lymphoid hyperplasia in response to infection.[155] The rearrangement has been reported to be detectable by PCR in the peripheral blood of up to 55 percent of the population, and the frequency of the rearrangement increases with age.[156] Cells carrying the translocation may represent a long-lived premalignant population that has the potential to progress to lymphoma with the accumulation of additional mutations.

Inactivation of p53 is unique in eliminating an important negative regulatory control on proliferation while making the cell more resistant to apoptosis in response to aberrant replication. The double-edged effect of p53 inactivation may explain why this mutation is seen frequently in a wide array of human malignancies and also why p53 inactivation is such a frequent target of early gene expression by oncogenic viruses.

APOPTOSIS AND CANCER THERAPY

Chemotherapeutic Resistance

One of the most important problems that arise in cancer patients undergoing treatment is the development of tumors with multidrug resistance. This can arise *de novo* but is especially prevalent in previously treated patients. The multidrug resistance phenotype can be explained in a minority of cases by up-regulation of the *mdr-1* gene, which encodes a cell membrane pump that can expel a defined collection of antineoplastic agents.[157] A more general mechanism of multidrug resistance has been elucidated that involves apoptosis control.

Traditionally, tumoricidal radiation and chemotherapy were thought to function by causing irreparable metabolic or physical damage to cancer cells, resulting in cell necrosis. However, studies of cells killed by radiation and any of a wide variety of antineoplastic agents have demonstrated that these modalities induce typical apoptotic changes in the cells.[158] Cells exposed to chemotherapy are not passively killed by the drug. Instead, most cells appear to die because intracellular surveillance mechanisms recognize the alterations of normal cell physiology caused by chemotherapy and induce apoptosis. These observations suggest that a major mechanism for chemotherapeutic resistance in tumors may result from the inhibition of apoptosis.

Studies of tumor cell lines in vitro as well as tumors arising *in vivo* have demonstrated the relevance of this idea. Overexpression of Bcl-2 or Bcl-x_L can increase tumor resistance to multiple chemotherapeutic agents and radiation.[159–164] Agents that have been tested in such assays represent essentially all major categories of antineoplastic drugs, including antimetabolites, anthracyclines, DNA crosslinking agents, topoisomerase inhibitors, and mitotic spindle inhibitors. Cells overexpressing Bcl-x_L that are exposed to chemotherapeutic agents arrest at the characteristic cell cycle stages where individual drugs are known to have their effects.[164] Subsequent removal of the chemotherapeutic agents from the media permits cell cycle progression and proliferation, confirming the viability of the treated cells. High levels of endogenous Bcl-x_L expression have been reported in tumor cells after exposure of those cells to chemotherapy. Bcl-x_L and Bcl-2 expression in neuroblastoma decreases apoptotic sensitivity to chemotherapy.[161,165] High-level Bcl-2 expression has been correlated with chemotherapeutic resistance in acute myeloid leukemia.[166,167]

Inactivation of p53 similarly has been associated with increased chemotherapeutic resistance, perhaps by the loss of p53-dependent apoptosis.[168] p53-independent mechanisms also can detect DNA damage, cause cell cycle arrest, and initiate apoptosis. Chemotherapeutic mutagens or radiation causes cell cycle arrest and apoptosis in tumors of p53-negative mice.[169] Expression of antiapoptotic control genes therefore may be a more potent mechanism of chemotherapeutic resistance than p53 inactivation.

Antiapoptotic Gene Expression and Mutation Rate

Overexpression of antiapoptotic genes in cancer cells abrogates a major protective mechanism against the expansion of cells that demonstrate abnormal cell cycle progression. Cells that suffer abnormal mitosis, chromosome loss, or major genomic mutation normally are prevented from attempting replication by cell cycle checkpoints that trigger apoptotic cell death. Up-regulation of antiapoptotic gene expression permits the survival and propagation of such mutant cells and thus would be expected to greatly augment the rate of accumulation of genetic errors. Since inhibition of apoptosis appears to be a common step in oncogenesis, this mechanism could explain the high degree of chromosomal instability characteristic of cancer cells.

Cancer treatments may further accelerate mutagenesis. DNA-damaging chemotherapeutic agents and radiation are inherently mutagenic. Cells exposed to high levels of these mutagens are killed unless apoptotic pathways are blocked. Antiapoptotic gene expression therefore may promote tumor evolution by allowing the propagation of chemotherapy-induced mutations.

Inhibition of apoptosis in cells exposed to chemotherapeutic agents may promote chromosomal aberrations. An example of this type of derangement is seen in cells exposed to vincristine or nocodazole, agents that inhibit mitotic spindle formation.[170] These agents induce cell cycle arrest and apoptosis in tumor cells. Cells overexpressing Bcl-x_L arrest but do not die in response to these agents and on drug removal begin to proliferate without completing mitosis, thus becoming polyploid. Loss of appropriate response to aberrant mitoses is thought to play an important role in the chromosomal instability characteristic of most advanced malignancies.[171]

Rational Cancer Treatment Design

As described here, apoptotic regulation has been found to be a critical determinant of tumorigenesis and the therapeutic responsiveness of tumors. One of the challenges that is only beginning to be addressed is the translation of this new perspective on cancer biology into meaningful changes in clinical practice. As the associations between patient outcome and the activity of various antiapoptotic genes become clearer, screening of tumors for the expression of apoptotic regulatory genes may help define prognostic categories and influence treatment decisions.

More fundamentally, the study of apoptotic mechanisms affected by malignancy offers an opportunity for the consideration of entirely new approaches to the treatment of cancer. The unexpected finding that most successful anticancer treatments, including radiotherapy, chemotherapy, and hormonal modulation, function by apoptotic induction has generated increasing interest in therapies specifically targeted to apoptotic pathways. Such treatment may have much less nonspecific toxicity than do traditional antineoplastic agents. Pilot studies of anti-Bcl-2 antibodies and antisense *bcl-2* oligonucleotides as anticancer agents are ongoing.[172,173] Disruption of LMP-1 signaling pathways could play an important role in the treatment of EBV-associated malignancies and lymphoproliferative disorders. Modification of apoptotic pathways by influencing the activity or accessibility of cell surface receptors has not been fully explored. Therapy designed to stimulate apoptosis in target cells may play an increasingly central role in the treatment of cancer.

CONCLUSIONS

A great deal of information about the regulation of apoptosis at the molecular level has been acquired in the years since its initial phenotypic description. In mammalian cells, although many levels of apoptotic regulation have been defined, much of the control appears to be concentrated in a central pathway consisting of highly evolutionarily conserved regulatory proteins. Determination of the apoptotic threshold of a cell depends on interactions between positive and negative signaling elements in this central apoptotic pathway. A number of external conditions, including the presence of growth factors, cytokines, and the membrane proteins of neighboring cells, influence the balance of the central apoptotic regulators through multiple cell surface receptors and intracellular signaling pathways.

The control of apoptosis is integral to many aspects of cancer biology. Apoptosis serves as an essential mechanism to prevent the proliferation of cells with potentially transforming mutations. As a corollary, inhibition of apoptosis may lead to the accumulation of cells with a higher mutation rate, thus accelerating malignant transformation. Cell cycle checkpoint controls play a critical role

in detecting aberrant cells and initiating apoptosis. Viral and cellular oncoproteins, by driving cell cycle progression, often are strong inducers of apoptosis. Most antineoplastic therapies function by triggering apoptosis in sensitive cells. Resistance to treatment can result from specific inhibition of apoptotic signaling. Apoptotic inhibition in tumor cells exposed to chemotherapy or radiation may increase mutation rate and hasten tumor evolution.

The study of apoptosis has not had a dramatic effect on clinical practice in oncology. However, the conceptual changes that have derived from apoptosis research have potentially wide clinical ramifications. We can look forward to many more trials of cancer therapy based on the modification of the controlling pathways of apoptotic regulation.

REFERENCES

1. Kerr JFR, Wyllie AH, Currie AR: Apoptosis: A basic biological phenomenon with wide-ranging implications in tissue kinetics. *Br J Cancer* **26**:239,1972.
2. Wyllie AH, Kerr JFR, Currie AR: Cell death: The significance of apoptosis. *Int Rev Cytol* **68**:251, 1980.
3. Thompson CB: Apoptosis in the pathogenesis and treatment of disease. *Science* **267**:1456, 1995.
4. Gougeon M-L, Montagnier L: Apoptosis in AIDS. *Science* **260**:1269, 1993.
5. Mountz JD, Wu J, Cheng J, Zhou T: Autoimmune disease: A problem of defective apoptosis. *Arthritis Rheum* **37**:1415, 1994.
6. Margolis RL, Chuang D-M, Post RM: Programmed cell death: Implications for neuropsychiatric disorders. *Biol Psychiatry* **35**:946, 1994.
7. Harrington EA, Fanidi A, Evan GI: Oncogenes and cell death. *Curr Opin Genet Dev* **4**:120, 1994.
8. Ellis RE, Yan J, Horvitz HR: Mechanism and function of cell death. *Annu Rev Cell Biol* **7**:663, 1991.
9. Raff MC: Social controls on cell survival and cell death. *Nature* **356**:397, 1992.
10. Oppenheim RW: Cell death during development of the nervous system. *Annu Rev Neurosci* **14**:453, 1991.
11. Fadok VA, Voelker DR, Campbell PA, Cohen JJ, Bratton DL, Henson PM: Exposure of phosphatidylserine on the surface of apoptotic lymphocytes triggers specific recognition and removal by macrophages. *J Immunol* **148**:2207, 1992.
12. Fadok VA, Savill JS, Haslett C, Bratton DL, Doherty DE, Campbell PA, Henson PM: Different populations of macrophages use either the vitronectin receptor or the phosphatidylserine receptor to recognize and remove apoptotic cells. *J Immunol* **149**:4029, 1992.
13. Hall SE, Savill JS, Henson PM, Haslett C: Apoptic neutrophils are phagocytosed by fibroblasts with participation of the fibroblast vitronectin receptor and involvement of a mannose/fructose-specific lactin. *J Immunol* **153**:3218, 1994.
14. Tsujimoto Y, Finger LR, Yunis J, Nowell PC, Croce CM: Cloning of the chromosome breakpoint of neoplastic B cells with the t(14;18) chromosome translocation. *Science* **226**:1097, 1984.
15. Tsujimoto Y, Gorman J, Cossman J, Jaffe E, Croce CM: The t(14;18) chromosome translocations involved in B-cell neoplasms result from mistakes in VDJ joining. *Science* **229**:1390, 1985.
16. Bakhshi A, Jensen JP, Goldman P, Wright JJ, McBride OW, Epstein AL, Korsmeyer SJ: Cloning the chromosomal breakpoint of t(14;18) human lymphomas: Clustering around JH on chromosome 14 and near a transcriptional unit on 18. *Cell* **41**:889, 1985.
17. Cleary ML, Sklar J: Nucleotide sequence of a t(14;18) chromosomal breakpoint in follicular lymphoma and demonstration of a breakpoint cluster region near a transcriptionally active locus on chromosome 18. *Proc Natl Acad Sci USA* **82**:7439, 1985.
18. Longo DL, DeVita VT, Jaffe ES, Mauch P, Urba WJ: Lymphocytic lymphomas, in DeVita VT, Hellman S, Rosenberg SA (eds): *Cancer: Principles and Practice of Oncology*, 4th ed.Philadelphia, Lippincott, 1993.
19. Vaux DL, Cory S, Adams JM: Bcl-2 gene promotes haemopoietic cell survival and co-operates with c-Myc to immortalize pre-B cells. *Nature* **335**:440, 1988.
20. Yang E, Korsmeyer SJ: Molecular thanatopsis: A discourse on the BCL2 family and cell death. *Blood* **88**:386, 1996.
21. Korsmeyer SJ: Bcl-2 initiates a new category of oncogenes: Regulators of cell death. *Blood* **80**:879, 1992.

22. Arends MJ, Wyllie AH: Apoptosis: Mechanisms and roles in pathology. *Int Rev Exp Pathol* **32**:223, 1991.

23. Horvitz HR, Shaham S, Hengartner MO: The genetics of programmed cell death in the nematode *Caenorhabditis elegans*. *Cold Spring Harbor Symp Quant Biol* **59**:377, 1994.

24. Ellis RE, Horvitz HR: Genetic control of programmed cell death in the nematode *C. elegans*. *Cell* **44**:817, 1986.

25. Hengartner MO, Ellis RE, Horvitz HR: Caenorhabditis elegans gene ced-9 protects cells from programmed cell death. *Nature* **356**:494, 1992.

26. Shaham S, Horvitz HR: Developing *Caenorhabditis elegans* neurons may contain both cell-death protective and killer activities. *Gene Dev* **10**:578, 1996.

27. Wu D, Wallen HD, Nunez G: Interaction and regulation of subcellular localization of CED-4 by CED-9. *Science* **275**:1126, 1997.

28. Chinnauyan AR, O'Rourke K, Lane BR, Dixit VM: Interaction of CED-4 with CED-3 and CED-9: a molecular framework for cell death. *Science* **275**:1122, 1997.

29. Seshagiri S, Miller LK: *Caenorhabditis elegans* CED-4 stimulates CED-3 processing and CED-3-induced apoptosis. *Curr Biol* **7**:455, 1997.

30. Chinnauyan AR, Shaudhary D, O'Rourke K, Koonin EV, Dixit VM: Role of CED-4 in the activation of CED-3. *Nature* **388**:728, 1997.

31. Irmler M, Hofmann K, Vaux D, Tschopp J: Direct physical interaction between the *Caenorhabditis elegans* "death proteins" CED-3 and CED-4. *FEBS Lett* **406**:189, 1997.

32. Hengartner MO, Horvitz HR: *C. elegans* cell survival gene ced-9 encodes a functional homolog of the mammalian proto-oncogene bcl-2. *Cell* **76**:665, 1994.

33. Vaux DL, Weissman IL, Kim SK: Prevention of programmed cell death in *Caenorhabditis elegans* by human bcl-2. *Science* **258**:1955, 1992.

34. Zou H, Benzel WJ, Liu X, Lutschg A, Wang X: Apaf-1, a human protein homologous to *C. elegans* CED-4, participates in cytochrome c-dependent activation of caspase-3. *Cell* **90**:405, 1997.

35. Yan J, Shahm S, Ledoux S, Ellis HM, Horvitz HR: The *C. elegans* cell death gene ced-3 encodes a protein similar to mammalian interleukin-1β-converting enzyme. *Cell* **75**:641, 1993.

36. Boise LH, Gonzalez-Garcia M, Postema CE, Ding L, Lindsten T, Turka LA, Mao X, Nunes G, Thompson CB: bcl-x, a bcl-2-related gene that functions as a dominant regulator of apoptotic cell death. *Cell* **74**:597, 1993.

37. Oltvai ZN, Milliman CL, Korsmeyer SJ: Bcl-2 heterodimerizes in vivo with a conserved homolog, Bax, that accelerates programmed cell death. *Cell* **74**:609, 1993.

38. Sedlak TW, Oltvai ZN, Yang E, Wang K, Boise LH, Thompson CB, Korsmeyer SJ: Multiple Bcl-2 family members demonstrate selective dimerizations with Bax. *Proc Natl Acad Sci USA* **92**:7834, 1995.

39. Farrow SN, White JHM, Martinou I, Raven T, Pun K-T, Grinham CJ, Martinou J-C, Brown R: Cloning of a bcl-2 homologue by interaction with adenovirus E1B 19K. *Nature* **374**:731, 1995.

40. Chittenden T, Harrington EA, O'Connor R, Flemington C, Lutz RJ, Evan GI, Guild BC: Induction of apoptosis by the Bcl-2 homologue Bak. *Nature* **374**:733, 1995.

41. Kiefer MC, Brauer MJ, Powers VC, Wu JJ, Umansky SR, Tomei LD, Barr PJ: Modulation of apoptosis by the widely distributed Bcl-2 homologue Bak. *Nature* **374**:736, 1995.

42. Yang E, Zha J, Jockel J, Boise LH, Thompson CB, Korsmeyer SJ: Bad, a heterodimeric partner for Bcl-x$_L$ and Bcl-2, displaces Bax and promotes cell death. *Cell* **80**:285, 1995.

43. Sato T, Hanada M, Bodrug S, Irie S, Iwama N, Boise LH, Thompson CB, Golemis E, Fong L, Wang H-G, Reed JC: Interactions among members of the Bcl-2 protein family analyzed with a yeast two-hybrid system. *Proc Natl Acad Sci USA* **91**:9238, 1994.

44. Kelekar A, Thompson CB: Bcl-2 family proteins: The role of the BH3 domain in apoptosis. *Trends Cell Biol* **8**:324, 1998.

45. Muchmore SW, Sattler M, Liang H, Meadows RP, Harlan JE, Yoon HS, Nettesheim D, Chang B, Thompson CB, Wong S, Ng S-C, Fesik SW: X-ray and NMR structure of human Bcl-x$_L$, an inhibitor of programmed cell death. *Nature* **381**:335, 1996.

46. Cramer WA, Heymann JB, Schendel SL, Deriy BN, Cohen FS, Elkins PA, Stauffacher CB: Structure-function of the channel-forming colicins. *Annu Rev Biophys Biomol Struct* **24**:611, 1995.

47. Monoghan P, Robertson D, Amos T, Dyer M, Mason D, Greaves M: Ultrastructural localizations of Bcl-2 protein. *J Histochem Cytochem* **40**:1819, 1992.

48. Krajewski S, Tanaka S, Takayama S, Schibler MJ, Fenton W, Reed JC: Investigation of the subcellular distribution of the bcl-2 oncoprotein: Residence in the nuclear envelope, endoplasmic reticulum, and outer mitochondrial membranes. *Cancer Res* **53**:4701, 1993.

49. Nguyen M, Miller DG, Yong VW, Korsmeyer SJ, Shore GC: Targeting of Bcl-2 to the mitochondrial outer membrane by a COOH-terminal signal anchor sequence. *J Biol Chem* **268**:25265, 1993.

50. Zamzami N, Marchetti P, Castedo M, Zanin C, Vayssiüre J-L, Petit PX, Kroemer G: Reduction in mitochondrial potential constitutes an early irreversible step of programmed lymphocyte death in vivo. *J Exp Med* **181**:1661, 1995.

51. Castedo M, Hirsch T, Susin SA, Zamzami N, Marchetti P, Macho A, Kroemer G: Sequential acquisition of mitochondrion and plasma membrane alterations during early lymphocyte apoptosis. *J Immunol* **157**:512, 1996.

52. Green DR, Reed JC: Mitochondria and apoptosis. *Science* **281**:1309, 1998.

53. Zamzami N, Marchetti P, Castedo M, Decaudin D, Macho A, Hirsch T, Susin SA, Petit PX, Mignotte B, Kroemer G: Sequential reduction of mitochondrial transmembrane potential and generation of reactive oxygen species in early programmed cell death. *J Exp Med* **182**:367, 1996.

54. Zamzami N, Susin SA, Marchetti P, Hirsh T, Gomez-Monterrey I, Castedo M, Kroemer G: Mitochondrial control of nuclear apoptosis. *J Exp Med* **183**:1533, 1996.

55. Liu X, Kim CN, Yang J, Jemmerson R, Wang X: Induction of apoptotic program in cell-free extracts: Requirement for dATP and cytochrome c. *Cell* **86**:147, 1996.

56. Vander Heiden MG, Chandel NS, Williamson EK, Schumacker PT, Thompson CB: Bcl-x$_L$ regulates the membrane potential and volume homeostasis of mitochondria. *Cell* **9**:627, 1997.

57. Yang J, Liu X, Bhalla K, Kim CN, Ibrado AM, Cai J, Peng TI, Jones DP, Wang X: Prevention of apoptosis by Bcl-2: Release of cytochrome c from mitochondria blocked. *Science* **275**:1129, 1997.

58. Kluck RM, Bossy-Wetzel E, Green DR, Newmeyer DD: The release of cytochrome c from mitochondria: A primary site for Bcl-2 regulation of apoptosis. *Science* **275**:1132, 1997.

59. Rosse T, Olivier R, Monney L, Rager M, Conus S, Fellay I, Jansen B, Borner C: Bcl-2 prolongs cell survival after Bax-induced release of cytochrome c. *Nature* **391**:496, 1998.

60. Huang DC, Adams JM, Cory S: The conserved N-terminal BH4 domain of Bcl-2 homologues is essential for inhibition of apoptosis and interaction with CED-4. *EMBO J* **17**:1029, 1998.

61. Li P, Nijhawan D, Budihardjo I, Srinivasula SM, Ahmad M, Alnemri ES, Wang X: Cytochrome c and dATP-dependent formation of Apaf-1/caspase-9 complex initiates an apoptotic protease cascade. *Cell* **91**:479, 1997.

62. Hu Y, Benedict MA, Wu D, Inohara N, Nunez G: Bcl-x$_L$ interacts with Apaf-1 and inhibits Apaf-1-dependent caspase-9 activation. *Proc Natl Acad Sci USA* **95**:4386, 1998.

63. Pan G, O'Rourke K, Dixit VM: Caspase-9, Bcl-x$_L$, and Apaf-1 form a ternary complex. *J Biol Chem* **273**:5841, 1998.

64. AkES, Livingston DJ, Nicholson DW, Salvesen G, Thornberry NA, Wong WW, Yuan J: Human ICE/CED-3 protease nomenclature. *Cell* **87**:171, 1996.

65. Nicholson, DW, Thornberry NA: Caspases: Killer proteases. *TIBS* **22**:299, 1997.

66. Talanian RV, Quinlan C, Trautz S, Hackett MC, Mankovich JA, Banach D, Ghayur T, Brady KD, Wong WW: Substrate specificities of caspase family proteases. *J Biol Chem* **272**:9677, 1997.

67. Van de Craen M, Vandenabeele P, Declercq W, Van den Brande I, Van Loo G, Molemans F, Schotte P, Van Criekinge W, Beyaert R, Fiers W: Characterization of seven murine caspase family members. *FEBS Lett* **403**:61, 1997.

68. Vincenz C, Dixit VM: Fas-associated death domain protein interleukin-1 beta-converting enzyme 2 (FLICE2), an ICE/Ced-3 homologue, is proximally involved in CD95- and p55-mediated death signaling. *J Biol Chem* **272**:6578, 1997.

69. Humke EW, Dixit VM: ERICE, a novel FLICE-activatable caspase. *J Biol Chem* **272**:15702, 1998.

70. Miura M, Zhu H, Rotello R, Hartwieg EA, Yuan J: Induction of apoptosis in fibroblasts by IL-1βconverting enzyme, a mammalian homolog of the *C. elegans* cell death gene ced-3. *Cell* **75**:653, 1993.

71. Rabizadeh S, LaCount DJ, Friesen, PD, Bredesen DE: Expression of the baculovirus p35 gene inhibits mammalian neuronal cell death. *J Neurochem* **61**:2318, 1993.

72. Duan H, Chinnaiyan AM, Hudson PL, Wing JP, He WW, Dixit VM: ICE-LAP3, a novel mammalian homologue of the *Caenorhabditis*

elegans cell death protein CED-3, is activated during Fas- and tumor necrosis factor-induced apoptosis. *J Biol Chem* **369**:621, 1996.

73. Walker NP, Talanian RV, Brady KD, Dang LC, Bump NJ, Ferenz CR, Franklin S, Ghayur T, Hackett MC, Hammill LD, Herzog L, Hugunin M, Houy W, Mankovich JA, McGuiness L, Orlewicz E, Paskind M, Pratt CA, Reis P, Summani A, Terranova M, Welch JP, Xiong L, Moller A, Tracey DE, Kamen R, Wong WW: Crystal structure of the cysteine protease interleukin-1 beta-converting enzyme: A (p20/p10)2 homodimer. *Cell* **78**:343, 1995.

74. Alnemri ES, Fernandes-Alnemri T, Litwack G: Cloning and expression of four novel isoforms of human interleukin-1 beta converting enzyme with different apoptotic activities. *J Biol Chem* **270**:4312, 1995.

75. Wang L, Miura M, Bergeron L, Zhu H, Yuan J: Ich-1, an Ice/ced-3-related gene, encodes both positive and negative regulators of programmed cell death. *Cell* **78**:739, 1994.

76. Fernandes-Alnemri T, Litwack G, Alnemri ES: Mch2, a new member of the apoptotic CED-3/ICE cysteine protease gene family. *Cancer Res* **55**:2737, 1995.

77. Duan K, Orth K, Chinnaiyan AM, Poirier GG, Froelich CJ, He W-W, Dixit VM: ICE-LAP6, a novel member of the ICE/Ced-3 gene family, is activated by the cytotoxic T cell protease granzyme B. *J Biol Chem* **271**:16720, 1996.

78. Woo M, Hakem R, Soengas MS, Duncan GS, Shahinian A, Kagi D, Hakem A, McCurrach M, Khoo W, Kaufman SA, Senaldi G, Howard T, Lowe SW, Mak TW: Essential contribution of caspase 3/CPP32 to apoptosis and its associated nuclear changes. *Genes Dev* **12**:806, 1998.

79. Fraser A, Evan G: A license to kill. *Cell* **85**:781, 1996.

80. Nagata S: Apoptosis by death factor. *Cell* **88**:355, 1997.

81. Rao L, Perez D, White E: Lamin proteolysis facilitates nuclear events during apoptosis. *J Cell Biol* **135**:1441, 1996.

82. Kayalor C, Ord T, Testa P, Zhong L, Bredsen DE: Cleavage of actin by interleukin 1β-converting enzyme to reverse DNase I inhibition. *Proc Natl Acad Sci USA* **93**:2234, 1996.

83. Widmann C, Gibson S, Johnson GL: Caspase-dependent cleavage of signaling proteins during apoptosis: A turn-off mechanism for anti-apoptotic signals. *J Biol Chem* **273**:7141, 1998.

84. Ravi R, Bedi A, Fuchs EJ, Bedi A: CD95 (Fas)-induced caspase-mediated proteolysis of NF-κB. *Cancer Res* **58**:882, 1998.

85. Chen L, Marechal V, Moreau J, Levine AJ, Chen J: Proteolytic cleavage of the mdm2 oncoprotein during apoptosis. *J Biol Chem* **272**:22966, 1997.

86. Tan X, Martin SJ, Green DR, Wang JYJ: Degradation of retinoblastoma protein in tumor necrosis factor- and CD95-induced cell death. *J Biol Chem* **272**:9613, 1997.

87. Janicke RU, Walker PA, Lin XY, Porter AG: Specific cleavage of the retinoblastoma protein by an ICE-like protease in apoptosis. *EMBO J* **15**:6969, 1996.

88. Casciola-Rosen L, Nicholson DW, Chong T, Rowan KR, Thornberry NA, Miller DK, Rosen A: Apopain/CPP32 cleaves proteins that are essential for cellular repair: A fundamental principle of apoptotic death. *J Exp Med* **183**:1957, 1996.

89. Cheng EH, Kirsch DG, Clem RJ, Ravi R, Kastan MB, Bedi A, Ueno K, Hardwick JM: Conversion of Bcl-2 to a Bax-like death effector by caspases. *Science* **278**:1966, 1997.

90. Clem RJ, Cheng EH, Karp CL, Kirsch DG, Ueno K, Takahashi A, Kastan MB, Griffin DE, Earnshaw WC, Veliuona MA, Hardwick JM: Modulation of cell death by Bcl-x_L through caspase interaction. *Proc Natl Acad Sci USA* **95**:554, 1998.

91. Lazebnik YA, Kaufmann SH, Disnoyers S, Poirer GG, Earnshaw WC: Cleavage of poly(ADP-ribose) polymerase by a proteinase with properties like ICE. *Nature* **371**:346, 1994.

92. Nicholson DW, Ali A, Thornberry NA, Vaillancourt JP, Ding CK, Gallant M, Gareau Y, Griffin PR, Labelle M, Lazebnik YA, Munday NA, Raju SM, Smulson ME, Yamin T-T, Yu VL, Miller DK: Identification and inhibition of the ICE/CED-3 protease necessary for mammalian apoptosis. *Nature* **376**:37, 1995.

93. Tewari M, Quan LT, O'Rourke K, Desnoyers S, Zeng Z, Beidler DR, Poirier GG, Salvesen GS, Dixit VM: Yama/CPP32 beta, a mammalian homolog of CED-3, is a CrmA-inhibitable protease that cleaves the death substrate poly(ADP-ribose) polymerase. *Cell* **81**:801, 1995.

94. Wang Z-Q, Auer B, Stingle L, Berghammer H, Haidacher D, Schweiger M, Wagner EF: Mice lacking ADPRT and poly(ADP-ribosyl)ation develop normally but are susceptible to skin disease. *Gene Dev* **9**:509, 1995.

95. Boise LH, Thompson CB: Bcl-x_L can inhibit apoptosis in cells that have undergone Fas-induced protease activation. *Proc Natl Acad Sci USA* **94**:3759, 1997.

96. Bazzoni F, Beutler B: The tumor necrosis factor ligand and receptor families. *N Engl J Med* **334**:1717, 1996.

97. Chinnaiyan AM, O'Rourke K, Tewari M, Dixit VM: FADD, a novel death domain-containing protein, interacts with the death domain of Fas and initiates apoptosis. *Cell* **81**:505, 1995.

98. Stanger BZ, Leder P, Lee T, Kim E, Seed B: RIP: A novel protein containing a death domain that interacts with FAS/Apo-1 (CD95) in yeast and causes cell death. *Cell* **81**:513, 1995.

99. Hsu H, Xiong J, Goeddel DV: The TNF receptor 1-associated protein TRADD signals cell death and NF-κB activation. *Cell* **81**:495, 1995.

100. Hsu H, Shu H-B, Pan M-G, Goeddel DV: TRADD-TRAF2 and TRADD-FADD interactions define two distinct TNF receptor 1 signal transduction pathways. *Cell* **84**:299, 1996.

101. Liu Z-G, Hsu H, Goeddel DV, Karin M: Dissection of TNF receptor 1 effector functions: JNK activation is not linked to apoptosis while NF-κB activation prevents cell death. *Cell* **87**:565. 1996.

102. Boldin MP, Goncharov TM, Goltsev YV, Wallach D: Involvement of MACH, a novel MORT/FADD-interacting protease, in Fas/APO-1-and TNF receptor-induced cell death. *Cell* **85**:803, 1996.

103. Muzio M, Chinnaiyan AM, Kischkel FC, O'Rourke K, Shevchenko A, Ni J, Scaffidi C, Bretz JD, Zhang M, Gentz R, Mann M, Krammer PH, Peter ME, Dixit VM: FLICE, a novel FADD-homologous ICE/CED-3-like protease, is recruited to the CD95 (Fas/Apo-1) death-inducing signaling complex. *Cell* **85**:817, 1996.

104. Rothe M, Wong SC, Henzel WJ, Goeddel DV: A novel family of putative signal transducers associated with cytoplasmic domain of the 75 kDa tumor necrosis factor receptor family. *Cell* **78**:681, 1994.

105. Mosialos G, Birkenbach M, Yalamanchili R, VanArsdale T, Ware C, Kieff E: The Epstein-Barr virus transforming protein LMP1 engages signaling proteins for the tumor necrosis factor receptor family. *Cell* **80**:389, 1995.

106. Chang G, Cleary AM, Ye Z, Hong DI, Lederman S, Baltimore D: Involvement of CRAF1, a relative of TRAF, in CD40 signaling. *Science* **267**:1494, 1995.

107. Hu HM, O'Rourke K, Boguski MS, Dixit VM: A novel RING finger protein interacts with the cytoplasmic domain of CD40. *J Biol Chem* **269**:30069, 1994.

108. Sato T, Irie S, Reed JC: A novel member of the TRAF family of putative signal transducing proteins binds to the cytoplasmic domain of CD40. *FEBS Lett* **358**:113, 1995.

109. Nakano H, Oshima H, Chung W, Williams-Abbott L, Ware CF, Yagita H, Okumura K: TRAF5, an activator of NF-κB and putative signal transducer for the lymphotoxin-β receptor. *J Biol Chem* **271**:14661, 1996.

110. Gedrich RW, Gilfillan MC, Duckett CS, VanDongen JL, Thompson CB: CD30 contains two binding sites with different specificities for members of the tumor necrosis factor receptor-associated factor family of signal transducing proteins. *J Biol Chem* **271**:12852, 1996.

111. Ishida T, Tojo T, Aoki T, Kobayashi N, Ohishi T, Watanabe T, Yamamoto T, Inoue J-I: TRAF5, a novel tumor necrosis factor receptor-associated factor family protein, mediates CD40 signaling. *Proc Natl Acad Sci USA* **93**:9437, 1996.

112. Cao Z, Xiong J, Takeuchi M, Kurama T, Goeddel: TRAF6 is a signal transducer for interleukin-1. *Nature* **383**:443, 1996.

113. Ishida T, Mizuchima S-I, Azuma S, Kobayashi N, Tojo T, Suzuki K, Aizawa S, Watanabe T, Mosalios G, Kieff E, Yamamoto T, Inoue J-I: Identification of TRAF6, a novel tumor necrosis factor receptor-associated factor protein that mediates signaling from an amino-terminal domain of the CD40 cytoplasmic region. *J Biol Chem* **271**:28745, 1996.

114. Rothe M, Sarma V, Dixit VM, Goeddel DV: TRAF2-mediated activation of NF-κB by TNF receptor 2 and CD40. *Science* **269**:1424, 1995.

115. Regnier CH, Tomasetto C, Moog-Lutz C, Chenard M-P, Wendling C, Basset P, Rio MC: Presence of a new conserved domain in CART1, a novel member of the tumor necrosis factor receptor-associated protein family, which is expressed in breast carcinoma. *J Biol Chem* **270**:25715, 1995.

116. Masson R, Regnier CH, Chenard MP, Wendling C, Mattei M-G, Tomasetto C, Rio M-C: Tumor necrosis factor receptor associated factor 4 (TRAF4) expression pattern during mouse development. *Mech Dev* **71**:187, 1998.

117. Clem RJ, Miller LK: Control of programmed cell death by the baculovirus genes p34 and iap. *Mol Cell Biol* **14**:5212, 1994.

118. Roy N, Mahadevan MS, McLean M, Shutler G, Yaraghi Z, Farahani R, Baird S, Besner-Johnston A, Lefebvre C, Kang X, Salih M, Aubry H, Tamai K, Guan X, Ioannou P, Crawford TO, de Jong PJ, Surh L,

Ikeda J-E, Korneluk RG, MacKenzie A: The gene for neuronal apoptosis inhibitory protein is partially deleted in individuals with spinal muscular atrophy. *Cell* **80**:167, 1995.

119. Rothe M, Pan M-G, Henzel WJ, Ayres TM, Goeddel DV: The TNFR2-TRAF signaling complex contains two novel proteins related to baculoviral inhibitor of apoptosis proteins. *Cell* **83**:1243, 1995.

120. Duckett CS, Nava VE, Gedrich RW, Clem RJ, VanDongen JL, Gilfillan MC, Shiels H, Hardwick JM, Thompson CB: A conserved family of cellular genes related to the baculovirus iap gene and encoding apoptosis inhibitors. *EMBO J* **15**:2685, 1996

121. Liston P, Roy N, Tamai K, Lefebvre C, Baird S, Cherton-Horvat G, Farahani R, McLean M, Ikeda JE, MacKenzie A, Korneluk RG: Suppression of apoptosis in mammalian cells by NAIP and a related family of IAP genes. *Nature* **379**:349, 1996.

122. Uren AG, Pakusch M, Hawkins CH, Puls KL, Vaux DL: Cloning and expression of apoptosis inhibitory protein homologs that function to inhibit apoptosis and/or bind tumor necrosis factor receptor-associated factors. *Proc Natl Acad Sci USA* **93**:4974, 1996.

123. Ray CA, Black RA, Kronheim SR, Greenstreet TA, Sleath PR, Salvesen GS, Pickup DJ: Viral inhibition of inflammation: Cowpox virus encodes an inhibitor of the interleukin-1β-converting enzyme. *Cell* **69**:597, 1992.

124. Boyd JM, Malstron S, Subramanian T, Venkatesh LK, Schaeper U, Elangovan B, Sa-Eipper C, Chinnadurai G: Adenovirus E1B 19 kDa and Bcl-2 proteins interact with a common set of cellular proteins. *Cell* **79**:341, 1994.

125. Henderson S, Huen D, Rowe M, Dawson C, Johnson G, Rickson A: Epstein-Barr virus-coded BHRF1 protein, a viral homologue of Bcl-2, protects human B cells from programmed cell death. *Proc Natl Acad Sci USA* **90**:8479, 1993.

126. Nielan JG, Lu Z, Afonzo L, Kutish GF, Sussman MD, Rock DL: An African swine fever virus gene with similarity to the proto-oncogene bcl-2 and the Epstein-Barr virus gene BHRF1. *J Virol* **67**:4391, 1993.

127. Liebowitz D, Kieff E: Epstein-Barr virus, in Roizman B, Whitley RJ, Lopez C (eds): *The Human Herpesviruses*. New York, Raven Press, 1993, p. 107.

128. Liebowitz D: Epstein-Barr virus and a cellular signaling pathway in lymphomas from immunosuppressed patients. *N Engl J Med* **338**:1413, 1998.

129. Henderson S, Rowe M, Gregory C, Croom-Carter D, Wang F, Longnecker R, Kieff E, Rickinson A: Induction of Bcl-2 expression by Epstein-Barr virus latent membrane protein 1 protects infected B cells from programmed cell death. *Cell* **65**:1107, 1991.

130. Pena J, Rudin CM, Thompson CB: A Bcl-x_L transgene promotes malignant conversion of chemically initiated skin papillomas. *Cancer Res* **58**:2111, 1998.

131. Evan G, Littlewood T: The role of c-Myc in cell growth. *Curr Opin Genet Dev* **3**:44, 1993.

132. Evan G, Wyllie A, Gilbert C, Littlewood T, Brooks M, Waters C, Penn L, Hancock D: Induction of apoptosis in fibroblasts by c-Myc protein. *Cell* **63**:119, 1992.

133. Langdon WY, Harris AW, Cory S: Growth of E mu-myc transgenic B-lymphoid cells in vitro and their evolution toward autonomy. *Oncogene Res* **3**:271, 1988.

134. Bissonnette RP, Echeverri F, Mahboubi A, Green DR: Apoptotic cell death induced by c-Myc is inhibited by bcl-2. *Nature* **359**:552, 1992.

135. Harrington EA, Bennett MR, Fanidi A, Evan GI: c-Myc-induced apoptosis in fibroblasts is inhibited by specific cytokines. *EMBO J* **13**:3286, 1994.

136. Dedera D, Waller E, LeBrun D, Sen-Majumdar A, Stevens M, Barsh G, Cleary M: Chimeric homeobox gene E2A-PBX1 induces proliferation, apoptosis and malignant lymphomas in transgenic mice. *Cell* **74**:833, 1993.

137. Tommasino M, Crawford L: Human papillomavirus E6 and E7: Proteins which deregulate the cell cycle. *Bioessays* **17**:509, 1995.

138. Pan H, Griep AE: Temporally distinct patterns of p53-dependent and p53-independent apoptosis during mouse lens development. *Gene Dev* **9**:2157, 1995.

139. Rao L, Debbas M, Sabbatini P, Hockenberry D, Korsmeyer S, White E: The adenovirus E1A proteins induce apoptosis, which is inhibited by the E1B 19-kDa and Bcl-2 proteins. *Proc Natl Acad Sci USA* **89**:7742, 1992.

140. Yew PR, Berk AJ: Inhibition of p53 transactivation required for transformation by adenovirus early 1B protein. *Nature* **357**:82, 1992.

141. Murray AW: The genetics of cell cycle checkpoints. *Curr Opin Genet Dev* **5**:5, 1995.

142. Vogelstein B: Cancer: A deadly inheritance. *Nature* **348**:681, 1990.

143. Kuerbitz SJ, Plunkett BS, Walsh WV, Kastan MB: Wild-type p53 is a cell cycle checkpoint determinant following irradiation. *Proc Natl Acad Sci USA* **89**:7491, 1992.

144. Shaw P, Bovey R, Tardy S, Sahli R, Sordat B, Costa J: Induction of apoptosis by wild-type p53 in a human colon tumor-derived cell line. *Proc Natl Acad Sci USA* **89**:4495, 1992.

145. Yonish-Rouach E, Resnitzky D, Lotem J, Sachs L, Kimchi A, Oren M: Wild-type p53 induces apoptosis of myeloid leukaemic cells that is inhibited by interleukin-6. *Nature* **352**:345, 1991.

146. Symonds H, Krall L, Remington L, Saenz-Robles M, Lowe S, Jacks T, Van Dyke T: p53-dependent apoptosis suppresses tumor growth and progression in vivo. *Cell* **78**:703, 1994.

147. Lowe SW, Schmitt EM, Smith SW, Osborne BA, Jacks T: p53 is required for radiation-induced apoptosis in mouse thymocytes. *Nature* **362**:847, 1993.

148. Clarke AR, Purdie CA, Harrison DJ, Morris RG, Bird CC, Hooper ML, Wyllie AH: Thymocyte apoptosis induced by p53-dependent and independent pathways. *Nature* **362**:849, 1993.

149. Miyashita T, Krajewski S, Krajewska M, Wang HG, Lin HK, Liebermann DA, Hoffman B, Reed JC: Tumor suppressor p53 is a regulator of bcl-2 and bax gene expression in vitro and in vivo. *Oncogene* **9**:1799, 1994.

150. Knudson CM, Tung KSK, Tourtellote WG, Brown GAJ, Korsmeyer SJ: Bax-deficient mice with lymphoid hyperplasia and male germ cell death. *Science* **270**:96, 1995.

151. Riley DJ, Lee EY-HP, Lee W-H: The retinoblastoma protein: More than a tumor suppressor. *Annu Rev Cell Biol* **10**:1, 1994.

152. Lee EY-HP, Chang C-Y, Hu N, Wang Y-CJ, Lai C-C, Herrup K, Lee W-H, Bradley A: Mice deficient for Rb are nonviable and show defects in neurogenesis and haematopoiesis. *Nature* **359**:288, 1992.

153. Jacks T, Fazeli A, Schmitt EM, Bronson RT, Goodell MA, Weinberg RA: Effects of an Rb mutation in the mouse. *Nature* **359**:295, 1992.

154. Amati B, Littlewood T, Evan G, Land H: The c-Myc protein induces cell cycle progression and apoptosis through dimerisation with Max. *EMBO J* **12**:5083, 1994.

155. Limpens J, de Jong D, van Krieken JH, Price CG, Young BD, van Ommen GJ, Kluin PM: Bcl-2/JH rearrangements in benign lymphoid tissues with follicular hyperplasia. *Oncogene* **6**:2271, 1991.

156. Liu Y, Hernandez AM, Shibata D, Cortopossi GA: BCL2 translocation frequency rises with age in humans. *Proc Natl Acad Sci USA* **91**:8910, 1994.

157. Gottesman MM, Pastan I: Biochemistry of multidrug resistance mediated by the multidrug transporter. *Annu Rev Biochem* **62**:385, 1993.

158. Lowe SW, Ruley HE, Jacks T, Housman DE: p53-dependent apoptosis modulates the cytotoxicity of anticancer agents. *Cell* **74**:957, 1993.

159. Miyashita T, Reed JC: bcl-2 gene transfer increases relative resistance of S49:1 and WEHI7.2 lymphoid cells to cell death and DNA fragmentation induced by glucocorticoids and multiple chemotherapeutic drugs. *Cancer Res* **52**:5407, 1992.

160. Walton MI, Whysong D, O'Connor PM, Hockenbery D, Korsmeyer SJ, Kohn KW: Constitutive expression of human bcl-2 modulates nitrogen mustard and camptothecin induced apoptosis. *Cancer Res* **53**:1853, 1993.

161. Dole M, Nunez G, Merchant AK, Maybaum J, Rode CK, Bloch CA, Castle VP: Bcl-2 inhibits chemotherapy-induced apoptosis in neuroblastoma. *Cancer Res* **54**:3253, 1994.

162. Fisher TC, Milner AE, Gregory CD, Jackman AL, Aherne GW, Hartley JA, Dive C, Hickman JA: bcl-2 modulation of apoptosis induced by anticancer drugs: Resistance to thymidylate stress is independent of classical resistance pathways. *Cancer Res* **53**:3321, 1993.

163. Miyashita T, Reed JC: Bcl-2 oncoprotein blocks chemotherapy-induced apoptosis in a human leukemia cell line. *Blood* **81**:151, 1993.

164. Minn AJ, Rudin CM, Boise LH, Thompson CB: Expression of Bcl-x_L can confer a multidrug resistance phenotype. *Blood* **86**:1903, 1995.

165. Dole MG, Jasty R, Cooper MJ, Thompson CB, Nunez G, Castle VP: Bcl-x_L is expressed in neuroblastoma cells and modulates chemotherapy-induced apoptosis. *Cancer Res* **55**:2576, 1995.

166. Lotem J, Sachs L: Regulation by bcl-2, c-Myc, and p53 of susceptibility to induction of apoptosis by heat shock and cancer chemotherapy compounds in differentiation-competent and -defective myeloid leukemic cells. *Cell Growth Diff* **4**:41, 1993.

167. Campos L, Rouault J-P, Sabido O, Oriol P, Roubi N, Vasselon C, Archimbaud E, Magaud J-P, Guyotat D: High expression of bcl-2 protein in acute myeloid leukemia cells is associated with poor response to chemotherapy. *Blood* **81**:3091, 1993.

168. Lowe SW, Bodis S, McClatchey A, Remington L, Ruley HE, Fisher DE, Housman DE, Jacks T: p53 status and the efficacy of cancer therapy in vivo. *Science* **266**:807, 1994.

169. Strasser A, Harris AW, Jacks T, Cory S: DNA damage can induce apoptosis in proliferating lymphoid cells via p53-independent mechanisms inhibitable by Bcl-2. *Cell* **79**:329, 1994.

170. Minn, AJ, Boise LH, Thompson CB: Expression of Bcl-x$_L$ and loss of p53 can cooperate to overcome a cell cycle checkpoint induced by mitotic spindle damage. *Gene Dev* **10**:2621, 1996.

171. Cahill DP, Lengauer C, Yu J, Riggins GJ, Willson JKV, Markowitz SD, Kinsler KW, Vogelstein B: Mutations of mitotic checkpoint genes in human cancers. *Nature* **392**:300, 1998.

172. Webb A, Cunningham D, Cotter F, Clark PA, di Stefano F, Ross P, Corbo M, Dziewanowska Z: BCL-2 antisense therapy in patients with non-Hodgkin lymphoma. *Lancet* **349**:1137, 1997.

173. Piche A, Grim J, Rancourt C, Gomez-Navarro J, Reed JC, Curiel DT: Modulation of Bcl-2 protein levels by an intracellular anti-Bcl-2 single-chain antibody increases drug-induced cytotoxicity in the breast cancer cell line MCF-7. *Cancer Res* **58**:2134, 1998.

Oncogenes

Morag Park

1. Oncogenes are altered forms of normal cellular genes called proto-oncogenes. In human cancers, proto-oncogenes are frequently located adjacent to chromosomal breakpoints and are targets for mutation. The products of proto-oncogenes are highly conserved in evolution and serve to regulate the cascade of events that maintains the ordered progression through the cell cycle, cell division, and differentiation. In the cancer cell, this ordered progression is partially lost when one or more of the components of this pathway are altered.

2. The control of normal cell growth and differentiation is mediated by the interaction of growth factors and cytokines with their membrane-bound receptors. This event triggers a cascade of intracellular biochemical signals that eventually results in the activation and repression of various genes. Proto-oncogene products have been shown to function at critical steps in these pathways and include proteins such as extracellular cytokines and growth factors, transmembrane growth factor receptors, cytoplasmic proteins that act to transmit the signal to the nucleus, and nuclear proteins that include transcription factors and proteins involved in the control of DNA replication.

3. Accumulating evidence suggests that the activation of several oncogenes and the inactivation of several growth-suppressor genes are necessary for acquisition of a complete neoplastic phenotype. It has been possible from experimental studies to subdivide oncogenes into several groups. One class of genes rescues cells from senescence and programmed cell death; they act as immortalizing genes that block cell differentiation. A second class of genes reduces growth factor requirements and induces changes in cell shape that result in a continuous proliferative response that is no longer regulated.

4. The use of transgenic mice is providing a powerful experimental approach to investigate the role of oncogenes in cancer. Oncogene expression can be directed to specific tissues, where a role for the oncogene in tumor formation in those tissues can be evaluated. Although transgenic mouse strains carrying a single oncogene generally show an increased incidence of neoplasia, oncogene expression usually precedes tumor formation by many months, and the tumors that result are frequently clonal, implying that other events are necessary. Examination of the secondary events in tumors from oncogene-bearing transgenic mice has confirmed the conclusions derived from in vitro studies

and has identified new oncogenes. By crossing two strains of oncogene-bearing mice, the consequence of multiple oncogenes on tumor incidence can be studied in a host capable of mounting a physiological response.

In the past 15 years, the study of oncogenes has considerably advanced our understanding of the molecular mechanisms leading to cancer. The application of techniques from many cancer research disciplines has led to the discovery of both dominantly acting transforming genes and of tumor-suppressor genes. The dominant transforming genes, collectively called *oncogenes*, are altered forms of normal cellular genes called *proto-oncogenes*. Proto-oncogenes are highly conserved in evolution, and their products are important regulators of normal cell growth and differentiation from primitive eukaryotes to humans. They are localized throughout the cell and regulate the cascade of events that serve to maintain the ordered progression through the cell cycle, cell division, or the differentiated state of the cell. The function of these genes is discussed later, but sites of their activity are represented conceptually in Fig. 11-1. In the normal cell, interaction of growth factors and cytokines with specific membrane receptors triggers a cascade of intracellular biochemical signals that result in the expression and repression of various genes. In a cancer cell, this ordered progression is partially lost when one or more of the components of this pathway becomes altered as an oncogene. Mutations that alter the structure, levels, or sites of expression of the gene products in this pathway have been shown to activate their oncogenic potential.

Just as the growth-promoting proto-oncogenes are thought to regulate the proliferation of normal cells, the actions of tumor-suppressor genes function normally to constrain cell growth. Genetic lesions that inactivate tumor-suppressor genes therefore free the cell from the growth constraints imposed by these genes. The end result of oncogene activation or suppressor gene inactivation is deregulated cell growth. Increasing evidence suggests that the acquisition of multiple sequential alterations involving both oncogenes and tumor-suppressor genes is generally required for the progression from the normal to a fully malignant phenotype. This review focuses on the identification, mechanisms of activation, and function of the oncogene/proto-oncogene class of growth regulators; tumor-suppressor genes are discussed in Chapter 12.

DISCOVERY OF ONCOGENES

The majority of oncogenes were initially isolated as altered forms of proto-oncogenes acquired (transduced) by RNA tumor viruses (v-*onc*). In 1909, Payton Rous discovered that transplantable sarcomas in chickens could be induced by a cell-free agent. The transforming agent was a retrovirus that had transduced part of a normal cellular gene called *src* (*sarcoma*). The virally transduced *src* gene (v-*src*) was altered by mutation compared with its cellular counterpart (c-*src*), rendering it constitutively activated. This discovery demonstrated that our cells harbor genes that, when abnormally activated, are capable of inducing tumorigenesis.[1,2] In the last 20 years, over 30 retroviruses have been isolated that induce tumors with short latency, each containing a different oncogene, and their transduced oncogenes have been shown to

A list of standard abbreviations is located immediately preceding the index. Additional abbreviations used in this chapter include: bcr = breakpoint cluster region, or gene at 22q11 involved in translocations producing the Philadelphia chromosome; CML = chronic myelogenous leukemia; c-*onc* = cellular oncogene; CSF-1R = macrophage colony-stimulating factor-1 receptor; EGFR = epidermal growth factor receptor; *env* = retroviral gene encoding protein components of the virion nucleoprotein core; LTR = long terminal repeat sequences encoding retroviral transcriptional control elements; MMTV = mouse mammary tumor virus; PDGFR = platelet-derived growth factor receptor; Ph = Philadelphia chromosome; *pol* = retroviral gene encoding reverse transcriptase; TGF = transforming growth factor; v-*onc* = viral oncogene.

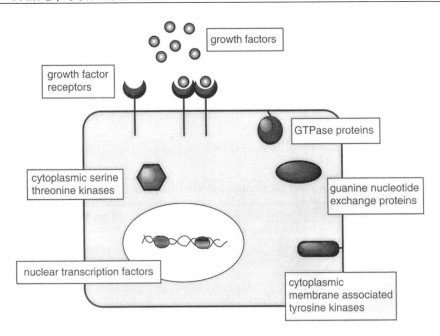

Fig. 11-1 Schematic representation of the cellular compartments where oncogene or proto-oncogene products are localized. These compartments include growth factors, transmembrane growth factor receptors, non-integral membrane-associated proteins of the *src* **tyrosine kinase gene family,** *ras* **GTPase gene family, guanine nucleotide exchange proteins plus serine threonine kinase onco-proteins localized in the cytoplasm, and nuclear transcription factors.**

have critical roles in cell transformation (Fig. 11-2).[3,4] Although retroviruses have not been shown to be etiologic agents involved in human cancer, they have provided useful insights into oncogene research. In addition to the acutely transforming retroviruses, slowly transforming retroviruses do not carry oncogenes but induce tumors by integrating themselves adjacent to a cellular gene and altering its transcriptional regulation (Fig. 11-2).[5] The presence of a provirus integrated in the same region of the cellular genome in independently derived tumors of the same histologic type has enabled investigators to identify new cellular genes that can be activated in specific tumor lineages. Following this strategy, many novel oncogenes have been discovered. An examination of human tumors by a variety of methods has revealed that many of the v-*onc* genes are also altered in human tumors.

DETECTION OF ONCOGENES IN HUMAN TUMORS

Evidence for a genetic role in cancer comes from multiple sources. Many of the cancer-prone syndromes, such as Fanconi syndrome, Bloom syndrome, and ataxia telangiectasia, show greatly increased chromosome instability.[6] Studies of colon cancer have shown that many cancers have accumulated multiple chromosome deletions and mutations.[7] The recent identification of the bacterial *mut*S and *mut*L DNA mismatch repair genes as genetic lesions that predispose individuals to colon cancer further supports the role of mutation in the generation of cancer.[8,9] To identify oncogenes in human tumors, several strategies have been developed. Oncogenes in human tumors were initially identified using DNA transfection techniques. The discovery that oncogenes are frequently activated by chromosomal translocations, however, has stimulated the isolation of genes that map to the breakpoints of nonrandom chromosomal rearrangement present in human tumors, as a method to identify new candidate oncogenes.

Detection of Oncogenes by DNA Transfection

The DNA transfection assay was developed to study and identify the transforming genes of RNA or DNA tumor viruses.[10] The cells used as recipients in most transfection experiments are NIH3T3 cells, which are mouse fibroblasts in origin and are maintained as contact-inhibited, nontumorigenic cell lines. Transformation of these cells by gene transfer is monitored by changes in cell morphology in culture and loss of contact inhibition, where cells overgrow the monolayer and form focal areas of dense layers

termed *foci*,[11] or by a modification of this technique in which the cells that have acquired transforming genes produce tumors in nude mice[12] (Fig. 11-3).

To assay for transforming genes, genomic DNA, prepared from human tumors or tumor cell lines, is transferred to recipient cells. Transfer of DNA-containing activated oncogenes will occasionally give rise to foci of morphologically altered cells that have tumorigenic properties. Foci or tumors thus obtained contain cells that are transformed as a result of incorporating human DNA containing an activated oncogene. Human repetitive DNA sequences located in the vicinity of the oncogene can be distinguished from mouse sequences and can be used to clone and isolate molecularly the DNA segment responsible for transformation of the NIH3T3 cells[13,14] (Fig. 11-3). Many of the human transforming genes identified in this manner are related to the *ras* family of oncogenes (Table 11-1). For instance, the transforming genes of a human bladder and lung carcinoma were shown to be homologous to the *ras* genes previously identified in the acute transforming retroviruses of the Harvey and Kirsten sarcoma viruses and were designated c-H-*ras* and c-K-*ras*,[15] respectively. In addition, a third *ras* gene family member was initially identified in a human neuroblastoma tumor cell line and human promyelocytic leukemia cell line and was designated N-*ras* (Table 11-1).[16]

Ras genes in human tumors have been shown to be activated by single point mutations predominantly involving codons 12, 13, and 61 (reviewed by Barbacid, 1987[17]). Although these mutations activate each of the *ras* genes as an oncogene in vitro, there is clear selectivity with regard to which *ras* homologue is mutationally activated in a given human cancer. Approximately 50 percent of colorectal cancers, 95 percent of pancreatic cancers, and 30 percent of lung adenocarcinomas harbor mutant Ki-*ras* genes, but mutant Ha-*ras* or N-*ras* genes are rarely detected in these cancers.[18] Similarly, about 25 percent of acute myelogenous leukemias and myelodysplastic syndromes contain mutant N-*ras* genes, but mutant Ha-*ras* and Ki-*ras* genes are rarely found. Moreover, mutant Ha-*ras* genes are rarely found in human tumors.[19] In most other tumor types (e.g., cancers of the breast, prostate, stomach, bladder, liver, and brain), however, *ras* mutations do not occur often, if at all. As *RAS* genes are ubiquitously expressed and presumably have similar functions in all cells, the basis for this tissue specificity is not understood.

Gene transfer studies have also led to the identification of a growing number of transforming genes that are not members of the *ras* gene family and that have not been previously identified in a

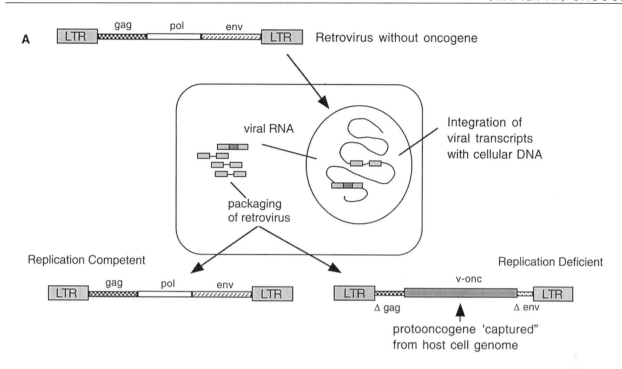

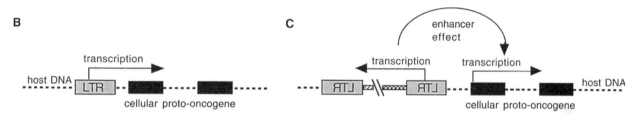

Fig. 11-2 Schematic representation of mechanisms of activation of a host gene by insertion of a provirus and the general structure of leukemia and leukosis and acute transforming retroviral genomes. A: Genome of a nondefective leukemia or leukosis retrovirus, infection of host cell, and integration into the host genome. The *gag* region encodes the internal structural proteins of the virion, the *pol* region encodes the virion RNA-dependent DNA polymerase (reverse transcriptase), and the *env* region encodes the proteins found on the surface of the virion envelope. LTR is the long terminal repeat that appears at each end of the integrated linear DNA forms. Within the LTR region are DNA sequences, which define the initiation site for RNA transcription and at the 3′ end encode a poly A addition site where the viral RNA polyadenylation occurs and transcription enhancer sequences that result in the production of high levels of transcripts. The LTR elements provide all of the necessary functions for eukaryotic transcription to take place and for the provirus to express genomic viral RNA. B and C: Two different configurations of inserted proviral DNA. Replication competent and replication defective viruses are produced. The genome of a replication-defective acute transforming retrovirus containing v-*onc* sequences is shown. Although substantial portions of *gag*, *pol*, and/or *env* may be deleted in acute transforming retroviruses, they still retain the terminal noncoding LTR regions. B: Insertion of a proviral LTR upstream of the first coding exon as observed with c-*myc*. This insertion results in a transcript that no longer contains sequences that regulate c-*myc* expression levels. The protein-coding domains (exons) of the normal host gene are in *solid black rectangles*. C: Integration of an intact provirus upstream (or downstream) from, for example, the *int 1* or *int 2* genes. This form of integration may not alter the gene product but generally results in increased transcription of that gene promoted by the transcriptional enhancing activity of the retroviral LTR.

retrovirus. These include multiple receptor tyrosine kinases (the *neu*, *met*, *trk*, *mas*, *erb*B-2/*HER2*, and *ret*), growth factors (*hst* and KS3 oncogenes), exchange factors that activate members of the Rho GTPase family, and multiple transcription factors (Table 11-1).

Identification of Oncogenes at Chromosomal Breakpoints

The chromosomal location of cellular proto-oncogenes determined by in situ hybridization has led to the identification of several proto-oncogenes at or near chromosomal translocation breakpoints.[20,21] In general, structural rearrangements that juxtapose two different chromosomal regions are thought to contain dominant transforming genes, whereas deletions or monosomies are thought to be the sites of recessive tumor-suppressor genes.

Recurrent tumor-specific chromosome translocations were first identified in cytogenetic analyses of leukemias and myelodysplasias and are considered to be involved in tumor development.[22,23] The tumor-specific chromosome abnormalities of leukemias and lymphomas are usually somatically acquired alterations. In some tumor types such as chronic myelogenous leukemia, the same translocations consistently appear, supporting the hypothesis that these events are a prerequisite for tumor induction. Where it has been possible to characterize and molecularly isolate the genes adjacent to translocation breakpoints, candidate genes implicated in tumor initiation and progression have been identified (Table 11-2). These alterations are discussed in more detail in other chapters.

In many cases, breaks occur within a gene on each of the participating chromosomes, resulting in the formation of a

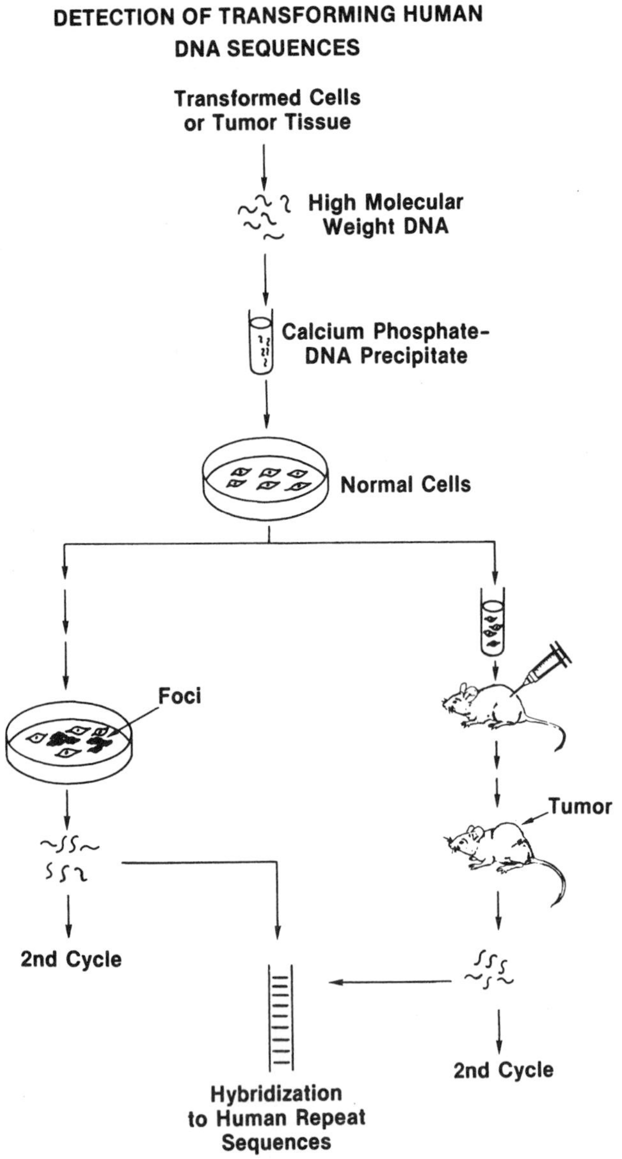

**DETECTION OF TRANSFORMING HUMAN
DNA SEQUENCES**

Fig. 11-3 NIH3T3 DNA transfection and/or transformation assay. High molecular weight DNA prepared from transformed cell or tumor DNA is precipitated with calcium phosphate and added to nontransformed mouse NIH3T3 cells. These cells are then assayed for tumor production in nude mice or are assayed for the appearance of foci. DNA is prepared from either primary foci or tumors and is subjected to a second cycle of transfection to facilitate the loss of additional nontransforming sequences that are transferred with the transforming gene. After several cycles of transfection, the majority of the foreign DNA in the focus or tumor corresponds to the transforming gene and can be isolated by recombinant DNA technology.

chimeric gene that encodes a fusion protein. An example of this includes chronic myelogenous leukemia (CML), which is a pluripotent stem cell disease characterized by the presence of a consistent translocation. The Philadelphia (Ph) chromosome translocation between chromosomes 9 and 22, t(9;22)(q34;qll)[24] is present in the leukemic cells of at least 95 percent of all CML patients.[25] The proto-oncogene c-abl, which is the normal cellular homologue of the oncogene v-abl of Abelson murine leukemic virus (A-MuLV) (Table 11-1) is translocated from chromosome 9, band q34, into the bcr gene on chromosome 22 at band q11.[26,27] This gives rise to a chimeric gene expressing a fusion protein containing the N-terminus derived from the Bcr protein and the C-terminus derived from the Abl protein (Fig. 11-4). The resulting chimeric protein has increased catalytic activity when compared with the normal protein and will transform cells in culture.[24]

Although many translocations give rise to a new protein, some, such as those involving the c-MYC and immunoglobulin genes on the chromosome translocations 2:14, 8:14, and 22:14 observed in lymphomas, result in altered regulation of the MYC gene (reviewed by Stanton et al, 1983[26]). Normally, the expression of this gene is tightly regulated, but, in cells where the translocation has occurred, the gene is constitutively expressed.

As a consequence of technical improvements, cytogenetic abnormalities have now been identified in solid tumors (reviewed by Cooper, 1996[27]). Such rearrangements are found in a high proportion of tumors, suggesting that they could provide much needed markers for use in diagnosis of sarcoma types. In addition to chromosomal rearrangements, frequent chromosomal abnormalities documented in solid tumors involve amplification or deletion of specific chromosomal regions.

Proto-oncogene Amplification

Cellular proto-oncogenes have been found in multiple copies in various tumors and transformed cell lines. The amplified proto-oncogene copies can occur in homogeneously staining chromosomal regions or double-minute chromosomes.[28,29] Oncogene amplification has also been observed by hybridization techniques in tumor cells in the absence of microscopic chromosomal changes. The mechanism of gene amplification is not fully understood, but illegitimate DNA replication occurring more than once during a single cell cycle could account for the increase in multiple segments (amplification units) of DNA from 200 to 2000 kb in size.[30]

All amplified proto-oncogenes express high levels of the corresponding RNA and protein and do not appear to be rearranged. The amplification unit containing the proto-oncogene DNA can be at a site distant from its normal locus as a heterogeneously staining region. The c-MYC gene was the first proto-oncogene shown to be amplified. In the promyelocytic leukemia cell line HL60, as well as in the primary tumor, 8 to 30 copies of c-MYC per cell were detected.[31,32] Other proto-oncogenes, including c-MYB, c-erbB (epidermal growth factor receptor or EGFR), HER-2 (also called c-erbB2 and corresponds to neu in the rat), and c-MYC family members, have also been shown to be amplified in certain tumors or tumor cell lines (Table 11-3). The presence of multiple copies of proto-oncogenes in tumor cells has been associated with poor prognosis. N-MYC, which was first identified as an amplified gene in a human neuroblastoma, is present in multiple copies in 40 percent of neuroblastomas, and its amplification correlates with more advanced stages of the disease.[33,34] Amplification of members of the MYC gene family (c-MYC, N-MYC, and L-MYC) in small-cell lung carcinomas also appears to be associated with the more malignant stages of the tumor.[35] The amplified proto-oncogene is frequently tumor specific; for example, N-MYC or c-MYC may be associated with the progression of neuroblastomas and small-cell lung carcinoma cells, the EGFR (c-erbB) gene has been found to be amplified in glioblastomas and several squamous carcinomas,[36,37] and the related HER-2 gene is often found amplified in adenocarcinomas[38] and in advanced, hormone-independent mammary tumors with a poor prognosis.[39,40] This suggests that increased expression of these proto-oncogenes plays a role in the development and progression of these tumors.

FUNCTIONS AND MECHANISMS OF ACTIVATION OF PROTO-ONCOGENE PRODUCTS

Conservation of Proto-oncogenes

Homologues of proto-oncogenes have been found in all multicellular animals studied thus far, and their widespread distribution in nature indicates that their protein products have essential

Table 11-1 Oncogenes

Oncogene	Lesion	Neoplasm	Proto-Oncogene
Growth factors			
v-sis		Glioma/fibrosarcoma	B-chain PDGF
int 2	Proviral insertion	Mammary carcinoma	Member of FGF family
KS3	DNA transfection	Kaposi sarcoma	Member of FGF family
HST	DNA transfection	Stomach carcinoma	Member of FGF family
int-l	Proviral insertion	Mammary carcinoma	Possible growth factor
Receptors lacking protein kinase activity			
mas	DNA transfection	Mammary carcinoma	Angiotensin receptor
Tyrosine kinases: integral membrane proteins, growth factor receptors			
EGFR*	Amplification	Squamous cell carcinoma	Protein kinase (tyr) EGFR
v-fms		Sarcoma	Protein kinase (tyr) CSF-1R
v-kit		Sarcoma	Protein kinase (tyr) stem cell factor R
v-ros		Sarcoma	Protein kinase (tyr)
MET	Rearrangement	MNNG-treated human osteocarcinoma cell line	Protein kinase (tyr) HGF/SFR
TRK	Rearrangement	Colon carcinoma	Protein kinase (tyr) NGFR
NEU	Point mutation	Neuroblastoma	Protein kinase (tyr)
	Amplification	Carcinoma of breast	
RET	Rearrangement	Carcinoma of thyroid Men 2A, Men 2B	Protein kinase (tyr) GDNFR
Tyrosine kinases: membrane associated			
SRC*		Colon carcinoma	Protein kinase (tyr)
v-yes		Sarcoma	Protein kinase (tyr)
v-fgr		Sarcoma	Protein kinase (tyr)
v-fps		Sarcoma	Protein kinase (tyr)
v-fes		Sarcoma	Protein kinase (tyr)
BCR/ABL*	Chromosome translocation	Chronic myelogenous leukemia	Protein kinase (tyr)
Membrane-associated G proteins			
H-RAS*	Point mutation	Colon, lung, pancreas carcinoma	GTPase
K-RAS*	Point mutation	Acute myelogenous leukemia thyroid carcinoma, melanoma	GTPase
N-RAS	Point mutation	Carcinoma, melanoma	GTPase
gsp	Point mutation	Carcinoma of thyroid	$G_6\alpha$
gip	Point mutation	Ovary, adrenal carcinoma	$G_1\alpha$
GEF family of proteins			
Dbl	Rearrangement	Diffuse B-cell lymphoma	GEF for Rho and Cdc42Hs
Ost		Osteosarcomas	GEF for RhoA and Cdc42Hs
Tiam-1	Metastatic and oncogenic	T lymphoma	GEF for Rac and Cdc42Hs
Vay	Rearrangement	Hematopoietic cells	GEF for Ras?
Lbc	Oncogenic	Myeloid leukemias	GEF for Rho
Serine/threonine kinases: cytoplasmic			
v-mos		Sarcoma	Protein kinase (ser/thr)
v-raf		Sarcoma	Protein kinase (ser/thr)
pim-1	Proviral insertion	T-cell lymphoma	Protein kinase (ser/thr)
Cytoplasmic regulators			
v-crk			SH-2/SH-3 adaptor
Nuclear protein family			
v-myc		Carcinoma myelocytomatosis	Transcription factor
N-MYC	Gene amplification	Neuroblastoma; lung carcinoma	Transcription factor
L-MYC	Gene amplification	Carcinoma of lung	Transcription factor
v-myb		Myeloblastosis	Transcription factor
v-fos		Osteosarcoma	Transcription factor API
v-jun		Sarcoma	Transcrption factor API
v-ski		Carcinoma	Transcription factor
v-rel		Lymphatic leukemia	Mutant NFκB
v-ets		Myeloblastosis	Transcription factor
v-erbA		Erythroblastosis	Mutant thioredoxin receptor

ABBREVIATIONS: CSF-1R = macrophage colony-stimulating factor-1 receptor; EGFR = epidermal growth factor receptor; FGF = fibroblast growth factor; GEF = guanine nucleotide exchange factor; GDNF = glial derived neurotropic factor; HGF/SF = hepatic growth factor/scatter factor; NGF = Nerve growth factor; PDGF = platelet-derived growth factor.

Table 11-2 Molecularly Characterized Neoplastic Rearrangements

Affected Gene	Translocation	Disease	Protein Type
Gene fusions			
c-ABL (9q34) BCR (22q11)	t(9;22) (q34;q11)	Chronic myelogenous leukemia and acute leukemia	Tyrosine kinase activated by B-cell receptor
PBX-1 (1q23) E2A (19p13.3)	t(1;19)(q23;p13.3)	Acute pre-B-cell leukemia	Homeodomain HLH
PML (15q21) RAR (17q21)	t(15;17) (q21;q11-22)	Acute myeloid leukemia	Zn finger
CAN (6p23) DEK (9q34)	t(6;9) (p23;q34)	Acute myeloid leukemia	No homology
REL	ins(2;12)	Non-Hodgkin lymphoma	NF-κB family
NRG	(p13;p11.2-14)		No homology
Oncogenes Juxtaposed with immunoglobulin loci			
c-MYC	t(8;14) (q24;q32) t(2;8) (p12;q24) t(8;22) (q24;q11)	Burkitt lymphoma, BL-ALL	HLH domain
BCL1 (PRADI?)	t(11;14) (q13;q32)	B-cell chronic lymphocyte leukemia	PRADI-G1 cyclin
BCL-2	t(14;18) (q32;21)	Follicular lymphoma	Inner mitochondrial membrane
BCL-3	t(14;19) (q32;q13.1)	Chronic B-cell leukemia	CDC10 motif
IL-3	t(5;14) (q31;q32)	Acute pre-B-cell leukemia	Growth factor
Oncogenes juxtaposed with T-cell receptor loci			
c-MYC	t(8;14) (q24;q11)	Acute T-cell leukemia	HLH domain
LYL-1	t(7;19) (q35;p13)	Acute T-cell leukemia	HLH domain
TAL-1/SCL/TCL-5)	t(1;14) (p32;q11)	Acute T-cell leukemia	HLH domain
TAL-2	t(7;9) (q35;q34)	Acute T-cell leukemia	HLH domain
Rhombotin 1/Ttg-1	t(11;14) (p15;q11)	Acute T-cell leukemia	LIM domain
Rhombotin 2/Ttg-2	t(11;14) (p13;q11) t(7;11) (q35;p13)	Acute T-cell leukemia	LIM domain
HOX-11	t(10;14) (q24;q11) t(7;10) (q35;q24)	Acute T-cell leukemia	Homeodomain
TAN-1	t(7;9) (q34;q34.3)	Acute T-cell leukemia	Notch homologue
Gene fusions in sarcomas			
FLI1, EWS	t(11;22) (q24;q12)	Ewing sarcoma	Ets transcription factor family
ERG, EWS	t(21;22) (q22;q12)	Ewing sarcoma	Ets transcription factor family
ATV1, EWS	t(7;21) (p22;q12)	Ewing sarcoma	Ets transcription factor family
ATF1, EWS	t(12;22) (q13;q12)	Soft tissue clear cell sarcoma	Transcription factor
CHN, EWS	t(9;22) (q22-31;q12)	Myxoid chondrosarcoma	Steroid receptor family
WT1, EWS	t(11;22) (p13;q12)	Desmoplastic small round cell tumor	Wilm tumor gene
SSX1, SSX2, SYT	t(X;18) (p11.2;q11.2)	Synovial sarcoma	HLH domain
PAX3, EKHR	t(2;13) (q37;q14)	Alveolar	Homeobox homologue
PAX7, EKHR	t(1;13) (q36;q14)	Rhabdomyosarcoma	Homeobox homologue
CHOP, TLS	t(12;16) (q13;p11)	Myxoid liposarcoma	Transcription factor
var, HMGI-C	t(var;12) (var;q13-15)	Lipomas	HMG DNA-binding protein
HMGI-C, ?	t(12;14) (q13-15)	Leiomomas	HMG DNA-binding protein
Oncogenes juxtaposed with other loci			
PTH deregulates PRADI	inv(11)(p15;q13)	Parathyroid adenoma	PRADI-GI cyclin
BTGI deregulates MYC	t(8;12)(q24;q22)	B-cell chronic lymphocytic leukemia	MYC-HLH domain

ABBREVIATIONS: HLH = helix-loop-helix structural domain; zn = zinc; HMG = high mobility group.

Normal Configuration of
Chromosomes 9 and 22

Rearranged Chromosome 9(9q+) & 22(Ph)

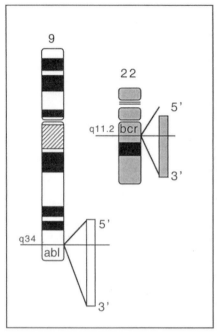

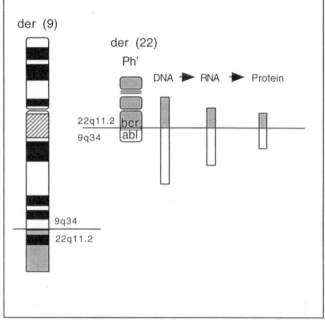

Fig. 11-4 Schematic representation of the chromosomes involved in the generation of the Philadelphia chromosome observed in more than 95 percent of chronic myelogenous leukemia (CML). A schematic presentation of the normal chromosomes 9 and 22, and of the chromosome translocations 9q+ and 22q− are shown. The c- *ABL* **proto-oncogene on the distal tip of chromosome 9q34 is translocated into the** *BCR* **locus on chromosome 22q11.2. This generates a chimeric gene that expresses a chimeric** *BCR-ABL* **messenger RNA and fusion protein.**

biologic roles. The more highly conserved domains of the protein are probably those that have a crucial structural and/or functional role, and characterization of their normal biochemical properties will provide insight into the contribution that an activated oncogene has to cell transformation. Understanding the mechanism of activation of each oncogene requires characterization of the proto-oncogene, a comparison of the changes that have occurred, and systematic testing of changes influencing the transforming potential.

There are essentially only three biochemical mechanisms by which proto-oncogenes act. One mechanism involves phosphorylation of proteins on serine, threonine, or tyrosine residues.[41] Proteins of this class transfer phosphate groups from adenosine triphosphate (ATP) to the side chain of tyrosine, serine, or threonine residues. Phosphorylation serves two basic purposes in signal transduction. In many instances, it changes the conformation and activates the enzymatic kinase activity of the protein. Secondly, phosphorylation of tyrosine residues generates docking

sites that recruit target proteins, which the activated kinase may phosphorylate. Thus, phosphorylation acts to potentiate signal transmission through the generation of complexes of signal-transducing molecules at specific sites in the cell where they are required to act. For example, activation of the catalytic activity of a receptor tyrosine kinase by its ligand leads to the formation of a complex of signaling proteins at the plasma membrane where the receptor is localized.

The second mechanism by which genes act to transmit signals is by GTPases.[42] The prototype for this class of proteins is the *ras* gene family. In a similar manner to the kinase gene family, Ras proteins function as molecular switches that are turned of and on via a regulated GDP/GTP cycle. Ras proteins have been implicated as key intermediates that relay the signal from upstream tyrosine kinases to downstream serine-threonine kinase pathways. Some of the conventional heterotrimeric G proteins can also transform cells when altered.[43,44] The third mechanism involves proteins that are localized in the nucleus. A large variety of proteins that control progress through the cell cycle and gene expression are encoded by proto-oncogenes, some of which may also be involved in DNA replication.[45,46] Thus, the relaxation of requirements of transformed cells for growth factors could be mediated by an activated oncogene at multiple levels of the signal transduction pathway.

Growth Factors

Growth factors are responsible for stimulating cells in a resting or G0 stage to enter the cell cycle. This mitogenic response occurs in two phases: a quiescent cell is stimulated to proceed into the G1 phase of the cell cycle by *competence factors* and then becomes committed to DNA synthesis by *progression factors* (Fig. 11-5).[47] Successful transition through the G1 phase requires sustained growth factor stimulation over a period of several hours. This is followed by a critical phase where the presence of a progression factor such as insulin growth factor I is required in addition to the

Table 11-3 Examples of Cellular Proto-Oncogenes Amplified in Human Tumors

Tumor	Oncogene	Amplification
Small-cell lung cancer	c-*myc*	Up to 80×
	N-*myc*	Up to 50×
	L-*myc*	Up to 20×
Neuroblastomas	N-*myc*	Up to 250×
Glioblastomas	c-*erb*B1 (EGFR)	Up to 50×
Mammary carcinoma	c-*erb*B2 (HER2)	Up to 30×
	c-*myc*	Up to 50×
	Cyclin D1	Up to 30×

ABBREVIATION: EGFR = endothelial growth factor receptor.

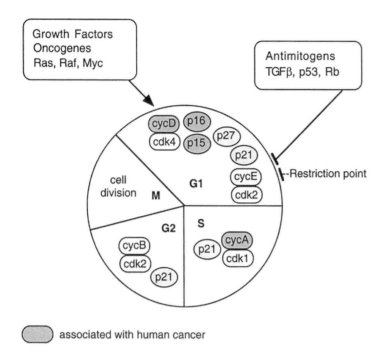

Fig. 11-5 Combinatorial interactions of cyclins and cyclin-dependent kinases (cdks) during the cell cycle. Progression from G0 through the restriction point in G1 requires the continued presence of growth factors. This requirement is overcome by oncogenes, such as Myc, Ras, or Raf, or tyrosine kinases. Progression through G1 can be blocked by antimitogens, TGFβ, or the p53 or Rb tumor-suppressor genes. Cyclins D and E in complexes with cdks are required for progression through G1 and entry into S phase. Cyclins A and B form complexes with cdk2 later in the cell cycle and are involved in progression from G2 to M. The activity of cyclin-D complexes can be inhibited by p15 and p16, thus preventing the advance of the cell from G1 to S. Other inhibitors of cyclin-dependent kinases, p21 and p27, can act throughout the cell cycle. Cyclins and inhibitors found altered in human cancers are shown in grey.

growth factor for successful progression through the cell cycle. This dual signal requirement may prevent accidental triggering of quiescent cells into the cell cycle by transient exposure to mitogenic growth factors. In some cell types, the absence of growth factor stimulation causes the rapid onset of programmed cell death (apoptosis).[48] Therefore, inappropriate expression of a growth factor may result in a constant stimulation of cell growth in addition to a block in cell differentiation.

There is now much evidence to support a role for growth factors and their receptors in the development of human malignancies. The first direct correlation of an oncogene with a growth factor was revealed from a computer-assisted comparison that showed that the amino acid sequence of the v-*sis* oncogene product was highly related to the B chain of platelet-derived growth factor (PDGF) (Table 11-1).[49] PDGF is released from platelets during clotting and is recognized as an important serum mitogen required for mesenchymal cell growth in culture. Connective tissue tumors such as sarcomas and glioblastomas have been shown to express PDGF, whereas their normal tissue counterparts did not.[50] Thus, in an autocrine fashion, the sarcoma and glial tumor cells appear to synthesize the mitogen to which they are normally responsive. On the other hand, no genetic alterations of the PDGF gene have yet been observed that would explain this synthesis. Until the mechanism underlying the expression of PDGF is clarified, it will be difficult to know whether this expression is a cause or an effect of neoplastic growth.

Int-2, whose expression is activated by mouse mammary tumor virus (MMTV) proviral insertion in mouse mammary carcinomas, the *KS3* oncogene identified in a Kaposi sarcomas, and *HST*, a transforming gene identified in a human stomach cancer by DNA transfection, are members of the basic or acidic fibroblast growth factor (FGF) family of related peptide mitogens. Basic FGFs are expressed by human melanoma cell lines but not by normal melanocytes that are dependent on bFGF to proliferate.[51,52] Similarly, transforming growth factor α (TGFα) is frequently produced by carcinomas that express high levels of the EGFR and appears to function as an autocrine in this system through stimulation of the EGFR.[53] Because many ligands and their receptors are not yet characterized, the contribution of autocrine growth stimulatory loops to human malignancies may be greater than is presently appreciated.

Growth Factor Receptors

Oncogenes derived from growth factor receptors confer on the cells the ability to bypass the growth factor requirement, rendering cells growth factor independent. By far, the largest number of receptor-derived oncoproteins are derived from growth factor receptors that have tyrosine kinase activity.

Tyrosine Protein Kinases. More than 40 different protein tyrosine kinases have been identified (Table 11-1).[54] These kinases are subdivided into two main categories: those, such as the EGFR, spanning the plasma membrane and those located in the cytoplasm, many of which are associated with the plasma membrane, such as c-Src (Fig. 11-6). All of the protein tyrosine kinases have sequence homology over a region of approximately 300 amino acids that has been defined as the *catalytic kinase domain*[55] (Fig. 11-6). This domain is responsible for catalyzing the transfer of the phosphate group of ATP to tyrosine residues during trans- and autophosphorylation. This kinase domain is also homologous to the Raf, ERK, and Mos protein members, which have phosphorylation specificity for serine and threonine.[56,57] Phosphorylation on tyrosine is a rare event in normal cells and accounts for only 0.05 percent of all protein phosphorylation, but tyrosine kinases regulate key events in signal transduction pathways that control cell shape and growth.[58]

Growth Factor Receptor Tyrosine Kinases. Many growth factors mediate their effects by means of receptors with tyrosine kinase activity. These receptors have an extracellular ligand-binding domain, a single transmembrane domain, and an intracellular catalytic domain responsible for transducing the signal[59] (Fig. 11-6). Binding of growth factors to cell surface receptors results in receptor dimerization and activation of their intrinsic tyrosine kinase, leading to intermolecular phosphorylation of each receptor on specific tyrosine residues.[60] This results in the recruitment of signaling molecules containing Src homology 2 (SH2) domains,[61] which recognize, in a sequence specific manner, short peptide segments containing phosphotyrosine within activated receptors[62–64] (Fig. 11-7). These include proteins with enzymatic activity, such as phospholipase Cγ (PLCγ), phosphatidylinositol 3-kinase (PI3K), and the GTPase-activating protein for p21Ras (p120GAP), and proteins that lack enzyme activity and function as adaptor proteins, such as Grb2. Collectively, they act to

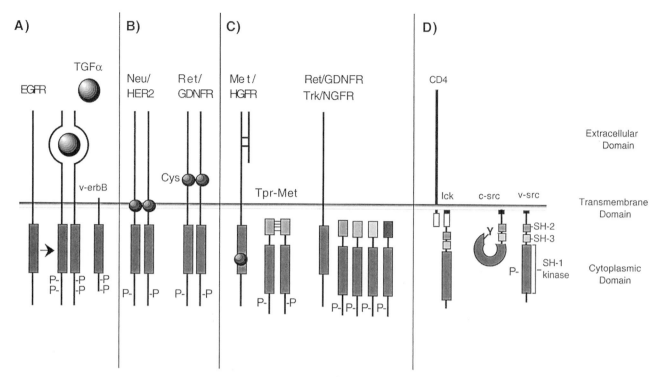

Fig. 11-6 Schematic comparison of structural features of cell surface growth factor receptor tyrosine kinases and membrane-associated tyrosine kinase oncogene products. The cytoplasmic tyrosine kinase domain is represented in grey (*src* homology 1 or SH-1), and SH-2 and SH-3 domains are indicated. A: Ligand binding to the epidermal growth factor receptor (EGFR) promotes receptor dimerization, activation of the kinase, and transphosphorylation of the receptor cytoplasmic domain on tyrosine residues, which then interact with SH-2 domain containing substrates and elicit an intracellular signal. The N- and C-terminal deletions, in addition to point mutations within critical domains of the molecule, that activate v-*erb*B are illustrated. Autocrine production of TGFβ in cells that express the EGFR results in constitutive activation of the EGFR. B: A single point mutation in the transmembrane domain of the *Neu/HER2* oncogene product is sufficient for ligand-independent activation. This mutation promotes receptor dimerization and kinase activation in the absence of ligand. Similarly, the loss of a single cysteine residue in the extracellular domain of the Ret receptor in multiple endocrine neoplasia type-2A syndrome results in a constitutively activated receptor. This mutation frees a cysteine residue that is normally involved in intrareceptor disulphide bond formation and enhances receptor dimerization presumably by the formation of intermolecular disulphide bonds promoting constitu-tive activation of the receptor catalytic activity. C: The gene rearrangements that activate the Met and Trk and Ret receptor-derived oncogene products. The majority of receptor oncogenes activated by gene rearrangement are fused with a protein domain capable of protein-protein interaction and thus mediate dimerization and constitutive activation of the kinase in the absence of ligand. D: The complex formed between CD4 and the Src family kinase Lck. The protein domains through which Lck and CD4 interact are represented as *open boxes* in these molecules. The c-Src kinase is maintained in an inactive conformation through the interaction of a negative regulatory phosphotyrosine residue in the C-terminus of c-Src with the Src SH-2 domain. The v-*src* oncogene is generated following deletion of this negative regulatory C-terminal tyrosine residue such that the kinase is now in an unconstrained conformation and is constitutively active. Following activation of many growth factor receptor tyrosine kinases, the c-Src SH-2 domain interacts with a phosphorylated tyrosine residue on the receptor with a greater affinity than its C-terminal phosphotyrosine residue (see Fig. 25-8). This relieves the negative regulation of c-Src and activates the kinase. EGF = epidermal growth factor; HGF/SF = hepatocyte growth factor-scatter factor; NGF = nerve growth factor; GDNF = glial cell derived nerve growth factor, TGFβ = transforming growth factor β.

transmit signals that mediate the pleiotrophic responses to growth factors (reviewed in Pawson, 1995[65] and Hunter, 2000[66]). PLCγ hydrolyzes phosphoinositols and thereby generates diacylglycerol and inositol-3-phosphate. PI3K phosphorylates phosphoinositides and generates putative second messengers for cytoskeletal rearrangements and cellular trafficking. By contrast, Grb2 lacks enzymatic activity and contains only SH2 and SH3 domains. SH3 domains also function as protein-protein interaction motifs and recognize proline-rich domains in other proteins.[67] Grb2 serves as an adaptor that binds to phosphotyrosines in activated receptors via its SH2 domain and recruits the Ras nucleotide exchange factors Son of sevenless (mSos-1 and mSos-2) to the receptor via its SH3 domain. Sos catalyzes exchange of GDP bound to Ras for GTP and is considered to be the most important step in Ras activation.[68,69] These proteins, through a series of protein-protein interactions, in part mediated through SH2 domains and SH3 domains, form signaling complexes downstream of receptor tyrosine kinases (reviewed by Pawson & Saxton, 1999[70]). Many of these signaling complexes regulate the activity of serine/threonine kinases, which in turn regulate through phosphorylation

the activity of transcription factors. A generalized scheme for receptor signaling is presented in Figure 11-7.

A number of oncogenes encode mutant forms of receptor tyrosine kinases. These include receptors for known factors, such as the epidermal growth factor receptor (EGFR) (v-*erb*B), colony-stimulating factor-1 receptor (CSF-1R) (v-*fms*), hepatocyte growth/scatter factor receptor (*met*), nerve growth factor receptor (*trk*), stem cell factor receptor (SCFR) (*kit*), neuroregulin receptor (Neu/HER2), glial derived neurotopic factor (GDNF) receptor (*ret*), and receptor-like proteins with unknown ligands (*ros*) (Table 25-1). In the receptor-related oncogenes so far examined, the structural changes that activate the transforming potential appear to deregulate the receptor kinase activity, and these oncoproteins transform by delivering a continuous ligand-independent signal (reviewed by Rodrigves & Park, 1994).[71] Receptors isolated as retrovirally transduced oncogenes, such as v-*erb*B (EGFR), v-*fms* (CSF-1R), and v-*kit* (SCFR) (Table 11-1), frequently sustain deletions of the extracellular ligand-binding domain in combination with other structural alterations, such as C-terminal deletions or mutations that remove negative regulatory

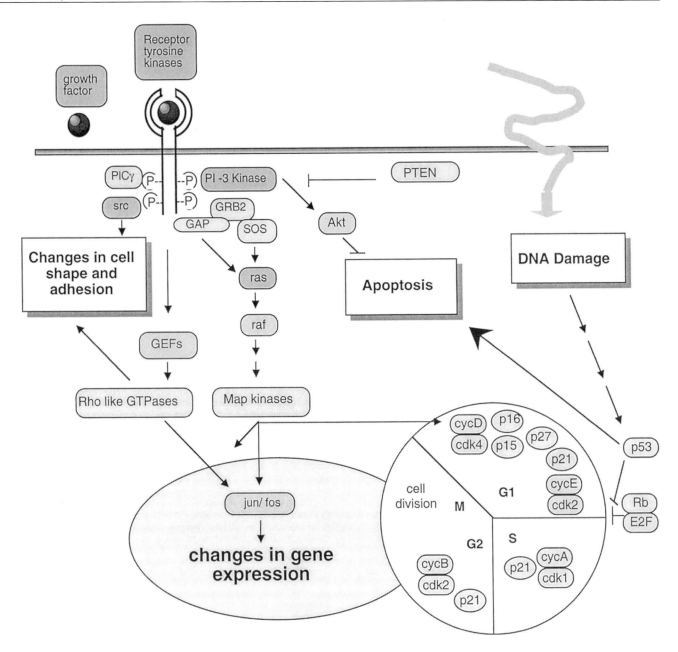

Fig. 11-7 Substrates and mitogenic signaling for receptor tyrosine kinases (RTKs). Activation of receptor tyrosine kinases by the binding of growth factors stimulates cross phosphorylation of their kinase domains. Substrates containing SH-2 domains bind to phosphorylated tyrosine residues on activated receptors. Substrates shown to directly interact with and become activated by or phosphorylated by RTKs; GAP (GTPase-activating protein), PLCγ (phospholipase Cγ), PI-3 kinase (phosphatidylinositol 3′ kinase), and Src (tyrosine kinase) are represented. The Grb2 adaptor protein that lacks enzymatic activity acts as a bridge to translocate the Sos guanine nucleotide exchange protein to the plasma membrane, where it stimulates the exchange of GDP for GTP, activating the Ras protein (see in detail in Fig. 25-8). Activation of Ras translocates the serine threonine kinase Raf to membrane, where it is activated by an unknown mechanism. Activated Raf then activates kinases of the MAP kinase pathway that stimulate the phosphorylation of transcription factors and expression of the *fos* and *jun* transcription factors. Secondary responses involve the breakdown of phosphatidylinositol 4,5 *bis*-phosphate into diacylglycerol (DAG) and inositol triphosphate (InsP3), which stimulate protein kinase C and calcium release, respectively. Components of the signal transduction pathway that have been identified as oncogenes are shown in grey.

domains and render the receptor catalytically active in the absence of ligand.[71])

Mutations that promote ligand-independent dimerization represent a general mechanism for oncogenic activation of receptor tyrosine kinases. A single point mutation in the transmembrane domain of the Neu/HER2 oncogene product is sufficient for ligand-independent activation. This mutation promotes receptor dimerization and kinase activation in the absence of ligand[72,73] (Fig. 11-6). Similarly, the loss of a single cysteine residue in the extracellular domain of the Ret receptor in multiple endocrine neoplasia type 2A syndrome results in a constitutively activated receptor. This mutation frees a cysteine residue that is normally involved in intrareceptor disulphide bond formation and enhances receptor dimerization by the formation of intermolecular disulphide bonds promoting constitutive activation of the receptor catalytic activity.[74,75] A similar mechanism has been demonstrated for the activation of the Neu/HER2 receptor in experimentally induced mammary neoplasias.[76] Alternatively, activation of the

Ret receptor in multiple endocrine neoplasia type 2B occurs by a single point mutation in the kinase domain that increases the basal kinase activity and alters the substrate specificity of the receptor, thus altering the signal transduction pathways activated by the receptor.[77,78]

A growing class of receptor tyrosine kinase oncogenes in human tumors, including *TRK, MET, RET*, and the platelet-derived growth factor receptor (*PDGFR*), are also rendered constitutively active following genomic rearrangements that juxtapose novel sequences derived from unrelated loci with the kinase domain of the receptor (Fig 11-7).[79] The majority of receptor oncogenes activated by gene rearrangement are fused with a protein domain capable of protein-protein interaction and thus mediate dimerization and constitutive activation of the kinase in the absence of ligand.[71] Receptor fusion oncogenes involving *RET* and *TRK* have been detected in papillary thyroid carcinomas.[80–82] In these tumors, both *RET* (10q11.2)[83] and *TRK* (1q21)[83] are rearranged with loci from the same chromosome, such as H4-ret (D10S170, Ptc) 10q21[83] and tropomyosin or tpr/trk (1q21-31).[84] Thus, small intrachromosomal deletions or inversions that are not readily detected cytogenetically may be a common event in the oncogenic activation of these receptor kinases in human tumors.

In addition to structural rearrangements, growth factor receptors are frequently amplified and overexpressed in human tumors. The EGFR is overexpressed in squamous cell carcinomas and gliomas,[36,37] Neu/HER2 in adenocarcinomas of the breast stomach and ovary,[38–40] *MET* (hepatocyte growth factor receptor, HGFR) in human stomach and some colon carcinomas,[85,86] and *bek*, a member of the FGFR family, in human stomach carcinomas[87] (Table 11-4).

Nonreceptor Protein Tyrosine Kinases. The protein products of v-*src*, v-*fes*, v-*fps*, v-*fgr*, v-*yes*, and *lck* are associated with the plasma membrane but are not transmembrane proteins (Fig. 11-6 and Table 11-1). Many of these proteins have a myristilated N-terminal glycine residue that promotes association with the plasma membrane. The cytoplasmic tyrosine protein kinase domain is in the C-terminus of the protein, and all of the tyrosine kinase oncogene proteins are homologous in this region. The *src* subfamily has additional regions of homology not found in the receptor family. These regions include two additional domains named *src* homology 2 and 3 (SH-2 and SH-3) (with SH-1 defined as the kinase domain) (Fig. 11-6).[88] As already discussed, the *src* homology 2 domain is highly conserved in proteins involved in signal transduction and recognizes phosphotyrosine residues, whereas the SH3 domain recognizes proline-rich motifs present in signaling proteins and cytoskeletal proteins.

Association of *src* family kinases with the plasma membrane is essential for their transforming activity. Mutation of the myristoylation signal in these proteins abolishes membrane association and transforming activity, indicating that their signal must be initiated at the plasma membrane, perhaps through interaction with other membrane-bound proteins.[56,89] Oncogenic activation of *src*-like kinases as retrovirally transduced oncoproteins occurs through the acquisition of point mutations and/or deletion of negative regulatory protein domains located at the C-terminus. These alterations generate oncoproteins that phosphorylate cellular proteins on tyrosine residues in an unregulated fashion and thus deliver a continuous, rather than a regulated, signal. The *src* or other *src*-like kinases are essential components of mitogenic signaling pathways downstream from receptor tyrosine kinases.[90] Moreover, *src* kinase activity is activated by receptor tyrosine kinases,[91] suggesting that *src* or *src*-like kinases would be activated in tumors where receptor tyrosine kinases are deregulated. Indeed, activation of c-*src* has been observed in mammary tumors in transgenic mice induced by an oncogenic Neu/HER2 receptor.[92]

The *abl* tyrosine kinase constitutes a separate family of nonreceptor tyrosine kinases that are localized to both the nucleus and the cytoplasm. The Bcr-Abl product has been implicated in the

pathogenesis of greater than 95 percent of CML. In a manner similar to receptor fusion oncoproteins, Bcr mediates oligomerization of Bcr-Abl, promoting constitutive activation of the Abl kinase[93] and association with downstream signaling molecules. Moreover, the Bcr-Abl oncoproteins are excluded from the nucleus, which may also prevent interactions with substrates that act to regulate cell growth negatively.[94]

Cytoplasmic Adaptor Proteins. The discovery that some oncogenes encode adaptor proteins that lack contain only SH2 and SH3 domains but lack any catalytic activity has enabled a more complete understanding of the role of these proteins in signal transduction. For example, the v-*crk* oncogene product[95] contains only SH2 and SH3 domains but causes an increase in tyrosine phosphorylated proteins in the cell.[96] Crk and other SH-2/SH-3 domain-containing adaptor proteins bind to phosphorylated tyrosine residues on activated receptor tyrosine kinases or other proteins via their SH2 domains and bind to other proteins via their SH3 domains. In this manner, they bring together heteromeric protein complexes that allow the subsequent phosphorylation of proteins in this complex by the kinase.[97,98] This phosphorylation event, in addition to dephosphorylation events, acts as a mechanism to relay the signal from the cell surface to the nucleus.

Proteins with GTPase Activity. The role of proteins with GTPase activity in tumorigenesis was first identified through the discovery of the *ras* oncogenes that encode a previously unknown form of GTPase. Three *ras* gene family members designated c-Ha-*ras*, c-Ki-*ras*, and N-*ras* involved in malignant transformation have been identified by their presence in rapidly transforming retroviruses and by DNA transfection. In normal cells, members of the *ras* family have been highly conserved throughout evolution and encode cytoplasmic proteins of 21,000 daltons (p21*ras*).[99] Ras proteins are posttranslationally targeted to the plasma membrane through a highly conserved sequence at their N- and C-termini. Membrane association is essential for function of Ras proteins. Certain domains in the Ras proteins are homologous to the subunit of trimeric G proteins, in regions involved in guanine nucleotide binding, and Ras proteins have been shown to bind guanine nucleotides (GTP and GDP).[99] The model proposed for the p21Ras proto-oncogene product is that it exists in equilibrium between two conformations: active, with GTP bound; and inactive, with GDP bound (Fig. 11-8).

In the past 10 years, components of signal transduction pathways have been elucidated and place Ras as a crucial regulator of cell shape, motility, and growth downstream from growth factor receptors (Fig. 11-7). Activation of Ras is coupled to ligand stimulation of growth factor receptors and is mediated by a guanine nucleotide exchange factor (GEF) (Sos). In the case of receptor tyrosine kinases, activation of Ras is mediated by binding of the Grb2 adaptor molecule via its SH2 domain to a specific phosphorylated tyrosine residue on the receptor. Grb2 pulls along the Sos protein, thus localizing it to the plasma membrane where its substrate Ras is localized. Sos then stimulates the exchange of GDP for GTP on Ras, converting Ras from an inactive to an active form[100,101] able to interact with an effector/substrate molecule(s)[102] (Fig. 11-8). Conversely, the inactivation of Ras is mediated in part by the intrinsic GTPase activity of Ras. Usually this activity is low; however, the GTPase activity is stimulated by a GTPase-activating protein GAP, which converts the active GTP-bound form of Ras into the inactive GDP-bound form.[103–105] GAP also contains an SH2 domain and is recruited by activated receptor tyrosine kinases to the plasma membrane.

The activation and inactivation of Ras proteins are carefully orchestrated. The conversion of Ras to the GTP-bound state enables it to interact with other proteins that function as downstream effectors for Ras. One effector for Ras is the serine-threonine kinase Raf. Activation of Ras recruits the Raf kinase to the membrane where it is activated. In turn, Raf activates a linear

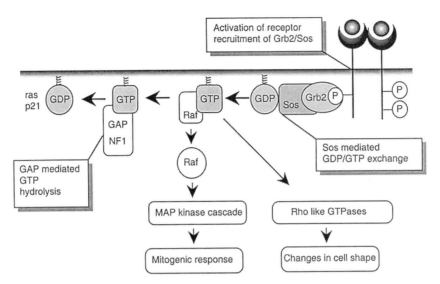

Fig. 11-8 Model for regulation of the Ras p21 product and for the GTPase-activating protein (GAP) as a downstream effector and regulator of *ras* activity. Ras is localized to the inner aspect of the plasma membrane. The alternating relaxed (GDP bound) and activated (GTP bound) states of the p21 Ras protein are shown in normal cells. Conversion of GDP- to GTP-bound forms is the rate-limiting step. Binding of the Grb2 adaptor protein to a specific tyrosine-phosphorylated residue on an activated (growth factor stimulated) receptor tyrosine kinase translocates the Sos guanine nucleotide exchange factor to the plasma membrane, where it stimulates the exchange of GDP for GTP on Ras. Activation of Ras alters its conformation and enables it to interact with and recruit the Raf serine-threonine kinase to the membrane where it becomes activated by an unknown (not Ras) mechanism. Activation of Raf activates the downstream MAP kinase signaling pathway involved in the mitogenic response. In addition, activation of Ras stimulates changes in cell shape and motility mediated through Rho-like GTPase proteins that are part of the Ras superfamily of small GTPase proteins. Inactivation of Ras is in part controlled by the intrinsic intrinsic Ras GTPase, catalyzed by GTPase-activating proteins (GAP and NF1). Oncogenic p21 Ras proteins with mutations at amino acid positions 12, 13, 59, or 61 remain in their active GTP-bound states and constitutively activate downstream signaling pathways.

signaling pathway involving a series of mitogen activated protein (MAP) kinases that culminates in the expression and activation of transcription factors Fos and Jun (Fig. 11-7). These in turn form the AP1 transcription factor that induces transcription of the c-*MYC* transcription factor, which in turn regulates genes whose products control cell cycle progression, culminating in one round of DNA replication and cell division.

The Raf protein kinase was independently isolated as a retrovirally transduced oncoprotein *v-raf* (Table 25-1). Inhibition of the Raf signaling pathway by specific inhibitors or through the use of dominant negatively interfering mutants[106] blocks transformation of fibroblasts in culture by an oncogenic Ras protein. In addition to Raf, transformation of cells by an oncogenic Ras also requires the activity of members of the Rho family of GTPases: Rho and Rac.[107,108] Members of the Rho family of GTPases are involved in rearrangements in the actin cytoskeleton and are thought to regulate the morphologic changes in cell shape associated with transformation of cells by Ras.[109,110]

The *RAS* oncogenes have been identified in a variety of tumors. As discussed previously, the oncogenic forms of Ras differ from their normal counterparts by mutations that result in amino acid substitutions at positions 12, 13, or 61 in the phosphate-binding domain of the protein (reviewed by Barbacid[111]). These oncogenic Ras proteins are locked in their active GTP-bound state through an increased exchange of GDP for GTP or through an inability to interact with or be dephosphorylated by GAPs.[112,113] They therefore have a reduced requirement for GDP/GTP exchange factors and no longer require activation by the Sos exchange factor.

Multiple GAP proteins that function to switch the Ras signal off have been identified. The p120 GAP and neurofibromin (NF1) were the first to be discovered. The p120 GAP appears to control the response of Ras to growth factor stimulation, whereas NF1 appears to control basal Ras activity.[114,115] In humans, loss of the GAP protein NF1 results in the disease neurofibromatosis type 1. Aspects of the disease can be explained in terms of elevated Ras-GTP and are thought to be the result of the loss of neurofibromin GAP activity.[116,117]

GTPase Exchange Factors

Support for Rho-like GTPases in cell transformation and tumorigenesis is also provided by the discovery that multiple independently isolated oncogenes act as exchange factors for Rho-type GTP-binding proteins. Dbl, Vav, Ect-2, Ost, Tiam, Lbc, Lfc, and Dbs were discovered by gene transfer methods by virtue of their ability to transform fibroblasts in culture[118] (Table 11-1). Tiam-1, which appears to directly influence the invasive capacity of T-lymphoma cells, was identified adjacent to a proviral insertion site in retrovirally induced invasive T-lymphoma varients.[119] The *DBL* oncogene was the first member of this family to be identified.[120] Amino acid sequence analysis revealed that Dbl shared homology with a yeast cell division cycle protein Cdc 24, which is an exchange protein for a yeast Rho-like small GTP-binding protein.[120] The homology was restricted to the domain of Cdc24 responsible for the GEF activity, and this result led to the discovery that Dbl is an exchange factor for a mammalian Rho-like protein (Cdc42).[121] All of the oncogenic exchange proteins for small GTP-binding proteins that have been identified, contain a similar domain that is now referred to as a Dbl homology domain. The Dbl domain is essential for the transforming activity of this class of oncogenes, suggesting that their exchange activity for Rho-like GTP-binding proteins is essential for transformation. A full characterization of the mechanism of oncogenic activation of this family of oncoproteins has not been achieved, but the deletion of N-terminal sequences of Dbl or Vav result in oncogenic activation.[122,123] These deletions may remove a negative regulatory domain that normally acts to regulate the GEF activities of these proteins. The current thinking is that Dbl and related proteins activate Rho-like GTP-binding proteins that play important roles in mediating various cytoskeletal reorganizations in cells. Unlike the signaling cascade in which the Ras GEF Sos participates, which binds to the adaptor protein Grb2 and translocates Sos to cell surface receptor tyrosine kinases to activate Ras in response to growth factors, the signaling complexes coupling Dbl-like GEFs to upstream components remain elusive.

Dbl-like GEFs act as exchange factors for members of the Rho family of small GTPases. These proteins are structurally related to the Ras family of GTPases. Members of the Rho family of small GTPases Rho, Rac, and Cdc42 are important regulators of the actin cytoskeleton. Microinjection of activated proteins into serum-starved fibroblasts demonstrates that Rho stimulates the organization of actin stress fibers, Rac stimulates the formation of lamellipodia, and Cdc42 induces filopodial formation.[124] Because of their effects on motile cytoskeletal structures, it is not hard to envision that inappropriate activation of Rho family of GTPases during tumorigenesis could affect whether a cell maintains a differentiated morphology or acquires a motile, invasive phenotype.

Cytoplasmic Serine-Threonine Protein Kinases

The serine-threonine kinases studied so far are soluble cytoplasmic proteins. This class includes the Mos, Cot, Pim-1, and Raf oncogenes in addition to protein kinase C (PKC) (Table 11-1). Oncogenic forms of the v-*raf* serine kinase have lost N-terminal regulatory sequences that lead to constitutive activation of the kinase activity and mitogenic MAP kinase pathway (Fig. 11-7). Phosphorylation of the c-Raf protein kinase is normally tightly regulated. Raf kinase activity is rapidly elevated when resting cells are stimulated by mitogens[125] (Fig. 11-7) or by another member of the serine-threonine kinase family, PKC. Several tumor promoters act via stimulation of the PKC family[126] and mediate activation of the Raf signaling pathway. Although a mutant form of PKCα has been detected as an oncogene and although overexpression of PKC can affect the growth of cells in culture,[127] mutant PKC enzymes are rare in human cancers.

Nuclear Protein Family

The products of oncogenes and proto-oncogenes localized to the nucleus are directly implicated in the control of gene expression involved in cellular proliferation and differentiation. Many of these have been shown to act as transcription factors and appear to be constitutively activated forms of their normal cellular counterparts (reviewed by Lewin, 1991[128]). For example, a complex between c-Jun[129] and c-Fos[130] corresponds to the mammalian transcription factor AP-l, which interacts following phorbol ester treatment or serum stimulation of cells with specific promoter elements to stimulate gene transcription.[131,132] The oncogenic Jun and Fos transcription factors carry mutations that lead to loss of negative regulatory elements, and these factors are now constitutively active.[133] In addition to loss of negative regulatory domains, some oncogenic transcription factors lose positive effector domains, resulting in *dominant negative* proteins that appear to prevent expression of genes required for cell differentiation.[134]

Since many nuclear oncogenes have been implicated in *trans*-activating and/or *trans*-repressing gene expression, it is possible that alteration of these genes either directly (activated c-*myc*, v-*jun*, or v-*erb*A) or indirectly (e.g., induction of their expression by an activated growth factor receptor) may lead to an imbalance in the delicate network of gene expression that regulates cell differentiation and growth control. Consistent with the hypothesis that nuclear oncogenes have central roles in events involved in cellular proliferation, the proto-oncogene forms of these genes are normally expressed in a variety of cell types during proliferation and have RNA and protein products with short half-lives. Because of the lability of the RNA and protein products, changes in transcription could lead to relatively rapid fluctuations in the steady-state levels of RNA and protein.[133] For example, c-*fos* and c-*myc* are expressed in replicating cells, but their expression is negligible in quiescent cells or during terminal differentiation.[134,135] When quiescent murine fibroblasts are stimulated with serum or growth factors to enter the Gl phase of growth, a transient increase in the levels of c-*myc*, c-*fos*, c-*jun*, and c-*myb* is observed (Fig. 11-5).[133–135] It is now accepted that these proto-oncogenes are required for cells to transit from a resting state (G0) to a state in which proliferation can proceed (Gl) (c-*fos*, c-*jun*, and c-*myc*) and to traverse specific points in the cell cycle.

The retroviruses that have transduced *myc*, *myb*, and *fos* express these genes in infected cells at levels higher than their cellular counterparts and in a nonregulated manner. Similarly, the amplification of the c-*MYC* locus in human tumors or the rearranged c-*MYC* locus in Burkitt lymphomas is no longer subjected to control, and these genes are expressed constitutively. Thus, the unregulated and/or ectopic expression of these genes in a differentiated cell substitutes for the growth factor requirement for quiescent cells to enter G1 and provides a constant proliferative signal in the absence of growth factors.

The identification of new oncogenes and tumor-suppressor genes can lead to the delineation of new signaling pathways involved in cancer. The recent dissection of the function of the adenomatous polyposis coli tumor suppressor and β-catenin has identified a critical role for these proteins in tumorigenesis. β-Catenin is found in two distinct multiprotein complexes in the cell. One complex located at the plasma membrane couples cadherins (calcium-dependent adhesion molecules) with the actin cytoskeleton, stabilizing cell-cell adhesion.[136] The other complex, which contains the adenomatosis polyposis coli (APC) protein, a serine-threonine kinase (glycogen synthase kinase 3β), and another protein called Axin, targets β-catenin for degradation.[137,138] In the absence of functional APC, β-catenin is not degraded and free β-catenin acts to enhance transcription through its interaction with a transcription factor: LEF1/TCF. This process is normally regulated by extracellular signals. Mutations in the APC gene that cause loss of function are found in multiple human tumors, thus stabilizing β-catenin and enhancing transcription.[139] Defects in the APC gene are responsible for inherited and sporadic forms of colon cancer and may account for up to 80 percent of the cancers in this tissue, implicating β-catenin-dependent signals as a key event in colon carcinogenesis.[140] Recently, mutations have also been identified in β-catenin that prevent its degradation induced by a wild-type APC protein.[141–143] These have been identified in human melanomas, hepatocellular carcinomas, cancers of the uterine and ovarian endometrium, and a small subset of colon cancers. Where studied, mutations in β-catenin and APC are mutually exclusive (reviewed by Polakis, 1999[144]). The APC gene is targeted for mutation in human colon cancer far more frequently than is β-catenin. This might relate to the specific dietary or environmental insults that give rise to these mutations. In contrast in experimentally induced intestinal tumors induced in rats, the majority contained mutations in β-catenin but not APC.[145] Once activated, β-catenin can constitutively interact with multiple different targets, thus sending persistent signals that override normal cell growth control. Activation of gene transcription through LEF/TCF is probably involved in the cancer process, as the proto-oncogene *myc* has recently been identified as one of the targets of the APC pathway.[146]

In addition to protein kinases acting as signal relays important for the control of cell growth and tumorigenesis, lipid kinases have emerged as controlling many cellular processes.[147,148] One subfamily of lipid kinases include phosphoinositide 3-kinases (PI3′K), which catalyze the addition of a phosphate molecule specifically to the 3-position of the inositol ring of phosphoinositides.[149] Phosphatidylinositol 3,4,5-phosphate acts as a ligand for some proteins that contain a phospholipid-binding PH domain.[150] One of these is a serine-threonine kinase (PDK1) that activates the Akt kinase.[151] Activation of Akt results in the phosphorylation of multiple proteins, some of which act to suppress apoptosis[152] whereas others stimulate a mitogenic response (Fig. 11-7).[153] Notably, the PI3′K and Akt gene β were identified as retroviral oncoproteins and the P13′K gene is amplified in human ovarian cancer.[154] In addition to enzymes that phosphorylate lipids, an enzyme called PTEN was recently identified that dephosphorylates PI-3,4,5. This acts to antagonize the activity of PI3′K, and loss of a functional PTEN gene has been demonstrated in multiple human tumors (reviewed by Cantley & Neel, 1999[154]).

COOPERATION BETWEEN ONCOGENES

Accumulating evidence suggests that the products of proto-oncogenes and growth-suppressor genes function in both common and parallel signaling pathways (reviewed by Weinberg, 1989[155]). The activation of cooperating oncogenes and the inactivation of growth-suppressor genes appear necessary for a complete neoplastic phenotype. Several events are required to influence aspects of the transformed phenotype: for example, cell shape, invasiveness, and anchorage-independent growth, in addition to blocking cell differentiation and driving a cell constantly through uncontrolled cell division. Transformation causes cells to acquire anchorage and/or serum independence, suggesting that oncogenes that cause anchorage-independent growth represent signaling molecules downstream from integrin-mediated adhesive events, whereas oncogenes causing serum independence are part of growth factor signaling pathways, and oncogenes inducing both are part of convergent pathways.[156]

Oncogenes and the Cell Cycle

The signals from the oncogenes described above converge on a control apparatus: the cell cycle clock that controls cell proliferation. The genomic changes and mutations observed in tumor cells are now considered to be the result of defects in checkpoints that control the cell cycle in response to DNA damage, defects in DNA replication, or chromosome attachment to the spindle (reviewed by Hartwell & Weinert, 1989[157]).

There are many regulated decision points required for a cell to progress through the cell cycle, and it is now clear that many of these are targets for oncogene action. Based on studies on yeasts and the conserved nature of the cell cycle components, the eukaryotic cell cycle is believed to be regulated at two major decision points: a point in G1 when a cell becomes committed to DNA synthesis and the G2 mitosis (M) boundary (Fig. 11-5) (reviewed by Murray, 1992[158]).

Many cells in vivo are in a quiescent state (G0) with unduplicated DNA. Growth-inhibitory signals are provided by soluble factors such as TGFβ, cell-to-cell contacts, and adhesion to extracellular matrix components,[159,160] whereas growth stimulatory signals are provided by growth factors. The balance between growth-inhibitory signals and growth stimulatory signals forces cells to make a decision to enter G1 and initiate cell division.[161] At a checkpoint in late G1 (the *restriction point*),[162] a cell decides whether the signals received are suitable for growth and progresses through G1 into S phase (Fig 11-5).

The transition through the restriction point in late G1 represents a critical point where a cell decides between continued proliferation and escape from the cell cycle. In recent years, it has become clear that the deregulation of this transition is critical to malignant growth. Cancer cells escape growth inhibition in several ways. One mechanism involves the activation of growth-promoting genes, growth factors, receptors, *RAS* genes, or nuclear oncoproteins that allow the cell to progress through G1, whereas a second mechanism involves the loss of receptors for growth-inhibitory genes such as TGFβ.[162] Once at the restriction point at the end of G1, the entry into S phase is governed through the activation of cyclin-dependent kinases. The G1 cyclins (D and E types) regulate the G1/S boundary, whereas mitotic cyclins (A and B types) regulate the G2/M transition (Fig. 11-5). Alterations in cyclins can cause transformation. Cyclin D1 was identified as the oncogene product of *PRAD1*, a gene rearranged in human parathyroid carcinomas[163] and expressed at high levels,[164] and as the product of the *bcl1* oncogene, a proviral integration site.[165] Cyclin D1 is amplified and its mRNA overexpressed in many tumor types.[166] Moreover, mice carrying a cyclin D1 transgene under the control of a mammary-specific promoter develop mammary hyperplasia and adenocarcinoma,[206] whereas overexpression of cyclin D1 and

c-*myc* in lymphoid cells of transgenic mice gives rise to lymphomas.[168,169]

The control of the G1-S checkpoint is regulated by the phosphorylation of the tumor-suppressor gene product Rb by cyclin D- and E-dependent kinases.[170] Phosphorylated Rb is unable to form complexes with E2F-type transcription factors, which are then free to induce transcription of S-phase-specific genes.[171] Regulation of this checkpoint is lost by several mechanisms. One involves the overexpression of cyclin D. Others involve the loss of function of the tumor-suppressor gene *Rb*, such that it no longer interacts with E2F, or loss of function of inhibitors of cyclin D (p16, p15).[172–174] Thus, the functional inactivation of *Rb* obtained either through the deregulated expression of cyclin D1, inactivation of inhibitors of cyclin D1 (p16, p15), or mutation in the *Rb* gene results in the loss of a cell cycle checkpoint and is thought to be an obligatory step for tumorigenesis.

The product of c-*mos*, a serine-threonine kinase, is also implicated in cell cycle control. It activates serine kinases of the MAP kinase family and is implicated in the reorganization of microtubules that lead to formation of the spindle pole during meiosis in oocytes.[175] The aberrant expression of *mos* in somatic cells leads to cells with 4N DNA content, possibly through interference with the assembly and positioning of the mitotic spindle.[176] Such an event could provide a mechanism for genetic instability that leads to the polyploid DNA content frequently observed in tumor cells.

Oncogenes and Cell Death

Whether in a normal tissue or in a tumor, the balance between cell death and proliferation governs the accumulation of cells. There is now evidence that induced suicide (apoptosis) is a major mechanism for the elimination of cells with DNA damage or an aberrant cell cycle, i.e., cells that are precursors for neoplastic changes. In contrast to *necrosis*, which represents a pathologic response to severe cellular injury, *apoptosis* is a cell's normal response to physiological signals or lack thereof (reviewed by Kerr & Harmon, 1996[177]). Apoptosis is an active process. Internucleosomal cleavage of DNA is a feature of apoptosis, and the resulting DNA ladder is used as an assay for apoptosis. Apoptotic cells can also be detected in tumors, either cytologically or by using molecular assays on tissue sections. Thus, cell death probably accounts for the slow growth rate of some tumors.

Some dominant oncogenes have been shown to exhibit a surprising biologic property: the ability to induce apoptosis. The c-*myc* proto-oncogene, whose expression is altered or deregulated in a large percentage of tumors, can promote apoptosis as well as proliferation.[178,179] Many cytokines are both survival and proliferation signals, suggesting that their receptors transduce signals that stimulate proliferation and entry into the cell cycle as well as inhibiting apoptosis. Thus, a mechanism coupling cell proliferation with apoptosis would provide a safety net for any proliferating cell when stimulated by a mitogen, or a mutation (amplified *myc*) would spontaneously induce cell death when it exhausted available cytokines (Fig 11-9).

Many of the signals that monitor the state of the cell in response to these distinct physiological signals converge on the p53 protein, which then signals the cell cycle clock to shut down until the problem, such as DNA damage is corrected, or alternatively will initiate cell death through apoptosis. The p53 tumor-suppressor gene (reviewed by Lane, 1992 Donehower & Bradley, 1993[180,181]) encodes a transcription factor that regulates the expression of proteins that negatively regulate the cyclin-dependent kinases required for cell cycle progression (reviewed by Hunter, 1993[182]). Thus, if induction of apoptosis were an automatic response to oncogene activation, then an increase in cell number would depend on active suppression of apoptosis.[183] This can be achieved through loss or mutation of p53, a frequent event in human cancers, where cells that sustain DNA damage or oncogene activation no longer trigger apoptosis.[180] Alternatively, the deregulated expression of the *bcl-2* oncogene mediates

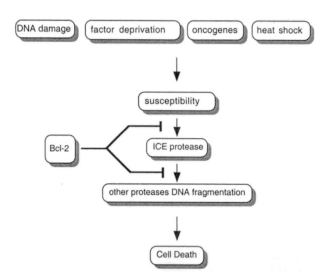

Fig. 11-9 Model for regulation of apoptosis by Bcl-2. Apoptosis is triggered by many agents, including DNA damage, factor deprivation, and oncogene activation (e.g., Myc and stress, such as heat shock). The ability of Bcl-2 to inhibit cell death caused by many different agents argues for the involvement of Bcl-2 in a final common pathway. This involves an ICE-like cysteine protease. Bcl-2 may suppress apoptosis by either preventing cleavage and activation of the cysteine protease proenzyme, interfering with proteolytic activity, or sequestering a target protein.

antiapoptotic effects and specifically blocks the ability of c-*myc* to induce apoptosis.[184,185]

The *Bcl*-2 oncogene was found at the junction of the chromosome 14;18 translocation in follicular lymphoma[186] (Table 11-1) and encodes a membrane-associated protein that is found in the endoplasmic reticulum and nuclear and outer mitochondrial membranes.[187] Although *BCL*-2 activation alone is not sufficient for follicular lymphoma formation, *BCL*-2 translocations appear to lead to cell immortalization and suggest an initiating role for *BCL*-2 in the etiology of tumors through prolonged cell survival. Bcl-2 is a member of a growing family of proteins that have been conserved throughout evolution and inhibits p53-mediated apoptosis induced by growth factor deprivation, deregulated *myc*, or genotoxic agents.[187,188] Since Bcl-2 can inhibit apoptosis induced by a wide variety of agents, the step regulated by Bcl-2 was thought to lie within a common final pathway. Indeed, Bcl-2 proteins inhibit the action of ICE-like proteases that trigger apoptosis (Fig 11-9).[189]

Experimental Evidence for Cooperating Oncogenes

It has been possible to subdivide the oncogenes further into two groups based on their phenotypes in DNA transfection assays performed in embryo fibroblast cells that have a finite life in culture. One class of genes rescues embryo fibroblasts from senescence, thus allowing cells to be continuously maintained in culture (*immortalization*), whereas the second class morphologically alters the rescued cells and renders them tumorigenic (*transformation*).[190-192] It was subsequently discovered that many of the oncogenes could be assigned to either the immortalization group or the transformation group. Furthermore, members of the immortalization group act synergistically with members of the transformation group to transform embryo fibroblasts; for example, foci of transformed cells appear when embryo fibroblasts are transfected with both v-H-*ras* and v-*myc* oncogenes.[190-191] The v-*myc* oncogene rescues cells from senescence and therefore belongs to the immortalization-complementation group, which includes the *myc* gene family and nuclear transcription factors *fos* and *jun* (Table 11-4). In this assay, the v-*ras* gene morphologically

transforms immortalized embryo fibroblasts and belongs to the transformation-complementation group.

NIH3T3 cells have properties similar to those of embryo fibroblast cells immortalized with a member(s) of the first complementation group, and therefore these cells are particularly useful in DNA transfection assays for identifying genes of the second complementation group (e.g., *ras*). In general, the protein products of the members of the first group are found in the nucleus and do not generally alter cell morphology or anchorage requirements but appear to immortalize cells. Conversely, products of the second group are found in the cytoplasm and, in most cases, are associated with the cytoplasmic side of the plasma membrane. These oncoproteins can reduce growth factor requirements, induce cell shape changes, and lead to anchorage-independent cell growth, but do not immortalize cells (reviewed in Hunter, 1997[193]).

TRANSGENIC MOUSE MODELS FOR CANCER

Compelling evidence for oncogene cooperation has also come from studies of transgenic mice.[194,195] Specific genes (*transgenes*) are introduced into the germ line of mice by microinjection of recombinant DNA into the male pronucleus of fertilized eggs. Progeny from implanted transgenic embryos are scored for the presence of the transgene by analysis of DNA extracted from the tail of the newborn animal. In this system, the action of activated oncogenes can be assessed in a host capable of mounting a physiological response to tumor formation.

Transgenic mouse strains carrying a single oncogene under the transcriptional control of ubiquitous promoter elements or tissue-specific promoter elements from heterologous genes generally show a strongly enhanced level of neoplasia or hyperplasia, but this frequently occurs only in specific tissues and not in all tissues expressing the oncogene. In many cases, oncogene expression precedes tumor formation by many months. Long latencies and variable penetrance may be observed; frequently, the tumors that do arise are both rare and clonal, inferring that other events are necessary.[197] Retroviruses carrying a single oncogene give rise to tumors, but this occurs largely through virus spread that recruits surrounding cells into forming a polyclonal tumor. Although chronic myelogenous leukemia may be initiated solely by Bcr-Abl expression, its chronic phase may actually represent a preneoplastic syndrome. In general, there is little evidence to support the concept that in vivo expression of a single oncogene can induce polyclonal tumors (reviewed by Frost et al, 1995[196]).

Tumor-prone transgenic mice provide insight into oncogene collaboration. Known or putative oncogenes can be tested for their ability to accelerate tumorigenesis. When two strains of oncogene-bearing mice are crossed, the tumor incidence is often greatly accelerated and increased. Moreover, an effective way to screen for many genes that can collaborate with the transgene is provided by insertional mutagenesis with a retrovirus that lacks an oncogene (Fig. 11-2). These viruses promote tumorigenesis by chance integration next to a cellular gene, altering its transcription. Consequently, sites of integration common to several tumors are used to identify genes that have contributed to the neoplastic process.

Studies with retroviruses and transgenic mice have identified eight genes that can cooperate with *myc* to transform lymphoid cells. In mice bearing a *myc* gene coupled to an immunoglobulin heavy-chain enhancer (Eu), constructed to mimic the translocations that occur in Burkitt lymphoma, B-lymphoid tumors invariably develop.[198] Tumor onset takes place randomly, however, and tumors are monoclonal in nature. Despite its proliferative signal, the deregulated expression of *myc* was not sufficient for full neoplastic transformation, and both the pre-B and B cells died rapidly if deprived of growth factors in culture. Thus, additional oncogenic mutations that can collaborate with the transgene are required. Doubly transgenic progeny from Eu-*myc* and Eu-N-*ras* mice rapidly developed B-cell tumors.[199] Thus, *myc* and *ras* are effective partners in leukomagenesis as well as other tumor types. In addition to *ras*, *myc* synergizes with the *raf* and *pim*-1 serine-threonine kinases in addition to the *abl* tyrosine kinase, the antiapoptotic gene *Bcl*-2, the transcription factor *bmi*-1, as well as mutations in the tumor-suppressor gene *p53*. Mutations in different genes are thought to provide complementary functions. For example, *myc* seems to prevent cells from becoming quiescent by overcoming the G1-S checkpoint, whereas *Bcl*-2 blocks apoptosis induced by expression of *myc* and others; for example, *ras*, *raf*, or *pim*-1 may decrease growth factor requirements.

The synergistic action of expression of v-Ha-*ras* and c-*myc* constructs also induces breast cancer when the transgenes are expressed in breast epithelia by using the mouse mammary tumor virus (MMTV) promoter/enhancer.[200] In all cases, however, tumors arise as clonal outgrowths, and nonmalignant cells expressing both oncogenes predominate. Moreover, *RAS* mutations are rare in human breast cancers. Instead, at least three proto-oncogenes have been implicated in human breast carcinogenesis. These include Myc, the HER2/Neu receptor tyrosine kinase, and Cyclin D1, each of which has been found amplified and overexpressed in human mammary tumors.[201,202] Similar transgenetic models for breast cancer have been made involving *myc*, *HER2/neu*, and cyclin D1 under the MMTV or whey acid protein promoter/enhancer.[203–206] Female transgenic mice from each of these systems develop mammary tumors, although it is apparent that events in addition to the transgene are usually required for tumor development.

TARGETING SIGNAL TRANSDUCTION PATHWAYS AS A METHOD FOR THERAPY

The high correlation of the clinical pattern of CML with the Phl chromosome and expression of the chimeric Bcr-Abl protein argue for a role of the *BCR-ABL* gene in the development of CML. Other cellular oncogenes have been implicated in the development of human neoplasia. The *HER*2 gene is amplified in mammary carcinomas with poor prognosis, and the *EGFR* (c-*erb*B) and c-*MYB* genes have been found to be amplified and overexpressed in certain tumors. The expression of the growth factor c-*sis* (B-chain PDGF) is increased in some human sarcoma and glioblastoma cell lines and tumors and may function as an autocrine for these tumors.

A major goal of new antitumor therapies involves interrupting the constitutive signals that drive tumor cell growth. The goal is to introduce agents that specifically turn off the signaling pathway(s) in a given tumor type. Signaling pathways can be inhibited by a variety of reagents, including small peptide-based mimics, antibodies, DNA encoding dominant negative proteins, antisense RNA, and target-specific RNA ribozymes. Most of the efforts to generate novel drugs aimed at signal transduction pathways are aimed at designing small molecules that act as specific inhibitors of enzymatic activity or protein-protein interactions interrupting the ability of docking proteins to interact with their receptor. Intensive efforts have therefore been invested in generating inhibitors of protein tyrosine kinase activity, and highly selective blockers have been synthesized.[207,208] Specific blockers for the EGFR have been shown to block the growth of solid tumors overexpressing EGFR,[209,210,211] although none of these studies reported complete eradication of the tumor. However, antibodies against the HER2/Neu receptor and EGF receptor are already in clinical trials as a treatment for breast cancer,[212] and cancers that overexpress the EGF receptor.[213] Complete tumor eradication was achieved in a JAK-2 kinase-driven pre-B-cell acute lymphoblastic leukemia model using an inhibitor of the JAK-2 kinase.[214] More importantly, no toxic side effects were observed. Specificity in these systems is, however, dependent on either the restricted expression of the oncogene primarily to tumor tissue, such as Jak-2, or an apparent decrease in the redundancy of growth factor-driven signaling pathways observed in human tumors.

Other targets are designed to inhibit proteins such as Ras and cyclin-dependent kinases that are involved in many mitogenic pathways. Specific inhibitors of cyclin-dependent kinases induce cell cycle arrest in the G1-S phase boundary of the cell cycle. Moreover, the frequency with which *ras* genes are activated in human tumors, and that gene's role as an important signal transducer for signals from protein tyrosine kinases, make it an ideal target for inhibitors. One effective strategy is based on the requirement of the Ras protein to first attach to the inner surface of the plasma membrane by linking to an isoprenyl group (farnesyl). A number of small molecules have been developed to inhibit this process in vivo,[215] and some of these inhibit the growth of Ras-transformed cells in vitro; however, the central nature of Ras action in normal cellular signaling pathways requires that inhibitors target only mutant Ras or Ras in tumor cells. Other strategies have been designed to interfere with the interaction of Ras with exchange proteins required for its activation. Other techniques involve gene therapy that is designed to introduce into tumor cells genes encoding dominant negative inhibitors of ras that produce a mutant protein that incorporates into and blocks the signaling pathway. Although these strategies have been used successfully in tumor cells in vitro, this approach awaits further development as a suitable anticancer therapy. As every tumor is usually driven by multiple signaling pathways, a combination of strategies may be essential for complete suppression of tumor growth. Considering that oncogenes were discovered only 20 years ago, the pace of recent developments in the molecular nature of their action has opened the gate to the ability to design specific inhibitors for each of these products.

SUMMARY

It is now accepted that cancer is a multistep process and that activation of oncogenes is involved in at least some steps of this pathway. Although the link between oncogene activation and initiation or progression of human cancer is complex, several oncogenes in human cancers have been identified. Thus, alterations to proto-oncogenes have been implicated in the genesis of human and animal tumors. The same rearrangements and mutations involving genes already identified by retroviral transduction have been found repeatedly in human and animal tumors. Clearly, the link between oncogene activation and development of human cancer is complex, but the discovery of oncogenes has provided a new method, particularly in hematologic malignancies, and now for sarcomas, for tumor diagnosis. Having sufficient information about the structure and function of the proteins encoded by dominant oncogenes will enable the design of specific inhibitors for each oncogene product and should ultimately lead to the development of new treatments for neoplastic disease.

REFERENCES

1. Stehlin D, Varmus HE, Bishop JM, Vogt PK: DNA related to the transforming gene(s) of avian sarcoma viruses is present in normal avian DNA. *Nature* **260**:170, 1976.
2. Temin HM: On the origin of genes for neoplasia: Clowes Memorial Lecture. *Cancer Res* **34**:2835, 1974.
3. Bishop JM: Enemies within: The genesis of retrovirus oncogenes. *Cell* **23**:5, 1982.
4. Aaronson SA: Growth factors and cancer. *Science* **254**:1146, 1991.
5. Hunter T, Karin M: The regulation of transcription by phosphorylation. *Cell* **70**:375, 1992.
6. Hanawalt PC, Sarasin A: Cancer-prone hereditary diseases with DNA processing abnormalities. *Trends Genet* **2**:124, 1986.
7. Vogelstein B, Fearon ER, Scott EK, Hamilton SR, Preisinger AC, Nakamura Y, White R: Allelotype of colorectal carcinomas. *Science* **244**:207, 1989.
8. Leach FSC, Nicolaides NC, Papadopoulos N, Liu B, Jen J, Parsons R, Peltomaki P, Sistonen P, Aaltonen LA, Nystrom-hahti M et al.: Mutations of a mutS homolog in hereditary non-polyposis colorectal cancer. *Cell* **75**:1215–25, 1993.

9. Fishel R, Lescoe MK, Rao MR, Copeland NG, Jenkins NA, Garber J, Kane M, Kolodner R: The human mutator gene homolog MSH2 and its association with hereditary nonpolyposis colon cancer. *Cell* **75**:1027, 1993 [erratum appears in *Cell* **77**:167, 1994].

10. Graham FL, Van der Eb AJ: A new technique for the assay of infectivity of human adenovirus 5 DNA. *J Virol* **52**:456, 1973.

11. Shih C, Weinberg RA: Isolation of a transforming sequence from a human bladder carcinoma cell line. *Cell* **29**:161, 1982.

12. Blair DG, Cooper CS, Oskarsson MK, Eader LA, Vande Woude G: New method for detecting cellular transforming genes. *Science* **218**:1122, 1982.

13. Goldfarb MP, Shimizu K, Perucho M, Wigler M: Isolation and preliminary characterization of a human transforming gene from T24 bladder carcinoma cells. *Nature* **296**:404, 1982.

14. Pulciani S, Santos E, Lauver AV, Long LK, Aaronson SA, Barbacid M: Oncogenes in solid human tumours. *Nature* **300**:539, 1982.

15. Parada LP, Tabin CJ, Shih C, Weinberg RA: Human EJ bladder carcinoma oncogene is homologue of Harvey sarcoma virus *ras* gene. *Nature* **297**:474, 1982.

16. Perucho M, Goldfarb MP, Shimizu K, Lama C, Pogh J, Wigler M: Human-tumor-derived cell lines contain common and different transforming genes. *Cell* **27**:467, 1981.

17. Barbacid M: *ras* Genes. *Annu Rev Biochem* **56**:779, 1987.

18. Bos JL: *ras* Oncogenes in human cancer: A review. *Cancer Res* **49**:4682, 1989 [erratum appears in *Cancer Res* **50**:1352, 1990].

19. Ahuja HG, Foti A, Bar-Eli M, Cline MJ: The pattern of mutational involvement of *RAS* genes in human hematologic malignancies determined by DNA amplification and direct sequencing. *Blood* **75**:1684, 1990.

20. Rowley JD: The critical role of chromosome translocations in human leukemias [Review, 94 references]. *Annu Rev Genet* **32**:495, 1998.

21. Rabbitts TH: Perspective: Chromosomal translocations can affect genes controlling gene expression and differentiation. Why are these functions targeted? [Review, 41 references]. *J Pathol* **187**:39, 1999.

22. Nowell PC, Rowley JD, Knudson AG Jr: Cancer genetics, cytogenetics: Defining the enemy within. *Nature Med* **4**:1107, 1998.

23. De Klein A, Van Kessel AG, Grosveld G, Bartram CR, Hagemeijer A, Bootsma D, Spurr NK, Heisterkamp N, Groffen J, Stephenson JR: Cellular oncogene is translocated to the Philadelphia chromosome in chronic myelocytic leukaemia. *Nature* **300**:765, 1982.

24. Wang JYJ: Abl tyrosine kinase in signal transduction and cell-cycle regulation. *Curr Opin Genet Dev* **3**:35, 1993.

25. Spencer CA, Groudine M: Control of c-*myc* regulation in normal and neoplastic cells. *Adv Cancer Res* **56**:1, 1991.

26. Stanton LW, Watt R, Marcu KB: Translocation, breakage and truncated transcripts of c-*myc* oncogene in murine plasmacytomas. *Nature* **303**:401, 1983.

27. Cooper CS: Translocations in solid tumours. *Curr Opin Genet Dev* **6**:71, 1996.

28. Alitalo K, Schwab M, Lin CC, Varmus HE, Bishop JM: Homogeneously staining chromosomal regions contain amplified copies of an abundantly expressed cellular oncogene (c-*myc*) in malignant neuroendocrine cells from a human colon carcinoma. *Proc Natl Acad Sci USA* **80**:1707, 1983.

29. Schwab M, Alitalo K, Klempnauer K-H, Varmus HE, Bishop JM, Gilbert F, Brodeur GM, Goldstein M, Trent J: Amplified DNA with limited homology to *myc* cellular oncogene is shared by human neuroblastoma cell lines and a neuroblastoma tumour. *Nature* **305**:245, 1983.

30. Schwab M: Oncogene amplification in solid tumors [Review, 46 references]. *Semin Cancer Biol* **9**:319, 1999.

31. Collins S, Groudine M: Amplification of endogenous *myc*-related DNA sequences in a human myeloid leukaemia cell line. *Nature* **298**:679, 1982.

32. Dalla-Favera R, Wong-Staal F, Gallo RC: *onc* Gene amplification in promyelocytic leukaemia cell line HL-60 and primary leukaemic cells of the same patient. *Nature* **299**:61, 1982.

33. Brodeur GM, Seeger RC, Schwab M, Varmus HE, Bishop JM: Amplification of N-*myc* in untreated human neuroblastomas correlates with advanced disease stage. *Science* **224**:1121, 1984.

34. Little CD, Nau MM, Carney DN, Gazdar AF, Minna JD: Amplification and expression of the c-*myc* oncogene in human lung cancer cell lines. *Nature* **306**:194, 1983.

35. Nau MM, Brooks BJ, Battey J, Sausville E, Gazdar AF, Kirsch IR, McBride OW, Bertness V, Hollis GF, Minna JD: L-*myc*, a new *myc*-related gene amplified and expressed in human small lung cancer. *Nature* **318**:69, 1984.

36. Yamamoto T, Kamat N, Kawano H, Shimizu S, Kuroki T, Toyoshima K, Rikimaru K, Nomura N, Ishizaki R, Pastan I, Gamou S, Shimizu N: High incidence of amplification of the epidermal growth factor receptor gene in human squamous carcinoma cell lines. *Cancer Res* **46**:414, 1986.

37. Reissmann PT, Koga H, Figlin RA, Holmes EC, Slamon DJ: Amplification and overexpression of the cyclin D1 and epidermal growth factor receptor genes in non-small-cell lung cancer. Lung Cancer Study Group. *J Cancer Res Clin Oncol* **125**:61, 1999.

38. Yokota J, Terada M, Toyoshima K, Sugimura T, Yamato T, Battifora H, Cline MJ: Amplification of the c-*erb*B-2 oncogene in human adenocarcinomas *in vivo*. *Lancet* **1**:765, 1986.

39. Zhou D, Battifora H, Yokota J, Yamamoto T, Cline MJ: Association of multiple copies of the C-*erb*B-2 oncogene with spread of breast cancer. *Cancer Res* **47**:6123, 1987.

40. Pegram MD, Pauletti G, Slamon DJ: *HER*-2/neu as a predictive marker of response to breast cancer therapy [Review, 39 references]. *Breast Cancer Res Treat* **52**:65, 1998.

41. Bishop JM: Molecular themes in oncogenesis. *Cell* **64**:235, 1991.

42. Bourne HR, Sanders DA, McCormick F: The GTPase superfamily: I. A conserved switch for diverse cell functions. *Nature* **348**:125, 1990.

43. Reuther GW, Der CJ: The Ras branch of small GTPases: Ras family members don't fall far from the tree [Review, 83 references]. *Curr Opin Cell Biol* **12**:157, 2000.

44. Medema RH, Bos JL: The role of p21ras in receptor tyrosine kinase signaling. *Crit Rev Oncogenesis* **4**:615, 1993.

45. Hunter T: Braking the cycle. *Cell* **75**:839, 1993.

46. Treisman R: Ternary complex factors: Growth factor regulated transcriptional activators. *Curr Opin Genet Dev* **4**:96, 1994.

47. Aaronson SA: Growth factors and cancer. *Science* **254**:1146, 1991.

48. Harrington EA, Fanidi A, Evan GI: Oncogenes and cell death. *Curr Opin Genet Dev* **4**:120, 1994.

49. Waterfield MD, Scrace GT, Whittle N, Stroobant P, Johnsson A, Wasteson A, Westermark B, Heldin CH, Huang JS, Deuel TF: Platelet-derived growth factor is structurally related to the putative transforming protein p28 sis of simian sarcoma virus. *Nature* **304**:35, 1983.

50. Shapiro WR, Shapiro JR: Biology and treatment of malignant glioma [Review, 66 references]. *Oncology (Huntington)* **12**:233 [Discussion 240, 246], 1998.

51. Halaban R, Langdon R, Birchall N, Cuomo C, Baird A, Scott G, Moellmann G, McGuire J: Basic fibroblast growth factor from human keratinocytes is a natural mitogen for melanocytes. *J Cell Biol* **107**:1611, 1988.

52. Yayon A, Ma YS, Safran M, Klagsbrun M, Halaban R: Suppression of autocrine cell proliferation and tumorigenesis of human melanoma cells and fibroblast growth factor transformed fibroblasts by a kinase-deficient FGF receptor 1: Evidence for the involvement of Src-family kinases. *Oncogene* **14**:2999, 1997.

53. Hoodless PA, Wrana JL: Mechanism and function of signaling by the TGF beta superfamily [Review, 160 references]. *Curr Top Microbiol Immunol* **228**:235, 1998.

56. Sagata N, Daar I, Oskarsson M, Showalter SD, Vande Woude GF: The product of the MOS proto-oncogene as a candidate initiator for oocyte maturation. *Nature* **245**:643, 1989.

57. Laird AD, Shalloway D: Oncoprotein signalling and mitosis [Review, 126 references]. *Cell Signal* **9**:249, 1997.

58. Hunter T: Protein kinases and phosphatases: The Yin and Yang of protein phosphorylation and signaling. *Cell* **80**:225, 1995.

59. Ullrich A, Schlessinger J: Signal transduction by receptors with tyrosine kinase activity. *Cell* **61**:203, 1990.

60. Schlessinger J, Ullrich A: Growth factor signaling by receptor tyrosine kinases. *Neuron* **9**:383, 1992.

61. Pawson T, Schlessinger J: SH2 and SH3 domains. *Curr Biol* **3**:434, 1993.

62. Cantley LC, Songyang Z: Specificity in protein-tyrosine kinase signaling [Review, 17 references]. *Adv Second Messenger Phosphoprotein Res* **31**:41, 1997.

63. Pawson T: Tyrosine kinases and their interactions with signalling proteins. *Curr Opin Genet Dev* **2**:4, 1992.

64. Fantl WJ, Escobedo JA, Martin GA, Turck CW, Del Rosario M, McCormick F, Williams LT: Distinct phosphotyrosines on a growth factor receptor bind to specific molecules that mediate different signaling pathways. *Cell* **69**:413, 1992.

65. Pawson T: Protein modules and signalling networks. *Nature* **373**:573, 1995.

66. Hunter T: Signaling: 2000 and beyond [Review, 93 references]. *Cell* **100**:113, 2000.

67. Rozakis-Adcock M, Fernley R, Wade J, Pawson T, Bowtell D: The SH2 and SH3 domains of mammalian Grb2 couple the EGF receptor to the Ras activator mSos1. *Nature* **363**:83, 1993.

68. Gale NW, Kaplan S, Lowenstein EJ, Schlessinger J, Bar-Sagi D: Grb2 mediates the EGF-dependent activation of guanine nucleotide exchange on Ras. *Nature* **363**:88, 1993.

69. McCormick F: *ras* GTPase activating protein: Signal transmitter and signal terminator. *Cell* **56**:5, 1989.

70. Pawson T, Saxton TM: Signaling networks: Do all roads lead to the same genes? [Comment] [Review, 21 references]. *Cell* **97**:675, 1999.

71. Rodrigues GA, Park M: Oncogenic activation of tyrosine kinases. *Curr Opin Genet Dev* **4**:15, 1994.

72. Weiner DB, Liu J, Cohen JA, Williams WV, Greene MI: A point mutation in the *neu* oncogene mimics ligand induction of receptor aggregation. *Nature* **339**:230, 1989.

73. Bargmann CI, Hung M-C, Weinberg RA: Multiple independent activations of the *neu* oncogene by a point mutation altering the transmembrane domain of pl85. *Cell* **45**:649, 1986.

74. Asai N, Iwasha T, Matsuyama M, Takahashi M: Mechanism of activation of the *ret* proto-oncogene by multiple endocrine neoplasia 2A mutations. *Mol Cell Biol* **15**:1613, 1995.

75. Saarma M, Sariola H, Pazchnis V: GDNF signalling through the Ret receptor tyrosine kinase. *Nature* **381**:789, 1996.

76. Siegel PM, Dankort DL, Hardy WR, Muller WJ: Novel activating mutations in the *neu* proto-oncogene involved in induction of mammary tumors. *Mol Cell Biol* **14**:7068, 1994.

77. Santoro M, Carlomango F, Romano A, Bottaro DP, Dathan NA, Grieco M, Fusco A, Vecchio G, Matoskova B, Kraus MH, Di Fiore PP: Activation of RET as a dominant transforming gene by germline mutations of MEN 2A and MEN 2B. *Science* **267**:381, 1995.

78. Carlson KM, Dou S, Chi D, Scavarda N, Toshima K, Jackson CE, Wells SA, Goodfellow PJ, Donis-Keller H: Single missense mutation in the tyrosine kinase catalytic domain of the RET proto-oncogene is associated with multiple endocrine neoplasia type 2B. *Proc Natl Acad Sci USA* **91**:1579, 1994.

79. Rodrigues G, Park M: Dimerization mediated by a leucine zipper oncogenically activates the met receptor tyrosine kinase. *Mol Cell Biol* **13**:6711, 1993.

80. Lanzi C, Borrello MG, Bongarzone I, Migliazza A, Fusco A, Grieco M, Santoro M, Gambetta RA, Zunino F, Porta GD, Pierotti MA: Identification of the product of two oncogenic rearranged forms of the RET proto-oncogene in papillary thyroid carcinomas. *Oncogene* **7**:2189, 1992.

81. Greco A, Pierotti MA, Bongarzone I, Pagliardini S, Lanzi C, Della Porta G: *Trk*-t1 is a novel oncogene formed by the fusion of *tpr* and *trk* genes in a human papillary thyroid carcinoma. *Oncogene* **7**:237, 1992.

82. Bounacer A, Wicker R, Caillou B, Cailleux AF, Sarasin A, Schlumberger M, Suarez HG: High prevalence of activating *ret* proto-oncogene rearrangements, in thyroid tumors from patients who had received external radiation. *Oncogene* **15**:1263, 1997.

83. Pierotti MA, Santoro M, Jenkins RB, Sozzi G, Bongarzone I, Grieco M, Monzini N, Miozzo M, Herrmann MA, Fusco A, Hay ID, Della Porta G, Vecchio G: Characterization of an inversion on the long arm of chromosome 10 juxtaposing D10S170 and RET and creating the oncogenic sequence RET/PTC. *Proc Natl Acad Sci USA* **89**:1616, 1992.

84. Martin-Zanca D, Barbacid M, Parada LF: Expression of the *trk* proto-oncogene is restricted to the sensory cranial and spinal ganglia of neural crest origin in mouse development. *Genes Dev* **4**:683, 1990.

85. Yonemura Y, Kaji M, Hirono Y, Fushida S, Tsugawa K, Fujimura T, Miyazaki I, Harada S, Yamamoto H: Correlation between over-expression of c-MET gene and the progression of gastric cancer. *Int J Oncol* **8**:555, 1996.

86. Vande Woude GF, Jeffers M, Cortner J, Alvord G, Tsarfaty I, Resau J: Met-HGF/SF: Tumorigenesis, invasion and metastasis [Review, 40 references]. *Ciba Found Symp* **212**:119 [Discussion 130, 148], 1997.

87. Porter AC, Vaillancourt RR: Tyrosine kinase receptor-activated signal transduction pathways which lead to oncogenesis [Review, 106 references]. *Oncogene* **17**:1343, 1998.

88. Pawson T: Non-catalytic domains of cytoplasmic protein-tyrosine kinases: Regulatory elements in signal transduction. *Oncogene* **3**:491, 1988.

89. Hunter T: Protein kinases and phosphatases: The Yin and Yang of protein phosphorylation and signaling. *Cell* **80**:225, 1995.

90. Twamley-Stein GM, Pepperkok R, Ansorge W, Courtneidge SA: The Src family tyrosine kinases are required for platelet-derived growth factor-mediated signal transduction in NIH 3T3 cells. *Proc Natl Acad Sci USA* **90**:7696, 1993.

91. Kypta RM, Goldberg Y, Ulug ET, Courtneidge SA: Association between the PDGF receptor and members of the src family of tyrosine kinases. *Cell* **62**:481, 1990.

92. Muthuswamy SK, Siegel PM, Dankort DL, Webster MA, Muller WJ: Mammary tumors expressing the *neu* proto-oncogene possess elevated c-Src tyrosine kinase activity. *Mol Cell Biol* **14**:735, 1994.

93. McWhirter JR, Galasso DL, Wang JYJ: A coiled-coil oligomerization domain of *Bcr* is essential for the transforming function of Bcr-Abl oncoproteins. *Mol Cell Biol* **13**:7587, 1993.

94. McWhirter JR, Wang JY: Activation of tyrosine kinase and microfilament-binding functions of c-*abl* by *bcr* sequences in *bcr/abl* fusion proteins. *Mol Cell Biol* **11**:1553, 1991.

95. Matsuda M, Mayer BJ, Fukui Y, Hanafusa H: Binding of transforming protein, P47gag-crk, to a broad range of phosphotyrosine-containing proteins. *Science* **248**:1537, 1989.

96. Mayer BJ, Hanafusa H: Association of the v-*crk* oncogene product with phosphotyrosine-containing proteins and protein kinase activity. *Proc Natl Acad Sci USA* **87**:2638, 1990.

97. Pawson T, Scott JD: Signaling through scaffold, anchoring, and adaptor proteins [Review, 72 references]. *Science* **278**:2075, 1997.

98. Pawson T, Saxton TM: Signaling networks: Do all roads lead to the same genes? [Comment] [Review, 21 references]. *Cell* **97**:675, 1999.

99. Barbacid M: *ras* Genes. *Annu Rev Biochem* **56**:779, 1987.

100. Egan SE, Giddings BW, Brooks MW, Buday L, Sizeland AM, Weinberg RA: Association of Sos Ras exchange protein with GRB2 is implicated in tyrosine kinase signal transduction and transformation. *Nature* **363**:45, 1993.

101. Downward J, Riehl R, Wu L, Weinberg RA: Identification of a nucleotide exchange-promoting activity for p21ras. *Proc Natl Acad Sci USA* **87**:5998, 1990.

102. Shields JM, Pruitt K, McFall A, Shaub A, Der CJ: Understanding Ras: "It ain't over 'til it's over" [Review, 55 references]. *Trends Cell Biol* **10**:147, 2000.

103. Trahey M, McCormick F: A cytoplasmic protein stimulates normal N-*ras* p21 GTPase, but does not affect oncogenic mutants. *Science* **238**:542, 1987.

104. Ellis C, Moran M, McCormick F, Pawson T: Phosphorylation of GAP and GAP-associated proteins by transforming and mitogenic tyrosine kinases. *Nature* **343**:377, 1990.

105. Boguski MS, McCormick F: Proteins regulating Ras and its relatives. *Nature* **366**:643, 1993.

106. Dudley DT, Pang L, Decker SJ, Bridges AJ, Saltiel AR: A synthetic inhibitor of the mitogen-activated protein kinase cascade. *Proc Natl Acad Sci USA* **92**:7686, 1995.

107. Qiu RG, Chen J, Kim D, McCormick F, Symons M: An essential role for Rac in Ras transformation. *Nature* **374**:457, 1995.

108. Khosravi-Far RSP, Clark GJ, Kinch MS, Der CJ: Activation of Rac1, RhoA and mitogen activated protein kinases is required for Ras transformation. *Mol Cell Biol* **15**:6443, 1995.

109. Hall A: Rho GTPases and the actin cytoskeleton [Review, 50 references]. *Science* **279**:509, 1998.

110. Nobes CD, Hall A: Rho GTPases control polarity, protrusion, and adhesion during cell movement. *J Cell Biol* **144**:1235, 1999.

111. Levinson AD: Normal and activated *ras* oncogenes and their encoded products. *Trends Genet* **2**:81, 1986.

112. Trahey M, McCormick F: A cytoplasmic protein stimulates normal N-*ras* p21 GTPase, but does not affect oncogenic mutants. *Science* **238**:542, 1987.

113. Clanton DJ, Hattori S, Shih TY: Mutations of the *ras* gene product p21 that abolish guanine nucleotide binding. *Proc Natl Acad Sci USA* **83**:5076, 1986.

114. Boguski MS, McCormick F: Proteins regulating Ras and its relatives. *Nature* **366**:643, 1993.

115. Henkemeyer M, Rossi DJ, Holmyard DP, Puri MC, Mbamalu G, Harpal K, Shih TS, Jacks T, Pawson T: Vascular system defects and neuronal apoptosis in mice lacking Ras GTPase-activating protein. *Nature* **377**:695, 1995.

116. Xu G, O'Connell P, Viskochil D, Cawthon R, Robertson M, Culver M, Dunn D, Stevens J, Gesteland R, White R, Weiss R: The neurofibromatosis type 1 gene encodes a protein related to GAP. *Cell* **62**:599, 1990.

117. Buchberg AM, Cleveland LS, Jenkins NA, Copeland NG: Sequence homology shared by neurofibromatosis type-1 gene and IRA-1 and

IRA-2 negative regulators of the RAS cyclic AMP pathway. *Nature* **347**:291, 1990.

118. Cerione RA, Zheng Y: The *Dbl* family of oncogenes. *Curr Opin Cell Biol* **8**:216, 1996.

119. Habets GGM, Scholtes EHM, Zuydgeest D, Van der Kammen RA, Stam JC, Berns A, Collard JG: Identification of an invasion-inducing gene, *Tiam*-1, that encodes a protein with homology to GDP-GTP exchangers for rho-like proteins. *Cell* **77**:537, 1994.

121. Ron D, Zannini M, Lewis M, Wickner RB, Hunt LT, Graziani G, Tronick SR, Aaronson SA, Eva A: A region of proto-*dbl* essential for its transforming activity shows sequence similarity to a yeast cell-cycle gene, *CDC24*, and the human breakpoint cluster gene, *bcr*. *New Biol* **3**:372, 1991.

120. Eva A, Aaronson SA: Isolation of a new human oncogene from a diffuse B-cell lymphoma. *Nature* **316**:273, 1985.

122. Katzav S: VAV: Captain Hook for signal transduction? *Crit Rev Oncogenesis* **6**:87, 1995.

123. Westwick JK, Lee RJ, Lambert QT, Symons M, Pestell RG, Der CJ, Whitehead IP: Transforming potential of Dbl family proteins correlates with transcription from the cyclin D1 promoter but not with activation of Jun NH2-terminal kinase, p38/Mpk2, serum response factor, or c-Jun. *J Biol Chem* **273**:16,739, 1998.

124. Hall A: Signal transduction pathways regulated by the Rho family of small GTPases [Review, 17 references]. *Br J Cancer* **80**:25, 1999.

125. Morrison DK, Kaplan DR, Rapp U, Roberts TM: Signal transduction from membrane to cytoplasm: Growth factors and membrane-bound oncogene products increase Raf-1 phosphorylation and associated protein kinase activity. *Proc Natl Acad Sci USA* **85**:8855, 1988.

126. Kikkawa U, Kishimoto A, Nishizuka Y: The protein kinase C family: Heterogeneity and its implications. *Annu Rev Biochem* **53**:31, 1989.

127. Housey GM, Johnson MD, Hsiao WLW, O'Brian CA, Murphy JP, Kirschmeier P: Overproduction of protein kinase C causes disordered growth in rat fibroblasts. *Cell* **52**:343, 1988.

128. Lewin B: Oncogenic conversion by regulatory changes in transcription factors. *Cell* **64**:303, 1991.

129. Rauscher III FJ, Cohen DR, Curran T, Bos TJ, Vogt PK, Bohmann D, Tjian R, Franza BR Jr: *Fos*-associated protein p39 is the product of the *jun* proto-oncogene. *Science* **240**:1010, 1988.

130. Bohmann D, Bos TJ, Admon A, Nishimura T, Vogt PK, Tjian R: Human proto-oncogene c-*jun* encodes a DNA binding protein with structural and functional properties of transcription factor AP-I. *Science* **238**:1386, 1987.

131. Distel RJ, Ro H-S, Rosen BS, Groves DL, Spiegelman BM: Nucleoprotein complexes that regulate gene expression in adipocyte differentiation: Direct participation of c-*fos*. *Cell* **49**:835, 1987.

132. Weinberger C, Thompson C, Ong E, Gruold, Evans R: The C-v-*erbA* gene encodes a thyroid hormone receptor. *Nature* **324**:641, 1986.

133. Greenberg ME, Ziff EB: Stimulation of mouse 3T3 cells induces transcription of the c-*fos* oncogene. *Nature* **311**:433, 1984.

134. Luscher B, Eisenman RN: New light on Myc and Myb. Part I. Myc. *Genes Dev* **4**:2025, 1990.

135. Muller R, Bravo R, Burckhardt J, Curran T: Induction of c-*fos* gene and protein by growth factors precedes activation of c-*myc*. *Nature* **312**:716, 1984.

136. Morin PJ: Beta-catenin signaling and cancer [Review, 88 references]. *Bioessays* **21**:1021, 1999.

137. Su LK, Vogelstein B, Kinzler KW: Association of the APC tumor suppressor protein with catenins. *Science* **262**:1734, 1993.

138. Rubinfeld B, Albert I, Porfiri E, Munemitsu S, Polakis P: Loss of beta-catenin regulation by the APC tumor suppressor protein correlates with loss of structure due to common somatic mutations of the gene. *Cancer Res* **57**:4624, 1997.

139. Shih IM, Yu J, He TC, Vogelstein B, Kinzler KW: The beta-catenin binding domain of adenomatous polyposis coli is sufficient for tumor suppression. *Cancer Res* **60**:1671, 2000.

140. Miyoshi Y, Nagase H, Ando H, Horii A, Ichii S, Nakatsuru S, Aoki T, Miki Y, Mori T, Nakamura Y: Somatic mutations of the APC gene in colorectal tumors: Mutation cluster region in the APC gene. *Hum Mol Genet* **1**:229, 1992.

141. Rubinfeld B, Robbins P, El-Gamil M, Albert I, Porfiri E, Polakis P: Stabilization of beta-catenin by genetic defects in melanoma cell lines [see Comments]. *Science* **275**:1790, 1997.

142. Morin PJ, Sparks AB, Korinek V, Barker N, Clevers H, Vogelstein B, Kinzler KW: Activation of beta-catenin-Tcf signaling in colon cancer by mutations in beta-catenin or APC [see Comments]. *Science* **275**:1787, 1997.

143. Takahashi M, Fukuda K, Sugimura T, Wakabayashi K: Beta-catenin is frequently mutated and demonstrates altered cellular location in azoxymethane-induced rat colon tumors. *Cancer Res* **58**:42, 1998.

144. Polakis P: The oncogenic activation of beta-catenin [Review, 71 references]. *Curr Opin Genet Dev* **9**:15, 1999.

145. Dashwood RH, Suzui M, Nakagama H, Sugimura T, Nagao M: High frequency of beta-catenin (ctnnb1) mutations in the colon tumors induced by two heterocyclic amines in the F344 rat. *Cancer Res* **58**:1127, 1998.

146. He TC, Sparks AB, Rago C, Hermeking H, Zawel L, Da Costa LT, Morin PJ, Vogelstein B, Kinzler KW: Identification of c-MYC as a target of the APC pathway [see Comments]. *Science* **281**:1509, 1998.

147. Fruman DA, Meyers RE, Cantley LC: Phosphoinositide kinases [Review, 153 references]. *Annu Rev Biochem* **67**:481, 1998.

148. Leevers SJ, Vanhaesebroeck B, Waterfield MD: Signalling through phosphoinositide 3-kinases: The lipids take centre stage [Review, 54 references]. *Curr Opin Cell Biol* **11**:219, 1999.

149. Vanhaesebroeck B, Leevers SJ, Panayotou G, Waterfield MD: Phosphoinositide 3-kinases: A conserved family of signal transducers [Review, 53 references]. *Trends Biochem Sci* **22**:267, 1997.

150. Fruman DA, Rameh LE, Cantley LC: Phosphoinositide binding domains: Embracing 3-phosphate [Review, 19 references]. *Cell* **97**:817, 1999.

151. Cohen P, Alessi DR, Cross DA: PDK1, one of the missing links in insulin signal transduction? *FEBS Lett* **410**:3, 1997.

152. Franke TF, Kaplan DR, Cantley LC, Toker A: Direct regulation of the *Akt* proto-oncogene product by phosphatidylinositol-3,4-bisphosphate [see Comments]. *Science* **275**:665, 1997.

153. Chang HW, Aoki M, Fruman D, Auger KR, Bellacosa A, Tsichlis PN, Cantley LC, Roberts TM, Vogt PK: Transformation of chicken cells by the gene encoding the catalytic subunit of PI 3-kinase. *Science* **276**:1848, 1997.

154. Cantley LC, Neel BG: New insights into tumor suppression: PTEN suppresses tumor formation by restraining the phosphoinositide 3-kinase/AKT pathway [Review, 76 references]. *Proc Natl Acad Sci USA* **96**:4240, 1999.

155. Weinberg RA: Oncogenes, anti-oncogenes, and the molecular bases of multistep carcinogenesis. *Cancer Res* **49**:3713, 1989.

156. Schwartz MA, Toksoz D, Khosravi-Far R: Transformation by Rho exchange factor oncogenes is mediated by activation of an integrin-dependent pathway. *EMBO J* **15**:6525, 1996.

157. Hartwell LH, Weinert TA: Checkpoints: Controls that ensure the order of cell cycle events. *Science* **246**:629, 1989.

158. Murray AW: Creative blocks: Cell cycle checkpoints and feedback controls. *Nature* **359**:599, 1992.

159. Attisano L, Wrana JL: Mads and Smads in TGF beta signalling [Review, 65 references]. *Curr Opin Cell Biol* **10**:188, 1998.

160. Massague J: TGF-beta signal transduction [Review, 290 references]. *Annu Rev Biochem* **67**:753, 1998.

161. Kimchi A, Wang X-F, Weinberg RA, Cheifetz S, Massagué J: Absence of transforming growth factor-β receptors and growth inhibitory responses in retinoblastoma cells. *Science* **240**:196, 1987.

162. Pardee AB: G1 events and regulation of cell proliferation. *Science* **246**:961, 1989.

163. Motokura T, Bloom T, Jueppner H, Ruderman J, Kronenberg H, Arnold A: A novel cyclin encoded by a *bcl*-1-linked candidate oncogene. *Nature* **350**:12,336, 1991.

164. Motokura T, Bloom T, Kim HG, Juppner H, Ruderman JV, Kronenberg HM, Arnold A: A novel cyclin encoded by a *bcl*1-linked candidate oncogene. *Nature* **350**:512, 1991.

165. Withers D, Harvey R, Faust J, Melnyk O, Carey K, Meeker T: Characterization of a candidate *bcl*-1 gene. *Mol Cell Biol* **11**:4846, 1991.

166. Motokura T, Arnold A: Cyclin D and oncogenesis. *Curr Opin Genet Dev* **3**:5, 1993.

167. Wang TC, Cardiff RD, Zukerberg L, Lees E, Arnold A, Schmidt EV: Mammary hyperplasia and carcinoma in MMTV-cyclin D1 transgenic mice. *Nature* **369**:669, 1994.

168. Bodrug S, Warner B, Bath M, Lindeman G, Harris A, Adams J: Cyclin D1 transgene impedes lymphocyte maturation and collaborates in lymphomagenesis with the *myc* gene. *EMBO J* **13**:2124, 1994.

169. Lovec H, Grzeschiczek A, Kowalski M, Moroy T: Cyclin D1/Bcl-1 cooperates with *myc* genes in the generation of B-cell lymphoma in transgenic mice. *EMBO J* **13**:3487, 1994.

170. Ewen ME: The cell cycle and the retinoblastoma protein family. *Cancer Metastasis Rev* **13**:45, 1994.

171. Nevins JR: E2F: A link between the Rb tumor suppressor protein and viral oncoproteins. *Science* **258**:424, 1992.

172. Hussussian CJ, Struewing JP, Goldstein AM, Higgins PA, Ally DS, Sheahan MD, Clark WHJR, Tucker MA, Dracopol NC: Germline p16 mutations in familial melanoma. *Nature Genet* **8**:15, 1994.

173. Kamb A, Shattuck-Eidens D, Beles R, Liu Q, Gruis NA, Drig W, Hussey C, Tran T, Miki Y, Weaver-Feldhaus J, et al: Analysis of the p16 gene (CDKN2) as a candidate for the chromosome 9p melanoma susceptibility locus. *Nature Genet* **8**:22, 1994.

174. Caldas C, Hanh SA, Da Costa LT, Redston MS, Schutze M, Seymour AB, Weinstein CL, Hruban RH, Yeo CJ, Kern SE: Frequent somatic mutations and homozygous deletions of the p16 (MTS1) gene in pancreatic adenocarcinoma. *Nature* Genet **8**:27, 1994.

175. Zhou R, Oskarsson M, Paules RS, Schulz N, Cleveland D, Vande Woude GF: Ability of the c-*mos* product to associate with and phosphorylate tubulin. *Nature* **350**:671, 1991.

176. Wang XM, Yew N, Peloquin JG, Vande Woude GF, Borisy GG: Mos oncogene product associates with kinetochores in mammalian somatic cells and disrupts mitotic progression. *Proc Natl Acad Sci USA* **91**:8329, 1994.

177. Kerr JFR, Harmon BV: Apoptosis: An historical perspective. *Curr Commun Cell Mol Biol* **3**:5, 1996.

178. Askew DS, Ashmun RA, Simmons BC, Cleveland JL: Constitutive c-*myc* expression in an IL-3-dependent myeloid cell line suppresses cell cycle arrest and accelerates apoptosis. *Oncogene* **6**:1915, 1991.

179. Evan GI, Wyllie AH, Gilbert CS, Littlewood TD, Land H, Brooks M, Waters CM, Penn LZ, Hancock DC: Induction of apoptosis in fibroblasts by c-*myc* protein. *Cell* **69**:119, 1992.

180. Lane DP: p53, guardian of the genome. *Nature* **358**:15, 1992.

181. Donehower LA, Bradley A: The tumor suppressor p53. *Biochim Biophys Acta* **1155**:181, 1993.

182. Hunter T: Braking the cycle. *Cell* **75**:839, 1993.

183. Bissonnette R, Echeverri F, Mahboubi A, Green D: Apoptotic cell death induced by c-*myc* is inhibited by *bcl*-2. *Nature* **359**:552, 1992.

184. Fanidi A, Harrington E, Evan G: Co-operative interaction between c-*myc* and *bcl*-2 can block drug-induced apoptosis. *Nature* **359**:554, 1992.

185. Hockenberry D, Nuñez G, Milliman C, Schreiber RD, Korsmeyer S: Bcl-2, an inner mitochondrial membrane protein blocks programmed cell death. *Nature* **348**:334, 1990.

186. Krajewski S, Tanaka S, Takayama S, Schibler M, Fenton W, Reed JC: Investigation of the subcellular distribution of the *Bcl*-2 oncoprotein: Residence in the nuclear envelope, endoplasmic reticulum, and outer mitochondrial membranes. *Cancer Res* **53**:4701, 1993.

187. Vaux DL, Weissman IL, Kim SK: Prevention of programmed cell-death in *Caenorhabditis elegans* by human *bcl*-2. *Science* **258**:1955, 1992.

188. Henderson S, Huen D, Rowe M, Dawson C, Johnson G, Rickinson A: Epstein-Barr virus-coded BHRF1 protein, a viral homolog of *Bcl*-2, protects human B-cells from programmed cell-death. *Proc Natl Acad Sci USA* **90**:8479, 1993.

189. Miura M, Zhu H, Rotello R, Hartwieg EA, Yuan J: Induction of apoptosis in fibroblasts by IL-1 beta-converting enzyme, a mammalian homolog of the *C. elegans* cell death gene ced-3. *Cell* **75**:653, 1993.

190. Parada LF, Land H, Weinberg RA, Wolfe D, Rotter V: Cooperation between gene encoding P53 tumour antigen and *ras* in cellular transformation. *Nature* **312**:648, 1984.

191. Yancopoulos GD, Nisen PD, Tesfaye A, Kohl NE, Goldfarb MP, Att FW: N-*myc* can cooperate with *ras* to transform normal cells in culture. *Proc Natl Acad Sci USA* **82**:5455, 1983.

192. Eliyahu D, Raz A, Gruss P, Givol D, Oven M: Participation of p53 cellular tumor antigen in transformation of normal embryonic cells. *Nature* **312**:647, 1984.

193. Hunter T: Oncoprotein networks [Review, 126 references]. *Cell* **88**:333, 1997.

194. Hanahan D: Transgenic mice as probes into complex systems. *Science* **246**:1265, 1989.

195. Adams JM, Cory S: Transgenic models of tumor development. *Science* **254**:1161, 1991.

196. Frost P, Hart I, Kerbel RS: Transgenic mice. *Cancer Metastasis Rev* **14**:77, 1995.

197. Quintanilla M, Brown K, Ramsden M, Balmain A: Carcinogen-specific mutation and amplification of Ha-*ras* during mouse skin carcinogenesis. *Nature* **322**:78, 1986.

198. Adams JM, Harris AW, Pinker CA, Corcoran LM, Alexander WS, Cory S, Palmiter RD, Brinster RL: The c-*myc* oncogene driven by immunoglobulin enhancers induces lymphoid malignancy in transgenic mice. *Nature* **318**:533, 1985.

199. Alexander WS, Bernard O, Cory S, Adams JM: Lymphomagenesis in Emu-*myc* transgenic mice can involve *ras* mutations. *Oncogene* **4**:575, 1989.

200. Sinn E, Muller W, Pattengale PK, Tepler I, Wallace R, Leder P: Coexpression of MMTV/v-Ha-*ras* and MMTV/c-*myc* genes in transgenic mice: Synergistic action of oncogenes *in vivo*. *Cell* **49**:465, 1987.

201. Lammie GA, Fantl V, Smith R, Schuuring E, Brookes R, Michalides R, Dickson C, Arnold A, Peters G: D11S287, a putative oncogene on chromosome 11q13, is amplified and expressed in squamous cell and mammary carcinomas and linked to BCL-1. *Oncogene* **6**:439, 1991.

202. Machotka SV, Garrett CT, Schwartz AM, Callahan R: Amplification of the proto-oncogenes int-2, c-erbB-2, and c-*myc* in human breast cancer. *Clin Chim Acta* **184**:207, 1989.

203. Cardiff RD, Muller WJ: Transgenic models of mammary tumorigenesis. *Cancer Surv* **16**:97, 1993.

204. Andres AC, Bchini O, Schubaur B, Dolder B, LeMeur M, Gerlinger P: H-*ras* induced transformation of mammary epithelium is favoured by increased oncogene expression or by inhibition of mammary regression. *Oncogene* **6**:771, 1991.

205. Wang TC, Cardiff RD, Zukerberg L, Lees E, Arnold A, Schmidt FV: Mammary hyperplasia and carcinoma in MMTV-cyclin D1 transgenic mice. *Nature* **369**:669, 1994.

206. Muller, W. J. Expression of activated oncogenes in the murine mammary gland: Transgenic models for human breast cancer. *Cancer Metastasis Rev* **10**:217, 1991.

207. Levitzki A, Gazit A: Tyrosine kinases inhibition: An approach to drug development. *Science* **267**:1782, 1995.

208. Gibbs JB, Oliff A: Pharmaceutical research in molecular oncology. *Cell* **79**:193, 1994.

209. Fry DW, Kraker AJ, McMichael A, Ambroso LA, Nelson JM, Leopold WR, Connors RW, Bridges AJ: A specific inhibitor of the epidermal growth factor receptor tyrosine kinase. *Science* **9**:1093, 1994.

210. Buchdunger E, Trinks U, Mett H, Regenass U, Muller M, Meyer T, McGlynn E, Pinna LA, Traxler P, Lydon NB: 4,5-Dianilinophthalimide: A protein-tyrosine kinase inhibitor with selectivity for the epidermal growth factor receptor signal transduction pathway and potent in vivo antitumor activity. *Proc Natl Acad Sci USA* **91**:2334, 1994.

211. Vincent PW, Bridges AJ, Dykes DJ, Fry DW, Leopold WR, Patmore SJ, Roberts BJ, Rose S, Sherwood V, Zhou H, Elliott WL: Anticancer efficacy of the irreversible EGFr tyrosine kinase inhibitor PD 0169414 against human tumor xenografts. *Cancer Chemother Pharmacol* **45**:231, 2000.

212. Shepard HM, Lewis GD, Sarup JC, Fendrly BM, Maneval D, Mordenti J, Figari I, Kotts CE, Palladino MAJR, Ullrich A: Monoclonal antibody therapy of human cancer: Taking the *HER*2 protooncogene to the clinic. *J Clin Immunol* **11**:117, 1991.

213. Baselga J, Mendelsohn J: Receptor blockade with monoclonal antibodies as anti-cancer therapy. *Pharmacol Ther* **64**:127, 1994.

214. Meydan N, Grunberger T, Dadi H, Shahar M, Arpaia E, Lapidot Z, Leader S, Freedman M, Cohen A, Gazit A, Roifman CM: Inhibition of recurrent human pre-B acute lymphoblastic leukemia by Jak-2 tyrosine kinase inhibitor. *Nature* **379**:645, 1996.

215. Kohl NE, Omer CA, Conner MW, Anthony NJ, Davide JP, Desolms SJ, Giuliani EA, Gomez RP, Graham SL, Hamilton K, et al: Inhibition of farnesyltransferase induces regression of mammary and salivary carcinoma in *ras* transgenic mice. *Nature Med* **1**:792, 1995.

Tumor-Suppressor Genes

Eric R. Fearon

Cancers arise as the result of an accumulation of inherited and somatic mutations in proto-oncogenes and tumor-suppressor genes. In contrast to the activating mutations that generate oncogenic alleles from proto-oncogenes, tumor-suppressor genes are targeted by loss-of-function mutations in cancer cells. A third class of mutated genes, with a rather more indirect role in cancer initiation and progression, has been identified; namely, the DNA-repair-pathway genes. Their inactivation in cancer is presumed to contribute to the development of mutations in other genes that directly affect cell proliferation and survival, such as the oncogenes and tumor-suppressor genes. Because DNA-repair genes are affected by loss-of-function mutations in cancer, they are often considered to represent a subset of the tumor-suppressor genes.

While a number of relatively straightforward approaches have enabled the identification of oncogenic alleles in cancer, identification of tumor-suppressor genes has proven more difficult. Somatic cell genetic studies provided early evidence that tumorigenicity was a recessive trait in many cancers. Based on such findings, the existence of tumor-suppressor genes was inferred. The somatic cell genetic approaches have provided a means to define specific chromosomal regions containing tumor-suppressor genes, even though few tumor-suppressor genes have been identified using the approaches.

Knudson's epidemiologic studies of retinoblastoma led to a proposal that has subsequently been termed the "two-hit hypothesis." In brief, Knudson proposed that two inactivating mutations were necessary for retinoblastoma development. The first mutation at the retinoblastoma susceptibility locus could be either a germ line or somatic mutation, while the second mutation was always somatic. Knudson's hypothesis not only illustrated the mechanisms through which inherited and somatic mutations might collaborate in tumorigenesis, but it linked the notion of recessive genetic determinants for cancer susceptibility to the findings from the somatic cell genetic studies.

To date, more than 20 tumor-suppressor genes have been localized and identified through various experimental approaches, often employed in concert. The approaches include cytogenetic studies of constitutional chromosomal alterations in cancer patients, linkage analyses to localize genes that predispose to cancer, and loss of heterozygosity (LOH) or allelic loss studies undertaken on matched pairs of normal and cancer tissue.

The authenticity of a tumor-suppressor gene is most clearly established by the identification of inactivating germ line mutations that segregate with cancer predisposition, coupled with the identification of somatic mutations inactivating the wild-type allele in the cancers arising in those with a germ line mutation. Supportive, but less convincing, evidence of a tumor-suppressor role for other genes may be presented, such as the identification of somatic, inactivating mutations in a gene in one or more types of cancer, or its decreased or absent expression in cancers. Largely because of the difficulties in assigning causal significance to any gene solely based on somatic alterations in its sequence and/or expression in cancers, genes not affected by inactivating, germ line mutations are most appropriately considered as candidate tumor-suppressor genes until additional data are available.

Powerful insights into the cellular functions of many tumor-suppressor proteins, such as pRb, p16, p53, and APC, have been obtained. It has become apparent that tumor-suppressor proteins function in a diverse array of signaling pathways and growth regulatory networks. In some cases, the protein products of tumor-suppressor genes and proto-oncogenes function in overlapping regulatory networks. Further studies of tumor-suppressor gene function will advance our understanding of cancer pathogenesis and the basis for the site-specific pattern of cancer often seen in individuals with germ line mutations in tumor-suppressor genes.

INTRODUCTION

Cancers arise, at least in part, as the result of two distinct, but linked, processes. The first process is mutation of cellular genes. The second process, termed clonal selection, promotes outgrowth of variant progeny with increased proliferative and survival properties. Two classes of genes—proto-oncogenes and tumor-suppressor genes—are affected by mutations in cancer cells. Oncogenes are distinguished by their harboring gain-of-function mutations that endow them with increased or novel function. In contrast, tumor-suppressor genes are affected by loss-of-function mutations. A third class of mutated genes with a more indirect role in cancer initiation and progression has been identified; namely, the DNA-repair-pathway genes. Because DNA-repair genes are affected by loss-of-function mutations in cancer, they are often considered to represent a subset of the tumor-suppressor genes. This chapter focuses predominantly on tumor-suppressor genes that appear to have direct effects on growth control. However, brief mention is made of some of the properties of the DNA-repair subset of tumor-suppressor genes. It also should be emphasized that the vast majority of mutations that contribute to the development and behavior of cancer are somatic and present only in the neoplastic cells of the patient. Although only a small subset of the mutations in a cancer cell are present in the germ line, when present, they not only predispose to cancer, but they can also be passed on to future generations. Studies of the mutations that underlie the highly penetrant inherited cancer syndromes have provided some of the most unique and compelling insights into tumor-suppressor genes and their role in cancer.

The relationship between proto-oncogenes and oncogenes and their functions in growth control and apoptosis have been extensively reviewed previously in Chapters 9, 10 and 11. More than 75 different proto-oncogenes have been identified through various experimental strategies.[1,2] In general, proto-oncogenes have critical roles in growth regulation, and their protein products are distributed throughout virtually all subcellular compartments. Point mutation, chromosomal rearrangement, or gene amplification of the proto-oncogene sequences generates the oncogenic variant alleles present in cancer.

The role of DNA-repair genes in cancer is extensively discussed in Chapters 13, 14 and 18. As noted above, the DNA-repair genes comprise a subset of the tumor-suppressor genes because they are affected by loss-of-function mutations in cancer.

Nevertheless, because of certain features they can be distinguished as a unique subset of the tumor-suppressor genes. Specifically, while protein products of many tumor-suppressor genes are likely to be directly involved in regulating cell growth or differentiation, many DNA-repair proteins are likely to have a more passive role in growth, differentiation, and cell survival. Their inactivation in tumor cells leads to the acquisition of a "mutator phenotype," with a resultant increased rate of mutations in other cellular genes. Because the accumulation of mutations in proto-oncogenes and tumor-suppressor genes appears to be rate-determining in tumorigenesis, the process of tumor progression is greatly accelerated by DNA-repair gene inactivation.

As is reviewed in subsequent chapters, enormous progress has been made in the identification of inherited and somatic mutations in tumor-suppressor genes. Therefore, the findings on the prevalence and nature of specific tumor-suppressor gene mutations in various cancer types are not summarized in any detail here. Rather, the primary aims of this chapter are to review the somatic cell, family, and loss of heterozygosity studies that established the existence of tumor suppressor genes; to provide an overview of the identification and function of selected tumor-suppressor genes; and to highlight some critical insights into cancer development provided by study of tumor-suppressor genes.

SOMATIC CELL GENETIC STUDIES

As reviewed in Chap. 11, the identification of oncogenic alleles in human tumors has been greatly facilitated by several of their features, including the prior identification of retroviral (*v-onc*) genes and the molecular cloning and characterization of novel oncogene sequences at translocation breakpoints.[1,2] In addition, the ability of certain oncogenes, such as activated *K-RAS* or *H-RAS* alleles, to generate tumorigenic properties when transferred to nontumorigenic recipient cells not only supports the critical role of oncogene mutations in cell transformation, but provides a straightforward functional approach for the identification of oncogenic alleles.[3–6]

In contrast, the direct identification of tumor-suppressor genes has proven far more difficult. For example, functional strategies for their identification have a number of theoretical and practical problems. Although the successful transfer of a functional copy of a tumor-suppressor gene to a tumor cell might be expected to revert aspects of its phenotype, the identification of such reverted cells in the midst of a background of fully transformed cells has proven to be a particularly arduous experimental task. Hence, the strategies for identification of tumor-suppressor genes and the mutations in these genes in human cancers have been more circuitous. Nevertheless, because somatic cell genetic studies provided early evidence supporting the existence of tumor-suppressor genes, the studies are reviewed here.

Harris and his colleagues were the first to demonstrate that the growth of murine tumor cells in syngeneic animals could be suppressed when the malignant cells were fused to nonmalignant cells.[7,8] However, tumorigenic revertants often arose when the hybrid cells were cultured for extended periods, and chromosome losses were found in the revertants. It was hypothesized, therefore, that malignancy was a recessive trait that could be suppressed in somatic cell hybrids. This proposal was further supported through studies of somatic cell hybrids from other rodent species and man.[8–10] Hybrids retaining both sets of parental chromosomes were suppressed for tumorigenic growth in athymic mice. Furthermore, it was demonstrated that the loss of specific chromosomes, and not simply chromosome loss in general, correlated with reversion. Tumorigenicity could be suppressed even if activated oncogenes, such as mutant *RAS* genes, were expressed in the hybrids.[11] Because the loss of specific chromosomes was associated with tumorigenic reversion, it was suggested that a single chromosome, and perhaps even a single gene, might be sufficient to suppress the tumorigenic growth of human cancer cells in nude mice. To directly test this hypothesis, single chromosomes were transferred from normal cells to cancer cells, using the technique of microcell-mediated chromosome transfer. As predicted, the transfer of specific human chromosomes suppressed the tumorigenic growth properties of various cancer cell lines.[12–17]

Although the tumorigenic phenotype can often be suppressed following single-chromosome transfer or cell fusion, other traits of the parental cancer cells, such as immortality and anchorage-independent growth, may be retained in the hybrids. Consistent with the notion that most malignant tumors arise from multiple genetic alterations, suppression of tumorigenicity might thus represent correction of only one of the alterations. Nevertheless, because the transferred genes suppressed at least some of the phenotypic properties seen in cancer cells, all genes that suppressed neoplastic growth properties in *in vitro* assays or *in vivo* tumor models have often been referred to collectively as tumor-suppressor genes. As is discussed below, this may be an overly broad definition of tumor-suppressor genes.

KNUDSON'S TWO-HIT HYPOTHESIS

Essentially concurrent with the somatic cell studies, Knudson undertook epidemiologic studies of retinoblastoma.[18] Although most cases of retinoblastoma are sporadic, in some families, autosomal dominant inheritance is seen. Knudson found that familial cases were more likely than sporadic cases to develop bilateral or multifocal disease. In addition, Knudson found that the familial and bilateral/multi-focal cases had, in general, an earlier age of onset. Knudson developed a model based largely on these observations.[18] In this model, he hypothesized that two "hits" or mutagenic events were necessary for retinoblastoma development in all cases (Fig. 12-1). In individuals with the inherited form of retinoblastoma, Knudson proposed that the first hit was present in the germ line, and thus in all cells of the body. However, inactivation of one allele of the susceptibility gene was insufficient for tumor formation, and a second somatic mutation was needed. Given the high likelihood of a somatic mutation occurring in at least one retinal cell during eye development, the dominant inheritance pattern of retinoblastoma in some families could be explained. In the non-hereditary form of retinoblastoma, both mutations were somatic and hypothesized to arise within the same

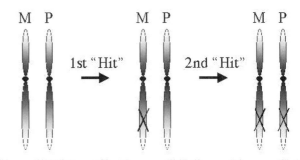

Fig. 12-1 Diagram of the Knudson "two-hit" hypothesis. Knudson proposed that two or more "hits" or mutagenic events were necessary for the development of retinoblastoma and perhaps other tumors. In individuals with inherited retinoblastoma, Knudson proposed the first hit in a retinoblastoma suppressor gene (*RB1*) was present in the germ line, predisposing all developing retino-blasts to cancer ("predisposed cells"). Inactivation of the second *RB1* allele resulted in retinoblastoma development. In the nonhereditary (sporadic) form of retinoblastoma, both *RB1* mutations were somatic. Consistent with retinoblastoma being rare in those who do not carry a germ line *RB1* mutation, there is a low probability that somatic mutations would inactivate both *RB1* in a single developing retinoblast. Knudson's hypothesis illustrated mechanisms through which inherited and somatic genetic changes might collaborate in tumorigenesis, and it postulated a role for recessive genetic determinants in human cancer.

Table 12-1 Germ line and Somatic Mutations in Tumor-Suppressor Genes and Functions of the Tumor-Suppressor Proteins

Gene	Associated Inherited Cancer Syndrome	Cancers With Somatic Mutations	Presumed Function of Protein
RB1	Familial retinoblastoma	Retinoblastoma, osteosarcoma, SCLC, breast, prostate, bladder, pancreas, esophageal, others	Transcriptional regulator; E2F binding
TP53	Li-Fraumeni syndrome	Approx. 50% of all cancers (rare in some types, such as prostate carcinoma and neuroblastoma)	Transcription factor; regulates cell cycle and apoptosis
p16/INK4A	Familial melanoma, familial pancreatic carcinoma	25–30% of many different cancer types (e.g., breast, lung, pancreatic, bladder)	Cyclin-dependent kinase inhibitor (i.e., cdk4 and cdk6)
p14^{Arf}(p19^{Arf})	?Familial melanoma?	Approx. 15% of many different cancer types	Regulates Mdm-2 protein stability and hence p53 stability; alternative reading frame of p16/INK4A gene
APC	Familial adenomatous polyposis coli (FAP), Gardner syndrome, Turcot syndrome	Colorectal, desmoid tumors	Regulates levels of β-catenin protein in the cytsol; binding to microtubules
WT-1	WAGR, Denys-Drash syndrome	Wilms tumor	Transcription factor
NF-1	Neurofibromatosis type 1	Melanoma, neuroblastoma	p21ras-GTPase
NF-2	Neurofibromatosis type 2	Schwannoma, meningioma, ependymoma	Juxtamembrane link to cytoskeleton
VHL	Von Hippel-Lindau syndrome	Renal (clear cell type), hemangioblastoma	Regulator of protein stability (e.g. HIFα)
BRCA1	Inherited breast and ovarian cancer	Ovarian (approx. 10%), rare in breast cancer	DNA repair; complexes with Rad 51 and BRCA2; transcriptional regulation
BRCA2	Inherited breast (both female and male), pancreatic cancer, ?others?	Rare mutations in pancreatic, ?others?	DNA repair; complexes with Rad 51 and BRCA1
MEN-1	Multiple endocrine neoplasia type 1	Parathyroid adenoma, pituitary adenoma, endocrine tumors of the pancreas	Not known
PTCH	Gorlin syndrome, hereditary basal-cell carcinoma syndrome	Basal-cell skin carcinoma, medulloblastoma	Transmembrane receptor for sonic hedgehog factor; negative regulator of smoothened protein
PTEN/MMAC1	Cowden syndrome; sporadic cases of juvenile polyposis syndrome	Glioma, breast, prostate, follicular thyroid, carcinoma, head and neck squamous carcinoma	Phosphoinositide 3-phosphatase; protein tyrosine phosphatase
DPC4	Familial juvenile polyposis syndrome	Pancreatic (approx. 50%), 10–15% of colorectal cancers, rare in others	Transcriptional factor in TGF-β signaling pathway
E-CAD	Familial diffuse-type gastric cancer	Gastric (diffuse type), lobular breast carcinoma, rare in other types (e.g., ovarian)	Cell-cell adhesion molecule
LKB1/STK1	Peutz-Jeghers syndrome	Rare in colorectal, not known in others	Serine/threonine protein kinase
EXT1	Hereditary multiple exostoses	Not known	Glycosyltransferase; heparan sulfate chain elongation
EXT2	Hereditary multiple exostoses	Not known	Glycosyltransferase; heparan sulfate chain elongation
TSC1	Tuberous sclerosis	Not known	Not known; cytoplasmic vesicle localization
TSC2	Tuberous sclerosis	Not known	Putative GTPase-activating protein for Rap1 and rab5; golgi localization
MSH2, MLH1 PMS1, PMS2 MSH6	Hereditary nonpolyposis colorectal cancer	Colorectal, gastric, endometrial	DNA mismatch repair

cell. Although each of the two hits could have been in different genes, Knudson later suggested that both hits might be at the same locus, inactivating both alleles of the retinoblastoma (*RB1*) susceptibility gene. Subsequently, loss of heterozygosity studies and definitive mutational analyses (see below) established this point. The significance of Knudson's hypothesis was two-fold: First, it illustrated the mechanisms through which inherited and somatic genetic changes might collaborate in tumorigenesis. Second, it linked the notion of recessive genetic determinants for human cancer to the somatic cell genetic studies.

APPROACHES TO IDENTIFY TUMOR-SUPPRESSOR GENES

Among the strategies successfully applied to the localization of tumor-suppressor genes are cytogenetic studies to identify constitutional chromosomal alterations in cancer patients; DNA linkage approaches to localize genes involved in inherited predisposition to cancer; and studies of chromosome regions affected by allelic loss (also termed loss of heterozygosity [LOH]) or, in some cases, loss of both alleles (termed homozygous deletion). The approaches ultimately require positional cloning methods to identify and isolate a tumor-suppressor gene from the chromosomal region or the thorough characterization of a positional candidate gene previously mapped to the region. Nevertheless, as summarized in Table 12-1, these strategies have been highly successful in identifying more than 20 tumor-suppressor genes.

Cytogenetic Studies Provide Clues to Tumor-Suppressor Gene Locations

Among the successful approaches to the localization of chromosomal regions that may contain tumor-suppressor genes have been cytogenetic studies carried out on peripheral blood lymphocytes from cancer patients. The rationale for such an approach is that chromosomal deletions, as well as some translocations, might be predicted to inactivate one of the two copies of a tumor-suppressor gene in the affected region. Unfortunately, only a very small subset of cancer patients has constitutional chromosomal deletions or rearrangements detectable by conventional cytogenetic techniques. Nevertheless, when noted, the chromosomal defects have proven extremely valuable for identifying regions likely to contain tumor-suppressor genes.

In upwards of 5 percent of patients with retinoblastoma, cytogenetic studies of peripheral blood lymphocytes or skin fibroblasts have revealed interstitial deletions involving band q14 of chromosome 13.[19] Similarly, some patients with the constellation of findings termed WAGR (for Wilms tumor, aniridia, genitourinary abnormalities, and mental retardation) have been found to have interstitial deletions of chromosome 11p13.[20] Cytogenetic studies of a mentally retarded man with hundreds of adenomatous intestinal polyps and no prior family history of polyposis revealed that the patient had an interstitial deletion involving chromosome 5q, suggesting that mutant alleles of a gene which predisposed to adenomatous polyps might map to chromosome 5q.[21] Furthermore, in some cancer patients, balanced translocations in constitutional cells have been noted, such as those involving chromosome 17q in a very small subset of patients with neurofibromatosis type 1 (NF-1), suggesting the presence of the *NF-1* gene on this chromosome.[22,23]

Linkage Analysis

Recurrent constitutional alterations of specific chromosomal regions in patients with a particular cancer type provide powerful evidence that cancer predisposition genes may reside there. Nevertheless, additional data are required to establish that the predisposition gene functions as a tumor suppressor (see below). Moreover, the identification of a single cancer patient with a constitutional deletion of a particular chromosomal region, such as the patient with the chromosome 5q deletion and polyposis, does not provide definitive proof that a Mendelian cancer predisposition gene maps to the region. In such cases, linkage analysis must be used to document that genetic markers from the implicated chromosomal region co-segregate with the inheritance of the disease phenotype in a number of large, multigenerational kindreds with a specific inherited cancer syndrome.

Localization of cancer predisposition genes for which a candidate chromosomal region has not yet been highlighted by cytogenetic studies can be accomplished using genome-wide linkage scans. Although linkage analysis can pinpoint the location of a cancer predisposition gene to a region much smaller than a chromosomal band, identification of the predisposition gene ultimately requires positional cloning approaches and/or detailed mutational analyses. In several cancer syndromes, including familial polyposis, von Hippel-Lindau syndrome, and neurofibromatosis type 2, further localization and eventual identification of each tumor-suppressor gene was greatly aided through studies of a subset of patients that had interstitial chromosomal deletions, which, while not detectable in conventional cytogenetic analyses, were readily detectable by techniques such as pulsed-field gel electrophoresis.[24–30]

Loss of Heterozygosity Studies

Cytogenetic studies of a subset of patients with retinoblastoma identified deletions involving chromosome band 13q14. Interestingly, in many patients with 13q14 deletions, levels of esterase D, an enzyme of unknown physiological function, were approximately half the levels seen in normal individuals.[31] This finding and further studies of families with inherited retinoblastoma established that the *esterase D* and *RB1* loci were genetically linked.[32] Subsequently, a child with inherited retinoblastoma was found to have esterase D levels approximately one-half of normal, although no chromosome 13 defects were seen in cytogenetic studies of his blood cells and skin fibroblasts.[33] Tumor cells from the patient had no esterase D activity, despite harboring a single copy of chromosome 13 that appeared intact by cytogenetic analysis. To explain the findings, it was proposed that the chromosome 13 retained in the tumor cells had a submicroscopic deletion of both the *esterase D* and *RB1* genes.[33] It was also suggested that cells with a defect in only one *RB1* allele had a normal phenotype. The effect of the predisposing mutation could, however, be unmasked by a second somatic event, such as loss of the chromosome 13 carrying the intact *RB1* gene. This proposal was entirely consistent with Knudson's two-hit hypothesis.

To establish the generality of these observations, others undertook studies of a panel of retinoblastomas using chromosome 13 DNA probes. On comparison of the marker patterns seen in paired normal and tumor samples, LOH or allelic loss of chromosome 13 was seen in greater than 60 percent of the studied tumors.[34] LOH of the 13q region containing the *RB1* locus resulted from various mechanisms (Fig. 12-2). In addition, through the study of inherited cases, it was shown that the *RB1* allele retained in the tumor cells was derived from the affected parent, and that the wild-type *RB1* allele had been lost.[35] These data established that the unmasking of a predisposing mutation at the *RB1* locus, whether the initial mutation had been inherited or had arisen somatically, occurred by the same chromosomal mechanisms.

Genetic analysis of somatically mutated alleles of tumor-suppressor genes can therefore supplement and reinforce information derived from analysis of germ line mutations. For example, LOH was found to target the chromosome 5q region implicated in predisposition to intestinal polyposis in a large fraction of sporadic adenomatous polyps and colorectal cancers.[36,37] Indeed, convincing evidence that a predisposition gene functions as a suppressor gene can be provided by data demonstrating that the chromosome harboring the wild-type allele of the gene is the target of LOH and the mutant allele is specifically retained in tumors. In the vast majority of cases, LOH affects many or all of the markers on the particular chromosomal arm carrying a predisposition and/or tumor-suppressor gene. For this reason, precise localization of a tumor-suppressor gene is rarely achieved by LOH analysis alone.

In addition to LOH affecting particular chromosome regions, a small fraction of cancers have deletions of both parental alleles in the region of a tumor-suppressor gene locus. Such deletion events are often termed homozygous deletions. If they are restricted in their extent, homozygous deletions can be particularly useful for pinpointing the location of a tumor-suppressor gene locus. The identification of homozygous deletions involving chromosome 13q12 and 18q21.1 sequences in certain pancreatic cancers proved instrumental in the localization and subsequent cloning of the *BRCA2* and *DPC4* tumor-suppressor genes, respectively.[38,39] Similarly, the identification of homozygous deletions of chromosome 10q23 sequences in brain, prostate, and breast cancers were critical in the identification of the *PTEN* gene.[40,41]

INSIGHTS INTO RATE-LIMITING MUTATIONS

Multiple mutations in oncogenes and tumor-suppressor genes are present in cancer cells. Distinguishing mutations that underlie cancer initiation from those likely contribute to tumor progression is a critical issue in the cancer genetics field. Most mutations that

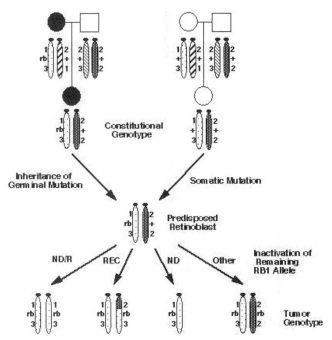

Fig. 12-2 Chromosomal mechanisms result in loss of heterozygosity for alleles at the retinoblastoma predisposition (*RB1*) locus at chromosome band 13q14. In the inherited setting (top left), the affected daughter inherits a mutant *RB1* allele (*rb*) from her affected mother and a normal *RB1* allele (+) from her father (constitutional genotype rb/+). DNA polymorphisms can distinguish the two copies of chromosome 13 in her normal cells (polymorphic alleles are designated by a number). Retinoblastoma arises after inactivation of the remaining wild-type *RB1* allele through these mechanisms: chromosome non-disjunction and reduplication of the remaining copy of chromosome 13 (ND/R); mitotic recombination (REC); non-disjunction (ND); and other more localization mutations that inactivate the remaining *RB1* allele (OTHER). In the non-inherited (sporadic) form of the disease, a somatic mutation arises in a developing retinal cell and inactivates one of the *RB1* alleles, and the remaining *RB1* allele is inactivated by one of the mechanisms shown. (Modified with permission from Cavenee W, Koufos A, Hansen M: Recessive mutant genes predisposing to human cancer. *Mutat Res* 168:3, 1986. The figure corresponds to Fig. 11-3 of Fearon ER: Oncogenes and tumor suppressor genes, in MD Abeloff, JO Armitage, AS Lichter, JE Niederhuber (eds). *Clinical Oncology.* New York: Churchill Livingstone, 1995.)

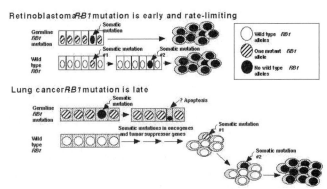

Fig. 12-3 Mutations in the retinoblastoma tumor-suppressor gene (*RB1*) contribute to inherited and sporadic cancers. The figure indicates that cell context affects the contribution of *RB1* mutations to cancer development. In individuals carrying a germ line mutation in one *RB1* allele, somatic inactivation of the remaining normal *RB1* allele is an early and rate-limiting event in retinoblastoma formation. Sporadic forms of retinoblastoma are also dependent on inactivation of both *RB1* alleles. Because somatic inactivation of both *RB1* alleles must occur in a single developing retinoblast before tumor formation can ensue, retinoblastoma is a rare disease in those who do not carry a germ line *RB1* mutation. A rather paradoxical finding is that those who carry a germ line *RB1* mutation are not highly predisposed to other cancer types, such as lung cancer, despite *RB1* mutations being frequently observed in sporadic forms of lung cancer (e.g., small cell lung carcinoma). These observations imply that *RB1* mutations are likely contributors to tumor progression rather than to tumor initiation in most cancer types, other than retinoblastoma and, perhaps, osteosarcoma. Possible explanations are that inactivation of both *RB1* alleles prior to the acquisition of other mutations in oncogenes or tumor-suppressor genes is not associated with any growth advantage, and perhaps *RB1* inactivation may even be associated with induction of apoptosis. (Figure modified with permission from Fig. 1 of Haber DA, Fearon ER: The promise of cancer genetics. *Lancet* 351 (suppl II):1, 1998.)

arise in somatic cells are likely to have little, if any, positive effect on cell growth and survival. In fact, many mutations may have detrimental or even lethal effects. Only a small fraction of mutations are associated with clonal selection, because mutations that promote clonal outgrowth must confer increased proliferative and improved survival properties upon affected cells. Those rare mutations that cause both significant expansion of a variant clone and a marked increase in the risk of malignant conversion of the clone's progeny are said to be "rate-limiting" for cancer development. The low frequency of mutations that can initiate the cancer process in a tissue is a critical bottleneck that presumably blocks or delays development of many cancers until late in adult life. However, after sustaining a rate-limiting mutation and successfully transiting the bottleneck, the generation of a highly expanded population of precancerous cells is essentially assured. Additional somatic mutations then arise in one or more of the precancerous cells and contribute to their progression to frank malignancy.

The role of rate-limiting mutations in cancer development is well illustrated in those individuals who carry inherited mutations in tumor-suppressor genes, such as the *RB1* and *APC* genes. Germ line inactivation of one *RB1* allele is not associated with any adverse effects per se. However, inactivation of the remaining functional *RB1* allele in developing retinoblasts initiates retino-

blastoma formation (Fig. 12-3). The likelihood that this second somatic event will occur in one or more developing retinoblasts of an individual with a germ line *RB1* mutation is very high, which explains why inherited retinoblastoma is often a highly penetrant, dominant syndrome, with cancers arising at an early age and often in a bilateral or multifocal pattern. Sporadic cases of retinoblastoma are also critically dependent on *RB1* inactivation (Fig. 12-3). However, in an individual lacking a germ line mutation of *RB1*, the likelihood is very low that both *RB1* alleles will be coincidentally inactivated by somatic mutation in a single, developing retinoblast. This accounts, therefore, for the low prevalence of retinoblastoma in the general population, as well as the disease's more common later onset and its unifocal presentation when it does occur.

Further support for the concept of rate-limiting mutations has been provided through studies of the *APC* gene. Germ line mutation of one *APC* allele in those individuals affected by familial adenomatous polyposis (FAP) predisposes to the development of hundreds to thousands of adenomatous polyps in the colon and rectum, and to a very high risk that one or more carcinomas will arise from the large population of adenomas.[42] In those with FAP, somatic mutation of the remaining wild-type *APC* allele leads to adenoma formation, indicating that the *APC* protein has a critical role in tumor suppression in intestinal epithelial cells. Similar to *RB1* inactivation in retinoblastoma, *APC* pathway inactivation may be a rate-limiting step in essentially all colorectal tumors, because more than 75 percent of sporadic colorectal adenomas and carcinomas have somatic mutations inactivating *APC* function.[42]

TISSUE-SPECIFIC EFFECTS OF GERM LINE MUTATIONS

In general, those individuals carrying a germ line mutation of a specific tumor-suppressor gene are predisposed to a limited spectrum of cancer types. This finding is puzzling for at least two reasons. First, most tumor-suppressor genes are expressed in many different adult tissues. Second, somatic mutations in certain tumor-suppressor genes are present in a broad spectrum of sporadic cancer types (Table 12-1). With respect to this latter point, children who carry a germ line mutation in the *RB1* gene have a very elevated risk of developing retinoblastoma, and a more modest risk of developing osteosarcoma, but no significantly increased risk of most common cancers. Thus, it is curious that somatic *RB1* mutations have been found and are believed critical in the development of many different cancer types, such as lung, breast, prostate, pancreas, and bladder cancer. Several potential explanations have been offered, and two are considered here. The *RB1* gene may be a primary controlling factor in retinoblast growth regulation, such that its inactivation leads to retinoblastoma. However, in other tissues, including lung or breast epithelial cells, *RB1* may have a less critical or even redundant role in growth control, and its inactivation may not promote neoplastic growth unless other mutations are also present (Fig. 12-3). An alternative, and perhaps equally tenable, proposal is that somatic inactivation of *RB1* may trigger programmed cell death or apoptosis in many cells types, unless other somatic mutations have arisen previously and altered the cell's ability to resist apoptosis following disruption of *RB1* function (Fig. 12-3).

TUMOR-SUPPRESSOR GENE FUNCTION

The protein products of tumor-suppressor genes have been implicated in a diverse array of cellular processes, including cell-cycle control, differentiation, cell-cell adhesion, apoptosis, and maintenance of genomic integrity. The presumed functions of selected tumor suppressor proteins are summarized in Table 12-1. Given the diversity of their functions, have any themes emerged? Yes, some have emerged. Perhaps the principal theme is that the protein products of tumor-suppressor genes often function in conserved signaling pathways. Moreover, in these signaling pathways, individual tumor-suppressor proteins function in concert with the products of other tumor-suppressor genes and proto-oncogenes.

One of the best studied of these regulatory networks is the one in which the *RB1* gene and its protein product pRb function.[43] The pRb protein appears to have an important role in regulating cell-cycle progression, presumably as a result of its ability to silence expression of E2F-target genes, such as those needed for the DNA synthetic (S) phase of the cell cycle. The functional activity of the pRb protein is correlated with its phosphorylation status, and the cyclin D1 protein and cyclin-dependent kinase 4 (cdk4) proteins regulate pRb phosphorylation. The p16 tumor-suppressor protein is a critical regulator of the activity of the cdk4/cyclin D1 complex. As noted above, a subset of sporadic cancers of various types have inactivating mutation in the *RB1* gene. In other cancers, the pRb functional pathway is inactivated as a result of mutations in other components of the pathway.[43] Many cancers that lack *RB1* mutations have inactivating mutations in the p16/INK4A gene. In others that lack *RB1* mutations, such as some breast cancers, gene amplification and overexpression of cyclin D1 is found. In other cancers, such as some glioblastomas and sarcomas, amplification and overexpression of the *CDK4* gene is frequently observed. The net effect of mutations in the pathway is to inactivate pRb function, including its ability to regulate expression of E2F-target genes (Fig. 12-4*A*).

Studies of other tumor-suppressor proteins have also supported the existence of regulatory networks in which tumor-suppressor gene and proto-oncogene protein products function. A critical function of the APC protein is regulation of β-catenin (β-cat) protein stability in the cytosol (Fig. 12-4*B*) (reviewed in reference 44). APC mutations result in increased levels of β-cat in the cell, and constitutive complexing of β-cat with transcription factors of the T-cell factor (Tcf) or lymphoid-enhancer factor (Lef) family, such as Tcf-4. When bound to Tcf/Lef factors, β-cat functions as a

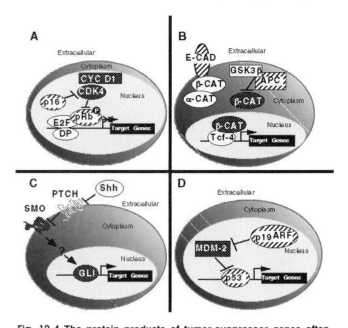

Fig. 12-4 The protein products of tumor-suppressor genes often function in conserved signaling pathways with other tumor-suppressor gene and oncogene protein products. Tumor-suppressor proteins are indicated with striped symbols and oncogene proteins with filled symbols. *A*, The pRb tumor-suppressor pathway. The protein product of the *RB1* gene, pRb, is regulated by phosphorylation. The hyperphosphorylated form of pRb is inactive and unable to bind to E2F and regulate transcription of E2F-target genes. The cyclin D1 (CYC D1) and cyclin-dependent kinase 4 (CDK4) proteins appear to have a critical role in regulating pRb phosphorylation. The p16 protein is a critical inhibitor of the activity of the CYC D1 and CDK4 complex. Inactivating mutations in the pRb or p16 tumor-suppressor proteins or activating mutations (e.g., gene amplification) of CYC D1 or CDK4 are present in the majority of cancers. *B*, The APC and E-cadherin tumor-suppressor pathways. The APC protein, in collaboration with glycogen synthase kinase 3β (GSK3β), has a critical role in regulating β-catein (β-CAT) protein stability in the cell. If APC is inactivated by mutation, or β-CAT is activated by mutation of its N-terminus, β-CAT levels cannot be appropriately regulated. β-CAT complexes with Tcf (T-cell factor) or Lef (lymphoid-enhancer factor) transcription factors, such as Tcf-4, and activates expression of Tcf-target genes (e.g., *c-MYC*). β-CAT also functions in E-cadherin (E-CAD) cell-cell adhesion, linking E-CAD to the cytoskeleton via its interaction with α-catenin (α-CAT). E-CAD functions as a tumor-suppressor gene, although it is not clear that the consequence of E-CAD inactivation is similar to that of APC inactivation; i.e., there are no data to demonstrate that E-CAD and APC function in a shared or common signaling pathway even though both proteins interact with β-CAT. *C*, The patched (*PTCH*) tumor-suppressor pathway. Germ line mutations in the *PTCH* gene are responsible for Gorlin syndrome and hereditary nevoid basal-cell cancer syndrome, in which affected individuals develop large numbers of basal-cell cancers, as well as medulloblastomas. The *PTCH* protein inhibits the activity of the smoothened (*SMO*) protein, and the sonic hedgehog (Shh) factor regulates *PTCH* activity. *SMO* functions to activate expression of the Gli transcription factor. Inactivating mutations in *PTCH*, or activating mutation in *SMO* or Gli, have been found in cancer, and are mutually exclusive. *D*, The p53 tumor-suppressor pathway. p53 functions as a transcription factor and regulates expression of a large number of target genes with roles in cell cycle control and apoptosis (e.g., p21, Bax). p53 protein stability is regulated by the MDM-2 protein, and MDM-2 protein stability is regulated by the p19^Arf (also known as p14^Arf) protein. Inactivating mutation in p53 are found in upwards of 50 percent of all human cancers. In some cancers, activating mutations in MDM-2 or inactivation of p19^Arf appear to have the same net consequence as p53 inactivation. (Figure modified with permission from Fig. 2 of Haber DA, Fearon ER. The promise of cancer genetics. *Lancet* 351 (suppl II):1, 1998.)

transcriptional coactivator, and, in cancers with APC mutations, Tcf transcriptional activity is deregulated. In a subset of the colorectal cancers lacking APC inactivation, activating (oncogenic) mutations in the β-cat protein have been found. These mutations render β-cat resistant to regulation by APC, and the mutant β-cat protein accumulates in the cell and deregulates Tcf transcription. While most Tcf-4-regulated genes remain to be identified, the *c-MYC* gene was recently suggested as a target of the APC/β-cat/Tcf-4 pathway, and mutations in APC or β-cat appear to result in transcriptional activation of *c-MYC*.[45] Other tumor-suppressor gene regulatory networks include the p53/mdm-2/p19[Arf] and Ptch/Smo/Gli networks (Figs. 12-4*C* and 12-4*D*).

CANDIDATE TUMOR-SUPPRESSOR GENES

The tumor-suppressor genes discussed above and summarized in Table 12-1 are noteworthy in that germ line-inactivating mutations in the genes are associated with inherited predisposition to cancer. The link between germ line mutation and inherited cancer provides incontrovertible evidence of the importance of the genes in tumorigenesis. In addition, as reviewed above, other findings, such as the demonstration of LOH of one allele of a tumor-suppressor gene and somatic mutation of the remaining allele in sporadic tumors, often support a more widespread role for many of the genes in cancer (Table 12-1). While many members of the tumor-suppressor gene class have been definitively linked to inherited cancer syndromes, it seems reasonable to suspect that germ line mutations in a number of tumor-suppressor genes may be associated with quite enigmatic cancer syndromes. Germ line mutations in yet other tumor-suppressor genes may fail entirely to predispose to cancer. Tumor-suppressor genes in this last group might still be frequently inactivated by somatic mutations in cancer. As such, the genes would be presumed to have important roles in cancer development, although their principal role might be in tumor progression rather than initiation. Nevertheless, because the compelling link between germ line mutations and inherited cancer might be lacking for some tumor-suppressor genes, the genes might be initially termed "candidate" tumor-suppressor genes to reflect uncertainties regarding their role in cancer development. Should further genetic and functional data bolster their candidacy, they might then be considered full-fledged tumor-suppressor genes.

Somatic Mutational Analysis as a Primary Approach to Tumor-Suppressor Gene Identification

An approach that has contributed significantly to the identification and characterization of tumor-suppressor genes is allelic loss or LOH studies. Consistent with Knudson's hypothesis, chromosomal regions frequently affected by LOH in one or more cancers have been proposed to contain inactivating mutations in a tumor-suppressor gene(s). For some of the chromosome regions frequently affected by LOH in one or more cancer types, no cancer predisposition genes have been localized to the affected regions. For other chromosome regions, although a tumor-suppressor gene with a role in a particular inherited cancer syndrome might have already been identified in the region, somatic mutations of the gene are rare or absent in sporadic cancers. Chromosomes 1p, 3p, 8p, 10q, 17q, 18q, and 22q are among the regions for which tumor-suppressor genes with important roles in sporadic cancer remain to be fully defined. Studies of candidate tumor-suppressor genes from several chromosome regions frequently affected by LOH in cancer are reviewed below, because the studies suggest that those who would hope to identify tumor-suppressor genes solely from LOH and somatic mutational analyses should proceed with caution.

Allelic losses of 18q are frequent in a number of cancers, including colorectal, pancreatic, gastric, and endometrial cancer.[37,46,47] It has been rather difficult to definitively localize the region(s) on 18q that contain the tumor-suppressor gene(s) solely through LOH analyses, because a large portion of 18q is often lost. However, in pancreatic and colorectal cancers, the common region of LOH appears to include chromosome bands 18q12.3 to 18q21.3. As noted above, the identification of homozygous deletions at chromosome band 18q21.1 in 20 to 25 percent of

pancreatic cancers was critical in the identification of the *DPC4* gene.[39] Subsequent studies revealed that *DPC4* encodes a transcription factor that functions in the TGF-β signaling pathway, and DPC4 is somatically mutated in about 50 percent of pancreatic cancers, in 10 to 15 percent of colorectal cancers, and in a small fraction of other cancer types.[48] In addition, the *DPC4* gene has been found to be mutated in the germ line of some patients with juvenile polyposis syndrome (JPS).[49] Those patients with JPS develop benign (hamartomatous) polyps of the intestinal tract and are at increased risk of colorectal and gastric cancer. Thus, because of its role in an inherited cancer syndrome and the sizable cohort of somatic, inactivating mutations found in sporadic pancreatic, colorectal, and gastric cancers, *DPC4* has been definitively established as a tumor-suppressor gene. Nevertheless, *DPC4* is only mutated in a subset of the pancreatic, colorectal, gastric, and other cancers with 18q LOH,[48,50] and the existence of other tumor-suppressor genes on chromosome 18q must be considered, including the *DPC4*-related gene known as *JV18-1/MADR2/SMAD2* and the *DCC* (deleted in colorectal cancer) gene.

Somatic, inactivating mutations in the *SMAD2* gene at 18q12.3 have been found in about 5 percent of colorectal cancers,[51,52] and *SMAD2* mutations are rare or absent in the majority of other cancer types studied.[48,53–56] *DCC* is an enormous gene that spans >1350 kb at 18q21.2, and the gene encodes a large transmembrane protein.[46] Somatic mutations in *DCC* have been detected in only a small subset of cancers,[46] although there are both theoretical and practical difficulties associated with screening for inactivating mutations in a gene the size of *DCC*. In the majority of colorectal cancers and cancer cell lines, *DCC* expression is markedly reduced or absent, consistent with the hypothesis that loss of *DCC* function may contribute to the cancer cell phenotype.[46] Nevertheless, in the majority of cases, the mutational and/or epigenetic mechanisms underlying loss of *DCC* expression remain to be determined. As a result of these uncertainties, it is not clear whether *DCC* inactivation is a causal factor in cancer development or a reflection of the cancer phenotype. Intriguingly, recent studies indicate that the *DCC* protein may induce apoptosis in some cell types, a function perhaps consistent with its possible role as a tumor-suppressor gene in certain cancer types.[57] Perhaps the principal lesson from the studies of chromosome 18q is that at least three different 18q genes that are affected by somatic, inactivating mutations in cancer have already been identified. Such findings illustrate the difficulties that may be encountered in definitive identification of the gene(s) targeted by a common LOH event. Furthermore, the findings with the *SMAD2* and *DCC* genes reinforce the point that, in the absence of other supporting data, such as the identification of germ line mutations in those with a cancer predisposition syndrome, a limited cohort of somatic alterations provides rather weak evidence to implicate any gene in cancer development.

Properties of selected candidate tumor-suppressor genes are summarized in Table 12-2. However, findings on the *MCC* and *FHIT* candidate tumor-suppressor genes are reviewed here to highlight additional problematic issues in the evaluation of candidate tumor-suppressor genes. In the search for the adenomatous polyposis coli (*APC*) gene at chromosome 5q21, a candidate tumor-suppressor gene, termed *MCC* (for mutated in colorectal cancer), was identified prior to the cloning of *APC*.[58] MCC was somatically mutated in 5 to 10 percent of colorectal cancers, and the mutations included missense mutations affecting conserved amino acids, splicing mutations, and gross rearrangement of the gene. In large part because the *APC* gene, and not *MCC*, was mutated in the germ line of those with familial polyposis, further studies on *MCC* have lagged. The *MCC* gene may have a role in some colorectal cancers. However, more definitive insights into the role of *MCC* in human cancer await the results of further studies.

The *FHIT* (fragile histidine triad) gene at chromosome 3p14.2 is a controversial candidate tumor-suppressor gene.[59–61] *FHIT* is a very large gene, spanning roughly 1000 kb, although it encodes a small protein of 147 amino acids that appears to function as a

Table 12-2 Selected Candidate Tumor-Suppressor Genes and Their Encoded Proteins

Gene	Cancers with Somatic Mutations	Protein Function	Comments
TGF-β type II R	RER + colorectal and gastric cancer, head and neck, lung, and esophageal squamous cell carcinoma	TGF-β receptor component	Both alleles inactivated in RER+ cancers with mutations; mutations less frequent in non-RER+ cancers; germ line variant allele proposed to be associated with "HNPCC-like" phenotype
BAX	RER+ colorectal	Pro-apoptotic factor	Mutations are heterozygous (1 allele) in the majority of cancers; ?genetically unstable microsatellite tract vs. specific target for inactivation?
FHIT	Lung, cervical, renal, others	Dinucleoside polyphosphate hydrolase	Mutations detected in 5–10% of cancers; majority of mutations affect noncoding sequences; aberrant splicing and reduced RNA and protein levels are common; ?genetically unstable locus vs. specific target for inactivation?
α-CAT	Some prostate and lung, ?others	Links E-cadherin cell-adhesion complex to cytoskeleton	Mutations present in a small fraction of cancers
DCC	Some colorectal, neuroblastoma, male germ cell cancer, gliomas, ?others?	Netrin-1 receptor component; regulates cell migration and apoptosis	Mutations rarely detected; decreased or absent expression is seen in >50% of a variety of cancer types
MADR2/SMAD2	Some colorectal	Transcription factor/signaling molecule in TGF-β pathway	Mutations in <5% of colorectal and other cancers (e.g., gastric)
CDX2	Rare mutations in colorectal	Homeobox transcription factor	Cdx2+/− knockout mice are predisposed to intestinal tumors; decreased Cdx2 protein expression in human and rodent colorectal tumors
MKK4	Rare mutations in pancreas, lung, breast and colorectal; ?others?	Stress- and cytokine-induced protein kinase	
PP2R1B	Lung, colorectal	Subunit of serine/threonine protein phosphatase 2A	Mutations are heterozygous in some cases
MCC	Rare mutations in colorectal	Not known	Mutations in about 5–10% of sporadic colorectal cancers

dinucleoside polyphosphate hydrolase. Somatic mutations at the FHIT locus have been identified in a number of different cancer types. However, in most cases, the mutations do not affect FHIT coding exons. The most consistent observations are that aberrant FHIT transcripts are found in cancer. While most aberrant FHIT transcripts appear to arise from alternative splicing and such transcripts have been found at low abundance in normal tissues, in several cancer types, the aberrant transcripts have been correlated with markedly reduced FHIT gene and protein expression. Hence, based on the somatic mutations observed at the FHIT locus and the aberrant expression of FHIT transcripts and protein, FHIT has been suggested as a tumor-suppressor gene. Unfortunately, some gaps exist in the data set needed to definitively establish FHIT as a tumor-suppressor gene. For instance, germ line mutations in FHIT have not yet been clearly linked to a cancer predisposition syndrome. It is also uncertain whether the limited cohort of somatic mutations in FHIT is a cause of cancer or a reflection of FHIT's location at a chromosome fragile site. Finally, the relationship of the biochemical action of the FHIT protein to its potential tumor suppression function remains to be more clearly established.

In summary, the results obtained thus far in studies of the SMAD2, DCC, MCC, and FHIT genes indicate that a cautious approach is both reasonable and appropriate for those investigators who hope to rely predominantly on LOH and somatic mutational analyses for identification and evaluation of tumor-suppressor genes.

Other Approaches to Identify Candidate Tumor-Suppressor Genes

Germ line inactivation of the mouse homologues of human tumor-suppressor genes has generated some useful new cancer models. Unfortunately, several mouse models of inherited cancer, includ-

ing mice with germ line Rb and Nf2 defects, do not manifest the tumor types seen in man, and, in fact, develop tumors not seen in humans with the corresponding defect.[62] Other mouse models, including mice heterozygous for defects in the homologues of the BRCA1, BRCA2, WT1, and VHL genes, fail to manifest an elevated rate of spontaneous tumors. Nevertheless, it seems reasonable to suggest that another approach for identification of candidate tumor-suppressor genes in human cancer is to carefully consider the tumor predisposition phenotypes seen in mouse "knockout" models. In fact, several knockout models display increased rates of spontaneous tumor development. For instance, gonadal stromal tumors develop in mice homozygous for inactivating mutations in α-inhibin, and intestinal tumors are seen in mice heterozygous for inactivating mutations in the Cdx2 homeobox gene. Mutations in α-inhibin have not been described in man, and somatic mutations in CDX2 are uncommon in colorectal cancers in man.[63] Thus, it seems likely that mouse knockout models may not always accurately predict the identities of tumor-suppressor genes that are frequently mutated in cancers arising in man. Nonetheless, the mouse models may still be of considerable utility for highlighting potential tumor-suppressor gene signaling pathways, and other genes in the pathway may be frequently mutated in human cancer.

Finally, there are some caveats concerning the premature designation of a gene as a tumor suppressor. An increasing number of genes that have decreased or absent expression in cancers are being discovered. These genes are sometimes termed tumor suppressors based simply on their decreased expression. Similarly, other genes that antagonize the tumorigenic or in vitro growth properties of cancer cell lines may be termed tumor suppressors. Undoubtedly, some of these genes may prove critical in growth regulation and may even be targets for loss-of-function mutations in human cancer. However, it should be remembered that the altered expression of many genes in cancers may not result from specific inactivation by mutational mechanisms, but may simply reflect the altered growth properties of cancer cells. Finally, as is the case for the retinoblastoma-related gene termed p107, the p53-related gene known as p73, and the p53 target gene known as *p21/WAF1/CIP1*, some genes may have particularly potent growth suppressive properties in cancer cells, but may be rarely, if ever, mutated in human cancer. In the end, it is the sum total of the mutational and functional data that establish whether a gene has a causal role in tumorigenesis and is appropriately designated as a tumor-suppressor gene.

SUMMARY

There is now compelling evidence to support the importance of tumor-suppressor genes in cancer. Evidence for the existence of tumor-suppressor genes emerged gradually from somatic cell genetic and epidemiologic studies, as well as studies of chromosome losses in tumor cells using cytogenetic and molecular genetic techniques. In the last decade, more than two dozen well-documented tumor-suppressor genes and a number of intriguing candidate tumor-suppressor genes have been identified. The genes are inactivated in the germ line in some cancer patients, and, in such cases, their inactivation strongly predisposes to cancer. Far more frequently, tumor-suppressor genes are inactivated by somatic mutations arising during tumor development. As is reinforced in subsequent chapters, although we have learned much about tumor-suppressor genes, much work remains. A more complete description of tumorigenesis will emerge with the identification of additional tumor-suppressor genes, the detailed characterization of their normal cellular functions, and the elucidation of germ line and somatic mutations that inactivate these genes in human tumors. These findings will provide new insights into cancer pathogenesis, and should prove crucial in improving the management and treatment of patients and families with cancer.

REFERENCES

1. Bishop JM: Molecular themes in oncogenesis. *Cell* **64**:235, 1991.
2. Rabbitts TH: Chromosomal translocations in human cancer. *Nature* **372**:143, 1994.
3. Shih C, Shilo BZ, Goldfarb MP, Dannenberg A, Weinberg RA: Passage of phenotypes of chemically transformed cells via transfection of DNA and chromatin. *Proc Natl Acad Sci USA* **76**:5714, 1979.
4. Parada LF, Tabin CJ, Shih C, Weinberg RA: Human EJ bladder carcinoma oncogene is homologue of Harvey sarcoma virus ras gene. *Nature* **297**:474, 1982.
5. Der CJ, Krontiris TG, Cooper GM: Transforming genes of human bladder and lung carcinoma cell lines are homologous to the ras genes of Harvey and Kirsten sarcoma viruses. *Proc Natl Acad Sci USA* **79**:3637, 1982.
6. Santos E, Tronick SR, Aaronson SA, Pulciani S, Barbacid M: T24 human bladder carcinoma oncogene is an activated form of the normal human homologue of BALB- and Harvey-MSV transforming genes. *Nature* **298**:343, 1982.
7. Ephrussi B, Davidson RL, Weiss MC, Harris H, Klein G: Malignancy of somatic cell hybrids. *Nature* **224**:1314, 1969.
8. Harris H: The analysis of malignancy in cell fusion: the position in 1988. *Can Res* **48**:3302, 1988.
9. Klinger HP: Suppression of tumorigenicity. *Cytogenet Cell Genet* **32**:68, 1982.
10. Stanbridge EJ, Der CJ, Doersen CJ, Nishimi RY, Peehl DM, Weissman BE, Wilkinson JE: Human cell hybrids: analysis of transformation and tumorigenicity. *Science* **215**:252, 1982.
11. Geiser AG, Der CJ, Marshall CJ, Stanbridge EJ: Suppression of tumorigenicity with continued expression of the c-Ha-ras oncogene in EJ bladder carcinoma-human fibroblast hybrid cells. *Proc Natl Acad Sci USA* **83**:5209, 1986.
12. Saxon PJ, Srivatsan ES, Stanbridge EJ: Introduction of human chromosome 11 via microcell transfer controls tumorigenic expression of HeLa cells. *EMBO J* **5**:3461, 1986.
13. Weissman BE, Saxon PJ, Pasquale SR, Jones GR, Geiser AG, Stanbridge EJ: Introduction of a normal human chromosome 11 into a Wilms' tumor cell line controls its tumorigenic expression. *Science* **236**:175, 1987.
14. Shimizu M, Yokota J, Mori N, Shuin T, Shinoda M, Terada M, Oshimura M: Introduction of normal chromosome 3p modulates the tumorigenicity of a human renal cell carcinoma cell line YCR. *Oncogene* **5**:185, 1990.
15. Trent JM, Stanbridge EJ, McBride HL, Meese EU, Casey G, Araujo DE, Witkowski CM, Nagle RB: Tumorigenicity in human melanoma cell lines controlled by introduction of human chromosome 6. *Science* **247**:568, 1990.
16. Oshimura M, Hugoh H, Koi M, Shimizu M, Yamada H, Satoh H, Barrett JC: Transfer of human chromosome 11 suppresses tumorigenicity of some but not all tumor cell lines. *J Cell Biochem* **42**:135, 1990.
17. Tanaka K, Oshimura M, Kikuchi R, Seki M, Hayashi T, Miyaki M: Suppression of tumorigenicity in human colon carcinoma cells by introduction of normal chromosome 5 or 18. *Nature* **349**:340, 1991.
18. Knudson AG: Mutation and cancer: Statistical study of retinoblastoma. *Proc Natl Acad Sci USA* **68**:820, 1971.
19. Francke U: Retinoblastoma and chromosome 13. *Cytogenet Cell Genet* **16**:131, 1976.
20. Francke U, Holmes LB, Atkins L, Riccardi VM: Aniridia-Wilms' tumor association: Evidence for specific deletion of 11p13. *Cytogenet Cell Genet* **24**:185, 1979.
21. Herrera L, Kakati S, Gibas L, Pietrzak E, Sandberg AA: Brief clinical report: Gardner syndrome in a man with an interstitial deletion of 5q. *Am J Med Genet* **25**:473, 1986.
22. Fountain JW, Wallace MR, Bruce MA, Seizinger BR, Menon AG, Gusella JF, Michels VV, Schmidt MA, Dewald GW, Collins FS: Physical mapping of a translocation breakpoint in neurofibromatosis. *Science* **244**:1085, 1989.
23. O'Connell P, Leach R, Cawthon RM, Culver M, Stevens J, Viskochil D, Fournier RE, Rich DC, Ledbetter DH, White R: Two von Recklinghausen neurofibromatosis translocations map within a 600 kb region of 17q11.2. *Science* **244**:1087, 1989.
24. Groden J, Thliveris A, Samowitz W, Carlson M, Gelbert LA, Joslyn G, Stevens J, Spirio L, Robertson M: Identification and characterization of the familial adenomatous polyposis coli gene. *Cell* **66**:589, 1991.
25. Joslyn G, Carlson M, Thliveris A, Albertsen H, Gelbert L, Samowitz W, Groden J, Stevens J, Spirio L, Robertson M: Identification of deletion mutations and three new genes at the familial polyposis locus. *Cell* **66**:601, 1991.
26. Kinzler K, Nilbert M, Su L, Vogelstein B, Bryan T, Levy D, Smith K, Preisinger A, Hedge P, McKechnie D, Rinniear R, Markham A, Groffen J, Boguski M, Altschul S, Horii A, Ando H, Miyoshi Y, Miki Y, Nishisho I, Nakamura Y: Identification of FAP locus genes from chromosome 5q21. *Science* **253**:661, 1991.
27. Nishisho I, Nakamura Y, Miyoshi Y, Miki Y, Ando H, Horii A, Koyama K, Utsunomiya J, Baba S, Hedge P: Mutations of chromosome 5q21 genes in FAP and colorectal cancer patients. *Science* **253**:665, 1991.
28. Latif F, Tory K, Gnarra J, Yao M, Duh FM, Orcutt ML, Stackhouse T, Kuzmin I, Modi W, Geil L, et al: Identification of the von Hippel-Lindau disease tumor suppressor gene. *Science* **260**:1317, 1993.
29. Trofatter JA, MacCollin MM, Rutter JL, Murrell JR, Duyao MP, Parry DM, Eldridge R, Kley N, Menon AG, Pulaski K, et al: A novel moesin-, ezrin-, radixin-like gene is a candidate for the neurofibromatosis 2 tumor suppressor. *Cell* **72**:791, 1993.
30. Rouleau GA, Merel P, Lutchman M, Sanson M, Zucman J, Marineau C, Hoang-Xuan K, Demczuk S, Desmaze C, Plougastel B: Alteration in a new gene encoding a putative membrane-organizing protein causes neuro-fibromatosis type 2. *Nature* **363**:515, 1993.
31. Sparkes RS, Sparkes MC, Wilson MG, Towner JW, Benedict W, Murphree AL, Yunis JJ: Regional assignment of genes for human esterase D and retinoblastoma to chromosome band 13q14. *Science* **208**:1042, 1980.
32. Sparkes RS, Murphree AL, Lingua RW, Sparkes MC, Field LL, Funderburk SJ, Benedict WF: Gene for hereditary retinoblastoma assigned to human chromosome 13 by linkage to esterase D. *Science* **219**:971, 1983.
33. Benedict WF, Murphree AL, Banerjee A, Spina CA, Sparkes MC, Sparkes RS: Patient with 13 chromosome deletion: evidence that the retinoblastoma gene is a recessive cancer gene. *Science* **219**:973, 1983.
34. Cavenee WK, Dryja TP, Phillips RA, Benedict WF, Godbout R, Gallie BL, Murphree AL, Strong LC, White RL: Expression of recessive alleles by chromosomal mechanisms in retinoblastoma. *Nature* **305**:779, 1983.

35. Cavenee WK, Hansen MF, Nordenskjold M, Kock E, Maumenee I, Squire JA, Phillips RA, Gallie BL: Genetic origin of mutations predisposing to retinoblastoma. *Science* **228**:501, 1985.

36. Solomon E, Voss R, Hall V, Bodmer WF, Jass JR, Jeffreys AJ, Lucibello FC, Patel I, Rider SH: Chromosome 5 allele loss in human colorectal carcinomas. *Nature* **328**:616, 1987.

37. Vogelstein B, Fearon ER, Hamilton S, Kern S, Preisinger A, Leppert M, Nakamura Y, White R, Smits A, Bos J: Genetic alterations during colorectal-tumor development. *N Engl J Med* **319**:525, 1988.

38. Schutte M, Rozenblum E, Moskaluk CA, Guan X, Hoque AT, Hahn SA, da Costa LT, de Jong PJ, Kern SE: An integrated high-resolution physical map of the DPC/BRCA2 region at chromosome 13q12. *Can Res* **55**:4570, 1995.

39. Hahn SA, Schutte M, Hoque AT, Moskaluk CA, da Costa LT, Rozenblum E, Fischer A, Yeo CJ, Hruban RH, Kern SE: DPC4, a candidate tumor suppressor gene at human chromosome 18q21.1. *Science* **271**:350, 1996.

40. Li J, Yen C, Liaw D, Podsypanina K, Bose S, Wang SI, Puc J, Miliaresis C, Rodgers L, McCombie R, Bigner SH, Giovanella BC, Ittmann M, Tycko B, Hibshoosh H, Wigler MH, Parsons R: PTEN, a putative protein tyrosine phosphatase gene mutated in human brain, breast, and prostate cancer [see comments]. *Science* **275**:1943, 1997.

41. Steck PA, Pershouse MA, Jasser SA, Yung WK, Lin H, Ligon AH, Langford LA, Baumgard ML, Hattier T, Davis T, Frye C, Hu R, Swedlund B, Teng DH, Tavtigian SV: Identification of a candidate tumour suppressor gene, MMAC1, at chromosome 10q23.3 that is mutated in multiple advanced cancers. *Nat Genet* **15**:356, 1997.

42. Kinzler KW, Vogelstein B: Lessons from hereditary colorectal cancer. *Cell* **87**:159, 1996.

43. Sellers WR, Kaelin WG Jr: Role of the retinoblastoma protein in the pathogenesis of human cancer. *J Clin Onc* **15**:3301, 1997.

44. Clevers H, van de Wetering M: TCF/LEF factor earn their wings. *Trends Genet* **13**:485, 1997.

45. He TC, Sparks AB, Rago C, Hermeking H, Zawel L, da Costa LT, Morin PJ, Vogelstein B, Kinzler KW: Identification of c-MYC as a target of the APC pathway. *Science* **281**:1509, 1998.

46. Cho KR, Fearon ER: DCC—linking tumour suppressor genes and altered cell surface interactions in cancer. *Eur J Cancer* **31A**:1055, 1995.

47. Hahn SA, Seymour AB, Hoque AT, Schutte M, da Costa LT, Redston MS, Caldas C, Weinstein CL, Fischer A, Yeo CJ and others: Allelotype of pancreatic adenocarcinoma using xenograft enrichment. *Can Res* **55**:4670, 1995.

48. Moskaluk CA, Kern SE: Cancer gets Mad: DPC4 and other TGFβ pathway genes in human cancer. *Biochimica et Biophysica Acta* **1288**:M31, 1996.

49. Howe JR, Roth S, Ringold JC, Summers RW, Jarvinen HJ, Tomlinson IP, Houlston RS, Bevan S, Mitros FA, Stone EM: Mutations in the SMAD4/DPC4 gene in juvenile polyposis. *Science* **280**:1086, 1998.

50. Schutte M, Hruban RH, Hedrick L, Cho KR, Nadasdy GM, Weinstein CL, Bova GS, Isaacs WB, Cairns P, Nawroz H, Sidransky D, Casero JRA, Meltzer PS, Hahn SA, Kern SE: DPC4 gene in various tumor types. *Can Res* **56**:2527, 1996.

51. Riggins GJ, Thiagalingam S, Rozenblum E, Weinstein CL, Kern SE, Hamilton SR, Willson JK, Markowitz SD, Kinzler KW, Vogelstein B: Mad-related genes in the human. *Nature Genet* **13**:347, 1996.

52. Eppert K, Scherer SW, Ozcelik H, Pirone R, Hoodless P, Kim H, Tsui LC, Gallinger S, Andrulis IL, Thomsen GH, Wrana JL, Attisano L: MADR2 maps to 18q21 and encodes a TGFbeta-regulated MAD-related protein that is functionally mutated in colorectal carcinoma. *Cell* **86**:543, 1996.

53. Uchida K, Nagatake M, Osada H, Yatabe Y, Kondo M, Mitsudomi T, Masuda A, Takahashi T: Somatic *in vivo* alterations of the *JV18-1* gene at 18q21 in human lung cancers. *Can Res* **56**:5583, 1996.

54. Maesawa C, Tamura G, Nishizuka S, Iwaya T, Ogasawara S, Ishida K, Sakata K, Sato N, Ikeda K, Kimura Y, Saito K, Satodate R: *MAD*-related genes on 18q21.1, *Smad2* and *Smad4*, are altered infrequently in esophageal squamous cell carcinoma. *Jpn J Can Res* **88**:340, 1997.

55. Kong X-T, Choi SH, Inoue A, Xu F, Chen T, Takita J, Yokota J, Bessho F, Yanagisawa M, Hanada R, Yamamoto K, Hayashi Y: Expression and mutational analysis of the *DCC*, *DPC4*, and *MADR2/JV18-1* genes in neuroblastoma. *Can Res* **57**:3772, 1997.

56. Ikezoe T, Takeuchi S, Kamioka M, Daibata M, Kubonishi I, Taguchi H, Miyoshi I: Analysis of the Smad2 gene in hematological malignancies. *Leukemia* **12**:94, 1998.

57. Mehlen P, Rabizadeh S, Snipas SJ, Assa-Munt N, Salvesen GS, Bredesen DE: The DCC gene product induces apoptosis by a mechanism requiring receptor proteolysis. *Nature* **395**:801, 1998.

58. Kinzler KW, Nilbert MC, Vogelstein B, Levy DB, Smith KJ, Preisinger AC, Hamilton SRH, Markham A, et al.: Identification of a gene located at chromosome 5q21 that is mutated in colorectal cancers. *Science* **251**:1366, 1991.

59. Sozzi G, Huebner K, Croce CM: FHIT in human cancer. *Adv Can Res* **74**:141-66: 1998.

60. Mao L: Tumor suppressor genes: does FHIT fit? *J Natl Canc Inst* **90**:412, 1998.

61. Le Beau MM, Drabkin H, Glover TW, Gemmill R, Rassool FV, McKeithan TW, Smith DI: An FHIT tumor suppressor gene? *Genes Chrom Canc* **21**:281, 1998.

62. Jacks T: Tumor suppressor gene mutations in mice. *Annu Rev Genet* **30**:603, 1996.

63. Wicking C, Simms LA, Evans T, Walsh M, Chawengsaksophak K, Beck F, Chenevix-Trench G, Young J, Jass J, Leggett B, Wainwright B: CDX2, a human homologue of Drosophila caudal, is mutated in both alleles in a replication error positive colorectal cancer. *Oncogene* **17**:657, 1998.

PART 3

FAMILIAL CANCER SYNDROMES

CHAPTER

13

Familial Cancer Syndromes: The Role of Caretakers and Gatekeepers

Kenneth W. Kinzler ■ *Bert Vogelstein*

The past decade has witnessed the elucidation of the specific genetic bases of nearly twenty inherited predispositions to cancer. This information not only is yielding immediate practical benefits in the form of genetic testing but also is providing important insights into mechanisms regulating cancer susceptibility.

The inheritance of a predisposition to a sporadic event such as tumor formation has always presented an interesting problem. The complexity of this problem is compounded by studies of the age dependence of cancer incidence and other studies that suggest that multiple genetic changes are required for cancer formation. This prompted Knudson to postulate that individuals with an autosomal dominant cancer susceptibility inherited one genetic alteration that was rate-limiting for tumor formation but that subsequent steps also were required for a tumor to form. Over the years, Knudson's hypothesis has been refined to include the idea that one of the key subsequent steps is a somatic, inactivating mutation of the wild-type allele inherited from the unaffected parent. Knudson's hypotheses have been confirmed abundantly within the last 20 years (e.g., *Rb* in retinoblastoma, Chap. 22; *APC* in colorectal cancer, Chap. 34), and concrete demonstrations of the multiple genetic events required for tumorigenesis have emerged (e.g., colorectal cancer, Chap. 34). The characterization of the genes underlying inherited predispositions to neoplasia also has provided important insights into the nature of tumor suppressor genes.

It appears that most tumor suppressor genes can be broadly divided into two groups, called *gatekeepers* and *caretakers*. Gatekeepers are genes that directly regulate the growth of tumors by inhibiting their growth or by promoting their death. The functions of these genes are rate-limiting for tumor growth, and as a result, both the maternal and paternal copies of these genes must be inactivated for a tumor to develop (Fig. 13-1). In accord with Knudson's hypothesis, predisposed individuals inherit one damaged copy of such a gene and as a result require only one additional mutation for tumor initiation. The identity of gatekeepers varies with each tissue such that inactivation of a given gene leads to specific forms of cancer predisposition. For example, inherited mutations of *APC* lead to colon tumors but not kidney cancers (see Chap. 34), whereas inherited mutations of *VHL* predispose to kidney cancers but not colon cancers (see Chap. 27). Because these gatekeeping genes are rate-limiting for tumor initiation, they must be mutated in sporadic cancers through somatic mutations as well as mutated in the germ line of predisposed individuals.

In contrast, inactivation of caretakers does not directly promote growth of tumors. Rather, inactivation of caretakers leads to a genetic instability that only indirectly promotes growth by causing an increased mutation rate. Because numerous mutations are required for the full development of a cancer, inactivation of caretakers, with the consequent increase in genetic instability, can

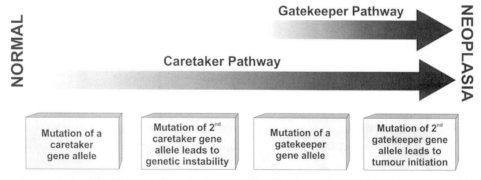

Fig. 13-1 Pathways to neoplasia. Inherited mutation of either a gatekeeper or caretaker can predispose an individual to neoplasia. However, additional genetic changes are required to convert a predisposed cell to a neoplastic cell. In the case of the caretaker pathway, three additional mutations generally are required. However, the genetic instability that follows inactivation of the second caretaker allele accelerates the accumulation of the latter mutations. In the case of the gatekeeper pathway, only one additional mutation (inactivation of the second gatekeeper allele) is required to initiate neoplasia. (Although the concepts depicted in this figure apply to all inherited cancer susceptibilities, variations do occur. For example, inherited mutations of both alleles of a caretaker gene occur in recessively inherited diseases such as xeroderma pigmentosum, and a single dominant negative mutation can substitute for two inactivating mutations of a caretaker gene).

greatly accelerate the development of cancers. Caretaker mutations in the germ line occur in two different forms. In dominantly inherited diseases (e.g., hereditary nonpolypsosis colorectal cancer; see Chap. 18), only one mutant allele of the caretaker is inherited; as with gatekeepers, the remaining allele of the caretaker gene must be mutated for a phenotypic defect (i.e., increased mutation rate) to be realized (see Fig. 13-1). In other cases, both alleles of the gene must be inherited in mutant form to cause susceptibility (e.g., *XP;* see Chap. 14). The targets of the accelerated mutagenesis that occurs in cells with defective caretakers are the gatekeeping tumor suppressor genes, other tumor suppressor genes (whose inactivation can lead to tumor progression), and oncogenes (genes whose activation leads to cancer). Somatic mutations of caretaker genes are only rarely found as initiating events in tumors arising in the general population, presumably because such mutations would still need to be followed by several other mutations in order for a tumor to initiate (see Fig. 13-1).

For the purposes of this book, we have divided cancer susceptibility syndromes into two forms, gatekeepers and caretakers, based on the predominant mechanism underlying the susceptibility. In some cases, the mechanism underlying the susceptibility is not completely characterized, and the assignments were made based on the best current evidence. For example, the *BRCA1* and *BRCA2* genes (see Chap. 33) have been hypothesized to function as caretakers in some studies and as gatekeepers in others; further research will be required to discriminate the true role of these genes in tumor suppression.

Nucleotide Excision Repair Syndromes: Xeroderma Pigmentosum, Cockayne Syndrome, and Trichothiodystrophy*

Dirk Bootsma ▪ *Kenneth H. Kraemer*
James E. Cleaver ▪ *Jan H. J. Hoeijmakers*

1. Three rare autosomal recessive syndromes are associated with a nucleotide excision repair (NER) defect: xeroderma pigmentosum (XP), Cockayne syndrome (CS), and the photosensitive form of trichothiodystrophy (TTD). A common denominator of all three conditions is an extreme sensitivity to sunlight. XP patients exhibit in addition to photosensitivity a greater than thousand-fold increased frequency of sunlight-induced skin cancers. Other features include progressive degenerative alterations of the skin and eyes and in some cases accelerated neurologic degeneration due to increased neuronal death. Patients with CS have a combination of sun sensitivity, short stature, severe neuro-logic abnormalities due to dysmyelination, cataracts, dental caries, a wizened appearance, and a characteristic bird-like facies. They do not display cancer predisposition. The hallmark of TTD is sulfur-deficient brittle hair and nails. Patients also have ichthyosis and many symptoms char-acteristic of CS. About half of TTD patients are hypersen-sitive to ultraviolet (UV) light, and they have a NER defect. As in CS, there are no indications for an increased risk of cancer. In addition to the preceding, rare patients showing combined XP-CS symptoms have been described.

2. The NER pathway removes a remarkably wide array of structurally unrelated DNA lesions. Among these are numerous helix-distorting chemical adducts induced by carcinogens such as benz[a]pyrene, as well as cyclobutane pyrimidine dimers (CPD) and [6-4]pyrimidine-pyrimidone photoproducts (6-4PP) produced in human skin by the shortwave UV component of the solar spectrum. This explains why patients with inherited deficiencies in the NER process display marked hypersensitivity to sun exposure. Defective repair also results in genetic instability leading to increased chromosome abnormalities and mutagenesis and in many cases predisposition to cancer. At least two NER subpathways exist: a rapid transcription-coupled repair (TCR) pathway responsible for the efficient elimination of lesions from the transcribed strand of active genes that permits rapid resumption of the vital process of transcrip-tion and for some lesions a less efficient global genome repair (GGR) subpathway that surveys the entire genome.

3. Complementation analysis by cell fusion has allowed a further genetic classification of XP, CS, and TTD patients. In XP, seven different complementation groups are distinguished, representing seven distinct defective genes involved in NER in XP: XP-A, -B, -C, -D, -E, -F, and -G. In addition, another class of XP patients (XP variant) appears to be deficient in a gene product that in normal cells permits semiconservative replication of previously damaged sites in the DNA template (postreplication repair). Similarly, complementation analysis has revealed two complementa-tion groups in CS, CS-A and CS-B, and three in TTD, of which two overlap with XP groups: TTD-A, XP-B, and XP-D. Patients with combined XP-CS have been assigned to three XP complementation groups: XP-B, XP-D and XP-G.

4. The NER defect in the cells of most XP and TTD patients is located in the core of the NER mechanism and affects both

---

*This text is a complete revision of Chapter 148, Xeroderma Pigmentosum and Cockayne Syndrome, in the 7th edition of *Metabolic and Molecular Bases of Inherited Diseases*. Part of this chapter is an updated version of Hoeijmakers JHJ: Human nucleotide excision repair syndromes: Molecular clues to unexpected intricacies, *Eur J Cancer* 30A(13):1912, 1994; used with permission from Elsevier Science, Ltd., The Boulevard, Lanfordlane, Kidlington OX5 1GB, UK.

A list of standard abbreviations is located immediately preceding the index. Nonstandard abbreviations used in this chapter include: XP = xeroderma pigmentosum; NER = nucleotide excision repair; CS = Cockayne syndrome; TTD = trichothiodystrophy; BER = base escision repair; TCR = transcription-coupled repair; GGR = global genome repair; UDS = unscheduled DNA synthesis; SCE = sister chromatid exchange; UVS = ultraviolet sensitivity; DDB = DNA damage-binding protein; MEFs = mouse embryonal fibroblasts.

transcription-coupled and global genome repair. In XP-C cells the defect is limited to the global genome repair system, whereas in CS only the transcription-coupled repair pathway is impaired.

5. All XP, CS, and TTD genes, except TTD-A and XP-variant, have been cloned, and their functions in the NER mechanism are known or in the process of being clarified. Disease-causing mutations have been identified in most of the corresponding genes.

6. Several of the protein (complexes) involved in NER participate in other DNA transactions as well. All NER genes associated with TTD:XP-B, XP-D, and TTD-A — are simultaneously implicated in basal transcription. The XP-F complex probably has a dual involvement in a mitotic recombination pathway, and later steps in NER are shared with replication. The notion of function sharing has important implications for the clinical consequences of inherited mutations in these NER proteins. It is likely that the symptoms, which are not easy to explain on the basis of an NER defect per se (e.g., the brittle hair and nerve dysmyelination), are caused by subtle insufficiencies in basal transcription.

7. Mouse models for NER deficiencies have been generated. They provide excellent tools for understanding the complex relationships between DNA repair defects and clinical consequences.

8. Prenatal diagnosis for XP, CS, and TTD is possible if an unequivocal NER defect or the responsible mutations in the family have been demonstrated.

The development and maintenance of life have critically depended on the evolvement of mechanisms that ensure genetic integrity and stability. DNA, the vital carrier of genetic information, is continually subject to undesired chemical alterations. Numerous environmental or endogenous compounds and various types of radiation, such as x-rays and ultraviolet (UV) light, induce a wide variety of lesions in the bases, sugars, or phosphates that make up the DNA. Obviously, such lesions (adducts, crosslinks, breaks, etc.) interfere with the proper functioning of the genome. An intricate network of single- and multistep DNA repair systems constitutes the main protecting barrier against the deleterious consequences of DNA injury. This is illustrated by the phenotype of inherited defects in one of these repair pathways. Invariably such disorders are associated with a characteristic hypersensitivity to a specific class of genotoxic agents. In addition, the DNA lesions that persist lead to cell malfunctioning and to enhanced mutagenesis because of the higher chance that mistakes are made on replication of a damaged template. Somatic mutagenesis is the initiator and driving force for the multistep process of carcinogenesis. Rare inborn disorders with hallmarks characteristic for repair defects or inadequate response to DNA damage comprise a class of *chromosomal instability syndromes.* Well-known examples are Fanconi anemia, ataxia telangiectasia, and Bloom syndrome, all of which display different manifestations of cancer proneness and increased sensitivity to specific mutagens. The prototype repair disorder, however, is xeroderma pigmentosum (XP), in which a defect in the nucleotide excision repair (NER) pathway underlies the pronounced predisposition to skin cancer and the characteristic photosensitivity of most patients. It clearly highlights the importance of the NER process. In the past decade, impressive progress has been made in unravelling the molecular intricacies of NER; for instance, all seven NER genes involved in XP (named *XP-A* through *XP-G*) have been cloned and their defect analyzed in patients; in addition, the core of the NER process has been reconstituted in vitro from purified components, which has enabled a stepwise dissection of the contribution of the various gene functions.

Genetic analysis of NER mutants and biochemical studies have provided evidence for the involvement of more than 20 gene products in the repair process. As discussed below, these proteins have been conserved to a remarkable degree throughout the over 1.2×10^6 years of eukaryotic evolution, underlining the fundamental importance of this process. This makes it likely that the mode of action of NER in lower eukaryotes, such as the baker's yeast *Saccharomyces cerevisiae,* is probably to a large extent similar to that in humans. On the other hand, clear differences have become apparent with the process in the prokaryotic model organism *Escherichia coli.*

Furthermore, intimate links between NER and other cellular processes have been disclosed, some of which were quite unexpected: Tight coordination of repair and cell cycle regulation exists: On encountering abnormally high levels of damage, a transient arrest in cell cycle progression is introduced before DNA replication or prior to cell division. This gives the repair machinery the opportunity to remove the lesions before they give rise to permanent, potentially catastrophic changes in the genetic material. In addition, connections with recombination, replication, chromatin dynamics, and the basic transcription apparatus have been unveiled.

For all the human NER syndromes and many of the NER genes, bona fide mouse models have been generated. This will be of great importance for clinical studies, for understanding the biologic relevance of the NER system, and for cancer research in general.

In this chapter the present knowledge of consequences of NER deficiency will be discussed. Besides XP, other disorders such as Cockayne syndrome (CS) and the remarkable hair disorder trichothiodystrophy (TTD) will be covered, since both are associated with repair deficiency as well. It will become clear that the relation between the molecular defect and the clinical symptoms appears straightforward in some cases. In other instances there is a beginning of understanding, and a great deal of mystery remains. For a comprehensive review of DNA damage and the intricate network of DNA repair systems in general, the interested reader is referred to Friedberg, Walker, and Siede.[1]

CLINICAL ASPECTS OF XP, CS, AND TTD

Xeroderma Pigmentosum

XP is a rare autosomal recessive disease. Affected patients (homozygotes) have sun sensitivity resulting in progressive degenerative changes of sun-exposed portions of the skin and eyes, often leading to neoplasia. Some XP patients have, in addition, progressive neurologic degeneration.[2] Obligate heterozygotes (parents) generally are asymptomatic.

History. *Xeroderma,* or "parchment skin," was the term given by Moritz Kaposi to the condition he observed in a patient in 1863 and reported in the dermatology textbook he wrote with Ferdinand von Hebra in 1874.[3] In 1882, the term *pigmentosum* was added to emphasize the striking pigmentary abnormalities. Eye involvement, including cloudiness of the cornea, was recognized by Kaposi. In 1883, Neisser reported two brothers with cutaneous XP and neurologic degeneration beginning in the second decade.[4] De Sanctis and Cacchione in 1932 described three siblings with cutaneous XP associated with microcephaly, progressive mental deterioration, dwarfism, and immature sexual development — the DeSanctis-Cacchione syndrome.[5]

Epidemiology. XP has been found in all races worldwide. The frequency is about 1 in 1 million in the United States and Europe[6] but is considerably higher in Japan (1 in 100,000)[7] and North Africa. In a literature survey of more than 800 patients,[2] there were nearly equal numbers of male (54 percent) and female (46 percent) patients. Consanguinity of the patient's parents was reported in 31 percent. Nearly 20 percent of the patients, including a high proportion of Japanese patients, had neurologic abnormalities.

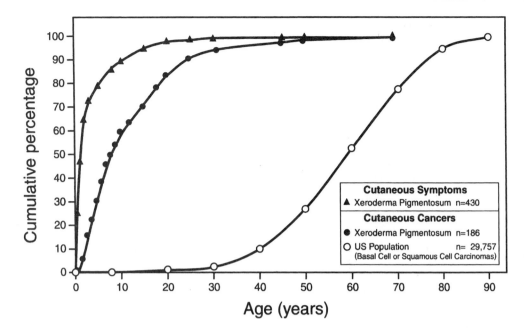

Fig. 14-1 Age at onset of XP symptoms. Age at onset of cutaneous symptoms (generally sun sensitivity or pigmentation) was reported for 430 patients. Age at first skin cancer was reported for 186 patients and is compared with age distribution for 29,757 patients with basal cell carcinoma or squamous cell carcinoma in the U.S. general population. (*From Kraemer et al.*[2] *Used by permission.*)

Symptoms. The median age of onset of symptoms is between 1 and 2 years. In 5 percent of the reported patients, onset of symptoms is delayed until after 14 years[2] (Fig. 14-1). Initial symptoms include abnormal reaction to sun exposure in 19 percent (including severe sunburn with blistering and persistent erythema on minimal sun exposure) (Table 14-1). However, many patients sunburn normally. Freckling occurs by 2 years of age in most of the patients. The cutaneous abnormalities are usually strikingly limited to sun-exposed areas of the body (Fig. 14-2). At an early stage, the skin appears similar to that seen in farmers and sailors after many years of sun exposure: areas of increased pigment alternating with areas of decreased pigment, which display atrophy and telangiectasia. A few patients who exhibit a wide spectrum of characteristic cutaneous and ocular findings have been unambiguously diagnosed as having XP, even though the erythematous response to sun exposure was normal.[6] This may be a distinctive feature of the form of XP known as *variant or pigmented xerodermoid*.[6]

Premalignant actinic keratoses and malignant and benign neoplasms develop.[2] The neoplasms are predominantly basal cell or squamous cell carcinomas (at least 45 percent of patients, many with multiple primary neoplasms) but also include melanomas (5 percent of patients), sarcomas, keratocanthomas, and angiomas. About 90 percent of the basal cell and squamous cell carcinomas occur on the face, head, and neck—the sites of greatest UV exposure. The median age of onset of first skin neoplasm is 8 years, nearly 50 years younger than that in the general population of the United States (see Fig. 14-1). This represents one of the largest reductions in age of onset of neoplasia documented for any recessive human genetic disease. The frequency of basal cell carcinomas, squamous-cell carcinomas, or melanomas of the skin is 2000 times greater than in the general population for patients under 20 years of age.[8] There is an approximate 30-year reduction in survival, with a 70 percent probability of surviving to age 40 years.[2] Many patients die of neoplasia.

Ocular abnormalities include photophobia, which may vary among patients from severe to absent; conjunctivitis of the interpalpebral (sun-exposed) area; ectropion (turning out of the lids) due to atrophy of the skin of the eyelids; exposure keratitis; and benign and malignant neoplasms of the lids, conjunctiva, and limbus (see Table 14-1). The distribution of ocular damage and neoplasms corresponds closely with the sites of UV exposure. The ocular neoplasms involve the anterior portion of the eye (lids, cornea, conjunctiva) almost exclusively. This portion of the eye

shields the posterior eye (uveal tract, retina) from UV radiation; visible light is the only radiation that reaches the photosensitive cells of the retina. The frequency of ocular neoplasms is greatly increased in patients under 20 years of age.[6] There is also a great increase in squamous cell carcinoma of the tip of the tongue, another sun-exposed portion of the body.

The 18 percent of XP patients with neurologic abnormalities have a sex ratio, reported age, frequency of ocular abnormalities, and frequency of cutaneous neoplasms similar to those of patients with only skin and eye involvement.[6] The neurologic symptoms vary in age of onset and severity but are characterized by

Table 14-1 Most Common Clinical Features of Xeroderma Pigmentosum

Skin abnormalities (usually limited to sun-exposed sites)
  Erythema and bullae (acute sensitivity in infancy)
  Freckles
  Xerosis (dryness) and scaling
  Areas of hyperpigmentation alternating with hyperpigmentation
  Telangiectasia
  Atrophy
  Benign lesion: actinic keratoses, keratocanthomas, angiomas, fibromas
  Malignant lesions: basal cell carcinoma, squamous cell carcinoma, melanoma

Ophthalmologic abnormalities (limited to anterior UV-exposed portion of the eye)
  Atrophy of lids
  Conjunctivitis with photophobia, lacrimation, edema
  Corneal abnormalities: keratitis, opacification, impaired vision
  Neoplasms of conjunctiva, cornea, and lids

Neurologic manifestations
  Microcephaly
  Low intelligence
  Progressive mental deterioration
  Progressive sensorineural deafness
  Abnormal motor activity
  Hyporeflexia or areflexia
  Primary neuronal degeneration

SOURCE: Adapted from Cleaver and Kraemer.[6] Used by permission.

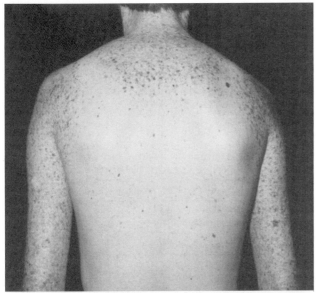

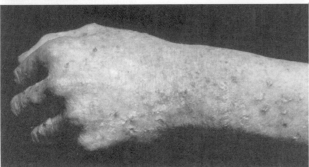

Fig. 14-2 Typical skin abnormalities in an adolescent XP patient (complementation group XP-C). *Top:* **Pigmentation abnormalities; freckling and dryness and atrophy visible at the sun-exposed areas of the skin.** *Bottom:* **Hand of same patient showing actinic keratosis and (pre)malignant lesions. (***Courtesy of Department of Dermatology, Erasmus University, Rotterdam.***)**

Table 14-2 Most Common Clinical Features of Cockayne Syndrome

Growth failure
 Decreased height and weight
 Decreased head circumference (microcephaly)

Neurologic manifestations
 Delayed psychomotor development
 Increased muscle tone
 Tremor
 Limb ataxia/incoordination
 Gait abnormality
 Hearing loss
 Calcification of basal ganglia of brain

Ophthalmologic abnormalities
 Cataracts
 Optic atrophy/hypoplasia
 Pigmentary retinopathy

Dental abnormalities: Caries

Skin abnormalities
 Photosensitivity
 Thin, dry hair

Cockayne Syndrome

CS is a rare, pleiotropic, autosomal recessive disorder with an extensive variation in symptoms and severity. Patients have cutaneous, neurologic, and somatic abnormalities (Table 14-2). Sun sensitivity of the skin is apparent in about three-fourths of affected individuals. In contrast to XP, CS patients do not have skin cancer predisposition. Since many patients exhibit multiple symptoms of premature aging, CS is also considered one of the progeroid disorders. The average age of death of reported patients is 12 years.

The first report on this condition by Cockayne appeared in 1936[6]: dwarfism with retinal atrophy and deafness. An extensive review, comprising 140 cases, was published by Nance and Berry in 1992.[12] These authors distinguish three clinically different classes of the disease: (1) a classic form (or CSI), which includes the majority of the patients, (2) a severe form (or CSII), characterized by early onset and severe progression of manifestations, and (3) a mild form, typified by late onset and slow progression of symptoms. Classical CS patients (CSI) (Fig. 14-3) show (1) growth failure (short stature), (2) neurodevelopmental and later neurologic dysfunction, (3) cutaneous photosensitivity (with or without thin or dry skin or hair), (4) progressive ocular abnormalities (such as progressive pigmentary retinopathy and/or cataracts), (5) hearing loss, (6) dental caries, and (7) a characteristic physical appearance (cachectic dwarfism, wizened facial appearance: bird-like facies). The last four criteria are more often registered in the older children. For diagnosis of CS in the infant, the presence of the first two criteria and a few of the other five criteria, together with biochemical and cellular evidence (UV sensitivity and DNA repair characteristics of CS in fibroblasts; see below), are required. Pathologic calcifications have been observed in the basal ganglia and at other locations in the central nervous system. Primary dysmyelination is an important feature seen in the nervous system of CS patients, in contrast to primary neuronal degeneration in XP. Often sexual development is impaired. The symptoms described above are much more severe and the onset much earlier in the CSII form of the disease. The characteristic facial and somatic appearance is present within the first 2 years of life. The prognosis is much worse than that of the classic CS patients. Death usually occurs by age 6 or 7. For details on the different forms of CS and further reference to other publications, the reader is referred to the review of Nance and Berry.[12]

progressive deterioration[9,10] (see Table 14-1). Diminished deep tendon reflexes and sensorineural deafness are frequent early abnormalities. In some patients, progressive mental retardation becomes evident only in the second decade of life. Patients with the DeSanctis-Cacchione syndrome have neurologic and somatic abnormalities beginning in the first years of life.[5] They have microcephaly, intellectual deterioration with loss of the ability to talk, and increasing spasticity with loss of ability to walk, leading to quadriparesis, in addition to dwarfism and immature sexual development. Among the few autopsies reported, the major finding is a primary neuronal degeneration with loss (or absence) of neurons, particularly in the cerebral cortex and cerebellum, without evidence of a storage process or inflammatory changes.[6] The severity of neurologic disease has been reported to correlate with the degree of sensitivity of cultured skin fibroblasts to UV inhibition of colony-forming ability.[11]

Evidence is presented for an increased risk of neoplasms in non-integumental tissues in individuals with XP.[8] However, more data are required to draw definite conclusions on this point. There are reports of patients with primary brain tumors (including two sarcomas), two with leukemia, two with lung tumors, and patients with gastric carcinomas.[6] Chemical carcinogens are suspected to play a role in these neoplasms, since cultured cells from XP patients are hypersensitive to certain DNA-binding chemical carcinogens that produce damaged DNA that is normally acted on by the NER system. These include benz[a]pyrene derivatives (found in cigarette smoke) and tryptophan pyrolysis products (found in charred food).[6]

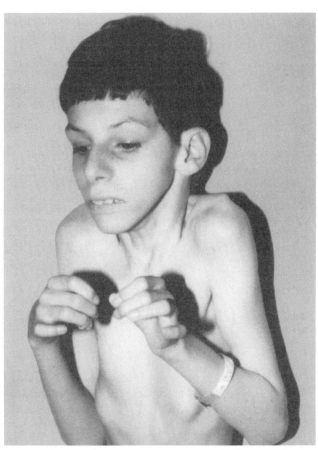

Fig. 14-3 Patient with CS. Growth failure, characteristic wizened facial appearance (bird-like facies), and skeletal deformation are visible. (*Photograph kindly provided by D. Atherton, Hospital for Sick Children, London. From Lehmann.[13] Used by permission.*)

Table 14-3 Main Clinical Symptoms of NER Syndromes

Clinical Symptoms	XP	XP-CS	CS	TTD
Photosensitivity	++	++	+*	+*
Abnormal pigmentation	++	+	−	−
Skin cancer	++	+	−	−
Progressive mental degeneration	−/+†	+	+	+
Neuronal loss	−/+†	−	−	−
Neurodysmyelination	−	++	+	+
Wizened facies	−	+	+	+
Growth defect	+/−†	+	+	+
Hypogonadism	−/+	+	+	+
Brittle hair and nails	−	−	−	+
Ichthyosis	−	−	−	+

* Also TTD and CS patients occur without photosensitivity and NER defect.
† These neurologic and growth defects are characteristic features of XP patients with the DeSanctis-Cacchione syndrome.

Trichothiodystrophy

TTD (sulfur-deficient brittle hair) is a rare autosomal recessive disorder. It represents a specific hair dysplasia associated with a variable range of abnormalities in organs derived from ectoderm and neuroendoderm (Fig. 14-4). About half the patients show photosensitivity of the skin that is due to a defect in NER.

The term *trichothiodystrophy* was introduced by Price in 1979.[14] The clinical hallmark of TTD is sulfur-deficient brittle hair, which is due to a reduced content of a class of matrix hair proteins that provide the hair shaft with its natural strength by crosslinking the keratin filaments. With polarizing light microscopy, a typical tiger tail pattern of the hair is visible. On scanning electron microscopy, the hair is flattened and irregular with longitudinal ridging and often somewhat twisted along the axis. Frequently, fractures are apparent, and the viscoelastic parameters of hair are different from controls.[15] The amino acid composition of the hair proteins is dramatically changed, with a strong reduction in cysteine and to a lesser extent proline, threonine, and serine residues and a concomitant relative increase in aspartic acid, methionine, phenylalanine, alanine, leucine, and lysine.[16] This is due to the strong reduction or complete absence of the class of ultra-high sulfur-rich matrix proteins, up to 30 percent of which are composed of cysteine residues that are involved in disulfide crosslinks. In addition, nails are dystrophic. Cutaneous signs include photosensitivity, ichthyosis, keratosis, erythema, and collodion baby. In many cases the brittle hair is associated with a heterogeneous complex of neuroectodermal abnormalities. Neurologic and developmental impairments within TTD are reminiscent of those found in CS. In a few cases, calcification of basal ganglia and dysmyelination[17–19] have been reported, as has been observed in CS (Table 14-3). Clinical manifestations and their severity vary extensively between TTD individuals. The broad spectrum of symptoms partly explains the confusing nomenclature in the literature for (probably) the same disease.[20,21] *PIBIDS* is an acronym for a specific combination of symptoms: photosensitivity, ichthyosis, brittle hair and nails, impaired intelligence, decreased fertility, and short stature. TTD also encompasses IBIDS, BIDS, and SIBIDS (osteosclerosis and IBIDS). Several other names have been used to describe patients in whom a number of the preceding features are present in combination with brittle hair: Pollitt, Tay, Amish brittle hair, Sabinas, and Marinesco-Sjögren syndromes and ONMR (onychotrichodysplasia, neutropenia, mental retardation). These patients, whether they have TTD or not, do not show photosensitivity and probably do not have a DNA repair defect. A practical classification scheme, based on a checklist of clinical abnormalities associated with TTD, is proposed by Tolmie et al.[19] and may be helpful in diagnosis of TTD patients.

A TTD patient has been described who lost his hair during an episode of pneumonia.[22] Within a period of a few months, the scalp hair returned. This peculiar phenomenon of hair loss after fever may be indicative of a thermosensitive mutation in the gene responsible for the disorder in these patients (see below).

Xeroderma Pigmentosum-Cockayne Syndrome Complex

A number of patients have been identified with clinical features of both XP and CS.[23–25] These patients had the cutaneous

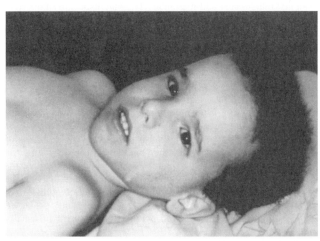

Fig. 14-4 Patient with TTD. Note the brittle hair as one of the crucial features of TTD. (*Photograph kindly provided by A. Sarasin, CNRS, Villejuif, France, and C. Blanchet-Bardon, Hopital Saint-Louis, Paris. From Lehmann.[13] Used by permission.*)

pigmentary and, in most cases, neoplastic features of XP along with the dwarfism, mental retardation, increased reflexes, and retinal degeneration typical of CS. They may correspond with the severe form of CS (CSII).

BIOCHEMICAL AND CELLULAR ASPECTS OF XP, CS, AND TTD

Production of Cellular Damage by Sunlight

Sunlight is the major environmental agent that is involved in many of the clinical symptoms of XP; it does so by damaging cutaneous cells. Understanding the biochemical defects in XP requires knowledge of the way the damaging wavelengths in sunlight are absorbed by macromolecules and the nature of the damage that is produced.

The wavelengths of sunlight reaching the surface of the earth extend into the near-UV region, the shortest detectable being about 290 nm. Shorter-wavelength UV (present in solar radiation in space) is blocked from reaching the ground by ozone and other components of the atmosphere. This lower limit slightly overlaps the upper region of the absorption spectra of nucleic acids and proteins. Energy in this region of overlap is absorbed by macromolecules in the skin, producing harmful effects that include erythema, burns, and actinic carcinogenesis.[26–28] Comparisons between direct sunlight and short-wavelength UV light (254 nm) indicate that sunlight in the midwestern United States is equivalent in germicidal activity to about 0.1 to 0.2 J/m² of surface per minute (J/m²min) of 254-nm UV light.[6,] Since normal human cells in culture have a D_{37}* of only about 3 to 5 J/m² of radiation at 254 nm, the direct exposure of human proliferating cells to sunlight can result in significant amounts of cell killing.

Radiation at the UV end of the sun's spectrum produces its biologic effects through absorption of quanta in molecules that have unsaturated chemical bonds, such as aromatic amino acids in proteins and purine and pyrimidine components of DNA and RNA. The action spectra for production of DNA damage (pyrimidine photoproducts), cell killing, production of aberrant chromosomes, and induction of unscheduled DNA repair synthesis (i.e., DNA synthesis not associated with the normal cell cycle; see below) are all similar, exhibiting maximum efficiency in wavelengths from 260 to 280 nm. Although there is negligible energy in this region of the sun's spectrum, there is sufficient overlap of the shortest end of the sun's spectrum with the longer-wavelength side of the absorption spectrum of DNA for significant photochemical reaction to occur. Shorter-wavelength UV is absorbed by the outer, nondividing layers of skin cells. An action spectrum of production of DNA damage in human skin shows a peak at about 302 nm.[6]

Two kinds of pyrimidine photoproducts are the most relevant type of damage induced in DNA by absorption of UV light. The most frequent is the cyclobutane pyrimidine dimer (Fig. 14-5). This is formed between adjacent pyrimidines in the same strand of DNA by the formation of two bonds between the 5 positions and between the 6 positions on the pyrimidine rings. An alternative dipyrimidine photoproduct is the [6-4]pyrimidine-pyrimidone product, mainly consisting of 5′TC or 5′CC (see Fig. 14-5), which is formed at lower rates than the cyclobutane dimer but is also important biologically. Various estimates suggest that the [6-4] photoproduct is formed at 10 to 50 percent of the frequency of cyclobutane dimers by low doses of 254-nm light. Numerous biologic effects, such as cell killing, production of chromosome aberrations, mutagenesis, and carcinogenesis, can be attributed to these photoproducts in DNA. Other photoproducts have biologic effects in some circumstances. These include the unstable cytosine

---

*The D_{37} is the dose required to reduce survival to 0.37 from the initial value of 1.0 and in target theory corresponds to the dose required to produce an average of one lethal hit on the sensitive target of an irradiated organism when the survival curve is exponential.

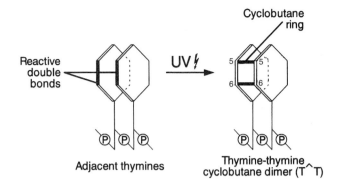

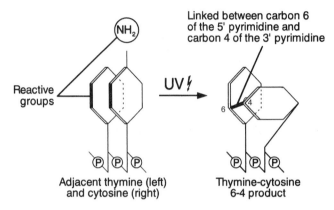

Fig. 14-5 Main UV-induced DNA lesions. *Top*: The cyclobutane pyrimidine dimer between adjacent thymines on the same strand of DNA. *Bottom*: [6-4] photoproduct between adjacent thymine and cytosine on same strand of DNA. Particularly the latter results in considerable distortion of the phosphodiester backbone of DNA.

hydrate, purine photoproducts, and at relatively high doses, locally denatured regions, DNA-protein crosslinks, and single-strand breaks.

Repair of Sunlight-Induced DNA Damage

At least three different biochemical repair systems operate in sunlight-exposed cells to safeguard DNA from permanent damage. These are excision repair, postreplication repair (which is more like a damage-tolerance mechanism), and photoreactivation. These systems have been found in bacteria, yeast, amphibians, fish, rodents, marsupials, and mammals. They are especially important in the skin, where they mend damage to DNA caused by UV light. Some of the repair systems also can mend damage to DNA caused by chemical carcinogens. These systems presumably protect internal tissues against the carcinogenic and mutagenic consequences of exposure to chemicals that damage DNA.

Excision repair is extremely versatile and can mend a large variety of UV light, x-ray, and chemically induced forms of damage to DNA.[6,29] Excision repair may be subdivided into NER and base excision repair (BER). The NER system, which will be discussed in the next section, excises damaged single strands of DNA and replaces them with a new sequence of bases, using as a template for base pairing the intact strand of DNA opposite the original damaged site. BER removes damaged bases, leaving the sugar-phosphate backbone of the DNA intact and creating an AP (apurinic or apyrimidinic) site. This site is subsequently converted into a strand break and repaired by short-patch repair of usually one or a few nucleotides.

Postreplication repair is not a damage-repair pathway per se but a damage-tolerance mechanism that solves the problem the replication machinery faces when it encounters a damage in the template. This poorly defined process has been studied best in *S.*

cerevisiae, where two subpathways have been distinguished.[30] The first is reinitiation of DNA replication at a more downstream location, leaving a gap opposite the lesion. After replication of the complementary strand, the newly copied information is used to fill in the gap in the other strand by recombination. This pathway is in principle error-free. The second subpathway induces translesion DNA replication. However, this process is error-prone and may be the main determinant of all damage-induced mutations. Very little is known about this pathway in mammals, and it is not sure whether it follows the same principal steps in higher species.

The third repair system, photoreactivation, simply reverts the damaged DNA to the normal chemical state without removing or exchanging any material from the DNA. This is accomplished by a single protein, photolyase, carrying two blue-light–harvesting chromophore cofactors that provide the energy for disrupting the dipyrimidine bonds. The photoreactivation system was thought to be specific for one form of damage induced by UV light — the cyclobutane pyrimidine dimer. A [6-4] photoproduct — specific photolyase was observed in *Drosophila* and various other organisms (*Xenopus,* plants) pointing to a widespread occurrence.[31] CPD-photoreactivation has been demonstrated in bacteria, yeast, fish, amphibians, and marsupials, but the existence and importance of this system in human tissue are still controversial.[6] Interestingly, two human genes were identified in the sequence data-base with significant overall homology to the *Drosophila* [6-4]-photolyase but even more to blue-light receptors in plants[31,32] that carry out a variety of blue-light–sensing functions. This renders it unlikely that the human genes are involved in DNA repair.

The NER System

NER is one of the major and most versatile repair mechanisms that operates in the cell. This universal system eliminates a remarkably diverse array of structurally unrelated lesions that range from UV-induced photoproducts (cyclobutane pyrimidine dimers and [6-4] photoproducts) to bulky and small chemical adducts as well as interstrand crosslinks. Thus it is not surprising that the NER process entails multiple steps and involves the concerted action of a number of proteins. The details of this repair mechanism are best understood in the case of the UvrABC system in the bacterium *E. coli.*[33–36] Briefly, at least six distinct steps can be discerned: (1) lesion recognition and (2) lesion demarcation, which involves

conformational changes in DNA, are carried out by the UvrA2B complex. (3) A complex of UvrB and UvrC incises the damaged strand on both sides of the lesion at some distance, leaving the nondamaged strand intact. (4) The damage-containing oligomer is removed by the helicase action of UvrD, followed by (5) gap-filling DNA synthesis by DNA polymerase I. The process is completed by (6) the sealing of the new DNA to the preexisting strand by DNA ligase. In principle, this mode of repair is error-free because it uses the nucleotide sequence information of the intact complementary DNA strand.

Although in outline and in concept quite simple, it is becoming increasingly apparent that the scheme of the NER repair mechanism as depicted above for *E. coli* represents a dramatic oversimplification, particularly when extrapolated to eukaryotes. This notion is based on a number of observations.

First, a minimum of two in-part overlapping NER subpathways have been discovered; these are represented schematically in Fig. 14-6. One subpathway, here referred to as *transcription-coupled repair (TCR),* deals with the complication that the vital process of transcription is blocked by lesions in the template. To cope with this urgent problem, TCR takes care for the complete elimination of injury in the transcribed strand of active structural genes.[37,38] This holds particularly for lesions for which repair otherwise would be too slow or inefficient. In this specialized NER subpathway, initial damage detection is thought to be carried out by RNA polymerase II, when it is blocked in front of a lesion. As part of the repair mechanism, the stalled RNA polymerase complex has to be displaced to give the repair machinery access to the injury. The process occurs in *E. coli* and eukaryotes. Another branch of the NER system — here designated *global genome repair (GGR)* — accomplishes removal of lesions in the entire genome. Damage recognition in this repair system is performed by a specific NER protein (complex) and is for many lesions (e.g., CPD lesions) — but not all (e.g., [6-4] photoproducts) — more slow and less efficient when compared with TCR. The efficiency of damage recognition by the GGR system varies strongly from lesion to lesion and also may vary with the chromatin conformation, the location in the genome, and the state of differentiation of the cell. This is not so surprising when one realizes the tremendous task that is faced by this system in continually surveilling the 2 m of DNA double helix in every mammalian nucleus for trace amounts of a diversity of lesions.

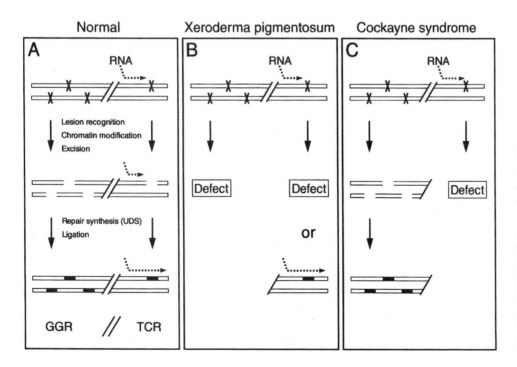

Fig. 14-6 NER pathways and defects in XP and CS. This simplified scheme shows in the left panel (normal cells) the transcription-coupled repair (TCR) pathway (*at right*) that mends lesions in the transcribed strand of active genes, and the global genome repair (GGR) pathway (*at left*) that deals with lesions in the remaining part of the genome. In XP (*center panel*), the genetic defect in most cases affects both mechanisms; in XP complementation group C, only GGR is impaired. In CS (*right panel*) the defect is opposite XP-C; only TCR is deficient.

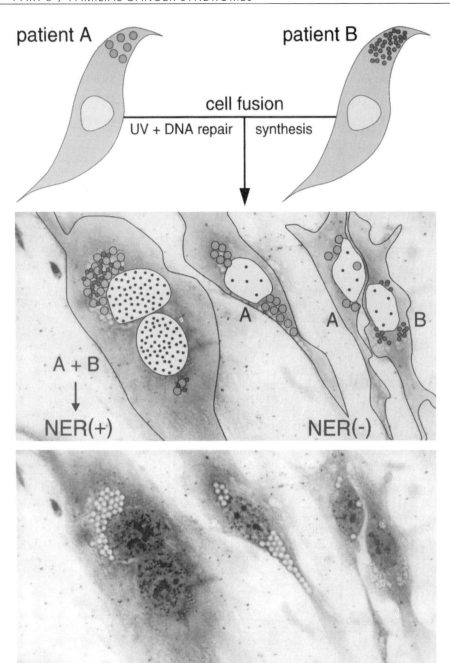

Fig. 14-7 Genetic heterogeneity in XP studied by cell fusion and UV-induced unscheduled DNA synthesis (UDS). *Top*: A schematic representation of the micrograph presented at the bottom. Cultured fibroblasts from two unrelated patients (A and B) were fused, exposed to UV light, pulse labeled with [³H]thymidine, fixed, and autoradiographed to visualize DNA repair synthesis (UDS). Cells of patient A are marked with engulfed large latex beads and those of patient B with small beads. This marking enables the identification of the fused cells containing nuclei of both patients (heterokaryons). If the patients are mutated in different DNA repair genes (gene *A* and gene *B*), the heterokaryon will be able to perform normal levels of DNA repair synthesis (UDS is visualized by wild-type levels of autoradiographic grains in the emulsion above the nuclei). In this case patients A and B belong to two different complementation groups. (*From the Department of Cell Biology and Genetics, Erasmus University, Rotterdam, W. Vermeulen and D. Bootsma.*)

NER is visualized under the microscope by the unscheduled DNA synthesis (UDS) test. Cultured fibroblasts are exposed to UV and briefly (2-3 h) incubated in [³H]thymidine-containing medium. Cells in G1 or G2 phase of the cell cycle become radioactively labeled by the gap-filling DNA-synthesis step of the NER process. Following autoradiography, the repair capacity of these cells can be quantified at the single-cell level. The UDS test has proven to be a powerful tool to measure NER in repair-proficient and -deficient cells (see Figs. 14-7 and 14-11).

NER Activity in XP, CS, and TTD Cells

Defective DNA excision repair in UV-irradiated skin fibroblasts from some XP patients was reported for the first time by Cleaver in 1968[39] and in skin in vivo by Epstein et al.[40] The NER defect in TTD cells was first reported by Stefanini et al.[41] The defect in most XP and TTD cells is reflected by decreased levels of UDS (Fig. 14-7). Measurement of UV-induced UDS is in fact required for a definitive diagnosis of NER-deficient XP and TTD. Different levels of UDS in unrelated XP patients suggested heterogeneity at the molecular level in this syndrome.[42] A number of XP patients have shown a normal response in the UDS test. They have been designated as *XP variants*[43] and were found to have a defect in the ill-defined postreplication repair process.[44] Similarly, various degrees of NER deficiency have been demonstrated among TTD patients, including normal DNA repair in approximately half of patients.[49]

UDS in CS cells is not significantly different from that in normal cells. However, by measuring NER separately in transcribed and nontranscribed strands of specific genes, a technique developed by the group of Hanawalt,[45] Venema et al.[46] have demonstrated deficient repair of the transcribed strand of active genes in CS cells (see Fig. 14-6). The less efficient GGR is still functional. Since TCR makes a relatively small contribution to the total repair synthesis, CS fibroblasts show near-normal levels of UDS. The TCR defect prevents the rapid recovery of RNA synthesis after UV exposure. This delayed recovery of

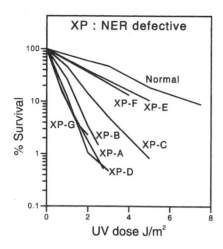
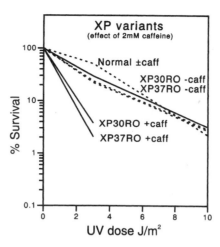
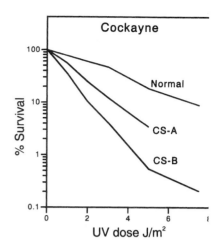

Fig. 14-8 UV-sensitivity of XP and CS cells. (*Left*) XP cells of different complementation groups. (*Center*) XP-variant cells in the presence and absence of caffeine. Caffeine sensitizes XP-variant cells to UV. (*Right*) CS cells. (*From the Department of Cell Biology and Genetics: Raams, Jaspers, and Hoeijmakers.*)

RNA synthesis and also of S-phase DNA synthesis in CS cells following UV exposure is used as a diagnostic criterion of CS[25,47,48] in combination with clinical symptoms.

Colony-Forming Ability of XP, CS, and TTD Cells

The number of cells in culture that can grow into colonies after UV irradiation can be used as an in vitro measurement of sensitivity. Heterogeneity in the response of fibroblasts of unrelated XP patients is evident (Fig. 14-8, left panel). In all cases, NER-deficient XP fibroblasts are more sensitive than normal cells, and those from patients who exhibit neurologic abnormalities are generally the most sensitive.[10]

XP cells are also more sensitive to carcinogenic chemicals creating bulky DNA adducts (including benz[a]pyrene) but are normal in response to DNA methylating agents and, with a few exceptions, to x-rays.[6]

Fibroblasts of XP-variants do not exhibit a significant increase of UV-sensitivity under standard test conditions. A dramatic increase in sensitivity becomes apparent if XP-variant cells are incubated in the presence of caffeine after UV exposure (see Fig. 14-8, middle panel). This effect of caffeine on UV-sensitivity may be used as a diagnostic test that is specific for the XP-variant type and much simpler than the demonstration of a defective post-replication repair.

The delayed recovery of RNA synthesis as a result of the TCR defect in CS cells probably causes the increased sensitivity in CS cells (see Fig. 14-8, right panel). An increasing number of patients have been diagnosed as probable CS cases who do not show photosensitivity.[12] Fibroblasts of these patients do not display increased sensitivity in the colony-formation test. Similar patterns of UV sensitivity are observed with fibroblast cultures of photosensitive and non-photosensitive TTD patients.[49] These non-photosensitive CS and TTD fibroblasts also behave like normal cells in UDS and in DNA- and RNA-synthesis recovery tests. These results suggest that these patients do not have a DNA repair defect and that their clinical symptoms have another cause. (For an explanation, see "Implications for Diagnosis" below.)

CS cells are also sensitive to UV-mimetic carcinogens such as 4NQO and *N*-acetoxy-*N*-2-acetyl-2-aminofluorene but not to monofunctional alkylating agents.[50]

Mutational Events in XP, CS, and TTD Cells

Cultured cells from most XP and CS patients have a normal karyotype. Distinctive spontaneous karyotypic changes characteristic for some diseases with a high cancer incidence, such as ataxia telangiectasia, Fanconi anemia, and Bloom syndrome,[21] are not seen in XP patients.

XP cells show a normal frequency of spontaneous sister chromatid exchanges (SCEs) but a greater than normal frequency after exposure to UV light and most chemical carcinogens.[6] Similarly, XP cells show more chromosome aberrations than normal cells after exposure to UV light and chemical carcinogens.[6]

The frequency with which cells resistant to 6-thioguanine, ouabain, diphtheria toxin, or other toxic chemicals are produced by irradiation with UV light or artificial sunlight or by exposure to chemical carcinogens is greater in all XP cells, including XP-variants, than in normal cells.[6] This implies that the genetic defects in XP cells confer increased mutability. In the XP-variant, the repair system has lost fidelity and so produces a high frequency of mutations. Evidence has been presented for increased transformation to anchorage independence (growth in suspension instead of attached to the bottom of a culture disk, which is considered to represent a step in the direction of neoplastic transformation) after UV irradiation of XP-variant cells compared with normal cells.[51]

Shuttle vector plasmids that are capable of autonomous replication in both mammalian cells and *E. coli* have been used for measuring the frequency and spectrum of mutations following exposure of transfected cells to DNA damage.[6] There were significantly fewer plasmids with tandem or multiple base substitution mutations or with single or tandem transversion mutations after transfection of UV-damaged plasmids in XP cells than in normal cells. With all cell lines, the predominant base substitution mutation was the G-C to A-T transition; i.e., the C mutated to a T. Thus, with these human cells, the major UV photoproduct, the TT cyclobutane dimer, is not the major premutagenic lesion. This finding is consistent with the A rule: a tendency of polymerases to insert adenines opposite noninstructional lesions. Thus insertion of A opposite TT dimers results in the correct pairing, whereas insertion of A opposite a C, involved in cyclobutane dimers and [6-4] photoproducts (see Fig. 14-5), results in G-C to A-T transitions.

UV-damaged viruses and plasmids also have been used as substrates to measure the capacity of NER-deficient cells to repair DNA damage by monitoring the extent of their biologic recovery, e.g., by their ability to propagate in bacterial hosts.[6] The extent of this host-cell reactivation by various cell types often parallels the ability to survive UV damage. Host-cell reactivation assays employing UV-damaged plasmids treated in vitro with CPD-photolyase (which selectively removes cyclobutane dimers) have been used to study repair of different types of photoproducts. While XP-A cells show poor repair of all types of photoproducts, CS cells have faulty repair of cyclobutane dimers but normal repair of non-dimer photoproducts.[52,53]

GENETIC ASPECTS OF XP, CS, AND TTD

Complementation Analysis of NER Deficiency Syndromes

The clinical heterogeneity in XP and the marked differences in cellular expression of the NER defect in terms of unscheduled DNA synthesis in different patients[42] were studied by using a cell fusion assay to investigate genetic heterogeneity in XP.[54] Heterokaryons formed between fibroblasts of different XP patients exposed to UV light either showed normal or nearly normal levels of UDS (i.e., patients complement each other's defects and therefore belong to different complementation groups; see Fig. 14-7) or exhibited the impaired levels of UDS seen in the unfused XP cells (i.e., patients are in the same complementation group). Each complementation group may represent a gene that, if mutated and in homozygous condition, causes XP (intergenic complementation).

A total of seven complementation groups have been identified in NER-deficient XP.[6] In comparison, at least 15 distinct genes involved in NER (the *RAD3* epistasis group) have been identified in *S. cerevisiae*. This difference is probably due to incompatibility of some defects with normal embryonic development.

By using the RNA-synthesis recovery test in cell fusion studies, the patients with CS (in its classic form, without XP features and/or without GGR deficiency) could be assigned to two complementation groups: CS-A and CS-B.[47,55]

The rare patients having the XP-CS complex were found to be members of complementation groups XP-B, -D, and -G.[24] There is also genetic overlap between XP and TTD, although the clinical features are very different. Almost all UV-sensitive TTD patients fall into the XP-D group.[49] Recently, one TTD family was found to belong to XP-B,[56] and a third kindred constitutes a distinct NER-deficient complementation group, TTD-A[41] not (yet) associated with XP.

Thus both genetic heterogeneity within and genetic overlap between all NER disorders is found. A specific subset of XP groups (notably XP-D and XP-B) is associated with extreme variability ranging from XP to CS to TTD. Therefore, these disorders may in fact be considered different manifestations of one heterogeneous clinical continuum.

Characteristics of Complementation Groups

Some of the properties of the XP and TTD complementation groups are summarized in Table 14-4.

XP Group A. Group A usually corresponds to the most severe clinical form of XP, in which there are both skin symptoms and central nervous system (CNS) disorders. Many patients exhibit manifestations from birth or early in life and correspond to the clinical category of the DeSanctis-Cacchione syndrome with progressive neurologic degeneration.[6]

Excision repair is generally very low (<2 percent of normal) in cells of most XP-A patients, and they are about 10 times more sensitive than normal to killing by UV irradiation or other UV-mimicking carcinogens (see Fig. 14-8). The genetic defect in this group interferes with both TCR and GGR.

There are exceptions to these general characteristics of group A cells. Cells from a British patient without CNS disorders (XP8LO) exhibited about 30 percent of normal cellular excision repair and higher survival after UV than other group A cells.[6] A 35-year-old Egyptian male (XP13CA) had the typical low level of unscheduled synthesis but was neurologically normal, had normal stature, and was fertile. Two other group A patients (XP12BE and XP1LO) also show milder neurologic abnormalities, whereas their cells are less UV sensitive than the majority in group A.[6] In one Italian family, group A siblings exhibited different clinical symptoms; only one had CNS signs.[6] In cell cultures, it appeared that the sibling without CNS disorder had, on average, higher repair due to a subpopulation of cells with normal repair mixed with typical group A cells. Therefore, although group A patients usually have the associated neurologic abnormalities of the DeSanctis-Cacchione syndrome, several are known who are neurologically normal or have less severe neurologic abnormalities.

XP Group B. For many years XP group B consisted only of 1 patient (XP11BE)[23] (Fig. 14-9). This patient died of acute hypertension at age 33. She had small stature, deafness, mental retardation, immature sexual development, premature senility, absence of subcutaneous fat, and optic nerve and retinal pigment degeneration characteristic of CS. She exhibited acute sun sensitivity, ocular changes, and multiple cutaneous malignancy at age 18, all typical of XP.

Two siblings (XP1BA and XP2BA) with mild features of XP and CS were recently assigned to XP-B.[58] Developmental abnormalities are nearly absent in these individuals, and neurologic symptoms became evident only after the second decade of life.[59]

A remarkable clinical variation is observed between these two XP-B families. The two siblings do not display any cutaneous malignancies despite a relatively advanced age for XP of more than 40 years, whereas patient XP11BE had skin tumors at 18

Table 14-4 Properties of XP, CS, and TTD Complementation Groups

Complementation Group	UV sensitivity	Residual UDS*	NER Activity TCR†	NER Activity GGR‡	Relative Frequency§	Skin Cancer	Neurologic Abnormalities	Clinical Phenotype
XP-A	+++	<5%	−	−	High	+	++	XP
XP-B	++	3–40%	−	−	3 families	+/−	++/+	XP/CS or TTD
XP-C	+	15–30%	+	−	High	+	−	XP
XP-D	++	15–50%	−	−	Intermediate	+/−	++/−	XP, XP/CS or TTD
XP-E	±	50%	?	?	Rare	+/−	−	XP
XP-F	+	15–30%	−	−	Rare	+/−	−/±	XP
XP-G	++	<5–25%	−	−	Rare	+/−	++/+	XP or XP/CS
TTD-A	+	10%	−	−	1 family	−	+	TTD
CS-A	+	Normal range	−	+	Intermediate	−	++	CS
CS-B	+	Normal range	−	+	High	−	++	CS
XP-V¶	+/±	Normal range	+	+	High	+/−	−	XP

*Unscheduled DNA synthesis, expressed as percentage of repair synthesis in normal cells.
† Transcription coupled repair.
‡Global genome repair.
§ The overall frequency of XP is between 10^{-5} to 10^{-6}; less than 500 cases have been classified.
¶XP-variant, defect in post-replication repair, proficient NER.

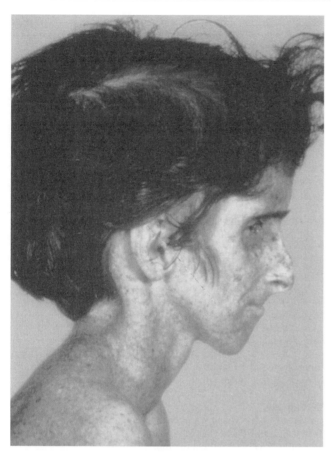

Fig. 14-9 XP patient (XP11BE). This patient, 28 years old, from complementation group B, exhibits skin, ocular, and neurologic characteristics that have been ascribed to both XP and CS. (*From Kraemer.*[57] *Used by permission.*)

years. Nevertheless, the level of UDS representing the repair defect is similar in both families (5–10 percent of NER-proficient cells) and affects both TCR and GGR. A new Slovenian 28 year-old patient with XP and CS features was assigned to this group, having the same residual UDS level (Bohnert, Jaspers, and Bootsma, unpublished observations).

The assignment to XP-B of two siblings (TTD4VI and TTD6VI) with relatively mild clinical features of TTD and moderately impaired NER characteristics (about 40 percent UDS)[56] extends the clinical heterogeneity within this complementation group.

XP Group C. Group C is one of the largest groups and is often referred to as the classic form of XP. The patients usually show only skin and eye disorders. These vary considerably in severity, depending on sun exposure. Patients of over 80 years of age have been diagnosed. Tumors of the tip of the tongue have been observed in several patients. A case of XP-C is presented in Fig. 14-2. The level of UDS varies between 15 and 30 percent of normal, and XP-C cells are less sensitive to killing by UV light and chemical carcinogens than cells from groups A and D (see Fig. 14-8). One characteristic of repair unique to this group is that the repair sites are clustered rather than random[60] due to a selective loss in the capacity to perform GGR in the presence of normal levels of TCR.[61] In this respect, this defect is opposite to the deficiency in the classic form of CS[46] (see Fig. 14-6).

One exceptional patient (XP1MI) exhibited symptoms of XP, systemic lupus erythematosus, microcephaly, and a marginal degree of mental retardation.[62] Cells from this patient had DNA repair levels typical for XP-C but were the most UV-sensitive in group C.[11] Two reported instances of CNS tumors in XP

patients—XP106LO and Hawaiian patient XP15BE—are in this group.[6]

XP Group D. This is a very interesting group because of the extensive clinical heterogeneity. Many XP-D patients have skin and neurologic abnormalities like those in group A, although the onset of the CNS disorders may be delayed until the second decade. Patients with a very mild photosensitivity also were found in this group (Jaspers and Bootsma, unpublished observations). In addition to these classic XP patients, almost all the photosensitive TTD patients have been assigned to this complementation group.[49,63] So far no reports on the occurrence of skin cancer within this group of XP-D TTD patients have appeared. Furthermore, five patients with the combined XP-CS complex of varying severity were found to belong to XP group D[6] (Jaspers and Bootsma, unpublished observations). Thus XP-D is a complex group involving diverse clinical syndromes.[64] GGR, measured as UDS, varies from 15 to over 70 percent, with no clear correlation with the clinical severity or type of symptoms. Some evidence suggests that the amount of UDS in the XP and XP-CS cases is higher than expected from the low amount of dimer excision observed in these cells and their sensitivity to cell killing (comparable with XP-A cells; see Fig. 14-8). This is perhaps due to better repair of [6-4] photoproducts in these cells.[6]

XP Group E. Patients in the rare group E exhibit mild skin symptoms and are neurologically normal.[23] The level of excision repair is high (> 50 percent of normal), and the level relative to normal cells increases with increasing UV dose. The cells are only slightly more sensitive than normal to UV damage (see Fig. 14-8). Patients have been reported from Europe and Japan. One XP-E patient (XP2RO) died from metastatic tumor of endothelial origin.

XP Group F. Most representatives of group F have been described in Japan.[65] The patients had acute sun sensitivity in infancy but relatively mild symptoms with late onset of skin cancer despite a substantially reduced level of repair. Two patients have been reported with neurologic deficits late in life. Excision repair was 15 to 30 percent of normal but increased to 60 percent with incubation and appears long-lasting. The cells seem to be more defective in repair of damage that occurs at rapid rates and at early times after irradiation such as [6-4] photoproducts.[6] They show an intermediate sensitivity to killing by UV light and a high degree of excision of pyrimidine dimers when measured at late times after irradiation. There was a marked enhancement of UV survival when cells were held in a density-inhibited condition after irradiation.[66]

XP Group G. Until 1996 this rare group comprised only eight patients, all from Europe and Japan,[24,67] but since then, at least seven additional patients have been identified from all continents (Jaspers and Bootsma, unpublished observations). The clinical symptoms vary from mild cutaneous and no neurologic abnormalities to severe dermatologic and neurologic impairment characteristic of XP. So far a skin tumor was reported in only one patient from Japan (XP31KO), which appeared at a relatively late age. UDS and survival levels are usually very low, but significant residual activity was observed in a few (e.g., XP31KO, 25 percent UDS). A rapidly growing subset of patients with very low UDS levels (2 percent or less) displays severe symptoms of CS already at birth; very often XP features do not become manifest (presumably due to continuous hospitalization and early demise). Occasionally, these infants were first thought to have a related disorder such as cerebro-oculofacial syndrome (COFS). The category of XP-CS patients is now in the majority within XP group G, but this may well represent a selection bias over the more standard XP patients, who are genetically scrutinized to a lesser extent. Interestingly, cells from some patients with either XP or XP-CS showed mild cellular hypersensitivity to ionizing radiation and/or hydrogen peroxide.[67,68] This sensitivity, pointing to a possible deficiency in the repair of oxidative radical damage, was suggested (at least partially) to underlie the severe clinical phenotypes in XP-G.[68,69]

XP-Variant. Patients in the variant group have mild to severe skin symptoms and usually have normal CNS functions. The variant form is found worldwide and is a frequently occurring and distinct group, even though it cannot often be identified clinically without cell culture studies. Originally defined as a clinically recognized XP without a defect in excision repair,[23,43] it also was described earlier under the clinical designation *pigmented xerodermoid*.[70] With careful clinical investigation, some patients in this group may be recognized by relatively mild symptoms and the absence of an enhanced erythematous response, but this is insufficient for unambiguous diagnosis, and other XP-variant patients may have severe clinical symptoms.[23]

The high level of mutagenesis with near-normal levels of cell survival after UV irradiation could be interpreted as an indication that the inherited disorder has made XP-variant cells error-prone.[6] The outstanding feature of this form of XP is that after UV irradiation, replication forks appear to stop or to be interrupted during semi-conservative replication at every site of DNA damage.[44] This is interpreted as a defect in postreplication repair.

Whether the variant group is homogeneous or has multiple subgroups is not known, but the clinical heterogeneity is suggestive. The pigmented xerodermoid family of Jung et al.,[70] although biochemically identical to other XP-variants, is unusual because no clinical symptoms were evident until after age 40, and patients lived into their eighties. These mild symptoms contrast with other variant families from comparable environments in whom the disease is quite severe.[6] One attempt at studying complementation between cells from different XP-variant patients indicated a single XP-variant group.[71]

TTD Group A. The cells of one TTD patient (TTD1BR) complemented cells from all seven XP complementation groups and apparently represents a third TTD complementation group (TTD-A) in addition to XP-B and XP-D.[41] This patient, first described in 1982,[72] has typical symptoms of TTD and has been sensitive to sunlight since early childhood. His clinical features are quite distinct from those associated with XP, showing no significant freckling or other pigmentary changes and no skin tumors.[41]

CS Complementation Groups. Complementation analysis has disclosed two groups in the classic form of CS: CS-A and CS-B. CS is clinically heterogeneous. The clinical differentiation among CS individuals, based on the age of onset and severity of the disease (CSI and CSII),[12] does not correlate with these two complementation groups. Clinical variation is further complicated by other syndromes, which resemble many of the traits observed in CS: CAMFAK (cataracts, microcephaly, failure to thrive, kyphoscoliosis) and COFS (cerebro-oculofacial syndrome). Assays of DNA repair have been normal in these syndromes.[12] In addition to these COFS and CAMFAK patients, who usually show no evidence of UV sensitivity,[12] there is an increasing group of other patients without clinical and cellular photosensitivity and with only some or various hallmarks of a CS diagnosis[12,73] (Jaspers and Bootsma, unpublished observations). In the absence of a suitable biochemical marker, the genetic relationship of these patients, as well as the CAMFAK and COFS patients, to CS remains to be established.

Two other patients with a CS-type DNA repair defect, assigned to CS complementation group B, exhibit only XP symptoms.[74] At the other side of the spectrum, there are individuals with clear CS hallmarks (dwarfism, mental retardation, deafness, and peculiar facies) but without a reduced post-UV RNA synthesis recovery and photosensitivity.[73]

UVS Syndrome. Two siblings were described with a sun-sensitive skin but no apparent clinical symptoms of CS or XP.[75] Accordingly, hypersensitivity and irreversible inhibition of transcription were found after UV exposure. The level of UDS was normal, a biochemical pattern grossly reminiscent of CS but also observed in some XP-D patients (Jaspers and Bootsma, unpublished observations). Careful genetic analysis revealed that these siblings belong to a separate category called *ultraviolet sensitive* (UVS) that is different from all XP and CS groups and XP-variants.[76]

These observations strengthen the notion that the syndromes XP, CS, and TTD are closely related biochemically and may be part of a broad clinical continuum.

Genetic Classification of Other Eukaryotic NER Mutants

The clinical and genetic heterogeneity in NER syndromes raised the question of whether the complementation groups represent single gene defects, inherited in a simple Mendelian fashion, or whether more than one genetic locus is involved in each patient.[77] Cloning of the responsible genes would give the answer.

An important first step on the way to cloning repair genes was the isolation of repair-deficient rodent mutant cell lines. Many of these cell lines are of Chinese hamster origin (CHO and V79 cell lines). So far complementation analysis of these UV-sensitive mutants has revealed at least 11 distinct complementation groups.[78,79] The main features are summarized in Table 14-5. The first five groups consist of cell lines that are extremely

Table 14-5 Properties of Rodent NER Complementation Groups

Group	Representative Mutant	Parental Strain*	Sensitivity†		Incision Deficiency	Correcting Human Gene	XP or CS Equivalent
			UV	MMC			
1	UV20, 43-3B	CHO	++	+++	Yes	ERCC1	Not identified
2	UV5, VH-1	CHO/V79	++	+	Yes	ERCC2	XP-D
3	UV24, 28-1	CHO	++	+	Yes	ERCC3	XP-B
4	UV41	CHO	++	+++	Yes	ERCC4	XP-F
5	UV135, Q31	CHO, mouse lymphoma	+(+)	±	Yes	ERCC5	XP-G
6	UV61, US46	CHO, mouse lymphoma	+	+	Partial	ERCC6	CS-B
7	VB11	V79	+	±	Partial	?	?
8	US31	Mouse lymphoma	+	+	?	ERCC8	CS-A
9	CHO4PV	CHO	+	+	Partial	—	?
10	CHO7PV	CHO	+	+	Partial	—	?
11	UVS1	CHO	+/++	+	Yes	ERCC11‡	XP-F

*CHO = Chinese hamster ovary.
†+: 2–5×; ++: 5–10×; +++: >10× wild-type sensitivity; MMC = mitomycin C.
‡ERCC11 and ERCC4 are probably identical.

sensitive to UV and bulky adducts and, in that respect, resemble the XP groups A, B, D, and G. Repair in the few representatives of the remaining groups (except group 11) appears to be only partially disturbed, as in CS-A and CS-B and in XP groups C, E, and F and UVS. A unique characteristic of groups 1 and 4 is their extreme sensitivity to crosslinking agents such as mitomycin C (MMC). This suggests that the NER genes affected in these mutants act in additional systems other than NER or respond to crosslink damage in DNA. Cell fusion studies performed by Thompson[80] showed that human genes could complement the rodent repair defects in these mutant cell lines.

Another relevant class of eukaryotic NER mutants is presented by the *RAD3* epistasis group of bakers yeast *S. cerevisiae.* At least 15 complementation groups have been identified in this category of UV-sensitive yeast mutants (for review, see ref. 36). The versatility of yeast genetics has permitted the cloning of almost all the corresponding genes. The strong parallels with the mammalian system that have emerged in recent years make this organism a relevant paradigm for human NER. As shown below, there is considerable overlap between the yeast and Chinese hamster mutants and the human NER syndromes. This overlap is represented by the sequence homology of DNA repair genes and proteins in yeast, *Drosophila,* and mammals including humans and is based on strong evolutionary conservation of DNA repair mechanisms. It emphasizes the important function of DNA repair in maintaining life.

Cloning of Human NER Genes

Different strategies have been followed to clone human NER genes. A time-consuming but successful procedure has been transfection of genomic DNA from repair-proficient human cells or from a chromosome-specific cosmid library to repair-deficient rodent mutants followed by UV selection of repair-competent, UV-resistant transformants. The correcting gene subsequently can be isolated via standard recombinant DNA techniques. This strategy has resulted in the cloning of the human excision repair cross-complementing (*ERCC*) genes that correct the rodent complementation groups 1 to 6: *ERCC1,*[81] *ERCC2,*[82] *ERCC3,*[83] *ERCC4,*[84] *ERCC5,*[85] and *ERCC6.*[86]

Their possible role in NER syndromes in humans can be investigated by DNA transfection of the cloned genes into cells of the different complementation groups of XP, CS, or TTD. Alternatively, the cDNA or the gene product can be microinjected into the nucleus or cytoplasm of cultured fibroblasts of NER-deficient patients. Introduction of the *ERCC2, ERCC3, ERCC5,* and *ERCC6* genes into human NER-deficient cells alleviated the specific defects in cells from XP-D,[87,88] XP-B,[89] XP-G,[90] and CS-B,[91] respectively. An example is presented in Fig. 14-10.

The cloning of the *XPG* and *CSB* genes nicely demonstrates the unexpected contribution of findings in related and sometimes unrelated fields of research. The serendipitous cloning of the *XPG* gene was based on the screening of a *Xenopus laevis* cDNA expression library with antiserum from a human patient with the autoimmune disease lupus erythematosis by Clarkson and co-workers (Geneva).[90] The isolated full-length frog and corresponding human cDNA turned out to be homologous to the yeast NER gene *RAD2.* The human cDNA was able to correct the defect in cells of an XP-G patient. Independently, the *ERCC5* gene was cloned and also found to be homologous to *RAD2.*[92] Extracts of ERCC5 and XP-G cells appeared both deficient in the same protein.[93] A possible role of the *ERCC6* gene in CS was suggested by an observation of Fryns et al. (Leuven) that a CS patient had a constitutional deletion of a region of chromosome 10 to which we had mapped *ERCC6.*[91,94]

Genomic DNA transfection directly to cultured cells of patients with NER syndromes has, with one notable exception,[95] been unsuccessful. The difficulty of isolating repair-competent transformants after transfection of repair-defective human cells is due to the low amount of DNA that stably integrates in the genome of these cells. Compared with rodent cells, approximately 30- to

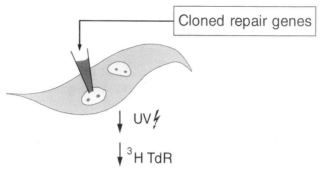

Cloned repair genes

UV

^{3}H TdR

Autoradiography to visualize UDS

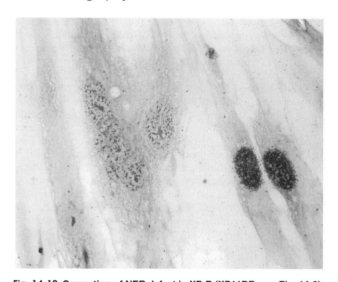

Fig. 14-10 Correction of NER defect in XP-B (XP11BE; see Fig. 14-9) multinuclear cells after microinjection of ERCC3 in one of the nuclei. *Top:* **Scheme of microinjection procedure.** *Bottom:* **DNA repair synthesis (UDS) is corrected to normal levels in the multinucleated cell after introduction of ERCC3 cDNA. The low UDS level of the mononuclear fibroblast (*left*) reflects the NER defect of XP11BE cells. The two heavily labeled fibroblasts at the right were in S phase. (*From the Department of Cell Biology and Genetics, Erasmus University Rotterdam, W. Vermeulen.*)**

more than 100-fold less DNA is integrated. This raises the number of cells required to be transfected to generate one genomic transformant containing a specific gene to extremely high levels (depending on gene length, to more than 10^9 cells[96]). Therefore, the one example of successful isolation of an NER gene, the gene defective in XP group A (*XPA*), by Tanaka and coworkers[95] via very large-scale genomic DNA transfection to XP-A cells was a formidable effort. They used an interspecies system (mouse DNA into human cells) to be able to identify and isolate the correcting (mouse) gene. This enabled the cloning of the human counterpart by cross-hybridization.

An alternative transfection approach has been the use of episomally replicating plasmid vectors carrying the Epstein-Barr virus replication origin and the gene for the Epstein-Barr virus nuclear antigen, *EBNA1.* With these vectors containing human cDNAs, the *XPC* gene was cloned by Legerski et al.[97] and the *CSA* gene by the group of Friedberg.[98] Fusion of CS-A cells with the only rodent mutant representing complementation group 8 and transfection of the cloned *CSA* gene in these rodent mutant cells revealed the identity of *CSA* and *ERCC8* (see ref. 99 and Table 14-5).

Sequence homology based on evolutionary conservation has been used for the cloning of several other (human) DNA repair genes in different manners. One method uses nucleotide sequence homology to cross species barriers. Attempts to use cloned yeast NER genes for the isolation of homologous human sequences by low-stringency cross-hybridization with human DNA libraries has resulted in the cloning of two human genes homologous to *S. cerevisiae RAD6: HHR6A* and *HHR6B*.[100] *RAD6* encodes a protein involved in ubiquitin conjugation and is implicated in postreplication repair and damage-induced mutagenesis. The yeast protein and its two human counterparts may exert their functions by modulating chromatin structure via histone ubiquitination.[101]

Alternatively, sequence conservation may permit the design of degenerate oligonucleotide primers based on conserved domains. These primers can be used for the cloning of homologous sequences by polymerase chain reaction (PCR) amplification. In this manner we have succeeded in cloning a human cDNA with clear homology to the yeast *RAD1* gene.[102] Subsequent transfection and microinjection experiments revealed that this human *RAD1* homologue corrected the DNA repair defects in rodent ERCC 4 and 11 mutants (revealing for the first time intragenic complementation between two rodent complementation groups) and XP-F fibroblasts.[102] Independently, the *ERCC4* gene was cloned by Thompson and collaborators (Livermore) by cosmid DNA transfection.[84]

These types of cloning strategies based on sequence conservation are enhanced by computerized database homology searching using powerful sequence-similarity search algorithms. The wealth of sequence information that is now available and will be even more so in the future as a result of the Human Genome Project and related efforts opens the possibility of identification of mammalian homologues of known relevant genes of lower species. This can be done by critical database screening based on conserved domains. Examples are two human genes homologous to the *S. cerevisiae* NER gene *RAD23: HHR23A* and *HHR23B*.[103] The same procedures also work in the other direction: from human DNA sequences to the isolation of homologues in lower eukaryotes. An example is the cloning of the *S. cerevisiae* counterpart of *CSB* (*ERCC6*): *RAD26*.[104]

Another obvious procedure for cloning genes starts with purification of the gene product, followed by designing nucleotide primers on the basis of a partial amino acid sequence obtained by microsequencing of the protein and cloning of the gene by PCR. A gene that may be involved in XP complementation group E was cloned in this manner. The purification and characterization of this DNA damage-binding protein (DDB) were reported by Hwang et al. (see ref. 105 and references therein) and the group of S. Linn.[106,107] Similarly, Hanaoka and collaborators purified the XPC protein (in a complex with another polypeptide that turned out to be HHR23B) and subsequently cloned the cDNAs.[103]

MAMMALIAN NER GENES: THEIR FUNCTION IN THE NER PATHWAY AND ROLE IN NER SYNDROMES

Candidates for the NER genes involved in all seven XP complementation groups have been molecularly cloned, although the gene responsible for XP-E is still uncertain. In 1999 the gene responsible for the variant form of XP has been cloned.[216,217] In addition, the two genes implicated in the classic form of CS have been isolated, and two of the three TTD (photosensitive form) genes have been identified. Futhermore, several human NER genes have been cloned for which no human NER complementation groups are known yet but for which either a rodent mutant or a yeast NER equivalent exists.

Using *in vitro* NER assay systems based on cell-free extracts (developed by the groups of Wood and Sancar[108,109]), several proteins known to be involved in DNA replication also have been demonstrated to participate in the incision and/or DNA synthesis step of the NER pathway. The core of the mammalian NER reaction was reconstituted successfully *in vitro* with (partly) purified components.[110,111] These *in vitro* systems provide valuable tools for studying the function of isolated repair proteins.

Computer-assisted comparison of the predicted amino acid sequence of the encoded proteins with known gene products

present in large databases has highlighted a striking functional resemblance with NER proteins of the yeast *RAD3* epistasis group. The extent of similarity suggests a golden rule: For each yeast NER protein there is a counterpart in humans, and vice versa. The conclusion must be that the entire NER mechanism is strongly conserved in all eukaryotes. The primary amino acid sequence also disclosed homology with functional protein domains, such as well-characterized DNA-binding and helix-unwinding sequence motifs. This type of information provided valuable clues to the biochemical activity of the encoded polypeptides. Finally, overproduction, purification, and enzymologic characterization have led to the elucidation of functional properties of several of the NER proteins and the identification of intricate complexes. Table 14-6 lists all mammalian NER genes cloned to date and summarizes their main properties.

In the following paragraphs the function of the genes involved in the NER syndromes will be discussed within the context of a model for the NER pathway that is based on currently available evidence, taking into account our still considerable ignorance. A schematic representation of the model for the multistep NER mechanism is depicted in Fig. 14-11.

Four subsequent phases are distinguished:

1. *Damage recognition.* How do cells identify lesions in the DNA? Which proteins are involved, and what is their specificity?
2. *Demarcation of the lesion.* Chromatin and DNA have to be made accessible to enzymes that will remove the damage.
3. *Dual incision.* Nicks have to be made at both sides of the lesion in the damaged strand only.
4. *Postincision events.* The damage-containing oligomer should be removed and the gap filled in by repair DNA synthesis, followed by ligation.

Damage Recognition (XPC-HHR23B, XPA, XPE?) (Fig. 14-11 and Table 14-6)

The first step in NER is expected to be the binding of a damage-recognition factor to the lesion, which enables the association of further repair components. Evidence for involvement of a protein complex composed of XPC and HHR23B in this step was presented by Sugasawa et al.[112] *In vivo*, the XPC protein is stably bound to HHR23B, one of the two human homologues of the yeast repair protein RAD 23.[103] XPC-HHR23B and XPC alone display a similar high affinity for both single- and double-stranded DNA and a preference for UV-damaged DNA.[103,113,114] *In vitro* experiments by Sugasawa et al.[112] revealed that XPC-HHR23B is the first actor in NER and capable of recruiting the rest of the repair machinery to the lesion.

Also XPA and XPE (or DDB) may be involved in damage recognition, since both proteins have a high affinity for UV-damaged DNA. The *XPA* gene specifies a protein with the sequence hallmarks of a DNA-binding Zn21-finger domain.[115] The gene product has been purified, and biochemical evidence confirmed that it is a zinc metalloprotein with affinity for double-stranded (ds) and single-stranded (ss) DNA.[116–118] A marked preference has been found for a number of lesions, including [6-4] photoproducts and Cs-Pt adducts but poor binding to cyclobutane pyrimidine dimers.[116,119] This parallels strikingly the preference of the NER pathway itself and is reminiscent of the lesion-binding spectrum of the *E. coli* UvrA2B complex. However, it also may reflect the limitations of *in vitro* studies, since in these assays the configuration of DNA is different from DNA packed into nuclear chromatin. Using the *in vitro* cell-free NER assay, the XPA product has been functionally assigned to a step in the pre-incision stage of the reaction.[108] These data are consistent with the idea that XPA is implicated in damage recognition. Studies of mutations in *XPA* demonstrated that an intact Zn-finger is indispensable for proper function of the protein.[118,120,121] The *S. cerevisiae* homologue of *XPA* is *RAD14*.[122] *RAD14* also binds preferentially to [6-4] photoproducts and chelates zinc.[123]

Table 14-6 Main Properties of Cloned Human NER Genes

Gene*	Chrom. Location	Size Protein (aa)†	Yeast Homologue	Protein Properties‡
XPA	9q34	273	RAD14	Zn^{2+}-finger, binds different types of damaged DNA, transient interaction with ERCC1, RPA and TFIIH(?) complex
XPB(ERCC3)	2q21	782	RAD25	$3' \rightarrow 5'$ DNA helicase, subunit of TFIIH, essential for transcription initiation
XPC	3p25.1§	940	RAD4	Complexed with HHR23B, strong damage-specific DNA binding, involved in global genome repair only, initiator of global genome repair
XPD(ERCC2)	19q13.2§	760	RAD3	$5' \rightarrow 3'$ DNA helicase, subunit of TFIIH, essential for transcription initiation
XPE	11	1140	Identified¶	Binds UV-damaged DNA, no causative mutations identified in complex with 48 kD, WD-repeat containing protein
XPF(ERCC4)	16p13.3	~905	RAD1	Also identical to ERCC11, complex with ERCC1 makes 5' incision, Y structure–specific endonuclease, dual function in recombination
XPG(ERCC5)	13q32-33	1186	RAD2	Y structure–specific endonuclease, makes 3' incision
CSA(ERCC8)	5	396	RAD28	5 WD-repeats, involved in transcription-coupled repair only
CSB(ERCC6)	10q11-21	1493	RAD26	DNA-dependent ATPase (helicase?), involved in transcription-coupled repair only, present in (elongating) RNA polymerase II complex
ERCC1	19q13.2§	297	RAD10	Partial homology to UvrC and many nucleases, complex with XPF makes 5' incision Y structure–specific endonuclease, dual function in recombination
HHR23A	19p13.2	363	RAD23	Ubiquitin-like N-terminus, 2 ubiquitin-associated domains
HHR23B	3p25.14§	409	RAD23	As HHR23A, fraction of HHR23B complexed with XPC, complex binds ssDNA and is involved in global genome repair only
p62^TFIIH	11p14-15.1	548	TFB1	Subunit of TFIIH, essential for transcription initiation
p52^TFIIH	6p21.3	513	TFB2	Subunit of TFIIH, essential for transcription initiation
p44^TFIIH	5q1.3	395	SSL1	DNA-binding Zn^{2+}-finger, subunit of TFIIH, essential for transcription initiation.
p34^TFIIH	12	303	TFB4	Zn^{2+}-finger, subunit of TFIIH, essential for transcription initiation.

*Not included in this table are the genes for protein involved in the DNA-synthesis step of the NER reaction, such as PCNA, RPA, RF-C, DNA ligase.
† aa: amino acids.
‡ Question marks indicate properties inferred but not proven.
§ The XPC and HHR23B genes are located on a common 650 kb M1ul fragment; ERCC1 and XPD(ERCC2) are less than 20 kb apart.

¶ A yeast gene encoding a product with clear overall homology to the XPE protein has been identified in the yeast genome database. In addition, a second human gene with significant similarity to XPE has been discovered (van der Spek, Hoeijmakers, unpublished results).

The other potential damage-recognition factor, DDB, was first identified in human cell lysates by specific retention with UV-damaged oligonucleotides.[124] This DDB activity is possibly implicated in XP-E, since it is absent in extracts derived from some, but not all, XP-E patients.[125,126] Microinjection of purified DDB transiently corrects the partial NER defect in XP-E cells that lack the DDB activity.[107] The DDB activity copurified with a heterodimeric complex consisting of 124- and 41-kDa proteins.[106,127] Mutations have been described to occur in the small subunit in DDB-deficient XP-E patients.[128] Structural homologues of the large subunit were found in a database search, including a DDB-like polypeptide in human and yeast (van der Spek and Hoeijmakers, unpublished observations) and *Caenorhabditis elegans*.[129] These gene products probably represent a novel class of DNA-binding proteins. It is tempting to speculate that the relatively mild DNA repair defect in XP-E cells is due to the fact that this second human *XPE*-like gene might be functionally redundant to the original human *XPE* gene. The XP-E correcting factor has a strong preference for binding to DNA containing [6-4] photoproducts but exhibits modest discrimination of cyclobutane pyrimidine dimers and no measurable affinity for psoralen-thymine monoadducts.[130] The striking abundance of the protein in normal cells (in the order of 10^5 copies per cell[106]) suggests that it has an additional function. A general characteristic of NER factors is that they seem to be present only in trace amounts. One possibility is that the XP-E correcting protein assists XPA in detection of some lesions, but direct interaction between these polypeptides has not been demonstrated.

Alternatively, evidence has been presented that XPA can transiently associate with the ERCC1-XPF incision complex by interaction with ERCC1,[131,132] while binding domains for RPA[133,134] and TFIIH[135,136] also have been reported (see below).

The network of protein-protein contacts between XPA and other core NER factors suggests that XPA has a central role in coordinating events in NER. The idea that XPA is the NER initiation factor[137] appears to be wrong. The work of Sugasawa et al.[112] demonstrates that XPC acts prior to XPA in vitro and serves to recruit the remainder of the NER machinery to the lesion.

XPC is the sole XP factor that is dispensable for TCR. Detection of the primary lesion in the transcription-coupled NER subpathway might be performed by RNA polymerase II. The transcription machinery probably subjects the DNA to a more rigorous test for intactness than achieved via the standard NER damage-recognition complex. This may explain why lesions that are poorly removed from the genome overall are efficiently eliminated by the TCR mode.

Demarcation of the Lesion (XPB, XPD) (Fig. 14-11 and Table 14-6).

By analogy with the *E. coli* system, it is plausible that after damage detection the DNA and chromatin have to be made accessible for recognition by the incision protein complex(es). This may involve the induction of a strongly kinked, locally unwound—but uniform for all lesions—DNA structure as observed with the UvrA2B complex, which overrides the aberrant lesion-specific conformation. By analogy with the recently described mechanism of action of *E. coli* photoreactivating enzyme, this may involve flipping out of the photoproduct from the DNA axis.[138]

By using *in vitro* repair systems, the groups of Wood[139] and Sancar[140] have shown that once lesions have been recognized, an open DNA complex is found by the coordinating activities of XPC-HHR23B, TFIIH, XPA, and RPA. TFIIH possesses bidirectional DNA unwinding activity and will be discussed in the next

Model for human NER mechanism

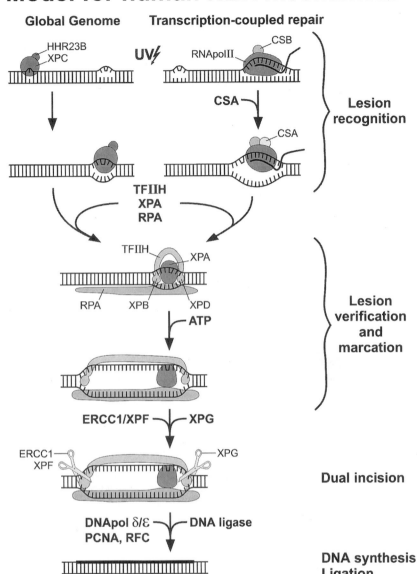

Fig. 14-11 Model for the first steps in the human NER mechanism. I-II: Damage recognition. II-III: Damage demarcation. III-IV: DNA unwinding. IV: Dual incision.

section. The RPA complex is composed of three single-stranded DNA binding proteins. It was found previously to participate in initiation and elongation of DNA replication and already shown to play a role prior or at the incision step in NER.[108,141] RPA may stabilize the unwound intermediate. XPA may account for correct positioning of the pre-incision complex, since it can bind the DNA lesion and interacts with both TFIIH and RPA.[133–135] In addition, XPG seems to stabilize this opened pre-incision complex.[139,140,142]

Both studies of Wood et al. and Sancar et al. indicate a two-step unwinding model with an ATP-dependent TFIIH-mediated initial opening and a subsequent extension of the open complex 5′ away from the lesion.

The Role of the TFIIH Transcription-Repair Complex (Fig. 14-11 and Table 14-6). Many parallels exist between XPD and XPB (and their yeast counterparts RAD3 and RAD25, also known as SSL2).[89] Based on identification of helicase motifs in the primary amino acid sequence Weeda et al.[89] proposed that both proteins form a complex with bidirectional helix-unwinding activity. As apparent below, this early idea has been corroborated

in later studies. The notion that null alleles of one or both genes in yeast,[143,144] *Drosophila*,[145] and mouse[146] are inviable indicates that these repair proteins must be involved in an additional process essential for viability. The nature of the latter was elucidated by a surprising discovery made by Egly and coworkers,[147] who were studying transcription initiation, an intricate process involving the concerted action of numerous products (for a review, see ref. 148). A multisubunit component required in a late stage of RNA polymerase II basal transcription initiation is TFIIH, previously also designated BTF2. It is a complex of at least nine polypeptides[149,150] (Table 14-7). The two largest subunits of this basal transcription factor were found to be the repair proteins XPB[147] and XPD.[151,152] Moreover, purified TFIIH corrects the XP-B, XP-D, and TTD-A repair defects *in vivo* as well as *in vitro*,[56,153] indicating the presence of at least three repair proteins in this transcription factor and a striking relationship with NER complementation groups involving TTD.

With the cell-free NER assay it also was shown that TFIIH stimulates NER activity.[153] Since in this assay neither transcription nor translation can occur, this stimulation suggests a direct involvement of TFIIH in the NER reaction. Correcting activities

Table 14-7 Main Properties of Human and Yeast TFIIH Components

Human Gene	Yeast Gene	Features/Function
XPB (ERCC3)	RAD25/SSL2	$3' \rightarrow 5'$ helicase
XPD (ERCC2)	RAD3	$5' \rightarrow 3'$ helicase
p62	TFB1	Unknown
p52	TFB2	Unknown
p44	SSL1	2 Zn^{2+}-fingers
Mo15/CDK7	Kin28	CDK-like kinase
p34	Scp34	SSL1-like Zn^{2+}-finger
cyclinH	cc11	Homology to cyclins
MAT1	TFB3	Ring Zn^{2+}-finger

of XP-B, XP-D, and TTD-A exactly co-elute with transcription and helicase activities of TFIIH.[56,153] NER-competent cell lysates and purified TFIIH fractions can be deprived of repair activity after immunoprecipitation with antibodies directed against some components of TFIIH (anti-XPB, -p62, -p44, -p43; see Table 14-7).[56,154] Furthermore, mutations in the yeast SSL1 and TFB1, yeast homologues of the human TFIIH subunits p44 and p62, give rise to a UV-sensitive phenotype consistent with a function in repair.[155]

These data suggest that the entire transcription initiation factor TFIIH is involved in NER. The dual functionality of the entire TFIIH complex is also evident from recent studies with yeast TFIIH.[156–159] Purified TFIIH displays the following activities and properties: a DNA-dependent ATPase, a protein kinase phosphorylating the C-terminus of the large subunit of RNA polymerase II, and a bidirectional DNA unwinding activity (see ref. 151 and references therein). The latter is due to the XPB ($3' \rightarrow 5'$) and the XPD ($5' \rightarrow 3'$) helicases. In addition, the TFIIH complex is endowed with two proteins (p44 and p34) containing one or more Zn^{2+}-finger domains that likely mediate DNA and/or protein-protein interactions[154] (see Table 14-7). Studies using *in vitro* transcription initiation assays have not fully established the role of TFIIH in transcription initiation. However, several plausible models can be advanced. The bidirectional helicase activity may be required for inducing a specific DNA conformation by locally opening the template[148] for loading RNA polymerase onto the transcribed strand. Alternatively, or in addition, the complex may promote promoter clearance.[160]

What can be the role of the TFIIH complex in NER? Since TFIIH repair mutants show defects in both TCR and GGR (see Table 14-4), the complex probably functions in the core of the NER reaction. Furthermore, it is reasonable to suppose that TFIIH catalyses a similar step in the context of NER and transcription initiation. Thus one of the options is that it induces a melted DNA conformation required for loading a NER incision complex onto the template and/or for altering the DNA conformation around the lesion in a manner similar to UvrA2B. Alternatively, or in addition, this complex may be involved in clearance of the damaged region, possibly including release of the damage-containing oligonucleotide and turnover of repair proteins (see Fig. 14-11).

Dual Incision (ERCC1/XPF Complex, XPG) (Fig. 14-11 and Table 14-5)

Following lesion demarcation, the actual incisions are performed by the structure-specific endonucleases XPG and ERCC1-XPF complex. XPG makes the 3′ incision and ERCC1-XPF the 5′ incision.[102,161,162]

The *XPG* gene is identical to the previously cloned human *ERCC5* gene and homologous to the yeast *RAD2* (see Table 14-6). XPG-mediated incisions always occur in one strand of duplex DNA at the 3′ side of a junction with single-stranded DNA. One single-stranded arm, protruding in either the 3′ or the 5′ direction, is necessary and sufficient for the correct positioning of XPG incisions.[163]

The ERCC1-XPF complex (also containing ERCC4 and ERCC11 correcting activities[164,165]) has a yeast counterpart comprising the RAD1 and the RAD10 protein. The RAD1-RAD10 complex possesses a single-stranded DNA-endonuclease activity that specifically cleaves the 3′ protruding single strand at the transition from a double- to single-strand region,[166–168] leading to the suggestion that this heterodimer makes the 5′ incision. The yeast complex is also implicated in intrachromosomal mitotic recombination.[168–170] Both processes encompass DNA incision as an obligatory step in their reaction mechanism.

In collaboration with Wood et al., we have shown that *ERCC4* and *XPF* (and probably *ERCC11*) are identical. Causative mutations and strongly reduced but still detectable XPF protein levels were identified in XP-F patients.[102] The incisions are made asymmetrically, with the 3′ incision 2 to 8 nucleotides and the 5′ incision 15 to 24 nucleotides away from the lesion, corresponding to the borders of the open complex.[171,173] The exact incision position seems to depend on the type of DNA lesion.[161,173,174] Although incisions occur near synchronously, consensus exists that the 3′ incision precedes the 5′ incision.[175]

Other factors are also required for an efficient excision of damaged DNA. One of them is the single-stranded binding protein complex RPA (see above). It plays a crucial role in nuclease positioning. Each side of the molecule, oriented on single-stranded DNA, interacts with a distinct nuclease. Bound to single-stranded DNA, the 3′ oriented side of RPA interacts with ERCC1-XPF and strongly stimulates its nuclease activity, whereas the 5′ oriented side of RPA does not interact with the complex and blocks ERCC1-XPF-mediated incision. RPA presumably contributes but is not sufficient to confer strand specificity to XPG (de Laat, Hoeijmakers et al., unpublished observations). These findings position RPA to the non-damaged strand of the opened NER intermediate. Given the intimate link between XPG and TFIIH,[176,177] TFIIH is an attractive candidate to be involved in XPG positioning as well.

Postincision Events (Fig. 14-11)

The final stages of the NER reaction should entail release of the damage-containing oligomer, turnover of the bound NER proteins, gap-filling DNA synthesis [used most frequently for assaying NER (UDS)], and sealing of the remaining nick by ligation. At present it is unknown which proteins carry out the first of these steps. Again, the TFIIH complex is a potential candidate because it harbors two helicases that could peel off the damage-containing 28-29-mer. Alternatively, it is possible that the DNA replication machinery carries out this reaction.

Use of the cell-free NER assay has permitted identification of the proliferating cell nuclear antigen (PCNA) as being required for the gap-filling DNA synthesis step.[108,178] PCNA is known to stimulate DNA polymerase delta and/or epsilon in regular DNA replication. The implication of PCNA in this part of the NER reaction mechanism suggests that the repair synthesis itself is mediated by any or both of these polymerases. The final sealing of the new DNA to the preexisting strand is thought to be carried out by DNA ligase I.

It is interesting to note that mutations in the ligase I gene can give rise to a UV-sensitive phenotype.[179] So far only one patient with a ligase I defect has been discovered, but it may well turn out that this individual (designated 46BR) belongs in a new category of NER-deficient patients.

So far we have dealt with steps in the core of the NER reaction. As mentioned earlier, two subpathways have been distinguished in NER: GGR and TCR. Gene functions specific for these subpathways are discussed in the following paragraphs. Finally, as discussed below, instead of a stepwise assembly of individual factors described earlier, evidence has been presented in the analogous yeast system for the existence of a preassembled "repairosome."[158] Furthermore, the preceding tentative model does not incorporate yet the chromatin dynamics that must play a part in vivo.

Steps Specific for the GGR Pathway (XPC) (Table 14-6)

Analysis of mutants has lead to the identification of at least three genes selectively implicated in the repair of the nontranscribed bulk of the genome: *RAD7* and *RAD16* in yeast[180] and *XPC* in humans.[181] The function of the XPC-HHR23B complex in damage recognition was described earlier. The XPC amino acid sequence displays significant homology to the yeast RAD4 protein.[97,103] However, *rad4* null mutants, in contrast to *XPC* mutants, are defective in both NER subpathways.[180] This may reflect a principal difference between mammals and yeast. A notable feature of the HHR23 proteins is the presence of an ubiquitin-like domain in the N-terminus.[103] In some other ubiquitin-fusion proteins this moiety is thought to function as a chaperone, facilitating complex formation. Hence this domain may perform a similar role in assembling the XPC-HHR23B complex. To date, no known human NER syndromes have been associated with the *HHR23B* gene, and a simple explanation might be that the highly homologous HHR23A protein diminished the effect of loss of HHR23B function.

In keeping with the golden rule derived from the striking correspondence between yeast and mammalian NER, it would be expected that human homologues of RAD7 and RAD16 exist and that they participate in the global repair process. The RAD7 sequence does not reveal any clue to its function.[182] The *RAD16* gene, however, encodes a protein containing a special type of DNA-binding Zn^{2+} finger and an extended region with strong homology to a specific subfamily of presumed DNA helicases.[183] Interestingly, CSB, a protein specific for TCR, is also equipped with such domains.[91] A characteristic of other members of this helicase subfamily is that they reside in multiprotein complexes. Genetic evidence in yeast suggests that the complex interacts with chromatin (see ref. 184 and references therein).

In this light, what is the role of these genes? One possibility, suggested elsewhere, is that they are involved in uncoupling essential NER components from the transcription machinery to make them available for GGR,[103] or vice versa when repair is finished, to allow recovery of RNA synthesis. The TFIIH transcription-repair complex is the most logical partner in this option. The CSA and CSB proteins might be involved in this process (see below). On the other hand, the RAD16 protein (complex?) may be implicated in altering chromatin structure required for global genome repair. Obviously, these speculations need to be experimentally investigated.

Steps Specific for TCR (CSA,CSB) (Table 14-6)

Two genes involved in TCR that are defective in CS are *CSA* and *CSB*. The protein sequence of CSA contains the consensus of five WD-repeats.[98] This type of motif is present in many proteins believed to possess a regulatory rather than a catalytic function.[185] Many of these WD-repeat proteins reside in multiprotein complexes. CSA is thought to associate with p44 (a component of TFIIH; see Table 14-7) and with CSB.[98]

CSB is a member of the closely related subfamily of putative DNA/RNA helicases, described earlier, to which RAD16 also belongs. A yeast homologue of this protein was unknown, but the sequence conservation seen for all other eukaryotic NER factors permitted bridging the large evolutionary gap between human and yeast. Like CSB, a yeast disruption mutant, designated *rad26*, displayed a selective defect in TCR.[104] Interestingly, inactivation of this NER subpathway in yeast does not induce a significant UV sensitivity, suggesting that this process is not very important for UV survival in yeast.

Hanawalt and Mellon[38] argued that in order to couple NER to transcription, the stalled RNA polymerase II complex has to retract or dissociate to allow access of repair proteins to the lesion.[186,187] It is possible that defects in this process underlie the total TCR defect in CS cells, implicating CSA and CSB in the release of RNA polymerase II from the damaged site. The role for CSA and CSB, with the latter found to be associated with elongating RNA polymerase II complexes,[186,188,189] is still matter for speculation.[190]

Higher-Order NER Complexes

Although most of the important players in mammalian NER are identified, it is not known yet how these factors assemble on a lesion and how they interact with each other. Several reports appeared in the literature dealing with proposed interactions between NER factors. However, many of these studies are based on associations either in a rather artificial environment (immobilized fusion proteins) or after overexpression in yeast (two-hybrid system). In both systems, transient or low-affinity interactions can be selected, which may not reflect the in vivo situation.

A central role for the XPA protein is likely in view of the very severe NER-deficient phenotype of XP-A cells. Biochemical studies with XPA suggest that this factor serves as an nucleation point in the repair reaction. Interaction of XPA (in addition to that with damaged DNA) has been described with ERCC1,[131,132,191] RPA,[133,134] and TFIIH.[135,136] Binding of both ERCC1 and RPA to XPA has a synergistic effect on the DNA damage-specific binding affinity of XPA.[134,191] RPA is claimed to interact with XPG,[134] whereas XPG and XPC may be associated with TFIIH.[152,177] Several of these assumed interactions depend on isolation conditions,[111] and variable or different results have been obtained by other laboratories.[56,110] Using specific isolation conditions, an NER supercomplex ("repairosome") was purified from yeast cells.[158] The majority of the different yeast NER factors are reported to reside in this "repairosome." However, this isolated complex still lacks some essential factors because it is not active in a reconstituted NER reaction. Also, the amount of each of the NER factors residing in this complex is not known.

Mouse Models for Genetic Defects in NER

Gene targeting by homologous recombination in totipotent embryonal stem (ES) cells permits the generation of mouse mutants in any cloned NER gene. This methodology enables the development of experimental animal models for all types of NER deficiencies and associated syndromes. Genes can be fully inactivated (knockout mutants), but it is also possible to reconstruct specific partially inactivating mutations encountered in patients in the mouse genome. The use of this genetic tool will have a major impact on clinical and fundamental research of the human NER syndromes and cancer in general. First, it will help in understanding the complex ramifications and biologic relevance of NER pathways particularly with respect to understanding the mechanisms of carcinogenesis, neurodegeneration, photoimmunology, and aging. Second, animal models for human NER syndromes will be instrumental for clinical research on these conditions, including diagnosis, prevention, and therapy. Furthermore, it may lead to the discovery of new disorders for NER genes for which no corresponding condition has been identified yet. In addition, it will help in disentangling the intricate genotype-phenotype relationships of CS and TTD. Crossing animals with different genetic lesions will permit the study of synergistic effects with other mechanisms implicated in genetic (in)stability, such as cell cycle control, complementary repair pathways, and apoptosis. Finally, since the NER system targets a very wide spectrum of DNA lesions, mice deficient in this pathway will be a valuable and sensitive model for assessing the genotoxic effect of known and unknown compounds.

The ERCC1 Mouse. The first NER-deficient mouse mutant was generated in the *ERCC1* gene,[192] one of the NER genes for which no parallel human syndrome is yet known.[193] Thus it was not *a priori* evident whether full inactivation of this function would be compatible with life, particularly since both the yeast and rodent mutants provide evidence for a dual involvement of this gene in an additional mitotic recombination repair pathway with unpredictable biologic impact, as noted previously. A functional knockout mutation appeared barely viable; indeed, most ERCC1-deficient embryos die in utero or perinatally, and the few mutants surviving are severely runted and usually die before weaning, i.e., within 4 weeks.[194] Recent evidence indicates that the genetic makeup influences the life span and embryonal death to a considerable extent; maximal life span is extended to several months in a C57B1/6 strain, and mutant embryonal death is postponed to the moment of birth in an FVB background.[194] This indicates that these two types of early death may have different causes. One of the causes of postnatal death is liver malfunction, probably due to increased nuclear aneuploidy. Elevated levels of aneuploid nuclei are also apparent in kidney, and there is ferritin deposition in spleen. Increased levels of p53 are reported in liver, brain, and kidney.[192] Subcutaneous fat is absent. As far as investigated, the neurologic status of the mice seems normal. Several of the preceding clinical features point to premature aging, possibly as a result of accumulation of unremoved endogenous DNA lesions. At the cellular level, replicative senescence is seen as well as increased spontaneous transformation.[194] As expected, mouse embryonal fibroblasts (MEFs) derived from the mutant mice display a total NER defect and are hypersensitive to UV and chemical genotoxins that are substrates of the NER pathway. In addition, there is cellular sensitivity to crosslinking agents, presumably as a consequence of an additional defect in one of the recombination repair pathways. In order to create a milder phenotype, a mouse mutant was designed in which only the very C-terminal 7 amino acids were deleted[194] (ERCC1*292; Fig. 14-12). However, apart from an extended life span to more than 6 months, most of the other features were very similar to those of the full knockout mice, indicating that the very last part of the protein is still important for its biologic functions. The signs of premature senescence observed in the ERCC1[2/2] suggest that accumulation of unrepaired DNA damage contributes to early aging. The ERCC1*292 mice were used in a carcinogenesis experiment. Cutaneous application of dimethylbenz[a]anthracene (DMBA) at a dose easily tolerated by XPA knockout mice (see below) caused death within 3 days, revealing an extreme sensitivity to genotoxins.[195] Apart from the UV sensitivity, the clinical picture is very different from any of the human NER syndromes. The lack of similarity between the mouse and the human NER mutants may, in part, reflect species differences, but the picture also may be compounded by the dual functionality of the ERCC1 protein. In this connection, a comparison of the severe clinical phenotype of ERCC1 mutant mice with that of XPA knockout mice (also harboring a complete NER defect) will be very instructive.

The XPA Mouse. A closer but still partial correspondence to the parallel human disease was noted with a mouse model for XP-A generated independently in two laboratories. Consistent with the human pathology, XPA knockout mice display cutaneous and ocular photosensitivity and a greatly increased susceptibility to UV- and DMBA-induced skin cancer.[195,196] However, in contrast to XP-A patients, knockout mutant mice appear physiologically normal, are fertile, and at the age of 18 months fail to develop the neuropathology characteristic of the human condition. One factor that should be taken into account in this regard is the difference in life span. The accelerated neurodegeneration observed in XP-A human patients is manifested over the course of several years, whereas such a time period cannot be reached in the mouse model. As in the case with ERCC1 in one genetic background, approximately half the XPA-deficient embryos died in the midfetal stage (with signs of anemia),[196] whereas in another background this phenomenon was absent.[195] XPA-deficient MEFs exhibited all parameters of a total NER deficiency. This indicates that the NER phenotype is as predicted and also as observed in ERCC1-deficient mice. The fact that, with respect to the NER defect, XPA and ERCC1 knockout mice are indistinguishable permits a valid comparison between these two phenotypes. Considering the additional function of ERCC1 in a mitotic recombination repair

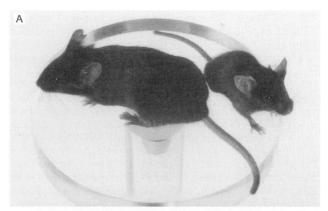

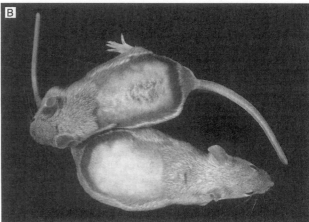

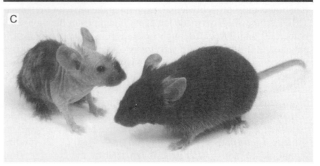

Fig. 14-12 Mouse models of NER syndromes. NER-deficient mice were obtained by targeting mouse embryonic stem cells with a DNA construct containing a mutated NER gene, followed by blastocyst injection and breeding germ-line chimeras. *Top:* ERCC1-mutant mouse showing growth defects (compare the small mutant mouse with its normal litter mate). This mouse is extremely sensitive to ultraviolet light and UV-mimicking agents. *Center:* Homozygous and heterozygous CSB mutant mouse representing a mouse model for CS. The UV-induced erythema on the skin reflects the severe UV sensitivity of this CSB2/2 mouse. *Bottom:* Homozygous TTD mutant showing brittle hair and other characteristic features of TTD. (*From the Department of Cell Biology and Genetics, Erasmus University, Rotterdam; G. Weeda, ERCC1 mouse, B. van der Horst, CSB mouse, and Jan de Boer, TTD mouse.*)

pathway, it is logical to conclude that the extra symptoms registered in the ERCC1-deficient mice, such as liver and kidney aneuploidy, growth retardation, and premature aging, are a consequence of a compromise of this second function.

The XPC Mouse. A phenotype very similar to XPA mice is observed in mice carrying an inactivating mutation in the *XPC* gene. As in the case of XP-C patients, a normal development and clear UV hypersensitivity and increased frequency of skin cancer were found.[197]

The CSB Mouse. We have mimicked a mutation of a known CS-B patient in the mouse genome.[198] Analysis of repair parameters in embryonic fibroblasts from the CSB mutant versus wild-type and heterozygous mice showed a specific loss of TCR. In agreement with the human syndrome, CSB-deficient mice are photosensitive (see Fig. 14-12). The other CS-like clinical features observed were mild, such as slightly retarded growth and neurologic (behavioral and motor coordination) abnormalities. Remarkably, when a GGR defect was introduced in CSB-deficient mice, a strong augmentation of the CS phenotype was observed. Such XPC/CSB and XPA/CSB double mutant mice exhibit a very severe growth retardation (75 percent), are unable to walk, and die around day 18. These observations suggest that a CS defect becomes exaggerated in the absence of GGR, pointing to accumulation of endogenous damage as a contributing factor to the CS symptoms.[190] In striking contrast to human CS, CSB-deficient mice appear clearly prone to skin cancer when exposed to UV light or to the chemical carcinogen DMBA.[198] Thus, in the mouse, intact GGR is not sufficient to protect from tumorigenesis. This finding could imply that CS patients may have a hitherto unnoticed cancer predisposition. Alternatively, the species difference in tumorigenesis could be due to the fact that, in humans compared with rodents, the GGR pathway is more potent in eliminating cyclobutane pyrimidine dimers, the major UV-induced lesion.[198]

Mouse Mutants in the TFIIH Subunits XPB and XPD. Like some of the other NER genes, the TFIIH complex has a dual functionality complicating the clinical outcome of a mutation in the genes involved. In the case of TFIIH, the second function entails initiation of basal transcription of all structural genes transcribed by RNA polymerase II. This is one of the most fundamental processes in the cell. Complete inactivation of such a function is most probably lethal, explaining the rarity of mutants in TFIIH genes. We have made knockout mutations in the mouse for both *XPB* and *XPD*. Although heterozygous mice were readily obtained, 2/2 mutants were selectively absent from the offspring. Death occurs at the two-cell stage when embryonal transcription has to start up.[146] This demonstrates that inactivation of these genes is lethal and that this is due to their role in transcription. More subtle mutations had to be made mimicking the phenotype-determining allele in the corresponding human patients. We have generated a mouse model for TTD by using a novel gene targeting strategy (gene-cDNA fusion targeting).[199] Part of the coding region of the mouse *XPD* gene is replaced by the corresponding part of the human cDNA that encodes the point mutation causing the disease in a TTD patient. The mice reflect to a remarkable extent the clinical symptoms of the TTD patient (see Fig. 14-12): brittle hair, developmental abnormalities, UV sensitivity, skin abnormalities, and reduced life span.[199] The same divergence between the CSB patient and the CSB model is observed in the case of TTD: The TTD mice show increased sensitivity to experimental induction of skin cancer by UVB and chemicals, whereas TTD patients do not show elevated cancer incidence (De Boer, Hoeijmakers et al., unpublished results).

IMPLICATIONS FOR DIAGNOSIS AND TREATMENT

Clinical Heterogeneity and Pleiotropy Associated with Mutations in TFIIH

It is clear that the spectrum of diseases linked with mutations in the TFIIH subunits *XPB, XPD,* and *TTDA* is remarkably heterogeneous and pleiotropic. It includes seemingly unrelated symptoms as photosensitivity, predisposition to skin cancer, brittle hair and nails, neurodysmyelination, impaired sexual development, ichthyosis, and dental caries. The rare XP group B consists of only 6 patients: 4 had the XP-CS complex and two had TTD. The more common group D is associated with classic XP, combinations of XP and CS, and TTD[56,58,200] (see Table 14-4). The clinical

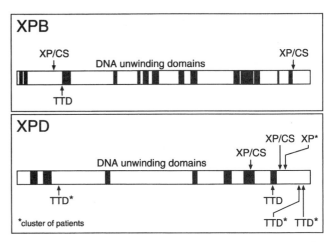

Fig. 14-13 Position of mutations in the *XPB* and *XPD* genes in patients with XP, XP-CS, and TTD. Clusters of different mutations causing TTD or XP were found at specific sites. (*From Broughton*[201] *and unpublished results.*)

variability in TTD is also apparent from the fact that at least seven disorders are thought to be identical or closely related to TTD. These include the following syndromes: Pollitt (MIM 275550), Tay (242170), Sabinas (211390), Netherton (256500), ONMR (258360), hair-brain (234050), and the Marinesco-Sjögren (248800) syndromes.[20,21] The occurrence of TTD in three distinct NER-deficient complementation groups argues against a chance association between genetic loci separately involved in NER and in brittle hair. Consistent with the idea that these processes are intimately connected is the recent identification of point mutations in the *XPD* and *XPB* genes in TTD patients[201,202] (Fig. 14-13) and the generation of TTD mice by introducing a specific mutation in the *XPD* gene.[199] The positions of the relatively large number of mapped XPD mutations and the three XPB mutations indicate that mutations resulting in XP, combined XP and CS (XP-CS), or TTD do not overlap (see Fig. 14-13). Therefore, these mutations may interfere with the functions of these genes in a specific manner, resulting in the three different phenotypes.

The Clinical Features Derived from the NER Defect

In striking contrast to the pleiotropy and clinical heterogeneity selectively associated with XP-B and XP-D, the symptoms seen in the most common XP groups, A (totally deficient in NER) and C (defective in the GGR subpathway) are much more uniform. They involve photosensitivity, pigmentation abnormalities, predisposition to skin cancer, and in the case of XP-A, accelerated neuro-degeneration (which is not associated with neurodysmyelination) but no CS and TTD symptoms. The gene products affected in these groups are not vital and therefore do not appear to be essential for basal transcription. This indicates that these forms of XP present the manifestations of a pure NER defect. The fact that XP-C is associated with a strong cancer predisposition suggests that the global genome subpathway is of major importance for preventing mutagenesis and carcinogenesis. This may provide a plausible explanation why, in CS, no significant cancer proneness is observed; CS patients still possess a potent GGR system. The TCR subpathway may be important for cell survival but less relevant for preventing mutagenesis, since it accomplishes—and only for some lesions—more rapid repair in only one of the strands of an active gene.

Evidence for the Involvement of Transcriptional Defects in CS and TTD

Mutations in subunits of the multifunctional and intricate TFIIH are envisioned to have multiple effects. The selective association of TFIIH with the peculiar forms of XP and the dual role of this complex in repair and transcription make it tempting to link the unexpected TTD and CS features with the additional transcription-related function of the NER genes involved. Indeed, it would be highly unlikely that all mutations in subunits of this bifunctional complex would only affect the repair function and leave the inherent transcriptional role entirely intact. This interpretation is supported by the phenotype of a *Drosophila ERCC3* mutant, *haywire*. This mutant displays UV sensitivity, CNS abnormalities, and impaired sexual development, as found in XP-B.[145] Spermatogenesis in *Drosophila* is very sensitive to the level of β_2-tubulin.[203] Mutations in the *Drosophila ERCC3* gene seem to affect β-tubulin expression, causing the male sterility.[145] It is therefore likely that expression of this gene in *Drosophila* (and, by inference, possibly in humans) is particularly sensitive to the level of transcription and thereby to subtle mutations in TFIIH. This could easily explain the immature sexual development found in TTD and CS. Expression of the myelin basic protein is known to be critically dependent on transcription. It has been demonstrated that reduced transcription of the myelin basic protein gene in mice causes neurologic abnormalities.[204] Thus the characteristic neurodysmyelination of CS and TTD[18,205] also may relate to suboptimal transcription of this or other genes involved in myelin sheath formation. Similarly, reduced transcription of genes encoding the class of ultrahigh-sulfur proteins of the hairshaft may account for the observed reduced cysteine content in the brittle hair of TTD patients[20] and TTD mice.[199] Experimental support for this hypothesis was obtained by the finding of reduced transcription of a skin-specific gene in the TTD mouse.[199] A comparable explanation is proposed for the poor enamelation of teeth in CS and TTD. Thus mutations in TFIIH that subtly disturb its transcription function may affect a specific subset of genes whose functioning critically depends on the level or fine-tuning of transcription. It is logical to suppose that strong secondary structures in a promoter requires full unwinding capacity, i.e., a maximally active complex, to permit efficient transcription. Recent studies indicate that the requirement for basal transcription factors may vary from promoter to promoter depending on the sequence around the initiation site, the topologic state of the DNA, and the local chromatin structure.[206] These mechanisms can readily explain the pronounced clinical heterogeneity even within families. Obviously, total inactivation of the transcription is lethal; this is consistent with the observation that deletion mutants of TFIIH subunits in yeast, *Drosophila*, and mice are inviable.[56,146] The narrow window of viable mutations also explains the rarity of these TFIIH-associated diseases.

As noted previously,[207] there are many parallels between CS and TTD, suggesting that they are manifestations of a broad clinical continuum. This is consistent with the finding that mutations in different subunits of the same (TFIIH) complex give rise to a similar set of CS and TTD features. Thus defects in *CSA* and *CSB* as well as *XPG* also may affect basal transcription because they give rise to a comparable phenotype (see also below).

Transcription and Repair/Transcription Syndromes

A tentative model proposed for the etiology of the defects in the conglomerate of CS, TTD, and related disorders is shown in Table 14-8. In this model, mutations in TFIIH subunits inactivating only the NER function result in an XP phenotype as observed in the classic patients of XP group D. If, in addition, the transcription function is subtly affected, the combination of XP and CS features is found. Theoretically, mutations causing a (still viable) transcription problem without NER impairment may be expected as well. Indeed, recently CS (-like) patients without an associated NER defect were identified.[73] This model fits with the observation of specific sites of mutations in XPB and XPD resulting in a XP, XP-CS, or TTD phenotype (see Fig. 14-13).

When CS features are due to mutations that cripple the transcription function of TFIIH, how can the differences between CS and TTD, i.e., the additional presence of brittle hair and nails in TTD, be rationalized? In view of the intrinsic properties of complexes such as TFIIH, it is likely that some mutations also will affect the stability of the complex. In fact, a significant proportion of TFIIH mutations in yeast yield a temperature-sensitive phenotype,[155] pointing to complex instability. It is feasible that such types of mutations also occur among TFIIH patients. As mentioned earlier, an exceptional TTD individual exhibited a reversible sudden, dramatic worsening of the brittleness of the hair formed during an episode of fever.[22] This fits with a human temperature-sensitive TFIIH mutation. Furthermore, it suggests that transcription of the genes for cysteine-rich matrix proteins of hair and nails is affected by TFIIH instability. In other cells, the steady-state levels of TFIIH may be sufficient, because *de novo* synthesis is high enough to cope with the reduced $t_{1/2}$ of the complex. However, the cysteine-rich matrix proteins are one of the last gene products produced in very large quantities in keratinocytes before they die. Thus the hallmark of TTD may be due to a TFIIH stability problem becoming overt in terminally differentiated cells that are exhausted for TFIIH before completion of their differentiation program.

Many TTD patients are not noticeably photosensitive and have normal NER.[73] According to the scheme in Table 14-8, these patients may have a TFIIH transcription and stability problem without concomitant impairment of the NER function of the

Table 14-8 Model for the Relation Between TFIIH Defects and Clinical Features

TFIIH-Related Disorder	NER	TFIIH Function* Transcription	TFIIH Function* Stability	Documented Gene Mutation
XP	−	+	+	*XPD*
XP-CS	−	+/−	+	*XPD, XPB, XPG*†
CS (photosensitive)	+/−‡	+/−	+	*CSA, CSB*†
CS (nonphotosensitive)§	+	+/−	+	?
TTD (photosensitive)	−	+/−	+/−	*XPD, XPB, TTDA*
TTD (nonphotosensitive)§	+	+/−	+/−	?

* Symbol designation: +, normal repair or transcription function or stability of TFIIH; +/−, partly affected function/stability; −, severely impaired function.
† TFIIH transcription may be indirectly affected by mutations in *XPG, CSA,* and *CSB*. In addition, *XPG* affects total NER; *CSA* and *CSB* affect only transcription-coupled repair.
‡ Only the NER subpathway of transcription-coupled repair is distributed.
§ CS patients without a NER defect have been identified[74] (Jaspers, Kleijer, and Hoeijmakers unpublished observations). There may be many disorders related to nonphotosensitive variants of TTD and CS such as Netherton syndrome, brain-hair syndrome, Pollitt syndrome, etc.

complex. These findings extend the implications to non-repair-defective disorders. Therefore, and in view of the model's pronounced heterogeneity, it is possible that the Sjögren-Larsson (MIM 270200), RUD (308200), ICE (146720), OTD (257960), IFAP (308205), CAM(F)AK (212540), Rothmund-Thomson (268400), KID (242150), and COF syndromes[21,56] also fall within this category. Interestingly, some of these diseases show occurrence of skin cancer.

When the CS features in TTD are due to a basal transcription problem, this also should apply to the other complementation groups with CS patients, i.e., CS-A, CS-B, and XP-G. Although the CSA, CSB, and probably the XPG proteins are not vital and therefore not essential for transcription, they may influence TFIIH functioning indirectly (see Table 14-8). For instance, CSA and CSB could have an auxiliary function for TFIIH in transcription and in transcription-coupled (but not global genome) repair. Some XP-G (XP-CS) patients are more severely affected than XP-A patients,[24] although the latter are, in general, more defective in NER, suggesting that XPG has an additional, nonrepair function. Consistent with these considerations, interactions between TFIIH components and the CS proteins have been claimed.[98,152,177]

In conclusion, these findings provide evidence for the presence of a wide class of disorders that can collectively be called *transcription syndromes*.[207] A prediction from this model is that these patients carry mutations in transcription factors that do not affect the NER process. This explanation introduces a novel concept into human genetics. It can be envisioned that similar phenomena are associated with subtle defects in translation, implying the potential existence of translation syndromes.

Patient Care

Treatment. Treatment of XP, CS, and TTD patients is purely symptomatic. The discovery of the molecular defects in these disorders has not (yet) resulted in specific modalities for treatment.

Treatment of XP patients is a multifaceted process involving early diagnosis, genetic counseling, patient and family education, and regular monitoring of the skin.[208] The diagnosis is suspected in patients with marked sun sensitivity, photophobia, and/or early onset of freckling. Laboratory tests of UV sensitivity of fibroblasts and of excision repair confirm the diagnosis. Genetic counseling is directed toward acquainting the patients and their parents with the inherited aspects of the disease and its rarity, the increased risk for parents (with the 25 percent probability that the disease will appear among subsequent offspring), and the improbability of the patients having affected children.[2,21,209]

Patients should be shielded from sunlight by protective measures, including wearing two layers of clothing, using long hairstyles, wearing broad-brimmed hats and UV-absorbing sunglasses with side shields, and using chemical sunscreens with sun protection factor (SPF) numbers of 15 or higher. Patients should avoid direct exposure to sunlight, especially during the peak UV hours (about 10 A.M. to 3 P.M. in the continental United States) and indirect UV light reflected from snow or water. Window glass and many plastic shields for fluorescent lamps will absorb UV radiation indoors. Known chemical carcinogens such as tobacco smoke should be avoided. Patients and their families should be taught to examine their skin and to recognize and bring to medical attention any lesions suspected to be malignant. Color photographs are often useful for follow-up.

Malignant skin neoplasms are treated as in patients who do not have XP by excision, electrodesiccation, and curettage, cryosurgery, or chemosurgery. XP patients have received x-ray therapy for malignant skin tumors and have had a normal response.[208] Dermabrasion or dermatome shaving has been used in patients with multiple tumors, permitting the epidermis to be repopulated by cells from the hair follicles, which are relatively shielded from sunlight.[208] Total removal of the skin of the face with grafting of skin from sun-shielded areas has been used in extreme cases. Oral retinoids have been shown to prevent new skin cancers in XP patients but have many severe side effects.[210]

Nance and Berry[12] mention several measures that can be taken in management of CS patients, including monitoring of treatable complications of this condition such as hypertension, hearing loss, and dental carries. As in XP, photosensitive CS patients should avoid excessive sun exposure and use sunscreens when outdoors. If the condition is compatible with life into the teens and twenties (in the case of CSI), the neurologic and neurosensory capacities should be assessed periodically. This assessment of intellectual, social, visual, and auditory skills can help in providing appropriate home and school services for the patient. Nance and Berry[12] also recommend physical therapy directed toward preventing contractures and maintaining ambulation in the older patient.

Although little is known about the treatment of TTD patients, the overlap of clinical symptoms in TTD and CS (neurologic and growth defects) indicates comparable management of patients suffering from these diseases.

Prenatal Diagnosis. Since the NER-deficiency syndromes have autosomal recessive inheritance, parents of an affected child face a high risk of recurrence (25 percent) in subsequent pregnancies. Prenatal diagnosis is possible if the deficiency has been demonstrated unequivocally in cultured skin fibroblasts of the index patient.

Early reports of prenatal diagnosis of XP concern the analysis of UDS in cultured amniocytes.[211,212] This approach allows a relatively rapid diagnosis within 1 or 2 weeks after amniocentesis in the sixteenth week, since only a few cells are needed for the autoradiographic assessment of UDS. A much earlier diagnosis is possible, however, by chronic villus sampling (CVS) in the tenth to twelfth weeks of pregnancy. Autoradiographic analysis of the early outgrowths of cells from the villi then allows a first-trimester diagnosis. Successful prenatal diagnoses using chorionic villus cells have been reported for XP and TTD.[22,213,214] The TCR defect in CS can be demonstrated indirectly by measuring the recovery of RNA or DNA synthesis after UV exposure of cultured cells. The reliability of this test for the (postnatal) diagnosis of CS using cultured skin fibroblasts has been shown extensively. Cases of prenatal diagnosis using amniocytes[48] and chorionic villus cells[213] have been reported. Because of the earlier stage of sampling, the use of chronic villus cells may be prefered, but the present experience for CS is very small. Therefore, if initial results on the chorionic villus cells suggest a normal fetus, it may be considered to confirm the diagnosis by amniocentesis. Mutation analysis using DNA from uncultured chorion villi would, in principle, allow reliable and early diagnosis. This requires knowledge of the gene involved and of the mutations in the family. In general, it may not be practical to search for these mutations in these rare diseases unless common mutations are known, as reported for Japanese XP-A patients.[215]

ACKNOWLEDGMENTS

We are indebted to all members of the DNA repair group of the Medical Genetics Centre South-West Netherlands (MGC) for valuable and stimulating discussions and for providing new information for this chapter. We thank Dr. W. J. Kleijer, Dr. M. F. Niermeijer, and Dr. P. C. Hanawalt for a thoughtful review of the manuscript and Rita Boucke (secretary), Mirko Kuit (photography), Wim Vermeulen, Koos Jaspers, Geert Weeda, Bert van der Horst, Wouter de Laat, and Jan de Boer for their help in preparing this chapter. The research of the MGC group is supported by the Dutch Cancer Society, the Netherlands Organization for Scientific Research (NWO) through the Foundations of Medical Sciences and Chemical Sciences, the Commission of the European Community, and the Louis Jeantet Foundation.

REFERENCES

1. Friedberg EC, Walker GC, Siede W: *DNA Repair and Mutagenesis.* Washington, ASM Press, 1995.
2. Kraemer KH, Lee MM, Scotto J: Xeroderma pigmentosum: Cutaneous, ocular and neurologic abnormalities in 830 published cases. *Arch Dermatol* **123**:241, 1987.
3. von Hebra F, Kaposi M: *On diseases of the Skin, Including the Exanthemata*, vol 3, trans by W. Tay. London, New Sydenham Society, 1874, p 252.
4. Neisser A: Ueber das Xeroderma pigmentosum (Kaposi) lioderma essentialis cum melanosi et telangiectasia. *Viertel Dermatol Syphil* 47, 1883.
5. DeSanctis C, Cacchione A: Lidiozia xerodermica. *Riv Sper Freniatr* **56**:269, 1932.
6. See reference(s) cited in: Cleaver JE, Kraemer KH: Xeroderma pigmentosum and Cockayne syndrome, in Scriver CR, Beaudet AL, Sly WS, Valle D (eds): *The Metabolic and Molecular Bases of Inherited Disease*, 7th ed. New York, McGraw-Hill, 1995, p 4393.
7. Takebe H, Nishigori C, Satoh Y: Genetics and skin cancer of xeroderma pigmentosum in Japan. *Jpn J Cancer Res (Gann)* **78**:1135, 1987.
8. Kraemer KH, Lee MM, Andrews AD, Lambert WC: The role of sunlight and DNA repair in melanoma and non-melanoma skin cancer: The xeroderma pigmentosum paradigm. *Arch Dermatol* **130**:1018, 1994.
9. Mimaki T, Itoh N, Abe J, Tagawa T, Sato K, Yabuuchi H, Takebe H: Neurological manifestations of xeroderma pigmentosum. *Ann Neurol* **20**:70, 1986.
10. Robbins JH, Brumback RA, Mendiones M, Barrett SF, Carl JR, Cho S, Denckla MB, Ganges MB, Gerber LH, Guthrie RA, Meer J, Moshell AN, Polinsky RJ, Ravin PD, Sonies BC, Tarone RE: Neurological disease in xeroderma pigmentosum: Documentation of a late onset type of the juvenile onset form. *Brain* **114**:1335, 1991.
11. Andrews AD, Barrett SF, Robbins JH: Xeroderma pigmentosum neurological abnormalities correlate with colony-forming ability after ultraviolet radiation. *Proc Natl Acad Sci USA* **75**:1984, 1978.
12. Nance MA, Berry SA: Cockayne syndrome: Review of 140 cases. *Am J Med Genet* **42**:68, 1992.
13. Lehmann AR: Nucleotide excision repair and the link with transcription. *Trends Biochem Sci* **20**:402, 1995.
14. Price VH, Odom RB, War WH, Jones FT: Trichothiodystrophy: Sulfur-deficient brittle hair as a marker for a neuroectodermal symptom complex. *Arch Dermatol* **116**:1378, 1980.
15. Tsambaos D, Nikiforidis G, Balas C, Marinoni S: Trichothiodystrophic hair reveals an abnormal pattern of viscoelastic parameters. *Skin Pharmacol* **7**:257, 1994.
16. van Neste DJJ, Gillespie JM, Marshall RC, Taieb A, de Brouwer B: Morphological and biochemical characteristics of trichothiodystrophy-variant hair are maintained after grafting of scalp specimens on to nuce mice. *Br J Dermatol* **128**:384, 1993.
17. Chen E, Cleaver JE, Weber CA, Packman S, Barkovich AJ, Koch TK, Williams ML, Golabi M, Price VH: Trichothiodystrophy: Clinical spectrum, central nervous system imaging, and biochemical characterization of two siblings. *J Invest Dermatol* **103**:154, 1994.
18. Peserico A, Battistella PA, Bertoli P: MRI of a very hereditary ectodermal dysplasia: PIBI(D)S. *Neuroradiology* **34**:316, 1992.
19. Tolmie JL, de Berker D, Dawber R, Galloway C, Gergory DW, Lehmann AR, McClure J, Pollitt JR, Stephenson JPB: Syndromes associated with trichothiodystrophy. *Clin Dysmorphol* **1**:1, 1994.
20. Itin PH, Pittelkow MR: Trichothiodystrophy: Review of sulfur-deficient brittle hair syndromes and association with the ectodermal dysplasias. *J Am Acad Dermatol* **22**:705, 1990.
21. McKusick VA: *Mendelian Inheritance in Man*, 11th ed. Baltimore, Johns Hopkins University Press, 1994.
22. Kleijer WJ, Beemer FA, Boom BW: Intermittent hair loss in a child with PIBI(D)S syndrome and trichothiodystrophy with defective DNA repair—Xeroderma pigmentosum group D. *Am J Med Gen* **52**:227, 1994.
23. Robbins JH, Kraemer KH, Lutzner MA, Festoff BW, Coon HG: Xeroderma pigmentosum: An inherited disease with sun sensitivity, multiple cutaneous neoplasms and abnormal DNA repair. *Ann Intern Med* **80**:221, 1974.
24. Hamel BCJ, Raams A, Schuitema-Dijkstra AR, Simons P, van der Burgt I, Jaspers NGJ, Kleijer WJ: Xeroderma pigmentosum-Cockayne syndrome complex: A further case. *J Med Genet* **33**:607, 1996.
25. Moriwaki SI, Stefanini M, Lehmann AR, Hoeijmakers JHJ, Robbins JH, Rapin I, Botta E, Tanganelli B, Vermeulen W, Broughton BC, Kraemer KH: DNA repair and ultraviolet mutagenesis in cells from a new patient with xeroderma pigmentosum group G and Cockayne syndrome resemble xeroderma pigmentosum cells. *J Invest Dermatol* **107**:647, 1996.
26. Setlow RB: The wavelengths in sunlight effective in producing skin cancer: A theoretical analysis. *Proc Natl Acad Sci USA* **71**:3363, 1974.
27. Epstein JH: Ultraviolet carcinogenesis. *Photophysiology* **5**:235, 1970.
28. Blum HF: *Carcinogenesis by Ultraviolet Light*. Princeton, NJ, Princeton University Press, 1959.
29. Cleaver JE: Repair processes for photochemical damage in mammalian cells, in Lett JT, Adler H, Zelle M (eds): *Advances in Radiation Biology*. New York, Academic Press, 1974, p 1.
30. Lawrence C: The Rad6 DNA repair pathway in *Saccharomyces cerevisiae*: What does it do and how does it do it? *Bioessays* **16**:253, 1994.
31. Todo T, Takemori H, Ryo H, Ihara M, Matsunaga T, Nikaido O, Sato K, Nomura T: A new photoreactivating enzyme that specifically repairs ultraviolet light-induced [6-4] photoproducts. *Nature* **361**:371, 1993.
32. Todo T, Ryo H, Yamamoto K, Toh H, Inui T, Ayaki H, Nomura T, Ikenaga M: Similarity among *Drosophila* [6-4] photolyase, a human photolyase homolog, and the DNA photolyase-blue-light photoreceptor family. *Science* **272**:109, 1996.
33. Sancar A, Sancar GB: DNA repair enzymes. *Annu Rev Biochem* **57**:29, 1988.
34. van Houten B: Nucleotide excision repair in *Escherichia coli*. *Microbiol Rev* **54**:18, 1990.
35. Grossman L, Thiagalingam S: Nucleotide excision repair, a tracking mechanism in search of damage. *J Biol Chem* **268**:16871, 1993.
36. Hoeijmakers JHJ: Nucleotide excision repair: I. From *E. coli* to yeast. *Trends Genet* **9**:173, 1993.
37. Bohr VA: Gene specific DNA repair. *Carcinogenesis* **12**:1983, 1991.
38. Hanawalt P, Mellon I: Stranded in an active gene. *Curr Biol* **3**:67, 1993.
39. Cleaver JE: Defective repair replication of DNA in xeroderma pigmentosum. *Nature* **218**:652, 1968.
40. Epstein JH, Fukuyama K, Reed WB, Epstein WL: Defect in DNA synthesis in skin of patients with xeroderma pigmentosum demonstrated in vivo. *Science* **168**:1477, 1970.
41. Stefanini M, Vermeulen W, Weeda G, Giliani S, Nardo T, Mezzina M, Sarasin A, Harper JL, Arlett CF, Hoeijmakers JHJ, Lehmann AR: A new nucleotide-excision-repair gene associated with the disorder trichothiodystrophy. *Am J Hum Genet* **53**:817, 1993.
42. Bootsma D, Mulder MP, Pot F, Cohen JA: Different inherited levels of DNA repair replication in xeroderma pigmentosum cell strains after exposure to ultraviolet irradiation. *Mutat Res* **9**:507, 1970.
43. Cleaver JE: Xeroderma pigmentosum: Variants with normal DNA repair and normal sensitivity to ultraviolet light. *J Invest Dermatol* **58**:124, 1972.
44. Lehmann AR, Kirk-Bell S, Arlett CF, Paterson MC, Lohman PHM, de Weerd-Kastelein EA, Bootsma D: Xeroderma pigmentosum cells with normal levels of excision repair have a defect in DNA synthesis after UV-irradiation. *Proc Natl Acad Sci USA* **72**:219, 1975.
45. Bohr VA, Smith CA, Okumoto DS, Hanawalt PC: DNA repair in an active gene: removal of pyrimidine dimers from the DHFR gene of CHO cells is much more efficient than in the genome overall. *Cell* **40**:359, 1985.
46. Venema J, Mullenders LHF, Natarajan AT, van Zeeland AA, Mayne LV: The genetic defect in Cockayne syndrome is associated with a defect in repair of UV-induced DNA damage in transcriptionally active DNA. *Proc Natl Acad Sci USA* **87**:4707, 1990.
47. Tanaka K, Kawai K, Kumahara Y, Ikenaga M, Okada Y: Genetic complementation groups in Cockayne syndrome. *Somat Cell Genet* **7**:445, 1981.
48. Lehmann AR, Francis AJ, Gianelli F: Prenatal diagnosis of Cockayne syndrome. *Lancet* **1**:486, 1985.
49. Stefanini M, Lagomarsini P, Giliani S, Nardo T, Botta E, Peserico A, Kleijer WJ, Lehmann AR, Sarasin A: Genetic heterogeneity of the excision repair defect associated with trichothiodystrophy. *Carcinogenesis* **14**:1101, 1993.
50. Wade MH, Chu EHY: Effects of DNA damaging agents on cultured fibroblasts derived from patients with Cockayne syndrome. *Mutat Res* **59**:49, 1979.
51. McCormick JJ, Kately-Kohler S, Watanabe M, Maher VM: Abnormal sensitivity of human fibroblasts from xeroderma pigmentosum variants to transformation to anchorage independence by ultraviolet radiation. *Cancer Res* **46**:489, 1986.

52. Barrett SF, Robbins JH, Tarone RE, Kraemer KH: Defective repair of cyclobutane pyrimidine dimers with normal repair of other DNA photoproducts in a transcriptionally active gene transfected into Cockayne syndrome cells. *Mutat Res* **255**:281, 1991.

53. Parris CN, Kraemer KH: Ultraviolet induced mutations in Cockayne syndrome cells are primarily caused by cyclobutane dimer photoproducts while repair of other photoproducts is normal. *Proc Natl Acad Sci USA* **90**:7260, 1993.

54. de Weerd-Kastelein EA, Keijzer W, Bootsma D: Genetic heterogeneity of xeroderma pigmentosum demonstrated by somatic cell hybridization. *Nature New Biol* **238**:80, 1972.

55. Lehmann AR: Three complementation groups in Cockayne syndrome. *Mutat Res* **106**:347, 1982.

56. Vermeulen W, van Vuuren AJ, Chipoulet M, Schaeffer L, Appeldoorn E, Weeda G, Jaspers NGJ, Priestley A, Arlett CF, Lehmann AR, Stefanini M, Mezzina M, Sarasin A, Bootsma D, Egly J-M, Hoeijmakers JHJ: Three unusual repair deficiencies associated with transcription factor BTF2(TFIIH): Evidence for the existence of a transcription syndrome. *Cold Spring Harbor Symp Quant Biol* **59**:317, 1994.

57. Kraemer KH: Xeroderma pigmentosum, in Demis DJ, McGuire J (eds): *Clinical Dermatology*, vol 4. Philadelphia, Harper & Row, 1980, p 1.

58. Vermeulen W, Scott RJ, Potger S, Muller HJ, Cole J, Arlett CF, Kleijer WJ, Bootsma D, Hoeijmakers JHJ, Weeda G: Clinical heterogeneity within xeroderma pigmentosum associated with mutations in the DNA repair and transcription gene ERCC3. *Am J Hum Genet* **54**:191, 1994.

59. Scott RJ, Itin P, Kleijer WJ, Kolb K, Arlett C, Muller H: Xeroderma pigmentosum-Cockayne syndrome complex in two new patients: Absence of skin tumors despite severe deficiency of DNA excision repair. *J Am Acad Dermatol* **29**:883, 1993.

60. Mansbridge JN, Hanawalt PC: Domain-limited repair of DNA in ultraviolet fibroblasts from xeroderma pigmentosum complementation group C, in Friedberg EC, Bridges BA (eds): *Cellular Responses to DNA Damage*. New York, Alan R Liss, 1983, p 195.

61. Venema J, van Hoffen A, Natarajan AT, van Zeeland AA, Mullenders LHF: The residual repair capacity of xeroderma pigmentosum complementation group C fibroblasts is highly specific for transcriptionally active DNA. *Nucleic Acids Res* **18**:443, 1990.

62. Hananian J, Cleaver JE: Xeroderma pigmentosum exhibiting neurological disorders and systemic lupus erythematosus. *Clin Genet* **17**:39, 1980.

63. Lehmann AR, Arlett CF, Broughton BC, Harcourt SA, Steingrimsdottir H, Stefanini M, Malcolm A, Taylor R, Natarajan AT, Green S: Trichiothiodystrophy, a human DNA repair disorder with heterogeneity in the cellular response to ultraviolet light. *Cancer Res* **48**:6090, 1988.

64. Wood RD: Seven genes for three diseases. *Nature* **350**:190, 1991.

65. Arase S, Kozuka T, Tanaka K, Ikenaga M, Takebe H: A sixth complementation group in xeroderma pigmentosum. *Mutat Res* **59**:143, 1979.

66. Nishigori C, Fujiwara H, Uyeno K, Kawaguchi T, Takebe H: Xeroderma pigmentosum patients belonging to complementation group F and efficient liquid recovery of ultraviolet damage. *Photodermatol Photoimmunol Photomed* **8**:146, 1991.

67. Vermeulen W, Jaeken J, Jaspers NGJ, Bootsma D, Hoeijmakers JHJ: Xeroderma pigmentosum complementation group G associated with Cockayne syndrome. *Am J Hum Genet* **53**:185, 1993.

68. Cooper PT, Nouspikel T, Clarkson S, Leadon S: Defective transcription-coupled repair of oxidative base damage in Cockayne syndrome patients from XP group G. *Science* **275**:990, 1997.

69. Nouspikel T, Lalle P, Leadon S, Cooper P, Clarkson S: A common mutational pattern in Cockayne syndrome patients from xeroderma pigmentosum group G: implications for a second XPG function. *Proc Natl Acad Sci USA* **94**:3116, 1997.

70. Jung EG: New form of molecular defect in xeroderma pigmentosum. *Nature* **228**:361, 1970.

71. Jaspers NGJ, Jansen-v.d., Kuilen G, Bootsma D: Complementation analysis of xeroderma pigmentosum variants. *Exp Cell Res* **136**:81, 1981.

72. Jorizzo JL, Atherton DJ, Crounse RG, Wells RS: Ichthyosis, brittle hair, impaired intelligence, decreased fertility and short stature (IBIDS syndrome). *Br J Dermatol* **106**:705, 1982.

73. Lehmann AR, Thompson AF, Harcourt SA, Stefanini M, Norris PG: Cockaynes syndrome: Correlation of clinical features with cellular sensitivity of RNA synthesis to UV irradiation. *J Med Genet* **30**:679, 1993.

74. Itoh T, Cleaver JE, Yamaizumi M: Cockayne syndrome complementation group B associated with xeroderma pigmentosum phenotype. *Hum Genet* **97**:176, 1996.

75. Itoh T, Ono T, Yamaizumi M: A new UV-sensitive syndrome not belonging to any complementation groups of xeroderma pigmentosum or Cockayne syndrome: Siblings showing biochemical characteristics of Cockayne syndrome without typical clinical manifestations. *Mutat Res* **314**:233, 1994.

76. Itoh T, Fujiwara Y, Ono T, Yamaizumi M: UVs syndrome, a new general category of photosensitive disorder with defective DNA repair, is distinct from xeroderma pigmentosum variant and rodent complementation group 1. *Am J Hum Genet* **56**:1267, 1995.

77. Lambert WC, Lambert MW: Co-recessive inheritance: a model for DNA repair, genetic disease and carcinogenesis. *Mutat Res* **145**:227, 1985.

78. Thompson LH, Busch DB, Brookman K, Mooney CL: Genetic diversity of UV-sensitive DNA repair mutants of Chinese hamster ovary cells. *Proc Natl Acad Sci USA* **78**:3734, 1981.

79. Collins AR: Mutant rodent cell lines sensitive to ultraviolet light, ionizing radiation and cross-linking agents: A comprehensive survey of genetic and biochemical characteristics. *Mutat Res* **293**:99, 1993.

80. Thompson LH: Somatic cell genetics approach to dissecting mammalian DNA repair. *Environ Mol Mutagen* **14**:264, 1989.

81. Westerveld A, Hoeijmakers JHJ, van Duin M, de Wit J, Odijk H, Pastink A, Wood RD, Bootsma D: Molecular cloning of a human DNA repair gene. *Nature* **310**:425, 1984.

82. Weber CA, Salazar EP, Stewart SA, Thompson LH: Molecular cloning and biological characterization of a human gene, ERCC2, that corrects the nucleotide excision repair defect in CHO UV5 cells. *Mol Cell Biol* **8**:1137, 1988.

83. Weeda G, van Ham RCA, Masurel R, Westerveld A, Odijk H, de Wit J, Bootsma D, van der Eb AJ, Hoeijmakers JHJ: Molecular cloning and biological characterization of the human excision repair gene ERCC-3. *Mol Cell Biol* **10**:2570, 1990.

84. Thompson LH, Brookman KW, Weber CA, Salazar EP, Reardon JT, Sancar A, Deng Z, Siciliano MJ: Molecular cloning of the human nucleotide-excision-repair gene ERCC4. *Proc Natl Acad Sci USA* **91**:6855, 1994.

85. Mudgett JS, MacInnes MA: Isolation of the functional human excision repair gene ERCC 5 by intercosmid recombination. *Genomics* **8**:623, 1990.

86. Troelstra C, Odijk H, de Wit J, Westerveld A, Thompson LH, Bootsma D, Hoeijmakers JHJ: Molecular cloning of the human DNA excision repair gene ERCC-6. *Mol Cell Biol* **10**:5806, 1990.

87. Weber CA, Thompson LH, Salazar EP: Characterization of ERCC2 and its correction of xeroderma pigmentosum group D, in *Proceedings of the American Association for Cancer Research Special Conference on Cellular Responses to Environmental DNA Damage, Banff, Canada.* December 1, 1991.

88. Flejter WL, McDaniel LD, Johns D, Friedberg EC, Schultz RA: Correction of xeroderma pigmentosum complementation group D mutant cell phenotypes by chromosome and gene transfer: involvement of the human ERCC2 DNA repair gene. *Proc Natl Acad Sci USA* **89**:261, 1992.

89. Weeda G, van Ham RCA, Vermeulen W, Bootsma D, van der Eb AJ, Hoeijmakers JHJ: A presumed DNA helicase encoded by ERCC-3 is involved in the human repair disorders xeroderma pigmentosum and Cockayne syndrome. *Cell* **62**:777, 1990.

90. Scherly D, Nouspikel T, Corlet J, Ucla C, Bairoch A, Clarkson SG: Complementation of the DNA repair defect in xeroderma pigmentosum group G cells by a human cDNA related to yeast RAD2. *Nature* **363**:182, 1993.

91. Troelstra C, van Gool A, de Wit J, Vermeulen W, Bootsma D, Hoeijmakers JHJ: ERCC6, a member of a subfamily of putative helicases, is involved in Cockayne syndrome and preferential repair of active genes. *Cell* **71**:939, 1992.

92. MacInnes MA, Dickson JA, Hernandez RR, Learmont D, Lin GY, Mudgett JS, Park MS, Schauer S, Reynolds RJ, Strniste GF, Yu JY: Human ERCC5 cDNA-cosmid complementation for excision repair and bipartite amino acid domains conserved with RAD proteins of *S. cerevisiae* and *S. pombe*. *Mol Cell Biol* **13**:6393, 1993.

93. O'Donovan A, Wood RD: Identical defects in DNA repair in xeroderma pigmentosum group G and rodent ERCC group 5. *Nature* **363**:185, 1993.

94. Fryns JP, Bulcke J, Verdu P, Carton H, Kleczkowska A, van den Berghe H: Apparent late-onset Cockayne syndrome and interstitial deletion of

the long arm of chromosome 10 [del(10)(q11.23q21.2)]. *Am J Med Genet* **40**:343, 1991.

95. Tanaka K, Satokata I, Ogita Z, Uchida T, Okada Y: Molecular cloning of a mouse DNA repair gene that complements the defect of group A xeroderma pigmentosum. *Proc Natl Acad Sci USA* **86**:5512, 1989.

96. Hoeijmakers JHJ, Odijk H, Westerveld A: Differences between rodent and human cell lines in the amount of integrated DNA after transfection. *Exp Cell Res* **169**:111, 1987.

97. Legerski R, Peterson C: Expression cloning of a human DNA repair gene involved in xeroderma pigmentosum group C. *Nature* **359**:70, 1992.

98. Henning KA, Li L, Iyer N, McDaniel L, Reagan MS, Legerski R, Schultz RA, Stefanini M, Lehmann AR, Mayne LV, Friedberg EC: The Cockayne syndrome group A gene encodes a WD repeat protein that interacts with CSB protein and a subunit of RNA polymerase II TFIIH. *Cell* **82**:555, 1995.

99. Itoh T, Shiomi T, Shiomi N, Harada Y, Wakasugi M, Matsunaga T, Nikaido O, Friedberg EC, Yamaizumi M: Rodent complementation group 8 (ERCC8) corresponds to Cockayne syndrome complementation group A. *Mutat Res* **362**:167, 1996.

100. Koken MH, Reynolds P, Jaspers-Dekker I, Prakash L, Prakash S, Bootsma D, Hoeijmakers JH: Structural and functional conservation of two human homologs of the yeast DNA repair gene RAD6. *Proc Natl Acad Sci USA* **88**:8865, 1991.

101. Jentsch S: The ubiquitin-conjugation system. *Annu Rev Genet* **26**:179, 1992.

102. Sijbers AM, de Laat WL, Ariza RR, Biggerstaff M, Wei YF, Moggs JG, Carter KC, Shell BK, Evans E, de Jong MC, Rademakers S, de Rooij J, Jaspers NGJ, Hoeijmakers JHJ, Wood RD: Xeroderma pigmentosum group F caused by a defect in a structure-specific DNA repair endonuclease. *Cell* **86**:811, 1996.

103. Masutani C, Sugasawa K, Yanagisawa J, Sonoyama T, Ui M, Enomoto T, Takio K, Tanaka K, van der Spek PJ, Bootsma D, Hoeijmakers JHJ, Hanaoka F: Purification and cloning of a nucleotide excision repair complex involving the xeroderma pigmentosum group C protein and a human homolog of yeast RAD23. *EMBO J* **13**:1831, 1994.

104. van Gool AJ, Verhage R, Swagemakers SMA, van de Putte P, Brouwer J, Troelstra C, Bootsma D, Hoeijmakers JHJ: RAD26, the functional S. cerevisiae homolog of the Cockayne syndrome B gene ERCC6. *EMBO J* **13**:5361, 1994.

105. Hwang BJ, Liao JC, Chu G: Isolation of a cDNA encoding a UV-damaged DNA binding factor defective in xeroderma pigmentosum group E cells. *Mutat Res* **362**:105, 1996.

106. Keeney S, Chang GJ, Linn S: Characterization of human DNA damage binding protein implicated in xeroderma pigmentosum E. *J Biol Chem* **268**:21293, 1993.

107. Keeney S, Eker APM, Brody T, Vermeulen W, Bootsma D, Hoeijmakers JHJ, Linn S: Correction of the DNA repair defect in xeroderma pigmentosum group E by injection of a DNA damage-binding protein. *Proc Natl Acad Sci USA* **91**:4053, 1994.

108. Shivji MKK, Kenny MK, Wood RD: Proliferating cell nuclear antigen is required for DNA excision repair. *Cell* **69**:367, 1992.

109. Sibghat-Ullah, Husain I, Carlton W, Sancar A: Human nucleotide excision repair in vitro: Repair of pyrimidine dimers, psoralen and cisplatin adducts by HeLa cell-free extract. *Nucleic Acids Res* **17**:4471, 1989.

110. Aboussekhra A, Biggerstaff M, Shivji MKK, Vilpo JA, Moncollin V, Podust VN, Protic M, Hubscher U, Egly J, Wood RD: Mammalian DNA nucleotide excision repair reconstituted with purified components. *Cell* **80**:859, 1995.

111. Mu D, Park C-H, Matsunaga T, Hsu DS, Reardon JT, Sancar A: Reconstitution of human DNA repair excision nuclease in a highly defined system. *J Biol Chem* **270**:2415, 1995.

112. Sugasawa K, Ng JMY, Masutani C, Iwai S, van der Spek PJ, Eker APM, Hanaoka F, Bootsma D, Hoeijmakers JHJ: Xeroderma pigmentosum group C protein complex is the initiator of global genome nucleotide excision repair. *Mol Cell* **2**: August, 1998.

113. Reardon J, Mu D, Sancar A: Overproduction, purification, and characterization of the XPC subunit of the human DNA repair excision nuclease. *J Biol Chem* **271**:19451, 1996.

114. Shivji MKK, Eker APM, Wood RD: DNA repair defect in xeroderma pigmentosum group C and complementing factor from HeLa cells. *J Biol Chem* **269**:22749, 1994.

115. Tanaka K, Miura N, Satokata I, Miyamoto I, Yoshida MC, Satoh Y, Kondo S, Yasui A, Okayama H, Okada Y: Analysis of a human DNA excision repair gene involved in group A xeroderma pigmentosum and containing a zinc-finger domain. *Nature* **348**:73, 1990.

116. Robins P, Jones CJ, Biggerstaff M, Lindahl T, Wood RD: Complementation of DNA repair in xeroderma pigmentosum group A cell extracts by a protein with affinity for damaged DNA. *EMBO J* **10**:3913, 1991.

117. Eker APM, Vermeulen W, Miura N, Tanaka K, Jaspers NGJ, Hoeijmakers JHJ, Bootsma D: Xeroderma pigmentosum group A correcting protein from calf thymus. *Mutat Res* **274**:211, 1992.

118. Miyamoto I, Miura N, Niwa H, Miyazaki J, Tanaka K: Mutational analysis of the structure and function of the xeroderma pigmentosum group A complementing protein. *J Biol Chem* **267**:12182, 1992.

119. Jones CJ, Wood RD: Preferential binding of the xeroderma pigmentosum group A complementing protein to damaged DNA. *Biochemistry* **32**:12096, 1993.

120. Asahina H, Kuraoka I, Shirakawa M, Morita EH, Miura N, Miyamoto I, Ohtsuka E, Okada Y, Tanaka K: The XPA protein is a zinc metalloprotein with an ability to recognize various kinds of DNA damage. *Mutat Res* **315**:29, 1994.

121. Miura N, Miyamoto I, Asahina H, Satokata I, Tanaka K, Okada Y: Identification and characterization of XPAC protein, the gene product of the human XPAC (xeroderma pigmentosum group A complementing) gene. *J Biol Chem* **266**:19786, 1991.

122. Bankmann M, Prakash L, Prakash S: Yeast RAD14 and human xeroderma pigmentosum group A DNA repair genes encode homologous proteins. *Nature* **355**:555, 1992.

123. Guzder SN, Sung P, Prakash L, Prakash S: Yeast DNA-repair gene RAD14 encodes a zinc metalloprotein with affinity for ultraviolet-damaged DNA. *Proc Natl Acad Sci USA* **90**:5433, 1993.

124. Chu G, Chang E: Xeroderma pigmentosum group E cells lack a nuclear factor that binds to damaged DNA. *Science* **242**:564, 1988.

125. Kataoka H, Fujiwara Y: UV damage-specific DNA protein in xeroderma pigmentosum complementation group E. *Biochem Biophys Res Commun* **175**:1139, 1991.

126. Keeney S, Wein H, Linn S: Biochemical heterogeneity in xeroderma pigmentosum complementation group E. *Mutat Res* **273**:49, 1992.

127. Hwang BJ, Chu G: Purification and characterization of a human protein that binds to damaged DNA. *Biochemistry* **32**:1657, 1993.

128. Nichols AF, Ong P, Linn S: Mutations specific to the xeroderma pigmentosum group E Ddb(—) phenotype. *J Biol Chem* **271**:24317, 1996.

129. Takao M, Abramic M, Moos M, Otrin VR, Wootton JC, Mclenigan M, Levine AS, Protic M: A 127 kDa component of a UV-damaged DNA-binding complex which is defective in some xeroderma pigmentosum group E patients is homologous to a slime mold protein. *Nucleic Acids Res* **21**:4111, 1993.

130. Reardon JT, Nichols AF, Keeney S, Smith CA, Taylor JS, Linn S, Sancar A: Comparative analysis of binding of human damaged DNA-binding protein (XPE) and *Escherichia coli* damage recognition protein (UvrA) to the major ultraviolet photoproducts T[CS]TT[Ts]TT[6-4]T and T[Dewar]T. *J Biol Chem* **268**:21301, 1993.

131. Li L, Elledge SJ, Peterson CA, Bales ES, Legerski RJ: Specific association between the human DNA repair proteins XPA and ERCC1. *Proc Natl Acad Sci USA* **91**:5012, 1994.

132. Park C-H, Sancar A: Formation of a ternary complex by human XPA, ERCC1 and ERCC4(XPF) excision repair proteins. *Proc Natl Acad Sci USA* **91**:5017, 1994.

133. Saijo M, Kuraoka I, Masutani C, Hanaoka F, Tanaka K: Sequential binding of DNA repair proteins RPA and ERCC1 to XPA in vitro. *Nucleic Acids Res* **24**:4719, 1996.

134. He Z, Henricksen LA, Wold MS, Ingles CJ: RPA involvement in the damage and incision step of nucleotide excision repair. *Nature* **374**:566, 1995.

135. Park C-H, Mu D, Reardon JT, Sancar A: The general transcription-repair factor TFIIH is recruited to the excision repair complex by the XPA protein independent of the TFIIE transcription factor. *J Biol Chem* **270**:4896, 1995.

136. Nocentini S, Coin F, Saijo M, Tanaka K, Egly J: DNA damage recognition by XPA protein promotes efficient recruitment of transcription factor II H. *J Biol Chem* **272**:22991, 1997.

137. Bootsma D, Kraemer KH, Cleaver JE, Hoeijmakers JHJ: Nucleotide excision repair syndromes: xeroderma pigmentosum, Cockayne syndrome and trichothiodystrophy, in Vogelstein B, Kinzler KW (eds): *The Genetic Basis of Human Cancer*. New York, McGraw-Hill, 1998, p. 245.

138. Park H-W, Kim S-T, Sancar A, Deisenhofer J: Crystal structure of DNA photolyase from *Escherichia coli*. *Science* **268**:1866, 1995.

139. Evans E, Moggs J, Hwang J, Egly J, Wood R: Mechanisms of open complex and dual incision formation by nucleotide excision repair factors. *EMBO J* **16**:6559, 1997.

140. Mu D, Wakasugi M, Hsu D, Sancar A: Characterization of reaction intermediates of excision repair nuclease. *J Biol Chem* **272**:28971, 1997.

141. Coverley D, Kenny MK, Lane DP, Wood RD: A role for the human single-stranded DNA binding protein HSSB/RPA in an early stage of nucleotide excision repair. *Nucleic Acids Res* **20**:3873, 1992.

142. Wakasugi M, Reardon J, Sancar A: The non-catalytic function of XPG protein during dual incision in human nucleotide excision repair. *J Biol Chem* **272**:16030, 1997.

143. Naumovski L, Friedberg EC: A DNA repair gene required for the incision of damaged DNA is essential for viability in *Saccharomyces cerevisiae*. *Proc Natl Acad Sci USA* **80**:4818, 1983.

144. Park E, Guzder S, Koken MHM, Jaspers-Dekker I, Weeda G, Hoeijmakers JHJ, Prakash S, Prakash L: RAD25, a yeast homolog of human xeroderma pigmentosum group B DNA repair gene is essential for viability. *Proc Natl Acad Sci USA* **89**:11416, 1992.

145. Mounkes LC, Jones RS, Liang B-C, Gelbart W, Fuller MT: A *Drosophila* model for xeroderma pigmentosum and Cockayne syndrome: Haywire encodes the fly homolog of ERCC3, a human excision repair gene. *Cell* **71**:925, 1992.

146. de Boer J, Donker I, de Wit J, Hoeijmakers JHJ, Weeda G: Disruption of the mouse XPD DNA repair/basal transcription gene results in preimplantation lethality. *Cancer Res* **58**:89, 1998.

147. Schaeffer L, Roy R, Humbert S, Moncollin V, Vermeulen W, Hoeijmakers JHJ, Chambon P, Egly J: DNA repair helicase: A component of BTF2 (TFIIH) basic transcription factor. *Science* **260**:58, 1993.

148. Conaway RC, Conaway JW: General initiation factors for RNA polymerase II. *Annu Rev Biochem* **62**:161, 1993.

149. Feaver WJ, Svejstrup JQ, Henry NL, Kornberg RD: Relationship of CDK-activating kinase and RNA polymerase II CTD kinase TFIIH/TFIIK. *Cell* **79**:1103, 1994.

150. Roy R, Adamczewski JP, Seroz T, Vermeulen W, Tassan J-P, Schaeffer L, Nigg EA, Hoeijmakers JHJ, Egly J: The MO15 cell cycle kinase is associated with the TFIIH transcription repair factor. *Cell* **79**:1093, 1994.

151. Schaeffer L, Moncollin V, Roy R, Staub A, Mezzina M, Sarasin A, Weeda G, Hoeijmakers JHJ, Egly JM: The ERCC2/DNA repair protein is associated with the class II BTF2/TFIIH transcription factor. *EMBO J* **13**:2388, 1994.

152. Drapkin R, Reardon JT, Ansari A, Huang JC, Zawel L, Ahn K, Sancar A, Reinberg D: Dual role of TFIIH in DNA excision repair and in transcription by RNA polymerase II. *Nature* **368**:769, 1994.

153. van Vuuren AJ, Vermeulen W, Ma L, Weeda G, Appeldoorn E, Jaspers NGJ, van der Eb AJ, Bootsma D, Hoeijmakers JHJ, Humbert S, Schaeffer L, Egly J-M: Correction of xeroderma pigmentosum repair defect by basal transcription factor BTF2(TFIIH). *EMBO J* **13**:1645, 1994.

154. Humbert S, van Vuuren AJ, Lutz Y, Hoeijmakers JHJ, Egly J-M, Moncollin V: Characterization of p44/SSL1 and p34 subunits of the BTF2/TFIIH transcription/repair factor. *EMBO J* **13**:2393, 1994.

155. Wang Z, Buratowski S, Svejstrup JQ, Feaver WJ, Wu X, Kornberg RD, Donahue TD, Friedberg EC: The yeast TFB1 and SSL1 genes, which encode subunits of transcription factor IIH, are required for nucleotide excision repair and RNA polymerase II transcription. *Mol Cell Biol* **15**:2288, 1995.

156. Feaver WJ, Svejstrup JQ, Bardwell L, Bardwell AJ, Buratowski S, Gulyas KD, Donahue TF, Friedberg EC, Kornberg RD: Dual roles of a multiprotein complex from S. cerevisiae in transcription and DNA repair. *Cell* **75**:1379, 1993.

157. Guzder SN, Sung P, Bailly V, Prakash L, Prakash S: RAD25 is a DNA helicase required for DNA repair and RNA polymerase II transcription. *Nature* **369**:578, 1994.

158. Svejstrup JQ, Want Z, Feaver WJ, Wu X, Bushnell DA, Donahue TF, Friedberg EC, Kornberg RD: Different forms of TFIIH for transcription and DNA repair: holo-TFIIH and a nucleotide excision repairosome. *Cell* **80**:21, 1995.

159. Wang Z, Svejstrup JQ, Feaver WJ, Wu X, Kornberg RD, Friedberg EC: Transcription factor b (TFIIH) is required during nucleotide excision repair in yeast. *Nature* **368**:74, 1994.

160. Okhuma Y: Multiple functions of general transcription factors TFIIE and TFIIH: Possible points of regulation by trans-acting factors. *J Biochem* **122**:481, 1997.

161. Matsunaga T, Mu D, Park C-H, Reardon JT, Sancar A: Human DNA repair excision nuclease: Analysis of the roles of the subunits involved in dual incisions by using anti-XPG and anti-ERCC1 antibodies. *J Biol Chem* **270**:20862, 1995.

162. O'Donovan A, Davies AA, Moggs JG, West SC, Wood RD: XPG endonuclease makes the 3′ incision in human DNA nucleotide excision repair. *Nature* **371**:432, 1994.

163. de Laat WL, Appeldoorn E, Jaspers NGJ, Hoeijmakers JHJ: DNA structural elements required for ERCC1-XPF endonuclease activity. *J Biol Chem* **273**:7835, 1998.

164. van Vuuren AJ, Appeldoorn E, Odijk H, Yasui A, Jaspers NGJ, Bootsma D, Hoeijmakers JHJ: Evidence for a repair enzyme complex involving ERCC1 and complementing activities of ERCC4, ERCC11 and xeroderma pigmentosum group F. *EMBO J* **12**:3693, 1993.

165. Biggerstaff M, Szymkowski DE, Wood RD: Co-correction of ERCC1, ERCC4 and xeroderma pigmentosum group F DNA repair defects in vitro. *EMBO J* **12**:3685, 1993.

166. Bardwell AJ, Bardwell L, Tomkinson AE, Friedberg EC: Specific cleavage of model recombination and repair intermediates by the yeast Rad1-Rad10 DNA endonuclease. *Science* **265**:2082, 1994.

167. Davies AA, Friedberg EC, Tomkinson AE, Wood RD, West SC: Role of the Rad1 and Rad10 proteins in nucleotide excision repair and recombination. *J Biol Chem* **270**:24638, 1995.

168. Fishman-Lobell J, Haber JE: Removal of nonhomologous DNA ends in double-strand break recombination: The role of the yeast ultraviolet repair gene RAD1. *Science* **258**:480, 1992.

169. Saffran WA, Greenberg RB, Thaler MS, Jones MM: Single strand and double strand DNA damage-induced reciprocal recombination in yeast: Dependence on nucleotide excision repair and RAD1 recombination. *Nucleic Acids Res* **22**:2823, 1994.

170. Schiestl RH, Prakash S: RAD10, an excision repair gene of *Saccharomyces cerevisiae* is involved in the RAD1 pathway of mitotic recombination. *Mol Cell Biol* **10**:2485, 1990.

171. Evans E, Fellows J, Coffer A, Wood RD: Open complex formation around a lesion during nucleotide excision repair provides a structure for cleavage by human XPG protein. *EMBO J* **16**:625 1997.

172. Huang JC, Svoboda DL, Reardon JT, Sancar A: Human nucleotide excision nuclease removes thymine dimers from DNA by incising the 22nd phosphodiester bond 5′ and the 6th phosphodiester bond 3′ to the photodimer. *Proc Natl Acad Sci USA* **89**:3664, 1992.

173. Moggs JG, Yarema KJ, Essigmann JM, Wood RD: Analysis of incision sites produced by human cell extracts and purified proteins during nucleotide excision repair of a 1,3- intrastrand d(GpTpG)-cisplatin adduct. *J Biol Chem* **271**:7177,1996.

174. Svoboda DL, Taylor JS, Hearst JE, Sancar A: DNA repair by eukaryotic endonuclease. *J Biol Chem* **268**:1931, 1993.

175. Mu D, Hsu DS, Sancar A: Reaction mechanism of human DNA repair excision nuclease. *J Biol Chem* **271**:8285, 1996.

176. Bardwell AJ, Bardwell L, Iyer N, Svejstrup JQ, Feaver WJ, Kornberg RD, Friedberg EC: Yeast nucleotide excision repair proteins rad2 and rad4 interact with RNA polymerase II basal transcription factor b (TFIIH). *Mol Cell Biol* **14**:3569, 1994.

177. Iyer N, Reagan MS, Wu K-J, Canagarajah B, Friedberg EC: Interactions involving the human RNA polymerase II transcription/nucleotide excision repair complex TFIIH, the nucleotide excision repair protein XPG, and Cockayne syndrome group B (CSB) protein. *Biochemistry* **35**:2157, 1996.

178. Nichols AF, Sancar A: Purification of PCNA as a nucleotide excision repair protein. *Nucleic Acids Res* **20**:2441, 1992.

179. Barnes DE, Tomkinson AE, Lehmann AR, Webster ADB, Lindahl T: Mutations in the DNA ligase 1 gene of an individual with immunodeficiencies and cellular hypersensitivity to DNA-damaging agents. *Cell* **69**:495, 1992.

180. Verhage R, Zeeman A, de Groot N, Gleig F, Bang D, van der Putte P, Brouwer J: The RAD7 and RAD16 genes are essential for repair of non-transcribed DNA in *Saccharomyces cerevisiae*. *Mol Cell Biol* **14**:6135, 1994.

181. Venema J, van Hoffen A, Karcagi V, Natarajan AT, van Zeeland AA, Mullenders LHF: Xeroderma pigmentosum complementation group C cells remove pyrimidine dimers selectively from the transcribed strand of active genes. *Mol Cell Biol* **11**:4128, 1991.

182. Perozzi G, Prakash S: RAD7 of *Saccharomyces cerevisiae*: Transcripts, nucleotide sequence analysis and functional relationship between the RAD7 and RAD23 gene products. *Mol Cell Biol* **6**:1497, 1986.

183. Bang DD, Verhage R, Goosen N, Brouwer J, Putte PVD: Molecular cloning of RAD16, a gene involved in differential repair in *Saccharomyces cerevisiae*. *Nucleic Acids Res* **20**:3925, 1992.

184. Wolffe AP: Switched-on chromatin. *Curr Biol* **4**:525, 1994.

185. Neer EJ, Schmidt CJ, Nambudripad R, Smith TF: The ancient regulatory-protein family of WD-repeat proteins. *Nature* **371**:297, 1994.

186. Selby C, Sancar A: Human transcription-repair coupling factor CSB/ERCC6 is a DNA-stimulatedATPase but is not a helicase and does not disrupt the ternary transcription complex of stalled RNA polymerase II. *J Biol Chem* **272**:1885, 1997.

187. Donahue BH, Yin S, Taylor J-S, Reines D, Hanawalt PC: Transcript cleavage by RNA polymerase II arrested by a cyclobutane pyrimidine dimer in the DNA template. *Proc Natl Acad Sci USA* **91**:8502, 1994.

188. Tantin D, Kansal A, Carey M: Recruitment of the putative transcription-repair coupling factor CSB/ERCC6 to RNA polymerase II elongation complexes. *Mol Cell Biol* **17**:6803, 1997.

189. van Gool A, Citterio E, Rademakers S, van Os R, Vermeulen W, Constantinou A, Egly J, Bootsma D, Hoeijmakers J: The Cockayne syndrome B protein, involved in transcription-coupled DNA repair, resides in a RNA polymerase II-containing complex. *EMBO J* **16**:5955, 1997.

190. van Gool A, van der Horst G, Citterio E, Hoeijmakers J: Cockayne syndrome: Defective repair of transcription? *EMBO J* **16**:4155, 1997.

191. Nagai A, Saijo M, Kuraoka I, Matsuda T, Kodo N, Nakatsu Y, Mimaki T, Mino M, Biggerstaff M, Wood RD, Sijbers A, Hoeijmakers JHJ, Tanaka K: Enhancement of damage-specific DNA binding of XPA by interaction with the ERCC1 DNA repair protein. *Biochem Biophys Res Commun* **211**:960, 1995.

192. McWhir J, Seldridge J, Harrison DJ, Squires S, Melton DW: Mice with DNA repair gene (ERCC-1) deficiency have elevated levels of p53, liver nuclear abnormalities and die before weaning. *Nature Genet* **5**:217, 1993.

193. van Duin M, Vredeveldt G, Mayne LV, Odijk H, Vermeulen W, Klein B, Weeda G, Hoeijmakers JHJ, Bootsma D, Westerveld A: The cloned human DNA excision repair gene ERCC-1 fails to correct xeroderma pigmentosum complementation groups A through I. *Mutat Res* **217**:83, 1989.

194. Weeda G, Donker I, de Wit J, Morreau H. Janssens R, Vissers CJ, Nigg A, van Steeg H, Bootsma D, Hoeijmakers JHJ: Disruption of mouse ERCC1 results in a novel repair syndrome with growth failure, nuclear abnormalities and senescence. *Curr Biol* **7**:427, 1997.

195. Nakane H, Takeuchi S, Yuba S, Saijo M, Nakatsu Y, Ishikawa T, Hirota S, Kitamura Y, Kato Y, Tsunoda Y, Miyauchi H, Horio T, Tokunaga T, Matsunaga T, Nikaido O, Nishimune Y, Okada Y, Tanaka K: High incidence of ultraviolet-B or chemical-carcinogen-induced skin tumours in mice lacking the xeroderma pigmentosum group A gene. *Nature* **377**:165, 1995.

196. de Vries A, van Oostrom CTM, Hofhuis FMA, Dortant PM, Berg RJW, de Gruijl FR, Wester PW, van Kreijl CF, Capel PJA, van Steeg H, Verbeek SJ: Increased susceptibility to ultraviolet-B and carcinogens of mice lacking the DNA excision repair gene XPA. *Nature* **377**:169, 1995.

197. Sands AT, Abuin A, Sanchez A, Conti CJ, Bradley A: High susceptibility to ultraviolet-induced carcinogenesis in mice lacking XPC. *Nature* **377**:162, 1995.

198. van der Horst GTJ, van Steeg H, Berg RJW, van Gool AJ, de Wit J, Weeda G, Morreau H, Beems RB, van Kreijl CF, de Gruijl FR, Bootsma D, Hoeijmakers JHJ: Defective transcription-coupled repair in Cockayne syndrome B mice is associated with skin cancer predisposition. *Cell* **89**:425, 1997.

199. De Boer J, de Wit, van Steeg H, Berg RJW, Morreau H, Visser P, Lehmann AR, Duran M, Hoeijmakers JHJ, Weeda G: A mouse model for the basal transcription/DNA repair syndrome: Trichothiodystrophy. *Mol Cell* **1**:981,1998.

200. Johnson RT, Squires S: The XPD complementation group. Insights into xeroderma pigmentosum, Cockaynes syndrome and trichothiodystrophy. *Mutat Res* **273**:97, 1992.

201. Broughton BC, Steingrimsdottir H, Weber CA, Lehmann AR: Mutations in xeroderma pigmentosum group D DNA repair/transcription gene in patients with trichothiodystrophy. *Nature Genet* **7**:189, 1994.

202. Weeda G, Eveno E, Donker I, Vermeulen W, Chevallier-Lagente O, Taïeb A, Stary A, Hoeijmakers JHJ, Mezzina M, Sarasin A: A mutation in the XPB/ERCC3 DNA repair transcription gene, associated with trichothiodystrophy. *Am J Hum Genet* **60**:320, 1997.

203. Kemphues KJ, Kaufman TC, Raff RA, Raff EC: The testis-specific beta-tubulin subunit in *Drosophila melanogaster* has multiple functions in spermatogenesis. *Cell* **31**:655, 1982.

204. Readhead C, Popko B, Takahashi N, Shine HD, Saavedra RA, Sidman RL, Hood L: Expression of a myelin basic protein gene in transgenic shiverer mice: Correction of the dysmyelinating phenotype. *Cell* **48**:703, 1987.

205. Sasaki K, Tachi N, Shinoda M, Satoh N, Minami R, Ohnishi A: Demyelinating peripheral neuropathy in Cockayne syndrome: A histopathologic and morphometric study. *Brain Dev* **14**:114, 1992.

206. Parvin JD, Sharp PA: DNA topology and a minimum set of basal factors for transcription by RNA polymerase II. *Cell* **73**:533, 1993.

207. Bootsma D, Hoeijmakers JHJ: DNA repair: Engagement with transcription. *Nature* **363**:114, 1993.

208. Kraemer KH, Slor H: Xeroderma pigmentosum. *Clin Dermatol* **3**:33, 1985.

209. Lynch HT, Anderson DE, Smith JL, Howell JB, Krush AJ: Xeroderma pigmentosum, malignant melanoma and congenital ichthyosis. *Arch Dermatol* **96**:625, 1967.

210. Kraemer KH, Digiovanna JJ, Moshell AN, Tarone RE, Peck GL: Prevention of skin cancer with oral 13-cisretinoic acid in xeroderma pigmentosum. *N Engl J Med* **318**:1633, 1988.

211. Ramsay CA, Coltart TM, Blunt S, Pawsey CA, Gianelli F: Prenatal diagnosis of xeroderma pigmentosum: Report of the first successful case. *Lancet* **2**:1109, 1974.

212. Halley DFF, Keijzer W, Jaspers NGJ, Niermeijer MF, Kleijer WJ, Boué A, Bootsma D: Prenatal diagnosis of xeroderma pigmentosum (group C) using assays of unscheduled DNA synthesis and postreplication repair. *Clin Genet* **16**:137, 1979.

213. Cleaver JE, Volpe JPG, Charles WC, Thomas GH: Prenatal diagnosis of xeroderma pigmentosum and Cockayne Syndrome. *Prenatal Diagn* **14**:921, 1994.

214. Sarasin A, Blanchet-Bardon C, Renault G, Lehmann A, Arlett C, Dumez Y: Prenatal diagnosis in a subset of trichothiodystrophy patients defective in DNA repair. *Br J Dermatol* **127**:485, 1992.

215. Matsumoto N, Saito N, Harada N, Tanaka K, Niikawa N: DNA-based prenatal carrier detection for group A xeroderma pigmentosum in a chorionic villus sample. *Prenatal Diagn* **15**:1675, 1995.

216. Masutani C, Kusumoto R, Yamada A, Dohmae N, Yokoi M, Yuasa M, Araki M, Iwai S, Takio K, Hanaoka F: The XPV (xeroderma pigmentosum variant) gene encodes human DNA polymerase eta. *Nature* **399**:700, 1999.

217. Johnson RE, Kondratick CM, Prakash S, Prakash L: hRAD30 mutations in the variant form of xeroderma pigmentosum. *Science* **285**:263, 1999.

CHAPTER 15

Ataxia-Telangiectasia

Richard A. Gatti

1. The diagnosis of ataxia-telangiectasia (A-T) is based primarily on clinical examination and should include progressive cerebellar ataxia with onset between 1 and 3 years of age. Ocular apraxia is a reliable diagnostic criterion after 3 years of age. Telangiectasias often are manifested several years after the onset of ataxia; the degree of telangiectasia is quite variable from family to family. Serum α-fetoprotein (AFP) is elevated in 95 percent of patients. Magnetic resonance imaging shows a dystrophic cerebellum. Karyotyping, if successful, reveals characteristic translocations involving chromosomes 14q11-12, 14q32, 7q35, and 7p14. Immunodeficiency and cancer, usually lymphoid, are observed in many A-T patients. Most patients have no measurable ATM (A-T mutated) protein in lysates of their cells or cell lines, while a few have small amounts.

2. Because A-T patients are radiosensitive, conventional doses of radiation therapy are contraindicated. In all young patients with lymphoid malignancies, an underlying diagnosis of A-T should be considered before one calculates doses of radiation or radiomimetic drugs.

3. The incidence of A-T is estimated at 1 per 40,000 live births in the United States. The carrier frequency was estimated at 1 percent; recent molecular studies support this early estimate. In some assays, carriers are indistinguishable from normal individuals. Despite this, female carriers are reported to be at a fivefold increased risk of breast cancer. Carriers may account for 5 percent of all cancer patients in the United States. Carriers are intermediate in their *in vitro* responses to ionizing radiation-induced DNA damage. Whether they are clinically more radiosensitive than normals is not known. Conventional wisdom suggests that exposure of A-T carriers to ionizing radiation should be minimized. However, mammograms are recommended, and the same age-dependent schedule as for noncarriers should be followed. Thus far, attempts to demonstrate an increased frequency of ATM mutations in breast cancer patients have not corroborated earlier epidemiologic observations. Given the lack of convincing data on cancer risks for A-T carriers, it is prudent to advise carriers only that the possibility of an increased cancer risk is still under investigation.

4. The ATM gene and gene product(s) are very large: 3056 amino acids, 350 kDa, a 13-kb transcript (and smaller, alternatively spliced products), and 66 exons that cover 150 kb of genomic DNA. ATM is expressed in all organs tested. ATM belongs to a large-molecular-weight family of protein kinases. Delayed or reduced expression of p53 in radiation-damaged A-T cells suggests that ATM interacts with proteins upstream of p53 in sensing double-strand break DNA damage. The ATM gene product also plays a role in gametogenesis, as part of the synaptonemal complex.

5. Seventy percent of ATM mutations result in a shortened (truncated) protein. These mutations are found over the entire gene and are best detected by mRNA-based techniques that first translate the mRNA to cDNA by RT-PCR before screening for mutations. The favored RT-PCR-based methods are PTT, REF, SSCP, and direct sequencing. Rapid assays that are DNA-based are being developed for the more common mutations, and for mutations that are common to particular ethnic populations, such as the Amish, Moroccan Jews, Sardinians, Italians, British, Costa Ricans, Norwegians, Poles, Turks, Iranians, and Hispanics.

6. Several related syndromes overlap with A-T. Nijmegen Breakage syndrome (NBS) Berlin Breakage syndrome (BBS) share t(7;14) translocations, radiosensitivity, immunodeficiency, and cancer susceptibility with A-T, but these patients do not have ataxia, telangiectasia, or elevated AFP. NBS/BBS patients are microcephalic and mentally retarded and sometimes have syndactyly or anal stenosis. NBS and BBS result from mutations in the same gene, *NBS1*, on chromosome 8q21. AT$_{Fresno}$ combines the A-T and NBS syndromes. AT$_{Fresno}$ patients have ATM mutations. Ninety percent of European NBS/BBS patients carry a 657del5 Slavic mutation. Patients with *hMre11* deficiency share the progressive ataxia, radiosensitivity, and t(7;14) chromosomal aberrations with A-T patients; however they have normal AFP, no telangiectasia, and a milder phenotype.

7. A-T is a very pleiotropic syndrome that stems from the defective functioning of a single gene—Purkinje cells degenerate and migrate abnormally in the cerebellum during prenatal development; the thymus remains embryonic; histology of most organs shows variability in nuclear size, i.e., nucleomegaly; and radiation hypersensitivity. The ATM gene product senses double-stranded DNA breaks, probably by phosphorylating pivotal molecules such as p53; when the ATM protein is defective, the signal to arrest the cell cycle is not given and DNA damage does not get properly repaired before the next replication cycle begins. A-T cells have G1, S, and G2/M checkpoint defects. In addition to phosphorylating p53, the ATM protein phosphorylates IkB-α, to release the transcription factor NFkB. It also interacts with RPA, Chk1, Chk2, Rb, c-abl, ATR, MLH1, and Rad51. Thus, by functioning as a hierarchical protein kinase, the ATM protein acts on both cell-cycle signaling and on the processing of double-strand DNA breaks, whether physiological, as in meiotic recombination and gene rearrangements, or nonphysiological double-strand breaks, as in the DNA damage caused by environmental agents.

8. Therapy for A-T patients remains restricted mainly to supportive care. Free-radical scavengers are recommended, such as vitamin E, α-lipoic acid, and coenzyme Q10. Daily folic acid may minimize chromosome breakage events. Physical therapy is extremely important to avoid debilitating contractures. Patients with frequent severe infections may require intravenous γ-globulin.

Now that the ataxia-telangiectasia (A-T) gene has been isolated, it seems more pertinent than ever to carefully review the changes that occur in the various physiological systems that are affected by

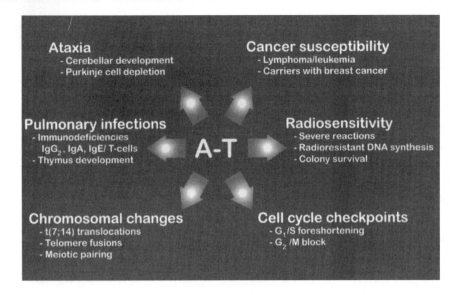

Fig. 15-1 The A-T syndrome.

A-T, trying to relate each facet of the syndrome to the functions of the gene. With the gene in hand, many new and old hypotheses are now testable. While it is clear that the gene functions both in the cytoplasm and in the nucleus, and that elucidating these functions is the present frontier of A-T research, the next frontier will involve translating how mistakes in single cells can misdirect the function and fate of entire cell lineages and result in cerebellar degeneration, thymic dystrophy, and tumor formation.

THE ATAXIA-TELANGIECTASIA SYNDROME

The A-T syndrome varies little from family to family in its late stages.[1-6] Its primary features include (a) progressive gait and truncal ataxia with onset from 1 to 3 years of age; (b) progressively slurred speech; (c) oculomotor apraxia, i.e., an inability to follow an object across the visual fields; (d) oculocutaneous telangiectasia, usually by 6 years of age; (e) elevated serum α-fetoprotein; (f) frequent infections, with accompanying serum and cellular immunodeficiencies; (g) susceptibility to cancer, usually leukemia or lymphoma; (h) hypersensitivity to ionizing radiation, contra-indicating the use of conventional doses of radiation therapy for cancer; and (i) reciprocal translocations that involve chromosomes 7 and 14 almost exclusively. Other features include premature aging and endocrine abnormalities. Fig. 15-1 highlights some of the major features of this complex syndrome.

Neurology and Neuropathology

The most obvious and disabling characteristic of the A-T syndrome is the progressive cerebellar ataxia. Shortly after learning to walk, A-T children begin to stagger. By 10 years of age, they are confined to a wheelchair for the remainder of their lives. The ataxia begins as purely truncal but within several years also involves peripheral coordination. Deep tendon reflexes are decreased or absent in older patients; plantar reflexes are upgoing or absent. Slurred speech and oculomotor apraxia are noted early. Both horizontal and vertical saccadic eye movements are affected. Writing is affected by 7 or 8 years of age. Choreoathetosis is found in almost all these patients. Myoclonic jerking and intention tremors are present in about 25 percent. Drooling is a frequent complaint. All teenage A-T patients need help dressing, eating, washing, and using the toilet. The neurologic status of some patients appears to improve between 3 and 7 years of age, and then begins to progress again; this is probably due to the rapid neurologic learning curve of young individuals. Muscle power is normal at first, but wanes with disuse, especially in the legs. Arm strength generally remains. Contractures in fingers and toes are common in older patients, but may be prevented through rigorous exercise.

The typical patient with A-T is of normal intelligence, although slow responses make it difficult to support this by timed IQ testing. Many American and British patients have finished high school with good grades; some have finished college or university. A few seem to be minimally retarded. Most patients have excellent memories.

The most obvious lesion in the central nervous system at postmortem examination is the paucity of Purkinje cells (PCs) in the cerebellum. About 10 years ago, my laboratory wished to determine whether these cells are absent from birth or degenerate afterward. Knowing that basket cells form only around preexisting PCs, we sought to visualize basket cells by Bielschowsky silver-staining. We showed that normal or nearly normal numbers of basket cells were present (Fig. 29-2). We therefore concluded that PC numbers must also have been normal or near normal at birth and degenerated after birth.[7,8]

We also found evidence suggesting that PC migration and arborization are not completely normal.[8] A significant number of ectopic PCs can be found in cerebellar sections from A-T patients from both undermigration and overmigration (Fig. 15-2). PCs make their last cell division at about 13 weeks of gestation and then begin to migrate toward the pial surface. Following the tracts of climbing fibers, they arrive at the single-cell PC layer during the fifth to seventh month of gestation. Thus, this lesion of ectopic PCs would most likely be expressed by the last trimester of pregnancy. This is the earliest known manifestation of the A-T defect.

It remains possible that PCs are not the primary A-T lesion and that the observed PC defects are due to other factors, such as an absence or abnormalities of supporting cells such as basket cells, mossy fibers, parallel fibers, climbing fibers, or glial cells. The frequent presence of choreoathetosis suggests that the basal ganglia, not the cerebellum, are the primary site of neuropathology in A-T. Anterograde or retrograde degeneration of PCs would then occur, with the underlying lesion being either afferent or efferent to the PCs. Becker-Catania, in our laboratory, was able to demonstrate the presence of ATM message in PCs, as well as in cells of the internal and external granular layers and in neurons of the dentate nucleus. ATM mRNA is seen in both healthy and affected tissues (Fig. 15-2). However, because most mutated ATM proteins would be truncated and unstable, the primary site of pathogenesis in the cerebellum remains unclear. This has important implications when considering where to target gene or cell therapy.

Changes also have been noted in the dentate and olivary nuclei. The medulla shows neuroaxonal dystrophy.[9] Degenerative changes are seen in the substantia nigra. Diffuse demyelination in the

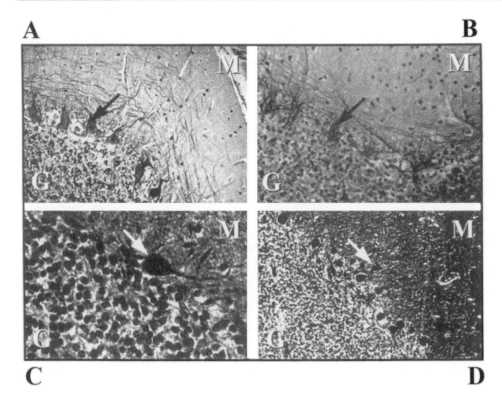

Fig. 15-2 Neuropathology. Photomicrographs of the cerebellum. M—molecular layer; G—granular cell layer. *A,* Bielschovsky stain of normal cerebellum (10×) showing basket cell fibers surrounding Purkinje cells (arrow). *B,* Bielschovsky stain of cerebellum from an A-T patient (10×) showing empty basket cells (arrow) in the Purkinje cell layer. *C, In situ* hybridization with ATM cDNA on normal infant cerebellum (40×) showing a Purkinje cell (arrow) with a positive peroxidase stain for ATM mRNA. *D, In situ* hybridization with ATM cDNA on cerebellum from an A-T patient (20×) showing ectopic (overmigrated) Purkinje cells (arrow) with a positive peroxidase stain for ATM mRNA. (Courtesy of S. Becker-Catania.)

posterior columns of the spinal cord was noted in some of the original autopsies[1] and is a progressive change. For further details of postmortem changes in A-T patients, consult the two lengthy reviews authored by Sedgwick and Boder.[2,5]

Nucleomegaly is a universal finding throughout the organs of A-T patients.[2,5] Nucleomegaly is best seen in organs where nuclear morphology is very regular, such as the hepatic cords and renal tubules. Here it is obvious that the size of the nucleus is extremely variable in A-T tissues, as compared to normal. Some nuclei are very large, hyperchromatic (dark staining), and irregular in shape. Nucleomegaly also is seen in association with normal aging and in viral lesions. Numerous studies, however, have failed to demonstrate virus or viral particles in A-T cells, including Gadjusek's attempt to inoculate primates with brain-tissue extracts from two A-T patients.[5] It is entirely possible that the nucleomegaly seen in A-T tissues results from defective cell-cycle checkpoints that lead to mitotic division without cell replication in random cells. Naeim *et al.*[10] demonstrated polyploidy (4n and 8n) in lymphoblastoid cell lines (LCLs) from A-T patients by flow cytometric cell-cycle analysis.

It was expected that by developing mouse strains in which the *atm* gene was made nonfunctional by one means or another, animal models would become available for dissecting the neuropathology of A-T. Unfortunately, at least five independent *atm* knockouts (atm-/-) have failed to show the severe progressive ataxia seen in A-T patients.[16,169,203,222,223,254,255] This observation limits the application of neuropathology findings in atm-/- mice to patients. Kuljis and Baltimore[254] described changes in the cerebellar cortex when the tissues were examined by electron microscopy. More recently, Borghesani *et al.*[203] described an atmy/y strain that survives beyond 1 year. The mice do not show a progressive ataxia; however, they do show significant changes in Pcs and they manifest motor learning deficits compatible with perturbed cerebellar function. Based on *in vitro* irradiation of yet another atm-/- strain, Herzog *et al.*[256] suggested that inappropriate cell death and apoptosis may underlie the abnormal neurologic development. All of these knockout strains show changes in radiosensitivity, immunologic development, and marked cancer susceptibility.

Telangiectasia

Fig. 15-3 shows a typical pattern of telangiectasia in a 12-year-old patient. Telangiectasias aid in diagnosis. Telangiectasias can be seen on the conjunctiva, as well as on the ears, over the bridge of the nose, in the antecubital fossae, and behind the knees in some patients. Occasional patients have them all over their bodies. Telangiectasias usually do not appear until about 4 to 6 years of age, and although they are a hallmark of the disorder, they sometimes do not become obvious for several years after the onset of ataxia. Elderly individuals without A-T occasionally have similar telangiectasias in many of the same places. Boder felt that telangiectasias appear in response to ultraviolet light exposure; however, that would not explain finding them behind the knee in some patients. About 5 percent of A-T patients never develop prominent telangiectasias. These tend to be patients with milder symptoms. Cafe-au-lait spots are found in almost all A-T patients but are not pathognomonic for just A-T.

Telangiectasias are composed of dilated capillaries. The pattern of these capillaries does not resemble a response to angiogenic factors; instead, it appears to be a response of endothelial cells to a dilatory stimulus. On the other hand, it is still possible that the propensity of A-T patients to develop tumors and form telangiectasias reflects a defective balance between activation of the p53 pathway, apoptosis, angiogenesis, and oxidative stress.[317,325] Van Meir *et al.* have shown that at least one pathway for inhibition of angiogenesis is through p53,[11] and that p53 expression and phosphorylation are reduced in A-T cells (see "Cell-Cycle Aberrations," below). Recent studies of gene

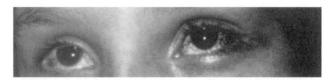

Fig. 15-3 Characteristic telangiectasias over the conjunctiva of a 12-year-old A-T patient.

expression arrays in several laboratories find that unstimulated A-T cells are already in an elevated state of oxidative stress. With rare exceptions,[1,12–15] telangiectasias are not found internally at surgery or at postmortem examination, nor do atm knockout mice manifest internal telangiectasias.[16] Amromin et al.[15] noted widely distributed gliovascular nodules in the cerebral white matter and, to a lesser extent, in the brain stem and spinal cord postmortem in a 32-year-old patient. These nodules consisted of dilated capillary loops, many with fibrin thrombi, with perivascular hemorrhages and hemosiderosis, surrounded by demyelinated white matter, reactive gliosis, and numerous atypical astrocytes. These nodules were not seen in the cerebellum and have not been observed in other postmortem examinations of younger patients.

Telangiectasia occasionally develop within the fields of prior radiation therapy, not only in A-T patients or carriers, but in apparently normal persons as well.[289] Telangiectasia are sometimes observed in the parents and sibs of A-T patients and may be a subtle manifestation of heterozygosity and radiosensitivity.

Radiosensitivity *In Vivo* and *In Vitro*

Over the past 30 years, radiation therapists have observed that when A-T patients with cancer are treated with conventional doses of ionizing radiation, they develop life-threatening sequelae characteristic of much higher doses.[17–21] This radiosensitivity can also be demonstrated *in vitro* using fibroblasts or lymphoblasts from A-T homozygotes, which are sensitive to ionizing radiation and to a variety of radiomimetic and free-radical-producing agents.[22,23,111] (Also see the discussion of colony survival assay under "Differential Diagnosis" below.)

Early radiosensitivity assays for A-T measured colony formation efficiency of fibroblasts. Cells are irradiated and then cultured, and the number of colonies that grow are scored after a measured period of incubation. Fibroblasts from A-T heterozygotes form colonies with an efficiency that is intermediate between A-T homozygosity and normal;[22] the same observation can be made using neocarzinostatin.[24] Despite this, colony-forming efficiency is not a reliable way to detect individual heterozygotes.[23–26] Many other methods have been tried to identify A-T heterozygotes, but none are reliable because the normal and heterozygous data sets overlap.[10,27–31] Recently, a "comet" assay has been described for identifying ATM heterozygotes by measuring DNA repair in peripheral blood lymphocytes (BPL) following 3 Gy of irradiation.[315.]

Now that genetic testing in families with prior affected patients can identify A-T heterozygotes (carriers) more easily, physicians are confronted with the dilemma of having to advise carriers about the risks of radiation exposure. Unfortunately, there are as yet no clinical studies on which to base such advice. For example, data are lacking on whether the *in vitro* radiosensitivity of heterozygotes has any clinical correlate; i.e., unusual reactions to standard radiologic procedures or increased cancer risk. One can only make the general recommendation that exposure to all types of ionizing radiation be minimized in persons suspected of being A-T carriers, e.g., both parents, remembering as well that two-thirds of the sibs of A-T patients are likely to be carriers. Whether routine dental x-rays should be recommended in A-T patients is also an unresolved issue.

ATM knockout mice that are heterozygous (atm +/−) do not show an abnormal response to total-body irradiation.[16] Some caveats: (a) Only one specific site in the ATM gene was disrupted in each of the knockout mice strains, and (b) knockout mouse models seldom mimic a human disease in all facets of the syndrome. Swift's epidemiologic data suggest that exposure of heterozygotes to myelograms and other diagnostic x-rays may increase their cancer risk.[32] There is also cause for concern about mammograms in female A-T carriers, who appear to be at an increased risk of breast cancer (see below). The recommendation at this writing is that mammograms be continued on the same age-dependent schedule used for noncarriers but that the most up-to-date mammography machines be employed to minimize exposure

to only a few rads. The added risk of cancer to such women is only slightly increased (from 1.5 in 100 from annual mammography screening doses in noncarriers to perhaps 2 in 100 in A-T carriers), and this should be compared to a 1 in 9 natural lifetime risk and the 30 percent reduction in mortality from annual mammography screening in women over age 40.[33–35]

Epidemiologic and radiosensitivity studies of A-T family members further suggest that many cancer patients may be receiving the wrong doses of radiotherapy—too much for A-T heterozygotes and too little for noncarriers.[33,34,36] Considering that 5 percent of cancer patients under 46 years of age may be A-T carriers and intermediate in their radiosensitivity,[37] this issue could involve many thousands of patients annually (see "Cancer Susceptibility," below). Some x-ray dosage regimens were first tested empirically on cadres of cancer patients, and if those cadres were to have contained up to 5 percent A-T carriers, one can easily imagine how radiation sequelae might be more apt to appear in the A-T carriers, thereby lowering the "safe" doses defined for everyone else. Once A-T carrier testing can be implemented on a wide scale, these issues may be resolved.

Although radiation damage to DNA has been used for many years as a laboratory tool for characterizing the phenotype of A-T cells, it should be remembered that A-T cells normally are not exposed to irradiation *in vivo*. Thus, the radiosensitivity of A-T cells is largely a laboratory artifact because irradiation damage mimics double-strand DNA breaks and tests the cells' abilities to rejoin these breaks in an orderly fashion. Because the complex A-T syndrome develops quite uniformly in most affected patients, the major substrate for ATM protein must be a naturally-occurring molecule(s) generated by an equally common event that causes double-strand DNA breaks. p53 is a good candidate for the major substrate,[198,199] while oxidative stress and the normal production of DNA-damaging free-radical products of metabolism are good candidates for the commonly-recurring and inciting event.[38,328,329] Although many attempts have been made to demonstrate defective DNA repair in A-T cells, this has not been convincingly defined.[39] Recent observations suggest that it is the *inability* to sense this damage that is defective in A-T cells, not the actual mechanisms of repair.[38,40]

When DNA synthesis of irradiated fibroblasts is measured, A-T homozygotes show a characteristic dose-response curve (Fig. 29-4) that is diagnostic of the disease.[82] This phenomenon is called radioresistant DNA synthesis (RDS) because, unlike normal cells which temporarily halt the synthesis of new DNA after irradiation damage, A-T cells simply continue into S phase of the cell cycle. Later experiments that attempted to complement RDS and other radiomimetic features of A-T cells by transfection found, however, that these phenomena often were dissociated.[6,83] Thus, RDS most likely reflects a cell-cycle checkpoint failure at S phase that is independent of other radiosensitivity phenotypes of A-T cells. Using RDS, heterozygous cells cannot be distinguished from normals.

The shape of the RDS curve (Fig. 15-4) for A-T cells has been insightfully interpreted by Painter[85,86] as having two components, one reflecting replicon initiation and the other reflecting chain elongation. The slope of the curve above 20 Gy determines the second component, and this slope does not differ in normal and A-T fibroblasts. The early component, however, is essentially missing from the A-T curves, suggesting that replicon initiation is quite abnormal. Painter further suggested that while in unirradiated normal cells initiation occurs synchronously at the origins of a cluster of replicons, and that in irradiated normal cells damage to one replicon inhibits the entire cluster, in irradiated A-T cells damage to one replicon inhibits only that replicon; i.e., the damage is not sensed or translated to the rest of the cluster, and chain elongation near the growing forks is not curbed. Thus, radiation to A-T cells blocks initiation of individual replicons rather than blocking the initiation of clusters of replicons.[39,85,86] Hand and Gautschi[87] provided evidence that one single-strand break may inactivate the initiation of as many as 100 replicons.

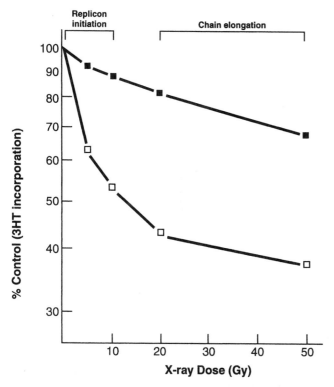

Fig. 15-4 Graph of radioresistant DNA synthesis (RDS) depicting theoretical targets of radiation at increasing doses of radiation. The major defect in A-T (black squares) is seen at very low radiation doses, affecting replicon initiation, while chain elongation appears normal in A-T, as depicted by the normal slope of that portion of the curve.

Although Painter's interpretation of the RDS curve was put forth over 10 years ago, it remains a very attractive hypothesis for explaining one facet of the pathogenesis of A-T. Atomic force microscopy analyses suggest that ATM protein can exist either as a monomer or as a tetramer in the repair of double-strand DNA breaks.[134,200–202,318]

Cancer Susceptibility

During their shortened lifetimes, 38 percent of A-T homozygotes develop a malignancy.[41] This represents a 61- and a 184-fold increase in European-American and African-American patients, respectively. Roughly 85 percent of these malignancies are either leukemia or lymphoma. In younger patients, an acute lymphocytic leukemia is most often of T-cell origin,[42,43] although the pre-B origin common to ALL of childhood (HLADR1, CD101, CD51, and CD191) has also been seen in A-T patients. When leukemia develops in older A-T homozygotes, it is usually an aggressive T-cell leukemia with a morphology similar to that of chronic lymphoblastic leukemia, hence the old name T-CLL;[42–45] T-cell prolymphocytic leukemia (T-PLL) is the equivalent modern nomenclature.[45,46] The leukemic cells often contain a translocation and/or inversion involving the T-cell receptor α-chain gene complex at 14q11-12[47–49] (see discussion of non-leukemic clonal expansions in A-T patients under "Chromosomal Instability," below). Myeloid leukemia is very uncommon in A-T patients. Lymphomas in A-T homozygotes, in contrast to leukemias, are common and are usually B-cell types, although T-cell lymphomas also have been observed. As A-T patients are living longer, more nonlymphoid cancers are being observed. Several of our older patients have developed breast cancer and melanoma. Cancers of the stomach and ovary have been reported.[5,42] When fibroids or leiomyomas are found in A-T females, a special effort should be made by the pathologist to quantitate high-power fields for mitotic

figures, because leiomyosarcomas of precocious onset have been reported.[50] For specific lists of other tumor types and frequencies, see references 41, 42, and 44.

A-T heterozygotes are also believed to be cancer-prone.[37] They are not clinically distinguishable from normal individuals. An increased incidence of breast cancer in female A-T heterozygotes has been reported in the United States, England, and Norway.[32,51–53] In the U.S. study, the risk of breast cancer was found to be fivefold higher among the mothers of A-T homozygotes than in a comparable female population.[32,52] Based on this observation, Swift *et al.* estimated that between 8 and 18 percent of all breast cancer patients may be A-T heterozygotes.[37] This would imply that ATM is the most common cancer susceptibility gene in the general population. While the issue is far from settled, many recent genetic studies of breast cancer cohorts have failed to find an increased frequency of mutations in the ATM gene,[54,55,257,258,306,331] with the exceptions of a report of an allelic variant at the ATM locus being associated through a rare HRAS1 allele in a stratified study of 66 sib pairs affected with breast cancer[260] and recent findings by Teraoka *et al.*[305] of 11 ATM mutations in 142 breast cancer patients versus only 1 in 81 controls. They used primarily denaturing high-power liquid chromatography (dHPLC); all mutations detected were of the missense type. Vorechovsky *et al.*[54] looked for ATM mutations in tumor tissue from 38 sporadic breast cancers. They first screened this material by single-stranded conformational polymorphism (SSCP) gels, and then sequenced any regions suspected of harboring mutations. They found no significant mutations. Spurr and coworkers[56] looked for a linkage to BRCA1 and BRCA2 in 63 early onset breast cancer families; 55 percent linked to BRCA1 and 45 percent linked to BRCA2. This implied that none linked to 11q22-23, as Wooster *et al.*[58] and Cortessis *et al.*[57] had reported earlier. However, because the epidemiologic data from A-T families suggested that the breast cancer seen among A-T mothers (who are obligate heterozygotes) peaks in the age group of 45 to 54,[52] and is not an early onset pattern, other studies have screened late-onset or sporadic breast cancers for ATM mutations. Using PTT, FitzGerald *et al.*[55] detected ATM mutations in 2 of 401 women with sporadic early onset breast cancer. They also found mutations in 2 of 202 control samples. Recently, Swift and coworkers[59] again noted an increased incidence of breast cancer in A-T heterozygotes who were identified by haplotyping members of extended A-T families.

The apparent paradox of (a) not finding many ATM mutations in breast cancer cohorts and (b) not finding A-T patients in the families of breast cancer patients with ATM mutations may be explained by the hypothesis that two types of A-T carriers may exist within the general population, those with nonsense (truncating) mutations and those with missense mutations, and each type of mutation may have a different Phenotype—both in the heterozygous and in the homozygous state. Heterozygous missense mutations might create a dominant negative situation,[330] whereby the defective copy of the ATM protein *binds* to substrates but cannot *phosphorylate* them, or vice versa. This would create a far more serious situation than a nonsense mutation that would not produce *any* stable defective protein. Most A-T patients have two truncating mutations. Homozygous missense mutations are extremely uncommon in A-T patients and some could even be lethal. Thus, it is possible that ATM missense carriers are more likely to be cancer prone than ATM nonsense carriers. (This hypothesis is developed further in reference 306.)

Several independent studies of ATM knockout mice have confirmed the extreme cancer susceptibility of atm−/− homozygotes; all atm−/− strains develop massive, widely metastasized malignant thymic lymphomas.[16,169,203,222,223,254,255] Heterozygous animals have not shown tumors, nor has breast cancer been observed in either homozygous or heterozygous animals.

Carter *et al.* reported significant loss of heterozygosity in sporadic breast cancers across chromosome 11q22-23[60] as did others.[267–270,297,298] Although this region includes the ATM gene (at 11q22.3-23.1) and the CHK1 gene (at 11q23.3),[271] it measures 35 cM and probably includes more than 1000 other genes as well. Thus, the contribution of ATM mutations to familial breast cancer appears to be low, with ATM perhaps playing a more important role in a sporadic, low-penetrance form of breast cancer.

The most frequently reported cancers in American A-T heterozygotes are breast, trachea/bronchus/lung, stomach, prostate, melanoma, and gallbladder.[32] In Italy and Costa Rica, gastric cancer has been especially noteworthy. Among 64 A-T parents and grandparents in Costa Rica, half of the 12 cancers reported were gastric cancer.[61] (Costa Rica ranks among the top three countries in the world for stomach cancer in the general population, making it difficult to interpret these observations.) In Italian families, 7 of 20 cancers in grandparents were gastric cancer.[62] Stomach cancer has been reported in homozygotes as well,[42,44] including two families in which both affected sibs developed stomach cancer. Despite this, Morrell et al.[41] did not note any increase in stomach cancers in A-T homozygotes.

Other recent observations move the cancer susceptibility association with A-T in new directions. Most individuals who develop T-PLL have ATM mutations in one or both alleles. While it was first thought that these patients represented constitutional A-T heterozygotes, the data are lacking to establish this.[259] Thus, these patients may be at no increased prior risk of cancer but simply develop an ATM mutation somatically. The ATM mutations found in T-PLL cells are mainly missense mutations,[84] unlike the predominantly nonsense mutations found in A-T patients[237]. However, if A-T heterozygotes acquire T-PLL by a second "hit"[84,129] on the ATM gene, this would then suggest that ATM can function as a tumor-suppressor gene, in addition to its growing list of other roles.[264]

Four reports link loss of ATM integrity to an aggressive subgroup of B-cell chronic lymphocytic leukemia (B-CLL) patients.[301-304] Approximately 40 percent of B-CLL patients have 11q deletions or fail to express ATM protein. Here again, where ATM mutations have been identified, they have been mainly missense types. Unfortunately, missense mutations are still very difficult to detect in such a large gene (see below).

A gain of chromosome 3q is present in many cancers, including cervical carcinomas, small cell lung carcinomas, head and neck squamous cell carcinomas, and embryonal rhabdomyosarcomas.[261] When microcell hybrids were transferred into a differentiation-competent myoblast cell line C2C12, the cells exhibited a nondifferentiating phenotype.[262] Selecting 3q candidate genes, ATR (AT- and rad3-related/FRAP-related protein 1) was tested. ATR is a protein kinase with strong homology to ATM.[71,72,233] It was found that forced expression of ATR resulted in a phenocopy of the 3q-containing microcell hybrids. ATR apparently inhibits MyoD, which is a marker for classifying sarcomas as rhabdosarcomas. ATR is thought to share functional overlap with ATM in cell-cycle progression[139,263] and may be phosphorylated by ATM. Like ATM, ATR phosphorylates the Serine 15 position on p53, albeit at a much-reduced level and at a slower rate.[199] Furthermore, overexpression of ATR corrects the defective radiation-induced S-phase checkpoint in A-T cells.[263] (ATR's relationship to ATM is further described in "Chromosomal Instability" below).

Cell-Cycle Aberrations

Important checkpoints monitor the progress of the cell cycle and prevent mutagenic damage to DNA from becoming fixed into future cell generations. The G1 checkpoint prevents replication of a damaged DNA template; the G2 checkpoint prevents segregation of damaged chromosomes.[64] Kastan et al.[65,66] showed that A-T cells have a delayed radiation-induced increase in p53, compared to normal cells. p53, dubbed the "guardian of the genome," acts to suppress normal cell-cycle progression at G1 until DNA repairs have been completed. (For reviews pertinent to p53 in A-T cells, see references 38, 40, and 67.) It accomplishes this by binding DNA at sequence-specific sites, thereby transcriptionally activating a signal-transduction cascade. In so doing, p53 functions as a

tumor suppressor. Cells from p53 knockout mice, lacking both normal alleles of p53 (p53−/−), fail to observe the G1 checkpoint; they do not experience G1 arrest after irradiation nor do they show neurologic abnormalities, immune defects, or problems with sterility,[40,67,68] as in A-T. The strong association of multiple types of cancer with p53 deficiency[67,74-77] further suggests that involvement of this pathway in apoptosis and in differentiation may help explain the increased frequency of cancer in A-T.

Interestingly, p53−/− mutants are not radiosensitive.[76,78] Thus, yet another mechanism must account for the radiosensitivity of A-T cells. Much work still needs to be done before the role of ATM proteins in intracellular signaling can be fully appreciated. For example, despite much evidence of the inefficiency of G1/S, S, and G2/M checkpoints in A-T cells, holding A-T cells in G0 for up to 7 days does not improve their postirradiation survival,[40] which suggests that even these checkpoint defects may not be the crucial common denominator underlying A-T pathogenesis. Evidence presented by Jung and et al.[79,80] using SV40-transformed fibroblasts, implicates the NF-kB and IkB-α proteins in ATM function; the ATM protein appears to phosphorylate IkB-α, thereby activating the transcription factor NF-kB.[81] These findings would also support observations of increased radiation-induced apoptosis in cell lines derived from A-T patients.[40,76,77] However, a recent report by Ashburner et al.[324] suggests that the constitutive activation of NFκB reported by Jung et al. may be due more to SV40-transformation than to the A-T phenotype. The phosphorylation of replication factor A (RPA) is also delayed in A-T cells after irradiation.[69,265] Three groups have independently shown that the Serine-15 position of p53 is selectively phosphorylated by ATM.[198,199,300] Further, Shafman et al.[70] have reported that c-abl binds to an SH3 domain on the ATM molecule.

Immunodeficiency

At postmortem examination, virtually every A-T homozygote has a small embryonic-like thymus.[12] In the late 1960s, and again in the early 1980s, many attempts were made to characterize the immunodeficiencies of A-T patients.[88] No single, consistent abnormality could be identified in all A-T patients; affected sibs often differ in the degree and profile of their immunodeficiencies. In a review of British patients, Woods and Taylor[89] noted normal immunologic function in 27 of 70 patients. Only 10 percent had severe immunodeficiencies.

When the genomic order of the IGH V, D, J, and H gene subfamilies was first described, we noted that the immunoglobulin (Ig) classes that were most frequently decreased in A-T patients were those with the greatest genomic distances between the variable (V) genes and the respective heavy-chain genes;[90] 60 to 80 percent of A-T homozygotes manifest an IgA, IgE, and/or IgG2 deficiency,[12,88,89-95,121,122] whereas serum levels of IgM, IgG1, and IgG3 are usually normal. This suggests that B cells from these patients have a maturational problem with Ig class switching, perhaps based on a recombinase-related deficiency. On a similar note, an increased proportion of T gamma/delta cells noted in one early study suggested a maturational delay in T cells; however, this was before normal T gamma/delta cell ranges had been clearly defined and has not been generally confirmed. IgM levels are occasionally extremely high (see below), which could be based on a similar defective maturational mechanism that arrests some B cells at the IgM-producing stage. However, when V(D)J recombination was examined in A-T cells, both signal and coding joint formation were normal.[96-98] Approximately half of A-T patients with immunodeficiencies have T-cell deficiencies. CD41/CD45RA1 (naive) T cells are decreased in some patients.[99] Responses to antigens are poor, especially allogeneic antigens.[12,88,100-105] T-cell cytotoxicity to influenza-infected target cells is reduced.[106] T lymphocytes show abnormally fast capping of FITC-labeled concanavalin A.[88] Markedly elevated cyclic AMP levels have been observed in T cells from A-T patients.[88] Neutrophil chemotaxis was reported to be decreased in some studies and normal in others. Similarly, NK cell activity and NK cell levels have been described as normal, decreased, or increased in various studies.[88,107,108,266] Some of these discrepancies no doubt reflect the transient immune status of patients with active infections. Although 91 percent of Costa Rican A-T patients had diminished PHA responses, 65 percent of them had the same mutation; thus, this sample would be skewed against some features and would favor others, and probably has only minimal bearing on patients around the world with other mutations. Further immunologic analyses of this cohort are under way. Knockout ATM mice have many of these same immune defects as A-T patients; T and B cell precursors in thymus and bone marrow, respectively, are present in normal numbers.[169]

Sanal *et al.*[275] have recently described a new form of immunodeficiency in A-T patients. IgG antibody responses to pneumococcal polysaccharide vaccine (serotypes 3, 6A, 7F, 14, 19F, and 23F) were studied in 29 classic A-T patients; in 22 patients (76 percent), no responses were observed. The remaining patients had responses to 1, 2, or 4 serotypes. Zeilin *et al.*[327] support this finding.

Hyper-IgM with Ataxia-Telangiectasia

Elevated serum IgM levels are fairly common in A-T patients,[100,277] arising perhaps as compensation for low IgA, IgE, and IgG2 levels. However, occasional A-T patients with classic symptoms have an extended syndrome that may include very high serum IgM levels, splenomegaly, lymphoadenopathy, neutropenia, thrombocytopenia, hypertension, renal anomalies, and congestive heart failure from high blood viscosity.[109,110] The latter symptoms were somewhat ameliorated by reducing blood volume, and further by splenomegaly. Steroids markedly improved three patients (unpublished, personal experience). The postirradiation colony survival assay (CSA)[111] in six of these families, although not easily quantifiable, suggests a level of radiosensitivity that is intermediate between that seen in normals and that seen in other A-T patients (see "Differential Diagnosis," below). In three families, ATM mutations have already been identified. It is of interest that in three families, the affected sibs were discordant for hyper-IgM.[278–280] Another patient was atypical in that depletion of cerebellar Purkinje cells was not seen, and ATM protein levels were normal.[109] In an Argentine family, the hyper-IgM followed treatment of the immunodeficiency with IVIg.[281] Thus, while hyper-IgM and A-T have been observed together in a number of families, the underlying pathology remains obscure and the observation of discordant sibs in three families suggests that the hyper-IgM represents a somatic, not a genetic, variation. Recently, Rosenblatt *et al.*[296] have provided some evidence that this hyper-IgM may be due to an up-regulation of the CD40 ligand gene.

α-Fetoprotein

Although elevated serum α-fetoprotein (AFP) levels can be very useful in confirming a suspected diagnosis of A-T, 5 to 10 percent of typical A-T patients have normal AFP levels. This is independent of race, sex, or complementation group, and is usually concordant in affected sibs. AFP levels do not increase with patient age.[89] Serum AFP levels still elevated from infancy sometimes can be misleading in children under 2 years of age in whom normal ranges have not been carefully defined by most clinical laboratories. Thus, it is best to avoid using AFP as a diagnostic criterion until after 2 years of age. Other causes of elevated AFP, such as liver disease, familial hyper-AFP[309,310] and the presence of a teratoma, are not likely to confound a diagnosis of A-T. Ishiguro *et al.*[115] showed that the lectin-binding profile of elevated AFPs from A-T patients was most likely of hepatic origin, and although no evidence of liver disease is present at postmortem examination, other liver proteins, such as serum glutamic-pyruvic transaminase (SGPT), serum glutamic-oxalacetic transaminase (SGOT), alkaline phosphatase, and carcinoembryonic antigen, are often increased as well.[90,112]

AFP is thought to have a suppressor effect on the developing immune system and on immune function.[112–114,311,312] The mechanisms by which AFP is elevated in sera of most A-T patients remains unclear but may involve the NFκB/IκBα complex and/or p53, both of which are phosphorylated by ATM.[79,80,98,199,300,313]

With the routine monitoring of AFP in amniotic fluid now in vogue, the question is occasionally asked whether amniotic AFP levels are elevated when the fetus has A-T. AFP levels are very high in all fetuses, peaking at about 13 weeks of gestation.[112] In two cases who had been diagnosed by prenatal testing, and in which a decision had been made by the parents not to terminate the pregnancies, amniotic AFP levels were measured and were within normal ranges. A cord blood AFP was elevated in one of these patients, and remained so over the next 3 years. (In the other patient, cord blood was not tested.) Thus, although the serum AFP level of a fetus is high, there appears to be no extravasation or secretion into the amniotic fluid of A-T-affected fetuses, as occurs in open neural tube defects and Down syndrome.

Chromosomal Instability

A-T homozygotes show nonrandom chromosomal aberrations in lymphocytes, such as translocations and inversions, which preferentially involve chromosomal breakpoints at 14q11, 14q32, 7q35, 7p14, 2p11, and 22q11.[43,117] These aberrations appeared to correlate generally with the regions of the T-cell receptor (TCR-α, β, and γ) and B-cell receptor (IGH, IGK, and IGL) gene complexes. Because these six sites contain the only gene complexes in the genome that are presently known to require site-specific gene rearrangement/recombination before expressing a mature protein, it was logical to examine V(D)J recombination mechanisms in A-T cells. As was noted above, signal and coding joint formation are both normal.[96–98] When we examined the chromosomes of fibroblasts from eight A-T homozygotes, all with typical 7:14 translocations in their lymphocytes, the fibroblast aberrations were totally random.[117,118] Hecht and Hecht studied almost 50,000 amniotic fluid cell metaphases; of 37 translocations in that non-A-T sample, none involved chromosomes 7 and 14.[119] This is intriguing when one considers that, like lymphocytes and lymphoblasts, fibroblasts and amniotic cells express the radiosensitivity defect, suggesting that the radiosensitivity is intrinsic to A-T cells, whereas the chromosome aberrations are secondary to chromosome movement and telomere clustering in the nucleus.[134] Heterozygotes show t(7;14) translocations in lymphocytes, but only in 1 to 2 percent of metaphases.[119]

In some patients, cell clones with the above breakpoints expand,[45,120] sometimes accounting for 100 percent of the lymphocytes that are karyotyped. Despite this, lymphocyte counts remain within the normal range for years thereafter. Some of these clones have been followed for 10 to 20 years by us and others.[48,118] These clones tend to evolve, with subclones adding new rearrangements, such as inv(14;14)(q11;q32), i(8q), and 6q-, in addition to many other smaller clones. Eventually, most such patients develop T-PLL, previously referred to as T-CLL (T-cell chronic lymphoblastic leukemia).[45,46] Affected sibs usually are not concordant for developing such clones, thus again implicating somatic influences superimposed on an A-T genotype.

These clonal expansions have allowed the breakpoint sites to be analyzed by molecular techniques. Three types of patients have been studied: (a) A-T patients with nonleukemic clones, (b) A-T patients with leukemic clones, and (c) non-A-T patients with similar cytogenetic translocations and T-PLL. Thanks to many years of perseverance by Taylor and coworkers[124] in trying to pinpoint the breakpoints of these translocations or inversions, a fascinating story is now emerging that is quite similar to that of myc in Burkitt lymphoma. The A-T expanded clones always juxtapose one of the TCR genes, usually TCRα, with another family of genes located proximal to, but not actually within, the B-cell receptor-gene complexes. The most common and best-studied translocations are those involving 14q11 (TCRα) and a breakpoint cluster region 10 Mb proximal to the IGH locus at 14q32. Within

400 kb, at least 8 such breakpoints have been identified in A-T patients with and without leukemia, and in several non-A-T patients with T-PLL. This region centers on the TCL-1 (T-cell leukemia-1) gene,[123] the 1.3-kb transcript of which is preferentially expressed in immature (and leukemic) B and T cells. Circulating mature T cells do not express this gene. Leukemia cells without the t(14;14) or inv(14;14) clones typically do not express TCL-1.[223]

An occasional A-T patient has a large t(X;14)(q28;q11) clone, including at least two that have developed T-CLL/T-PLL and one without leukemia when last studied.[45] The breakpoints at Xq28 cluster to within a few kilobases in a region of 70 kb proximal to the factor VIII gene. This region contains the genes c6.1A and c6.1B. (The latter gene is believed to be the crucial one in these translocations, because two of the breakpoints fall within the first exon of c6.1B, also known as MTCP1, "mature T-cell proliferation-1."[124–126]) Most interesting, c6.1B has homology with TCL-1 (40 percent identity, 60 percent similarity) and is a mitochondrial protein.[127] TCL-1 and MTCP-1 also share three-dimensional structure. TCL-1 prevents apoptosis and is p53-independent. Because TCRα/TCL-1 translocations do not by themselves cause leukemia, another factor must interact with the protein product or products that result from the translocations. Based on the recent finding that most non-AT patients with T-PLL have ATM mutations in one or both alleles, the ATM protein is a likely candidate for this role.[84] Despite this, leukemia cells from an occasional A-T/T-PLL patient do not show abnormal TCL-1 expression, suggesting that yet other genes are involved in this pathway from clonal expansion to leukemia.

Inherited cytogenetic defects involving translocations or deletions at 11q22-23 have not been observed in A-T homozygotes, even though karyotypes of >500 patients have been examined worldwide. Many cytogenetic reports on children with suspected A-T return with the statement "insufficient metaphases for analysis." This problem occurs because the necessary lymphocyte response to mitogens, such as phytohemagglutinin (PHA), is often weak or delayed in A-T patients, and when cell cultures are harvested routinely at 48 h, few cells are dividing. Harvest results can be improved by using a double-dose of mitogen and harvesting at 72 h or at several time points.

Telomeric fusions are observed frequently in A-T patients, which is a provocative finding considering the strong homology between ATM and the yeast Tel-1 mutant gene.[71] Tumor cells and senescent cells of normal persons can also show such fusions.[133] Pandita et al.[130] showed that although the telomeres of A-T cell lines are shorter than normal cells, telomerase activity was normal. Metcalfe et al.[135] demonstrated significant telomere shortening in A-T peripheral blood lymphocytes (PBLs). PBLs from 20 A-T patients showed an average loss of 95 ± 23 bp (base pairs) per year of age, compared to a loss of 35 ± 9 bp per year in normals. The preleukemic T-cell clones described above showed an even greater loss of 158 ± 9 bp per year and are especially prone to show telomeric fusions. Recently, as the biochemistry of telomere maintenance is being unravelled,[134] it appears that the Ku70/85 heterodimeric complex is physically bound to telomeres in yeast. Ku protects telomeres from nucleases and recombinases. Cells without Ku do not repair double-strand breaks or perform gene rearrangements for T or B cell maturation; Ku-deficient mutants display telomere shortening. In mammalian cells, Ku is the DNA-binding subunit of a large enzyme, DNA-dependent protein kinase (DNA-PK$_{cs}$), which is a member of the large-molecular-weight protein kinase family that also includes ATM.[71,72] The Ku complex interacts with the Rad50/Mre11/Xrs2/Brca1 complex for nonhomologous end-joining.[134] Xrs2 (yeast) was recently identified as the human Nijmegen Breakage syndrome protein, nibrin[201,202] (See discussion of "Related Syndromes" below.) The Rad50/Mre11/NBS1 complex, together with Ku and Brca1, is required for the telomerase pathway of end maintenance. The Rad50/Mre11/NBS1/Brca1 complex may be the exonuclease that provides the single-strand substrate required for telomerase

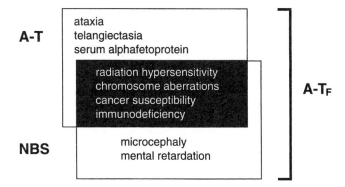

Fig. 15-5 Overlapping A-T and NBS syndromes combine to form the AT$_{Fresno}$ syndrome.

activity. ATM interacts with the Rad50/Mre11/NBS1/Brca1 complex by phosphorylating both Brca1[299] and nibrin.[307] This would explain the overlap of symptoms between A-T and NBS (Fig. 15-5). Patients lacking hMre 11 protein have recently been described and closely resemble A-T patients in that they manifest progressive ataxia, t(7;14) translocations, and radiosensitivity. ATM protein expression is normal; nibrin and Rad50 expression are diminished.[308]

Accelerated telomeric shortening is probably a characteristic of all rapidly dividing A-T cells. It is of further interest that telomeric shortening is associated with senescence of CD282/CD81 T cells in AIDS patients and centenarians.[136] In both situations, this may account for waning T-cell immunity. A similar mechanism might explain the abnormal development and function of the immune system in A-T patients. Thus, the precocious onset of cancers such as basal cell carcinoma,[2] leiomyosarcoma,[50] and T-PLL[124] may reflect the basic propensity of their cells to accelerate telomere shortening and a waning immunity due not so much to poor V(D)J joining but to telomere shortening and senescence. This would also provide a p53-independent, radiation-independent pathway to cancer susceptibility in A-T patients.

When the ATM gene was isolated and sequenced, it was noted to have its strongest homology to the yeast tel1 gene, primarily through sharing a region of PI-3 kinase homology, and secondarily through sharing weak homology with rad3.[137–141] (Reference 141 contains a comprehensive analysis of homologies between kinase, rad3, RH3, and FRB domains.) Absence of tel1 results in telomere shortening. Rad3 is a fission yeast gene containing helicase motifs that is required for G2 arrest after DNA damage.[142,143] Of the large family of genes sharing PI-3 kinase homology with ATM, only tel1, mec1 (another yeast gene), and mei41 (of *Drosophila*) also share some rad3 homology. (The rad3 homology of tel1 is admittedly weak.) A growing body of evidence suggests that tel1, mec1, and ATM perform overlapping functions. Of the three, only mec1 is an essential gene. In yeast, mec1 (mitosis entry checkpoint) is required for regulation of the S/M and G2/M checkpoints,[144] the rate of ongoing S phase in response to damage,[145] and meiotic recombination.[145,146] Cells with mutations in mec1 (also called ESR1 or SAD3) proceed directly to mitosis when DNA replication is inhibited with hydroxyurea and are unable to delay the onset of mitosis (G2/M) on induction of DNA damage.[147] Rad53 is also regulated by MEC1 and Tel1.[147] Although tel1 mutants are not radiosensitive and mec1 mutants are, tel1/mec1 double-mutants somehow synergize to increase the sensitivity to DNA damage from ionizing radiation and radiomimetic drugs.[141] The human homologue of mec1, called ATR (AT-related Rad3-related) or FRP1 (FRAP-related protein), was recently cloned and maps to chromosome 3q22-q24.[141,148] It plays a reciprocal role to ATM on synapsing chromosomes during meiotic recombination,[139] localizing to the nonsynapsed portion of the chromosomes and interacting with Rad51 and BRCA1. RPA and chk1 also colocalize with ATR on late pachynema chromosomes.[271,272] RPA binds to single-stranded DNA, and probably facilitates formation of recombination intermediates.[273,274] (ATR is also discussed under "Cancer Susceptibility" above.)

Complementation Groups

Fusion of fibroblasts from unrelated patients will often correct or "complement" their radiosensitivity, as measured by RDS.[149–151,204] Five complementation groups have been defined (Groups A, C, D, E, and V1).[151] The first four groups are phenotypically identical and can be distinguished from one another only by complementation studies. It was unclear whether these complementation groups represented several distinct A-T genes, perhaps forming part of a common enzymatic pathway or coding for parts of a common multimeric molecule, or, alternatively, whether the complementation groups represented intragenic mutations of a single gene. It was also possible that complementation was a nongenetic phenomenon. In 1988, we localized the gene for A-T Group A (ATA) to chromosome 11q22-23.[152] In 1991, in a collaboration with Shiloh's lab, A-T Group C (ATC) was localized to the same region, also by linkage analysis.[153] Between 1990 and 1994, 26 genes were shown to complement A-T fibroblasts; none were localized to chromosome 11q23.1.[6,40,154,155] No convincing evidence for genetic heterogeneity was ever found in the linkage analysis studies despite such expectations. In 1995, when Savitsky et al.[72] identified part of a single gene (ATM), mutations were found for all four major complementation groups. Most interesting is that one homozygous mutation is present in both a Group C patient and a Group E patient, suggesting either that complementation groups in A-T are somewhat artifactual or that assigning patients to complementation groups is somewhat error-prone. To date, no laboratory has confirmed whether the cells from these two patients complement each other. Most likely this reflects that complementation group assignment by fusion of A-T fibroblasts is extremely tedious and that no laboratory has performed such studies since around 1990. Varying chromosomal ploidy between fused (4N) and nonfused (2N) cells also may have accounted for what appeared to be "complementation".

Complementation of A-T cells by gene transfections was a commonly used approach to cloning the gene. Many genes complemented various facets of the radiophenotype. These complementing genes presumably interact in some way with the ATM gene, the protein, or the signal transduction pathway. Some may bypass the ATM block in A-T cells, and they might provide exciting therapeutic opportunities for replacement therapy in A-T patients.[156] Despite the lack of success in cloning the A-T gene by complementation analyses, and the existing confusion about how intragenic mutations might complement, complementation may eventually provide a useful way of identifying functional domains in the ATM molecule.

Genetics

A-T is transmitted as an autosomal recessive disease.[1–6] The incidence of A-T has been estimated at 1 in 40,000 to 100,000 live births, while the gene frequency is believed to be as high as 3 percent of the general population.[4,163] Recent studies of breast cancer in several large populations have provided convincing data in support of an ≈1 percent carrier frequency.[55,258,282] All races are affected by A-T. Despite the A-T gene's affecting so many different and apparently unrelated systems, the disease is inherited in each family as a single autosomal recessive gene defect. It is unclear why, in an autosomal recessive disorder, so many of the parents of British, Italian, and American patients are unrelated. This is borne out by the recent finding that most A-T patients worldwide are compound heterozygotes; i.e., they have different paternal and maternal mutations.[72,157] In the rare instances where two patients share a common mutation, their haplotypes usually differ, indicating independent origins for the mutation. The large size of the gene certainly provides a large target for new mutations. Recent studies suggest that gametogenesis is abnormal in ATM knockout mice[16] and that mitotic and meiotic recombination is

increased in A-T patients.[76,158] Furthermore, as was discussed above, the ATM gene shares homology with mec1 (yeast) and mei41 (*Drosophila*),[40,141] and both are meiotic-recombination defective mutants.[40,159] Whether this would affect heterozygous parents in A-T families sufficiently to influence the incidence of affected fetuses remains to be clarified. Recombination fractions in A-T families (i.e., in the parents) were normal across a 40 cM range of chromosome 11q22-23.[161]

Claims that "A-T is not always a recessive disorder"[45,160] are misleading and belie the consortium experience of having localized the ATM gene to the proper 400-kb genomic segment using a mathematical model that assumed autosomal recessive inheritance of a single gene and included 176 families. Families that do *not* link to 11q22-23 should be considered to carry mutations in other genes and to likely represent other syndromes. New names will have to be given to such "AT-like" disorders (see "Related Syndromes," below).

The rate of spontaneous mutations is unknown. Of the 176 consortium families, however, all but seven linked to chromosome 11q23.1.[161,162] Follow-up studies have found mutations in the ATM gene in six of these families. (A seventh family may be due to uniparental disomy.) Thus, linkage analyses of 175 families did not detect spontaneous mutations. Using the ratio of 5:176 and a gene frequency estimate of 0.01, mutation rate estimates approximate $1.5-3 \times 10^{-4}$ percent. This is rather high even for a large gene. Of course, if the ATM gene product really affects gametogenesis,[16,139,169] it may be inappropriate to apply standard genetic algorithms, which are based on the Hardy-Weinberg equilibrium, to the existing epidemiologic data.[163,164] It may also be that some young patients succumb to malignancies before a diagnosis of A-T can be recognized, further skewing the data. Furthermore, recent studies of ATM mutations in A-T patients versus cancer patients from non-AT families suggest that the frequencies of truncating versus missense ATM mutations may differ in the general population (See "Cancer Susceptibility" above).[306]

Endocrine Defects

Very little research has been done on endocrine defects in A-T patients. This may change, considering that ATM knockout mice have problems with both spermatogenesis and ovulation.[16,39,169] Gonadal streaks, absent or hypoplastic ovaries, dysgerminomas, and undeveloped fallopian tubes have been observed at postmortem examination in both mice[16] and human patients.[2] Laboratory tests of pituitary function reveal no consistent abnormality.

In stark contrast to the earlier statement that "female hypogonadism with sexual infantilism is found consistently [in A-T patients],"[2,5] most female patients followed by the author have normal menstrual cycles, and although menstruation sometimes starts late, cycles come at regular intervals. There is no other evidence as to whether these patients ovulate normally. Anecdotally, some long-lived female patients may have entered menopause prematurely. Others report very irregular cycles. Most male patients develop normal secondary sex characteristics. Some of these patients can have erections and even ejaculate. Studies of sperm haplotyping on semen from several A-T patients have documented that some actually produce sperm. None have fathered a child. One report of a putative female A-T patient having borne a child is clouded because this woman lived beyond 50 years, which is very atypical for A-T, and a similarly affected sib also demonstrated remarkable dexterity while already in her thirties (she worked in a knitware factory). In contrast, female NBS patients manifest very severe endocrine defects, most showing little or no development of secondary sex characteristics and markedly elevated (prepubertal) follicle-stimulating hormone (FSH) and luteinizing hormone (LH) levels.[283]

Some patients develop insulin-resistant diabetes, usually in the late teens. This is characterized by hyperglycemia without glycosuria or ketosis.[165,166] Other forms of diabetes, such as juvenile diabetes mellitus and late-onset diabetes, have been frequently observed among nonaffected members of A-T families. A genetic imprinting model has been considered, but this would not explain the pattern of diabetes in these families. Telomere silencing of subtelomeric genes, such as the insulin gene, might be an alternative hypothesis.[134]

Premature Aging

Many of the chromosomal instability syndromes, such as A-T, Fanconi anemia, xeroderma pigmentosum, and Bloom syndrome, show progeroid features.[167] Young A-T patients often have strands of gray hairs and develop keratoses; precocious basal cell carcinoma has been reported.[2,42] Some of these findings may reflect either premature menarche or the accelerated shortening of telomeres described above[135] (see "Chromosomal Instability"). However, thymic dystrophy and lymphoid depletion are also characteristic of aging and may be secondary to recombination defects during T-cell maturation rather than to telomeric shortening. Autoantibody formation is also found in both aging populations and A-T patients[9,168,170] (see the discussion in reference 170).

Postmortem examinations of older patients show progeric changes, such as neurofibrillary tangles in large neurons of the cerebral cortex, hippocampus, basal ganglia, and spinal cord, similar to those seen in Alzheimer disease.[15] Lipofuscin granules have been found in many neurons, in satellite cells of the dorsal ganglia, and in Schwann cells. Further, Marinesco bodies seen in the pigmented neurons of the substantia nigra in A-T patients are considered signs of precocious aging.[171]

Other Findings

Among Costa Rican families with classical A-T, about 40 percent of patients have clubbing of the fingertips, a finding that is usually associated with poorly oxygenated blood supply. These A-T children do not have cardiac defects. Most, but not all, live in San José, which is 3700 feet above sea level, not high enough to aggravate most cardiac or pulmonary problems. The mutations in these families have all been identified, and the clubbing does not associate with a particular mutation (see "Patient Mutations," below). It is possible that as part of their A-T syndrome these patients also have a pulmonary abnormality that compromises the oxygenation of their blood, such as microscopic arteriovenous fistulas or an anomalous bronchial tree.[197] However, this is purely speculative; at this writing, there is no explanation for the clubbing in Costa Rican A-T patients.[61]

Many of the Costa Rican patients also have hypertrichosis (excessive body hair).[61] This has been noted in other A-T patients as well.[5] Considering the diverse endocrinologic abnormalities that have been described in A-T patients (and in ATM knockout mice), hypertrichosis could reflect a mild hormonal imbalance in some patients.

Swift et al.[32] observed a fourfold increase of ischemic heart disease among female A-T carriers. Thus, while heterozygotes are at a 3.2-fold increased mortality risk, only 44 percent and 35 percent of the deaths (men and women, respectively) observed by Swift et al. were attributable to cancer; 34 percent and 35 percent of the deaths (men and women, respectively) were attributable to heart disease.

Related Syndromes

The related Nijmegen Breakage syndrome (NBS)[172] and the Berlin Breakage syndrome (BBS),[173] respectively assigned to complementation groups V1 and V2, do not show ataxia and do not link to chromosome 11q23.[162,174,175] These syndromes found their way into the A-T literature because cells from these patients manifest the 7;14 translocations and radioresistant DNA synthesis that are typical of A-T cells. These patients are also cancer susceptible and immunodeficient. Telangiectasias are absent, and the serum AFP level is normal. NBS patients have birdlike facies, microcephaly, and mental retardation (A-T patients typically are not mentally retarded). BBS very closely resembles NBS, and when the NBS1

gene was cloned in 1998, both BBS and NBS patients had mutations in that gene. NBS1 is on chromosome 8q11.[253] The NBS1 protein, nibrin, is absent from cell lysates of both NBS and BBS patients. NBS and BBS are now considered to be a single disorder. Because new evidence suggests that ATM phosphorylates nibrin,[307] in the Rad50/Mre11/nibrin complex, it would follow that the A-T and NBS phenotypes might overlap and that these genes might complement radioresistant synthesis.[151] Why NBS cells complement the radioresistant DNA synthesis of BBS is again a mystery of complementation experiments. Only a handful of BBS patients have been described in the literature. They have most of the signs and symptoms of NBS, with the possible addition to the syndrome of syndactyly, anal atresia, and hypospadias. Most of the reported NBS and BBS families have been of eastern Europe origin and carry the 657del5 mutation.[176–178,283,284]

AT$_{Fresno}$ (AT$_F$) combines the classical A-T syndrome with NBS (Fig. 15-5).[179] Whenever microcephaly and mental retardation are seen in an otherwise classical A-T patient, diagnosis of AT$_F$ should be suspected. However, because AT$_F$ families link to chromosome 11q23.1 and ATM mutations have been found in four AT$_F$ families, the clinical importance of this diagnostic distinction is presently unclear. Furthermore, the same ATM mutations found in two AT$_F$ families have also been observed in classic A-T patients. If a second modifier gene were involved, it would have to link to the 11q22-23 region as well.

Many other reports describe patients who do not meet all the diagnostic criteria for A-T discussed above.[180–182,189,308,314] Many of these reports describe: (1) very young patients (when the A-T syndrome would not yet be fully expressed), (2) transient ataxias (some possibly infectious), (3) probable A-T patients without telangiectasias,[162,183,184] (4) patients with normal AFP levels, or (5) those with nearly normal immunologic parameters. Recent screening for ATM mutations in such "variant" families in the international consortium (families that were categorically excluded from the linkage analyses so as to avoid contaminating the positional cloning data) suggests that most of these were A-T. In several families with classically affected patients, prominent telangiectasias have been noted in members who do not have ataxia and who do not carry the two affected ATM haplotypes.[162] Some of these persons are bona fide A-T heterozygotes.

Other families have been described with intermediate radiosensitivity, a parameter that is difficult to quantitate; nonetheless, in some hands, this must be considered a quantifiable result that will probably relate in some way to the sites of ATM mutations in those families or to mutations in other genes that link to the 11q22-23 region[308,318] (see "Correlating Phenotypes with Genotypes," below). Undoubtedly, other radiosensitive individuals exist whose symptoms partially overlap the A-T syndrome. It will be interesting to learn whether these patients have leaky ATM mutations or mutations in other genes that interact with the ATM protein.

Differential Diagnosis

The most difficult challenge in making a diagnosis of A-T involves very young patients. The most common misdiagnosis is cerebral palsy, especially when there is a spastic component to the child's movements. With time, however, a diagnosis of A-T becomes clear when the ataxia is notably progressive, eye movements demonstrate poor tracking, and speech becomes slurred. The absence of telangiectasia at this stage should not weigh against a diagnosis of A-T. Family history may be helpful if a prior child exists with similar signs and symptoms and the parents are related. Both factors should certainly raise suspicion about a hereditary disorder, and A-T is the most common hereditary early-onset progressive ataxia. The presence or absence of cancer in the family generally is not helpful, for it can be interpreted in many ways. Laboratory studies should include serum AFP, a cytogenetic search for t(7;14) translocations, in vitro radiosensitivity (see below), and an immunologic evaluation. Recent evidence suggests that ATM protein levels in lysates of A-T cells are very low or absent in most classical patients; these can be measured semi-quantitatively by Western blotting. In those bona fide A-T patients with ATM protein (∼20%), the function is assumed to be compromised. This need not be limited to just the p53 kinase function; defects in alternative splicing, DNA binding, or tissue specificity could also have similar phenotypic effects.

Even if some of the above tests are not informative, a diagnosis of A-T may still be valid for these following reasons: (a) The AFP remains normal throughout life in 5 percent of patients. As was discussed above, the serum AFP is occasionally elevated in normal children under 2 years of age, and thus is not a reliable test until after that age. (b) A cytogenetic search for t(7;14) translocations or clones is often unsuccessful in A-T patients because a poor mitogenic response makes it difficult to find enough good-quality metaphases for analysis (see "Chromosomal Instability," above). Even if sufficient metaphases are found, the translocations are sometimes missed. Radiation-induced and bleomycin-induced breakage studies may be helpful, but they seldom contribute to making the diagnosis because of overlap between normal and A-T ranges.[89] (c) The immunologic evaluation is normal in some A-T patients. Whether it becomes progressively more abnormal in older A-T patients is debatable (see "Immunodeficiency," above). The response to allogeneic cells, the mixed lymphocyte response, is quite abnormal in some patients; however, this is a very laborious and costly test that is hard to quantitate without extensive controls and is therefore difficult to justify for strictly clinical purposes.

A MRI (magnetic resonance imaging) of the cerebellum will usually reveal marked dystrophy in children over 4 years of age (Fig. 15-6). Newer techniques for imaging the cerebellum are also being evaluated. These include functional MRI and PET (positron emission tomography) scanning;[231,232] however, both depend heavily on patient cooperation and may not be applicable to very young children. Furthermore, PET scanning uses radioactive tracers, and although the exposure doses are very small, they could theoretically contribute to cancer risk, especially in the bladder where the radioisotope accumulates rapidly during the procedure. When risk-benefit ratios are considered for procedures using ionizing radiation, difficult judgments must be made.

The most dangerous diagnostic situation for a young A-T patient occurs when cancer is the presenting symptom. Fortunately, this does not occur very often. Anecdotally, one child had a cerebellar astrocytoma removed at 27 months of age, but his unsteady gait actually worsened postoperatively. His clinicians

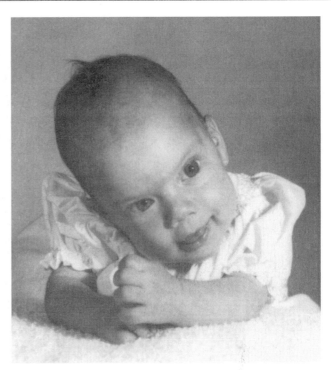

Fig. 15-7 Head-tilting in a 6-month-old infant with A-T. Staggering was not noted until she began to walk.

were quite concerned and confused by the persistent ataxia until several years later, when the patient's younger sister began to stagger as well and a diagnosis of A-T was made on both children. Because the astrocytoma was totally resectable, no consideration was given to further therapy with chemotherapeutic agents or radiation. The patient died more than 20 years later without any sequelae of the cancer or surgery. Other children have not been so fortunate,[17–19] presenting with a malignancy and receiving conventional doses of irradiation because it was not realized that they were suffering from A-T, only to suffer iatrogenic deaths. The late Dr. Boder claimed that she could make a diagnosis of A-T in any child under 2 years of age. While this is a challenging claim, it is certainly true that most young A-T patients do have at least some suspicious neurologic findings at a very early age. On questioning, mothers sometimes volunteer that they noted head tilting or swaying in these infants (Fig. 15-7). Thus, it is prudent for pediatric oncologists and radiation oncologists to rule out the diagnosis of A-T before treating *any* young child with cancer, either by obtaining a complete history and performing a careful neurologic examination with this in mind, or by obtaining a neurologic consultation as part of the workup.

While the presence of hypersensitivity to ionizing radiation is a laboratory hallmark of the disease, clinical testing for this has not been readily available, primarily because most radiosensitivity assays use fibroblasts, and establishing fibroblasts in A-T patients is painful and labor intensive. With this in mind, Huo *et al.*[111] laboratory established the CSA, a clonogenic assay that evaluates the colony survival fraction of LCLs from patients after the cells have received 1 Gy of ionizing irradiation.[111] From a single 10-ml heparinized blood sample (that should be shipped without refrigeration), cells are transformed with Epstein-Barr virus. Once a stable cell line is established, the cells are plated in two cell concentrations on 96-well tissue culture trays that are irradiated (or not irradiated) and returned to an incubator for 10 days, at which point the number of wells containing colonies larger than 32 cells is scored and compared to the colony survival fractions of normal cells. Unlike other colony survival assays, the CSA conditions were selected so that heterozygotes would score as normals, which allows for more reliable detection of A-T homozygotes (Fig. 15-8). Recently, two referred patients with

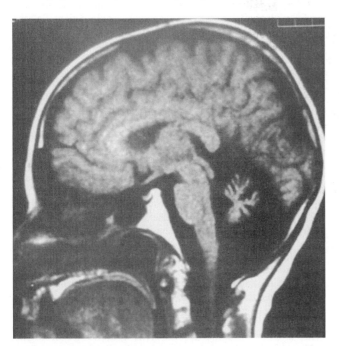

Fig. 15-6 Magnetic resonance imaging of a 6-year-old A-T patient showing markedly reduced size of the cerebellar shadow.

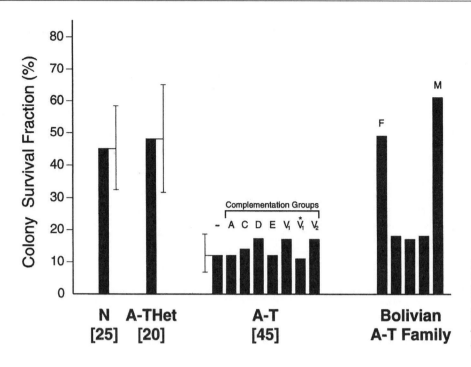

Fig. 15-8 Colony survival assay (CSA) measures radiosensitivity of LCLs from patients with A-T, A-T heterozygotes, normals, and a Bolivian family with three affected children, following 1 Gy of irradiation. Also included are results from patients with NBS (V1), BBS (V2), and AT$_F$ (V1*).

normal CSA results on repeated testing were subsequently found to have the typical (GAA)n expansions of Friedreich ataxia on chromosome 9q13. Although the differential diagnosis between Friedreich ataxia (FRDA) and A-T is usually not difficult — FRDA is a later-onset ataxia (usually around puberty) and most FRDA patients have hypertrophic cardiomyopathy (by ECG testing), whereas A-T patients generally do not have cardiac problems — this experience served to underscore the value of using radiosensitivity to confirm a suspected early diagnosis of A-T. FRDA patients have normal CSA results.[111,185] Patients from all complementation groups, including NBS and BBS, have the same markedly reduced CSA levels. Human Mre11 deficiency patients[308] are also radiosensitive but have not yet been tested by CSA

Abnormal facies other than the slowly developing smile, or masklike expression of many A-T patients, should raise suspicion about other diagnoses. Severe mental retardation and inability to speak at an appropriate age are also uncharacteristic of A-T. Mental retardation is seen more commonly in lower socioeconomic-level families and countries, perhaps because they lack the resources needed to keep A-T patients in the mainstream of family and community life, whereby they must learn to respond to various personal challenges. The absence of oculomotor apraxia by 5 years of age is also strong evidence against the diagnosis of A-T.

Ataxia is common to a variety of other hereditary disorders:[186] (a) as a major feature with progressive ataxia — hMre11 deficiency[308] β-lipoprotein abnormalities selective vitamin E deficiency, hexosaminidase deficiency (GM2), and cholesterolosis; (b) as a major feature with intermittent ataxia — urea-cycle defects, maple syrup urine disease, isovaleric acidosis, 2-hydroxyglutaric aciduria, Hartnup disease, pyruvate dysmetabolism, and mitochondrial disease; and (c) as a minor feature of Niemann-Pick syndrome, metachromatic leukodystrophy, multiple sulfatase deficiency, late-onset globoid cell leukodystrophy, adrenoleukodystrophy, sialidosis type 1, and ceroid lipofuscinosis. The latter can be diagnosed only by biopsy of the conjunctiva or brain. Most of the other listed disorders will show abnormalities in urinary amino acids, lysosomal hydrolases, or very long chain fatty acids. Retinitis pigmentosa, deafness, polyneuropathy, and ataxia characterize Refsum disease.[187] Non-hereditary ataxia may result from an acute infection or from a posterior fossa tumor. (For further information, see reference 5.)

Determining whether a new patient's ataxia has been inherited in a dominant or a recessive manner can aid in distinguishing A-T

from olivopontocerebellar atrophy and any of the spinocerebellar ataxias, all of which are dominant disorders. The familial pattern for age at onset of the ataxia is also helpful, because few other familial ataxias present in early childhood as A-T does. While an occasional case of early-onset FRDA might be mistaken for A-T on this basis, neurologic examination will reveal spinal cord ataxia with a positive Romberg sign, and, in the laboratory, homozygosity for a (GAA)n expansion in the first intron of the FRDA gene is easily diagnosed[188,316]; FRDA cells are also not radiosensitive.[111]

Determining whether two mutations exist within the ATM gene of a child suspected of having A-T is the most definitive way of establishing a diagnosis. At this writing such an approach is just becoming feasible (see "Patient Mutations," below). In families of certain ethnic backgrounds, rapid DNA assays can be performed for mutations that are common in that population. By first haplotyping the DNA of a suspected A-T patient in the chromosome 11q22-23 region, previously described haplotypes carrying mutated ATM genes can be identified. However, unless the patient is homozygous for a mutation — which is very unlikely unless the parents are consanguineous — a second mutation must still be sought. This requires a great deal of effort either by mRNA/cDNA/RT-PCR-based screening assays or by a systematic genomic search of the 66 exons of the ATM gene. Even this approach is not 100 percent effective in finding all mutations, because some lie deep within introns and others require analysis of both genomic DNA and mRNA. Eventually, we hope to determine the mutations and affected haplotypes for most A-T families. This database will expedite both the diagnosis of A-T and prenatal diagnosis.

Aicardi et al.[189] described a group of 14 patients with a late-onset progressive ataxia, choreoathetosis, and oculomotor apraxia without frequent infections or telangiectasia. The AFP was normal and a search for t(7;14) translocations was negative. Aicardi suggested that these children suffered from "an unusual type of spinocerebellar degeneration," probably not A-T. However, it would be informative to determine whether any of those patients are radiosensitive, for example, by CSA.

Prenatal Diagnosis

With the fine mapping of the ATM gene, a set of highly informative genetic markers was developed that now allows accurate haplotyping within families, with basically 100 percent reliability of the fetus either being affected or not being affected, i.e., less than 1 percent recombination between ATM and the markers used. The finding of only a single A-T gene for all complementation groups also simplifies this diagnostic approach. This is in contrast to earlier attempts to perform prenatal diagnoses by trying to quantitate spontaneous chromosome breakage[89,109-193] (see the discussion in reference 150), assessing radiation-induced chromosomal damage of amniocytes or fetal fibroblasts, or performing RDS, all of which were misleading at one time or another (anonymous oral communications). One hopes that these approaches have by now been abandoned.

Prenatal diagnosis by haplotyping relies on a prior affected child to (a) establish a firm diagnosis of A-T and (b) identify the two affected chromosome 11q23.1 segments (i.e., haplotypes) carrying the ATM gene.[192] Figure 15-9 illustrates haplotyping and how it was possible to determine that the first cousin of an affected patient was not affected. A definitive diagnosis was possible only because a prior affected cousin existed in a consanguineous family. It is of paramount importance that the diagnosis of A-T in the prior affected member be confirmed before attempting haplotyping for prenatal diagnosis. The markers we use today are all within 1 percent recombination of the ATM gene: D11S1817,[194] D11S1819,[194] NS22,[285] D11S2179,[195] and D11S1818.[194] Two of these markers are within the ATM gene itself, thereby circumventing the need for reporting the risk of recombination separating the testing markers from the actual ATM gene. Most of this testing can be performed before conception, i.e., preconceptional testing. Once a DNA sample is available from the fetus, either from growing amniocytes or from a chorionic villous biopsy, the entire haplotyping can be completed within a week. With new "molecular beacons" this will become even more streamlined.[298] Because abortion guidelines vary with the country or state of residence of the mother, we ask for the referring laboratory's deadline for reporting the results of prenatal diagnosis to the family, rather than for the due date or the date of last menses. In keeping with modern guidelines for genetic testing, the results are conveyed to the family by a genetic counselor.

Therapy

No effective therapy exists for halting the progression of the ataxia.[2,5,196] Clinical trials are under way to test the efficacy of myoinositol, *N*-acetylcysteine, and L-dopa on general symptoms. To date, preliminary data have been disappointing. (For a review of other AT-related medications, see reference 196.) Vitamin E has been prescribed by some A-T specialists for years, based on anecdotal information from Dr. Elena Boder.[15] Recent studies suggesting that A-T cells may be in a constant state of increased oxidative stress make it likely that most antioxidants or free-radical scavengers might counteract some of the progressive neurological deterioration of A-T patients.[38,317,325,326,327] Thus, vitamin E continues to be recommended; α-lipoic acid and coenzyme Q10 may also slow the deterioration. Folic acid may formation further help to minimize chromosomal fragility and the formation of double-strand DNA breaks. All of the above dietary supplements are available without a prescription.

Areas of great concern to the health of A-T patients are pulmonary infections and malignancy. Pulmonary infections usually are due to the normal spectrum of microbes and are treatable by conventional approaches. Opportunistic infections do not occur in A-T patients as they do in patients with other immuno-deficiency disorders (with the possible exception of mycobacterium). Malignancies must be treated with great care to avoid conventional doses of radiation therapy or radiomimetic agents. If possible, neurotoxic chemotherapeutic agents should be avoided.

Not all A-T patients manifest frequent pulmonary or sinus infections. Those with chronic bronchiectasis are best treated in the same way as patients with cystic fibrosis: routine chest percussion, postural drainage, and generally aggressive pulmonary hygiene. Periodic pulmonary function studies may assist in monitoring infection-prone patients. In older patients, pulmonary

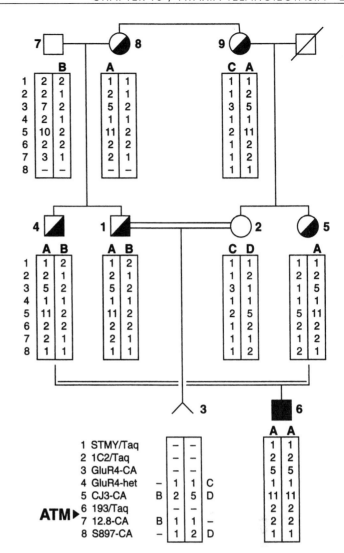

Fig. 15-9 Prenatal testing to determine whether a fetus (3) is affected. By history, two brothers had married two sisters who were their first cousins. One couple (4 and 5) had an affected child (6), prompting the second couple (1 and 2) to seek prenatal testing. However, testing before conception would have identified the mother (2) as a noncarrier, thereby circumventing any further testing on the fetus. Haplotype [A] carries the affected ATM gene. The genetic markers that are currently being used for prenatal testing are given in the text.

infections are the major cause of failing health and death. Increasing bulbar dysfunction may predispose to aspiration pneumonia. In addition to appropriate antibiotics, intravenous γ-globulin every 3 to 4 weeks may reduce the frequency of infections in infection-prone patients. There is some indication that the lungs of A-T patients may not be anatomically normal. Pump *et al.*[197] made a latexlike impression of one lung (using a substance called Vultex moulage [General Latex and Chemicals Ltd., Verdun, Quebec]) from a single A-T patient. They found bronchiectatic changes in many parts of the lung, with saccular dilatations throughout the bronchi.

Perhaps the most effective impact on care that the physician can make is to strongly encourage the parents of young A-T patients to institute an aggressive and engaging physical exercise program aimed at enhancing lung function, preventing contractures, and avoiding positional kyphoscoliosis. Almost all patients who have been denied such care develop severe contractures of the feet and hands. These become apparent in the late teens. An annual assessment by a physical therapist allows this care to be customized.

Speech therapy is also effective, not in arresting the progression of the dysarthria, but in minimizing the frustration felt by the patients when they cannot be understood by peers. Increased social interaction generally improves speech clarity.

Some of the neurologic symptoms, such as ataxia, drooling, and tremors, can be partially relieved by various agents.[196] Buspirone, a serotonergic 5-hydroxytryptophan agonist, is active in some types of cerebellar ataxia.[253] Amantadine improves balance and coordination and minimizes drooling in some patients. Postural tremors may be reduced by baclofen, a GABA inhibitor, or propranolol and other β blockers, while cerebellar tremors and myoclonus may respond to low doses of clonazepam or valproic acid. However, these agents sometimes increase the ataxia, drowsiness, or depression. Methyl scopolamine or propantheline hydrochloride are sometimes effective in reducing drooling. Ligating the salivary ducts can also alleviate drooling. This may also reduce the risk of aspiration pneumonia.

When radiation therapy is planned for treating a malignancy in an A-T patient, doses should be reduced by approximately 30 percent. Some chemotherapeutic agents, especially alkylating agents, probably should also be used in reduced doses. It has been suggested that topoisomerase inhibitors should be avoided. Unfortunately, there is only anecdotal literature on the important and recurring issue of oncologic treatment of A-T patients.

Occasionally, the possibility of bone marrow transplantation arises, usually because a young A-T patient has developed leukemia and has an HLA-compatible sib to serve as a potential donor. Despite several such attempts over the past 20 years, the author is unaware of a single transplant with convincing documentation of long-term engraftment. This could be for several reasons, the most compelling of which is the difficulty of establishing a safe but effective regimen for delivering the marrow-ablating irradiation or chemotherapy for the reasons given above. In general, hyperfractionation of radiation doses would seem prudent under such circumstances if this need were to arise. There is, of course, only a remote possibility that bone marrow transplantation would alter the cerebellar degeneration.[286,287] Hematopoietic stem cell transplantation might reduce the need for complete ablation but probably would also reduce the chances of a full immunologic engraftment. Neural stem cell engraftment may eventually become an important therapeutic alternative.

Many A-T patients have been immunized inadvertently for smallpox, polio, and varicella, with no apparent sequelae. Nevertheless, natural varicella infections are often quite severe. Thus, contrary to the general warning that patients with immunodeficiencies not be given live vaccines, varicella immunization is advisable for patients whose immune status is satisfactory.

Prognosis

Most A-T patients in the United States live well beyond 20 years. Many are now in their thirties. This is a major change from just a few years ago when it was unusual for these patients to live beyond their teenage years. Unfortunately, this is still true in many countries, for reasons that are unknown. However, the improved survival in the United States may be related to better nutrition, better diagnostics, better treatment of pulmonary infections and malignancies, and more aggressive physical therapy. There is hope among A-T investigators that the young children being diagnosed today will benefit from some currently undiscovered therapy before their neurologic status becomes irreversible.

MOLECULAR GENETICS

Our laboratory utilized a large Amish pedigree, that included four branches of the family with living affected members, to localize the ATM gene to 11q22-23 in 1988.[152,205] This family was later assigned by Jaspers and coworkers to complementation group A.[150–151,204] To our initial surprise, when lod scores from all A-T families were added together, regardless of complementation

group assignments, the cumulative lod scores increased.[152,206,207] This suggested that either (a) the complementation group genes were all clustered in the 11q22-23 region, (b) most of the families were of similar complementation groups (Groups A and C were thought to include over 80 percent of the typed families), (c) the complementation groups represented intragenic mutations, or (d) complementation typing with A-T fibroblasts did not reflect Mendelian inheritance. In all our subsequent linkage analyses over the next 7 years, we never found any convincing evidence for genetic heterogeneity.[18,206–208] The cloning of a single gene for all complementation groups corroborated these early interpretations.

Subsequent to our initial report localizing the A-T gene to 11q22-23,[152] many reports followed that confirmed and extended that observation.[153,161,162,181,206–221] In the final linkage studies of 169 bona fide families that had been entered into a 9-country consortium, over 40 genetic markers were tested. The location score curve peaked at D11S535 with a lod score of 73. The 2-lod support region containing the A-T locus was a 500-kb interval beginning 150-kb proximal to S384 and ending just short of S1294. If we counted the number of families with recombinants in the candidate region, the same 500-kb region of common overlap

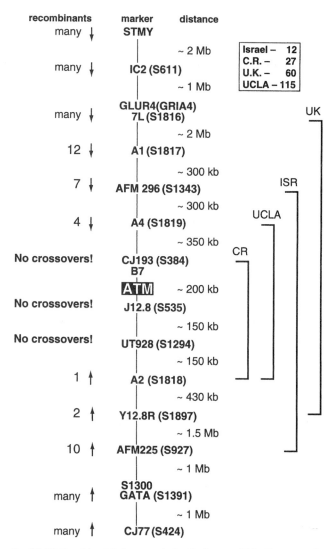

Fig. 15-10 Combined linkage and physical map of 11 cM surrounding the ATM gene. The map is based on the combined linkage analysis of 249 families (59 CEPH and 190 A-T) and pulsed-field gel analyses.[220] Also depicted are the most likely regions for the ATM gene that were based on the number of families from the respective consortium members (see box and brackets at right). On the left, the number of recombinants in the consortium families is given. The position of the ATM gene on this map was added later.

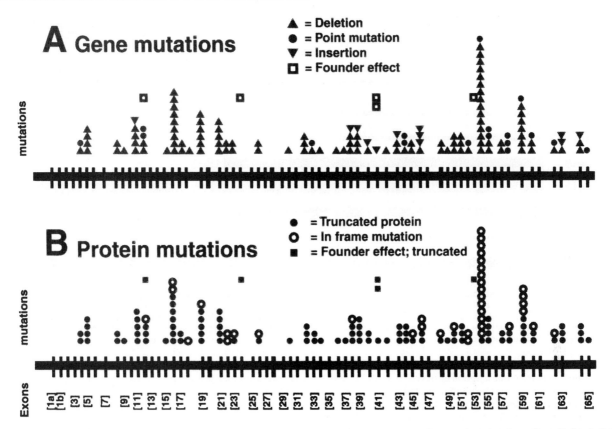

A Gene mutations

▲ = Deletion
● = Point mutation
▼ = Insertion
□ = Founder effect

mutations

B Protein mutations

● = Truncated protein
○ = In frame mutation
■ = Founder effect; truncated

mutations

Exons [1a][1b] [3] [5] [7] [9] [11][13] [15][17] [19] [21][23] [25] [27] [29] [31] [33] [35] [37][39] [41] [43][45] [47] [49][51] [53][55] [57] [59] [61] [63] [65]

Fig. 15-11 Spectrum of 120 ATM mutations based on studies of cDNA from cells of patients from many countries. *A*, Mutations seen in related (or probably related, because they share haplotypes) families are indicated only once (by boxes) to avoid biasing the distribution. The exact position of many of these mutations will be revised once the genomic mutation sites have been defined. *B*, The majority of mutations result in truncated ATM proteins. (For an updated version of this figure, see Web site: http://www.vmre-search.org/atm.htm.)

could be appreciated. The accuracy of these positional cloning experiments depended heavily on the construction of an accurate genetic map (Fig. 15-10).

From 1993 to 1995, detailed YAC, BAC, and cosmid maps were made of the candidate region by several of the consortium laboratories, and, using these genomic segments, many transcripts from many cDNA libraries were isolated. Five recovery methods were used, including exon trapping,[224] the only method that did not depend on whether the A-T gene was being expressed in any particular library. Each of the recovered transcripts had to be sequenced so that PCR primers could be designed and used to amplify and screen for mutations, using cDNAs from 100 A-T patients as templates for the PCRs. In 1993, several labs found a large transcript, E14/CAND3/NPAT, which was ubiquitously expressed, thus qualifying it as a good candidate A-T gene. Despite very thorough searches of CAND3 for mutations in over 100 A-T patients, using SSCP, heteroduplex analysis (HA), density gradient gel electrophoresis (DGGE), and direct cDNA sequencing, no mutations were found. In 1995, the ATM gene was isolated by the Israeli members of the consortium[72,73] from within the 500-kb region defined by the linkage analyses. E14/CAND3/NPAT was only 544 bp upstream of the initiation site for ATM, oriented in the opposite transcriptional direction and sharing a common promoter.[225–227] Although this gene also contains a kinase domain, its function remains unknown.

The ATM Gene

The ATM gene transcript is 13 kb (9054 nt of ORF), with 66 exons, the largest being exon 12 with 372 nucleotides (nt) (GDB accession numbers U82828, U26455, X91196, U40887-40918, and U33841, as well as the reports of Savitsky *et al.*,[72,140] Rasio *et al.*,[228] Uziel *et al.*,[229] Byrd *et al.*,[225] Vorechovsky *et al.*,[54]

Pecker *et al.*,[230] and Platzer *et al.*[251]). It has a molecular weight of 350 and is a member of a family of high-molecular-weight protein kinases.[72,139–141,233] Northern blots reveal expression in all tissues, with several transcripts of 10.5 (fibroblasts), 6.2, and 4.9 kb. Recent studies by Rotman and coworkers[194,319] indicate that a considerable amount of alternative splicing occurs at the 5′ end. The 3′ portion of the gene has strong homology to yeast and mammalian phosphatidylinositol 3-kinases, as well as to DNA-PK. Thus, ATM appears to play a major role as an intracellular signal transducer that gives warning to the cell, via cell-cycle checkpoints, of DNA damage that must be repaired before the next cell division. However, as was discussed above, another role for the ATM protein remains to be elucidated, one that is p53-independent and probably involves replicon initiation and meiotic pairing during gametogenesis. A leucine zipper domain around exon 27 suggests that the ATM protein may form homo- or heterodimers and bind DNA. When this region of the gene was transfected into normal cells, the normal cells developed an A-T phenotype, which suggests a dominant negative effect for the leucine zipper region.[288,330] An SH₃ domain (residues 1373 to 1382) binds c-abl in response to DNA damage.[70]

Patient Mutations

Over 400 mutations in the ATM gene have been identified (Fig. 15-11).[72,157,222,225,234,235,237,252,289,321–323] A Web site has been created for tracking those already published: http://www.vmresearch.org/atm.htm. Intially these laboratories used a variety of screening approaches; restriction endonuclease fingerprinting (REF), SSCP followed by single-strand sequencing, protein truncation testing (PTT), and conformation sensitive gel electrophoresis (CSGE).[157] Each screening approach strongly biases the types of mutations found. Almost all the early work used mRNA

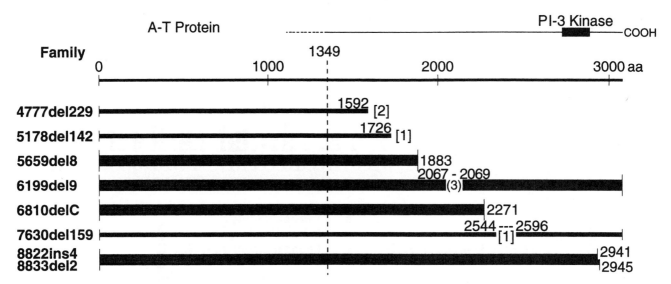

Fig. 15-12 Depiction of theoretical protein truncations based on cDNA and genomic mutations and their relationship to the most conserved portion of the PI-3 kinase domain. Bracketed numbers represent deleted exons; numbers in parentheses represent deleted codons. While most deletions result in truncation of the protein, a few do not create frameshifts, and presumably the protein continues to be translated downstream from the deletion, thereby including the presumably important PI-3 kinase domain. Thick bars represent patients with homozygous mutations. Such patients can now be analyzed for phenotype-genotype correlations (see Table 15-3).

as a template (via reverse transcription of mRNA to cDNA). About 70 percent of ATM mutations result in truncated proteins, most of which affect splice sites;[222,252] these types of mutations are detected efficiently by PTT, which is still the method of choice if live cells are available as a source of RNA. Platzer et al.[251] used dye terminator methodology to directly sequence 27.3 kb of DNA on each of 72 patients; only 50 percent of mutations were detected. A comparative discussion of mutation detection strategies for ATM is beyond the scope of this chapter. (For further details, see references 236 and 237.)

Because the 3′ half of the ATM gene was sequenced first, the distribution of mutations shown in Fig. 15-11 is slightly biased against finding equal numbers of mutations in the 5′ half. Most A-T patients are compound heterozygotes. One potential hotspot (approximately 15 percent of mutations) was identified, in exon 54.[235] Exon 54 is just proximal to the PI-3 kinase homology domain, and, therefore, mutations in this region could be especially important. In screening cDNAs, two types of changes were observed here: c2544del159nt and c2546del9nt, both of which resulted in in-frame deletions in cDNA (for example, see mutation 7630del159nt in Fig. 15-12 which deletes 53 amino acids). (The numbers prefacing a cDNA change indicates the first codon to be affected.) The genomic mutation that causes the 159nt-exon 54 to be skipped during splicing may appear anywhere within that genomic region. For example, three genomic mutations are now known to cause a splicing deletion of exon 54: 7788G > A, 7926A > C, and IVS53-2A > C. (Many of the published cDNA changes have not been updated in the literature with the corresponding genomic mutations.) Further studies of exon 54 similarly indicate that many of the 15 patients from around the world with the 7636del9 (c2547del9) mutation share a common haplotype and they are mainly of Irish-English background.[252,289] Thus, the putative exon 54 hotspot contains at least four different mutations and many of the patients are probably distantly related; i.e., the frequency of the 7636del9 mutation should be counted only once for this lineage.

Because of the marginal effect that the 7636del9 in-frame mutation might have on the predicted protein—i.e., it would delete three amino acids (codons 2547–49)—it could be argued that this represents a polymorphism and not a true mutation. Wright et al.[235] addressed this issue by screening 75 parents of CEPH families; no examples of this mutation were found. Lavin et al.[320] introduced this mutation into atm−/− cell and it did not

restore a normal phenotype, except for a small amount of ATM protein.

Vorechovsky et al.[54] found 7 similar unique DNA changes in a group of 38 breast tumors that were not observed in paired blood samples or in an extended sampling of 224 unrelated chromosomes. These are "rare allelic variants" (RAVs). Considering together the prediction that 1 in every 500 bp in the human genome is "mutated," and the 150-kb genomic size of the ATM gene, one would expect to find 300 polymorphic sites within the ATM gene. Those changes that obviously affect coding or splicing regions are mostly mutations, certainly those detected by PTT would truncate the protein.[157,252] However, it has been increasingly difficult to interpret the biological effects of so-called "silent mutations" and "missense mutations," as well as the effects of changes found deep within introns, in cases where RNA is not also available for analysis. A "silent mutation" that leads to a splicing defect is shown in Fig. 15-13. In this example, a genomic 2250G > A mutation does not change the amino acid (AAG and AAA are both lysine codons); however, the cDNA-based PTT indicates that this "silent" mutation results in a more deleterious 126 nt deletion.

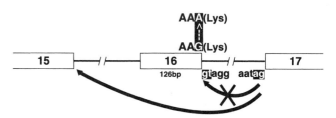

Fig. 15-13 Genomic mutation 2250G > A at the end of exon 16 would not result in a change of the lysine at codon 709. The G > A transition is a "silent mutation." However, protein truncation testing (PTT) demonstrates that this mutation results in a 126-nt deletion in the cDNA. This perturbs the donor splice site of exon 16 and causes the acceptor site to skip upstream to the donor site of exon 15, thereby deleting exon 16. Because the deletion does not result in a frameshift, downstream translation of the truncated protein should not be affected. However, western blotting of lysates from the cells of this patient, failed to show any ATM protein. Thus, what might appear from genomic analysis to be an insignificant mutation is in fact a deleterious one, as evidenced by the characteristic A-T phenotype of two unrelated homozygous patients with this mutation.

mutation "418": 5762+1126 a-->g (c1921ins137nt)

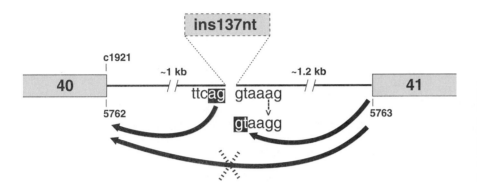

Fig. 15-14 Mutation IVS40+1126A > G inserts an artificial 137-bp exon into the mRNA by creating a new donor splice site 5 nucleotides upstream of the mutation (at IVS40+1122) and taking advantage of an existing potential acceptor splice site further upstream (for further details, see reference 239).

Because the last nucleotide in an exon is a "G" 79 percent of the time,[238] the G > A change most likely disturbs the splice donor site for exon 16 so that the splice acceptor site at exon 17 skips upstream to the next acceptable splice donor site, that of exon 15. This deletes the 126 nt of exon 16, thereby truncating the protein by 42 amino acids. Mutation IVS40 + 1126A > G, described by McConville et al.,[239] is an example of how a change deep within intron 40 leads to the formation of a new artifical exon (Fig. 15-14). The expanded mRNA apparently results in a "leaky" mutation that is associated with a somewhat milder phenotype (see "Correlating Phenotypes with Genotypes" below).

Castellvi-Bel et al.[323] have detected 10 conventional polymorphisms (Table 15-1) and 2 RAVs (Table 15-2). Udar et al.[285] have identified an additional complex microsatellite repeat within the ATM gene. Given the low frequency of RAVs in general populations, they must represent rather recent changes in the genome. Another microsatellite repeat, DNA11S2179 was described by Vanagaite et al.[195] Because we have only screened approximately 23 kb (or 15 percent) of the genomic region containing the ATM gene, we would have expected to find about 45 (0.15 × 300) unique DNA changes. Combining the seven RAVs described by Vorechovsky et al.[54] with our 34 polymorphisms, this estimate compares favorably with the 41 polymorphisms actually found to date. Undoubtedly, other investigators will find additional DNA changes within introns of the gene that are not mutations; i.e., they do not compromise the integrity of the ATM protein. If large populations of cancer patients are to be screened using only DNA, some significant "mutations" may be misinterpreted as insignificant, and polymorphisms may be mistaken as mutations. Indeed, within the Internet Web site for ATM mutations in A-T homozygotes, [http://www.vmresearch.org/atm.htm], roughly 60 percent of patients have only one allele defined, strongly suggesting that present mutation detection methods do not detect a large proportion of ATM mutations. Perhaps some of these mutations reside in the 3′UT region, a region that has not yet been screened because of the great difficulty of distinguishing mutations from polymorphisms. This limitation will also mask potential genotype-phenotype correlations.

In an almost independent effort to localize the A-T gene without segregation analysis (in the event that meiotic recombination might be increased in A-T—a chromosomal breakage syndrome, after all—and the linkage results might mislead the positional cloning experiments), we utilized a subset of 27 Costa Rican families to track ancestral haplotypes,[223] a form of linkage disequilibrium analysis and "identity by descent" analysis. Even before the cloning of the gene, it was possible to establish that only a single gene was responsible for all of the Costa Rican families by pairing each of the Costa Rican haplotypes with a different one (Fig. 15-15). We further reasoned that the patients carrying

Table 15-1 Common Polymorphisms in the *ATM* Gene

	Allelic frequency (N ~ 100)
10807A > G	72:28
IVS3−122T > C	55:45
IVS4 + 36insAA	61:39
IVS6 + 70delT	71:29
IVS16−34C > A	75:25
IVS22−77T > C	72:28
IVS24−9delT	86:14
IVS25−15delA	63:37
5557G > A	75:25
IVS48−69insATT	61:39
IVS62−55T > C	69:31

Table 15-2 "Rare Allelic Variants" in the *ATM* Gene

	Allelic frequency (%) (N ~ 100)
10677G > C	1
10742G > T	0.5
10819G > T	0.5
10948A > G	1
IVS3−300G > A	4
IVS7−28T > C	0.5
IVS8−24del5	1
IVS13−137T > C	1
IVS14−55T > G	5
1986T > C	0.5
IVS20 + 27delT	1
IVS23−76T > C (28% in IRAT)	0
IVS25−35T > A	3
IVS27−65T > C	2
IVS30−54T > C	0.5
4362 A > C	0.5
IVS38−8T > C	6
5793T > C	1
IVS47−11G > T	0.5
IVS49−16T > A	0.5
IVS53 + 34insA	1
IVS60−50delTTAGTT	0.5
IVS62 + 8A > C	2
IVS62−65G > A	0.5

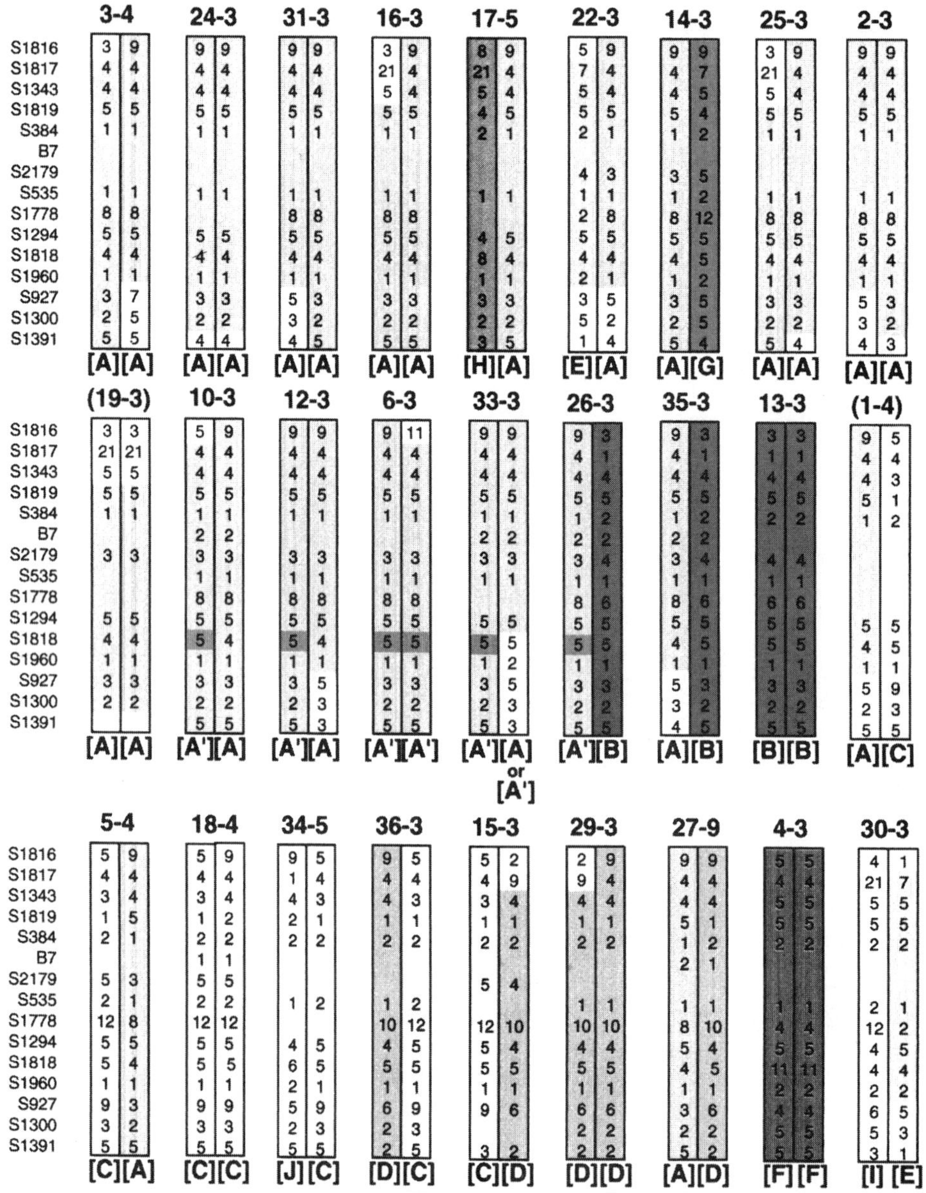

Markers (rows, top to bottom): S1816, S1817, S1343, S1819, S384, B7, S2179, S535, S1778, S1294, S1818, S1960, S927, S1300, S1391

Row 1 patients: 3-4 [A][A], 24-3 [A][A], 31-3 [A][A], 16-3 [A][A], 17-5 [H][A], 22-3 [E][A], 14-3 [A][G], 25-3 [A][A], 2-3 [A][A]

Row 2 patients: (19-3) [A][A], 10-3 [A'][A], 12-3 [A'][A], 6-3 [A'][A'], 33-3 [A'][A] or [A'], 26-3 [A'][B], 35-3 [A][B], 13-3 [B][B], (1-4) [A][C]

Row 3 patients: 5-4 [C][A], 18-4 [C][C], 34-5 [J][C], 36-3 [D][C], 15-3 [C][D], 29-3 [D][D], 27-9 [A][D], 4-3 [F][F], 30-3 [I][E]

Fig. 15-15 Haplotyping of 27 Costa Rican A-T patients defined by genotyping with 15 markers across 7 cM flanking the most likely region for the later-cloned ATM gene. The most prominent haplotype, haplotype [A], was found in 19 patients (70 percent), 12 of whom were homozygous for this haplotype. Subsequent studies have confirmed that these patients all carry an identical mutation, as demonstrated by the assay shown in Fig. 29-14. As different descendants of the original carrier inherited haplotype [A], the genomic region that remained associated with the true region of the gene was reduced by random recombination. Thus, "ancestral haplotyping" provided further localization of the gene. Furthermore, by pairing the 10 haplotypes observed in these families, it was possible to predict that a single gene was causing the syndrome (with the exception of haplotype [F], which was never observed paired with another haplotype).

haplotype [A] were carrying the same mutation. We later confirmed this and found that roughly two-thirds of these purportedly "unrelated" families shared the same mutation on the same affected haplotype (haplotype [A] in Fig. 15-15). Inferred (ancestral) recombination events involving this common haplotype in earlier generations also allowed us to further localize the candidate region for the gene. Nine other haplotypes were identified within the Costa Rican population. We have identified the mutations and developed rapid DNA screening tests for seven Costa Rican mutations.[221,252,290] Together, these tests identify >99 percent of ATM mutations in that country. Such rapid screening tests take less than a day to screen hundreds of DNAs (Fig. 15-16). This provides an opportunity to compare the clinical symptoms of multiple patients with the same mutation; indeed, some of the patients are homozygous for this mutation. It also allows >99 percent of A-T carriers to be identified in Costa Rica.

Our laboratory has taken this approach in other ethnic populations as well.[252] A peculiar 3245ATC > TGAT mutation accounts for 55 percent of Norwegian patients[252] and has been traced to a single common ancestor who lived from 1684 to 1755 and had eight children.[293] Despite the appearance of breast cancer in several of the extant branches of this extended family, the frequency of the 3245ATG > TGAT mutation was not increased in Norwegian breast cancer patients from the same region. Rapid screening tests are now available for Amish (1563delAG), Moroccan Jews (103C > T),[291] Sardinian (3894insT), Mennonites (5932G > T), and other genetic isolates. Some of these mutations are represented as boxes in Fig. 15-11 because they are founder-effect defects; i.e., they are common to multiple patients from presumably related families. As can be seen in Table 15-3, we also have observed five recurring defects in Polish families that represent 30 percent of Polish A-T patients, four mutations that

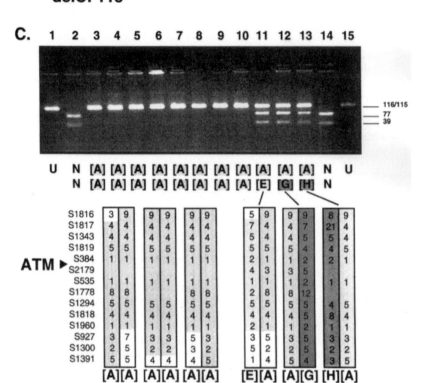

Fig. 15-16 Example of a rapid assay for the Costa Rican haplotype [A] mutation, a deletion of a "C" at position 5908 that destroys a Sau3A1 recognition site. Thus, in haplotype [A] homozygotes, a 115-bp PCR fragment is seen on agarose gels. A 116nt fragment is also seen in compound heterozygotes who carry another ATM mutation as well.

encompass 55 percent of Iranian families, and five mutations that encompass > 25 percent of Turkish patients. In the United Kingdom, 11 mutations represent 73 percent of mutations found in A-T patients.[289] In Japan, only two mutations encompass ~50 percent of patients. Founder-effect mutations are also being identified among Hispanic A-T patients by comparing over 100 families from Spain, Brazil, Mexico, Argentina, and Puerto Rico to those of Costa Rica and the United States.

Correlating Phenotypes with Genotypes

Correlating phenotypes with genotypes requires that the mutations of a large number of patients first be defined. Because most nonconsanguineous A-T patients have two distinct mutations, such studies further require that both mutations be defined before the symptoms can be compared. Another major caveat for this aspect of A-T research is that although most patients have two stable forms of mutated ATM mRNA in LCLs and PBLs, as demonstrated by the extensive analyses with RNA-based assays, cells from most patients do not appear to contain any stable ATM protein — even when small deletions occur. This makes it somewhat difficult to conceptualize how specific mutations will affect phenotypes.

Nonetheless, 14 families from the British Midlands were described with "late-onset ataxia" and intermediate radiosensitivity.[219,239] They share a common chromosome 11q23.1 haplotype ("418") that was identified during the positional cloning studies and before the shared phenotype was appreciated. The report describes a very interesting 137-bp insertion into the mRNA (a new exon!) coupled with a point mutation that enhances the

efficiency of an abnormal ("cryptic") splice site (see Fig. 15-14). Each patient has a different second mutation, and this has not been defined in all cases. This subset of families could provide interesting insights about phenotype-genotype relationships; however, the "late-onset ataxia" data are not convincingly homogeneous, given in Table 1 of that report[239] as years 8, 3, 3, 3, 5, 2, 2.5, 2.5, 1.8, 12, and 1.5. Considering that the average age at onset is characteristically between 1 and 3 years, only 4 of the 12 patients would qualify as "late-onset". Furthermore, we have a family with three affected siblings who are heterozygous for the same "418" mutation; their ages at onset were 8 months, 18 months, and 3 years. Thus, it is difficult to draw any convincing phenotype/genotype correlations with such mutations unless a substantial number of patients can be identified who are homozygous for that mutation. the McConville et al.[239] report lacks a single patient who is homozygous for this mutation. On the other hand, the author's suggestion that a small subset of patients may exist with two "mild" ATM mutations that do not lead to clinically obvious A-T deserves further study.

In collaboration with Sanal and coworkers (unpublished), we have studied a family in which all four sibs are affected with A-T. Because the parents are first cousins, the children are homozygous for their mutation at 6199del9, which deletes three amino acids at codons 2067–2069, well before the region of strongest homology with PI3-K (see Fig. 15-12). Table 15-4 describes the partial phenotypes of these four sibs and gives a preview of phenotype-genotype analyses. Note that this mutation is not associated with infections or immunodeficiencies in this family. The same mutation has not been seen in any other family to date.

Table 15-3 ATM Mutations in Ethnic Populations

Ethnicity	Mutation	Frequency (%)	Rapid assay
Costa Rica			
[A]	5908C≥T	56	Yes
[B]	IVS63del17 kb	7	Yes
[C]	7449G > A(del70)	12	Yes
[D]	4507C > T	12	Yes
[E]	8264del5	4	Yes
[F]	1120C > T	2	Yes
Poland			
[A]	IVS53-2A > C(del 159)	9	Yes
[B]	6095G > A(del89)	7	Yes
[C]	7010delGT	4.5	Yes
[D]	5932G > T(del88)	4.5*	Yes
[E]	5546gelT	4.5	—
Italy			
[A]	7517del4	20	Yes
[B]	3576G > A	7	—
[S1]	3894insT	Sardinia (>95%)	Yes
[S2]		Sardinia (<5%)	—
United Kingdom†			
[FM1-11]		73	—
[FM7]	5762ins137	18‡	Yes
[FM10]	7636del9	15§	Yes
North African Jews¶	103C > T	>99	Yes
Amish	1563delAG	>99	Yes
Utah Mormon			
[1]	IVS32-12A > G	—	—
[2]	8494C > T	—	—
[3]	IVS62 + 1G > A	—	—
African American			
[1]	IVS16-10T > G	—	—
[2]	2810insCTAG	—	—
[3]	7327C > T	—	—
[4]	7926A > C	—	—
Japan			
[A]	7883del5	25	Yes
[B]	IVS33 + 2T > C	25	—
Norway			
[A]	3245ATC > TGAT	55	Yes
Turkey	5 mutations	31	—
Iran	4 mutations	55	—
Brazil	4 mutations	60	—
Argentina	2 mutations	25	—
Spain	2 mutations	23	—
Amer-Hispanic	2 mutation	15	—

*Also found in Mennonites.
†Based on reference 289
‡Milder phenotype?
§Widely disseminated
¶Based on Reference 291

Table 15-4 Phenotypes of Four Consanguineous Hemozygous Affected Siblings with Mutation 6199del9 [deleted codons 2067–2069 (haplotypes in parentheses)]

	Sib 1	Sib 2	Sib 3	Sib 4
	(AC)	(AC)	(AC)	(AC)
Ataxia onset (year)	1	2.5	2	0.5
Walked unaided until (year)	7	7	9	7
Telangiectasia onset (year)	4	4	2.5	4
Dysarthria onset (year)	2	2.5	2.5	3
Gray hairs	0	0	0	0
Frequent infections	0	0	0	0
Serum immunoglobulins	N	N	N	N
α-fetoprotein (ng/ml)	54	30	16	—

Epilogue

Each of the first eight A-T workshops has painstakingly brought us a little closer to understanding this complex disorder. Summaries were published for most of the workshops,[240–244,292,332] and books were published based on the first,[245] second,[246] fifth,[247] and sixth[248] workshops. The recorded comments and discussions that followed the presentations at the 1984 workshop (ATW2) are still very pertinent to much of today's research.[246]

In 1981 (ATW1), a better phenotype was described in preparation for linkage studies. In 1984 (ATW2), the neurodegenerative nature of A-T was clarified by the presence of basket cell "footprints,"[7,8] and plans for positional cloning continued. By 1987 (ATW3), as part of that approach, many key families around the world had been assigned to complementation groups, primarily through the work of Jaspers and coworkers.[150,151] In 1989 (ATW4), formal presentations and confirmations were made regarding the localization of an A-T gene to chromosome 11q22-23.[152] A higher-resolution map of distal chromosome 11 was already under way,[209,248] taking advantage of the burgeoning new genome projects around the world, such as the CEPH linkage mapping consortium in Paris.[203] However, at that time, most investigators felt that the A-T gene would be cloned not by the slower positional cloning approach but by more direct transfection and complementation experiments. Indeed, a candidate A-T gene (ATDC) isolated by this method was much discussed at ATW5 (1992).[249,250] It was already becoming clear, however, that ATDC was not the true gene, and complementational cloning was potentially misleading. The ATW6 (1994) workshop confirmed both of these conclusions, for by then 26 cDNA clones had been found to complement RDS, radiomimetic sensitivity, or both, but none localized to 11q22-23.[6,63,154,244]

In 1995, the gene was cloned purely by positional cloning.[72] A scientific logjam was broken! Many new investigators entered the field of A-T research to make antibodies, to construct full-length cDNAs, and to develop functional assays. Once again, however, from what was to have been the pinnacle, many new peaks were sighted. ATW7 addressed new mutations, the failure of many investigators to find an increase in the frequency of ATM mutations in breast cancer patients, the pathology of the knockout mice, the molecules with which the ATM protein interacts, and the recent cloning of the NBS1 gene.[202] ATW8[332] brought together >200 scientists to review the many complex facets of A-T biology, as well as to establish the validity of using p53 phosphorylation at serine 15 as a functional and specific assay for the ATM protein. Three major stumbling blocks still have to be addressed: (a) the lack of a progressive ataxia in the knockout mice, which almost negates this model for unraveling the neuropathology of A-T; (b) the lack of sufficient amounts of purified ATM protein for functional and structural studies; and (c) an effective therapeutic approach.

Another report suggests that patients who have *some* ATM protein in their cell lysates may have milder or variant phenotypes.[294] This remains to be confirmed and depends to some extent on the ability of a laboratory to reliably quanititate the protein levels. In our hands, 81 percent of classic A-T patients (101 of 124) do not have any measurable protein; in the remaining <19 percent, the protein level is present but almost always reduced.[295]

ACKNOWLEDGMENTS

This chapter is dedicated to Drs. Elena Boder and Robert Sedgwick, both of whom died in 1995 knowing that the ATM gene had finally been cloned. Almost 40 years had elapsed since their seminal observations and descriptions of the A-T syndrome. I thank them for having provided me with almost 30 years of enlightenment on A-T, their encouragement to persevere in the linkage studies, and their insights and efforts in identifying new families for our research.

The positional cloning project was initiated with funding from three major grants between 1984 and 1986 from the Ataxia-Telangiectasia Medical Research Foundation: to Richard Gatti (Los Angeles), to Yosef Shiloh (Tel Aviv), and to N. J. G Jaspers (Rotterdam). For additional support we thank the Department of Energy (ER60548) (1987 to 1999), the American Cancer Society (CD-328), the National Cancer Institute (CA16042), the North Atlantic Treaty Organization (ARW920385), the Ataxia-Telangiectasia Medical Trust-UK, the Ataxia-Telangiectasia Children's Project, the Joseph Drown Foundation, the Andrew Norman Foundation, the Eric Lightner Memorial Fund, and the Harry Ringel Foundation. We acknowledge Ken Lange and his four generations of graduate students in biomathematics for devising new analytic approaches in response to each obstacle we encountered, which ensured constant progress in the positional cloning of the gene. Last and most important, the A-T patients, their families, and the referring immunologists and neurologists must be acknowledged for their continuing cooperation in innumerable blood drawings, skin biopsies, and clinical discussions.

REFERENCES

1. Boder E, Sedgwick RP: Ataxia-telangiectasia: A familial syndrome of progressive cerebellar ataxia, oculocutaneous telangiectasia and frequent pulmonary infection. *Pediatrics* **21**:526, 1958.
2. Sedgwick RP, Boder E: Ataxia-telangiectasia, in Vinken PJ, Bruyn GW (eds): *Handbook of Clinical Neurology*, vol. 14. Amsterdam, North-Holland, 1972, pp 267–339.
3. Boder E: Ataxia-telangi: ectasia: An overview, in Gatti RA, Swift M (eds): *Ataxia-Telangiectasia: Genetics, Neuropathology, and Immunology of a Degenerative Disease of Childhood*. New York, Liss, 1985, pp 1–63.
4. Gatti RA, Boder E, Vinters HV, Sparkes RS, Norman A, Lange K: Ataxia-telangiectasia: An interdisciplinary approach to pathogenesis. *Medicine* **70**:99, 1991.
5. Sedgwick RP, Boder E: Ataxia-telangiectasia, in de Jong JMBV (ed): *Handbook of Clinical Neurology*, vol. 16, *Hereditary Neuropathies and Spinocerebellar Atrophies*. Amsterdam, Elsevier, 1991, pp 347–423.
6. Shiloh Y: Ataxia-telangiectasia: Closer to unraveling the mystery. *Eur J Hum Genet* **3**:116, 1995.
7. Gatti RA, Vinters HV: Cerebellar pathology in ataxia-telangiectasia, in Gatti RA, Swift M (eds): *Ataxia-Telangiectasia: Genetics, Neuropathology, and Immunology of a Degenerative Disease of Childhood*. New York, Liss, 1985, pp 225–232.
8. Vinters HV, Gatti RA, Rakic P: Sequence of cellular events in cerebellar ontogeny relevant to expression of neuronal abnormalities in ataxia-telangiectasia, in Gatti RA, Swift M (eds): *Ataxia-Telangiectasia: Genetics, Neuropathology, and Immunology of a Degenerative Disease of Childhood*. New York, Liss, 1985, pp 233–255.
9. Aguilar MJ, Kamoshita S, Landing BH, Boder E, Sedgwick RP: Pathological observations in ataxia-telangiectasia: A report on 5 cases. *J Neuropathol Exp Neurol* **27**:659, 1968.
10. Naeim A, Repinski C, Huo Y, Hong J-H, Chessa L, Naeim F, Gatti RA: Ataxia-telangiectasia: Flow cytometric cell cycle analysis of lymphoblastoid cell lines in G2/M before and after gamma-irradiation. *Mod Pathol* **7**:587, 1994.
11. Van Meir EG, Polverini PJ, Chazin VR, Su Huang H-J, de Tribolet N, Cavenee WK: Release of an inhibitor of angiogenesis upon induction of wild-type p53 expression in glioblastoma cells. *Nat Genet* **8**:171, 1994.
12. Peterson RD, Kelly WD, Good RA: Ataxia-telangiectasia: Its association with a defective thymus, immunological-deficiency disease, and malignancy. *Lancet* **1**:1189, 1964.
13. Centerwall WR, Miller MM: Ataxia-telangiectasia and sinopulmonary infections: A syndrome of slowly progressive deterioration in childhood. *Am J Dis Child* **95**:385, 1958.
13a. Sourander P, Bonnevier JO, Olsson Y: A case of ataxia-telangiectasia with lesions in the spinal cord. *Acta Neurol Scand* **42**:354, 1966.
14. Thieffry S, Arthuis M, Farkas-Barceton E, Vinh LeT: L'ataxia-telangiectasia: Une observation anatomo-clinique familiale. *Ann Pediatr* **13**:749, 1966.
15. Amromin GD, Boder E, Teplitz R: Ataxia-telangiectasia with a 32-year survival: A clinicopathological report. *J Neuropathol Exp Neurol* **38**:621, 1979.
16. Barlow C, Hirotsune S, Paylor R, Liyanage M, Eckhaus M, Collins F, Shiloh Y, Crawley JN, Tied T, Tagle D, Wynshaw-Boris A: Atm-deficient mice: A paradigm of ataxia-telangiectasia. *Cell* **86**:159, 1996.
17. Gotoff SP, Aminmokri E, Liebner EJ: Ataxia-telangiectasia. Neoplasia, untoward response to x-irradiation, and tuberous sclerosis. *Am J Dis Child* **114**:617, 1967.
18. Morgan JL, Holcomb TM, Morrissey RW: Radiation reaction in ataxia-telangiectasia. *Am J Dis Child* **116**:557, 1968.
19. Cunliffe PN, Mann JR, Cameron AH, Roberts KD, Ward HWC: Radiosensitivity in ataxia-telangiectasia. *Br J Radiol* **48**:374, 1975.
20. Abadir R, Hakami N: Ataxia-telangiectasia with cancer. An indication for reduced radiotherapy and chemotherapy does. *Br J Radiol* **56**:343, 1983.
21. Hart RM, Kimler BR, Evans RG, Park CH: Radiotherapeutic management of medulloblastoma in a pediatric patient with ataxia-telangiectasia. *Int J Radiat Oncol Biol Phys* **13**:1237, 1987.
22. Taylor AMR, Harnden DG, Arlett CF, Harcourt SA, Lehmann AR, Stevens S, Bridges BA: Ataxia-telangiectasia: A human mutation with abnormal radiation sensitivity. *Nature* **258**:427, 1975.
23. Shiloh Y, Tabor E, Becker Y: In vitro phenotype of ataxia-telangiectasia fibroblast strains: Clues to the nature of the "AT DNA lesion" and the molecular defect in AT, in Gatti RA, Swift M (eds): *Ataxia-telangiectasia: Genetics, Neuropathology, and Immunology of a Degenerative Disease of Childhood*. New York, Liss, 1985, pp 111–121.
24. Shiloh Y, Tabor E, Becker Y: The response of ataxia-telangiectasia homozygous and heterozygous skin fibroblasts to neocarzinostatin. *Carcinogenesis* **3**:815, 1982.
25. Paterson MC, Mac Farlane SJ, Gentner NE, Smith BP: Cellular hypersensitivity to chronic gamma-radiation in cultured fibroblasts from ataxia-telangiectasia heterozygotes, in Gatti RA, Swift M (eds): *Ataxia-Telangiectasia: Genetics, Neuropathology, and Immunology of a Degenerative Disease of Childhood*. New York, Liss, 1985, pp 73–87.
26. Weeks DE, Paterson MC, Lange K, Andrais B, Davis RC, Yoder F, Gatti RA: Assessment of chronic gamma radiosensitivity as an in vitro assay for heterozygote identification of ataxia-telangiectasia. *Radiation Res* **128**:90, 1991.
27. Parshad R, Sanford KK, Jones GM, Tarone RE: G2 chromosomal radiosensitivity of ataxia-telangiectasia heterozygotes. *Cancer Genet Cytogenet* **14**:163, 1985.
28. Parshad R, Sanford KK, Jones GM: Chromosomal radiosensitivity during the G2 cell cycle period of skin fibroblasts from individuals with familial cancer. *Proc Natl Acad Sci USA* **82**:5400, 1985.
29. Shiloh Y, Parshad R, Frydman M, Sanford KK, Portnoi S, Ziv Y, Jones GM: G2 chromosomal radiosensitivity in families with ataxia-telangiectasia. *Hum Genet* **84**:15, 1989.
30. Rosin MP, Ochs HD, Gatti RA, Boder E: Heterogeneity of chromosomal breakage levels in epithelial tissue of ataxia-telangiectasia homozygotes and heterozygotes. *Hum Genet* **83**:133, 1989.
31. Scott D, Jones LA, Elyan SAG, Spreadborough A, Cown R, Ribiero G: Identification of A-T heterozygotes, in Gatti RA, Painter RB (eds): *Ataxia-Telangiectasia*. Heidelberg, Springer-Verlag, 1993, pp 101–116.
32. Swift A, Morrell D, Massey RB, Chase CL: Incidence of cancer in 161 families affected by ataxia-telangiectasia. *N Engl J Med* **325**:1831, 1991.
33. Norman A, Kagan AR, Chan SL: The importance of genetics for the optimization of radiation therapy. *Am J Clin Oncol* **11**:84, 1988.
34. Norman A, Withers R: Recommendation about radiation exposure for A-T heterozygotes in Gatti RA, Painter RB (eds): *Ataxia-Telangiectasia*. Heidelberg, Springer-Verlag, 1993, pp 137–142.
35. Law J: Patient dose and risk in mammography. *Brit J Radiol* **64**:360, 1991.

36. Peterson RDA, Funkhouser JD, Tuck-Miller CM, Gatti RA: Cancer susceptibility in ataxia-telangiectasia, in *Leukemia*. New York, Macmillan, 1992, pp 8–13.

37. Swift M, Sholman L, Perry M, Chase C: Malignant neoplasms in the families of patients with ataxia-telangiectasia. *Cancer Res* **36**:209, 1976.

38. Rotman G, Shloh Y: The ATM gene and protein: Possible roles in genome surveillance, checkpoint controls and cellular defense against oxidative stree. *Cancer Surv* **29**:285, 1997.

39. Painter R: Altered DNA synthesis in irradiated and unirradiated ataxia-telangiectasia cells, in Gatti RA, Swift M (eds): *Ataxia-Telangiectasia: Genetics, Neuropathology, and Immunology of a Degenerative Disease of Childhood*. New York, Liss, 1985, pp 89–100.

40. Meyn MS: Ataxia-telangiectasia and cellular responses to DNA damage. *Cancer Res* **55**:5991, 1995.

41. Morrell D, Cromartie E, Swift M: Mortality and cancer incidence in 263 patients with ataxia-telangiectasia. *J Natl Cancer Inst* **77**:89, 1986.

42. Spector BD, Filipovich AH, Perry GS, Kersey JH: Epidemiology of cancer in ataxia-telangiectasia, in Bridges BA, Harnden DG (eds): *Ataxia-Telangiectasia: Cellular and Molecular Link between Cancer, Neuropathology and Immune Deficiency*. New York, Wiley, 1982, pp 103–107.

43. Hecht F, Koler RD, Rigas DA, Dahnke G, Case M, Tisdale V, Miller RW: Leukaemia and lymphocytes in ataxia-telangiectasia. *Lancet* **2**:1193, 1966.

44. Gatti RA, Good RA: Occurrence of malignancy in immunodeficiency diseases. *Cancer* **28**:89, 1971.

45. Taylor AMR, Metcalfe JA, Thick J, Mak Y-F: Leukemia and lymphoma in ataxia-telangiectasia. *Blood* **87**:423, 1996.

46. Foon KA, Gale RP: Is there a T-cell form of chronic lymphocytic leukaemia? *Leukemia* **6**:867, 1992.

47. Hollis RJ, Kennaugh AA, Butterworth SV, Taylor AMR: Growth of chromosomally abnormal T cell clones in ataxia-telangiectasia patients is associated with translocation at 14q11 — a model for other T cell neoplasia. *Hum Genet* **76**:389, 1987.

48. Russo G, Isobe M, Gatti RA, Finan J, Batuman O, Huebner K, Nowell PC, Croce CM: Molecular analysis of a t(14;14) translocation in leukemic T-cells of an ataxia-telangiectasia patient. *Proc Natl Acad Sci USA* **86**:602, 1989.

49. Davey MP, Bertness V, Nakahara K, Johnson JP, McBride OW, Waldmann TA, Kirsch IR: Juxtaposition of the T-cell receptor alpha-chain locus (14q11) and a region (14q32) of potential importance in leukemogenesis by a 14;14 translocation in a patients with T-cell chronic lymphocytic leukemia and ataxia-telangiectasia. *Proc Natl Acad Sci USA* **85**:9287, 1988.

50. Gatti RA, Nieberg R, Boder E: Uterine tumors in ataxia-telangiectasia. *Gynecol Oncol* **32**:257, 1989.

51. Pippard EC, Hall AJ, Baker DJP, Bridges BA: Cancer in homozygotes and heterozygotes of ataxia-telangiectasia and xeroderma pigmentosum in Britain. *Cancer Res* **48**:2929, 1988.

52. Swift M, Reitnauer PJ, Morrell D, Chase CL: Breast and other cancers in families with ataxia-telangiectasia. *N Engl J Med* **316**:1289, 1987.

53. Borresen A-L, Andersen TI, Tretli S, Heiberg A, Moller P: Breast cancer and other cancers in Norwegian families with ataxia-telangiectasia. *Genes Chrom Cancer* **2**:339, 1990.

54. Vorechovsky I, Rasio D, Luo L, Monaco C, Hammarstrom L, Webster DB, Zaloudik J, Barbanti-Brodano G, James M, Russo G, Croce CM, Negrini M: The ATM gene and susceptibility to breast cancer: Analysis of 38 breast tumors reveals no evidence for mutation. *Cancer Res* **56**:2726, 1996.

55. FitzGerald MG, Bean JM, Hegde SR, Unsal H, MacDonald DJ, Harkin DP, Finkelstein DM, Isselbacher KJ, Haber DA: Heterozygous ATM mutations do not contribute to early onset of breast cancer. *Nat Genet* **15**:307, 1997.

56. Spurr NK, Kelsell CP, Mavrakis E, Bryant SP, Crockford G, Bishop DT: Genetic heterogeneity in UK breast and ovarian cancer families. *Am J Hum Genet* **S57**:A5, 1995.

57. Cortessis V, Ingles S, Millikan R, Diep A, Gatti RA, Richardson L, Thompson WD, Paganini-Hill A, Sparkes RS, Haile RW: Linkage analysis of DRD2, a marker linked to the ataxia-telangiectasia gene, in 64 families with premenopausal bilateral breast cancer. *Cancer Res* **53**:5083, 1993.

58. Wooster R, Easton DF, Ford D, Mangion J, Ponder BAJ, Peto J, Stratton M: The A-T gene does not make a major contribution to familial breast cancer, in Gatti RA, Painter RB (eds): *Ataxia-Telangiectasia*. Heidelberg, Springer-Verlag, 1993, pp 127–136.

59. Athma P, Rappaport R, Swift M: Molecular genotyping shows that ataxia-telangiectasia heterozygotes are predisposed to breast cancer. *Cancer Genet Cytogenet* **92**:130, 1996.

60. Carter SL, Negrini M, Baffa R, Illum DR, Rosenberg AL, Schwartz GF, Croce CM: Loss of heterozygosity at 11q22-23 in breast cancer. *Cancer Res* **54**:6270, 1994.

61. Porras O, Arguendas O, Arata M, Barrantes M, Gonzalez L, Saenz E: Epidemiology of ataxia-telangiectasia in Costa Rica, in Gatti RA, Painter RB (eds): *Ataxia-Telangiectasia*. Heidelberg, Springer-Verlag, 1993, pp 199–208.

62. Chessa L, Fiorilli M: Epidemiology of ataxia-telangiectasia in Italy, in Gatti RA, Painter RB (eds): *Ataxia-Telangiectasia*. Heidelberg: Springer-Verlag, 1993, pp 191–198.

63. Lohrer HD: Regulation of the cell cycle following DNA damage in normal and ataxia-telangiectasia cells. *Experentia* **52**:316, 1996.

64. Hartwell LH, Weinert TA: Checkpoints: Controls that ensure the order of cell cycle events. *Science* **246**:629, 1989.

65. Kastan MB, Zhan Q, El-Deiry WS, Carrier F, Jacks Y, Walsh WV, Plunkett BS, Vogelstein B, Fornace AJ: A mammalian cell cycle checkpoint pathway utilizing p53 and GADD45 is defective in ataxia-telangiectasia. *Cell* **71**:587, 1992.

66. Kastan MB: Ataxia-telangiectasia: defective in a p53-dependent signal transduction pathway, in Gatti RA, Painter RB (eds): *Ataxia-Telangiectasia*. Heidelberg, Springer-Verlag, 1993, pp 163–173.

67. Donehower LA, Harvey M, Stagle BL, McArthur MJ, Montgomery CA, Butel JS, Bradley A: Mice deficient for p53 are developmentally normal but susceptible to spontaneous tumors. *Nature* **356**:215, 1992.

68. Purdie CA, Harrison DJ, Peter A, Dobbie L, White S, Howie SE, Salter DM, Bird CC, Wyllie AH, Hooper ML: Tumour incidence, spectrum and ploidy in mice with a large deletion in the p53 gene. *Oncogene* **9**:603, 1994.

69. Liu VF, Weaver DT: The ionizing radiation-induced replication protein A phosphorylation response differs between ataxia-telangiectasia and normal human cells. *Mol Cell Biol* **13**:7222, 1993.

70. Shafman T, Khanna KK, Kedar P, Spring K, Kozlov S, Yen T, Hobson K, Gatei M, Zhang N, Watters D, Egerton M, Shiloh Y, Kharbanda S, Kufe D, Lavin MF: Interaction between ATM protein and c-Abl in response to DNA damage. *Nature* **387**:520, 1997.

71. Lavin MF, Khanna KK, Beamish H, Spring K, Watters D, Shiloh Y: Relationship of the ataxia-telangiectasia protein ATM to phosphoinositide 3-kinase. *Trends Biol Sci* **20**:382, 1995.

72. Savisky K, Bar-Shira A, Gilad S, Rotman G, Ziv Y, Vanagaite L, Tagle DA, Smith S, Uziel T, Sfez S, Ashkenazi M, Pecker I, Frydman M, Harnik R, Patanjali SR, Simmons A, Clines GA, Sartiel A, Gatti RA, Chessa L, Sanal O, Lavin MF, Jaspers NGJ, Taylor MR, Arlett CF, Miki T, Weissman SM, Lovett M, Collins FS, Shiloh Y: A single ataxia-telangiectasia gene with a product similar to PI-3 kinase. *Science* **268**:1749, 1995.

73. Nowak R: Discovery of AT gene sparks biomedical research bonanza. *Science* **268**:1700, 1995.

74. Hartwell LH, Kastan MB: Cell cycle control and cancer. *Science* **266**:1821, 1994.

75. Vogelstein B: A deadly inheritance. *Nature* **348**:681, 1990.

76. Meyn MS, Strasfeld L, Allen C: Testing the role of p53 in the expression of genetic instability and apoptosis in ataxia-telangiectasia. *Int J Radiat Biol* **66**:S141, 1994.

77. Lowe SW, Ruley HE, Jacks T, Housman DE: P53-dependent apoptosis modulates the cytotoxicity of anticancer agents. *Cell* **74**:957, 1993.

78. Lee JM, Bernstein A: P53 mutations increase resistance to ionizing radiation. *Proc Natl Acad Sci USA* **90**:5742, 1993.

79. Jung M, Zhang Y, Dritschilo A: Correction of radiation sensitivity in ataxia-telangiectasia cells by a truncated IkB-α. *Science* **268**:1619, 1995.

80. Jung M, Kondratyev A, Lee SA, Dimtchev A, Dritschilo A: ATM gene product phosphorylates IkB-α. *Canc Res* **57**:24, 1997.

81. Thanos D, Maniatis T: NF-kB: A lesson in family values. *Cell* **80**:529, 1995.

82. Painter RB, Young BR: Radiosensitivity in ataxia-telangiectasia: A new explanation. *Proc Natl Acad Sci USA* **77**:7315, 1980.

83. Thacker J: Cellular radiosensitivity in ataxia-telangiectasia. *Int J Radiat Biol* **66**:S87, 1994.

84. Vorechovsky I, Luo L, Dyer MJS, Catovsky D, Amlot PL, Yaxley JC, Foroni L, Hammarstrom L, Webster DB, Yuille MAR: Clustering of missense mutations in the ataxia-telangiectasia gene in a sporadic T-cell leukaemia. *Nat Genet* **17**:96, 1997.

85. Painter RB: Inhibition of mammalian cell DNA synthesis by ionizing radiation. *Int J Radiat Biol* **49**:771, 1986.

86. Painter RB: Radiobiology of ataxia-telangiectasia, in Gatti RA, Painter RB (eds): *Ataxia-Telangiectasia*. Heidelberg, Springer-Verlag, 1993, pp 257–268.

87. Hand R, Gautschi JR: Replication of mammalian DNA in vitro: Evidence for initiation from fiber autoradiography. *J Cell Biol* **82**:485, 1979.

88. Gatti RA, Bick MB, Tam CF, Medici MA, Oxelius V-A, Holland M, Goldstein AL, Boder E: Ataxia-telangiectasia: A multiparameter analysis of eight families. *Clin Immunol Immunopathol* **23**:501, 1982.

89. Woods CG, Taylor AMR: Ataxia-telangiectasia in the British Isles: The clinical and laboratory features of 70 affected individuals. *Q J Med New Series* **298**:169, 1992.

90. Gatti RA: Ataxia-telangiectasia: A neuroendocrine-immune disease? Alternative models of pathogenesis, in Fabris N, Garaci E, Hadden J, Mitchison, NA (eds): *Immunoregulation*. New York, Plenum, 1983, pp 385–398.

91. Thieffry S, Arthuis M, Aicardi J, Lyon G: L'ataxie-telangiectasie. *Rev Neurol* **105**:390, 1961.

92. Oxelius V-A, Berkel AI, Hanson LA: IgG2 deficiency in ataxia-telangiectasia. *N Engl J Med* **306**:515, 1982.

93. Rivat-Peran L. Buriot D, Salier J-P, Rivat C, Dumitresco S-M, Griscelli C: Immunoglobulins in ataxia-telangiectasia: Evidence for IgG4 and IgA2 subclass deficiencies. *Clin Immunol Immunopathol* **20**:99, 1981.

94. Ammann AJ, Cain WA, Ishizaka K, Hong R, Good RA: Immunoglobulin E deficiency in ataxia-telangiectasia. *N Engl J Med* **281**:469, 1969.

95. Polmar SH, Waldmann TA, Balestra ST, Jost M, Terry WD: Immunoglobulin E in immunologic deficiency disease. *J Clin Invest* **51**:326, 1972.

96. Hsieh C-L, Lieber MR: Lymphoid V(D)J recombination: Accessibility and reaction fidelity in normal and ataxia-telangiectasia cells, in Gatti RA, Painter RB (eds): *Ataxia-Telangiectasia*. Heidelberg, Springer-Verlag, 1993, pp 143–154.

97. Hsieh CL, Arlett CF, Lieber MR: V(D)J recombination in ataxia-telangiectasia, Bloom's syndrome and a DNA ligase I-associated immunodeficiency disorder. *J Biol Chem* **268**:20105, 1993.

98. Kirsch IR: V(D)J recombination and ataxia-telangiectasia: A review. *Int J Radiat Biol* **66**:S97, 1994.

99. Paganelli R, Scala E, Scarselli E, Ortolani C, Cossarizza A, Carmini D, Aiuti F, Fiorilli M: Selective deficiency of CD41/CD45RA1 lymphocytes in patients with ataxia-telangiectasia. *J Clin Immunol* **12**:84, 1992.

100. Eisen AH: Delayed hypersensitivity in ataxia-telangiectasia. *N Engl J Med* **272**:801, 1965.

101. Oppenheim JJ, Barlow M, Waldmann TA, Block JB: Impaired in vitro lymphocyte transformation in patients with ataxia-telangiectasia. *Br Med J* **2**:330, 1966.

102. Leiken SI, Bazelon M, Park KH: In vitro lymphocyte transformation in ataxia-telangiectasia. *J Pediatr* **68**:477, 1966.

103. Epstein WL, Fudenberg HH, Reed WB, Boder E, Sedggwick RP: Immunologic studies in ataxia-telangiectasia. *Int Arch Allergy* **30**:15, 1966.

104. Hosking G: Ataxia telangiectasia. *Dev Med Child Neurol* **24**:77, 1982.

105. Waldmann TA, Misiti J, Nelson DL, Kraemer KH: Ataxia-telangiectasia: A multisystem hereditary disease with immunodeficiency, impaired organ maturation, x-ray hypersensitivity, and a high incidence of neoplasia. *Ann Intern Med* **99**:367, 1983.

106. Nelson DL, Biddison WE, Shaw S: Defective in vitro production of influenza virus-specific cytotoxic T lymphocytes in ataxia-telangiectasia. *J Immunol* **130**:2629, 1983.

107. Weaver M, Gatti RA: Lymphocyte subpopulations in ataxia-telangiectasia, in Gatti RA, Swift M (eds): *Ataxia-Telangiectasia: Genetics, Neuropathology, and Immunology of a Degenerative Disease of Childhood*. New York, Liss, 1985, pp 309–314.

108. Peter HH: The origin of human NK cells: An ontogenic model derived from studies in patients with immunodeficiencies. *Blut* **46**:239, 1983.

109. Sanal O, Ersoy F, Tezcan I, Gogus S: Ataxia-telangiectasia presenting as hyper IgM syndrome, in Chapel HM, Levinsky JR, Webster ADB (eds): *Progress in Immune Deficiency*, vol III. London, Royal Society of Medicine, 1991.

110. Thiele EA, Bonilla F, Rosen F, Riviello JI: Ataxia telangiectasia associated with the hyper-IgM syndrome. San Francisco, International Neurology Conference, Sept. 9–11, 1994.

111. Huo YK, Wang Z, Hong J-H, Chessa L, McBride WH, Perlman SL, Gatti RA: Radiosensitivity of ataxia-telangiectasia X-linked agammaglobulinemia and related syndromes. *Cancer Res* **54**:2544, 1994.

112. McFarlin DE, Strober W, Waldmann TA: Ataxia-telangiectasia. *Medicine* **51**:281, 1972.

113. Waldmann TA, McIntire KR: Serum alpha-fetoprotein levels in patients with ataxia-telangiectasia. *Lancet* **2**:112, 1972.

114. Yamashita T, Nakane A, Watanabe T, Miyoshi I, Kasai M: Evidence that alpha-fetoprotein suppresses the immunological function in transgenic mice. *Biochem Biophy Res Commun* **201**:1154, 1994.

115. Ishiguro T, Taketa K, Gatti RA: Tissue of origin of elevated alpha-fetoprotein in ataxia-telangiectasia. *Dis Markers* **4**:293, 1986.

116. Gatti RA, Aurias A, Griscelli C, Sparkes RS: Translocations involving chromosomes 2p and 22q in ataxia-telangiectasia. *Dis Markers* **3**:169, 1985.

117. Kojis TL, Gatti RA, Sparkes RS: The cytogenetics of ataxia-telangiectasia. *Cancer Genet Cytogenet* **56**:143, 1992.

118. Kojis TL, Schreck RR, Gatti RA, Sparkes RS: Tissue specificity of chromosomal rearrangements in ataxia-telangiectasia. *Hum Genet* **83**:337, 1989.

119. Hecht F, Hecht BK: Ataxia-telangiectasia breakpoints in chromosome rearrangements reflect genes important to T and B lymphocytes, in Gatti RA, Swift M (eds): *Ataxia-Telangiectasia: Genetics, Neuropathology, and Immunology of a Degenerative Disease of Childhood*. New York, Liss, 1985, pp 189–195.

120. Hecht F, McCaw BK, Koler RD: Ataxia-telangiectasia—Clonal growth of translocation lymphocytes. *N Engl J Med* **289**:286, 1972.

121. Berkel AI: Studies of IgG subclasses in ataxia-telangiectasia patients. *Monogr Allergy* **29**:100, 1986.

122. Roifman CM, Gelfand EW: Heterogeneity of the immunological deficiency in ataxia-telangiectasia: Absence of a clinical-pathological correlation, in Gatti RA, Swift M (eds): *Ataxia-Telangiectasia: Genetics, Neuropathology, and Immunology of a Degenerative Disease of Childhood*. New York, Liss, 1985, pp 273–285.

123. Virgilio L, Narducci MG, Isobe M, Billips LG, Cooper MD, Croce CM, Russo G: Identification of the TCL1 gene involved in T cell malignancies. *Proc Natl Acad Sci USA* **91**:12530, 1994.

124. Taylor AMR, Lowe PA, Stacey M, Thick J, Campbell L, Beatty D, Biggs P, Formstone CJ: Development of T cell leukaemia in an ataxia-telangiectasia patient following clonal selection in t(X;14) containing lymphocytes. *Leukemia* **6**:961, 1992.

125. Kenwrick S, Llevinson B, Taylor S, Shapiro A, Gitschier J: Isolation and sequence of two genes associated with a CpG island 59 of the factor VIII gene. *Hum Mol Genet* **1**:179, 1992.

126. Soulier J, Madni A, Cacheux V, Rosenwajg M, Sigaux F, Stern M-H: The MTCP-1/c6-1B gene encodes for a cytoplasmic 8kd protein overexpressed in T cell leukaemia bearing a t(X;14) translocation. *Oncogene* **9**:3565, 1994.

127. Madani A, Soulier J, Schmid M, Plichtova R, Lerme F, Gateau-Roesch O, Garnier J-P, Pla M, Sigaux F, Stern M-H: The 8 kd protein of the putative oncogene MTCP-1 is a mitochondrial protein. *Oncogene* **10**:2259, 1995.

128. Fu T, Virgilio L, Narducci MG, Facciano A, Russo G, Croce CM: Characterisation and localisation of the TCL-1 oncogene product. *Cancer Res* **54**:6297, 1994.

129. Knudsen AG: Hereditary cancer, oncogenes, and antioncogenes. *Cancer Res* **45**:1437, 1985.

130. Pandita TK, Pathak S, Geard C: Chromosome and associations, telomeres and telomerase activity in ataxia-telangiectasia cells. *Cytogenet Cell Genet* **71**:86, 1995.

131. Moyzis RK, Buckingham JM, Cram LS, Dani M, Deaven LL, Jones MD, Meyne J, Ratliff RL, Wu J-R: A highly conserved repetitive DNA sequence (TTAGGG)n, present in the telomeres of human chromosomes. *Proc Natl Acad Sci USA* **85**:6622, 1988.

132. Kipling D, Cooke HJ: Beginning or end? Telomere structure, genetics and biology. *Hum Mol Genet* **1**:3, 1992.

133. De Lange T, Shiue L, Myers RM, Cox DR, Naylor SL, Killery AM, Varmus HE: Structure and variability of human chromosome ends. *Mol Cell Biol* **10**:518, 1990.

134. Shore D: Telomeres–Unstickky ends. *Science* **281**:1818, 1998.

135. Metcalfe JA, Parkhill J, Campbell L, Stacey M, Biggs P, Byrd PJ, Taylor AMR: Accelerated telomere shortening in ataxia-telangiectasia. *Nat Genet* **13**:350, 1996.

136. Effros RB, Allsopp R, Chiu C-P, Hausner MA, Hirji K, Wang L, Harley CB, Villeponteau B, West MD, Giorgi JV: Shortened telomeres in the expanded CD28-CD81 cell subset in HIV disease implicate replicative senescence in MIV pathogenesis. *AIDS* **10**:F17, 1996.

137. Enoch T, Norbury C: Cellular responses to DNA damage: Cell cycle checkpoints, apoptosis and the roles of p53 and ATM. *Trends Biol Sci* **20**:426, 1995.

138. Lehmann AR, Carr AM: The ataxia-telangiectasia gene: A link between checkpoint controls, neurodegeneration and cancer. *Trends Genet* **11**:375, 1995.

139. Keegan KS, Holtzmann DA, Plug AW, Christenson ER, Brainerd EE, Flaggs G, Bentley NJ, Taylor EM, Meyn MS, Moss SB, Carr AM, Ashley T, Hoekstra MF: The Atr and Atm protein kinases associate with different sites along meiotically pairing chromosomes. *Genes Dev* **10**:2423, 1996.

140. Savitsky K, Sfez S, Tagle DA, Ziv Y, Sartiel A, Collins FS, Shiloh Y, Rotman G: The complete sequence of the coding region of the ATM gene reveals similarity to cell cycle regulators in different species. *Hum Mol Genet* **4**:2025, 1995.

141. Cimprich KA, Shin TB, Keith CT, Schreiber SL: cDNA cloning and gene mapping of a candidate human cell cycle checkpoint protein. *Proc Natl Acad Sci USA* **93**:2850, 1996.

142. Al-Khodairy F, Carr AM: DNA repair mutants defining G2 checkpoint pathways in Schizosaccharomyces pombe. *EMBO J* **11**:1343, 1992.

143. Seaton BL, Yucel J, Sunnerhagen P, Subramani P: Isolation and characterization of S. pombe rad3 gene involved in the DNA damage and DNA synthesis checkpoints. *Gene* **119**:83, 1992.

144. Weinert TA, Kiser GL, Hartwell LH: Mitotic checkpoint genes in budding yeast and the dependence of mitosis on DNA replication and repair. *Genes Dev* **8**:652, 1994.

145. Paulovich AG, Hartwell LH: A checkpoint regulates the rate of progression through S phase in S. cerevisiae in response to DNA damage. *Cell* **82**:841, 1995.

146. Kato R, Ogawa H: An essential gene, ESR1, is required for mitotic cell growth, DNA repair and meiotic recombination in Saccharomyces cerevisiae. *Nucleic Acids Res* **22**:3104, 1994.

147. Sanchez Y, Desany BA, Jones WJ, Liu Q, Wang B, Elledge SJ: Regulation of RAD53 by the ATM-like kinases MEC1 and TEL1 in yeast cell cycle checkpoint pathways. *Science* **271**:357, 1996.

148. Morrow DW, Tagle DA, Shiloh Y, Collins FS, Hieter P: TEL1, an S. cerevisiae homolog of the human gene mutated in ataxia-telangiectasia, is functionally related to the yeast checkpoint gene MEC1. *Cell* **82**:831, 1995.

149. Jaspers NGJ, Bootsma D: Genetic heterogeneity in ataxia-telangiectasia studies by cell fusion. *Proc Natl Acad Sci USA* **79**:2641, 1982.

150. Jaspers NGJ, Painter RB, Paterson MC, Kidson C, Inoue T: Complementation analysis of ataxia-telangiectasia, in Gatti RA, Swift M (eds): *Ataxia-Telangiectasia: Genetics, Neuropathology, and Immunology of a Degenerative Disease of Childhood.* New York, Liss, 1985, pp 147–162.

151. Jaspers NGJ, Gatti RA, Baan C, Linssen PCML, Bootsma D: Genetic complementation analysis of ataxia-telangiectasia and Nijmegen breakage syndrome: A survey of 50 patients. *Cytogenet Cell Genet* **49**:259, 1988.

152. Gatti RA, Berkel I, Boder E, Braedt G, Charmley P, Concannon P, Ersoy F, Foroud T, Jaspers NGJ, Lange K, Lathrop GM, Leppert M, Nakamura Y, O'Connell P, Paterson M, Salser W, Sanal O, Silver J, Sparkes RS, Susi E, Weeks DE, Wei S, White R, Yoder F: Localization of an ataxia-telangiectasia gene to chromosome 11q22-23. *Nature* **336**:577, 1988.

153. Ziv Y, Rotman G, Frydman M, Dagan J, Cohen T, Foroud T, Gatti RA, Shiloh Y: The ATC (ataxia-telangiectasia Group C) locus localizes to chromosome 11q22-q23. *Genomics* **9**:373, 1991.

154. Meyn MS, Lu-Kuo JM, Herzing LBK: Expression cloning of multiple human cDNAs that complement the phenotypic defects of ataxia-telangiectasia Group D fibroblasts. *Am J Hum Genet* **53**:1206, 1993.

155. Gatti RA, Nakamura Y, Nussmeier M, Susi E, Shan W, Grody WW: Informativeness of VNTR genetic markers for detecting chimerism after bone marrow transplantation. *Dis Markers* **7**:105, 1989.

156. Fritz E, Elsea SH, Patel PI, Myen MS: Overexpression of a truncated human topoisomerase III partially corrects multiple aspects of the ataxia-telangiectasia phenotype. *Proc Natl Acad Sci USA* **94**:4538, 1997.

157. Telatar M, Wang Z, Udar N, Liang T, Bernatowska-Matuszkiewicz E, Lavin M, Shiloh Y, Concannon P, Good RA, Gatti RA: Ataxia-telangiectasia: Mutations in ATM cDNA detected by protein-truncation screening. *Am J Hum Genet* **59**:40, 1996.

158. Meyn MS: High spontaneous intrachromosomal recombination rates in ataxia-telangiectasia. *Science* **260**:1327, 1993.

159. Muriel WJ, Lamb JR, Lehmann AR: UV mutation spectra in cell lines from patients with Cockayne's syndrome and ataxia-telangiectasia, using the shuttle vector pZ189. *Mutat Res* **254**:119, 1991.

160. Woods CG, Bunday SE, Taylor AMR: Unusual features in the inheritance of ataxia-telangiectasia. *Hum Genet* **84**:555, 1990.

161. Lange E, Corresen A-L, Chen X, Chessa L, Chiplunkar S, Concannon P, Dandekar S, Gerken S, Lange K, Liang T, McConville C, Polakow J, Porras O, Rotman G, Sanal O, Sheikhavandi S, Shiloh Y, Sobel E, Taylor M, Telatar M, Teraoka S, Tolun A, Udar N, Uhrhammer N, Vanagaite L, Wang Z, Wapelhorst B, Yang H-M, Yang L, Ziv Y, Gatti RA: Localization of an ataxia-telangiectasia gene to a 500-kb interval on chromosome 11q23.1: Linkage analysis of 176 families in an international consortium. *Am J Hum Genet* **57**:112, 1995.

162. Gatti RA, Lange E, Rotman G, Chen S, Uhrhammer N, Liang T, Chiplunkar S, Yang L, Udar N, Dandekar S, Sheikhavandi S, Wang Z, Yang U-M, Polakow J, Elashoff M, Telatar M, Sanal O, Chessa L, McConville C, Taylor M, Shiloh Y, Porras O, Borresen A-L, Wegner R-D, Curry C, Gerken S, Lange K, Concannon P: Genetic haplotyping of ataxia-telangiectasia families localizes the major gene to an 850-kb region on chromosome 11q23.1. *Int J Radiat Biol* **66**:S57, 1994.

163. Swift M, Morrell D, Cromartie E, Chamberlin AR, Skolnick MH, Bishop DT: The incidence and gene frequency of ataxia-telangiectasia in the United States. *Am J Hum Genet* **39**:573, 1986.

164. Swift M: Genetics and epidemiology of ataxia-telangiectasia, in Gatti RA, Swift M (eds): *Ataxia-Telangiectasia: Genetics, Neuropathology, and Immunology of a Degenerative Disease of Childhood.* New York, Liss, 1985, pp 133–144.

165. Barlow MH, McFarlin ED, Schalch DS: An unusual type of diabetes mellitus with marked hyperinsulinism in patients with ataxia telangiectasia. *Clin Res* **13**:530, 1965.

166. Schalch DS, McFarlin DE, Barlow MH: An unusual form of diabetes mellitus in ataxia telangiectasia. *N Engl J Med* **282**:1396, 1970.

167. Gatti RA, Walford RL: Immune function and features of aging in chromosomal instability syndromes, in Segre D, Smith L (eds): *Immunologic Aspects of Aging.* New York, Marcel Dekker, 1981, pp 449–465.

168. Terplan KL, Krauss RF: Histopathologic brain changes in association with ataxia-telangiectasia. *Neurology* **19**:446, 1969.

169. Xu Y, Ashley T, Brainerd EE, Bronson RT, Meyn MS, Baltimore D: Targeted disruption of ATM leads to growth retardation, chromosomal fragmentation during meiosis, immune defect, and thymic lymphoma. *Genes Dev* **10**:2411, 1996.

170. Herndon RM: Selective vulnerability in the nervous system, in Gatti RA, Swift M (eds): *Ataxia-Telangiectasia: Genetics, Neuropathology, and Immunology of a Degenerative Disease of Childhood.* New York, Liss, 1985, pp 257–267.

171. Kamoshita S, Aguilar MJ, Landing BH: Precocious aging in ataxia-telangiectasia: Pathological evidence in the central nervous system, in *Proceedings of the First International Congress of Child Neurology.* Toronto, 1975.

172. Weemaes CMR, Hustinx TWJ, Scheres JMJC, Van Munster PJJ, Bakkeren JAJM, Taalman RDFM: A new chromosomal instability disorder: The Nijmegen breakage syndrome. *Acta Paediatr Scand* **70**:557, 1981.

173. Wegner RD, Metzger M, Hanefeld NG, Jaspers J, Baan C, Magdorf K, Kunze J, Sperling K: A new chromosomal instability disorder confirmed by complementation studies. *Clin Genet* **33**:20, 1988.

174. Stumm M, Seemanova E, Gatti RA, Sperling K, Reis A, Wegner R-D: The ataxia-telangiectasia variant genes 1 and 2 show no linkage to the AT candidate region on chromosome 11q22-23. *Am J Hum Genet* **57**:960, 1995.

175. Saar K, Chrzanowska KH, Stumm M, Jung M, Nurnberg G, Wienker TF, Seemanova E, Wegner R-D, Reis A, Sperling K: The gene for ataxia-telangiectasia-variant (Nijmegen breakage syndrome) maps to a 1 cM interval on chromosome 8q21. *Am J Hum Genet* **60**:605, 1997.

176. Taalman RDFM, Hustinx TWJ, Weemaes CMR, Seemanova E, Schmidt A, Passarge E, Scheres JMJC: Further delineation of the Nijmegen breakage syndrome. *Am J Med Genet* **32**:425, 1989.

177. Burgt I, Chrzanowska K, Smeets D, Weemaes C: Nijmegen breakage syndrome. *J Med Genet* **33**:153, 1996.

178. Chrzanowska KH, Kleijer WJ, Krajewska-Walasek M, Bialecka M, Gutkowska A, Goryluk-Kozakiewicz B, Michalkiewicz J: Eleven Polish patients with microcephaly, immunodeficiency and chromosomal instability: The Nijmegen breakage syndrome. *Am J Med Genet* **57**:462, 1995.

179. Curry CJR, O'Lague P, Tsai J, Hutchinson HT, Jaspers NGJ, Wara D, Gatti RA: AT$_{Fresno}$: A phenotype linking ataxia-telangiectasia with the Nijmegen breakage syndrome. *Am J Hum Genet* **45**:270, 1989.

180. Gatti RA: Ataxia-telangiectasia: genetic studies, in Griscelli C, Gupta S (eds): *New Concepts in Immunodeficiency.* Chichester, UK, Wiley, 1993, pp 203–229.

181. Lange E, Gatti RA, Sobel E, Concannon P, Lange K: How many A-T genes? in Gatti RA, Painter RB (eds): *Ataxia-Telangiectasia*. Heidelberg, Springer-Verlag, 1993, pp 37–54.

182. Taylor AMR, McConville CM, Woods GW, Byrd PJ, Hernandez D: Clinical and cellular heterogeneity in ataxia-telangiectasia, in Gatti RA, Painter RB (eds): *Ataxia-Telangiectasia*. Heidelberg, Springer-Verlag, 1993, pp 209–233.

183. Maserati E, Ottoline A, Veggiatti P, Lanzi G, Pasquali F: Ataxia without telangiectasia in two sisters with rearrangements of chromosomes 7 and 14. *Clin Genet* **34**:283, 1988.

184. Byrne E, Hallpike JF, Manson JI, Sutherland GR, Thong YH: Progressive multisystem degeneration with IgE deficiency and chromosomal instability. *J Neurol Sci* **66**:307, 1984.

185. Regueiro JR, Porras O, Lavin M, Gatti RA: Ataxia-Telangiectasia. A primary immunodeficiency revisited. *Allergy Immunol Clin North Am,* In press.

186. Harding A: *The Inherited Ataxias and Related Disorders*. London, Churchill Livingstone, 1984.

187. Bird TD: Hereditary motor sensory neuropathies: Charcot-Marie-Tooth syndrome. *Neurol Clin North Am* **7**:9, 1989.

188. Campuzano V, Montermini L, Molto MD, Pianese L, Cossee M, Cavalcanti F, Monros E, Rodius F, Duclos F, Monticelli A, Zara F, Canizares J, Koutnikova H, Bidichandani SI, Gellera C, Brice A, Trouillas P, De Michele G, Filla A, De Frutos, Palau F, Patel PI, Di Donato S, Mandel J-L, Cocozza S, Koenig M, Pandolfo M: Friedreich's ataxia: Autosomal recessive disease cased by an intronic GAA triplet repeat expansion. *Science* **271**:1423, 1996.

189. Aicardi J, Barbosas C, Andermann E, Andermann F, Morcos R, Ghanem Q, Fukuyama Y, Awaya Y, Moe P: Ataxia-ocular motor apraxia: A syndrome mimicking ataxia-telangiectasia. *Ann Neurol* **24**:497, 1988.

190. Jaspers NGJ, van der Kraan M, Linssen PCML, Macek M, Seemanova E, Kleijer WJ: First-trimester prenatal diagnosis of the Nijmegen breakage syndrome and ataxia-telangiectasia using an assay of radioresistant DNA synthesis. *Prenat Diagn* **10**:667, 1990.

191. Gianelli F, Avery JA, Pembrey ME, Blunt S: Prenatal exclusion of ataxia-telangiectasia, in Bridges BA, Harnden DG (eds): *Ataxia-Telangiectasia: Cellular and Molecular Link between Cancer, Neuropathology and Immune Deficiency*. New York, Wiley, 1982, pp 393–407.

192. Gatti RA, Peterson KL, Novak J, Chen X, Yang-Chen L, Liang T, Lange E, Lange K: Prenatal genotyping of ataxia-telangiectasia. *Lancet* **342**:376, 1993.

193. Kleijer WJ, van der Kraan M, Los FJ, Jaspers MGJ: Prenatal diagnosis of ataxia-telangiectasia and Nijmegen breakage syndrome by the assay of radioresistant DNA synthesis. *Int J Radiat Biol* **66**:S167, 1994.

194. Rotman G, Savitski K, Vanagaite L, Bar-Shira A, Ziv Y, Gilad S, Vchenik V, Smith S, Shiloh Y: Physical and genetic mapping at the ATA/ATC locus on chromosome 11q22-23. *Int J Radiat Biol* **66**:S63, 1994.

195. Vanagaite L, James MR, Rotman G, Savitsky K, Var-Shira A, Gilad S, Ziv Y, Uchenik V, Sartiel A, Collins FS, Sheffield VC, Richard CW III, Weissenbach J, Shiloh Y: A high-density microsatellite map of the ataxia telangiectasia locus. *Hum Genet* **95**:451, 1995.

196. Perlman SL: Treatment of ataxia-telangiectasia, in Gatti RA, Painter RB (eds): *Ataxia-Telangiectasia*. Heidelberg, Springer-Verlag, 1993, pp 269–278.

197. Pump KK, Dunn HG, Meuwissen H: A study of the bronchial and vascular structures of a lung from a case of ataxia-telangiectasia. *Dis Chest* **47**:473, 1965.

198. Banin S, Moyal L, Shieh S-Y, Taya Y, Anderson CW, Chessa L, Smorodinsky NI, Prives C, Reiss Y, Shiloh Y, Ziv Y: Enhanced phosphorylation of p53 by ATM in response to DNA damage. *Science* **281**:1675, 1998.

199. Canman CE, Lim D-S, Cimprich KA, Taya Y, Tamai K, Sakaguchi K, Appella E, Kastan MB, Siliciano JD: Activation of the ATM kinase by ionizing radiation and phosphorylation of p53. *Science* **281**:1677, 1998.

200. Hendrickson EA: Insights from model systems: Cell-cycle regulation of mammalian DNA double-strand-break repair. *Am J Hum Genet* **61**:795, 1997.

201. Carney JP, Maser RS, Olivares H, Davis EM, Le Beau M, Yates JR, Hays L, Morgan WF, Petrini JHJ: The hMre11/hRad50 protein complex and Nijmegen breakage syndrome: Linkage of double-strand break repair to the cellular DNA damage response. *Cell* **93**:477, 1998.

202. Varon R, Vissinga C, Platzer M, Cerosaletti KM, Chrzanowska KH, Saar K, Beckmann G, Seemanova E, Cooper PR, Nowak NJ, Stumm M, Weemaes CMR, Gatti RA, Wilson RK, Digweed M, Rosenthal A, Sperling K, Concannon P, Reis A: Nibrin, a novel DNA double-strand break repair protein, is mutated in Nijmegen Breakage Syndrome. *Cell* **93**:467, 1998.

203. Borghesani PR, Alt FA, Bottaro A, Davidson L, Aksoy S, Rathbun GA, Roberts TM, Swat W, Segal RA, Gu Y: Abnormal development of Purkinje cells and lymphocytes in *Atm* mutant mice. *Proc Natl Acad Sci USA* In press.

204. Murnane JP, Painter RB: Complementation of the defects in DNA synthesis in irradiated and unirradiated ataxia-telangiectasia cells. *Proc Natl Acad Sci USA* **79**:1960, 1982.

205. Gatti RA, Shaked R, Wei S, Koyama M, Salser W, Silver J: DNA polymorphism in the human THY-1 gene. *Hum Immunol* **22**:145, 1988.

206. Sanal O, Wei S, Foroud T, Malhotra U, Concannon P, Charmley P, Salser W, Lange K, Gatti RA: Further mapping of an ataxia-telangiectasia locus to the chromosome 11q23 region. *Am J Hum Genet* **47**:860, 1990.

207. Foroud T, Wei S, Ziv Y, Sobel E, Lange E, Chao A, Goradia T, Huo Y, Tolun A, Chessa L, Charmley P, Sanal O, Salman N, Julier C, Lathrop GM, Concannon P, McConville C, Taylor M, Shiloh Y, Lange K, Gatti RA: Localization of an ataxia-telangiectasia locus to a 3-cM interval on chromosome 11q23: Linkage analyses of 111 families by an international consortium. *Am J Hum Genet* **49**:1263, 1991.

208. Sanal O, Lange E, Telatar M, Sobel E, Salazar-Novak J, Ersoy F, Concannon P, Tolun A, Gatti RA: Ataxia-telangiectasia-linkage analysis of chromosome 11q22-23 markers in Turkish families. *FASEB J* **6**:2848, 1992.

209. Charmley P, Foroud T, Wei S, Concannon P, Weeks DE, Lange D, Gatti RA: A primary linkage map of the human chromosome 11q22-23 region. *Genomics* **6**:316, 1990.

210. Charmley P, Nguyen J, Wei S, Gatti RA: Genetic linkage analysis and homology of syntenic relationships of genes located on human chromosome 11q. *Genomics* **10**:608, 1991.

211. Concannon P, Malhotra U, Charmley P, Reynolds J, Lange K, Gatti RA: Ataxia-telangiectasia gene (ATA) on chromosome 11 is distinct from the ETS-1 gene. *Genomics* **46**:789, 1990.

212. Wei S, Rocchi M, Archidiacono N, Sacchi N, Romeo G, Gatti RA: Physical mapping of the human chromosome 11q23 region containing the ataxia-telangiectasia locus. *Cancer Genet Cytogenet* **46**:1, 1990.

213. McConville CM, Byrd PJ, Ambrose HJ, Taylor AMR: Genetic and physical mapping of the ataxia-telangiectasia locus on chromosome 11q22-23. *Int J Radiat Biol* **66**:545, 1994.

214. McConville CM, Formstone CJ, Hernandez D, Thick J, Taylor AMR: Fine mapping of the chromosome 11q22-23 region using PFGE, linkage and haplotype analysis: Localization of the gene for ataxia-telangiectasia to a 5 cM region flanked by NCAM/DRD2 and STMY/CJ52.75, ph2.22. *Nucleic Acids Res* **18**:4334, 1990.

215. McConville C, Woods CG, Farrall M, Metcalfe JA, Taylor AMR: Analysis of 7 polymorphic markers at chromosome 11q22-23 in 35 ataxia-telangiectasia families: Further evidence of linkage. *Hum Genet* **85**:215, 1990.

216. McConville CM, Byrd PJ, Ambrose H, Stankovic T, Ziv Y, Bar-Shira A, Vanagaite L, Rotman G, Shiloh Y, Gillett GT, Riley JH, Taylor AMR: Paired STSs amplified from radiation hybrids, and from associated YACs, identify highly polymorphic loci flanking the ataxia-telangiectasia locus on chromosome 11q22-23. *Hum Mol Genet* **2**:969, 1994.

217. Cornelis F, James M, Cherif D, Tokino T, Davies J, Girault D, Bernard C, Litt M, Berger R, Nakamura Y, Lathrop M, Julier C: Precise localization of a gene responsible for ataxia-telangiectasia on chromosome 11q, in Gatti RA, Painter RB (eds): *Ataxia-Telangiectasia*. Heidelberg, Springer-Verlag, 1993, pp 23–36.

218. Oskato R, Bar-Shira A, Vanagaite L, Ziv Y, Ehrlich S, Rotman G, McConville CM, Chakravarti A, Shiloh Y: Ataxia-telangiectasia: Allelic association with 11q22-23 markers in Moroccan-Jewish patients. *Am J Hum Genet* **53**:A1055, 1993.

219. Taylor AMR, McConville CM, Rotman G, Shiloh Y, Byrd PJ: A haplotype common to intermediate radiosensitivity variants of ataxia-telangiectasia in the UK. *Int J Radiat Biol* **66**:S35, 1994.

220. Uhrhammer N, Concannon P, Huo Y, Nakamura Y, Gatti RA: A pulsed-field gel electrophoresis map in the ataxia-telangiectasia region of chromosome 11q22.3. *Genomics* **20**:278, 1994.

221. Uhrhammer N, Lange E, Porras O, Naeim A, Chen X, Sheikhavandi S, Chiplunkar S, Yang L, Dandekar S, Liang T, Patel N, Udar N, Concannon P, Gerken S, Shiloh Y, Lange K, Gatti RA: Sublocalization of an ataxia-telangiectasia gene distal to D11S384 by ancestral haplotyping in Costa Rican families. *Am J Hum Genet* **57**:103, 1995.

222. Teraoka S, Telatar M, Becker-Catania S, Liang T, Onegut S, Tolun A, Chessa L, Sanal O, Bernatowska E, Gatti RA, Concannon P: Splicing defects in the ataxia-telangiectasia gene, ATM: under lying mutations and phenotypic consequences. *Am J Hum Genet* **64**:1617, 1999.

223. Croce CM: Role of TCL1 and ALL1 in human leukemias and development. *Cancer Res* **59**:177s, 1998.

224. Buckler AJ, Chang DD, Graw SL, Brook JD, Haber DA, Sharp PA, Housman DE: Exon amplification: A strategy to isolate mammalian genes based on RNA splicing. *PNAS* **88**:4005, 1991.

225. Byrd PJ, McConville CM, Cooper P, Parkhill J, Stankovic T, McGuire GM, Thick JA, Taylor AMR: Mutations revealed by sequencing the 59 half of the gene for ataxia-telangiectasia. *Hum Mol Genet* **5**:145, 1996.

226. Imai T, Yamauchi M, Seki N, Sugawara T, Saito T, Matsuda Y, Ito H, Nagase T, Nomua N, Hori T: Identification and characterization of a new gene physically linked to the ATM gene. *Genome Res* **6**:439, 1996.

227. Chen X, Yang L, Udar N, Liang T, Uhrhammer N, Xu S, Bay JO, Wang Z, Dandakar U, Chiplunkar S, Klisak I, Telatar M, Yang H, Concannon P, Gatti RA: CAND3: A ubiquitously-expressed gene immediately adjacent and in opposite transcriptional orientation to the ATM gene at 11q23.1. *Mamm Genome* **8**:129, 1997.

228. Rasio D, Negrini M, Croce CM: Genomic organization of the ATM locus involved in ataxia-telangiectasia. *Cancer Res* **55**:6053, 1995.

229. Uziel T, Savitsky K, Platzer M, Ziv Y, Helbitz T, Nehls M, Boehm T, Rosenthal A, Shiloh Y, Rotman G: Genomic organization of the ATM gene. *Genomics* **33**:317, 1996.

230. Pecker I, Avrahan KB, Gilbert DJ, Savitsky K, Rotman G, Harnik R, Fukao T, Schrock E, Hirotsune S, Tagle DA, Collins FS, Wynshow-Boris A, Ried T, Copeland NG, Jenkins NA, Shiloh Y, Ziv Y: Identification and chromosomal localization of atm, the mouse homolog of the ataxia-telangiectasia gene. *Genomics* **35**:39, 1996.

231. Gao J-H, Parsons LM, Bowers JM, Xiong J, Li J, Fox PT: Cerebellum implicated in sensory acquisition and discrimination rather than motor control. *Science* **272**:545, 1996.

232. Barinaga M: The cerebellum: Movement coordinator or much more? [editorial overview]. *Science* **272**:482, 1996.

233. Keith CT, Schreiber SL: PIK-related kinases: DNA repair, recombination, and cell cycle checkpoints. *Science* **270**:50, 1995.

234. Gilad S, Khosravi R, Shkedy D, Uziel T, Ziv Y, Savitsky K, Rotman G, Smith S, Chessa L, Jorgensen TJ, Harnik R, Frydman M, Sanal O, Portnoi S, Goldwicz Z, Jaspers MGJ, Gatti RA, Lenoir G, Lavin M, Tatsumi K, Wegner RD, Shiloh Y, Bar-Shira A: Predominance of null mutation in ataxia-telangiectasia. *Hum Mol Genet* **5**:433, 1996.

235. Wright J, Teraoka S, Onengut S, Tolun A, Gatti RA, Ochs HD, Concannon P: A high frequency of distinct ATM mutations in ataxia-telangiectasia. *Am J Hum Genet* **59**:839, 1996.

236. Forrest S, Cotton R, Landegren U, Southern E: How to find all those mutations. *Nat Genet* **10**:375, 1995.

237. Concannon P, Gatti RA: Diversity of ATM gene mutations detected in patients with ataxia-telangiectasia. *Hum Mutat* **10**:100, 1997.

238. Hawkins JD: *Gene Structure and Expression*, 2d ed. Cambridge, UK, Cambridge University Press, 1991, p 127.

239. McConville CM, Stankovic T, Byrd PJ, McGuire GM, Yao Q-Y, Lennox GG, Taylor AMR:Mutations associated with variant phenotypes in ataxia-telangiectasia. *Am J Hum Genet* **59**:320, 1996.

240. Gatti RA: Ataxia-telangiectasia: Immune dysfunction is one of many defects. *Immunol Today* **5**:121, 1984.

241. Lehmann A, Jaspers NJG, Gatti RA: Ataxia-telangiectasia: Meeting report. *Cancer Res* **47**:4750, 1987.

242. Lehmann AR, Jaspers NGJ, Gatti RA: Meeting report: Fourth International Workshop on Ataxia-Telangiectasia. *Cancer Res* **49**:6162, 1989.

243. Taylor AMR, Jaspers NGJ, Gatti RA: Meeting report: Fifth International Workshop on Ataxia-Telangiectasia. *Cancer Res* **53**:438, 1993.

244. Gatti RA, McConville CM, Taylor AMR: Meeting report. Sixth International Workshop on Ataxia-Telangiectasia. *Cancer Res* **54**:6007, 1994.

245. Bridges BA, Harnden DG (eds): *Ataxia-Telangiectasia: A Cellular and Molecular Link between Cancer, Neuropathology, and Immune Deficiency.* Chichester, UK, Wiley, 1982, p 1–402.

246. Gatti RA, Swift M (eds): *Ataxia-Telangiectasia: Genetics, Neuropathology, and Immunology of a Degenerative Disease of Childhood.* New York, Liss, 1985.

247. Gatti RA, Painter RB (eds): *Ataxia-Telangiectasia*, vol 77. NATO ASI Series. Heidelberg, Springer-Verlag, 1993.

248. Julier C, Nakamura Y, Lathrop M, O'Connell P, Leppert M, Litt M, Mohandas T, Lalouel J-M, White R: Detailed map of the long arm of chromosome 11. *Genomics* **7**:335, 1990.

249. Kapp LN, Painter RB, Yu L-C, van Loon N, Richard CW, James MR, Cox DR, Murnane JP: Cloning of a candidate gene for ataxia-telangiectasia group D. *Am J Hum Genet* **51**:45, 1992.

250. Kapp LN, Murnane JP: Cloning and characterization of a candidate gene for A-T complementation Group D, in Gatti RA, Painter RB (eds): *Ataxia-Telangiectasia.* Heidelberg, Springer-Verlag, 1993, pp 7–22.

251. Platzer M, Rotman G, Bauer D, Uziel T, Savitsky K, Bar-Shira A, Gilad S, Shiloh Y, Rosenthal A: Ataxia-telangiectasia locus: Sequence analysis of 184 kb of human genomic DNA containing the entire ATM gene. *Genome Res* **7**:592, 1997.

252. Telatar M, Teraoka S, Wang Z, Chun HH, Liang T, Castellvi-Bel S, Udar N, Borresen-Dale A-L, Chessa L, Bernatowska-Matuszkiewicz E, Porras O, Watanabe M, Junker A, Concannon P, Gatti RA: Ataxia-telangiectasia: Identification and detection of founder mutations in the ATM gene in ethnic populations. *Am J Hum Genet* **62**:86, 1998.

253. Trouillas P, Xie J, Adeleine P: Buspirone, a serotonergic 5-HT1A agonist, is active in cerebellar ataxia. A new fact in favor of the serotonergic theory of ataxia. *Prog Brain Res* **114**:589, 1997.

254. Kuljis RO, Xu Y, Aguila MC, Baltimore D: Degeneration of neurons, synapses, and neuropil and glial activation in a murine Atm knockout model of ataxia-telangiectasia. *Proc Natl Acad Sci USA* **94**:12688, 1997.

255. Westphal CH, Rowan S, Schmaltz C, Elson A, Fisher DE, Leder P: atm and p53 cooperate in apoptosis and suppression of tumorigenesis, but not in resistance to acute radiation toxicity. *Nat Genetics* **16**:397, 1997.

256. Herzog K-H, Chong MJ, Kapsetaki M, Morgan JI, McKinnon PJ: Requirement for ATM in ionizing radiation-induced cell death in the developing central nervous system. *Science* **280**:1089, 1998.

257. Bay J-O, Grancho M, Pernin D, Presneau N, Rio P, Tchirkov A, Uhrhammer N, Verrelle P, Gatti RA, Bignon Y-J: No evidence for constitutional ATM mutation in breast/gastric cancer families. *Intl J Oncol* **12**:1385, 1998.

258. Chen J, Birksholtz GC, Lindblom P, Rubio C, Lindblom A: The role of ataxia-telangiectasia heterozygotes in familial breast cancer. *Cancer Res* **58**:1376, 1998.

259. Luo L, Lu F-M, Hart S, Foroni L, Rabbani H, Hammarstrom L, Webster ADB, Vorechowsky I: Ataxia-telangiectasia and T-cell leukemias: no evidence for somatic ATM mutation in sporadic T-ALL or for hypermethylation of the ATM-NPAT/E14 bidirectional promoter in T-PLL. *Cancer Res* **58**:2293, 1998.

260. Larson GP, Zhang G, Ding S, Foldenauer K, Udar N, Gatti RA, Neuberg D, Lunetta KL, Ruckdeschel JC, Longmate J, Flanagan S, Krontiris TG: An allelic variant at the ATM locus is implicated in breast cancer susceptibility. *Genet Testing* **1**:165, 1998.

261. Forozan F, Karthu R, Kononen J, Kallionieni A, Kallioniemi OP: Genome screening by comparative genomic hybridization. *Trends Genet* **13**:405, 1997.

262. Smith L, Liu SJ, Goodrich L, Jacobson D, Degnin C, Bentley N, Carr A, Flaggs G, Keegan K, Hoekstra M, Thayer M: Duplication of ATR inhibits MyoD, induces aneuploidy and eliminates radiation-induced G1 arrest. *Nat Genet* **19**:39, 1998.

263. Cliby WA, Roberts CJ, Cimprich KA, Stringer CM, Lamb JR, Schreiber SL, Friend SH: Overexpression of a kinase-inactive ATR protein causes sensitivity of DNA-damaging agents and defects in cell cycle checkpoints. *EMBO J* **17**:159, 1998.

264. Stilgenbauer S, Schaffner C, Litterst A, Liebisch P, Gilad S, Bar-Shira A, James MR, Lichter P, Dohner H: Evidence for ATM as a tumor suppressor gene in T-prolymphocytic leukemia. *Nat Med* **3**:1155, 1997.

265. Hendricksen LA, Carter T, Dutta A, Wold MS: Phosphorylation of human replication protein A by the DNA-dependent protein kinase is involved in the modulation of DNA replication. *Nucleic Acids Res* **24**:3107, 1996.

266. Rivero ME, Porras O, Leiva I, Pacheco A, Regueiro JR: Phenotypical and functional characterization of herpes virus saimiri-immortalized T cells from ataxia-telangiectasia patient [abstract #61]. Clermont-Ferrand, France: Seventh International Workshop on Ataxia-Telangiectasia, November 22–24, 1997.

267. Gabra H, Watson VJE, Taylor KJ, Mackay J, Leonard RC, Steel CM, Porteous DJ, Smyth JF: Definition and refinement of a region of loss of heterozygosity at 11q23.3-q24.3 in epithelial ovarian cancer associated with poor prognosis. *Cancer Res* **56**:950, 1996.

268. Koreth J, Bakkenist CJ, McGee J: Allelic deletions at chromosome 11q22-q23.1 and 11q25-qterm are frequent in sporadic breast but not colorectal cancers. *Oncogene* **14**:431, 1997.

269. Nanashima A, Tagawa Y, Tasutake T, Fujise N, Kashima K, Nakagoe T, Ayabe H: Deletion of chromosome 11 and development of colorectal carcinoma. *Cancer Detect Prev* **21**:7, 1997.

270. Hui AB, Lo KW, Leung SF, Choi PH, Fong Y, Lee JC, Huang DP: Loss of heterozygosity on the long arm of chromosome 11 in nasopharyngeal carcinoma. *Cancer Res* **56**:3225, 1996.

271. Flaggs G, Plug AW, Dunks KM, Mundt KE, Ford JC, Quiggle MRE, Taylor EM, Westphal CH, Ashley T, Hoekstra MF, Carr AM: Atm-dependent interactions of a mammalian Chk1 homolog with meiotic chromosomes. *Curr Biol* **7**:977, 1997.

272. Plug AW, Peters AHFM, Xu Y, Keegan KS, Hoekstra MF, Baltimore D, de Boer P, Ashley T: ATM and RPA in meiotic chromosome synapsis and recombination. *Nat Genet* **17**:457, 1997.

273. Baumann P, Benson FE, West SC: Human Rad51 protein promotes ATP-dependent homologous pairing and strand transfer reactions in vitro. *Cell* **87**:757, 1996.

274. Cox MM, Lehman IR: recA protein-promoted DNA strand exchange: Stable complexes of recA protein and single-stranded DNA formed in the presence of ATP and single-stranded DNA-binding protein. *J Biol Chem* **257**:8523, 1982.

275. Sanal O, Smeets D, Aksoy Y, Beerket AI, Ersoy F, Gariboglu S, Metin A, Ogus H, Weemaes C, Yel L: Heterogenicity in ataxia-telangiectasia: Various laboratory features of 47 patients [abstract #47]. Clermont-Ferrand, France: Seventh International Workshop on Ataxia-Telangiectasia, November 22–24, 1997.

276. Schubert R, Kappenhagen N, Royer N, Zielen S: Ongoing apoptosis of lymphocytes in patients with ataxia-telangiectasia. [abstract #66]. Clermont-Ferrand, France: Seventh International Workshop on Ataxia-Telangiectasia, November 22–24, 1997.

277. Fiorilli M, Businco L, Pandolfi F, Paganelli R, Russo G, Aiuti F: Heterogeneity of immunological abnormalities in ataxia-telangiectasia. *J Clin Immunol* **3**:135, 1983.

278. Porras O: Personal communication. oral 1997

279. Pastorino AC, Almeida AG, Dias MJM, Jacob CMA, Duarte AJS, Grumach AS: Ataxia-telangiectasia. Aspectos clinico-laboratoriasis de 11 pacientes. *Latin American Group for Immunodeficiency meeting.* Sao Paolo, Brazil, Sept 3–5, 1998.

280. Sanal O, Berkel AI, Ersoy F, Tezcan I, Topaloglu H: Clinical variants of ataxia-telangiectasia. In: Ataxia-telangiectasia, in Gatti RA, Painter RB (eds): *Ataxia-Telangiectasia. NATO ASI series.* Berlin, Springer-Verlag, 1993, pp 183–187.

281. Bezrodnik L, Krasovec S, Gaillard MI, Rivas EM: Sindrome de ataxia telangiectasia: presentacion de 9 pacientes. *Latin American Group for Immunodeficiency meeting.* Sao Paolo, Brazil, Sept 3–5, 1998.

282. Vorechovsky I, Luo L, Lindblom A, Negrini M, Webster DB, Croce CM, Hammarstrom L: ATM mutations in cancer families. *Cancer Res* **56**:4130, 1996.

283. Chrzanowska K, Krajewska-Walasek M, Bernatowska E, Kostyk E, Midro AT, Metera M, Bialecka M, Gregorek H, Michalkiewicz J, Brrzeziinska A, Rozynek A: Polish patients with Nijmegen breakage syndrome. *Clinical and genetic studies.* Disease Marters **14**:31, 1998.

284. Cerosaletti KM, Lange E, Stringham HM, Weemaes CMR, Smeets D, Solder B, Belohradsky BH, Taylor AMR, Marnes P, Elliott A, Komatsu K, Gatti RA, Boehnke M, Concannon P: Fine localization of the Nijmegen breakage syndrome gene to 8q21: Evidence for a common founder haplotype. *Am J Hum Genet* **63**:125, 1998.

285. Udar N, Farzad S, Taj -Q, Bay J-Q, Gatti RA: NS22, a high polymorphic marker with the ATM gene. *Am J Med Genet* **82**:287, 1999.

286. Krivit W, Sung JH, Shapiro EG, Lockman LA: Microglia: The effector cell for reconstitution of the central nervous system following bone marrow transplantation for lysosomal and peroxisomal storage diseases. *Cell Transplant* **4**:385, 1995.

287. Unger ER, Sung JH, Manivel JC, Chenggis ML, Blazar BR, Krivitt W. Male donor-derived cells in the brains of female sex-mismatched bone marrow transplant recipients: A Y-chromosome specific in situ hybridization study. *J Neuropathol Exp Neurol* **52**:460, 1993.

288. Lim DS, Kirsch DG, Lee A, Rhodes N, Gilmer T, Kastan MB: Functional interactions between ATM and adapting proteins [abstract #526]. *AACR Proc* **39**:S77, 1998.

289. Stankovic T, Kidd AMJ, Sutcliffe A, McGuire GM, Robinson P, Weber P, Bedenham T, Bradwell AR, Easton DF, Lennox GG, Haites N, Byrd PJ, Talyor AMR: ATM mutations and phenotypes in ataxia-telangiectasia families in the British Isles: Expression of mutant ATM and the risk of leukemia, lymphoma, and breast cancer. *Am J Hum Genet* **62**:334, 1998.

290. Telatar M, Wang Z, Castellvi-Bel S, Tai L-Q, Sheikhavandi S, Regueiro JG, Porras O, Gatti RA: A model for ATM heterozygote identification in a large population: Four founder-effect ATM

291. Gilad S, Bar-Shira A, Harnik R, Shkedy D, Ziv Y, Shosravi R, Brown K, Vanagaite L, Xu G, Frydman M, Lavin MF, Hill D, Tagle DA, Shiloh Y: Ataxia-telangiectasia: Founder effect among North African Jews. *Hum Mol Genet* **5**:2033, 1996.

292. Uhrhammer N, Bay J-O, Bignon Y-J: Seventh International Workshop on Ataxia-Telangiectasia. *Cancer Res* **58**:3480, 1998.

293. Laake K, Telatar M, Geitvik GA, Hansen RO, Heiberg A, Andresen AM, Gatt RA, Borresen-Dale A-L: Identical mutation in 55% of the ATM alleles in 11 Norwegian AT families: Evidence for a founder effect. *Eur J Hum Genet* **6**:235, 1998.

294. Gilad S, Chessa L, Khosravi R, Russel P, Galanty Y, Piane M, Gatti RA, Jorgensen TJ, Shiloh Y, Bar-Shira A: Genotype-phenotype relationships in ataxia-telangiectasia and variants. *Am J Hum Genet* **62**:551, 1998.

295. Becker-Catania SG, Chen G, Hwang MJ, Wang Z, Sun X, Sanal O, Bernatowska-Matuszkiewicz E, Chessa L, Lee EYH-P, Gatti RA: ATM protein expression, mutations, radiosensitivity and clinical phenotype in 124 ataxia-telangiectasia pateients. Submitted.

296. Rosenblatt HM, Brown B, Parikh N, Jorczak A: Abnormal up-regulation of CD-40 ligand (CD40L) in patients with ataxia-telangiectasia (AT) and elevated serum IGM levels [abstract #5336]. *FASEB J* **12**:A922, 1998.

297. Laake K Odegard A, Andersen Tl, Bukholm lK, Karesen R, Nesland JM, Ottestad L, Shiloh Y, Borresen-Dale A-L: Loss of heterozygosity at 11q23.1 in breast carcinomas: indication for involvement of a gene distal and close to ATM. *Gene Chrom Cancer* **18**:175, 1997.

298. Tyagi S, Bratu DP, Kramer FR: Multicolor molecular beacons for allele discrimination. *Nature Biotech* **16**:49, 1998.

299. Cortez D, Wang Y, Qin J, Elledge SJ: Requirement of ATM-dependent phosphorylation of Brca1 in the DNA damage response to double-strand breaks. *Science* **286**:1162, 1999.

300. Khanna KK, Keating KE, Kozlov S, Scott S, Gatei M, Hobson K, Taya Y, Gabrielli B, Chan D, Less-Miller SP, Lavin MF: ATM associates with and phosphorylates p53: Mapping the region of interaction. *Nat Genet* **20**:398, 1998.

301. Fegen C, Robinson H, Thompson P, Whittaker JA, White D: Karyotypic evolution in CLL: Identification of a new sub-group with deletions of 11q and advanced or progressive disease. *Leukemia* **9**:2003, 1995.

302. Starostik P, Manshouri T, O'Brien S, Freireich E, Kantarjian H, Lerner S, Keating M, Albitar M: The ATM gene is deleted in a subgroup of B-cell chronic lymphocytic leukemia. *Proceedings of the American Society of Hematology, Dec 8-10, 1997, San Diego, Calif.* (abst 396, p 90a).

303. Stankovic T, Weber P, Stewart G, Bedenham T, Byrd PJ, Moss PA, Taylor AM: Inactivation of ataxia telangiectasia mutated gene in B-cell chronic lymphocytic leukaemia. *Lancet* **353**:26, 1999.

304. Bullrich F, Tasio D, Kitada S, Starostik P, Kipps T, Keating M, Albitar M, Reed JC, Croce CM: ATM mutations in B-cell chronic lymphocytic leukemia. *Cancer Res* **59**:2427, 1999.

305. Teraoka SN, Malone KE, Doody D, Suter NM, Ostrander EA, Daling JR, Concannon P: Increased frequency of ATM mutations in breast carcinoma patients with early onset disease and positive family history. *Cancer* **92**:479, 2001.

306. Gatti RA, Tward A, Concannon P: Cancer risk in ATM heterozygotes: a model of phenotypic and mechanistic differences between missense and truncating mutations. *Molec Genet Metab* **69**:419, 1999.

307. Zhao S, Yuan FS-S, Weng Y-C, Lin Y-L, Hsu H-C, Lin S-Cj, Gerbino E, Song M-H, Zdzienicka MZ, Gatti RA, Shay J, Ziv Y, Shiloh Y, Lee EY-HP: A functional link between ATM kinase and NBS1 in the DNA damage response. *Nature* In press.

308. Stewart GS, Maser RS, Stankovic T, Bressan Da, Kaplan Ml, Jaspers NGJ, Raams A, Byrd PJ, Petrini JHJ, Taylor AMR: The DNA double-strand break repair gene hMRE11 is mutated in individuals with an ataxia-telangiectasia-like disorder. *Cell* **99**:577, 1999.

309. Greenberg F, Rose E, Alpert E: Hereditary persistence of alpha-fetoprotein. *Gastroenterology* **98**:1083, 1990.

310. McVey JH, Michaelides K, Hansen LP, Ferguson-Smith M, Tilghman S, Krumlauf R, Tuddenham EGD: A G > A substitution in an HNF 1 binding site in the human α-fetoprotein gene is associated with hereditary persistence of α-fetoprotein (HPAFP). *Human Molec Genet* **2**:379, 1993.

311. Murgita RA, Wigzell H: The effects of mouse alpha-fetoprotein on T-cell-dependent and T-cell-independent immune response in vivo. *Scand J Immunol* **5**:1215, 1976.

312. Murgita RA, Anderson LC, Sherman MS: Effects of human alpha-fetoprotein on human B and T lymphocyte proliferation in vitro. *Clin Exp Immunol* **33**:347, 1978.

313. Lee KC, Crowe AJ, Barton MC: P53-mediated repression of alpha-fetoprotein gene expression by specific DNA binding. *Mol Cell Biol* **19**:1279, 1999.

314. Hernandez D, McConville CM, Stacey M, Woods, CG, Brown MM, Shutt P, Rysiecki G, Taylor AMR: A family sowing no evidence of linkage between the ataxia telaphigectasia Taylor AMR: A family showing no evidence of linkage between the ataxia telaphigectasia gene and chromosome 11q22-23. *J Med Genet* **30**:135, 1993.

315. Djozenova CS, Schindler D, Stopper H, Hoehn H, Flentje M, Oppitz U: Identification of ataxia telangiectasia heterozygotes, a cancer-prone population, using the single-cell gel electrophoresis (Comet) assay. *Lab Invest* **79**:699, 1999.

315. Geschwind DH, perlman S, Grody W, Telatar M, Montermini L, pandolfo M, Gatti RA: Friedreich's ataxia GAA repeat expansion in patients with recessive or sporadic ataxia. *Neurology* **49**:1004, 1997.

317. Lavin MF: Radiosensitivity and oxidative signalling in ataxia telangiectasia: An update. *Radiother Oncol* **47**:113, 1998.

318. Smith GCM, Cary RB, Lakin ND, Hann BC, Teo S-H, Chen DJ, Jackson SP: Purification and DNA binding properties of the ataxia-telangiectasia gene product ATM. *Proc Natl Acad Sci USA* **96**:11134, 1999.

319. Savitsky K, Platzer M, Uziel T, Gilad S, Sartiel A, Rosenthal A, Elroy-Stein O, Shiloh Y, Rotman G: Ataxia-telangiectasia: Structural diversity of untranslated sequences suggests complex post-transcription regulation of ATM gene expression. *Nucleic Acids Res* **25**:1678, 1997.

320. Lavin M: Written personal communication. 1999.

321. Broeks A, de Klein A, Floore AN, Muijtjens M, Kleijer WJ, Jaspers NG, van't Veer LJ: ATM germline mutations in classical ataxia-telangiectasia patients in the Dutch population. *Hum Mutat* **12**:330, 1998.

322. Sandoval N, Platzer M, Rosenthal A, Dork T, Bendix R, Skawran B, Stuhrmann M, Wegner R-D, Sperling K, Banin S, Shiloh Y, Baumer A, Mernthaler U, Sennefelder H, Brohm M, Weber BHF, Schindler D: Characterization of ATM gene mutations in 66 ataxia telangiectasia families. *Hum Mol Genet* **8**:69, 1999.

323. Castellvi-Bel S, Sheikhavandi S, Telatar M, Tai L-Q, Hwang M, Wang Z, Yang Z, Cheng R, Gatti RA: New mutations, polymorphisms, and rare variants in the ATM gene detected by a novel strategy. *Hum Mutat* **14**:156, 1999.

324. Ashburner BP, Shackelford RE, Baldwin AS, Paules RS: Lack of involvement of ataxia telangiectasia mutated (ATM) in regulation of nuclear factor-κB (NF-κB) in human diploid fibroblasts. *Cancer Res* **59**:5456, 1999.

325. Reichenback J, Schubert R, Schwan C, Muller K, Bohles HJ, Zielen S: Anti-oxidative capacity in patients with ataxia telangiectasia. *Clin Exp Immunol* **117**:535, 1999.

326. Battisti C, Formichi P, Federico A: Vitamin E serum levels are normal in ataxia telangiectasia (Louis-Bar disease). *J Neurol Sci* **141**:114, 1996.

327. Zielen S, Schubert R, Schindler D, Buehring l: Patients with A-T are unable to produce lgG antibodies to pneumococcal polysaccharides. International Workshop on Ataxia-Telangiectasia, Nov 22-24, 1997, Clermont-Ferrand, France (abst 41).

328. Cornforth MW, Bedford JS: On the nature of a defect in cells from individuals with ataxia-telangiectasia. *Science* **227**:1589, 1985.

329. Meyn MS: Ataxia-telanigectasia, cancer and the pathobiology of the ATM gene. *Clin Genet* **55**:289, 1999.

330. Morgan SE, Lovly C, Pandita TK, Shiloh Y, Kastan MB: Fragments of ATM which have dominant-negative or complementing activity. *Mol Cell Biol* **17**:2020, 1997.

331. Shafman TD, Levitz S, Nixon AJ, Gibans L-A, Nichols KE, Bell DW, Ishioka C, Isselbacher KJ, Gelman R, Garber J, Harris JR, Haber DA: Prevalence of germline truncating mutations in ATM in women with a second breast cancer after radiation therapy for a contralateral tumor. *Genes Chrom Cancer*. In press.

332. Lavin MF, Concannon P, Gatti RA: Eighth International Workshop on Ataxia-Telangiectasia (ATW8). *Cancer Res* **59**:3845, 1999.

Bloom Syndrome

James German ▪ *Nathan A. Ellis*

1. Clinically, Bloom syndrome (BS) features (a) proportional dwarfism, usually accompanied by (b) a sun-sensitive erythematous skin lesion limited to the face and dorsa of the hands and forearms, (c) a characteristic facies and head configuration, and (d) immunodeficiency, often associated with otitis media and pneumonia. (e) Affected males fail to produce spermatozoa, and females although sometimes fertile experience an unusually early cessation of menstrual cycles. (f) Excessive numbers of well-circumscribed areas of dermal hypo- and hyperpigmentation are present. (g) The three major complications are chronic lung disease, diabetes mellitus, and — by far the most important and most frequent — cancer.

2. BS is a genetically determined trait that is transmitted in a straightforward autosomal recessive fashion, with mutations at a single locus, *BLM*, being responsible. Various mutations at *BLM* are segregating in human populations, but the same phenotype (BS) is produced by either homozygosity or compound heterozygosity of those so far identified. The mutations are predominantly null alleles, but missense mutations have been detected also. BS is rare in all populations, but in the Ashkenazi Jewish population, one particular mutant allele, a 6-base pair (bp) deletion and 7-bp insertion that results in premature translation termination, has, through founder effect, reached a relatively high carrier frequency of approximately 1 percent; in 31 percent of all persons with BS, one or both parents are Ashkenazi Jews.

3. The genome is abnormally unstable in the somatic cells of persons with BS. Mutations arise spontaneously and accumulate in numbers manyfold greater than normal, including both microscopically visible chromatid gaps, breaks, and rearrangements and mutations at specific loci. Exchanges take place excessively between chromatids, usually at what appear to be homologous sites. One consequence of this hyperrecombinability is the reduction to homozygosity of constitutionally heterozygous loci distal to the points of exchange. The hyperrecombinability in persons with BS who are genetic compounds can lead to reversion at *BLM* itself: crossing-over between the two different mutated sites within *BLM* can result in the generation of a functionally normal gene, and thereby correction of the cellular phenotype of the somatic cells that comprise the progeny of the cell in which the recombinational event had occurred.

4. Many of the clinical characteristics of BS may be viewed as direct or indirect consequences of the hypermutability and/or hyperrecombinability. It is postulated to be a major causative factor in BS's small size by way of the induction of factors that either inhibit further cell division or promote cell death. A major consequence is proneness to neoplasia; BS more than any other known human state predisposes to the development of cancer of the types and sites that affect the general population, and at unusually early ages. BS thus is the prototype of a class of disease that may be referred to as the somatic mutational disorders.

5. Diagnosis of BS is based on clinical observation; the phenotype is striking. Laboratory confirmation ordinarily is by cytogenetic demonstration of the characteristically increased tendency of chromatid exchange to take place. BS is the only condition known that features a greatly increased rate of sister-chromatid exchange (SCE). Blood lymphocytes in short-term culture are suitable for demonstrating this. Under certain circumstances, diagnosis can be confirmed by demonstrating mutation(s) in *BLM*.

6. With respect to the clinical management of BS, measures to increase the size have not been found. Protection from the sun, especially during infancy and childhood, is valuable in reducing the facial skin lesion severity. Regarding the proneness to cancer, greater than normal surveillance for carcinoma is indicated in persons who reach adulthood; however, because many are the sites and types of neoplasia that may arise, devising a surveillance program in BS is a particularly challenging matter, for both the affected person and the physician.

7. The mapping of *BLM* to chromosome band 15q26.1 and its subsequent molecular isolation identified a nuclear protein that contains a 350-amino acid domain consisting of 7 motifs characteristic of DNA and RNA helicases. The helicase domain of the BLM protein is 40 to 45 percent identical to the helicase domain present in the RecQ subfamily of DNA helicases. Although DNA-dependent adenosine triphosphatase (ATPase) and DNA-duplex-unwinding activities have been demonstrated for several RecQ helicases, including BLM, the nucleic acid substrates these proteins act upon in the cell are unknown. Whatever these substrates are, the molecular and genetic evidence implicates the RecQ helicases in the cellular mechanisms that maintain genomic stability. Therefore, the biochemical, molecular, and functional characterization of BLM, a protein not known earlier in mammalian cells, promises to provide fundamental understanding of how stability of the genome is maintained in somatic cells.

Homozygosity or compound mutant heterozygosity at *BLM*, a gene distal on chromosome No. 15, results in a striking phenotype known as Bloom syndrome (BS).[1–4, 5 and references cited therein] A constant clinical feature of BS, and one that makes a lasting impression on the observer, is a well-proportioned small size. The additional constant feature, but one not apparent from physical observation of the affected person, is instability of the genome; BS somatic cells accumulate more mutations than any other cell type known, apparently at any and every part of the genome. The genomic instability, which is of a characteristic type and to some extent recognizable through the microscope as "chromosome breakage,"[6,7] doubtless is responsible for the most important complication of BS, namely cancer.

BS's rarity explains its obscurity as an entity in clinical medicine; in contrast, the remarkable genomic instability and consequent hypermutability of the BS cell and the dramatic cancer proneness of the affected individual have awarded it prominence among students of mutation, DNA synthesis, DNA repair, and recombination, and among human biologists interested in the developmental consequences of mutation in somatic cells, including the consequences of somatic crossing-over which is greatly increased in BS. This chapter describes the clinical entity and its genetics; summarizes what is known of the hyperrecombinability and hypermutability of BS cells, including the microscopically visible chromosome breakage, the feature that first called attention to BS as an important clinical entity and experimental model; and summarizes its molecular genetics and recently acquired information about the protein encoded by *BLM*.

Diagnosing BS is always a momentous occasion because the physician who identifies a person with BS simultaneously identifies a person who, along with the other few persons alive with this very rare disorder, is at a far greater risk than anyone else of developing one or many of the cancers of the standard sites and types that affect humans, and at an unusually early age. Cancer emerges excessively in BS because throughout intrauterine and postnatal life an excessive number of mutations of various types and sites arise and accumulate in the somatic cells. However, some, possibly most, of the clinical features of BS other than the cancer proneness also are attributable to this genomic instability. Consequently, BS is the prototype of a class of human disease that can be referred to as the *somatic mutational disorders*.[4,8]

Thus, despite BS being exceedingly rare, it takes on inordinate significance in both academic medicine and human biology for two reasons. First, it displays dramatically the clinical consequences of an excessive somatic mutation rate. Any abnormality present in a person with BS, even though it may not be a recognized or recurring feature of the syndrome, is brought under suspicion of being etiologically a consequence of mutation, either directly or indirectly. Second, the BS cell and *BLM*, the BS gene, constitute valuable experimental materials in cell biology. It has been clear for a long time that the protein encoded by the BS gene must be of pivotal importance in the maintenance of genomic stability of somatic cells. Now its exact role there can be defined because with the cloning of the gene, molecular reagents have become available to investigate directly the function of the BLM protein.

THE CLINICAL ENTITY

Unreported data held in the files of the 168 persons who comprise the Bloom's Syndrome Registry are the source of most of the information presented here.[9] The Registry is comprised of the vast majority of persons ever diagnosed with BS up to 1991 (when it arbitrarily was closed to new accessions), and as far as can be determined is an unbiased representation of this very rare entity (Table 16-1). The mean age of those alive in the Registry is 21.6 years (range, 4 to 46 years), and the mean age at death has been 23.6 years (range, <1 to 49 years). Published clinical information from the Registry about BS, including photographs of affected persons, is found in references 1 to 5.

The predominating and constant clinical features of BS are listed as 1 and 2 below. Only the first, however, is obvious from physical observation:

1. An overall *small body size* with fairly normal proportioning except for a slightly disproportionately small brain/head accompanied by dolichocephaly. Subcutaneous fatty tissue is disproportionately sparse. The several fetuses whose size has been monitored by sonography have been much smaller than expected for their ages. The mean birth weight for males is 1906 g (range, 930 to 3400) and for females 1810 g (range, 920 to 2667). The mean adult height for men is 147.5 cm (range, 130 to 162), and for women is 138.6 cm (range, 122 to 151) (Fig. 16-1).
2. An enormous *predisposition to cancer*, of many cell types and sites.

Eleven additional features that may or may not be present in persons with BS and that vary in severity are the following

Table 16-1 Composition of the Population in the Bloom's Syndrome Registry

	No.	Age* (yr.) Mean	Age* (yr.) Range
Persons affected with BS			
Alive	108 (64%)	21.6	4–46
Dead	60 (35%)	23.6	<1–49
Total affected persons	168		
Families			
With 1 affected with BS	116 (83%)		
With 2 affected with BS	22 (16%)		
With 3 affected with BS	0 (0%)		
With 4 affected with BS	2 (1%)		
Total families	140		
Dwelling places of persons			
North America	83		
Europe	41		
Asia Minor	16		
Japan	12		
Meso- & South America	11		
Australia	3		
North Africa	2		
Ethnic origins of families			
European, non-Jewish	66		
Mixed	34**		
German	11		
Italian	9		
Dutch/Flemish	6		
British	5		
Other	4		
Jewish	42		
Ashkenazi***	41		
Non-Ashkenazi	1		
Japanese	10		
South American Mixed	6		
African American	4		
Turkish	4		
Arab Mohammedan	2		
Mexican Mestizo	2		
Gypsy	1		
*Consanguinity****			
Non-Jewish	31/105 families		
Ashkenazi Jewish*****	2/35 families		
Non-Ashkenazi Jewish	1/1 families		

NOTE: 114 of the 168 registered persons have been examined personally by at least one registrar, i.e., by the late David Bloom, James German, and, or, Eberhard Passarge.
*Age at present if living; age at death if dead.
**Most non-Jewish Americans, Canadians, and Australians are classified "Mixed."
***One or both parents.
****Of the parents of affected individuals.
*****Both parents.

(ordinarily, the presence of several of these serves to distinguish BS from other disorders that feature a striking degree of growth deficiency):

3. A *characteristic facies* (Fig. 16-2). The face is somewhat keel-shaped because of the small narrow cranium, malar hypoplasia, nasal prominence, and small mandible. The ears may be protuberant and unusually prominent.
4. *Hypersensitivity to sunlight* of the areas of the skin ordinarily exposed to the sun during infancy, i.e., the face and the dorsa of the hands and forearms.
5. Patchy areas of *hyper- and hypopigmentation of the skin.*

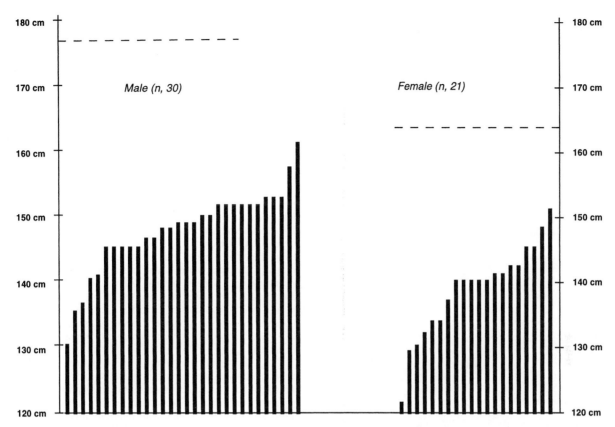

Fig. 16-1 Distribution of known heights (tops of vertical bars) of persons in the Registry who have reached the age of 20 years. (Dashed lines show the means for normal adults.)

6. A *characteristic voice*, high-pitched and of a somewhat coarse, squeaky timbre.

7. A variable degree of *vomiting and diarrhea* during infancy, that often rapidly leads to life-threatening dehydration. Their basis is obscure. Also, a large proportion of affected infants and young children show a profound *lack of interest in eating*. The gastrointestinal problems, along with the repeated respiratory tract and ear infections, make infancy a trying period for many parents of children with BS.

8. *Diabetes mellitus*, as yet neither well characterized clinically nor studied experimentally (Table 16-2). Diabetes has been diagnosed in 20 of the 168 persons in the Registry (11.9 percent), at a mean age of 24.9 years (range, 11 to 40 years). Although the diabetes of BS in many ways resembles standard late-onset, noninsulin-dependent diabetes, it has not yet been studied sufficiently to permit such classification; six of the diabetics in the Registry required insulin therapy; ketoacidosis occurred in several of the diabetics, and diabetic retinopathy was documented in one.

9. *Infertility*, although four exceptional women have given birth to seven normal, healthy babies. At least after puberty the testes are abnormally small. Women cease menstruating unusually early.

10. *Immunodeficiency* of a generalized type, ranging from mild and essentially asymptomatic to severe, manifested by recurrent respiratory tract infections complicated by otitis media and pneumonia.[10] In 20 percent of cases, at least one life-threatening bacterial infection of the respiratory tract that would have led to early death in the preantibiotic era is recorded. Inadequately treated lung infections may lead to bronchiectasis and crippling chronic lung disease that in five instances has been fatal, becoming the second commonest cause of death, next after cancer (Table 16-2). Serious middle-ear infections have occurred in 29 percent of persons with BS, which may decrease auditory acuity. Although not known to

be on an infectious basis, a mild, sometimes recurring, idiopathic hepatitis has been reported in several affected individuals, and evidence of liver toxicity is common when cancer chemotherapy is administered.

11. A slightly excessive incidence of *minor anatomic anomalies*, including mildly anomalous digits, pilonidal dimples, wedges of altered color of the irides, and, curiously, obstructing anomalies of the urethra, this last being of major clinical importance in several cases.

12. *Restricted intellectual ability.* Intelligence in BS is judged (usually without testing) sometimes to be average but much more often low-average. When limitation does exist, it varies widely in degree from moderate to frankly deficient. It is impossible to predict early in life whether a person with BS will have some degree of mental deficiency or be normal. Although two affected individuals have been frankly deficient mentally, several others have completed college, two obtaining masters degrees. However, even when testing indicates normal intelligence, there tends to be a poorly defined and unexplained learning disability and short attention span. Characteristically this is associated with an inability to develop a normally wide array of interests. From earliest childhood, the person with BS typically exhibits a charming, pleasant personality, but fails to mature from a childlike judgment and gullibility and (perhaps fortunately, in view of the grim specter of early neoplasia) maintains a seemingly inordinate optimism. Several affected persons have displayed unusually poor memory.

13. Any one of an array of seemingly *unrelated clinical entities or features*. Each of these has occurred in only one or a few individuals, and they are not to be considered part of BS itself. They include hyperlipidemia, congenital thrombocytopenia, chronic idiopathic thrombocytopenic purpura, hypothyroidism, idiopathic hepatitis, mild anemia, and, in some cases, a poorly defined dyserythropoiesis, asthma, arthritis (in one case

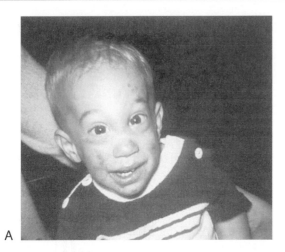

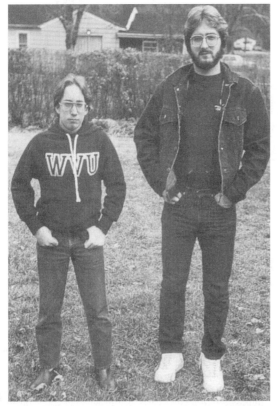

Fig. 16-2 51(KeMc) in the Bloom's Syndrome Registry manifests the major clinical features of BS. His birthweight was 2160 g and his birth length 44.5 cm. He exhibited striking dolichocephaly and hypoplastic malar areas. Within the first year of life, a moderate to severe photosensitive erythematous skin lesion appeared that was limited to the face and hands. He also had a recurring fissure of the lower lip. *A.* 51(KeMc) at about 18 months showing the facial skin lesion. *B.* On left, 51(KeMc) at age 17, exhibiting small body size (height 147 cm, weight 41 kg) and the facial skin lesion, and on right, his unaffected brother at age 19. The unaffected brother is just under 6 feet tall. 51(KeMc), who is healthy at age 27, was successfully treated for acute undifferentiated leukemia at age 12.

severe and accompanied by psoriasis), acanthosis nigricans, and Legg-Perthes disease.

The Skin in BS

In BS, two unrelated skin lesions coexist:

A Sun-Sensitive Facial Lesion. The clinically more important skin lesion of BS is a sun-sensitive erythema that is limited almost

exclusively to the face, usually unassociated with dyspigmentation. The cheeks and nose are the areas most often affected, explaining an early erroneous confusion by dermatologists of BS and lupus. In exceptionally severe cases, the erythema does extend to the ears, sides, and back of the neck, the suprasternal area, and, very rarely and in mild degree, onto the shoulders or upper chest. The dorsa of the hands and forearms may be mildly affected. However, effectively ruling out the diagnosis, BS is any prominent erythematous, telangiectatic lesion that affects the trunk, lower extremities, arms, or buttocks even though the face might also be affected.

The clinical onset of the facial skin lesion usually is as persistent erythema that follows the infant's first significant exposure to sunlight, which most often has been during the first or second summer of life. In one exceptional case, the lesion did not appear until age 12. The sun-sensitive skin lesion varies in severity and may be absent. The severity of the erythema when present ranges from a faint blush during the summertime to a disfiguring, flaming red lesion of irregular distribution over the bridge of the nose, cheeks, and other facial areas. Crying may accentuate what appears on first examination to be a minimal or absent lesion. The lower eyelids often are hyperemic, and atrophy of the lower lid with loss of eyelashes is common. In many cases, blistering and encrustation and a recurring fissure of the lower lip during summertime become a particularly aggravating aspect of the lesion.

The severity and extent of the skin lesion usually is apparent by early childhood. Often parents intuitively protect a child from the sun when they realize that hypersensitivity is present, which may explain the failure of progression in severity at later ages in many cases. Similarly, in sibships with multiple affected children, the rigorous protection from the sun of later-born affecteds is associated with a mild or absent skin lesion. Ordinarily, if there is to be a significant skin lesion, it makes its appearance during the first two years of life. (It is not congenital as originally described — "congenital telangiectatic erythema resembling lupus erythematosus in dwarfs."[11]) Although some form of sun sensitivity quite clearly exists early in life in BS, the few objective tests of nonfacial skin that have been carried out by dermatologists have failed either to characterize the defect or even detect its existence. Furthermore, several adults with BS report that they enjoy sunbathing and tanning, and that they are unaware of sun-hypersensitivity of other than facial skin. However, the lesion in the area that was symptomatic early in life persists, as does its continued accentuation by sun-exposure.

Usually, careful examination of the affected area reveals an accompanying telangiectasia, varying in degree from minimal to prominent. It usually is absent during infancy. Even when the erythema is minimal to absent, careful examination often reveals a faint degree of telangiectasia at the margin of the upper lip or about the nose or cheeks. In severe cases, the erythema and telangiectasia are accompanied by irregular patches of atrophic skin and dyspigmentation. In 6 of the 168 registered cases, prominent telangiectasia of the bulbar conjunctiva — as prominent as in the entity ataxia-telangiectasia — has been present, but not correlated with the severity of the skin lesion.

The pathogenesis of the sun-sensitive skin lesion of BS is obscure. Histologic study has been made in a few cases but has contributed little to an understanding of the pathogenesis; biopsy is not indicated for diagnostic purposes. In males, the lesion is more severe than in females, and relatively greater underdiagnosis of BS itself in females probably contributes to their slight under-representation in the Bloom's Syndrome Registry — 93 males versus 75 females.

A Non-Sun-Sensitive Lesion Not Limited to the Face. A second skin abnormality exists in BS, clinically and presumably pathogenetically completely different from the sun-sensitive lesion. It consists of prominent well-circumscribed areas of hyperpigmentation — the café-au-lait spots of normal people but

Table 16-2 The Serious Medical Complications in the 168 Persons in the Bloom's Syndrome Registry

	Number of Persons Affected	Death from the Complication	Age at diagnosis (yrs)	
			Mean	Range
Chronic lung disease	7	5		
Diabetes mellitus	20	0	24.9	11–40
Cancer*				
Persons with 1 or > 1 primaries	71	50	24.7	2–48
Persons with 2 or > 2 primaries	19			
Persons with 3 or > 3 primaries	5			
Persons with 4 or > 4 primaries	3			
Persons with 5 primaries	2			

*A total of 100 cancers diagnosed, in 71 of the 168 persons in the Registry.[12]

present in BS in excessive numbers and often quite extensive. These lesions may appear anywhere on the body, but are most commonly found on the trunk. The hyperpigmented lesions vary in diameter from a few millimeters to many centimeters, in an occasional person being linear and extending over the back of the thorax. Most often, the several hyperpigmented lesions tend to have similar degrees of brownness, but an occasional spot may be considerably darker than the others. Sometimes the brownish spots, large as well as small, are found in a localized cluster. Well-demarcated hypopigmented areas also are highly characteristic of BS but usually are less conspicuous than the hyperpigmented lesions. Exceptionally, a hypopigmented area can, like a hyperpigmented one, be extensive and cover an area many centimeters in diameter. In affected individuals of sub-Saharan African ancestry, the hyperpigmented and especially the hypopigmented areas are more prominent than in lighter-complexioned persons, some appearing quite black and others strikingly white. It usually is in early childhood, rather than in infancy, that the pigmentary changes are first noted.

Neoplasia[4,12]

At any time in the life of a person with BS, a neoplasm is much more likely to appear than in other people of the same age. The four most impressive aspects of the neoplasia proneness of BS are the great frequency with which both benign (not discussed further here) and malignant neoplasia arise, the wide variety of anatomic sites and cellular types, the exceptionally early age at which neoplasms become clinically apparent, and the frequency with which multiple neoplasms arise in one person (Table 16-2).

The first 100 cancers that arose in BS after it was recognized as a clinical entity in 1954 are listed in Table 16-3 along with the age ranges at which they were diagnosed. The distribution of sites and types of cancers in BS resembles that in the general population (however, with a few interesting exceptions, e.g., prostate), but in BS, they arise at a greatly increased frequency, and in the case of the carcinomata and acute myelogenous leukemias, they arise decades earlier than expected. The mean age at diagnosis of cancer has been 24.7 years (range, 2 to 48 years). It has been responsible for the death of 50 of the 60 persons in the Registry who have died.

Because of this remarkable excess in BS of the cancers that affect other people, BS has been chosen as a model. The study of BS at the cellular, chromosomal, and DNA levels should facilitate the analysis of the changes responsible for the initiation and progression of the generality of human cancer. The hypotheses in such work are that among the mutations that arise in BS cells are those responsible, as in other people, not just for neoplastic

transformation but also for progression of a transformed clone into clinical cancer; and that the changes that arise abnormally frequently in BS cells very probably include those responsible for these processes in other people. In BS, these changes take place spontaneously; in others they may also be spontaneous during normal cell metabolism — very possibly this is the usual situation in human cancer — or they may be the effects of environmental mutational agents.

The inherited mutations responsible for the phenotype BS are in a category different from those that arise at the loci mutated in, for example, retinoblastoma, Wilms tumor, and familial polyposis coli. When mutated, those cell proliferation-controlling loci become so-called cancer genes and can represent one step of many in cancer's initiation and progression. In contrast, homozygosity or compound heterozygosity for BS-causing mutation(s) at *BLM* constitutes *a mutator genotype*. In BS cells, the somatic mutations that must occur for clinical cancer to emerge were not inherited through the germ line, but they are far more likely to arise spontaneously than in cells of other people because BS is a mutator phenotype. It also is noteworthy that in BS, every cell in the body capable of further division is at the high risk of neoplastic transformation.

Somatic mutation at *BLM* is not itself known to be of significance as a step in either cancer initiation or progression. That a somatic mutation can give rise to a genetically unstable cell lineage that is of etiologic significance in cancer is a concept that derives from the study of sporadic cancer as well as hereditary nonpolyposis colorectal cancer (HNPCC), and, therefore, the development through somatic mutation of a lineage "with Bloom syndrome" is an interesting formal possibility, evidence for which could be sought.

Thus, the basis for the predisposition to cancer in BS doubtless is the remarkably excessive genomic instability featured by BS cells. The immunodeficiency of BS quite conceivably contributes to the cancer proneness, but its role in progression is difficult to determine because of the major role played by mutation.

GENOMIC INSTABILITY

The enzymatic systems that carry out the fundamental processes of the replication and transmission of the genetic material from generation to generation, of both germ-line and somatic cells, are diverse and complex. To ensure fidelity, these systems incorporate multiple mechanisms to maintain genomic stability, including (a) proofreading capacities of the DNA polymerases and replication machinery; (b) mechanisms that allow the DNA replication

Table 16-3 The First 100 Cancers Recorded in the Bloom's Syndrome Registry[12], Showing the Age Groups at Time of Diagnosis

Class & type	Age Group 0–10	11–20	21–30	31–40	41–50	Total
Rare tumors* (n = 5)						
Medulloblastoma	1					1
Wilms tumor	2					2
Osteogenic sarcoma	1	1				2
Leukemia, acute (n = 22)						
Lymphocytic	4	2	1			7
Myelogenous	1	1	3	1		6
Biphenotypic		1		1		2
Other or unspecified	1	3	2	1		7
Lymphoma (n = 22)						
Non-Hodgkin	4	6	6	3	1	20
Hodgkin disease		2				2
Carcinoma (n = 51)						
Skin		2	3	3		8
Auditory canal, external			1	1		2
Tongue, posterior			1	1	2	4
Esophagus, squamous				3		3
Esophagus, adeno					1	1
Stomach			1	1		2
Colon						
Cecum, ascending			1	2		3
Hepatic flexure transverse		1		2	1	4
Descending, sigmoid, rectum			1	5		6
Tonsil				1		1
Larynx; epiglottis			2	1		3
Lung				1		1
Uterus						
Cervix		1	3			4
Corpus					1	1
Breast			1	5	1	7
Metastatic, primary site unknown			1			1
Totals	14	20	27	32	7	100

*A meningioma was diagnosed at age 9 in one registered individual. Two Wilms tumors and a retinoblastoma diagnosed at 5 months, 22 months, and 2 years of age, respectively, are known to have occurred in children with BS who are known to the Registry, but not officially registered.

complex to idle at damaged DNA in a way that permits repair; (c) mechanisms that allow the bypass of the damaged DNA altogether (*trans*-lesion synthesis); (d) repair enzymes that recognize damaged DNA and either repair the damage directly or recruit other enzymes to carry that out; (e) proteins that signal to the cell the presence of DNA damage and that prevent the cell's traversing its cycle prior to repair; and (f) systems that package and condense the chromatin and that ensure the proper segregation of the chromosomes at mitosis. These systems maintain genomic stability and act to prevent errors that might lead, on the one hand, to unscheduled cell death or, on the other, to abnormal, unregulated cellular proliferation.

Genetically determined defects in the systems that maintain genomic stability and ensure fidelity of replication have been identified in many model organisms, and also in the human. In human genetics, genomic instability first was recognized through microscopic observation of chromosomal abnormalities—chromosome breakage—in cultured cells from individuals with certain rare syndromes, first in BS and later in Fanconi anemia, ataxia-telangiectasia, the Nijmegan breakage syndrome, Werner syndrome, and xeroderma pigmentosum (in the last, only after ultraviolet light irradiation). In all of these syndromes, the cytogenetic abnormalities are accompanied by an increase in the rate of spontaneous somatic mutations, mutagen-induced mutations, or both. This hypermutability provides an explanation for the predisposition to some type of cancer, a feature shared by all these syndromes. These clinical entities, along with several others that lack chromosome breakage but that are characterized by some form of genomic instability at the molecular level (e.g., HNPCC), fall under the rubric already proposed, somatic mutational disorders.

When the chromosomes in BS cells that are proliferating in culture but otherwise untreated are examined microscopically, an abundance of gaps, breaks, and structural rearrangements in the chromosomes is found.[7] However, the difference from normal is quantitative, and similar lesions in the chromosomes are present in untreated cells from other people, just much less frequently. The two most characteristic cytogenetic abnormalities (1 and 2 below) are the result of a strikingly increased tendency in BS somatic cells for exchange to take place between DNA strands, probably at the time they replicate during the S phase of the cell-division cycle:

1. The exchanges may be between a chromatid of each of the two homologues of a chromosome pair (e.g., between the two Nos. 1 or the two Nos. 19), the points of exchange being at seemingly homologous regions of the chromatids involved. At the mitosis that follows, such an interchange is detectable microscopically as a symmetrical, four-armed configuration—a quadriradial (QR)—composed of the pair of chromosomes between which the interchange had taken place (Fig. 16-3). Or,

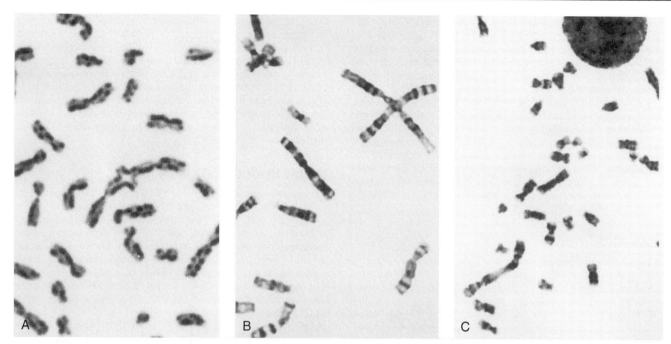

Fig. 16-3 *A.* A portion of a Bloom syndrome lymphocyte metaphase. The cell had been cultured in BrdU-containing medium to make possible the differential staining (light or dark) of sister chromatids; alternating regions of light and dark staining signify exchanges between sister chromatids (SCEs). The number of SCEs in cells from normal persons averages <10/metaphase, whereas BS lymphocytes show (as here) 60 to 90/metaphase or more; a greatly elevated SCE frequency is diagnostic of BS. Also present in this cell is a quadriradial (QR) configuration, the result of an interchange between chromatids of the No. 1 chromosomes. QRs affecting homologous regions of the homologous chromosomes are present in approximately 1% of BS blood T lymphocytes, but they also are found on rare occasions in cells from healthy persons without BS. Both QRs and SCEs can be induced in normal cells by exposure to certain DNA-damaging agents, as in *B*; BS cells, already with an elevated constitutional number of such lesions, show an excessive response to such agents. B. G-banded metaphase chromosomes showing a QR, the result of a chromatid interchange at the proximal portions of the long arms of the No. 1 chromosomes. The cell, from a healthy person without BS, had been exposed *in vitro* to mitomycin C several hours before it entered mitosis. QRs of this type are present in excessive number in untreated cells from persons with BS. *C.* G-banded metaphase chromosomes of a BS lymphocyte showing a telomere association, possibly the result of a chromatid interchange (equivalent to those that resulted in the QRs in *A* and *B*) that had taken place near the ends of the short arms of the No. 1 chromosomes. (Reprinted with permission from German J: Bloom syndrome: A mendelian prototype of somatic mutational disease. *Medicine* 72:393, 1993.)

2. The exchanges may be intrachromosomal, between the two sister chromatids of one chromosome. The consequence of these exchanges also are microscopically visible in appropriately treated cells — SCEs (Fig. 16-3A). In cells from non-BS individuals, a mean of fewer than 10 SCEs/metaphase is found; in striking contrast, BS cells characteristically have from 50 to 100 SCEs/metaphase depending on the type of cell examined, but highest in blood lymphocytes in short-term culture.

Submicroscopic mutations also are increased in BS. BS cells taken directly from the circulating blood have a dramatic increase over normal in the number of mutations they have accumulated at the coding loci that have been studied extensively, namely, the locus on the X chromosome that encodes the enzyme HPRT, the glycophorin A locus on chromosome No. 4 that determines the MN blood type, and the HLA locus on chromosome No. 6.[4,13,14] The types of mutations that have been detected include somatic crossing-over.[15] Other evidence of the genomic instability of BS cells, at least *in vitro*, is excessive mutation at regions of the genome composed of repeat sequences.[16–18]

DIAGNOSIS

Any cell type that can be brought into mitosis by the cytogeneticist can be employed to rule a clinical diagnosis of BS in or out. Blood lymphocytes stimulated to enter cell cycling by phytohemagglutinin are most often used, but freshly aspirated bone marrow cells or long-term cultures of skin fibroblasts or of embryonic/fetal cells also can be examined. The two most valuable indicators of BS are (a) the demonstration of the symmetric QR interchange configuration in untreated cells and (b) the greatly increased number of SCEs in cells allowed to pass two cell cycles in medium containing BrdU (Fig. 16-3). BS is the only disorder known to feature an increased rate of SCE.

BS should be considered whenever severe intrauterine growth deficiency is encountered and cannot be explained, especially if the deficiency extends into infancy and childhood. Also, BS might well be considered in small but well-proportioned children or adults with a sun-sensitive, erythematous skin lesion that is limited to the face even if their growth deficiency is of only moderate degree. Correspondingly, a normal birth weight with a postnatal length/height not less than the third percentile for normals, militate strongly against the diagnosis BS.

Therefore, an SCE analysis is indicated in both children and adults with unexplained growth deficiency (i.e., BS should be included in the differential diagnosis). Although SCE screening has not yet been carried out, so that its value is unknown, an SCE analysis will possibly identify persons with BS in unusually small members of the following groups of individuals even when a characteristic skin lesion is lacking: persons with excessive numbers of café-au-lait spots, usually accompanied by hypopigmented spots; persons with unexplained immunodeficiency; children or adults with an unexplained restriction on intelligence; persons in whom diabetes mellitus develops later than the usual age of onset of type I and earlier than that of type II; infertile men with abnormally small testes for which no explanation can be found, and possibly women with an exceptionally early onset of menopause; children or adults who develop clinical neoplasia. It is unknown how valuable a routine SCE analysis would be for unusually small persons who develop cancer but who lack BS's facial lesion; however, in the Registry, 7 of the 71 individuals with BS who developed cancer (Table 16-2) were recognized to have BS only at the time or after a cancer was diagnosed. Only then was the significance of their small size, unusual facies, or facial skin lesion recognized by some physicians who knew of BS.

BS doubtless is underdiagnosed. Many cases of it long remain in diagnostic wastebaskets such as idiopathic intrauterine growth retardation, "primordial dwarfism," and "failure to thrive" until an informed physician requests an SCE analysis. Some patients are erroneously considered to have some rare disorder other than BS; for example, 10 of the 168 persons with proven BS in the Bloom's Syndrome Registry were thought possibly or definitely to have Russell-Silver dwarfism until cytogenetic study provided the correct diagnosis.

GENETICS

Clinical BS is the phenotype that results from the inheritance from each parent of a mutation at *BLM*, the BS gene, which is located in chromosome band 15q26.1.[19] Individuals heterozygous for mutations at *BLM* ("carriers") are normally developed and healthy. With respect to the germ line, however, where the BS protein attaches transiently during meiotic prophase to synapsed chromosome bivalents,[20,21] the only study available points to an effect of heterozygosity for *BLM* mutation.[22]

Mutation(s) at *BLM* appears to segregate in most if not all human populations, but in all, BS is very rare. Only in Ashkenazi Jews is mutation at *BLM* known to have reached a relatively high frequency; a population survey of BS in Israel in 1971 and 1972 indicated a heterozygote frequency greater than 1 in 120. The recent identification of a 6-bp deletion and a 7-bp insertion in exon 10 of *BLM* (see below), referred to as *blm^Ash*, now has permitted a more accurate determination of the frequency of carriers in that major subgroup of Jewry: survey of New York City Ashkenazi Jews conducted in collaboration with the Department of Medical Genetics of Mt. Sinai Hospital Medical School sets the number at 1 in 107.[23] In other surveys, similar estimates of the allele frequency of *blm^Ash* have been obtained.[24–26]

The mutated loci on the two No. 15 chromosomes in any given individual with BS may correctly be suspected to be identical — homozygous — when that person's parents are consanguineous or when the parents both are Ashkenazi Jews. In those two situations the mutations at *BLM* are usually identical by virtue of their descent from a common ancestor who was a carrier of a BS mutation.[19,27] In addition to homozygosity, two unlike mutations sometimes are inherited and are responsible for BS; such individuals are referred to as genetic compounds, or said to have compound heterozygosity. The phenotype BS seems to be the same regardless of whether the mutant *BLM* loci are or are not inherited from a common ancestor. As becomes apparent below, the majority of the many BS-associated mutations at *BLM* are essentially nulls for the encoded protein.

The carrier of a BS mutation ordinarily is identified only after having become the parent of a child with BS. Molecular isolation of *BLM* now does provide another means of heterozygote detection among other relatives of persons with BS, as well as in the population at large.[23,28] The risk of other children with BS is 1 in 4 after an affected child is born to a union of proven heterozygotes. Pregnancies at risk can be tested by sonography and cytogenetics. In families in which each of the two mutated *BLM* alleles has been defined at the molecular level, direct sequence determination can be performed. However, if the two mutated *BLM* alleles have not been identified, haplotype analysis can be carried out.

MOLECULAR GENETICS OF *BLM*

The chromosome abnormalities observed in BS cells noted earlier pointed to a defect in some fundamental process of DNA metabolism that helps maintain genomic stability. Retarded replication-fork progression and abnormal replicational intermediates, but the absence of defects in known DNA-repair systems, implicated a disturbance of the process of DNA replication itself.[4] Biochemical studies of a number of enzymes that participate in replication and repair did reveal abnormalities in the enzymatic activities of DNA ligase I, topoisomerase II in BrdU-treated cells, uracil DNA glycosylase, O^6-methylguanine methyltransferase, N-methylpurine DNA glycosylase, and superoxide dismutase. However, none of these abnormalities, though often demonstrable, identified the primary defect in BS; they appear to be phenotypic consequences of the BS mutation. Because the identification of the primary defect promised to reveal an important component in nucleic acid metabolism, a positional cloning strategy was undertaken to isolate *BLM*—as a result of which a previously unknown protein in mammalian cells was identified.[28]

Localization of *BLM* to 15q26.1[19]

A limited amount of evidence from cell hybridization studies had suggested that BS is a single-gene disorder.[29] The first step in the positional cloning effort to isolate the gene was to identify linkages between *BLM* and mapped polymorphic markers. Introduction of a normal human chromosome 15 by microcell-mediated chromosome transfer was shown to correct toward normal the high-SCE phenotype of a BS cell line.[30] Subsequently, homozygosity mapping demonstrated tight linkage between *BLM* and *FES*.[19] *FES* already had been localized by *in situ* hybridization to 15q26.1. Linkage in most of these families was detected thereafter[27] at five additional highly polymorphic DNA markers that flank *FES* (depicted in Fig. 16-4). Thus, homozygosity mapping permitted assignment of *BLM* to a 2-cM interval that includes *FES*.

Founder Effect in Ashkenazi Jews with Bloom Syndrome[3,27]

As mentioned earlier, BS is more common in the Ashkenazi Jewish than in any other known population.[3] Several of the polymorphic microsatellite loci found to be tightly linked to *BLM* by homozygosity mapping were genotyped in affected and

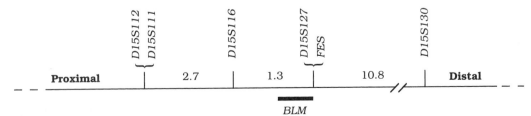

Fig. 16-4 Map positions of six highly polymorphic DNA markers on chromosome 15 linked to *BLM*. The loci shown above the line representing chromosome 15 were employed in homozygosity mapping (genetic map distances in cM). Braced loci have not been separated by recombinational analysis. *FES* and *D15S127* are separated by 30 kb (see Fig. 16–6). The location of *BLM* is represented by the thick line between DNA markers *FES/D15S127* and *D15S116*.

unaffected individuals from the Ashkenazi Jewish population. A striking allele association between *blm^Ash* and one of the six alleles at *FES*, specifically allele C3, and between *blm^Ash* and two related alleles of the CA-repeat locus *D15S127* [a locus that is 30 kilobases (kb) proximal to *FES*], specifically alleles 145 bp and 147 bp, was detected in Ashkenazi Jews with BS.[27] (The association of *blm^Ash* with two alleles rather than one at *D15S127* is assumed to result from recurrent mutation at *D15S127*, producing toggling between the 145- and 147-bp alleles.)

This linkage disequilibrium confirmed the linkage results from homozygosity mapping and provided strong support for a founder-effect hypothesis to explain the increased incidence of BS in the Ashkenazim relative to other populations. By one historical model, a chromosome that bore *blm^Ash* in the genome of a postulated "founder" was carried into Eastern Europe several centuries ago as the Jews, along with many others, migrated there. Subsequently, *blm^Ash* and its flanking chromosomal segments increased in frequency in the Jews there as a result of genetic drift. In other words, today Ashkenazi Jews with BS inherit their mutated *BLM* gene identical by descent from a common ancestor who lived possibly 30 generations ago, making the parents of such individuals distant cousins. Definitive evidence for the founder-effect hypothesis has been obtained by mutational analysis of the mutated *BLM* in the majority of Ashkenazi Jewish persons ever diagnosed BS (presented below).

Evidence for Allelic Heterogeneity at *BLM*[31]

A strikingly elevated SCE rate is uniquely characteristic of BS cells and is present in all cell types examined: mitogen-stimulated blood T and B lymphocytes in short-term culture; Epstein-Barr virus-transformed lymphocytes in long-term culture; cells from the bone marrow in short-term culture; cultured diploid fibroblasts, including fibroblasts from skin, amniotic fluid, chorionic villi, and surgical specimens; and aneuploid SV40-transformed fibroblasts in long-term culture. All persons with BS have high-SCE cells. However, an important, and until recently unexplained, exception was recognized over two decades ago[128]: a small number of blood lymphocytes with a normal SCE rate circulate in the blood in a minority of persons with BS. In these persons, the frequency of low-SCE cells detected in short-term cultures of phytohemagglutinin-stimulated T lymphocytes ranges from under 1 percent to in excess of 50 percent (the highest level recorded in the Registry being 75 percent). The low-SCE cells are considered functionally normal because cell hybrids formed by a low-SCE BS cell and a high-SCE BS cell have a low-SCE phenotype,[29] just as do cell hybrids formed between a low-SCE cell from a normal person and a high-SCE BS cell.[32]

This enigmatic high-SCE/low-SCE mosaicism was investigated by comparing its incidence in subpopulations of persons with BS sorted according to whether or not *BLM* was known to have been inherited identical by descent. A striking negative correlation emerged:[31] In persons with BS whose parents share a common ancestor, the case in persons born either to consanguineous parents or to two Ashkenazi Jewish parents (approximately one-half the BS families), a population of low-SCE cells is almost never found; conversely, the mosaicism occurs almost exclusively in persons with BS whose parents are not known to share a common ancestor. Because those who share a common ancestor almost all inherit the identical mutation at *BLM*, the negative correlation was interpreted to mean that emergence of low-SCE cells in BS depends in some way on the preexistence of compound heterozygosity, i.e., on having two different mutated *BLM* alleles. A corollary to this was that BS is genetically heterogeneous. That multiple mutations are present at *BLM* now has been confirmed by mutational analysis of *BLM* in different persons with BS (see below, and Table 16-4).

Somatic Intragenic Recombination[33]

The population cytogenetic data just summarized[31] indicated that high-SCE/low-SCE mosaic persons are genetic compounds. The requirement of compound heterozygosity, when considered along with the known high rate of homologous recombination taking place in BS somatic cells as compared to normal cells, suggested that a specific form of crossing-over that was not known to occur in higher organisms, namely, intragenic recombination, explains the mosaicism in some persons with BS. Somatic crossing-over between the paternally derived and the maternally derived mutated sites within *BLM* could generate a functionally wild-type *BLM* that would correct the high-SCE phenotype of a BS cell (Fig. 16-5). By this model, the newly generated, functionally wild-type gene on one chromosome No. 15 could segregate at mitosis with either the nonrecombinant chromatid of the other chromosome No. 15—allele losses distal to *BLM* then would ensue (i.e., reduction to homozygosity)—or with the recombinant chromatid that now carries a doubly mutant *BLM*—allele losses distal to *BLM* would not ensue.

Evidence supporting the intragenic recombination model was obtained by genotype analysis of 12 loci syntenic with *BLM*—6 proximal and 6 distal to it—in 11 persons who exhibited the high-SCE/low-SCE mosaicism.[33] In 5 of the 11 persons examined, polymorphic loci on chromosome 15q distal to *BLM* that were heterozygous in their high-SCE cells had become homozygous in their low-SCE cells, whereas loci proximal to *BLM* that were heterozygous on 15q had remained heterozygous. In the remaining six persons, loci both proximal and distal to *BLM* that were heterozygous in their high-SCE cells had remained heterozygous in their low-SCE cells. These observations indicate that intragenic recombination between the two different mutated alleles at *BLM* is a mechanism that can generate a functionally wild-type *BLM* gene (Fig. 16-5). Thus, the low-SCE lymphocytes present in the blood of mosaic persons can be the progeny of a somatic stem cell in which such an intragenic recombination event had occurred.

After identification of the *BLM* gene, characterization of the majority of mutations present in persons with BS (described below) revealed a second mechanism by which high-SCE/low-SCE mosaicism could be generated.[34] In two of the persons in which heterozygosity had been maintained distal to the *BLM* locus in low-SCE compared to the high-SCE cells, the causative mutation detected in the DNA from the high-SCE cells was homozygous. One person was constitutionally homozygous for the mutation *BLM*1544insA* and the other person for the mutation *BLM*2702G → A*. Analysis of the DNAs from the low-SCE cells showed that a normal allele at *BLM* had been reconstituted by back mutation—in one person by deletion of an A base that had been inserted and in the other person by nucleotide substitution of a normal G base for a mutant A base. Thus, bona fide back mutation becomes the second important mechanism by which mosaicism can be generated, having occurred in the cells of 2 of the 11 persons examined from whom both low-SCE and high-SCE cells were available. Determination of the constitutional *BLM* mutations in the 10 other persons with BS who had exhibited high-SCE/low-SCE mosaicism and from whom constitutional DNA was available for mutational analysis revealed homozygosity for the mutation *BLM*1544insA* in one suggesting that back mutation had occurred in this person and for the *blm^Ash* mutation in an Ashkenazi Jewish person. In this Jewish person, however, it is unlikely that back mutation was the molecular mechanism by which mosaicism was generated, because *blm^Ash* is a complex insertion/deletion mutation that leads to a +1 frameshift. Rather, we suggest that a single-base deletion occurred just proximal to the site of *blm^Ash* that compensated for the frameshift event at the expense of several out-of-frame amino acids being inserted into the protein. Compensatory frameshift has been demonstrated as a mechanism that can generate mosaicism in a person with Fanconi anemia;[35] unfortunately, low-SCE cell lines from the mosaic person homozygous for *blm^Ash* are unavailable to test this hypothesis.

Isolation and Mutational Analysis of *BLM*[36]

The availability of the five low-SCE cell lines just mentioned, in which somatic intragenic recombination had led to reduction to

Table 16-4 Representative BLM Mutations Identified in Persons with Bloom Syndrome (August 31, 1996)[a]

Identification[b]	Ancestry	Zygosity of the Mutation[c]	Nucleotide Change[d]	Protein Change[e]
Missense mutations				
139(ViKre)[g]	Mixed European	Heterozygous	2015A > G	Q672R
31(CaDe)[g]	Dutch	Heterozygous	2015A > G	Q672R
40(DoRoe)	Mixed European	Homozygous	2702G > A	C901Y[f]
113(DaDem)	Italian	Homozygous	3164G > C	C1055S
Nonsense mutations				
97(AsOk)	Japanese	Homozygous	557-559delCAA	S186X
112(NaSch)	Mixed European	Heterozygous	814A > T	K272X
98(RoMo)[g]	Mixed European	Heterozygous	1090A > T	R364X
81(MaGrou)	French Canadian	Homozygous	1784C > A	S595X
11(IaTh)[g]	Mixed European	Heterozygous	1933C > T	Q645X
61(DoHop)	Mixed European	Homozygous	1933C > T	Q645X
NRI(ErBor)[g]	Mixed European	Heterozygous	1933C > T	Q645X
NR8(KeSol)[g]	Mixed European	Heterozygous	1933C > T	Q645X
51(KeMc)	Mixed European	Homozygous	2098C > T	Q700X
Frameshift mutations				
93(YoYa)	Japanese	Homozygous	1544insA (1618insA)	514+1 > X
15(MaRo)	Ashkenazi Jewish	Homozygous	2207-2212delATCTGAinsTAGATTC[h]	735+4 > X
42(RaFr)	Ashkenazi Jewish	Homozygous	2207-2212delATCTGAinsTAGATTC[h]	735+4 > X
107(MyAsa)	Ashkenazi/Sephardic	Homozygous	2207-2212delATCTGAinsTAGATTC[h]	735+4 > X
NR2(CrSpe)	Ashkenazi Jewish	Homozygous	2207-2212delATCTGAinsTAGATTC[h]	735+4 > X
126(BrNa)	Ashkenazi/Sephardic	Heterozygous	2207-2212delATCTGAinsTAGATTC[h]	735+4 > X
Exon-skipping mutations				
126(BrNa)	Ashkenazi/Sephardic	Heterozygous	Skips exon 2[i]	[i]
112(NaSch)	Mixed European	Heterozygous	Skips exon 6[j]	362+4 > X
Exonic deletion				
92(VaBia)	Italian	Homozygous	Skips exons 11 & 12[k]	769+1 > X

[a]Mutation screening reported in this table was carried out on 25 persons with BS from whom cell lines were available. Total RNA was prepared by using Trizol (Gibco BRL). Mutations in the RNA product of BLM were detected by RT-PCR followed by single-stranded conformation polymorphism (SSCP) analysis[26], by an RNase cleavage assay (unpublished observations) marketed by Ambion, or by both techniques. The mutations were then identified by direct sequencing of PCR-amplified cDNA and confirmed by sequencing of the genomic DNA.

[b]Bloom's Syndrome Registry designations. Mutation has gone undetected in only one person with BS of the 25 examined, namely, 140(DrKas). Mutations in four persons from whom a cell line was available are not reported here.

[c]In all persons studied, zygosity of the mutation was confirmed by analysis of the genomic DNA. Similarly, mutations were confirmed in available parents.

[d]Standard nomenclature (from Antonarakis SE: Recomendation for a nomenclature system for human gene mutations. Nomenclature Working Group. *Hum Mutat* 11:1, 1998) has been used to indicate the genetic alteration in the gene. In parentheses, the nucleotide positions are as identified in the *BLM* cDNA H1-5'.[26]

[e]Standard nomenclature has been used to indicate the alteration in the gene product except in the case of frameshift mutation. The effect of a frameshift is shown by first indicating the number of BLM amino acid residues that are incorporated followed by the number of out-of-frame residues that are incorporated until a stop codon is reached (denoted by an X).

[f]This missense mutation formally could be a polymorphism.

[g]In this heterozygote, the other mutated *BLM* allele has yet to be determined or is not reported here.

[h]This mutation also is known as *blm^Ash* and is described as a 6-bp deletion and 7-bp insertion at nucleotide 2281 in the *BLM* cDNA.

[i]An RT-PCR product with a smaller-than-normal size was detected by agarose gel electrophoresis. Sequencing of the abnormal fragment identified a deletion of exon 2, cDNA nucleotides 71 to 172. Sequence analysis of genomic DNA amplified with oligonucleotide primers flanking exon 2 revealed a G-to-T transversion in the 5' splice site (GT to TT). Splicing out of exon 2 removes the initiator methionine for BLM. Use by the ribosome of the next downstream ATG would result in the generation of a small out-of-frame peptide.

[j]An RT-PCR product with a smaller-than-normal size was detected by agarose gel electrophoresis. Sequencing of the abnormal cDNA fragment identified a deletion of exon 6, nucleotides 1162 to 1294. Sequence analysis of genomic DNA amplified with oligonucleotide primers flanking exon 6 revealed an A to G transition at the third position of the 5' splice site. Splicing of exons 5 and 7 results in the addition of 4 out-of-frame amino acids followed by premature termination.

[k]The mutation present in 92 (VaBia) was assigned incorrectly in reference [26] as a G to C at nucleotide position 2596 in the *BLM* cDNA. Subsequently, a deletion of exons 11 and 12—nucleotides 2382 to 2629 in the *BLM* cDNA—was detected by RT-PCR analysis, and its existence was confirmed in genomic DNA by Southern blot analysis and PCR as a 6126-bp deletion confirmed by DNA sequencing. Splicing of exons 10 and 13 results in the addition of 1 out-of-frame amino acid followed by premature termination.

homozygosity at loci distal but not proximal to *BLM*,[33] provided an efficient strategy to determine the exact location of *BLM*. The objective became to identify (a) the most proximal polymorphic locus that was constitutionally heterozygous and that had been reduced to homozygosity in the five low-SCE cell lines and (b) the most distal polymorphic locus that had remained constitutionally heterozygous in them. *BLM* would have to be in the short interval defined by the reduced and the unreduced, i.e., still heterozygous, markers. The power of this approach, termed *somatic crossover-point (SCP) mapping*, would be limited only by the density of polymorphic loci available in the immediate vicinity of the gene.

As mentioned earlier, *BLM* had been localized by homozygosity mapping to a 2-cM interval flanking *FES*. A 2-Mb yeast artificial chromosome (YAC) and P1 contig encompassing *FES* was constructed, and the required, closely spaced, polymorphic DNA markers in the contig were identified.[37] *BLM* then was assigned by SCP mapping to an interval in this contig of only 250 kb in size that was bounded by the polymorphic loci *D15S1108* and *D15S127* (Fig. 16-6). Then a cosmid clone (referred to as 905) that was present in the 250-kb interval was used to isolate by direct selection an 849-bp clone from a fibroblast cDNA library. By hybridization and RT-PCR techniques, this cDNA clone, in turn,

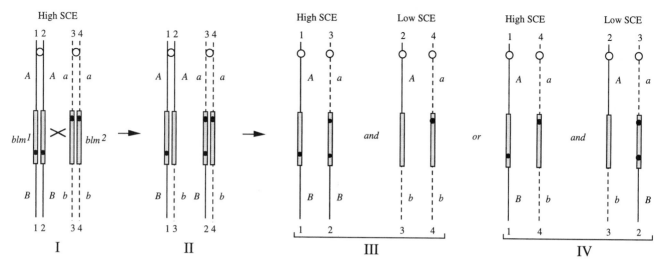

High SCE — I — II — High SCE — Low SCE — III — High SCE — Low SCE — IV

Fig. 16-5 Model to generate a wild-type *BLM* locus via somatic intragenic recombination: *I*, The two pairs of sister chromatids of the homologous chromosome Nos. 15 in a G2 somatic cell of a BS genetic compound (*blm¹/blm²*) are numbered 1-1 to 4-4. Each of the two mutations in *BLM* (the hatched rectangle), represented by black dots, one inherited from each parent, is at a different site in the gene. Flanking markers proximal to and distal to the mutated loci are heterozygous *A/a* and *B/b*. *II*, After homologous interchange between chromatids 2-2 and 3-3 at a point between the sites of mutation within *BLM* (the X in *I*), a wild-type gene is reconstituted on chromatid 2-3 that corrects to normal the high-SCE phenotype of BS cells. Simultaneously, the distal marker *b* becomes associated with the wild-type gene on chromatid 2-3. *III* and *IV*, By segregational events at mitosis, two pairs of daughter cells are possible. If chromatids 2-3 and 4-4 cosegregate to the same daughter cell, the distal marker becomes homozygous *b/b* (the diagram on the right side of *III*). On the other hand, if chromatid 2-3 and 3-2 cosegregate, the distal marker remains heterozygous *b/B* (the diagram on the right side of *IV*). The proximal marker remains heterozygous *A/a* in both cases. In the sister cells, segregation of chromatids 1-1 and 3-2 (the diagram on the left side of *III*) or of chromatids 1-1 and 4-4 (the diagram on the left side of *IV*) do not give rise to a low-SCE phenotype. (*Note*: Cells of heterozygous carriers of a mutation at *BLM*, viz. *blm*/BLM parents of persons with BS, display a low-SCE rate.) (Figure reprinted from Ellis NA, Lennon DJ, Proytcheva M, Alhadeff B, Henderson EE, German J: Somatic intragenic recombination within the mutated locus *BLM* can correct the high-SCE phenotype of Bloom syndrome cells. *Am J Hum Genet* 57:1019, 1995.)

was used to isolate many additional cDNAs from fibroblast, lymphoblastoid, and HeLa cells. A 4437-bp cDNA sequence, referred to as H1-5′, that contained a long open reading frame encoding a 1417-amino acid protein was defined. By Southern blot analysis of genomic DNA and of sequences cloned in the YACs, P1s, and cosmids of the contig, the H1-5′ sequences hybridized to single-copy sequences spanning about 100 kb of the genome. (The complete genomic sequences of this region are available in the DNA sequence database at the National Center for Biotechnology Information.) A 4.5-kb transcript was identified by northern blot analysis of total RNAs prepared from various human cells proliferating *in vitro*. Northern analysis of seven lymphoblastoid cell lines derived from seven unrelated persons with BS revealed three cell lines in which the levels of messenger ribonucleic acid (mRNA) that hybridized to labeled H1-5′ sequences were five- to tenfold less than those in control normal cell lines. In addition, there was a fourth cell line in which both the mRNA levels were reduced and the length of the mRNA was approximately 200 bp shorter than the normal mRNA molecule. Because it is known that mutations that produce premature translation termination often reduce mRNA stability, the abnormalities in mRNA levels here suggested that the gene encoding these mRNAs was mutated. Northern analysis was subsequently performed on over 30 BS cell lines, and steady-state levels of *BLM* mRNAs are reduced in the cell lines that were found to contain protein truncating mutations in both alleles of *BLM*.

Mutations in the H1-5′ sequences were sought in persons with BS. Initially, analysis was carried out using reverse transcriptase (RT)-PCR and single-stranded conformation polymorphism (SSCP) on RNA from 13 BS lymphoblastoid cell lines. In 10 of 13 cell lines examined, 7 different mutations were detected. Five of the seven mutations led to premature translation termination, and two were amino acid substitutions at highly conserved residues (see below and Table 16-4). Using additional mutation-searching methods, including an RNAse cleavage assay (marketed by Ambion), the protein truncation test, PCR-restriction enzyme

analysis, Southern blot analysis, DNA-high-performance liquid chromatography (D-HPLC) heteroduplex analysis, and DNA sequencing, we have identified 64 unique mutations in 124 of the 133 persons with BS examined. The mutations listed in Table 16-4 are representative, but eventually a complete report of the mutational analysis will be made. Ten of the 64 mutations are amino acid substitutions made at conserved residues the alteration of which putatively disturbs the enzymatic activity of the protein (see below); 20 are nonsense mutations; 21 are oligonucleotide insertions or deletions that cause frameshifting and premature translation termination immediately downstream of the mutation; 9 are mutations at splice sites, some of which by northern or RT-PCR analyses are known to disturb the proper splicing of the mRNA; and 4 are deletions of 1 or more exons. In the 10 missense alleles, the open reading frame is maintained, but in the remaining 54 mutant alleles the open reading frame is in some way disrupted.

Each of 46 of the 64 mutations that have been identified in persons with BS was detected in but a single person (in either the homozygous or heterozygous state), whereas 18 were recurrent, each having been identified in two or more unrelated persons. The most common of the recurrent mutations was *blm^Ash*, which was detected in 70 of the 240 alleles present in the 124 unrelated persons in whom mutations were identified. The next most common mutation was the allele *BLM*1933C → T*, a nonsense mutation that putatively results in truncation of the protein at codon 645 (see Table 16-4; also unpublished observations); 24 alleles were found in 18 unrelated persons of non-Jewish European ancestry. Eight of the 18 recurrent mutations were detected in a range of 10 to 3 unrelated persons, and the remaining 8 mutations were detected in only 2 unrelated persons. Most of the 18 recurrent mutations clustered in different populations, including Ashkenazi Jews, non-Jewish European North American, non-Jewish mixed European, Italian, German, Japanese, Brazilian, and Mexican. All the mutations arose in interbreeding populations with one exception: the allele *BLM*1544insA*, which consists of an insertion of an A base in a run of nine A bases, was identified in

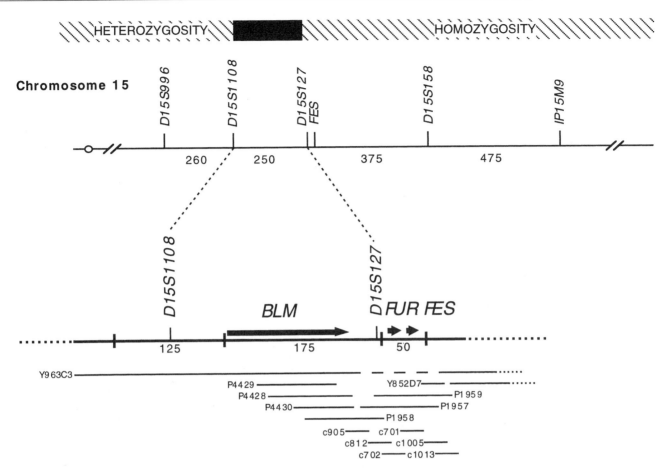

Fig. 16-6 SCP mapping of BLM. Genetic map of the *BLM* region of 15q. On the upper horizontal line, the order and distances (shown in kb) between the polymorphic microsatellite loci were estimated by long-range-restriction mapping.[37] The distance between *D15S127* and *FES* (not indicated) was determined to be 30 kb by restriction enzyme mapping of a cosmid contig. Vertical lines indicate the position of the marker loci, and the circle represents the centromere. The interval between loci *D15S1108* and *D15S127* is expanded below the map. Vertical lines intersecting mark the unmethylated CpG-rich regions identified by long-range-restriction mapping, and arrows indicate the direction of transcription of three genes in the region. Certain YACs, P1s, and cosmids (Y, P, and c, respectively) from the contig are depicted by horizontal lines underneath the map.[37] Dashes on the YAC lines indicate internal deletions. At the top of the figure, the horizontal crosshatched bar to the right indicates regions distal to *BLM* that had become homozygous. The minimal region to which *BLM* was thus assigned by SCP mapping is represented in black. (Figure reprinted slightly modified from Ellis NA, Groden J, Ye T-Z, Straughen J, Lennon DJ, Ciocci S, Proytcheva M, German J: The Bloom's syndrome gene product is homologous to RecQ helicases. *Cell* 83:655, 1995.)

four Japanese and an African American, possibly representing independent mutation in the Japanese and the African populations.

Forty-nine persons were heterozygous for mutation at *BLM*, and 75 were homozygous. The predominant explanation for persons being homozygous at *BLM* is founder effect: (a) In 26 families, the parents were cousins, and therefore these persons inherited *BLM* identical by descent from an ancestor common to each parent. (b) In 25 families, the parents of the person with BS were Ashkenazi Jews[38] (in one of these Jewish families, the parents were cousins, so that the family was counted twice in this enumeration); these persons inherited *blm^Ash* also identical by descent from an ancestor common to each parent, even though the ancestor would have lived many generations ago. (c) In the remaining 25 families, the parents did not know they were related. Theoretically, mutations could be identical because of independent mutational events. Yet, founder effect was manifestly the cause in many of these families, because in 18 of them the mutations had been identified in other unrelated persons. For example, 4 persons were homozygous for *BLM*1933C → T*, 4 for *blm^Ash*, and the remaining 10 were homozygous for less common, but nonetheless recurrent, mutations. Altogether, these results suggested that these various recurrent mutations were transmitted by ancestors some of whom lived many generations ago and others who lived relatively recently. Finally, the mutation survey indicates that founder effect has taken place repeatedly and in many different places, at different times in history, and in different populations.

Two unusual examples are these: (a) In one of the exon-skipping mutations, the initiator AUG was not present in the cDNA; the next downstream AUG is out of frame, probably resulting in failure to produce normal *BLM* product. (b) In one of the genomic deletions, the last three exons of *BLM* were deleted, resulting in the loss of the polyadenylation-addition signal. Presumably, the RNA polymerase continues to transcribe until it meets with an intergenic sequence that can serve as a polyadenylation-addition signal, or until it transcribes through a downstream gene—one that is transcribed in the same direction as *BLM*—and terminates transcription at the end of that gene. Whatever the affects are of losing the polyadenylation-addition signal, the putative protein could contain no more than 1250 amino acids of *BLM*. As is discussed below, domains necessary for the proper function and expression of *BLM* extend at least to amino acid residue 1334; consequently, even if the proteins are expressed from mutant alleles that lack the last 100 or so amino acids, they are predicted to be non-functional. As mentioned above, northern analysis was performed on over 30 BS cell lines, and the mRNAs from alleles encoding *BLM* proteins with premature translation termination were expressed at reduced levels. Therefore, the effects of the mutations at *BLM* comprised both deficiencies in expression at the message level and deficiencies in protein expression and function.

In our mutational analysis of persons with BS, we identified both mutant *BLM* alleles in 116 persons, a single mutant allele in 8, and no mutant alleles in 9. The possible reasons for failing to identify mutations in 17 persons are the following: (a) the mutation(s) went undetected for technical reasons; (b) the person with BS has a mutation in a different gene, i.e., there is locus heterogeneity in BS; and (c) the person was incorrectly diagnosed BS. Incorrect diagnosis is probably not the reason for failing to find mutations in these 17 persons, because, in addition to the characteristic clinical features being present, a cytogenetic study confirmed the diagnosis of BS for all these persons. Certainly, in the eight persons in whom a single mutation with *BLM* was detected, we missed the other allele for technical reasons. The mutation may be in a part of the gene that was not sequenced, or it may be difficult to detect by sequencing or Southern analysis. In the nine persons in whom no mutant allele was detected, locus heterogeneity is a possibility; however, because the number of persons in whom no mutant allele detected is similar to the number in whom only a single allele was detected, our having missed the mutation is the probable explanation. One way to distinguish these possibilities would be to introduce a normal *BLM* gene into a high-SCE cell from a person in whom mutation in *BLM* went undetected and to test that transformed cell for high numbers of SCEs: if low-SCEs were observed, then a mutation in *BLM* is probably present; if high-SCEs were observed (noncomplementation), then mutation in some other gene is probable.

DNA samples from 155 parents were available from 89 unrelated persons with BS, and each of them carried one of the alleles present in his or her child, indicating that no *de novo* mutations were identified. In addition to the 64 manifestly BS-causing *BLM* mutations detected, we identified 17 polymorphic or rare variants that for different reasons we classified as nonBS-causing (absence of amino acid substitution, frequency in unaffected persons, presence in persons with two manifestly BS-causing mutations, or ability to complement the high-SCE phenotype of BS cells when introduced into a normal *BLM* cDNA and expressed in BS cells, as is explained further below).

In summary, from the extensive mutational analyses that we have performed, six conclusions are drawn: (a) The discovery of mutations in the H1-5′ sequence in persons with BS proves that the gene that had been isolated is *BLM*. (b) That multiple mutations exist in the gene confirms the allelic heterogeneity at *BLM* predicted from the Registry cytogenetics.[31] (c) The identification of 54 premature-translation-termination mutations, many of which are homozygous in persons with BS, demonstrates that loss of function of the *BLM* protein is the major underlying cause of the clinical syndrome. (d) Null mutations at *BLM* are not cell-lethal.[28] (e) Most if not all of the recurrent *BLM* mutations are present via founder effect in persons with BS not known to be related. (f) In addition, because mutations in *BLM* have been detected in nearly all of the persons with BS who were examined, the clinical entity is defined at the molecular level by mutation at *BLM*; BS-causing mutations of loci other than *BLM* either do not exist or are very rare. A corollary to these observations is that the known missense alleles probably functionally are null mutations. The clinical outcome of having a mutation that confers partial or novel *BLM* protein function would be an interesting finding but is currently unknown.

During the initial mutational analysis of four persons with Ashkenazi Jewish ancestry, the aforementioned 6-bp deletion and 7-bp insertion mutation at nucleotide 2281 was detected—*blm^Ash*. Fortuitously, this mutation introduces a *Bst*NI site that can be detected by restriction enzyme digestion in DNA amplified by PCR of both cDNA and genomic DNA.[39] Fifty-eight of 60 chromosomes derived from Ashkenazi Jewish persons with BS that have been examined contain this *Bst*NI site; i.e., transmit this one mutation.[38] This confirms the hypothesis that founder effect is the explanation for the elevated frequency of BS in the Ashkenazi

Jewish population.[3] Assay for the *Bst*NI site in genomic DNA samples from all persons with BS available through the Registry reveals a conspicuous absence of *blm^Ash* from all of the 49 non-Jewish persons with Northern European ancestry who were examined, as well as from all of the 8 Italians, 8 Japanese, 4 North Americans with African ancestry, 4 Turks, 4 Brazilians, an Argentinean, a Portuguese, a Spaniard, a Persian Jew, a Lebanese, and an Indian.

However—and completely unexpectedly—the *blm^Ash* mutation turned up in six of the eight unrelated persons with BS examined from American families that were of Spanish ancestry.[38] These six persons were born into Catholic families that for many generations have lived in El Salvador, Mexico, or the American Southwest; these families were unaware of Jewish ancestry, although one family reports an oral tradition of their being a distant ancestor of the maternal grandmother of the proposita who was "a Sephardi."

The unexpected finding of *blm^Ash* in only this one particular group of non-Jews supports the following hypothesis:[38] *blm^Ash* was a mutation at *BLM* that was segregating in the Jews of Spain in the fifteenth century, probably at a low frequency, as do various *BLM* mutations in many non-Jewish populations today. Sometime during the colonization of the Americas by Spain after the expulsion of the Sephardim in 1492 by Ferdinand and Isabella, a Spanish Jew who had been converted to Christianity, a converso, and who by chance was heterozygous for *blm^Ash* migrated to New Spain. This person transmitted *blm^Ash* to his or her descendants. By this hypothesis, two different founder effects pertaining to *blm^Ash* have been identified: the one long-recognized that took place in Eastern Europe and another one that took place in New Spain. From the available genetic evidence, the exact historical path(s) of *blm^Ash* into both the Ashkenazim and the Sephardim cannot be delineated. However, our observations in the genetics of BS point to the existence of a common ancestor of, or to admixture between, these two major Jewish populations. More broadly, they are examples of the impact of migration and genetic drift on the formation of human populations.

MOLECULAR BIOLOGY OF THE BLM PROTEIN

Homology searching of the amino acid sequence databases revealed that the 1417-amino acid protein encoded by the *BLM* cDNA sequence contains homology to RecQ helicases (Fig. 16-7), a subfamily of DExH box-containing DNA and RNA helicases.[28] The RecQ helicases are members of a much larger group of proteins that contain seven amino acid motifs that are present in most DNA and RNA helicases. These same motifs are present also in a large number of proteins that are not DNA or RNA helicases; some of these proteins are known to have DNA-dependent ATPase activity and have functions in "chromatin remodeling." Consequently, the seven motifs probably form an evolutionarily conserved protein fold(s) that uses the energy released from ATP hydrolysis to manipulate DNA-protein complexes.

Helicases are defined biochemically by two activities: (a) they are DNA- or RNA-dependent ATPases and (b) with ATP and Mg^{++} as cofactors they catalyze the unwinding of duplex nucleic acids. Because nucleic acids are predominantly in a duplex form in the cell, helicases are active in all processes in nucleic acid metabolism that require access to single-stranded molecules, namely, DNA replication, DNA repair, recombination, RNA transcription, and protein translation. Given that *BLM* and the other RecQ helicases that have been tested are bona fide DNA helicases (see below), there are two fundamental questions that need to be addressed: What function(s) does *BLM* and the other RecQ helicases perform in the cell? and What are the cellular and organismal mechanisms that operate in the molecular pathogenesis of mutants of the RecQ helicases? Recent biochemical and genetic studies have approached these two questions: the biochemists have determined the specific substrates on which the RecQ helicases are active and the other proteins that interact physically and

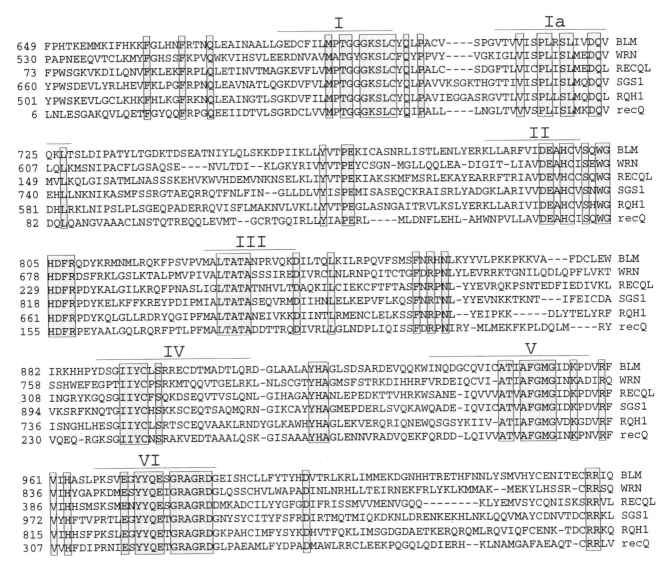

Fig. 16-7 Alignment of the amino acid sequences in the domains containing the seven helicase motifs (I, Ia, II, III, IV, V, and VI) of selected RecQ helicases. Sequence alignments were performed by the Megalign computer program (DNAStar). Numbers at left indicate the amino acid positions in each protein, and gene product names are at the right. Identities present in all six selected proteins are boxed. Overlined sequences mark the seven helicase motifs in the helicase domain. The DExH box is in helicase motif II. (Reprinted with permission from Ellis, NA, German J: Molecular genetic of Bloom's syndrome. *Hum Mol Genet* 5:1457, 1996.)

functionally with the RecQ helicases; the geneticists have determined the functions that are defective in cells containing mutations of the RecQ helicases. Some of the recent experimental evidence and important insights into RecQ function are discussed in the following sections.

The RecQ Gene Family

The Bacterial RecQ Helicase. The RecQ helicases comprise a large family of genes. Although there are some completely sequenced bacterial species that lack an recQ+ gene, the evolutionary conservation of these helicases is impressive, they being present in eubacteria, yeasts, and all metazoans that have been examined. Originally, *recQ* was isolated as a mutation in *E. coli* that generated resistance to thymineless death and was identified as a member of the RecF pathway of DNA recombination.[40] In appropriately marked bacterial strains, *recQ* mutants are hyporecombinogenic, which strongly suggested that RecQ carries out a step in DNA recombination. Purified RecQ has DNA-dependent ATPase and ATP-dependent DNA strand-displacement activities, which define it as a DNA helicase.[41] A function for RecQ in separation of DNA single strands is

suggested by the fact that RecQ can enter and unwind a supercoiled circular DNA duplex, and that it can stimulate the activity of *E. coli* topoisomerase III (Topo III) to catenate double-stranded DNA duplexes.[42] (The functional interaction between RecQs and Topo IIIs is an important theme of RecQ helicase biology that is revisited several times in this section.) Together with RecA and SSB (single-stranded DNA-binding) proteins, purified RecQ can catalyze the formation or dissolution of recombination intermediates *in vitro*.[43]

Genetic evidence has suggested that RecQ can inhibit "illegitimate" recombination events, i.e., events between molecules that are only partially homologous.[44] RecQ functions in the repair of gapped DNA molecules by a recombination pathway that is associated with crossing-over of flanking DNA sequences.[45] There is genetic evidence that the RecF pathway and, by extension, RecQ operate during DNA replication to ensure the eventual continuation of replication complexes that have stalled, e.g., when they have encountered sites of DNA damage such as cyclopyrimidine dimers.[46] Further evidence for an association of RecQ function with replication came from the study of bacterial strains in which palindromic DNA sequences had been inserted into the chromosome.[47] After the replication fork has passed through the palindrome, the DNA putatively makes a hairpin structure on the lagging strand that inhibits DNA synthesis. The structures probably are converted into DNA double-strand breaks and these breaks are then repaired by recombination. RecQ is active in this pathway of recombination repair. Thus, RecQ functions in various repair pathways that employ recombination-based DNA replication to maintain the integrity of the genome. Theoretically, RecQ may function in a number of nonexclusive processes: it could provide substrate for RecA to promote the formation of joint molecules that produce recombination events; it could disrupt joint molecules that are in some way improperly formed; and it could be active in influencing the kinds of recombination products that are formed (products with or without crossing-over of flanking DNA sequences).

The *Saccharomyces cerevisiae* RecQ Helicase. In *S. cerevisiae*, where the entire genomic DNA sequence is known, there is a single RecQ family member. This gene, *SGS1*, was first identified as a mutation that is a slow-growth suppressor of a cell containing a mutation in its Topo III (*TOP3*) gene.[48] The structure of Sgs1p (the protein) differs from *E. coli*'s RecQ in an important way: RecQ is a 610-amino acid protein with an N-terminal helicase domain (approximately 300 amino acids) and a C-terminal domain postulated to function in nucleic acid binding. These two domains are both highly positively charged, consistent with their binding to DNA. Sgs1p, on the other hand, is a 1447-amino acid protein that, in addition to the helicase and C-terminal domains, contains a highly negatively charged N-terminal domain (approximately 650 amino acids). In its structure, *BLM* resembles Sgs1p in having a negatively charged N-terminal domain (650 amino acids) along with positively charged helicase and C-terminal domains. These N-terminal domains have no recognized amino acid homologies to each other or to any other proteins in the database.

Topo IIIs are type IA topoisomerases that act by breaking and rejoining DNA via an enzyme-DNA intermediate in which a protein tyrosine forms an ester bond with a 5'-phosphoryl group in DNA.[49] In *S. cerevisiae*, cells mutant in the *TOP3* gene not only proliferate slowly but also have greatly elevated recombination frequencies, e.g., at the rDNA locus, near telomeres, and in diploids at genes marked by heteroallelic mutations.[50] *Top3* mutants sporulate poorly and have a defect in the formation of recombinant DNA molecules.[51] Suppression of these phenotypes by deletion of *SGS1* suggests that Top3p and Sgs1p interact physically. Supporting this possibility, *SGS1* was identified by *TOP3* in a yeast two-hybrid screen.[48] Biochemical investigations have shown that interaction between Sgs1p and Top3p is mediated via the N-terminal 170 amino acids or so of Sgs1p,[52–54] and expression of an Sgs1p that is deleted for this interaction domain fails to complement the hyperrecombination phenotype of *sgs1* null cells (see below).[55] In addition to interaction with Top3p, Sgs1p interacts physically with Top2p;[56] however, the region of Sgs1p that binds Top2p is more proximal to the helicase domain than the region that binds Top3p. Finally, *sgs1/top1* double mutants exhibit a slow-growth phenotype that neither single mutant exhibits.[57] Thus, with three topoisomerases in yeast, Sgs1p has genetic interactions, physical interactions, or both.

Phenotypes of Mutations of *SGS1*. As with *E. coli* RecQ, Sgs1p possesses DNA-dependent ATPase and DNA strand-displacement activities.[57] Mutations in *SGS1* confer multiple genetic and cellular defects: *sgs1* mutant cells feature slow growth, increased chromosome mis-segregation in both mitosis and meiosis,[56,58] and an approximately fifteenfold increase in spontaneous recombination and a twentyfold increase in gross chromosomal rearrangements.[58,59] However, the frequency of recombination events in meiosis[60] and those induced by gamma or ultraviolet irradiation[61] are reduced. Diploids, but not haploids, are hypersensitive to ionizing radiation, suggesting that the cells have a defect in recombination repair of double-strand breaks.[61] Cells doubly

mutant for *sgs1* and *srs2*, another DNA helicase the absence of which causes radiation-sensitivity, have a low plating efficiency[62] ("synthetic lethality," probably caused by increased cell death) that is suppressed by mutations in *rad51*, *rad55*, and *rad57*, which all are factors that operate in homologous recombination.[61] These observations suggest that the functions of Sgs1p and Srs2p are overlapping, and that together they are essential; because the lethality is suppressed by mutations in the recombination apparatus, the lethality may be caused by aberrant recombination. In the absence of telomerase, *sgs1* cells cannot maintain their telomeres by recombination.[63–65] It has been suggested that Sgs1p acts to suppress recombination, for example, in highly repetitive DNA sequences,[48] and genetic evidence suggests that Sgs1p, like RecQ, can inhibit illegitimate recombination;[59,66] expression of a normal *BLM* cDNA in *sgs1* cells can complement that defect partially.[66]

Sgs1p levels are highest during S phase, and *sgs1* cells are defective in the activation of an intra-S phase checkpoint.[67] By immunofluorescence and cell fractionation experiments, Sgs1p together with Rad53p, which functions in the intra-S checkpoint, co-localize to 40 to 50 percent of replication foci, and MEC1-dependent phosphorylation of Rad53p is defective in *sgs1 rad24* double mutants.[67] (Rad24p also signals to Rad53p via an independent pathway.) These data point to a function for Sgs1p in DNA replication.

Similar to RecQ, the genetic functions ascribed to Sgs1p include a triad of interrelated functions: repair of DNA double-strand breaks, recombination, and DNA replication. Double-strand breaks that arise during DNA replication are thought to be repaired by a recombination event between the sister chromatids, and such a recombination event presumably can lead to crossing-over of flanking DNA sequences. In a mammalian cell, presumably a recombination event such as this would be microscopically visible as an SCE. It is a significant fact that the only other mutation of mammalian cells known that increases SCE levels dramatically as in BS is mutation of the *XRCC1* gene.[129] *XRCC1* encodes a ligase III-associated accessory factor that is active in the base excision-repair pathway. This pathway, the final step of which is ligation of a single-stranded DNA nick, repairs DNA that is damaged by the normal oxidative processes within the cell. A nick will be converted into a DNA double-strand break if a replication fork should happen to come by before ligation of the nick is completed. If a nick is encountered by the replication fork on the leading strand, then the chromosome is broken and the replication fork collapses, requiring restart. If the nick is encountered on the lagging strand, again the chromosome is broken, but the replication fork need not collapse. In both cases, the broken chromosome is likely to be mended by a recombination event between the sister chromatids. Putting together the data from bacteria and yeast, we conclude that absence of RecQ helicase function can result in increased recombination in two nonexclusive ways: (a) there is an increase in DNA structures or lesions that stimulates recombination and (b) RecQ helicases act in the regulation of recombination by influencing the outcome of exchanges events.

The *Schizosaccharomyces pombe* RecQ Helicase. In *S. pombe*, an *SGS1*-like *recQ* gene, referred to as *rqh1+*, is present that was identified by one mutation, *rad12*, which causes hypersensitivity to ultraviolet (UV) irradiation, and by a second mutation, *hus2*, which causes hypersensitivity to hydroxyurea.[68,69] These mutations also confer hyperrecombination and chromosome-nondis-junction phenotypes similar to those in *S. cerevisiae sgs1*. The chromosomes appear to be trapped on the metaphase plate, the sister chromatids being unable to separate, and the cell wall dissects the chromosomes to give a "cut"-like phenotype. Molecular genetic evidence points to a function for rqh1+ protein in maintaining replication-fork integrity when DNA damage or fork-progression inhibition occurs during S phase,[68,69] and possibly a function in signaling to the cell-cycle-control machinery.[70] *rqh1* defects can be suppressed by expression in the mutant cells of a bacterial resolvase that cleaves Holliday junctions,[71] implying that either rqh1+ protein functions in the normal processing of recombination intermediates or that its absence leads to the formation of aberrant recombination intermediates which cannot be processed in time for completion of cell division.

Another remarkable similarity to the situation in *S. cerevisiae* is the genetic and physical interactions between *rqh1+* and *top3+*. top3 mutants in *S. pombe* are viable for only a limited number of cell generations, and, like *rqh1* mutants, they exhibit a "cut"-like phenotype, which signifies aberrant chromosome segregation. Consistent with a conserved interaction between the RecQ proteins and Topo IIIs, *rqh1* mutation suppresses the *top3* lethal phenotype.[72,73] Altogether, the observations support the hypothesis that the RecQ proteins and Topo IIIs together facilitate sister-chromatid separation at the sites of termination of DNA replication.[48] The combined genetic and biochemical evidence points to possible roles for RecQ proteins in three critical processes: (a) the repair, by recombination, of breaks or lesions that are encountered by the replication fork; (b) the suppression of illegitimate recombination events; and (c) the separation of sister chromatids.

The cloning of *rqh1+* uncovered another feature of the domain structure of the RecQ family. Immediately C-terminal of their central helicase domains, rqh1+ and *BLM* both contain a segment of 200 amino acids with approximately 20 percent identity that is referred to as the C-terminal extended homology region. The other RecQ family members mentioned above contain this region, but in pair-wise comparisons, the homology varies both in the number of amino acids and in the percent of identity.[74] Additionally, by homology searching of the protein databases, a second motif was identified C-terminal of the C-terminal extended homology region.[75] This motif, called the HRDC (for *h*elicase and *RNAaseD* C-terminal domain), is implicated in DNA binding.[75] Because mutation in the C-terminal extended homology region can destroy helicase activity (see below), and because the HRDC is proposed to act in DNA binding, these regions may play a role in the recognition of specific substrates.

Mammalian RecQ Helicases. In addition to *BLM*, mammalian cells have four other *recQ*-like genes: *RECQL1*, *WRN*, *RECQL4* (also referred to as *RTS*), and *RECQL5*. The protein encoded by *RECQL1* consists of 659 amino acids; RECQL1 was isolated as a major ATPase of HeLa cells and was shown to have DNA helicase activity.[76,77] The cellular role of RECQL1 is unknown. *WRN*, the gene that when mutated results in Werner syndrome (WS)—defined clinically by premature aging (see Chap. 19)—encodes a 1432-amino acid product having domain structures similar to that of Sgs1p and BLM.[78] WRN is a DNA helicase,[79,80] but, unlike BLM or the other known RecQ helicases, WRN contains a 5′ to 3′ exonuclease activity in its N-terminal domain.[81] This difference in their N-terminal domain structures and functions could explain, in part, why clinical BS bears essentially no resemblance to clinical WS. WS does predispose to certain rare neoplasms. WS cells exhibit what has been called "variegated translocation mosaicism:"[82] although excessive chromosome breakage as seen in BS is not present, fibroblasts cultured from WS skin grow as clones, each clone marked by a distinctive chromosome translocation.[82,83] WS cells also exhibit an increased frequency of mutations at the *HPRT* locus, which mostly are deletions. Thus, the identification of *WRN* may have established a connection between the aging process and the maintenance of genomic stability. Correspondingly, the *sgs1* mutation in yeast gives a premature aging phenotype.[84,85] The *RECQL4* and *RECQL5* genes were identified by searching the cDNA sequence database.[86] *RECQL4* mutations were identified in some persons diagnosed with the Rothmund-Thomson syndrome.[87] For *BLM* and *WRN* we know that absence of a normal allele leads to genomic instability. For the two other RecQ members, *RECQL1* and *RECQL5*, although there is no information to suggest that mutations in them produce viable phenotypes, it is possible that unexplained entities caused by such already are known in clinical medicine.

Structure and Function of the BLM Helicase

Biochemical Analyses of BLM. Homology to the RecQ helicases strongly suggested that BLM itself is a DNA helicase. To demonstrate that BLM has this activity, it was expressed with a C-terminal hexahistidine tag in *S. cerevisiae*, partially purified by nickel-chelation chromatography, and tested in conventional assays for DNA-dependent ATPase and strand-displacement activities.[88,89] BLM is not a highly processive helicase, being unable to unwind efficiently more than 250 base-paired nucleotides.[90] In the presence of single-stranded binding protein RPA, with which BLM can physically interact *in vitro*, BLM's processivity is increased several-fold. More striking, however, is the preference of BLM for substrates that resemble recombination intermediates. BLM can bind and unwind a number of all such DNA substrates tested, including G4 DNA (a tetrameric DNA structure that can form between runs of guanines, at least *in vitro*),[91] Holliday junctions,[92] and D-loops (joint molecules).[93] When other purified RecQ helicases were tested on these substrates, including RecQ itself, they efficiently unwound them,[94–96] suggesting that the helicases' specificities for these substrates likely are contained within the conserved helicase and possibly the C-terminal domains. The fact that these DNA structures are unwound by the RecQ helicases has been viewed as support for an "antirecombinogenic" function, one that *de facto* is defective in the hyperrecombinogenic mutant cell.

In the 124 persons with BS in whom the 64 different mutations have been identified, 5 of the 10 missense mutations identified alter amino acid residues in the helicase domain. One mutation replaces the glutamine at residue 672 with an arginine (Q672R; see Table 16-4); this glutamine lies 10 amino acid residues N-terminal of the helicase motif I and is conserved in almost all RecQ helicases (see Fig. 16-7). Two mutations have been identified in motif IV, one in motif V, and one at a conserved histidine residue between motifs V and VI (our unpublished observations). We expect that all five of these amino acid substitutions reduce or destroy BLM's helicase activity. Experimentally, the Q672R mutation was introduced into a *BLM* cDNA expression construct, the mutant BLM was produced in yeast, and the partially purified protein was assayed for helicase activity: indeed, BLM Q672R protein has reduced DNA-dependent ATPase activity and lacks detectable DNA strand-displacement activity.[89]

In addition to finding mutations within the BLM helicase domain, a cluster of 5 amino acid substitutions has been found in one particular 50-amino acid stretch of the RecQ C-terminal extended homology region (reference 97 and our unpublished observations). The first of these mutations that has been studied in some detail replaces a conserved cystine at residue 1055 with a serine (C1055S). This amino acid substitution was introduced experimentally into a *BLM* cDNA expression construct, the mutant *BLM* then was produced in yeast, and the partially purified protein was assayed for helicase activity; the BLM C1055S protein lacks detectable ATPase and DNA strand-displacement activities.[89] A similar result was obtained when this mutation was introduced at the same position of the mouse *Blm* gene.[74] (Mouse and human *BLM* genes are highly conserved throughout this region.) Given the clustering of the amino acid substitutions in the C-terminal extended homology region of BLM, we predict that the other mutations in this region have similar effects on BLM's helicase activity. The observation that *BLM* mutations in persons with BS ablate its helicase activity is interpreted to mean that the helicase activity is indispensable for the protein's normal function.

Antibodies to an N-terminal segment of BLM have been raised in rabbits, and a protein of apparent molecular weight 180-kDa has been identified by western blot analysis of fibroblast, lymphoblastoid, and HeLa cells. This 180-kDa molecule is absent from all the BS cell lines homozygous for premature translation-termination mutations that have been examined.[89,98] This indicates that the 180-kDa molecule is BLM, the BS protein. Simultaneously, it demonstrates that these anti-BLM antibodies are useful for characterizing BLM, for defining its location in the cell, and for identifying proteins with which BLM may interact.

Complementation Studies with Normal and Mutated *BLM* genes. With the BLM antibodies available, it has been possible to introduce a *BLM* cDNA expression construct into BLM-lacking BS cells and determine whether BLM becomes detectable by western blot analysis and cellular immunofluorescence. Therefore, the normal *BLM* expression construct was transfected into SV40-transformed BS fibroblasts (cell line GM08505). This cell line is derived from a diploid fibroblast line homozygous for *blm*^Ash; it lacks detectable BLM protein and it has the high-SCE phenotype of BS. Transfection of *BLM* restores the 180-kDa BLM molecule to GM08505 cells and concomitantly reduces the SCE rate of these cells from a mean of 58 SCEs per 46 chromosomes to a mean of 23.[98] The same level of SCE reduction has been observed when normal cells are hybridized to GM08505 cells or when a normal chromosome 15 is introduced into these cells by chromosome-mediated gene transfer,[30] which is not completely to the level seen in non-SV40-transformed non-BS fibroblasts. Consequently, the transfected *BLM* cDNA functions in GM08505 cells to reduce SCEs as efficiently as the *BLM* gene when in its normal chromosomal location; similar correction results have been reported by others.[99]

These complementation experiments have allowed the development of a system for studying structure-function relationships of BLM. Two BS-causing mutations mentioned above — the helicase-negative Q672R and the C1055S amino acid substitutions — were introduced experimentally into the *BLM* cDNA and transfected into GM08505 cells. Although a 180-kDa molecule was detectable by western blot analysis after transfection and cloning of the cells, albeit present at levels lower than when normal *BLM* cDNA is transfected, expression of the mutant BLM proteins failed to reduce the high-SCE rate of these cells.[89] These results indicate that the helicase activity of BLM is required for its function in suppressing SCEs.

The intracellular localization of BLM has been determined by employing BLM antibodies and the indirect immunofluorescence microscopy technique in the study of various BS and non-BS cell lines. BLM protein is present in the nucleus of all proliferating cells examined save those from persons with BS. Consistent with BLM's presence in the nucleus, transient transfections of constructs in which amino acids C-terminal of residue 1341 were deleted demonstrate that BLM protein contains a nuclear localization signal (NLS) in its last 100 amino acids. Examination of the sequences there disclosed a bipartite NLS at residues 1334 to 1349, as found in numerous other nuclear proteins (e.g., DNA polymerase α and Topoisomerase II).[100] The WRN helicase contains an NLS at a similar location (residues 1370 to 1376).[101] Because the NLSs of BLM and WRN are at the C-termini, premature translation-termination mutations N-terminal of the NLSs render the proteins nonfunctional via the mutant protein's inability to be moved into the nucleus. Supporting this observation is the finding of a protein-truncating mutation in the *BLM* of a person with BS that encodes a BLM abnormal only in lacking its 175 C-terminal amino acids (our unpublished observation).

Cell Biological Analyses of BLM. A number of observations have been made with respect to BLM protein in non-BS cells: First, its steady-state levels varies in the different cell types examined. For example, a normal fibroblast has an average of approximately 4000 molecules of BLM per cell, an SV40-transformed fibroblast 25,000 molecules, and a HeLa cell 50,000 molecules (our unpublished observations). These differences in quantity also are apparent by western blot analysis and indirect immunofluorescence microscopy. Second, cells that are out of cycle, such as serum-deprived fibroblasts or unstimulated blood lymphocytes, express very little BLM protein.[102] Third, the abundance of BLM that is detectable microscopically varies greatly in unsynchronized cells; western blot and microscopic analyses of synchronized cells shows that BLM is lowest in early G1 phase of the cell cycle and reaches a maximum by late S/G2 phases.[102–105] Fourth, BLM is present in the nucleus in at least two distributions: (a) diffuse, finely granular microspeckles that can vary in local concentration from region to region within the nucleus, and (b) bright, punctate foci that range in size from 0.2 to 1.0 μm and in number from 3 to 20. These bright foci were identified as the PML nuclear bodies (PML-NBs),[106] which are identified with antibodies to the PML protein. In untreated cycling cells, BLM can be observed by immunofluorescence microscopy in the PML-NBs in almost all cells in which BLM protein is detectable. In transformed cells, in which the levels of BLM are relatively higher than in untransformed cells, the fraction of cells in which BLM and PML are colocalized exceeds 90 percent, and greater than 90 percent of the foci in these cells contain both proteins. At metaphase, the PML-NBs persist after breakdown of the nuclear membrane, whereas BLM protein becomes homogeneous and diffuse throughout the "cytoplasm" (excluded from the condensed chromosomes).[105] This reorganization of BLM is correlated with a hyperphosphorylation of BLM that is ATM-dependent, suggesting that the binding of BLM to chromatin or nuclear matrix is controlled by phosphorylation.[107] Concentrations of BLM are sometimes observed in nucleoli, at telomeres, and at or near some replication foci, transiently or under certain treatment conditions (e.g., γ-irradiation), and further investigations are required to determine the significance of these observations.

The PML-NBs represent a major site for the concentration of BLM protein. The functional significance of this focal concentration of BLM is unknown; however, evidence is accumulating that implicates the PML-NBs in the biological responses to DNA damage. Besides BLM, a number of other proteins that function in DNA-damage responses have been localized to the PML-NBs, including p53,[108,109] hypophosphorylated Rb,[110] the RAD50/MRE11/NBS1 complex,[111,112] Topo IIIα (there are two Topo IIIs known in humans Topo IIIα and Topo IIIβ),[113,114] RAD51,[115,116] and RPA.[105,115] In mouse PML-null cells, in which the PML-NBs are disrupted, the levels of SCEs are increased twofold.[106]

Protein-Protein Interactions Involving BLM. Just as Sgs1p and rqh1+ interact with yeast Topo III, BLM was shown to interact physically by immunoprecipitation and far-western blot analyses with mammalian Topo IIIα.[113,114] The region of BLM that mediates the interaction has been mapped to the first 133 amino acids of the protein, demonstrating that despite the lack of homology between Sgs1p and BLM at their N-termini, they both contain Topo IIIα-binding domains that are localized to the same region.[117] Topo IIIα is localized to the PML-NBs in normal cells, whereas, in BS cells that contain null mutations of *BLM*, Topo IIIα is not localized there.[113,114] In BS cells that express a Green Fluorescent Protein (GFP)-tagged normal BLM protein, Topo IIIα is relocalized to the PML-NBs, but in BS cells that express a GFP-BLM in which the Topo IIIα interaction domain has been removed by deletion of amino acids 1–132 (GFP-BLM 133–1417), Topo IIIα fails to localize to the PML-NBs.[117] Moreover, localization of Topo IIIα to the PML-NBs in normal cells can be inhibited by overexpressing a fragment of BLM consisting of the interaction domain (1–132). These results show that BLM recruits Topo IIIα to the PML-NBs. In addition, SCE levels in BS cells that express the GFP-BLM 133–1417 fragment are significantly higher than in cells that express normal GFP-BLM, implicating the action of the BLM-Topo IIIα complex in the regulation of SCEs.[117]

BLM interacts directly with RAD51 by yeast two-hybrid and far-western blot analyses.[116] RAD51 localizes to PML-NBs in a small percentage of asynchronously poliferating cells, but after γ-irradiation, a significant proportion of the foci that are "induced" contain RAD51, BLM, and PML.[115,116] In the SV40-transformed BS fibroblast cell line GM08505, RAD51 is present in the PML-NBs constitutively.[116] Antibodies to RAD51 can immunoprecipitate BLM in extracts of cells blocked in S-phase with aphidicolin. These data suggest that BLM functions in recombination-based repair of double-strand breaks in somatic cells.

In addition to a function in somatic cells, the infertility of persons with BS implicates BLM in gametogenesis. BLM adjoins the paired chromosomes in the zygotene-leptotene stages of meiotic prophase, which is when crossing-over is taking place.[20,21] BLM appears on the chromosomes slightly after RAD51 appears there; similarly, it leaves them after RAD51 has left.[21] These data suggest that BLM performs a function in meiotic recombination that follows the function of RAD51. RAD51 presumably acts in the formation of joint molecules in the molecular steps prior to establishment of the Holliday junction. Because BLM is active on Holliday junctions *in vitro*,[92] the data suggest that BLM acts on the joint molecules formed by RAD51. Possibly, the BLM-Topo IIIα complex clears the paired chromosomes of incorrectly formed joint molecules, which are not normally resolved by other mechanisms.

Gel filtration and electron microscopic analyses of purified BLM protein shows that BLM forms tetrameric and hexameric ring structures.[118] A purified N-terminal fragment of BLM consisting of amino acids 1 to 431 also can form hexameric structures, suggesting that the N-terminus is important for the homo-oligomerization of the protein.[119] Coincidentally, the N-terminal 415 amino acids of BLM are cleaved by caspase 3 in cells undergoing apoptosis; the C-terminal fragment that is generated by cleavage maintains helicase activity.[120] Further structural analyses are needed to determine whether BLM homo-oligomerization is critical for its enzymatic activity.

Mutations in *BLM* in Other Model Genetic Systems. Analysis of *BLM* genes in metazoans other than humans has provided a number of additional clues into BLM function. During the evolution of multicellular organisms, the genes encoding the RecQ helicases were duplicated multiple times. Six RecQ genes have been identified in *Arabidopsis thaliana*, four in *Caenorhabditis elegans*, three in *Drosophila melanogaster*,[121] two so far in *Xenopus laevis*,[122] and one in chicken; except for *A. thaliana*, each species named is known to contain a *BLM* homolog. In a screen for mutagen sensitivity, two mutants of *D. melanogaster* were isolated in a gene referred to as *mus390* that now have been identified as different null mutations in the fly homolog of *BLM*.[123] Besides sensitivity to methylmethane sulfonate (MMS), the female flies are sterile and the males partially so. The frequency of nullo-X and XY sperm is increased, probably resulting from mis-segregation events in cell divisions preceding meiotic prophase. In addition, male offspring of *mus309* mutants lost portions of the Y chromosome, which resulted in male sterility. Introduction of an additional copy of the *Ku70* gene partially compensated for the *blm* defect.

A mutant of chicken *BLM* has been prepared in DT40 lymphoblastoid cells,[124] in which system gene replacement by homologous recombination using recombinant DNA is highly efficient. The mutant cells exhibit many similarities to BS cells, including increases in the frequency of targeted integration events and isochromatid breaks and, characteristically, SCEs. The hyperrecombination in the *BLM* mutants is dependent on the recombination machinery, because *BLM/RAD54* double mutants exhibit greatly reduced levels of SCEs compared to *BLM* single mutants.

Mouse strains with different mutations in *Blm* have been produced by homologous recombination and embryonic stem cell technology.[125,126] Embryonic fibroblasts derived from mouse mutants that have a targeted disruption of *Blm* exhibit the high-SCE phenotype characteristic of BS, indicating that Blm protein function is defective. The homozygous null animals display embryonic lethality, dying at day 13.5, developmentally delayed and anemic.[125] As a possible explanation for the developmental delay, excessive apoptosis was detected in the postimplantation mutant embryos. Mouse mutants produced by insertion of additional No. 3 exons of *Blm* are born alive but small, and they exhibit increased cancer susceptibility, providing a potentially useful mouse model for BS.[126]

MANAGEMENT

Growth

A means of increasing growth in BS is unknown. Infants and young children with BS are notoriously poor eaters. Gastro-esophageal reflux has been demonstrated in several infants. The course ordinarily followed in a child with BS is to set nutritious food before the child, supplement it with a multiple vitamin preparation, and just let the child eat as the appetite dictates. Nonvolitional feeding of infants with BS is under investigation in a few centers, by, for example, surgically placed intragastric feeding tubes, and some promising results are being obtained in the four children so treated.

Growth hormone production when estimated in BS usually is found in the normal to low-normal range. A few affected persons have been treated with growth hormone, usually without much effect. (That a few men with BS have reached 5 feet or slightly more in height [Fig. 16-1] without any specific treatment is unexplained.) Although more information on the possibly beneficial effect of growth hormone with respect to final body size in BS is desirable, reports of cancer that has arisen during or following its administration, including in BS, usually deter trials.

The Skin

Avoidance of the sun and the regular use of a hat or bonnet and sun-screening ointments control the facial skin lesion of BS best. Especially advisable are measures that limit sun exposure in the first few years of life, judging from the observation that in most cases the severity of the skin lesion appears to be established at that time.

Cancer

Although knowledge of the cancer proneness of BS quite naturally is distressing to an affected family, such knowledge can be lifesaving. Here, information is withheld from neither affected adults nor the parents of affected children. Families and patients handle this information well if it is presented to them appropriately by the physician or geneticist in charge, i.e., in comprehensible and useful terms. It can be presented in the context of the already great frequency of cancer in the general population, and then supplemented by an explanation of the basis for the inordinate increase and its prematurity in the person with BS. That the risk, although always more than in other people, is relatively much less at the early ages can be emphasized, as well as the shift of type toward carcinoma after adulthood is reached.[12] The potential value such knowledge of the cancer proneness provides to an affected person also can be emphasized, and some idea of practical and effective surveillance programs to be instituted at different ages can be provided. In this way, the physician who makes the diagnosis also, in lieu of treatment in the usual sense, offers a modus operandi.

Until the prognosis of leukemia if diagnosed and treated in its earliest stages can be shown to be better than treatment initiated after the disease becomes symptomatic, periodic hematologic surveillance of children with BS is not recommended. However, for adults with BS, close and long-term contact with an internist or clinic knowledgeable about BS is highly advisable. An unusual degree of attention then will be paid to symptoms that in other persons might properly be ignored, but that in BS will permit early diagnosis of carcinoma, where surgical excision still provides the best chance of cure. (Among symptoms and signs that already have led to early diagnosis of cancer in persons in the Registry — sometimes, but unfortunately not always, lifesaving — are these: hoarseness [laryngeal carcinoma]; pain in the side of the throat [posterior lingual carcinoma]; mild dysphagia [esophageal carcinoma]; red blood-staining in the feces [carcinoma of the lower large bowel]; a lump in the breast palpable by the patient; a positive Papanicolaou smear [cervical carcinoma-*in-situ*]; lower abdominal pain [uterine adenocarcinoma]; unexplained recurring abdominal discomfort [pelvic lymphoma; adenocarcinoma of the colon]; intussusception [lymphoma of the small bowel]; and, abrupt onset of convulsions [meningioma] or headache [medulloblastoma].) After the age of 20, annual visits with the internist seem advisable with at least annual screening by conventional methods for carcinoma of the breast, cervix, and colon.

In the treatment of the cancers that arise in persons with BS, consideration is given to the hypersensitivity such persons usually show to many of the DNA-damaging chemicals in standard regimens of therapy. Several persons with BS have shown severe damage or destruction of the bowel mucosa and bone marrow, sometimes lethal. Although specific recommendations of dosage of chemotherapeutic agents in BS cannot be given, doses approximately half the standard dose of the DNA-damaging agents have usually been tolerated, and in several have proven adequate for cure. Ionizing irradiation has been tolerated seemingly normally in the usual dosage.

The "management" of a person with BS is not to be viewed by his or her physician as of little value just because normal body size cannot be prescribed for nor cancer prevented. Knowledge of the correct diagnosis and an understanding of the condition are of inestimable value to parents of affected persons. Also, the affected individual benefits both physically and emotionally when in the hands of someone who knows the correct diagnosis, understands the syndrome itself, and is able to communicate accurate information about it both appropriately and wisely, including its important complications.

CONCLUDING COMMENTS

Since 1960, when its clinical and laboratory investigation began, rare BS has been a source of important, as well as very interesting, biological information, as reviewed here. The new things that can be learned from BS depend to a considerable extent on technical advances. First, experimental laboratory observation of the chromosomes of BS cells supplemented by long-term contact with affected individuals provided *some of the earliest and firmest evidence that chromosome mutation is etiologic in human cancer.* Cytogenetics complemented by molecular biology also showed that *somatic crossing-over can take place in mammalian cells.* Most recently, recombinant DNA technology applied to the study of BS, still in conjunction with clinical investigation, notably the use in the laboratory of cell lines derived from families about whom reliable clinical and genetic information had been accumulated, has brought to light *a protein not previously known to exist in mammalian cells.* With the identification of BLM as a protein important in DNA metabolism, but one that is not lethal when absent from the nucleus in humans (in mice it is), the BS cell and the BS gene in themselves become *valuable experimental material.* Now the nucleic acid enzymologist and molecular biologist can employ them to investigate little understood, if not previously completely obscure, nuclear mechanisms by which the genetic material is manipulated — and manipulated properly if genomic stability is to be maintained. For, a major consequence for the cell of absence from it of the normal functioning of the *BLM* gene product is an unacceptably high rate of mutation, including hyperrecombination. (Definition of the role of BLM in the germ line has just begun, but clinical observations in BS supplemented by some preliminary laboratory information indicate that it is an important one, probably — judging from the cytogenetics of BS somatic cells — concerned with *the control of meiotic recombination.*)

The identification of BLM coincides temporally with that of other "new" proteins such as WRN (absent in Werner syndrome), ATM (absent or abnormal in ataxia-telangiectasia), nibrin (absent in the Nijmegan breakage syndrome), and the Fanconi anemia proteins. All these proteins were introduced into cell biology via intensive investigation in several laboratories of a group of rare, recessively transmitted phenotypes that, although clinically dissimilar, have for heuristic purposes been lumped together for the past 30 years as "chromosome-breakage syndromes."[127] The several proteins concerned with DNA repair (some of which deal with transcription as well) that are absent or abnormal in xeroderma pigmentosum, Cockayne syndrome, and trichothiodystrophy are often advantageously grouped with those abnormal in the classic "breakage" syndromes. The continued study of this recently recognized group of proteins will provide increasingly detailed understanding of cellular mechanisms by which stability of the genome is maintained, and quite possibly also will bring to light some previously unrecognized mutational mechanisms.

Some of this information is of direct and immediate value in the clinical management of the disease states themselves. This is fortunate for the affected persons and families, many of whom have become steadfast — essential — partners with the clinical investigators and their colleagues at the laboratory bench, both in defining accurately and then in understanding their conditions. However, in the broader sense, these rare disorders can be viewed as models for the cell biologist to find out new things. Their greatest importance, therefore, is in providing fundamental understanding in an area of biology that until relatively recently had not even been recognized as something to be studied — *how the genome of somatic cells is guarded against change, and what the consequences of somatic mutation can be.*

REFERENCES

1. German J: Bloom's syndrome. I. Genetical and clinical observations in the first twenty-seven patients. *Am J Hum Genet* **21**:196, 1969.
2. German J: Bloom's syndrome. II. The prototype of genetic disorders predisposing to chromosome instability and cancer, in German J (ed): *Chromosomes and Cancer.* New York, John Wiley, 1974, p 601.
3. German J: Bloom's syndrome. VIII. Review of clinical and genetic aspects, in Goodman RM, Motulsky AG (eds): *Genetic Diseases Among Ashkenazi Jews.* New York, Raven Press, 1979, p 121.
4. German J: Bloom syndrome: A mendelian prototype of somatic mutational disease. *Medicine* **72**:393, 1993.
5. German J: Bloom's syndrome, in Cohen PR, Kurzrock R (eds): *Genodermatoses with Malignant Potential,* Philadelphia, W. B. Saunders, 1995, pp 7–18. Dermatologic Clinics, Vol 13.
6. German J: Genes which increase chromosomal instability in somatic cells and predispose to cancer, in Steinberg AG, Bearn AG (eds): *Progress in Medical Genetics,* vol. VIII. New York, Grune & Stratton, 1972, p 61.
7. Ray JH, German J: The cytogenetics of the "chromosome-breakage syndromes," in German J (ed): *Chromosome Mutation and Neoplasia.* New York, Alan R. Liss, 1983, p 135.
8. German J: Bloom's syndrome XVII. A genetic disorder that displays the consequences of excessive somatic mutation, in Bonne-Tamir B, Adam A (eds): *Genetic Diversity Among Jews.* New York, Oxford University Press, 1992, p 129.
9. German J, Passarge E: Bloom's syndrome. XII. Report from the Registry for 1987. *Clin Genet* **35**:57, 1989.
10. German J: The immunodeficiency of Bloom syndrome, in Ochs HD, Smith JCIE, Puck J (eds): *Primary Immunodeficiency Diseases. A Molecular and Genetic Approach.* New York, Oxford University Press, 1999, p 335.
11. Bloom D: Congenital telangiectatic erythema resembling lupus erythematosus in dwarfs. *Am J Dis Child* **88**:754, 1954.
12. German J: Bloom's syndrome. XX. The first 100 cancers. *Cancer Genet Cytogenet* **93**:101, 1997.
13. Tachibana A, Tatsumi K, Masui T, Kato T: Large deletions at the *HPRT* locus Associated with the mutator phenotype in a Bloom's syndrome lymphoblastoid cell line. *Mol Carcinog* **17**:41, 1996.
14. Kusunoki Y, Hayashi T, Hirai Y, Kushiro J, Tatsumi K, Kurihara T, Zghal M, Kamoun MR, Takebe H, Jeffreys A, et al: Increased rate of spontaneous mitotic recombination in T lymphocytes from a Bloom's

syndrome patient using a flow-cytometric assay at HLA-A locus. *Jpn J Cancer Res* **85**:610, 1994.

15. Groden J, Nakamura Y, German J: Molecular evidence that homologous recombination occurs in proliferating human somatic cells. *Proc Natl Acad Sci U S A* **87**:4315, 1990.

16. Groden J, German J: Bloom's syndrome. XVIII. Hypermutability of a tandem-repeat locus. *Hum Genet* **90**:360, 1992.

17. Foucault F, Buard J, Praz F, Jaulin C, Stoppa-Lyonnet D, Vergnaud G, Amor-Gueret M: Stability of microsatellites and minisatellites in Bloom syndrome, a human syndrome of genetic instability. *Mutat Res* **362**:227, 1996.

18. Kaneko H, Inoue R, Yamada Y, Sukegawa K, Fukao T, Tashita H, Teramoto T, Kashara K, Takami Kondo N: Microsatellite instability in B-cell lymphoma originating from Bloom syndrome. *Int J Cancer* **69**:480, 1996.

19. German J, Roe AM, Leppert M, Ellis NA: Bloom syndrome: An analysis of consanguineous families assigns the locus mutated to chromosome band 15q26.1. *Proc Natl Acad Sci U S A* **91**:6669, 1994.

20. Walpita D, Plug AW, Neff NF, German J, Ashley T: Bloom syndrome protein (BLM) colocalizes with replication protein A in meiotic prophase nuclei of mammalian spermatocytes. *Proc Natl Acad Sci U S A* **96**:5622, 1999.

21. Moens PB, Freire R, Tarsounas M, Spyropoulos B, Jackson SP: Expression and nuclear localization of BLM, a chromosome stability protein mutated in Bloom's syndrome, suggest a role in recombination during meiotic prophase. *J Cell Sci* **113**:663, 2000.

22. Martin RM, Rademaker A, German J: Chromosomal breakage in human spermatozoa, a heterozygous effect of the Bloom syndrome mutation. *Am J Hum Genet* **53**:1242, 1994.

23. Li L, Eng C, Desnick B, German J, Ellis NA: Frequency of *blm^Ash*, the mutation responsible for the high frequency of Bloom's syndrome in the Ashkenazim. *Mol Genet Metab* **64**:286, 1998.

24. Shahrabani-Gargir L, Shomrat R, Yaron Y, Orr-Urtreger A, Groden J, Legum C: High frequency of a common Bloom syndrome Ashkenazi mutation among Jews of Polish origin. *Genet Test* **2**:293, 1998.

25. Oddoux C, Clayton CM, Nelson HR, Ostrer H: Prevalence of Bloom syndrome heterozygotes among Ashkenazi Jews. *Am J Hum Genet* **64**:1241, 1999.

26. Roa BB, Savino CV, Richards CS: Ashkenazi Jewish population frequency of the Bloom syndrome gene 2281 delta 6ins7 mutation. *Genet Test* **3**:219, 1999.

27. Ellis NA, Roe AM, Kozloski J, Proytcheva M, Falk C, German J: Linkage disequilibrium between the *FES, D15S127,* and *BLM* loci in Ashkenazi Jews with Bloom syndrome. *Am J Hum Genet* **55**:453, 1994.

28. Ellis NA, Groden J, Ye T-Z, Straughen J, Lennon DJ, Ciocci S, Proytcheva M, German J: The Bloom's syndrome gene product is homologous to RecQ helicases. *Cell* **83**:655, 1995.

29. Weksberg R, Smith C, Anson-Cartwright L, Maloney K: Bloom syndrome: A single complementation group defines patients of diverse ethnic origin. *Am J Hum Genet* **42**:816, 1988.

30. McDaniel LD, Schultz RA: Elevated sister chromatid exchange phenotype of Bloom syndrome cells is complemented by human chromosome 15. *Proc Natl Acad Sci U S A* **89**:7968, 1992.

31. German J, Ellis NA, Proytcheva M: Bloom's syndrome. XIX. Cytogenetic and population evidence for genetic heterogeneity. *Clin Genet* **49**:223, 1996.

32. Bryant EM, Hoehn H, Martin GM: Normalization of sister chromatid exchange frequencies in Bloom's syndrome by euploid cell hybridization. *Nature* **279**:795, 1979.

33. Ellis NA, Lennon DJ, Proytcheva M, Alhadeff B, Henderson EE, German J: Somatic intragenic recombination within the mutated locus *BLM* can correct the high-SCE phenotype of Bloom syndrome cells. *Am J Hum Genet* **57**:1019, 1995.

34. Ellis NA, Ciocci S, German J: Back mutation can produce phenotype reversion in Bloom syndrome somatic cells. *Hum Genet* **108**:167, 2001.

35. Waisfisz Q, Morgan NV, Savino M, de Winter JP, van Berkel CG, Hoatlin ME, Ianzano L, Gibson RA, Arwert F, Savoia A, Mathew CG, Pronk JC, Joenje H: Spontaneous functional correction of homozygous Fanconi anaemia alleles reveals novel mechanistic basis for reverse mosaicism. *Nat Genet* **22**:379, 1999.

36. Ellis NA, German J: Molecular genetics of Bloom's syndrome. *Hum Mol Genet* **5**:1457, 1996.

37. Straughen J, Ciocci S, Ye T-Z, Lennon DN, Proytcheva M, Goodfellow P, German J, Ellis NA, Groden J: Physical mapping of the Bloom syndrome region by the identification of YAC and P1 clones from human chromosome 15 band q26.1. *Genomics* **33**:118, 1996.

38. Ellis NA, Ciocci S, Proytcheva M, Lennon D, Groden J, German J: The Ashkenazi Jewish Bloom syndrome mutation *blm^Ash* is present in non-Jewish Central Americans. *Am J Hum Genet* **63**:1685, 1998.

39. Straughen J, Johnson J, McLaren D, Proytcheva M, Ellis NA, German J, Groden J: A rapid method for detecting the predominant Ashkenazi Jewish mutation in the Bloom's syndrome gene. *Hum Mut* **11**:175, 1998.

40. Nakayama H, Nakayama K, Nakayama R, Irino N, Nakayama Y, Hanawalt PC: Isolation and genetic characterization of a thymineless death-resistant mutant of *Escherichia coli* K12: identification of a new mutation (*recQ1*) that blocks the RecF recombination pathway. *Mol Gen Genet* **195**:474, 1984.

41. Umezu K, Nakayama K, Nakayama H: *Escherichia coli* RecQ protein is a DNA helicase. *Proc Natl Acad Sci U S A* **87**:5363, 1990.

42. Harmon FG, DiGate RJ, Kowalczykowski SC: RecQ helicase and topoisomerase III comprise a novel DNA strand passage function: A conserved mechanism for control of DNA recombination. *Mol Cell* **3**:611, 1999.

43. Harmon FG, Kowalczykowski SC: RecQ helicase, in concert with RecA and SSB proteins, initiates and disrupts DNA recombination. *Genes Dev* **12**:1134, 1998.

44. Hanada K, Ukita T, Kohno Y, Saito K, Kato J, Ikeda H: RecQ DNA helicase is a suppressor of illegitimate recombination in *Escherichia coli*. *Proc Natl Acad Sci U S A* **94**:3860, 1997.

45. Kusano K, Sunohara Y, Takahashi N, Yoshikura H, Kobayashi I: DNA double-strand break repair: Genetic determinants of flanking crossing-over. *Proc Natl Acad Sci U S A* **91**:1173, 1994.

46. Courcelle J, Carswell-Crumpton C, Hanawalt PC: *recF* and *recR* are required for the resumption of replication at DNA replication forks in *Escherichia coli*. *Proc Natl Acad Sci U S A* **94**:3714, 1997.

47. Cromie GA, Millar CB, Schmidt KH, Leach DR: Palindromes as substrates for multiple pathways of recombination in *Escherichia coli*. *Genetics* **154**:513, 2000.

48. Gangloff S, McDonald JP, Bendixen C, Arthur L, Rothstein R: The yeast type I topoisomerase top3 interacts with Sgs1, a DNA helicase homolog: A potential eukaryotic reverse gyrase. *Mol Cell Biol* **14**:8391, 1994.

49. Wang JC: DNA topoisomerases. *Annu Rev Biochem* **65**:635, 1996.

50. Wallis JW, Chrebet G, Brodsky G, Rolfe M, Rothstein R: A hyper-recombination mutation in *S. cerevisiae* identifies a novel eukaryotic topoisomerase. *Cell* **58**:409, 1989.

51. Gangloff S, de Massy B, Arthur L, Rothstein R, Fabre F: The essential role of yeast topoisomerase III in meiosis depends on recombination. *EMBO J* **18**:1701, 1999.

52. Bennett RJ, Noirot-Gros MF, Wang JC: Interaction between yeast sgs1 helicase and DNA topoisomerase III. *J Biol Chem* **275**:26898, 2000.

53. Duno M, Thomsen B, Westergaard O, Krejci L, Bendixen C: Genetic analysis of the Saccharomyces cerevisiae Sgs1 helicase defines an essential function for the Sgs1-Top3 complex in the absence of SRS2 or TOP1. *Mol Gen Genet* **264**:89, 2000.

54. Fricke WM, Kaliraman V, Brill SJ: Mapping the DNA topoisomerase III binding domain of the Sgs1 DNA helicase. *J Biol Chem* **276**:8848, 2001.

55. Mullen JR, Kaliraman V, Brill SJ: Bipartite structure of the SGS1 DNA helicase in *Saccharomyces cerevisiae*. *Genetics* **154**:1101, 2000.

56. Watt PM, Louis EJ, Borts RH, Hickson ID: Sgs1: A eukaryotic homolog of *E. coli* RecQ that interacts with topoisomerase II *in vivo* and is required for faithful chromosome segregation. *Cell* **81**:253, 1995.

57. Lu J, Mullen JR, Brill SJ, Kleff S, Romeo AM, Sternglanz R: Human homologues of yeast helicase. *Nature* **383**:678, 1996.

58. Watt PM, Hickson ID, Borts RH, Louis EJ: SGS1, a homologue of the Bloom's and Werner's syndrome genes, is required for maintenance of genome stability in *Saccharomyces cerevisiae*. *Genetics* **144**:935, 1996.

59. Myung K, Datta A, Chen C, Kolodner RD: SGS1, the *Saccharomyces cerevisiae* homologue of *BLM* and WRN, suppresses genome instability and homologous recombination. *Nat Genet* **27**:113, 2001.

60. Miyajima A, Seki M, Onoda F, Shiratori M, Odagiri N, Ohta K, Kikuchi Y, Ohno Y, Enomoto T: Sgs1 helicase activity is required for mitotic but apparently not for meiotic functions. *Mol Cell Biol* **20**:6399, 2000.

61. Gangloff S, Soustelle C, Fabre F: Homologous recombination is responsible for cell death in the absence of the Sgs1 and Srs2 helicases. *Nat Genet* **25**:192, 2000.

62. Lee SK, Johnson RE, Yu SL, Prakash L, Prakash S: Requirement of yeast SGS1 and SRS2 genes for replication and transcription. *Science* **286**:2339, 1999.

63. Johnson FB, Marciniak RA, McVey M, Stewart SA, Hahn WC, Guarente L: The *Saccharomyces cerevisiae* WRN homolog Sgs1p participates in telomere maintenance in cells lacking telomerase. *EMBO J* **20**:905, 2001.

64. Huang P, Pryde FE, Lester D, Maddison RL, Borts RH, Hickson ID, Louis EJ: SGS1 is required for telomere elongation in the absence of telomerase. *Curr Biol* **11**:125, 2001.

65. Cohen H, Sinclair DA: Recombination-mediated lengthening of terminal telomeric repeats requires the Sgs1 DNA helicase. *Proc Natl Acad Sci U S A* **98**:3174, 2001.

66. Yamagata K, Kato J, Shimamoto A, Goto M, Furuichi Y, Ikeda H: Bloom's and Werner's syndrome genes suppress hyperrecombination in yeast sgs1 mutant: Implication for genomic instability in human diseases. *Proc Natl Acad Sci U S A* **95**:8733, 1998.

67. Frei C, Gasser SM: The yeast Sgs1p helicase acts upstream of Rad53p in the DNA replication checkpoint and colocalizes with Rad53p in S-phase-specific foci. *Genes Dev* **14**:81, 2000.

68. Murray JM, Lindsay HD, Munday CA, Carr AM: Role of Schizosaccharomyces pombe RecQ homolog, recombination, and checkpoint genes in UV damage tolerance. *Mol Cell Biol* **17**:6868, 1997.

69. Stewart E, Chapman CR, Al-Khodairy F, Carr AM, Enoch T: rqh1+, a fission yeast gene related to the Bloom's and Werner's syndrome genes, is required for reversible S phase arrest. *Embo J* **16**:2682, 1997.

70. Davey S, Han CS, Ramer SA, Klassen JC, Jacobson A, Eisenberger A, Hopkins KM, Lieberman HB, Freyer GA: Fission yeast rad12+ regulates cell cycle checkpoint control and is homologous to the Bloom's syndrome disease gene. *Mol Cell Biol* **18**:2721, 1998.

71. Doe CL, Dixon J, Osman F, Whitby MC: Partial suppression of the fission yeast rqh1(−) phenotype by expression of a bacterial Holliday junction resolvase. *EMBO J* **19**:2751, 2000.

72. Goodwin A, Wang SW, Toda T, Norbury C, Hickson I: Topoisomerase III is essential for accurate nuclear division in *Schizosaccharomyces pombe*. *Nucleic Acids Res* **27**:4050, 1999.

73. Maftahi M, Han CS, Langston LD, Hope JC, Zigouras N, and Freyer GA: The top3(+) gene is essential in and the lethality associated with its loss is caused by Rad12 helicase activity. *Nucleic Acids Res* **27**:4715, 1999.

74. Bahr A, De Graeve F, Kedinger C, Chatton B: Point mutations causing Bloom's syndrome abolish ATPase and DNA helicase activities of the BLM protein. Oncogene **17**:2565, 1998.

75. Morozov V, Mushegian AR, Koonin EV, Bork P: A putative nucleic acid-binding domain in Bloom's and Werner's syndrome helicases. *Trends Biochem Sci* **22**:417, 1997.

76. Puranam KL, Blackshear PJ: Cloning and characterization of *RECQL*, a potential human homologue of the *Escherichia coli* DNA helicase RecQ. *J Biol Chem* **269**:29838, 1994.

77. Seki M, Miyazawa H, Tada S, Yanagisawa J, Yamaoka T, Hoshino S, Ozawa K, Eki T, Nogami M, Okumura K, Taguchi H, Hanaoka H, Enomoto T: Molecular cloning of cDNA encoding human DNA helicase Q1 which has homology to *Escherichia coli* RecQ helicase and localization of the gene at chromosome 12p12. *Nucleic Acids Res* **22**:4566, 1994.

78. Yu C-E, Oshima J, Fu Y-H, Wijsman EM, Hisama F, Alisch R, Matthews S, Nakuro J, Miki T, Ouais S, Martin GM, Mulligan J, Shellenberg GD: Positional cloning of the Werner syndrome gene. *Science* **272**:258, 1996.

79. Gray MD, Shen JC, Kamath-Loeb AS, Blank A, Sopher BL, Martin GM, Oshima J, Loeb LA: The Werner syndrome protein is a DNA helicase. *Nat Genet* **17**:100, 1997.

80. Suzuki N, Shimamoto A, Imamura O, Kuromitsu J, Kitao S, Goto M, Furuichi Y: DNA helicase activity in Werner's syndrome gene product synthesized in a baculovirus system. *Nucleic Acids Res* **25**:2973, 1997.

81. Huang S, Li B, Gray MD, Oshima J, Mian IS, Campisi J: The premature aging syndrome protein, WRN, is a 3′ → 5′ exonuclease. *Nat Genet* **20**:114, 1998.

82. Hoehn H, Bryant EM, Au K, Norwood TH, Bowman H, Martin GM: Variegated translocation mosaicism in human skin fibroblast cultures. *Cytogenet Cell Genet* **15**:282, 1975.

83. Schonberg S, Niermeijer MF, Bootsma D, Henderson E, German J: Werner's syndrome: Proliferation in vitro of clones of cells bearing chromosome translocations. *Am J Hum Genet* **36**:387, 1984.

84. Sinclair DA, Mills K, Guarente L: Accelerated aging and nucleolar fragmentation in yeast sgs1 mutants. *Science* **277**:1313, 1997.

85. Sinclair DA, Guarente L: Extrachromosomal rDNA circles — a cause of aging in yeast. *Cell* **91**:1033, 1997.

86. Kitao S, Ohsugi I, Ichikawa K, Goto M, Furuichi Y, Shimamoto A: Cloning of two new human helicase genes of the *RecQ* family: Biological significance of multiple species in higher eukaryotes. *Genomics* **54**:443, 1998.

87. Kitao S, Shimamoto A, Goto M, Miller RW, Smithson WA, Lindor NM, Furuichi Y: Mutations in RECQL4 cause a subset of cases of Rothmund-Thomson syndrome. *Nat genet* **22**:82, 1999.

88. Karow JK, Chakraverty RK, Hickson ID: The Bloom's syndrome gene product is a 3′-5′ DNA helicase. *J Biol Chem* **272**:30611, 1997.

89. Neff NF, Ellis NA, Ye TZ, Noonan J, Huang K, Proytcheva M, Sanz M: The DNA helicase activity of BLM is necessary for the correction of the genomic instability of Bloom syndrome cells. *Mol Biol Cell* **10**:665, 1999.

90. Brosh RM Jr, Li JL, Kenny MK, Karow JK, Cooper MP, Kureekattil RP, Hickson ID, Bohr VA: Replication protein A physically interacts with the Bloom's syndrome protein and stimulates its helicase activity. *J Biol Chem* **275**:23500, 2000.

91. Sun H, Karow JK, Hickson ID, Maizels N: The Bloom's syndrome helicase unwinds G4 DNA. *J Biol Chem* **273**:27587, 1998.

92. Karow JK, Constantinou A, Li JL, West SC, Hickson ID: The Bloom's syndrome gene product promotes branch migration of Holliday junctions. *Proc Natl Acad Sci U S A* **97**:6504, 2000.

93. van Brabant AJ, Ye T, Sanz M, German J, Ellis NA, Holloman WK: Binding and melting of D-loops by the Bloom syndrome helicase. *Biochemistry* **39**:14617, 2000.

94. Bennett RJ, Keck JL, Wang JC: Binding specificity determines polarity of DNA unwinding by the Sgs1 protein of *S. cerevisiae*. *J Mol Biol* **289**:235, 1999.

95. Fry M, Loeb LA: Human Werner syndrome DNA helicase unwinds tetrahedral structures of the Fragile X syndrome repeat sequence d(CGG)n. *J Biol Chem* **274**:12797, 1999.

96. Sun H, Bennett RJ, Maizels N: The Saccharomyces cerevisiae Sgs1 helicase efficiently unwinds G-G paired DNAs. *Nucleic Acids Res* **27**:1978, 1999.

97. Foucault F, Vaury C, Barakat A, Thibout D, Planchon P, Jaulin C, Praz F, Amor-Guert M: Characterization of a new BLM mutation associated with a topoisomerase II alpha defect in a patient with Bloom's syndrome. *Hum Mol Genet* **6**:1427, 1997.

98. Ellis NA, Proytcheva M, Sanz MM, Ye TZ, German J: Transfection of *BLM* into cultured Bloom syndrome cells reduces the SCE rate toward normal. *Am J Hum Genet* **65**:1368, 1999.

99. Giesler T, Baker K, Zhang B, McDaniel LD, Schultz RA: Correction of the Bloom syndrome cellular phenotypes. *Somat Cell Mol Genet* **23**:303, 1997.

100. Kaneko H, Orii KO, Matsui E, Shimozawa N, Fukao T, Matsumoto T, Shimamoto A, Furuichi Y, Hayakawa S, Kasahara K, Kondo N: *BLM* (the causative gene of Bloom syndrome) protein translocation into the nucleus by a nuclear localization signal. *Biochem Biophys Res Commun* **240**:348, 1997.

101. Matsumoto T, Shimamoto A, Goto M, Furuichi Y: Impaired nuclear localization of defective DNA helicases in Werner syndrome. *Nat Genet* **16**:335, 1997.

102. Kawabe T, Tsuyama N, Kitao S, Nishikawa K, Shimamoto A, Shiratori M, Matsumoto T, Anno K, Sato T, Mitsui Y, Seki M, Enomoto T, Goto M, Ellis NA, Ide T, Furuichi Y, Sugimoto M: Differential regulation of human RecQ family helicases in cell transformation and cell cycle. *Oncogene* **19**:4764, 2000.

103. Gharibyan V, Youssoufian H: Localization of the Bloom syndrome helicase to punctate nuclear structures and the nuclear matrix and regulation during the cell cycle: Comparison with the Werner's syndrome helicase. *Mol Carcinog* **26**:261, 1999.

104. Dutertre S, Ababou M, Onclercq R, Delic J, Chatton B, Jaulin C, Amor-Gueret M: Cell cycle regulation of the endogenous wild type Bloom's syndrome DNA helicase. *Oncogene* **19**:2731, 2000.

105. Sanz MM, Proytcheva M, Ellis NA, Holloman WK, German J: BLM, the Bloom's syndrome protein, varies during the cell cycle in its amount, distribution, and co-localization with other nuclear proteins. *Cytogenet Cell Genet* **91**:217, 2000.

106. Zhong S, Hu P, Ye TZ, Stan R, Ellis NA, Pandolfi PP: A role for PML and the nuclear body in genomic stability. *Oncogene* **18**:7941, 1999.

107. Ababou M, Dutertre S, Lecluse Y, Onclercq R, Chatton B, Amor-Gueret M: ATM-dependent phosphorylation and accumulation of endogenous *BLM* protein in response to ionizing radiation. *Oncogene* **19**:5955, 2000.

108. Fogal V, Gostissa M, Sandy P, Zacchi P, Sternsdorf T, Jensen K, Pandolfi PP, Will H, Schneider C, Del Sal G: Regulation of p53 activity in nuclear bodies by a specific PML isoform. *EMBO J* **19**:6185, 2000.

109. Guo A, Salomoni P, Luo J, Shih A, Zhong S, Gu W, Paolo Pandolfi P: The function of PML in p53-dependent apoptosis. *Nat Cell Biol* **2**:730, 2000.

110. Alcalay M, Tomassoni L, Colombo E, Stoldt S, Grignani F, Fagioli M, Szekely L, Helin K, Pelicci PG: The promyelocytic leukemia gene product (PML) forms stable complexes with the retinoblastoma protein. *Mol Cell Biol* **18**:1084, 1998.

111. Wu G, Lee WH, Chen PL: NBS1 and TRF1 colocalize at promyelocytic leukemia bodies during late S/G2 phases in immortalized telomerase-negative cells. Implication of NBS1 in alternative lengthening of telomeres. *J Biol Chem* **275**:30618, 2000.

112. Lombard DB, Guarente L: Nijmegan breakage syndrome disease protein and MRE11 at PML nuclear bodies and meiotic telomeres. *Cancer Res* **60**:2331, 2000.

113. Johnson FB, Lombard DB, Neff NF, Mastrangelo MA, Dewolf W, Ellis NA, Marciniak RA, Yin Y, Jaenisch R, Guarente L: Association of the Bloom syndrome protein with topoisomerase IIIalpha in somatic and meiotic cells. *Cancer Res* **60**:1162, 2000.

114. Wu L, Davies SL, North PS, Goulaouic H, Riou JF, Turley H, Gatter KC, Hickson ID: The Bloom's syndrome gene product interacts with topoisomerase III. *J Biol Chem* **275**:9636, 2000.

115. Bischof O, Kim SH, Irving J, Beresten S, Ellis NA, Campisi J: Regulation and localization of the Bloom syndrome protein in response to DNA damage. *J Cell Biol* **153**:367, 2001.

116. Wu L, Davies SL, Levitt NC, Hickson ID: Potential role for the *BLM* helicase in recombinational repair via a conserved interaction with RAD51. *J Biol Chem* **267**:19375, 2001.

117. Hu P, Beresten S, van Brabant A, Ye T-Z, Pandolfi P-P, Johnson FB, Guarente L, Ellis NA: Evidence for BLM and Topoisomerase IIIα interaction in genomic stability. *Hum Mol Genet* **10**:1287, 2001

118. Karow JK, Newman RH, Freemont PS, Hickson ID: Oligomeric ring structure of the Bloom's syndrome helicase. *Curr Biol* **9**:597, 1999.

119. Beresten SF, Stan R, van Brabant AJ, Ye T, Naureckieme S, Ellis NA: Purification of overexpressed hexahistidine-tagged BLM N431 as oligomeric complexes. *Protein Expr Purif* **17**:239, 1999.

120. Bischof O, Galande S, Farzane F, Kohwi-Shigematsu T, Campisi J: Selective cleavage of BLM, the Bloom syndrome protein, during apoptotic cell death. *J Biol Chem* **276**:12068, 2001.

121. Kusano K, Berres ME, Engels WR: Evolution of the RECQ family of heliacases: A Drosophila homolog, *Dmblm*, is similar to the human Bloom syndrome gene. *Genetics* **151**:1027, 1999.

122. Liao S, Graham J, Yan H: The function of Xenopus Bloom's syndrome protein homolog (xBLM) in DNA replication. *Genes Dev* **14**:2570, 2000.

123. Kusano K, Johnson-Schlitz DM, Engels WR: Sterility of Drosophila with mutations in the Bloom syndrome gene—complementation by Ku70. *Science* **291**:2600, 2001.

124. Wang W, Seki M, Narita Y, Sonoda E, Takeda S, Yamada K, Masuko T, Katada T, Enomoto T: Possible association of BLM in decreasing DNA double strand breaks during DNA replication. *EMBO J* **19**:3428, 2000.

125. Chester N, Kuo F, Kozak C, O'Hara CD, Leder P: Stage-specific apoptosis, developmental delay, and embryonic lethality in mice homozygous for a targeted disruption in the murine Bloom's syndrome gene. *Genes Dev* **12**:3382, 1998.

126. Luo G, Santoro IM, McDaniel LD, Nishijima I, Mills M, Youssoufian H, Vogel H, Schultz RA, Bradley A: Cancer predisposition caused by elevated mitotic recombination in Bloom mice. *Nat Genet* **26**:424, 2000.

127. German J: Chromosomal breakage syndromes. *Birth Defects: Original Article Series* **5**:117, 1969.

128. German J, Schonberg S, Louie E, Chaganti RSK: Bloom's syndrome. IV. Sister-chromotid exchanges in lymphocytes. *Amer J Hum Genet* **29**:248, 1977.

129. Caldecott KW, McKeown CK, Tucker JD, Ljungquist S, Thompson LH: An interaction between the mammalian DNA repair protein XRCC1 and DNA ligase III. *Mol Cell Biol* **14**:68, 1994.

Fanconi Anemia

Arleen D. Auerbach ■ *Manuel Buchwald* ■ *Hans Joenje*

1. Fanconi anemia (FA) is an autosomal recessive disorder that is characterized clinically by diverse congenital abnormalities and a predisposition to bone marrow failure and malignancy, particularly acute myelogenous leukemia (AML). FA patients exhibit extreme clinical heterogeneity and may have abnormalities in any major organ system. It is recognized that the FA phenotype is so variable, with considerable overlap with the phenotypes of a variety of genetic and nongenetic diseases, that diagnosis on the basis of clinical manifestations alone is difficult.

2. FA is found in all races and ethnic groups and has been widely reported to have a carrier frequency of 1 in 300. This estimate was based on the incidence of affected individuals before the full spectrum of the FA phenotype was recognized. The true gene frequency is likely to be considerably higher than this; a low estimate would result from an incomplete ascertainment of cases before the widespread application of chromosomal breakage tests for FA diagnosis. Up to 0.5 percent of the general population may be heterozygous at an FA locus.

3. Hypersensitivity of FA cells to the clastogenic (chromosome-breaking) effect of crosslinking agents provides a unique cellular marker for the disorder. This is used as a diagnostic criterion because of the difficulty of diagnosing FA on the basis of clinical manifestations alone. Comparative studies have led to the choice of diepoxybutane (DEB) as the agent most widely used for FA diagnosis. The crosslinking test can be used to identify preanemic patients as well as patients with aplastic anemia or leukemia who may or may not have the physical stigmata associated with FA.

4. The hypersensitivity of FA cells to crosslinking agents has been used to assess complementation in somatic cell hybrids. Complementation groups usually are considered to represent distinct disease genes, and for FA the genes for six groups (A, C, D2, E, F, and G) have so far been identified and mapped. The first FA gene isolated by expression cloning methodology (*FANCC*, alias *FAC*) mapped to chromosome 9q22.3 by *in situ* hybridization. *FANCA* (alias *FAA*) was mapped by linkage of the disease in FA-A families to microsatellite markers positioned close to the telomere of chromosome 16 (16q24.3). *FANCD2*, mapped originally as FA-D by microcell-mediated chromosome transfer, has been localized to chromosome 3p25.3. *FANCG* is identical with the previously isolated human gene *XRCC9*, which was mapped to 9p13. *FANCE* and *FANCF*, both isolated by expression cloning, were mapped to 6p21-22 and 11p15 respectively. Considerable variability in the prevalence of the different complementation groups has been observed among various ethnic

groups. Overall, FA-A is the most prevalent group, accounting for approximately 65 percent of all FA cases.

5. A cDNA expression cloning procedure was adapted and used successfully to clone the gene defective in FA-C cells (*FANCC*). The *FANCC* coding region contains 14 exons and leads to a predicted protein of 558 amino acids. The predicted structure of FANCC does not resemble that of any known protein and has no obvious functional domains. The protein is found primarily in the cytoplasm, although approximately 10 percent is in the nucleus. FANCC appears to play a direct role in protecting cells against the damage produced by crosslinking agents.

6. Homologous recombination in embryonic stem (ES) cells has been used to target the endogenous *Fancc* locus, with the consequent removal of exon 8 or exon 9. These cells have been used to derive strains of mice (*Fancc*$^{-/-}$) in which no active Fancc protein is produced. The mutant mice show the characteristic FA sensitivity to crosslinkers but do not demonstrate any morphologic or hematopoietic phenotypes up to 1 year of age. In addition to the cellular sensitivity, the principal phenotype of *Fancc*$^{-/-}$ mice is decreased fertility of both male and female animals. This phenotype appears to be a more severe version of similar disease-related complications in FA patients.

7. *FANCA* was cloned by two parallel approaches. One was essentially the same as that used to clone *FANCC*. A cDNA clone was identified that corrected the crosslink hypersensitivity of FA-A cells but not that of FA-C cells. *FANCA* also was identified through positional cloning of the 16q24.3 region. The defective gene was identified by fine mapping, contig isolation, and exon trapping. *FANCA* codes for a predicted protein of 1455 amino acids that has no strong homologies to known proteins. On the basis of a predicted nuclear localization signal, the protein may be localized to the nucleus. The gene contains 43 exons spanning approximately 80 kb. More than 70 mutations in *FANCA* have been described worldwide. The heterogeneity of the mutation spectrum and the frequency of intragenic deletions present a considerable challenge for the molecular diagnosis of FA-A.

8. *Fanca-/-* mice have now been generated and characterized. The animals appear viable, have no developmental or hematological abnormalities, but show reduced fertility. Embryonic fibroblasts derived from the Fanca-deficient mice exhibited spontaneous and +crosslink-induced chromosomal instability very similar to the phenotype of human FA cells. The deduced mouse Fanca protein shares 81 percent sequence similarity and 66 percent identity with the human protein. In spite of the species difference, the murine Fanca cDNA was fully capable of correcting the defect of human FA-A lymphoblasts.

9. A cDNA representing the FA-G gene *FANCG* was isolated from the same expression library used for the functional cloning of *FANCC* and *FANCA*. The 2.5 kb complementing cDNA was identified as identical to human *XRCC9*, a novel

---

A list of standard abbreviations is located immediately preceding the index. Nonstandard abbreviations used in this chapter include: FA = Fanconi anemia; AML = acute myelogenous leukemia; DEB = diepoxybutane; MMC = mitomycin C; MDS = myelodysplastic syndrome; BM = bone marrow.

gene defined by its capacity to partially complement the MMC-sensitive Chinese hamster mutant UV40. *FANCE* and *FANCF* were also isolated from this expression library. The encoded FANCG/XRCC, FANCE and FANCF proteins have no sequence similarities to any other known protein or motifs that could point to a molecular function.

10. Complementation group D is heterogeneous; positional cloning has identified a gene on 3p (*FANCD2*) that complements the hypersensitivity of some (FA-D2), but not other (FA-D1), cell lines in this group. FANCD2 is the only FA protein so far identified that is conserved in nonvertebrate species such as *A. thaliana*, *C. elegans*, and *D. melanogaster*; however the function of these homologs is also unknown. FANCA, FANCC, FANCF, and FANCG proteins are required for the activation of the FANCD2 protein to a monoubiquitinated isoform, and normal activated FANCD2 colocalizes with the breast cancer susceptibility protein, BRCA1, in ionizing radiation–induced foci and in synaptonemal complexes of meiotic chromosomes. Most of the recent studies of FA proteins have focused on subcellular localizations and mutual interactions.

11. Transplantation with hematopoietic stem cells from bone marrow or umbilical cord blood currently offers the only possibility for a cure for bone marrow failure in FA as well as a possible cure for or prevention of leukemia. Recent analyses of HLA-matched sibling transplants show that increased survival is associated with younger age, less severe hematologic disease, and absence of malignant transformation.

Fanconi anemia (FA) is an autosomal recessive disorder that is characterized clinically by diverse congenital abnormalities and a predisposition to bone marrow failure and malignancy, particularly acute myelogenous leukemia (AML).[1–3] FA patients exhibit extreme clinical heterogeneity and may have abnormalities in any major organ system.[4] Clinical heterogeneity in FA is both interfamilial and intrafamilial; there is a lack of concordance for specific congenital malformations among affected siblings, and even monozygotic twins may exhibit phenotypic heterogeneity.[5] FA cells exhibit an abnormally high level of chromosomal breakage and are hypersensitive to both the cytotoxic and the clastogenic effects of DNA crosslinking agents such as diepoxybutane (DEB) and mitomycin C (MMC).[6–9] The relationship of this DNA instability to the potential for FA patients to develop cancer is unknown.

It is recognized that the FA phenotype is so variable, with considerable overlap with the phenotypes of a variety of genetic and nongenetic diseases, that a correct diagnosis on the basis of clinical manifestations alone is difficult.[10,11] Although the pathophysiology of the syndrome is unknown, diagnosis of FA has been facilitated by the study of DEB-induced chromosomal breakage, which provides a unique marker for the FA genotype.[12–15] This cellular characteristic can be used as a diagnostic test to identify preanemic patients as well as patients with aplastic anemia or leukemia who may or may not have the classic physical stigmata associated with FA.[16]

The clinical variability of FA may be in part dependent on the existence of considerable genetic heterogeneity. A minimum of seven complementation groups have been identified through somatic cell studies, and at least four of these groups (FA-A, FA-C through FA-G) represent independent genetic loci for which genes have been cloned.[17–20] Analysis of patients mutant in the first FA gene to be cloned (*FANCC*) has shown that some of the clinical variability in this group of patients can be accounted for by the different *FANCC* mutations present.[21–23] Further heterogeneity may be attributed to specific genetic events as more of the genes are identified and more patients are analyzed.

Biochemical studies of cells from FA patients have led to a large volume of literature that includes considerable variability in the reproducibility of the results. In hindsight, it can be seen that many of these studies have inadvertently mixed cells from different complementation groups, since the cells under study were not classified.[24] Nevertheless, reproducible phenotypes involving processes that can be explained by defects in DNA repair, oxygen sensitivity, growth factor homeostasis, apoptosis, and cell cycle regulation now are known to be characteristic of FA cells.[25,26] The specific defects in each complementation group are not known.

The procedures for the cloning of FA genes initially exploited the increased sensitivity of FA cells to MMC or DEB. While early studies using genomic DNA were unsuccessful, the use of episomal cDNA libraries led to the identification of *FANCC*, the gene defective in FA patients of group C.[27] A similar approach has led to the identification of *FANCA*,[28] *FANCG*, *FANCF*, and *FANCE*, in that order. The *FANCA* gene, which is defective in the majority of FA patients, was also identified by the positional cloning approach,[29] as was *FANCD2*. Thus one can expect that during the next few years considerable progress will be made in our understanding of the fundamental defects in FA and their relationship to the development of the FA phenotype. The reader interested in additional material on FA is referred to the book *Fanconi Anemia: Clinial, Cytogenetic and Experimental Aspects*.[30] A chapter on FA in *Aplastic Anemia Acquired and Inherited* offers a comprehensive review of the literature on the clinical aspects of syndrome.[4] Reviews on FA also have been published recently.[24–26,31–34]

CLINICAL ASPECTS ON FA

Historical Perspective

In 1927, Fanconi described a family in which three male children between the ages of 5 and 7 years had pancytopenia and birth defects.[35] On the basis of his observations in this family and others, Fanconi's chief criteria for the diagnosis of FA included pancytopenia, hyperpigmentation, skeletal malformations, small stature, urogenital abnormalities, and familial occurrence. According to Fanconi, Naegeli suggested in 1931 that the term *Fanconi's anemia* be used to describe such patients.[1] Fanconi's observations formed the basis of the chief criteria for the diagnosis of FA for many years. Consideration of FA in the differential diagnosis of a patient manifesting clinical features of the syndrome depends on the clinician's concept of the FA phenotype. Most patients reported in textbooks and in the literature present a clinical picture similar to that of the original patients described by Fanconi. In a study comparing the frequencies of congenital anomalies among FA probands and their affected siblings, Glanz and Fraser observed that there was a significant reduction in the incidence of congenital anomalies among affected siblings compared with probands.[10] Affected siblings with milder phenotypic features were diagnosed after the diagnosis of FA in another affected family member, not because of their phenotypic presentation. In fact, patients with bone marrow failure who completely lacked congenital malformations, who were previously described as having the Estren-Damenshek syndrome, were found in the same sibships as classic FA.[10,36,37] In a survey of black African children with FA and associated congenital malformations, more than 90 percent of diagnoses were delayed until the development of hematologic abnormalities.[38] The delay in diagnosis in the majority of FA patients with congenital malformations indicates the need for an increased awareness among physicians of the clinical features associated with the syndrome.[11] It has been recognized that the FA phenotype is extremely variable and that congenital malformations in FA may involve any of the major organ systems. FA patients may present with *v*ertebral anomalies, *a*nal atresia, *t*racheoesophageal fistula, and *r*adial (*l*imb), *r*enal, and *c*ardiac abnormalities. These abnormalities constitute the *VATER* or *VACTERL* syndrome; thus there is considerable overlap of FA with these syndromes. Other syndromes with phenotypic overlap with FA include Holt-Oram syndrome, thrombocytopenia absent radius (TAR), Baller-Gerold syndrome, velocardiofacial syndrome, Diamond-Blackfan anemia, and dyskeratosis congenita. Abnormalities of the central nervous system, gastrointestinal system, and skeletal system (in addition to radial ray defects) have been added to the FA phenotype.[11]

Incidence

FA is found in all races and ethnic groups and is widely cited as having a carrier frequency of 1 in 300.[2] This estimate was based on the incidence of affected individuals in New York State in 1971, before recognition of the full spectrum of the FA phenotype. The true gene frequency is likely to be considerably higher than this; a low estimate would result from an incomplete ascertainment of cases before the widespread application of DEB testing for FA diagnosis.[13] Up to 0.5 percent of the general population may be heterozygous for the FA gene. Generally applicable methods for carrier screening are not available, since heterozygotes cannot be detected by the DEB test, and DNA methods for carrier screening are not available for FA complementation groups other than FA-C. The frequency of FA varies among ethnic populations; some have a particularly high incidence because of a founder effect. The heterozygote frequency has been estimated at 1 in 100 in South African Afrikaans and 1 in 89 (specifically for the IVS4 mutation in *FANCC*) in individuals of Ashkenazi Jewish descent.[39,40] The incidence of individuals affected with FA also is high in certain ethnic groups, such as Turkish and Saudi Arabian, in which consanguineous marriages are common.

Variable Expressivity

A recent analysis of congenital malformations among siblings with FA revealed that there is both interfamilial and intrafamilial phenotypic variation in the specific types of congenital malformations among affected siblings.[5] Fifty-three sibships composed of 120 siblings were analyzed. Even the two sets of monozygotic (MZ) twins described in this report were phenotypically discordant. In MZ twin pair 1, the fetuses were examined after pregnancy termination as a result of prenatal diagnosis performed because of the presence of two prior affected siblings in the pedigree. Twin A had a bifid thumb, whereas twin B had no physical stigmata of FA. The proband in this sibship had duodenal atresia, whereas the other affected sibling had no congenital abnormalities. In MZ twin pair 2, 15-year-old girls with FA, twin A had unilateral absence of the radius, bilateral absent thumbs, and an absent right clavicle. Twin B had a bifid right thumb, a hypoplastic left thumb, and an absent left clavicle. However, the analysis showed that the occurrence of malformations among FA siblings is nonrandom; siblings usually were concordant for the presence or absence of multiple congenital malformations. Also, an analysis of hematologic abnormalities in FA demonstrated a concordance in the findings in sibships; the age at detection of hematologic abnormalities in probands and siblings was correlated ($p = 0.006$).[41] To explain the clinical heterogeneity in FA, it has been postulated that the phenotypic features of an affected individual depend on the specific FA mutation, somatic DNA instability, other genes, and environmental factors. Thus FA may be caused by genes that directly or indirectly affect morphogenesis.

DIAGNOSTIC CRITERIA

Crosslinker Hypersensitivity

Diagnosis of FA on the basis of clinical manifestations often is difficult and unreliable owing to the considerable overlap of the FA phenotype with those of a variety of genetic and nongenetic diseases.[42–44] Schroeder *et al.* first suggested the use of spontaneous chromosomal breakage as a cellular market for FA;

Table 17-1 Summary of Major Congenital Malformations Observed in IFAR Patients

Abnormality	All FA Patients (percent)
Radial ray	49.1
Other skeletal	21.6
Renal and urinary tract	33.8
Male genital	19.7
Gastrointestinal	14.3
Heart	13.2
Hearing loss	11.3
Central nervous system	7.7

however, longitudinal studies of chromosome instability in FA patients have shown a wide variation in the frequency of baseline breakage within the same individual, ranging from no breakage to high levels.[6,45] Numerous studies of the sensitivity of FA cells to a variety of DNA crosslinking agents have been performed over the past 27 years.[7,8,12,13,16,46–48] Hypersensitivity of FA cells to the clastogenic (chromosome-breaking) effect of crosslinking agents provides a unique cellular marker for the disorder. Comparative studies have led to the choice of DEB as the agent most widely used for FA diagnosis.[16,49] Extensive experience with the DEB test has demonstrated the sensitivity, specificity, and reproducibility of the results.[13,16] Crosslinker hypersensitivity can be used to identify preanemic patients as well as patients with aplastic anemia or leukemia who may or may not have the physical stigmata associated with FA (Tables 17-1 through 17-6 and Figs. 17-1, 17-2 and 17-3).

Clinical Features

The International Fanconi Anemia Registry. More than 800 cases of FA have been reported in varying detail in the literature, and these cases have been reviewed by Young and Alter.[4] The cases in the literature, particularly those reported before the present decade, were reported when aplastic anemia or leukemia developed in individuals with characteristic physical abnormalities; thus reviews in the literature are biased toward the most severe clinical cases. The literature also contains cases diagnosed on the basis of physical manifestations alone, without confirmation by DEB testing; some of these cases are now known to be misdiagnosed. The International Fanconi Anemia Registry (IFAR) was established at the Rockefeller University in 1982 to collect clinical, genetic, and hematologic information from a large number of FA patients in order to study the full spectrum of clinical features of the disease.[50] The primary source of case material for the IFAR is physician reporting. Once a potential case is identified, an IFAR questionnaire form is completed by the referring physician, and copies of laboratory reports and other patient records are obtained with the consent of the patient or guardian. Diagnosis of FA is confirmed by study of chromosomal

Table 17-2 Radial Ray Abnormalities in IFAR Patients

Bilateral Radial Ray Defect	Unilateral Radial Ray Defect
Absent radii and thumbs	Absent radius and thumb
Absent radius and bilateral thumb abnormality	Hypoplastic radius and thumb abnormality
Hypoplastic radii and bilateral thumb abnormality	Absent thumb
Bilateral absent thumbs	Hypoplastic thumb
Bilateral hypoplastic thumb	Bifid thumb
Unilateral absent thumb, contralateral abnormal thumb	Other
Unilateral hypoplastic thumb, contralateral abnormal thumb	Other

Table 17-3 Other Skeletal Malformations Reported in IFAR Patients

Abnormality	All FA Patients (percent)
Congenital hip	6.6
Vertebral	3.2
Scoliosis	3.2
Rib	3.0
Clubfoot	1.4
Sacral agenesis (hypoplasia)	1.1
Perthes disease	1.1
Sprengel deformity	1.1
Genu valgum	0.8
Leg length discrepancy	0.5
Kyphosis	0.5
Spina bifida	0.3
Navicular aplasia	0.3
Brachydactyly	0.3
Arachnodactyly	0.3
Metacarpal (other than first)	0.3
Craniosynostosis	0.3
Humeral abnormality	0.3
Short toes	0.3
Upper thoracic spine	0.3

Table 17-5 Central Nervous System Abnormalities Reported in IFAR Patients

Abnormality	All FA Patients (percent)
Hydrocephalus or ventriculomegaly	4.6
Absent septum pellucidum, corpus callosum	1.4
Neural tube defect	0.8
Migration defect	0.8
Arnold-Chiari malformation	0.5
Moyamoya	0.5
Single ventricle	0.3

anemia patients tested (81 percent), including short stature, GH insufficiency, hypothyroidism, glucose intolerance, hyperinsulinism and/or overt diabetes mellitus.[52] Significantly, hyperinsulinemia was present in 72 percent of subjects tested and spontaneous overnight growth hormone secretion was abnormal in all patients tested ($n = 13$). The mean height was greater than 2 SD below the reference mean (SDS of -2.33 ± 0.27). Patients in groups FA-A and FA-G were relatively taller than the group as a whole (but still below the mean for the general population), while those in FA-C had a significantly reduced height for age (Table 17-7). Those patients with endocrine dysfunction are more likely to have short stature. These data indicate that short stature is an integral feature of Fanconi anemia, but that superimposed endocrinopathies further impact on growth. The demonstration of abnormal endogenous GH secretion may demonstrate an underlying hypothalamic-pituitary dysfunction that results in poor growth.

Major Congenital Malformations. In a survey of the clinical findings obtained from the IFAR, a number of congenital malformations associated with FA have been described. A review of these data indicated that the FA phenotype is more variable than was previously recognized. Gastrointestinal, central nervous system, and skeletal malformations in FA patients, previously not included as part of the FA phenotype, were observed.[11] Major congenital malformations reported in IFAR patients are summarized in Tables 17-1 through 17-5. This analysis showed that most

breakage induced by DEB or another crosslinking agent. Clinical information from the IFAR has been analyzed for phenotypic features and hematologic abnormalities, and the results have been reported in the literature.[3,11,13,41,51] The purpose of some of these reports was to address the need for earlier diagnosis of FA by increasing the awareness of clinicians of the complete phenotypic spectrum of the syndrome. Currently, there are over 700 patients in the IFAR with a diagnosis of FA confirmed in the United States. Most IFAR patients live in the United States, Canada, or Brazil. Large numbers of subjects and long follow-up make this database unique compared with literature reports. However, there are potential limitations, such as selective reporting and incompleteness and inaccuracy of data reporting. Approximately 10 percent of the patients were examined at the Rockefeller University Hospital or affiliated institutions, which provides a check on the accuracy of data reporting. Summaries of the phenotypic features and hematologic manifestations of FA presented here are taken from the IFAR. Tables 17-1 through 17-6 and Figs. 17-1 through 17-3 show some of the clinical features manifested by the FA patients examined.

Growth Parameters and Endocrine Abnormalities. Endocrinopathies are a common feature of Fanconi anemia, primarily manifesting as glucose/insulin abnormalities, growth hormone (GH) insufficiency and hypothyroidism. In a recent study, endocrine abnormalities were found in 44 of the 54 Fanconi

Table 17-4 Gastrointestinal Malformations Reported in IFAR Patients

Abnormality	All FA Patients (percent)
Anorectal	5.1
Duodenal atresia	4.6
Tracheoesophageal fistula	3.5
Esophageal atresia	1.4
Annular pancreas	1.4
Intestinal malrotation	1.1
Intestinal obstruction	1.1
Duodenal web	0.5
Biliary atresia	0.3
Foregut duplication cyst	0.3

Table 17-6 Minor Anomalies and Mild Malformations Reported in IFAR Patients

Abnormality	Specific Types
Skin pigmentation	Café-au-lait spots, hyperpigmentation, hypopigmentation
Eye	Short palpebral fissures (microphthalmia), almond-shaped palpebral fissures, hypertelorism, hypotelorism, epicanthal folds
Nose	Flattened nasal bridge, nasal pit
Ear, minor	Low set, protruding, minor helix abnormality
Oral cavity	Arched palate, geographic tongue, thin upper lip
Face	Triangular face, facial asymmetry, facial flattening
Neck	Webbing of neck, low hairline
Hand	Thenar hypoplasia, clinodactyly of fifth digit, syndactyly of fingers, hyperextensible thumbs, arachnodactyly, contractures
Foot	Syndactyly of toes, wide space between first and second toes, pes planus, hypoplastic toenails
Prominent forehead	
Other	Sacral dimple, frontal hair upsweep, chest asymmetry, pectus excavatum

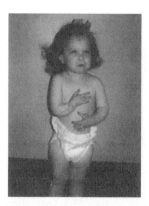

Fig. 17-1 A 2-year-old male of Ashkenazi Jewish ancestry who demonstrates physical features associated with FA. The photograph was taken after surgery on his hands. Before the surgery, the right hand exhibited a hypoplastic radius and absent thumb, whereas the left hand had a hypoplastic thumb. The patient exhibits growth retardation, dysmorphic facial features, microphthalmia, microcephaly, and café-au-lait spots; he also has a kidney abnormality, undescended testes, and a small penis. This patient is homozygous for the IVS4+4 A > T mutation in *FANCC*.

FA patients with congenital malformations are not diagnosed until after the onset of hematologic abnormalities; delayed diagnosis may be due to lack of physician awareness of the phenotypic spectrum of FA. From a developmental standpoint, it is interesting that radial ray abnormalities in FA patients can be bilateral or unilateral (see Table 17-2). Even patients with bilateral abnormalities usually exhibit asymmetry, with their limbs having different specific anomalies[13] (see Table 17-2 and Fig. 17-1).

Minor Malformations. Approximately one-third of FA patients do not manifest congenital malformations[11] (see Fig. 17-2). In these patients the diagnosis of FA generally is made only after a patient presents with clinical symptoms of hematologic dysfunction; the mean age of diagnosis in this group is considerably older than that for FA patients with malformations. FA patients without congenital malformations frequently have alterations in growth parameters, with height, weight, or head circumference below the fifth percentile. Other very common findings in these patients are skin pigmentation abnormalities and/or microphthalmia. Minor anomalies and mild malformations reported among FA patients lacking major malformations are listed in Table 17-6.[51] It is noteworthy that many FA patients have distinctive facial characteristics, including microphthalmia and small facial size (see Fig. 17-3). Increased awareness of the facial anomalies as

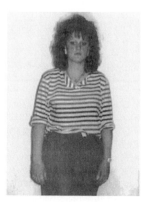

Fig. 17-2 A 17-year-old female with normal phenotypic features. She was diagnosed with FA at age 12 on the basis of hematologic abnormalities and a positive DEB test. She also exhibited short stature and café-au-lait spots. She died at age 21 of AML. This patient is the product of a consanguineous marriage and was homozygous for the Q13X mutation in exon 1 of *FANCC*.

well as the complete spectrum of minor malformations in FA by clinicians should allow an earlier diagnosis to be made in patients without congenital anomalies.

Fertility. Older females have irregular menses, and menopause usually starts during the fourth decade. Fifteen percent of females cited in the literature or reported to the IFAR who reached at least 16 years of age and were not receiving androgen therapy had at least one pregnancy.[4,53] Thus pregnancy can occur in FA, although it often is associated with complications such as progression of bone marrow failure and preeclampsia. Genital malformations and hypoplastic gonads are common findings in males with FA[54] (see Table 17-1). There are extremely few reported cases of affected males having offspring.[55] Results of semen analysis on several males in the IFAR showed abnormal spermatogenesis, with very low sperm counts.

Hematologic Manifestations. An analysis of hematologic data from 388 patients with FA reported to the IFAR showed that hematologic abnormalities were detected in 332 persons at a median age of 7 years (range, birth to 31 years).[41] Actuarial risk of developing a hematologic abnormalities by 40 years of age was 98 percent; actuarial risk of death from hematologic causes was 81 percent by 40 years of age. Initial hematologic findings were diverse; thrombocytopenia associated with an elevated hemoglobin F (HbF) level and macrocytosis usually preceded the onset of anemia or neutropenia. In some cases, patients presented with myelodysplastic syndrome (MDS) or AML without a prior diagnosis of aplastic anemia. Thrombocytopenia and pancytopenia often were associated with decreased bone marrow (BM) cellularity. Actuarial risk of clonal cytogenetic abnormalities during BM failure was 67 percent by 30 years of age. Fifty-nine patients developed MDS and/or AML; actuarial risk of MDS and/or AML by 40 years of age was 52 percent.

In a recent study of genotype-phenotype correlations in FA-C patients, it was shown that the *FANCC* genotype affects clinical outcome and allows division of these patients into three groups: (1) patients with the IVS4 mutation ($n = 26$), (2) patients with at least one exon 14 mutation (R548X or L554P) ($n = 16$), and (3) patients with at least one exon 1 mutation (322delG or Q13X) and no known exon 14 mutation ($n = 17$).[56] Individuals with IVS4 or exon 14 mutations had a significantly earlier onset of hematologic abnormalities and poorer survival compared with exon 1 patients and with the non-FA-C IFAR population. Sixteen of the 59 FA-C patients (27 percent) have developed AML. The incidence of leukemia in each of the FA-C subgroups ranges from 19 to 37 percent. The median age at diagnosis of leukemia is younger in the IVS4 and exon 14 groups compared with the exon 1 group (10.8 and 15.9 years versus 21.9 years). Twenty-eight of the 59 FA-C patients have died. Leukemia was the cause of death in 13 of those 28 (46 percent). Three patients with a history of leukemia have survived; one patient was recently diagnosed, and two are in remission after BM transplantation.

These data indicate an extraordinarily high risk of BM failure and AML in persons with FA and underscore the potential use of FA as a model of BM failure and leukemia development. Recent preliminary data have suggested an increased frequency of *FANCC* sequence variants in children with sporadic AML.[57] Study of a larger series of AML patients and controls, together with analysis of epidemiologic data, is required to substantiate this interesting finding.

Nonhematologic Malignancies. Patients with FA have an increased cancer predisposition. In addition to the extraordinarily high frequency of AML in FA patients (actuarial risk of 52 percent for the development of MDS and/or AML by 40 years of age),[41] FA patients have been reported to exhibit malignancies of a variety of organ systems, most commonly gastrointestinal and gynecologic[4,58] (Table 17-8). The high incidence of nonhematologic malignancy in FA patients is especially striking

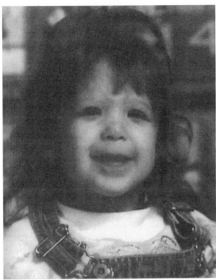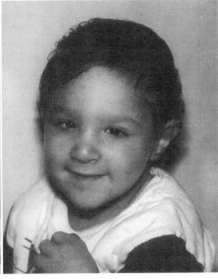

Fig. 17-3 Two unrelated FA patients exhibiting typical facial features of FA. Note microphthalmia and elfinlike facies. These patients are of Ashkenazi Jewish ancestry and are homozygous for the IVS4+4 A>T mutation in FANCC, but similar facial features frequently are seen in genetically diverse FA patients.

because of the predicted early death from hematologic causes associated with the syndrome (median estimated survival is 23 years; actuarial risk of death from hematologic causes is 81 percent by 40 years of age). Thus patients are unusually young when they develop cancer, and the incidence of malignancy probably would be considerably higher if patients had a longer life expectancy. Most of the nonhematologic tumors in FA patients are squamous cell carcinomas. Liver tumors, mostly hepatocellular carcinomas, are also common in FA. Most of these tumors occur in patients who have been treated with androgen therapy for BM failure. Discontinuation of androgens may lead to resolution of the liver tumors.[4]

GENETIC HETEROGENEITY

Complementation Groups

The hypersensitivity of FA cells to crosslinking agents has been used to assess the complementation of the cellular defect in somatic cell hybrids. Successful complementation is considered indicative of the existence of various genes causing FA, as has been performed previously for xeroderma pigmentosum through the analysis of heterokaryons.[59] The most successful approach has involved the use of Epstein-Barr virus-immortalized lymphoblastoid cell lines. Such studies have revealed an extensive degree of genetic heterogeneity. In the first systematic study, lymphoblastoid cell lines from seven unrelated FA patients were investigated.[18] A HPRT-ouab-resistant derivative of one of these cell lines (HSC72) was used as a universal fusion partner in hybridizations with the other cell lines, allowing selective outgrowth of hybrids in culture medium containing hypoxanthine-aminopterin-thymidine (HAT) plus ouabain. MMC sensitivity versus resistance of the hybrids was used as a criterion for complementation. Two groups of cell lines could be distinguished among the seven studied: three that

failed to complement the reference cell line HSC72 in fusion hybrids (termed A) and three that fully complemented the defect (termed B or non-A). The correction of the drug sensitivity phenotype was confirmed by the analysis of both spontaneous and MMC-induced chromosomal breakage.

The three non-A cell lines subsequently were marked with dominant drug resistance markers that were introduced by stable transfection with plasmids conferring hygromycin or neomycin resistance and allowed the selection of fusion hybrids generated from combinations of these cell lines. Since all possible combinations yielded crosslinker-resistant hybrids, each non-A cell line apparently represented a separate complementation group: FA-B, FA-C, and FA-D.[17] This analysis was taken a step further by means of the generation of doubly marked derivatives of the three non-A cell lines and analysis of complementation after fusion with cell lines from another 13 FA patients.[19] All cell lines except one failed to complement only one reference group cell line and therefore could be classified as belonging to an existing group. Mutation screening in four patients who had been assigned to the C group by complementation analysis revealed mutations in *FANCC*, supporting the validity of the complementation analysis. A single cell line (EUFA130) derived from a patient of Turkish ancestry complemented all four existing groups and therefore represented a fifth complementation group, FA-E.[19] Subsequently, group E, defined as "different from groups A-D,"[60] appeared heterogeneous and could be split up into at least four distinct groups, designated FA-E, FA-F, FA-G and FA-H.[20] Recently the sole representative of the eighth FA complementation group (FA-H) was reassigned to group A,

Table 17-8 Nonhematologic Malignancies in FA Patients

Type	Specific Variety	No. (n=800)
Oropharyngeal	Gingiva, tongue, jaw, mandible, pharynx	17
Gastrointestinal	Esophagus, stomach, anus, colon	13
Gynecologic	Vulva, cervix, breast	9
Central nervous system	Medulloblastoma, astrocytoma	5
Other	Skin, renal, bronchial, lymphoma	6

SOURCE: Adapted from Young NS, Alter BP: Clinical features of Fanconi's anemia, in Young NS, Alter BP (eds): *Aplastic Anemia Acquired and Inherited.* Philadelphia, Saunders, 1994, p 275. Eight hundred patients reported in the literature are reviewed. Cancers exclude leukemia and liver tumors. The latter tumors are associated with androgen therapy.

Table 17-7 Height SDS by Complementation Group

	Ht SDS	p-value
Overall	−2.35±0.29	—
FA-A	−1.55±0.45	0.08
FA-C	−3.44±0.86	0.01
FA-C (IVS4)	−4.50±0.88	0.0006
FA-G	−2.01±0.78	0.93

SOURCE: From Wanjrajch et al.[52] Used by permission.

reducing the number of groups and genes from eight to seven.[60a] Complementation group D has recently been shown to be heterogeneous, consisting of at least two genes, *FANCD1* and *FANCD2*, as positional cloning has identified a gene (*FANCD2*) that complements the MMC-sensitivity and was found to be mutated in some (PD20 and VU008), but not other cell lines in group D, including the reference cell line (HSC62).[60b] The localization of group FA-D to chromosome 3p was based on microcell fusion studies with cell line PD20; thus *FANCD2* is on chromosome 3p, while the chromosomal location of *FANCD1* is not yet determined.

One Gene per Group?

Complementation groups usually are considered to represent distinct disease genes. However, in another autosomal recessive chromosomal instability disorder, ataxia-telangiectasia, this assumption has not been borne out, since mutations were found in a single gene (*ATM*) in patients previously assigned to four different complementation groups.[61] For FA, however, at least five complementation groups (A, C, E, F and G) must represent distinct genes on the basis of their separate positions in the human genetic map, while group D represents at least two groups (*FANCD1* and *FANCD2*). The first FA gene isolated by expression cloning methodology (*FANCC*) mapped to chromosome 9q22.3 by *in situ* hybridization, whereas different map positions were established for *FANCA*, *FANCD2*, and *FANCE*, *FANCF*, and *FANCG*. A consortium of investigators used a panel of nine FA families classified as FA-A by complementation analysis to map the *FANCA* locus to 16q24.3.[62] A genomewide search using microsatellite markers led to the initial linkage to D16S520. More refined analysis, including other FA families, led to a lod score of 8.01 at $\theta = 0.00$ to marker D16S305. This finding was independently replicated by the results of a genomewide scan using homozygosity mapping to identify genes causing FA.[63] This study was performed using 23 inbred families from the IFAR. Complementation studies were not performed in these patients, but families known to belong to FA-C were excluded from the family set. Significant genetic heterogeneity ($p = 0.0013$) was shown with marker D16S520 (maximum lod score = 6.08; $\alpha = 0.66$). Simultaneous search analysis suggested several additional chromosomal regions that were not the locations for FA-C and FA-D that could account for a small fraction of FA in the family set, but sample size was insufficient to provide statistical significance. Fine genetic mapping using multipoint linkage analysis with a test of heterogeneity showed $Z_{max} = 27.16$, $\theta = 0.00$, $\alpha = 0.73$ at D16S303, the most telomeric marker on chromosome 16q. The mapping panel for this study included 50 multiplex or consanguineous families from the IFAR selected only on the basis of being non-group C.[64]

Microcell-mediated chromosome transfer was used to map the gene for FA-D (now called FA-D2) to the short arm of chromosome 3, 3p22-26,[65] while cloned genes for groups FA-E, F and G map to chromosomes 6p21.2-21.3, 11p15, and 9p13 respectively. These data suggest that for FA the one group = one gene concept does seem to hold up.[66] Results from the complementation studies thus strongly suggest that at least eight distinct genes (*FANCA* though *FANCG*, and including *FANCD1* and *FANCD2*), when defective, can cause FA. Of these, *FANCB* and *FANCD1* have not yet been identified.

Relative Prevalence of Complementation Groups

Cell fusion studies are a time-consuming and labor-intensive means of determining the genetic subtype of FA patients. Consequently, only a limited number of patients have been analyzed by functional complementation analysis, and the results may well be biased depending on the different ethnic backgrounds of the patients analyzed. The figures reported in a cumulative European-U.S.-Canadian survey based on 47 patients indicate 66 percent to be group A, 4.3 percent to be B, 12.7 percent to be C, 4.3 percent to be D, and 12.7 percent to be E (non-A-D).

Group E now consists of groups E-G. Results of a fine mapping study based on a racially and ethnically diverse mapping panel of 50 non-C IFAR families indicated that 73 percent of these families were in group A.[64] This result is based on the fraction of families showing linkage to marker D16S303, the most telomeric marker on chromosome 16q, which is known be very close to the location of *FANCA* on the physical map.[29] Since approximately 15 percent of IFAR patients are in group C, FA-A accounts for about 62 percent of patients in the IFAR. FA-G is estimated to account for ~10 percent of all IFAR patients. Thus FA-E and FA-F are relatively rare in this registry comprised primarily of patients living in the United States, Canada, and Brazil.[64a]

It is clear that different populations may have widely different pictures. The IVS4+4 A>T splice site mutation in *FANCC* is responsible for most cases of FA in the Ashkenazi Jewish population.[21,22] In a study of over 3000 Jewish individuals, primarily of Ashkenazi descent, the frequency of IVS4 carriers was shown to be 1 in 89.[40] The high carrier frequency of the IVS4 mutation places FA-C in the group of so-called Jewish genetic diseases, which includes Tay-Sachs, Gaucher, and Canavan diseases, among others. With a carrier frequency of more than 1 percent and simple testing available, the IVS4 mutation merits inclusion in the battery of tests routinely provided to the Jewish population. Group C also is relatively prevalent among Dutch patients, mainly exhibiting the exon 1 frameshift 322delG, whereas group A is the prevalent complementation group represented in Italy as well as in the Afrikaans-speaking population of South Africa.[60,62,67] The most frequent pathogenic mutations in *FANCG* found in the IFAR population are: IVS11+1G>C (French-Acadian); IVS8-2A>G (Portuguese-Brazilian); 1794-1803del (Northern European); IVS3+1G>C (Korean/Japanese); and 1184-1194del (Northern European).[64a] Somatic cell hybidization analysis of 21 consecutively sampled patients, mainly from Germany and The Netherlands, found all complementation groups represented. We are virtually ignorant about complementation groups in the relatively large Asian populations, even though FA has been encountered in people of Chinese, Korean, Japanese, and Indian ancestry (Auerbach, unpublished IFAR data). Once the genes for the different complementation groups have been identified, the relative prevalences of the groups in different parts of the world can begin to be estimated through mutation screening methods.

THE BASIC DEFECT IN FA

Defining the basic defect in FA has been complicated by the extensive genetic heterogeneity present in the disease. The bulk of the biochemical literature has been derived from the analysis of unclassified FA cell lines. If the fundamental defect is different in the various complementation groups, this could lead to the inadvertent analysis of two or more basic defects simultaneously. This may explain some of the difficulties encountered by different laboratories in reproducing each other's results. At present, hypotheses to account for the pleiotropic FA phenotype postulate abnormalities in DNA repair, oxygen metabolism, growth factor homeostasis, and cell cycle regulation.[24-26,34]

DNA Repair

FA has been considered a DNA repair disorder in which the defect(s) lie in the repair of DNA crosslinks, thus explaining the increased sensitivity of FA cells to DNA crosslinking agents, hypomutability, and increased frequency of forming deletions.[68-73] Defects in DNA repair would cause abnormal cell replication in hematopoietic, osteogenic, and other cells and would lead to the developmental defects. However, biochemical studies of DNA repair defects in FA cells have been inconclusive or contradictory.[24,25] This may represent the confounding effect of studying cells from different complementation groups or the fact that repair deficiencies may be secondary to the primary (proximate) basic defect. The most convincing evidence for a DNA repair defect is in FA-A, where cell extracts are defective in incising crosslinked DNA and have lower amounts of a protein that binds to interstrand crosslinks.[74,75] In contrast, in FA-C it has been suggested that the defect lies in the initial induction of crosslinks, not in the subsequent repair phase.[76] In a recent study, FA cells exhibited inappropriately elevated levels of homologous recombination activity.[77] Defects in blunt DNA end-joining, which can be corrected by transfection of *FANCC*, have been reported in FA-C.[78] Similarly, defects in double-strand break processing are characteristic of FA-B and FA-D cells.[79] In addition, FA group C and D cells exhibited an elevated frequency of aberrant rearrangements generated during V(D)J recombination, again consistent with excessive degradation of DNA ends during repair of double-strand breaks.[80] Since double-strand breaks are frequently produced during fundamental cellular processess such as replication, repair, and recombination, these studies suggest a mechanism for the elevated chromosomal breakage and deletion proneness in FA.

Oxygen Toxicity

It has been suggested that the FA phenotype may arise from defects in oxygen metabolism.[81] This would explain the sensitivity of the growth of FA cells to ambient oxygen, which is reflected in increased chromosomal aberrations and as accumulation of cells in the G2 phase of the cell cycle.[82–84] The increased sensitivity to oxygen could be due either to increased production of toxic intermediates (e.g., free radicals) or to their decreased removal.[85–87] The sensitivity of FA cells to DNA crosslinking agents may result from aberrant handling of reactive metabolities produced during intracellular activation.[81,88] The increased sensitivity to ambient oxygen also could affect the growth of FA cells *in vivo*, including those in the hematopoietic cell lineages. However, introduction of *FANCC* cDNA into FA-C lymphoblasts does not alter their oxygen sensitivity.[89] This result is consistent with the view that the oxygen sensitivity is a secondary feature of the basic defect, since SV40-transformed FA fibroblasts are not oxygen-sensitive but still retain their hypersensitivity to DNA crosslinkers.[90] The possible involvement of cytochrome P450 in spontaneous and induced chromosomal breaks has been suggested.[91]

Growth Factor Homeostasis

The nearly universal BM failure and the high incidence of congenital malformations in FA patients have led to suggestions that the FA genes function directly in cellular growth and/or differentiation.[26,92,93] Antisense oligonucleotides complementary to FANCC mRNA inhibit the *in vitro* clonal growth of normal erythroid and granulocyte-macrophage progenitor cells, even in the presence of exogenous growth factors.[94] Similarly, peripheral blood CD34+ cells isolated from an FA-C patient and transduced with a recombinant adeno-associated virus containing the FANCC cDNA exhibit a 5- to 10-fold increase in the number of progenitor colonies formed in vitro.[95] FA fibroblasts grow slower and senesce more rapidly than do matched controls and demonstrate ultrastructural and physiological changes characteristic of cells from aged individuals.[9,96,97] The FA gene products may play a role in regulating the levels of growth factors, many of which act in both hematopoiesis and osteogenesis.[98] Addition of interleukin-6 (IL-6) to FA lymphoblast cultures reduces the sensitivity of those cells to MMC and DEB and decreases the number of chromosomal breaks.[99] Increased amounts of tumor necrosis factor-α (TNFα) have been reported in FA cell cultures and in patient serum samples, and anti-TNFα antibodies partially correct the chromosomal fragility of FA cells.[99–101] Recent evidence that double-stranded RNA-dependent protein kinase (PKR) is constitutively activated in FANCC-/-cells suggests that PKR has a role in mediating the hypersensitivity of FA-C cells to TNFα, interferon γ (IFNγ) and to double-stranded RNA.[101a] Since PKR is inducible by both TNFα and IFNγ and also can influence fas activity and

activate caspase 3 and 8, PKR may be involved in the signaling pathway leading to excessive apoptosis in FA cells.

Cell Cycle Regulation/Apoptosis

The basic defect may directly cause the known abnormalities of cell cycle regulation seen in FA cells.[102] More specifically, it has been suggested that FA cells may be defective in apoptosis, or programmed cell death, implicated in the G2 arrest and death of cells treated with DNA crosslinking agents.[103,104] The high variability of the FA phenotype, including lack of concordance between identical twins, suggests that the FA gene products may function in a cellular process such as apoptosis.[5] Such a relationship is also implied by the involvement of apoptosis in hematopoiesis and in embryonic development, i.e., formation of the forelimb, which is abnormal in many FA patients.[105,106] The role of FANCC in apoptosis has been investigated by various groups and is discussed in more detail below.

The primary defects in FA probably involve one (or more) of the previously mentioned biologic systems. The FA gene products could function as separate steps in the same pathway (e.g., growth factor homeostasis) or could be in different pathways (e.g., some in DNA repair and others in oxygen metabolism), or all products could be part of a multiprotein complex involved in one pathway (e.g., DNA repair). Each of these models would be expected to lead to a set of similar phenotypes in the various patients.[107] An intriguing recent observation is the elevation of *MxA*, one of the interferon-inducible genes, in cells of four FA complementation groups and its reduction in complemented FA-C cells.[108] This would suggest that the FA subtypes converge onto a final common pathway related to interferon signaling.

IDENTIFICATION OF THE FA GENES

In view of the difficulties in defining the basic defect in FA through biochemical analysis of FA cells, various groups have attempted to clone the defective genes directly. The first approach used to identify the FA genes involved correcting the MMC sensitivity of FA cells by introducing genomic DNA from normal cells (marker rescue) and then isolating the complementing DNA. This procedure has been used to isolate the normal human version of several mutant genes in ultraviolet (UV)- and MMC-sensitive Chinese hamster ovary (CHO) cells.[59] The genes so identified are called *ERCC* (*e*xcision *r*epair *c*ross-*c*omplementing) and are the human homologues of the mutant *CHO* genes. They show similarities to bacterial and yeast repair genes, suggesting their direct role in similar processes in mammalian cells.[109–111] Several *ERCC* genes were shown subsequently to be equivalent to xeroderma pigmentosum genes.[34,112] With respect to FA, partial complementation of the MMC-sensitive phenotype of both FA-A and FA-D cells using mouse DNA was reported, but these initial studies did not lead to the identification of an FA gene.[114–116] To overcome the disadvantages of the preceding method for the cloning of FA genes, a cDNA expression cloning procedure was adapted and used successfully to initially clone the gene defective in FA-C cells (*FANCC*) and, more recently, *FANCA* and *FANCG*.

Cloning of *FANCC*

The cDNA expression system uses the pREP4 vector, based on the regulatory sequences of the Epstein-Barr virus that allow it to function as an episomal shuttle vector between bacterial and human cells.[117] A cDNA library constructed in pREP4 was used to clone a set of cDNAs that specifically complemented the MMC and DEB sensitivity of FA-C cells.[27] After transfection of the cDNA library into HSC536 (FA-C) cells and selection in MMC and/or DEB, the low-molecular-weight DNA was isolated from populations of growing cells. Eight candidate cDNAs were detected in the various pools and were tested individually for their ability to specifically complement the cellular defect of FA-C

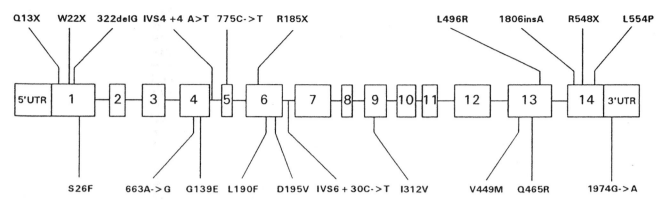

Fig. 17-4 Nucleotide sequence changes in the *FANCC* gene. A schematic diagram of the 14 coding exons of the gene is provided, with the pathogenic mutations shown above and polymorphisms shown below the diagram.[195] (*Data are from Refs. 21, 22, 27, and 195–200.*)

cells. A set of complementing cDNAs was identified that coded for the same predicted ORF. Alternate forms of the cDNA contain three alternative 3′ UTRs, each terminated by a consensus polyadenylation signal, in combination with one of two 5′ UTRs. The 5′ UTRs reflect the presence of alternative transcriptional start sites spliced to a common downstream exon, since they all possess suitable splice donor sites only at the 3′ end.[27,118,119] The murine, rat, and bovine cDNAs also are characterized by multiple 3′ UTRs.[120,121] Their significance is not known. The FA-C cells used in the selection of the FANCC cDNA carry a mutation predicted to produce an L554P substitution that inactivates the cDNA.[27,122] The second mutant allele of this cell line leads to a deletion of 327 bp that eliminates all putative ATG start codons, leading to a nonfunctional transcript.[123] *FANCC* was localized to 9q22.3 by *in situ* hybridization.[17] The mapping of *FANCC* was confirmed by genetic analysis of known FA-C patients.[21,22] Analysis of these patients led to the identification of frameshift, splicing, amino acid substitutions, and chain termination mutations. In some cases (e.g., IVS4+4 A >T) no protein is detected, whereas in others (e.g., L554P) a protein of normal size is seen.[21,22,124,125] Thus a number of protein modifications lead to the FA phenotype, suggesting that all alterations abrogate *FANCC* function. Figure 17-4 summarizes known mutations and polymorphic sequence variations in *FANCC*. Mutations and polymorphisms in *FANCC* are listed in the Fanconi Anemia Mutation Database at *http://www.rockefeller.edu/fanconi/mutate/.*

Features of *FANCC*

The *FANCC* coding region contains 14 exons and leads to a predicted protein of 558 amino acids.[27] The noncoding 5′ exons, now called −1, −1a, and −1b, have suitable splice signals as their 3′ ends but not at their 5′ ends.[27,118,119] The region upstream of exon −1 has promoter activity in transfection assays using a luciferase reporter gene.[119] All 17 exons have been mapped to phages isolated from a genomic library; the minimum size of *FANCC* is 150 kb, since two introns are not completely defined.[126] The 3′ terminal half of the mouse gene was isolated as a step toward the development of the *Fancc^-/-* mouse model; the human and mouse genes are strikingly similar in this region.[127] The mouse ORF shows 79 percent amino acid similarity to the human.[120] The mouse and rat genes have been mapped, the former in close proximity to the flexed-tail locus.[128]

Function of FANCC

The predicted structure of FANCC (and Fancc) does not resemble that of any known protein. The protein is found primarily in the cytoplasm, although approximately 10 percent is in the nucleus.[124,129,130] The predicted ORF codes for a 63-kDa protein (558 amino acids) with a preponderance of hydrophobic amino

acids but no predicted transmembrane domains.[27] No functional motifs have been identified within the protein that could serve as clues to its biologic role.[27] Comparison of the primary sequences of the human, mouse, rat, and bovine proteins does not reveal, apart from putative phosphorylation sites, any obvious regions of higher homology, thus precluding identification of more instructive functional domains.[121] The FA cellular phenotype of increased sensitivity to MMC can be recreated by introducing *FANCC* antisense oligonucleotides into wild-type cells, suggesting that FANCC plays a direct role in protecting cells against the cytotoxic and clastogenic action of this compound.[94]

In vitro transcription and translation of the cDNA produce a protein with an apparent molecular weight of 60 kDa, and a protein of similar size is immunoprecipitated from lymphoblasts or transfected cells using anti-FANCC antibodies.[117,124,129] The predicted protein has no obvious nuclear localization motifs and, as determined by immunofluorescence and subcellular fractionation, appears to be primarily cytoplasmic.[124,129] Targeting of FANCC to the nucleus renders it incapable of correcting the MMC sensitivity of FA-C cells.[76] Immunoprecipitation of FANCC from cell extracts has identified a set of associated cytoplasmic proteins of approximately 70, 50, and 30 kDa.[131] The existence of FANCC-binding proteins is also supported by the fact that overexpression of the L554P mutant protein in normal cells leads to an FA-like phenotype, suggesting that the presence of elevated levels of an inactive mutant protein sequesters other proteins.[125] The 50-kDa protein appears to be an amino truncated form of FANCC that reinitiates at amino acid 55.[23] The molecular chaperone GRP94 binds to FANCC and modulates its intracellular expression.[132]

The cytoplasmic localization of FANCC has led to studies aimed at determining whether the protein has a function in apoptosis. Initial studies have focused on the possible role of FANCC in MMC-mediated apoptosis. Results suggest that FA-C cells may have a generalized defect in apoptosis that is mediated by treatment with MMC or gamma radiation and may involve a failure to induce p53, although conflicting results regarding p53 have been reported.[133–135] Human MO7e and mouse 32D cells expressing FANCC constitutively show a significant delay in cell death compared with the neomycin controls after IL-3 deprivation.[136–138] Thus FANCC appears to play a role in the apoptotic pathway of hematopoietic cells, a role consistent with its cytoplasmic localization as well as its increased expression in hematopoietic precursors. A hypothesis that could explain these observations is that the normal role of FANCC is to modulate the apoptosis that may occur during normal fluctuation of growth factors levels in the marrow microenvironment.[105] More hemopoietic cells will die in FA-C patients than in normal individuals and, with time, will lead to hemopoietic failure. Direct involvement of FANCC in cell cycle regulation has been implied by its direct interaction with a cyclin-dependent kinase (cdc2) which, in turn, regulates G2 progression.[139] However, cell cycle checkpoints do not appear affected in FA-C cells.[140]

Patterns of *FANCC* and *Fancc* Expression

The analysis of gene expression can yield two essential pieces of information about gene function: the sites and levels where the gene functions and the mechanisms that mediate expression. In the case of FA-C, the pleiotropic phenotype of patients and the presence of three putative transcription start sites of the gene point to complex regulation.[27,118,119] Both the human and mouse genes are expressed ubiquitously at low levels in adult tissues.[27,120] Analysis of Fancc expression, using polymerase chain reaction (PCR)-derived cDNA libraries from single hemopoietic cells, shows that higher levels of expression can be detected in less differentiated (multilineage progenitors) than in more differentiated cells (single-lineage progenitors). During mouse embryogenesis, Fancc expression is high in undifferentiated mesenchymal cells 8 to 10 days postconception. Starting at 13 days, expression becomes restricted to regions with rapidly replicating chondro- and osteoprogenitors (e.g., perichondrium), a pattern that persists to later stages (15–19.5 days), except in regions where differentiation has taken place (e.g., hypertrophic chondrocytes of the epiphyseal growth plate). As bone development proceeds, expression is seen in osteogenic and hematopoietic cells in the zone of calcification.[141]

Cloning of *FANCA*

FANCA was cloned by two parallel approaches. One was essentially the same as that used to clone *FANCC*.[27] HSC72 (FA-A) cells were transfected and selected in hygromycin and MMC. A surviving cell population was obtained that exhibited a wild-type level of resistance to MMC and was fully cross-resistant to DEB and *cis*-diamminedichloroplatinum(II). Only one clone was identified that corrected crosslinker hypersensitivity of FA-A cells but not of FA-C cells. Screening of a bacterial artificial chromosome library with the cDNA yielded a positive clone that was used to localize the gene by fluorescence *in situ* hybridization; a signal was observed at the telomere of chromosome 16q, which is the genetic map location established for *FANCA*, thus strengthening the candidacy of this cDNA.[62] To obtain further proof of the identity of the candidate cDNA, cell lines from FA patients classified as FA-A by complementation analysis were screened for mutations in this gene. Various sequence variations were encountered in patients from different ancestral backgrounds; these variations were likely to be pathogenic on the basis of their severity and their segregation with the disease in three informative multiplex families. These data confirmed that the cDNA indeed represented the *FANCA* gene.[28]

The alternative approach used was positional cloning. Subsequent to the mapping of the FA-A locus to 16q24.3, a consortium was established with the objective of cloning the *FANCA* gene as well as a putative breast cancer tumor suppressor gene that maps to the same region of chromosome 16q.[62,63] The candidate region of 16q24.3 was narrowed by further linkage studies and by allelic association analysis. The preliminary physical map of the critical region was developed by screening a gridded chromosome 16 cosmid library with sequence tagged sites and expressed sequence tags. An integrated cosmid contig of about 650 kb was obtained. The cosmids were used for exon trapping and direct selection of cDNAs. Products obtained from the direct selection were used to probe high-density gridded cDNA clones, resulting in the identification of a clone that contained a poly(A) tail and was located at the 3′ end of a candidate gene. An overlapping cDNA clone was then identified; together these two clones gave a combined sequence of 2.3 kb. Exon trapping identified potential additional exons, which were used to extend the sequence by RT-PCR and to screen cDNA libraries for larger clones. One of these was found to be partially deleted in an Italian FA-A patient

and was investigated in more detail as a candidate for the *FANCA* gene. Several additional mutations, all of which would be expected to disrupt the function of the protein, were observed in FA-A patients of various ethnic origins.[29] The sequence of this putative *FANCA* cDNA was found to be virtually identical to the cDNA isolated from an expression library, as described previously.

Features of *FANCA*

FANCA has an open reading frame of 4365 bp predicted to encode a protein of 1455 amino acids (~163 kd).[28,29] The gene contains 43 exons ranging from 34 to 188 bp[142] and spans ~80 kb between microsatellites D16S3026 and D16S303.[29] There are no homologies to any known protein that might suggest a function for FAA. Sequence analysis has identified two overlapping nuclear localization signals, as well as a partial leucine-zipper consensus domain, but neither of these domains has yet been demonstrated to be functional.

Over 70 mutations in *FANCA* have been reported worldwide.[28,29,143–148] These include missense, nonsense, splicing, and frameshift mutations, which are widely distributed over the gene. A large number of the mutations are microdeletions/microinsertions associated with short direct repeats or homonucleotide tracts, a type of mutation thought to be generated by a mechanism of slipped-strand mispairing during DNA replication.[143] The sequence CCTG (CAGG), observed to be a hot spot for homologous recombination leading to mutations in a large number of human genes, is found in the vicinity of some mutations in *FANCA*. In addition, the TTC repeat (MboII restriction site) motif, another hot spot for spontaneous deletions, is also associated with microdeletions/microinsertions in *FANCA*.[143] Very few *FANCA* mutations are shared between affected individuals. The two most common mutations, 3788-3790del and 1115-1118del, are carried on about 5 and 2 percent of *FANCA* alleles, respectively.[143] 3788-3790del, a common mutation demonstrating a founder effect in the Brazilian population, appears in a variety of ethnic groups. The mutation spectrum of *FANCA* also includes a variety of large genomic deletions that are difficult to detect by PCR-based screening methods. The presence of numerous *Alu* repeat elements in *FANCA* suggests that *Alu*-mediated recombination might be an important mechanism for the generation of *FANCA* mutations.[146–148] The heterogeneity of the mutation spectrum and the frequency of intragenic deletions make the molecular diagnosis of FA a formidable task. The assignment of complementation group based on screening of FA patients for mutations in *FANCA* will be much less useful than it was for *FANCC*.[21,40,56] A more practical method for initial identification of FA-A patients may be to use retroviral gene transfer into primary T-lymphocytes or lymphoblastoid cell lines, as recently described.[149–151] The subsequent identification of the specific mutations in a family, a step necessary in order to offer rapid prenatal diagnosis and carrier detection as well as genetic counseling, will offer a significant challenge. Mutations and polymorphisms in *FANCA* are listed in the Fanconi Anemia Mutation Database at *http://www.rockefeller.edu/fanconi/mutate/*. Figure 17-5 summarizes the spectrum of known mutations in *FANCA*.

The presence of sequence-specific hypermutable regions in *FANCA* suggests that *FANCA* may have a higher mutation rate than the genes for the other FA complementation groups, which would explain why FA-A accounts for approximately two-thirds of all FA patients.[143] This also raises the possibility that *FANCA* may be susceptible to increased somatic mutation, which would have implications for FA-A heterozygotes. The FA cellular phenotype of genomic instability predisposes FA cells to malignant transformation and a very high cancer incidence in FA patients. The epidemiologic and molecular implications of the hypothesis of increased somatic mutation in *FANCA* increasing the cancer risk of *FANCA* heterozygotes are currently being tested. So far there is no evidence to implicate a mutated

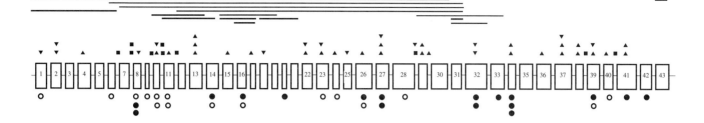

— LARGE DELETION
▲ MICRODELETION / MICROINSERTION
○ POLYMORPHISMS IN THE CODING SEQUENCE
● MISSENSE MUTATION
■ SPLICE SITE ALTERATION
▼ NONSENSE MUTATION

Fig. 17-5 Spectrum of ∼85 mutations in the *FANCA* gene. A schematic diagram of the 43 coding exons of the gene is provided, with large deletions, microdeletions/microinsertions, and nonsense mutations shown above and missense mutations and polymorph- isms in the coding sequence shown below the diagram.[142] (*Data are from Refs. 28, 29, and 143–148.*) Specific mutations and polymorphisms in *FANCA* are listed in the Fanconi Anemia Mutation Database at *http://www.rockefeller.edu/fanconi/mutate/.*

FANCA gene in breast tumors with loss of heterozygosity at 16q24.3.[152]

Cloning of *FANCG*

A cDNA representing the group G gene, *FANCG,* was recently isolated by expression library transfection of a lymphoblast cell line derived from an FA-G patient.[153] The 2.5-kb complementing cDNA insert was identified as human *XRCC9,* a recently described novel gene defined by its capacity to partially cross-complement the MMC-sensitive Chinese hamster mutant.[154,155]

XRCC9 is localized to chromosome band 9p13,[154] a region reported to harbor a non-A,B,C,D FA gene.[156] Proof that this gene indeed represented the *FANCG* gene came from the presence of pathogenic mutations in four unrelated FA patients. Other mutations have since been described.[64a,156a,156b] FA-G is the first proven example of a FA complementation group with a counterpart among experimentally obtained hamster cell mutants selected on the basis of sensitivity to DNA damaging agents. The encoded protein has no sequence similarities to any other known protein, including FANCA and FANCC, has no functional motifs, and has no apparent nonmammalian homologs. Thus, *FANCG* is yet another FA gene with an enigmatic function. The recently described partial nuclear localization of FANCA and FANCC as well as FANCA and FANCG indicates that at least part of the FA pathway is confined to the nucleus.[130,157,157a,157b]

Cloning of *FANCE* and *FANCF*

In the year 2000 two more FA genes were identified by expression cloning, *FANCF* and *FANCE.*[157c,157d] Both encode novel proteins, like the previously found FA genes. The 42 kD FANCF protein had an interesting motif also found in ROM, a double stranded RNA binding protein in prokaryotes. However, disruption by targeted mutagenesis of *FANCF* revealed that the motif was probably not functional as in ROM.[157d] The predicted FANCE protein (60 kD) also lacks significant homologies to other proteins but has two nuclear localization consensus motifs strongly suggesting FANCE to be a nuclear protein. Immunoprecipitation and cell fractionation studies have revealed that FANCA, FANCC, FANCE, FANCF, and FANCG proteins can form a multiprotein complex that functions in the nuclear compartment of the cell.[157e,157f]

Cloning of *FANCD2*

Complementation group D is heterogeneous. Positional cloning has identified a gene (*FANCD2*) that complements the MMC-sensitivity of some (FA-D2), but not other (FA-D1), cell lines in this group.[60b] The gene present in the cell lines that are complemented by *FANCD2* show sequence variations consistent with mutations, whereas no such sequence variations in *FANCD2* have been shown in cell lines that are not complemented. *FANCD2* is different from the other FA genes in that strong homologies are observed to genes in species such as *A. thaliana, C. elegans,* and *D. melanogaster.* Cells from both D subgroups are similar, in that the complex between FANCA, C, F, and G forms normally, unlike the case of cells from the other FA groups. FANCD2 is not posttranslationally modified in the absence of FANCA, B, C, E, F, or G, whereas absence of FANCD1 results in normal modification. This suggests that FANCD1 acts in parallel, or downstream, to FANCD2. Activated FANCD2 protein has been reported to colocalize with the breast cancer susceptibility protein, BRCA1, in synaptonemal complexes of meiotic chromosomes and in ionizing radiation–induced foci.[157g] Other BRCA1-associated proteins in these nuclear foci include tumor suppressors; DNA damage repair proteins MSH2, MSH6, MLH1, ATM, and BLM; and the RAD50-MRE11-NBS1 protein complex.[157h] Thus the association of FANCD2 with BRCA1 in these foci suggests FA proteins may also play a role in maintenance of genomic integrity during the process of DNA replication and repair.

ANIMAL MODELS

FA-C

Mouse models of human disease can be useful in a variety of studies, including the development of novel therapies. Flexed-tailed mice have been considered as possible models for FA-C, since the *f* locus is positioned close to *Fancc.*[128] However, flexed-tail mice do not have an increased sensitivity to MMC.[158] Either the flexed-tail mouse is not mutated at the *Fancc* locus or the mutation is mild. Since no natural mouse mutations in the *Fancc* locus are known, a murine model must be developed experimentally. Homologous recombination in embryonic stem (ES) cells has been used to target the endogenous *Fancc* locus with the consequent removal of exon 8 or exon 9.[159,160] These cells have been used to derive strains of mice (*Fancc[-/-]*) in which no active Fancc protein is produced. The mutant mice show the characteristic FA sensitivity to DNA crosslinking agents but do not demonstrate any morphologic phenotypes or hematopoietic failure to 1 year of age.[161,162]

In addition to the cellular sensitivity to DNA crosslinking agents, the principal phenotype of *Fancc[-/-]* mice is markedly decreased fertility of both male and female animals.[159,160] This phenotype appears to be a more severe version of similar complications seen in FA patients (see "Fertility" above). Male mice have testicular atrophy, degeneration of seminiferous tubules, low numbers of mature sperm, and epithelial sloughing in the epididymis. These results suggest that *Fancc* plays a role in sperm maturation. Females cannot carry embryos beyond days 9 to 10 of gestation. Analysis of a small number of *Fancc⁻/⁻* females shows ovarian hypoplasia and/or abnormal decidua, suggesting that the defect is physiological.

The mild hematologic and morphologic phenotype of *Fancc⁻/⁻* mice perhaps is surprising given the abundant levels of *Fancc* expression during embryogenesis, especially in early mesenchyme and zones of endochondral ossification and in early hematopoietic progenitors. On the other hand, treatment of *Fancc⁻/⁻* mice with chronic, low doses of MMC leads to profound pancytopenia, detected both by a striking acellularity of the marrow cavity and loss of progenitors in *in vitro* assays, and subsequent death.[163] Hematopoietic progenitor cells from *Fancc⁻/⁻* mice are hypersensitive to interferon-γ (IFN-γ)[160,163] as well as TNFα and macrophage inflammatory protein-1α, both with respect to growth and apoptosis.[165] Recently, transgenic mice overexpressing human FANCC were created.[166] Experiments with these *FANCC*-transgenic mice implicate FANCC in the regulation of apoptosis mediated by the Fas death receptor. These various studies suggest a role for *FANCC* in bone marrow homeostasis. Thus these FA-C mouse models promise to be useful in helping us understand the *in vivo* role of *FANCC* as well as in testing new therapies.

FA-A

Fanca-/- mice have now been generated and characterized.[166a] The animals appear viable, have no developmental or hematological abnormalities, but show reduced fertility. Embryonic fibroblasts derived from the Fanca-deficient mice showed spontaneous chromosomal instability and are hypersensitive for the clastogenic effect of mitomycin C, very similar to the phenotype of human FA cells. The deduced mouse Fanca protein shares 81 percent sequence similarity and 66 percent identity with the human protein.[166b] In spite of the species difference the murine Fanca cDNA was fully capable of correcting the defect of human FA-A lymphoblasts.

DIAGNOSIS AND TREATMENT

The DEB Test

The clinical variability in FA is so great that diagnosis must be based on a laboratory test that measures the sensitivity of cells to chromosomal breakage induced by crosslinking agents.[13,16] Comparative studies have led to the choice of DEB as the agent most widely used for FA diagnosis because of reports of false-positive and false-negative diagnoses when other agents are used. It is recommended that patients have a peripheral blood sample tested at birth if they have congenital malformations known to be associated with FA.[11] All siblings of FA patients also should be screened routinely, because a lack of concordance of phenotype in affected siblings makes clinical diagnosis unreliable even within sibships.[5] Peripheral blood is the preferred tissue for the diagnosis of FA, since the sample is easy to obtain and work with and the results of the analysis of crosslinker-induced chromosome breakage can be obtained within 3 to 4 days. Data from DEB testing indicate that there is great variability in the degree of hypersensitivity in FA patients, although there is no overlap with the normal range[13] (Fig. 17-6). Approximately 10 percent of patients with a positive crosslinker test appear to have two populations of lymphocytes; the majority of crosslinker-treated cells examined have no chromosomal breakage, whereas the remainder exhibit the high number of breaks and exchanges typical of FA patients.[13] Interestingly, there is no correlation between the degree of crosslinker hypersensitivity and the presence or absence of birth defects in FA patients.

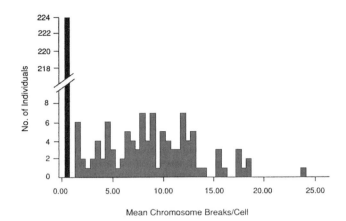

Fig. 17-6 DEB-induced chromosomal breakage in peripheral blood lymphocytes from patients studied at Rockefeller University. Solid bar: 5 DEB-insensitive (non-FA) patients; hatched bars: 5 DEB-sensitive (FA) patients. There is no overlap in the range for the two groups when data are expressed as mean chromosome breaks per cell. Note heterogeneity in the degree of hypersensitivity of FA patients. (*From Auerbach et al.[13] Used by permission.*)

The chromosomal breakage test also can be applied to the study of fetal cells obtained by chorionic villus sampling (CVS), amniocentesis (AFC), or percutaneous umbilical blood sampling (PUBS).[14,15] Prenatal testing for FA in North American pregnancies with a known 1 in 4 recurrence risk (in couples who have had a previously affected child) tested from 1978 through March 1998 are as follows: 80 CVS, 78 AFC, 158 total (28 FA, 130 normal).[167] These results are consistent with the expected ratio. Results from CVS sometimes are uncertain; in these cases it is recommended that PUBS be performed to clarify the diagnosis. The protocols used for both prenatal and postnatal diagnosis of FA using the DEB test are described in detail in *Current Protocols in Human Genetics*.[168]

Hematologic Mosaicism

Two sets of observations suggest that a proportion of FA patients may exhibit hematologic mosaicism. First, two cell types are occasionally detected in chromosomal breakage tests of cross-linker-treated PHA-stimulated peripheral blood lymphocytes, one demonstrating an FA phenotype and the other demonstrating a normal one.[13,169] In addition, lymphoblastoid cell lines derived from FA patients may be DEB/MMC-resistant.[170] Apparently, in a proportion of blood cells from such mosaic patients the disease phenotype has reverted to normal. The origin of such a reversion in an MMC-resistant lymphoblastoid cell line from a female FA-C patient has been determined recently. This patient was compound heterozygous for two frameshift mutations, one in exon 1 (322delG) and the other in exon 14 (1806insA). Because of mitotic recombination in the phenotypically reverted cells, both mutations are now present in the same allele, whereas the other one has lost its mutation.[171] This phenomenon also has been described in lymphoblast lines from patients with Bloom syndrome and has been correlated with a presumed hyperrecombination phenotype of Bloom syndrome cells.[172] Another mechanism demonstrated to give rise somatic mosaicism in FA is the introduction of compensatory mutations. In three cases in which the FA patients were homozygous for dissimilar mutations, a different type of compensatory change in lymphocytes was found in each.[172a] Two of these individuals had frameshift mutations in *FANCA* that were compensated for by downstream mutations. The third case is perhaps the most interesting: A pair of FA siblings, homozygous for the *FANCC* missense mutation 1749G > T, independently developed the same compensatory mutation, 1748C > T. Although a milder phenotype has been suggested in FA patients with somatic mosaicism, subjects with revertant mosaicism frequently develop bone marrow failure and leukemia.[172b] Thus the question remained whether genetic reversion ever occurs in the pluripotent lympho-hematopoietic stem cell. If the reversion occurred not only in lymphocytes but also in hematopoietic stem cells, it would serve as a "natural model"of gene therapy for this disease. In order to identify the cellular origin of the genotypic reversion, each lympho-hematopoietic and stromal cell lineage was examined in an FA patient with a 2815-2816ins19 mutation in *FANCA* and known lymphocyte somatic mosaicism.[172c] DNA extracted from individually plucked peripheral blood T cell colonies and marrow colony-forming unit-granulocyte-macrophage (CFU-GM) and burst-forming unit-erythroid (BFU-E) revealed absence of the maternal *FANCA* exon 29 mutation in 74.0 percent, 80.3 percent and 86.2 percent of colonies, respectively. These data, together with absence of the *FANCA* exon 29 mutation in EBV-transformed B cells and its presence in fibroblasts, indicate that genotypic reversion, most likely due to gene conversion, originated in a lympho-hematopoietic stem cell and not solely in a lymphocyte population. Contrary to a predicted increase in marrow cellularity resulting from reversion in a hematopoietic stem cell, pancytopenia was progressive. Additional evaluations revealed a deletion of 11q21 in 3 of 20 bone marrow metaphase cells. Using interphase fluorescence *in situ* hybridization (FISH) with an MLL gene probe mapped to band 11q23 to identify CFU-GM and BFU-E cells with the 11q21 deletion, the abnormal clone was limited to colonies with the *FANCA* exon 29 mutation. This subsequent development of a clonal cytogenetic abnormality in nonrevertant cells suggests that *ex vivo* correction of hematopoietic stem cells by gene transfer may not be sufficient for providing lifelong stable hematopoiesis in patients with FA.

Treatment

Allogeneic hematopoietic cell transplantation using stem cells from BM or umbilical cord blood currently offers the only proven treatment with the potential possibility for a cure for correcting the BM failure in FA patients as well as a possible cure or prevention of leukemia. Nontransplantation treatment strategies include androgen therapy (most commonly oxymetholone initiated at 2 mg/kg/day, which provides improvement in peripheral blood counts in about 50 percent of FA patients treated.[4] However, even patients who exhibit a good initial response to androgens usually become refractory to this treatment in time and eventually require blood cell and platelet transfusions to maintain adequate peripheral blood counts. Complications of androgen therapy include virilization, acne, liver toxicity, and liver tumors. If either of the latter two complications occur, alternative therapies have to be investigated. Treatment with hematopoietic growth factors may provide improvement in white blood counts but generally does not result in significant improvement in red blood cell or platelet counts.[173–175] Granulocyte colony-stimulating factor (G-CSF) treatment was associated with the occurrence of monosomy 7 in the BM of some patients; long-term administration of this drug requires close monitoring for the development of MDS or leukemia. The use of gene therapy for treatment of FA-C currently is under investigation in a phase I clinical trial at the National Institutes of Health.[177] In this approach, hematopoietic progenitor cells from an FA-C patient are collected by aphoresis, transduced *ex vivo* with an retroviral vector containing a normal *FANCC* cDNA, and reinfused into the patient.[176,178] The aim of this approach is to provide hematopoietic reconstitution with a genetically normalized pool of stem cells. Unfortunately, current methods of targeting retroviral vectors to primitive human stem cells are extremely inefficient.[177] There is no evidence of a long-term cure for any genetic disease achieved by this method; thus it seems unlikely that gene therapy will provide a cure for FA in the near future.

Early experience with BM transplantation for FA showed a poor outcome that was primarily due to regimen-related toxicity; the use of a specially designed pretransplant conditioning protocol that considers the hypersensitivity of FA cells to DNA crosslinking agents including cyclophosphamide greatly improved the results of transplantation in patients with an unaffected HLA-identical sibling available as a donor.[179–182] Recent analysis of 151 HLA-matched sibling transplants for FA from the multicenter International Bone Marrow Registry (IBMTR) and 18 HLA-matched sibling transplants for FA from Cincinnati shows that increased survival is associated with younger age, less severe hematologic disease, and absence of malignant transformation.[183,184] However, only 30 to 40 percent of patients in need of therapy have an HLA-matched family donor. Experience has indicated that many families will pursue future pregnancies in hopes of having a nonaffected HLA-matched sibling to provide a source of hematopoietic stem cells for transplantation.[185] Preimplantation diagnosois of unaffected HLA-matched embryos is also being investigated as an option for families in which the FA mutations are known, but no pregnancies have yet been achieved in FA families using this technology. Although the results of unrelated BM transplants are inferior to those using an HLA-matched sibling, such transplants may be the only option for a patient with severe hematologic disease or evidence of malignant transformation.[151,154]

In vitro studies have shown that there are a sufficient number of stem/progenitor cells in cord blood for hematopoietic reconstitution; this has led to the use of umbilical cord blood as an alternative to in place of BM as a source of transplantable stem cells.[186] To test whether umbilical cord blood from an HLA-identical sibling could be used for transplantation, one would first need to harvest the cord blood at the birth of an individual known to be histocompatible and not affected with hematopoietic disease. Cord blood was used successfully for the first time in a clinical trial in 1988 to treat a patient affected with FA.[187,188] Subsequently, the Placental Blood Program was established at the New York Blood Center in 1992 to test the feasibility of using banked placental blood from unrelated donors for transplantation.[189] Since 1988, there have been an estimated 500 related and unrelated donor umbilical cord blood transplants.[190] The results of phase I clinical trials using both matched and mismatched (up to three mismatched antigens with high-resolution typing) unrelated donor umbilical cord blood from the Placental Blood Program for transplantation have shown that this source of transplantable hematopoietic stem cells has a high probability of donor engraftment and a low risk of severe acute graft-versus-host disease.[191,192] Several FA patients were included in these trials. Since most FA patients do not have a matched sibling or unrelated donor from the National Marrow Donor Program (NMDP) or other international BM donor pools, the availability of an alterative source of stem cells for hematopoietic reconstitution may be a breakthrough in the treatment of FA. Although the results of unrelated hematopoietic stem cell transplants are inferior to those using an HLA-matched sibling, such transplants may be the only option for a patient with severe hematologic disease or evidence of malignant transformation.[183,193,194]

ACKNOWLEDGMENTS

We gratefully acknowledge the contribution of the many physicians who referred patients to the IFAR and the students, fellows, and collaborators who have contributed to research in Fanconi anemia. Most of all we acknowledge the fortitude and commitment of patients with FA and their families for their continuous support of FA research.

Work in the laboratory of ADA was supported in part by grant HL 32987 from the National Institutes of Health, and by General Clinical Research Center grants RR00102 from the National Institutes of Health to the Rockefeller University Hospital and RR-06020 to The New York Hospital-Cornell Medical Center. Work in the laboratory of MB was supported by grants from the Canadian Institutes of Health Research and the National Cancer Institute of Canada. Work in the laboratory of HJ was supported by the Dutch Cancer Society, the Netherlands Organization for Scientific

Research (NWO), the Commission of the European Union (contracts PL 931562, CT 963784), and FARF and FA patient support groups in Europe.

REFERENCES

1. Fanconi G: Familial constitutional panmyelocytopathy, Fanconi's anemia (F.A.): I. Clinical aspects. *Semin Hematol* **4**:233, 1967.
2. Swift M: Fanconi's anemia in the genetics of neoplasia. *Nature* **230**:370, 1971.
3. Auerbach AD, Allen RG: Leukemia and preleukemia in Fanconi anemia patients: A review of the literature and report of the International Fanconi Anemia Registry. *Cancer Genet Cytogenet* **51**:1, 1991.
4. Young NS, Alter BP: Clinical features of Fanconi's anemia, in Young NS, Alter BP (eds): *Aplastic Anemia Acquired and Inherited*. Philadelphia, Saunders, 1994, p 275.
5. Giampietro PF, Verlander PC, Maschan A, Davis JG, Auerbach AD: Fanconi anemia: A model for somatic gene mutation during development. *Am J Med Genet* **52**:36, 1994.
6. Schroeder TM, Anschultz F, Knoff A: Spontane Chromosomenaberrationen bei familiarer Panmyelopathie. *Humangenetik* **1**:194, 1964.
7. Sasaki MS, Tonomura A: A high susceptibility of Fanconi's anemia to chromosome breakage by DNA cross-linking agents. *Cancer Res* **33**:1829, 1973.
8. Auerbach AD, Wolman SR: Susceptibility of Fanconi's anaemia fibroblasts to chromosome damage by carcinogens. *Nature* **261**:494, 1976.
9. Weksberg R, Buchwald B, Sargent P, Thompson MW, Siminovitch L: Specific cellular defects in patients with Fanconi anemia. *J Cell Physiol* **101**:311, 1979.
10. Glanz A, Fraser FC: Spectrum of anomalies in Fanconi anaemia. *J Med Genet* **19**:412, 1982.
11. Giampietro PF, Adler-Brecher B, Verlander PC, Pavlakis SG, Davis JG, Auerbach AD: The need for more accurate and timely diagnosis in Fanconi anemia: A report from the International Fanconi Anemia Registry. *Pediatrics* **91**:1116, 1993.
12. Auerbach AD, Adler B, Chaganti RSK: Prenatal and postnatal diagnosis and carrier detection of Fanconi anemia by a cytogenetic method. *Pediatrics* **67**:128, 1981.
13. Auerbach AD, Rogatko A, Schroeder-Kurth TM: International Fanconi Anemia Registry: Relation of clinical symptoms to diepoxybutane sensitivity. *Blood* **73**:391, 1989.
14. Auerbach AD, Sagi M, Adler B: Fanconi anemia: Prenatal diagnosis in 30 fetuses at risk. *Pediatrics* **76**:794, 1985.
15. Auerbach AD, Zhang M, Ghosh R, Pergament E, Verlinsky Y, Nicholas H, Bot EJ: Clastogen-induced chromosomal breakage as a marker for first trimester prenatal diagnosis of Fanconi anemia. *Hum Genet* **73**:86, 1986.
16. Auerbach AD: Fanconi anemia diagnosis and the diepoxybutane (DEB) test (editorial). *Exp Hematol* **21**:731, 1993.
17. Strathdee CA, Duncan AMV, Buchwald M: Evidence for at least four Fanconi anemia genes including *FACC* on chromosome 9. *Nature Genet* **1**:196, 1992.
18. Buchwald M, Clarke C, Ng J, Duckworth-Rysiecki, Weksberg R: Complementation and gene transfer studies in Fanconi anemia, in Schroeder-Kurth TM, Auerbach AD, Obe G (eds): *Fanconi Anemia: Clinical, Cytogenetic and Experimental Aspects*. Heidelberg, Springer-Verlag, 1989, p 228.
19. Joenje H, Lo Ten Foe, JR, Ostra AB, van Berkel CGM, Rooimans MA, Schroeder-Kurth T, Wagner R-D, et al: Classification of Fanconi anemia patients by complementation analysis: Evidence for a fifth genetic subtype. *Blood* **86**:2156, 1995.
20. Joenje H, Oostra AB, Wijker M, Di Summa F, Van Berkel C, Ebell W, Van Weel M, et al: Evidence for at least eight Fanconi anemia genes. *Am J Hum Genet* **61**:940, 1997.
21. Verlander PC, Lin JD, Udono MU, Zhang Q, Gibson RA, Mathew CG, Auerbach AD: Mutation analysis of the Fanconi anemia gene *FACC*. *Am J Hum Genet* **54**:595, 1994.
22. Whitney MA, Saito H, Jakobs PM, Gibson RA, Moses RE, Grompe MA: A common mutation in the *FACC* gene causes Fanconi anaemia in Ashkenazi-Jewish individuals. *Nature Genet* **4**:202, 1993.
23. Yamashita T, Wu N, Kupfer G, Corless C, Joenje H, Grompe M, D'Andrea AD: The clinical variability of Fanconi anemia (type C) results from expression of an amino terminal truncated Fanconi

24. anemia complementation group C polypeptide with partial activity. *Blood* **87**:4424, 1996.
24. Buchwald M, Moustacchi E: Is Fanconi anemia caused by a defect in the processing of DNA damage? *Mutat Res* **408**:75, 1998.
25. Dos Santos CC, Gavish H, Buchwald M: Fanconi anemia revisited: Old ideas and new advances. *Stem Cell* **12**:142, 1994.
26. Liu JM, Buchwald M, Walsh CE, Young NS: Fanconi anemia and novel strategies for therapy. *Blood* **84**:3995, 1994.
27. Strathdee CA, Gavish H, Shannon W, Buchwald M: Cloning of cDNAs for Fanconi anaemia by functional complementation. *Nature* **356**:763, 1992.
28. Lo Ten Foe, JR, Rooimans MA, Bosnoyan-Collins L, Alon N, Wijker M, Parker L, Lightfoot J, et al: A cDNA for the major Fanconi anemia gene, *FANCA*. *Nature Genet* **14**:320, 1996.
29. The Fanconi Anaemia Breast Cancer Consortium: Positional cloning of the Fanconi anaemia group A gene. *Nature Genet* **14**:324, 1996.
30. Schroeder-Kurth TM, Auerbach AD, Obe G: *Fanconi Anemia: Clinical, Cytogenetic and Experimental Aspects*. Heidelberg, Springer-Verlag, 1989.
31. Joenje H, Mathew C, Gluckman E: Fanconi anemia research: Current status and prospects. *Eur J Cancer* **31A**:268, 1995.
32. D'Andrea A, Grompe M: Molecular biology of Fanconi anemia: Implication for diagnosis and therapy. *Blood* **90**:1725, 1997.
33. D'Apolito M, Zelante L, Savoia A: Molecular basis of Fanconi anemia. *Haematologica* **83**:533, 1998.
34. Auerbach AD, Verlander PC: Disorders of DNA replication and repair. *Curr Opin Pediatr* **9**:600, 1997.
35. Fanconi G: Familääre infantile perniziosaartige Anämie (pernizioses Blutbild und Konstitution). *Jahrb Kinderh* **117**:257, 1927.
36. Estren S, Dameshek W: Familial hypoplastic anemia of childhood: Report of eight cases in two families with beneficial effect of splenectomy in one case. *Am J Dis Child* **73**:671, 1947.
37. Dallapiccola B, Alimena G, Brinchi V, Isacchi G, Gandini E: Absence of chromosome heterogeneity between classical Fanconi's anemia and the Estren Dameshek type. *Cancer Genet Cytogent* **2**:349, 1980.
38. Macdougall LG, Greeff MC, Rosendorff J, Bernstein R: Fanconi anemia in black African children. *Am J Med Genet* **36**:408, 1990.
39. Rosendorff J, Bernstein R, Macdougall L, Jenkins T: Fanconi anemia: Another disease of unusually high prevalence in the Afrikaans population in South Africa. *Am J Med Genet* **2**:793, 1987.
40. Verlander PC, Kaporis A, Liu Q, Zhang Q, Seligsohn U, Auerbach AD: Carrier frequency of the IVS4+4 A >T mutation of the Fanconi anemia gene *FANCC* in the Ashkenazi Jewish population. *Blood* **86**:4034, 1995.
41. Butturini A, Gale RP, Verlander PC, Adler-Brecher B, Gillio AP, Auerbach AD: Hematologic abnormalities in Fanconi anemia: An International Fanconi Anemia Registry study. *Blood* **84**:1650, 1994.
42. Giampietro PF, Auerbach AD, Elias ER, Gutman A, Zellers N, Davis JD: A new recessive syndrome characterized by increased chromosomal breakage and several features which overlap with Fanconi anemia. *Am J Med Genet* **78**:70, 1998.
43. Poole SR, Smith ACM, Hays T, McGavran L, Auerbach AD: Monozygotic twin girls with congenital malformations resembling Fanconi anemia. *Am J Med Genet* **42**:780, 1992.
44. Milner RGD, Khallour KA, Gibson R, Hajianpour A, Matthew CG: A new autosomal recessive anomaly mimicking Fanconi's anemia phenotype. *Arch Dis Child* **68**:101, 1993.
45. Schroder TM, Tilgen D, Kruger J, Vogel F: Formal genetics of Fanconi's anemia. *Hum Genet* **32**:257, 1976.
46. Schuler D, Kiss A, Fabian F: Chromosomal peculiarities and in vitro examinations in Fanconi's anaemia. *Humangenetik* **7**:314, 1969.
47. Cervenka J, Arthur D, Yasis C: Mitomycin C test for diagnostic differentiation of idiopathic aplastic anemia and Fanconi anemia. *Pediatrics* **67**:119, 1981.
48. Poll EHA, Arwert F, Joenje H, Eriksson AW: Cytogenetic toxicity of antitumor platinum compounds in Fanconi's anemia. *Hum Genet* **61**:228, 1982.
49. Schroeder-Kurth TM, Zhu TH, Hong Y, Westphal I: Variation in cellular sensitivities among Fanconi anemia patients, non-Fanconi anemia patients, their parents and siblings, and control probands, in Schroeder-Kurth TM, Auerbach AD, Obe G (eds): *Fanconi Anemia: Clinical, Cytogenetic and Experimental Aspects*. Heidelberg, Springer-Verlag, 1989, p 105.
50. Auerbach AD, Rogatko A, Schroder TM: International Fanconi Anemia Registry (IFAR): First report, in Schroeder TM, Auerbach

AD, Obe G (eds): *Fanconi Anemia, Clinical Cytogenetic and Experimental Aspects.* Heidelberg, Springer-Verlag, 1989, p 3.

51. Giampietro PF, Verlander PC, Davis JG, Auerbach AD: Diagnosis of Fanconi anemia in patients without congenital malformations: An International Fanconi Anemia Registry Study. *Am J Med Genet* **68**:58, 1997.

52. Wajnrajch MP, Gertner JM, Huma Z, Popovic J, Lin K, Verlander PC, Batish SD, Giampietro PF, Davis JG, New MI, Auerbach AD: Evaluation of growth and hormonal status in patients referred to the International Fanconi Anemia Registry. *J Pediatrics* In Press, 2000.

53. Alter BP, Frissora CL, Halperin DS, Freedman MH, Chitkara U, Alvarez E, Lynch L, et al: Fanconi's anemia and pregnancy. *Br J Haematol* **77**:410, 1991.

54. Bargman GJ, Shahidi NT, Gilbert EF, Opitz JM: Studies of malformation syndromes of man: XLVII. Disappearance of spermatogonia in the Fanconi anemia syndrome. *Eur J Pediatr* **125**:162, 1977.

55. Liu JM, Auerbach AD, Young NS: Fanconi anemia presenting unexpectedly in an adult kindred with no dysmorphic features. *Am J Med* **91**:555, 1991.

56. Gillio AP, Verlander PC, Batish SD, Giampietro PF, Auerbach AD: Phenotypic consequences of mutations in the Fanconi anemia *FANCC* gene: An International Fanconi Anemia Registry study. *Blood* **90**:58, 1997.

57. Awan A, Taylor GM, Gokhale DA, Dearden SP, Witt A, Stevens RF, Birch JM, et al: Increased frequency of Fanconi anemia group C genetic variants in children with sporadic acute myeloid leukemia. *Blood* **91**:4813, 1998.

58. Alter BP: Fanconi's anemia and malignancies. *Am J Hematol* **53:99, 1996.**

59. Thompson LH: Properties and applications of human DNA repair genes. *Mutat Res* **247**:213, 1991.

60. Joenje H, for EUFAR: Fanconi anemia complementation groups in Germany and the Netherlands. *Hum Genet* **97**:280, 1996.

60a. Joenje H, Levitus M, Waisfisz Q, D'Andrea AD, Garcia-Higuera I, Pearson T, Van Berkel CGM, et al: Complementation analysis in Fanconi anemia: assignment of the reference FA-H patient to group A. *Am J Hum Genet* **67**:759, 2000.

60b. Timmers C, Taniguchi T, Hejna J, Reifsteck C, Lucas L, Bruun D, Thayer M, et al: Positional cloning of a novel Fanconi anemia gene, *FANCD2. Mol Cell* **7**:241, 2001.

61. Savitsky K, Bar-Shira A, Gilad S, Rotman G, Ziv Y, Vanagaite L, Tagle DA, et al: A single ataxia telangiectasia gene with a product similar to P1-2 kinase. *Science* **268**:1749, 1995.

62. Pronk JC, Gibson RA, Savoia A, Wijker M, Morgan NV, Melchionda S, Ford D, et al: Localisation of the Fanconi anaemia complementation group A gene to chromosome 16q24.3. *Nature Genet* **11**:338, 1995.

63. Gschwend M, Levran O, Kruglyak L, Ranade K, Verlander PC, Shen S, Faure S, et al: A locus for Fanconi anemia on 16q determined by homozygosity of mapping. *Am J Hum Genet* **59**:377, 1996.

64. Levran O, Fann C, Erlich T, Ott J, Auerbach AD: Linkage analysis of Fanconi anemia: Refinement of the FANCA locus at 16q24.3. *Am J Hum Genet* **59**:A225, 1996.

64a. Auerbach AD, Greenbaum J, Batish SD, Giampietro P, Verlander PC: The Fanconi anemia gene *FANCG*: spectrum of mutations and phenotype correlations. *Am J Hum Genet* **65(Suppl)**:A282, 1999.

65. Whitney M, Thayer M, Reifsteck C, Olson S, Smith L, Jakobs PM, Leach R, et al: Microcell mediated chromosome transfer maps the Fanconi anemia group D gene to chromosome 3p. *Nature Genet* **11**:341, 1995.

65a. Timmers CD, Hejna JA, Reifsteck C, Olson SB, Moses RE, Thayer MJ, Grompe M: Positional cloning of the Fanconi anemia complementation group D (*FANCD*) gene. *Am J Hum Genet* **65**(Suppl):A20, 1999.

66. Buchwald M: Complementation groups: One or more per gene? *Nature Genet* **11**:228, 1995.

67. Savoia A, Zatterale A, Del Principe D, Joenje H: Fanconi anemia in Italy: High prevalence of complementation group A in two geographic clusters. *Hum Genet* **97**:599, 1996.

68. Setlow RB: Repair deficient human disorders and cancer. *Nature* **271**:713, 1978.

69. Ishida R, Buchwald M: Susceptibility of Fanconi's anemia lymphoblasts to DNA cross-linking and alkylating agents. *Cancer Res* **42**:4000, 1982.

70. Fujiwara Y, Tatsumi M, Sasaki MS: Cross-link repair in human cells and its possible defect in Fanconi's anemia cells. *J Mol Biol* **113:635, 1977.**

71. Papadopoulo D, Guillouf C, Mohrenweiser H, Moustacchi E: Hypomutability in Fanconi anemia cells is associated with increased deletion frequency at the HPRT locus. *Proc Natl Acad Sci USA* **87**:8383, 1990.

72. Guillouf C, Laquerbe A, Moustacchi E, Papadopoulo D: Mutagenic processing of psoralen monoadducts differ in normal and Fanconi anemia cells. *Mutagenesis* **8**:355, 1993.

73. Laquerbe A, Moustacchi E, Fuscoe JC, Papadopoulo D: The molecular mechanism underlying formation of deletions in Fanconi anemia cells may involve a site-specific recombination. *Proc Natl Acad Sci USA* **92**:831, 1995.

74. Lambert MW, Tsongalis GJ, Lambert WC, Hang B, Parrish DD: Defective DNA endonuclease activities in Fanconi's anemia, complementation group A, cells. *Mutat Res* **273**:57, 1992.

75. Lambert M, Tsongalis G, Lambert W, Parrish D: Correction of the DNA repair defect in Fanconi anemia complementation groups A and D cells. *Biochem Biophys Res Commun* **230**:587, 1997.

76. Youssoufian H: Cytoplasmic localization of FANCC is essential for the correction of a pre-repair defect in Fanconi anemia group C cells. *J Clin Invest* **97**:2003, 1996.

77. Thyagarajan B, Campbell C: Elevated homologous recombination activity in Fanconi anemia fibroblasts. *J Biol Chem* **272**:23328, 1997.

78. Escarceller M, Buchwald M, Singleton BK, Jeggo PA, Jackson SP, Moustacchi E, Papadopoulo D: Fanconi anemia C gene product plays a role in the fidelity of blunt DNA end-joining. *J Mol Biol* **279**:375, 1998.

79. Escarceller M, Rousset S, Moustacchi E, Papadopoulo D: The fidelity of double strand breaks processing is impaired in complementation groups B and D of Fanconi anemia, a genetic instability sydrome. *Somat Cell Mol Genet* **23**:401, 1997.

80. Smith J, Andrau JC, Kallenbach S, Laquerbe A, Doyen N, Papadopoulo D: Abnormal rearrangements associated with V(D)J recombination in Fanconi anemia. *J Mol Biol* **281**:815, 1998.

81. Joenje H, Gille JJP: Oxygen metabolism and chromosomal breakage, in Schroeder-Kurth TM, Auerbach AD, Obe G (eds): *Fanconi Anemia: Clinical, Cytogenetic and Experimental Aspects.* Berlin, Springer-Verlag, 1989, p 174.

82. Schindler D, Hoehn H: Fanconi anemia mutation causes cellular susceptibility to ambient oxygen. *Am J Human Genet* **43**:429, 1988.

83. Joenje H, Arwert F, Eriksson AW, de Koning J, Oostra AB: Oxygen-dependence of chromosomal aberrations in Fanconi's anemia. *Nature* **290**:142, 1981.

84. Poot M, Gross O, Epe B, Pflaum M, Hoehn H: Cell cycle defect in connection with oxygen and iron sensitivity in Fanconi anemia lymphoblastoid cells. *Exp Cell Res* **222**:262, 1996.

85. Korkina LG, Samochatova EV, Maschan AA, Suslova TB, Cheremisina ZP, Afanasev IB: Release of active oxygen radicals by leukocytes of Fanconi anemia patients. *J Leukoc Biol* **52**:357, 1992.

86. Gille JJP, Wortelboer HM, Joenje H: Antioxidant status of Fanconi anemia fibroblasts. *Hum Genet* **77**:28, 1987.

87. Porfirio B, Ambroso G, Giannella G, Isacchi G, Dallapiccola B: Partial correction of chromosome instability in Fanconi anemia by desferrioxamine. *Hum Genet* **83**:49, 1989.

88. Clarke A, Philpott N, Gordon-Smith E, Rutherford T: The sensitivity of Fanconi anemia group C cells to apoptosis induced by mitomycin C is due to oxygen radical generation, not DNA crosslinking. *Br J Hematol* **96**:240, 1997.

89. Joenje H, Youssoufian H, Kruyt FAE, dos Santos CC, Wevrick R, Buchwald M: Expression of the Fanconi anemia gene *FANCC* in human cell lines: Lack of effect of oxygen tension. *Blood Cells Mol Dis* **21**:182, 1995.

90. Saito H, Hammond AT, Moses RE: Hypersensitivity to oxygen is a uniform and secondary defect in Fanconi anemia cells. *Mutat Res* **294**:255, 1993.

91. Ruppitsch W, Meisslitzer C, Hirsh-Kauffmann M, Schweiger M: The role of oxygen metabolism for the pathological phenotype of Fanconi anemia. *Hum Genet* **99**:710, 1997.

92. Chaganti RSK, Houldsworth J: Fanconi anemia: A pleiotropic mutation with multiple cellular and developmental abnormalities. *Ann Genet* **34**:206, 1991.

93. Rosselli F, Sanceau J, Wietzerbin J, Moustacchi E: Abnormal lymphokine production: A novel feature of the genetic disease Fanconi anemia. *Hum Genet* **89**:42, 1992.

94. Segal GM, Magenis RE, Brown M, Keeble W, Smith TD, Heinrich MC, Bagby GC: Repression of Fanconi anemia gene (FACC) inhibits growth of hematopoietic progenitor cells. *J Clin Invest* **94**:846, 1994.

95. Walsh CE, Nienhuis AW, Samuski RJ, Brown MG, Miller JL, Young NS, Liu JM: Phenotypic correction of Fanconi anemia in human hematopoietic cells with a recombinant adeno-associated virus vector. *J Clin Invest* **94**:1440, 1994.

96. Elmore E, Swift M: Growth of cultured cells from patients with Fanconi anemia. *J Cell Physiol* **87**:229, 1975.

97. Willingale-Theune J, Schweiger M, Hirsh-Kauffman M, Meek AE, Paulin-Levasseur M, Traub P: Ultrastructure of Fanconi anemia fibroblasts. *J Cell Sci* **93**:651, 1989.

98. Centrella M, McCarthy TL, Canalis E: Growth factors and cytokines, in Hall BK (ed): *Bone*, vol 4. Boca Raton, FL, CRC Press, 1992.

99. Bagnara GP, Bonsi L, Strippoli P, Ramenghi U, Timeus F, Bonifazi F, Bonafe M, et al: Production of interleukin 6, leukemia inhibitory factor and granulocyte-macrophage colony stimulating factor by peripheral blood mononuclear cells in Fanconi's anemia. *Stem Cells* **11**(suppl 2):137, 1993.

100. Rosselli F, Sanceau J, Gluckman E, Wietzerbin J, Moustacchi E: Abnormal lymphokine production: A novel feature of the genetic disease Fanconi anemia: II. In vitro and in vivo spontaneous production of tumor necrosis factor alpha. *Blood* **84**:1216, 1994.

101. Schultz JC, Shahidi NT: Tumor necrosis factor alpha overproduction in Fanconi's anemia. *Am J Hematol* **42**:196, 1993.

101a. Pang Q, Keeble W, Diaz J, Christianson TA, Fagerlie S, Rathbun K, Faulkner GR, O'Dwyer M, Bagby GC Jr: Role of double-stranded RNA-dependent protein kinase in mediating hypersensitivity of Fanconi anemia complementation group C cells to interferon gamma, tumor necrosis factor-alpha, and double-stranded RNA. *Blood* **97**:1644, 2001.

102. Kubbies M, Schindler D, Hoehn H, Schinzel A, Rabinovitch PS: Endogenous blockage and delay of the chromosome cycle despite normal recruitment and growth phase explain poor proliferation and frequent endomitosis. *Am J Hum Genet* **37**:1022, 1985.

103. Raff MC: Social controls on cell survival and cell death. *Nature* **356**:397, 1992.

104. Sorensen CM, Barry MA, Eastman A: Analysis of events associated with cell cycle arrest at G2 phase and cell death induced by cisplatin. *J Natl Cancer Inst* **82**:749, 1990.

105. Koury MJ: Programmed cell death (apoptosis) in hematopoiesis. *Exp Hematol* **20**:391, 1992.

106. Jiang H, Kocklar DM: Induction of tissue transglutamine and apoptosis by retinoic acid in the limb bud. *Teratology* **46**:333, 1992.

107. Carreau M, Buchwald M: Fanconi's anemia: What have we learned from cloning the genes? *Mol Med Today* **4**:201, 1998.

108. Li Y, Youssoufian H: MxA overexpression reveals a common genetic link in four Fanconi anemia complementation groups. *J Clin Invest* **100**:2873, 1997.

109. van Duim M, de Wit J, Odjik H, Westerveld A, Yasui A, Koken MHM, Hoeijmakers JHJ, Bootsma D: Molecular characterization of the human excision repair gene ERCC-1: cDNA cloning and amino acid homology with the yeast repair gene RAD6. *Proc Natl Acad Sci USA* **88**:8865, 1991.

110. Westerveld A, Hoeijmakers JHJ, van Duin M, de Wit J, Odjik H, Pastink A, Wood RD, Bootsma D: Molecular cloning of a human DNA repair gene. *Nature* **310**:425, 1984.

111. Weber CA, Salazar EP, Stewart SA, Thompson LH: Molecular cloning and biological characterization of a human gene, *ERCC2*, that corrects the nucleotide excision repair defect in CHO UV5 cells. *Mol Cell Biol* **8**:1137, 1988.

112. Wevrick R, Buchwald M: Mammalian DNA-repair genes. *Curr Opin Gen Dev* **3**:470, 1993.

113. Mudgett JS, MacInnes MA: Isolation of the functional human excision repair gene ERCC5 by intercosmid recombination. *Genomics* **8**:623, 1990.

114. Diatloff-Zito C, Rosselli F, Heddle J, Moustacchi E: Partial complementation of the Fanconi anemia defect upon transfection by heterologous DNA. *Hum Genet* **86**:151, 1990.

115. Buchwald M, Clarke C: DNA-mediated transfer of a human gene that confers resistance to mitomycin C. *J Cell Phys* **148**:472, 1991.

116. Diatloff-Zito C, Duchaud E, Viegas-Piquignot E, Fraser D, Moustacchi E: Identification and chromosomal localization of a DNA fragment implicated in the partial correction of the Fanconi anemia group D cellular defect. *Mutat Res* **307**:33, 1994.

117. Groger RK, Morrow DM, Tykocinski ML: Directional antisense and sense cDNA cloning using Epstein-Barr virus episomal expression vectors. *Gene* **81**:285, 1989.

118. Parker L: Analysis of the 5′ end of human *FANCC*. M.Sc. thesis, University of Toronto, 1995.

119. Savoia A, Centra M, Lanzano L, de Cillis GP, Zelante L, Buchwald M: Characterization of the 5′ region of the Fanconi anemia group C gene. *Hum Mol Genet* **4**:1231, 1995.

120. Wevrick R, Clarke CA, Buchwald M: Cloning and analysis of the murine Fanconi anemia group C cDNA. *Hum Mol Genet* **2**:655, 1993.

121. Wong, JCY, Alon N, Buchwald M: Cloning of the bovine and rat Fanconi anemia group C cDNAs. *Mammalian Genome* **8**:522, 1997.

122. Gavish H, dos Santos CC, Buchwald M: Leu554-Pro substitution completely abolishes complementing activity of the Fanconi anemia (FACC) protein. *Hum Mol Genet* **2**:123, 1993.

123. Parker L, dos Santos C, Buchwald M: A mutation (delta 327) in the Fanconi anemia group C gene generates a novel transcript lacking the first two coding exons. *Hum Mutat* Suppl 1:S275, 1998.

124. Yamashita T, Barber DL, Zhu Y, Wu N, D'Andrea AD: The Fanconi anemia polypeptide FACC is localized to the cytoplasm. *Proc Natl Acad Sci USA* **91**:6712, 1994.

125. Youssoufian H, Li Y, Martin ME, Buchwald M: Induction of Fanconi anemia cellular phenotype in human 293 cells by overexpression of a mutant *FANCC* allele. *J Clin Invest* **97**:957, 1996.

126. Savoia A, Centra M, Ianzano L, Zelante Z, Buchwald M: Genomic structure of Fanconi anemia complementation C (*FANCC*) gene polymorphisms. *Mol Cell Probes* **10**:213, 1996.

127. Chen M, Tomkins D, Auerbach W, McKerlie C, Youssoufian H, Liu L, Gan O, Carreau M, Buchwald M: Inactivation of *Fancc* in mice produces inducible chromosomal instability and reduced fertility reminiscent of Fanconi anemia. *Nature Genet* **12**:448, 1996.

128. Wevrick R, Barke JE, Szpirer C, Buchwald M: Mapping of the murine and rat *Facc* genes and assessment of flexed-tail as a candidate mouse homolog of Fanconi anemia group C. *Mammal Gen* **4**:440, 1993.

129. Youssoufian H: Localization of Fanconi anemia C protein to the cytoplasm of mammalian cells. *Proc Natl Acad Sci USA* **91**:7975, 1994.

130. Hoatlin ME, Christianson TA, Keeble WW, Hammond AT, Zhi Y, Heinrich MC, Tower PA, Bagby GC: The Fanconi anemia group C gene product is located both in the nucleus and cytoplasm of human cells. *Blood* **91**:1418, 1998.

131. Youssoufian H, Auerbach AD, Verlander PC, Steimle V, Mach B: Identification of cytosolic proteins that bind to the Fanconi anemia polypeptide FACC in vitro: Evidence of a multimeric complex. *J Biol Chem* **270**:9876, 1995.

132. Hoshino T, Wang J, Devetten MP, Iwata N, Kajigawa S, Wise RJ, Liu JM, Youssoufian H: Molecular chaperone GRP94 binds to the Fanconi anemia group C protein and regulates its intracellular expression *Blood* **91**:4379, 1998.

133. Kruyt FA, Dijkmans LM, van den Berg TK, Joenje H: Fanconi anemia genes act to suppress a cross-linker-inducible p53-independent apoptosis pathway in lymphoblast cell lines. *Blood* **87**:938, 1996.

134. Rosselli F, Ridet A, Soussi T, Duchaud E, Alapetite C, Moustacchi E: p53-dependent pathway of radio-induced apoptosis is altered in Fanconi anemia. *Oncogene* **10**:9, 1995.

135. Kupfer GM, D'Andrea AD: The effect of the Fanconi anemia polypeptide, FANCC, upon p53 induction and G2 checkpoint regulation. *Blood* **88**:1019, 1996.

136. Avanzi GC, Lista P, Giovinazzo B, Miniero R, Sagli G, Benetton G, Coda R, et al: Cattoretti G, Pegoraro L: Selective growth response to IL-3 of a human leukaemic cell line with megakaryoblastic features. *Br J Hematol* **69**:359, 1988.

137. Metcalf D: Multi-CSF-dependent colony formation by cells of a murine hematopoietic cell line: Specificity and action of multi-CSF. *Blood* **65**:357, 1985.

138. Cumming RC, Liu JM, Youssoufian H, Buchwald M: Suppression of apoptosis in hematopoietic factor-dependent cell lines by expression of the FANCC gene. *Blood* **88**:4558, 1996.

139. Kupfer GM, Naf D, Suliman A, Pulsipher M, D'Andrea AD: The Fanconi anemia polypeptide, FANCC, binds to the cyclin-dependent kinase cdc2. *Blood* **90**:1047, 1997.

140. Heinrich MC, Hoatlin ME, Zigler AJ, Silvey KV, Bakke AC, Keeble WW, Zhi Y, et al: DNA cross-linker-induced G2/M arrest in group C Fanconi anemia lymphoblasts reflects normal checkpoint function. *Blood* **91**:275, 1998.

141. Krasnoshtein F, Buchwald M: Development expression of the *Fancc* gene correlates with congenital defects in Fanconi anemia patients. *Hum Mol Genet* **5**:85, 1996.

142. Ianzano L, d'Apolitol M, Centra M, Savino M, Levran O, Auerbach AD, Clenton-Jansen A-M, et al: The genomic organization of the Fanconi anemia group A (*FANCA*) gene. *Genomics* **41**:309, 1997.

143. Levran O, Erlich T, Magdalena N, Gregory JJ, Batish SD, Verlander PC, Auerbach AD: Sequence variation in the Fanconi anemia gene *FANCA*. *Proc Natl Acad Sci USA* **94**:13051, 1997.

144. Levran O, Doggett, NA, Auerbach AD: Identification of *Alu*-mediated deletions in the Fanconi anemia gene *FANCA, Hum Mutat* **12**:145, 1998.

145. Savino M, Ianzano L, Strippoli P, Ramenghi U, Arslanian A, Bagnara GP, Joenje H, et al: Mutations of the Fanconi anemia group A gene (*FANCA*) in Italian patients. *Am J Hum Genet* **61**:1246, 1997.

146. Wijker M, Morgan NV, Herterich S, van Berkel CGM, Tipping AJ, Gross HJ, Gille JJP, et al: Heterogeneous spectrum of mutations in the Fanconi anaemia group A gene. *Eur J Hum Genet* **7**:52, 1999.

147. Centra M, Memeo E, d'Apolito M, Savino M, Ianzano L, Notarangelo A, Liu J, et al: Fine exon-intron structure of the Fanconi anemia group A (*FANCA*) gene and characterization of two genomic deletions. *Genomics* **51**:463, 1998.

148. Morgan NM, Tipping AJ, Joenje H, Mathew CG: High frequency of large Intragenic Deletions in the Fanconi anemia group A gene *Am J Hum Genet* **65**:1330, 1999.

149. Hanenberg H, Batish SD, Vieten L, Verlander PC, Williams D, Auerbach AD: Phenotypic correction of primary T cells from patients with Fanconi anemia with retroviral vectors as a diagnostic tool. (submitted).

150. Fu K-L, Lo Ten Foe JR, Joenje H, Rao KW, Liu JM, Walsh C: Functional correction of Fanconi anemia group A hematopoietic cells by retroviral gene transfer. *Blood* **90**:3293, 1997.

151. Pulsipher M, Kupfer GM, Naf D, Suliman A, Lee JS, Jakobs P, Grompe M, et al: Subtyping analysis of Fanconi anemia by immunoblotting and retroviral gene transfer. *Mol Med* **4**:468, 1998.

152. Cleton-Jansen A-M, Moerland EW, Pronk JC, van Berkel C, Apostolou S, Crawford J, Savoia A, Auerbach AD, et al: Mutation analysis of the Fanconi anaemia A gene in breast tumors with loss of heterozygosity at 16q24.3. *Br J Cancer* **79**:1049, 1999.

153. De Winter JP, Waisfisz Q, Rooimans MA, Van Berkel CGM, Bosnoyan-Collins L, Alon N, Carreau M, et al: The Fanconi anemia group G gene is identical with human *XRCC9*. *Nature Genet* **20**:281, 1998.

154. Liu N, Lamerdin JE, Tucker JD, Zhou Z-Q, Walter CA, Albala JS, Busch DB, Thompson LH: The human XRCC9 gene corrects chromosomal instability and mutagen sensitivities in CHO UV40 cells. *Proc Natl Acad Sci USA* **94**:9232, 1997.

155. Busch DB, Zdzienicka MZ, Natarajan AT, Jones NJ, Overkamp WJI, Collins A, Mitchell DL, et al: A CHO mutant, UV40, that is sensitive to diverse mutagens and represents a new complementation group of mitomycin C sensitivity. *Mutat Res* **363**:209, 1996.

156. Saar K, Schindler D, Wegner R-D, Reis A, Wienker F, Hoehn H, Joenje H, et al: Localisation of a Fanconi anaemia gene to chromosome 9p. *Eur J Hum Genet* **6**:501, 1998.

156a. Yamada T, Tachibana A, Shimizu T, Mugishima H, Okubo M, Sasaki MS: Novel mutations of the *FANCG* gene causing alternative splicing in Japanese Fanconi anemia. *J Hum Genet* **45**:159, 2000.

156b. Demuth I, Wlodarski M, Tipping AJ, Morgan NV, de Winter JP, Thiel M, Gräsl S, et al: Spectrum of mutations in the Fanconi anaemia group G gene, FANCG/XRCC9. *Eur J Hum Genet* **8**:861, 2000.

157. Kupfer GM, Naf D, Suliman A, Pulsipher M, D'Andrea AD: The Fanconi anemia proteins, FANCA and FANCC, interact to form a nuclear complex. *Nature Genet* **17**:487, 1997.

157a. Waisfisz Q, de Winter JP, Kruyt FA, de Groot J, van der Weel L, Dijkmans LM, Zhi Y, Arwert F, Scheper RJ, Youssoufian H, Hoatlin ME, Joenje H: A physical complex of the Fanconi anemia proteins FANCG/XRCC9 and FANCA. *Proc Natl Acad Sci (USA)* **96**:10320, 1999.

157b. Garcia-Higuera I, Kuang Y, Denham J, D'Andrea AD: The Fanconi anemia proteins FANCA and FANCG stabilize each other and promote the nuclear accumulation of the Fanconi anemia complex. *Blood* **96**:3224, 2000.

157c. De Winter JP, Rooimans MA, Van der Weel L, Van Berkel CGM, Alon N, Bosnoyan-Collins L, De Groot J, et al: The Fanconi anaemia gene FANCF encodes a novel protein with homology to ROM. *Nature Genet* **24**:15, 2000.

157d. De Winter JP, Léveillé F, Van Berkel CGM, Rooimans MA, Van der Weel L, Steltenpool J, Demuth I, et al: Isolation of a cDNA representing the Fanconi anemia complementation group E gene. *Am J Hum Genet* **67**:1306, 2000.

157e. De Winter JP, Van der Weel L, De Groot J, Stone S, Waisfisz Q, Arwert F, Scheper RJ, et al: The Fanconi anemia protein FANCF forms a nuclear complex with FANCA, FANCC and FANCG. *Hum Mol Genet* **9**:2665, 2000.

157f. Medhurst AL, Huber PAJ, Waisfisz Q, de Winter JP, Mathew CG: Direct interactions of the five known Fanconi anaemia proteins suggest a common functional pathway. *Hum Molec Genet* **10**:423, 2001

157g. Garcia-Higuera I, Taniguchi T, Ganesan S, Meyn MS, Timmers C, Hejna J, Grompe M, D'Andrea AD: Interaction of the Fanconi anemia proteins and BRCA1 in a common pathway. *Mol Cell* **7**:249, 2001.

157h. Wang Y, Cortez D, Yazdi P, Neff N, Elledge SJ, Qin J: BASC, a super complex of BRCA1-associated proteins involved in the recognition and repair of aberrant DNA structures. *Genes & Development* **14**:927, 2000.

158. Urlando C, Krasnoshtein F, Heddle JA, Buchwald M: Assessment of the flexed-tail mouse as a possible model for Fanconi anemia: Analysis of mitomycin C-induced micronuclei. *Mutat Res* **370**:99, 1996.

159. Chen M, Tomkins D, Auerbach W, McKerlie C, Youssoufian H, Liu L, Gan O, et al: Inactivation of *Fancc* in mice produces inducible chromosomal instability and reduced fertility reminiscent of Fanconi anemia. *Nature Genet* **12**:448, 1996.

160. Whitney MA, Royle G, Low MJ, Kelly MA, Axthelm MK, Reifsteck C, Olson S, et al: Germ cell defects and hematopoietic hypersensitivity to gamma-interferon in mice with a targeted disruption of the Fanconi anemia C gene. *Blood* **88**:49, 1996.

161. Otsuki T, Wang J, Demuth I, Digweed M, Liu J: Assessment of mitomycin C sensitivity in Fanconi anemia complementation group C gene (Fac) knock-out mouse cells. *Int J Hematol* **67**:243, 1998.

162. Tomkins DJ, Care M, Carreau M, Buchwald M: Development and characterization of immortalized fibroblastoid cell lines from an FA(C) mouse model. *Mutat Res* **408**:27, 1998.

163. Carreau M, Gan O, Liu L, Doedens M, McKerlie C, Dick JE, Buchwald M: FAC regulates regeneration of early and commited hematopoietic progenitors after DNA damage. *Blood* **91**:2737, 1998.

164. Rathbun RK, Faulkner GR, Ostroski MH, Christianson TA, Hughes G, Jones G, Cahn R, et al: Inactivation of the Fanconi anemia group C gene augments interferon-gamma-induced apoptotic responses in hematopoietic cells. *Blood* **90**:974, 1997.

165. Haneline LS, Broxmeyer HE, Cooper S, Hangoc G, Carreau M, Buchwald M, Clapp WC: Multiple inhibitory cytokines induce deregulated progenitor growth and apoptosis in hematopoietic cells from *Fancc*-/- mice. *Blood* **91**:4092, 1998.

166. Wang J, Otsuki T, Youssoufian H, Lo Ten Foe J, Kim S, Devetten M, Yu J, et al: Overexpression of the Fanconi anemia group C gene (FAC) protects hematopoietic progenitors from death induced by Fas-mediated apoptosis. *Cancer Res* **58**:3538, 1998.

166a. Cheng NC, Van de Vrugt HJ, Van der Valk MA, Oostra AB, Krimpenfort P, De Vries Y, Joenje H, Berns A, Arwert F: Mice with a targeted disruption of the Fanconi anemia homolog Fanca. *Hum Mol Genet* **9**:1805, 2000.

166b. Van de Vrugt HJ, Cheng NC, de Vries Y, Rooimans MA, De Groot J, Scheper RJ, Zhi Y, et al: Cloning and characterization of murine Fanconi anemia group A gene: Fanca protein is expressed in lymphoid tissues, testis, and ovary. *Mammalian Genome* **11**: 326–331, 2000.

167. Auerbach AD: Prenatal diagnosis of Fanconi anemia, in New MI (ed.): *Proceedings of the Diagnosis and Treatment of the Unborn Child Conference* Italy, Idelson Publishing Company, 1998 p 27–35.

168. Auerbach AD: Diagnosis of Fanconi anemia by diepoxybutane analysis, in Dracopoli NC, Haines JL, Korf BR, Moir DT, Morton CC, Seidman CE, Seidman JG, Smith DR (eds): *Current Protocols in Human Genetics.* New York, Current Protocols, 1994, p 8.7.1.

169. Kwee ML, Poll EHA, van de Kamp JJP, De Koning H, Eriksson AW, Joenje H: Unusual response to bifunctional alkylating agent in a case of Fanconi anemia. *Hum Genet* **64**:384, 1983.

170. Auerbach AD, Koorse RE, Ghosh R, Venkatraj VS, Zhang M, Chiorazzi N: Complementation studies in Fanconi anemia, in Schroder TM, Auerbach AD, Obe G (eds): *Fanconi Anemia, Clinical, Cytogenetic and Experimental Aspects.* Heidelberg, Springer-Verlag, 1989, p 213.

171. Lo Ten Foe JR, Kwee ML, Rooimans, MA, Oostra AB, Veerman AJP, Pauli RM, Shahidi NT, et al: Somatic mosaicism Fanconi anemia: molecular basis and clinical significance. *Eur J Hum Genet* **5**:137, 1997.

172. Ellis NA, Lennon DJ, Proytcheva M, Alhadeff B, Henderson EE, German J: Somatic intragenic recombination within the mutated locus BLM can correct the high sister-chromatid exchange phenotype of Bloom syndrome cells. *Am J Hum Genet* **57**:994, 1995.

172a. Waisfisz Q, Morgan NV, Savino M, de Winter JP, van Berkel CG, Hoatlin ME, Ianzano L, et al: Spontaneous functional correction of homozygous Fanconi anaemia alleles reveals novel mechanistic basis for reverse mosaicism. *Nat Genet* **22**:379–383, 1999.

172b. MacMillan ML, Auerbach AD, Davies SM, DeFor TE, Gillio A, Giller R, Harris R, et al: Hematopoietic cell transplantation in patients with Fanconi anemia using non-genotypically identical donors: results of a TBI dose escalation trial. *Brit J Haematol* **109**:121, 2000.

172c. Gregory JJ, Wagner JE, Verlander PC, Levran O, Batish SD, Eide C, Steffenhagen A, Hirsch B, Auerbach AD: Somatic mosaicism in Fanconi anemia: evidence of genotypic reversion in lympho-hematopoietic stem cells. *Proc Natl Acad Sci (USA)* **98**:2532, 2001.

173. Rackoff WR, Orazi A, Robinson CA, et al: Prolonged administration of granulocyte colony-stimulating factor (Filgrastim) to patients with Fanconi anemia: A pilot study. *Blood* **88**:1588, 1996.

174. Guinan EC, Lopez KD, Huhn RD, Felser JM, Nathan DG: Evaluation of granulocyte-macrophage colony-stimulating factor for treatment of pancytopenia in children with Fanconi anemia. *Pediatrics* **124**:144, 1994.

175. Scagni P, Saracco P, Timeus F, Farinasso L, Dall'Aglio M, Bosa EM, Crescenzio N, et al: Use of recombinant granulocyte colony-stimulating factor in Fanconi's anemia. *Haematologica* **83**:432, 1998.

176. Walsh CE, Grompe M, Vanin E, Buchwald M, Young NS, Nienhuis AW, Liu JM: A functionally active retrovirus vector for gene therapy in Fanconi anemia group C. *Blood* **84**:453, 1994.

177. Walsh CE, Mann MM, Emmons RVB, Wang S, Liu JM: Transduction of CD34-enriched human peripheral and umbilical cord blood progenitors using a retroviral vector with the Fanconi anemia group C gene. *J Invest Med* **43**:379, 1995.

178. Liu JM: Gene transfer for the eventual treatment of Fanconi's anemia. *Semin Hematol* **35**:168, 1998.

179. Gluckman E, Devergie A, Schaison G, Bussel A, Berger R, Sohier J, Bernard J: Bone marrow transplantation in Fanconi anemia. *Br J Haematol* **45**:557, 1980.

180. Berger R, Bernheim A, Gluckman E, Gisselbrecht C: In vitro effect of cyclophosphamide metabolites on chromosomes of Fanconi anaemia patients. *Br J Haematol* **45**:565, 1980.

181. Auerbach AD, Adler B, O'Reilly RJ, Kirkpatrick D, Chaganti RSK: Effect of procarbazine and cyclophosphamide on chromosome breakage in Fanconi anemia cells: Relevance to bone marrow transplantation. *Cancer Genet Cytogent* **9**:25, 1983.

182. Gluckman E, Devergie A, Dutreix J: Bone marrow transplantation for Fanconi's anemia, in Schroder-Kurth TM, Auerbach AD, Obe G (eds): *Fanconi Anemia: Clinical, Cytogenetic and Experimental Aspects.* Berlin, Springer-Verlag, 1989, p 60.

183. Gluckman E, Auerbach AD, Horowitz MM, Sobocinski KA, Ash RC, Bortin MM, Butturini A, et al: Bone marrow transplantation for Fanconi anemia. *Blood* **86**:2856, 1995.

184. Kohli-Kumar M, Morris C, DeLaat C, Sambrano J, Masterson M, Mueller R, Shahidi NT, et al: Bone marrow transplantation in Fanconi anemia using matched sibling donors. *Blood* **94**:2050, 1994.

185. Auerbach AD: Umbilical cord blood transplants for genetic disease: Diagnostic and ethical issues in fetal studies. *Blood Cells* **20**:303, 1994.

186. Broxmeyer HE, Douglas GW, Hangoc G, Cooper S, Bard J, English D, Arny M, Boyse EA: Human umbilical cord blood as a potential source of transplantable hematopoietic stem/progenitor cells. *Proc Natl Acad Sci USA* **86**:3828, 1989.

187. Gluckman E, Broxmeyer HE, Auerbach AD, Friedman HS, Douglas GW, Devergie A, Esperou H, et al: Hematopoietic reconstitution in a patient with Fanconi's anemia by means of umbilical-cord blood from an HLA-identical sibling. *N Engl J Med* **321**:1174, 1989.

188. Kohli-Kumar M, Harris RE, Broxmeyer HE, Shahidi N, Auerbach AD, Harris RE: Cord blood transplant in Fanconi anemia. *Br J Haematol* **85**:419, 1993.

189. Rubinstein P, Rosenfield RE, Adamson JW, Stevens CE: Stored placental blood for unrelated bone marrow reconstitution. *Blood* **81**:1679, 1993.

190. Cairo MS, Wagner JE: Placental and/or umbilical cord blood: An alternative source of hematopoietic stem cells for transplantation. *Blood* **90**:4665, 1997.

191. Kurtzberg J, Laughlin M, Graham ML, Smith C, Olson JF, Halperin E, Ciocci G, Carrier C, Stevens CE, Rubinstein P: Placental blood as a source for hematopoietic stem cells for transplantation into unrelated recipients. *N Engl J Med* **335**:157, 1996.

192. Wagner JE, Rosenthal J, Sweetman R, Shu XO, Davies SM, Ramsay NKC, McGlave PB, Sender L, Cairo MS: Successful transplantation of HLA-matched and HLA-mismatched umbilical cord blood from unrelated donors: Analysis of engraftment and acute graft-versus-host disease. *Blood* **88**:795, 1996.

193. Davies SM, Kahn S, Wagner JE, Arthur DC, Auerbach AD, Ramsay NKC, Weisdorf DJ: Unrelated donor bone marrow transplantation for Fanconi anemia. *Bone Marrow Transplant* **17**:43, 1996.

194. Wagner JE, Davies SM, Auerbach AD: Hematopoietic cell transplant in the treatment of Fancoini anemia, in Forman SJ, Blume KG, Thomas, ED (eds), *Hematopoietic Cell Transplantation*, 2d ed. Malden, MA, Blackwell Science, 1998.

195. Gibson RA, Buchwald M, Roberts RG, Mathew CG: Characterization of the exon structure of the Fanconi anemia group C gene by vectorette PCR. *Hum Mol Genet* **2**:35, 1993.

196. Gibson RA, Hajianpoujr A, Murer-Orlando M, Buchwald M, Mathew CG: A nonsense mutation and exon skipping in the Fanconi anemia group C gene. *Hum Mol Genet* **2**:797, 1993.

197. Gibson RA, Morgan NV, Goldstein LH, Pearson IC, Kesterton IP, Foot NJ, Jansen S, et al: Novel mutations and polymorphisms in the Fanconi anemia group C gene. *Hum Mutat* **8**:140, 1996.

198. Lo Ten Foe JR, Rooimans MA, Joenje H, Arwert F: A novel frameshift mutation (1806insA) in exon 14 of the Fanconi anemia C gene, FAC. *Hum Mutat* **7**:264, 1996.

199. Lo Ten Foe JR, Barel MT, Tuss P, Digweed M, Arwert F, Joenje H: Sequence variations in the Fanconi anaemia gene, FAC: pathogenicity of 1806insA and R548X and recognition of D195V as a polymorphic variant. *Hum Genet* **98**:522, 1996.

200. Lo Ten Foe JR, Kruyt FAC, Zweekhorst MBM, Pals G, Gibson RA, Mathew CG, Joenje H, Arwert F: Exon 6 skipping in the Fanconi anemia C gene associated with a nonsense/missense mutation (775C > T) in exon 5. *Hum Mutat* Suppl. 1:S25, 1998.

CHAPTER 18

Hereditary Nonpolyposis Colorectal Cancer (HNPCC)

C. Richard Boland

Colorectal cancer is a fairly common disease of Western populations with a typical onset at about age 70 years. The international epidemiology of this disease suggests that environmental factors, probably dietary, are the most important influences for the high prevalence of this disease in certain countries.[1] Woven into the epidemiologic fabric for colorectal cancer is an important influence of genetic factors. Individuals who have even one first-degree relative with colorectal neoplasia (i.e., either cancers or adenomatous polyps) have an increased risk for these tumors themselves, which will appear earlier in life.[2-4] The familial risk increases when there is more than one family member involved or cancers occur before age 50.[3,4]

The most readily distinguished form of familial risk is the autosomal dominant genetic disease familial adenomatous polyposis (FAP). This disease has a distinctive phenotypic syndrome characterized by a large number of precursor adenomatous polyps in the colon and occurs in about 1 in 10,000 births. This is completely unrelated to the more common autosomal dominant colon cancer syndrome termed *hereditary nonpolyposis colorectal cancer* (HNPCC). HNPCC is due to an inactivating germ-line mutation in one of the DNA mismatch repair (MMR) genes (see below). This disease has no antecedent clinical phenotype until a cancer develops and was a controversial entity until the biologic basis of this disease was discovered in 1993.[5-8] Patients with HNPCC are at increased risk for cancers of the colon, endometrium, small intestine, ovary, stomach, urinary tract, brain, and some other, but not all, epithelial organs.[9-12] The mean age to develop colorectal cancer is in the early to mid-40's; however, many tumors occur in the 20's and even in teenagers. Although population-based surveys have not been completed, HNPCC may be the most common form of familial predisposition to cancer.[13-22] Now that the genetic basis of this disease has been elucidated, and the involvement of non-colonic cancers clearly demonstrated, it may be advised to refer to the disease as "Lynch syndrome" when a germ-line mutation in a DNA MMR gene has been identified in a family, and use "HNPCC" for familial clusters of colon cancer without an identifiable germ-line mutation,

FAMILY HISTORY AND COLORECTAL CANCER

The hereditary aspects of colon cancer are complex. The age-adjusted relative risk of developing colorectal cancer in individuals with one affected first-degree relative is 1.72 compared with those without such a family history. This risk rises to 2.75 when there are two or more affected first-degree relatives, and the relative risk increases as the family history occurs in younger relatives,

reaching 5.37 when the affected siblings are between 30 and 44 years of age.[3] Similarly, the relative risk for colorectal cancer is 1.78 for the first-degree relatives of patients with adenomatous polyps. The relative risk of cancer rises to 2.59 when the sibling is less than 60 years old and 3.25 when a sibling and parent are both affected.[4] This modest increase in risk, which worsens with increasing familial involvement and earlier age tumors, cannot be attributed solely to HNPCC. In all likelihood, several genetic risk factors play a partial role, as do dietary and other environmental influences. The challenge in defining HNPCC families has been to recognize the disease in the face of a large background incidence of colorectal cancer and the occasional clusters of sporadic tumors in families.

THE HISTORY OF HNPCC

The historical roots of HNPCC can be traced back to the end of the nineteenth century when a University of Michigan pathologist, A. S. Warthin, recognized a cluster of cancers in the family of his seamstress.[23,24] His patient's family was large and has been reported five times during the twentieth century, serving as the prototype for HNPCC.[25-29] Following this lead, Lynch documented family histories on this and other families, and by the 1970s, it became clear that the medical histories of several large families strongly suggested the involvement of an autosomal dominant disease that gave rise to early-onset cancers with a predisposition for proximal colonic involvement and cancers in certain other organs.[29-32]

Prior to identification of the genes for this disease, ascertainment was limited by the need for large families with a high degree of involvement. Two different subsets of families were identified. *Lynch syndrome I* (or *site-specific familial colorectal cancer*) was attached to those families which only manifested colorectal cancers. *Lynch syndrome II* (or *cancer family syndrome*) was assigned to families that also had tumors of other organs, principally of the female genital tract.[31] Over time, it has emerged that these are not distinct syndromes, but there may be specific mutations that predispose to cancers at extracolonic sites. In fact, one common mutation in *hMLH1* has been reported to result in a reduced frequency of extracolonic tumors.[33]

To cope with the uncertainties surrounding HNPCC, the International Collaborative Group on Hereditary Non-Polyposis Colorectal Cancer convened in 1991 to develop clinical criteria to standardize the study of this disease.[34] The "Amsterdam criteria" are listed in Table 18-1 but appear to be overly restrictive and do not take into account the possibility of later-onset variants, the implications of noncolonic tumors, or the limitations imposed by small family size or incomplete data recovery. Not all HNPCC families, diagnosed genetically, meet the Amsterdam criteria.

HNPCC has attracted interest not only because of its impact in clinical medicine; the genetic basis of this disease has led to the understanding of a unique pathogenetic mechanism for tumor

---

A list of standard abbreviations is located immediately preceding the index. Nonstandard abbreviations used in this chapter include: FAP = familial adenomatous polyposis; HNPCC = hereditary nonpolyposis colorectal cancer; MMR = mismatch repair; MSI = microsatellite instability; RER = replicative error; MSS = microsatellite stable.

Table 18-1 Amsterdam Criteria for HNPCC

1. At least three affected relatives with verified colorectal cancer
2. At least one is a first-degree relative of the other two
3. FAP is excluded
4. At least two successive generations affected
5. One colon cancer at < 50 years of age

development. The history surrounding the identification of the HNPCC genes and the unique type of genomic instability associated with these tumors has been reviewed in detail elsewhere.[24,35]

CLINICAL MANIFESTATIONS OF HNPCC

HNPCC is an autosomal dominantly inherited genetic disease characterized by an increased risk for cancers of the colon, rectum, and a number of other organs (Table 18-2). Endometrial cancer is nearly as common as colorectal cancers in some registries[36,37] and is a key component of the HNPCC phenotype. Small intestinal cancers are extremely rare in the general population, but the risk for these is greatly increased in HNPCC patients. These remain unusual tumors even in this setting, but they have an early age of onset (49 years), may present with obstructive symptoms like colorectal tumors, and appear to be associated with a better prognosis than what would be expected in the general population.[38]

Between 60 and 70 percent of colorectal cancers occur proximal to the splenic flexure.[23] There is an increased risk of synchronous and metachronous cancers of the colon, rectum, and other organs. Multiple adenomatous polyps of the colon and microadenomas, such as are seen in FAP, do not occur in HNPCC. Although the incidence of adenomatous polyps may be slightly increased in HNPCC patients,[39,40] this does not entirely explain the greatly increased incidence of carcinomas. It has been suggested that a higher rate of progression from adenoma to carcinoma is the major factor accounting for the cancer predisposition in HNPCC (Table 18-3).

There appears to be no significant increase in risk for cancer of the lung, breast, prostate, bladder, bone marrow, larynx, or brain if one ascertains tumors from clinical collections of families and compares them against population-based estimates.[12] The use of genetic techniques has provided insight into the extracolonic tumors that occur in HNPCC. An excess of gastric cancer occurs in members of affected families, and both intestinal and diffuse-type tumors may be found. The mean age of diagnosis of gastric cancer in these families is 56 years. Not all the gastric cancers have the characteristic hypermutability of HNPCC, so it is not necessarily the case that all of these tumors are attributable to the syndrome.[41] There are anecdotal accounts of early-onset breast cancers in HNPCC kindreds, and the report of convincing genetic evidence for the appearance of an HNPCC-related breast cancer in one case indicates that this tumor may occasionally occur in this setting.[42] Brain cancers, including a wide pathologic spectrum, have been reported to occur in 3.35 percent of a Dutch HNPCC registry.[43] Other tumors occurring with an increased relative risk include urinary tract tumors and ovarian cancer.

The prevalence of HNPCC in the general population is unknown. This is complicated by the fact that there is a 5 to 6 percent lifetime prevalence of colorectal cancer in North America, and it is at least this high in much of western Europe. Various estimates of prevalence have been attempted, as listed in Table 18-4.[15–20,44] The apparent proportion of families with HNPCC (based on a history of multiple cancers in the family) is approximately 3 to 4 percent of all colorectal cancers (with one remarkable outlier study from Finland[18]). These estimates predict a prevalence of HNPCC in the population of approximately 2 per 1000 persons; however, this is probably an underestimate because of limitations in family size (which limits recognition), historical recall (which is inaccurate), penetrance (which is undetermined), and involvement of organs other than the colon (which have not been considered in these studies). A more realistic estimate for the frequency of HNPCC in the general population may be much higher but is probably less than some estimates that have been as high as 1 per 200.

The diagnosis of HNPCC is made clinically by taking a family history. Even a single first-degree relative who develops a colorectal or endometrial cancer at a very young age raises this possibility. A subset of HNPCC families is easier to recognize by virtue of a constellation of findings that constitute the Muir-Torre variant.[45,46] This syndrome consists of all of the features of HNPCC plus sebaceous gland tumors (adenomas, epitheliomas,

Table 18-2 Estimates of Cancer Risk by Organ Site in HNPCC

Cancer Site	Lifetime Risk	Relative Risk	Median Age
Any cancer by age 70	91% (men), 69% (women)[36]		
Colon or rectum	74% (men), 30% (women)[36]		46 yrs[9]
With *hMLH1* mutations	80%		41 yrs[37]
With *hMSH2* mutations	80%		44 yrs[37]
Endometrium	20% (by age 70)[113]	(vs. 3% risk in the general population)	46 yrs[9]
	42% (by age 70)[36]		
	61% (*hMSH2* mutations)[37]		
	42% (*hMLH1* mutations)[37]		
Stomach		4.1[9]	54 yrs[9]
With *hMLH1* mutations		4.4[37]	
With *hMSH2* mutations		19.3[37]	
Ovaries		3.5[9]	40 yrs[9]
With *hMLH1* mutations		6.4[37]	
With *hMSH2* mutations		8.0[37]	
Small intestine		25[9]	53 yrs[9]
With *hMLH1* mutations		292[37]	
With *hMSH2* mutations		103[37]	
Hepatobiliary system		4.9[9]	66 yrs[9]
Kidney		3.2[9]	66 yrs[9]
Ureter		22	56 yrs[9]
Kidney/ureter (*hMSH2* mutations)		75.3[37]	

Table 18-3 Adenomatous Polyps of the Colon in HNPCC (Clinical Diagnoses of HNPCC)

A. Lanspa et al., Nebraska patients[39]

	HNPCC Patients* (N = 44, Mean Age 42.4)	Control Patients (N = 88, Mean Age 44.4)
Adenomatous polyps	30% (13/44)	11% (10/88)
Proximal colonic adenomas	18% (8/44)	1% (1/88)
Multiple colonic adenomas	20% (9/44)	4% (4/88)

B. Jass et al., New Zealand patients[40]

	HNPCC Patients	Age-Matched Autopsy Controls
Men <50 years old	30% (3/10)*	5% (2/42)
Women <50 years old	44% (4/9)†	5% (1/21)
Men 50–69 years old	66% (2/3)	36% (16/44)
Women 50–69 years old	100% (1/1)	12% (1/8)
Men >70 years old	None available	46% (13/28)
Women >70 years old	None available	33% (5/15)

*$p = 0.015$ vs. Controls (by χ^2).
†$p = 0.0075$ vs. Controls (by χ^2).

and carcinomas) and keratoacanthomas. The latter is a keratin-filled skin tumor that occurs in sun-exposed areas. Basal and squamous cell carcinomas also occur in Muir-Torre syndrome. Although these skin tumors are unusual manifestations of HNPCC, this diagnosis should be considered in any patient who has more than one skin tumor of this variety. To date, almost all Muir-Torre syndrome families who have had germ-line mutations identified have been linked to *hMSH2*.[47–49]

The pathologic features of colorectal neoplasms in HNPCC (Fig. 18-1) are somewhat unique.[23,50–52] As mentioned, the tumors occur at early ages, and most are in the proximal colon. Using typical pathologic criteria, 37 percent of colorectal cancers in HNPCC will be classified as poorly differentiated,[23] which would suggest that the tumors will behave aggressively. Contrary to this, colorectal cancers in HNPCC have a better outcome than sporadic tumors matched for stage.[23] Colorectal cancers in HNPCC are significantly more likely to be diploid or near-diploid compared with sporadic tumors.[53,54] In one flow cytometry study, 68 percent of HNPCC cancers were diploid, and 90 percent were diploid or near-diploid with a DNA index less than 1.27.[54] Over 35 percent of colorectal cancers in HNPCC are mucinous carcinomas.[23] HNPCC tumors (as well as other colorectal cancers with the MSI phenotype) are more likely to be exophytic, larger, look poorly differentiated, show focal or predominant mucin production, and show an intense Crohn-like reaction of tumor-infiltrating lympho-

cytes.[55] The combined pathologic features mentioned above should increase one's suspicion of HNPCC, even if found outside familial clusters of colorectal cancer.

THE HNPCC GENES

hMSH2: The First HNPCC Gene

The discovery of the HNPCC genes is an interesting story of excellent basic science research, fierce competition among several laboratories interested in the problem, and in some instances unusual good fortune.[24] It had been proposed by Loeb in the 1980s that a "hypermutable phenotype" would be necessary to account for all the mutations that seemed to be present in most cancers.[56,57] No mechanism was available to account for this at that time.

In 1993, three laboratories working independently reported that an unusual form of somatic mutation occurred in 12 to 15 percent of colorectal cancers. The mutations were insertions or deletions of simple repetitive elements that make up microsatellite sequences (see below). Each laboratory added to the interpretation. A group led by Perucho used an arbitrarily primed polymerase chain reaction (PCR) looking for genomic amplifications or deletions that might be present in colorectal cancers.[58] Instead, they noted that 12 percent of colorectal cancers harbored somatic deletions that altered the lengths of the microsatellite sequences.

Table 18-4 Prevalence of HNPCC in the Population

Ascertainment Method	Age Limit	Locale	Proportion of Families Estimated to Have HNPCC	Reference
Record search	70	Finland	3.8%	15
Patient recall	None	Italy	3.9%	16
Death certificates	None	UK	4.0%	17
Record search	50	Finland	30.0%	18
Record search	55	Ireland	6.0%	19
Patient recall	50	Canada	3.1%	20
Genetic testing	—	Finland	2%	75

NOTE: All estimates (except ref. 75) are based on family histories (not genetic diagnoses) and required 3 or more family members with colorectal cancer. These are probably underestimates (see text).

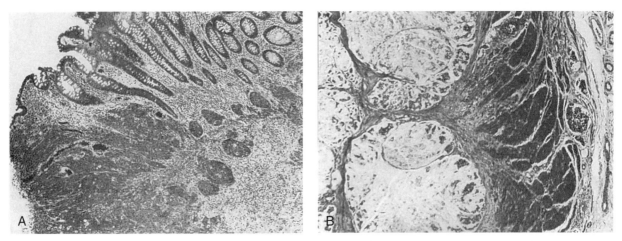

Fig. 18-1 Histopathology of HNPCC. *A.* **Poorly differentiated carcinoma without evidence of a glandular formation. The tumor cells have round regular nuclei. Such a tumor would be typically interpreted to be highly aggressive. (***Courtesy of T. Smyrk, M.D., Omaha, Nebraska.***)** *B.* **Mucinous adenocarcinoma is characteristic of more than one-third of colon cancers in HNPCC. (***Courtesy of T. Smyrk, M.D., Omaha, Nebraska.***)**

Their approach permitted them to estimate that affected tumors carried more than 10^5 of these types of mutations. They also noted that tumors with these "ubiquitous somatic mutations at simple repetitive sequences" had unique features that distinguished them from most colorectal cancers, and they proposed that this represented a novel form of carcinogenesis.[5]

Another group led by Thibodeau also was looking for genetic losses at tumor suppressor gene loci using PCR-based amplification of microsatellite sequences and recognized that *microsatellite instability* (initially called MIN but, by consensus, now abbreviated MSI[59]) was significantly correlated with tumors of the proximal colon. MSI was inversely related with loss of heterozygosity on chromosomes 5q, 17p, and 18q and positively correlated with improved patient survival. This group proposed that 28 percent of colorectal cancers developed through this unique mechanism of genomic instability.[6]

A third group, representing a multinational collaboration that included Vogelstein in the United States and de la Chapelle in Finland, performed a genome-wide search for a genetic locus of HNPCC. Using two large kindreds, one such locus was mapped to

2p15-16.[7] Microsatellite markers had been used to map the locus. Pursuing the hypothesis that the HNPCC gene would be a tumor suppressor gene, they looked for loss of heterozygosity in the tumors, using the microsatellites as targets. They also found insertion or deletion mutations at the repetitive sequences, which they termed the *replicative error* (RER) *phenotype.*[8] All three groups brought unique insights to bear on the issue, and together they illuminated for the first time the nature of HNPCC and discovered a novel mechanism for carcinogenesis.

The next step forward in solving the HNPCC riddle came unexpectedly from laboratories focused on yeast genetics who had not previously ventured into human genetics, let alone hereditary colon cancer. The characteristic mutational pattern (i.e., MSI) published in the autoradiograms used to resolve the amplified microsatellites by the preceding three groups resembled the mutational pattern seen in bacteria and yeast that had lost genes required for DNA MMR (Fig. 18-2). The microbial DNA MMR systems were complex and involved several genes of the Mut HLS mismatch repair pathway.[60,61] The system, which consists of several proteins working together in a complex, repairs errors in

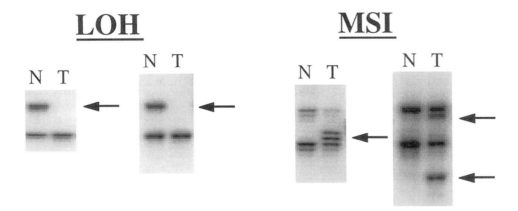

Fig. 18-2 Autoradiogram demonstrating microsatellite instability. A repetitive and polymorphic DNA sequence (microsatellite) is amplified by the polymerase chain reaction (PCR), and the normal tissue (N), if informative, provides two amplicons. On the left are two examples of loss of heterozygosity (LOH), in which one of the PCR products has been deleted from the genome of the tumor tissue (T) and lost from the autoradiogram, as indicated by the arrows. On the right are two examples of microsatellite instability (MSI), in which the length of the PCR product has been altered by an insertion or deletion mutation in the microsatellite sequence and the appearance of new bands on the autoradiogram (*arrows*). In the examples of MSI, residual normal DNA has been amplified along with the DNA from the neoplasm.

Table 18-5 The HNPCC Genes

HNPCC Gene	Chromosomal Location	*E. coli* Homologue	cDNA Size	Genomic Structure	Protein
hMSH2	2p 15-16	MutS	2727 bp	16 exons ~73 kb	934 aa's 106 kD
hMSH6	2p 15-16	MutS	4245	10 exons	1360 aa's 160 kD
hMLH1	3p 21	MutL	2268 bp	19 exons ~58 kb	756 aa's 85 kD
hPMS1	2q 31	MutL	2795 bp	—	932 aa's
hPMS2	7p 22[1]	MutL	2586 bp	15 exon ~16 kb	862 aa's 96 kD

DNA replication that occur during S phase that result in single-base-pair mismatches or mispaired loops that occur at repetitive sequences such as microsatellites. Strand et al. demonstrated that mutations in three yeast genes involved in DNA MMR (*PMS1, MLH*, and *MSH2*) led to 100- to 700-fold increases in mutations at poly(GT) sequences and, based on what had been reported in colorectal cancer, specifically suggested that these genes might be the loci sought by those studying HNPCC.[62] In a remarkably short period of time, investigating groups led by Kolodner[63] and Vogelstein[64] reported that a human *MutS* homologue (*hMSH2**) could be found on chromosome 2p. Germ-line mutations of this gene in HNPCC families demonstrated that it was responsible for the disease.[64] *hMSH2* was the second homologue found in the human genome related to the bacterial *MutS* or *yMHS* gene. Subsequently, at least 8 human homologues of the *MutS* genes have been found.

The genetics of HNPCC are somewhat complex but follow the paradigms of other tumor suppressor genes. HNPCC is inherited as an autosomal dominant characteristic when an inactivating germ-line mutation occurs in *hMSH2* or certain other DNA MMR genes. Resultingly, every somatic cell carries one inactivated copy and one wild-type copy of the MMR gene. With certain notable exceptions,[65] the phenotype at the cellular level or for the individual is normal but is susceptible to loss of the wild-type allele in a target tissue,[66] which leads to a hypermutable phenotype (MSI). The hypermutable cell then is susceptible to the accumulation of mutations at a greatly accelerated rate, which may then result in clonal expansion and the neoplastic phenotype. Thus a germ-line mutation at *hMSH2* leaves an individual susceptible to the development of hypermutability, which then facilitates the rapid accumulation of other mutations that are permissive of a neoplastic phenotype. There is not yet a suitable explanation for why specific organs are at selective risk to develop cancer. Certain germ-line mutations appear to have a *dominant negative* effect, in which heterozygous cells are themselves hypermutable. In this instance, MMR deficiency may be detected in phenotypically normal cells.[65]

Other HNPCC Genes: *hMLH1, hPMS1, hPMS2, and hMSH6*

Shortly after the first HNPCC locus was mapped to 2p, a second HNPCC locus was mapped to 3p in a Scandinavian kindred.[67] Based on the paradigm that led from 2p to *hMSH2*, these same two groups turned their attention to the *MutL* gene of *E. coli* (and the yeast *MutL* homologue). This research led to three human homologues, now termed *hMLH1, hPMS1*, and *hPMS2*, located on 3p, 2q, and 7p, all of which have be linked to HNPCC families.[68-70]

The identification of the DNA MMR genes and their linkage to HNPCC families led to a sharp increase in interest in the field and the identification of numerous families with inactivating germ-line mutations. *hMSH2* and *hMLH1* account for the majority of families with HNPCC and in roughly equal proportions.[71-75] Smaller numbers of families have HNPCC on the basis of mutations and *hPMS2*, and one family has been found with a germ-line mutation in *hPMS1*.[70] A dominant negative germ-line mutation in *hPMS2* has been identified that raises new possibilities for tumor development.[76] Two HNPCC families have been reported who have germ-line mutations in *hMSH6*, a gene that encodes for a protein that heterodimerizes with the hMSH2 protein.[77-79] In each of these families, the cancers had MSI at mono- and di-nucleotide repeat sequences. The genes known to give rise to HNPCC are listed in Table 18-5.

Can HNPCC Occur in the Absence of MSI?

A single, somewhat atypical family has been reported that stretches the borders of what constitutes HNPCC. Loss of the DNA MMR system results in a tissue that is hypermutable but not necessarily neoplastic as such. Several genes with potential tumor suppressor activity have been identified that contain repetitive sequences in their coding regions. The first of these to be identified was the type II receptor of transforming growth factor (TGF) β_1 (*TGFβ_1RII,* or *RII*). Members of a kindred with several cases of colorectal cancer shared an inactivating germ-line mutation in *RII*, and as expected, the tumors lacked MSI. Neither of two mutation-carrying offspring (ages 57 and 48) of an affected individual have developed cancers, and no other tumors have been found in the gene carriers. In one of the colon cancers, loss of heterozygosity was found at the *RII* locus. The clinical implications of this finding remain to be established.[80]

THE CELLULAR AND MOLECULAR BIOLOGY OF HNPCC

It is necessary to become familiar with the DNA MMR system to fully understand the implications of HNPCC. Cancers develop in HNPCC when the DNA MMR system fails. As described, DNA MMR requires the concerted action of several proteins. Loss of any component of the system will inactivate, to some degree, the repair system.

The DNA MMR System

The DNA MMR system is illustrated schematically in Fig. 18-3.[81-84] During the synthesis of a new strand of DNA, many of the replication errors are immediately corrected by the 3' to 5' exonuclease activity of DNA polymerase. The combined activities of all the proofreading functions reduce the rate of replication errors to approximately 1 per 10^{12} base pairs. It is estimated that 99.9 percent of the mutations that escaped the proofreading activity of DNA polymerase are repaired by the MMR system, particularly single-base-pair mismatches and "loop outs" of unpaired bases, which tend to occur during reannealing of the new and template strands at repetitive sequences such as

*The *Escherichia coli* gene is called *MutS*, the yeast homologue is called the *MutS homologue* or *yMSH*, and the human homologues are called *hMSH* genes.

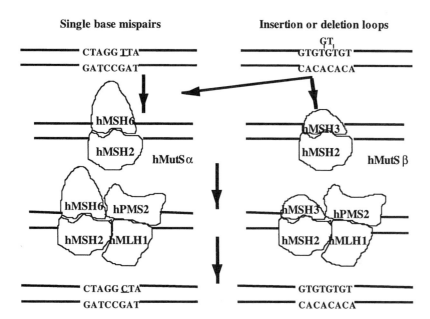

Fig. 18-3 DNA mismatch repair. During new strand synthesis, DNA polymerase may create mismatches, which will deform the newly formed DNA double helix. The newly synthesized strand transiently has gaps. The *hMutSα* complex (made up of *hMSH2* and *hMSH6*) recognizes the mismatch during S or G2 in the cell cycle and binds to it. The *hMHS2-hMSH6* complex has a particular affinity for recognition of single-base-pair mismatches. A second heteroduplex called *hMutSβ*, made up of *hMSH2* and *hMSH3*, has the additional ability to recognize and bind to loop-outs created at misaligned repetitive sequences that may occur at microsatellites. Some overlap may occur in these recognition affinities. There is no evidence for a functional *hMSH2* homoduplex. The *hMutLα* complex (made up of *hMLH1* and *hPMS2*) binds to the DNA mismatch-*hMutSα* complex in order to discriminate the strand containing the error. The role of *hPMS1* is not yet determined. After recognition of the mismatch, the complex accomplishes long patch excision, resynthesis, and ligation.

microsatellites. Commonly affected microsatellite sequences include mononucleotide repeats (such as A_n or G_n) and dinucleotide repeats (such as $\{CA/GT\}_n$).

A newly synthesized mispair will deform the double helix of DNA, creating a physical aberration. The deformed DNA strand is recognized and bound by a complex made up of a heterodimer of hMSH2 and either hMSH6 (initially called the *GT binding protein,* or GTBP)[85] or hMSH3. The hMSH2-hMSH6 heteroduplex is called hMutSα and favors binding to single-base-pair mismatches, and the hMSH2-hMSH3 heteroduplex is called hMutSβ and favors recognition of loop-outs that occur during misalignment of newly synthesized repetitive sequences such as microsatellites.[81–83] The regulation of the individual components of the DNA MMR system is currently not understood.

After the recognition complex binds to a DNA mismatch, the repair system must identify which of the two DNA strands represents the original template and which is the newly synthesized — and therefore erroneous — strand. This is achieved by the recruitment to the complex of a second heterodimer, made up of hMLH1 and hPMS2 (together called hMutLα), which binds to the DNA mispair-hMutSα/β complex; the full complex identifies the newly synthesized DNA strand, perhaps by virtue of gaps that remain between newly synthesized Okazaki segments. In lower organisms, newly synthesized strands are recognized by the transient absence of methylation. It is not known whether this mechanism also participates in the human MMR system. The repair system also requires the activity of several other enzymes, including helicase II, the DNA pol III holoenzyme, DNA ligase, single-stranded DNA-binding protein, and other DNA exonucleases. The DNA MMR system excises the newly synthesized strand from the point of its recognition (presumably the gap) back to the mismatch and then fully resynthesizes it.[60,61,83,84] This process is also known as *long patch excision,* which distinguishes it from another system (*short patch excision*) that repairs different types of DNA abnormalities (see Chap. 14). This process is probably even more complex in humans, and additional components of the system will likely be reported in the future.[86,87]

Understanding the DNA MMR system began with studies in *E. coli* and its Mut HLS system. In yeast, six *MutS* homologues (*yMSH1, yMSH2, yMSH3, yMSH4, yMSH5,* and *yMSH6*) and four *MutL* homologues (*yPMS1, yMLH1, yMLH2,* and *yMLH3*) have been identified.[60,88] *yMSH2-, yPMS1-,* and *yMLH1*-mutant strains of *Saccharomyces cerevisiae* undergo destabilization of microsatellite sequences during replication, as do the *MutL* and *MutS* mutants of *E. coli.* The human DNA MMR system is probably

more complex, but at this time, mutations in only five of the involved genes are known to cause Lynch syndrome.

The genomic instability at microsatellite sequences was the initial finding that suggested that DNA MMR was inactivated in HNPCC tumors. The phenotype for cells carrying one mutant and one wild-type DNA MMR gene is normal. A second, somatic event occurs that results in inactivation of the wild-type allele, inactivating the DNA MMR system, which permits a hypermutable phenotype.[66] As mentioned earlier, the hMutS complex has two variants that may serve to add specificity to the recognition of DNA alterations. An issue that remains unclear is whether there is heterogeneity in the hMutLα complex that can further modify the repair system. Several *hPMS2*-related genes have been found on chromosome 7, the function of which remains unknown,[89] and these are potential candidates for additional participants in human DNA MMR.

The *hMSH2* gene encodes a protein with a relative mass of 106,000 that may be found immunohistochemically in the nucleus of a variety of tissues. In the intestinal tract, hMSH2 expression is limited to the replicating compartment of the crypt unit.[90,91] Most benign and malignant colorectal tumors express hMSH2 protein throughout the neoplastic tissue. Tumors from patients with germline mutations in *hMSH2* do not express the protein, consistent with the "two hit" mechanism of gene inactivation.[91] In cultured cells, expression of the hMSH2 protein is regulated based on progression through the cell cycle. Levels remain relatively low in resting cells but are induced when progression through the cell cycle toward mitosis occurs.[92]

Knockout Models

Mice deficient in DNA MMR genes have been developed using knockout techniques. Hemizygous mice (i.e., the equivalent of HNPCC) have an apparently normal phenotype in all the MMR knockout models. Somewhat surprisingly, MSH2-deficient mice have a seemingly normal embryonic development but are at high risk for developing lymphomas at an early age. Nullizygous cells from these animals have a mutator phenotype and are relatively tolerant of methylation damage, and nullizygous animals do not spontaneously develop tumors of the colon or other sites characteristically affected in HNPCC.[93] However, it has been reported that MSH2-deficient mice develop a very high incidence of intestinal neoplasms (mostly small intestinal) if they survive beyond 6 months, that 7 percent develop keratoacanthoma-like skin lesions, and all die by 1 year.[94] Interestingly, 70 percent of the intestinal tumors had inactivation of the *APC* gene.

Mice with knockouts in *MLH1*, *PMS1*, and *PMS2* have surprisingly few tumors,[95] which may reflect differences in structure of the colorectal tumor suppressor genes between the mice and humans. This explanation is supported by the observation that hypermutability can be found in the tissues of mice deficient in PMS2.[96] Mice nullizygous for *PMS2* (which do not develop intestinal neoplasms) crossed with *Min* mice (which are heterozygous for the mouse equivalent of the *APC* gene) develop more adenomas of the small intestines than do the *Min* mice.[97] These findings underscore the interaction among the genes involved in the development of colorectal cancer.

An *MSH6* knockout mouse has been developed. Cells without MSH6 activity are defective in the repair of single-base-pair mismatches, but repair of insertion/deletion mismatches was not impaired, as one may have predicted based on the yeast model. Nullizygous animals are at greatest risk for lymphomas, rather than colorectal cancers, and these tumors did not demonstrate MSI.[98]

Knockout mice with no *MLH1* genes have the MSI phenotype, have no DNA MMR activity in cell extracts, and are sterile due to defective spermatogenesis.[99,100] MLH1-deficient spermatocytes show numerous prematurely separated chromosomes and meiotic pachytene arrest. Male mice defective at the *PMS2* locus have abnormal chromosome synapses in meiosis and are highly prone to the development of sarcomas and lymphomas.[101] None of the knockout mice or the heterozygotes of these models develop a syndrome that closely resembles HNPCC.

THE PATHOPHYSIOLOGY OF HNPCC TUMORS

Most sporadic colorectal cancers develop through a mechanism that involves loss of relatively large chromosomal segments, which is thought to represent the deletion of wild-type tumor suppressor genes from the nucleus.[102] A proportion of sporadic colorectal cancers (perhaps 15 percent) and nearly all HNPCC-related cancers progress through a different mechanism, with MSI. MSI is inversely correlated with loss of heterozygosity of chromosomes 5q, 17p, and 18q.[6] In sporadic colorectal cancers, over half show mutations in the *K-RAS* oncogene.

What Growth-Controlling Genes Are Altered in HNPCC Cancers?

One of the initial reports indicated that mutations at *K-RAS*, *APC*, and *p53* were at least as common in HNPCC colon cancers as in sporadic ones.[7] One of the other initial investigations in the area reported that *K-RAS* and *p53* mutations were significantly less

frequent in tumors with MSI but did not look for *APC* mutations.[5] The third of these initial groups did not look for point mutations in *APC*, *K-RAS*, or *p53* but noted an inverse relationship between MSI and loss of heterozygosity at 5q, 17p, and 18q.[6] A failure to microdissect the neoplastic tissue from infiltrating stroma or inflammatory cells (which can be considerable in these tumors) could lead to a systematic underestimate of cancer-associated mutations. This concern notwithstanding, one group has reported an inverse relationship between MSI and *p53* mutations in colon cancer cell lines,[103] and two groups reported a significant reduction in the incidence of mutations in *APC*, *p53*, and *K-RAS-2* in HNPCC colon cancers.[104,105] Additionally, immuno-histochemical detection of the p53 protein in colorectal tissues is a surrogate for point mutations in the gene, since these mutations often stabilize the gene product. There is an inverse relationship between MSI and p53 immunostaining, which supports the contention that *p53* mutations may be less common in colon cancers with MSI.[106] One group has reported that the putative inverse relationship between MSI and *p53* mutations may not obtain in distal colorectal cancers.[107] This area still requires additional clarification.

An analysis of 101 colon cancers led the Vogelstein group to conclude that *APC* mutations were present in colorectal tumors with or without MSI, but that in MSI there was a significant predilection for frameshift mutations at repetitive sequences, particularly in polyadenine tracts.[108] At this point in time, the data suggest that most colorectal neoplasia begins with inactivation of the *APC* gene whether or not the tumor has MSI. However, the genetic events after *APC* inactivation may diverge thereafter depending on the mechanism underlying the genomic instability, which will select for specific genes in multistep tumor progression (Fig. 18-4).

The genomic instability seen at microsatellites in human colorectal neoplasms is an early event and can be found in the adenomatous polyps that serve as precursors to cancer in HNPCC.[109] Although MSI has been described in phenotypically normal human lymphocytes in unusual instances,[65] the mucosa in the colons from most patients with HNPCC does not show this abnormality.[110] The adenomatous polyps associated with sporadic tumors with MSI, or those in HNPCC, also have MSI, unlike sporadic adenomas, which rarely do.[109,111] The proportion of microsatellite loci that are mutated increases with progression from adenoma to carcinoma in both instances.[111,112]

In one series of cancers from patients with HNPCC, 95 percent showed the MSI phenotype, regardless of stage. In contrast, this type of genomic instability was found in only 3 percent of early

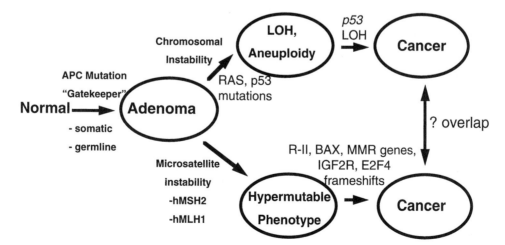

Fig. 18-4 Dual pathways for tumor development. The initial pathway for multistep carcinogenesis is depicted as the "chromosomal instability" at the top and involves LOH at tumor suppressor genes. The lower pathway (MSI) or the "mutator pathway" involves a unique destabilizing mechanism and inactivation of different genes, although both result in cancer. Both pathways may begin with an inactivating mutation at the *APC* locus, but the mutations leading to the lower pathway are those which would be expected with the loss of DNA MMR activity. These very distinct mechanisms lead to a similar pathologic result.

sporadic tumors (i.e., adenomas or intramucosal carcinomas) and 13 to 24 percent of sporadic invasive cancers. MSI has been reported in 35 percent of the liver metastases, suggesting that loss of the MMR system may play a role in tumor progression.[104]

One survey reported that 16 percent of sporadic colorectal cancers and 86 percent of colorectal cancers from HNPCC patients had MSI, including all patients in which a germ-line mutation in *hMSH2* was found. This lesion (i.e., MSI) was present in only 3 percent of 33 sporadic colorectal adenomas but in 57 percent of 14 adenomas associated with HNPCC. In addition, MSI was present in all the extracolonic cancers derived from HNPCC patients.[113] Although MSI has been described in phenotypically normal lymphocytes in patients with certain germ-line mutations in a DNA MMR gene,[65] the normal-appearing mucosa in the colons of patients with HNPCC does not show this abnormality.[110]

MSI in Non-HNPCC Tumors

MSI was first described in colorectal cancers not selected on the basis of a suspicion for HNPCC. Depending on the criteria used, 12 to 28 percent of colorectal cancers have MSI.[5–7] MSI is neither characteristic of colorectal cancer, limited to tumors of this organ, nor limited to HNPCC. MSI can be found in gastric cancers, endometrial cancers, ovarian tumors, urinary bladder tumors, non-small-cell lung cancers, small-cell lung cancers, breast cancers, and other tumors. In some instances, inactivation of a DNA MMR gene can be found, but this is not always the case. In some colon cancers, MSI can be found in association with loss of heterozygosity at one of the DNA MMR gene loci.[66] In the overwhelming majority of instances, there are no germ-line mutations at any of the known HNPCC loci when MSI is found.

As mentioned, a sizable minority of all sporadic colorectal cancers have MSI, and most of these are unrelated to HNPCC. Most of these tumors do not express hMHL1 immunohistochemically.[114,115] The mechanism responsible for silencing the *hMLH1* gene is frequently hypermethylation of promoter sequences in its 5′ upstream regulatory region.[116–119] Treating cultured tumor cells with 5-azacytidine can restore expression of hMLH1.[117–118] Hypermethylation and silencing of the *hMSH2* gene have not been found.[117,119]

Somatic Mutations Unique to Tumors with MSI

The finding of a type of hypermutability that was unrelated to the type of genomic instability seen in sporadic colorectal cancers (i.e., that manifested by widespread loss of heterozygosity) led to speculation that a distinct molecular pathway was responsible for HNPCC and related tumors.[35] An increased rate of mutation at the *hprt* locus was found in colorectal cancer cell lines that had MSI.[120] A recognition that MSI was associated with a disproportionate hypermutability at microsatellite sequences prompted several laboratories to look for repetitive sequences in the coding regions of genes that might be involved in growth control, with the speculation that these sequences would be at increased risk to experience a frameshift in a cell with MSI, resulting in a loss of function for the gene product.

The paradigm of this process was established on the identification of inactivating mutations in the type II transforming growth factor (TGF) β_1 receptor (called *RII*) in colon cancer cells with MSI.[121] TGFβ_1 signaling results in an inhibition of growth in colorectal epithelium.[122] Two repetitive sequences were found in coding regions of *RII*, a $(CA)_3$ and an A_8 sequence. Mutations in *RII* were concentrated on the A_8 sequence in MSI tumors and not found in non-MSI tumors. In each instance, the mutation resulted in loss of the RII transcript expression and a failure of cells to bind or respond to the TGFβ ligand. This is of particular importance because the TGFβ system inhibits the growth of colonic epithelial cells, and loss of this system in tumors with MSI represents a critical escape from growth control. Similar inactivating mutations in the *RII* gene have been found in gastric cancer cell lines and resected gastric carcinoma specimens; the mutations usually occur in a coding polyadenine tract.[123] It appears that inactivating

Table 18-6 Growth Regulatory Genes Mutated in Colorectal Cancers with MSI (Somatic Mutations in HNPCC)

GeneTarget	Repetitive Genetic Sequence	Frequency of Mutation in Colorectal Cancers with MSI or HNPCC	Reference
TGFβ₁ RII	A_8	85–90%(MSI)	121, 123, 124, 125
IGF IIR	G_8	9% of MSI tumors, 1/8 HNPCC tumors	126
Bax	G_8	51–54% (MSI); 52% in HNPCC	127, 130, 131
MSH6	C_8	33% in HNPCC	131
MSH3	A_8	52% in HNPCC	128, 129, 131, 132
E2F4	$(CAG)n$	65% (MSI)	129, 133
APC	Several	(See text)	108

mutations in growth-regulating genes may be a key mechanism by which tumors with MSI become neoplastic. These mutations are not commonly found in adenomas and may represent relatively late events in the multistep progressive neoplastic process in the evolution of a tumor in HNPCC.[124,125]

Additional genes that may be involved in growth control also contain repetitive sequences in coding regions, which puts them at risk for mutation when the DNA MMR system is inactivated. Several of these have been found to be mutated in some proportion of HNPCC tumors, including the insulin-like growth factor II (IGF-II) receptor (which acts "in series" with *RII* in TGFβ signaling), *BAX, hMSH3, hMSH6,* and *E2F4;* the genes and the hypermutable sequences are listed in Table 18-6.[124,126–133] The requirement for involvement of any of these genes in the evolution of a tumor with MSI and the sequence of events involved remains to be determined. Of particular interest, two of the genes are themselves DNA MMR genes: *hMSH3* and *hMSH6.* This raises the possibility of a cascade of events in which a partial loss of DNA MMR activity could lead to mutations in other MMR genes and amplify the genomic instability.[134]

MSI and Resistance to Cytotoxic Drugs. Inactivation of the DNA MMR system is associated with increased resistance to DNA alkylation, which is toxic to wild-type cells.[135] Restoration of the DNA MMR system in a colon cancer cell line defective at the *hMLH1* locus increases sensitivity to alkylation and restores the G2/M cell cycle checkpoint.[136,137] The DNA MMR system also is required for transcription-coupled DNA repair.[138] These findings imply additional growth advantages for tumor cells defective in DNA MMR, since the G2/M checkpoint may be bypassed in these cells, and an additional level of mutation repair is lost. Evidence is accumulating that DNA MMR-defective cells may be relatively resistant to cytotoxic chemotherapy used to treat cancer.[136,137,139–143] Cell lines have been identified that are deficient for each of the major human DNA MMR genes, which provide valuable models for study.[144] All these observations have come from experiments on cultured cells, and the clinical implications of this have not yet been tested on patients.

MSI and Neoplasia in Ulcerative Colitis. MSI is commonly seen in cancers associated with ulcerative colitis, as well as the dysplasias that antedate these tumors.[145] An intronic polymorphism in the *hMSH2* gene is more common in patients who develop colitis-associated neoplasia than in control patients with or without colitis.[146] Moreover, MSI may be found in the non-neoplastic colonic mucosa from patients with chronic ulcerative colitis.[147] It has not yet been confirmed whether inactivation of the DNA MMR system is an essential part of tumor development in chronic inflammation.

Table 18-7 Frequency of Specific Germ-Line Mutations in HNPCC

HNPCC Gene	Frequency/Proportion of Families[64]
hMSH2	31%
hMLH1	33%
hPMS1	Rare (one family)
hPMS2	4%
GTBP (hMSH6)	Rare (a few families)
Undetermined loci	32%

THE DIAGNOSIS AND MANAGEMENT OF HNPCC

Identification of the role of the DNA MMR system in the genesis of HNPCC provided a breakthrough in the premorbid diagnosis of the disease. Although many more proteins participate in the DNA MMR system, as a practical issue, two of the genes — *hMSH2* and *hMLH1* — appear to account for most Lynch syndrome diagnoses (Table 18-7). Unfortunately, the nature of the genes and the heterogeneity of the mutational spectrum have limited the clinical practicality of sequencing for germ-line mutations.

Testing for MSI: MSI-H, MSH-L, and MSS

Insight into the pathophysiology and genetic basis of HNPCC has provided multiple strategies for making this diagnosis. It is possible to screen for HNPCC by observing MSI in a tumor specimen. Guidelines for MSI testing were drawn up at a consensus workshop on HNPCC and have been referred to as the *Bethesda guidelines*[148] (Table 18-8). Furthermore, another workshop has led to the identification of a verified panel of consensus microsatellite loci that can ensure uniformity of diagnosis between laboratories.[59] According to these guidelines, five markers are considered to be a suitable panel to determine the presence of MSI. These microsatellite loci include two poly-adenine sequences (*BAT25* and *BAT26*) and three dinucleotide repeats (*D2S123, D5S346,* and *D17S250*).

If two or more microsatellite amplifications demonstrate microsatellite instability (compared with normal tissue from that patient), the tumor is called *MSI-H,* for high-frequency MSI. This group of tumors is phenotypically indistinguishable from HNPCC colon cancers, although the sporadic tumors are (by definition) not accompanied by germ-line mutations in a DNA MMR gene. Other markers may be shown to be equally useful, but these markers have been carefully validated, have undergone comparisons between reference laboratories, and are the currently recommended panel for MSI testing.[149,150] If none of five microsatellite markers shows instability, the tumor is considered to be *microsatellite stable* (MSS). The use of additional markers in these tumors is unlikely to be helpful.[149,150] If only one of five markers shows a frameshift mutation, this is termed *MSI-L,* for low-frequency MSI. The MSS and MSI-L tumors share the same phenotypic characteristics, distinct from the MSI-H group. In the case of ambiguous amplifications (or non-informative analyses), additional markers have been suggested, although in most instances five markers are adequate.[59] Some proportion of MSS tumors will show microsatellite instability in a small fraction of tested loci (i.e., < 10 percent) if a very large number is analyzed. The implications of this are not yet clear, and it is not evident that there are any distinctions to be made between the MSS and MSI-L tumor groups, or what *MSI-L* represents.

Screening Populations for HNPCC

Several groups have used methods other than direct sequencing to diagnose HNPCC. A group in the Netherlands used denaturing gradient gel electrophoresis (DGGE) to more rapidly screen for sequence aberrations and found germ-line mutations in *hMSH2* or

Table 18-8 The Bethesda Guidelines for Testing of Colorectal Tumors for MSI[148]

1. Individuals with cancer in families that meet the Amsterdam criteria
2. Individuals with two HNPCC-related cancers including synchronous and metachronous colorectal cancer or associated extracolonic cancers*
3. Individuals with colorectal cancer and a first-degree relative with colorectal cancer and/or HNPCC-related extracolonic cancer and/or a colorectal adenoma; one of the cancers diagnosed at age less than 45, the adenoma at age less than 40
4. Individuals with colorectal cancer or endometrial cancer diagnosed at age less than 45
5. Individuals with right-sided colorectal cancer with an undifferentiated pattern (solid/cribriform) on histopathology diagnosed at age less than 45†
6. Individuals with signet-ring-cell-type colorectal cancer diagnosed at age less than 45‡
7. Individuals with adenomas diagnosed at age less than 40

*Endometrial, ovarian, gastric, hepatobiliary, small bowel, transitional cell carcinoma of the renal pelvis or ureter.
†*Solid/cribriform* defined as poorly undifferentiated carcinoma composed of irregular solid sheets of large eosinophilic cells and containing small glandlike spaces.
‡Composed of more than 50% signet-ring cells.

hMLH1 in 47 of 184 (26 percent) suspected cancer families based on the history of multiple tumors among relatives.[74] This study recognized the predictive value of including endometrial cancer in the clinical diagnosis of families with HNPCC.

A large clinical study from Finland screened over 500 consecutive colorectal cancers for MSI, and if instability was noted at two or more of seven tested microsatellites, the patient was referred for sequencing of *hMSH2* and *hMLH1*.[75] Using these criteria, 63 of 509 (12 percent) tumors showed MSI, but only 10 of 63 (16 percent) of those with MSI had a germ-line mutation detected, and half of these came from a known founder mutation that is common in Finland. The authors estimated that at least 2 percent of their colorectal cancer patients had HNPCC. This and all other studies are limited to the extent that all the relevant HNPCC genes are known and by the inherent problems in finding all the genetic mechanisms by which these genes might be inactivated.

Making a Definitive Diagnosis of HNPCC

Although 92 percent of HNPCC-associated colon cancers have MSI,[72] only a minority of tumors with MSI come from HNPCC families.[151] Direct sequencing of the DNA MMR genes is a possible strategy to make the diagnosis of HNPCC, but the number of exons involved and the relative absence of "founder mutations" make this clinically impractical. Knowledge of the critical loci for HNPCC makes linkage analysis a possible approach, but multiple affected family members must be available for testing, and the diagnostic power is limited.[152] The large fraction of inactivating germ-line mutations in *hMSH2* that result in a truncated protein suggest that an *in vitro* transcription/translation assay may be clinically useful. This latter approach provided a positive test in about half of patients who met the Amsterdam criteria for HNPCC.[153]

Direct sequencing of the exons in *hMSH2* and *hMLH1* is a direct, if labor-intensive, approach to diagnosis. At this time, the full spectrum of disease-producing germ-line mutations and innocuous polymorphisms has not been catalogued, which may complicate the interpretation of DNA sequence data. Analyses based on harvesting RNA from lymphocytes is complicated by the observation that both *hMSH2* and *hMLH1* may undergo alternative splicing that will generate different messages and proteins, which

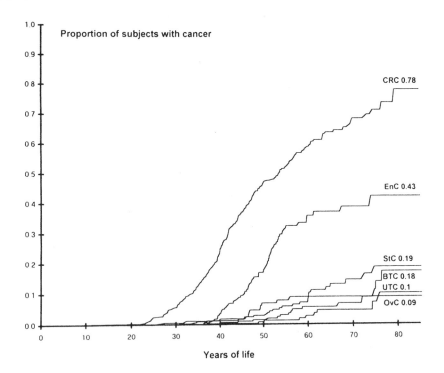

Fig. 18-5 Lifetime risk of different cancers in hereditary nonpolyposis colorectal cancer (HNPCC) syndrome. Lines represent estimates for colorectal cancer (CRC), endometrial cancer (EnC), stomach cancer (StC), biliary tract cancers (BTC), ureteral cancers (UTC), and ovarian cancers (OvC). (*From Aarnio et al.[161]*)

may complicate interpretation.[154–156] Unfortunately, the range of germ-line mutations in *hMSH2* and *hMLH1* is wide and includes insertions, deletions, nonsense mutations, and missense mutations.[72] These considerations make screening for a germ-line diagnosis in HNPCC a daunting undertaking. Nonetheless, when a mutation is correctly identified in a family, direct sequencing or *in vitro* transcription/translation will be highly reliable for other at-risk members of that family. In exceptional instances, founder mutations may be responsible for a large proportion of familial colon cancer in a specific geographic region with a relatively immobile population.[157,158]

Several published lists of germ-line mutations are available,[87,159] but an Internet site has been established to catalog and continuously update these mutations (*http://www.nfdht.nl/database/mdbchoice.htm*). This site contains a database for HNPCC pathologic germ-line mutations and intragenic polymorphisms and permits the submission of novel mutations.

Finding the germ-line mutation in an individual family has important implications. First, it permits the physician and genetic counselor to increase the certainty with which a diagnosis is made. Half those at risk will be informed that they did not inherit a high risk for cancer, and half will be informed with certainty of their risks, for which a surveillance program should be initiated.

Cancer Risk in HNPCC

The lifetime risk for cancer in HNPCC can only be estimated at this time (see Table 18-2). Cumulative risk for colorectal cancer has been estimated to range from 30 to 78 percent and endometrial cancer from 20 percent[161] to 43 percent for women[161] (Fig. 18-5 and Table 18-2). Patients with HNPCC must be identified because of the extremely high risk for metachronous cancers after successful treatment of the index tumor.[161] Patients with *hMLH1*-associated HNPCC in Finland have a significantly better survival rate when compared with patients with sporadic colorectal cancers[162] (Fig. 18-6). It is not known whether this observation is generally applicable to all *hMLH1* and *hMSH2*-associated HNPCC families.

Management of Patients with HNPCC

Once HNPCC patients are identified, a screening program consisting of colonoscopy or barium enema and sigmoidoscopy significantly reduces the rate of tumor development and death in patients with HNPCC[163] (Fig. 18-7). The observation that a screening program actually lowered the colorectal cancer incidence rates in family members with HNPCC suggests that the adenomatous polyps in this disease may be more prone to malignant transformation than adenomas in the general population and that their removal is an important part of a prevention program. Compared with sporadic cancers, at the time of diagnosis a lower stage of disease is commonly present in HNPCC, significantly fewer distant metastases are present, and survival is significantly better.[164,165] Colorectal lesions (including all adenomas) are detected in as many as 41 percent of asymptomatic patients who are referred for colonoscopy, but compliance with screening is surprisingly difficult.[166] Some reports have suggested that half the adenomas and perhaps as many of the early carcinomas in HNPCC are flat, making them a challenge for the

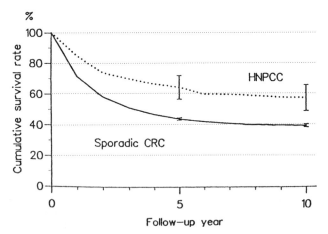

Fig. 18-6 Better survival rates in patients with *MLH1*-associated hereditary colorectal cancer. (*From Sankila et al.[162] Used by permission.*)

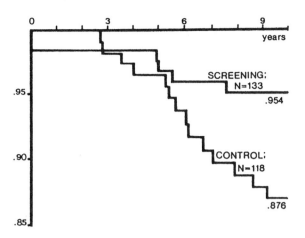

Fig. 18-7 Screening reduces colorectal cancer rate in families with hereditary nonpolyposis colorectal cancer. (*From Jarvinen et al.*[163] Used by permission.)

colonoscopist and very difficult lesions for detection radiographically.[167]

When a young individual (i.e., less than 45 years of age) develops colorectal cancer, this raises the concern that the patient and patient's relatives are at increased risk for HNPCC. One study suggested that the relative risk for colorectal cancer in the close relatives of such patients is increased five-fold and may be even higher for female relatives.[168] MSI is significantly more likely to occur in the colorectal cancers of young patients and can be found in 58 percent of patients under 35 years of age, even when the family history does not suggest HNPCC.[169] Even in such patients, less than half will have detectable germ-line mutations in the known DNA MMR genes.

The following approach might be followed to identify HNPCC. A careful family history should be taken in all patients who develop a cancer. A full pedigree should be drawn, and critical information should include all relatives who develop tumors, the organs affected, the age of first cancer, the occurrence of multiple cancers, and the ages reached by individuals who did not develop cancer. When the Amsterdam criteria are met, HNPCC is very likely. Under these circumstances, the *in vitro* transcription/translation assay for premature truncating mutations in *hMSH2* or *hMLH1* will provide a diagnosis in about half of families.[153] When available, tumor tissue can be valuable. Microsatellite analysis may be performed from paraffin-embedded tissues. Patients with HNPCC are likely to have MSI at multiple loci. If no MSI is found, the likelihood of HNPCC is substantially reduced, since perhaps 5 percent of such cancers lack this. Sporadic colorectal cancers are common, and phenocopies may occur in some families; in this instance, testing for MSI might be helpful. If available, direct sequencing of the DNA MMR genes is the gold standard for diagnosis, but some alterations—particularly missense mutations—may be ambiguous and difficult to interpret.

Although the rodent models suggest that inactivation of each of the DNA MMR genes is associated with a unique phenotype, there is less information of this type in human populations. One study has suggested that minor variations in non-colorectal cancers may be found between *hMSH2* and *hMLH1* families.[170] The Muir-Torre syndrome has been linked only to *hMSH2* mutations thus far.[48,49] Of interest, not all kindreds with the mutations found in some Muir-Torre syndrome families will necessarily develop the characteristic skin tumors.

TREATMENT OF HNPCC

When an HNPCC patient presents with an invasive cancer, the appropriate treatment is to perform a subtotal colectomy with an ileosigmoid or ileorectal anastamosis. The increased risk for tumor development in the rest of the colon mandates aggressive surgical treatment, but the ability to screen the rectum for recurrent disease makes a total proctocolectomy unnecessary. If a patient should present with an invasive rectal cancer, a total proctocolectomy may be required. The risk of rectal cancer in a patient with HNPCC after a rectal-sparing operation is approximately 12 percent at 12 years.[171] One report suggested that patients with *hMHS2* mutations had a 28 percent risk of rectal cancer, compared with an 8 percent risk in *hMLH1* patients.[172] The annual rate of metachronous colorectal cancer for their patients was 2.1 percent for *hMLH1* patients, 1.7 percent for *hMSH2* patients, and 0.33 percent for patients with sporadic cancers. When the diagnosis is known at the time of surgery, it is recommended that the proximal colon be removed, even if it is free of neoplasia, to simplify surveillance and protect the patient against the need for a second laparotomy or a missed diagnosis of a proximal cancer.

Patients who are identified in the presymptomatic stage by genetic testing should be informed that their lifetime risk for colorectal cancer may be as high as 80 to 90 percent and that surveillance colonoscopy every 3 years can significantly reduce morbidity and mortality. The occurrence of "interval cancers" in patients who have undergone surveillance at 2- to 3-year intervals has prompted some to argue for more aggressive surveillance, perhaps on an annual basis, because of the unique natural history of these tumors.[173] Surveillance colonoscopy every 2 to 3 years will increase the patient's life expectancy and is less expensive than waiting for signs or symptoms of a colorectal tumor.[174] A task force report from the Cancer Genetics Studies Consortium has recommended colonoscopy every 1 to 3 years beginning at age 20 to 25 in individuals known to have HNPCC.[175] Screening for endometrial carcinoma should begin at 25 to 35 years of age, but the optimal means of surveillance is not yet certain. There is no consensus on screening for cancer of other organs, since the risks are much lower outside the colon and uterus. Some patients will elect surgical removal of the colon and/or uterus (and perhaps ovaries) when informed of the risks of cancer and the limitations of screening; these decisions will depend on the level of risk the patient is willing to assume and his or her attitude about the screening tests. There is insufficient evidence at this time to estimate the effectiveness of screening tests, and some cautious patients may prefer prophylactic surgery.

The age of onset of tumors can be variable within an HNPCC family, leading to the misperception of a "skipped generation," which should be taken into account when managing families.[176] In the same vein, a retrospective study has indicated that in only 40 percent of patients was a family history available that suggested HNPCC when it was actually encountered.[177] In such families, the presence of a villous adenoma in a young patient should heighten the clinical suspicion for HNPCC, and perhaps such a lesion should be interpreted with the same implications as a cancer.

There are no known medical treatments for patients with HNPCC. Aspirin may play an important protective effect against the development of sporadic colorectal cancer; however, its impact on HNPCC is unknown. No other interventions or dietary modifications have been demonstrated to have a beneficial effect in this disease.

ACKNOWLEDGMENTS

This work was supported by Grant RO1-72851 and The Research Service of the Department of Veterans Affairs.

REFERENCES

1. Boland CR: Neoplasia of the gastrointestinal tract, in Yamada T (ed): *Textbook of Gastroenterology*, vol 24, 2d ed. Philadelphia, Lippincott, 1995, pp 578–595.
2. Cannon-Albright LA, Skolnick MH, Bishop DT, et al: Common inheritance of colonic adenomatous polyps and associated colorectal cancers. *N Engl J Med* **319**:533, 1988.

3. Fuchs CS, Giovannucci EL, Colditz GA, et al: A prospective study of family history and the risk of colorectal cancer. *N Engl J Med* **331**:1669, 1994.

4. Winawer SJ, Zauber AG, Gerdes H, et al: Risk of colorectal cancer in the families of patients with adenomatous polyps. The National Polyp Study Workgroup. *N Engl J Med* **334**:82, 1996.

5. Ionov Y, Peinado MA, Malkhosyan S, et al: Ubiquitous somatic mutations in simple repeated sequences reveal a new mechanism for colonic carcinogenesis. *Nature* **363**:558, 1993.

6. Thibodeau SN, Bren G, Schaid D: Microsatellite instability in cancer of the proximal colon. *Science* **260**:816, 1993.

7. Peltomaki P, Aaltonen LA, Sistonen P, et al: Genetic mapping of a locus predisposing to human colorectal cancer. *Science* **260**:810, 1993.

8. Aaltonen LA, Peltomaki P, Leach FS, et al: Clues to the pathogenesis of familial colorectal cancer. *Science* **260**:812, 1993.

9. Lynch HT, Lanspa S, Smyrk T, Boman B, Watson P, Lynch J: Hereditary nonpolyposis colorectal cancer (Lynch syndromes I & II): Genetics, pathology, natural history, and cancer control, part I. *Cancer Genet Cytogenet* **53**:143, 1991.

10. Lynch HT, Ens J, Lynch JF, et al: Tumor variation in three extended Lynch syndrome II kindreds. *Am J Gastroenterol* **83**:74, 1988.

11. Vasen HFA, Offerhaus GJA, den Hartog Jager FCA, et al: The tumor spectrum in hereditary non-polyposis colorectal cancer: a study of 24 kindreds in the Netherlands. *Int J Cancer* **46**:31, 1990.

12. Watson P, Lynch HT: Extracolonic cancer in hereditary nonpolyposis colorectal cancer. *Cancer* **71**:677, 1993.

13. St. John DJB, McDermott FT, Hopper Jl, et al: Cancer risk in relatives of patients with common colorectal cancer. *Ann Intern Med* **118**:785, 1993.

14. Houlston RS, Murday V, Harocopos C, et al: Screening and genetic counselling for relatives of patients with colorectal cancer in a family cancer clinic. *Br Med J* **301**:18, 1990.

15. Mecklin J-P, Jarvinen JH, Aukee S, et al: Screening for colorectal carcinoma in cancer family syndrome kindreds. *Scand J Gastroenterol* **22**:449, 1987.

16. Ponz de Leon M, Sassatelli R, Sacchetti C, et al: Familial aggregation of tumors in the three year experience of a population-based colorectal cancer registry. *Cancer Res* **49**:4344, 1989.

17. Stephenson BM, Finan PJ, Gascoyne J, et al: Frequency of familial colorectal cancer. *Br J Surg* **78**:1162, 1991.

18. Mecklin J-P: Frequency of hereditary colorectal cancer. *Gastroenterology* **93**:1021, 1987.

19. Kee F, Collins BJ: How prevalent is cancer family syndrome? *Gut* **32**:309, 1991.

20. Westlake PJ, Bryant HE, Huchcroft SA, et al: Frequency of hereditary nonpolyposis colorectal cancer in southern Alberta. *Dig Dis Sci* **36**:1441, 1991.

21. Kee F, Collins BJ: Families at risk of colorectal cancer: who are they? *Gut* **33**:787, 1992.

22. Mecklin J-P, Jarvinen HJ, Peltokallio P: Cancer family syndrome: Genetic analysis of 22 Finnish kindreds. *Gastroenterology* **90**:328, 1986.

23. Lynch HT, Smyrk TC, Watson P, et al: Genetics, natural history, tumor spectrum, and pathology of hereditary nonpolyposis colorectal cancer: An updated review. *Gastroenterology* **104**:1535, 1993.

24. Marra G, Boland CR: Hereditary nonpolyposis colorectal cancer (HNPCC): The syndrome, the genes, and an historical perspective. *J Natl Cancer Inst* **87**:1114, 1995.

25. Warthin AS: Heredity with reference to carcinoma. *Arch Intern Med* **12**:546, 1913.

26. Warthin AS: The further study of a cancer family. *J Cancer Res* **9**:279, 1925.

27. Warthin AS: Heredity of carcinoma in man. *Ann Intern Med* **4**:681, 1931.

28. Hauser IJ, Weller CV: A further report on the cancer family of Warthin. *Am J Cancer* **27**:434, 1936.

29. Lynch HT, Krush AJ: Cancer family "G" revisited: 1895-1970. *Cancer* **27**:1505, 1971.

30. Lynch HT, Shaw MW, Magnuson CW, et al: Hereditary factors in two large midwestern kindreds. *Arch Intern Med* **117**:206, 1966.

31. Boland CR, Troncale FJ: Familial colonic cancer in the absence of antecedent polyposis. *Ann Intern Med* **100**:700, 1984.

32. Boland CR: Familial colonic cancer syndromes. *West J Med* **139**:351, 1983.

33. Jager A, Bisgaard M, Myrhoj T, et al: Reduced frequency of extracolonic cancers in hereditary nonpolyposis colorectal cancer families with monoallelic hMLH1 expression. *Am J Hum Genet* **61**:129, 1997.

34. Vasen HFA, Mecklin J-P, Khan PM, et al: The International Collaborative Group on hereditary non-polyposis colorectal cancer. *Dis Colon Rectum* **34**:424, 1991.

35. Kinzler KW, Vogelstein B: Lessons from hereditary colorectal cancer. *Cell* **87**:159, 1996.

36. Dunlop MG, Farrington SM, Carothers AD, et al: Cancer risk associated with germline DNA mismatch repair gene mutations. *Hum Mol Genet* **6**:105, 1997.

37. Vasen H, Wijnen J, Menko F, et al: Cancer risk in families with hereditary nonpolyposis colorectal cancer diagnosed by mutation analysis. *Gastroenterology* **110**:1020, 1996.

38. Rodriguez-Bigas MA, Vasen H, Lynch H, et al: Characteristics of small bowel carcinoma in hereditary nonpolyposis colorectal carcinoma. *Cancer* **83**:240, 1998.

39. Lanspa ST, Lynch HT, Smyrk TC, et al: Colorectal adenomas in the Lynch syndromes: Results of a colonoscopy screening program. *Gastroenterology* **98**:1117, 1990.

40. Jass JR, Stewart SM: Evolution of hereditary non-polyposis colorectal cancer. *Gut* **33**:783 1992.

41. Aarnio M, Salovaara R, Aaltonen LA, et al: Features of gastric cancer in hereditary non-polyposis colorectal cancer syndrome. *Int J Cancer* **74**:551, 1997.

42. Risinger JI, Barrett JC, Watson P, et al: Molecular genetic evidence of the occurrence of breast cancer as an integral tumor in patients with the hereditary nonpolyposis colorectal carcinoma syndrome. *Cancer* **77**:1836, 1996.

43. Vasen HF, Sanders EA, Taal BG, et al: The risk of brain tumors in hereditary non-polyposis colorectal cancer (HNPCC). *Int J Cancer* **65**:422, 1996.

44. Mecklin J-P, Jarvinen HJ, Aukee S, Elomaa I, Karajalainen K: Screening for colorectal carcinoma in cancer family syndrome kindreds. *Scand J Gastroenterol* **22**:449, 1987.

45. Lynch HT, Lynch PM, Pester J, et al: The cancer family syndrome: Rare cutaneous phenotypic linkage of Torre's syndrome. *Arch Intern Med* **141**:607, 1980.

46. Lynch HT, Fusaro RM, Roberts L, et al: Muir-Torre syndrome in several members of a family with a variant of cancer family syndrome. *Br J Dermatol* **113**:295, 1985.

47. Honchel R, Halling KC, Schaid DJ, et al: Microsatellite instability in Muir-Torre syndrome. *Cancer Res* **54**:1159, 1994.

48. Kolodner RD, Hall NR, Lipford J, et al: Structure of the human MSH2 locus and analysis of two Muir-Torre kindreds for msh2 mutations. *Genomics* **24**:516, 1994.

49. Kruse R, Lamberti C, Wang Y, et al: Is the mismatch repair deficient type of Muir-Torre syndrome confined to mutations in the hMSH2 gene? *Hum Genet* **98**:747, 1996.

50. Kee F, Patterson CC, Collins BJ, et al: Histologic characteristics and outcome of familial non-polyposis colorectal cancer. *Scand J Gastroenterol* **26**:419, 1991.

51. Jass JR, Smyrk TC, Stewart SM, et al: Pathology of hereditary non-polyposis colorectal cancer. *Anticancer Res* **14**:1631, 1994.

52. Mecklin J-P, Sipponen P, Jarvinen HJ: Histopathology of colorectal carcinomas and adenomas in cancer family syndrome. *Dis Colon Rectum* **29**:849, 1986.

53. Frei JV: Hereditary nonpolyposis colorectal cancer (Lynch syndrome): II. Diploid malignancies with prolonged survival. *Cancer* **69**:1108, 1992.

54. Kouri M, Laasonen A, Mecklin J-P, et al: Diploid predominance in hereditary nonpolyposis colorectal carcinoma evaluated by flow cytometry. *Cancer* **65**:1825, 1990.

55. Kim H, Jen J, Vogelstein B, et al: Clinical and pathological characteristics of sporadic colorectal carcinomas with DNA replication errors in microsatellite sequences. *Am J Pathol* **145**:148, 1994.

56. Loeb LA: Mutator phenotype may be required for multistage carcinogenesis. *Cancer Res* **51**:3075, 1991.

57. Loeb LA: Microsatellite instability: Marker of a mutator phenotype in cancer. *Cancer Res* **54**:5059, 1994.

58. Peinado MA, Malkhosyan S, Velazquez, et al: Isolation and characterization of allelic losses and gains in colorectal tumors by arbitrarily primed polymerase chain reaction. *Proc Natl Acad Sci USA* **89**:10065, 1992.

59. Boland CR, Thibodeau SN, Hamilton SR, et al: A National Cancer Institute workshop on microsatellite instability for cancer detection and familial predisposition: Development of international criteria for the determination of microsatellite instability in colorectal cancer. *Cancer Res* (in press).

60. Fishel R, Kolodner RD: Identification of mismatch repair genes and their role in the development of cancer. *Curr Opin Genet Dev* **5**:382, 1995.

61. Kolodner RD: Mismatch repair: mechanisms and relationship to cancer susceptibility. *TIBS* **20**:397, 1995.

62. Strand M, Prolla TA, Liskay RM, Petes TD: Destabilization of tracts of simple repetetive DNA in yeast by mutations affecting DNA mismatch repair. *Nature* **365**:274, 1993.

63. Fishel R, Lescoe MK, Rao MRS, et al: The human mutator gene homolog MSH2 and its association with hereditary nonpolyposis colon cancer. *Cell* **75**:1027, 1993.

64. Leach FS, Nicolaides NC, Papadopoulos N, et al: Mutations of a mutS homolog in hereditary nonpolyposis colorectal cancer. *Cell* **75**:1215, 1993.

65. Parsons R, Li G-M, Longley M, et al: Mismatch repair deficiency in phenotypically normal human cells. *Science* **268**:738, 1995.

66. Hemminki A, Peltomaki P, Mecklin J-K: Loss of the wild type MLH1 gene is a feature of hereditary nonpolyposis colorectal cancer. *Nature Genet* **8**:405, 1994.

67. Lindblom A, Tannergard P, Werelius B, et al: Genetic mapping of a second locus predisposing to hereditary non-polyposis colon cancer. *Nature Genet* **5**:279, 1993.

68. Bronner CE, Baker SM, Morrison PT, et al: Mutation in the DNA mismatch repair gene homologue hMLH1 is associated with hereditary non-polyposis colon cancer. *Nature* **368**:258, 1994.

69. Papadopoulos N, Nicolaides NC, Wei YF, et al: Mutation of a mutL homolog in hereditary colon cancer. *Science* **263**:1625, 1994.

70. Nicolaides NC, Papadopoulos N, Liu B, et al: Mutations of two PMS homologues in hereditary nonpolyposis colon cancer. *Nature* **371**:75, 1994.

71. Liu B, Nicolaides NC, Markowitz S, et al: Mismatch repair gene defects in sporadic colorectal cancers with microsatellite instability. *Nature Genet* **9**:48, 1995.

72. Liu B, Parsons R, Papadopoulos N, et al: Analysis of mismatch repair genes in hereditary non-polyposis colorectal cancer. *Nature Med* **2**:169, 1996.

73. Luce MC, Marra G, Chauhan DP, et al: In vitro transcription/ translation assay for the screening of hMLH1 and hMSH2 mutations in familial colon cancer. *Gastroenterology* **109**:1368, 1995.

74. Wijnen JT, Vasen H, Khan PM, et al: Clinical findings with implications for genetic testing in families with clustering of colorectal cancer. *N Engl J Med* **339**:511, 1998.

75. Aaltonen LA, Salovaara R, Kristo P, et al: Incidence of hereditary nonpolyposis colorectal cancer and the feasibility of molecular screening for the disease. *N Engl J Med* **338**:1481, 1998.

76. Nicolaides N, Littman S, Modrich P, et al: A naturally occurring hPMS2 mutation can confer a dominant negative mutator phenotype. *Mol Cell Biol* **18**:1635, 1998.

77. Acharya S, Wilson T, Gradia S, et al: hMSH2 forms specific mispair-binding complexes with hMSH3 and hMSH6. *Proc Natl Acad Sci USA* **93**:13629, 1996.

78. Miyaki M, Konishi M, Tanaka K, et al: Germline mutation of MSH6 as the cause of hereditary nonpolyposis colorectal cancer. *Nature Genet* **17**:271, 1997.

79. Akiyama Y, Sato H, Yamada T, et al: Germ-line mutation of the hMSH6/GTBP gene in an atypical hereditary nonpolyposis colorectal cancer kindred. *Cancer Res* **57**:3920, 1997.

80. Lu SL, Kawabata M, Imamura T, et al: HNPC associated with germline mutation in the TGF-β type II receptor gene. *Nature Genet* **19**:17, 1998.

81. Cooper DL, Lahue RS, Modrich P: Methyl-directed mismatch repair is bidirectional. *J Biol Chem* **268**:11823, 1993.

82. Kunkel TA: Misalignment-mediated DNA synthesis errors. *Biochemistry* **29**:8003, 1990.

83. Modrich P: Mechanisms and biological effects of mismatch repair. *Annu Rev Genet* **25**:229, 1991.

84. Sancar A: DNA repair in humans. *Annu Rev Genet* **29**:69, 1995.

85. Drummond JT, Li G-M, Longley MJ, et al: Isolation of an hMSH2-p160 heterodimer that restores DNA mismatch repair to tumor cells. *Science* **268**:1909, 1995.

86. Umar A, Boyer JC, Kunkel TA: DNA loop repair by human cell extracts. *Science* **266**:814, 1994.

87. Marra G, Boland CR: DNA repair and colorectal cancer. *Gastroenterol Clin North Am* **25**(4):**755, 1996.**

88. Marsischky GT, Filosi N, Kane MF, et al: Redundancy of *Saccharomyces cerevisiae* MSH3 and MSH6 in MSH2-dependent mismatch repair. *Genes Dev* **10**:407, 1996.

89. Nicolaides NC, Carter KC, Shell BK, et al: Genomic organization of the human PMS2 gene family. *Genomics* **30**:195, 1995.

90. Wilson TM, Ewel A, Duguid JR, et al: Differential cellular expression of the human MSH2 repair enzyme in small and large intestine. *Cancer Res* **55**:5146, 1995.

91. Leach FS, Polyak K, Burrell M, et al: Expression of the human mismatch repair gene hMSH2 in normal and neoplastic tissues. *Cancer Res* **56**:235, 1996.

92. Marra G, Chang CL, Laghi LA, Chauhan DP, Young D, Boland CR: Expression of the human MutS homolog 2 (hMSH2) protein in resting and proliferating cells. *Oncogene* **13**:2189, 1996.

93. de Wind N, Dekker M, Berns A, et al: Inactivation of the mouse Msh2 gene results in mismatch repair deficiency, methylation tolerance, hyperrecombination, and predisposition to cancer. *Cell* **82**:321, 1995.

94. Reitmair AH, Redston M, Cai JC, et al: Spontaneous carcinomas and skin neoplasms in Msh2-deficient mice. *Cancer Res* **56**:3842, 1996.

95. Prolla TA, Baker SM, Harris AC, et al: Tumour susceptibility and spontaneous mutation in mice deficient in Mlh1, Pms1 and Pms2 DNA mismatch repair. *Nature Genet* **18**:276, 1998.

96. Narayanan L, Fritzell JA, Baker SM, et al: Elevated levels of mutation in multiple tissues of mice deficient in the DNA mismatch repair gene Pms2. *Proc Natl Acad Sci USA* **94**:3122, 1997.

97. Baker SM, Harris AC, Tsao JL, et al: Enhanced intestinal adenomatous polyp formation in Pms2; Min Mice. *Cancer Res* **58**:1087, 1998.

98. Edelmann W, Yang K, Umar A, et al: Mutation in the mismatch repair gene Msh6 causes cancer susceptibility. *Cell* **92**:467, 1997.

99. Edelmann W, Cohen PE, Kane M, et al: Meiotic pachytene arrest in MLH1-deficient mice. *Cell* **85**:1125, 1996.

100. Baker SM, Plug AW, Prolla TA, et al: Involvement of mouse Mlh1 in DNA mismatch repair and meiotic crossing over. *Nature Genet* **13**:336, 1996.

101. Baker SM, Bronner CE, Zhang L, et al: Male mice defective in the DNA mismatch repair gene PMS2 exhibit abnormal chromosome synapsis in meiosis. *Cell* **82**:309, 1995.

102. Fearon ER, Vogelstein B: A genetic model for colorectal tumorigenesis. *Cell* **61**:759, 1990.

103. Cottu PH, Muzeau F, Estreicher A, et al: Inverse correlation between RER$^+$ status and p53 mutation in colorectal cancer cell lines. *Oncogene* **13**:2727, 1996.

104. Konishi M, Kikuchi-Yanoshita R, Tanaka K, et al: Molecular nature of colon tumors in hereditary nonpolyposis colon cancer, familial polyposis, and sporadic colon cancer. *Gastroenterology* **111**:307, 1996.

105. Losi L, Ponz de Leon M, Jiricny J, et al: K-ras and p53 mutations in hereditary non-polyposis colorectal cancers. *Int J Cancer* **74**:94, 1997.

106. Kim H, Jen J, Vogelstein B, et al: Clinical and pathological characteristics of sporadic colorectal carcinomas with DNA replication errors in microsatellite sequences. *Am J Pathol* **145**:148, 1994.

107. Ilyas M, Tomlinson IP, Novelli MR, et al: Clinico-pathological features and p53 expression in left-sided sporadic colorectal cancer with and without microsatellite instability. *J Pathol* **179**:370, 1996.

108. Huang J, Papadopoulos N, McKinley AJ, et al: APC mutations in colorectal tumors with mismatch repair deficiency. *Proc Natl Acad Sci USA* **93**:9049, 1996.

109. Shibata D, Peinado MA, Ionov Y, et al: Genomic instability in repeated sequences is an early somatic event in colorectal tumorigenesis that persists after transformation. *Nature Genet* **6**:273, 1994.

110. Willliams GT, Geraghty JM, Campbell F, et al: Normal colonic mucosa in hereditary non-polyposis colorectal cancer shows no generalised increase in somatic mutation. *Br J Cancer* **71**:1077, 1995.

111. Jacoby RF, Marshall DJ, Kailas S, et al: Genetic instability associated with adenoma to carcinoma progression in hereditary colon cancer. *Gastroenterology* **109**:73, 1995.

112. Shibata D, Navidi W, Salovaara R, et al: Somatic microsatellite mutations as molecular tumor clocks. *Nature Med* **2**:676, 1996.

113. Aaltonen LA, Peltomaki P, Mecklin J-P, et al: Replication errors in benign and malignant tumors from hereditary nonpolyposis colorectal cancer patients. *Cancer Res* **54**:1645, 1994.

114. Thibodeau SN, French AJ, Roche PC, et al: Altered expression of hMSH2 and hMLH1 in tumors with microsatellite instability and genetic alterations in mismatch repair genes. *Cancer Res* **56**:4836, 1996.

115. Thibodeau SN, French AJ, Cunningham JM, et al: Microsatellite instability in colorectal cancer: Different mutator phenotypes and the principal involvement of hMLH1. *Cancer Res* **58**:1713, 1998.

116. Kane MF, Loda M, Gaida GM, et al: Methylation of the hMLH1 promoter correlates with lack of expression of hMLH1 in sporadic

colon tumors and mismatch repair-defective human tumor cell lines. *Cancer Res* 57:808, 1997.

117. Herman JG, Umar A, Polyak K, et al: Incidence and functional consequences of hMLH1 promoter hypermethylation in colorectal carcinoma. *Proc Natl Acad Sci USA* 95:6870, 1998.

118. Veigl ML, Kasturi L, Olechnowicz J, et al: Biallelic inactivation of hMLH1 by epigenetic gene silencing, a novel mechanism causing human MSI cancers. *Proc Natl Acad Sci USA* 95:8698, 1998.

119. Cunningham JM, Christensen ER, Tester DJ, et al: Hypermethylation of the hMLH1 promoter in colon cancer with microsatellite instability. *Cancer Res* 58:3455, 1998.

120. Eshleman JR, Lang EZ, Bowerfind GK, et al: Increased mutation rate at the hprt locus accompanies microsatellite instability in colon cancer. *Oncogene* 10:33, 1995.

121. Markowitz S, Wang J, Myeroff L, et al: Inactivation of the type II TGF-β receptor in colon cancer cells with microsatellite instability. *Science* 268:1336, 1995.

122. Alexandrow M, Moses HL: Transforming growth factor β and cell cycle regulation. *Cancer Res* 55:1452, 1995.

123. Myeroff LL, Parsons R, Kim SJ, et al: A transforming growth factor β receptor type II gene mutation common in colon and gastric but rare in endometrial cancers with microsatellite instability. *Cancer Res* 55:5545, 1995.

124. Akiyama Y, Iwanaga R, Saitoh K, et al: Transforming growth factor β type II receptor gene muations in adenomas from hereditary nonpolyposis colorectal cancer. *Gastroenterology* 112:33, 1997.

125. Grady WM, Rajput A, Myeroff L, et al: Mutation of the type II transforming growth factor-β receptor is coincident with the transformation of human colon adenomas to malignant carcinomas. *Cancer Res* 58:3101, 1998.

126. Souza R, Appel R, Yin J, et al: Microsatellite instability in the insulin-like growth factor II receptor gene in gastrointestinal tumours. *Nature Genet* 14:255, 1996.

127. Rampino N, Yamamoto H, Ionov Y, et al: Somatic frameshift mutations in the BAX gene in colon cancers of the microsatellite mutator phenotype. *Science* 275:967, 1997.

128. Akiyama Y, Tsubouchi N, Yuasa Y: Frequent somatic mutations of hMSH3 with reference to microsatellite instability in hereditary nonpolyposis colorectal cancer. *Biochem Biophys Res Commun* 236:248, 1997.

129. Ikeda M, Orimo H, Moriyama H, et al: Close correlation between mutations of E2F4 and hMSH3 genes in colorectal cancers with microsatellite instability. *Cancer Res* 58:594, 1998.

130. Yagi OK, Akiyama Y, Nomizu T, et al: Proapoptotic gene BAX is frequently mutated in hereditary nonpolyposis colorectal cancers but not in adenomas. *Gastroenterology* 114:268, 1998.

131. Yamamoto H, Sawai H, Weber TK, et al: Somatic frameshift mutations in DNA mismatch repair and proapoptosis genes in hereditary nonpolyposis colorectal cancer. *Cancer Res* 58:997, 1998.

132. Yin J, Kong D, Wang S, et al: Mutation of hMSH3 and hMSH6 mismatch repair genes in genetically unstable human colorectal and gastric carcinomas. *Hum Mutat* 10:474, 1997.

133. Yoshitaka T, Matsubara N, Ikeda M, et al: Mutations of E2F-4 trinucleotide repeats in colorectal cancer with microsatellite instability. *Biochem Biophys Res Commun* 227:553, 1996.

134. Perucho M: Microsatellite instability: The mutator that mutates the other mutator. *Nature Med* 2:630, 1996.

135. White RL, Fox MS: Genetic consequences of transfection with hetero-duplex bacteriophage lambda DNA. *Mol Gen Genet* 141:163, 1975.

136. Koi M, Umar A, Chauhan DP, et al: Human chromosome 3 corrects mismatch repair deficiency and microsatellite instability and reduces N-methyl-N'nitro-N-nitrosoguanidine tolerance in humancolon tumor cells with homozygous hMLH1 mutation. *Cancer Res* 54:4308, 1994.

137. Hawn MT, Umar A, Carethers JM, et al: Evidence for a connection between the mismatch repair system and the G2 cell cycle checkpoint. *Cancer Res* 55:3721, 1995.

138. Mellon I, Rajpal DK, Koi M, et al: Transcription-coupled nucleotide excision repair deficiency associated with mutations in human mismatch repair genes. *Science* 272:557, 1996.

139. Carethers JM, Chauhan DP, Fink D, Nebel S, Bresailer RS, Howell SB, Boland CR: Mismatch repair proficiency and *in vitro* response to 5-fluorouracil. *Gastroenterology* 117:123, 1999.

140. Aebi S, Kurdi-Haidar B, Gordon R, et al: Loss of DNA mismatch repair in acquired resistance to cisplatin. *Cancer Res* 56:3087, 1996.

141. Duckett DR, Drummond JT, Murchie AIH, et al: Human MutSa recognizes damaged DNA base pairs containing O^6-methylthymine, or the cisplatin-d(GpG) adduct. *Proc Natl Acad Sci USA* 93:6443, 1996.

142. Fink D, Nebel S, Norris PS, et al: The effect of different chemotherapeutic agents on the enrichment of DNA mismatch repair-deficient tumour cells. *Br J Cancer* 77:703, 1998.

143. Aebi S, Kurdi-Haidar B, Gordon R, et al: Loss of DNA mismatch repair in acquired resistance to cisplatin. *Cancer Res* 56:3087, 1996.

144. Boyer JC, Umar A, Risinger JI, et al: Microsatellite instability, mismatch repair deficiency, and genetic defects in human cancer cell lines. *Cancer Res* 55:6063, 1995.

145. Suzuki H, Harpaz N, Tarmin L, et al: Microsatellite instability in ulcerative colitis-associated colorectal dysplasias and cancers. *Cancer Res* 54:4841, 1994.

146. Brentnall TA, Rubin CE, Crispin DA, et al: A germline substitution in the human MSH2 gene is associated with cancer and high grade dysplasia in ulcerative colitis. *Gastroenterology* 109:151, 1995.

147. Brentnall TA, Crispin DA, Bronner MP, et al: Microsatellite instability is present in non-neoplastic mucosa from patients with longstanding ulcerative colitis. *Cancer Res* 56:1237, 1996.

148. Rodriguez-Bigas MA, Boland CR, Hamilton SR, et al: A National Cancer Institute workshop on hereditary nonpolyposis colorectal cancer syndrome: Meeting highlights and Bethesda guidelines. *J Natl Cancer Inst* 89:1758, 1997.

149. Bocker T, Diermann J, Friedl W, et al: Microsatellite instability analysis: A multicenter study for reliability and quality control. *Cancer Res* 57:4739, 1997.

150. Dietmaier W, Wallinger S, Bocker T, et al: Diagnostic microsatellite instabilty: Definition and correlation with mismatch repair protein expression. *Cancer Res* 57:4749, 1997.

151. Samowitz WS, Slattery ML, Kerber RA: Microsatellite instability in human colonic cancer is not a useful clinical indicator of familial colorectal cancer. *Gastroenterology* 109:1765, 1995.

152. Froggatt NJ, Koch J, Davies R, et al: Genetic linkage analysis in hereditary non-polyposis colon cancer syndrome. *J Med Genet* 32:352, 1995.

153. Luce MC, Marra G, Chauhan DP, et al: In vitro transcription/translation assay for the screening of hMLH1 and hMSH2 mutations in familial colon cancer. *Gastroenterology* 109:1368, 1995.

154. Hall NR, Taylor GR, Finan PJ, et al: Intron splice acceptor site sequence variation in the hereditary non-polyposis colorectal cancer gene hMSH2. *Eur J Cancer* 30A:1550, 1994.

155. Charbonnier F, Martin C, Scotte M, et al: Alternative splicing of MLH1 messenger RNA in human normal cells. *Cancer Res* 55:1839, 1995.

156. Xia L, Shen W, Ritacca F, et al: A truncated hMSH2 transcript occurs as a common variant in the population: Implications for genetic diagnosis. *Cancer Res* 56:2289, 1996.

157. Lahti MN, Sistonen P, Mecklin JP, et al: Close linkage to chromosome 3p and conservation of ancestral founding haplotype in hereditary nonpolyposis colorectal cancer families. *Proc Natl Acad Sci USA* 91:6054, 1994.

158. Lahti MN, Kristo P, Nicolaides NC, et al: Founding mutations and Alu-mediated recombination in hereditary colon cancer. *Nature Med* 1:1203, 1995.

159. Peltomaki P, Vaden H, et al: Mutations predisposing to hereditary nonpolyposis colorectal cancer: Database and results of a collaborative study. *Gastroenterology* 113:1146, 1997.

160. Watson P, Vasen HFA, Mecklin JP, et al: The risk of endometrial cancer in hereditary nonpolyposis colorectal cancer. *Am J Med* 96:516, 1994.

161. Aarnio M, Mecklin JP, Aaltonen LA, et al: Life-time risk of different cancers in hereditary nonpolyposis colorectal cancer (HNPCC) syndrome. *Int J Cancer* 64:430, 1995.

162. Sankila R, Aaltonen LA, Jarvinen HJ, et al: Better survival rates in patients with MLH1-associated hereditary colorectal cancer. *Gastroenterology* 110:682, 1996.

163. Jarvinen HJ, Mecklin JP, Sistonen P: Screening reduces colorectal cancer rate in families with hereditary nonpolyposis colorectal cancer. *Gastroenterology* 108:1405, 1995.

164. Watson P, Lin KM, Rodriguez-Bigas MA, et al: Colorectal carcinoma survival among hereditary nonpolyposis colorectal carcinoma family members. *Cancer* 83:259, 1998.

165. Percesepe A, Benatti P, Roncucci L, et al: Survival analysis in families affected by hereditary nonpolyposis colorectal cancer. *Int J Cancer* 71:373, 1997.

166. Ponz de Leon M, Casa GD, Benatti P, et al: Frequency and type of colorectal tumors in asymptomatic high-risk individuals in families with hereditary nonpolyposis colorectal cancer. *Cancer Epidemiol Biomark Prevent* 7:639, 1998.

167. Watanabe T, Muto T, Sawada T, et al: Flat adenoma as a precursor of colorectal carcinoma in hereditary nonpolyposis colorectal carcinoma. *Cancer* **77**:627, 1996.
168. Hall NR, Finan PJ, Ward B, et al: Genetic susceptibility to colorectal cancer in patients under 45 years of age. *Br J Surg* **81**:1485, 1994.
169. Liu B, Farrington SM, Petersen GM, et al: Genetic instability occurs in the majority of young patients with colorectal cancer. *Nature Med* **1**:348, 1995.
170. Vasen HFA, Wijnen JT, Menko FH, et al: Cancer risk in families with hereditary nonpolyposis colorectal cancer diagnosed by mutation analysis. *Gastroenterology* **110**:1020, 1996.
171. Rodriguez-Bigas MA, Vasen HF, Pekka-Mecklin J, et al: Rectal cancer risk in hereditary nonpolyposis colorectal cancer after abdominal colectomy. International Collaborative Group on HNPCC. *Ann Surg* **225**:202, 1997.
172. Lin KM, Shashidharan M, Ternent CA, et al: Colorectal and extracolonic cancer variations in MLH1/MSH2 hereditary nonpoly-posis colorectal cancer kindreds and the general population. *Dis Colon Rectum* **41**:428, 1998.
173. Vasen HFA, Nagengast FM, Khan PM: Interval cancers in hereditary non-polyposis colorectal cancer (Lynch syndrome). *Lancet* **345**:1183, 1995.
174. Vasen H, van Ballegooijen M, Buskens E, et al: A cost-effectiveness analysis of colorectal screening of hereditary nonpolyposis colorectal carcinoma gene carriers. *Cancer* **82**:1632, 1998.
175. Burke W, Petersen G, Lynch P, et al: Recommendations for follow-up care of individuals with an inherited predisposition to cancer. *JAMA* **277**:915, 1997.
176. Menko FH, Te Meerman GJ, Sampson JR: Variable age of onset in hereditary nonpolyposis colorectal cancer: Clinical implications. *Gastroenterology* **104**:946, 1993.
177. Mecklin JP, Jarvinen HJ: Clinical features of colorectal carcinoma in cancer family syndrome. *Dis Colon Rectum* **29**:160, 1986.

Werner Syndrome

Gerard D. Schellenberg ■ Tetsuro Miki
Chang-En Yu ■ Jun Nakura

1. Werner syndrome (WS) is a rare autosomal recessive disorder that is observed in many different ethnic groups. Prevalence estimates range from 1 in 22,000 to 1 in 1 million. All cases of WS are inherited and result from mutations in a single gene.
2. WS is characterized clinically by the premature appearance of cataracts, scleroderma-like skin pathology, short stature, graying hair and hair loss, and a general appearance of premature aging. More variable features include adult-onset diabetes mellitus, hypogonadism, osteoporosis, osteosclerosis, soft tissue calcification, hyperkeratosis, ulcers on the feet and ankles, premature vascular disease, elevated rates of some neoplasms, a hoarse high-pitched voice, and flat feet. Subjects often appear 20 to 30 years older than their chronologic age, and WS may be a model disease for accelerated aging. The mean age at death is 47 years, with the leading cause being neoplasia, followed by myocardial infarcts and cerebral vascular incidents.
3. WS subjects are at increased risk for a variety of neoplasms. This increased risk results primarily from an increase in non-epithelial-derived cancers and is not an across-the-board elevation in all common cancers. Soft tissue sarcomas, osteosarcomas, melanomas, and thyroid cancer are the predominant forms of cancer.
4. The gene for WS (*WRN*), located on chromosome 8p12, has been cloned and encodes a 1432-amino acid protein (WRNp) that has homology to the super-family of DExH box DNA and RNA helicases; WRNp has the seven motifs found in this class of protein, including the ATP-binding and Mg^{2+}-binding motifs. Outside the helicase domain, WRNp is homologous to an RNase D motif that may indicate a $3' \rightarrow 5'$ proofreading exonuclease activity.
5. Mutations have been identified in the *WRN* gene in all WS subjects studied. All the mutations result in a predicted truncated protein, the result of either a nonsense mutation or mutations leading to a frameshift. One splice-junction mutation is found in 50 to 60 percent of Japanese WS subjects. WS appears to be the result of loss of function of WRNp. No missense WS mutations have been found.
6. *In vitro*, WRNp is a functional $3' \rightarrow 5'$ DNA helicase. The *in vivo* function of WRNp is not known. WS is a genomic instability syndrome with elevated rates of chromosomal translocation and deletions and an elevated somatic cell mutation rate. This mutator phenotype, resulting from the loss of WRNp, could be a defect in an as yet unidentified DNA repair system, a defect in DNA replication initiation, or a defect in some other aspect of DNA metabolism that requires DNA unwinding.

Werner syndrome (WS) is a rare autosomal recessive disease first described in 1904 by Otto Werner in his doctoral thesis.[1,2] As a medical student in an ophthalmologic clinic, Werner saw a family with two brothers and two sisters, ages 31, 36, 38, and 40 years, with bilateral cataracts, sclerodermal skin changes, hyperkeratosis, and ulcers on the feet and ankles. He observed that one 36-year-old gave "the impression of extreme senility," thus hinting in this early work at the potential connection between WS and accelerated aging.[2] In 1934, Oppenheimer and Kugel[3] extended the description of the disease and gave it the eponym *Werner's syndrome*. Thannhauser, in a classic article published in 1945, described many of the clinical features now associated with WS.[4]

The WS phenotype is complex, age-dependent, and variable (Figs. 19-1 and 19-2). Affected subjects are typically normal throughout childhood and early adolescence, with the only symptoms being growth retardation occurring at or near puberty. Beginning in the second and third decades of life, graying and loss of hair begin, and scleroderma-like changes occur typically on the face, legs, and feet. In the fourth and subsequent decades, WS individuals develop many of the diseases that are common in the elderly, including arteriosclerotic vascular disease, neoplasms, diabetes mellitus, osteoporosis, and bilateral cataracts (for reviews of the clinical features of WS, see refs. 4 through 9). WS individuals often are described as having a "senile" appearance and look 20 to 30 years older than their true chronologic age.

Over the past 20 to 30 years, the biochemistry, cell biology, and genetics of WS have been studied intensively. The vigor with which this disorder has been pursued is not based on its importance to public health, since WS is quite rare. The physical appearance of premature aging and other clinical features led to the proposal that WS is a partial model of accelerated human aging.[10] Parallels between WS and aging are also based on *in vitro* studies of cell growth potential. In fibroblasts from normal subjects, the number of doublings a culture is capable of before senescence occurs is inversely proportional to the age of the donor; cultures from children have a cumulative cell-doubling capacity of approximately 50 divisions, whereas cultures from elderly donors are capable of only 30 to 40 divisions.[7,11] In contrast, WS fibroblasts have a very limited potential for division, with a mean cumulative doubling of only 12.4.[7,12] Thus WS has been studied in the hope that WS also may provide clues to how aging processes contribute to susceptibility to some of the common diseases of old age.

Another feature of WS is an elevated risk for a wide variety of cancers[13] and that WS cells exhibit genomic instability. Genomic instability has been demonstrated both *in vitro* and *in vivo* as an elevated somatic cell mutation rate,[14–17] as well as increased rates of random chromosomal breakage, deletions, and rearrangements.[18–24] A number of other inherited disorders also exhibit the combination of genomic instability and elevated cancer risks (see Chaps. 14, 15, 16, and 18 for discussions of xeroderma pigmentosum, ataxia-telangiectasia, Bloom syndrome, and hereditary nonpolyposis colorectal cancer, respectively). The study of WS and other inherited cancer-susceptibility disorders may provide additional clues to the mechanisms of cancer development.

A list of standard abbreviations is located immediately preceding the index. Nonstandard abbreviations used in this chapter include: WS = Werner syndrome; HA = hyaluronic acid; VTRP = variable transcription repeat; YAC = yeast artificial chromosome.

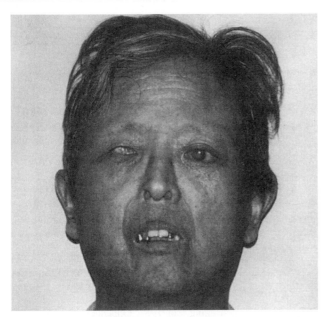

Fig. 19-1 A 51-year-old Japanese WS patient (definite diagnosis by the criteria in Table 19-3) with a known *WRN* mutation. See refs. 3, 4, 6, 38, and 128 for other photographs of WS subjects.

Positional cloning methods have been used to identify the gene responsible for WS[25] (the *WRN* gene). This gene encodes a predicted protein homologous to a superfamily of enzymes termed *helicases* that unwind double-stranded RNA or DNA into single strands. Now that the *WRN* gene has been identified, it should be possible to design experimental approaches to directly address questions concerning the relationship of WS to aging and age-related disease processes.

CLINICAL ASPECTS OF WS

Prevalence

Prevalence estimates for WS are difficult to obtain because the disorder is extremely rare, a fact that makes case finding difficult. Also, since the appearance of the full phenotypic spectrum of WS is not complete until the third and fourth decades of life (average age at diagnosis is 38.7 years[6]), younger subjects may be missed. Two methods have been used to generate prevalence and gene-frequency estimates. The first is case counting in defined populations. This method depends on case identification by community physicians. Since WS is rare and many physicians may not be familiar with the disorder, underdiagnosis may result, and the true prevalence may be underestimated. Also, the number of cases actually identified is typically small, making the estimates inaccurate. The second method for estimating prevalence is based on comparing consanguinity rates in the parents of WS subjects to estimates of consanguinity rates in the general population.[26,27] This method depends on accurate estimates of consanguinity in the general population. Consanguinity rates are difficult to measure and may vary even within an ethnic group or country, depending on whether the cases come from rural or urban settings.[28] Case-counting methods have yielded estimates ranging from 1 in 95,000 to 1 in 455,000 (Table 19-1), corresponding to allele frequencies of 0.0032 and 0.0015, respectively.[5,29] Prevalence estimates based on consanguinity rates range from 1 in 22,000 to 1 in 1 million, corresponding to allele frequencies of 0.0067 and 0.001, respectively.[5,6,29] Now that the gene has been cloned, populations can be screened directly for specific mutations,[25] and direct measurements of carrier frequencies can be obtained. In a preliminary study, 178 Japanese control subjects were screened for the most common Japanese WS mutation (mutation 4 in Table 19-2) by direct DNA sequencing. This mutation appears to account

for 50 to 60 percent of all Japanese WS cases. A single heterozygote was identified, yielding an allele frequency of 0.0027 with a 95 percent upper confidence limit of 0.008.[25] Based on a mutation frequency of 60 in Japanese WS cases, the allele frequency in the Japanese population for all WS alleles should be approximately 0.0045. This frequency estimate is within the range of estimates (0.001–0.0067) obtained by the methods described

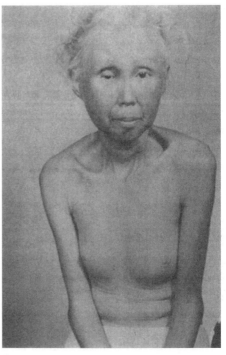

A

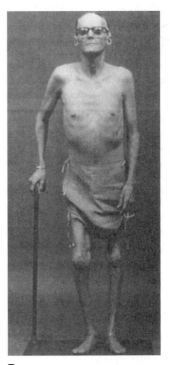

B

Fig. 19-2 *A.* A 48-year-old Japanese woman with WS (case 1 in Epstein et al.[6]). *B.* A 51-year-old Caucasian man with WS. Subject has typical thin limbs with normal trunk with scleroderma-like skin atrophy of the lower legs and feet. *C.* Skin atrophy of the feet and ankles. *D,E.* Ulcers on the ankles.

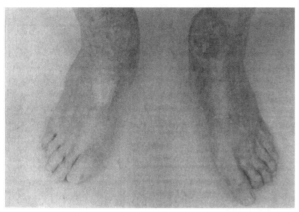

C

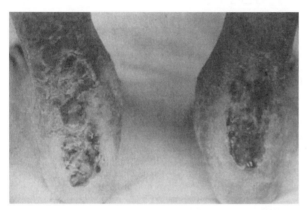

D

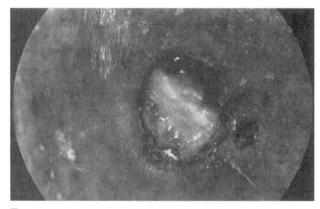

E

Fig. 19-2 (Continued)

above. Additional studies with a larger sample are needed to establish reliable allele frequency estimates for WS mutations.

Fraction of WS That Is Due to Inherited Factors

There is no evidence that WS is genetically or etiologically heterogeneous. The genetic mapping studies discussed below

suggest that WS in different ethnic groups is caused by the same locus on chromosome 8.[30–32] Subsequent identification of the gene permitted mutational analysis; to date, mutations in this gene, either in the homozygous state or as compound heterozygotes, have been identified in all the patients studied[25,33–37] (see Table 19-2). Thus all WS appears to be inherited. No WS phenocopies have been documented. The existence of new mutations on a heterozygous background cannot be ruled out. While a subject's environment may influence the expression of various components of the WS phenotype, there is no evidence that there is sporadic WS induced by environmental factors.

Diagnostic Criteria

There are no generally accepted standard diagnostic criteria for WS, although several have been used in research. The clinical picture of WS has been developed from case studies of subjects who are frequently in their thirties or forties. Since an early diagnosis usually is not possible, the onset of features such as growth cessation and graying of the hair is estimated retrospectively, depends on the subject's recollections, and may not be precise. Further, cohorts of WS subjects have not been followed longitudinally until death with subsequent autopsies; thus estimates of late-onset features such as vascular disease, diabetes mellitus, and neoplasms may be low. Estimates of the prevalence of a particular feature can vary considerably. For example, estimates of the percentage of WS patients with vascular disease vary from 25 percent[6] to 100 percent.[29] This variability may reflect the ages of the patient groups studied, different environmental influences (e.g., diet), or differing genetic backgrounds in different ethnic groups. Despite the limitations of the data collected, the clinical description of WS discussed below is remarkably consistent across the large numbers of WS cases that have been described in the literature. The reader is referred to Epstein et al.[6] for an excellent detailed description of the clinical and pathologic findings in a large number of WS subjects.

Two different criteria for diagnosis have been used in research on WS. The criteria used by Nakura et al.[32] (Table 19-3) consist of six primary features found in most WS subjects and an additional nine symptoms found less consistently. A diagnosis of "definite" requires all six cardinal symptoms and two of the less frequent features. "Probable" WS requires the first three cardinal signs and any two others. One limitation of these criteria is that hyaluronic acid analysis is not routinely available. Also, while parental consanguinity is a useful indicator of recessive inheritance, the majority of Caucasian subjects (64 percent[6]) and many Japanese subjects (20–32 percent[38,39]) are not from consanguineous families. Goto and coworkers[5] used a similar set of criteria (Table 19-4), and a diagnosis of WS requires that a subject have three of the four major symptom groups.

Features Found in Most Patients

Cataracts. The most constant feature of WS is cataracts (see Fig. 19-1), which are present in 94 to 100 percent of the subjects[6,7,39] (see Table 19-3). Cataracts typically appear in the third decade of life. In different case-review studies, the observed mean age at appearance was between 23 years[39] and 30 years.[6] Cataracts are usually bilateral, although they may be at different stages of development in each eye, and are typically indistinguishable from those seen in elderly subjects (see ref. 6 for a detailed review of ocular pathologies).

Table 19-1 Estimates of Prevalence Rates for WS

Population	Case-Counting-Based Estimates	Consanguinity-Based Estimates	Reference
Caucasian (Sardinian)	1/95,000 to 1/203,000	1/93,000 to 1/455,000	29
Japanese	1/300,000 to 1/500,000	1/22,000 to 1/370,000	5
Mostly Caucasian		1/45,000 to 1/1,000,000	6

Table 19-2 Summary of *WRN* Mutations

Mutation	Codon	Exon	Type of Mutation	Nucleotide Sequence	Comment	Predicted Protein Length
None	—	—	—	—	—	1432
1	1165	30	Substitution	CAG (Gln) to T*A*G (terminator)	Nonsense	1164
2	1305	33	Substitution	CGA (Arg) to T*G*A (terminator)	Nonsense	1304
3	1230–1273	32	4-bp deletion	ACAG deleted	Deletion/frameshift	1245
4	1047–1078	26	Substitution	tag-GGT to ta*c*-GGT	Substitution at a splice-donor site, exon 26 excluded	1060
A	369	9	Substitution	CGA (Arg) to TGA (terminator)	Nonsense	368
B	889	22	Substitution	CGA (Arg) to TGA (terminator)	Nonsense	888
C	759–816	20	Substitution	GAG-gta to CAG-tta	Substitution at splice-receptor site	760
D	389	9	1-bp deletion	AGAG (Arg) to GAG (Glu)	Frameshift	391
E	697–942	19–23	Deletion (> 15 kb)	—	Genomic deletion	1186
F	1154–1191	30	Deletion of exon 30 from WRN cDNA	—	—	1157
G	1104–1128	28	Deletion of exon 28 from the WRN cDNA	—	—	1138
H	426	10	4-bp insertion	ATCT inserted	Insertion/frameshift	429
I	696	18	105-bp insertion	—	Insertion/frameshift	708
J	697–942	19–23	Deletion of exons 19–23 from the WRN cDNA	—	Deletion/frameshift	704
K	1149	29	1-bp deletion	GAG (Glu) to GGC (Gly)	Deletion/frameshift	1160
L	1154	30		tttgttcagATT to ttagTTCAGATT	Altered splice site, frameshift	1165
M	463	11	Substitution	TAT (Tyr) TAA (terminator)	Nonsense	462
N	168	5	2-bp deletion	AAG (Lys) to GCT (Ala)	Frameshift	176

NOTE: Mutations A–N were not numbered due to different numbers being assigned to different mutations in published descriptions.

Table 19-3 Signs of WS

Feature	Mean Age of Onset (years)	Onset Range (years)	Number of Patients Affected (%)
Cardinal signs			
1. Bilateral cataracts	23–30	10–46	94–100
2. Dermatological pathology (tight skin, atrophic skin, pigmentary alterations, ulceration, hyperkeratosis, regional subcutaneous atrophy), characteristic "bird" facies	23, 25	5–42	86–100
3. Short stature	13	10–20	86–100
4. Consanguinity (3d cousin or greater) or affected sibling	N.A.	N.A.	68
5. Premature graying and/or thinning of scalp hair	20–21	5–42	80–100
6. Positive hyaluronic acid test	N.A.D.	N.A.D	100
Further signs and symptoms			
1. Diabetes mellitus	30–34[6,39]	10–55	44–67*
2. Hypogonadism (secondary sexual underdevelopment, diminished fertility, testicular or ovarian atrophy)	N.A.	N.A.	
3. Osteoporosis	N.A.D.	N.A.D.	33–100
4. Osteosclerosis of distal phalanges of fingers and/or toes (X-ray diagnosis)	N.A.D.	N.A.D.	N.A.D.
5. Soft tissue calcification	N.A.D.	N.A.D.	25–53
6. Premature atherosclerosis (e.g., history of myocardial infarction)	N.A.D.	N.A.D.	25–100
7. Mesenchymal neoplasms, rare neoplasms, or multiple neoplasms	N.A.D.	20–64†	N.A.D.
8. Voice changes (high-pitched squeaky or hoarse voice)	21–27	10–40	50–100
9. Flat feet	N.A.D.	N.A.D.	

NOTE: Diagnostic criteria are reproduced from Nakura et al.[32] (with permission from *Genomics*) and categories are as follows: definite, all cardinal signs, (number 6 when available) and any two others; probable, the first three cardinal signs and any two others; possible, either cataracts or dermatological alterations and any four others; exclusion, onset of signs and symptoms before adolescence (except short stature) or a negative hyaluronic acids test.

Data on prevalence estimates of symptoms and onset means are primarily from several case-report summaries.[6,29,39–43] as summarized by Tollefsbol and Cohen[7] and from Goto.[50] N.A.D., no available data; N.A., not applicable.
*Percent affected given includes subjects with impaired glucose tolerance.
†Range given is for all cancers.

Table 19-4 WS Diagnostic Criteria of Goto*

1. Characteristic habitus and stature	Short stature
	Low body weight
	Thin limbs with a stocky trunk
	Beak-shaped nose
2. Premature senescence	Birdlike appearance
	Loss of hair
	Skin hyperpigmentation
	Hoarse voice
	Diffuse arteriosclerosis
	Juvenile bilateral cataracts
	Osteoporosis
3. Scleroderma-like skin changes	Atrophic skin and muscle
	Hyperkeratosis
	Telangiectasia
	Tight skin over the bones of the feet
	Skin ulcers
	Localized calcification
4. Endocrine abnormalities	Diabetes mellitus
	Hypogonadism

*A diagnosis of WS requires three of the four criteria listed in the table.

SOURCE: Adapted from Goto et al.[30] Used by permission.

Dermatologic Pathology. By the second decade of life, most WS subjects have skin with a scleroderma-like appearance. The skin is tight, shiny, and smooth as a result of both dermal atrophy and loss of underlying connective tissue, muscle, and subcutaneous fat tissue.[4,6,38,49] Sites of abnormal skin include the upper and lower limbs; the ankles and feet are particularly severely affected. Atrophy of facial tissues results in the typical "birdlike" appearance with a sharp nose but relatively full cheeks. Hyperkeratosis also occurs, often resulting in ulcers on the feet and ankles. Ulceration can be severe (see Fig. 19-2), causing gangrene; amputation is sometimes required. Other skin abnormalities include general hyperpigmentation, areas of hypopigmentation, telangiectasia (36 percent of subjects), nail deformity (42 percent of subjects), and in general, thin, dry skin.

Stature and Habitus. Short stature is another feature typical of WS and is observed in most subjects (86–100 percent[38,39,50]). In Japanese subjects, males range in height from 137 to 161 cm (mean, 151–153 cm) and females range from 122 to 151 cm (mean, 131.7–144.2 cm). Non-Japanese (primarily Caucasian[6]) subjects are somewhat taller, with reported means of 157 cm (5 ft 1 in) and 146 cm (4 ft 9 $\frac{1}{2}$ in) for males and females, respectively. Growth arrest appears during early adolescence (between 10 and 20 years) and appears to result from the lack of a growth spurt at puberty. The short stature is accompanied by low body weight. While many body features are proportional to the subject's size, a consistent feature is thin limbs with a stocky trunk, which are observed in 76 to 100 percent of the subjects studied.[38,39] Muscle atrophy in the limbs is consistently observed. Despite the short stature, thyroid-stimulating hormone and growth hormone levels appear to be normal in adults.[39]

Graying and Loss of Hair. The hair of WS subjects often begins to turn gray in late adolescence, although gray hair can appear as early as 5 years of age.[6,38,39] This feature is perhaps one of the earliest symptoms (see Table 19-3). With time, the hair often becomes completely white. Loss of scalp and eyebrow hair and loss of eyelashes occur along with graying of the hair. The combination of the sparse gray or white hair and the dermal atrophy described above gives WS subjects the physical appearance of someone 20 to 30 years older than their chronologic age.

Excess Urinary Hyaluronic Acid. Excess hyaluronic acid (HA) in WS subjects' urine has been repeatedly observed.[38–43] Urinary HA was first identified in the analysis of urine for the connective tissue breakdown product, acid glycosaminoglycans. While acid glycosaminoglycan levels were normal, HA was high. HA levels are also elevated in Hutchinson-Gilford syndrome (progeria),[40] another disorder often mentioned as an accelerated aging disorder. HA is absent or is present in low levels in normal subjects.[44]

Features Found in a Subset of Patients

The following signs and symptoms are observed in a subset of patients. As was discussed earlier, the frequencies of some of these features may represent underestimates. In terms of morbidity and mortality, vascular disease and cancers are the most important; cancers, followed by myocardial and cerebrovascular accidents, are the most common causes of premature death (the average age at death for all causes is 47 years[6]).

Hypogonadism. Secondary sexual underdevelopment is a fairly common finding in WS subjects, occurring in 66 percent[39] to 96 percent[29] of the subjects studied. In males, small genitalia and sparse pubic hair are common though not universal. WS women have poorly developed genitalia with small uteruses. In about half the women studied, breasts were small, atrophic, or underdeveloped.[6] Both men and women with hypogonadism have had children, although fertility is reduced. The onset of menses ranges from 9 to 20 years (mean, 13.9 years; $n = 35$). Menstruation frequently ceases prematurely (18–45 years; mean, 33 years) before menopause.[6]

Osteoporosis and Soft Tissue Calcification. Osteoporosis is observed in a subset of WS subjects, often occurring most dramatically in the lower limbs, feet, and ankles and to a lesser extent in the upper limbs and spine. The rest of the trunk and the skull typically show less severe or no osteoporosis. In case series of Japanese and Caucasian subjects who were typically about 40 years of age, 33 to 41 percent of subjects showed evidence of loss of bone mass. The exception to this observed prevalence was a study of WS in Sardinians in which all subjects ($n = 6$) showed osteoporosis.[29] Soft tissue calcification is observed in WS often around the Achilles tendon and the knee and elbow tendons and in the ligaments and tissues surrounding these areas. Soft tissue calcification of the hands and feet was also observed.

Diabetes Mellitus. A diabetic tendency is observed in 44 to 70 percent of WS subjects.[6,7,38,39,45,50] In one study of oral glucose tolerance, 55 percent were categorized as having diabetes mellitus and another 22 percent had impaired glucose tolerance. Fasting glucose levels are elevated in only a subset of patients with abnormal glucose tolerance tests, indicating that in WS, diabetes is mild; symptoms of polyuria, polydipsia, pruritus, and weight loss are rarely found.[6] Hyperglycemia is typically treated by dietary restriction. Complications typical of diabetes (nephropathy, retinopathy, and neuropathy) have not been reported for WS. Since some WS subjects show no diabetic tendencies, factors other than mutations in the *WRN* gene must contribute to the appearance of diabetes in these subjects.

Vascular Disease. Premature generalized vascular disease is a common feature in WS and accounts for 15 percent of the deaths in WS subjects.[50] Between 70 and 90 percent of patients show hypercholesterolemia and hypertriglyceridemia,[9,46,47] and most were classified (WHO criteria) as having type IIb hyperlipidemia. Vascular calcification is observed, most frequently in the legs and feet. Clinical evidence of vascular disease was reported in 25 to 100 percent of WS subjects (average, 42 percent); the symptoms were abnormal electrocardiograms, congestive heart failure, angina, and infarction. In one autopsy series, all the subjects exhibited atherosclerosis beyond that expected for normal individuals of the same age.[6] Calcification of coronary arteries and of the leaflets or rings of the mitral and/or aortic valves occurs in some subjects.

Neoplasia. WS subjects have an elevated risk of developing a wide variety of carcinomas and sarcomas,[6,13,23,48] and malignancies are the leading cause of death (80 percent).[50] The reported case histories of a large number of Japanese and Caucasian WS subjects have been comprehensively reviewed with respect to the prevalence of cancers.[13] In WS patients there was an over-representation of nonepithelial cancer; the ratio of epithelial to nonepithelial cancer was 1:1 versus 10:1 in the general population.[49] The most common cancers in the Japanese WS subjects were soft tissue sarcomas, osteosarcomas, melanomas, and thyroid carcinomas; together these accounted for 57 percent of cancers in WS patients versus 2 percent in the general Japanese population. Conservative estimates based on the incidence rates of these cancers in the general population and an estimated population of 5000 WS subjects in Japan (probably a considerable overestimate) suggest that the incidence of soft tissue sarcomas is at least 20-fold higher in WS patients than in the general Japanese population. Acral lentiginous melanoma of the feet and nasal mucosa, the predominant form of melanoma observed in Japanese WS subjects, is extremely rare in Japan (0.16 cases per 100,000 people per year).[51] The osteosarcomas were also in excess of expected rates, with an unusual age distribution; 12 of the 13 cases observed occurred between the ages of 35 and 64 years, unlike the typical occurrence in the general population, where the incidence of osteosarcomas is highest in late adolescence. The thyroid carcinomas observed included both papillary (8 of 21 cases) and follicular carcinomas (10 of 21 cases). While papillary thyroid carcinomas are relatively common among the Japanese, follicular carcinomas are less common[52,53] and are proportionally in excess in WS subjects. In addition to the cancers mentioned earlier, a strikingly wide spectrum of isolated cases of other carcinomas is observed. Benign meningiomas may be common in WS; in a case series of 147 neoplasias reported by Goto and coworkers,[13] there were 15 benign meningiomas. Whether this represents an elevated frequency among WS patients is not known.

The elevation in cancer incidence in WS is not simply an increase in all forms of neoplasms but rather a selective increase in some relatively rare cancers. Thus WS is not an exact mimic of aging in terms of neoplasms. Conspicuously missing from the spectrum of cancers elevated in WS are some of the common epithelial malignancies, particularly prostate cancer, which in normal populations is very common in elderly men.

Central Nervous System. Early studies suggested that the central nervous system is not affected in most WS subjects.[6,54] However, more recent work with more modern methods and older subjects indicates that by 40 years of age, 40 percent of subjects have brain atrophy, as determined by computed tomographic (CT) and magnetic resonance imaging (MRI) analyses.[50,55] Mild senile dementia was reported in 21 percent of the patients studied.[39] Single cases of extensive cerebral atrophy[55] and a case of spastic parapataresis with polyneuropathy have been reported.[56] Neuropathologic data are limited; initial autopsies of two intellectually normal WS subjects, 51 and 57 years of age, using standard histologic methods, did not reveal Alzheimer disease-type changes (senile plaques or neurofibrillary tangles) typically associated with normal aging.[57] More recently, these same 2 patients were examined using more sensitive silver and immunohistologic methods using antibodies to the Alzheimer Aβ protein and hyperphosphorylated tau, the principal components of Alzheimer-type amyloid and neurofibrillary tangles, respectively. For the older subject, in the temporal and frontal lobes, and in the hippocampus, extensive Aβ deposits were found. The amyloid load was similar to that observed in Alzheimer disease patients and was greater than that observed in aged normal controls.[58] Tau pathology was not significantly different from controls. Additional

autopsies of WS patients who die after the age of 40 are needed to determine how severely the brain is affected.

Other Clinical Features of WS. In addition to the symptoms listed above, a subset (percent affected) of WS subjects have the following findings: flat feet (92 percent), irregular teeth (42 percent), hyperreflexia (79 percent), and a hoarse, high-pitched voice (83 percent; mean age of onset 21–27 years) caused by thickening and ulceration of the vocal cords.[4–7,9,38,39,50]

THE WS GENE

Pattern of Inheritance

The first cases of WS reported by Otto Werner in 1904 were familial, and subsequently, numerous pedigrees with multiple affected siblings were described. The parents of WS subjects are rarely affected, although several pedigrees with parent-child WS pairs exist.[5,9] Thannhauser in 1945 suggested that the inheritance of WS is recessive because of the high rate of consanguinity in the families of WS patients.[4] Elevated rates of consanguinity have been observed consistently in studies of both Japanese and Caucasians. Another line of evidence that WS is recessive is provided by segregation analysis. Epstein et al.[6] estimated that the percentage of affected offspring produced by unaffected parents range from 17.9 ± 2.5 percent to 26.5 ± 3.2 percent, depending on the method used to correct for ascertainment bias. These estimates are close to the 25 percent value expected for a recessively inherited disease. Thus WS is clearly a recessively inherited disorder, a conclusion subsequently supported by mutational analysis of WS subjects.[25] WS is found equally in both sexes, and there is no birth-order effect.[6]

Genetic Localization of the WS Gene

By the end of the 1980s, extensive *in vitro* biochemical and biologic studies had not revealed the primary defect responsible for WS. Fortunately, genetic mapping methods and resources had been sufficiently developed,[59,60] making localization of disease loci for inherited disorders highly feasible provided that a sufficient number of families could be identified.

The *WRN* locus was localized initially by using a combination of 8 outbred families and 13 consanguineous pedigrees, all from Japan.[30] Markers spanning much of the genome were analyzed by conventional maximum-likelihood methods; markers at 8p11.1-21.1 (Fig. 19-3) showed significant cosegregation with the WS phenotype. This localization was confirmed by homozygosity mapping methods[61,62] using primarily single affected subjects from a series of Japanese consanguineous families.[31] Significant positive-linkage results also were obtained with a panel of nine non-Japanese WS subjects who were primarily Caucasians.[32]

Initial mapping studies placed the *WRN* locus in a broad region from D8S137 to ANK1,[30–32,63,64] an interval spanning 16.6 cM[65,66] (see Fig. 19-3). Assignment of the *WRN* locus to this interval was based both on observed recombinants and on multipoint analysis.[32] Marker D8S339 was the closest marker showing the least recombination with WS. The D8S137-ANK1 interval contained relatively few known genes, which included heregulin (*HRB*), fibroblast growth factor receptor 1 (*FGFR1*), and DNA polymerase-β. *FGFR1* and *HRG* were excluded by recombination events between these genes and WS in affected subjects. The *pol*-β gene was excluded by DNA sequence analysis (no mutations were found[67]) and by radiation hybrid mapping, which placed the gene outside the D8S137-ANK1 region.[66]

High-Resolution Mapping of the *WRN* Gene

Fine mapping of the *WRN* locus became possible when short tandem repeat polymorphism (STRP) markers in linkage disequilibrium with WS were identified.[68] The first marker found that showed linkage disequilibrium with WS was at the glutathione reductase (*GSR*) gene. *GSR* had previously been assigned to

Chromosome 8

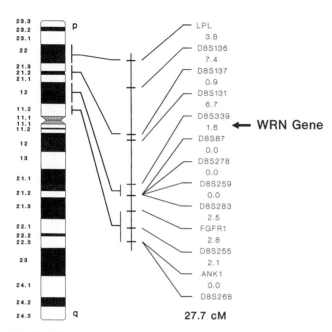

Fig. 19-3 Genetic map of the *WRN* region of chromosome 8. Genetic distances are sex-equal and are given in centimorgans (cM). The total length of the map is given at the bottom. (*From Oshima et al.*[66] *Used by permission.*)

chromosome 8 by somatic cell hybrid mapping but had not been mapped to a specific region of the chromosome. During the process of mapping *GSR* as a candidate gene, two STRP loci were identified in a cosmid clone containing the gene; in a group of 17 Japanese subjects, both STRP's had alleles that were in linkage disequilibrium ($p = 0.0025–0.001$) with the WS gene.[68] Subsequent analysis of other markers in the region demonstrated that D8S339 also was in disequilibrium with *WRN* in the same group of families, an observation confirmed in other studies.[69] *GSR* and D8S339 were subsequently found to be separated by approximately 200 kb (Fig. 19-4). Other markers flanking *GSR* and D8S339, including the clusters D8S131-D8S137 and D8S278-D8S87-D8S259-D8S283, were not in linkage disequilibrium with *WRN*.

To refine the location of the *WRN* gene, chromosome walking methods were used to clone DNA flanking D8S339/*GSR*. A yeast artificial chromosome (YAC) contig was constructed, using *GSR* as a starting point, and the contig was used as a source of cloned DNA for the identification of an additional 18 additional STRP loci[70–72] (see Fig. 19-4). Genotype data from these markers were used in three different approaches in an attempt to narrow the *WRN* region. First, the markers were used to define recombinants in WS pedigrees. Definitive recombinants were identified at D8S2194/D8S2192 and at D8S2186. Second, the markers were tested for linkage disequilibrium to identify the boundaries of the region of linkage disequilibrium. In Japanese kindreds, markers D8S2196 and D8S2162 and many markers in between were in linkage disequilibrium with *WRN*, while D8S2194-D8S2192 and D8S2186 as well as more distant flanking markers (D8S131-D8S137 and D8S278-D8S259-D8S87-D8S283) were not.[73,74] Third, because markers in this region are in disequilibrium with *WRN*, many of the subjects studied are presumed to be descendants of a common ancestor and thus should share a definable common haplotype. The genotype data from markers spanning the region were used to define a common ancestral haplotype and determine where ancestral recombinants had disrupted that haplotype.[68,74] The combined approach using these three methods yielded an

interval of approximately 1.2 megabases (Mb) that contained the *WRN* gene.

Positional Cloning of the *WRN* Gene

The *WRN* gene was identified by positional cloning methods,[25] with the effort focused on the 1.2-Mb region indicated by the preceding genetic studies. The YAC contig was converted to P1 clones, which are less prone to deletion and rearrangement artifacts. The P1 clones were used as a source of DNA to identify genes in the region, using exon trapping,[75] cDNA selection methods (hybridization of cDNA libraries to YAC and P1 clones[76]), and DNA sequence analysis (comparison of DNA sequence with the DNA sequence databases of known genes and potential expressed sequence-tagged sites). Each of these methods yielded gene fragments that were then used to isolate full-length cDNA clones for each gene in the *WRN* region. These candidates were screened for mutations by reverse-transcriptase polymerase chain reaction (RT-PCR) methods or direct DNA sequence analysis of genomic DNA. A total of 10 genes were characterized and screened for mutations before the *WRN* gene was identified. These were *GSR*, protein phosphatase 2 catalytic subunit β (*PPP2CB*), general transcription factor IIEβ (*GTF2E2*), a β-tubullin pseudogene 1 (*TUBBP1*), and six previously unidentified genes of unknown function.

The *WRN* gene was identified initially as a match between the genomic DNA of a P1 and 245-bp sequence in the expressed sequence tag database.[25] This short sequence was used to identify a 5.2-kb full-length cDNA clone that encodes a predicted protein of 1432 amino acids. The same gene also was identified by exon trapping. Comparison of the DNA sequence to known genes revealed a striking homology to genes in the super-family of DNA and RNA helicases (Fig. 19-5). Thus WS joins a list of inherited disorders caused by mutations in helicase genes. These disorders are xeroderma pigmentosum, complementation groups B[77] and D (helicases ERCC2 and ERCC3, respectively[78–82]), trichothiody-strophy (ERCC2[83,84]), Cockayne syndrome (helicase ERCC6,[85]), Bloom syndrome,[86] and X chromosome-linked α-thalassemia mental retardation syndrome.[87,88]

WRN Mutations

During initial characterization of the gene, four mutations were identified in the 3′ end[25] (see Table 19-2). Two (mutations 1 and 2) were single-base substitution nonsense mutations that result in truncated proteins of 1164 and 1060 amino acids, respectively, compared with 1432 for the normal protein. Mutation 3 is a 4-bp deletion resulting in a frameshift and a predicted truncated protein. This mutation was observed in a single Syrian family. Mutation 4 is a single base-pair intronic substitution at a splice junction that results in skipping of an exon and a frameshift, producing a truncated protein (see Fig. 19-5). The first four mutations identified were in the 3′ end of the gene, and all leave the helicase consensus domain intact. This bias resulted from the 3′ being available for mutational analysis first. Since the helicase region contains the ATPase region of the protein and presumably is the enzymatic component of the helicase, 3′-truncated proteins could still retain DNA/RNA-unwinding activity.

To screen the middle and the 5′ end of the gene, the genomic structure of *WRN* was determined. The gene consists of 35 exons, with the coding region beginning in the second exon.[33,35] The gene spans at least 100 kb, although the actual size of the gene is unknown. Five additional mutations (A–E, Table 19-2) were identified in the remainder of the gene. Two additional nonsense mutations and a splice-junction mutation were found. Another mutation is a 1-bp deletion that results in a frameshift and a premature stop codon. Mutation E is a large genomic deletion (0.15 kb) that probably occurred by a recombination event between two highly homologous Alu elements that are separated by 15 kb. Two of these mutations result in predicted truncated protein products that do not contain the helicase domains.

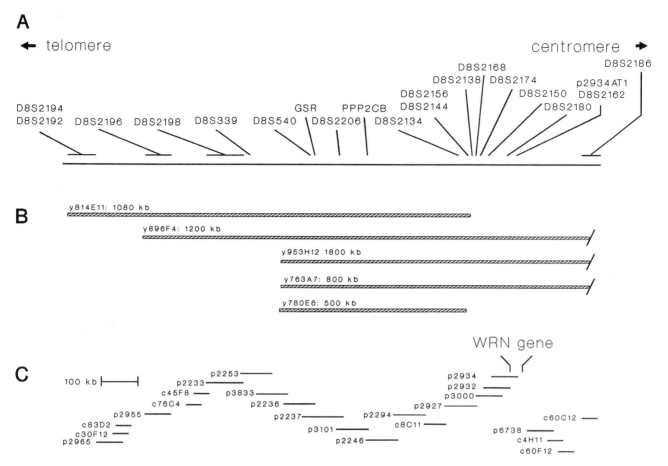

Fig. 19-4 Genetic markers, YACs, P1, and cosmid clones used in the positional cloning of the *WRN* gene. *A.* STRP loci. *B.* YAC clones. *C.* P1 clones (beginning with a *p*) and cosmid clones (beginning with a *c*). The size scale in kilobase units (kb) given in *C* also applies to *A* and *B*. (*Reproduced from Yu et al.[72] Used by permission.*)

To date, a total of 19 WS mutations[25,33,35–37] have been identified (see Table 19-2). All mutations, whether point mutations, insertions, or deletions, result in a predicted truncated protein product, and no missense mutations have been identified. The predicted truncated WRN proteins from the different mutations range in length from 176 to 1304 amino acids, with some retaining the helicase domain and others consisting only of the N-terminal end of the protein. Compound heterozygotes exist

for a number of different WS mutations. Despite the variety of predicted protein products and combinations of mutant alleles, there is no evidence that the severity of the disease correlates with the type of mutation observed.[35,89] Thus differential phenotype-genotype relationships may be subtle and difficult to detect and will require additional work. Heterozygotes (normal allele/WS mutation) do not appear to manifest any characteristics of WS, and some live past the age of 90. Presently, no other disease has been

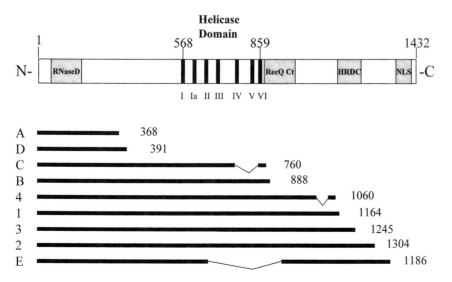

Fig. 19-5 The WS helicase. *A.* Schematic diagram of WRNp with the seven helicase motifs (I–VI) shown as solid bars. *B.* WS mutations: Bars indicate extent of translation of mutated WS alleles. Numbers to the right of the bars indicate the length of the mutated protein product. Breaks indicate skipped exons. All mutations result in production of a truncated protein due to nonsense mutations, frame shift mutations or skipped exons due to splice site mutations or genomic deletions.

associated with *WRN* mutations. In particular, subjects with Hutchinson-Gilford syndrome, a progeroid syndrome with a childhood onset, do not have *WRN* mutations.[90]

Pathogenic Mechanism of *WRN* Mutations

A common mechanism may exist for all *WRN* mutations. WRNp is localized primarily to the nucleus of cells.[91,92] This localization can be demonstrated either by cell fractionation methods or by generating a green-fluorescent protein (GFP) WRN fusion protein with GFP attached to the N-terminus of WRNp.[91] All WS mutations result in predicted truncated proteins that are missing 128 or more amino acids of the C-terminal end (see Table 19-2). When WS mutations are introduced into the GFP-WRNp fusion proteins, truncated proteins are produced that lack the C-terminus. Only the normal fusion protein goes to the nucleus, while all the C-terminus–deficient fusion proteins remain in the cytoplasm. This work shows that the C-terminus of WRN contains a nuclear localization signal that is missing in all WS mutation proteins. Assuming that the biologic function of the WRN protein is in the nucleus, *WRN* mutations keep the protein from reaching the site of its normal function, even if the enzymatic helicase portion of the molecule is intact and functional. Within the nucleus, WRNp may be localized to the nucleolus in human but not in murine cells.[92] This observation is intriguing because the yeast helicase SGS1p, which is partially homologous to WRNp, is also localized in the nucleolus, and mutations in SGS1p shorten life span and result in other age-related phenotypes in yeast.[93]

A second consequence of WS mutations is that the levels of WRN mRNA are reduced in mutation homozygotes to 30 percent compared with normal homozygotes.[94] The reduced levels are presumably due to reduced mRNA stability. In heterozygotes, WRN mRNA is less than the expected 65 percent, suggesting there may be some feedback regulation of transcription, mRNA processing, or mRNA degradation.

Origins of *WRN* Mutations

The existence of common Japanese founders was confirmed by mutational analysis. Among Japanese subjects, 50 to 60 percent had the same mutation (mutation 4).[33,35,89] Most of these subjects had the 141-bp allele at *GSR* that was overrepresented in WS patients compared with controls (frequency, 0.40 and 0.07, respectively) and therefore was responsible for the linkage disequilibrium observed at *GSR*. Further, for two highly polymorphic STRP loci within the *WRN* gene (D8S2162 and p2934AT1; see Fig. 19-4), haplotypes were identical for all mutation 4 carriers tested. In Japanese subjects, a second mutation (mutation A in Table 19-2) is also common in Japanese subjects, with a mutation frequency of 17.5 percent. Haplotype analysis suggests that this mutation is also the result of a common founder.[35] Mutations 2 and A are found in both Japanese and Caucasian subjects. For both mutations, different haplotypes for STRP markers within the *WRN* gene were observed in Caucasian versus Japanese subjects, suggesting an independent origin.[33] However, a common ancient founder cannot be completely ruled out, since intragenic recombination or mutations at the STRP loci cannot be excluded.

In Vitro WRNp Studies

The predicted sequence of WRNp indicates that it is a member of a super-family of DExH box DNA and RNA helicases. These DNA- and RNA-unwinding proteins share a common structure of seven motifs (I, Ia, II, III, IV, V, and VI) ranging in size from approximately 15 to 25 amino acids.[95] Motif I contains a nucleotide-binding site, and motif II has the DExH sequence of a Mg^{2+}-binding site (DEAH in the *WRN* gene); these sites presumably participate in the hydrolysis of ATP that occurs as the enzyme unwinds a double-stranded DNA or RNA helix. WRNp shows homology to these seven motifs in helicases from a wide variety of organisms, including *Escherichia coli* (recQ), *Saccharomyces cerevisiae* (SgS1), *Caenorhabditis elegans* (F18C5C), and

humans (RECQL).[25] The region of shared homology is in the center of WRNp, spanning amino acids 540 to 963. The sequences in between the seven motifs are not conserved, although the spacing between motifs is highly conserved. The homology between the predicted protein and other helicases strongly suggests that WRNp is a functional helicase.

Other domains shared with other proteins are more subtle than the helicase homology region. In the N-terminal end, between amino acids 59 and 105, is a domain shared with RNase D (called the *RNase D domain*) that is also found in the $3' \rightarrow 5'$ proofreading exonuclease domain of bacterial DNA polymerase.[96,97] This RNase D domain is not found in SGS1p or in the Bloom syndrome helicase (BLMp). Thus the WRN protein may have an exonuclease activity, although this has not been directly demonstrated. In the C-terminal end, from approximately amino acids 1150 to 1229, is another domain homologous to a different region of RNase D called the *helicase and RNase D C-terminal (HRDC) domain*. HRDC is found in some helicases including reqQ (*E. coli*), SGS1 (yeast), and BLM (human) and in RNases including RNase D (*E. coli*) and a number of eukaryotic homologues.[98] The HDRC domain is not required for helicase or RNase activities because not all helicases or RNases have this domain. The N-terminal end is highly acidic, containing 109 glutamate or aspartate residues, including one segment with 14 amino acids in a stretch of 19S. There is a 27-amino acid tandem repeat sequence beginning at amino acid 424 in the protein. The mouse and rat WRN homologues do not contain this repeat.[99]

The prediction from the WRNp sequence that WRNp is a helicase[25] has been confirmed recently by functional studies.[100–102] WRNp generated in an insect cell-baculovirus system can unwind double-stranded DNA (dsDNA) in an ATP-dependent process, and ATP hydrolysis is dsDNA-dependent. Mutation 4 (see Table 19-2) that has the helicase domain but lacks 242 amino acids from the C-terminus and is missing the HRDC domain still retains helicase activity. However, WRNp with a $^K577^M$ mutation at a highly conserved amino acid in the helicase I motif does not have helicase activity. The preferred polarity of WRNp helicase activity is $3' \rightarrow 5'$. RNA-DNA heteroduplexes are also unwound but with a lower efficiency than for DNA homoduplexes. As seen with other helicases, DNA unwinding activity is enhanced by the addition of single-strand DNA binding proteins from a number of different sources, with human single-strand binding protein being the most effective.[102]

WRNp and WS

The normal function of WRNp is unknown. It could function to unwind DNA during replication, repair, transcription, or any number of other DNA transactions requiring duplex unwinding. Other helicases function as part of multiprotein complexes. For example, ERCC2 and ERCC3, which are defective in xeroderma pigmentosum, are part of the RNA polymerase II basal transcription factor (TFIIH).[101] ERCC6, the helicase defective in Cockayne syndrome group B subjects, interacts with the product of the CSA gene, which is mutated in Cockayne syndrome group A subjects.[102] CSA in turn interacts with TFIIH. Thus the Cockayne syndrome helicase also may interact with TFIIH. By analogy to these other helicases, WRNp may interact with other proteins in a complex to perform its normal function in DNA metabolism. Since the N-terminal and C-terminal ends of each of these helicases are unique, presumably protein-protein interactions are dependent on the nonhelicase segments of the protein. Isolation of the other proteins that complex with WRNp will be critical to understanding the function of this helicase.

Previous studies of the biology of WS have yielded limited information on the potential function of WRNp. Two different lines of evidence indicate that WS cells have a mutator phenotype. First, both *in vitro* and *in vivo* studies show an elevated mutation rate using the hypoxanthine phosphoribosyltransferase gene as a reporter locus.[14–17] Characterization of the types of mutations that occur in WS cells indicates that the proportion of deletion mutations is higher than expected. These deletions may occur by nonhomologous recombination, since sequences of the deletions are not homologous.[17] The second indication of genomic instability is the elevated rate of random chromosomal rearrangements in WS cells, again observed both *in vitro* and *in vivo*.[18-23]

The WS mutator phenotype could result from defective DNA repair. For xeroderma pigmentosum and Cockayne syndrome, helicase defects result in faulty nucleotide excision repair and strand-specific transcription-coupled repair, respectively. Defective DNA repair in WS cells has been difficult to reproducibly demonstrate. Unscheduled DNA synthesis[105-107] and post-ultraviolet (UV) irradiation cell survival[108] are not defective in WS cells, and there is no increased sensitivity to a variety of DNA-damaging agents, including bleomycin, *cis*-dichlorodiamine platinum, diepoxybutane, isonicotinic acid hydrazide, 1-methyl-3-nitro-1-nitrosoguanidine, hydroxyurea, and methyl methanesulfonate.[107-113] Cells from WS subjects are sensitive to the DNA damaging agent 4-nitro-quinline-1-oxide (4NQO), and cells from heterozygotes have a level of sensitivity intermediate to normal individuals and WS subjects, suggesting a DNA repair defect. WS cell proliferation was more sensitive than normal cells to the topoisomerase I inhibitor camptothecin.[114] For topoisomerase II inhibitors, ellipticine and amsacrine do not differentially affect WS cell proliferation, while both positive and negative results have been reported with etoposide.[112,113] Mismatch repair is normal in Epstein-Barr virus-transformed lymphoblastoid cell lines but may be reduced in SV40-transformed fibroblastoid cell lines, although additional work is needed to confirm this finding.[115] Microsatellite length stability is not reduced,[116] and sister-chromatid exchange, with or without treatment with clastogens, is not elevated in WS cells.[110,118,117] To date, no specific DNA repair system has been associated with the loss of WRNp function.

Other alterations in DNA metabolism have been reported. For DNA synthesis, reduced chain-elongation rates[105] and increased distances between synthesis initiation sites[119,120] have been reported. This reduced rate of DNA synthesis could be responsible for the prolonged S phase observed in WS cells.[119,121] DNA ligation may be abnormal in WS cells.[122,123] While the rate of ligation is not altered, the accuracy of ligation events is reduced, suggesting a possible mechanism for generating mutations. Elevated rates of homologous recombination also have been reported.[124] Whether the WRN helicase defect is directly responsible for any of these alterations in DNA handling remains to be determined. The primary mechanism by which defective helicase mutations give rise to the WS phenotype also remains to be determined.

Model Organisms and WRNp Function

Recent work in model organisms has provided information about the normal function of WRNp. In yeast, the WRNp homologue Sgs1p is a suppressor of illegitimate recombination between nonhomologous or short homologous DNA sequences. In SGS1 loss-of-function mutants, genomic instability and a hyperrecombination occur.[125] The hyperrecombination phenotype can be partially suppressed by either WRNp or BLMp.[126] Thus the genomic instability observed in WS subjects could be due to processes related to illegitimate recombination.

In *Xenopus laevis,* a helicase called FFA-1 for focus-forming activity-1 was identified that is a homologue of WRNp and is required for DNA replication initiation.[127] FFA-1 is an ATP- and dsDNA-dependent helicase. DNA replication is initiated when an ssDNA-binding protein called *replication protein A* and FFA-1 bind to a specific DNA sequence that serves as an origin of replication. The gene for FFA-1 was cloned and shown to encode a 1436-amino acid protein that contains the 7 helicase motifs found in WRNp and other RecQ-type helicases. In addition, unlike Sgs1p, RecQ, and other helicases, FFA-1 is homologous to WRNp across the entire length of protein, not just in the helicase, HRDC, and RNase D domains. FFA-1 is 66 percent similar and 50 percent identical to WRNp. Thus WRNp may be involved in DNA

replication initiation, which is consistent with previous work demonstrating altered DNA synthesis in WS cells.[105,119-121] However, WRNp is probably not required for all DNA synthesis because WS mutations most likely result in the complete loss of function of WRNp, and other paralogues must exist in humans that can substitute for WRNp in DNA replication initiation.

RECENT IMPLICATIONS OF IDENTIFICATION OF THE *WRN* GENE FOR DIAGNOSIS

The diagnosis of WS can now potentially be confirmed definitively by mutational analysis of the *WRN* gene; WS subjects should be either homozygous or compound heterozygotes for mutations in this gene. In work to date, mutations have been identified in all subjects studied, including some with diagnoses of "probable" and "possible."[33] The mutational analysis confirms the usefulness of the clinical criteria outlined in Tables 19-3 and 19-4. The principal advantage of mutational analysis is that the diagnosis can be made at a young age, when WS is first suspected. In contrast, the mean age at diagnosis using clinical criteria is 37 years, because in some patients some of the defining symptoms do not develop until the third and fourth decades of life. Screening the *WRN* gene for mutations in Japanese subjects is simplified because one mutation accounts for 60 percent of the WS cases and two others make up an additional 33 percent. In Caucasians, it is not known what the frequencies of the different WS mutations are. Since the gene has 34 coding exons, complete analysis of the entire gene for a subject is expensive. The development of an *in vitro* protein-truncation assay for WS should facilitate mutation detection. Because WS is such a rare disorder, it is unlikely that mutation screening will become universally available.

ACKNOWLEDGMENTS

We thank Thomas D. Bird, Mary T. Ersek, and Raymond J. Monnat for reading the text before publication. We also thank Charles J. Epstein for making some of the photographs available. This work was funded in part by grant RO1 AG12019 (GDS) from the National Institute on Aging. We also thank the WS subjects who participated in the research described here.

REFERENCES

1. Werner CWO: Udber kataract in Verbindung mit Sclerodermie. *Doctoral dissertation,* Kiel, Schmidt & Klarnig, West Germany, 1904.
2. Werner O (trans H Hoehn): On cataract in conjunction with scledema. *Adv Exp Med Biol* **190**:1, 1985.
3. Oppenheimer BS, Kugel VH: Werner's syndrome, a heredofamilial disorder with scleroderma, bilateral juvenile cataracts, precocioius graying of the hair and endocrine stigmatization. *Trans Assoc Am Phys* **49**:358, 1934.
4. Thannhauser SJ: Werner's syndrome (progeria of the adult) and Rothmund's syndrome: Two types of closely related heredofamilial atrophic dermatoses with juvenile cataracts and endocrine features: A critical study with five new cases. *Ann Intern Med* **23**:559, 1945.
5. Goto M, Tanimoto K, Horiuchi Y, Sasazuki T: Family analysis of Werner's syndrome: A survey of 42 Japanese families with a review of the literature. *Clin Genet* **19**:8, 1981.
6. Epstein CJ, Martin GM, Schultz A, Motulsky AG: Werner's syndrome: A review of its symptomatology, natural history, pathologic features, genetics, and relationship to the natural aging process. *Medicine* **45**:177, 1966.
7. Tollefsbol TO, Cohen HJ: Werner's syndrome: An underdiagnosed disorder resembling premature aging. *Age* **7**:75, 1984.
8. Jacobson HG, Rifkin H, Zucker D: Werner's syndrome: A clinical entity. *Radiology* **74**:373, 1960.
9. Zucker-Franklin D, Rifkin H, Jacobson HG: Werner's syndrome: An analysis of ten cases. *Geriatrics* **23**:123, 1968.
10. Martin GM: Genetic syndromes in man with potential relevance to the pathobiology of aging. *Birth Defects* **14**:5, 1978.
11. Hayflick L: The limited *in vitro* lifetime of human diploid cell strains. *Exp Cell Res* **37**:614, 1965.

12. Martin GM, Sprague CA, Epstein CJ: Replicative life-span of cultivated human cells. *Lab Invest* **23**:86, 1970.

13. Goto M, Miller RW, Ishikawa Y, Sugano H: Excess of rare cancers in Werner syndrome (adult progeria). *Epidemiol Biomarkers Prevent* **5**:239, 1996.

14. Fukuchi K, Tanaka K, Nakura J, Kumahara Y, Uchida T, Okada Y: Elevated spontaneous mutation rate in SV40 Werner syndrome fibroblast cell lines. *Somat Cell Mol Genet* **11**:303, 1985.

15. Fukuchi K, Martin GM, Monnat RJ: Mutator phenotype of Werner syndrome is characterized by extensive deletions. *Proc Natl Acad Sci USA* **86**:5893, 1989.

16. Fukuchi K, Tanaka K, Kumahara Y, Maramo K, Pride M, Martin GM, Monnat RJ: Increased frequency of 6-thioguanine-resistant peripheral blood lymhocytes in Werner syndrome patients. *Hum Genet* **84**:249, 1990.

17. Monnat RJ, Hackmann AFM, Chiaverotti TA: Nucleotide sequence analysis of human hypoxanthine phosphoribosyltransferase (HPRT) gene deletions. *Genomics* **13**:777, 1992.

18. Hoehn H, Bryant EM, Au K, Norwood TH, Boman H, Martin GM: Variegated translocation mosaicism in human skin fibroblast cultures. *Cytogenet Cell Genet* **15**:282, 1975.

19. Salk D, Hoehn H, Martin GM: Cytogenetics of Werner's syndrome cultured in skin fibroblasts: Variegated translocation mosaicism. *Hum Genet* **62**:16, 1982.

20. Salk D: Werner's syndrome: A review of recent research with an analysis of connective tissue metabolism, growth control of cultured cells, and chromosomal aberrations. *Hum Genet* **62**:1, 1982.

21. Salk D, Au K, Hoehn H, Martin GM: Cytogenetics of Werner's syndrome cultured skin fibroblasts: Variegated translocation mosaicism. *Cytogenet Cell Genet* **30**:92, 1981.

22. Scappaticci S, Cerimele D, Fraccaro M: Clonal structural chromosomal rearrangements in primary fibroblast cultures and in lymphocytes of patients with Werner's syndrome. *Hum Genet* **62**:16, 1982.

23. Salk D, Au K, Hoehn H, Martin GM: Cytogenetic aspects of Werner syndrome. *Adv Exp Med Biol* **190**:541, 1985.

24. Morita K, Nishigori C, Sasaki MS, Matsuyoshi N, Ohta K, Okamoto H, Ikai K, et al: Werner's syndrome: Chromosome analyses of cultured fibroblasts and mitogen-stimulated lymphocytes. *Br J Dermatol* **136**:620, 1997.

25. Yu CE, Oshima J, Fu YH, Wijsman EM, Hisama F, Alisch R, Matthews S, et al: Positional cloning of the Werner's syndrome gene. *Science* **272**:258, 1996.

26. Barrai I, Mi MP, Morton NE, Yasuda N: Estimation of prevalence under incomplete selection. *Am J Hum Genet* **17**:221, 1965.

27. Dahlberg G: Methods for population genetics. *Am J Biol* **25**:90, 1950.

28. Neal JV, Kodani MB, Brewer R, Anderson RC: The incidence of consanguineous matings in Japan: Remarks on the estimation of comparative gene frequencies and the expected rate of induced recessive mutations. *Am J Hum Genet* **1**:156, 1949.

29. Cerimele D, Cotton F, Scappaticci S, Rabbiosi G, Borroni G, Sanna E, Zei G, et al: High prevalence of Werner's syndrome in Sardinia: Description of six patients and estimates of the gene frequency. *Hum Genet* **62**:25, 1982.

30. Goto M, Weber J, Woods K, Drayna D: Genetic linkage of Werner's syndrome to five markers on chromosome 8. *Nature* **355**:735, 1992.

31. Schellenberg GD, Martin GM, Wijsman EM, Nakura J, Miki T, Ogihara T: Homozygosity mapping and Werner's syndrome. *Lancet* **339**:1002, 1992.

32. Nakura J, Wijsman EM, Miki T, Kamino K, Yu CE, Oshima J, Fukuchi K, et al: Homozygosity mapping of the Werner syndrome locus (WRN). *Genomics* **23**:600, 1994.

33. Yu CE, Oshima J, Wijsman EM, Nakura J, Miki T, Puissan C, Matthews S, et al: Werner's syndrome collaborative group: Mutations in the consensus helicase domains of the Werner's syndrome gene. *Am J Hum Genet* **60**:330, 1997.

34. Meisslitzer C, Ruppitsch W, Weirichschwaiger H, Weirich HG, Jabkowsky J, Klein G, Schweiger M, Hirschkauffmann M: Werner syndrome: Characterization of mutations in the WRN gene in an affected family. *Eur J Hum Genet* **5**:364, 1997.

35. Matsumoto T, Imamura O, Yamabe Y, Kuromitsu J, Tokutake Y, Shimamoto A, Suzuki N, Satoh M, Kitao S, Ichikawa K, Kataoka H, Sugawara K, Thomas W, Mason B, Tsuchihashi Z, Drayna D, Sugawara M, Sugimoto M, Furuchi Y, Goto M: Mutation and haplotype analyses of the Werner's syndrome gene based on its genomic structure: Genetic epidemiology in the Japanese population. *Hum Genet* **100**:123 1997.

36. Goto M, Imamura O, Kuromitsu J, Matsumoto T, Yamabe Y, Tokutake Y, Suzuki N, et al: Analysis of helicase gene mutations in Japanese Werner's syndrome. *Hum Genet* **9**:191, 1997.

37. Oshima J, Yu CE, Piussan C, Klein G, Jabkowski J, Balci S, Miki T, et al: Homozygous and compound heterozygous mutations at the Werner syndrome locus. *Hum Mol Genet* **5**:1909, 1996.

38. Goto M, Horiuchi Y, Tanimoto K, Ishii T, Nakashima H: Werner's syndrome: Analysis of 15 cases with a review of the Japanese literature. *J Am Geriatr Soc* **26**:341, 1978.

39. Murata K, Nakashima H: Werner's syndrome: Twenty-four cases with a review of the Japanese medical literature. *J Am Geriatr Soc* **30**:303, 1982.

40. Kieras FJ, Brown WT, Houck GE, Zebrower M: Elevation of urinary hyaluronic acid in Werner's syndrome and progeria. *Biochem Med Metab Biol* **36**:276, 1986.

41. Tokunaga M, Futami T, Wakamatsu E, Endo M, Yosizawa Z: Werner's syndrome as "hyaluronuria." *Clin Chim Acta* **62**:89, 1975.

42. Goto M, Murata K: Urinary excretion of macromolecular acidic glycosaminoglycans in Werner's syndrome. *Clin Chim Acta* **85**:101, 1978.

43. Murata K: Urinary acidic glycosaminoglycans in Werner's syndrome. *Experimentia* **38**:313, 1982.

44. Varada DP, Cifonelli JA, Dorfman A: The acid mucopolysaccharides in normal urine. *Biochem Biophys Acta* **141**:103, 1967.

45. Imura H, Nakao Y, Kuzuya H, Okamoto M, Okamoto M, Yamada K: Clinical, endocrine and metabolic aspects of the Werner syndrome compared with those of normal aging. *Adv Exp Med Biol* **190**:171, 1985.

46. Mori S, Yokote K, Morisaki N, Saito Y, Yoshida S: Inheritable abnormal lipoprotein metabolism in Werner's syndrome similar to familial hypercholesterolemia. *Eur J Clin Invest* **20**:137, 1990.

47. Goto M, Kato Y: Hypercoagulable state indicates an additional risk factor for atherosclerosis in Werner's syndrome. *Thromb Haemost* **73**:576, 1995.

48. Sato K, Goto M, Nishioka K, Arima K, Hori N, Yamashita N, Fujimoto Y, Nanko H, Olwawa K, Ohara K: Werner's syndrome associated with malignancies: Five cases with a survey of case histories in Japan. *Gerontology* **34**:212, 1988.

49. Miller RW, Myers MH: Age distribution of epithelial and non-epithelial cancers. *Lancet* **2**:1250, 1983.

50. Goto M: Hierarchical deterioration of body systems in Werner's syndrome: Implications for normal ageing. *Mech Age Dev* **98**:239, 1997

51. Elwood JM: Epidemiology and control of melanoma in white populations and in Japan. *J Invest Dermatol* **92**:214, 1989.

52. Sampson RJ, Key CR, Buncher CR, Iijima S: Thyroid carcinoma at autopsy in Hiroshima and Nagasaki: I. Prevalence of thyroid cancer at autopsy. *JAMA* **209**:65, 1969.

53. Correa P, Chen VW: Endocrine gland cancer. *Cancer* **75**:338, 1995.

54. Postiglione A, Soricelli A, Covelli EM, Iazzetta N, Ruocco A, Milan G, Santoro L, Alfano B, Brunetti A: Premature aging in Werner's syndrome spares the central nervous system. *Neurobiol Aging* **17**:325, 1996.

55. Kakigi R, Endo C, Neshige R, Kohno H, Kuroda Y: Accelerated aging in the brain in Werner's syndrome. *Neurology* **42**:922, 1992.

56. Umehara F, Abe M, Nagawa M, Izumo S, Arimura K, Matsumuro K, Osame M: Werner's syndrome associated with spastic paraparesis and peripheral neuropathy. *Neurology* **43**:1252, 1993.

57. Sumi SM: Neuropathology of the Werner syndrome. *Adv Exp Med Biol* **190**:215, 1985.

58. Leverenz JB, Yu CE, Schellenberg GD: Aging-associated neuropathology in Werner syndrome. *Acta Neuropathol* **96**:421, 1998.

59. Weissenbach J, Gyapay G, Dib C, Vignal A, Morissette J, Millasseau P, Vaysseix G, Lathrop M: A second generation linkage map of the human genome. *Nature* **359**:794, 1993.

60. NIH/CEPH Collaborative Mapping Group: A comprehensive genetic linkage map of the human genome. *Science* **258**:148, 1992.

61. Lander ES, Botstein D: Homozygosity mapping: A way to map human recessive traits with the DNA of inbred children. *Science* **236**:1567, 1987.

62. Smith CAB: Detection of linkage in human genetics. *J R Stat Soc B* **15**:153, 1953.

63. Ye L, Nakura J, Mitsuda N, Fujioka Y, Kamino K, Ohta T, Jinno Y, Niikawa N, Miki T, Ogihara T: Genetic association between chromosome 8 microsatellite (MS8-134) and Werner syndrome (WRN): Chromosome microdissection and homozygosity mapping. *Genomics* **28**:566, 1995.

64. Thomas W, Rubenstein M, Goto M, Drayna D: A genetic analysis of the Werner syndrome region on human chromosome 8p. *Genomics* **16**:685, 1993.

65. Tomfohrde J, Wood S, Schertzer M, Wagner MJ, Wells DE, Parrish J, Sadler LA, Blanton SH, Daiger SP, Wang ZY, Wilkie PJ, Weber JL: Human chromosome linkage map based on short tandem repeat polymorphisms: Effect of genotyping errors. *Genomics* **14**:144, 1992.

66. Oshima J, Yu CE, Boehnke M, Weber JL, Edelhoff S, Wagner MJ, Wells DE, Wood S, Disteche CM, Martin GM, Schellenberg GD: Integrated mapping analysis of the Werner syndrome region of chromosome 8. *Genomics* **23**:100, 1994.

67. Chang M, Burmer GC, Sweasy J, Loeb LA, Edelhoff S, Disteche CM, Yu CE, Anderson L, Oshima J, Nakura J, Miki T, Kamino K, Ogihara T, Schellenberg GD, Martin GM: Evidence against DNA polymerase beta as a candidate gene for Werner syndrome. *Hum Genet* **93**:507, 1994.

68. Yu C, Oshima J, Goddard KAB, Miki T, Nakura J, Ogihara T, Fraccaro M, Piussan C, Martin GM, Schellenberg GD, Wijsman EM: Linkage disequilibrium and haplotype studies of chromosome 8p 11.1.1 markers and Werner's syndrome. *Am J Hum Genet* **55**:356, 1994.

69. Kihara K, Nakura J, Ye L, Mitsuda N, Kamino K, Zhao Y, Fujioka Y, Miki T, Ogihara T: Carrier detection of Werner's syndrome using a microsatellite that exhibits linkage disequilibrium with the Werner's syndrome locus. *Jpn J Hum Genet* **39**:403, 1994.

70. Ye L, Nakura J, Mitsuda N: A highly polymorphic dinucleotide repeat at the D8S1222 locus. *Jpn J Hum Genet* **40**:287, 1995.

71. Nakura J, Ye L, Kihara K, Yamagata H, Mamino K, Nakamura Y, Miki T, Ogihara T: Two dinucleotide repeat polymorphisms at the D8S1442 and D8S1443 loci. *Jpn J Hum Genet* **40**:281, 1995.

72. Yu CE, Oshima J, Hisama F, Matthews S, Trask BJ, Schellenberg GD: A YAC, P1 and cosmid contig and 17 new polymorphic markers for the Werner's syndrome region at 8p12. *Genomics* **35**:431, 1996.

73. Goddard KAB, Yu CE, Oshima J, Miki T, Nakura J, Piussan C, Martin GM, Schellenberg GD, Wijsman EM: International Werner's syndrome collaborative group: Toward localization of the Werner syndrome gene by linkage disequilibrium and ancestral haplotyping: Lessons learned from analysis of 35 chromosome 8p11.1.1 markers. *Am J Hum Genet* **58**:1286, 1996.

74. Nakura J, Miki T, Ye L, Mitsuda N, Zhao Y, Kihara K, Yu CE, et al: Narrowing the position of the Werner syndrome locus by homozygosity analysis: Extension of homozygosity analysis. *Genomics* **36**:130, 1996.

75. Parimoo S, Kolluri R, Weissman S: cDNA selection from total yeast DNA containing YACs. *Nucleic Acids Res* **21**:4422, 1993.

76. Weeda G, van Ham RCA, Vermeulen W, Bootsma D, van der Eb AJ, Hoeijmakers JHJ: A presumed DNA helicase encoded by ERCC is involved in the human repair disorders xeroderma pigmentosa and Cockayne's syndrome. *Cell* **62**:777, 1990.

77. Broughton BC, Thompson AF, Harcourt SA, Vermeulen W, Hoeijmakers JHJ, Botta E, Stefanini M, King MD, Weber CA, Cole J, Arlett CF, Lehmann AR: Molecular and cellular analysis of the DNA repair defect in a patient in xeroderma pigmentosum complementation group D who has the clinical features of xeroderma pigmentosum and Cockayne syndrome. *Am J Hum Genet* **56**:167, 1995.

78. Flejter WL, McDaniel LD, Johns D, Friedberg EC, Schultz RA: Correction of xeroderma pigmentosum complementation group D mutant cell phenotypes by chromosome and gene transfer: Involvement of the human ERCC2 DNA repair gene. *Proc Natl Acad Sci USA* **89**:261, 1992.

79. Frederick GD, Amirkhan RH, Schultz RA, Friedberg EC: Structural and mutational analysis of the xeroderma pimentosum group D (XPD) gene. *Hum Mol Genet* **3**:1783, 1994.

80. Takayama K, Salazar EP, Broughton BC, Lehmann AR, Sarasin A, Thompson LH, Weber CA: Defects in the DNA repair and transcription gene ERCC2(XPD) in trichothiodystrophy. *Am J Hum Genet* **58**:263, 1996.

81. Sung P, Bailly V, Weber C, Thompson LH, Prakash L, Prakash S: Human xeroderma pigmentosum group D gene encodes a DNA helicase. *Nature* **365**:852, 1993.

82. Broughton BC, Steingrimsdottir H, Weber CA, Lehmann AR: Mutations in the xeroderma pigmentosum group D DNA repair/transcription gene in patients with trichothiodystrophy. *Nature Genet* **7**:189, 1994.

83. Takayama K, Salazar EP, Broughton BC, Lehmann AR, Sarasin A, Thompson LH, Weber CA: Defects in the DNA repair and transcription gene ERCC2(XPD) in trichothiodystrophy. *Am J Hum Genet* **58**:263, 1996.

84. Troelstra C, van Gool A, Wit JD, Vermeulen W, Bootsma D, Hoeijmakers JHJ: ERCC6, a member of a subfamily of putative helicases, is involved in Cockayne's syndrome and preferential repair of active genes. *Cell* **71**:939, 1992.

85. Ellis NA, Groden J, Ye TZ, Straughen J, Lennon DJ, Ciocci S, Proytcheva M, German J: The Bloom's syndrome gene product is homologous to RecQ helicases. *Cell* **83**:655, 1995.

86. Stayton CL, Dabovic B, Gulisano M, Gecz J, Broccoli V, Giovanazzi S, Bossolasco M, Monaco L, Rastan S, Boncinelli EE, Bianchi M, Consalez GG: Cloning and characterization of a new human Xq13 gene, encoding a putative helicase. *Hum Mol Genet* **3**:1957, 1994.

87. Ion A, Telvi L, Chaussain JL, Galacteros F, Valayer J, Fellous M, McElreavey K: A novel mutation in the putative DNA helicase XH2 is responsible for male-to-female sex reversal associated with an atypical form of the ATR syndrome. *Am J Hum Genet* **58**:1185, 1996.

88. Miki T, Nakura J, Ye L, Mitsuda N, Morishima A, Sato N, Kamino K, Ogihara T: Molecular and epidemiological studies of Werner syndrome in the Japanese population. *Mech Age Dev* **98**:255, 1997.

89. Oshima J, Brown WT, Martin GM: No detectable mutations at Werner helicase locus in progeria. *Lancet* **348**:1106, 1996.

90. Matsumoto T, Shimamoto A, Goto M, Furuichi Y: Impaired localization of defective DNA helicases in Werner's syndrome. *Nature Genet* **16**:335, 1997.

91. Marciniak RA, Lombard DB, Johnson FB, Guarente L: Nucleolar localization of the Werner syndrome protein in human cells. *Proc Natl Acad Sci USA* **95**:6887, 1998.

92. Sinclair DA, Mills K, Guatente L: Accelerated aging and nuceolar fragmentation in yeast sgs1 mutants. *Science* **277**:1313, 1997.

93. Yamabe Y, Sugimoto M, Satoh M, Suzuki N, Sugawara M, Goto M, Furuichi Y: Down-regulation of the defective transcripts of the Werner's syndrome gene in the cells of patients. *Biochem Biophys Res Commun* **236**:151, 1997.

94. Gorbalenya AE, Koonin EV, Donchenko AP, Blinov VM: Two related superfamilies of putative helicases involved in replication, repair and expression of DNA and RNA genomes. *Nucleic Acids Res* **17**:4713, 1989.

95. Mushegian AR, Bassett DE, Boguski MS, Bork P, Koonin EV: Positionally cloned human disease genes: patterns of evolutionary conservation and functional motifs. *Proc Natl Acad Sci USA* **94**:5831, 1997.

96. Lombard DB, Guarente L: Cloning the gene for Werner syndrome: A disease with many symptoms of premature aging. *Trends Genet* **12**:283, 1996.

97. Morozov V, Mushegian AR, Koonin EV, Bork P: A putative nucleic acid-binding domain in Bloom's and Werner's syndrome helicases. *TIBS* **22**:417, 1997.

98. Imamura O, Ichikawa K, Yamabe Y, Goto M, Sugawara M, Furuchi Y: Cloning of a mouse homologue of the Werner syndrome gene and assignment to 8A4 by flourescence in situ hybridization. *Genomics* **41**:298, 1997.

99. Gray MD, Shen JC, Kamathloeb AS, Blank A, Sopher BL, Martin GM, Oshima J, Loeb LA: The Werner syndrome protein is a DNA helicase. *Nature Genet* **17**:100, 1997.

100. Suzuki N, Shimamoto A, Imamura O, Kuromitsu J, Kitao S, Goto M, Furuichi Y: DNA helicase activity in Werner's syndrome gene product synthesized in a baculovirus system. *Nucleic Acids Res* **25**:2973, 1997.

101. Shen JC, Gray MD, Oshima J, Loeb LA: Characterization of Werner syndrome protein DNA helicase activity: Directionality, substrate dependence and stimulation by replication protein A. *Nucleic Acids Res* **26**:2879, 1998.

102. Schaeffer L, Roy R, Humbert S, Moncollin V, Vermeulen W, Hoeijmakers JHJ, Chambon P, Egly JM: DNA repair helicase: A component of BTF2 (TFIIH) basic transcription factor. *Science* **260**:58, 1993.

103. Henning KA, Li L, Lyer N, McDaniel LD, Reagan MS, Legerski R, Schultz RA, Stefanini M, Lehmann AR, Mayne LV, Friedberg EC: The Cockayne syndrome group A gene encodes a WD repeat protein that interacts with CBS protein and a subunit of RNA polymerase II TFIIH. *Cell* **82**:555, 1995.

104. Fujiwara Y, Higashikawa T, Tatsumi M: A retarded rate of DNA replication and normal level of DNA repair in Werner's syndrome fibroblast cultures. *J Cell Physiol* **92**:365, 1977.

105. Higashikawa T, Fujiwara Y: Normal level of unscheduled DNA synthesis in Werner's syndrome fibroblasts in culture. *Exp Cell Res* **113**:438, 1978.

106. Stefanini M, Scappaticci S, Lagomarsini P, Borroni G, Berardesca E, Nuzzo F: Chromosome instability in lymphocytes from a patient with

Werner's syndrome is not associated with DNA repair defects. *Mutat Res* **219**:179, 1989.

107. Saito H, Moses RE: Immortalization of Werner syndrome and progeria fibroblasts. *Exp Cell Res* **192**:373, 1991.

108. Arlett CF, Harcourt SA: Survey of radiosensitivity in a variety of human cell strains. *Cancer Res* **40**:926, 1980.

109. Gebhart E, Schnizel M, Ruprecht KW: Cytogenetic studies using various clastogens in two patients with Werner syndrome and control individuals. *Hum Genet* **70**:324, 1985.

110. Gebhart E, Bauer R, Raub U, Schinzel M, Ruprecht KW, Jonas JB: Spontaneous and induced chromosomal instability in Werner syndrome. *Hum Genet* **80**:135, 1988.

111. Okada M, Goto M, Furuichi Y, Sugimoto M: Differential effects of cytotoxic drugs on mortal and immortalized B-lymphoblastoid cell lines from normal and Werner's syndrome patients. *Biol Pharm Bull* **21**:235, 1998.

112. Elli R, Chessa L, Antonelli A, Petrinelli P, Ambra R, Marcucci L: Effects of topoisomerase II inhibition in lymphoblasts from patients with progeroid and "chromosome instability" syndromes. *Cancer Genet Cytogenet* **87**:112, 1996.

113. Ogburn CE, Oshima J, Poot M, Chen R, Hunt KE, Gollahon KA, Rabinovitch PS, Martin GM: An apoptosis-inducing genotoxin differentiates heterozygotic carriers from Werner helicase mutations from wild-type and homozygous mutants. *Hum Genet* **101**:12, 1997.

114. Bennett SE, Umar A, Oshima J, Monnat RJ, Kunkel TA: Mismatch repair in extracts of Werner syndrome cell lines. *Cancer Res* **57**:2956, 1997.

115. Brooks-Wilson AR, Emond MJ, Monnat RJ: Unexpectedly low loss of heterozygosity in genetically unstable Werner syndrome cell lines. *Genes Chrom Cancer* **18**:133, 1997.

116. Melaragno MI, Pagni D, Smith MDC: Cytogenetic aspects of Werner's syndrome lymphocyte cultures. *Mech Age Dev* **78**:117, 1995.

117. Gawkrodger DJ, Priestley GC, Vijayalamix, Ross JA, Narcisi P, Hunter JAA: Werner's syndrome. *Arch Dermatol* **121**:636, 1985.

118. Takeuchi F, Hanaoka F, Goto M, Akaoka I, Hori T, Yamada M, Miyamoto T: Altered frequency of initiation sites of DNA replication in Werner's syndrome cells. *Hum Genet* **60**:365, 1982.

119. Hanaoka F, Takeuchi F, Matsumura T, Goto M, Miyamoto T, Tamada M: Decrease in the average size of replicons in a Werner syndrome cell line by a simian virus 40 infection. *Exp Cell Res* **144**:463, 1983.

120. Poot M, Hoehn H, Runger TM, Martin GM: Impaired S-phase transit of Werner syndrome cells expressed in lymphoblastoid cell lines. *Exp Cell Res* **202**:267, 1992.

121. Runger TM, Sobotta P, Dekant B, Moller K, Bauer C, Kraemer KH: *In vivo* assessment of DNA ligation efficiency and fidelity in cells from patients with Franconi's anemia and other cancer-prone hereditary disorders. *Toxicol Lett* **67**:309, 1993.

122. Runger TM, Bauer C, Dekant B, Moller K, Sobotta P, Czemy C, Poot M, Martin GM: Hypermutable ligation of plasmid DNA ends in cells from patients with Werner syndrome. *J Invest Dermatol* **102**:45, 1994.

123. Cheng RZ, Murano S, Kurz B, Shmookler Reis RJS: Homologous recombination is elevated in some Werner-like syndromes but not during normal or *in vitro* senescence of mammalian cells. *Mutat Res* **237**:259, 1990.

124. Watt PM, Hickson ID, Borts RH, Louis EJ: SGS1, a homologue of the Bloom's and Werner's syndrome genes, is required for maintenance of genome stability in *Saccharomyces cerevisiae*. *Genetics* **144**:935, 1996.

125. Yamagata K, Kato J, Shimamoto A, Goto M, Furuichi Y, Ikeda H: Bloom's and Werner's syndrome genes suppress hyperrecombination in yeast sgs1 mutant: Implication for genomic instability in human diseases. *Proc Natl Acad Sci USA* **95**:8733, 1998.

126. Yan H, Chen C.-Y, Kobayashi R, Newport J: Replication focus-forming activity 1 and the Werner syndrome gene product. *Nature Genet* **19**:375, 1998.

127. Adoue DPF: Werner's syndrome. *N Engl J Med* **337**:977, 1997.

Peutz-Jeghers Syndrome

Lauri A. Aaltonen

1. The typical features of Peutz-Jeghers syndrome (PJS) are mucocutaneous melanin pigmentation and gastrointestinal polyposis.
2. Peutz-Jeghers polyps are hamartomas characterized by a stromal tree-like pattern of smooth muscle tissue.
3. PJS patients are predisposed to cancer. An excess of gastrointestinal as well as extraintestinal cancers has been reported in PJS families. The cancer predisposition is less focused than in many other cancer-susceptibility syndromes.
4. The major predisposing gene is *LKB1*. *LKB1* mutations are found in most but not all PJS patients. At present it is unclear whether more predisposing loci exist.
5. LKB1 is a serine/threonine kinase, but detailed information on its function is at present not available. The germ-line mutations associated with tumorigenesis are usually of an inactivating nature, suggesting a role as a tumor suppressor.

The syndrome is named after Peutz and Jeghers, the discoverers of the disease. The first report was by Peutz in 1921,[1] followed by work by Jeghers et al. in 1949.[2] The major hallmarks of Peutz-Jeghers syndrome (PJS) are mucocutaneous melanin pigmentation and intestinal hamartomatous polyposis.[3] PJS patients appear to be at increased risk of cancer (Table 20-1). Especially malignant tumors of the gastrointestinal tract, breast, uterine cervix, and ovary may be associated with the disease.[4-6] Benign ovarian (such as granulosa cell tumor, sex cord tumor with annular tubules) and testicular (Sertoli cell tumor) lesions are relatively frequently found in PJS.[3] Since PJS is a rare disorder, considerably more rare than, for example, familial adenomatous polyposis, it has been difficult to evaluate the cancer spectrum and risk levels typical for PJS. Giardiello et al.[4] reported an 18-fold lifetime risk of malignancy in PJS. Boardman et al.[5] reported a similar relative risk for women, but in their study the risk for men was only 6.2. Gastrointestinal cancer and gynecologic malignancies in particular, as well as breast cancer, were associated with PJS in this study.

Germ-line mutations in a serine/threonine kinase gene *LKB1* (also called *STK11*) located on chromosome 19p 13.3 recently have been shown to underlie a major proportion of PJS cases.[7] *LKB1* is believed to act as a tumor suppressor gene,[7,8] and detailed functional analyses are underway to evaluate the role and partners of LKB1 in cell growth control and development.

CLINICAL ASPECTS

Incidence

The incidence of the PJS is difficult to evaluate, since even in countries with a nationwide adenomatous polyposis registry little attention has been paid to hamartomatous polyposis syndromes, and careful registration and evaluation of this group of patients have not been performed. Based on the experience of polyposis registries, PJS is clearly more rare than familial adenomatous

polyposis, which is believed to be the most common polyposis syndrome, with a carrier frequency of 1 in 5000 to 10,000 live births.[3] A frequency of 1 in 8300 to 1 in 29,000 live births has been estimated.[9] The relatively frequent complications due to bowel obstruction today can be adequately treated surgically. Thus the syndrome is likely to have a smaller impact on biologic fitness now than some decades ago.

Since the molecular background of the PJS has been revealed recently, it is likely that more attention will be focused on PJS, and more light may be shed on the issue of its incidence. Molecular analyses also may reveal cases that do not fulfill the present diagnostic criteria. One difficulty is that although PJS is considered an autosomal dominant disease, patients frequently lack a PJS family history. Future molecular analyses should reveal the background of such patients, but initial results suggest that germ-line *LKB1* defects also play a role in "sporadic" PJS.[10] Interestingly, *de novo* mutations appear to be frequent in PJS patients without a family history.[11] This may reflect the improved biologic fitness of PJS patients, and PJS in the future may be somewhat more common through this effect.

Diagnostic Criteria and Histologic Features

PJS has two clinical hallmarks: mucocutaneous melanin pigmentation and hamartomatous intestinal polyposis. The pigmentation is most often present in and around the mouth but also on hands and feet and axillary pits.[3] The significance of the pigmentation as a key feature of the syndrome is clear, but the presence of similar melanin spots in up to 15 percent of the normal population hampers the use of this sign in clinical practice.[12] The degree of

Table 20-1 Cancer Cases Reported in Patients with Peutz-Jeghers Syndrome.

Gastrointestinal	
Esophagus	1
Stomach	16
Small intestine	22
Large intestine	26
Pancreas	8
Extraintestinal	
Breast	17
Uterine cervix	10
Ovary	7
Uterus	2
Fallopian tube	1
Testis	1
Prostate	1
Lung	9
Thyroid	2
Leiomyosarcoma	2
Gall bladder	1
Liver	1
Basal cell	1
Osteosarcoma	1
Multiple myeloma	1

SOURCE: Data from Hemminki[6,7] and Boardman et al.[5]

A list of standard abbreviations is located immediately preceding the index. Nonstandard abbreviations used in this chapter include: PJS = Peutz-Jeghers syndrome; LOH = loss of heterozygosity.

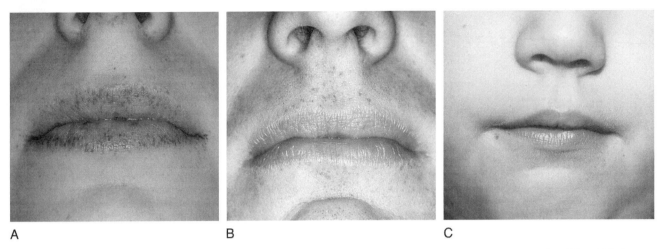

Fig. 20-1 *A.* Typical perioral pigmentation in a Peutz-Jeghers patient. *B, C.* Perioral pigmentation in a 31-year-old patient (B) and his 6-year-old daughter (*C*) illustrates the variation in pigmentation even within a family and the difficulty in relying on pigmentation in PJS diagnostics.

pigmentation varies greatly, even within a family (Fig. 20-1). In a subset of the PJS patients the pigmentation diminishes with age, and some never display it.

The presence of intestinal Peutz-Jeghers polyposis is the diagnostic feature of PJS. Peutz-Jeghers polyps are hamartomatous lesions that have pathognomonic histologic characteristics (Fig. 20-2). In contrast to juvenile polyps, for example, Peutz-Jeghers polyps display a core of a prominent tree-like smooth muscle cell structure that extends into the lamina propria. The overlying folded epithelium contains histologically normal cells without features of neoplasia.[3] The number of polyps in PJS is low as compared with familial adenomatous polyposis and varies greatly from zero to dozens of lesions. A single Peutz-Jeghers polyp without a PJS family history or other features of the syndrome may well be a sporadic lesion. Although the polyps may occur anywhere in the gastrointestinal tract, the small intestine is the most commonly affected part of the bowel. PJS patients commonly also display hyperplastic and adenomatous polyps, but the diagnosis is based on the pathognomonic histology of Peutz-Jeghers polyps. Neoplastic changes sometimes may arise in the Peutz-Jeghers polyps themselves.[13–15]

While it is clear that pigmentation without any other signs of the syndrome is not a good indicator of PJS (see Fig. 20-1) and that, similarly, one Peutz-Jeghers polyp without family history of PJS may be a sporadic lesion, it is less clear how one should evaluate the family members of diagnosed PJS patients. A recent study that identified a locus predisposing to PJS suggested that all individuals carrying the affected haplotype had one of the two

cardinal features of PJS.[8] This was slightly unexpected, since PJS-like pigmentation is not rare in the normal population,[12] and many of the relatives displaying pigmentation did not display a prominent polyposis.[8] This emphasizes that pigmentation as evaluated by an experienced physician is a useful clue, but nevertheless, pigmentation as the only sign should be interpreted with caution. The current diagnostic criteria are: (1) three or more histologically confirmed Peutz-Jeghers polyps; or (2) any number of Peutz-Jeghers polyps with family history of PJS; or (3) characteristic, prominent, mucocutaneous pigmentation (see Fig. 20-1A as an example) with family history of PJS; or (4) any number of Peutz-Jeghers polyps and characteristic, prominent, mucocutaneous pigmentation.

The ultimate diagnostic laboratory test is the detection of a *LKB1* germ-line mutation.[7] The mutations are usually truncating, which facilitates interpretation of the results. When a mutation in a particular family has been detected, the relatives who are willing to undergo genetic testing can be analyzed with reasonable efficiency.

Differential Diagnosis

The different polyposis syndromes have overlapping clinical features. Polyps of mixed histologic subtypes (e.g., adenoma, hyperplastic polyp, hamartoma) are seen relatively commonly in PJS patients, and careful histologic evaluation of the removed lesions is essential. The striking phenotype of familial adenomatous polyposis with typically hundreds or thousands of adenomas is usually easily distinguishable from the other

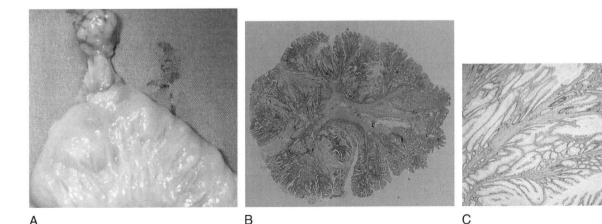

Fig. 20-2 *A.* A hamartomatous Peutz-Jeghers polyp. *B.* Histologic view of the lesion. *C.* Microscopical view. Note the smooth muscle cell core of the polyp.

polyposis syndromes including PJS. The two other major hamartomatous polyposis syndromes, Cowden syndrome and juvenile polyposis, are more difficult in this regard. Detection of lesions displaying the pathognomonic polyp core with arborizing smooth muscle pattern forms the basis of the PJS diagnosis.

GENETIC LOCI

Loci for Hereditary PJS

Few genetic loci have been implicated in PJS. A study by Amos et al.[16] found evidence for linkage on chromosome 1 in a large U.S. kindred, but further genotyping analyses did not support the finding (Amos, personal communication). In 1997, Hemminki et al.[8] used a novel approach to reveal a predisposing locus. Malignant tumors often display multiple genetic alterations that tend to occur during tumor development and in part drive the process. Benign tumors, such as hamartomatous polyps, are likely to harbor many fewer molecular changes. It was hypothesized that by studying multiple polyps from a single Peutz-Jeghers patient, genetic loci associated with early development of these lesions might be revealed. Indeed, the short arm of chromosome 19 appeared to be deleted in some of the polyps. This result was confirmed by microdissection and polymerase chain reaction (PCR) assays; loss of heterozygosity (LOH) experiments using 19p microsatellite markers demonstrated the loss of the wild-type (maternal) chromosome in a subset of the polyp cells. The same markers were used for genetic linkage analysis in a collection of twelve PJS families, and conclusive evidence of linkage was obtained. These experiments showed that a PJS susceptibility gene that is likely to have a tumor suppressor function resided in 19p.[8]

However, not all families display 19p linkage. A small subset of the families has been demonstrated to be incompatible with linkage to 19p,[17] and in one PJS family, evidence of linkage to chromosome 19q has been reported.[18]

Sporadic Tumors and Chromosome 19p

The PJS locus on 19p is not one of the most common targets of chromosomal deletions during sporadic tumor progression. In some tumor types, such as adenoma malignum of the uterine cervix, pancreatic cancer, and chronic myelocytic leukemia, 19p deletions appear to be relatively common.[19–21] Interestingly, adenoma malignum is a rare tumor that appears to be associated with PJS.[6] Avizienyte et al.[22] detected LOH at D19S886 in 13 of 50 (26 percent) colorectal carcinomas. A paper by Dong et al.[23] reported LOH at the locus D19S886 and/or D19S883 in 10 of 19 (53 percent) colorectal cancers, but no LOH in 25 informative colorectal adenomas.

MUTATIONS OF SERINE/THREONINE KINASE GENE *LKB1* UNDERLIE PJS

The gene for PJS was identified through positional cloning.[7] The effort was greatly facilitated by the fact that the target area in chromosome 19p determined by linkage results was covered by a physical map.[24] Researchers working at and in collaboration with the Lawrence Livermore National Laboratory had constructed a cosmid contig that soon spanned across the whole region of interest.

After mapping the PJS locus through comparative genomic hybridization[25] and targeted linkage analysis, Hemminki et al.[7] first reduced the target area by creating novel polymorphic microsatellite and biallelic markers and analyzing the families displaying critical recombinations. In this way the area was reduced to 800 kb. Genes and expressed sequence tags that mapped to the region of interest were analyzed for mutations in PJS families using reverse-transcriptase (RT) PCR and sequencing. Since these efforts produced only negative findings, the researchers performed direct cDNA selection experiments to derive novel transcripts that map to the area. Multiple candidate

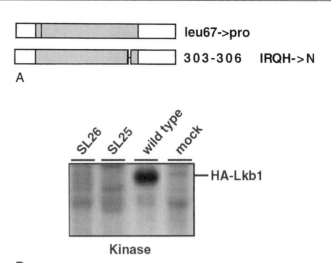

Fig. 20-3 Functional analysis of LKB1 kinase activity. *A.* The mutations in SL25 (missense change, leu67 → pro) and SL 26 (in-frame deletion of 9 bases, 303–306 IRQH → N), respectively. The kinase domain is shaded. *B.* The results of an autophosphorylation assay. While the wild-type LKB1 is capable of autophosphorylation, the missense mutation in SL25 and the in-frame deletion of 9 bp in SL26 have resulted in a protein that displays no kinase activity.

sequences were isolated from this gene-rich area. One of these represented the *LKB1* gene, a previously cloned gene that had not been mapped to a chromosomal locus. The full-length *LKB1* cDNA had been reported in 1996 as a Gen Bank submission by Dr. Nezu.[26]

Mutation analysis of the *LKB1* cDNA soon revealed multiple truncating mutations in PJS patients. Eleven of the 12 patients used in the PJS gene search displayed a mutation. The changes segregated with the disease phenotype and were absent in multiple control individuals.[7] Subsequent work has shown that approximately 60 percent of unselected PJS patients display *LKB1* mutations.[10,12] The difference is likely due to patient selection; the samples used in the initial mutation screen were derived from scrutinized 19p-linked PJS families.

LKB1 encodes a 432-amino-acid protein that through sequence homology was predicted to act as a serine/threonine kinase. The gene appears to be ubiquitously expressed, with especially prominent expression in the pancreas and testis.[7] Mutations in kinase genes had been described in association with hereditary cancer earlier, but this was the first time that inactivating mutations in such a gene were reported. The detailed function of LKB1 remains to be clarified. The gene has no human homologues but is highly homologuous to a *Xenopus* cytoplasmic serine/threonine kinase *XEEK1.*[27] XEEK1 is expressed only during the very first days of embryonic life and may be involved in early development. XEEK1 is capable of autophosphorylation. Recent work has demonstrated that the same is also true for LKB1[10] (Fig. 20-3). It is likely that autophosphorylation is not the main function of the gene, and yeast double-hybrid experiments and other assays should provide further data on how LKB1 is involved in cell growth regulation and which proteins are its substrates and upstream effectors.

Somatic Mutations in *LKB1*

Bignell et al.[28] reported absence of mutations in sporadic breast cancers. Avizienyte et al.[22] studied a set of colonic, testicular, cervical, and lung cancers, as well as sarcomas and myeloma and melanoma cell lines. One missense mutation was found in a testicular cancer as well as in a lung cancer, and one mutation leading to frameshift and truncating protein product was detected in an adenocarcinoma of the uterine cervix.[29] Subsequently, the missense mutation detected in a testicular cancer was shown to in part but not completely abolish the kinase function of the LKB1 protein.[10] Tomlinson et al.[30] reported the absence of *LKB1* mutations in colorectal and ovarian cancers. Park et al.[31] found little evidence of *LKB1* involvement in gastric carcinomas; only 1 of 23 samples displayed a missense mutation. Two of the 23 tumors were reported to display somatic nucleotide changes that did not lead to amino acid substitutions.

To summarize, most reports thus far have found little evidence of somatic mutational inactivation of *LKB1,* although clearly in a few tumor cases somatic inactivation of *LKB1* has been seen. *LKB1* mutations may play a more prominent role in tumor types that have not yet been examined.

Animal Models

Animal models for PJS are not yet available, but multiple research groups are at present working toward a mouse model. *Xenopus Xeek1* mutants also could serve as a model organism. Since the *Xenopus LKB1* homologue *Xeek1* is expressed in early embryos, and since the knockout mice for the other hamartomatous polyposis genes *PTEN*[32] and *SMAD4/DPC4*[33] failed to develop, a conditional knockout mouse might serve research better than a conventional knockout animal. The animal models are expected to reveal data on LKB1 function in development as well as tumorigenesis.

IMPLICATIONS FOR DIAGNOSIS

The discoveries on the molecular background of PJS will allow identification of at-risk individuals in a subset of the families. Predictive testing always should be associated with appropriate genetic counseling, and testing should be performed only after obtaining informed consent.

First, the genetic defect in a particular family should be detected through *LKB1* germ-line analysis of a typically affected patient.[7] Since *LKB1* is a relatively small gene, genomic sequencing of the nine coding exons[28] consisting of 1299 nucleotides is recommended. Since no mutation analysis technique is complete, and since locus heterogeneity still is a possibility in PJS, a negative mutation analysis result gives little information. Since the current mutation detection rate in PJS patients in whom no linkage information is available is not much more than 50 percent,[10] the option that the analyses will not reveal a mutation should be explained carefully to the patient before a sample is derived and analyzed. This issue is different, of course, in families segregating a characterized mutation, where unambiguous results can be obtained.

Unlike in Bannayan-Riley-Ruvalcaba syndrome,[34] PJS patients without a family history of the disease often have a *LKB1* germ-line defect, and thus these patients and their relatives also may benefit from molecular analyses.

Most *LKB1* defects appear to be truncating, and interpretation of the mutation analysis result is not problematic in such cases. However, a subset of the changes consists of small in-frame deletions or missense mutations. The autophosphorylation function of LKB1 may in the future provide clues to the functional significance of such *LKB1* variants.[10] If an allele encoded by a particular mutation displays a defect in the autophosphorylation assay, it is likely to be pathogenic. A result indicating normal kinase function would be difficult to interpret, since other functions of LKB1 are not known.

IMPLICATIONS FOR TREATMENT

Accurate diagnosis of PJS is important in view of cancer prevention. The at-risk individuals appear to need surveillance for at least gastrointestinal and gynecologic tumors, as well as breast cancer. The unraveling of the molecular background of the various hamartomatous syndromes may well contribute to the management of patients in the future. Ideally, the molecular analyses could clarify the particular predisposing defect in a patient, and tumor prevention measures could be targeted to the sites at greatest risk. Considering the complex and overlapping clinical features of the hamartomatous polyposis syndromes, molecular methods for exact diagnosis and evaluation of tumor risk would be welcome. However, molecular epidemiologic studies should first characterize the cancer risks associated with the different genetic defects. Owing to the rarity of the syndromes, this can be achieved only through collaborative efforts.

The ultimate goal of the molecular research conducted is to prevent tumors in susceptible individuals through clarifying the exact mechanisms of tumor predisposition.

ACKNOWLEDGMENTS

Drs. Järvinen, Salovaara, and Ylikorkala are acknowledged for providing the figures.

REFERENCES

1. Peutz JL: A very remarkable case of familial polyposis of mucous membrane of intestinal tract and accompanied by peculiar pigmentations of skin and mucous membrane. (in Dutch). *Ned Tijdschr Geneeskd* **10**:134, 1921.
2. Jeghers H, McKusick VA, Katz KH: Generalized intestinal polyposis and melanin spots of the oral mucosa, lips and digits. *N Engl J Med* **241**:992, 1949.
3. Phillips RKS, Spigelman AD, Thomson JPS: *Familial Adenomatous Polyposis and Other Polyposis Syndromes.* London, Edward Arnold, 1994.
4. Giardiello FM, Welsh SB, Hamilton SR, Offerhaus GJ, Gittelsohn AM, Booker SV, Krush AJ, Yardley JH, Luk GD: Increased risk of cancer in the Peutz-Jeghers syndrome. *New Engl J Med* **316**:1511, 1987.
5. Boardman LA, Thibodeau SN, Schaid DJ, Lindor NM, McDonnell SK, Burgart LJ, Ahlquist Da, Podratz KC, Pittelkow M, Hartmann LC: Increased risk for cancer in patients with the Peutz-Jeghers syndrome. *Ann Intern Med* **128**:896, 1998.
6. Hemminki A: Inherited predisposition to gastrointestinal cancer: The molecular backgrounds of Peutz-Jeghers syndrome and hereditary nonpolyposis colorectal cancer. Academic dissertation, University of Helsinki, 1998.
7. Hemminki A, Markie D, Tomlinson I, Avizienyte E, Roth S, Loukola A, Bignell G, Warren W, Aminoff M, Höglund P, Järvinen H, Kristo P, Pelin K, Ridanpää M, Salovaara R, Toro T, Bodmer W, Olschwang S, Olsen AS, Stratton Mr, de la Chapelle A, Aaltonen lA:A serine/ threonine kinase gene defective in Peutz-Jeghers syndrome. *Nature* **391**:184, 1998.
8. Hemminki A, Tomlinson I, Markie D, Järvinen H, Sistonen P, Björkqvist A-M, Knuutila S, Salovaara R, Bodmer W, Shibata D, de la Chapelle A, Aaltonen LA: Localization of a susceptibility locus for Peutz-Jeghers syndrome to 19p using comparative genomic hybridization and targeted linkage analysis. *Nature Genet* **15**:87, 1997.
9. Finan MC, Ray MK: Gastrointestinal polyposis syndromes. *Dermatol Clin* **7**:419, 1989.
10. Ylikorkala A, Avizienyte E, Tomlinson IPM, Tiainen M, Roth S, Loukola A, Hemminki A, Johansson M, Sistonen P, Markie D, Neale K, Phillips R, Zauber P, Twama T, Sampson J, Järvinen H, Mäkelä TP, Aaltonen La: Mutations and impaired function of LKB1 in familial and non-familial Peutz-Jeghers syndrome and a sporadic testicular cancer. *Hum Mol Genet* **8**:45, 1999.
11. Westerman AM, Entius MM, Boor PP, Koole R, de Baar E, Offerhaus GJ, Lubinski J, Lindhout D, Halley DJ, de Rooij FW, Wilson JH: Novel Mutations in the LKB1/STK11 gene in Dutch Peutz-Jeghers families. *Hum Mutat* **13**:476, 1999.
12. Westerman AM, Chong YK, Entius MM, Wilson JHP, van Velthuysen, Lindhout D, Offerhaus GJA: The diagnostic value of mucocutaneous pigmentations in Peutz-Jeghers Syndrome. Abstract book, first joint meeting, ICG-HNPCC & LCPG, 1997, p 23.
13. Hizawa K, Iida M, Matsumoto T, Kohrogi N, Yao T, Fujishima M: Neoplastic transformation arising in Peutz-Jeghers polyposis. *Dis Colon Rectum* **36**:953, 1993.
14. De Facq L, De Sutter J, De Man M, Van der Spek P, Lepoutre L: A case of Peutz-Jeghers syndrome with nasal polyposis, extreme iron deficiency anemia, and hamartoma-adenoma transformation: Management by combined surgical and endoscopic approach. *Am J Gastroenterol* **90**:1330, 1995.

15. Defago MR, Higa AL, Campra JL, Paradelo M, Uehara A, Torres Mazzucchi MH, Videla R: Carcinoma in situ arising in a gastric hamartomatous polyp in a patient with Peutz-Jeghers syndrome. *Endoscopy* **28**:267, 1996.

16. Bali D, Gourley IS, McGarrity TJ, Spencer CA, Howard L, Frazier ML, Lynch PM, Seldin MF, Amos CI: Peutz-Jeghers syndrome maps to chromosome 1p. In American Society of Human Genetics, abstract 1067, 1995.

17. Olschwang S, Markie D, Seal S, Neale K, Phillips R, Cottrell S, Ellis I, Hodgson S, Zauber P, Spigelman A, Iwama T, Loff S, McKeown C, Marchese C, Sampson J, Davies S, Talbot I, Wyke J, Thomas G, Bodmer W, Hemminki A, Avizienyte E, de la Chapelle A, Aaltonen LA, Stratton M, Houlston R, Tomlinson I: Peutz-Jeghers disease: Most families compatible with linkage to 19p13.3, but evidence for a second locus at a different site. *J Med Genet* **35**:42, 1997.

18. Mehenni H, Blouin J-L, Radhakrishna U, Bhardwaj SS, Bhardwaj K, Dixit VB, Richards KF, Bermejo-Fenoll A, Leal AS, Raval RC, Antonarakis SE: Peutz-Jeghers syndrome: Confirmation of linkage to chromosome 19p13.3 and identification of a potential second locus, on 19q13.4. *Am J Hum Genet* **61**:1327, 1997.

19. Lee JY, Dong SM, Kim HS, Kim HS, Kim SY, Na EY, Shin MS, Lee SH, Park WS, Kim KM, Lee YS, Jang JJ, Yoo NJ: A distinct region of chromosome 19p13.3 associated with the sporadic form of adenoma malignum of the uterine cervix. *Cancer Res* **58**:1140, 1998.

20. Hoglund M, Gorunova L, Andren-Sandberg A, Dawiskiba S, Mitelman F, Johansson B: Cytogenetic and fluorescence in situ hybridization analyses of chromosome 19 aberrations in pancreatic carcinomas: Frequent loss of 19p13.3 and gain of 19q13.1-13.2. *Genes Chromosomes Cancer* **21**:8, 1998.

21. Mori N, Morosetti R, Lee S, Spira S, Ben-Yehuda D, Schiller G, Landolfi R, Mizoguchi H, Koeffler HP: Allelotype analysis in the evolution of chronic myelocytic leukemia. *Blood* **90**:2010, 1997.

22. Avizienyte E, Roth S, Loukola A, Hemminki A, Lothe RA, Stenwig AE, Fosså SD, Salovaara R, Aaltonen LA: Somatic mutations in LKB1 are rare in sporadic colorectal and testicular tumors. *Cancer Res* **58**:2087, 1998.

23. Dong SM, Kim KM, Kim SY, Shin MS, Na EY, Lee SH, Park WS, Yoo NJ, Jang JJ, Yoon CY, Kim JW, Kim SY, Yang YM, Kim SH, Kim CS, Lee JY: Frequent somatic mutations in serine threonine kinase 11/Peutz-Jeghers syndrome gene in left-sided colon cancer. *Cancer Res* **58**:3787, 1998.

24. Ashworth LK: An integrated metric physical map of human chromosome 19. *Nature Genet* **11**:422, 1995.

25. Kallioniemi A, Kallioniemi O-P, Sudar D, Rutovitz D, Gray JW, Waldman F, Pinkel D: Comparative genomic hybridization for molecular cytogenetic analysis of solid tumors. *Science* **258**:818, 1992.

26. Nezu J: Molecular cloning of a novel serine/threonine protein kinase expressed in human fetal liver (direct submission to GenBank). In http://www.ncbi.nlm.nih.gov/irx/cgi-bin/birx_doc?genbank+65606, 1996.

27. Su J-Y, Erikson E, Maller JL: Cloning and characterization of a novel serine/threonine protein kinase expressed in early *Xenopus* embryos. *J Biol Chem* **271**:14430, 1996.

28. Bignell GR, Barfoot R, Seal S, Collins N, Warren W, Stratton MR: Low frequency of somatic mutations in the LKB1/Peutz-Jeghers syndrome gene in sporadic breast cancer. *Cancer Res* **58**:1384, 1998.

29. Avizienyte E, Loukola A, Roth S, Hemminki A, Salovaara R, Arola J, Bützow R, Husgafvel-Pursiainen K, Tarkkanen M, Kokkola A, Järvinen H, Aaltonen LA: LKB1 somatic mutations in sporadic tumors. *Am J Pathol* **154**:677, 1999.

30. Wang ZJ, Taylor F, Churchman M, Norbury G, Tomlinson I: Genetic pathways of colorectal carcinogenesis rarely involve the PTEN and LKB1 genes outside the inherited hamartoma syndromes. *Am J Pathol* **153**:363, 1998.

31. Park WS, Moon YW, Yang YM, Kim YS, Kim YD, Fuller BG, Vortmeyer AO, Fogt F, Lubensky IA, Zhuang Z: Mutations of the STK11 gene in sporadic gastric carcinoma. *Int J Oncol* **13**:601, 1998.

32. Di Cristofano A, Pesce B, Cordon-Cardo C, Pandolfi PP: Pten is essential for embryonic development and tumor suppression. *Nature Genet* **19**:348, 1997.

33. Takaku K, Oshima M, Miyoshi H, Matsui M, Seldin MF, Taketo MM: Intestinal tumorigenesis in compound mutant mice of both Dpc4 (Smad4) and Apc genes. *Cell* **92**:645, 1998.

34. Carethers JM, Furnari FB, Zigman AF, Lavine JE, Jones MC, Graham GE, Teebi AS, Huang HJ, Ha HT, Chauhan DP, Chang CL, Cavenee WK, Boland CR: Absence of PTEN/MMAC1 germ-line mutations in sporadic Bannayan-Riley-Ruvalcaba syndrome. *Cancer Res* **58**:2724, 1998.

Juvenile Polyposis Syndrome

James R. Howe

1. Juvenile polyposis (JP) is an autosomal dominant syndrome characterized by multiple hamartomatous polyps of the gastrointestinal (GI) tract. Patients may have juvenile polyps of the stomach, small intestine, and/or colon. The diagnosis of JP is made by having more than five juvenile polyps in the colon, juvenile polyps throughout the GI tract, or one or more juvenile polyps in the setting of a family history of JP. Patients with other genetically distinct syndromes may also have hamartomatous polyps, and these conditions need to be excluded by careful history and physical examination. Due to the association of juvenile polyps with several heterogeneous syndromes, it is likely that there are multiple genes that predispose to JP.

2. Approximately 20 to 50 percent of JP cases are familial, with the remainder arising *de novo*. As many as 20 percent of patients may have associated anomalies, which are more common in sporadic cases. Patients with JP are at approximately 50 percent risk for the developing GI cancers, the majority of which are colorectal cancers, but they are also at risk for upper GI cancers.

3. The pathologic features of juvenile polyps are dilated, cystic glands, infiltration of the lamina propria by inflammatory cells, and an overabundance of stroma. Larger polyps may also contain adenomatous areas; adenocarcinoma has also been described within juvenile polyps. Although the exact mechanism of carcinogenesis is unclear, it has been suggested that the changes seen in the lamina propria are brought about through *landscaper defects,* where changes in this tissue layer lead to an environment predisposing to neoplastic transformation of the overlying epithelium.

4. Loss of heterozygosity studies have revealed a tumor-suppressor locus for JP on chromosome 10q22, with the minimal region of overlap defining a 3-cM region approximately 7 cM centromeric to the *PTEN* gene. Germ line *PTEN* mutations have been described in four unrelated patients with JP, but it is possible that some of these patients had Cowden syndrome.

5. A gene for JP has been mapped to chromosome 18q21.1 by genetic linkage analysis, within an interval containing the two tumor-suppressor genes *DCC* and *DPC4 (SMAD4).* Germ line mutations in one of these genes, *SMAD4*, have been found in 6 of 10 familial and sporadic JP patients. In familial cases, these mutations segregated with the JP phenotype, and all were predicted to cause truncation of the SMAD4 protein, resulting in loss of its C-terminus required for oligomerization.

6. The *SMAD4* gene consists of 11 exons and encodes for 552 amino acids. SMAD4 is a common mediator for the transforming growth factor-β, activin, and bone morphogenetic protein signaling pathways. The SMAD4 protein associates with other SMAD proteins following their phosphorylation by activated receptors, then translocates to the nucleus where it regulates transcription through direct binding to specific DNA sequences. SMAD4 is required for differentiation of the mesoderm and visceral endoderm during embryogenesis; transgenic mice with *SMAD4* and *Apc* mutations have polyps with stromal proliferation reminiscent of juvenile polyps.

HISTORY

The first clearly documented juvenile polyp was reported by Diamond in 1939, in a 30-month-old girl with a prolapsing polyp of the rectum. Although Diamond described the polyp as an adenoma, photomicrographs show a juvenile polyp.[1] Helwig gave an excellent pathologic description of juvenile polyps in 1946, and differentiated these "adenomas" in children from those of adults by their showing "foci in which the glandular structures are embedded in a stroma of cellular connective tissue infiltrated with inflammatory cells".[2] Ravitch reported an 18-month-old male who died postoperatively after exploration for an intussusception, and who, at autopsy, was found to have adenomatous polyps from stomach to anus.[3] Review of these photomicrographs reveals that this patient actually had generalized juvenile polyposis. Juvenile polyps later became known as a distinct form of colonic polyps through the work of Horilleno, Eckert, and Ackerman in 1957,[4] and Morson in 1962.[5] McColl and associates coined the term *juvenile polyposis coli* in 1964, to differentiate patients with multiple juvenile polyps from those with either adenomatous polyposis or solitary juvenile polyps.[6] Smilow, Pryor, and Swinton described a clear familial pattern of JP in a three-generation kindred in 1966. They hypothesized an autosomal dominant inheritance, reported one affected family member with colon cancer, and did not believe there was adequate evidence to suggest that juvenile polyps had malignant potential.[7] Veale and coworkers also noted the familial association of juvenile polyps, and described seven cases of JP in four families. Despite 14 other members of these families having developed colorectal cancer, they also did not suggest that juvenile polyps might predispose to malignancy.[8] The conclusions of these groups that JP was a benign condition, albeit complicated in some cases by GI bleeding and congenital anomalies, were supported by previous studies in solitary juvenile polyps. Roth and Helwig followed 60 children (with a mean followup of 6.4 years) and 27 adults (for a mean followup of 10.6 years) diagnosed with juvenile polyps, and found that no cases of GI cancer developed in these patients.[9] For nearly a decade, it was believed that both solitary juvenile polyps and polyps from JP patients were hamartomas with no malignant potential.

In 1975, however, a kindred was described in which 10 family members had JP of the stomach and/or colon, and 11 family members had developed GI carcinoma. The authors believed that the same gene causing JP was also likely to predispose to GI cancer, but they were careful not to suggest that these malignancies developed within juvenile polyps.[10] Since this report, there have been many accounts of GI malignancy developing in patients with JP, including colon cancer,[10–19] stomach cancer,[10,19,20] and pancreatic cancer.[10,21] The risk of developing colorectal cancer in affected family members has been estimated to be from as low as 9 percent[15] to as high as 68 percent,[22] and these patients are also at risk for cancers of the upper GI tract.[23]

Our understanding of the genetics of JP has been confounded somewhat by the association of juvenile polyps with several heterogeneous genetic syndromes. The first suggestion of a chromosomal localization for JP was reported by Jacoby and colleagues as a result of cytogenetic[24] and loss of heterozygosity (LOH) studies[25] in 1997. Howe and associates described the first locus to be identified by genetic linkage analysis in 1998,[26] and JP patients were reported with germ line mutations of two different tumor-suppressor genes in 1998.[27,28]

CLINICAL ASPECTS

Incidence

The prevalence of juvenile polyps is considered to be 1 to 2 percent of the population, but the vast majority of these cases are solitary juvenile polyps and not cases of JP. The average age of diagnosis of solitary juvenile polyps is 3 to 5 years, and these polyps are usually sloughed into the stool and do not recur.[4,9] Helwig found incidental juvenile polyps in 5 of 449 autopsies performed on consecutive patients less than 21 years of age.[2] Toccalino and colleagues found 50 cases of juvenile polyps in 4000 pediatric gastroenterologic consultations (1.25 percent) over a 6-year-period in Argentina.[29] Sulser and associates found 3 cases of juvenile polyps in 90 consecutive patients with polyps (all 3 patients were adults: 2 with solitary polyps, and 1 with approximately 100 polyps).[30] Restrepo and coworkers performed autopsies on 508 patients over 10 years of age from Medellin, Colombia, and found 12 cases of juvenile polyps (2.4 percent). This number would have undoubtedly been higher if individuals aged 0 to 10 years were included.[31]

Restrepo and associates also compared the number of adenomatous and hamartomatous GI polyposis patients seen in 763 cases of colonic polyps from Cali and Medellin, Colombia over a 30-year-period. They found 27 cases of JP (most patients having between 25 and 100 polyps), 14 cases of familial adenomatous polyposis (FAP), and 10 patients with Peutz-Jeghers syndrome. Thirteen of 27 JP cases could be traced to 5 families (2 were suggestive of being familial), and in 12 patients, JP appeared to arise *de novo*.[32] Juvenile polyposis was the most common GI polyposis syndrome seen in this population, which has been described in other developing nations, such as Nigeria.[33] In contrast, Burt and colleagues suggested that the incidence of JP is less than Peutz-Jeghers syndrome, which they estimated to be one-tenth as common as FAP.[34] Because FAP has an incidence of 1 in 8000 live births, Burt et al. would place the incidence of JP at approximately 1 in 100,000. The incidence estimates from Restrepo and Burt vary by a factor of 10: Restrepo found JP to be more common than FAP, but could have been biased by the presence of several JP families from a small geographic region or by other factors unique to developing countries. Chevrel and coworkers from France suggested that JP represented 10 percent of cases of GI polyposis, which they reported had an incidence of 1 in 16,000.[35] Because JP is relatively rare and there are no data available from population-based registries, a more reliable estimate of the incidence of JP is not possible.

Diagnostic Criteria

The criteria currently accepted for diagnosing JP were described by Jass and associates in 1978, and are met by patients with (a) more than five juvenile polyps of the colorectum; (b) juvenile polyps throughout the GI tract; or (c) any number of juvenile polyps with a family history of JP.[36] Howe and colleagues have also suggested that members of JP families with either affected offspring or a history of GI cancer should be considered as affected, even in the absence of histologic demonstration of juvenile polyps.[26] In larger pedigrees, it is often found that members of earlier generations have never had endoscopic screening confirming the presence of juvenile polyps, but have died of GI cancer and had affected offspring.[8,23]

It is important to recognize that these criteria define JP of the GI tract, but not necessarily the more narrow definitions of sporadic or familial JP, for they do not take into account the association of JP with other specific and genetically heterogeneous syndromes, including Cowden syndrome (CS; MIM 158350), Bannayan-Ruvalcaba-Riley syndrome (BRR; MIM 153480), Gorlin syndrome (or basal cell nevus syndrome, BCNS; MIM 109400), and hereditary mixed polyposis syndrome (HMPS; MIM 601228). Patients with CS have benign and malignant lesions of the breast, thyroid, skin (trichilemmomas), and mucous membranes; 40 to 60 percent may have hamartomatous intestinal polyps.[37] Nelen and colleagues mapped the gene for CS to 10q22-24,[38] and Liaw and associates identified germ line mutations in the *PTEN* gene.[39] The clinical manifestations of BRR are hamartomatous GI polyposis, macrocephaly, pseudopapilledema, multiple lipomas, and enlarged penis with speckled pigmentation of the glans. Germ line mutations in these patients have also been found in the *PTEN* gene, suggesting that CS and BRR are allelic conditions.[40] Patients with Gorlin syndrome may have multiple basal cell nevi, palmar pits (also seen in CS), medulloblastoma, mental retardation, ophthalmologic anomalies, and multiple skeletal abnormalities. The incidence of hamartomatous GI polyps appears to be low, however, with large reviews by Gorlin,[41] Evans,[42] and Shanley and collaborators making no mention of GI tract involvement.[43] However, there have been case reports of Gorlin syndrome patients with hamartomatous polyps of the stomach.[44,45] This disorder was mapped to chromosome 9q22.3-31,[46] and found to be caused by germ line mutations in the human *PTC* gene.[47,48] To date, only one family has been well documented with HMPS, in which affected family members have atypical juvenile polyps, colonic adenomas, and colorectal carcinoma, with no extracolonic manifestations.[49] Thomas and coworkers mapped the gene for HMPS in this family to chromosome 6q.[50]

Patients with Cronkhite-Canada syndrome (MIM 175500) have acquired, generalized GI polyposis in which gastric polyps are indistinguishable from juvenile polyps in the stomach, but in which colonic polyps tend to be sessile rather than pedunculated.[51] Distinguishing between this syndrome and JP is aided by Cronkhite-Canada being nonfamilial, of adult onset, and accompanied by diffuse pigmentation, alopecia, and onchorotrophia.[52,53] Although the polyps seen in patients with Peutz-Jeghers syndrome (PJS; MIM 175200) are also hamartomatous, they differ from juvenile polyps in that they contain muscle bundles in the head and stalk of the polyps, whereas juvenile polyps do not have this muscle within their expanded lamina propria. Patients with PJS have pigmented lesions on the lips and buccal mucosa, and may have polyps throughout the GI tract, but these are most commonly found in the small intestine.[54] Hemminki and collaborators established linkage of PJS to markers on chromosome 19p13 in 1997,[55] and germ line mutations were identified soon thereafter in the *LKB1* gene.[56]

Because of the overlap of these clinical syndromes involving JP, patients should be classified as having JP if they meet any of the diagnostic criteria suggested by Jass, *and* do not meet the diagnostic criteria for CS, BRR, BCNS, HMPS, or Cronkhite-Canada syndrome. This task may be troublesome in sporadic cases where there is a higher association with other anomalies, and may even be difficult in families with multiple affected members due to incomplete penetrance or variable expression. Eventually, these syndromes will be more accurately classified by the germ line defects responsible for each case.

Subtypes of Juvenile Polyposis

Sachatello categorized JP patients into three groups to highlight differences in phenotype: (a) juvenile polyposis of infancy; (b) juvenile polyposis coli, to designate those with colonic involvement only; and (c) generalized juvenile polyposis.[57] The latter two groups may be somewhat artificial, for even within families with generalized juvenile polyposis, many members may have colonic involvement only. Hizawa and colleagues have suggested a fourth entity, juvenile polyposis of the stomach, based on 3 patients they followed for 1, 7, and 30 years who had not developed polyps outside the stomach.[58] In a large kindred from Iowa originally described by Stemper, Kent, and Summers,[10] long-term followup of 29 affected family members revealed that 27 had juvenile polyps or cancer of the colorectum, while 11 (38 percent) had polyps or cancer of the upper GI tract. However, only 17 patients had endoscopic or radiologic evaluation of the upper GI tract (65 percent of those screened for this component of the disease had upper GI involvement).[23] Therefore, there is variable expression of the extent of GI tract involvement within families with the same germ line defect. Many of the families reported in the literature have either not been screened for upper GI involvement, or have had few members and no long-term follow-up. This makes it difficult to determine whether juvenile polyposis coli, generalized juvenile polyposis, and juvenile polyposis of the stomach are truly discrete entities or result from variable expression of the same genetic defect.

Juvenile polyposis of infancy has a biologic behavior that appears to be somewhat different from these other subgroups. The patient with generalized juvenile polyposis described by Ravitch presented with diarrhea since birth, malnutrition, anemia, edema, and digital clubbing, and died at 18 months of age following operation for intussusception.[3] Soper and Kent described an infant with macrocephaly and no family history of polyposis who had diarrhea from 3 months of age. The infant later developed hypoalbuminemia, rectal prolapse, and intussusception related to polyposis of the small intestine and colon. He died at age 18 months after reoperation for progressive deterioration, although colectomy was not performed.[59] Gourley and coworkers believed that the hypoalbuminemia seen in a similar patient was due to protein-losing enteropathy, based upon the improvement in serum protein levels after removal of 12 juvenile colonic polyps.[60] Sachatello and colleagues reviewed the literature and reported another infant with small and large intestinal JP with a ventricular septal defect, hepatosplenomegaly, hypoalbuminemia, digital clubbing, diarrhea, duplication of the left renal pelvis and ureter, and a bifid uterus and vagina.[57] They proposed a non-sex-linked recessive inheritance because there was no family history of polyposis in these patients. Of the seven patients reviewed, only one survived beyond 2 years of age,[61] perhaps due to early subtotal colonic resection. Sachatello believed that JP of infancy warranted a separate subgroup to highlight the unfavorable prognosis seen in these patients.[57]

Associated Conditions

One unusual condition, which has been described concurrently with JP, is ganglioneuromatous proliferation within polyps. Donnelly, Sieber, and Yunis described a 9-year-old male with sporadic JP who had both juvenile polyps and polyps with ganglioneuromatous proliferation; only one polyp was found with both of these elements present.[62] Weidner, Flanders, and Mitros reported a 16-year-old male with sporadic JP and ganglioneuromatosis of both normal colonic mucosa and within juvenile polyps.[63] Pham and Villanueva gave an account of a 25-year-old with sporadic JP with eight polyps removed over a 1-year period in which three polyps demonstrated ganglioneuromatous proliferation within the lamina propria.[64] The only familial cases were described in a father and three children with diffuse, polypoid ganglioneuromatosis and epithelial changes resembling JP.[65] None of the patients in these four reports were known to have a family

history of MEN2B or neurofibromatosis. Mendelsohn and Diamond believed that the ganglioneuromatous proliferation resulted in the formation of juvenile polyps in their patients, and emphasized that ganglion cells are not normally present within the lamina propria.[65] Whether excess trophic factors are being produced in these polyps causing neural differentiation, or that they result from changes in the same or different genes predisposing to JP, has not been resolved.

The association of JP with features of hereditary hemorrhagic telangiectasia has been depicted as a separate entity (MIM 175050). Cox and colleagues described a mother and daughter with generalized JP, digital clubbing, blanching lesions on the buccal mucosa, and pulmonary arteriovenous malformations. The mother had three normal siblings and a normal son, and there was no family history of either JP or hereditary hemorrhagic telangiectasia.[66] Conte and associates reported a man dying at age 36 of metastatic adenocarcinoma of the colon, pulmonary arteriovenous malformation, hypertrophic pulmonary osteoarthropathy, and digital clubbing. His son and daughter both presented with rectal bleeding and were found to have multiple juvenile polyps in the ileum and colon in their colectomy specimens. They also had pulmonary arteriovenous malformations, hypertrophic pulmonary osteoarthropathy, and digital clubbing.[67] Three similar cases of sporadic JP, digital clubbing, and hypertrophic osteoarthropathy have also been described; two had pulmonary arteriovenous malformations,[68,69] while the other did not.[70] Cox and coworkers suggested that the simultaneous occurrence of these disorders was likely to result from a new autosomal dominant syndrome rather than new mutations in genes predisposing to both hereditary hemorrhagic telangiectasia and JP.[66] Conversely, none of the patients described with hereditary hemorrhagic telangiectasia and germ line mutations of the endoglin gene on 9q33-34,[71,72] or of the activin receptor-like kinase 1 gene from the pericentromeric region of chromosome 12,[73] have been specifically noted to have JP.

The majority of cases of familial JP thus far reported have not had extraintestinal manifestations. Hofting, Pott, and Stolte reviewed 272 JP patients reported in the literature and determined the rate of extraintestinal anomalies to be 11 percent.[74] A similar review of 218 patients (83 familial cases, 73 sporadic, 62 unknown) by Coburn and associates estimated the incidence of congenital malformations to be 15 percent, with reports of 17 cardiothoracic, 12 central nervous system, 8 soft tissue, 5 GI, and 4 genitourinary anomalies.[75] Bussey, Veale, and Morson reported that the incidence of associated congenital anomalies in the 50 patients in the St. Mark's Registry was approximately 20 percent, with the majority occurring in sporadic patients, who accounted for about 75 percent of cases.[76] Because sporadic cases presumably arise through new mutation, these patients are more likely to have deletions or mutations involving more than just the JP gene.

The first description of JP by McColl and colleagues in 1964 reported 11 cases from 8 families, in which 4 sporadic cases had congenital anomalies. One patient had macrocephaly, hypertelorism, and polydactyly; another had intestinal malrotation (transverse colon below the jejunum), cryptorchidism, mild communicating hydrocephalus, and a Meckel's diverticulum with fecal fistula; another had a mesenteric lymphangioma; and the fourth's cecum was found in a subhepatic position and had episodes of acute porphyria.[6,8] In 27 cases of JP from Colombia (15 familial, 12 sporadic), 4 patients (3 familial, 1 sporadic case) had congenital cardiac anomalies. One patient had tetralogy of Fallot and his second cousin had coarctation of the aorta; another patient had subvalvular aortic stenosis and familial congenital lymphedema, and the other had an atrial septal defect.[32] Walpole and Cullity reported a patient with sporadic generalized JP with macrocephaly, cryptorchidism, digital clubbing, and mental retardation, who ultimately died of pancreatic cancer at age 19.[21] Lipper and associates described a patient with sporadic JP and spina bifida.[77] Jarvinen's review of 18 patients in the Finnish

Polyposis Registry revealed one with a ventricular septal defect and another with panhypopituitarism.[78] Watanabe and colleagues reported a brother and sister who were found to have juvenile polyps of the stomach only, whose mother had died at age 37 of metastatic gastric carcinoma. Both children were noted to be of low intelligence and have brown hair (as did their mother, who was of normal intelligence), which is unusual in the Japanese population.[79]

Desai and colleagues studied the anomalies associated with 23 patients considered to have JP, consisting of 17 sporadic cases and 2 members each from 3 families. They suggested that two patients actually had Gorlin syndrome, two had Bannayan-Riley-Ruvalcaba syndrome, and one had associated hereditary hemorrhagic telangiectasia (and two others were suspected but not all diagnostic criteria were present). Extracolonic abnormalities were detected in 17 of 23 (78 percent) patients. Sixteen patients had skeletal abnormalities (13 hypertelorism, 9 macrocephaly, 5 broad hands, 3 digital clubbing, 1 polydactyly, 1 cleft palate), 13 had dermatologic manifestations (5 telangiectasia, 2 penile pigmentation, 2 nevi, 2 freckles, 1 basal cell cancer, 1 skin pits, 1 palmar nodules), 5 had mental retardation (3 also had hydrocephalus), 4 had cryptorchidism, 2 had ventricular septal defects (both closing without intervention), and 1 had an intestinal malrotation.[80] This study was clouded somewhat by the inclusion of patients with other distinct clinical syndromes.

PATHOLOGY

Horilleno, Eckert, and Ackerman performed a comprehensive review of juvenile polyps by examining the pathologic features of 55 cases of nonfamilial colorectal polyps presenting to St. Louis Children's Hospital between 1935 and 1955. Three-fourths were located within the rectum and 15 percent were in the sigmoid colon, which was probably biased by the fact that sigmoidoscopy was the only endoscopic technique available at the time.[4] Seventy-three percent had solitary polyps, and of the 15 children with more than 1 polyp, 10 had 2, 3 had 3, and 2 had more than 3 polyps. Mestre later showed that with colonoscopic evaluation, 53 percent of children had multiple polyps, of which 60 percent were proximal to the sigmoid colon.[81] Grossly, Horilleno noted that 75 percent of the polyps had pedicles, while 25 percent were sessile, and most measured 1 to 1.5 cm in size (range: 0.3 to 4.0 cm). The external surfaces of the polyps were generally smooth, although finely granular, and smaller polyps were friable while larger polyps were firm (Fig. 21-1). Their shape was commonly disclike, or in some cases, spherical or mushroom-shaped. They were gray, brown, or red in color, which was related to the density of connective tissue within them or recent hemorrhage. On gross sectioning, the polyps usually had a central fibrous region and small peripheral cysts filled with mucin; areas of hemorrhage were common.[4]

Microscopically, there are three distinguishing features of juvenile polyps: (a) dilated, cystic spaces lined by glandular epithelium; (b) infiltration by inflammatory cells (lymphocytes, plasma cells, eosinophils, and polymorphonuclear cells); and (c) overabundance of stromal elements all occurring within the lamina propria (Fig. 21-3). These polyps are classified as hamartomatous, to distinguish them from the adenomatous polyps seen in FAP. Hamartomas are defined as abnormal arrangements of tissues that are normally found at a particular site, and hamartomatous intestinal polyps have been divided into the juvenile and Peutz-Jeghers types. Juvenile polyps differ from the polyps seen in Peutz-Jeghers syndrome in that they are devoid of smooth muscle coursing through the stalk and head of the polyps, while the latter have branching of muscular bundles in these regions.[82] Juvenile polyps have also been referred to as "retention polyps" in the past, referring to the cystic glandular spaces filled with mucin.[5] The histologic features of gastric juvenile polyps are similar to those of colonic juvenile polyps, although the lamina propria is usually less inflamed and the cysts are less prominent. Juvenile polyps of the

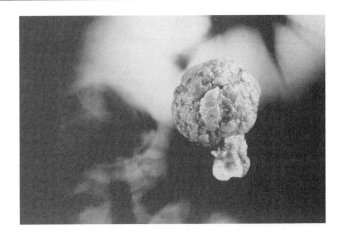

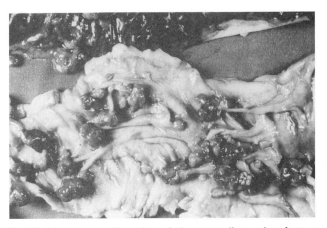

Fig. 21-1 Large juvenile polyp of the ascending colon from a member of the Iowa JP kindred, superimposed upon the patient's barium enema (above). This polyp was removed endoscopically (photo courtesy of R.W. Summers). Multiple juvenile polyps of the intestine at autopsy in a 20-year-old member of the Iowa JP kindred who died of duodenal cancer (below). Note the hypervascular, bosselated appearance, and pedunculated nature of these polyps.

stomach tend to be multiple, diffuse, and less pedunculated than colonic polyps (Fig. 21-2), and can be difficult to differentiate from hyperplastic polyps and those seen in the Cronkhite-Canada syndrome.[51,83]

Another frequent microscopic finding in juvenile polyps is the loss of epithelium at the surface and replacement by fibrin. Based on these findings, Horilleno and associates speculated that juvenile polyps were caused by trauma to the epithelium from feces, resulting in hyperplasia of the mucous glands, inflammation, and deposition of connective tissue. Fibrin could cover these denuded surfaces, sealing the glands and thus creating retention cysts.[4] Roth and Helwig concurred with this theory on the formation of solitary juvenile polyps, and went on to suggest that the polyps develop stalks as they enlarge and are pulled into the fecal stream. They ultimately infarct by twisting on their pedicle, and are sloughed into the stool.[9] Morson believed instead that juvenile polyps were hamartomas of the intestinal mucosa not involving the muscularis mucosae, because of their different appearance relative to inflammatory polyps, their onset in infancy or childhood, and their natural history.[5] Franzin and associates compared the histologic features of 24 juvenile polyps and 27 inflammatory polyps removed from patients with ulcerative colitis, Crohn disease, or after various interventions (such as ureterosigmoidostomy or polypectomy for adenomas). They concluded that these two groups of polyps were very similar, composed of granulation tissue covered by a thin layer of epithelium, and therefore agreed

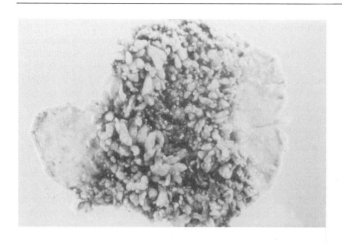

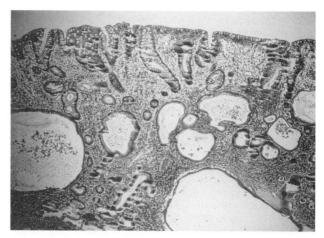

Fig. 21-3 Photomicrograph of a colonic juvenile polyp that demonstrates the characteristic features of cystically dilated glands and strikingly expanded lamina propria with a pronounced inflammatory infiltrate.

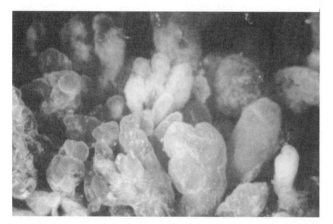

Fig. 21-2 Juvenile polyps of the stomach in a member of the Iowa kindred in a subtotal gastrectomy specimen (above). These polyps are diffuse with some antral sparing. The gastric polyps tend to be thick finger- or leaflike projections and may appear edematous. Unlike the intestinal polyps, they are not usually pedunculated (below; photos courtesy of F.A. Mitros and J.A. Benda).

with the hypothesis of an inflammatory origin for juvenile polyps.[84]

These speculations were based on observations made in solitary juvenile polyps, not in patients meeting the diagnostic criteria for JP. Grossly and microscopically, solitary juvenile polyps are indistinguishable from those in patients with JP. However, the multiplicity of polyps seen in JP patients suggests a germ line defect, while solitary juvenile polyps are likely to arise from two somatic mutations, as Knudson hypothesized in retinoblastoma.[85] Subramony and colleagues looked at normal colonic mucosa and juvenile polyps of various sizes in eight members of a JP family who underwent colectomy. The number of polyps in each specimen varied from 3 to greater than 50, and 6 of 8 specimens also had areas of nodular colonic mucosa. Normal mucosa showed an infiltration of inflammatory cells in the superficial one-third of the lamina propria, with no changes in the glandular elements, but there was significant variability from different areas of the colon. Other areas showed mild abnormalities in the colonic crypts. Foci of nodular colorectal mucosa without discrete polyps had a dense inflammatory infiltrate without surface erosion, which appeared to be the cause of the elevation of the mucosa. Polyps less than 1 cm in size had typical features of juvenile polyps, some with superficial ulceration and granulation tissue. Those 1 to 2.9 cm in size were usually pedunculated, with areas of mild to moderate dysplasia of the glands. Polyps larger than 3 cm were usually mixed (having features of both adenomatous and juvenile polyps) and had moderately dysplastic

epithelium. The largest polyp examined had mixed features of villous adenoma and juvenile polyp, with areas of severe dysplasia, and focal invasive adenocarcinoma in the adenomatous portion of the polyp. The authors concluded that the origin of these polyps was due to an unknown inflammatory stimulus, similar to that proposed for solitary polyps,[4,9] but that they should not be considered as hamartomatous, which implies no malignant potential.[86]

Mechanisms of Neoplastic Transformation in Juvenile Polyps

As discussed above, the belief that juvenile polyps were originally thought to be hamartomas with no malignant potential gradually gave way to the knowledge that patients with juvenile polyps were at increased risk for GI cancer, with numerous reports demonstrating this association. One issue which is less clear is whether juvenile polyps themselves actually develop into adenocarcinoma, or whether patients with JP are predisposed to both juvenile polyps and intestinal cancers, which arise through different precursor lesions. Giardiello and colleagues noted that two sporadic and five familial JP patients they studied had adenomatous epithelium within colorectal juvenile polyps.[87] They found 13 similar cases described in the literature, suggesting that juvenile polyps may undergo adenomatous change and thereby be at risk for progression to carcinoma.

To date, there have been two reports of adenocarcinoma developing in a juvenile polyp and three cases of carcinoma *in situ* within juvenile polyps. Liu and associates gave the first description of carcinoma within a juvenile polyp, in a 16-year-old boy with a solitary 4.5-cm juvenile colonic polyp with foci of signet ring carcinoma, capillary-lymphatic invasion, and metastasis to one lymph node.[11] Subramony and colleagues noted a case of invasive adenocarcinoma within adenomatous elements of a mixed villous and juvenile polyp.[86] Longo and coworkers gave an account of a patient with sporadic JP who at age 4 had a juvenile polyp removed with dysplasia, at age 6 with adenomatous changes, and at age 19 with a focus of intramucosal carcinoma in a juvenile polyp.[69] Ramaswamy, Elhosseiny, and Tchertkoff reported a 19-year-old patient who was found to have hundreds of juvenile polyps at total colectomy, some of which displayed adenomatous changes with severe epithelial dysplasia, as well as foci of carcinoma *in situ*.[14] Jones, Hebert, and Trainer reported a 24-year-old man with hematochezia and no family history of polyposis, who had four juvenile polyps removed, three with adenomatous changes, and one showing intramucosal carcinoma.[17] In 1979, Goodman, Yardley, and Milligan hypothesized that juvenile polyps develop from inflamed hyperplastic polyps, which then may develop an adenomatous focus, which becomes progressively dysplastic, and finally undergoes malignant transformation.[12] This view was supported by Grigioni and coworkers, who described a patient similar to that of Goodman et al. with hyperplastic polyps, juvenile polyps, juvenile polyps with adenomatous change, adenomas, and adenocarcinoma.[88] Jass thought that it was unlikely that cancer developed from solitary adenomas in JP. This was based on the fact that of 1032 polyps removed from 80 JP patients, only 21 were adenomas without juvenile features, and that dysplasia was a frequent finding within juvenile polyps.[36]

Kinzler and Vogelstein proposed a new class of cancer susceptibility genes based on the example provided by JP, which they designated as "landscaper" genes. These genes act indirectly, as opposed to gatekeeper and caretaker genes, which regulate cell growth or are involved in DNA-mismatch repair. This model is based on observations that both histologic and genetic changes in juvenile polyps appear to predominantly involve cells in the lamina propria,[25] yet patients with JP are at risk for epithelial malignancies. Kinzler and Vogelstein hypothesized that the germ line defects in JP patients may create an abnormal stromal environment predisposing the overlying epithelium to neoplastic transformation, perhaps through the production of paracrine factors.[89]

Risk of Gastrointestinal Malignancy

Estimates of the risk for developing colorectal or GI cancer in JP patients have varied widely. In a review published in 1984, Jarvinen and Franssila calculated that the risk of colorectal cancer was 9 percent, with 9 cases of colorectal cancer developing in 102 patients with familial and sporadic JP. Thirty-three additional cases of GI cancers in these 19 families were not included because these individuals did not have juvenile polyps documented.[15] Hofting et al.[74] and Coburn et al.[75] reviewed the literature and found a 17 to 18 percent incidence of GI cancer. Examination of 87 JP patients from the St. Mark's polyposis registry revealed 18 (20.7 percent) cases of colorectal cancer.[36] Many patients from these families had undergone colectomy, which probably reduced their risk of developing cancer, and Jass estimated that the cumulative risk of colorectal cancer might be as high as 68 percent by the age of 60 years.[22]

Howe et al. reported the long-term follow-up of the Iowa kindred, which had been first described in 1975,[10] consisting of 117 known members, 29 of whom had been diagnosed with either juvenile polyps or GI cancer.[23] Of these 29 patients, 16 developed GI cancer for an overall incidence of 55 percent. Eleven of these 29 (38 percent) developed colorectal cancer, and 6 (21 percent) had upper GI cancers (4 stomach, 1 duodenum, 1 pancreas). The median age of diagnosis of colorectal cancer was 42.0 years (range: 17.4 to 68.2 years) and 57.6 years (range: 20.8 to 72.8 years) for upper-GI cancer. The definition used for affected differed from previous studies in that family members with a history of GI cancer were also defined as being affected, even in the absence of a histologic diagnosis of juvenile polyps. Many of these individuals had died of advanced cancers in the earlier part of this century, and 12 of the 16 with cancer either also had documented juvenile polyps or had offspring with JP. This paper also reviewed previous reports of 131 familial JP patients from 22 families,[7,8,11–18,20,21,23,32,36,69,79,86–88,90–93] and found 42 cases of colorectal cancer (31.5 percent), 15 of stomach cancer (11.3 percent), and 1 case each of pancreatic and duodenal cancer (0.75 percent). Overall, 58 of these 131 patients (44.4 percent) developed GI cancer, confirming a significant predisposition to cancer in JP.[23]

GENETICS

Pattern of Inheritance

The observation that familial JP was an autosomal dominant disorder in 1966[7,8] has been confirmed over the following decades.

Twenty to 50 percent of cases have a family history,[74–76] while the remaining cases presumably arise *de novo* from new mutations, rather than recessive inheritance as hypothesized by Sachatello.[57] The mean age at diagnosis has varied between studies, with Veale estimating it at 4.5 years in sporadic cases and 9.5 years in familial cases.[8] Coburn's review of the literature, including both sporadic and familial cases, found a mean age of diagnosis of 18.5 years,[75] while Howe et al. reported the mean age at presentation to be 30.5 years in the Iowa kindred.[23] The age of diagnosis is clearly influenced by whether patients are detected by screening endoscopy, or whether they present with symptoms, and thus far there have been no reliable prospective or retrospective studies to carefully determine the age of onset. For these reasons, the age-related penetrance in JP is also unknown, but there is evidence to suggest that it is incomplete by middle age. Howe et al. reported that one member of the Iowa kindred inheriting a predisposing germ line mutation was asymptomatic and has had both negative upper and lower endoscopy at the age of 44.5 years.[94] There is variable expression in terms of upper and lower GI polyposis within and between families, and the association of multiple juvenile polyps with a variety of genetic conditions suggest that there is significant genetic heterogeneity, with multiple chromosomal loci influencing the development of these polyps. A slight preponderance of cases in males have been described in some reports (17 of 23 by Desai,[80] 15 of 27 by Restrepo,[32] 80 of 149 by Coburn[75]), but the sex distribution in the Iowa kindred was essentially equal (14 males of 29).[23]

Cytogenetic and Loss of Heterozygosity (LOH) Studies

In 1997, Jacoby and colleagues reported a 4-year-old patient with multiple colonic juvenile polyps, hypoplastic ears, tricuspid insufficiency, widely spaced canthi, and who was < 5th percentile for head circumference, height, and weight. On cytogenetic analysis, this patient was noted to have an interstitial deletion of 10q22.3-q24.1, leading the authors to hypothesize that this region contained a tumor-suppressor gene associated with JP.[24] Based on the findings in this patient, they evaluated this region for LOH in juvenile polyps from 13 unrelated JP patients (5 of whom had less than 5 polyps) and 3 with solitary juvenile polyps. The marker *D10S219* was deleted in 39 of 47 (83 percent) polyps from these 16 patients and the minimal region of overlap of all deletions was an approximately 3-cM region between markers *D10S219* and *D10S1696*. They next performed fluorescent *in situ* hybridization on tissue sections from juvenile polyps using a cosmid clone mapping near this region, and compared the staining in epithelial versus lamina propria cells. They found that 30 of 39 (77 percent) polyps examined had somatic deletions from 10q, predominantly within lymphocytes and macrophages in the lamina propria. These findings suggested the presence of a tumor-suppressor gene predisposing to juvenile polyps on 10q22 (named *JP1*),[25] in the same vicinity as the locus recently mapped for Cowden syndrome.[38]

Linkage Studies

Prior to these reports, linkage studies in familial JP had been limited to one study that had excluded *APC* and *MCC* as the gene for JP in an Australian family.[95] After Jacoby's report of 10q deletions in juvenile polyps, Marsh and associates genotyped 4 microsatellite markers from this region on 47 members of 8 JP families, and were able to exclude linkage of the JP gene by multipoint lod scores less than − 2.0 over the entire putative *JP1* interval. Howe et al. genotyped 43 members (13 affected, 24 at-risk, 6 spouses) of the Iowa kindred using 5 microsatellite markers from this region and also found no evidence for linkage.[26]

In the latter study, markers were also examined from the regions of several genes known to play an important role in either the development of sporadic colorectal cancer or hamartomatous polyps. These included *MSH2* (2p16), *MLH1* (3p21), *MCC*, *APC*

(5q21-22), *HMPS* (6q21), *JP1, PTEN* (10q22-24), *KRAS2* (12p12), *TP53* (17p13), *DCC* (18q21), and *LKB1* (19p13), as well as *CDKN2* (9q21). No evidence for linkage was found with markers from most of these regions, but linkage was detected with markers from 18q21. Genotyping and linkage analysis with 27 microsatellite markers from 18q21 resulted in lod scores > 3.0 with 7 different markers, with a maximum lod score of 5.00 (at $\theta = 0.001$) with the marker *D18S1099*. Haplotype analysis revealed five affected individuals with recombination events, allowing for localization of the JP gene to an 11.9-cM interval between markers *D18S1118* and *D18S487* on 18q21.1.[28] This interval was known to contain two tumor-suppressor genes, *DCC* (deleted in colorectal carcinoma[96]), and *DPC4* (deleted in pancreatic cancer 4, also known as *SMAD4*[97]), and was also known to be commonly deleted in both sporadic colorectal[96] and pancreatic carcinomas.[98] This is the only locus for JP identified by linkage thus far, but efforts continue to identify additional loci for this apparently genetically heterogeneous syndrome.

PTEN Mutations on 10q23

The *PTEN* gene on 10q23 is a tumor-suppressor gene that is frequently mutated in glioblastomas, prostate cancers, and breast cancers, with homology to tyrosine phosphatases and the protein tensin.[99,100] It has also been shown to be the predisposing locus for both CS[39] and BRR[40] (see Chap. 45 for more detail on the *PTEN* gene). There have been two reports describing *PTEN* mutations in JP patients.[27,101] Lynch and colleagues reported a R334X germ line mutation in two members of a family believed to have both CS and JP. The affected father had a history of small intestinal cancer, skin lesions, and macrocephaly, while his affected son also had skin lesions, macrocephaly, and small intestinal and colonic polyps. Eng and Ji have suggested that these patients might be more accurately classified as having CS.[102] Olschwang and associates reported *PTEN* mutations in 3 of 14 patients presenting with GI bleeding and > 10 juvenile polyps. One patient had a deletion at codon 232 leading to a premature stop at codon 255, was 74 years of age with upper and lower GI juvenile polyps, had a laryngeal cancer treated by radiotherapy 2 years earlier, and a heterogeneous thyroid nodule. Another patient, 10 years of age with generalized JP (with no extraintestinal manifestations of CS), was found to have a M35R substitution, while a third patient was 14 years old with colonic JP (and no family history of CS or BRR) with a mutation in a splice donor site of exon 6.[27] Eng and Ji believed the first patient was suggestive of having CS, and made the point that CS could not be ruled out in the other two patients (aged 10 and 14 years) because the penetrance is < 10 percent below the age of 15 years. These authors cautioned that the diagnosis of JP should be made after exclusion of other syndromes such as CS and BRR, and if *PTEN* mutations were found in these patients, then a high index of suspicion for the diagnosis of CS or BRR should be maintained.[102]

This recommendation was also influenced by two studies in which *PTEN* mutations were not found in JP patients. Riggins and associates sequenced the *PTEN* gene in 11 patients with familial JP and found no mutations.[103] Marsh and coworkers found no *PTEN* mutations in members of 14 JP families and 11 sporadic cases, and concluded that *PTEN* was either not a predisposing gene for JP or that it was only involved in a small group of cases. Furthermore, they raised the possibility that if there were a susceptibility locus on 10q22-24, as suggested by Jacoby,[25] then the 3 cM region as proposed for *JP1* is 7 cM centromeric to the *PTEN* gene.[104] In summary, mutations of *PTEN* or another nearby gene on 10q22-24 may be responsible for a subset of patients with JP, but it is important to rule out CS or BRR in these patients because approximately 80 percent of CS patients and 60 percent of BRR patients have *PTEN* mutations[105] and may also have hamartomatous polyps. Patients with CS need to be followed closely for the development of breast and thyroid neoplasms, while JP patients do not.

SMAD4 Mutations on 18q21.1

The finding of linkage to chromosome 18q21.1 in an interval containing two tumor-suppressor genes thought to play a role in the development of GI cancers led us to screen these genes for mutations in affected members of the Iowa JP kindred. After sequencing all 11 exons of *SMAD4* and 14 of 29 *DCC* exons, a 4 base-pair (bp) deletion was found in exon 9 of the *SMAD4* gene. All 13 affected members of this kindred had this deletion, as did 4 of 26 individuals at-risk, while 7 spouses and 242 control patients did not (Fig. 21-4). The maximum 2-point lod score of this deletion with the JP phenotype in this family was 5.79 at $\theta = 0.00$. This deletion occurred between nucleotides 1244 and 1247 (codons 414 to 416) and resulted in a frameshift, creating a new stop codon at the end of exon 9 (codon 434).[28]

To further study the importance of the *SMAD4* gene in JP, all exons were sequenced in eight other unrelated patients. The same 4 bp deletion in exon 9 was also found in affected members of JP families from Mississippi (originally described by Subramony et al.[86]) and Finland.[28] Since this report, an additional Caucasian kindred from Texas has also been found with the same deletion. The sharing of this common deletion from exon 9 raises the possibility that these kindreds may either have a common ancestor or that this region is a mutational hotspot. Genotyping of members of all four families with several markers from 18q21 revealed that there was no shared haplotype between these families for markers closest to the *SMAD4* gene, suggesting that this area in exon 9 is indeed more susceptible to mutation.[106]

In the six other unrelated patients studied, four had the wild-type sequence for all exons of the *SMAD4* gene. One patient with sporadic generalized JP was found to have a 2 bp deletion at codon 348 of exon 8, which caused a frameshift and stop at codon 350.

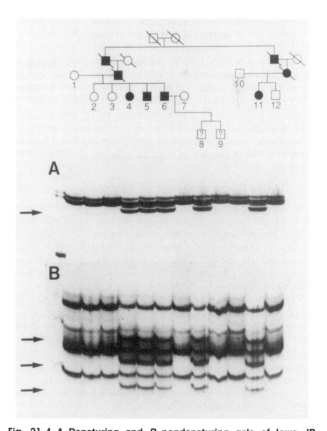

Fig. 21-4 *A* Denaturing and *B* nondenaturing gels of Iowa JP kindred members showing the exon 9 PCR product. Affected individuals 4, 5, 6, and 11, as well as one at-risk (8), all have an extra band (arrow in *A*) on denaturing gels that is produced by the 4-bp deletion. The mutant allele is also seen as a shift by SSCP analysis (arrows in *B*; reproduced from Howe et al.[28] with permission).

Table 21-1 *SMAD4* Sequencing Results in 10 Unrelated JP Patients

Patient	Type	Codon (exon)	Nucleotide Change	Predicted Effect	Control Pts.
I-13*	Familial	414–416 (9)	4 bp deletion	Frameshift, stop at codon 434	0/242
M-1*	Familial	414–416 (9)	4 bp deletion	Frameshift, stop at codon 434	0/242
T-1*	Familial	414–416 (9)	4 bp deletion	Frameshift, stop at codon 434	0/242
JP 5/1*	Familial	414–416 (9)	4 bp deletion	Frameshift, stop at codon 434	0/242
JP 11/1	Sporadic	348 (8)	2 bp deletion	Frameshift, stop at codon 350	0/101
JP 10/1	Sporadic	229–231 (5)	1 bp insertion	Frameshift, stop at codon 235	0/101
JP 6/1	Sporadic	—	—	—	
JP 4/1	Familial	—	—	—	
JP 1/1	Sporadic‡	—	—	—	
JP 2/13†	Familial	—	—	—	

* Sequence variant segregates with JP phenotype in respective family (13, 5, 5, and 2 affecteds with the mutation in the Iowa, Mississippi, Texas, and JP 5 Finnish kindreds, respectively).
† Multipoint lod score of 1.00 with chromosome 18q21 markers in this family (6 affected, 11 normals).

‡ JP 1/1 has a brother with colon cancer but no family members with documented JP (modified and reprinted from Howe et al.[28] by permission).

Another patient with sporadic JP diagnosed at age 6 with 30 to 40 colonic juvenile polyps had a 1 bp insertion between codons 229 and 231 of exon 5. This mutation, which added a guanine to six sequential guanines, caused a frameshift and stop at codon 235.[28] A summary of the results of *SMAD4* sequencing in these patients is shown in Table 21-1.

Fraction of Cases due to *SMAD4* and *PTEN*

There is little doubt that there is genetic heterogeneity in JP patients, but the degree of this heterogeneity and the number of genes involved remain to be defined. As discussed above, we have found *SMAD4* mutations in 60 percent of the familial and sporadic cases thus far examined. However, no evidence for linkage to 18q21 markers has been seen in other JP families, and gel shifts were observed in only 1 of 20 unrelated individuals studied by conformation-sensitive gel electrophoresis of the *SMAD4* gene.[107] It would, therefore, appear that the frequency of *SMAD4* mutations in JP patients might range from as low as 23 percent to as high as 60 percent. The role of *PTEN* mutations in JP remains to be clarified. Riggins et al.[103] and Marsh et al.[104] found no mutations in 36 sporadic and familial cases, while Olschwang and coworkers found 3 of 14 (21 percent) of their patients had germ line *PTEN* mutations.

The *SMAD4* Gene and Human Tumors

Hahn and associates identified a new tumor-suppressor locus by virtue of the fact that approximately 90 percent of pancreatic cancers had deletions of chromosome 18q and 30 percent had homozygous losses within a common interval on 18q21.1, which did not include the *DCC* gene.[98] They found three expressed sequences from this region, one of which showed significant homology to the *Drosophila Mad* (*m*others *a*gainst *d*ecapentaplegic) gene. This gene was named *DPC4* based on its being the fourth deletion locus described in pancreatic cancers, and it encodes for a 552 amino acid protein. Somatic mutations of this gene were found in 6 of 27 pancreatic cancers without homozygous deletions on 18q21, implicating it as a tumor suppressor predisposing to pancreatic cancer.[97] *DPC4* is now referred to as *SMAD4*, a nomenclature that combines the terms for the homologous *Mad* genes in *Drosophila melanogaster* and *sma* genes in *Caenorhabditis elegans*.[108]

Subsequent studies have shown that the rates of *SMAD4* mutations are modest in other GI tumors, and are distinctly uncommon in extraintestinal tumors. Thiagalingam and coworkers found loss or mutation of *SMAD4* in 5 of 18 colorectal carcinoma cell lines exhibiting 18q loss. These tumors were taken from a panel of 55 tumors with 18q loss (out of a total of 100 colorectal tumors), suggesting an overall mutation rate of approximately 15 percent.[109] Tagaki and associates found 5 *SMAD4* mutations in 31 primary colorectal cancers, for a total mutation rate of 16 percent.[110] MacGrogan and colleagues found *SMAD4* mutations in 4 of 21 (19 percent) primary colorectal carcinomas and cell lines.[111] Hoque and coworkers found LOH on 18q21 and a *SMAD4* mutation in one of six (17 percent) colitis-associated colorectal cancers.[112] Lei and collaborators found no mutations of *SMAD4* in 10 gastric, 10 esophageal, and 10 colitis-associated colorectal cancers.[113] Powell and coworkers found one case with inactivation of both copies of *SMAD4* (one deleted and the other with nonsense mutation at codon 334) in a panel of 35 gastric adenocarcinomas.[114] Hahn and colleagues reported 5 mutations in 32 (16 percent) carcinomas of the biliary tract, even though they only examined exons 8 through 11.[115] Moskaluk and colleagues sequenced the *SMAD4* gene from members of 11 families with familial pancreatic cancer (defined as 2 affected first-degree relatives) and found no mutations in these patients. They speculated that this situation could be similar to that seen in Li-Fraumeni syndrome, in which affected family members have germ line mutations of the *p53* gene but do not develop colorectal cancers, while sporadic colorectal cancers have a high rate of *p53* mutation.[116]

Schutte and associates analyzed 64 non-GI tumors (11 prostate, 8 breast, 8 ovary, 7 bladder, 6 hepatocellular carcinoma, 6 lung cancers, 5 head and neck carcinomas, 4 melanomas, 3 osteosarcomas, 3 renal cell carcinomas, 2 glioblastomas, and 1 medulloblastoma) displaying 18q loss for sequence changes in the *SMAD4* gene, and found only 2 alterations, 1 in a breast and the other in an ovarian cancer. They concluded that another tumor-suppressor gene from 18q might be involved in the development of these tumors.[117] Kim and coworkers found 2 mutations in head and neck tumors derived from cell lines of 11 patients and 20 primary tumors (6 percent).[118] MacGrogan and collaborators found no mutations in 45 primary and metastatic prostate cancers.[111]

Function of the *SMAD4* Gene

The SMAD4 protein is the common mediator involved in the transforming growth factor-β (TGF-β), activin, and bone morphogenetic protein (BMP) signal-transduction pathways. Members of the TGF-β superfamily initiate a wide spectrum of effects on a variety of cell types, including cell differentiation, proliferation, and apoptosis.[119,120] Currently, there are eight known *SMAD* genes in vertebrates. The SMAD2 and SMAD3 proteins function as cytoplasmic effectors in the TGF-β and activin pathways. Their counterparts in the BMP pathway are SMAD1, SMAD5, and possibly SMAD8. SMAD6 and SMAD7 function as inhibitors of all three pathways by binding to type I receptors and interfering with phosphorylation.[120]

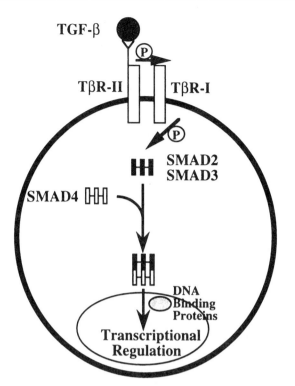

Fig. 21-5 Overview of the TGF-β signaling pathway. TGF-β binds to TβR-II, which then phosphorylates TβR-I, thereby activating it. TβR-I then phosphorylates SMAD2 or SMAD3, allowing them to form homo-oligomers or hetero-oligomers with SMAD4. Hetero-oligomeric complexes of SMAD4 with SMAD2 or SMAD3 associate with DNA-binding proteins. These complexes then bind to sequences in the promoter regions of genes under TGF-β control, regulating their transcription.

An overview of the sequence of proteins involved in the TGF-β signaling pathway is shown in Fig. 21-5. TGF-β binds to plasma membrane serine/threonine kinases, and, specifically, to the type II TGF-β receptor (TβR-II). This then complexes with the type I receptor (TβR-I), causing phosphorylation in a serine- and threonine-rich domain of TβR-I.[121] These activated type I receptors phosphorylate cytoplasmic monomers of SMAD2 or SMAD3, allowing these to form oligomers and to associate with SMAD4 monomers or oligomers.[122,123] Hetero-oligomers of SMAD2 or SMAD3 and SMAD4 then migrate to the nucleus and regulate transcription in conjunction with DNA-binding proteins.[124]

The mechanism by which this transcriptional regulation occurs is just beginning to be understood. Within the nucleus, the SMAD4 protein appears to bind directly to DNA,[125] and it has been shown that both SMAD3 and SMAD4 efficiently bind the 8-bp nucleotide sequence GTCTAGAC.[126] Another sequence that binds SMAD3 and SMAD4 (AG(C/A)CAGACA, dubbed the "CAGA box") has been described at positions -730, -580, and -280 within the plasminogen activator inhibitor-1 promoter, which is strongly inducible by TGF-β. Experiments cloning CAGA boxes upstream of various promoters resulted in markedly increased responses to TGF-β, and mutations within these sites decreased these responses.[127] The recently identified human DNA-binding protein *hFAST-1* also appears to bind to specific DNA sequences in response to TGF-β in the presence of SMAD2 and SMAD4.[128] In *Xenopus*, it has been proposed that FAST-1 binds to the C-terminus region of SMAD2, and SMAD4 stabilizes these proteins by binding to SMAD2.[129] This complex appears to be required for transcription of TGF-β and activin target genes, which is achieved by hFAST-1 and SMAD4 associating with their sequence-specific binding elements.[128]

The majority of *SMAD4* mutations thus far described in human cancers have been between codons 330 and 526,[97,110,117,118] within several highly conserved domains. This C-terminus of *SMAD4* is important in the formation of *SMAD4* homo-oligomers (initially believed to be homo-trimers), which then form hetero-oligomers with other SMAD proteins.[122] Recently, it has been suggested that the majority of intracellular SMAD4 is found in the form of monomers rather than homo-trimers, and that SMAD4 competes with SMAD2 and SMAD3 in the formation of hetero-trimer complexes.[123] It has been demonstrated that mutations which disrupt SMAD4 homo- and hetero-oligomerization lead to loss of TGF-β superfamily induced signaling pathways.[130] Lagna and associates showed that loss of the terminal 38 amino acids of SMAD4 leads to a dominant negative effect on the induction of mesoderm in *Xenopus* embryos by SMAD2, and that mutant and wild-type proteins form oligomers which may be responsible for their loss of activity.[131]

Zhou and colleagues constructed heterozygous and homozygous *SMAD4* deletions by homologous recombination in the colorectal cancer cell line HCT116, which has a truncating mutation of TβR-II and requires restoration of this gene in order to mediate TGF-β signaling. When TβR-II was reintroduced into these cells, cell lines with heterozygous *SMAD4* deletions generated an equal response to TGF-β as cell lines without deletion, while those having homozygous deletions had no signaling. Similar results were observed when an activated TβR-I receptor (TβR-I[T204D]) was introduced into these cells, or when they were stimulated by the addition of activin. Furthermore, the proliferation of cell lines in which a functional TβR-II gene had been introduced was substantially decreased in the parental cell line, and in those with heterozygous *SMAD4* deletions, when placed in medium containing TGF-β. Similar cell lines with homozygous *SMAD4* deletions had a significantly lower level of growth inhibition. These results indicated that *SMAD4* mutation was a potential mechanism by which tumor cells could escape the antiproliferative effects of TGF-β.[132]

Animal Models

Generation of transgenic mice with heterozygous and homozygous inactivation of *Smad4* has added insight into the role of this gene in embryogenesis and tumor formation. Sirard and colleagues created *Smad4* mutant embryonic stem cells by homologous recombination, using a construct replacing exons 8 and 9 with a neomycin resistance gene. They followed 25 *Smad4* heterozygous mutant $(+/-)$ mice for 11 months, and found no increase in tumors relative to wild-type mice, suggesting that loss of the other allele was necessary for tumor development. *Smad4* homozygous mutant $(-/-)$ mice died *in utero*, predominantly at 7.5 days of embryogenesis. These embryos manifested impaired growth, with poor separation of embryonic and extraembryonic boundaries. Histologic comparison of wild-type and $-/-$ embryos at 6.5 days revealed that $-/-$ embryos had no mesoderm formation, as well as abnormal development of the visceral endoderm. This defect in gastrula formation could be rescued by aggregation with tetraploid embryonic cells, but the resulting embryos had impaired development of anterior structures.[133] Yang and coworkers confirmed these findings using a similar model, and concluded that Smad4 is necessary for epiblast proliferation, egg-cylinder formation, and induction of the mesoderm.[134]

Takaku and associates created transgenic mice by homologous recombination using a construct disrupting the *Smad4* gene within exon 1, and generated compound *Smad4/Apc* mutant mice, taking advantage of the fact that these genes are approximately 30 cM apart on mouse chromosome 18. *Smad4* $-/-$ mutant mice died in utero, while *Smad4* $+/-$ mutants were viable, fertile, and had no histologic abnormalities within their intestines or pancreas relative to wild-type litter mates. Compound *Apc*$^{\Delta716}$ and *Smad4* heterozygous mutant mice had only about 12 percent of the number of intestinal polyps seen in *Apc*$^{\Delta716}$ $+/-$ mice, but their average size was larger (1 to 2 mm vs. 0.5 mm). Fifty-three percent also had epidermoid cysts, and 20 percent developed adenocarcinoma of the ampulla of Vater, which was not seen in *Apc* or *Smad4* +/− mice. Intestinal polyps from the compound mutant mice also showed stromal proliferation similar to that observed in juvenile polyps, and an increased incidence of malignant tumors relative to *Apc*$^{\Delta 716}$ +/− mice. Examination of tumor DNA from compound heterozygous mutant mice revealed that adenocarcinomas had lost the wild-type chromosome 18 and reduplicated the compound mutant chromosome.[135] Together, these studies demonstrate that *Smad4* most likely functions as a tumor-suppressor gene, for heterozygous mutants did not display increased numbers of tumors and were phenotypically normal. Furthermore, formation of tumors may require somatic mutations in addition to loss of *Smad4*, as seen in polyps of *cis*-compound *Smad4/Apc* mutants, which had histologic changes reminiscent of those seen in JP patients.

Mutations of Other Genes in the TGF-β Pathway

Mutations within the TβR-II gene have been demonstrated in 90 percent of tumors with microsatellite instability, occurring within a 10-bp polyadenine tract of this gene.[136–138] Restoration of functional TβR-II expression in deficient cell lines reduces their tumorigenicity in cell cultures and nude mice.[139] There has been one report of a germ line mutation at codon 315 (T315M) of TβR-II in an hereditary colorectal cancer family without microsatellite instability, which suggests that mutations outside the polyadenine tract in this gene may be another mechanism for the development of colorectal cancer, independent of defects in DNA mismatch-repair.[140]

SMAD2 has been mapped to chromosome 18q21.1 approximately 3 Mb centromeric to the *SMAD4* gene, appears to be ubiquitously expressed,[141] and consists of 11 exons and 467 amino acids.[142] It may play a role in the development of sporadic colorectal cancers, but mutations within *SMAD2* appear to be infrequent in these tumors. Analysis of *SMAD2* in 18 colorectal cancer cell lines revealed homozygous loss in one tumor, and a truncated protein in another.[143] Of 66 sporadic colorectal carcinomas, 4 (6 percent) were found with missense mutations in *SMAD2*. Adjacent normal mucosa from these patients did not have these mutations, indicating that these events were somatic within the tumors. No germ line mutations of *SMAD2* were identified in a panel of 15 patients with a strong family history of colorectal cancer or early age of onset.[142]

SMAD3 has been mapped to chromosome 15q21-22,[143] and consists of 9 exons and 424 amino acids.[144] Examination of 167 cancer cell lines (70 colorectal, 22 breast, 22 brain, 15 lung, 12 pancreas, 8 head and neck, 6 ovary, 4 esophagus, 4 stomach, and 4 prostate) by *in vitro* synthesized protein assays for SMAD3, found no truncated proteins in any of these tumor lines.[145] Study of the *SMAD3* gene in 35 sporadic and 15 HNPCC colorectal cancers revealed no mutations, but 2 of 17 informative tumors showed LOH from this region.[144] These studies suggest that both *SMAD2* and *SMAD3* may not significantly contribute to colorectal carcinogenesis, but do not address the question as to whether alterations in these genes contribute to the development of hamartomatous polyps.

Currently, little is known about *SMAD6* and *SMAD7* except that they are inhibitory through their binding to type I receptors, thus interfering with phosphorylation of downstream SMAD proteins. They both have high homology to other *SMAD* genes in their C-terminus, but appear to lack conserved regions in their amino-terminal domains common to other *SMAD* genes.[120,145] *SMAD6* encodes a 235 amino acid protein, and has been localized to chromosome 15q21-22, the same region as the *SMAD3* gene.[143,145] SMAD7 has been shown to inhibit TGF-β signaling by binding to the type I receptor and preventing the phosphorylation of SMAD2. A truncated SMAD7 protein demonstrated loss of this inhibition.[146] Although it has not yet been demonstrated, it is conceivable that other mutations could lead to stable binding with type I receptors and sustained inhibition of the antiproliferative effects of TGF-β.

IMPLICATIONS FOR DIAGNOSIS AND TREATMENT

Genetic Testing

Genetic testing of at-risk members of JP families has the potential to significantly improve the current method of presymptomatic diagnosis, which consists of periodic upper and lower screening endoscopy. Compliance with this regimen has been poor for insurance reasons, and because it is uncomfortable, relatively expensive, and needs to be repeated every 1 to 3 years.[94] DNA testing would simplify initial screening by requiring a single blood sample, and theoretically would allow noncarriers to avoid repetitive endoscopy. Health care resources could then be focused on the close surveillance of carriers and the early detection of their GI neoplasms.

The major problem with genetic testing for JP is the potential for genetic heterogeneity. As mentioned earlier, patients must be carefully evaluated clinically and pathologically to exclude other conditions associated with hamartomatous polyps, and even then, these associations may go undetected due to incomplete penetrance or variable expression. If the diagnostic criteria for JP are satisfied, then we begin with single-stranded conformational polymorphism (SSCP) and sequencing of all exons of the *SMAD4* gene in an affected member of the kindred. If mutations are identified, the sequence changes are examined for their potential biologic significance, and then SSCP or sequencing is used to determine whether these changes are present in other family members. Whether germ line mutations predispose to the JP phenotype is confirmed by its segregation with all affected family members and the absence of similar changes in a large number of control subjects. If no mutations are detected in *SMAD4*, then the *PTEN* gene is sequenced in an affected family member. If a mutation is found, then the rest of the family is examined for that exon, and all family members with mutations must be followed closely for the development of GI cancers, as well as for those of the thyroid and breast. If mutations are not found in either *SMAD4* or *PTEN* genes, then presymptomatic genetic testing is considered nondiagnostic. These families are then made a part of ongoing linkage studies attempting to identify other loci predisposing to JP.

The small number of mutations reported thus far limit our ability to estimate what percent of JP cases will be detected by sequencing these two genes. As discussed earlier, *SMAD4* mutations may be responsible for anywhere from 23 to 60 percent of cases,[28] while *PTEN* mutations may account for 0 to 21 percent of cases.[27,103,104] Other genes will undoubtedly emerge as the search for additional JP loci continues, which will improve our ability to provide genetic testing. The confusion regarding the classification of certain patients with hamartomatous polyposis should also be resolved in the near future, as they are categorized according to the specific germ line mutations present in each individual.

Genetic Counseling and Clinical Management

Genetic counseling should be offered to all JP patients, to make them are aware of the autosomal dominant nature of this syndrome, its spectrum of expression, and the risk for malignancy. Frequently encountered old myths, such as the recommendation to not have children, should be dispelled and replaced by patient education. Indications for screening endoscopy, endoscopic polypectomy, and surgical treatment also need to be discussed. Finally, the current status of genetic testing and the possibility of nondiagnostic results should be explored. The considerable experience with genetic testing for other GI cancer syndromes provides excellent models on which we base our approach for genetic counseling in JP, as reviewed by Petersen and Boyd for FAP[147] and Lynch, Smyrk, and Lynch in HNPCC.[148]

Adult patients found to have germ line mutations in *SMAD4* or *PTEN* must be notified that they have inherited an abnormality in a gene predisposing to JP.[149] Patients with positive genetic tests should have upper and lower endoscopy performed at this time to determine whether they currently have polyps, whether these require intervention, and to decide on the interval for future screening. Screening endoscopy should begin in the early second decade in asymptomatic patients, because the earliest age of cancer diagnoses that we have seen have been at 17.4 years for colorectal and 20.5 years for upper GI cancers.[23] Patients who develop symptoms of hematochezia, melena, rectal prolapse, intussusception, or frequent abdominal pain should have baseline endoscopy performed at the time these symptoms are recognized. If endoscopy is negative for polyps, screening should be carried out every 1 to 3 years as long as these patients remain asymptomatic. When polyps are encountered, they should be removed endoscopically to decrease the chance for malignant transformation and to help avoid the bleeding and anemia frequently seen in these patients. These patients should have annual endoscopy until the GI tract is free of polyps, then every 1 to 3 years thereafter. Although some authors have advocated subtotal colectomy in affected patients,[19] this may not be necessary if patients agree to periodic follow-up. Subtotal colectomy or total colectomy with ileoanal pull-through is recommended in patients who are likely to be lost to follow-up, have large polyps that cannot be removed endoscopically, have recurrent episodes of significant GI bleeding or protein-losing enteropathy, or have severe dysplasia or adenocarcinoma on biopsy. The diffuse nature of gastric polyposis makes endoscopic polypectomy impractical, and, therefore, symptomatic patients require subtotal or total gastrectomy.

Patients with nondiagnostic genetic test results should be screened by endoscopy every 3 years while asymptomatic and free of polyps. Patients with negative genetic test results should be screened for colon cancer as recommended for the normal population, and until further experience with these patients accumulates, we also recommend intermittent screening (such as every 5 to 10 years until the age of 50) to guard against the unlikely event of an error in genetic testing. Children should participate in genetic counseling sessions to learn about the condition that runs in their family, but the issue of at what age children should be informed of testing results remains controversial. In FAP, although the vast majority of parents questioned wanted to have their children tested at birth, most did not think they should be told until they were old enough to understand.[150] Accordingly, as long as children remain asymptomatic, it may be best to delay giving the results of genetic testing to patients until they begin screening endoscopy in adolescence. Other important issues to be discussed with families in any genetic testing scenario include how test results could change the patient's insurability, as well as the possibility of detecting nonpaternity. With the current pace of advances in the molecular biology of cancer, we expect that presymptomatic genetic testing will become the important first step in the life-long management of patients with JP.

REFERENCES

1. Diamond M: Adenoma of the rectum in children: Report of a case in a thirty-month-old girl. *Am J Dis Child* **57**:360, 1939.
2. Helwig EB: Adenoma of the large bowel in children. *Am J Dis Child* **72**:1946.
3. Ravitch MM: Polypoid adenomatosis of the entire gastrointestinal tract. *Ann Surg* **128**:283, 1948.
4. Horrilleno EG, Eckert C, Ackerman LV: Polyps of the rectum and colon in children. *Cancer* **10**:1210, 1957.
5. Morson BC: Some peculiarities in the histology of intestinal polyps. *Dis Colon Rectum* **5**:337, 1962.
6. McColl I, Bussey HJR, Veale AMO, Morson BC: Juvenile polyposis coli. *Proc Roy Soc Med* **57**:896, 1964.
7. Smilow PC, Pryor CA, Swinton NW: Juvenile polyposis coli: A report of three patients in three generations of one family. *Dis Colon Rectum* **9**:248, 1966.
8. Veale AMO, McColl I, Bussey HJR, Morson BC: Juvenile polyposis coli. *J Med Genet* **3**:5, 1966.
9. Roth SI, Helwig EB: Juvenile polyps of the colon and rectum. *Cancer* **16**:468, 1963.
10. Stemper TJ, Kent TH, Summers RW: Juvenile polyposis and gastrointestinal carcinoma. *Ann Intern Med* **83**:639, 1975.
11. Liu T-H, Chen M-C, Tseng H-C: Malignant change of juvenile polyp of colon. *Chin Med J* **4**:434, 1978.
12. Goodman ZD, Yardley JH, Milligan FD: Pathogenesis of colonic polyps in multiple juvenile polyposis. *Cancer* **43**:1906, 1979.
13. Rozen P, Baratz M: Familial juvenile colonic polyposis with associated colon cancer. *Cancer* **49**:1500, 1982.
14. Ramaswamy G, Elhosseiny AA, Tchertkoff V: Juvenile polyposis of the colon with atypical adenomatous changes and carcinoma in situ. *Dis Colon Rectum* **27**:393, 1984.
15. Jarvinen HJ, Franssila KO: Familial juvenile polyposis coli: Increased risk of colorectal cancer. *Gut* **25**:792, 1984.
16. Baptist SJ, Sabatini MT: Coexisting juvenile polyps and tubulovillous adenoma of colon with carcinoma in situ: Report of a case. *Hum Pathol* **16**:1061, 1985.
17. Jones MA, Hebert JC, Trainer TD: Juvenile polyp with intramucosal carcinoma. *Arch Path Lab Med* **111**:200, 1987.
18. Bentley E, Chandrasoma P, Radin R, Cohen H: Generalized juvenile polyposis with carcinoma. *Am J Gastroenterol* **84**:1456, 1989.
19. Scott-Conner CEH, Hausmann M, Hall TJ, Skelton DS, Anglin BL, Subramony C: Familial juvenile polyposis: Patterns of recurrence and implications for surgical management. *J Am Coll Surg* **181**:407, 1995.
20. Yoshida T, Haraguchi Y, Tanaka A, Higa A, Daimon Y, Mizuta Y, Tamaki M, et al: A case of generalized juvenile gastrointestinal polyposis associated with gastric carcinoma. *Endoscopy* **20**:33, 1988.
21. Walpole IR, Cullity G: Juvenile polyposis: A case with early presentation and death attributable to adenocarcinoma of the pancreas. *Am J Med Genet* **32**:1, 1989.
22. Jass JR: Juvenile polyposis, in Phillips RKS, Spigelman AD, Thomson JPS (eds). *Familial Adenomatous Polyposis and Other Polyposis Syndromes.* London: Edward Arnold, 1994, p 203.
23. Howe JR, Mitros FA, Summers RW: The risk of gastrointestinal carcinoma in familial juvenile polyposis. *Ann Surg Oncol* **5**:751, 1998.
24. Jacoby RF, Schlack S, Sekhon G, Laxova R: Del(10)(q22.3q24.1) associated with juvenile polyposis. *Am J Med Genet* **70**:361, 1997.
25. Jacoby RF, Schlack S, Cole CE, Skarbek M, Harris C, Meisner LF: A juvenile polyposis tumor suppressor locus at 10q22 is deleted from nonepithelial cells in the lamina propria. *Gastroenterology* **112**:1398, 1997.
26. Howe JR, Ringold JC, Summers RW, Mitros FA, Nishimura DY, Stone EM: A gene for familial juvenile polyposis maps to chromosome 18q21.1. *Am J Hum Genet* **62**:1129, 1998.
27. Olschwang S, Serova-Sinilnikova OM, Lenoir GM, Thomas G: PTEN germ-line mutations in juvenile polyposis coli. *Nat Genet* **18**:12, 1998.
28. Howe JR, Roth S, Ringold JC, Summers RW, Jarvinen HJ, Sistonen P, Tomlinson IPM, et al: Mutations in the SMAD4/DPC4 gene in juvenile polyposis. *Science* **280**:1086, 1998.
29. Toccalino H, Guastavino E, De Pinni F, O'Donnell JC, Williams M: Juvenile polyps of the rectum and colon. *Acta Paediatr* **62**:337, 1973.
30. Sulser H, Deyhle P, Clavadetscher P, Ammann P: Juvenile dickdarm-schleimhautpolypen bei erwachsenen. *Schweiz Med Wschr* **106**:107, 1976.
31. Restrepo C, Correa P, Duque E, Cuello C: Polyps in a low-risk colonic cancer population in Colombia, South America. *Dis Colon Rectum* **24**:29, 1981.
32. Restrepo C, Moreno J, Duque E, Cuello C, Amsel J, Correa P: Juvenile colonic polyposis in Colombia. *Dis Colon Rectum* **21**:600, 1978.
33. Williams AO, Prince DL: Intestinal polyps in the Nigerian African. *J Clin Pathol* **28**:367, 1975.
34. Burt RW, Bishop DT, Lynch HT, Rozen P, Winawer SJ: Risk and Surveillance of individuals with heritable factors for colorectal cancer. *Bull WHO* **68**:655, 1993.
35. Chevrel J-P, Amouroux J, Gueraud J-P: Trois cas familiaux de polypose juvenile. *Chirurgie* **101**:708, 1975.
36. Jass JR, Williams CB, Bussey HJR, Morson BC: Juvenile polyposis — A precancerous condition. *Histopathology* **13**:619, 1988.
37. Gentry WC Jr, Eskritt NR, Gorlin RJ: Multiple hamartoma syndrome (Cowden disease). *Arch Dermatol* **109**:521, 1974.
38. Nelen MR, Padberg GW, Peeters EAJ, Lin AY, van den Helm B, Frants RR, Coulon V, et al: Localization of the gene for Cowden disease to chromosome 10q22-23. *Nat Genet* **13**:114, 1996.
39. Liaw D, Marsh DL, Li J, Dahia PLM, Wang SI, Zheng Z, Bose S, et al: Germ line mutations of the PTEN gene in Cowden disease, an inherited breast and thyroid cancer syndrome. *Nat Genet* **16**:64, 1997.

40. Marsh DJ, Dahia PLM, Zheng Z, Liaw D, Parsons R, Gorlin RJ, Eng C: Germline mutations in PTEN are present in Bannayan-Zonana syndrome. *Nat Genet* **16**:333, 1997.

41. Gorlin RJ: Nevoid basal-cell carcinoma syndrome. *Medicine (Baltimore)* **66**:98, 1987.

42. Evans DG, Ladusans EJ, Rimmer S, Burnell LD, Thakker N, Farndon PA: Complications of the naevoid basal cell carcinoma syndrome: Results of a population-based study. *J Med Genet* **30**:460, 1993.

43. Shanley S, Ratcliffe J, Hockey A, Haan E, Oley C, Ravine D, Martin N, et al: Nevoid basal cell carcinoma syndrome: Review of 118 affected individuals. *Am J Med Genet* **50**:282, 1994.

44. Scully RE, Galdabini JJ, McNeely BU: Case records of the Massachusetts General Hospital. Weekly clinicopathological exercises. Case 14-1976. *N Engl J Med* **294**:772, 1976.

45. Schwartz RA: Basal-cell-nevus syndrome and gastrointestinal polyposis. *N Engl J Med* **299**:49, 1978.

46. Farndon PA, Del Mastro RG, Evans DG, Kilpatrick MW: Location of gene for Gorlin syndrome. *Lancet* **339**:581, 1992.

47. Hahn H, Wicking C, Zaphiropoulous PG, Gailani MR, Shanley S, Chidambaram A, Vorechovsky I, et al: Mutations of the human homolog of *Drosophila* patched in the nevoid basal cell carcinoma syndrome. *Cell* **85**:841, 1996.

48. Johnson RL, Rothman AL, Xie J, Goodrich LV, Bare JW, Bonifas JM, Quinn AG, et al: Human homolog of patched, a candidate gene for the basal cell nevus syndrome. *Science* **272**:1668, 1996.

49. Whitelaw SC, Murday VA, Tomlinson IPM, Thomas HJW, Cottrell SE, Ginsberg A, Bukofzer S, et al: Clinical and molecular features of the hereditary mixed polyposis syndrome. *Gastroenterology* **112**:327, 1997.

50. Thomas HJW, Whitelaw SC, Cottrell SE, Murday VA, Tomlinson IPM, Markie D, Jones T, et al: Genetic mapping of the hereditary mixed polyposis syndrome to chromosome 6q. *Am J Hum Genet* **58**:770, 1996.

51. Burke AP, Sobin LH: The pathology of Cronkhite-Canada polyps. A comparison to juvenile polyposis. *Am J Surg Pathol* **13**:940, 1989.

52. Cronkhite LW, Canada WJ: Generalized gastrointestinal polyposis: an unusual syndrome of polyposis, pigmentation, alopecia, and onychatrophia. *N Engl J Med* **252**:1011, 1955.

53. Daniel ES, Ludwig SL, Lewin KJ, Ruprecht RM, Rajacich GM, Schwabe AD: The Cronkhite-Canada syndrome. An analysis of clinical and pathologic features and therapy in 55 patients. *Medicine (Baltimore)* **61**:293, 1982.

54. Spigelman AD, Phillips RKS: Peutz-Jeghers syndrome, in Phillips RKS, Spigelman AD, Thomson JPS (eds). *Familial Adenomatous Polyposis and Other Polyposis Syndromes.* London: Edward Arnold, 1994, p 188.

55. Hemminki A, Tomlinson I, Markie D, Jarvinen H, Sistonen P, Bjorkqvist AM, Knuutila S, et al: Localization of a susceptibility locus for Peutz-Jeghers syndrome to 19p using comparative genomic hybridization and targeted linkage analysis. *Nat Genet* **15**:87, 1997.

56. Hemminki A, Markie D, Tomlinson I, Avizienyte E, Roth S, Loukola A, Bignell G, et al: A serine/threonine kinase gene defective in Peutz-Jeghers syndrome. *Nature* **391**:184, 1998.

57. Sachatello CR, Hahn IL, Carrington CB: Juvenile gastrointestinal polyposis in a female infant: Report of a case and review of the literature of a recently recognized syndrome. *Surgery* **75**:107, 1974.

58. Hizawa K, Iida M, Yao T, Aoyagi K, Fujishima M: Juvenile polyposis of the stomach: Clinicopathological features and its malignant potential. *J Clin Pathol* **50**:771, 1997.

59. Soper RT, Kent TH: Fatal juvenile polyposis of infancy. *Surgery* **69**:692, 1971.

60. Gourley GR, Odell GB, Selkurt J, Morrissey J, Gilbert E: Juvenile polyps associated with protein-losing enteropathy. *Dig Dis Sci* **27**:941, 1982.

61. Ray JE, Heald RJ: Growing up with juvenile gastrointestinal polyposis: report of a case. *Dis Colon Rectum* **14**:375, 1971.

62. Donnelly WH, Sieber WK, Yunis EJ: Polypoid ganglioneurofibromatosis of the large bowel. *Arch Pathol* **87**:537, 1969.

63. Weidner N, Flanders DJ, Mitros FA: Mucosal ganglioneuromatosis associated with multiple colonic polyps. *Am J Surg Pathol* **8**:779, 1984.

64. Pham BN, Villanueva RP: Ganglioneuromatous proliferation associated with juvenile polyposis coli. *Arch Path Lab Med* **113**:91, 1989.

65. Mendelsohn G, Diamond MP: Familial ganglioneuromatous polyposis of the large bowel. Report of a family with associated juvenile polyposis. *Am J Surg Pathol* **8**:515, 1984.

66. Cox KL, Frates RC Jr, Wong A, Gandhi G: Hereditary generalized juvenile polyposis associated with pulmonary arteriovenous malformation. *Gastroenterology* **78**:1566, 1980.

67. Conte WJ, Rotter JI, Schwartz AG, Congleton JE: Hereditary generalized juvenile polyposis, arteriovenous malformations and colonic carcinoma. *Clin Res* **30**:93A, 1982.

68. Baert AL, Casteels-Van Daele M, Broeckx J, Wijndaele L, Wilms G, Eggermont E: Generalized juvenile polyposis with pulmonary arteriovenous malformations and hypertrophic osteoarthropathy. *AJR Am J Roentgenol* **141**:661, 1983.

69. Longo WE, Touloukian RJ, West B, Ballantyne GH: Malignant potential of juvenile polyposis coli. *Dis Colon Rectum* **33**:980, 1990.

70. Simpson EL, Dalinka MK: Association of hypertrophic osteoarthropathy with gastrointestinal polyposis. *AJR Am J Roentgenol* **144**:983, 1985.

71. McAllister KA, Lennon F, Bowles-Biesecker B, McKinnon WC, Helmbold EA, Markel DS, Jackson CE, et al: Genetic heterogeneity in hereditary haemorrhagic telangiectasia: possible correlation with clinical phenotype. *J Med Genet* **31**:927, 1994.

72. McAllister KA, Grogg KM, Johnson DW, Gallione CJ, Baldwin MA, Jackson CE, Helmbold EA, et al: Endoglin, a TGF-beta binding protein of endothelial cells, is the gene for hereditary haemorrhagic telangiectasia type 1. *Nat Genet* **8**:345, 1994.

73. Johnson DW, Berg JN, Baldwin MA, Gallione CJ, Marondel I, Yoon S-J, Stenzel TT, et al: Mutations in the activin receptor-like kinase I gene in hereditary haemorrhagic telangiectasia type 2. *Nat Genet* **13**:189, 1996.

74. Hofting I, Pott G, Stolte M: Das Syndrom der Juvenilen Polyposis. *Leber Magen Darm* **23**:107, 1993.

75. Coburn MC, Pricolo VE, DeLuca FG, Bland KI: Malignant potential in intestinal juvenile polyposis syndromes. *Ann Surg Oncol* **2**:386, 1995.

76. Bussey HJR, Veale AMO, Morson BC: Genetics of gastrointestinal polyposis. *Gastroenterology* **74**:1325, 1978.

77. Lipper S, Kahn LB, Sandler RS, Varma V: Multiple juvenile polyposis: A study of the pathogenesis of juvenile polyps and their relationship to colonic adenomas. *Hum Pathol* **12**:804, 1981.

78. Jarvinen HJ: Juvenile gastrointestinal polyposis. *Probl Gen Surg* **10**:749, 1993.

79. Watanabe A, Nagashima H, Motoi M, Ogawa K: Familial juvenile polyposis of the stomach. *Gastroenterology* **77**:148, 1979.

80. Desai DC, Murday V, Phillips RKS, Neale KF, Milla P, Hodgson SV: A survey of phenotypic features in juvenile polyposis. *J Med Genet* **35**:476, 1998.

81. Mestre JR: The changing pattern of juvenile polyps. *Am J Gastroenterol* **81**:312, 1986.

82. Jass JR: Pathology of polyposis syndromes with special reference to juvenile polyposis, in Utsunomiya J, Lynch HT (eds). *Hereditary Colorectal Cancer.* Tokyo: Springer-Verlag, 1990, p 343.

83. Mitros FA: Personal communication. Sept 1, 1998.

84. Franzin G, Zamboni G, Dina R, Scarpa A, Fratton A: Juvenile and inflammatory polyps of the colon-a histological and histochemical study. *Histopathology* **7**:719, 1983.

85. Knudson AG Jr, Hethcote HW, Brown BW: Mutation and childhood cancer: A probabilistic model for the incidence of retinoblastoma. *Proc Natl Acad Sci U S A* **72**:5116, 1975.

86. Subramony C, Scott-Conner CEH, Skelton D, Hall TJ: Familial juvenile polyposis. Study of a kindred: Evolution of polyps and relationship to gastrointestinal carcinoma. *Am J Clin Pathol* **102**:91, 1994.

87. Giardiello FM, Hamilton SR, Kern SE, Offerhaus GJA, Green PA, Celano P, Krush AJ, et al: Colorectal neoplasia in juvenile polyposis or juvenile polyps. *Arch Dis Child* **66**:971, 1991.

88. Grigioni WF, Alampi G, Martinelli G, Piccaluga A: Atypical juvenile polyposis. *Histopathology* **5**:361, 1981.

89. Kinzler KW, Vogelstein B: Landscaping the cancer terrain. *Science* **280**:1036, 1998.

90. Grotsky HW, Rickert RR, Smith WD, Newsome JF: Familial juvenile polyposis coli: A clinical and pathologic study of a large kindred. *Gastroenterology* **82**:494, 1982.

91. Sassatelli R, Bertoni G, Serra L, Bedogni G, Ponz de Leon M: Generalized juvenile polyposis with mixed pattern and gastric cancer. *Gastroenterology* **104**:910, 1993.

92. Hofting I, Pott G, Schrameyer B, Stolte M: Familiare juvenile polyposis mit vorwiegender magenbeteiligung. *Z Gastroenterol* **31**:480, 1993.

93. Sharma AK, Sharma SS, Mathur P: Familial juvenile polyposis with adenomatous-carcinomatous change. *J Gastroenterol Hepatol* **10**:131, 1995.

94. Howe JR, Ringold JC, Hughes J, Summers RW: Direct genetic testing for *SMAD4* mutations in patients at risk for juvenile polyposis. In preparation. *Surgery* **126**:162, 1999.

95. Leggett BA, Thomas LR, Knight N, Healey S, Chenevix-Trench G, Searle J: Exclusion of APC and MCC as the gene defect in one family with familial juvenile polyposis. *Gastroenterology* **105**:1313, 1993.

96. Fearon ER, Cho KR, Nigro JM, Kern SE, Simons JW, Ruppert JM, Hamilton SR, et al: Identification of a chromosome 18q gene that is altered in colorectal cancers. *Science* **247**:49, 1990.

97. Hahn SA, Shutte M, Shamsul Hoque ATM, Moskaluk CA, da Costa LT, Rozenblum E, Weinstein CL, et al: DPC4, a candidate tumor suppressor gene at human chromosome 18q21.1. *Science* **271**:350, 1996.

98. Hahn SA, Shamsul Hoque ATM, Moskaluk CA, da Costa LT, Scutte M, Rozenblum E, Seymour AB, et al: Homozygous deletion map at 18q21.1 in pancreatic cancer. *Cancer Res* **56**:490, 1996.

99. Li J, Yen C, Liaw D, Podsypanina K, Bose S, Wang SI, Puc J, et al: PTEN, a putative protein tyrosine phosphatase gene mutated in human brain, breast, and prostate cancer. *Science* **275**:1943, 1997.

100. Steck PA, Pershouse MA, Jasser SA, Yung WK, Lin H, Ligon AH, Langford LA, et al: Identification of a candidate tumour suppressor gene, MMAC1, at chromosome 10q23.3 that is mutated in multiple advanced cancers. *Nat Genet* **15**:356, 1997.

101. Lynch ED, Ostermeyer EA, Lee MK, Arena JF, Ji H, Dann JKS, et al: Inherited mutations in PTEN that are associated with breast cancer, Cowden disease, and juvenile polyposis. *Am J Hum Genet* **61**:1254, 1997.

102. Eng C, Ji H: Molecular classification of the inherited hamartoma polyposis syndromes: Clearing the muddied waters. *Am J Hum Genet* **62**:1020, 1998.

103. Riggins GJ, Hamilton SR, Kinzler KW, Vogelstein B: Normal PTEN gene in juvenile polyposis. *NOGO* **1**:1, 1997.

104. Marsh DJ, Roth S, Lunetta KL, Hemminki A, Dahia PLM, Sistonen P, Zheng Z, et al: Exclusion of PTEN and 10q22-24 as the susceptibility locus for juvenile polyposis syndrome. *Cancer Res* **57**:5017, 1997.

105. Marsh DJ, Coulon V, Lunetta KL, Rocca-Serra P, Dahia PL, Zheng Z, Liaw D, et al: Mutation spectrum and genotype-phenotype analyses in Cowden disease and Bannayan-Zonana syndrome, two hamartoma syndromes with germline PTEN mutation. *Hum Mol Genet* **7**:507, 1998.

106. Howe JR, Wagner B, Amos C, Ringold JC, Roth S, Aaltonen LA: Haplotype analysis of a common Smad4 exon 9 deletion in juvenile polyposis families. In preparation.

107. Houlston R, Bevan S, Williams A, et al: Mutations in DPC4 (Smad4) cause juvenile polyposis syndrome, but only account for a minority of cases. *Hum Mol Genet* **7**:1907, 1998.

108. Derynck R, Gelbart WM, Harland RM, Heldin CH, Kern SE, Massague J, Melton DA, et al: Nomenclature: vertebrate mediators of TGF-β family signals. *Cell* **87**:173, 1996.

109. Thiagalingam S, Lebauer C, Leach FS, Schutte M, Hahn SA, Overhauser J, Willson SA, et al: Evaluation of candidate tumour suppressor genes on chromosome 18 in colorectal cancers. *Nat Genet* **13**:343, 1996.

110. Takagi Y, Kohmura H, Futamura M, Kida H, Tanemura H, Shimokawa K, Saji S: Somatic alterations of the DPC4 gene in human colorectal cancers in vivo. *Gastroenterology* **111**:1369, 1996.

111. MacGrogan D, Pegram M, Slamon D, Bookstein R: Comparative mutational analysis of DPC4(Smad4) in prostatic and colorectal carcinomas. *Oncogene* **15**:1111, 1997.

112. Hoque ATMS, Hahn SA, Schutte M, Kern SE: DPC4 gene mutation in colitis associated neoplasia. *Gut* **40**:120, 1997.

113. Lei P, Zou T-T, Shi Y-Q, Zhou X, Smolinski KN, Yin J, Souza RF, et al: Infrequent DPC4 gene mutation in esophageal cancer, gastric cancer and ulcerative colitis-associated neoplasms. *Oncogene* **13**:2459, 1996.

114. Powell SM, Harper JC, Hamilton SR, Robinson CR, Cummings OW: Inactivation of Smad4 in gastric carcinomas. *Cancer Res* **57**:4221, 1997.

115. Hahn SA, Bartsch D, Schroers A, Galehdari H, Becker M, Ramaswamy A, Schwarte-Waldhoff I, et al: Mutations of the DPC4/Smad4 gene in biliary tract carcinoma. *Cancer Res* **58**:1124, 1998.

116. Moskaluk CA, Hruban RA, Schutte M, Lietman AS, Smyrk T, Fusaro L, Fusaro R, et al: Genomic sequencing of DPC4 in the analysis of familial pancreatic cancer. *Diagn Mol Pathol* **6**:85, 1997.

117. Schutte M, Hruban RH, Hedrick L, Cho KR, Nadasdy GM, Weinstein CL, Bova GS, et al: DPC4 in various tumor types. *Cancer Res* **56**:2527, 1996.

118. Kim SK, Fan Y, Papadimitrakopoulou V, Clayman G, Hittelman WN, Hong WK, Lotan R, et al: DPC4, a candidate tumor suppressor gene, is altered infrequently in head and neck squamous cell carcinoma. *Cancer Res* **56**:2519, 1996.

119. Massague J: TGFβ signaling: Receptors, transducers, and Mad proteins. *Cell* **85**:947, 1996.

120. Heldin C-H, Miyazono K, Ten Dijke P: TGFβ signaling from cell membrane to nucleus through SMAD proteins. *Nature* **390**:465, 1997.

121. Wrana JL, Attisano L, Wieser R, Ventura F, Massague J: Mechanism of activation of the TGF-beta receptor. *Nature* **370**:341, 1994.

122. Shi Y, Hata A, Lo RS, Massague J, Pavletich NP: A structural basis for mutational inactivation of the tumor suppressor Smad4. *Nature* **388**:87, 1997.

123. Kawabata M, Inoue H, Hanyu A, Imamura T, Miyazono K: SMAD protein exist as monomers in vivo and undergo homo- and hetero-oligomerization upon activation by serine/threonine kinase receptors. *EMBO J* **17**:4056, 1998.

124. Liu F, Pouponnot C, Massague J: Dual role of the Smad4/DPC4 tumor suppressor in TGF-β-inducible transcriptional complexes. *Genes Dev* **11**:3157, 1997.

125. Yingling JM, Datto MB, Wong C, Frederick JP, Liberati NT, Wang XF: Tumor suppressor Smad4 is a transforming growth factor beta-inducible DNA binding protein. *Mol Cell Biol* **17**:7019, 1997.

126. Zawel L, Dai JL, Buckhaults P, Zhou S, Kinzler KW, Vogelstein B, Kern SE: Human Smad3 and Smad4 are sequence-specific transcription activators. *Mol Cell* **1**:611, 1998.

127. Dennler S, Itoh S, Vivien D, ten Dijke P, Huet S, Gauthier JM: Direct binding of Smad3 and Smad4 to critical TGF beta-inducible elements in the promoter of human plasminogen activator inhibitor-type 1 gene. *EMBO J* **17**:3091, 1998.

128. Zhou S, Zawel L, Lengauer C, Kinzler KW, Vogelstein B: Characterization of human FAST-1, a TGF-β and activin signal transducer. *Mol Cell* **2**:121, 1998.

129. Chen X, Weisberg E, Fridmacher V, Watanabe M, Naco G, Whitman M: Smad4 and FAST-1 in the assembly of activin-responsive factor. *Nature* **389**:85, 1997.

130. Wu RY, Zhang Y, Feng XH, Derynck R: Heteromeric and homomeric interactions correlate with signaling activity and functional cooperativity of Smad3 and Smad4/DPC4. *Mol Cell Biol* **17**:2521, 1997.

131. Lagna G, Hata A, Hemmati-Brivanlou A, Massague J: Partnership between DPC4 and SMAD proteins in TGF-β signaling pathways. *Nature* **383**:832, 1996.

132. Zhou S, Buckhaults P, Zawel L, Bunz F, Riggins G, Le Dai J, Kern SE, et al: Targeted deletion of Smad4 shows it is required for transforming growth factor beta and activin signaling in colorectal cancer cells. *Proc Natl Acad Sci U S A* **95**:2412, 1998.

133. Sirard C, de la Pompa JL, Elia A, Itie A, Mirtsos C, Cheung A, Hahn S, et al: The tumor suppressor gene Smad4/Dpc4 is required for gastrulation and later for anterior development of the mouse embryo. *Genes Dev* **12**:107, 1998.

134. Yang X, Li C, Xu X, Deng C: The tumor suppressor SMAD4/DPC4 is essential for epiblast proliferation and mesoderm induction in mice. *Proc Natl Acad Sci U S A* **95**:3667, 1998.

135. Takaku K, Oshima M, Miyoshi H, Matsui M, Seldin MF, Taketo MM: Intestinal tumorigenesis in compound mutant mice of both DPC4 (Smad4) and APC genes. *Cell* **92**:645, 1998.

136. Markowitz S, Wang J, Myerhoff L, Parsons R, Sun L, Lutterbaugh J, Fan RS, et al: Inactivation of the type II TGF-β receptor in colon cancer cells with microsatellite instability. *Science* **268**:1336, 1995.

137. Parsons R, Myeroff LL, Liu B, Willson JKV, Markowitz SD, Kinzler KW, Vogelstein B: Microsatellite instability and mutations of the transforming growth factor β type II receptor gene in colorectal cancer. *Cancer Res* **55**:5548, 1995.

138. Samowitz WS, Slattery ML: Transforming growth factor-β receptor type 2 mutations and microsatellite instability in sporadic colorectal adenomas and carcinomas. *Am J Pathol* **151**:33, 1997.

139. Wang J, Sun L, Myeroff L, Wang X, Gentry LE, Yang J, Liang J, et al: Demonstration that mutation of the type II transforming growth factor beta receptor inactivates its tumor suppressor activity in replication error-positive colon carcinoma cells. *J Biol Chem* **270**:22044, 1995.

140. Lu S-L, Kawabata M, Imamura T, Akiyama Y, Nomizu T, Miyazono K, Yuasa Y: HNPCC associated with germline mutation in the TGF-β type II receptor gene. *Nat Genet* **19**:17, 1998.

141. Nakao A, Roijer E, Imamura T, Souchelnytskyi S, Stenman G, Heldin C-H, ten Dijke P: Identification of Smad2, a human Mad-related protein in the transforming growth factor-beta signaling pathway. *J Biol Chem* **272**:2896, 1997.

142. Eppert K, Scherer SW, Ozcelik H, Pirone R, Hoodless P, Kim H, Tsui L-C, et al: MADR2 maps to 18q21 and encodes a TGFB-regulated

MAD-related protein that is functionally mutated in colorectal carcinoma. *Cell* **86**:543, 1996.

143. Riggins GJ, Thiagalingam S, Rozenblum E, Weinstein CL, Kern SE, Hamilton SR, Willson JKV, et al: Mad-related genes in the human. *Nature Genet* **13**:347, 1996.

144. Arai T, Akiyama Y, Okabe S, Ando M, Endo M, Yuasa Y: Genomic structure of the human Smad3 gene and its infrequent alterations in colorectal cancers. *Cancer Lett* **122**:157, 1998.

145. Riggins GJ, Kinzler KW, Vogelstein B, Thiagalingam S: Frequency of Smad gene mutations in human cancers. *Cancer Res* **57**:2578, 1997.

146. Hayashi H, Abdollah S, Qiu Y, Cai J, Xu Y-Y, Grinnell BW, Richardson MA, et al: The MAD-related protein Smad7 associates with the TGF-β receptor and functions as an antagonist of TGF-β signaling. *Cell* **89**:1165, 1997.

147. Petersen GM, Boyd PA: Gene tests and counseling for colorectal cancer risk: Lessons from familial polyposis. *Monogr Natl Cancer Inst* **17**:67, 1995.

148. Lynch HT, Smyrk T, Lynch J: An update of HNPCC (Lynch syndrome). *Cancer Genet Cytogenet* **93**:84, 1997.

149. Pelias MZ: Duty to disclose in medical genetics: A legal perspective. *Am J Med Genet* **39**:347, 1991.

150. Whitelaw S, Northover JM, Hodgson SV: Attitudes to predictive DNA testing in familial adenomatous polyposis. *J Med Genet* **33**:540, 1996.

Retinoblastoma

Irene F. Newsham ▪ *Theodora Hadjistilianou*
Webster K. Cavenee

1. Retinoblastoma is the most common intraocular malignancy in children, with a worldwide incidence between 1 in 13,500 and 1 in 25,000 live births. The presenting signs and symptoms include leukokoria, strabismus, low-vision orbital cellulitis, unilateral mydriasis, and heterochromia. The disease can be unifocal or multifocal and unilateral or bilateral. The average age of diagnosis is 12 months for bilateral and 18 months for unilateral cases, and 90 percent of affected individuals are diagnosed before age 3 years. Unusual manifestations of this disease include late onset retinoblastoma, 13q-deletion syndrome, retinoma, trilateral retinoblastoma, and second-site primary tumors, including osteosarcoma, Ewing sarcoma, leukemia, and lymphoma.

2. Early diagnosis and treatment are of primary importance in the survival of retinoblastoma patients. A variety of diagnostic approaches are used, including computed tomography (CT), magnetic resonance imaging (MRI), ultrasonography, and fine-needle aspiration biopsy (FNAB). Each has advantages, and when used in combination, they can establish the proper disease classification. Effective methods for the treatment of retinoblastoma tumors include enucleation, external-beam irradiation, episcleral plaques, xenon arc and argon laser photocoagulation, cryotherapy, and chemotherapy. The choice of treatment depends on several factors, such as multifocal or unifocal disease, site and size of the tumor, diffuse or focal vitreous seeding, age at diagnosis, and histopathologic findings.

3. Retinoblastoma has served as the prototypic example of a genetic predisposition to cancer. It is estimated that 60 percent of cases are nonhereditary and unilateral, 15 percent are hereditary and unilateral, and 25 percent are hereditary and bilateral. A model encompassing these findings suggests a requirement for as few as two stochastic mutational events for tumor formation. The first of these events can be inherited through the germ line or can be somatically acquired, whereas the second occurs somatically in either case and leads to a tumor that is doubly defective at the retinoblastoma locus. Cytogenetic analyses have demonstrated the involvement of a genetic alteration in a gene for negative growth regulation at chromosome band 13q14. This model has been tested and confirmed using restriction-fragment-length polymorphisms (RFLP) for loci on chromosome 13. These studies have shown that the second wild-type retinoblastoma allele may be lost by several somatic mutational mechanisms, including mitotic nondisjunction with loss of the wild-type chromosome, mitotic nondisjunction with duplication of the mutant chromosome, mitotic recombination between the RB1 locus and the centromere, and other regionalized events, such as deletion and point mutation.

4. The 200-kb genomic locus for RB1 has been isolated, and its exon/intron structure has been characterized. Current molecular technology has allowed the identification of a variety of aberrations in this locus in retinoblastoma patients and their tumors at the DNA, RNA, and protein levels. RB1 alterations also have been detected in a variety of clinically related second-site primary tumors and nonrelated tumors, including osteosarcoma, breast carcinoma, and small-cell lung carcinoma. The ability to detect mutations in RB1 coupled with the isolation of polymorphic sequences within the gene locus, has further extended the prenatal risk assessment for this pediatric tumor.

5. The RB1 locus is transcribed into a 4.7-kb mRNA with a corresponding protein product of 110 kDa that is ubiquitously expressed in normal human and rat tissues, including brain, kidney, ovary, spleen, liver, placenta, and retina. The p110^{RB} protein is differentially phosphorylated, and the unphosphorylated form is found predominantly in the G1 stage of the cell cycle, with an initial phosphorylation occurring at the G1/S boundary. This protein can be physically complexed with a number of viral and cellular proteins. SV40 large T antigen, adenovirus E1A protein, and papillomavirus E7 protein all contain conserved regions that are required for binding with the p110^{RB} protein. The same regions appear to be necessary for the transforming function of the viral proteins.

6. Intracellular proteins whose function are mediated by the retinoblastoma protein have been isolated from complexes formed *in vitro* using pRB "pocket-binding" affinity chromatography columns against different cell lysates. Transcription factors DRTF and E2F have been isolated, and their physical and functional relationships to the retinoblastoma protein have been assessed. Other cellular proteins identified in these complexes include cyclin D1, p16, and the RB-like proteins p107 and p130. Interestingly, the complexing of these factors to p110^{RB} has also been shown to oscillate in a cell cycle-dependent manner, thereby linking the tumor-suppressing function of the retinoblastoma protein with transcriptional regulation.

CLINICAL ASPECTS AND TREATMENT OF RETINOBLASTOMA

Epidemiology

Retinoblastoma is the most common intraocular malignancy in children. In 1964, Francois[1] reported an incidence varying from 1 in 34,000 to 1 in 14,000 births and noted a steady increase in the frequency of occurrence of the tumor between 1927 and 1960. A number of studies support this finding and indicate a worldwide incidence of 1 in 3500 to 1 in 25,000, with no significant difference between the sexes or races.[2–9] An apparent mortality rate for blacks 2.5 times greater than that for whites has been reported, but seems to be attributable to delays in diagnosis rather than a higher disease incidence.[10] In general, there seems to be little correlation of disease incidence with geographic location. However, in some populations (e.g., Jamaicans, Nigerians, Haitians),[11] apparently higher incidence rates have been observed for what appears to be the unilateral sporadic form of retinoblastoma; this may suggest an environmental modification of the probability of tumor formation.[12]

Presenting Signs and Symptoms

Differential Diagnosis. In the majority of cases, the first sign at presentation is the characteristic cat's-eye reflex, which is usually noted by the child's parents or pediatrician. This white, pink-white, or yellow-white pupillary reflex, termed leukokoria, results from replacement of the vitreous by the tumor or by a tumor growing in the macula[13,14] (Fig. 22-1). Another common symptom, strabismus (exotropia or esotropia), can occur alone when small macular tumors interfere with vision, or can be associated with leukokoria. It is not uncommon to find after an accurate patient history is taken that strabismus occurred some months before leukokoria.

Less frequent presenting signs for retinoblastoma are red, painful eye with secondary glaucoma, low-vision orbital cellulitis, unilateral mydriasis, and heterochromia.[15] Sometimes the tumor can be difficult to differentiate from a variety of simulating lesions, such as persistent hyperplastic primary vitreous, retrolental fibroplasia, Coats disease, *toxocara canis* infection, retinal dysplasia, and chronic retinal detachment.[16,17] In 265 patients with pseudoretinoblastoma, persistent hyperplastic primary vitreous, followed by retrolental fibroplasia and posterior cataract, was the most common simulating condition.[18] Of 136 children with suspected retinoblastoma reported to the Ocular Oncology Service of the Wills Eye Hospital in Philadelphia between 1974 and 1978, 60 had retinoblastoma and 76 had simulating lesions, the most frequent being ocular toxocariasis (26 percent), persistent hyperplastic primary vitreous (20 percent), and Coats disease (16 percent). Despite these complications, most simulating lesions can be distinguished through modern diagnostic methods (described later in this chapter) or after a careful history of the family and the affected child.[16,17,19]

A complete workup for such a patient includes an ophthalmologic examination; a systemic, pediatric, and radiographic evaluation; and, more recently, genetic studies (Table 22-1).[17,19,20] At fundus examination, the disease can be unifocal or multifocal; in bilateral cases, usually one eye is in a more advanced stage, while the contralateral eye has one or more tumor foci (Fig. 22-1B). Furthermore, fundus examination of the first-degree relatives may also document the presence of a retinoma or a regressed retinoblastoma and indicate a potential hereditary basis for the tumor.

The average age at diagnosis is 12 months for bilateral retinoblastoma and 18 months for unilateral cases, with 90 percent of the patients diagnosed before age 3. Several factors may influence the time of diagnosis and therapy,[21,22] including (a) ignorance of the revealing signs, (b) difficulty in ophthalmoscopic examination

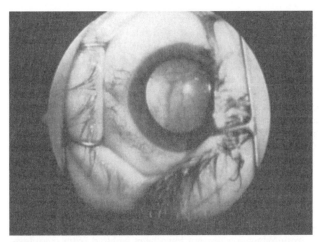

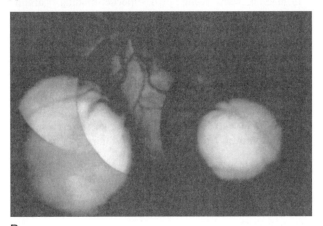

Fig. 22-1 Presenting signs of retinoblastoma. *A,* Leukokoria: exophytic retinoblastoma, overlying retinal detachment, clear lens, and visible retinal blood vessels. *B,* Multifocal retinoblastoma. (Courtesy of R. Frezzotti, MD, Director of the Institute of Ophthalmological Sciences, University of Siena, Italy.)

Table 22-1 Clinical and Laboratory Assessment for Retinoblastoma Patients

Ophthalmologic examination
  Binocular indirect ophthalmoscopy with scleral indentation (child, parents, siblings, relatives)
  Site and dimensions of the tumor(s)
  Necrosis, calcification
  Degree of vascularization, hemorrhage
  Vitreous "seeding"
  Retinal detachment
  Fundus photography and drawing of the lesion(s)
  Slit-lamp examination
  Pseudohypopion, hyphema
  Corneal and lens transparency
  Rubeosis iris
  Corneal diameter (buphthalmos)
  Pupil, anisocoria
  Tonometry
  Ecography (calcification, biometry)
  Aqueous and vitreous cytology and enzymology—fine-needle aspiration biopsy
Systemic examination
Radiographic examination
  Skull x-ray
  Computed tomography (orbits and brain with and without contrast enhancement)
  Magnetic resonance imaging (orbits and brain)
Pediatric examination
  Bone marrow biopsy
  Lumbar puncture (cerebrospinal fluid examination)
  Serologic tests (toxocara)
  Neurologic evaluation
  Electroencephalogram
Genetic studies
  Esterase D
  High-resolution chromosome analysis—karyotyping
  DNA analysis of blood and tumor tissues

(age of the patient, level of transparency of the media, full mydriasis, and scleral indentation), (c) socioeconomic situation, (d) unusual clinical manifestations, and (e) multiple consultants.

Unusual Clinical Manifestations

Late Retinoblastoma. It is an exceptional instance when retinoblastoma presents after the age of 7, and the older the child, the more unusual the first signs of the disease. These unusual manifestations include orbital cellulitis and edema of the lids; hypopyon, hyphema, iris heterochromia, and keratitis (anterior segment); and vitreous opacification, retinal cysts, vitreous hemorrhage, and endophthalmitis (posterior segment).[23] Atypical uveitis in an older child, particularly if associated with secondary glaucoma and a poor response to corticosteroids, may be the first manifestation of a late retinoblastoma[24] (Fig. 22-2A). Repetitive diagnostic anterior chamber paracentesis may yield negative results.[23] Among 618 cases of retinoblastoma in older children, 41 (6.6 percent) were misdiagnosed as primary ocular inflammations.[25]

Sometimes retinoblastoma can resemble a panophthalmitis, which is frequently seen as a reaction to a necrotic uveal melanoma.[26] Pseudohypopyon as a result of retinoblastoma cells settled in the anterior chamber is another rare sign of the disease (Fig. 22-2B). A diffuse, infiltrating retinoblastoma can present with hypopyon or a severe anterior uveitis.[27,28] The term *diffuse infiltrated retinoblastoma* has been used to describe a form of the

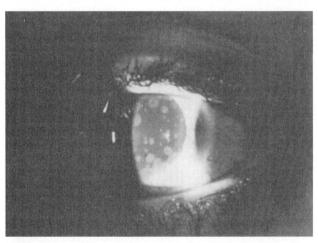

A

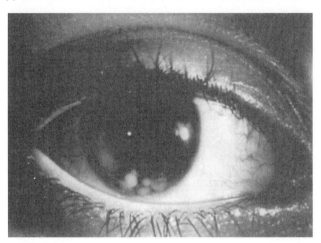

B

Fig. 22-2 Unusual manifestations of retinoblastoma. *A,* Pseudo-uveitis in retinoblastoma. *B,* Nodules at the pupillary margin and pseudohypopyon caused by a retinoblastoma. (Courtesy of R. Frezzotti, MD, Director of the Institute of Ophthalmological Sciences, University of Siena, Italy.)

tumor in which no well-defined exophytic or endophytic mass is evident. This retinoblastoma pattern frequently produces aqueous and vitreous seeding, particularly in older children,[27,29–32] and seems to have a low potential for malignancy, although there is still controversy on this point.[27,28] Furthermore, cystic retinoblastoma, presumably a variant of the diffuse infiltrating type, tends to simulate uveitis and presents with clinically visible cysts.[33,34]

Associated Clinical Abnormalities

13q-Deletion Syndrome. The 13q-deletion syndrome includes sporadic retinoblastoma in association with moderate growth and mental retardation, a broad, prominent, nasal bridge, a short nose, ear abnormalities, and muscular hypotonia.[35,36] Niebuhr and Ottosen also reported seven cases of retinoblastoma associated with systemic abnormalities (mental retardation, microcephaly, genital malformations, and ear abnormalities) in a review of 13q deletions and 13 ring chromosomes.[37] Such a karyotypic analysis prompted by the presentation of dysmorphic features can facilitate early detection of a deletion in the long arm of chromosome 13. Subsequent ophthalmoscopic examination can identify the retinoblastoma at an earlier stage.[38]

Retinoma. The term *retinoma* has been used to denote a benign tumor of retinocytic origin. Although the origins of this entity are obscure, it has been proposed that it arises from a mutation in the retinoblastoma susceptibility gene in a well-differentiated retinocyte and leads to a hyperplastic nodule of differentiated cells.[39] Retinomas are composed of apparently benign cells that show photoreceptor differentiation with no evidence of necrosis or mitotic activity, but with numerous rosettes.[40] Characteristically, retinomas have at least two of the following characteristics: irregular translucent retinal mass, calcification, and pigment epithelium migration and proliferation (Fig. 22-3A). Histopathologic and immunohistochemical studies suggest that retinomas are primary benign tumors, not regressed retinoblastomas. Malignant transformation of retinomas is quite rare, although some cases have been reported, notably a 7-year-old girl who developed an undifferentiated retinoblastoma 3 years after the diagnosis of a retinoma.[41,42]

Various physiological conditions (including reduced blood supply and necrosis, calcium [as an inhibitor of tumor growth], and host immune defense mechanisms) could be implicated in the spontaneous regression of retinoblastoma (Fig. 22-3B). Often, bulbi with intraocular calcification are the final physical embodiment of a spontaneously regressed retinoblastoma.[43] These phthisis bulbi can be attributed to tumor necrosis after ocular ischemia but cannot explain the retinoma, because the vascular supply in these lesions is intact.[44] On the basis of the available data, it appears that the term *regressed retinoblastoma* should be reserved to describe shrunken, calcified, phthisical eyes, whereas retinoma should be used to refer to nonprogressive retinal lesions that are highly associated with retinoblastoma but lack a malignant pattern.[45]

Trilateral Retinoblastoma. Bader and coauthors[46] coined the term *trilateral retinoblastoma* to describe the association between bilateral retinoblastoma and midline brain tumors, usually in the pineal region. Similar observations had been reported by Jensen and Miller[10] and Jakobiec et al.,[47] and had suggested that involvement of the pineal gland (third eye) represents a further point of origin for multicentric retinoblastoma rather than a second primary tumor.[48] In patients with hereditary retinoblastoma, both the pineal and the retina may contain susceptible cells. Because these pineal tumors may be indistinguishable from well-differentiated retinoblastomas, they are also called *ectopic retinoblastomas.*[46] It is possible that pineal tumors have been misinterpreted as intracranial spread of retinoblastoma,[49] whereas the advent of CT scanning and MRI has facilitated more accurate diagnoses. This is clinically important, because an ectopic intracranial retinoblastoma requires adequate therapy to the whole neuraxis,

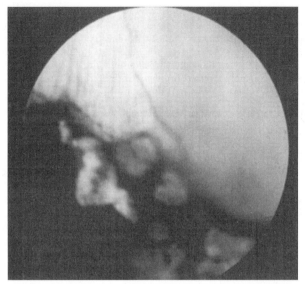

A

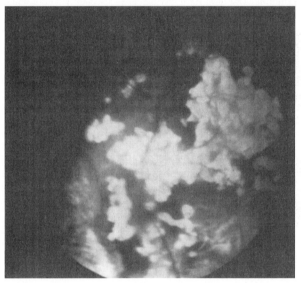

B

Fig. 22-3 Abnormalities associated with retinoblastoma. *A,* Retinoma: translucent retinal mass and pigment epithelium migration and proliferation. *B,* Spontaneously regressed retinoblastoma. (Courtesy of R. Frezzotti, MD, Director of the Institute of Ophthalmological Sciences, University of Siena, Italy.)

as well as high-dose equivalent radiotherapy to the primary tumor. Intrathecal therapy with methotrexate should also be considered.[50]

Second Malignant Tumors. The term *second site primary malignant tumor* refers to nonmetastatic tumors arising in disease-free patients successfully treated for the initial disease. Some of the tumors found in association with retinoblastoma include osteosarcoma, fibrosarcoma, chondrosarcoma, epithelial malignant tumors, Ewing sarcoma, leukemia, lymphoma, melanoma, brain tumors, and pinealoblastoma. These second tumors have been classified into five groups:[51] (a) tumors appearing in the irradiated area; (b) tumors appearing outside and remote from the irradiated area; (c) tumors in patients not receiving radiotherapy; (d) tumors that cannot be characterized as primary or metastases; and (e) tumors appearing in members of retinoblastoma families who are free of retinal tumors.

Reese, Merriam, and Martin[52] reported the first two cases of second tumors in 55 retinoblastoma patients treated with external radiation and surgery. These patients presented with a maxillary

sinus sarcoma and a rhabdomyosarcoma of the temporal muscle. A similar case of mixed-cell fibrosarcoma has been reported by Frezzotti and Guerra.[53] A causal relationship between radiation therapy and secondary tumors has been suggested.[54–56] However, from the reported series of cases, two important observations have emerged: (a) The great majority of children in whom second neoplasms developed had suffered bilateral retinoblastoma, and (b) the incidence of second neoplasms in this group of children was similar whether or not they received radiation. These conclusions have been supported by studies that have reported the incidence of second nonocular tumors and analyzed the effect of radiation therapy. Osteogenic sarcomas have been the most common second-site neoplasms in all the published series. Derkinderen,[57] Lueder,[58] Draper,[59] and their colleagues found low rates of development of second tumors and are in agreement that the incidence increases with radiation therapy. Abramson *et al.* reported the incidence of second tumors in patients with hereditary retinoblastoma and found a frequency of 20 percent at 10 years, 50 percent at 20 years, and 90 percent at 30 years after diagnosis.[60] Somewhat lower rates have been recorded by other authors. For example, in a series of 215 bilateral retinoblastomas, second tumors developed in 4.4 percent of the patients during the first 10 years of follow-up, in 18.3 percent after 20 years, and in 26.1 percent after 30 years.[61]

Histopathology

Retinoblastoma occurs either as an intraocular mass between the choroid and the retina (exophytic) or as a bulge from the retina toward vitreous (endophytic). However, most of the advanced tumors examined showed both patterns of growth. Retinoblastoma rarely spreads superficially (1 percent), forming no mass and invading the whole retina (diffuse infiltrating retinoblastoma).

The tumor is histologically characterized by the presence of rosettes and fleurettes, which are believed to represent maturation and differentiation of the neoplastic cells. Rosettes are spherical structures (circular in section) constituted by uniform cuboidal or short columnar cells arranged in an orderly fashion around a small round lumen (Flexner-Wintersteiner rosette) or without any lumen (Homer-Right rosette). The latter type can often be found in other neuroectodermal tumors, such as medulloblastomas. Fleurettes are arranged in the opposite way, with short and thin stromal axes surrounded by fairly differentiated neoplastic cells with the apical part facing the externum, resembling the shape of a flower (Fig. 22-4*A*). Often the tumor appears highly necrotic, with the surviving cells positioned around blood vessels, creating structures called pseudorosettes. Calcified foci can be found in areas of necrosis, as can debris from nucleic acids, giving rise to basophilic vessel walls.[62,63]

A retinoblastoma tumor is capable of spreading outside the bulb through the eye coats, invading the choroid and the sclera. It is the invasion of this highly vascularized choroid that represents an effective vehicle for distant metastasis (Fig. 22-4*B*), and such choroid invasion is directly correlated with a poor prognosis. Invasion also can involve the optic nerve and meningeal space, providing access to the central nervous system. Growth patterns and other histologic parameters (such as pseudorosettes, necrosis, and calcification), although necessary for the identification of the tumor itself, do not seem to offer much information in regard to the prognosis. The degree of differentiation and the number of mitoses show a weak correlation with the prognosis; however, stronger relationships exist with invasion of the choroid and sclera. In particular, progressive invasion of the eye coats, even in the horizontal plane, is highly informative in determining the prognosis.[64,65]

Diagnosis

Because many of the symptoms described above are clearly not specific to retinoblastoma and because early surgical or conservative treatment is of primary importance in the survival of these patients, it is imperative to confirm these impressions by

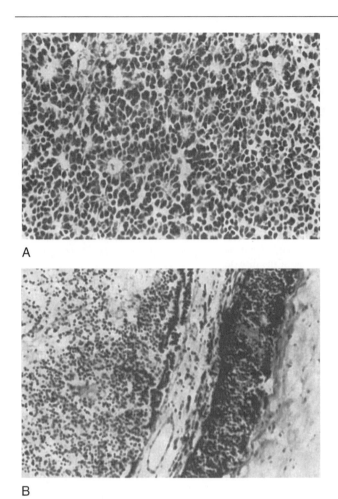

A

B

Fig. 22-4 Histopathology of retinoblastoma. *A,* A well-differentiated retinoblastoma showing rosettes and fleurettes (hematoxylin-eosin, 100). *B,* Low-differentiated retinoblastoma infiltrating the choroid and sclera (hematoxylin-eosin, 100). (Courtesy of P. Toti, MD, Institute of Anatomic Pathology, University of Siena, Italy.)

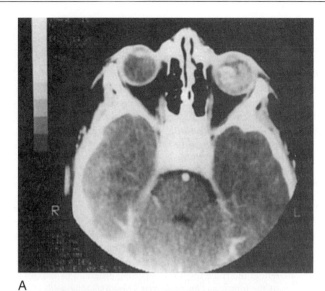

A

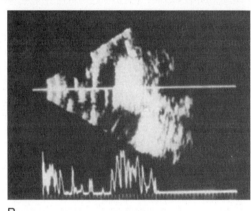

B

Fig. 22-5 Diagnostic tools for retinoblastoma. *A,* CT scan: retinoblastoma filling the whole vitreous cavity with typical calcifications (Courtesy of C. Venturi, MD, Department of Neuroradiology, University of Siena, Italy). *B,* B scan technique. The echogram shows a lesion with an irregular oval shape and dense acoustic tissue. High attenuation of ultrasound is occurring, with the shadowing of the echoes coming from the orbital tissue. The tumor has developed in the vitreous and occupies it almost entirely. (Courtesy of E. Motolese, MD, Institute of Ophthalmological Sciences, University of Siena, Italy.)

examination. There are a variety of diagnostic tools available for this, including CT, MRI, ultrasonography, and FNAB. The application and advantages of each procedure are briefly discussed below.

Computed Tomography and Magnetic Resonance Imaging. CT is a valuable adjunct in the differential diagnosis, staging, and treatment of retinoblastoma.[66,67] Intraocular calcification in children under 3 years of age is highly suggestive of a retinoblastoma. Some studies have reported that the degree of calcification appeared to depend on tumor size, with the smallest tumor showing calcification 8 mm in diameter and 4 mm in thickness[68,69] (Fig. 22-5*A*). However, in children more than 3 years of age confusion may arise from some simulating lesions, including retinal astrocytoma, retrolental fibroplasia, toxocariasis, and optic-nerve-head drusen, which can also produce calcifications.[68–70] Thus, CT is often coupled with MRI to better detect subtle scleral invasion, infiltrative spread along the optic nerve, subarachnoid seeding, or involvement of the central nervous system through direct tumor extension or by metastasis.[71] Furthermore, MRI appears to be more sensitive in the differential diagnosis of lesions simulating retinoblastoma[70,72,73] and in the evaluation of the degree of tumor differentiation.[74]

The role of both CT and MRI in staging and therapy is of great importance in accurately determining extraocular disease such as intracranial metastasis, retrobulbar spread, orbital recurrence, and secondary tumors, and it is often on the basis of these diagnostic results that further treatment (radiotherapy and/or chemotherapy) is planned. Still, subtle optic nerve involvement cannot be predicted reliably.[68] By using CT as a diagnostic tool, Danziger

and Price[75] proposed the division of retinoblastoma cases into three groups: grade I tumors are high-density masses with calcification in any part of the eyeball; grade II tumors are high-density masses involving the optic nerve and orbital soft tissue but with rare calcifications; and grade III tumors are intracranial or extraorbital high-density masses showing marked contrast enhancement. These classifications further aid in the determination of appropriate therapeutic measures.

Ultrasonography. Ultrasonography is another diagnostic technique that can distinguish the type of growth for retinoblastoma and related tumor types. Endophytic and exophytic growths show variations in the ultrasonographic context of both A and B scanning techniques.

B Scan Technique. In the case of an endophytic growth, the retinoblastoma appears as a single or, more often, a multiple lesion on the retinal plane. The tumors are monolobate or multilobate and have a roundish or irregular oval shape, with dense acoustics and variable homogeneity (Fig. 22-5*B*). A discrete attenuation of the ultrasound occurs, with the shadowing of the echoes coming from the orbital tissue. The attenuation is considerable if, as is often the case, areas of calcification are found inside the tumor mass.[76] The tumor itself may develop within the vitreous chamber and occupy it almost entirely, and, at times, areas of pseudocysts may be found in front of and/or in the context of the neoplastic mass, thus making it difficult to recognize the lesion.[77] Nevertheless, the attenuation of the ultrasound is considerable.

With the exophytic growth, the diagnosis is harder to establish, especially if the tumor is analyzed during the initial stage. It is easily confused with the high echogenic portion of the sclera, while no significant evidence of it appears on the retinal plane. The only significant noticeable sign is a certain attenuation of the ultrasound coming from the orbital tissue, with a display on the echogram that simulates the acoustic shadow of the optic nerve, but does not resemble it in topography and size.[77]

A Scan Technique. In the case of an endophytic tumor growth, a standardized A scan tracing shows an opening peak that appears at high or medium reflectivity but is never maximal. This is the case because the internal retinal surface is considerably compromised and heterogeneous, thus attenuating the contrast that exists at the vitreous-retinal interface level. The opening peak can be maximal, however, if the tumor has an exophytic growth as long as the layer of the limiting internal membrane and the nerve fibers are not disintegrated by the growth of the tumor.[77,78]

In the opposite case, a peak at high reflectivity found during a subsequent checkup may reveal a peritumorous satellite area, even if small and confined, rather than an opening peak of the tumor. The internal structure of the tumor usually appears quite regular at medium-high reflectivity and at medium reflectivity in the case of a retinoblastoma with no calcifications.[77] Vitreous activity with the absence of seeding is minor in retinoblastoma before photocoagulation, while afterward it is possible to find juxtalesional vitreous echoes at medium reflectivity and, sometimes, areas of peritumorous retinal fissions.[79]

Invasion of the sclera entails the loss of its homogeneity as an acoustic interface and causes a decrease in the reflectivity of the closing scleral peak that may be mistaken for the retinal echoes of the same tumor. This represents an important ultrasonographic sign, which can determine the margins and posterior borders of the lesion. In the A and B scanning methods, the calcifications are characteristically evident even when the amplitude appears reduced. Furthermore, suspicion of invasion of the optic nerve is indicated by the presence in the nervous tissue of an ultrasonographic tracing that reproduces the features of a retinoblastoma in an A scan.

Fine-Needle Aspiration Biopsy. The cytologic approach to the study of retinoblastoma has become particularly relevant as the techniques for obtaining tumor material have improved. Specimens from the posterior chamber can be obtained by using vitrectomy techniques in addition to anterior chamber paracentesis for cytologic and enzymologic evaluation of the aqueous. Aqueous and vitreous aspiration for cytologic studies may be useful in differentiating retinoblastoma from the previously described simulating conditions.

The use of fine-needle biopsy in ophthalmology, originally introduced by Schyberg for the diagnosis of orbital tumors, was utilized in the diagnosis of intraocular neoplasms by Jakobiec et al.[80] and extended to the diagnosis of intraocular and extraocular retinoblastoma by Char and Miller.[81] This approach is not recommended as a routine procedure for retinoblastoma and generally is reserved for children who present with unusual manifestations or for differentiating an orbital recurrence of retinoblastoma from a second malignant neoplasm.[81] A limbal approach is used for anterior segment tumors, whereas a via pars plana approach after opening of the conjunctiva, scleral diathermy, and 1.5-mm sclerotomy is used for posterior tumors.[82,83] Complications that may occur with the use of fine-needle biopsy include intraocular hemorrhage, retinal detachment, and recurrence in the orbit or along the intraocular needle tract. Although tumoral-cell seedings within the scleral needle tracks after biopsy

are controversial,[84,85] this possibility suggests that fine-needle biopsy be limited to patients who present diagnostic uncertainties. These patients include older children with suspected retinoblastoma and rather atypical findings and children with orbital masses who previously have been treated for retinoblastoma.[86–88]

Therapy

If a retinoblastoma or a related ocular tumor is discovered at an early stage and diagnostic tools have appropriately classified the type, there are several current and effective methods for treatment, including enucleation, external-beam irradiation, episcleral plaques, xenon arc and argon laser photocoagulation, cryotherapy, and chemotherapy. The choice of treatment depends on factors such as (a) multifocal or unifocal disease, (b) site and size of the tumor, (c) diffuse or focal vitreous seeding, (d) age of the child, and (e) histopathologic findings. Therefore, an appropriate therapeutic approach greatly depends on accurate staging of the disease.

Staging and Classification. The most widely used staging system for retinoblastoma, which was proposed by Reese and Ellsworth,[89] is based on the ophthalmoscopic evaluation of the tumor extension and generally is limited to patients with intraocular retinoblastoma. Pratt extended this system to include intraocular and extraocular extension of the disease.[90] Another system is based on an accurate evaluation of the histopathologic findings.[91] Most recently, a pretreatment TNM classification has been introduced that also addresses the importance of visual acuity in addition to patient survival and ocular extension.[92] Table 22-2 presents the different criteria for these classification systems.

Enucleation. Enucleation is the standard treatment in unilateral cases and for the more severely affected eye in bilateral ones. An attempt to save the eye is worthwhile only when there is hope for useful vision and no risk of a systemic prognosis.[93] Generally there are several major indications that call for the nonconservative removal of the diseased eye. These tumor characteristics include (a) a large mass involving more than 50 percent of the retina associated with retinal detachment, (b) a buphthalmic painful eye, (c) a phthisical eye (in bilateral cases), and (d) unsuccessful conservative treatment (radiotherapy with or without chemotherapy and photocoagulation). Regardless of which of the various enucleation techniques is used, the procedure should be performed with the least trauma possible for the patient while avoiding scleral perforation, and at least 10 mm of the optic nerve should be resected.[94] After enucleation, the use of an implant is recommended for both cosmetic reasons and to stimulate orbital growth. Usually a conformer is used for 2 to 3 days directly after surgery, followed by a temporary insert prosthesis (about 1 week after enucleation) after complete healing of the surgical incision.[13]

External Irradiation. Retinoblastoma is a highly radiosensitive tumor, and the first attempt at its treatment with x-rays occurred in 1903.[95] External-beam irradiation, utilizing gamma rays from a linear accelerator, is now the most commonly used treatment for intraocular and orbital disease. This technique is indicated when (a) in unilateral retinoblastoma cases there is a large tumor not involving the macula and optic nerve, (b) in bilateral retinoblastoma cases there are advanced tumors in both eyes, or in the remaining eye when multiple tumors or diffuse vitreous seeding is present, and (c) in orbital tissue, where histopathologic studies of the enucleated eye and optic nerve document an invasion of the optic nerve, scleral invasion, or orbital recurrence.[13]

The goal of external irradiation in retinoblastoma is to sterilize the entire retina and vitreous of malignant cells with the best possible visual prognosis. A dose generally considered to be optimally therapeutic is 4000 rad fractionated into about 20 doses over a 3- to 4-week period. At the Utrecht Retinoblastoma Center, a highly accurate irradiation method has been developed,[96] based on the temporal approach, which ensures precise delivery of a

Table 22-2 Classification Systems for Retinoblastoma

Reese-Ellsworth Classification	Pratt Classification	Standard Classification	TNM Classification
Group I: Very favorable prognosis A: Solitary tumor, less than 4 dd* in size, at or behind the equator B: Multiple tumors, none more than 4 dd in size, at or behind the equator	I: Tumor (unifocal or multifocal) confined to the retina A: Occupying 1 quadrant or less B: Occupying 2 quadrants or less C: Occupying more than 50% of the retinal surface	Stage I: Lesions amenable to local therapy Stage II: Lesions unsuitable for conservative local therapy but still confined to the eye—subdivisions based on histologic assessment of the eye	T1: Tumor or tumors 10 dd or less in largest diameter T1a: Macula not involved T1b: Macula involved T2: Tumor or tumors larger than 10 dd involving up to half the retina T2a: Macula not involved T2b: Macula involved
Group II: Favorable prognosis A: Solitary lesion, 4–10 dd at or behind the equator B: Multiple lesions, 4–10 dd at or behind the equator	II: Tumor (unifocal or multifocal) confined to the globe A: With vitreous seeding B: Extending to optic-nerve head C: Extending to choroid D: Extending to choroid and optic-nerve head E: Extending to emissaries	N0: No invasion of the optic nerve N1: Invasion up to or into the lamina cribrosa N2: Invasion beyond the lamina cribrosa resection line free N3: Optic nerve involved up to the resection line	T3: Tumor or tumors involving more than half the retina T4: Extraretinal or orbital extension T4a: Invasion of optic nerve T4b: Invasion of choroidea, corpus ciliare, iris, or anterior chamber T4c: Scleral involvement T4d: Two or more a–c
Group III: Doubtful prognosis A: Any lesion anterior to the equator B: Solitary tumor larger than 10 dd behind the equator	III: Extraocular extension of tumor (regional) A: Extending beyond cut end of optic nerve (including subarachnoid extension) B: Extending through sclera into orbital contents C: Extending to choroid and beyond cut end of optic nerve (including subarachnoid extension) D: Extending though sclera into orbital contents and beyond cut end of optic nerve (including subarachnoid extension)	C0: No choroidal invasion C1: Superficial involvement of the choroid up to half of its thickness C2: Full-thickness choroidal invasion C3: Scleral invasion, including tumor in the emissary vessels C4: Extrascleral invasion	N: Regional lymph nodes NX: Minimum requirements to assess the regional lymph nodes cannot be met N0: No evidence of regional lymph node involvement N1: Evidence of involvement of regional lymph nodes
Group IV: Unfavorable prognosis A: Multiple tumors, some larger than 10 dd B: Any lesion extending anteriorly to the ora serrata		Stage III: Local spread beyond the eye without hematogenous metastases 1: Orbital tumors 2: Preauricular or cervical nodes 3: Central nervous system disease	M: Distant metastases M0: No evidence of distant metastases M1: Evidence of distant metastases (can be subdivided according to the organs involved)
Group V: Very unfavorable prognosis A: Massive tumors involving over 50% of the retina B: Vitreous seeding	IV: Distant metastases A: Extending through optic nerve to brain B: Blood-borne metastases to soft tissue and bone C: Bone-marrow metastases	Stage IV: Hematogenous metastases	

*dd denotes disk diameter; one dd = 1.6 mm.

uniform radiation dose to the whole retina or vitreous with maximal sparing of the lens. Accurate positioning of the collimated field is obtained by magnetic fixation of the eye to the beam-defining collimator by a low-vacuum contact lens. Because the eye is fixed in the isocenter of the accelerator, rotation of the gantry directs the beam. Other centers have adopted this technique and have confirmed the extreme precision and sharp-beam profile that can be obtained.[97,98]

Four regression patterns after radiation for retinoblastoma have been described by Reese and Ellsworth[99] and by Buys et al.[101] These patterns are described as follows: type I—characterized by calcification, marked alterations of the retinal pigment epithelium, and the cottage cheese aspect; type II—the tumor is shrunken in size and adopts a gray, translucent appearance (fish flesh); type III—a combination of the patterns seen for types I and II; and type IV—represented by the typical pattern after cobalt-plaque treatment, with complete destruction of the tumor and choroid; the white scar represents the sclera underlying the tumor.

Buys et al. found that the most common type of regression at the first evaluation was type III (43.8 percent). However, after a

minimum of 7 years, a decrease in this pattern was found (from 43.8 to 36 percent). It was also reported that the type II patterns can turn into any one of the other types over a number of years. Furthermore, a correlation seems to exist between the size of the tumor and the regression pattern.[101]

As with most procedures, complications can arise after external irradiation. They are divided into immediate, usually reversible complications and late, usually irreversible complications. The most severe complications are growth retardation of the orbital region, dry-eye syndrome caused by the reduced or absent lacrimal secretion, radiation cataract, iris atrophy, vascular changes, and retinal exudates (radiation retinopathy).[102]

Episcleral Plaques. The use of radon seed brachytherapy for the conservative treatment of retinoblastoma was introduced in 1929. In 1948, Stallard developed radioactive applicators using radium, and these applications were later modified to use ^{60}Co. Later techniques expanded to include ^{125}Ie, ^{192}Ir, and ^{106}Ru eye plaques, which are now all used routinely in the focal treatment of the disease.[103] Many treatment centers have a preference for ^{125}I

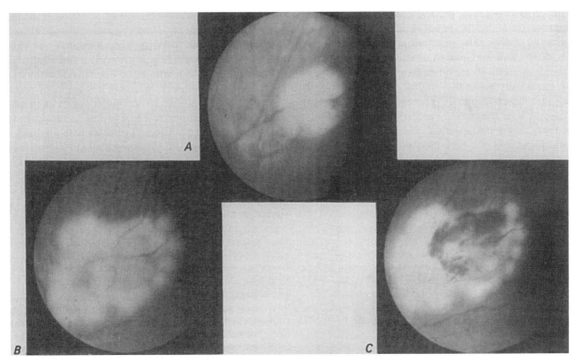

Fig. 22-6 Regression patterns for retinoblastoma after photocoagulation. *A,* A small retinoblastoma. *B,* After indirect xenon-arc photocoagulation. *C,* After direct xenon-arc photocoagulation. (Courtesy of R. Frezzotti, MD, Director of the Institute of Ophthalmological Sciences, University of Siena, Italy.)

plaques because orbital tissues can be shielded with a gold-plaque carrier, ridge plaques can limit the spread of radiation to the nerve and foveal region, and there is less radiation exposure for the patient and the assisting staff.[104] Regardless of the type used, the episcleral plaque technique is highly advantageous compared with other forms of therapy because the procedure time is short while the dose of irradiation is delivered directly to the tumor, minimizing radiation effects to the extraocular structures.

The use of radioactive scleral plaques as a primary treatment is particularly successful for medium-size tumors no greater than 12 mm in diameter and more than 3 mm from the optic disk or macula.[105] Scleral plaques are also useful as a secondary treatment for recurrent or new tumors which are impossible to control using photo- or cryocoagulation. The regression patterns seen after plaque treatment appear to be identical to those described for external-beam irradiation (types I, II, and III). However, a type IV radiation regression pattern characterized by complete destruction of the tumor choroid and all vessels, leaving a white scleral patch, has been observed only after cobalt plaque treatment.[100]

Photocoagulation. In 1955, Meyer-Schwickerath developed a photocoagulation technique using a xenon arc in which retinoblastomas are surrounded by a ring of coagulation placed in the normal retina before the tumor tissue itself is treated.[106] The experience of others[104,107–110] suggests that the success of photocoagulation is due to the destruction of the retinal blood supply, not to its effect on the tumor itself or on the underlying choroid. The best results have occurred with tumors up to 4 to 5 disk diameters in size, with an elevation of 4 diopters,[111,112] although tumors up to 6 or more disk diameters have also been treated successfully in this way.[107,108] Indications, contraindications, and results of photocoagulation appear to be disparate. There are different opinions regarding the size, elevation, site, and clinical conditions in which retinoblastoma should be treated with photocoagulation.[109] Photocoagulation has been suggested as a primary approach for small and moderate retinoblastomas posterior to the equator and for the treatment of recurrent or new tumors after external radiotherapy or radioactive plaques.[108] Photocoagulation is not appropriate when tumors lie directly on the optic nerve or when there is vitreous seeding.

Complications arising from the use of photocoagulation may include occasional retinal hemorrhage; retinal traction; retinal folds; macular distortion; iris damage; corneal edema; and/or cataract (caused by inadvertent iris heating or energy absorption by preexisting opacities). The regression patterns observed after photocoagulation treatment depend on the size and elevation of the tumor (Fig. 22-6). Furthermore, it appears that vascularization of the tumor can influence sensitivity to xenon photocoagulation.[107] After photocoagulation, small tumors appear as a flat avascular pigmented scar. Larger tumors may present marked coarctation, reduced vascularization, and a translucent gray appearance similar to that described as fish flesh. However, both of these regression patterns closely resemble those of types I and II after radiotherapy.

Cryocoagulation. Cryotherapy[113] for retinoblastoma can be used as a primary or supplementary treatment after other conservative therapeutic attempts and can be effective in clinical situations involving new or recurrent tumors after irradiation therapy or in tumors anterior to the equator in eyes that have not been treated.[114] Cryotherapy can be successful on tumors up to 3.5 mm in diameter and 2.0 mm in thickness, but more than one treatment may be necessary.[115]

Vitreous base tumors are very rarely cured with cryocoagulation alone.[116] Localization of the tumor is obtained by indentation with a cryoprobe under indirect ophthalmoscopy. Tumors are frozen with applications of $-80°C$ for 30 to 60 s, and the treatment is typically repeated three times.[117] Cryotherapy destroys the tumor by direct intracellular and intravascular formation of microcrystals. The most frequent complications after cryotherapy are conjunctival and lid edema.

Chemotherapy. To date, chemotherapy has played only a secondary role in the treatment of retinoblastoma, because good control can be achieved with more local treatment. There is also a relative paucity of randomized studies on the efficacy of chemotherapy compared with other therapeutic procedures, and this is further complicated by a lack of suitable markers for the detection of minimal residual disease.[57,59,60,118] The first to use a chemotherapeutic agent in retinoblastoma treatment was Kupfer, who obtained partial regression of a retinal tumor mass by using nitrogen mustard.[119] After this preliminary experience, other antitumor drugs, especially vincristine and cyclophosphamide, were used alone or in combination in several situations, such as in association with radiotherapy for advanced disease[120,121] to reduce the mortality caused by micrometastatic disease[120-127] and with locally advanced disease or distant metastasis.[128-130] Especially in the last group of patients, sequential chemotherapy protocols or courses of intensive chemotherapy followed by autologous bone marrow transplantation have given encouraging results. Despite these achievements, the role of antiblastic chemotherapy in the treatment of retinoblastoma remains controversial, and the only generally accepted indications for it are orbital or metastatic disease, trilateral retinoblastoma, and salvage therapy for relapses in the residual eye. More controversial indications include shrinkage of the neoplastic mass, optic nerve infiltration beyond the lamina cribrosa, and choroidal infiltration (whole thickness and/or ciliary body invasion) with or without optic nerve involvement up to the lamina cribrosa. This mode of therapy still awaits homogeneous staging and therapeutic criteria to evaluate its general efficacy.[131,132]

THE GENETICS OF RETINOBLASTOMA

Retinoblastoma has served as the prototypic example of the genetic predisposition to cancer.[133] Although the majority of tumors occur with no preceding family history, the inherited form of the disease has been extensively documented.[134-136] The familial disease is transmitted, with few exceptions, as a typical Mendelian autosomal dominant trait with virtually full penetrance. It has been estimated from epidemiologic data[137] that about 60 percent of cases are nonhereditary and unilateral, 15 percent are hereditary and unilateral, and 25 percent are hereditary and bilateral.

Although there are examples of apparent nonpenetrance among antecedent or collateral relatives of familial retinoblastoma patients, among descendants of such patients penetrance is nearly complete.[137] There have been a few pedigrees reported in which the disease seems to have truly skipped a generation, in other words being transmitted from grandparent to grandchild via an unaffected parent. Retrospective analysis of families of retinoblastoma probands has yielded several examples of presumed obligate carriers who did not develop the disease. Examination of a number of retinoblastoma pedigrees[15,135-139] showed apparent nonpenetrance in 52 of 128 families either through multiply affected sibships with both parents unaffected or through other affected relatives (such as cousins and aunts) with unaffected intervening relatives. In contrast, when pooled data from published sources were used to determine the segregation ratio among the offspring of familial retinoblastoma patients, it was observed that bilaterally affected parents had 49 percent affected offspring, as is

expected for a dominantly inherited disease with complete penetrance, whereas unilaterally affected parents had 42 percent affected offspring, indicating some lack of penetrance.[139] These data were relevant to the proposal of a host resistance model by which heritable resistance factors to a predisposing gene are minimal in bilaterally affected individuals, intermediate in unilaterally affected individuals, and maximal in unaffected carriers.[139]

One proposed model[133,137] encompasses the observations that familial cases are generally multifocal and bilateral, whereas sporadic cases typically present with unilateral unifocal disease of later diagnosis. According to the model, as few as two stochastic mutational events are required for tumor formation, the first of which can be inherited through the germ line (in heritable cases) or can occur somatically in individual retinal cells (in nonheritable cases). The second event occurs somatically in either case and leads to tumor formation in each doubly defective retinal cell. This empirically based hypothesis has been supported by direct experimental scrutiny using molecular genetic approaches.

Cytogenetics

The involvement of genetic alteration in the first step of this pathway of oncogenesis has been supported by cytogenetic analysis which has shown that a small proportion of patients carry a microscopically visible deletion of one chromosome 13 homologue in all their constitutional cells. Since the first such report,[140] more than 30 deletions have been described occurring in a small percentage of retinoblastoma cases;[141-143] the common region of overlap of such deletions is chromosome 13, band q14.[144,145] An example of such a deletion of one constitutional chromosome 13 homologue is illustrated in Fig. 22-7. In the context of the two-hit model, such deletions could act as the first hit and, when they are germinal, could confer the risk of tumor formation in an autosomal dominant manner. Evidence that the same locus is involved in retinoblastoma cases that lack an apparent chromosomal deletion was provided through the demonstration of tight genetic linkage between the retinoblastoma and esterase D loci,[146] the latter being a moderately polymorphic isozymic enzyme whose encoding locus also maps to 13q14.[147]

Furthermore, cytogenetic analysis has provided important information concerning the occasional occurrence of apparent nonpenetrance in some retinoblastoma families. A large kindred has been reported in which unilateral retinoblastoma was transmitted by a number of unaffected individuals. Each affected individual carried the same constitutional deletion involving 13q14, whereas the unaffected carriers had a balanced insertional translocation involving the same region.[148] This and other related reports of chromosomal translocations, inversions, or deletions in transmitting parents[148,150] provide a clear biologic basis for segregation distortion without invoking nonpenetrance. In addition, two reports describe individuals who carry a constitutional

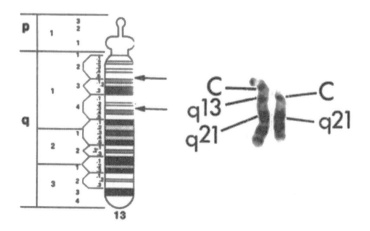

Fig. 22-7 Chromosome 13 deletion in constitutional cells from a patient with retinoblastoma. The idiogram of chromosome 13 to the left indicates the two breakpoints (arrows) of the interstitial deletion. To the right is a G-banded partial karyotype with the normal homologue on the left (centromere, C, bands q13 and q21 indicated) and the deleted homologue on the right (centromere and q21 band indicated). Only one chromosome homologue is altered. Hence, this aberration may represent the first and predisposing event in the child. (Courtesy of David Ledbetter, Baylor College of Medicine, Houston.)

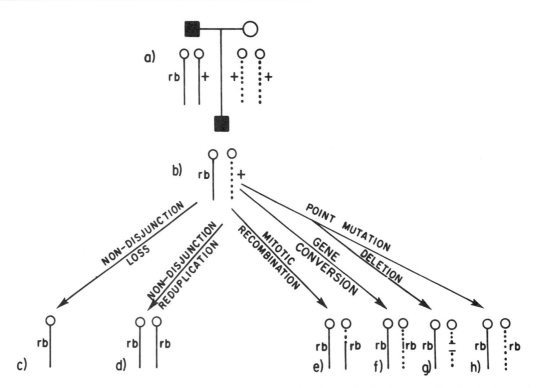

Fig. 22-8 Chromosomal mechanisms that could reveal recessive mutations. In this example, an affected male (a) who carries a recessive defect at the RB1 locus on chromosome 13, designated rb, in all his cells mates with a genotypically wild-type, +, female. One of their children (b) inherits the defective chromosome 13 from his father and so is rb/+ at the RB1 locus in all his cells. A tumor in his retinal cells may develop by eliminating the dominant wild-type allele at the RB1 locus by the mechanisms required to effect the tumor cell genotype shown schematically in c to h. (Reprinted by permission from Cavenee et al., *Nature,* vol. 305, p. 779, copyright 1983, Macmillan Journals, Limited.)

deletion involving 13q14 but have no signs of retinoblastoma at age 5[151] or 25 years.[152] Whether a significant proportion of unaffected carriers can be accounted for by such mechanisms remains to be demonstrated. Another theoretical explanation for isolated multiply affected sibships with unaffected parents is parental mosaicism. Chromosomal mosaicism for deletions involving 13q14 was reported in one series in lymphocytes from 5 to 50 sporadic retinoblastoma patients.[153] In these cases, a significant proportion of retinal cells must have carried the deletion; alternatively, if relatively few retinoblasts carried the deletion, an individual could be at low risk for expressing the disease, but at high risk for its transmission. The increasing resolution of cytogenetic technology and the use of DNA probes for loci in the immediate vicinity of the retinoblastoma locus (gene symbol RB1) have also allowed the detection of more subtle genomic rearrangements that were undetectable previously and have shed light on individuals carrying nonpenetrant mutations in the retinoblastoma susceptibility locus (see below).

The presence of 13q14 deletion in patients without mental retardation or major anomalies,[154] and in familial cases in which transmission might appear to be autosomal dominant,[155] suggests that high-resolution chromosome analysis should be done in all patients with retinoblastoma. When a deletion is found in a proband, parental studies should be considered to rule out deletion, insertional translocation, or mosaicism.

Molecular Genetics

Specific predictions of the nature of the second tumor-eliciting event in the two-step model on oncogenesis[133,137] have been proposed:[156] (a) The autosomal dominant hereditary form of retinoblastoma, in the absence of a gross chromosomal deletion, involves the same genetic locus that is involved in cases showing large deletions of chromosome 13. Thus, the first step in the pathway toward tumorigenesis in these cases is a submicroscopic

mutational event at the RB1 locus. (b) The same genetic change that has occurred as a germ-line mutation in hereditary retinoblastoma occurs as a somatic genetic alteration of the RB1 locus in a retinal cell in nonhereditary retinoblastoma. (c) The second step in tumorigenesis in both heritable and nonhereditable retinoblastoma involves somatic alteration of the normal allele at the RB1 locus in such a way that the mutant allele is unmasked. Thus, the first mutation in this process, although it may be inherited as an autosomal dominant trait at the organism level, is in fact a recessive defect in the individual retinal cell.

The model that arises from these considerations is shown in Fig. 22-8. It outlines specific chromosomal mechanisms that should allow phenotypic expression of a recessive germinal mutation of the RB1 locus (Fig. 22-8A). This aberration is inherited by an individual who thus carries such a mutation in all somatic as well as germ-line cells (Fig. 22-8B). Any additional event that results in homozygosity or hemizygosity for the mutant allele (that is, the RB1 locus is mutant on both chromosome 13 homologues) will result in a tumor clone. Several chromosomal mechanisms can be imagined in this process: (a) mitotic non-disjunction with loss of the wild-type chromosome (Fig. 22-8C), resulting in hemizygosity at all loci on chromosome 13; (b) mitotic nondisjunction with duplication of the mutant chromosome (Fig. 22-8D), resulting in homozygosity at all loci on the chromosome; (c) mitotic recombination (Fig. 22-8E) between the RB1 locus encoding the mutant allele and the centromere, resulting in heterozygosity at loci in the proximal region and homozygosity throughout the rest of the chromosome, including the RB1 locus; and (d) several other more regionalized events such as gene conversion (Fig. 22-8F), deletion (Fig. 22-8G), or mutation (Fig. 22-8H). Both nonheritable and hereditable retinoblastoma could arise through the appearance of homozygosity at the RB1 locus, the difference being two somatic events in the former instance and one germinal event and one somatic event in the latter instance.

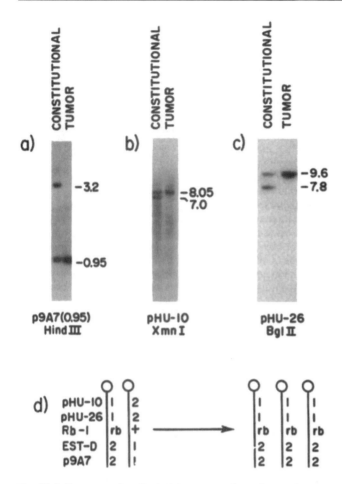

a) p9A7(0.95)
HindIII
−3.2
−0.95

b) pHU-10
XmnI
−8.05
−7.0

c) pHU-26
Bgl II
−9.6
−7.8

d)
pHU-10	1	2		1	1	1
pHU-26	1	2		1	1	1
Rb-1	rb	+		rb	rb	rb
EST-D	2	1		2	2	2
p9A7	2	1		2	2	2

Fig. 22-9 Homozygosity effected by segregation of one chromosome 13 homologue with duplication of the remaining one. *A,* Results obtained when *Hind*III-digested DNA was hybridized to p9A7, which contains an insert homologous to a locus on chromosome 13 mapping between band q22 and the terminus of the long arm. B, The pattern obtained when *Xmn*I-digested DNA was hybridized to the insert fragment derived from the plasmid pHU10, which is homologous to a locus on chromosome 13 mapping between bands q12 and q22. C, The pattern obtained when *Bgl*III-digested DNA was hybridized to the insert fragment isolated from the plasmid pHU26, which is homologous to a locus on chromosome 13 mapping between bands q12 and q22. D, A diagram incorporating these data with previous analysis of the esterase D alleles present and the karyotype of the two samples from patient Rb-409. (Reprinted by permission from Cavenee et al., *Nature,* vol. 305, p. 780, copyright 1983, Macmillan Journals, Limited.)

The approach that has been taken to examine these hypotheses relies on the variability of DNA sequences among humans, which results in inherited differences in restriction-endonuclease recognition sites. In this approach, segments of the human genome are isolated in recombinant DNA form, and the loci homologous to these probe segments are tested for their encompassing restriction-endonuclease recognition sequences, which vary between unrelated individuals. Two types of such variation have been defined. The first, and most abundant, results from simple base-pair changes within the recognition-site sequence for a particular restriction endonuclease and yields alleles of greater (when the effect of the mutation is loss of a site) or lesser (when the effect of the mutation is gain of a site) length.[157] The second type results from the insertion or deletion of varying numbers of blocks of like DNA sequence into or out of the genomic locus.[158] Practically, the net result is the observation of two alleles at the locus encompassing a site change (presence or absence of the site) or numerous alleles at a locus subject to insertion or deletion of larger segments of DNA, respectively. In either case, however, any given individual

will reveal only two alleles at the locus, one from the paternally derived chromosome and one from the maternally derived homologue. In all cases examined to date, these types of markers have been shown to behave in family studies in the manner that would be predicted for simple Mendelian codominant alleles. Recombinant DNA probes for loci mapped along the length of human chromosome 13 have been isolated, characterized,[159,160] and used in multilocus analysis to detect alterations in the somatic genotypes of tumors compared with the germ-line genotype of the individuals harboring these tumors.[156,161,162] A reasonably large series of retinoblastoma cases has been examined in this manner; examples are illustrated in Fig. 22-9 and Fig. 22-10.

Nondisjunction and Duplication. The mechanism depicted in Fig. 22-8*D*, in which, together with the nondisjunctional loss of the wild-type chromosome, the mutant chromosome is duplicated, would be difficult to detect cytogenetically or by quantitation of esterase D activity. However, with the use of codominant DNA markers, these events were detected as a loss of one allele at each informative locus on the chromosome. The patient described in Fig. 22-9 was found to be heterozygous at the ESD locus and showed no visible abnormality of either chromosome 13. An examination of tumor tissue from this individual again showed no abnormalities of chromosome 13 except that in addition to the expected two copies of the chromosome, another copy was present as a translocation involving chromosomes 13 and 14. However, the tumor cells exhibited only one of the two isozymic types of the esterase D enzyme—the allele from the father. It was proposed[163] that this resulted from somatic inactivation of the maternally derived allele of the ESD locus on one homologue of chromosome 13.

Constitutional and tumor cells derived from this patient were tested with seven recombinant DNA probes. Three of the probes revealed heterozygosity in the germ-line tissue: p9A7, which maps in the region 13q22-qter, and pHU26 and pHU10, both of which map in the region 13q12-q22. In each of these cases (Fig. 22-9A to C), although both codominant alleles were present in the germ line, only one allele at each locus was present in the tumor, and this allele was derived in each case from the chromosome 13 inherited from the father. A reasonable interpretation of these results is diagrammed in Fig. 22-9D. Rather than somatic inactivation of the ESD locus on one chromosome 13 homologue, these data are consistent with the complete loss of the entire maternally derived chromosome accompanied by duplication of the paternally derived chromosome. It is likely that this chromosome carried a *de novo* germinal mutation, because the father showed no evidence of retinoblastoma, but the subject was bilaterally affected. It is also possible that one or two of the chromosomes 13 in the tumor were derived by mitotic exchange between the wild-type mutant chromosomes (as diagrammed in Fig. 22-8*E*) so that an original mutant chromosome and a recombinant chromosome (or two) were maintained. If this had happened, the point of interchange must have been proximal to the region detected by the most proximal marker locus, because all the markers, including esterase D (which maps to 13q14), show reduction to homozygosity in the tumor.

Mitotic Recombination. Another possible mechanism by which part of a pair of chromosomes may become homozygous, although not previously observed in humans, is illustrated in Fig. 22-8*E*. A somatic, or mitotic, recombination between the mutant and wild-type chromosome homologues, with subsequent segregation, can result in a cell that maintains heterozygosity at loci proximal to the breakpoint of the recombinational event, but shows homozygosity at loci distal to such a breakpoint. An instance of this mechanism was presented in patient Rb-412.[156] The germ-line cells from this person had been determined to be heterozygous at the ESD locus as well as heterozygous for a quinacrine-staining satellite heteromorphism on the short arm of chromosome 13. An examination of the tumor cells derived from this patient showed the presence of

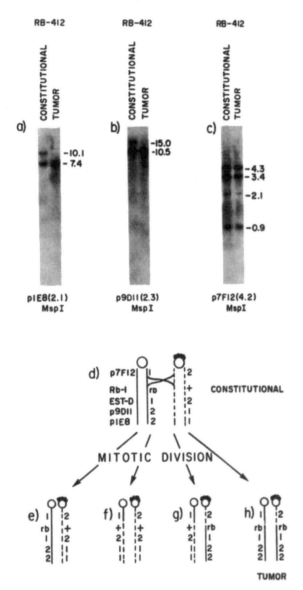

Fig. 22-10 Homozygosity effected by a mitotic recombination event. A, The pattern obtained when the hybridization probe was p1E8, which is homologous to a locus on chromosome 13 mapping between band q22 and the terminus of the long arm. **B,** Results obtained when the hybridization probe was p9D11, which is homologous to a locus on chromosome 13 mapping to band q22. **C,** Results obtained with the hybridization probe p7F12, which is homologous to a locus on chromosome 13 mapping between bands q12 and q14. **D,** Diagram showing inferred haplotypes on each chromosome derived from karyology, esterase D determinations, and these data. The cap on the chromosome homologues represented by the dashed lines denotes a fluorescent-staining heterochromatic region. In this figure, the point of crossover must lie between the RB1 and 7F12 loci and is shown occurring between chromatids of the chromosome 13 homologue at the four-strand stage of mitotic chromosome replication. **E–H,** Diagram of the four possible combinations of wild-type and recombinant homologues. Possibilities **E** to **G** result in a phenotypically wild-type cell. The allelic data shown in **H** corresponds to the experimental data and results in homozygosity for the mutant (rb) allele at the RB1 locus. (Reprinted by permission from Cavenee et al., *Nature,* vol. 305, p. 781, copyright 1983, Macmillan Journals, Limited.)

both types of satellite staining, but only one isozymic form of esterase D. A reasonable interpretation of these data[162] was that both chromosomes 13 were present in their entirety in the Rb-412 tumor and that a somatic inactivation of one of the isozymic forms of esterase D had occurred during tumor formation. Alternatively,

a mitotic recombination event occurring between the centromere and the ESD locus, as was described above, could generate chromosomes consistent with these results. Germ-line and tumor genotypes of this patient were examined at chromosome 13 loci defined by seven DNA probes (Fig. 22-10). Three of the markers were heterozygous in skin fibroblasts from Rb-412: p1E8, which maps distal to 13q22; p9D11, which maps at 13q22; and p7F12, which maps between the RB1 locus and the centromere. The tumor tissue from this patient showed a loss of one allele at the 9D11 and 1E8 loci, whereas the 7F12 locus remained heterozygous (Fig. 22-10C). An interpretation of these results, taken together with the satellite heteromorphism and esterase D data described above, is illustrated in Fig. 22-10D and suggests that a recombination event took place between the mutant and wild-type chromosomes 13 in the cell that gave rise to the tumor. The crossover point was between the 7F12 and the RB1 loci, and each locus distal to the RB1 locus became homozygous. Between RB1 and the terminus of the short arm, however, two markers maintained both the maternal and paternal haplotypes.

Data similar to those shown in Figs. 22-9 and 22-10 have been obtained in more than 75 percent of the retinoblastoma tumors examined. They provide experimental support for the proposed recessive model of oncogenesis,[133,137,156] by which predisposing mutations are revealed by elimination of the homologous wild-type locus through chromosomal segregation or recombination rather than simple point mutation. The supposition that it was the chromosome 13 homologue carrying the wild-type RB1 allele that was lost during the process of tumorigenesis was tested by comparing constitutional and tumor genotypes of patients with familial retinoblastoma.

The model described in Fig. 22-8 demands that the chromosomes 13 remaining in the tumors of such children be derived from the affected parent. The analysis[163] of one such case, KS2H, is shown in Fig. 22-11. This child was constitutionally heterozygous at the HU26 locus. His retinoblastoma tumor tissue (Rb-KS2H) showed only the longer allele at this locus. His unaffected parent, KS2C, was constitutionally heterozygous at this locus, while his affected parent, KS2F, was homozygous for the longer allele. Therefore, the proband must have inherited the shorter allele at the locus from his unaffected parent, and it was this chromosome that was lost in the tumor. The chromosome remaining in the tumor was inherited from his affected parent and must be the one carrying the initial predisposing mutation at RB1. In this family, the proband inherited the predisposition to retinoblastoma from his father, KS2F, who had inherited it from his mother, KS2G (Fig. 22-11B). He obtained the shorter allele from his unaffected mother and the longer allele from his affected father. It is the latter chromosome that must contain the mutant RB1 locus, and it was this chromosome which was retained in the child's tumor. Corroborating evidence of this interpretation was obtained by examining genotypic combinations at other loci on chromosome 13 in other members of the family. Assignment of the alleles at each of these loci, in combination with those for HU26, and a consideration of the allelic combinations from the grandparents (KS2A, KS2B, and KS2G), parents (KS2C and KS2F), child (KS2H), and child's tumor (Rb-KS2H) made it possible to infer chromosomal haplotypes (Fig. 22-11B). The proband (KS2H) inherited a nonrecombinant chromosome from his paternal grandmother (KS2G) through his father (KS2F) and a recombinant chromosome from his mother (KS2C). It appears that the chromosome retained in the tumor (Rb-KS2H) was inherited from his affected grandmother (KS2G) through his affected father (KS2F). In other inherited cases examined, the prediction that the chromosome 13 derived from the affected parent would be retained in the tumor has also been confirmed.

It is noteworthy that although the unmasking of predisposing mutations at the RB1 locus occurs in mechanistically similar ways in sporadic and heritable retinoblastoma patients, only the latter carry the initial mutation in each of their cells. Patients with heritable disease also seem to be at greatly increased risk for the

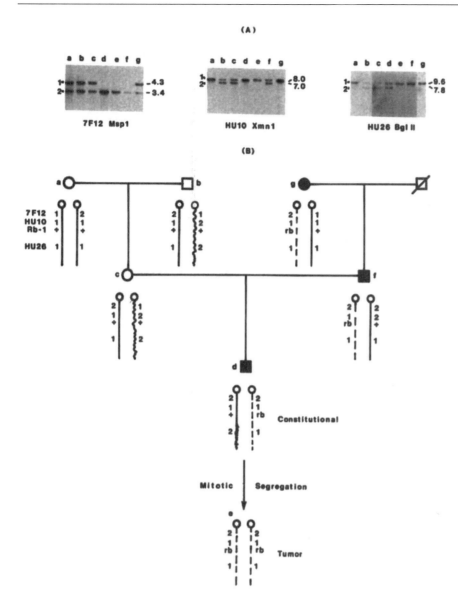

Fig. 22-11 Loss of germ line heterozygosity in a hereditary retinoblastoma tumor. *A*, DNA was isolated from peripheral blood leukocytes from each of the indicated individuals and from a primary tumor biopsy from the proband KS2H. The DNA was digested with the indicated restriction endonucleases, separated by electrophoresis through 0.8% agarose gels, transferred to nylon membranes, and hybridized to the indicated probes homologous to loci on human chromosome 13. The family members are designated: (a) KS2A, (b) KS2B, (c) KS2C, (d) KS2H, (e) Rb-KS2H (tumor), (f) KS2F, and (g) KS2g. *B*, Pedigree Rb-KS2 and inferred chromosome 13 haplotypes at the 7F12, HU10, RB1, and HU26 loci. Filled symbols = individuals with retinoblastoma; dashed line = nonrecombinant chromosome; straight and wavy lines = recombinant chromosome. (Reprinted by permission from Cavenee et al., *Science* 228:501, 26 April 1985, copyright 1985, American Association for the Advancement of Science.)

development of second-site primary tumors, particularly osteogenic sarcoma.[164] A testable corollary of the model outlined above is that this high propensity is not merely fortuitous but is genetically determined by the predisposing RB1 mutation. This notion of pathogenetic causality in the clinical association between these two rare tumor types was tested by determining the constitutional and osteosarcoma genotypes at RFLP loci on chromosome 13. The data indicated that osteosarcomas arising in retinoblastoma patients had become homozygous specifically around the chromosomal region carrying the RB1 locus.[165] Furthermore, the same chromosomal mechanisms eliciting losses of constitutional heterozygosity were observed in sporadic osteosarcomas, suggesting a genetic similarity in pathogenetic causality. These findings are of obvious relevance to the interpretation of human mixed-cancer families, as they suggest differential expression of a single pleiotropic mutation in the etiology of clinically associated cancer of different histologic types.

A likely explanation for the association between retinoblastoma and osteosarcoma is that both tumors arise subsequent to chromosomal mechanisms, which unmask recessive mutations. This may involve either one common locus that is involved in normal regulation of differentiation of both tissues or separate loci that are located closely within chromosome region 13q14. In either

case, germ-line deletions of the retinoblastoma locus may also affect the osteosarcoma locus. Deletions are likely to be an important form of predisposing mutations at the RB1 locus, because a considerable fraction of bilateral retinoblastoma patients carry visible constitutional chromosome deletions[141–143] and submicroscopic deletions have been detected by reduction of esterase D activity.[147]

These epidemiologic, genetic, cytogenetic, and molecular genetic studies provided data with which to make specific predictions about the nature of the RB1 locus that have been useful in its molecular isolation. First, any candidate gene should map to the 13q14.1 region of the genome. Second, by analogy with other human diseases, such as Duchenne muscular dystrophy,[166] chronic granulomatous disease,[167] and several of the hemoglobinopathies, at least a proportion of mutations at the RB1 locus should be submicroscopic deletions. Third, a comparison of normal and tumor tissues from heritable cases should show hemizygous aberrancy in the former and homozygous defects in the latter. Fourth, even in the absence of detectable genomic alterations, defects in the mRNA transcribed from the locus or the protein products translated from the mRNA should be detected in tumors.

To provide DNA probes for landmark locations within 13q14, metaphase chromosomes 13 were sorted using a fluorescence-activated cell sorter, and portions of this were used in the derivation of a chromosome-enriched recombinant DNA library.[168] Several unique sequence probes were isolated from this library, and their physical location were determined by *in situ* hybridization to metaphase chromosomes and by determining hybridization dosage in normal cells from retinoblastoma patients with cytogenetically visible deletions of chromosome 13. One such probe, termed H3-8, was localized to the region 13q14.1, thus fulfilling the first criterion listed above.[169] When this probe was used to determine the genomic organization of its cognate locus in retinoblastoma tumors, 2 of 37 showed hybridization patterns consistent with homozygous deletion,[170] thus fulfilling the second criterion. In addition, these deletions were shown to arise either germinally or somatically in bilateral or unilateral disease, respectively,[170] thereby fulfilling the third criterion. The H3-8 probe was used to isolate larger, overlapping segments of DNA, and a unique sequence subfragment of one of these segments was used as a hybridization probe to determine the genomic organization of the approximately 200-kb locus and the transcription pattern of its 4.7-kb mRNA in tumor and normal tissues. Several provocative findings arose. First, deletions that were entirely contained within the locus were observed in some cases. Further characterization of the complete RB1 genomic sequence[171] allowed a rigorous and complete cataloging of the different mutations that affect the gene in retinoblastoma tumors. Simple Southern blot hybridizations have identified submicroscopic deletions involving various regions of the gene in up to 40 percent of tumor tissues or constitutional cells from individuals

affected by retinoblastoma.[169,170,172–174] Application of the polymerase chain reaction amplification technique coupled with DNA sequencing and RNase protection assays has increased the proportion of retinoblastomas with measurable RB1 locus alterations by detecting subtle exonic and intronic base changes.[175,176] Figure 36-12 schematically represents some of the characterized retinoblastoma mutations.

Recently, epigenetic mechanisms of mutagenesis involving methylation have also been discovered for RB1. Typical of "housekeeping genes," Rb has a small CpG island that encompasses the promoter region. Fujita and colleagues[177] studied the methylation status of CpGs in the 5′ promoter region of RB1 using methylation-sensitive restriction enzymes. They discovered altered methylation in 9.3 percent (13 of 140) of unilateral sporadic cases, but only 1 percent (1 of 101) of bilateral hereditary tumors. These tumor-associated alterations affected regions as small as the RB1 promoter itself to as large as 5.5 kb extending into the first intron, inhibiting binding of transcription factors and resulting in reduction of Rb expression.[178] Thus, aberrant methylation can act as the functional equivalent of a genetic loss-of-function mutation for Rb. Hypermethylation of promoter regions in other tumor suppressor genes has also been reported, the most notable being p16 on chromosome 9p. p16 is frequently hypermethylated in several cancer lines and also in 20 to 40 percent of primary tumors.[179,180] CpG dinucleotides also occur throughout the coding region of the Rb gene, suggesting that they, too, may be susceptible targets for alteration. In Rb tumors, most

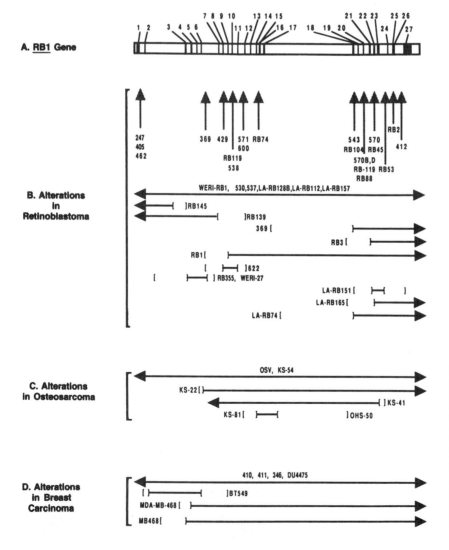

Fig. 22-12 Genomic alteration in the RB1 gene for retinoblastoma and associated tumors. RB1 gene alterations are designated as they appeared in their respective primary references. ↔ = complete deletion of the RB1 locus; [ ]→, ←[ ], and [ ]-[ ] = partial deletion of the RB1 locus, where one or both deletion endpoints occur within the bracketed area in the genomic sequence. Vertical hatched arrows indicate the position of small deletions/point mutations characterized by PCR/DNA sequencing or RNase protection assays. (Reprinted by permission from Gennett and Cavenee, *Brain Pathology* 1:25–32, copyright 1990, ISN Journals.)

common point mutations have been found to be C-to-T transitions, occurring at CGA (arginine) codons. One study determined that as many as 69 percent of the single-base substitutions found in 119 patients occurred at CGA codons and led to premature terminations. Thus, the mutational spectra for Rb suggests methylated CpGs are common and important targets of mutation.[181]

The extensive size of the genomic locus has made complete sequence analysis of RB1 alleles a labor-intensive approach, and so alterations at the transcription level have been pursued to increase the sensitivity of detection of mutations in the locus. When transcription patterns were first analyzed in tumor tissue, no apparent RNA transcript was detected in retinoblastomas or osteosarcomas, although normal-size mRNA was present in retinal cells and several other tissue types (see "Biochemical Characterization of the Retinoblastoma Gene Product" below). These results have been extended by several other groups,[177,178] and transcripts of aberrant size have been identified in tumors previously shown to contain normal genomic structure, thus fulfilling the last criterion listed above. Investigations of RB1 gene alterations at both the DNA and RNA levels cumulatively reveal a strong correlative relationship between lack of the RB1 gene product and the appearance of retinoblastoma tumors. In addition, both DNA and RNA alterations appear to be common in both sporadic and heritable disease, as would be expected from the genetic model discussed earlier.

In addition to cancers such as osteosarcoma, which are clinically related to retinoblastoma, other tumors have been found to have aberrancies of the retinoblastoma gene. The involvement of RB1 in these tumors is inferred from alterations in the gene structure itself or as loss of heterozygosity for DNA markers in the 13q14 region surrounding the RB1 gene. Some examples of such alterations found in osteosarcomas and breast carcinomas are shown in Fig. 22-12. Molecular analysis of small cell lung carcinomas has revealed RB1 structural abnormalities in approximately 15 percent of cases,[179] and loss of heterozygosity for chromosome 13 has been detected in about 25 percent of breast cancers and their derived cell lines analyzed to date.[180,181] A more detailed analysis of the involvement of loss of heterozygosity for chromosome 13 in tumors has been compiled[182] and clearly shows that not all tumors result from direct or indirect alteration of the RB1 locus. However, the cumulative data suggest that RB1 is pleiotropically active, and subsets of tumors may share a common pathogenetic mechanism, which results from unmasking mutations that affect the tumor-suppressing function of RB1.

The observations described above satisfy all the physical criteria for the identity of the RB1 locus as a tumor-suppressor gene. As in all cases of "reverse genetics," however, proof of this requires biochemical and functional analysis. The nature of this gene and the effect its elimination has on oncogenesis rely on the cell biologic and biochemical approaches described below. Its isolation alone, however, constitutes a powerful example of the reverse genetics approach to gene identification through physical and genetic mapping.

Genetic Complementation. The genetic model requiring sequential inactivating mutations and structural evidence in its support suggests that retinoblastoma and its genetically associated tumors arise through loss of function of the RB1 locus. One prediction of this line of reasoning is that the replacement of wild-type RB1 function into cells which lack that function should have normalizing effects on at least parts of the tumorigenic phenotype. This has been directly addressed through the introduction of the wild-type gene into retinoblastoma (the WERI-Rb27 line) and osteosarcoma (the SaOS-2 line) cells through recombinant retroviral vector transfer and assessment of morphology, growth rate, or tumorigenic capability.[183]

Neither type of cell was affected in any capacity after infection by the vector carrying an irrelevant luciferase (Lux) gene. However, after the introduction of the vector carrying the Rb cDNA, two separate morphologies were apparent in the affected

populations: One was flattened and greatly enlarged and represented 90 to 95 percent of the population, while the remainder was composed of small cells and mimicked uninfected cells. This suggested that these two RB$^+$-reconstituted cell lines differed from the RB$^-$ parental lines in their morphology and cell division rates, which correlated with the presence of the expression of wild-type RB. Subcutaneous injection of Lux- and RB$^+$-reconstituted cells into nude mice resulted in palpable tumors only in those injected with Lux-infected cells, indicating that induction of wild-type p110^{RB} protein expression was capable of suppressing tumorigenicity in both retinoblastomas and osteosarcomas. Similar suppression of tumorigenicity has been demonstrated after the introduction of these retroviral RB$^+$ vectors into bladder[184] and prostate[185] carcinoma cells, although the effect of reconstituted RB expression on their morphology and growth rate was less dramatic.

There is also evidence that the location of injection may create environments that are more or less suited for tumor growth. In fact, some cancer cells incapable of forming tumors when injected subcutaneously are able to do so when grafted into the anterior chamber of the rodent eye.[186] When retinoblastoma cells used in the retroviral reconstitution experiments were assayed in this site,[187] the malignant WERI-Rb27 parental line formed tumors 40 days after inoculations of 10^3 to 10^4 cells (compared to the 10^7 cells required in subcutaneous injections). Also, 11 of 14 RB^1-reconstituted clones were unable to form tumors. Evaluation of the levels of pp110^{RB} showed that they resulted from the growth of a small fraction of uninfected parental cells such that the tumor cells were unable to express the RB1 protein. All this suggests that pp110^{RB} can function to suppress the tumorigenic phenotype in retinoblastoma cell lines, as predicted by the model.

Other experiments with the breast cancer cell line MDA-468-S4 and retinoblastoma cell lines WERI-RB1 and Y79 have provided less support for the tumor-suppressing ability of p110^{RB}.[188] In these studies, expression of exogenous p110^{RB} did not alter growth rate or cloning efficiency in the breast cancer cell line, whereas reintroduction of Rb into both RB cell lines reduced colony formation but had no effect on morphology, growth rate, or tumorigenicity. In clear contrast to the studies described above, the reconstituted retinoblastoma cell line formed intraocular tumors with the same efficiency as did the RB^2 parental cell lines. These tumors, formed in the anterior chamber of the eye, were excised from the mice and expanded in culture. All the tumor cells recovered showed expression of p110^{RB} at levels similar to those of the original parental clones, indicating that tumor formation was not due to loss of function of the transferred RB1 gene. These experiments suggest that tumorigenesis is not deterred by replacement of a normal RB1 allele or expression of RB in homozygously RB-defective cells. Certainly, this confusing situation and the role of p110^{RB} in the tumorigenic process require further exploration.

Prenatal Diagnosis

Advantage has been taken of the increasingly precise molecular elucidation of genomic alterations in retinoblastoma tumors to provide conceptual and methodologic approaches to the assignment of disease risk.[189,190] These methods are either indirect and linkage-based[189] or direct[190] in their detection of genetic defects.

The first approach used polymorphic restriction-fragment-length alleles as linkage markers to deduce genotypes at the RB1 locus in the children of retinoblastoma gene carriers. This method takes advantage of neutral DNA sequence variation in the population, which results in the variable presence of bacterial restriction-endonuclease recognition sites at loci on chromosome 13. This approach had three major limitations. First, most of the loci identified by RFLP[159,160] were genetically distant from the RB1 locus,[191] and, consequently, the reliability of the method was reduced by the occurrence of meiotic recombination. Second, the population frequencies of alleles of these loci were such that only a fraction of families were informative. Third, the method required

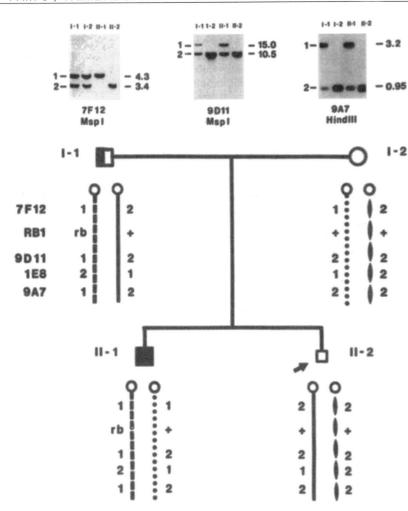

Fig. 22-13 Pedigree of a familial retinoblastoma case that shows no evidence of meiotic recombination. Closed symbols = bilaterally affected family members; half-closed symbols = unilaterally affected members; open symbols = unaffected members. Arrows indicate the family member for whom diagnosis before illness was performed; the indications of the presence or absence of disease are based on subjects' status at their most recent ophthalmic examination. Inferred alleles at the retinoblastoma (RB1) locus are designated rb for a mutant allele and + for a wild-type allele. The circles with vertical lines below them that are shown under each family member symbol represent the member's two constitutional chromosome 13 homologues. The numbers beside each chromosome symbol represent the allelic form of each locus. The vertical order of loci within each family is the same as that shown under the symbol for its I-1 member. The data illustrate the power of information about a first child in discriminating which chromosome a second child has inherited from the affected parent. (Reprinted from Cavenee et al., *New England Journal of Medicine*, vol. 314, pp. 1201–1207, 1986, by permission.)

an affected parent and a first child to define the haplotypic phase. Therefore, analysis was restricted to nuclear families in which informative allelic combinations could be discerned at loci flanking the RB1 locus.

The family described in Fig. 22-13 illustrates how parental haplotypes of chromosome 13 can be deduced through the analysis of the parents and an affected first child. In this example, the first child (II-I) inherited the predisposition for retinoblastoma (Fig. 22-13*B*) and the longer alleles at the 7F12 and 9D11 loci (Fig. 22-13*A*) from his affected father. The fetus (II-2), however, inherited the alternative chromosome 13, which carried the shorter alleles at the 7F12 and 9D11 loci. Because the 7F12 and 9D11 loci flank the RB1 locus at recombination distances of approximately 12 and 30 percent, respectively, the fetus will have inherited the predisposition for retinoblastoma only if two meiotic crossovers occurred between these two loci. The risk estimate for the development of retinoblastoma by this child arises from the conjoint probability of two such crossing-over events. Because the parental haplotype was inferred from the first child, these risk estimates must also consider crossovers in both children, giving a joint probability of 84 percent that retinoblastoma will not develop in the second child. At age 8 years, this child showed no signs of the disease, in accordance with this prediction.

There were several major limitations to this initial approach. First, chromosome 13 haplotypes could not be determined in the carrier parent unless there was either one affected grandparent or one previously affected child, or unless the first unaffected child had passed the age for development of retinoblastoma (which is 7 years or more). Second, there was a chance that gene carriers

would remain unaffected because of the somewhat less than absolute penetrance of these predisposing mutations. Third, relatively few and incompletely informative markers for chromosome 13 had been isolated, and these markers were not, for the most part, tightly linked to the RB1 locus. This resulted in risk estimates that were much less precise than desired and allowed only a very few clinical decisions to be based solely on these analyses. Most of these limitations could be minimized if several highly informative and closely linked markers were isolated. The isolation of a cDNA for the closely linked gene esterase D[192,193] allowed an RFLP with better allele frequencies than the protein polymorphism at the same locus. Clearly, the most desirable situation in this regard is the ability to determine the gene defect directly in individual retinoblastoma cases. This is particularly important in counseling families with a single case of bilateral retinoblastoma, because in most instances linkage-based analysis can be used only if there is more than one affected family member. There was a similar need for direct determination of mutations of the RB1 locus in cases of sporadic unilateral retinoblastoma; such patients constitute more than 50 percent of all retinoblastoma cases, and about 10 percent of them carry germ-line mutations.

The isolation of the retinoblastoma susceptibility gene has allowed these goals to be reached, because, as was previously mentioned, the predictive value of RFLP analysis increases in direct proportion to the proximity of informative marker loci to the disease locus. Intragenic polymorphisms are, of course, the best of this class, and so far five independent intragenic RFLPs have been described.[194] Four of these polymorphisms were due to restriction-site alterations for KpnI, XbaI, MboII, and TthIII, and a fifth was due to length variability in the number of tandem repeats of a 50-bp sequence that resulted in eight distinct alleles. The inheritance pattern of these polymorphisms in 13 families with heritable retinoblastoma showed cosegregation of alleles with the disease locus. Furthermore, because of their location within the gene itself, inference errors arising from undetected meiotic recombination within the gene are much reduced in comparison with even the nearest flanking polymorphic probe. As more sequence data have become available, these intragenic polymorphisms have been adapted from standard Southern protocols to PCR amplification methods.[195–197]

These modern approaches to risk assessment may still be complicated somewhat by parental bias in the origin of RB1 mutations. Evidence has been provided that paternal gametogenesis confers a higher mutation rate on the RB1 locus.[198,199] The examination of sporadic bilateral retinoblastoma cases showed that disease arises subsequent to a new germ-line mutation in the paternal allele, followed by somatic alteration or loss of the maternally derived wild-type allele in 13 of 14 cases. In contrast, the examination of sporadic unilateral retinoblastoma tumors showed that only 4 of 10 unilateral tumors retained the allele derived from the father. This suggests that mutations in the RB1 locus occur more commonly during spermatogenesis, or that the paternal chromosome in the early embryo is at a higher risk for mutation. Similar analysis of 13 sporadic osteosarcomas showed that 12 were preferentially mutated in the paternal allele.[200] Considering the clinical association between heritable retinoblastoma and second-site primary tumors such as osteosarcoma, the mechanisms which result in germ-line mutations in retinoblastoma probably are also responsible for producing sporadic related diseases.

Genomic imprinting is one mechanism that might explain the unusual imbalance in mutation and retention of the paternal allele of specific retinoblastomas and related tumors. This is a process, described as epigenetic allele inactivation, that is dependent on the gamete of origin.[201] Imprinted alleles may act as mutated alleles but differ from mutations in the classical sense in that they show a preference for inheritance from only one sex. Consistent with this is the analysis of polymorphic markers on chromosome 13q in parents of patients with sporadic retinoblastoma, which showed that three of three bilateral tumors retained the paternal chromosome (in accordance with previous studies) and that seven of eight unilateral tumors also did so.[202] The discrepancy between the parental biases shown in this report and those discussed above may be explained by the imprinting process being superimposed on the genetic background of the patient.

Although the pattern of inheritance for retinoblastoma suggests 90 percent penetrance,[203] cases of transmitted, nonpenetrant mutations of the RB1 locus have been described (see "Molecular Genetics," above), and these asymptomatic mutations may have an impact on the accuracy of DNA diagnostics. DNA analysis at the level afforded by current technologies offers the possibility of discriminating in unaffected offspring noncarriers from asymptomatic carriers of a nonpenetrant mutation. For example, screening of the RB1 coding structure using exon-by-exon single-stranded conformation polymorphism (SSCP) analysis utilizes the sequence-dependent migration of single-stranded DNA through gel matrices. Such experiments have revealed abnormalities in exon 20, as well as in the promoter region of RB1.[204,205] The former were determined to be single-base changes resulting in amino acid substitutions. The discovery of these alterations suggests that they might serve to reduce the functional efficiency of the retinoblastoma gene product rather than ablate its suppressing ability altogether. It is interesting to note that these studies may suggest the potential existence of different sets of functional mutations in retinoblastoma—and that these groups may, in turn, define differentially functioning regions of the gene product itself. Such predictions require a full characterization of the biochemical role of the retinoblastoma gene product in both normal and tumorigenic cells.

BIOCHEMICAL CHARACTERIZATION OF THE RETINOBLASTOMA GENE PRODUCT

After the documentation of the types of mutations and rearrangements of the RB1 locus in retinoblastomas and other tumors, an understanding of their significance required an understanding of the normal biologic and biochemical function of the protein that locus encoded. The impetus and basis for this was the prior determination of the genomic structure for RB1 and the isolation and sequencing of its 4.7-kb mRNA described above. Analysis of the tissue specificity of RB1 mRNA expression showed ubiquitous presence in normal human and rat tissues, including brain, kidney, ovary, spleen, liver, placenta, and retina. This surprising result was augmented by the demonstration that genomic DNA sequences homologous to human RB1 cDNA were present in a variety of organisms. The sequences were measurably divergent among vertebrates, with homology decreasing as a function of the distance from humans along the evolutionary tree.[177] Thus, although the tumors elicited by inherited mutations of the RB1 locus are relatively narrow in type, its broad tissue expression and species conservation suggested a common and potentially pivotal role in the growth or differentiation of cell types of a variety of ontogenies. Moreover, these observations raise the possibility of interaction of the RB1 gene or its product with others to provide tissue specificity.

The Retinoblastoma Protein

Sequence analysis of an initial cDNA clone provided a great deal of predictive information about the nature and features of the RB1 protein product:[177] it was 816 amino acids in length, had an estimated molecular mass of 94 kDa, and contained 10 dispersed potential glycosylation sites and a leucine zipper (indicated by the presence of periodic leucine residues every seventh position in an alpha helix,[206] which is thought to be important for dimerization of proteins) within exon 20. Furthermore, the region containing amino acids 663 to 716 contains 14 prolines among its 54 residues. Such proline-rich regions have been observed in the nuclear oncogenes, *c-myc* and *c-myb*.[207] The subsequent isolation of several full-length 4.7-kb cDNA clones[172] showed that the initial size estimate of 94 kDa was based on a sequence missing 236 of the 5′-most amino acids, whereas the full-length sequence resulted in a predicted protein of about 110 kDa with the same structural motifs inferred from the first analysis.

Transcriptional analysis of the gene identified three potential sites of initiation at nucleotide positions 11, 144, and 151.[208] Deletion analysis of the 59 RB gene sequences indicated that the region between nucleotides 2154 and 1186 possessed promoter function, with a critical initiating subregion of nucleotides 113 to 1183. Identified enhancer-like sequences included interferon-responsive elements, heat-shock elements, and three Sp1 transcription-factor-binding regions at nucleotides 2291, 176, and 1123.[209]

These transcriptional and translational features led to the suggestion that the RB1 gene product might be a nucleic acid-binding protein that exerts its tumor-suppressor activity through the regulation of transcription of a variety of cellular proteins. In 1987, Lee and coworkers[210] prepared rabbit antiserums against a trpE-RB fusion protein and purified an anti-RB antibody that precipitated a protein of 110,000 to 114,000 daltons. These reagents led to the uncovering of several other interesting features. First, there was no evidence of glycosylation despite such potential sites in the sequence. Second, subcellular fractionation of ^{35}S-methionine-labeled cells into nuclear, cytoplasmic, and membrane fractions, showed that 85 percent of the RB1 protein resided in the nucleus, a location that was further substantiated by immunohistochemical staining with the anti-RB antibody. In fact, the RB protein was shown to be retained on and eluted from single-stranded DNA cellulose columns. Third, when cells were metabolically labeled with ^{32}P-phosphoric acid, the anti-RB antibody immunoprecipitated ^{32}P-labeled protein which was shown to be identical to the RB protein (pp110RB). Finally, analyses of pp110RB expression and its phosphorylation have led to insights into the mechanisms by which it exerts its effects in normal cells and more general ideas about how tumor cells can bypass controls on their proliferation.

Involvement of pp110RB in the Cell Cycle

Phosphorylation of pp110RB. The process of cell proliferation can be subdivided into discrete stages of quiescence (G0), preparation for DNA replication (G1), DNA duplication (S), preparation for mitosis (G2), and actual cell division (M). The traverse of a cell from the G0/G1 through mitosis (M) stages is designated as one cell cycle. Much of what is known about the events that positively and negatively regulate the intricate pathways of this cycle have been deciphered using cell-division cycle (cdc) mutants in yeast.[211] The genetics and biochemistry of these mutants have led to a reasonably detailed view of the complex steps, which, in combination, control the nuclear and cytoplasmic events involved in normal cell proliferation. A great deal of evidence has been accumulated showing that cells of a variety of types require a substantial lag time to progress through a number of substages within G1, regardless of whether the cycling arises from stimulation out of the quiescent G0 stage or from the completion of a previous cell cycle. It is during these substages of G1 that proliferation and cellular differentiation are initiated and controlled, and it appears that the switches for entry into or exit from G1 are the main determinants of postembryonic cell proliferation.[212] Thus, it seems quite reasonable to propose that genes with tumor-suppressor function, such as RB1, may function as negative control elements in the process. Further, it may be that the inactivation of such a gene allows defective cells to traverse the stages of the cell cycle under conditions of growth that would be insufficient for the proliferation of normal cells.[211,213]

One way to achieve functional inactivation of the RB1 gene is to mutate it in such a way that the synthesis of p110RB is reduced, or its degradation is increased. This was tested by determining the steady-state amount of p110RB protein in the different phases of the cell cycle[214] through fluorescent staining of cellular p110RB and DNA in conjunction with flow cytometry. The results showed that the amount of p110RB per cell increased as cells progressed through the cell cycle, such that cells in later G2/M stages immediately before cell division contained approximately twice as much p110RB as cells entering G1. Further, p110RB had an invariant half-life of about 10 h, and pulse labeling of synchronized cells showed that p110RB was synthesized in both quiescent and proliferative phases. These data suggested that the antiproliferative activity of the protein is not regulated in normal cells at the transcriptional level or the translational level.

The first indication that posttranslational modification of the RB protein is involved in cell-cycle control was provided by the uncovering of a correlation in several cell types between cell-cycle stage and the phosphorylation state of the protein.[214,215] Cell lysates prepared from quiescent or cycling cells (human umbilical vein endothelial cells, primary T lymphocytes, cells of a human breast cancer, and HeLa cells) showed an apparent size shift from p110RB in the quiescent cells to pp112–114RB in proliferating cells (Fig. 22-14). Treatment of the latter lysates with potato acid phosphatase reduced the more slowly migrating protein species (p112–p114RB) to the same mobility as the p110RB species, suggesting that the former were actually multiply phosphorylated forms of the latter protein species.

The timing of the p110RB to pp112–114RB transition was concurrent with the initiation of incorporation of radioactive thymidine into cellular DNA. Quantitation of the relative abundance of the higher-molecular-weight phosphorylated proteins to their nascent protein products showed that G1 (resting) cells had a 10:1 p110RB:pp112–114RB ratio while G2/M (cycling) cells had a 1:1 ratio. After mitosis and cell division, the ratio returned to 10:1.[216] Regardless of the enzymatic mechanism involved, it is clear that phase-specific phosphorylation and dephosphorylation

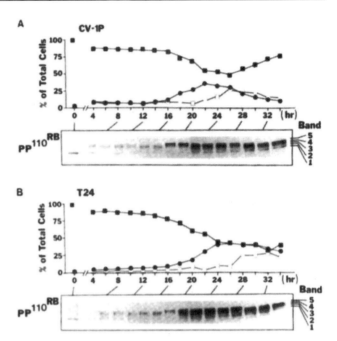

Fig. 22-14 Oscillation of phosphorylation of the p110RB protein during the different stages of the cell cycle. CV-1P cells (*A*) and T24 cells (*B*) were synchronized in G0/G1 by density arrest and then allowed to enter the cell cycle by sparsely replating cells in fresh medium. Equal numbers of cells were seeded into about 50 culture dishes (3×10^6 cells per dish) and were allowed to grow to time points of 18 to 34 h. One entire plate was harvested for each lane on the Western blot. A second batch of dishes (1.5×10^6 cells per dish) was plated 16 h later than the first and was harvested for hours 2 to 16. Again, each lane contained cells from one plate. At 2-h intervals after replating, cells were collected for cell cycle distribution analysis and RB protein determination. The percentage of cells in G1 (filled squares), S (filled circles), and G2/M (open squares) at each indicated time was determined by flow cytometry. RB protein was analyzed by immunoprecipitation followed by immunoblotting; five RB bands could be distinguished. The sudden change in signal intensity in CV-1P and T24 cells is due both to a decrease in the number of cells seeded for hours 2 to 16 and to random variability in the counting of different batches. (Reprinted by permission from Chen et al., *Cell*, vol. 58, pp. 1193–1198, copyright 1989, Cell Press.)

of the RB protein occurs during the cell cycle and proliferation. Mapping tryptic phosphopeptides of the human protein showed that the phosphorylation was on serine and threonine, but not tyrosine residues, which suggests the possibility of cell-cycle regulation by serine/threonine protein kinases.[217] One candidate is cdc2, a protein kinase that is known to be important in yeast at the G1/S and G2/M phases,[218] and which has been isolated in a protein complex that is capable of activating DNA synthesis in G1 cell extracts.[219] Lin *et al.*[217] found that human cdc2 phosphorylates each of the tryptic p110RB phosphopeptides *in vitro* and *in vivo,* and the consensus target sequence for cdc2 phosphorylation[220] (Basic/Polar-Ser/Thr-Pro-X-Basic) occurs eight times within the p110RB protein. Together these studies strongly suggest that human cdc2 is involved in regulating the cell-cycle phosphorylation of p110RB protein. It is also possible that other cdc2-like kinases exist in the cell and play a role in the process as well.

Changes in the phosphorylation state of the RB protein also have been linked to cellular differentiation. Unlike proliferating cells, which actively cycle and divide, terminally differentiated cells cease normal cellular division and are shunted into a G0/G1 quiescent-like state. The effects of the induction of cellular differentiation on the phosphorylation status of p110RB have been analyzed in several leukemic cell lines, which could be induced to differentiate after treatment with phorbol esters or retinoic acid. Monoblastic U937 and HL-60 showed a marked dephosphorylation of p110[RB] after differentiation,[221,222] and similar treatment of other partially responsive cells led to a coordinate level of p110[RB] phosphorylation. These experiments have led to several models for the function played by phosphorylation of p110[RB] in G0/G1.[223] The first is that p110[RB] regulates a cellular block which prevents exit from G1 by blocking the initiation of DNA synthesis. Phosphorylation of p110[RB] would render it inactive, thereby releasing the cell from its negative regulation and allowing the cell to progress through a full cell cycle. An alternative model depicts the dephosphorylation of RB as a subcellular event that communicates the precise time for cell cycle exit (i.e., from M to G1/G0). As such, dephosphorylation may be part of a signaling pathway in which intracellular or extracellular factors switch G1 cells into the quiescent stage (G0). One relevant addition to the cell-cycle stage effect of p110[RB] is the recent demonstration that it undergoes three separate rounds of phosphorylation in T lymphocytes stimulated to proliferate with the mitogen phytohemagglutinin A.[224] The first occurs in middle to late G1, as was described earlier, the second during S phase, and the third in G2/M. Because these modifications occur at different locations on the protein, it is possible that p110[RB] actually has several different

proliferation-controlling functions. The complexity of function that phosphorylation of p110[RB] produces at the cellular level is further enhanced by more recent demonstrations that this protein can be physically complexed with a number of viral and cellular proteins.

Cyclin D1, p16, and pp110. Recent developments in our understanding of the components of the cell cycle have strengthened the central role the Rb protein plays in growth regulation. One of the most important checkpoints in mammalian cells in late G1, deemed the restriction point, has many positive and negative controllers, including pp110. These key controllers include cyclins (A, D1-3, E, etc.) cyclin-dependent kinases (cdk2, 4, 6, etc.), and cyclin-dependent kinase inhibitors (p16, p15, etc.).[225] At the biochemical level, the kinase complexes of cyclin D1-cdk4 or cdk6 promote progression through late G1 by phosphorylating the retinoblastoma protein product. The Rb phosphorylation described above can be negatively regulated by cdk4/6I or p16INK/CDKN2 (henceforth referred to as p16) (Fig. 22-15). Thus, it appears that the normal biochemical pathway that regulates progression through G1 can be disrupted by

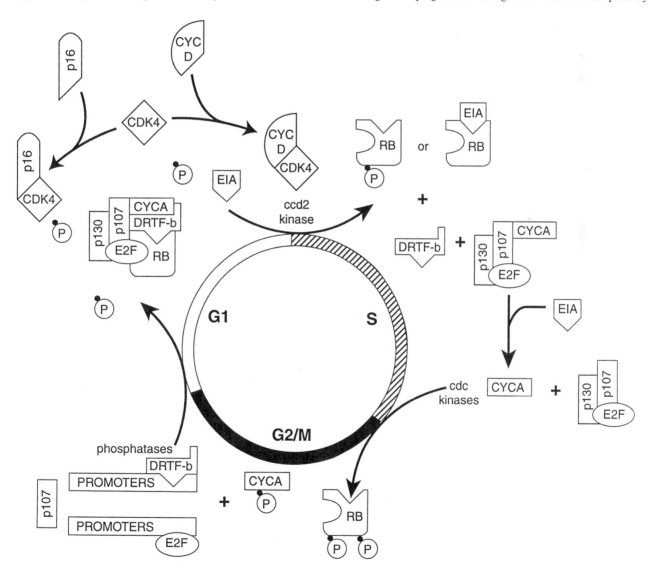

Fig. 22-15 Cell-cycle-dependent binding of cellular proteins to p110[RB]. The cell-cycle stage-dependent complexing and dissociation of cellular proteins are schematically represented. DRTF and E2F are transcription factors that have been shown to bind to p110[RB] at the G1 stage of the cell cycle. On phosphorylation of the protein at the G1/S boundary, these transcriptional factors are released from the complex. Phosphorylation of p110[RB] appears to be controlled by a family of cdc kinases that are active at both the G1/S and G2/M boundaries. E1A has also been shown to bind p110[RB], thereby dissociating DRTF and E2F from the G1 complex in much the same manner as occurs when p110[RB] is phosphorylated. At the completion of the cell cycle, phosphatases dephosphorylate p110[RB], thus allowing the protein to sequester E2F and DRTF back into their inactive complexed forms. Cyc A = cyclin A.

abnormalities targeted at any one of these specific components. As discussed at length throughout this chapter, pRb itself can be inactivated by mutation, deletion, methylation, and viral sequestration (see "Viral Oncoproteins," below).

In addition, cell-cycle components such as cyclin D1, whose encoding locus resides at 11q13, can be amplified or rearranged and overexpressed in tumor cells.[225–227] D-type cyclins and their associated cdks (4 and 6) are able to bind to pp110 through an N-terminal LXCXE motif.[228–230] In fact, Rb[230] and E2F[231] are the only known substrates for cycD/cdk4 complexes *in vitro,* and this complex phosphorylates most of the sites *in vivo* on the retinoblastoma protein. Their interaction is strengthened by their apparent involvement in a negative feedback loop where hypo-phosphorylated Rb seems to stimulate cyclin D1 transcription, and D1 and D1/cdk4 complexes are down-regulated in Rb-deficient cells[231–234] (Fig. 22-15).

Negative regulators active at the G1/S boundary, such as the cdk inhibitors, can also be altered in tumors. One such inhibitor, p16, appears to function normally by down-modulating the phosphorylating activity of its target kinases cdk4[235] and cdk6[236] by binding in competition with cyclin D1. p16 has been found deleted, mutated, or silenced by promoter methylation in a majority of tumor cell lines[237–241] and in a variety of tumors,[242–248] albeit in a much smaller fraction. p16 is elevated in cells that lack functional Rb, suggesting that Rb may suppress p16 expression,[249,250] the reciprocal of what is found for Rb and cyclin D1. This speaks to the positive (cyclin D1) and negative (p16) regulatory roles displayed by each of these cell cycle components and suggests that the pleiotropic tissue specificity of the tumors in which RB1 inactivation occurs may be at the fundamental level of governing cell growth. It further suggests that the cyclin D1-cdk4-p16 pathway operates upstream of pRB, as both the G1-accelerating function of cyclin D1-ckd4 and growth suppression by p16 require functional pRB.

The inverse correlation and reciprocity of function between cell-cycle controllers and Rb are clearly demonstrated in adult small cell lung carcinomas (SCLCs) and non-small cell lung carcinomas (NSCLCs). The Rb gene has been shown to be a common target for somatic mutations.[179] The frequency of absent or aberrant Rb protein expression for SCLC tumors is 90 percent and 15 percent for NSCLC.[251] Several recent studies that have examined the loss of p16 gene expression in these tumor types found a striking inverse correlation. The absence of p16 was a rare event in SCLC,[252,253] with 80 to 100 percent of cell lines and primary tumors displaying a p16+/pRb − phenotype. In contrast, the majority of NSCLCs (67 to 100 percent) analyzed lacked detectable p16 protein, rendering them p16 −/Rb+.[252–254] In one study,[252] cyclin D1 was observed to be overexpressed in most cell lines, suggesting that this alteration may be a common early event in both lung-tumor subtypes. However, this controversial model of the role of cyclin D1 as the earliest mutational event has not been substantiated in other studies examining lung[255] or esophageal carcinomas.[226] Nonetheless, the data clearly demonstrate that the p16-Rb pathway is inactivated in both SCLC and NSCLC at a very high frequency, but that the targets of the inactivating mutational events are distinct, depending on the subtype of lung tumor analyzed.

pp110^RB Protein Complexes

Viral Oncoproteins. At about the same time the oscillation of pp110^RB phosphorylation within the cell cycle was being uncovered, an unexpected link between this negative growth regulator and the cellular transforming capacities of the viral oncoproteins of polyomaviruses (SV40), adenoviruses (Ad-2 and AD-5), and papillomaviruses (HPV-16) was reported. Each of these DNA tumor viruses encodes a set of proteins, some of which are capable of disrupting the normal regulation of cellular proliferation, leading to *in vitro* transformation of cells and establishment of the tumorigenic phenotype. For example, the E1A protein of oncogenic adenoviruses is capable of immortaliz-

ing primary cells and mediating transcription, negatively and positively, for both viral and cellular genes.[256] Furthermore, the E1A of infected cells can be coimmunoprecipitated with a set of host-cell proteins of various molecular weights. The large T oncoprotein of SV40 is a nuclear phosphoprotein of 708 amino acids, which is necessary for cellular transformation by the virus.[257] It typically functions in concert with the SV40 small t protein product, but when expressed at high levels, it can perform all the functions required for transformation. Finally, the protein product of the E7 open-reading frame of human papillomaviruses of types associated with progressive cervical neoplasia is also capable of immortalizing cells *in vitro.*[258] The functional similarities between these oncoproteins are also mirrored to some extent in their amino acid sequences and predicted higher-order structures. For example, deletion and mutation studies have shown that small segments of the SV40 T protein (between residues 105 and 114)[259,260] or the E1A protein (between residues 121 and 139)[261] are required for transforming capacity; these regions are structurally homologous. Comparisons of the amino acid sequences of E7 and E1A revealed a similar relationship between the NH2 terminus of E7 and the two conserved regions in E1A.[262] These similarities have led to the prediction that these regions may bind cellular proteins that actively participate in and/or cooperate with the transforming properties of large T, E1A, and E7.[206]

Several lines of evidence point to the retinoblastoma gene product as one such cellular protein. As was mentioned above, earlier studies had shown the E1A protein to be complexed with a variety of cellular proteins, and one of these proteins had a molecular mass of about 110 kDa.[263] Using various monoclonal antibodies raised against large T, E1A, and p110^RB, as well as polyclonal antibodies raised against E7, *in vitro* immunoprecipitation from cell lysates showed coprecipitation of the p110^RB with each of the oncoproteins from a variety of cell lines transformed by viral infection or their normal counterparts.[264–266] The presence of p110^RB in these complexes was further confirmed by the demonstration of the expected protein fragments generated by partial proteolysis using staphylococcus V8 protease.

The extent to which these associations represented functional relationships in which both partners are active participants in a common regulatory pathway has also been documented. The analysis of a series of mutant species of large T and E1A proteins revealed that mutations affecting the sequences necessary for transformation also affected the ability of the oncoprotein to form complexes with p110^RB.[259,260,265,267] Examples of the effect mutations of large T have on p110^RB binding are shown in Fig. 22-16. Because one function of these viral oncoproteins appears to be the creation of a cellular environment that is permissive for DNA synthesis, it may be that one of their modes of action involves sequestration of the antiproliferative p110^RB, such that viral infection releases the cell from its negative regulation by RB, allowing it to inappropriately or more frequently enter S phase. An examination of the data derived from immunoprecipitations with large T showed that lysates from ^32P-labeled cells contained phosphorylated T but not phosphorylated pp110^RB.[268] An RB species did, however, coprecipitate with the anti-T antibody and was shown by densitometric analysis of gel electrophoresis patterns to be p110^RB, the unphosphorylated form. This protein species was the only form of p110^RB consistently bound to T, even though immunoprecipitation of the same lysates with an anti-RB antibody demonstrated the simultaneous existence of the other phosphorylated forms, that is, p112–114RB. Binding of large T to the unphosphorylated form held true for a stably SV40-transformed derivative of the cells used in the previous experiments, indicating that viral transformation does not alter the overall state of RB protein phosphorylation. These studies also showed that newly synthesized T did not immediately bind to p110^RB, and this led to the hypothesis that the structure of T must change in some way to facilitate its successful heterologous binding. In fact, when large T from synchronized ^35S-labeled cell

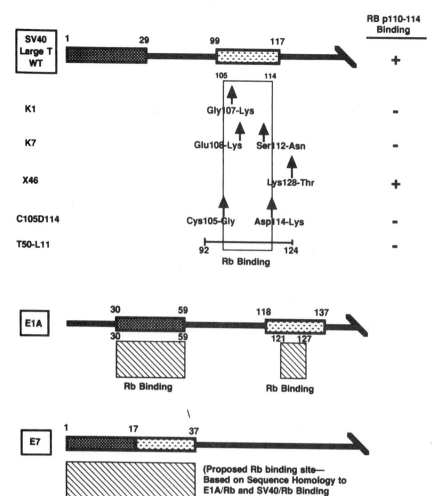

Fig. 22-16 Binding sites for the retinoblastoma protein in SV40 large T antigen, adenovirus E1A, and papillomavirus E7 proteins. The sequences of several SV40 large T mutants are shown with their corresponding p110^{RB}-binding properties; + = T antigen was capable of complexing with the retinoblastoma protein; − = complex formation was abolished by the mutation. Regions in E1A and E7 necessary for binding p110^{RB} assessed by similar mutational analyses are also depicted.

lysates was examined by sucrose gradients, it was determined that newly synthesized large T proteins existed as monomers and over the course of the cell cycle gradually oligomerized;[268] only after oligomerization was the oncoprotein capable of binding to p110^{RB}. This is supported by the SV40 mutant 5080 (Fig. 22-16) that carries a Pro$_{584}$-Leu substitution, which renders it transformation-deficient[270] and inefficient for oligomerization;[271] it also fails to coprecipitate with the RB protein.[269] It is possible that such oligomer-forming behavior is a process by which large T can bind to more than one protein involved in cellular growth regulation. It is tantalizing to note that regions of E1A and T involved in binding p110^{RB} also interact with at least one cellular protein, p107.[272,273] Whatever the reason for the multiple oncoproteins binding to p110^{RB}, the data together support a model in which the unphosphorylated form of RB (p110^{RB}) is the species active in growth suppression. It follows that binding by E1A, E7, or large T would serve to inactivate the growth suppression normally exerted by pRB. Further, in the absence of viral infection, it is the phosphorylation of the RB protein that serves to override growth suppression and allows cell division to take place.

Retinoblastoma Protein-Binding Sites. Binding of viral oncoproteins to p110^{RB} and the subsequent release of these infected cells from negative growth control suggested that there may be cellular proteins with analogous properties. These proteins might be sequestered by p110^{RB} and be maintained in an inactivated form until phosphorylation of p110^{RB} makes them available for proliferation or transcriptional/translational uses. To determine the regions in the RB gene that are required for binding of the viral

oncoproteins and potentially other cellular regulatory proteins, a systematic series of deletion mutants were generated in the p110^{RB} coding regions.[274,275] Polypeptide products generated through *in vitro* protein synthesis systems were analyzed for their ability to bind and coimmunoprecipitate SV40 large T or E1A. The data showed two distinct noncontiguous regions in p110^{RB} necessary for complexing with these oncoproteins; these regions included amino acid residues 393 to 572 and residues 646 to 772. It was further determined that a spacer region of undefined length between these two blocks was required to maintain this binding integrity.

Comparison of these binding regions with many of the naturally occurring RB mutations revealed striking similarities. The mutations displayed in Fig. 22-17 are naturally occurring examples from retinoblastomas, as well as other tumors commonly found to be mutated for RB1 (see the discussion above). Each of these mutants was in some way affected in a region essential for the binding of E1A and large T. The absence of p110^{RB} binding, using mutant proteins of cells from bladder carcinoma,[276] small-cell-lung carcinoma,[277] prostate carcinoma,[278] and osteosarcoma,[279] has been confirmed by *in vitro* immunoprecipitation experiments. This is strong evidence that the regions that normally bind to viral-transforming proteins are also involved in naturally mutated RB proteins in tumorigenic cells.

Cellular-Binding Proteins. The viral oncoprotein-binding data suggested the existence of intracellular proteins whose function is mediated by binding to the RB protein or whose binding mediates the function of the RB protein itself. Several approaches have been

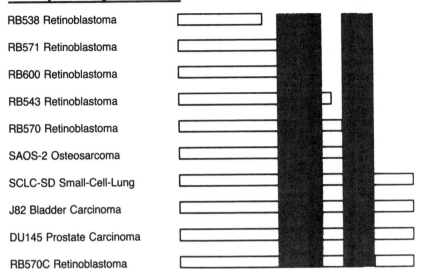

Fig. 22-17 Comparison of binding sites of EB to E1A/SV40 T antigen with naturally occurring RB1 mutations. This comparison includes RB1 mutations characterized in retinoblastoma, osteosarcoma, bladder carcinoma, and prostate carcinoma cells. The solid boxes at the top of the figure represent the regions of RB essential for binding to E1A and SV40 T antigen. The stippled regions indicate the positions of the binding regions relative to the RB sequences present in the naturally occurring mutants (open boxes). Amino acid sequences that are essential for binding to E1A and SV40 T are absent in each mutant. (Reprinted by permission from Hu et al., *EMBO J* 9(4):1147–1155, copyright 1990, Oxford University Press.)

used to search for these putative cellular components, and each has been in some way based on complementarity to the viral oncoprotein-binding regions. One line of experimentation involved screening a human lung fibroblast cDNA expression library with a 60-kDa recombinant RB protein. This analysis identified two individual cDNAs—RBP-1 and RBP-2280—whose products bound specifically to antimouse pRB monoclonal antibodies, although neither cross-hybridized with the other. Northern analyses of lung mRNA revealed 5.2- and 4.3-kb transcripts homologous to RBP-1, whereas RBP-2 detected a 6.0-kb transcript. DNA sequencing of these cDNAs indicated no homologies to known protein sequences except that each contained a 10-amino acid motif that mimicked the p110[RB]-binding domain.

A second approach utilized *in vitro* immunoprecipitation techniques. For these experiments, excess free p110[RB] was added to drive the reaction equilibrium toward complex formation with subsequent coprecipitation of these RB complexes with anti-RB antibodies.[280–281] A 56-kDa pRB fusion protein containing both regions necessary for the binding of T antigen to the C terminus stoichiometrically precipitated a 46-kDa protein from HeLa cells. Competition studies with large T antigen and the addition of p56 kDa RB protein containing deletion/insertion mutations, indicate that this 46-kDa cellular protein is directly associated with the recombinant p56 kDa RB protein through its T-binding domains.

The most successful approach to date for isolating cellular RB complexing proteins involves generating glutathione-S-transferase pRB fusion proteins, which then are used as protein-affinity chromatography agents against different cell lysates. The pRB portion of these proteins contains the minimal conserved region required for binding of SV40 large T and adenovirus E1A oncoproteins. When cellular lysates of the retinoblastoma cell line WERI-Rb27 were passed over affinity columns of fusion proteins that included regions of RB necessary for SV40 T-antigen binding, several cellular proteins, ranging in size from 25 to 146 kDa, were retained.[282] Similar-sized proteins could be separated from extracts of a variety of tumor cell lines. Each of the proteins was found primarily in the cellular nucleus, and at least one, of 68 to 72 kDa, displayed apparently S-phase-dependent binding behavior.

The function of the proteins isolated in each of these ways became clear through analyses of their physical relationship to p105[RB] and their effect on cellular transcription. DRTF is a sequence-specific transcription factor found in different forms (DRTF-b or DRTF-a) as embryonal carcinoma stem cells differentiate.[283,284] DRTF-b migrates faster than does DRTF-a in band-shift assays, suggesting that the DRTF-b complex is missing one or more protein components found in DRTF-a. To determine whether this transcription factor interacted with the tumor-suppressor RB product p110[RB], E1A protein was added to cell lysates of the embryonic stem-cell line F9. Using band-shift-binding assays, it was shown that E1A sequestered a protein from the DRTF-a complex, creating the DRTF-b form, an effect dependent on the E1A-conserved regions 1 and 2 that were previously determined to be necessary for transformation. Monoclonal antibodies to RB produced a similar shift from DRTF-a to DRTF-b, leading to the conclusion that p110[RB] is part of the DRTF transcription complex and providing a link between tumor-suppressor activity and control of gene transcription.

Because E1A affected the complexing of p110[RB] into DRTF, E1A-associated proteins were analyzed to see if they were part of the same complex. One such protein, cyclin A, like p110[RB], varies in mass amount during the mitotic phase of the cell cycle. The addition of an anticyclin A antibody to DRTF complexes caused a disruption of the RB-containing DRTF-a complex, but not a disruption of the RB-deficient DRTF-b complex.[285] Furthermore, the RB-deficient DRTF-b complex could complex with p110[RB] only when cyclin A was added, thus indicating that cyclin A facilitated the sequestering of RB into the DRTF complex. A consideration of the binding characteristics of DRTF, RB, and cyclin A in light of the cell-cycle regulation of the latter two, suggests that DRTF has an important cell-specific role in regulating the transcription of genes whose protein products are required for progression through the cell cycle (Fig. 22-15). Such coordinated behavior could provide a molecular mechanism by which viral and cellular transforming oncoproteins might act in part to sequester RB from DRTF-a. This would have the effect of freeing the transcriptionally active DRTF-b form, which is no longer under the negative regulation of p110[RB].

These experiments show that Rb probably functions in growth control and differentiation through interactions with a variety of cellular proteins. Other interacting proteins in this category include RIZ[286], Myo D[287], c-Abl[288], MDM2[289], and E2F[286–289] (described below). The transcriptional activators hBRG1/hBRM have also been functionally linked with pRB. hBRG1 (human brahma-related gene 1 protein) and its family member hBRM are the mammalian homologues of the yeast SNF2/SWI2 transcriptional activator and the Drosophila brahma protein. These proteins are thought to restructure chromatin and facilitate the function of specific transcription factors. All share a domain that is also found in many nuclear proteins, such as the E1A-binding protein p300.[290] hBRG1 interacts only with hypophosphorylated pp110^{RB} through the same LXCXE motif found in other pRB-interacting proteins described in this chapter.[291] This suggests that these transcriptional activators are rendered nonfunctional in G1 by their association with pRB and are released upon phosphorylation of the retinoblastoma protein.

E2F is another sequence-specific transcription factor that was initially identified as a cellular factor involved in the regulation of the adenovirus early E2 gene by the E1A protein. Using a glutathione-S-transferase protein fused to the 379 to 792 binding domain residues of p110^{RB} and a degenerate mixture of 62-bp DNA oligonucleotides, Chittenden et al.[292] attempted to determine whether any pRB pocket-binding cellular protein had sequence-specific DNA-binding activity. After several rounds of enrichment, two oligonucleotides were found to be the major components in the selected population. More than 80 percent of the sequenced oligonucleotides shared a class 1 TTTGGCGGG consensus sequence, while 15 percent contained a class 2 ATTTGCGCGGG consensus sequence. Comparison of these with other known sequence-binding sites uncovered a strong similarity to the binding site of E2F (TTTCGCGC). One interpretation of this study is that E2F binds specifically to the p110^{RB} product. Isolation of two cDNAs encoding E2F or E2F-like proteins (one of which corresponds to RBP-1, as was discussed earlier)[293,294] should provide the reagents needed to test this hypothesis.

Further studies determined that E2F was associated with the unphosphorylated form of p110^{RB} present in the G1 phase of the cell cycle near the G1-S border.[295,296] This behavior is consistent with the recruitment of unphosphorylated p110^{RB} into the DRTF complex and suggests that E2F can play a role in transcription or regulation, either alone or in concert with other proteins in the DRTF factor. Furthermore, as E2F is released upon entry into S phase, it can be found complexed with cyclin A; an E2F-cyclin A complex may be cooperatively released upon phosphorylation of p110^{RB} in the S phase of the cell cycle. The function of the RB/E2F in G1 phase transition is becoming more clearly defined. The complex is active in silencing the E1A promoter when bound to an E2F binding site.[297] In this form, RB/E2F inhibits the function of other promoter elements, such as enhancers, thereby causing transcription to cease. On phosphorylation of p110^{RB} or the addition of E1A, E2F is released and becomes a positive transcriptional element. Thus, positive and negative regulation of transcription is linked not only to E2F but also to the phosphorylation cycle of the retinoblastoma-suppressor gene. All these experiments are consistent with a model in which p110^{RB} controls the transcription of genes that contain E2F sites in their promoters, are cyclically expressed in relation to the cell cycle, and are important for cell proliferation.

RB can also suppress the growth of cells (mass increase), as well as their proliferation. Genes regulated by E2F are transcribed by RNA polymerase (pol) II, suggesting that Rb can specifically control proliferation through E2F. How Rb inhibits cell growth might be explained by the recent discovery that Rb can also regulate transcription by pol I and pol III.[303] These polymerases regulate the synthesis of rRNA and tRNA, and, therefore, their inhibition can repress the level of protein synthesis. As the rate of growth can be shown to be directly proportional to the rate of protein accumulation, Rb regulation of pol I and pol III may be the means by which it regulates cell growth.

pp110^{RB} Protein Family Members. An intriguing aspect of the E2F studies described above is the independent association of E2F with both cyclin A and p110^{RB}, even though neither of the latter two contains known structural similarities. Isolation of p107, a retinoblastoma-like protein, has shed light on this confusing phenomenon.[298] Anti-p107 antibodies precipitated p107 together with a few other cellular proteins, the most abundant being cyclin A and another being E2F. The demonstration that this p107 protein is a component of the E2F-cyclin A complex provided the structural basis for its binding behavior. It appears that p107 mediates the indirect binding of E2F to cyclin A, which explains how E2F can bind the structurally dissimilar p110^{RB} and cyclin A proteins.

Another member of this family of proteins, p130, was recently isolated, increasing the complexity of this growth regulation pathway. p130 shares 50 percent identity with p107 and has homology to pp110^{RB} in the pocket-binding domain.[299] Several studies show that this is the same p130 protein found associated with adenovirus E1A.[300,301] Both p107 and p130 bind to the viral oncoproteins and share the spacer region between the two subunits of the pocket-binding domain. This spacer region mediates their interaction with cyclins A and E.[302,303] Because these pRb-related proteins can bind to E2F,[300] they also exhibit growth-suppressing properties similar to those seen with pRB.[303] Interestingly, p130 has been mapped to the long arm of chromosome 16 in a region known to undergo allelic deletion and translocation in another pediatric cancer, Wilms' tumor.[304–306] This suggests that these Rb-related family members should be studied further for mutations in adult tumors not altered for either Rb or p16, and examined for their potential role as tumor-suppressor genes in the fashion described above for the retinoblastoma gene.

Retinoblastoma Mouse Models

The retinoblastoma genotypes and related phenotypes described throughout this chapter paint a somewhat paradoxical picture of the function of RB1. The p110^{RB} protein seems to play a central role in the regulation of the cell-cycle activity common to all cells, yet germ-line mutations in RB1 predispose individuals to a very specific spectrum of tumors. Thus, it remains unclear whether p110^{RB} serves solely as a barrier against specific tumorigenesis or actually plays an important role in normal cellular development. One approach, which has been undertaken to resolve and define these issues for RB1, involves the generation and analysis of animal models such as homozygous mutant (Rb −/−) knockout or transgenic mice. By creating mouse embryonic stem cell lines manipulated genetically to a null status at the RB1 locus and fusing these cell lines with normal blastocyst-stage mouse embryos, mice heterozygous for the mutant Rb allele (Rb+/−) are generated. These predisposed heterozygous mice can be observed for signs of increased tumor incidence and phenotypic abnormalities as well as backcrossed to generate homozygous Rb −/− progeny whose development and tumor profiles should help define the role RB1 in the normal cell.

Several Rb −/− mice have been engineered with insertional mutations in the regions of exons 3–4[305] and exon 20.[306] Observations of these mice and the progeny of their backcrosses were strikingly similar and unexpected. Most notable was the absence of any retinoblastomas or retinomas in the over 200 Rb+/− mice observed. These mice are genotypically equivalent to humans who inherit a mutated RB1 allele and are inevitably diagnosed, at greater than 90 percent penetrance, with retinoblastoma tumors. This systemic difference is further exemplified by the high incidence of brain tumors[306] and pituitary adenocarcinomas[305] exhibited in these Rb+/− animals after 8 to 10 months of observation. Molecular analysis of these tumors reveals loss of the remaining wild-type Rb allele, providing evidence that the two-hit hypothesis described in this chapter for humans also holds for these heterozygous mouse tissues.

Backcrosses of Rb+/− mice did not produce the expected 25 percent Rb −/− progeny. In fact, these Rb −/− embryos were not viable past approximately 13 days of gestation,[305,306] precluding the ability to study pRb[110] function in normal development. However, chimeric animals partially composed of Rb-deficient cells were viable and showed a widespread contribution of these mutant cells to all adult tissues and normal development of most tissues, including the retina and erythrocytes.[307] This indicates that Rb function is not required for the differentiation of cells in many adult tissues. When nonviable Rb −/− embryos were examined pathologically, significant defects in the brain and blood-forming tissues were discovered. There was massive cell death in the central nervous system tissues, which was highest in the hindbrain. An apparent block in hepatic erythropoiesis most likely accounts for the observation that 65 to 90 percent of red blood cells remain nucleated.

The results from these mouse models do little to solve the Rb paradox, but they do suggest that there may be fundamental systemic differences in the function of pRb in mouse and human tissues. Despite these discrepancies, it is clear that Rb does not play a critical role in regulating cell division or cell differentiation up to the thirteenth day of gestation of the mouse. One explanation for the lack of retinoblastoma tumors in Rb+/− animals is that the population of susceptible target cells in the relatively small mouse eye is below the threshold required for tumorigenesis to occur. However, retinoblastomas have been observed in transgenic mice expressing SV40 T antigen (see "Viral Oncoprotein," above).[308] Thus, there may be a requirement for additional genetic alterations to occur for retinoblastoma tumors to appear in the mouse. Alternatively, in the absence of Rb expression, a Rb-related protein such as p107 or p130 (see "pp110^{RB} Protein Family Members," above) might provide an analogous function in most tissues, preempting a role for p110^{RB} in tumorigenesis in the mouse.

Rb −/− cells isolated from early viable embryos provide a source for a variety of cell types that can be used to look in more detail at the function of Rb at the cellular level. Most importantly, these cells do not possess the multitude of other genetic lesions present in most human tumor cell genomes that might confuse or mask the precise role the pRb loss plays in tumorigenesis. Preliminary observations on Rb −/− fibroblasts show a shorter G1 phase of the cell cycle and a smaller cell size than in the wild type.[309] In addition, although most cell-cycle-regulated genes analyzed show no temporal or quantitative differences, cyclin E is derepressed earlier in G1 than is the case in wild-type cells. Cyclin E, found associated with cdk2, is one of the components responsible for phosphorylating pRb in late G1.[225] Studies utilizing double heterozygote and/or knockout mice for Rb and E2F support this theory. These studies revealed that the Rb1(−/−); E2F1(−/−) double mutant genotype is lethal, suggesting inactivation of E2F1 is not sufficient to rescue the lethal Rb1(−/−) phenotype.[316] Clearly, E2F deregulation is only one mechanism by which pRb1 functions to regulate cell growth *in vivo*. Further studies utilizing a number of other tissue types as well as cells from doubly Rb and p53 mutant mice[310–313] will no doubt add to our understanding of the role Rb plays in normal cellular function, as well as how it cooperates with other cellular oncogenes and tumor-suppressor genes with which it shares cellular control pathways.

ACKNOWLEDGMENTS

The authors are grateful to Prof. R. Frezzotti for his support and constructive criticisms and Dr. E. Motolese and Dr. G. Addabbo for assistance with sections of this review. Thanks also to Ms. C. Mallia for secretarial assistance. The work cited in this review was partly supported by a National Research Council (Italy) grant on retinoblastoma, #9000111.

REFERENCES

1. Francois J: Recent data on the heredity of retinoblastoma, in Boniuk M (ed): *Ocular and Adnexal Tumors*. St. Louis: Mosby, 1964.
2. Beck K, Jensen OA: Bilateral retinoblastoma in Denmark. *Arch Ophthalmol* **39**:561, 1961.
3. Hemmes GF, Tfsdscar J, Francois J: in Boniuk M (ed): *Ocular and Adnexal Tumors*. St. Louis: Mosby, 1964, p 123.
4. Albert DM, Lahav M, Lesser R, Craft J: Recent observations regarding retinoblastoma. *Trans Ophthal Mol Soc UK* **94**:909, 1974.
5. Berkow RL, Freshman JK: Retinoblastoma in Navajo Indian children. *Am J Dis Child* **137**:137, 1983.
6. Devesa SA: The incidence of retinoblastoma. *Am J Ophthalmol* **80**:263, 1975.
7. Sanders BM, Draper GJ, Kingston JE: Retinoblastoma in Great Britain 1969–80: Incidence, treatment, and survival. *Br J Ophthalmol* **75**:567, 1988.
8. Matsunaga E: Genetic epidemiology of retinoblastoma, in Lynch HP III, Hirayama T (eds): *Genetic Epidemiology of Cancer*. Boca Raton, FL: CRC, 1987, p 119.
9. Mahoney MC, Burnett WS, Majerovics A, Tanenbaum H: The epidemiology of ophthalmic malignancies in New York State. *Ophthalmology* **97**:1143, 1990.
10. Jensen RD, Miller RW: Retinoblastoma: Epidemiologic characteristics. *N Engl J Med* **285**:307, 1971.
11. Bras G, Cole H, Ashmeade-Dyer A, Walter DC: Report on 151 childhood malignancies observed in Jamaica. *J Natl Cancer Inst* **43**:417, 1969.
12. Parkin DM, Stiller CA, Draper GJ, Bieber C: The international incidence of childhood cancer. *Int J Cancer* **42**:511, 1988.
13. Frezzotti R, Bardelli AM, Fois A, Lasorella G, Acquaviva A, Hadjistilianou T, Bernardini C: Retinoblastoma: Terapie conservative del retinoblastoma, in Frezzotti R (ed): *Patologie Clinica e Terapia delle malattie dell' Orbita*. Ralazione 65° Congresso S.O.I., Siena 5–8, 1985, p 405.
14. Senft S, Al-Kaft A, Bergquist G, Jaafar M, Nasr A, Hidayat A, Sackey K, Cothier E: Retinoblastoma: The Saudi Arabian experience. *Ophthalmol Paediatr Genet* **9(2)**:115, 1988.
15. Ellsworth RM: The practical management of retinoblastoma. *Trans Am Ophthalmol Soc* **67**:461, 1969.
16. Francois J: Differential diagnosis of leukocoria in children. *Ann Ophthalmol* **10**:1375, 1978.
17. Shields JA, Augsburger JJ: Current approaches to the diagnosis and management of retinoblastoma. *Surv Ophthalmol* **25**:347, 1981.
18. Howard GM, Ellsworth RM: Differential diagnosis of retinoblastoma: A statistical study of 500 children. *Am J Ophthalmol* **60**:610, 1965.
19. Balmer A, Gailloud CL, Uffer S, Munier F, Pescia G: Retinoblastome et pseudoretinoblastome: Etude diagnostique. *Klin Mbl Augenheilk* **192**:589, 1988.
20. Murphree L, Rother C: Retinoblastoma, in Ryan SR (ed): *Retina*. St. Louis: Mosby, 1989, p 515.
21. Balmer A, Gailloud C: Retinoblastoma: Diagnosis and treatment. *Dev Ophthalmol* **7**:36, 1983.
22. Haik GB, Siedlecki A, Ellsworth RM, Sturgis-Buckhait L: Documented delays in the diagnosis of retinoblastoma. *Ann Ophthalmol* **17**:731, 1985.
23. Binder PS: Unusual manifestations of retinoblastoma. *Am J Ophthalmol* **77(5)**:674, 1974.
24. Richards WW: Retinoblastoma simulating uveitis. *Am J Ophthalmol* **65(3)**:427, 1968.
25. Stafford W, Yanoff M, Parnell BL: Retinoblastoma initially misdiagnosed as primary ocular inflammation. *Arch Ophthalmol* **82**:771, 1969.
26. Rozansky VM: A necrotic retinoblastoma simulating panophthalmitis. *Surv Ophthalmol* **9**:381, 1964.
27. Morgan G: Diffuse infiltrating retinoblastoma. *Br J Ophthalmol* **55**:600, 1971.
28. Garner A, Kanski JJ, Kinnear F: Retinoblastoma: Report of a case with minimal retinal involvement but massive anterior segment spread. *Br J Ophthalmol* **71**:858, 1987.
29. Schofield PB: Diffuse infiltrating retinoblastoma. *Br J Ophthalmol* **44**:35, 1960.
30. Nicholson DH, Norton EWD: Diffuse infiltrating retinoblastoma. *Trans Am Ophthalmol Soc* **78**:265, 1980.
31. Shields JA, Shields CL, Eagle RC, Blair CJ: Spontaneous pseudohypopyon secondary to diffuse infiltrating retinoblastoma. *Arch Ophthalmol* **106**:1301, 1988.

32. Shields CL, Shields JA, Shah P: Retinoblastoma in older children. *Ophthalmology* **98**:395, 1991.

33. Ginsberg J, Spaulding A, Asburg T: Cystic retinoblastoma. *Am J Ophthalmol* **80(5)**:930, 1975.

34. Ohnishi Y, Yamana Y, Minei M, Yoshitomi F: Snowball opacity in retinoblastoma. *Jpn J Ophthalmol* **26**:159, 1982.

35. Allderdice PW, Davis JG, Miller OJ: The 13q-deletion syndrome. *Am J Hum Genet* **21**:499, 1969.

36. Francke U, King F: Sporadic bilateral retinoblastoma and 13q-chromosome deletion. *Med Pediatr Oncol* **2**:379, 1976.

37. Niebuhr E, Ottosen J: Ring chromosome D(13) associated with multiple congenital malformations. *Ann Genet* **16**:157, 1973.

38. Seidman DJ, Shields JA, Augsburger JJ, Nelson LB, Lee ML, Sciorra LJ: Early diagnosis of retinoblastoma based on dysmorphic features and karyotype analysis. *Ophthalmology* **94**:663, 1987.

39. Gallie BL, Ellsworth RM, Abramson DH, Phillips RA: Retinoma: Spontaneous regression of retinoblastoma or benign manifestation of the mutation. *Br J Cancer* **45**:513, 1982.

40. Margo C, Hidayat CA, Kopelman J, Zimmerman LE: Retinocytoma: A benign variant of retinoblastoma. *Arch Ophthalmol* **101**:1519, 1983.

41. Eagle RC, Shields JA, Donoso L, Milner RS: Malignant transformation of spontaneously regressed retinoblastoma, retinoma/retinocytoma variant. *Ophthalmology* **96**:1389, 1989.

42. Abramson DH: Retinoma, retinocytoma, and the retinoblastoma gene [editorial]. *Arch Ophthalmol* **101**:1517, 1983.

43. Khodadoust AA, Roozitalab HM, Smith RE, Green WR: Spontaneous regression of retinoblastoma. *Surv Ophthalmol* **21**:467, 1977.

44. Aaby AA, Price RL, Zakov ZN: Spontaneously regressing retinoblastoma, retinoma or retinoblastoma group O. *Am J Ophthalmol* **96**:315, 1983.

45. Gallie BL, Phillips RA, Ellsworth RM, Abramson DH: Significance of retinoma and phthisis bulbi for retinoblastoma. *Ophthalmology* **89**:1393, 1982.

46. Bader JL, Miller RN, Meadows AT, Zimmerman LE, Champion LAA, Voute PA: Trilateral retinoblastoma. *Lancet* **582**:8194, 1980.

47. Jakobiec FA, Tso M, Zimmerman LE, Danis P: Retinoblastoma and intracranial malignancy. *Cancer* **39**:2048, 1977.

48. Dudgeon J, Lee WR: The trilateral retinoblastoma syndrome. *Trans Ophthalmol Soc UK* **103**:523, 1983.

49. Zimmerman LE, Burns RP, Wankum G, Tully R, Esterly JA: Trilateral retinoblastoma: Ectopic intracranial retinoblastoma associated with bilateral retinoblastoma. *Paediatr Ophthalmol Strabismus* **19(6)**:320, 1982.

50. Kingston JE, Plowman PN, Hungerford JL: Ectopic intracranial retinoblastoma in childhood. *Br J Ophthalmol* **69**:742, 1985.

51. Francois J, De Sutter E, Coppieters R, De Bie S: Late extraocular tumors in retinoblastoma survivors. *Ophthalmologica (Basel)* **181**:93, 1980.

52. Reese AB, Merriam GR, Martin HE: Treatment of bilateral retinoblastoma by irradiation and surgery: Report on 15 years results. *Am J Ophthalmol* **32**:175, 1949.

53. Frezzotti R, Guerra R: Sarcoma following irradiated retinoblastoma. *Arch Ophthalmol* **70**:471, 1963.

54. Forrest AW: Tumors following radiation about the eye. *Trans Am Acad Ophthalmol Otolaryngol* **65**:694, 1961.

55. Soloway HB: Radiation induced neoplasms following curative therapy for retinoblastoma. *Cancer* **19**:1984, 1966.

56. Sagerman RH, Cassady R, Tretter P, Ellsworth R: Radiation induced neoplasia following external beam therapy for children with retinoblastoma. *Am J Roentgenol Radium Ther Mucl Med* **105**:529, 1969.

57. Derkinderen DJ, Koten JW, Wolterbeek R, Beemer FA, Tan KE, Den Otter W: Non-ocular cancer in hereditary retinoblastoma survivors and relatives. *Ophthalmic Paediatr Genet* **8**:23, 1987.

58. Leuder GT, Judisch GF, O'Gorman TW: Second non-ocular tumors in survivors of heritable retinoblastoma. *Arch Ophthalmol* **104**:372, 1986.

59. Draper GJ, Sanders BM, Kingston JE: Second primary neoplasms in patients with retinoblastoma. *Br J Cancer* **53**:661, 1986.

60. Abramson DH, Ellsworth RM, Kitchin FD, Tung G: Second non-ocular tumors in retinoblastoma survivors: Are they radiation-induced? *Ophthalmology* **91**:1351, 1984.

61. Roarty JD, McLean IW, Zimmerman LE: Incidence of second neoplasms in patients with bilateral retinoblastoma. *Ophthalmology* **95**:1583, 1988.

62. Sang DN, Albert DM: Retinoblastoma: Clinical and histopathologic features. *Hum Pathol* **13**:133, 1982.

63. Brown DH: The clinicopathology of retinoblastoma. *Am J Ophthalmol* **97**:189, 1984.

64. Tosi P, Cintorino P, Toti V, Ninfo V, Montesco MC, Frezzotti R, Radjistilianou T, Acquaviva A, Barbini P: Histopathological evaluation for the prognosis of retinoblastoma. *Ophthalmic Paediatr Genet* **10**:173, 1987.

65. Kopelman JE, McLean IW, Rosenberg SH: Multivariate analysis of risk factors of metastasis in retinoblastoma treated by enucleation. *Ophthalmology* **94**:371, 1987.

66. Goldberg L, Danziger A: Computer tomographic scanning in the management of retinoblastoma. *Am J Ophthalmol* **84(3)**:380, 1977.

67. De Nicola M, Salvolini V: La risonanza magnetica nucleare e la tomografia assiale computerizzata nel retinoblastoma, in *Tumori Intraoculari. International Symposium Intraocular Tumors.* Palermo, Italy: Medical Books, 1990, p 43.

68. Char DH, Hedges TR, Norman D: Retinoblastoma: CT diagnosis. *Ophthalmology* **91**:1347, 1984.

69. Arrigg PG, Hedges RT, Char DH: Computed tomography in the diagnosis of retinoblastoma. *Br J Ophthalmol* **67**:558, 1983.

70. Mafee MF, Goldberg MF, Greenwald MJ, Schulman J, Malmed A, Flanders AE: Retinoblastoma and simulating lesions: Role of CT and MR imaging. *Radiol Clin North Am* **25(4)**:667, 1987.

71. Schulman JA, Peyman G, Mafee MF, Laurence L, Bauman AE, Goldman A: The use of magnetic resonance imaging in the evaluation of retinoblastoma. *J Pediatr Ophthalmol Strabismus* **23**:144, 1986.

72. Mafee MF, Goldberg MF, Cohen SB, Gotsis ED, Safran M, Chekuri L, Raofi B: Magnetic resonance imaging versus computed tomography of leukocoric eyes and use of in vitro proton magnetic resonance spectroscopy of retinoblastoma. *Ophthalmology* **96**:965, 1989.

73. Haik BG, Saint Louis L, Smith ME, Ellsworth RM, Abramson DH, Cahill P, Deck M, Coleman DJ: Magnetic resonance imaging in the evaluation of leukocoria. *Ophthalmology* **92**:1143, 1985.

74. Benhamou E, Borges J, Tso MOM: Magnetic resonance imaging in retinoblastoma and retinocytoma: A case report. *J Paediatr Ophthalmol Strabismus* **26**:276, 1989.

75. Danziger A, Price HI: CT findings in retinoblastoma. *Am J Radiol* **133**:695, 1979.

76. Coleman DJ, Lizzi FC, Jack PL: *Ultrasonography of the Eye and Orbit.* Philadelphia: Lea & Febiger, 1977, p 209.

77. Sampaolesi R, Zacrate J: Errors in the diagnosis of retinoblastoma, in *Ultrasound in Ophthalmology. Proceedings of the 11th S.I.D.U.O. Congress.* Kluwer Academic, 1986, p 189.

78. Ossolning KC: *Proceedings of the 10th Course and Workshop on Clinical Echo-Ophthalmology.* Vienna, December 12–15, 1973.

79. Motolese E, Addabbo G: Diagnosi ecografica delle neoplasie oculari. Atti Convegno interdisciplinare problemi oculari nell'infanzia. Siena 14–15 ottobre, 1988. *Boll Ocul* **68(5)**, 1989.

80. Jakobiec FA, Coleman DJ, Chattock A, Smith M: Ultrasonically guided needle biopsy and cytologic diagnosis of solid intraocular tumors. *Ophthalmology* **86**:1662, 1979.

81. Char DH, Miller TR: Fine needle biopsy in retinoblastoma. *Am J Ophthalmol* **97**:686, 1984.

82. Shields JA: Diagnostic approaches to intraocular tumors, in *Diagnosis and Management of Intraocular Tumors.* St. Louis: Mosby, 1983.

83. Midena E, Segato T, Piermarocchi S, Boccato P: Fine-needle aspiration biopsy in ophthalmology. *Surv Ophthalmol* **29**:410, 1985.

84. Augsburger JJ, Shields JA, Folberg R, Lang W, O'Hara BJ, Claricci J: Fine-needle aspiration biopsy in the diagnosis of intraocular cancer. *Ophthalmology* **92**:39, 1985.

85. Karcioglu ZA, Gordon R, Karcioglu G: Tumor seeding in ocular fine-needle aspiration biopsy. *Ophthalmology* **92**:1763, 1985.

86. Frezzotti R, Tosi P, Bardelli AM, Cintorino M, Hadjistilianou T: Cytologic diagnosis of retinoblastoma. *Proceedings I International Symposium on Ophthalmic Cytology,* Parma, Italy, October 9, 1987.

87. Arora R, Betharia SM: Fine-needle aspiration of paediatric orbital tumors. *Orbit* **7(2)**:115, 1988.

88. Frezzotti R, Hadjistilianou T, Greco G, Bartolomei A, Pannini S, Minacci C, Disanto A, Cintorino M: L'agobiopsia (FNAB) nella diagnosi differenziale delle neoplasie oculari ed orbitarie. *Atti LXIX Congresso S.O.I.* Rome, Oct. 12–15, 1989.

89. Reese AM, Ellsworth RM: Management of retinoblastoma. *Ann N Y Acad Sci* **114**:958, 1964.

90. Pratt CB: Management of malignant solid tumors in children. *Pediatr Clin North Am* **19(4)**:1141, 1972.

91. Stannard C, Lipper S, Sealy R, Sevel D: Retinoblastoma: Correlation of invasion of the optic nerve and choroid with prognosis and metastases. *Br J Ophthalmol* **63**:560, 1979.

92. Rosengren B, Monge OR, Flage T: Proposal of new pretreatment clinical TNM-classification of retinoblastoma. *Acta Oncol* **28**(4):547, 1989.

93. Shields JA, Shields CL, Sivalingam V: Decreasing frequency of enucleation in patients with retinoblastoma. *Am J Ophthalmol* **108**:185, 1989.

94. Ellsworth RM: Orbital retinoblastoma. *Trans Am Ophthalmol Soc* **72**:79, 1974.

95. Hilgartner HL: Report of a case of double glioma treated with X-ray. *Tex J Med* **18**:322, 1903.

96. Schipper J: An accurate and simple method for megavoltage radiation therapy of retinoblastoma. *Radiothes Oncol* **1**:31, 1983.

97. Harnett AN, Hungerford J, Lambert G, Hirst A, Darlinson R, Hart B, Trodd TC, Plowman P: Modern lateral external beam (lens sparing) radiotherapy for retinoblastoma. *Ophthalmic Paediatr Genet* **8**(1):53, 1987.

98. McCormick B, Ellsworth RM, Abramson DH: Results of external beam radiation for children with retinoblastoma: A comparison of two techniques. *J Pediatr Ophthalmol* **26**:239, 1989.

99. Reese AB, Ellsworth RM: The evaluation and current concept of retinoblastoma therapy. *Trans Am Acad Ophthalmol Otolaryngol* **67**:164, 1963.

100. Buys RJ, Abramson DH, Ellsworth RM, Haik B: Radiation regression patterns after cobalt plaque insertion for retinoblastoma. *Arch Ophthalmol* **101**:1206, 1983.

101. Abramson DH, Gerardi CM, Ellsworth RM, McCormick B, Sussman D, Turner L: Radiation regression patterns in treated retinoblastoma: 7 to 21 years later. *J Paediatr Ophthalmol Strabismus* **28**(2):108, 1991.

102. MacFaul PA, Bedford MA: Ocular complications after therapeutic irradiation. *Br J Ophthalmol* **54**:237, 1970.

103. Lommatzch PK: Die Anwendung von Betastrahlen mit 106 Ur/106 Rh Applikatoren bei dei Behandlung des Retinoblastomas. *Klin Monatsbl Augenheilkd* **156**:662, 1970.

104. Char DH: Retinoblastoma therapy, in *Clinical Ocular Oncology*. New York: Churchill Livingstone, 1989, p 207.

105. Shields J, Giblin ME, Shields C, Macroe AM, Karlsson V: Episcleral plaque radiotherapy for retinoblastoma. *Ophthalmology* **96**:530, 1989.

106. Meyer-Schwickerath G: The preservation of vision by treatment of intraocular tumors with light coagulation. *Arch Ophthalmol* **66**:458, 1961.

107. Frezzotti R, Hadjistilianou T: Is retinoblastoma vascularization a prognostic factor for xenon photocoagulation and for radiosensitivity? *Orbit* **7**(2):101, 1988.

108. Hadjistilianou T, Greco G, Frezzotti R: Photocoagulation therapy of retinoblastoma. *Orbit* **9**(4):283, 1990.

109. Abramson DH: The focal treatment of retinoblastoma with emphasis on xenon arc photocoagulation. *Acta Ophthalmol* **67**(suppl 194):6, 1989.

110. Shields JA, Shields CL, Parsons H, Giblin ME: The role of photocoagulation in the management of retinoblastoma. *Arch Ophthalmol* **108**:205, 1990.

111. Hopping W, Meyer-Schwickerath G: Light coagulation treatment in retinoblastoma, in Boniuk M (ed): *Ocular and Adnexal Tumors*. St. Louis: Mosby, 1964.

112. Hopping W, Schmitt G: The treatment of retinoblastoma. *Mod Probl Ophthalmol* **13**:106, 1977.

113. Lincoff H, McLean J, Long R: The cryosurgical treatment of intraocular tumors. *Am J Ophthalmol* **63**:389, 1967.

114. Abramson DH, Ellsworth RM, Rozakis GW: Cryotherapy for retinoblastoma. *Arch Ophthalmol* **100**:1253, 1982.

115. Shields JA, Parson H, Shields CL, Giblin ME: The role of cryotherapy in the management of retinoblastoma. *Am J Ophthalmol* **108**:260, 1989.

116. Molteno ACB, Griffiths JS, Marcus PB, Van Der Watt JJ: Retinoblastoma treated by freezing. *Br J Ophthalmol* **55**:492, 1971.

117. Rubin ML: Cryopexy for retinoblastoma. *Am J Ophthalmol* **66**:870, 1968.

118. White L: The role of chemotherapy in the treatment of retinoblastoma. *Retina* **3**:194, 1983.

119. Kupfer C: Retinoblastoma treated with intravenous nitrogen mustard. *Am J Ophthalmol* **36**:1721, 1953.

120. Haye C, Schlienger B: La chimiotherapie des tumers de la retine. *Bull Mem Soc Franc Ophthalmol* **92**:119, 1980.

121. Zucher JM, Lemercier N, Schlienger P, Marguilis E, Haye C: Chemotherapeutic conservative management in twenty-three patients with locally extended bilateral retinoblastoma. *Eur J Clin Oncol* **10**:1, 1982.

122. Wolff JA, Boesel CP, Dyment PG, Ellsworth RM, Gallie B, Hammond D, Leiken SL, Maurer HS, Tretter PK, Wara WM: Treatment of retinoblastoma. A preliminary report. *Int Cong Series* **570**:364, 1981.

123. Pratt CB: Management of malignant solid tumors in children. *Pediatr Clin North Am* **19**(4):1141, 1972.

124. Howarth C, Meyer D, Hustu O, Johnson WW, Shanks E, Pratt C: Stage-related combined modality treatment of retinoblastoma. *Cancer* **45**:851, 1980.

125. Acquaviva A, Barberi L, Bernardini C, D'Ambrosio A, Lasorella G: Medical therapy in retinoblastoma in children. *J Neurosurg Sci* **26**(1):49, 1982.

126. Zelter M, Gonzales G, Schwartz L, Gallo G, Schvartzman, Damel A, Sackmann MF: Treatment of retinoblastoma: Results obtained from a prospective study of 51 patients. *Cancer* **61**:153, 1988.

127. Akiyama K, Iwasaki M, Amemiya T, Yanai M: Chemotherapy for retinoblastoma. *Ophthalmic Paediatr Genet* **10**(2):111, 1988.

128. Pratt CB, Kun LE: Response of orbital and central nervous system metastases of retinoblastoma following treatment with cyclophosphamide/doxorubicin. *Pediatr Hematol Oncol* **4**:125, 1987.

129. Hungerford J, Kingston J, Plowman N: Orbital recurrence of retinoblastoma. *Ophthalmic Paediatr Genet* **8**:63, 1987.

130. Saarinen UM, Sariola N, Hovi L: Recurrent disseminated retinoblastoma treated by high-dose chemotherapy, total body irradiation, and autologous bone marrow rescue. *Am J Hematol Oncol* **13**(4):315, 1991.

131. White L: Chemotherapy in retinoblastoma: Current status and future directions. *Am J Pediatr Hematol Oncol* **13**(2):189, 1991.

132. White L: Chemotherapy in retinoblastoma: Where do we go from here? *Ophthalmic Paediatr Genet* **12**(3):115, 1991.

133. Hethcote HW, Knudson AGIR: Model for the incidence of embryonal cancers: Application to retinoblastoma. *Proc Natl Acad Sci U S A* **75**:2453, 1978.

134. Falls HF, Neel JV: Genetics of retinoblastoma. *Arch Ophthalmol* **151**:197, 1951.

135. Schappert-Kimmiiser J, Hemmes GD, Nijiland R: The heredity of retinoblastoma. *Ophthalmologica* **151**:197, 1966.

136. Vogel F: Neue untersuchunger zur genetik des retinoblastoms. *Z Menschl Vereh Konstit Lehre* **34**:205, 1957.

137. Knudson AGJR: Mutation and cancer: Statistical study of retinoblastoma. *Proc Natl Acad Sci U S A* **68**:820, 1971.

138. Macklin MT: A study of retinoblastoma in Ohio. *Am J Hum Genet* **12**:1, 1960.

139. Matsunaga E: Hereditary retinoblastoma: Delayed mutation or host resistance? *Am J Hum Genet* **30**:406, 1978.

140. Lele KP, Penrose LS, Stallard HB: Chromosome deletion in a case of retinoblastoma. *Ann Hum Genet* **27**:171, 1963.

141. Chaum E, Ellsworth RM, Abramsom DH, Haik BG, Kitchin FD, Chaganti RSK: Cytogenetic analysis of retinoblastoma: Evidence for multifocal origin and in vivo gene amplification. *Cytogenet Cell Genet* **38**:82, 1984.

142. Turleau C, de Grouchy U, Chavin-Coi IN F, Junien C, Seger J, Schieinger P, Leblanc A, Haye C: Cytogenetic forms of retinoblastoma: Their incidence in a survey of 66 patients. *Cancer Genet Cytogenet* **16**:321, 1985.

143. Squire J, Gallie BL, Phillips RA: A detailed analysis of chromosomal changes inheritable and non-heritable retinoblastoma. *Hum Genet* **70**:291, 1985.

144. Francke U: Retinoblastoma and chromosome 13. *Cytogenet Cell Genet* **16**:131, 1976.

145. Ward P, Packman S, Loughman W, Sparkes M, Sparkes RS, McMahon A, Gregory T, Ablin A: Location of the retinoblastoma susceptibility gene(s) and the human esterase D locus. *J Med Genet* **21**:92, 1984.

146. Sparkes RS, Murphree AL, Lingua RW, Sparkes MC, Field LL, Funderburk SJ, Benedict WF: Gene for hereditary retinoblastoma assigned to human chromosome 13 by linkage analysis to esterase D. *Science* **219**:971, 1983.

147. Sparkes RS, Sparkes MC, Wilson MG, Towner JW, Benedict WF, Murphree AL, Yunis JJ: Regional assignment of genes for esterase D and retinoblastoma to chromosome band 13q14. *Science* **208**:1042, 1980.

148. Strong LC, Riccardi VM, Ferrell RD, Sparkes RS: Familial retinoblastoma and chromosome 13 deletion transmitted via an insertional translocation. *Science* **213**:1501, 1981.

149. Sparkes RS, Muller H, Klisak I: Retinoblastoma with 13q-chromosomal deletion associated with maternal paracentric inversion of 13q. *Science* **203**:1027, 1979.

150. Riccardi VM, Hittner HM, Francke U, Pippin S, Holmquist GP, Kretzer FL, Ferrell R: Partial triplication and deletion of 13q: Study of

a family presenting with bilateral retinoblastoma. *Clin Genet* **15**:332, 1979.

151. Warburton D, Anyane-Yeboa K, Taterka P: Deletion of 13q14 without retinoblastoma: A case of non-penetrance. *Am J Hum Genet* **39**:A137, 1986.

152. Wilson WG, Carter BT, Conway BP, Atkin JF, Watson BA, Sparkes RS: Variable manifestations of deletion (13)(q14.1-q14.3) in two generations. *Am J Hum Genet* **39**:A47, 1986.

153. Motegi T: High rate of detection of 13q14 deletion mosaicism among retinoblastoma patients (using more extensive methods). *Hum Genet* **61**:95, 1982.

154. Wilson WG, Campochiaro PA, Conway BP, Sudduth KW, Watson BA, Sparkes RS: Deletion (13)(q14.1-q14.3) in two generations: Variability of ocular manifestations and definition of the phenotype. *Am J Med Genet* **28**:675, 1987.

155. Fukushima Y, Kuroki Y, Ito T, Kondo I, Nishigaki I: Familial retinoblastoma (mother and son) with 13q14 deletion. *Hum Genet* **77**:104, 1987.

156. Cavenee WK, Dryja TP, Phillips RA, Benedict WF, Godbout R, Gallie BL, Murphree AL, Strong LC, White RL: Expression of recessive alleles by chromosomal mechanisms in retinoblastoma. *Nature* **305**:779, 1983.

157. Barker D, Schaefer M, White RL: Restriction sites containing CpG show a higher frequency of polymorphism in human DNA. *Cell* **36**:131, 1984.

158. Wyman AR, White RL: A highly polymorphic locus in human DNA. *Proc Natl Acad Sci U S A* **77**:6754, 1980.

159. Cavenee WK, Leach RJ, Mohandas T, Pearson P, White RL: Isolation and regional localization of DNA segments revealing polymorphic loci from human chromosome 13. *Am J Hum Genet* **36**:10, 1984.

160. Dryja TP, Rapaport JM, Weichselbaum R, Bruns GAP: Chromosome 13 restriction fragment length polymorphisms. *Hum Genet* **65**:320, 1984.

161. Dryja TP, Cavenee WK, White RL, Rapaport JM, Peterson R, Albert DM, Bruns GAP: Homozygosity of chromosome 13 in retinoblastoma. *N Engl J Med* **310**:550, 1984.

162. Godbout R, Dryja TP, Squire JA, Gallie BL, Phillips RA: Somatic inactivation of genes on chromosome 13 is a common event in retinoblastoma. *Nature* **304**:550, 1983.

163. Cavenee WK, Hansen MF, Nordenskjold M, Kock E, Maumenee I, Squire JA, Phillips RA, Gallie BL: Genetic origin of mutations predisposing to retinoblastoma. *Science* **228**:501, 1985.

164. Abramson DH, Ellsworth RM, Kitchin FD, Tung G: Second nonocular tumors in retinoblastoma survivors: Are they radiation-induced? *Ophthalmology* **99**:1351, 1984.

165. Hansen MF, Koufos A, Gallie BL, Phillips RA, Fodstad O, Brogger A, Gedde-Dahl T, Cavenee WK: Osteosarcoma and retinoblastoma: A shared chromosomal mechanism revealing recessive predisposition. *Proc Natl Acad Sci U S A* **82**:6216, 1985.

166. Monaco AP, Bertelson CJ, Middlesworth W, Colletti C-A, Aldridge J, Fischbeck KH, Bartlett R, Pericak-Vance MA, Roses AD, Kunkel LM: Detection of deletions spanning the Duchenne muscular dystrophy locus using a tightly linked DNA segment. *Nature* **316**:842, 1985.

167. Royer-Pokora B, Kunkel LM, Monaco AP, Goff SC, Newburger PE, Baehner PL, Cole FS, Curnutte JT, Orkin SH: Cloning the gene for an inherited human disorder — chronic granulomatous disease — on the basis of its chromosomal location. *Nature* **322**:32, 1986.

168. Lalande M, Dryja TP, Schreck RR, Shipley J, Flint A, Latt SA: Isolation of human chromosome 13-specific DNA sequences cloned from flow sorted chromosomes and potentially linked to the retinoblastoma locus. *Cancer Genet Cytogenet* **13**:283, 1984.

169. Lalande M, Donlon T, Petersen R, Lieberparb R, Manter S, Latt SA: Molecular detection and differentiation of deletions in band 13q14 in human retinoblastoma. *Cancer Genet Cytogenet* **23**:151, 1986.

170. Dryja TP, Rapoport JM, Joyce JM, Petersen RA: Molecular detection of deletions involving band q14 of chromosome 13 in retinoblastomas. *Proc Natl Acad Sci U S A* **83**:7391, 1986.

171. Bookstein R, Lee EY-HP, To H, Young L-J, Sey T, Hayes R, Friedmann T, Lee W-H: Human retinoblastoma susceptibility gene: Genomic organization and analysis of heterozygous intragenic deletion mutants. *Proc Natl Acad Sci U S A* **85**:2210, 1988.

172. Friend SH, Bernards R, Rogelj S, Weinberg RA, Rapoport JM, Albert DM, Dryja TP: A human DNA segment with properties of the gene that predisposes to retinoblastoma and osteosarcoma. *Nature* **323:643, 1986.**

173. Fung Y-KT, Murphree A, Tang A, Qian J, Hinrichs S, Benedict W: Structural evidence for the authenticity of the human retinoblastoma gene. *Science* **236**:1657, 1987.

174. Horsthemke B, Gregor V, Barnert H, Hopping W, Passarge E: Detection of submicroscopic deletions and a DNA polymorphism at the retinoblastoma locus. *Hum Genet* **76**:257, 1987.

175. Dunn J, Phillips R, Zhu X, Becker A, Gallie B: Mutations in the RB1 gene and their effect on transcription. *Mol Cell Biol* **9**:4596, 1989.

176. Yandell D, Campbell T, Dayton S, Petersen R, Walton D, Little J, McConkie-Rosell A, Buckley E, Dryja T: Oncogenic point mutations in the human retinoblastoma gene: Their application to genetic counseling. *N Engl J Med* **321**:1639, 1989.

177. Lee W-H, Bookstein R, Hong F, Young L-J, Shew J-Y, Lee EY-HP: Human retinoblastoma susceptibility gene: Cloning, identification, and sequence. *Science* **235**:1394, 1987.

178. Horowitz J, Park S-H, Bogenmann E, Cheng J-C, Yandell D, Kaye F, Minna J, Dryja T, Weinberg R: Frequent inactivation of the retinoblastoma anti-oncogene is restricted to a subset of human tumor cells. *Proc Natl Acad Sci U S A* **87**:2775, 1990.

179. Harbour J, Lai S-L, Whang-Peng J, Gazdar A, Minna J, Kaye F: Abnormalities in structure and expression of the human retinoblastoma gene in SCLC. *Science* **242**:263, 1988.

180. Tang A, Varley J, Chakroborty S, Murphree A, Fung Y-KT: Structural rearrangement of the retinoblastoma gene in human breast carcinoma. *Science* **242**:263, 1988.

181. Bookstein R, Lee EY-HP, Peccei A, Lee W-H: Human retinoblastoma gene: Long-range mapping and analysis of its deletion in a breast cancer cell line. *Mol Cell Biol* **9**:1628, 1989.

182. Seizinger B, Klinger H, Junien C, Nakamura Y, Lebeau M, Cavenee W, Emanual B, Ponder B, Naylor S, Mitelman R, Louis D, Menon A, Newsham I, Decker J, Laelbing M, Henry IV, Deimling A: Report of the committee on chromosome and gene loss in human neoplasia. *Cytogenet Cell Genet* **58**:1080, 1991.

183. Huang H-JS, Yee J-K, Shew J-Y, Chen P-L, Bookstein R, Friedmann T, Lee EY-HP, Lee W-H: Suppression of the neoplastic phenotype by replacement of the RB gene in human cancer cells. *Science* **242**:1563, 1988.

184. Takahashi R, Hashimoto T, Xu H-J, Matsui T, Mikki T, Bigo-Marshall H, Aaronson S, Benedict W: The retinoblastoma gene functions as a growth and tumor suppressor in human bladder carcinoma cells. *Proc Natl Acad Sci U S A* **88**:5257, 1991.

185. Bookstein R, Shew J-Y, Chen P-L, Scully P, Lee W-H: Suppression of tumorigenicity of human prostate carcinoma cells by replacing a mutated RB gene. *Science* **247**:712, 1990.

186. Niederkorn J, Streilein J, Shaddock J: Deviant immune responses to allogeneic tumors injected intracamerally and subcutaneously in mice. *Invest Ophthalmol Vis Sci* **20**:355, 1981.

187. Madreperla S, Whittum-Hudson J, Prendergast R, Chen P-L, Lee W-H: Intraocular tumor suppression of retinoblastoma gene-reconstituted retinoblastoma cells. *Cancer Res* **51**:6381, 1991.

188. Muncaster M, Cohen B, Phillips R, Gallie B: Failure of RB1 to reverse the malignant phenotype of human tumor cell lines. *Cancer Res* **52**:654, 1992.

189. Cavenee WK, Murphree AL, Shull MS, Benedict WF, Sparkes RS, Kock E, Nordenskjold M: Prediction of familial predisposition to retinoblastoma. *N Engl J Med* **314**:1201, 1986.

190. Horsthemke B, Barnert HJ, Greger V, Passarge E, Hopping W: Early diagnosis in hereditary retinoblastoma by detection of molecular deletions at gene locus. *Lancet* **28**:511, 1987.

191. Leppert M, Cavenee W, Callahan P, Holm T, O'Connell P, Thompson K, Lathrop GM, Lalouel J-M, White R: A primary genetic map of chromosome 13q. *Am J Hum Genet* **39**:425, 1986.

192. Lee EY-HP, Lee WH: Molecular cloning of the human esterase D gene, a genetic marker for retinoblastoma. *Proc Natl Acad Sci U S A* **83**:6337, 1986.

193. Squire J, Dryja TP, Dunn J, Goddard A, Hoffman T, Musarella M, Willard HF, Becker AJ, Gallie BL, Phillips RA: Cloning of the esterase D gene: A polymorphic probe closely linked to the retinoblastoma locus on chromosome 13. *Proc Natl Acad Sci U S A* **83**:6573, 1986.

194. Wiggs J, Nordenskjold M, Yandell D, Rapaport J, Grondin V, Janson M, Werelius B, Peterson R, Craft A, Riedel K, Liberfarb R, Walton D, Wilson W, Dryja TP: Prediction of risk of hereditary retinoblastoma using DNA polymorphisms within the retinoblastoma gene. *N Engl J Med* **318**:151, 1988.

195. Vaughn G, Toguchida J, McGee T, Dryja T: PCR detection of the TthIII 1 RFLP within the retinoblastoma locus by PCR. *Nucleic Acids Res* **18**:4965, 1990.

196. McGee T, Cowley G, Yandell D, Dryja T: Detection of the Xba I RFLP within the retinoblastoma locus by PCR. *Nucleic Acids Res* **18**:207, 1990.

197. Scharf S, Bowcock A, McClure G, Klitz W, Yandell D, Erlich H: Amplification and characterization of the retinoblastoma gene VNTR by PCR. *Am J Hum Genet* **50**:371, 1992.

198. Dryja T, Mukai S, Petersen R, Rapaport J, Walton D, Yandell D: Parental origin of mutations of the retinoblastoma gene. *Nature* **339**:556, 1989.

199. Zhu X, Dunn J, Phillips R, Goddard A, Paton K, Becker A, Gallie B: Preferential germline mutation of the paternal allele in retinoblastoma. *Nature* **340**:313, 1989.

200. Toguchida J, Ishizaki K, Sasaki M, Hakamura Y, Ikenaga M, Kato M, Sugimot M, Kotoura Y, Yamamuro T: Preferential mutation of paternally derived RB gene as the initial event in sporadic osteosarcoma. *Nature* **338**:156, 1989.

201. Sapeinza C: Genome imprinting and dominance modification. *Ann N Y Acad Sci* **564**:24, 1989.

202. Leach R, Magewu N, Buckley J, Benedict W, Rother C, Murphree A, Griegels, Rajewsky M, Jones P: Preferential retention of paternal alleles in human retinoblastoma: Evidence for genomic imprinting. *Cell Growth Diff* **1**:401, 1990.

203. Vogel W: Genetics of retinoblastoma. *Hum Genet* **52**:1, 1979.

204. Onadim Z, Hogg A, Baird P, Cowell J: Oncogenic point mutations in exon 20 of the RB1 gene in families showing incomplete penetrance and mild expression of the retinoblastoma phenotype. *Proc Natl Acad Sci U S A* **89**:6177, 1992.

205. Sakai T, Ohtani N, McGee T, Robbins P, Dryja T: Oncogenic germ-line mutations in Sp1 and ATF sites in the human retinoblastoma gene. *Nature* **353**:83, 1991.

206. Landshulz WH, Johnson PF, McKnight SL: The leucine zipper: A hypothetical structure common to a new class of DNA binding proteins. *Science* **240**:1759, 1988.

207. Patthy L: Evolution of the proteases of blood coagulation and fibrinolysis by assembly from modules. *Cell* **41**:657, 1985.

208. Hong FD, Huang H-JS, To H, Young L-JS, Oro A, Bookstein R, Lee EY-HP, Lee W-H: Structure of the human retinoblastoma gene. *Proc Natl Acad Sci U S A* **86**:5502, 1989.

209. Jones NC, Rigby PWJ, Ziff EB: Trans-acting protein factors and the regulation of eukaryotic transcription: Lessons from studies on DNA tumor viruses. *Gene Dev* **2**:267, 1988.

210. Lee W-H, Shew J-Y, Hong FD, Sery TW, Donoso LA, Young L-J, Bookstein R, Lee EY-HP: The retinoblastoma susceptibility gene encodes a nuclear phosphoprotein associated with DNA binding activity. *Nature* **329**:642, 1987.

211. Cross F, Weintraub H, Roberts J: Simple and complex cell cycles. *Annu Rev Cell Biol* **5**:341, 1989.

212. Pardee AB: G1 events and regulation of cell proliferation. *Science* **246**:605, 1989.

213. Pardee AB: Molecules involved in proliferation of normal and cancer cells: Presidential address. *Cancer Res* **47**:1488, 1987.

214. Mihara K, Cao X-R, Yen A, Chandler S, Driscoll B, Murphree AL, Tang A, Fung Y-KT: Cell cycle-dependent regulation of phosphorylation of the human retinoblastoma gene product. *Science* **246**:1300, 1989.

215. Decaprio JA, Ludlow JW, Lynch D, Furukawa Y, Griffin J, Liwnica-Worms H, Huang C-M, Livingston DM: The product of the retinoblastoma susceptibility gene has properties of a cell cycle regulatory element. *Cell* **58**:1085, 1989.

216. Buchkovich K, Duffy LA, Harlow E: The retinoblastoma protein is phosphorylated during specific phases of the cell cycle. *Cell* **58**:1097, 1989.

217. Lin BT-Y, Gruenwald S, Morla AO, Lee W-H, Wang JYJ: Retinoblastoma cancer suppressor gene product is a substrate of the cell cycle regulator cdc2 kinase. *EMBO J* **10**:857, 1991.

218. Nurse P, Thuriaux P, Nasmyth K: Genetic control of the cell division cycle in the fission yeast Schizosaccharomyces pombe. *Mol Gen Genet* **146**:167, 1976.

219. D'Urso G, Marraccino RL, Marshak DR, Roberts JM: Cell cycle control of DNA replication by a homologue from human cells of the p34c-src protein kinase. *Science* **250**:786, 1990.

220. Shenoy S, Choi J-K, Bagrodia S, Copeland TD, Maller JL, Shalloway D: Purified maturation promoting factor phosphorylates pp60c-src at the sites phosphorylated during fibroblast mitosis. *Cell* **57**:763, 1989.

221. Chen P-L, Scully P, Shew J-Y, Wang JYJ, Lee W-H: Phosphorylation of the retinoblastoma gene product is modulated during the cell cycle and cellular differentiation. *Cell* **58**:1193, 1989.

222. Furukawa Y, Decaprio JA, Freedman A, Kanakura Y, Nakamura M, Ernst TJ, Livingston DM, Griffin JD: Expression and state of phosphorylation of the retinoblastoma susceptibility gene product in cycling and noncycling human hematopoietic cells. *Proc Natl Acad Sci U S A* **87**:2770, 1990.

223. Cooper JA, Whyte P: RB and the cell cycle: Entrance or exit? *Cell* **58**:1009, 1989.

224. Decaprio JA, Furukawa Y, Ajchenbaum F, Griffin JD, Livingston DM: The retinoblastoma-susceptibility gene product becomes phosphory-lated in multiple stages during cell cycle entry and progression. *Proc Natl Acad Sci U S A* **89**:1795, 1992.

225. Hunter T, Pines J: Cyclins and cancer: II. Cyclin D and CDK inhibitors come of age. *Cell* **79**:573, 1994.

226. Jinag W, Kahn SM, Tomita N, Zhang Y-J, Lu SH, Weinstein IB: Amplification and expression of the human cyclin D gene in esophageal cancer. *Cancer Res* **52**:2980, 1992.

227. Motokura T, Arnold A: Cyclins and oncogenesis. *Biochim Biophys Acta* **1155**:63, 1993.

228. Dowdy SF, Hinds PW, Louie K, Reed S, Arnold A, Weinberg RA: Physical interaction of the retinoblastoma protein with human D cyclins. *Cell* **73**:499, 1993.

229. Ewen ME, Sluss HK, Sherr CJ, Matshushime H, Kato J, Livingston DM: Functional interactions of the retinoblastoma protein with mammalian D-type cyclins. *Cell* **73**:487, 1993.

230. Kato J, Matsushime H, Hiebert SW, Ewen ME, Sherr CJ: Direct binding of cyclin D to the retinoblastoma gene product (pRb) and pRb phosphorylation by the cyclin D-dependent kinase CDK4. *Genes Dev* **7**:331, 1993.

231. Fagan R, Flint KJ, Jones N: Phosphorylation of E2F-1 modulates its interaction with the retinoblastoma gene product and the adenoviral E4 19-kDa protein. *Cell* **78**:799, 1994.

232. Bates S, Parry D, Bonetta L, Vousden K, Dickson C, Peters G: Absence of cyclin D/cdk complexes in cells lacking functional retinoblastoma protein. *Oncogene* **9**:1633, 1994.

233. Mller H, Lukas J, Schneider A, Warthoe P, Bartek J, Ellers M, Strasu M: Cyclin D1 expression is regulated by the retinoblastoma protein. *Proc Natl Acad Sci U S A* **91**:2945, 1994.

234. Tam SW, Theodoras AM, Shay JW, Draetta GF, Pagano M: Differential expression and regulation of cyclin D1 protein in normal and tumor human cells: Association with Cdk4 is required for cyclin D1 function in G1 progression. *Oncogene* **9**:2663, 1994.

235. Serrano M, Hannon GJ, Beach D: A new regulatory motif in cell-cycle control causing specific inhibition of cyclin D/CDK4. *Nature* **366**:704, 1993.

236. Hannon GI, Beach D: p15INK4B is a potential effector of TGF-B-induced cell cycle arrest. *Nature* **371**:257, 1994.

237. Kamb A, Gruis NA, Weaver-Feldhaus J, Lie Q, Harshman K, Tavtigian SV, Stockert E, Day RSI, Johnson BE, Skolnick MH: A cell cycle regulator potentially involved in genesis of many tumor types. *Science* **264**:436, 1994.

238. Nobori T, Miura K, Wu DJ, Lois A, Takabayashi K, Carson DA: Deletions of the cyclin-dependent kinase-4 inhibitor gene in multiple human cancers. *Nature* **368**:753, 1994.

239. Merlo A, Herman JG, Mao L, Lee DJ, Gabrielson E, Burger PC, Baylin SB, Sidransky D: 59 CpG island methylation is associated with transcriptional silencing of the tumour suppressor p16/CDKN2/ MTS1 in human cancers. *Nat Med* **1**:686, 1995.

240. Costello JF, Berger MS, Huang H-JS, Cavenee WK: Silencing of p16/CDKN2 expression in human gliomas by methylation and chromatin condensation. *Cancer Res* **56**:2405, 1996.

241. Arap W, Kishikawa R, Furnari FB, Cavenee WK, Huang H-JS: Replacement of the p16/CDKN2 gene suppresses human glioma cell growth. *Cancer Res* **55**:1351, 1995.

242. Bonetta L: Open questions on p16. *Nature* **370**:180, 1994.

243. Cairns P, Mao L, Merlo A, Lee DJ, Schwab D, Eby Y, Tokino K, van der Riet P, Blaugrund JE, Sidransky D: Rates of p16 (MTS1) mutations in primary tumors with 9p loss. *Science* **265**:415, 1994.

244. Kamp A, Liu Q, Harshman K, Tavtigian S: Rates of p16 (MTS1) mutations in primary tumors with 9p loss. *Science* **265**:416, 1994.

245. Spruck CHI, Gonzalex-Sulueta M, Shibata A, Simoneay AR, Lin M-F, Gonzales F, Tsai YC, Jones PA: p16 gene in uncultured tumours. *Nature* **370**:183, 1994.

246. He J, Olson JJ, James CD: Lack of p16INK4 or retinoblastoma protein (pRb) or amplification-associated overexpression of cdk4 is observed in distinct subsets of malignant glial tumors and cell lines. *Cancer Res* **55**:4833, 1995.

247. Mori T, Miura K, Aoki T, Nishihara T, Mori S, Nakamura M: Frequent somatic mutation of MTS1/CDK4 (multiple tumor suppressor/cyclin-dependent kinase 4 inhibitor) gene in esophageal squamous cell carcinoma. *Cancer Res* **54**:3396, 1994.

248. Caldas C, Hahn SA, da Costa LT, Redston MS, Schutte M, Seymour AB, Weinstein CK, Hruban RH, Yeo CJ, Kern SE: Frequent somatic mutations and homozygous deletions of the p16 (MTS1) gene in pancreatic adenocarcinoma. *Nat Genet* **8**:27, 1994.

249. Parry D, Bates S, Mann DJ, Peters G: Lack of cyclin D/Cdk complexes in RB-negative cells correlates with high levels of p16INK4/MTS1 tumour suppressor gene product. *EMBO J* **14**:503, 1995.

250. Li Y, Nichols MA, Shay JW, Xiong Y: Transcriptional repression of the D-type cyclin-dependent linases inhibitor p16 by the retinoblastoma susceptibility gene product, pRb. *Cancer Res* **54**:6078, 1994.

251. Shimizu E, Coxon A, Otterson GA, Steinberg SM, Kratzke RA, Kim YW, Fedorko J, Oie H, Johnson B, Mulsine JL, Minna JD, Gazdar AF, Kaye FJ: RB protein status and clinical correlation from 171 cell lines representing lung cancer, extrapulmonary small cell carcinoma, and mesothelioma. *Oncogene* **9**:2441, 1994.

252. Shapiro GI, Edwards CD, Kobzik L, Godleski J, Richars W, Sugarbaker DJ, Rollins BJ: Reciprocal Rb inactivation and p16INK4 expression in primary lung cancers and cell lines. *Cancer Res* **55**:505, 1995.

253. Otterson GA, Kratzke RA, Coxon A, Kim YW, Kaye FJ: Absence of p16INK4 protein is restricted to the subset of lung cancer lines that retains wild-type RB. *Oncogene* **9**:3375, 1994.

254. Sakaguchi M, Fuji Y, Hirabayashi H, Yoon H-E, Komoto Y, Oue T, Kusafuka T, Okada A, Matsuda H: Inversely correlated expression of p16 and Rb protein in non-small cell lung cancers: An immunohistochemical study. *Int J Cancer* **65**:442, 1996.

255. Schauer IE, Siriwardana S, Langan TA, Sclarani RA: Cyclin Da overexpression vs. retinoblastoma inactivation: Implications for growth control evasion in non-small cell and small cell lung cancer. *Proc Natl Acad Sci U S A* **91**:7827, 1994.

256. Berk A: Adenovirus promoters and E1A transactivation. *Annu Rev Genet* **20**:45, 1986.

257. Livingston DM, Bradley MK: Review: The simian virus 40 large T antigen—A lot packed into a little. *Mol Biol Med* **4**:63, 1987.

258. Zur Hausen H, Schneider A, in Howley PM, Salzman MP (eds): *The Papovaviridae, vol 2: The Papillomaviruses*. New York: Plenum, 1987, pp 245–263.

259. Cherington V, Brown M, Paucha E, St. Louis J, Spiegelman BM, Roberts TM: Separation of simian virus 40 large T-antigen-transforming and origin-binding functions from the ability to block differentiation. *Mol Cell Biol* **8**:1380, 1988.

260. Clayton CE, Murphy D, Lovett M, Rigby PWJ: A fragment of the SV40 T-antigen gene transforms. *Nature* **299**:59, 1982.

261. Whyte P, Ruley HE, Harlow E: Two regions of the adenovirus early region 1A proteins are required for transformation. *J Virol* **62**:257, 1988.

262. Phelps WC, Yee CL, Munger K, Howley PM: The human papilloma type 16 E7 gene encodes transactivation and transformation functions similar to those of adenovirus E1A. *Cell* **53**:539, 1988.

263. Harlow E, Whyte P, Franza BR Jr, Schley C: Association of adenovirus early-region 1A proteins with cellular polypeptides. *Mol Cell Biol* **6**:1579, 1986.

264. Whyte P, Buchkovich KJ, Horowitz JM, Friend SH, Raybuck M, Weinberg RA, Harlow E: Association between an oncogene and an antioncogene: The adenovirus E1A proteins bind to the retinoblastoma gene product. *Nature* **234**:124, 1988.

265. Decaprio JA, Ludlow JW, Figge J, Shew J-Y, Huang C-M, Lee W-H, Marsilio E, Paucha E, Livingston DM: SV40 large tumor antigen forms a specific complex with the product of the retinoblastoma susceptibility gene. *Cell* **54**:275, 1988.

266. Dyson N, Howley PM, Munger K, Harlow E: The human papilloma virus-16 E7 oncoprotein is able to bind to the retinoblastoma gene product. *Science* **243**:934, 1989.

267. Kalderon D, Smith AE: In vitro mutagenesis of a putative DNA binding domain of SV40 large T. *Virology* **139**:109, 1984.

268. Ludlow JW, Decaprio JA, Huang C-M, Lee W-H, Paucha E, Livingston DM: SV40 large T antigen binds preferentially to an underphosphorylated member of the retinoblastoma susceptibility gene product family. *Cell* **56**:57, 1989.

269. Ludlow JW, Shon J, Pipas JM, Livingston DM, Decaprip JA: The retinoblastoma susceptibility gene product undergoes cell cycle-dependent dephosphorylation and binding to and release from SV40 large T. *Cell* **60**:387, 1990.

270. Peden KWC, Srinivasan A, Parber JM, Pipas JM: Mutants with changes within or near a hydrophobic region of simian virus 40 large tumor antigen are defective for binding cellular protein p53. *Virology* **168**:13, 1989.

271. Tack LC, Cartwright CA, Wright JH, Eckhard W, Peden KWC, Srinivasan A, Pipas JM: Properties of a simian virus 40 mutant T antigen substituted in the hydrophobic region: Defective ATP-ase and oligomerization activities and altered phosphorylation accompany an inability to complex with cellular p53. *J Virol* **63**:3362, 1989.

272. Dyson N, Buchovich K, Whyte P, Harlow E: The cellular 107K protein that binds to adenovirus E1A also associates with the large T antigens of SV40 and JC virus. *Cell* **58**:249, 1989.

273. Ewen ME, Ludlow JW, Marsilio E, Decaprio JA, Millikan RC, Cheng SH, Paucha E, Livingston DM: An N-terminal transformation-governing sequence of SV40 large T antigen contributes to the binding of both p110^RB and a second cellular protein, p120. *Cell* **58**:257, 1989.

274. Hu Q, Dyson N, Harlow E: The regions of the retinoblastoma protein needed for binding to adenovirus E1A or SV40 large T antigen are common sites for mutations. *EMBO J* **9**(4):1147, 1990.

275. Huang S, Wang N-P, Tseng BY, Lee W-H, Lee EH-YP: Two distinct and frequently mutated regions of retinoblastoma protein are required for binding to SV40 T antigen. *EMBO J* **9**(6):1815, 1990.

276. Horowitz J, Yandell DW, Park S-H, Canning S, Whyte P, Buchkovich K, Harlow E, Weinberg RA, Dryja TP: Point mutational inactivation of the retinoblastoma antioncogene. *Science* **243**:937, 1989.

277. Shew J-Y, Ling N, Yang X, Fodstad O, Lee W-H: Antibodies detecting abnormalities of the retinoblastoma susceptibility gene product (pp110^RB) in osteosarcomas and synovial sarcomas. *Oncogene Res* **4**:205, 1989.

278. Bookstein R, Shew J-Y, Chen P-L, Scully P, Lee W-H: Suppression of tumorigenicity of human prostate carcinoma cells by replacing a mutated RB gene. *Science* **247**:712, 1990.

279. Shew J-Y, Lin BT-Y, Chen P-L, Tseng BY, Yang-Feng TL, Lee W-H: C-terminal truncation of the retinoblastoma gene product leads to functional inactivation. *Proc Natl Acad Sci U S A* **87**:6, 1990.

280. Defeo-Jones D, Huang PS, Jones RE, Haskell KM, Vuocolo GA, Hanobik MG, Huber HE, Oliff A: Cloning of cDNAs for cellular proteins that bind to the retinoblastoma gene product. *Nature* **352**:251, 1991.

281. Huang S, Lee W-H, Lee EY-HP: A cellular protein that competes with SV40 T antigen for binding to the retinoblastoma gene product. *Nature* **350**:160, 1991.

282. Kaelin WG, Pallas DC, Decaprio JA, Kaye FJ, Livingston DM: Identification of cellular proteins that can interact specifically with the T/E1A-binding region of the retinoblastoma gene product. *Cell* **64**:521, 1991.

283. Partridge JF, Lathangue NB: A developmentally regulated and tissue-dependent transcription factor complexes with the retinoblastoma gene product. *EMBO J* **10**:3819, 1991.

284. Bandara LR, Lathangue NB: Adenovirus E1A prevents the retinoblastoma gene product from complexing with a cellular transcription factor. *Nature* **351**:494, 1991.

285. Bandara LR, Adamczewski JP, Hunt T, Lathangue NB: Cyclin A and the retinoblastoma gene product complex with a common transcription factor. *Nature* **352**:249, 1991.

286. Buyse IM, Shao G, Huang S: The retinoblastoma protein binds to RIZ, a zinc-finger protein that shares an epotope with the adenovirus E1A protein. *Proc Natl Acad Sci U S A* **92**:4467, 1995.

287. Gu W, Schneider JW, Condorelli G, Kaushal S, Mahdavi V, Nadal-Ginard B: Interaction of myogenic factors and the retinoblastoma protein mediates muscle cell commitment and differentiation. *Cell* **72**:309, 1993.

288. Welch PJ, Wang JYJ: Abrogation of retinoblastoma protein function by c-Abl through tyrosine kinase-dependent and -independent mechanisms. *Mol Cell Biol* **15**:5542, 1995.

289. Xiao Z-X, Chen J, Levine AJ, Modjtahedi N, Xing J, Sellers WR, Livingston DM: Interaction between the retinoblastoma protein and the oncoprotein MDM2. *Nature (London)* **375**:694, 1995.

290. Eckner R, Ewen ME, Newsome D, Gerdes M, DeCaprio JA, Lawrence JB, Lingston DM: Molecular cloning and functional analysis of the adenovirus E1A-associated 300-kD protein (p300) reveals a protein with properties of a transcriptional adaptor. *Genes Dev* **8**:869, 1994.

291. Strober BE, Dunaief JL, Sushovan G, Goff SP: Functional interactions between the hBRM/hBRG1 transcriptional activators and the pRB family of proteins. *Mol Cell Biol* **16**:1576, 1996.

292. Chittenden T, Livingston DM, Kaelin WG: The T/E1A-binding domain of the retinoblastoma product can interact selectively with a sequence-specific DNA-binding protein. *Cell* **65**:1073, 1991.

293. Helin K, Lees JA, Vidal M, Dyson N, Harlow E, Fattaey A: A cDNA encoding a pRB-binding protein with properties of the transcription factor E2F. *Cell* **70**:337, 1992.

294. Kaelin WG, Krek W, Sellers WR, Decaprio JA, Ajchenbaum F, Fuchs CS, Chittenden T, Li Y, Farnham PJ, Blanar MA, Livingston DM, Flemington EK: Expression cloning of a cDNA encoding a retinoblastoma-binding protein with E2F-like properties. *Cell* **70**:351, 1992.

295. Chellappan SP, Hiebert S, Mudry JM, Horowitz JM, Nevins JR: The E2F transcription factor is a cellular target for the RB protein. *Cell* **65**:1053, 1991.

296. Bagchi S, Weinmann R, Raychaudhuri P: The retinoblastoma protein copurifies with E2F-I, and E1A-regulated inhibitor of the transcription factor E2F. *Cell* **65**:1063, 1991.

297. Weintraub SJ, Prater CA, Dean DC: Retinoblastoma protein switches the E2F site from positive to negative element. *Nature* **358**:259, 1992.

298. Ewen ME, Xing Y, Lawrence JB, Livingston DM: Molecular cloning, chromosomal mapping, and expression of the cDNA for p107, a retinoblastoma gene product-related protein. *Cell* **66**:1155, 1991.

299. Hannon GJ, Demetrick D, Beach D: Isolation of the Rb-related p130 through its interaction with CDK2 and cyclins. *Genes Dev* **7**:2378, 1993.

300. Cobrinik D, Whyte P, Peeper DS, Jacks T, Weinberg RA: Cell cycle-specific association of E2F with the p130 E1A-binding protein. *Genes Dev* **7**:2392, 1993.

301. Li Y, Graham C, Lacy S, Duncan AMV, Whyte P: The adenovirus E1A-associated 130-kD protein is encoded by a member of the retinoblastoma gene family and physically interacts with cyclins A and E. *Genes Dev* **7**:2366, 1993.

302. Ewen ME, Faha B, Harlow D, Livingston D: Interaction of p107 with cyclin A independent of complex formation with viral oncoproteins. *Science* **255**:85, 1992.

303. Zhu L, van der Heuvel K, Fattaey A, Ewen M, Livingston D, Dyson N, Harlow E: Inhibition of cell proliferation by p107, a relative of the retinoblastoma protein. *Genes Dev* **7**:1111, 1993.

304. Maw MA, Grundy PE, Millow LJ, Eccles MR, Dunn RS, Smith PJ, Feinberg AP, Law DJ, Paterson MC, Telzerow PE: A third Wilms' tumor locus on chromosome 16q. *Cancer Res* **52**:3094, 1992.

305. Slater RM, Mannens MM: Cytogenetics and molecular genetics of Wilms' tumor of childhood. *Cancer Genet Cytogenet* **61**:111, 1992.

306. Newsham I, Röhrborn-Kindler A, Daub D, Cavenee WK: A constitutional BWS-related t(11;16) chromosome translocation occurring in the same region of chromosome 16 implicated in Wilms' tumors. *Gene Chrom Cancer* **12**:1, 1995.

307. Jacks T, Faxeli A, Schmitt EM, Bronson RT, Goodell MA, Weinberg RA: Effects of an Rb mutation in the mouse. *Nature* **359**:295, 1992.

308. Lee EY-HP, Chang CY, Hu N, Wang Y-CJ, Lai C-C, Herrup K, Lee W-H, Bradley A: Mice deficient for Rb are nonviable and show defects in neurogenesis and haematopoiesis. *Nature* **359**:288, 1992.

309. Williams BO, Schmitt EM, Remington L, Bronson RT, Albert DM, Weinberg RA, Jacks T: Extensive contribution of Rb-deficient cells to adult chimeric mice with limited histopathological consequences. *EMBO J* **13**:4251, 1994.

310. Windle JJ, Albert DM, O'Brien JM, Marcus DM, Disteche CM, Bernards, Mellon PL: Retinoblastoma in transgenic mice. *Nature* **343**:665, 1990.

311. Herrera RE, Sah VP, Williams BO, Makela TP, Weinberg RA, Jacks T: Altered cell cycle kinetics, gene expression, and G1 restriction point regulation in Rb-deficient fibroblasts. *Mol Cell Biol* **16**:2402, 1996.

312. Harvey M, Vogel H, Lee EY-HP, Bradley A, Donehower LA: Mice deficient in both p53 and Rb develop tumors primarily of endocrine origin. *Cancer Res* **55**:1146, 1995.

313. Williams BO, Remington L, Albert DM, Mukai S, Bronson RT, Jacks T: Cooperative tumorigenic effects of germline mutations in Rb and p53. *Nat Genet* **7**:480, 1994.

Li-Fraumeni Syndrome

David Malkin

1. The Li-Fraumeni syndrome (LFS) is a rare autosomal dominantly inherited disorder. It is characterized by the diagnosis of bone or soft tissue sarcoma at an early age in an individual who has one first-degree relative with early onset cancer and a second close relative with early onset cancer or sarcoma diagnosed at any age.
2. Families in which the classic phenotype of the syndrome is not expressed completely are termed Li-Fraumeni syndrome-like (LFS-L) and are represented by many different features. Common to all these families is the occurrence of a variety of cancers of a distinct histopathologic type.
3. Germ-line alterations of the *p53* tumor-suppressor gene located on chromosome 17p13 have been observed in the majority of LFS families and in a proportion of LFS-L families. This gene encodes a 53-kDa nuclear phosphoprotein that is composed of 393 amino acids. Genetic alterations primarily result from base-pair substitutions that result in missense mutations. These changes are among the most frequently observed genetic abnormalities in human cancer. Somatic inactivation of *p53* occurs through base-pair substitutions or binding to other cellular proteins or to certain DNA tumor virus proteins.
4. The p53 protein binds specific DNA sequences and appears to be a transcription factor that may regulate the expression of other growth regulatory genes in a positive or negative manner. The antiproliferative effect of wild-type p53 is exerted at a checkpoint control site before G1/S of the cell cycle, with G2/M and the mitotic spindle being other potential targets. p53 mediates apoptosis and plays an important role in modulating the cellular response to DNA damage induced by ultraviolet (UV) irradiation or γ-irradiation and certain chemotherapeutic agents.
5. *p53* mutations are not observed in all classic LFS families. Germ-line *p53* mutations are seen in a small number of patients and families with cancer phenotypes that only superficially resemble LFS. Other mechanisms of *p53* inactivation may occur in some clinical settings, and other genes involved in cell cycle regulation may be altered in *p53* wild-type families.
6. Mouse models of *p53* deficiency have been created. These *p53* knockouts exhibit an increased rate of development of a spectrum of tumors, including lymphomas and sarcomas. Transgenic *p53* mice have been generated that have a tumor phenotype distinct from that of the *p53*-deficient animals. Mice heterozygous for a deleted *p53* allele exhibit an intermediate phenotype in that the rate of tumor formation is slower than that of the *p53*-null animals yet faster than that of wild-type littermates. These mice have been used as *in vivo* models to analyze p53 function and dysfunction in the setting of interventions with chemotherapy, radiation therapy, or teratogenic agents.
7. Predictive genetic testing for carriers of mutant *p53* is available in research settings in a few centers. The interpretation of results with respect to diagnostic capabilities and options for therapeutic intervention is under scrutiny. The value of such screening is tempered by the need to evaluate risk, counseling issues, the need for informed consent, and regulations on testing.

Studies of hereditary cancer clusters have led to the identification of genes critical to both carcinogenesis and normal development. The Li-Fraumeni syndrome (LFS) is a rare familial cancer syndrome that represents the paradigm of human cancer predisposition to multiple childhood and adult onset neoplasms. Before identification of a specific genetic defect that was inherited in a significant proportion of LFS families, it could not be definitely established that such a diverse spectrum of tumors could result from the alteration of a specific gene as a presumptive initiating event. The span of time from the initial clinical description of a family with this constellation of tumors to identification of germ-line alterations of the *p53* tumor-suppressor gene in many families was 20 years. The realization of a genetic link resulted from expertise in classic genetic epidemiology and the molecular biology of sporadic tumorigenesis and in many ways represented the realization of the development of the now burgeoning field of molecular epidemiology. The link between an extremely rare clinical phenotype (LFS) with alterations of perhaps the most commonly altered gene in human cancer (*p53*) points out the value of studying rare genetic phenotypes. These studies have led to a clearer understanding of the role *p53* plays in cell cycle control as well as to a cloudier picture of the way in which the LFS phenotype is derived in the absence of *p53* alterations. The generation of mouse models of deficient *p53* or altered *p53* functions has provided an opportunity to study not only the tumorigenic effects of this genotype but also the potential results of therapeutic, carcinogenic, and teratogenic interventions in tissues harboring an altered *p53* allele.

In addition to expanding our knowledge of cell cycle control, the study of these LFS families formed the early foundations on which recommendations and guidelines could be established to develop and monitor genetic testing programs for predisposition to both early and late onset disease. The models developed for other genetic diseases have been helpful as guides, but the unique imprecise nature of human carcinogenesis and the *p53*-LFS association require complex interactions among several disciplines.

The genetics of LFS and the complex roles of *p53* are still being elucidated. A vast literature has been generated about this gene, and characterizations of its roles in clinical genetics and clinical medicine are relatively early in their development. Future editions of this textbook will continue to clarify the relationship between the LFS phenotype and its variable genotype.

CLINICAL ASPECTS

Historical Perspective

In 1969, Li and Fraumeni reported the results of a retrospective survey of 280 medical records and 418 death certificates of

---

A list of standard abbreviations is located immediately preceding the index. Nonstandard abbreviations used in this chapter include: LFS = Li-Fraumeni syndrome; LFS-L = Li-Fraumeni syndrome-like; PCNA = poliferating cell nuclear antigen; ADCC = Adrenocortical carcinoma; ES = embryonic stem

childhood rhabdomyosarcoma patients diagnosed in the United States.[1,2] Five families were identified in whom siblings or cousins had been diagnosed with a childhood sarcoma. A high concentration of cancers of diverse types was observed in the ancestral line of one parent in each family. The most frequent of these cancers were soft tissue sarcomas, early onset breast cancers, and other early onset cancers. In fact, three of the mothers of the index children had developed breast cancer before 30 years of age. Other frequently occurring tumors included acute leukemias, brain tumors, and carcinoma of the lung, pancreas, and skin in first- and second-degree relatives and adrenocortical carcinoma in siblings. By making assumptions about family size, the authors estimated that among this series of childhood probands, considerably fewer than one pair of affected siblings would have been expected by chance. The occurrence of cancer in both a parent and a child in these families suggested the possibility of vertical transmission of an oncogenic agent through generations of genetically susceptible individuals.[1] Although it was implied, inherited predisposition on an exclusively genetic basis was not shown directly.

Within the first few years after these initial reports, several other phenotypically similar families were described in which unusual clusterings of cancers were observed.[3–6] In particular, Lynch and colleagues, in describing these pedigrees, coined the term *SBLA syndrome*. The letters represented what the authors considered the principal component tumors: sarcoma (*S*), breast and brain cancer (*B*), leukemia, lung, and laryngeal cancer (*L*), and adrenocortical carcinoma (*A*).[7] Although this terminology was initially prevalent, the syndrome is now more commonly known as the *Li-Fraumeni syndrome*.

It was suggested from the original reports that the familial occurrence of neoplasms originating at discordant sites might represent a counterpart of the tendency for a single individual to develop multiple primary tumors.[1,2] In fact, subsequent epidemiologic studies have confirmed that the neoplasms in LFS tend to develop in children and young adults, often as multiple primary cancers in affected individuals.[8] These studies also provided evidence to indicate that genetic predisposition is a primary causative factor. A follow-up study of the original four families found that over a 12-year period, 10 of the 31 surviving family members had developed 16 additional cancers, in comparison with less than 1 expected from general population rates.[9] These 16 malignancies were of the same types that had been observed originally and included 5 breast cancers, 4 soft tissue sarcomas, and 2 central nervous system tumors. Even after exclusion of the sarcomas that had arisen in the radiation fields of previous tumors, the remaining number of cancers still represented a significant excess above the expected (12 observed, 0.5 expected). Furthermore, 12 of these 16 cancers (primarily sarcomas and breast carcinomas) occurred in family members who had survived their original cancers. Analysis of 200 affected LFS family members in 24 families demonstrated a relative risk of occurrence of a second neoplasm of 5.3, with a cumulative probability of a second cancer occurrence of 57 percent at 30 years postdiagnosis of a first cancer. Over 70 percent of subsequent cancers were component cancers of LFS. The high frequency of second cancers with the same histopathologic diagnosis as types originally described in these families supported the argument in favor of genetic predisposition.

Defining the Classic LFS

Ascertainment biases have complicated interpretation of the original description and subsequent reports of LFS kindreds. These biases develop from the preferential attention given to the most dramatically affected kindreds, the possibility of chance occurrence of cancer in rare families (phenocopies), the uncertainty of the prevalence of the syndrome in the general population, and uncertainties in defining the spectrum of cancers in the syndrome and ultimately in characterizing the penetrance of the predisposing gene or genes.[10] The first attempt to formulate a "definition" of the syndrome was presented by Li and colleagues

Li-Fraumeni Syndrome "Classic" Pedigree

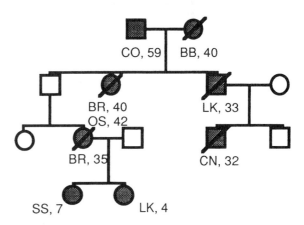

Fig. 23-1 Classic Li-Fraumeni syndrome pedigree. Notable features include the presence of a sarcoma before age 45 years and at least two first-degree relatives with cancer before age 45. In addition, multiple primary tumors occur in an affected member. Note also should be made of the presence of tumors less typical of the component neoplasms of LFS. The pattern of inheritance best fits an autosomal dominant model. BB 5, bilateral breast cancer; BR 5, breast cancer; CN 5, brain tumor; CO 5, colon cancer; LK 5, leukemia; SS 5, soft tissue sarcoma; OS 5, osteosarcoma.

in 1988, based on a prospective analysis of the characteristic component tumors and other detailed information on 24 kindreds.[11] To be eligible for this study, each kindred was required to conform to the following criteria: (1) a bone or soft tissue sarcoma diagnosed under 45 years of age in an individual who was then designated the proband, (2) one first-degree relative of the proband with cancer diagnosed before 45 years of age, and (3) one first- or second-degree relative of the proband in the same lineage with cancer before age 45 years or sarcoma diagnosed at any age.

These criteria have until recently found wide acceptance as a clinical definition of the syndrome, and families that adhere to these criteria have been referred to as having "classic" LFS. Such a family is illustrated in Fig. 23-1. This extensive study revealed continued expression of the dominantly inherited syndrome among young family members. Within the 24 families, 151 blood relatives had developed cancer, and of these cancers, 119 (79 percent) were diagnosed before the age of 45, compared with 10 percent of all cancers in this age range in the general population. Of note, excess occurrences were predominantly confined over time to the six previously described cancer types: breast carcinomas, soft tissue sarcomas, osteosarcomas, leukemias, brain tumors, and adrenocortical carcinomas. Adrenocortical carcinomas were confined to children under 14 years of age. Multiple primary tumors occurred in 15 family members, with the second and subsequent cancers also representing the principal tumor types. The analysis failed to implicate any additional tumors as components of the syndrome. However, subsequent analysis of many families at several major centers as well as in relatively isolated settings has identified cases that resemble the "classic" syndrome yet, in lacking one particular criterion or being associated with other, less frequently observed cancers, fail to meet the most stringent interpretation of the definition.[12–16] Several tumors are now considered to be associated with LFS, including germ-cell tumors,[17] melanoma,[17,18] and prostate and pancreatic cancer.[19] Families with these component tumors have been referred to as *extended LFS*.[20]

Defining LFS-like Families

Several families have been identified which demonstrate the clustering of tumors seen in typical extended LFS families but do not conform to the classic definition. These families have been defined in more than one way, reflecting the confusion arising from the lack of a definitive causative association in all cases. Eeles and colleagues defined *Li-Fraumeni-syndrome-like* (LFS-L) as the clustering of two different tumors seen in extended LFS in individuals who are first- or second-degree relatives with respect to each other and are affected at any age.[20] Birch et al.[16] have suggested that an age restriction of under 60 years be imposed because estimates of age-specific cancer risk in classic LFS are elevated up to but not beyond this point.[10] Further molecular epidemiologic studies are required to clarify the distinction between LFS and LFS-L and to determine the importance of perceived or actual differences.

GENETIC ASPECTS

Classic Genetic Analysis

Williams and Strong[21] and Lustbader et al.[13] performed segregation analyses in hospital-based series of survivors of childhood soft tissue sarcoma patients. Among the first-degree relatives of children in the series, 34 cancers occurred (21 expected), with the excess being predominantly breast cancers and sarcomas diagnosed at a young age. The relatives at the most elevated risk were those of children with soft tissue sarcomas diagnosed at young ages, with sarcomas of embryonal histologic subtype, and with multiple primary sarcomas.[12,19,21] It became evident that the cancer distribution in the families was most compatible with a rare autosomal dominant gene, the gene frequency being equal to 0.00002, or 1 in 50,000. The penetrance was estimated to be almost 50 percent by 30 years and 90 percent by 60 years of age.[21] This point becomes significant for any potential revisions to the original classic definition in that the age limit for tumor occurrence has been increased from 45 years, as established in 1988, to the current 60 years, as recommended by participants in the Third Workshop on Collaborative, Interdisciplinary Studies of *p53* and Li-Fraumeni Syndrome in 1996. The relative risk of developing cancer in children who carried the gene or genes was estimated to be 100 times the background rate. Although the age-specific penetrance was somewhat higher in females, this phenomenon was thought to be due to the occurrence of breast cancer. Maternal and paternal lineages appear to contribute equally to the evidence favoring a dominant gene.[13] These calculations generally have held up to the test of time, even as the genetic etiology of the syndrome has become apparent. Nevertheless, despite the careful phenotypic and statistical study of the syndrome, it became clear that the identification of a defective gene or genes conferring a predisposition in carriers within these families would assist in clarifying the definition of the syndrome.

Searching for an Etiologic "Agent"

Early attempts to isolate the LFS gene or genes were hampered by a variety of factors. The rarity, ambiguity of definition, and infrequent recognition of the syndrome, along with the high mortality among affected family members, significantly reduced the number of available informative tissue and blood samples. Cancers occurring in relatives who were not gene carriers were not histopathologically distinct from cancers in gene carriers. Consistent constitutional karyotypic alterations do not occur in these families, precluding a specific chromosomal site on which to focus a search for the responsible gene. Precancerous conditions such as benign adenomas and associated phenotypic malformations are not characteristic of LFS families and therefore cannot be used to map genes in the same fashion that the presence of aniridia (absence of the iris) was useful in the localization of the Wilms' tumor gene (*WT1*) to chromosome 11p13.[22-24]

Early cytogenetic, immunologic, serologic, and other attempts to determine the biologic basis of LFS were largely uninformative.[25] A report of two families suggested an association of HLA tissue type B12 with the disorder,[6] yet no follow-up of this observation is available. Studies of fibroblast cell lines from affected members of one family showed reduced cell killing by graded doses of ionizing radiation, and apparent activation of the c-*raf*-1 oncogene was reported in one of these lines.[26] However, fibroblasts from other families have demonstrated a normal cytotoxic response.[27] More recently, normal skin fibroblasts derived from affected LFS patients have been shown to exhibit features consistent with immortalization in the absence of stimulation by exogenous oncogenic or viral factors.[28] These features of altered morphology, aneuploidy, anchorage-independent growth, and an extended life span in culture appeared to occur spontaneously.[29] Furthermore, these spontaneously immortalized cells also have been shown to form tumors in nude mice when transformed by an activated Ha-*ras* oncogene,[30] perhaps suggesting that alterations in other genes, including the tumor-suppressor genes, enhance susceptibility to *ras*-induced transformation.

MOLECULAR BIOLOGY OF *p53*

The *p53* Tumor-Suppressor Gene

Comparisons between the frequencies of familial tumors, in particular retinoblastoma and Wilms tumor,[31-33] and their sporadic counterparts led Knudson *et al.*[34] to suggest that the familial forms of some cancers could be explained by the inheritance of constitutional mutations in growth-limiting genes. The resulting inactivation of these genes could facilitate cellular transformation. Inactivations of these growth-limiting, or tumor-suppressor, genes result from mutations in both alleles or a mutation in one allele followed by a loss of or reduction to homozygosity in the second as well as functional or structural alterations of the transcribed message or protein product. Mutant tumor-suppressor genes may be found in either germ cells or somatic cells. In germ cells they arise spontaneously in the gamete or are transmitted from generation to generation within a family.

Alterations of the *p53* tumor-suppressor gene and its encoded protein are the most frequently encountered genetic events in human malignancy.[35-38] The human gene, located on the short arm of human chromosome 17 band 13,[39] is approximately 20 kb in length, yields a 2.8-kb mRNA transcript, and encodes a 53-kDa nuclear phosphoprotein[40] composed of 393 amino acids. The gene contains 11 exons, only the first of which is noncoding. Analysis of the nucleotide and amino acid sequences demonstrates five evolutionarily conserved domains from *Xenopus* to human.[41] Attempts to identify *p53*-like genes in invertebrates such as sea urchins, yeast, and worms have been unsuccessful. The conserved regions are regarded as being essential for the normal function of the wild-type protein. The first conserved domain is contained within the noncoding exon 1; the other four are encompassed by codons 129–146, 171–179, 234–260, and 270–287 in exons 4, 5, 7, and 8, respectively[41] (Fig. 23-2). Several properties of the p53 protein are indicated by the presence of two DNA-binding domains,[42] two SV40 large tumor-antigen (T-Ag) binding sites,[43,44] a nuclear localization signal,[45] an oligomerization domain,[46,47] and several phosphorylation sites.[48]

The p53 protein was identified initially in SV40-transformed cells, where it was thought to be a transformation-specific protein, or tumor antigen, because of its apparent interaction with the large T antigen of the SV40 virus.[40,49] This virus, which is found in monkeys, is a member of the polyomavirus family. These viruses encode viral T-antigen proteins, which are synthesized immediately after infection. The proteins are responsible for the loss of cell growth control that is induced by the virus both *in vitro* and *in vivo*. Transfection assays in rat fibroblast NIH 3T3 cells initially suggested that *p53* was an oncogene because it was capable of immortalizing these cells by itself or of transforming them in conjunction with the *ras* oncogene.[50-52] It was demonstrated subsequently that only mutant forms of p53 conferred these biologic properties, whereas the wild-type protein actually suppressed transformation.[53] Furthermore, it was shown that sequence differences and substantial gene rearrangements occurred in Friend leukemia virus-infected erythroleukemia cells,

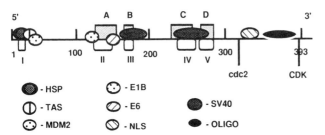

Fig. 23-2 Structural features of the *p53* gene and its encoded protein. The gene encodes a 53-kDa nuclear phosphoprotein. The 393 amino acids are spread over 11 exons. The transcription activation site (TAS), heat shock protein binding site (HSP), SV40 large T antigen binding sites (SV40), nuclear localization signal (NLS), oligomerization domain (OLIGO), and phosphorylation sites (P) all identify potential functional regions. The five evolutionarily conserved domains (HCD I-V) correspond closely to the regions most frequently mutated in sporadic cancer [hotspot regions (HSR A-D)]. Sites of binding of the extracellular E1B 55-kDa protein of adenovirus type 5 (E1B) and the E6 gene product of human papillomavirus types 16 and 18 (E6) are also indicated, as is the position of the MDM2 gene product-binding site (MDM2).

suggesting that an altered form of p53 was involved in the transformation process. Analysis of two colorectal tumors demonstrated allelic deletions of chromosome 17p and expressed high levels of p53 mRNA from the remaining allele. The second allele was shown to harbor a point mutation that changed a valine to alanine at residue 143 in one tumor and changed arginine to histidine at codon 175 in the other.[53a] These observations provided a practical illustration of the Knudson two-hit hypothesis and subsequently were extended by the demonstration of a variety of amino acid substitutions in several different tumor types.[53b] These exciting reports, coupled with the fact that the introduction of wild-type p53 protein blocks the growth of many transformed cells,[54,55] suggest that the normal function of p53 is in fact that of a growth suppressor.[56]

The p53 protein consists of five primary structural regions (see Fig. 23-2). First, an acidic N-terminus acts as a transcriptional activating domain if placed in apposition to DNA through the DNA-binding domain. Second, the internal highly conserved hydrophobic proline-rich region appears to be important in maintaining the overall structural integrity of the protein. Third, the DNA-binding region between amino acid residues 120 and 290 recognizes a DNA sequence motif containing two contiguous or closely spaced monomers 59-(purine)3C(A/T)(A/T)G-(pyrimidine)3-39.[56a,57] Fourth, the highly charged basic region at the C-terminus is required for the formation of homologous p53 tetrameric complexes.[58] Fifth, a nuclear transport sequence spanning codons 316 to 325 aids the protein's localization into the nucleus.[59] p53 is multiply phosphorylated by at least four protein kinases, with two sites being at the N-terminus, which is phosphorylated by a casein kinase I-like enzyme[60] and DNA-dependent protein kinase.[61] The other phosphorylation sites are at the C-terminus, at position 315, phosphorylated by p34cdc2 kinase, and CKII at codon 392, phosphorylated by casein kinase II.[62] The latter enzyme phosphorylates many substrates, including both transcription factors and DNA-binding proteins. The casein kinase II site also acts as a binding site for a ribosomal RNA moiety. These structural features all support the cell cycle control role of p53 activity (see below).

The p53 protein binds specific DNA sequences and appears to be a transcription factor that may regulate the expression of other growth regulatory genes in either a positive or negative manner.[63,64] The introduction of wild-type p53 protein into a variety of transformed cell types inhibits their growth, most likely by blocking progression of cells through the cell cycle late in the G1 phase of cell replication at a checkpoint control site before G1/S.[65-68] Recent evidence also suggests that the antiproliferative

effect of p53 may involve cell cycle regulation at the G2/M restriction point.[69-72] Cells lacking wild-type p53 display an attenuated G2 checkpoint response. The addition of methylxanthines such as caffeine, which are known to disrupt cell cycle arrest at the G2 checkpoint, leads to increased sensitivity of cultured cells to both radio- and chemotherapy.[73,74] Because cells lacking functional p53 have already lost the ability to arrest in G1, the loss of the G2 checkpoint seems to have an additive effect. This observation implies that p53-negative tumor cells may be more responsive to a combination of DNA-damaging agents and agents that abrogate the G2 checkpoint. As a component of a spindle checkpoint, p53 may ensure the maintenance of diploidy during cell cycle progression.[75] p53 may actively participate in maintaining genomic stability through regulation of centrosome duplication or as a monitor that limits centrosome overproduction.[76] Although p53 may not play a major role in the S-phase recombinational events leading to sister chromatid formation,[77] suggesting that conversion of radiation damage to chromatin lesions is independent of p53, the time to peak levels of chromosomal damage is shorter in p53-deficient cells. This observation is consistent with kinetic differences based on specific p53 genotypes. These kinetic differences also have been observed in p53-deficient LFS-derived lymphocytes.[78]

Other functions of p53 are suggested by experiments demonstrating that reentry of resting cells into the cell cycle can be blocked by the introduction of anti-p53 antibodies or antisense p53 cDNA fragments.[79,80] p53 may potentiate cell differentiation in this manner. Early work suggested that wild-type p53 could be involved in restricting precursor cell populations by mediating apoptosis, or programmed cell death, in the absence of appropriate differentiation or proliferation signals.[81,82] In p53-deficient thymocytes, substantial resistance to apoptotic induction by radiation was observed compared with wild-type littermates.[83,84] These observations were corroborated in solid tumors in nude mice subjected to radiation or chemotherapy.[85] Strikingly, acquired resistance could be induced by repeated low doses of radiation, with acquired *p53* mutations being observed in 50 percent of tumors. The relative degree of radioresistance and apoptosis seems to be cell type-specific, for in colorectal carcinoma cells lines and head and neck squamous cell cancer cell lines lacking functional p53,[86,87] significant differences in response compared with wild-type counterparts could not be demonstrated.

As suggested earlier, cells that either lack *p53* gene expression or overexpress mutant p53 do not exhibit G1 arrest. The fidelity of DNA repair during cell cycle arrest may play a role in the capacity of cells to tolerate radiation injury and therefore have an impact on radiation sensitivity. It has been reported in this context that p53 may play a role in the cellular response to γ-radiation damage, ultraviolet light, or certain chemotherapeutic drugs through inhibition of DNA synthesis[84,85,88-93] after DNA damage and thereby provide a cell cycle "checkpoint."[94,95] This response is particularly effective in the setting of double-strand DNA breaks. The *in vitro* effect has been observed in vivo in SCID mice carrying xenografts treated with either adriamycin or γ-irradiation.[96]

Transcriptional targets of *p53* include *mdm-2*, a gene that is commonly amplified in human sarcomas and is involved in a negative regulatory system that terminates a cell's response to DNA damage.[97,98] Other targets include a cyclin of unknown function called *cyclin G1*[99]; Bax, a promoter of apoptosis[100]; GADD45, a DNA repair protein[101]; and p21CIP1/WAF1 a multifunctional regulatory and the best candidate to date for the control of cell cycle arrest.[102-104] The abundant increases in p53 protein expression induced by ionizing radiation lead to the transcription of p21CIP1/WAF1. This inhibits cyclin-dependent kinase activity, which is in turn required for entry into S phase and DNA replication. Furthermore, p21CIP1/WAF1 also binds and inhibits a subunit of DNA polymerase called *poliferating cell nuclear antigen* (PCNA) directly,[105] thereby blocking DNA replication.

GADD45 is also induced by stresses that arrest cell growth or agents that induce DNA damage. Like p21[CIP1/WAF1], GADD45 has been shown to bind PCNA to induce excision repair of damaged DNA by a poorly understood mechanism.[106] p53 also binds ERCCC3, an excision repair molecule that recognizes and removes damaged DNA segments.[107] Taken together, these observations suggest that p53 may inhibit DNA replication through p21 while simulating DNA repair through GADD45 or ERCC3 simultaneously.

Structural analysis of the p53 core-DNA co-crystal using x-ray diffraction,[108] as well as the oligomerization domain using multidimensional nuclear magnetic resonance (NMR) spectroscopy,[109,109a] suggests that several highly conserved amino acid residues within the central core form actual contacts at the minor or major grooves of the DNA helix. Furthermore, each monomeric unit of p53 interacts with another subunit; the resulting dimer in turn interacts with another dimer, forming a four-helix bundle or p53 tetramer. It is believed that this cooperative binding greatly facilitates interactions with p53 response elements.[110]

Inactivation of p53 function occurs via several mechanisms. The occurrence of missense mutations, deletions, or nonsense mutations of the gene prevents the protein from oligomerizing and forming tetrameric complexes that can bind specific DNA sequences.[111] In fact, representative mutants from each of the four mutation hotspot regions (see Fig. 23-2.) have been tested for binding to p53-binding sites *in vitro* and for activation of p53-binding site reporter gene expression *in vivo* and *in vitro*. The majority of mutants lose the ability to bind p53-binding sites and therefore cannot activate expression of adjacent reporter genes.[56,112–114] Some mutations alter the conformation of the p53 protein, exposing epitopes that may alter certain functional properties. Because these properties are found in only a fraction of *p53* mutants, they are unlikely to be central to *p53* function. Nevertheless, the possibility remains that subtle genetic changes induce conformational alterations that affect the structure of functionally important domains distant from the mutation sites.[111] The impact of subtle genetic changes to *p53* may be exemplified by recent suggestions that a commonly observed polymorphism may in fact not be functionally neutral. Conformational changes of a mutant molecule also can affect wild-type molecules complexed with the mutant form within tetramers, preventing the complex from binding to DNA and transcriptionally activating reporter genes.[112,114,115] In fact, the vast majority of *p53* mutations are missense in nature,[116] accounting for upward of 85 percent of reported gene alterations. This observation is in stark contrast to many other genes in which variably sized deletions, alterations, or splice site defects are reported.

Inactivation of the p53 protein through binding of other cellular proteins also may prevent normal binding and thus prevent transcriptional activation.[117,118] Some of the DNA tumor virus genes, including SV40 T antigen, the *E1B* gene of adenovirus, and the *E6* gene of human papillomavirus, encode proteins that bind to p53. In cells that coexpress one of these viral oncoproteins along with p53, expression of p53-inducible reporter genes cannot be activated.[118] This inhibition of expression may be critical for viral replication and/or cell transformation. Disruption of normal p53 function also may be altered by alteration of *mdm-2*, a cellular gene that was identified originally by virtue of its amplification in a spontaneously transformed mouse cell line.[97,98,117,119] The Mdm-2 gene product binds to p53, resulting in inhibition of the ability of p53 to transactivate genes adjacent to p53-binding sites. At least in human sarcomas, the amplification of *Mdm-2* may lead to consequent overexpression of Mdm-2, which probably interferes with p53 activity.[97,120] Finally, p53 interactions with other tumor-suppressor genes have been observed. Interaction with the Wilms' tumor gene (*WT1*) in transfected cells modulates the ability of each protein to transactivate its targets.[121] Coincident mutations in *p53* and the retinoblastoma susceptibility gene (*RB1*) cooperate in transformation of certain cell types in mice.[122,123]

Tumor suppressors frequently have functional and structural cousins. Recent work suggests that p53 belongs to a larger group of related proteins. First, the gene *p73* was discovered to encode a protein sequence similar to that of p53, particularly in the core DNA-binding domain. *p73* is localized to chromosome 1p36.33 in a region frequently deleted in a wide range of tumors including neuroblastoma, breast cancer, melanoma, and hepatocellular carcinoma. Expression of a single copy of the wild-type gene in the absence of mutations of the remaining allele has been observed in several tumor types, although initial speculation that *p73* was a novel tumor suppressor gene that may be imprinted has not been validated. p73 may be functionally similar to p53 in that when overexpressed, it activates transcription of p53-responsive genes (i.e., p21[CIP1]) and inhibits cell growth in a p53-like manner by inducing apoptosis. In distinction to p53, p73 is not induced following exposure to UV radiation, nor do p73-deficient mice develop cancer. The sequence and functional similarities between p53 and p73 make the latter an obvious candidate to examine both as a potential predisposing gene in wt-p53 LFS and LFS-L families, as well as a modifier of cellular phenotype in *p53*-mutant individuals. It ultimately also will be important to examine whether p73 alterations modify the response of LFS cell lines to DNA-damaging agents. Similarly, isolation of two proteins, p51 and p40, encoded by the alternatively spliced mRNA products of a gene located on chromosome 3q28 offers further opportunities to study functionally and structurally related p53 homologues. Although the p51 sequence more closely resembles that of p73 rather than p53, p51 expression in Saos-2 cells leads to suppression of colony formation, as well as apoptotic cell death and activation of p21[CIP1]. Somatic mutations of the gene are rare (examined to date in nonsarcomatous tumors including neuroblastoma, brain tumors, and carcinoma of lung, pancreas, liver, breast and colon), suggesting that inactivation of p51 may occur through alternative mechanisms. *p51* and *p73* may serve as backup genes whose expression is induced by the loss of p53 function, or *p51* and *p73* may provide tumor-suppressor functions in cells lacking p53. The potential for germ-line alterations in genes that are structurally similar to *p53* to play a role in human carcinogenesis in the absence of *p53* alterations is intriguing and an area of intense study. Furthermore, p51/p63-deficient mice develop a spectrum of developmental abnormalities that closely resemble the human phenotype EEC (ectrodactyly, ectodermal dysplasia, cleft lip) in which germline p63 mutations have been identified. Humans and mice deficient in this gene are not at apparent increased susceptibility to cancer.[123a]

Therefore, although the precise functions of p53 are not clear, models have been proposed to account for the many observations summarized above.[94,124] In a cell with normal p53, levels of the protein rise in response to DNA damage mediated by pRB1,[125] and the cell arrests before the G1/S transition. At this point, genomic repair or apoptosis ensues, with the mechanism being determined by the transforming oncoprotein or oncoproteins. In cells in which the p53 pathway has been inactivated by gene mutations or by host or viral oncoprotein interactions, G1 arrest does not occur and damaged DNA is replicated. During mitosis, the presence of damaged DNA results in mutation, aneuploidy, mitotic failure, and cell death. p53 alterations are necessary but not sufficient for the ultimate cancer that arises from these malignant clones, since other genetic events are clearly required.

Patient Mutations

Inactivating mutations of the *p53* gene and disruptions of the p53 protein have been associated with some fraction of virtually every sporadically occurring malignancy. Included among these are osteosarcomas,[126] soft tissue sarcomas,[127] rhabdomyosarcomas,[128] leukemias,[129,130] brain tumors,[131] and carcinomas of the lung[132] and breast.[133] Together, these tumors account for more than two-thirds of the cancers in selected series of LFS families[2,11,134] (Fig. 23-3). Transgenic mice that overexpress mutant alleles of the *p53* gene in the presence of two wild-type alleles produce offspring

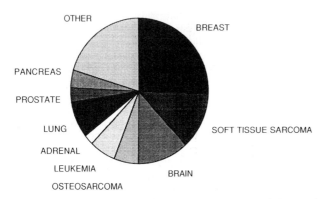

Fig. 23-3 Relative incidence of tumor types by age in 24 Li-Fraumeni syndrome families. The frequencies are confounded by the means of ascertainment, in this case through the proband, who has a sarcoma and who was therefore excluded from the tabulations. (*Adapted from Garber et al.[10] Used by permission.*)

Location of Human Germline *p53* Mutations

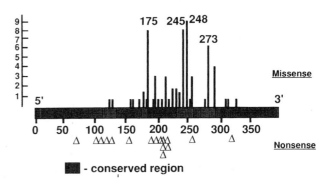

Fig. 23-4 Sites and frequency of reported human germ-line *p53* mutations. The horizontal axis represents the codon number; the vertical axis indicates the number of reported mutations. Missense mutations are designated above the *p53* cartoon, while nonsense mutations are seen below the cartoon. It is noteworthy that the four most frequently cited amino acid residues are at codons 175, 245, 248, and 273—not dissimilar to acquired mutations.

with a high incidence of osteosarcoma, lung adenocarcinoma, lymphoma, and rhabdomyosarcoma.[135]

Based on these observations, five LFS families were studied to determine whether *p53* played any role in the occurrence of cancer in affected family members. Base-pair mutations were identified in the germ line of affected members in each of the five families studied.[136] These missense mutations were all found within one highly conserved region of the gene, affecting codons 245, 248 (two families), 252, and 258 of the *p53* gene. In fact, subsequent analysis of one of the families revealed the codon 252 change to be artifactual; a 2-bp deletion was identified at codon 184 in exon 5.[137] This observation raises concerns with respect to the application of research technology in gene analysis to the clinical setting, as will be discussed below. Tumors in affected individuals who were tested had lost the remaining wild-type allele.[136] Furthermore, analysis of one of these families, using a highly polymorphic DNA sequence telomeric of *p53*, confirmed the cosegregation of the abnormal *p53* allele with the polymorphism. Unaffected members could be identified as gene carriers, suggesting that they might be at risk of developing cancer at a later date. After this initial report, a sixth classic LFS family was reported with another constitutional mutation in the same region as the previously identified ones.[137] In this family, however, one affected member was not a carrier of the mutant gene, suggesting that the mechanism of tumor formation in this individual did not involve *p53*. The apparent clustering of germ-line *p53* mutations in a short span of 14 codons within a highly conserved domain initially sparked much speculation about its possible significance, with suggestions that germ-line mutations may be restricted and that other mutations may be lethal in this context.[138] However, extensive analysis of other classic LFS families and subsequently several clinical scenarios of LFS-L phenotypes demonstrated the wide spectrum of germ-line *p53* mutations that were not dissimilar to those observed in sporadic tumors (Fig. 23-4).

Several families that fit the operative definition of LFS have been studied. Isolated families with germ-line *p53* mutations have been reported.[139,140] However, one study of eight families from the Manchester registry in England suggested that mutations of the *p53* gene would not be found in all classic LFS families.[141] Only two of these families were shown initially to carry germ-line mutations when only exon 7 was examined. Further analysis of other exons has still demonstrated the apparent absence of mutations within exons 5 to 8 in some of these families.[142] Ongoing studies suggest that not all classic LFS families have detectable germ-line mutations of the *p53* gene. In one quite typical Li-Fraumeni kindred, although no *p53* gene mutations were identified, overexpression of wild-type p53 was observed, suggesting that the biologically or biochemically altered protein yielded a similar phenotype to the mutant gene, perhaps by one of

the several mechanisms described above.[143] Subsequent analysis of this family has in fact confirmed the presence of a point mutation. This observation again points out the evolution of technologic improvements in studying the genetics of LFS. Evidence from several studies conducted in the United States, France, and the United Kingdom[16,144,145] suggests that the actual frequency of germ-line *p53* mutations in classic LFS families is somewhere between 50 and 70 percent. In the French series, germ-line *p53* mutations were particularly associated with families in which a young child was affected with rhabdomyosarcoma, while in the U.K. series the mutations appeared to be associated with families that included children with rhabdomyosarcoma and/or adrenocortical carcinoma. It is likely that as the clinical definition is expanded, the rate of germ-line *p53* mutations observed will increase.

The lack of 100 percent concordance between *p53* mutations and the classic phenotype may be explained in several ways. It is possible that post-translational *p53* alterations, as described previously,[143,146] occur more frequently than has been found to date. Recently, mutations outside the most commonly cited hotspot regions have been identified, particularly in the oligomerization domain.[146a] Presumably, more of these types of mutations will be discovered as these regions of the gene are analyzed more extensively. Evidence for endogenous promoter defects leading to aberrant expression of the p53 message has been sought with inconclusive success. Complete *p53* deletion, the effects of modifier genes, or alterations of other genes that may influence the phenotype generated by the presence of a specific germ-line *p53* alteration also have been postulated. Several groups have examined the potential causal association of inherited mutations in other tumor-suppressor genes with LFS. To date, these studies have been noninformative for germline alterations of PTEN, p16[INK4a], and p19[Arf]. Other genes involved in p53-mediated cellular growth regulation have also been examined. The recent observation of heterozygous germline mutations in the checkpoint kinase h*CHK2* in one LFS and one LFS-like family suggests an alternative mechanism for functional p53 inactivation.[146b] This gene is the human homolog of the yeast Cds1 and Rad53 G2 checkpoint kinases that are involved in preventing entry into mitosis in response to DNA damage.[146c] Although the checkpoint kinase pathway genes may be implicated in cancer predisposition in this setting, their impact is somewhat controversial in light of more recent findings indicating a lack of functional alterations of h*CHK2* in LFS patients lacking germline p53 mutations.[146d,146e] Despite these gaps, the high frequency of germ-line *p53* mutations in LFS families and the tight association of tumor formation in p53-deficient mice (see below) confirm a causal association of germ-line *p53* alterations and cancer predisposition.

Patient Mutations: Non-LFS

As DNA screening techniques improved, it became possible to analyze large populations of patients for constitutional abnormalities of the *p53* gene. Several recent studies have demonstrated that certain groups of "high risk" patients and their families carry germ-line *p53* mutations that presumably predispose them to the development of their respective malignancies. Germ-line *p53* mutations may be inherited from a parent who is healthy at the time when cancer is diagnosed in the child. Numerous studies of non-LFS patients and families have helped characterize the genetic heterogeneity of the p53 carrier state.

A striking feature of LFS kindreds is the high frequency, approaching 50 percent, of affected members who develop multiple primary neoplasms.[9] One multicenter study demonstrated germ-line mutations of the *p53* tumor-suppressor gene in leukocyte DNA from 4 of 59 patients (6.8 percent) who had survived second cancers but did not have family histories compatible with LFS.[147] Although one mutation at codon 248 in exon 7 was identical to that previously implicated in LFS,[136] three other mutations at codons 273, 282, and 325 had not been reported previously in the germ line. In addition to implicating codons outside the classically defined conserved regions of the *p53* gene, this study demonstrated the occurrence of germ-line *p53* mutations in patients with cancers not commonly represented among LFS component tumors. These included non-Hodgkin lymphoma, colon and gastric carcinoma, and neuroblastoma. A subsequent analysis of four patients with multifocal osteosarcoma and no family history of cancer demonstrated one apparently *de novo* germ-line *p53* mutation.[148] A similar analysis of patients with multifocal glioma demonstrated a very high frequency of germ-line *p53* mutations, although several of these individuals had family histories consistent with LFS or LFS-L.[148a] This observation suggests that other cancer patients who present with multiple nonfamilial tumors carry germ-line *p53* mutations.

An extensive analysis of 196 patients with malignant sarcomas was reported along with the second tumor study cited earlier.[149] Exons 2 through 11 were screened, thereby encompassing the complete coding region of the gene as well as less frequently evaluated regions. Eight of these 196 (4 percent) harbored germ-line *p53* mutations, and 5 of the 8 mutations were identified in patients from families with a high incidence of cancer. Both missense and nonsense germ-line mutations were found. The nonsense mutations arose as a result of a single-base frameshift mutation involving an insertion in two cases, a two-base deletion in one case, and the direct creation of a stop codon in one case. All occurred in codons outside the conserved domains (codons 71–72, 151–152, and 209–210), and all presumably yield a truncated p53 protein. Novel mutations, as well as the passage of a mutant allele for generations in at least one family, also were observed. In these cases, as in the previously described study, the affected individual presented a history that was not entirely consistent with LFS. This study also confirmed the observation of neutral polymorphisms within the *p53* sequence that must be evaluated carefully to rule out their disease-associated potential. One of these, at codon 213 in exon 6 (a nonconserved region), has been identified frequently in sporadic tumors.[116,127] Finally, this study pointed out the vagaries of the clinical definition of LFS in that one family with definitive germ-line inheritance of *p53* mutations had an excess of gastric carcinoma, a tumor that is thought to be rare in the operative definition of the syndrome. However, this family is from Japan, a country with a significantly higher incidence of gastric carcinoma than exists in North American or European populations. Other factors, both genetic and environmental, may influence the types of tumors that arise in patients who are carriers of the same *p53* germ-line mutations.

Although sarcomas and multiple primary cancers in affected patients constitute the most consistent characteristic features of the LFS phenotype, certain other cancers are also commonly represented. Among these, early onset breast cancer is most frequently encountered. However, little is known about the frequency of germ-line *p53* mutations in breast cancer patients outside families with classic LFS. Using a hydroxylamine mismatch base-pair technique, 5 families with early onset breast cancer were screened for constitutional mutations in all 11 exons of the *p53* gene.[150] No mutations were identified in these families, suggesting that *p53* probably did not play a significant role in the genesis of hereditary early onset breast cancer. These observations are also supported by another study that screened 25 breast cancer families in which no germ-line mutations of the gene were found in exons 5 through 9.[151] Nevertheless, in a third study, 1 of 67 unselected breast cancer patients and 1 of 40 early onset breast cancer patients were found to be carriers of mutant *p53*.[152] The mutation found in the unselected patient was at codon 181 (exon 5). The patient's pedigree showed a strong family history of cancer, although it did not quite fit the classic definition of LFS, since the relative with sarcoma was 47 years old (i.e., older than 45) at the time of diagnosis. In addition, studies of other family members as well as functional studies of the mutant gene suggest that this codon 181 mutation may be functionally silent and may not impart any increased cancer risk.[153] By contrast, the mutation found in the early onset breast cancer patient was at codon 245, a highly conserved amino acid. The identical mutation was identified in the patient's mother, who also had breast cancer. These findings suggest that germ-line *p53* mutations occur rarely in early onset breast cancer outside of LFS families and are corroborated by similar results reported elsewhere.[154] It is clear that other genetic events are responsible for the genesis of this familial cancer clustering. In fact, two genes for early onset hereditary breast cancer have been isolated, *BRCA1* and *BRCA2*, and intense efforts are in progress to fully characterize the mutational spectrum, genotype-phenotype correlation, and clinical implications of these genes. In light of the enormous efforts in characterizing the *BRCA* genes, it must be kept in mind that perhaps 1 percent of familial breast cancer may be due to germ-line *p53* mutations—a not insubstantial frequency.

Initial surveys of patients ascertained solely by the presence of a neoplasm that is a component tumor of LFS have yielded interesting observations. Adrenocortical carcinoma (ADCC) occurs rarely in the pediatric cancer population.[155] However, in LFS kindreds it is not uncommon to encounter at least one affected individual with this tumor.[11,16] Analysis of five patients with ADCC demonstrated inherited germ-line *p53* mutations in three.[156] Each of the families had cancer constellations that were consistent with LFS. In a survey of children with apparently sporadic adrenocortical carcinoma, 3 of 6 (50 percent) harbored germ-line *p53* mutations, and in one the alteration was demonstrated to be inherited from the child's mother, who subsequently developed breast cancer.[157] Subsequent studies have suggested that, in fact, the frequency of low penetrant p53 mutations may approach 80 percent in children with ADCC.[157a]

Two studies of childhood sarcoma patients confirmed the presence of germ-line *p53* mutations in a small fraction of those who lacked striking family histories of cancer. Among 235 children with osteosarcoma, 7 (3 percent) were found to carry mutations, and 3 of these 7 lacked a family history of cancer.[158] A similar survey of 33 childhood rhabdomyosarcoma patients identified 3 (9 percent) with germ-line *p53* mutations.[159] Although no association between the presence of mutations and histopathologic subtype or tumor grade was noted, it was of interest that the average age at onset of the tumors in children carrying germ-line *p53* mutations was lower than that of children with wild-type *p53* ($p < 0.06$), suggesting that the biologic nature of the tumors may be different.

A screen of primary lymphoblasts from 25 pediatric patients with acute lymphoblastic leukemia identified *p53* mutations in 4, one of whom was shown to harbor the mutation (in exon 8) in the remission marrow, suggesting its germ-line origin.[160] The

Table 23-1 Types of *p53* Mutations Found in the Germ Line

Mutation	Li-Fraumeni Syndrome, %	Li-Fraumeni Like Syndrome, %
Missense	70	84
Transition	81	67
Transversion	19	33
CpG site	69	4
Nonsense	4	4
Insertion/deletion	26	12

Table 23-2 Estimated Frequency of Germ-Line *p53* Mutations in Specific Cancer Patients and Families

Clinical Phenotype	Mutation Frequency, %
LFS and ADCC	75−100
LFS	50−85
LFS variant	10−30
Multisite cancer (non-LFS)	0−20
Sporadic ADCC	40−70
Sporadic rhabdomyosarcoma	5−15
Osteosarcoma	1−10
Second neoplasms	5−15
Early onset breast cancer	1

proband's family history was consistent with LFS. An analysis of primary lymphoblasts in affected members of 10 familial leukemia pedigrees identified two families in which nonhereditary *p53* alterations were present.[161] These included a 2-bp deletion in exon 6 in one and a codon 248 missense mutation in the other. Therefore, although leukemia represents a common component tumor of LFS, it appears that germ-line mutations of *p53* in primary leukemia patients are rare events. However, it is possible that when such alterations do exist in the germ line, they are potentially associated with an increased risk of secondary acute myelogenous leukemia related to prior treatment of the primary cancer with topoisomerase inhibitors.[162]

Most published germ-line *p53* mutations occur in the conserved regions of the gene and are missense in nature. There are no obvious differences in the mutation types or sites between LFS and LFS-L families. Approximately 75 percent are transitions, and the majority of these occur at CpG dinucleotides (Table 23-1). Transversions and occasional base-pair deletions or insertions also have been described. Three examples of intronic mutations have been reported. A novel germ-line *p53* splice-acceptor site mutation was found in a family that closely resembles the breast-ovarian cancer syndrome and in which the proband had a choroid plexus carcinoma.[163] This mutation, involving a single-base substitution in intron 5, results in deletion of exon 6 and creation of a frameshift leading to a premature stop codon in exon 7 that is thought to yield significant disruptions of the message. Another report identified a point mutation in the splice donor site of intron 4, leading to an aberrant larger transcript that could be detected in both tumor and constitutional DNA.[164] The third example is somewhat more unusual in that the mutation, detected in intron 5, consisted of a deletion of an 11-bp sequence that involved a region of splicing recognition. Like the first example, this deletion resulted in deletion of exon 6 and a premature stop codon in exon 7.[165] All three pedigrees resembled LSF but were more consistent with the LFS-L phenotype.

Whether specific germ-line *p53* mutations are more penetrant and are associated with different cancer phenotypes has not been resolved. Studies of possible correlations between mutation type and cancer phenotype are limited by the relative lack of fully characterized families. Furthermore, the influence of external factors on the development of malignancy in carriers is also unknown. One would expect that exposure to occupational or environmental carcinogens will contribute to the precise determination of cancer type and age at onset. At least superficially, however, it does not appear that the pattern of germ-line alterations of *p53* differs significantly from that of somatic mutations. Perhaps as more genotype-phenotype studies are performed, a distinctive pattern will emerge.

The studies described above clearly demonstrate that patients with germ-line *p53* mutations cannot be identified solely by a review of the family's history of cancer. The method by which the proband was ascertained will influence the frequency of carriers in the study population (Table 23-2). It has been shown that germ-line *p53* mutations may be inherited from a parent who has no clinical evidence of cancer at the time the disease is diagnosed in the child. A tumor may arise in a child before one does in the

parent as a result of the presumed stochastic acquisition of one or more additional genetic abnormalities in the cell that give rise to the malignant clone. Multicenter studies are in progress to determine the frequency of germ-line *p53* mutations in patients afflicted with other component tumors of LFS. These, as well as studies of non-LFS cancer-prone families, will help characterize the genetic heterogeneity of the *p53* carrier status.

Molecular Genetic Approaches to LFS Patients

As both the biologic and biochemical characteristics of *p53* have been elucidated, it also has been important to attempt to establish the functional significance of germ-line *p53* mutations and the structural features of the corresponding mutant p53 proteins. In addition, before associating a germ-line *p53* mutation with the development of cancer, one must carefully determine its functional significance. In one particularly extensive analysis, seven distinct *p53* mutations identified from LFS families were studied.[153] Oligonucleotide-directed mutagenesis of the *p53* cDNA was performed to generate mutant clones that could then be subcloned into expression vectors for transfection assays. The structural properties of the germ-line *p53* mutants showed a high degree of variability. However, with the exception of one mutant, at codon 181, none of the germ-line mutants retained all the structural features of the wild-type protein. Six of seven missense mutations disrupted the growth inhibitory properties and structure of the wild-type p53 protein. One mutation, at codon 181, was not recognized by the antibody PAb240, which recognizes an epitope specific for a mutant conformation,[166] and did not appear to alter the ability to suppress cell growth when transfected into Saos-2 osteosarcoma cells. Genetic analysis of this mutation demonstrated that it was not always associated with the development of cancer in the family from which it was derived. The mutation was not present in a member of the kindred who had developed two cancers, and the codon 181 mutant gene, not the normal allele, was somatically lost in tumor tissue from a cancer in another relative. It thus became apparent that certain germ-line mutations of *p53* might change the amino acid sequence in a conserved domain yet not be associated with an increased cancer risk.[153]

The functional significance of heterozygous germ-line mutations in members of LFS families also has been examined through the expression of the mutant *p53* allele in normal skin fibroblasts.[167] It was observed that both normal and mutant p53 RNA is expressed at low levels. In contrast to the transfection studies, the normal skin fibroblasts provide a system in which both wild-type and mutant *p53* alleles are naturally expressed at similarly low levels without potentially interfering dosage effects. Based on the studies demonstrating that mutant *p53* may inactivate the transcriptional activity of the wild-type protein, it has been postulated that direct analysis of the transcriptional activity of p53 expressed in fibroblasts or lymphocytes should permit the detection of inactivating germ-line mutations.[168] Using a short-term biologic assay in which p53 cDNA was amplified from cells and cloned into a eukaryotic expression vector that was then transfected with a reporter plasmid for the transcriptional activity of p53 into Saos-2 cells lacking p53, analysis of transcriptional activation could be performed. This assay demonstrated transcriptional activity in two of five and three of five clones from two LFS patients, respectively, indicating the presence of both wild-type and mutant p53 in these cells. The rapidity and apparent sensitivity of this assay suggest that it may be valuable as a functional screen. Yet another functional assay has been described that takes advantage of the fact that plasmids can be generated by homologous recombination *in vivo* in the yeast *S. cerevisiae*.[169] By this method, p53 is tested for its ability to activate transcription from a promoter containing p53-binding sites in these yeast. Cotransformation of a p53 PCR product and a cut promoter-containing plasmid results in repair of the plasmid with the PCR product *in vivo* and constitutive expression of full-length human p53 protein in the yeast. Clones that have repaired the plasmid are selected on media lacking leucine, and subsequent screening for histidine prototrophy identifies colonies that contain transcriptionally active p53.[169] This assay has the advantage of being rapid (less than 5 days) and having few steps, although it does assume that cancer-causing mutations of *p53* are defective in transactivation. Subsequent improvements in the efficiency of this assay have increased the spectrum of mutants, including temperature-sensitive forms that can be functionally evaluated.[170] Nevertheless, even this assay will miss mutant p53 if one considers growth arrest that is not dependent on transcriptional activation as the functional yardstick.

The combined value of appropriate multiple functional assays, standard DNA sequence analysis, and careful evaluation of the inheritance pattern of a potential mutation cannot be overestimated in conferring a significant level of confidence to the clinical relevance of a germ-line *p53* gene sequence alteration with respect to the patient's disease or the risk to unaffected relatives.

Animal Models

Transgenic animals that carry distinct deregulated oncogenes develop tumors that appear to be cell-type-specific. Because of difficulties in studying the effects of the genetic defects and potential interventions in humans, the development of mouse models that reflect the human genotype provides formidable tools with which to study the role of natural germ-line *p53* mutations in carcinogenesis and perhaps to develop treatment regimens. To better study *p53 in vivo*, several mouse models have been created that either lack functional p53 or express dominant-negative mutant alleles that inhibit wild-type p53 function. These animals have been used to study the interactions of p53 with other cell cycle regulatory elements that function in a p53-dependent or -independent manner. Furthermore, studies of both germ-line and somatic alterations in p53 in mice have greatly enhanced our understanding of the pathobiologic role of this gene in carcinogenesis.

The first attempt to determine the *in vivo* role of p53 in neoplasia involved generating *p53* transgenic mice that carry transgenes encoding for a p53 protein that differs from wild-type p53 either by a ^{193}Arg → Pro or by a ^{135}Ala → Val substitution.[135] The transgenes are under the transcriptional control of the endogenous promoter, and the mice carry the normal wild-type *p53* complement. Thus they weakly resemble the human *p53* genotype, although neither mutation has been implicated in LFS. The transgene was expressed in a wide range of tissues, yet tumors (primarily osteosarcomas, lymphomas, and adenocarcinomas of the lung) occur in only 20 percent of the mice, suggesting the presence of intrinsic tissue-specific differences. These mice provided a model with which to analyze the interactions of genetic and environmental factors in influencing cancer predisposition. For example, on infection of the *p53* transgenics with the polychythemia-inducing strain of Friend leukemia virus (FV-P), the animals progressed to the late stage of erythroleukemia more rapidly than did normal mice.[171] In addition, Friend leukemic cell lines derived from the *p53* transgenic mice overproduce mutant

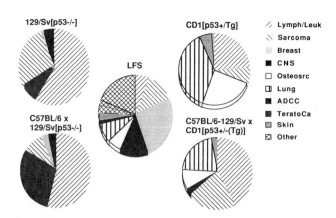

Fig. 23-5 Spectrum of tumors in *p53* mouse models compared with the human LFS phenotype. Not all tumors are represented; rather, those most frequently encountered with the category "other" contain isolated reports within specific mouse models. The particular mouse strain and the *p53* genotype are indicated above each pie.

p53 protein and demonstrate a high rate of rearrangement of the *ets*-related *Spi-1* oncogene, as had been reported previously in similar lines derived from nontransgenic animals. Thus p53 appears to play a rate-limiting role in the progression of the disease, with its mutant form present as an early event that accelerates neoplastic transformation. This transgenic model in fact contributed to the hypothesis that the tumor spectrum in LFS may arise from the transmission of a mutant *p53* gene (Fig. 23-5).

Because p53 is implicated in cell cycle control, it was proposed that this protein may be essential for normal embryonic development.[172] Although p53 is virtually ubiquitously expressed in murine tissues, its relatively short half-life of 20 min (wild-type conformation) yields generally low total protein levels. The amount of p53 mRNA expressed in developing mouse embryos reaches a maximum at 9 to 11 days, after which levels fall markedly.[173] Homologous recombination has been used in mouse embryonic stem (ES) cells to derive null alleles of *p53*.[172,174,175] Two models have been developed from the replacement with a neo^r cassette of exons 2 through 6 of the gene.[174,175] The third model includes an insertion of a *pol*II promoter-driven neo^r cassette into exon 5, together with a deletion of 350 nucleotides of intron 4 and 106 nucleotides of exon 5.[172] None of the *p53*$^{-/-}$ mice express detectable intact or truncated mRNA or protein. The mutant *p53* allele has been established in the germ line of chimeric mice with mixed inbred (C57Bl/6 × 129/Sv),[172,175] pure 129/Sv,[176] or 129/Ola[174,176] backgrounds. In all these situations, spontaneous development of different tumor types, principally lymphomas and sarcomas, occurred in more than 75 percent of the animals before 6 months of age. In heterozygotes (*p53*$^{+/-}$), tumor development, predominantly sarcoma, is delayed. Nevertheless, by 18 months of age, approximately 50 percent have developed neoplasms. Interestingly, multiple primary tumors have been noted in approximately 30 percent of the tumor-bearing *p53*$^{-/-}$ mice. In all mouse backgrounds, virtually none of the *p53*$^{+/+}$ animals had developed tumors by 18 months of age.

The importance of genetic background in influencing specific tumor type is best exemplified by the occurrence of unusual cancers, including pineoblastomas and islet-cell tumors, in *p53*$^{-/-}$ mice crossed with mice heterozygous for an *RB1* mutation in exon 3 of that gene.[122,123] In addition to these unusual tumor phenotypes, these mice had decreased viability and demonstrated other uncharacteristic pathologies, including bronchial epithelial hyperplasia and retinal dysplasia. Interestingly, in this situation the mechanism by which the *RB1* allele was knocked out may be significant in the cancer phenotype that is derived from the intercross. Deletion of exon 20 of *RB1* when crossed with $p53^{-/-}$ animals yields animals with a variety of endocrine tumors, including pituitary adenomas, medullary carcinoma of the thyroid, and parathyroid carcinomas, in addition to the previously mentioned islet-cell tumors.[123] Surprisingly, no pineoblastomas are found. In both intercross models, the accumulation of abnormal genetic events results in an increased rate of tumorigenesis. Thus, as the number of null alleles of each tumor-suppressor gene is increased, the age at onset decreases and the rate of tumorigenesis increases.

The relative lack of strain-to-strain variability in the *p53*-null-induced phenotype suggests that the *p53* genotype is important in dictating phenotype. Evidence from other genetic crosses supports this premise. For example, adenomatous polyposis coli (APC)-mutant (*Min*) mice develop bowel adenomas with malignant potential. This malignant phenotype demonstrates great strain-to-strain variability, and in fact, the development of malignant tumors is accelerated and modified when they are outbred to different genetic backgrounds, in particular to one carrying a modifier of *Min* termed *Mom*-1.[177] It is likely that similar or other variations of the *p53*-null-induced phenotype can be induced in a like manner by the interaction of modifier genes that play a role in the development of p53-induced tumors.

The interaction of genetic events in early embryonic development has been facilitated by the use of *p53*-null animals. As was described earlier, amplification of the *mdm*-2 gene product is thought to represent an alternative mechanism for preventing p53 function in tumor development. Recently, it was shown that Mdm-2-null mice are not viable, being embryonically lethal near the time of implantation.[178] However, when mice heterozygous for *mdm*-2 were crossed with those heterozygous for *p53*, viable progeny homozygous for both *p53* and *mdm*-2 were obtained.[178,179] These observations suggest that a critical *in vivo* function of Mdm-2 is the negative regulation of p53 activity.

Provocative studies have tested whether the tumorigenic activity of a mutant *p53* allele is altered by the presence or absence of wild-type p53 in vivo. Mice carrying the ^{135}Ala → Val mutant transgene were crossed with p53-deficient mice.[180] The mutant p53-Tg accelerated tumor formation in $p53^{+/-}$ but not $p53^{-/-}$ mice, suggesting that this loss-of-function mutation had a dominant negative effect with respect to tumor incidence and cell growth rates. Although the tumor spectrum was similar in transgenic and nontransgenic mice, the transgenice mice showed a predisposition to lung adenocarcinomas. Thus, a given p53 alteration may have distinct tissue specificity with respect to its tumorigenic potential. It will ultimately be of interest to extend this approach to other alleles that behave differently *in vivo* or *in vitro*. At least one group[181] is trying to establish mouse models to study tumor-derived p53 mutants *in vivo* that would establish a more precise model of LFS and clarify the role played by point mutant forms of altered p53 as distinct from the null genotype.

In some strains, $p53^{-/-}$ mice become colonized with pathogens, suggesting that p53 deficiency may be associated with a poorer prognosis after infection with common low-virulence organisms or viruses.[175] In all strains, the $p53^{-/-}$ state is compatible with normal murine development, although the yield of $p53^{-/-}$ offspring from heterozygous crosses varies from 16.6 to 23 percent.[172,175] This apparent increase in fetal loss has been correlated in part by demonstration of fetal exencephaly in a subset of animals,[182] yet it does not mirror the human counterpart in that fetal loss is not characteristic of human LFS families.[183] This may in fact be related to the fact that humans harboring *p53* mutations are heterozygous, whereas the mice are homozygously deleted of *p53* alleles. Thus the presence of one wild-type *p53* allele in a human may be sufficient to ensure fetal viability.

p53-deficient mice are more sensitive to the effects of certain carcinogenic agents.[184] Mice exposed to dimethylnitrosamine (DMN) developed liver hemangiosarcomas more rapidly than did similarly treated $p53^{+/+}$ animals.[184] $p53^{-/-}$ mice treated with an initiator, dimethylbenzanthracene (DMBA), and a promoter, 12-*O*-tetradecanoyl-phorbol-13-acetate (TPA), showed a more rapid rate of malignant progression of skin papillomas to carcinomas compared with their $p53^{+/+}$ counterparts. These studies help distinguish whether *p53* mutations play rate-limiting or tissue-specific roles in the tumor progression pathway.

p53-deficient mice have been used to evaluate the effects of environmental factors on both tumorigenesis and development. p53-deficient and transgenic mice exposed to sublethal doses of γ-irradiation develop tumors, predominantly sarcomas, earlier than do untreated animals.[92,93] This susceptibility is associated with a twofold increase in the accumulation of radiation-induced double-strand DNA breaks compared with what is seen in $p53^{+/+}$ animals. Using *p53*-transgenic mice, it has been demonstrated that the presence of *p53* mutations does not alter the latency period of chronic ultraviolet B-induced squamous cell carcinoma but does significantly increase the number of tumors and the propensity for multiple tumor formation.[185] Although p53 protein was undetectable in the keratinocytes of the untreated mice, it was elevated in 93 percent of skin tumors derived from the treated animals. These studies confirm that p53 prevents the accumulation of cells sustaining radiation-induced or chemically induced DNA damage.

It has been demonstrated that caloric restriction inhibits the development of spontaneous lymphoma in C57BL/6 mice.[186] Such treatment of $p53^{-/-}$ mice modulates spontaneous tumorigenesis, delaying the onset of tumor formation by a median of 16 weeks in *ad libitum* fed mice and 25 weeks in calorie-restricted animals.[187] It is thought that dietary perturbations can influence the outcome of a genomic liability such as the accelerated tumorigenesis demonstrated in p53-deficient mice. Given the important role of p53 in cell cycle control, a p53-deficient state would be expected to deregulate the differentiation and development and yield aberrant morphogenesis and embryonic lethality. In fact, studies of the effects of the teratogen and DNA-damaging carcinogen benzo[*a*]pyrene[188] and the anticonvulsant and teratogenic drug phenytoin[189] on pregnant p53-deficient mice demonstrated a two- to fourfold increase in the incidence of *in utero* fetal resorption (death), teratogenicity, and postpartum lethality over $p53^{+/+}$ controls. These observations provide substantial support for the embryoprotective role of p53.

The cumulative data from these studies indicate that loss or alterations of *p53* may accelerate prior tumor predisposition, that the rate and spectrum of development of some cancers may be strain-dependent, and that normal murine development is possible even in the absence of p53. Certain similarities exist between the various *p53* mouse models and LFS families in that a p53-related transformation pathway leads to development of a wide spectrum of cancers. Inheritance of one mutant and one wild-type *p53* allele in affected members of LFS families is more analogous to the $p53^{+/-}$ or p53-Tg mice that developed tumors at a relatively slower rate. However, none of these animal models presents a completely accurate reflection of the LFS genotype in that the vast majority of documented human germ-line *p53* mutations are missense in nature, with less than 10 percent being nonfunctional. Although the transgenic mice carry point mutations, the ^{135}Ala and ^{193}Arg mutations have not been reported in the human germ line. Although null alleles are valuable tools, their effects reflect the complete absence of gene function, a phenomenon that is not generally observed in the human syndrome. Changes at the nucleotide level would represent a more exact model and are being developed. Finally, although the tumor spectrum in current *p53*-altered mice is highly variable, none of these mice spontaneously mimic the human phenotype in its preponderance of sarcomas and breast cancers, except when the animals are radiated. Furthermore, the lymphomas predominant in mice are seen only rarely in LFS. Although these differences could be species-dependent, it is reasonable to suspect that specific mutations influence tumor development and yield a more accurate human phenotype. This hypothesis is substantiated by the recent studies of *p53*-null crosses exemplifying the *in vivo* role of p53 in distinct pathways of cell cycle control. The *Mdm-2*-null mouse that results in an early embryonic lethal phenotype is rescued by deletion of *p53* in that double-homozygous null mice are viable. A shift in tumor phenotype resulting from cooperativity of mutations is demonstrated in the intercrosses of *Min* mice and p53-deficient mice, highlighting the striking tissue-specific differences in the tumor-suppressor effects of p53.[190] Mice that overexpress a c-*myc* transgene stochastically develop clonal tumors — a relatively low incidence of T-cell lymphomas.[191] Lymphoma development is dramatically accelerated by the synergistic activity of the *p53*-null mutation in intercrosses,[192] while no significant increase in tumor incidence was seen in *myc* mice carrying a single-function *p53* allele. These studies, although making a strong case for the biochemical and functional interactions of *p53* with other genes crucial to tumor formation, also leave the way open to the analysis of similar synergistic effects that might be observed with a spectrum of *p53* point mutations yielding disrupted p53 function rather than the null allele that yields no function whatsoever. The tumors derived from these mice, carrying point mutations, will most closely resemble spontaneous tumors that can be studied for biochemical interactions and response to therapy. It also will be possible to evaluate *in vivo* the effect of coexistence of mutant and wild-type p53 and the functional influence of one on the other.

LABORATORY SCIENCE MEETS CLINICAL PRACTICE

Several important issues exist as a result of the identification of germ-line mutations of the *p53* tumor-suppressor gene in rare cancer-prone families. These include ethical concerns about predictive testing in unaffected members of LFS and LFS-L families, selection of patients to be tested, and selection of practical and accurate laboratory techniques to definitively identify *p53* mutations. In addition, the development of pilot testing programs and evaluation of the roles of interventions based on testing results have to be considered.

For several reasons, *p53* testing is still not believed to be appropriate for the general population, particularly in light of the demonstrably low carrier rate. Even in the general cancer population, the prevalence of germ-line *p53* mutations will be a fraction of 1 percent. Although the sensitivity and specificity of screening methods have improved with the advent of automated DNA sequence analysis and functional assays, both false-positive and false-negative results have been noted.

Even within the high-risk population, problems are apparent. It is unclear why the same germ-line *p53* mutation can give rise to different cancer phenotypes, and it is not clear if in families that do not have classic LFS the cancer risks from *p53* mutation are as high as they are in LFS.[20] Because 85 percent of all missense mutations described in the germ line occur in exons 5, 7, and 8 of the gene, predictive testing must include those regions. However, most centers are now sequencing the entire coding region of *p53* as well as the flanking splice-acceptor sites to increase the likelihood of identifying less common alterations.

Recommendations for multicenter research studies that incorporate a multidisciplinary approach to surveying, screening, and testing were established in 1992[193] and are being updated. These initial recommendations, although specifically addressing *p53* testing in LFS, could be applied to a number of other cancer-predisposition gene testing programs. In fact, both the American Society of Clinical Oncology[194] and the American Society of Human Genetics[195] have developed policy statements that include brief references to *p53* testing. Although the interpretation of who should be tested remains open, certain common recommendations are stated, including the necessity that cancer risk counseling be part of the mission of clinical oncologists, the need for informed consent, formats for regulation of genetic testing, and continued efforts to address research issues.

The component malignancies of LFS are for the most part exceedingly difficult to cure, with the possible exception of early-detected breast cancer, childhood acute lymphoblastic leukemia, and rare germ-cell tumors of the testis. Although the prognosis for component solid tumors improves with earlier stage at diagnosis, only mammography screening for breast cancer has been shown to reduce mortality.[196] Its efficacy under age 50 (the predominant risk in LFS) is disputed. Furthermore, the potential theoretical risk of repeated low-dose radiation from such screening methods to tissue that harbors altered p53 has not been carefully scrutinized in this setting. Chemopreventive trials are under way, but the rarity of the germ-line mutant *p53* carrier state makes studies of these patients impractical.

Despite the many drawbacks of predictive testing for *p53* at this time, the possibility of reducing the marked loss of human potential resulting from the death of a child or young adult makes further pilot research efforts worthwhile. To this end, further studies of the role of p53 in the development of human cancer, the development of more accurate testing techniques, and the development of novel animal models will continue to be important.

REFERENCES

1. Li FP, Fraumeni JF Jr: Soft tissue sarcomas breast cancer and other neoplasms: A familial cancer syndrome? *Ann Intern Med* **71**:747, 1969.
2. Li FP, Fraumeni JF Jr: Rhabdomyosarcoma in children: Epidemiologic study and identification of a familial cancer syndrome. *J Natl Cancer Inst* **43**:1365, 1969.
3. Bottomley RH, Trainer AL, Condit PT: Chromosome studies in a cancer family. *Cancer* **28**:519, 1971.
4. Lynch HT, Krush AJ, Harlan WL, Sharp EA: Association of soft tissue sarcoma, leukemia, and brain tumors in families affected with breast cancer. *Am J Surg* **39**:199, 1973.
5. Blattner WA, McGuire DB, Mulvihill JJ, Lampkin BC, Hananian J, Fraumeni JF Jr: Genealogy of cancer in a family. *JAMA* **241**:259, 1979.
6. Pearson ADJ, Craft AW, Ratcliffe JM, Birch JM, Morris-Jonese PH, Roberts DF: Two families with the Li-Fraumeni cancer family syndrome. *J Med Genet* **19**:362, 1982.
7. Lynch HT, Mulcahy GM, Harris RE, Guirgis HA, Lynch JF: Genetic and pathologic findings in a kindred with hereditary sarcoma, breast cancer, brain tumors, leukemia, lung, laryngeal, and adrenal cortical carcinoma. *Cancer* **41**:2055, 1978.
8. Draper GJ, Sanders BM, Kingston JE: Second primary neoplasms in patients with retinoblastoma. *Br J Cancer* **53**:661, 1986.
9. Li FP, Fraumeni JF Jr: Prospective study of a family cancer syndrome. *JAMA* **247**:2692, 1982.
10. Garber JE, Goldstein AM, Kantor AF, Dreyfus MG, Fraumeni JF Jr, Li FP: Follow-up study of twenty-four families with Li-Fraumeni syndrome. *Cancer Res* **51**:6094, 1991.
11. Li FP, Fraumeni JF Jr, Mulvihill JJ, Blattner WA, Dreyfus MG, Tucker MA, Miller RW: A cancer family syndrome in twenty-four kindreds. *Cancer Res* **48**:5358, 1988.
12. Birch JM, Hartley AL, Blair V, et al: Cancer in the families of children with soft tissue sarcoma. *Cancer* **66**:2239, 1990.
13. Lustbader ED, Williams WR, Bondy ML, Strom S, Strong LC: Segregation analysis of cancer in families of childhood soft-tissue sarcoma patients. *Am J Hum Genet* **51**:344, 1992.
14. Hartley AL, Birch JM, Kelsey AM, Marsden HB, Harris M, Teare MD: Malignant melanoma in families of children with osteosarcoma, chondrosarcoma and adrenal cortical carcinoma. *J Med Genet* **24**:664, 1987.
15. Hartley AL, Birch JM, Tricker K, Wallace SA, Kelsey AM, Harris M, Morris Jones PH: Wilms tumor in the Li-Fraumeni cancer family syndrome. *Cancer Genet Cytogenet* **67**:133, 1993.
16. Birch JM, Hartley AL, Tricker KJ, et al: Prevalence and diversity of constitutional mutations in the p53 gene among 21 Li-Fraumeni families. *Cancer Res* **54**:1298, 1994.
17. Hartley AL, Birch JM, Kelsey AM, Marsden HB, Harris M, Teare MD: Are germ cell tumors part of the Li-Fraumeni cancer family syndrome? *Cancer Genet Cytogenet* **42**:221, 1989.
18. Garber JE, Liepman MK, Gelles EJ, Corson JM, Antman KH: Melanoma and soft tissue sarcoma in seven patients. *Cancer* **66**:2432, 1990.

19. Strong LC, Stine M, Norsted TL: Cancer in survivors of childhood soft tissue sarcoma and their relatives. *J Natl Cancer Inst* **79**:1213, 1987.

20. Eeles RA: Germ line mutations in the p53 gene, in Ponder BAJ, Cavenee WK, Solomon E (eds): *Cancer Surveys,* vol 25: *Genetics and Cancer: A Second Look.* Cold Spring Harbor, NY, Cold Spring Harbor Laboratory Press, 1995, p 101.

21. Williams WR, Strong LC: Genetic epidemiology of soft tissue sarcomas in children, in Muller H, Weber W (eds): *Familial Cancer.* 1st International Research Conference on Familial Cancer. Basel, Karger, 1985, p 151.

22. Call KM, Glaser T, Ito CY, Buckler AJ, Pelletier J, Haber DA, Rose EA, Kral A, Yeger H, Lewis WH, Jones C, Housman DE: Isolation and characterization of a zinc finger polypeptide gene at the human chromosome 11 Wilms tumor locus. *Cell* **60**:509, 1990.

23. Gessler M, Poustka A, Cavenee W, Neve RL, Orkin SH, Bruns GAP: Homozygous deletion in Wilms tumors of a zinc-finger identified by chromosome jumping. *Nature* **343**:774, 1990.

24. Huang A, Campbell CE, Bonetta L, McAndrews-Hill MS, Coppes MJ, Williams BRG: Tissue, developmental, and tumor-specific expression of divergent transcripts in Wilms tumor. *Science* **250**:991, 1990.

25. Li FP: Cancer families: Human models of susceptibility to neoplasia. *Cancer Res* **48**:5381, 1988.

26. Bech-Hansen NT, Sell BM, Lampkin BC, Blattner WA, McKeen EA, Fraumeni JF Jr, Paterson MC: Transmission of in vitro radioresistance in a cancer-prone family. *Lancet* **1**:1135, 1981.

27. Chang EH, Pirollo KF, Zou ZQ, Cheung HY, Lawler EL, Garner R, White E, Bernstein WB, Fraumeni JF Jr, Blattner WA: Oncogenes in radioresistant, noncancerous skin fibroblasts from a cancer-prone family. *Science* **237**:1036, 1987.

28. Little JB, Nove J, Dahlberg WK, Troilo P, Nichols WW, Strong LC: Normal cytotoxic response of skin fibroblasts from patients with Li-Fraumeni cancer syndrome to DNA-damaging agents in vitro. *Cancer Res* **47**:4229, 1987.

29. Bischoff FZ, Strong LC, Yim SO, Pratt DR, Siciliano MJ, Giovanella BC, Tainsky MA: Tumorigenic transformation of spontaneously immortalized fibroblasts from patients with a familial cancer syndrome. *Oncogene* **7**:183, 1991.

30. Bischoff FZ, Yim SO, Pathak S, Grant G, Siciliano MJ, Giovanella BC, Strong LC, Tainsky MA: Spontaneous abnormalities in normal fibroblasts from patients with Li-Fraumeni cancer syndrome: Aneuploidy and immortalization. *Cancer Res* **50**:3234, 1990.

31. Knudson AG: Mutation and cancer: Statistical study of retinoblastoma. *Proc Natl Acad Sci USA* **68**:820, 1971.

32. Knudson AG, Strong LC: Mutation and cancer: A model for Wilms tumor of the kidney. *J Natl Cancer Inst* **48**:313, 1972.

33. Knudson AG, Strong LC, Anderson DE: Hereditary cancer in man. *Prog Med Genet* **9**:13, 1973.

34. Comings DE: A general theory of carcinogenesis. *Proc Natl Acad Sci USA* **70**:3324, 1973.

35. Caron de Fromentel C, Soussi T: TP53 suppressor gene: A model for investigating human mutagenesis. *Gene Chromos Cancer* **4**:1, 1992.

36. Harris CC: p53: At the crossroads of molecular carcinogenesis and risk assessment. *Science* **262**:1980, 1993.

37. Harris CC, Hollstein M: Clinical implications of the p53 tumor suppressor gene. *N Engl J Med* **329**:1318, 1993.

38. Hollstein M, Sidransky D, Vogelstein B, Harris CC: p53 mutations in human cancers. *Science* **253**:49, 1991.

39. McBride OW, Merry D, Givol D: The gene for human p53 cellular tumor antigen is located on chromosome 17 short arm (17p13). *Proc Natl Acad Sci USA* **83**:130, 1986.

40. Lane DP, Crawford LV: T antigen is bound to a host protein in SV40-transformed cells. *Nature* **278**:261, 1979.

41. Soussi T, Caron de Fromentel C, May P: Structural aspects of the p53 protein in relation to gene evolution. *Oncogene* **5**:945, 1990.

42. Foord OS, Bhattacharya P, Reich Z, Rotter V: A DNA binding domain is contained in the C-terminus of wild-type p53 protein. *Nucleic Acids Res* **19**:5191, 1991.

43. Fields S, Jang SK: Presence of a potent transcription activating sequence in the p53 protein. *Science* **249**:1046, 1990.

44. Jenkins JR, Rudge K, Currie GA: Cellular immortalization by a cDNA clone encoding the transformation associated phosphoprotein p53. *Nature* **312**:651, 1984.

45. Addison C, Jenkins JR, Sturzbecher H-W: The p53 nuclear localization signal is structurally linked to a p34^{cdc2} kinase motif. *Oncogene* **5**:423, 1990.

46. Milner J, Medcalf EA: Cotranslation of activated mutant p53 with wild-type drives the wild-type p53 protein into the mutant conformation. *Cell* **65**:765, 1991.

47. Stenger JE, Mayr GA, Mann K, Tegtmeyer P: Formation of stable p53 homotetramers and multiples of tetramers. *Mol Carcinogen* **5**:102, 1992.

48. Meek DW, Eckhart W: Phosphorylation of p53 in normal and simian virus 40-transformed NIH 3T3 cells. *Mol Cell Biol* **8**:461, 1988.

49. Linzer DIH, Levine AJ: Characterization of a 54K dalton cellular antigen present in SV40 transformed cells and uninfected embryonal carcinoma cells. *Cell* **17**:43, 1979.

50. Eliyahu D, Michalovitz D, Eliyahu S, Pinhasi-Kimhi O, Oren M: Wild-type p53 can inhibit oncogene-mediated focus formation. *Proc Natl Acad Sci USA* **86**:8763, 1984.

51. Jenkins JR, Chumakov P, Addison C, Sturzbecher HW, Wode-Evans A: Two distinct regions of the murine p53 primary amino acid sequence are implicated in stable complex formation within simian virus 40 antigen. *J Virol* **62**:3903, 1988.

52. Rovinski B, Benchimol S: Immortalisation of rat embryo fibroblasts by the cellular p53 oncogene. *Oncogene* **2**:445, 1988.

53. Hinds PW, Finlay CA, Levine AJ: Mutation is required to activate the p53 gene for cooperation with the ras oncogene and transformation. *J Virol* **63**:739, 1989.

53a. Baker SJ, Fearon ER, Nigro JM, Hamilton SR, Preisinger AC, Jessup JM, van Tuinen P, Ledbetter DH, Barker DF, Nakamura Y, White R, Vogelstein B: Chromosome 17 deletions and p53 gene mutations in colorectal carcinomas. *Science* **244**:217, 1989.

53b. Nigro JM, Baker SJ, Preisinger AC, Jessup JM, Hostetter R, Cleary K, Bigner SH, Davidson N, Baylin S, Devilee P, Glover T, Collins FS, Weston A, Modali R, Harris CC, Vogelstein B: Mutations in the p53 gene occur in diverse human tumor types. *Nature* **342**:705, 1989.

54. Baker SJ, Markowitz K, Fearon ER, Wilson JKV, Vogelstein B: Suppression of human colorectal carcinoma cell growth by wild-type p53. *Science* **249**:1912, 1990.

55. Diller L, Kassel J, Nelson CE, Gryka MA, Litwack G, Gebhardt MA, Friend SH: p53 functions as a cell cycle control protein in osteosarcomas. *Mol Cell Biol* **10**:5772, 1990.

56. Levine AJ, Momand J, Finlay CA: The p53 tumor suppressor gene. *Nature* **351**:453, 1991.

56a. El-Deiry WS, Kern SE, Pientenpol JA, Kinzler KW, Vogelstein B: Definition of a consensus binding site for p53. *Nature Genet* **1**:45, 1992.

57. Funk WD, Park DT, Karas RH, Wright WE, Shay JW: A transcriptionally active DNA-binding site for p53 protein complexes. *Mol Cell Biol* **12**:2866, 1992.

58. Iwabuchi K, Li B, Bartel P, Fields S: Use of the two-hybrid system to identify the domain of p53 involved in oligomerization. *Oncogene* **8**:1693, 1993.

59. Shaulsky G, Goldfinger N, Ben-Zeev A, Rotter V: Nuclear accumulation of p53 is mediated by several nuclear localization signals and plays a role in tumorigenesis. *Mol Cell Biol* **10**:6565, 1990.

60. Milne DM, Palmer RH, Campbell DG, Meek DW: Phosphorylation of the p53 tumor-suppressor protein at three N terminal sites by a novel casein kinase I-like enzyme. *Oncogene* **7**:1316, 1992.

61. Lees-Milner SP, Chen Y, Anderson CW: Human cells contain a DNA-activated protein kinase that phosphorylates simian virus 40 T-antigen, mouse p53, and the human Ku autoantigen. *Mol Cell Biol* **9**:3982, 1990.

62. Meek DW, Simon S, Kikkawa U, Eckhart W: The p53 tumor suppressor proteins is phosphorylated at serine 389 by casein kinase II. *EMBO J* **9**:3253, 1990.

63. Finlay CA, Hinds PW, Levine AJ: The p53 proto-oncogene can act as a suppressor of transformation. *Cell* **57**:1083, 1989.

64. Vogelstein B, Kinzler KW: p53 function and dysfunction. *Cell* **70**:523, 1992.

65. Mercer WE, Shields MT, Lin D, Appella E, Ullrich SJ: Growth suppression induced by wild-type p53 protein is accompanied by selective down-regulation of proliferating cell-nuclear antigen expression. *Proc Natl Acad Sci USA* **88**:1958, 1991.

66. Baker SJ, Markowitz K, Fearon ER, Wilson JKV, Vogelstein B: Suppression of human colorectal carcinoma cell growth by wild-type p53. *Science* **249**:1912, 1990.

67. Diller L, Kassel J, Nelson CE, Gryka MA, Litwack G, Gebhardt MA, Friend SH: p53 functions as a cell cycle control protein in osteosarcomas. *Mol Cell Biol* **10**:5772, 1990.

68. Michalovitz D, Halevy O, Oren M: Conditional inhibition of transformation and of cell proliferation by a temperature-sensitive mutant of p53. *Cell* **62**:671, 1990.

69. Paules RS, Levedakou EN, Wilson SJ, Innes CL, Rhodes N, Tlsty TD, Galloway DA, Donehower LA, Tainsky MA, Kaufmann WK: Defective G2 checkpoint function in cells from individuals with familial cancer syndrome. *Cancer Res* **55**:1763, 1995.

70. Guillof C, Rosselli F, Krisnaraju K, Moustacchi E, Hoffmann B, Liebermann DA: p53 involvement in control of G2 exit of the cell cycle: Role in DNA damage-induced apoptosis. *Oncogene* **10**:2263, 1995.

71. Stewart N, Hicks GG, Paraskevas F, Mowat M: Evidence for a second cell cycle block at G2/M by p53. *Oncogene* **10**:109, 1995.

72. Wang Y, Prives C: Increased and altered DNA binding of human p53 by S and G2/M but not G1 cyclin-dependent kinases. *Nature* **376**:88, 1995.

73. Fan S, Smith MK, Rivet DJ, Duba D, Zhan Q, Kohn K, Fornace AJ, O'Connor PM: Disruption of p53 function sensitizes breast cancer MCF-7 cells to cisplatin and pentoxifylline. *Cancer Res* **55**:1649, 1995.

74. Powell SN, DeFrank JS, Connell P, Eogen M, Preffer F, Dombkowski D, Tang W, Friend S: Differential sensitivity of p53(2) and p53(1) cells to caffeine-induced radiosensitization and override of G2 delay. *Cancer Res* **55**:1643, 1995.

75. Cross SM, Sanchez CA, Morgan CA, Schimke MK, Ramel S, Idzerda RL, Raskind WH, Reid BJ: A p53-dependent mouse spindle checkpoint. *Science* **267**:1353, 1995.

76. Fukasawa K, Choi T, Kuriyama R, Rulong S, Vande Woude GF: Abnormal centrosome amplification in the absence of p53. *Science* **271**:1744, 1996.

77. Bouffler SD, Kemp CJ, Balmain A, Cox R: Spontaneous and ionizing radiation-induced chromosomal abnormalities in p53-deficient mice. *Cancer Res* **5**:3883, 1995.

78. Parshad R, Price FM, Pirollo KF, Chang EH, Sandford KK: Cytogenetic responses to G2 phase X-irradiation in relation to DNA repair and radiosensitivity in cancer prone family with Li-Fraumeni syndrome. *Radiat Res* **136**:236, 1993.

79. Funk WD, Park DT, Karas RH, Wright WE, Shay JW: A transcriptionally active DNA-binding site for p53 protein complexes. *Mol Cell Biol* **12**:2866, 1992.

80. Eliyahu D, Raz A, Gruss P, Givol D, Oren M: Participants of p53 cellular tumor antigen in transformation of normal embryonic cells. *Nature* **312**:646, 1984.

81. Yonish-Rouach E, Resnitzky D, Lotem J, Sachs L, Kimchi A, Oren M: Wild-type p53 induces apoptosis of myeloid leukemic cells that is inhibited by interleukin-6. *Nature* **352**:345, 1991.

82. Shaw P, Bovey R, Tardy S, Sahli R, Sordat B, Costa J: Induction of apoptosis by wild-type p53 in a human colon tumor-derived cell line. *Proc Natl Acad Sci USA* **89**:4495, 1992.

83. Clarke AR, Purdie CA, Harrison DJ, Morris RG, Bird CC, Hooper ML, Wyllie AH: Thymocyte apoptosis induced by p53-dependent and independent pathways. *Nature* **362**:849, 1993.

84. Lowe SW, Schmitt EM, Smith SW, Osborne BA, Jacks T: p53 is required for radiation-induced apoptosis in mouse thymocytes. *Nature* **362**:847, 1993.

85. Lowe SW, Ruley HE, Jacks T, Housman DE: p53-dependent apoptosis modulates the cytotoxicity of anticancer agents. *Cell* **74**:957, 1993.

86. Slichenmeyer WJ, Nelson WG, Slebos RJ, Kastan MB: Loss of a p53-associated G1 checkpoint does not decrease cell survival following DNA damage. *Cancer Res* **53**:4164, 1993.

87. Brachman DG, Beckett M, Graves D, Haraf D, Vokes E, Weichselbaum RR: p53 mutation does not correlate with radio-sensitivity in 24 head and neck cancer cell lines. *Cancer Res* **53**:3667, 1993.

88. Maltzman W, Czyzk L: UV irradiation stimulates levels of p53 cellular tumor antigen in nontransformed mouse cells. *Mol Cell Biol* **4**:1689, 1984.

89. Kuerbitz SJ, Beverly SP, Walsh WV, Kastan MB: Wild-type p53 is a cell cycle checkpoint determinant following irradiation. *Proc Natl Acad Sci USA* **89**:7491, 1992.

90. Kastan MB, Onyekwere O, Sidransky D, Vogelstein B, Craig RW: Participation of p53 protein in the cellular response to DNA damage. *Cancer Res* **51**:6304, 1991.

91. Yamaizumi M, Sugano T: UV-induced nuclear accumulation of p53 is evoked through DNA damage of actively transcribed genes independent of the cell cycle. *Oncogene* **9**:2775, 1994.

92. Lee JM, Abrahamson JLA, Kandel R, Donehower LA, Bernstein A: Susceptibility to radiation-carcinogenesis and accumulation of chromosomal breakage in p53-deficient mice. *Oncogene* **9**:3731, 1994.

93. Lee JM, Bernstein A: p53 mutations increase resistance to ionizing radiation. *Proc Natl Acad Sci USA* **90**:5742, 1993.

94. Lane DP: p53, guardian of the genome. *Nature* **358**:15, 1992.

95. Zambetti GP, Levine AJ: A comparison of the biological activities of wild-type and mutant p53. *FASEB J* **7**:855, 1993.

96. Lowe LW, Bodis B, McCarthy A, Remington LH, Ruley E, Fisher D, Housman DE, Jacks T: p53 can determine the efficacy of cancer therapy in vitro. *Science* **266**:807, 1994.

97. Barak Y, Juven T, Haffner R, Oren M: mdm-2 expression is induced by wild-type p53 activity. *EMBO J* **12**:461, 1993.

98. Wu X, Bayle H, Olson D, Levine AJ: The p53-mdm2 autoregulatory feedback loop. *Gene Dev* **7**:1126, 1993.

99. Okamoto K, Beach D: Cyclin G is a transcriptional target of the tumor suppressor protein p53. *EMBO J* **13**:4816, 1994.

100. Myashita T, Reed TC: Tumor suppressor p53 is a direct transcriptional activator of the numan bax gene. *Cell* **80**:293, 1995.

101. Kastan MB, Zhan Q, El-Deiry WS, Carrier F, Jacks T, Walsh WV, Plunkett BS, Vogelstein B, Fornace AJ: A mammalian cell cycle checkpoint pathway utilizing p53 and GADD45 is defective in ataxia-telangiectasia. *Cell* **71**:587, 1992.

102. Harper JW, Adami GR, Wei N, Keyomarsi K, Elledge SJ: The p21 Cdk-interacting protein Cip1 is a potent inhibitor of G1 cyclin-dependent kinases. *Cell* **75**:805, 1993.

103. Xiong Y, Hannon GJ, Zhang H, Casso D, Kobayashi R, Beach D: p21 is a universal inhibitor of cylcin kinases. *Nature* **366**:701, 1993.

104. Gu Y, Turck CW, Morgan DO: Inhibition of CDK2 activity *in vivo* by an associated 20K regulatory subunit. *Nature* **366**:707, 1993.

105. Pines J: p21 inhibits cyclin shock. *Nature* **369**:520, 1994.

106. Smith ML, Chen I-T, Zhan Q, Bae I, Chen C-Y, Glimer TM, Kastan MB, O'Connor PM, Fornace AJ Jr: Interaction of the p53-regulated protein GADD45 with proliferating cell nuclear antigen. *Science* **266**:1376, 1994.

107. Wang XW, Forrester K, Yeh H, Feitelson MA, Gu JR, Harris CC: Hepatitis B virus X protein inhibits p53 sequence-specific DNA binding, transcriptional activity, and association with transcription factor ERCC3. *Proc Natl Acad Sci USA* **91**:2230, 1994.

108. Cho Y, Gorina S, Jeffrey PD, Pavletich NP: Crystal structure of a p53 tumor suppressor-DNA complex: Understanding tumorigenic mutations. *Science* **265**:346, 1994.

109. Clore GM, Omichinski JF, Sakaguchi K, Zambrano N, Sakamoto H, Appella E, Gronenborn AM: High-resolution structure of the oligomerization domain of p53 by multidimensional NMR. *Science* **265**:386, 1994.

109a. Lee W, Harvey TS, Yin Y, Yau P, Litchfield D, Arrowsmith CH: Solution structure of the tetrameric minimum transforming domain of p53. *Struct Biol* **1**:877, 1994.

110. Prives C: How loops, b sheets, and a helices help us to understand p53. *Cell* **78**:543, 1994.

111. Vogelstein B, Kinzler KW: X-rays strike p53 again. *Nature* **370**:174, 1994.

112. Farmer G, Bargonetti J, Zhu H, Friedman P, Prywes R, Prives C: Wild-type p53 activates transcription in vitro. *Nature* **358**:83, 1992.

113. Kern SE, Kinzler KW, Bruskin A, Jarosz D, Friedman P, Prives C, Vogelstein B: Identification of p53 as a sequence-specific DNA-binding protein. *Science* **252**:1708, 1991.

114. Kern SE, Pientenpol JA, Thiagalingam S, Seymour A, Kinzler KW, Vogelstein B: Oncogenic forms of p53 inhibit p53-regulated gene expression. *Science* **256**:827, 1992.

115. Milner J, Medcalf EA: Cotranslation of activated mutant p53 with wild-type p53 protein drives the wild-type p53 protein into the mutant conformation. *Cell* **65**:765, 1991.

116. Cariello NF, Cui L, Beroud C, Soussi T: Database and software for the analysis of mutations in the human p53 gene. *Cancer Res* **54**:4454, 1994.

117. Momand J, Zambetti GP, Olson DC, George D, Levine AJ: The mdm-2 oncogene product forms a complex with the p53 protein and inhibits p53-mediated transactivation. *Cell* **69**:1237, 1992.

118. Sheffner M, Werness BA, Huibregste JM, Levine AJ, Howley PM: The E6 oncoprotein encoded by human papillomavirus types 16 and 18 promotes the degradation of p53. *Cell* **63**:1129, 1990.

119. Fakharzadeh SS, Trusko SP, George DL: Tumorigenic potential associated with enhanced expression of a gene that is amplified in a mouse tumor cell line. *EMBO J* **10**:1565, 1991.

120. Oliner JD, Kinzler KW, Meltzer PS, George DL, Vogelstein B: Amplification of a gene encoding a p53-associated protein in human sarcomas. *Nature* **358**:80, 1992.

121. Maheswaran S, Park S, Bernard A, Morris JF, Rauscher FJ, Hill DE, Haber DA: Physical and functional interaction between WT1 and p53 proteins. *Proc Natl Acad Sci USA* **90**:5100, 1993.

122. Williams BO, Remington L, Albert DM, Mukai S, Bronson RT, Jacks T: Cooperative tumorigenic effects of germ line mutations in Rb and p53 proteins. *Nature Genet* **7**:480, 1994.

123. Harvey M, Vogel H, Lee EYHP, Bradley A, Donehower LA: Mice deficient in both p53 and Rb develop tumors primarily of endocrine origin. *Cancer Res* **55**:1146, 1995.

123a. Celli J, Duijf P, Hamel BC, Bamshad M, Kramer B, Smits AP, Newbury-Ecob R, Hennekam RC, Van Buggenhout G, van Haeringen A, Woods CG, van Essen AJ, de Waal R, Vriend G, Haber DA, Yang A, McKeon F, Brunner HG, van Bokhoven H: Heterozygous germline mutations in the p53 homolog p63 are the cause of EEC syndrome. *Cell* **99**:143, 1999.

124. Shimamura A, Fisher DE: p53 in life and death. *Clin Cancer Res* **2**:435, 1996.

125. Hansen R, Reddel R, Braithwaite A: The transforming oncoproteins determine the mechanism by which p53 suppresses cell transformation: pRB-mediated growth arrest or apoptosis. *Oncogene* **11**:2535, 1995.

126. Miller CW, Aslo A, Tsay C, Slamon D, Ishizaki K, Toguchida J: Frequency and structure of p53 rearrangements in human osteosarcoma. *Cancer Res* **50**:7950, 1990.

127. Toguchida J, Yamaguchi T, Ritchie B, Beauchamp RL, Dayton SH, et al: Mutation spectrum of the p53 gene in bone and soft tissue sarcomas. *Cancer Res* **52**:6194, 1992.

128. Felix CA, Kappel CC, Mitsudomi T, Nau MM, Tsokos M, et al: Frequency and diversity of p53 mutations in childhood rhabdomyosarcoma. *Cancer Res* **52**:2243, 1992.

129. Slingerland JM, Minden MD, Benchimol S: Mutation of the p53-gene in human myelogenous leukemia. *Blood* **77**:1500, 1991.

130. Prococimer M, Rotter V: Structure and function of p53 in normal cells and their aberrations in cancer cells: Projection of the hematologic cell lineages. *Blood* **84**:2391, 1994.

131. Mashiyama S, Murakami Y, Yoshimoto T, Sekiya T, Hayashi K: Detection of p53 gene mutations in human brain tumors by single-strand conformation polymorphism analysis of polymerase chain reaction products. *Oncogene* **6**:1313, 1991.

132. Takahashi T, Nan MM, Chiba I, Buchhagen DL, Minna JD: p53: A frequent target for genetic abnormalities in lung cancer. *Science* **246**:491, 1989.

133. Osborne RJ, Merlo GR, Mitsudomi T, Venesio T, Liscia DS, et al: Mutations in the p53 gene in primary human breast cancers. *Cancer Res* **51**:6194, 1991.

134. Malkin D: p53 and the Li-Fraumeni syndrome. *Biochem Biophys Acta* **1198**:197, 1994.

135. Laviguer A, Maltby V, Mock D, Rossant J, Pawson T, Bernstein A: High incidence of lung, bone, and lymphoid tumors in transgenic mice overexpressing mutant alleles of the p53 oncogene. *Mol Cell Biol* **9**:3982, 1989.

136. Malkin D, Li FP, Strong LC, Fraumeni JF Jr, Nelson CE, Kim DH, Kassel J, Gryka MA, Bischoff FZ, Tainsky MA, Friend SH: Germ line p53 mutations ina familial syndrome of breast cancer, sarcomas, and other neoplasms. *Science* **250**:1233, 1990.

137. Malkin D, Friend SH: Correction: A Li-Fraumeni syndrome mutation. *Science* **259**:878, 1993.

137a. Srivastava S, Zou Z, Pirollo K, Blattner W, Chang EH: Germ line transmission of a mutated p53 gene in a cancer-prone family with Li-Fraumeni syndrome. *Nature* **348**:747, 1990.

138. Vogelstein B: A deadly inheritance. *Nature* **348**:681, 1990.

139. Law JC, Strong LC, Chidambaram A, Ferrell RE: A germ line mutation in exon 5 of the p53 gene in an extended cancer family. *Cancer Res* **51**:6385, 1991.

140. Metzger AK, Sheffield VC, Duyk G, Daneshuar L, Edwards MSB, Cogen PH: Identification of a germ line mutation in the p53 gene in a patient with intracranial ependymoma. *Proc Natl Acad Sci USA* **88**:7825, 1991.

141. Santibanez-Koref MF, Birch JM, Hartley AL, Morris-Jones PH, Craft AW, et al: p53 germ line mutations in Li-Fraumeni syndrome. *Lancet* **338**:1490, 1991.

142. Birch JM: Germ line mutations in the p53 tumor suppressor gene: Scientific, clinical and ethical challenges. *Br J Cancer* **66**:424, 1992.

143. Barnes DM, Hanby AM, Gillett CE, Mohammed S, Hodson S, Bobrow LG, Leigh IM, Purkis T, MacGEoch C, Spur AM, Bartek J, Vojtesek B, Picksley SM, Lane DP: Abnormal expression of wild-type p53 protein in normal cells of a cancer family patient. *Lancet* **340**:259, 1992.

144. Frebourg T, Barbier N, Yan Y-X, Garber JE, Dreyfus M, Fraumeni JF Jr, Li FP, Friend SH: Germ line p53 mutations in 15 families with Li-Fraumeni syndrome. *Am J Hum Genet* **56**:608, 1995.

145. Brugieres L, Gardes M, Moutou C, Chompret A, Meresse V, et al: Screening for germ line p53 mutations in children with malignant tumor and a family history of cancer. *Cancer Res* **53**:452, 1993.

146. Birch JM, Heighway J, Teare MD, Kelsey AM, Hartley AL, Tricker KJ, Crowther D, Lane DP, Santibanez-Koref MF: Linkage studies in a Li-Fraumeni family with increased expression of p53 protein but no germ line mutation in p53. *Br J Cancer* **70**:1176, 1994.

146a. Varley JM, McGown G, Thorncroft M, Cochrane S, Morrison P, Woll P, Kelsey AM, Mitchell ELD, Boyle J, Birch JM, Evans DGR: A previously undescribed mutation within the tetramerization domain of TP53 in a family with Li-Fraumeni syndrome. *Oncogene* **12**:2437, 1996.

146b. Bell DW, Varley JM, Szydlo TE, Kang DH, Wahrer DC, Shannon KE, Lubratovich M, Verselis SJ, Isselbacher KJ, Fraumeni JF, Birch JM, Li FP, Garber JE, Haber DA: Heterozygous germ line hCHK2 mutations in Li-Fraumeni syndrome. *Science* **286**:2528, 1999.

146c. Hirao Z, Kong YY, Marsuoka S: DNA damage-induced activation of p53 by the checkpoint kinase Chk2. *Science* **287**:1824, 2000.

146d. Sodha N, Williams R, Mangion J, Bullock SL, Yuille MR, Eeles RA: Screening hCHK2 for mutations. *Science* **289** (5478):359, 2000.

146e. Boyle JM, Spreadborough A, Greaves MJ, Birch JM, Scott D: Chromosome instability in fibroblasts derived from Li-Fraumeni syndrome families without TP53 mutations. *Br J Cancer* **83**:1136, 2000.

147. Malkin D, Jolly KW, Barbier N, Look AT, Friend SH, Gebhardt MC, Andersen TI, Borresen A-L, Li FP, Strong LC: Germ line mutations of the p53 tumor suppressor gene in children and young adults with second malignant neoplasms. *N Engl J Med* **326**:1309, 1992.

148. Iavarone A, Mattay KK, Steinkirchner TM, Israel MA: Germ line and somatic p53 gene mutations in multifocal osteogenic sarcoma. *Proc Natl Acad Sci USA* **89**:4207, 1992.

148a. Kyritsis AP, Bondy ML, Xiao M, Berman EL, Cunningham JE, Lee PS, Levin VA, Saya H: Germ line p53 gene mutations in subsets of glioma patients. *J Natl Cancer Inst* **86**:344, 1994.

149. Toguchida J, Yamaguchi T, Dayton SH, Beauchamp RL, Herrera GE, Ishizaki K, Yamamuro T, Meyers PA, Little JB, Sasaki MS, Weichselbaum RR, Yandell DW: Prevalence and spectrum of germ line mutations of the p53 gene among patients with sarcoma. *N Engl J Med* **326**:1301, 1992.

150. Prosser J, Elder PA, Condie A, MacFayden I, Steel CM, Evans HJ: Mutations in p53 do not account for heritable breast cancer: A study in five affected families. *Br J Cancer* **63**:181, 1991.

151. Warren W, Eeles RA, Ponder BAJ, Easton DF, Averill D, Ponder MA, Anderson K, Evans AM, DeMars R, Love R, Dundas S, Stratton MR, Trowbridge P, Cooper CS, Peto J: No evidence for germ line mutations in exons 5-9 of the p53 gene in 25 breast cancer families. *Oncogene* **7**:1043, 1992.

152. Borresen A-L, Andersen TI, Garber J, Barbier N, Thorlacius S, Eyfjord J, Ottestad L, Smith-Sorensen B, Hovig E, Malkin D, Friend SH: Screening for germ line TP53 mutations in breast cancer patients. *Cancer Res* **52**:3234, 1992.

153. Frebourg T, Barbier N, Kassel J, Ng YS, Romero P, Friend SH: A functional screen for germ line p53 mutations based on transcriptional activation. *Cancer Res* **52**:6976, 1992.

154. Sidransky D, Tokino T, Helzlsouer K, Zehnbauer B, Rausch G, Shelton B, Prestigiacomo L, Vogelstein B, Davidson N: Inherited p53 gene mutations in breast cancer. *Cancer Res* **52**:2984, 1992.

155. Loriaux DL, Cutler GB Jr: Diseases of the adrenal glands, in Kohler PO (ed): *Clinical Endocrinology*. New York, Wiley, 1986, p 157.

156. Sameshima Y, Tsunematsu Y, Watanabe S, Tsukamoto T, Kawaha K, et al: Detection of novel germ line p53 mutations in diverse cancer prone families identified by selecting patients with childhood adrenocortical carcinoma. *J Natl Cancer Inst* **84**:703, 1992.

157. Wagner J, Portwine C, Rabin K, Leclerc J-M, Narod SA, Malkin D: High frequency of germ line p53 mutations in childhood adrenocortical cancer. *J Natl Cancer Inst* **86**:1707, 1994.

157a. Varley JM, McGown G, Thorncroft M, James LA, Margison GP, Forster G, Evans DG, Harris M, Kelsey AM, Birch JM: Are there low-penetrance TP53 alleles? Evidence from childhood adrenocortical tumors. *Am J Hum Genet* **65**:995, 1999.

158. McIntyre JF, Smith-Sorensen B, Friend SH, Kassel J, Borresen A-L, Yan YX, Russo C, Sato J, Barbier N, Miser J, Malkin D, Gebhardt MC: Germline mutations of the p53 tumor suppressor gene in children with osteosarcoma. *J Clin Oncol* **12**:925, 1994.

159. Diller L, Sexsmith E, Gottlieb A, Li FP, Malkin D: Germ line p53 mutations are frequently detected in young children with rhabdomyosarcoma. *J Clin Invest* **95**:1606, 1995.

160. Felix CA, Nau MM, Takahashi T, Mitsudomi T, Chiba I, Poplack DG, Reaman GH, Cole DE, Letterio JJ, Whang-Peng J, Knutsen T, Minna JD: Hereditary and acquired p53 mutations in childhood acute lymphoblastic leukemia. *J Clin Invest* **89**:640, 1992.

161. Felix CA, D'Amico D, Mitsudomi T, Nau MM, Li FP, Fraumeni JF Jr, Cole DE, McCalla J, Reaman GH, Whang-Peng J, Knutsen T, Minna JD, Poplack DG: Absence of hereditary p53 mutations in 10 familial leukemia pedigrees. *J Clin Invest* **90**:653, 1992.

162. Felix CA, Hosler MR, Provisor D, Salhany K, Sexsmith EA, Slater DJ, Cheung NKV, Winick NJ, Strauss EA, Heyn R, Lange BJ, Malkin D: The p53 gene in pediatric therapy-related leukemia and myelodysplasia. *Blood* **10**:4376, 1996.

163. Jolly KW, Malkin D, Douglass EC, Brown TF, Sinclair AE, Look, AT: Splice-site mutation of the p53 gene in a family with hereditary breast-ovarian cancer. *Oncogene* **9**:97, 1994.

164. Warneford SG, Wilton LJ, Townsend ML, Rowe PB, Reddell RR, Dalla-Pozza L, Symonds G: Germ line splicing mutation of the p53 gene in a cancer-prone family. *Cell Growth Differ* **3**:839, 1992.

165. Felix CA, Strauss EA, D'Amico D, Tsokos M, Winter S, Mitsudomi T, Nau MM, Brown DL, Leahey AM, Horowitz ME, Poplack DG, Costin D, Minna JD: A novel germ line p53 splicing mutation in a pediatric patient with a second malignant neoplasm. *Oncogene* **8**:1203, 1993.

166. Gannon JV, Greaves R, Iggo R, Lane DP: Activating mutations in p53 produce common conformation effects: A monoclonal antibody specific for the mutant form. *EMBO J* **9**:1591, 1990.

167. Srivastava S, Tong YA, Devadas K, Zou A-Q, Sykes VW, Chang EW: Detection of both mutant and wild-type p53 protein in normal skin fibroblasts and demonstration of a shared second hit on p53 in diverse tumors from a cancer-prone family with Li-Fraumeni syndrome. *Oncogene* **7**:987, 1992.

168. Frebourg T, Kassel J, Lam KT, Gryka MA, Barbier N, Andersen TI, Borresen A-L, Friend SH: Germ line mutations of the p53 tumor suppressor gene in patients with high risk for cancer inactivate the p53 protein. *Proc Natl Acad Sci USA* **89**:6413, 1992.

169. Ishioka C, Frebourg T, Yan Y-X, Vidal M, Friend SH, Schmidt S, Iggo R: Screening patients for heterozygous p53 mutations using a functional assay in yeast. *Nature Genet* **5**:124, 1993.

170. Flaman JM, Frebourg T, Moreau V, Charbonnier F, Martin C, Chappuis P, Sappino AP, Limacher IM, Bron L, Benhatter J: A simple p53 functional assay for screening cell lines, blood and tumors. *Proc Natl Acad Sci USA* **92**:3963, 1995.

171. Lavigueur A, Bernstein A: p53 transgenic mice: Accelerated erythroleukemia induction by Friend virus. *Oncogene* **6**:2197, 1991.

172. Donehower LA, Harvey M, Slagle BL, McArthur MJ, Montgomery CA, Butel J, Bradley A: Mice deficient for p53 are developmentally normal but susceptible to spontaneous tumors. *Nature* **356**:215, 1992.

173. Rogel A, Popliker M, Webb C, Oren M: p53 cellular tumor antigen: Analysis of mRNA levels in normal cell adult tissues, embryos, and tumors. *Mol Cell Biol* **5**:2851, 1985.

174. Purdie CA, Harrison DJ, Peter A, Dobbie L, White S, Howie SEM, Salter DM, Bird CC, Wyllie AH, Hooper ML, Clarke AR: Tumor incidence, spectrum and ploidy in mice with a large deletion in the p53 gene. *Oncogene* **9**:603, 1994.

175. Jacks T, Remington L, Williams BO, Schmitt EM, Halachmi S, Bronson RT, Weinberg RA: Tumor spectrum analysis in p53 mutant mice. *Current Biol* **4**:1, 1994.

176. Harvey M, McArthur MJ, Montgomery CA Jr, Bradley A, Donehower LA: Genetic background alters the spectrum of tumors that develop in p53-deficient mice. *FASEB J* **7**:849, 1993.

177. Dietrich WF, Lander ES, Smith JS, Moser AR, Gould KA, Luongo C, Borenstein N, Dove W: Genetic identification of Mom-1, a major modifiar locus affecting Min-induced intestinal neoplasia in the mouse. *Cell* **75**:631, 1993.

178. Montes de Oca Luna R, Wagner DS, Lozano G: Rescue of embryonic lethality in mdm-2-deficient mice by deletion of p53. *Nature* **378**:203, 1995.

179. Jones SN, Roe AE, Donehower LA, Bradley A: Rescue of embryonic lethality in Mdm-2-deficient mice by absence of p53. *Nature* **378**:206, 1995.

180. Harvey M, Vogel H, Morris D, Bradley A, Bernstein A, Donehower LA: A mutant p53 transgene accelerates tumor development in heterozygous but not nullizygous p53-deficient mice. *Nature Genet* **9**:305, 1995.

181. Liu G, Montes de Oca Luna R, Lozano G: Establishing mouse models to study tumor derived p53 mutants in vivo: Cancer genetics and tumor suppressor genes. *Cold Spring Harbor Lab Meeting* **172**: 1996.

182. Sah VP, Attardi LD, Mulligan GJ, Williams BO, Bronson RT, Jacks T: A subset of p53-deficient embryos exhibit exencephaly. *Nature Genet* **7**:480, 1994.

183. Hartley AL, Birch JM, Blair V, Kelsey AM, Morris-Jones PH: Fetal loss and infant deaths in families of children with soft-tissue sarcoma. *Int J Cancer* **56**:646, 1994.

184. Harvey M, McArthur MJ, Montgomery CA Jr, Butel JS, Bradley A, Donehower LA: Spontaneous and carcinogen-induced tumorigenesis in p53-deficient mice. *Nature Genet* **5**:225, 1993.

185. Li G, Ho VC, Berean K, Tron VA: Ultraviolet radiation induction of squamous cell carcinomas in p53 transgenic mice. *Cancer Res* **55**:2070, 1995.

186. Koizumi A, Tsudada M, Wada Y, Masuda H, Weindruch R: *J Nutr* **122**:1446, 1992.

187. Hursting SD, Perkins SN, Phang JM: Calorie restriction delays spontaneous tumorigenesis in p53-knockout transgenic mice. *Proc Natl Acad Sci USA* **91**:7036, 1994.

188. Nicol CJ, Harrison ML, Laposa RR, Gimelshtein IL, Wells PG: A teratologic suppressor role for p53 in benzo[a]pyrene-treated transgenic p53-deficient mice. *Nature Genet* **10**:181, 1995.

189. Laposa RR, Chan KC, Wiley MJ, Wells PG: Evidence for DNA damage and teratological suppressor genes in the initiation of and resistance to chemical teratogenesis: phenytoin teratogenicity in p53-deficient mice. *Toxicologist* **15**:161, 1995.

190. Clarke AR, Cummings MC, Harrison DJ: Interaction between murine germ line mutations in p53 and APC predisposes to pancreatic neoplasia but not to increased intestinal malignancy. *Oncogene* **11**:1913, 1995.

191. Stewart M, Cameron E, Campbell M, McFarlane R, Toth S, Lang K et al: Conditional expression and oncogenicity of c-myc linked to a CD2 gene dominant control region. *Int J Cancer* **53**:1023, 1993.

192. Blyth K, Terry A, O'Hara M, Baxter EW, Campbell M, Stewart M, Donehower LA, Onions DE, Neil JC, Cameron ER: Synergy between a human c-myc transgene and p53 null genotype in murine thymic lymphomas: Contrasting effects of homozygous and heterozygous p53 loss. *Oncogene* **10**:1717, 1995.

193. Li FP, Garber JE, Friend SH, Strong LC, Patenaude AF, Juengst ET, Reilly PR, Corea P, Fraumeni JF Jr: Recommendations on predictive testing for germ line p53 mutations among cancer-prone individuals. *J Natl Cancer Inst* **84**:1156, 1992.

194. American Society of Clinical Oncology: Statement of the American Society of Clinical Oncology: Genetic testing for cancer susceptibility. *J Clin Oncol* **14**:1730, 1996.

195. American Society of Human Genetics: Statements of the American Society of Human Genetics on genetic testing for breast and ovarian cancer predisposition. *Am J Hum Genet* **55**:i, 1994.

196. Shapiro S: Determining the efficacy of breast cancer screening. *Cancer* **63**:1873, 1989.

Wilms Tumor

Daniel A. Haber

1. Wilms tumor is a pediatric kidney cancer that can arise sporadically or in children with congenital syndromes conferring genetic susceptibility. In addition, some 10 percent of children with Wilms tumor present with bilateral cancers, evidence of a predisposing genetic lesion.

2. The genetic loci associated with the development of Wilms tumor have been identified by analysis of gross karyotype abnormalities in children with Wilms-associated syndromes, as well as by molecular analyses of DNA losses in tumor specimens. A genetic locus on chromosome 11 band p13 has been linked to Wilms tumor arising in the context of aniridia and abnormalities of genitourinary development (e.g., WAGR syndrome). A second locus on chromosome 11 band p15 is associated with hemihypertrophy (e.g., Beckwith-Wiedemann syndrome) and predisposition to Wilms tumor and other pediatric neoplasms. A third Wilms locus has been mapped recently to chromosome 17q12-21.

3. The *WT1* gene, mapping within the 11p13 genetic locus, was isolated in 1990. It encodes a transcription factor whose expression is strictly developmentally regulated in the normal kidney. Like the fetal kidney cells from which they appear to originate, most Wilms tumors express high levels of WT1 protein. However, in a fraction of Wilms tumors, *WT1* is either deleted or mutated to an inactive form, consistent with its characterization as a tumor suppressor gene. Reintroduction of wild-type WT1 into a Wilms tumor cell line with an aberrant endogenous *WT1* transcript results in inhibition of cell growth.

4. Inactivation of *WT1* in one germ-line allele confers a high degree of susceptibility to Wilms tumor, which is triggered by loss of the second *WT1* allele in somatic tissues. Hemizygosity for *WT1* in the germ line also results in a variable degree of developmental abnormalities in the genitourinary tract, more prominent in males than in females. Moreover, specific point mutations within the DNA-binding domain of *WT1* result in a dominant negative phenotype, characterized by severe abnormalities in sexual and renal development (Denys-Drash syndrome). In the mouse, hemizygous inactivation of *WT1* is not associated with genitourinary defects or tumor predisposition. However, homozygous inactivation of *WT1* leads to failure of renal and gonadal development, as well as to malformations of the heart and diaphragm.

5. The protein encoded by *WT1* belongs to a class of zinc-binding transcription factors, with multiple variants produced by alternative splicing. The four DNA-binding zinc finger domains of WT1 are disrupted by the variable insertion of three amino acids (KTS) between zinc fingers 3 and 4. Germ-line mutations that affect the KTS splice donor site, reducing the relative expression of the *WT1*(+KTS) splice variant, are associated with Frasier syndrome, characterized by abnormalities in sexual and renal differentiation. The uninterrupted zinc finger domains of WT1(−KTS) recognize

the DNA consensus sequence 5′-GCGTGGGAGT-3′. WT1(−KTS) represses transcription from many GC-rich promoters, but more recent studies of endogenous target genes have suggested that it may function as a transcriptional activator of genes involved in renal and gonadal differentiation programs. Ectopic expression of *WT1*(−KTS) also triggers myelo-monocytic differentiation in hematopoietic progenitors. The WT1(+KTS) isoform demonstrates reduced DNA binding and has been postulated to play a role in pre-mRNA processing, based on its distinct subnuclear localization. Characterization of the normal pathways involved in *WT1* function and of any potential interactions with other Wilms tumor genes may lead to a better understanding of normal kidney development and tumorigenesis.

Wilms tumor, or nephroblastoma, is a pediatric kidney cancer that can present either as a sporadic case or in the setting of genetic predisposition. Both epidemiologic studies of tumor incidence and early genetic studies pointed to the presence of one or more genes whose loss was associated with tumor development. The isolation of the first of these genes, *WT1*, has led to the discovery of a tumor suppressor gene encoding a transcription factor with a striking kidney-specific pattern of expression. Mutations in *WT1* have been linked both to the formation of Wilms tumor and to a range of developmental abnormalities in genitourinary development. The characterization of this gene and the ongoing search for the other Wilms tumor genes provide a key to understanding the basis of normal kidney development and tumorigenesis.

HISTOLOGY

The histologic characteristics of Wilms tumor are complex, consistent with its classification as a primitive, multilineage malignancy of renal stem cells.[1] The classic description is that of a "triphasic" tumor, including blastemal, epithelial, and stromal components (Fig. 24-1). All these components are thought to be derived from the malignant stem cell, although genetic evidence of shared lineage has not been demonstrated. Wilms tumors can vary in the predominance of one histologic component over the others, and some tumors show evidence of further multilineage differentiation, with the presence of muscle or neural elements. Clinical prognosis does not appear to be affected by the histologic appearance of the tumors, with the exception of anaplastic variants that have a more aggressive course.[2] Tumors with triphasic histology characteristic of Wilms tumor may arise outside the kidney. Such "extrarenal" Wilms tumors have been reported from a number of sites, primarily the pelvis and abdomen.[3] Although Wilms tumor is primarily a cancer of children under 5 years of age, it also has been reported in young adults. The histology of these tumors is similar to that of classic Wilms tumor seen in young children, leading to the suggestion that they arise from a small number of renal stem cells that have persisted into adulthood.

The relationship between Wilms tumor and normal renal development is best illustrated by the persistent nephrogenic rests seen within the normal kidney of children with Wilms tumor.[4,5] These lesions, also called *precursor lesions, persistent metaneph-*

A list of standard abbreviations is located immediately preceding the index.

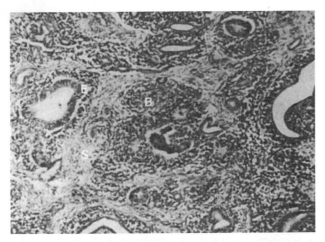

Fig. 24-1 Wilms tumor histology. The classic triphasic histologic pattern includes areas of primitive blastemal cells (B), epithelial cells (E), and stromal cell components (S). Tumors also can contain areas of further differentiation along muscle and rarely neural lineages. Expression of the *WT1* tumor suppressor gene appears restricted to the epithelial and blastemal components of Wilms tumors. (*Photomicrograph, hematoxylin and eosin stain, provided by Dr. Nancy Harris, Department of Pathology, Massachusetts General Hospital, Boston, Massachusetts.*)

ric blastema, nephroblastomatosis or *nodular renal blastema* are comprised of primitive blastemal cells with varying degrees of differentiation. They are usually less than 1 cm in diameter but rarely can become massive, compressing the normal kidney and easily mistaken for a genuine tumor. Although foci of Wilms tumor can arise within a large nephrogenic rest, the precursor lesions themselves do not appear to be malignant, and some have been shown to regress when followed noninvasively. Nephrogenic rests are present in the normal kidney at birth but are rarely found after 1 year of age. In contrast, virtually all children with genetic susceptibility to Wilms tumor have one or more such lesions within otherwise normal kidney. In these children, nephrogenic rests may represent the effect of a constitutional mutation predisposing to abnormal renal development, the first step toward the formation of Wilms tumor. In support of this notion is the observation that nephrogenic rests located in the periphery of a renal lobe, so-called perilobar rests, are found more frequently in the kidneys of children whose genetic susceptibility to Wilms tumor is associated with the locus on chromosome 11p15. Nephrogenic rests located within the renal lobe, known as intralobar rests, are smaller and less well defined histologically and are seen more commonly in the kidneys of children with evidence of a genetic lesion at the chromosome 11p13 locus.[5] However, even in the absence of genetic predisposition, some 30 percent of children with apparently sporadic Wilms tumor have nephrogenic rests within the normal surrounding kidney. Molecular evidence indicates that these nephrogenic rests harbor the same mutation in *WT1* as that found in the accompanying Wilms tumor, suggesting that both the tumor and the precursor lesion are derived from the same renal stem cell in which the tumor suppressor gene was mutated.[6]

CLINICAL FEATURES

Nephroblastosis was first described in 1899 by a German physician, Max Wilms, as a uniformly fatal cancer of children. With the use of modern multimodality therapy, the treatment of Wilms tumor has advanced dramatically, with a reported cure rate of 90 percent by the National Wilms Tumor Study Group.[7] Wilms tumor usually arises by age 5, with equal incidence between sexes and among different ethnic groups. In children with genetic susceptibility, the age of incidence is usually under 2 years, and frequent screening by renal ultrasound is recommended. The usual

presenting feature is that of an abdominal mass, with an adrenal malignancy such as neuroblastoma as the main differential diagnostic consideration. Initial preoperative evaluation is directed at excluding the presence of pulmonary metastases, local spread into the inferior vena cava, or involvement of draining lymph nodes. The surgical management of Wilms tumor calls for skill and experience, requiring resection of the affected kidney, exploration of the inferior vena cava, and lymph node dissection. Of utmost importance is examination of the contralateral kidney for any synchronous tumor. The occurrence of bilateral tumors in some 10 percent of patients is an indication of genetic susceptibility to Wilms tumor, but it cannot be excluded by a negative family history or the absence of associated congenital abnormalities. Most children with bilateral tumors have no prior evidence of genetic risk, and genetic studies to date have indicated that most of these children may harbor *de novo* germ-line mutations.[8,9] In the presence of bilateral Wilms tumors, most surgeons will perform a full nephrectomy on the side with the larger tumor and a partial nephrectomy on the other side, attempting to preserve as much renal function as possible.

Postoperative treatment of Wilms tumor with chemotherapy and radiation therapy is evolving as multi-institutional groups adjust the recommended regimens so as to improve the effectiveness and lower the toxicity of treatment.[10] Most children who fit into favorable prognostic groups based on tumor histology and stage are treated with chemotherapy including actinomycin D and vincristine. Radiation therapy in addition to chemotherapy is reserved for patients with anaplastic tumors or cancers of advanced stage. Wilms tumor appears to be very sensitive to chemotherapy drugs, and even patients with advanced metastatic disease have an excellent cure rate. The incidence of secondary malignancies in children cured of Wilms tumor is low and appears to be treatment-related, consisting primarily of soft tissue sarcomas arising within the radiation field and acute leukemia attributed to the use of alkylating agents and radiation therapy.[11] Genetic predisposition to Wilms tumor is only rarely associated with susceptibility to other tumor types, such as gonadoblastoma in Denys-Drash syndrome or adrenal carcinoma and hepatocellular carcinoma in Beckwith-Wiedemann syndrome. In the absence of such congenital syndromes, the great majority of children treated for Wilms tumor are fertile when they reach reproductive age, and the risk of Wilms tumor arising in their offspring has been found to be very low.[12]

THE KNUDSON MODEL IN WILMS TUMOR

Much of the conceptual basis for the genetic study of tumor suppressor genes was laid by Knudson in a series of epidemiologic studies of retinoblastoma, Wilms tumor, and neuroblastoma.[13–15] These childhood tumors are remarkable in that 10 to 30 percent of affected children present with bilateral or multicentric cancers. Bilateral tumors have an age of onset that is 1 to 2 years earlier than that of unilateral cancers, and in the case of the eye tumor retinoblastoma, they are often associated with a positive family history. By comparing the incidence of unilateral versus bilateral retinoblastomas in patients with a positive family history, Knudson found that the data fit the Poisson distribution for a single rare event. Thus these individuals, who had inherited one genetic mutation, only required one additional "genetic hit" in the target tissues to develop a tumor (Fig. 24-2). Given the number of target cells at risk for the second hit, multiple tumors are common, and they tend to arise early in life. In contrast, in the absence of genetic predisposition, two rare independent events are required for tumor formation, hence a low incidence of tumors, which are unilateral and which present at a later age. In addition to the difference in the mean age of tumor development between inherited and sporadic cases, the rate of decline in the incidence of new tumors is also predicted by the Knudson "two-hit" model. In genetically predisposed individuals, the age of onset declines exponentially, consistent with the exponential rate of differentiation of susceptible nephroblasts. In contrast, in sporadic cases, a more delayed

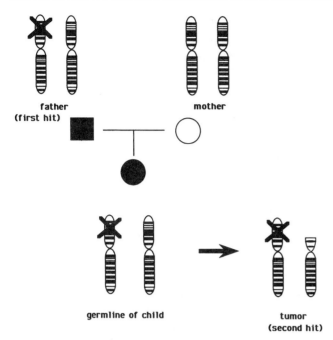

father
(first hit)

mother

germline of child

tumor
(second hit)

Fig. 24-2 Schematic representation of the Knudson model. Based on epidemiologic analyses of the age of incidence and number of tumors observed in children with genetic predisposition versus those with sporadic tumors, Knudson and Strong[12-14] predicted that two rate-limiting "hits" are required for tumorigenesis. This hypothesis has evolved with the detection of allelic losses in tumors and the concept of recessive oncogenes or tumor suppressor genes.[18,22] Thus a mutation present either in the germ line or in the germ cells of a parent constitutes the first hit. The child born with such a mutation in the germ line requires only one additional hit in the target tissue to trigger tumorigenesis. The relatively high frequency of this second hit explains the early age of onset of tumors and the fact that they are often bilateral. In contrast, a child without a germ-line mutation requires two independent rare events within the target tissue in order to achieve two rate-limiting hits. The low probability of two independent mutations at the same locus explains the later onset of tumors in sporadic cases and the fact that they are unilateral. In most cases of Wilms tumor, the initial hit results from a point mutation or a small deletion within the target tumor suppressor gene, while the second hit consists of a gross chromosomal deletion or non-disjunction event. These large chromosomal events can be identified by the loss of restriction fragment length polymorphisms (RFLP) in the affected locus (so-called loss of heterozygosity), thus providing a clue to the presence of a tumor suppressor gene.

decline in the incidence of new tumors is noted, suggesting that the second genetic lesion depends on the variable timing of the initial mutation.

The predictions of the Knudson model were first confirmed by the cloning of the retinoblastoma susceptibility gene, *RB1*.[16-18] Indeed, the two genetic hits represent the inactivation of the two alleles of this tumor suppressor gene.[19-22] The first hit appears to be most commonly a mutation or small deletion that is found in the germ line of predisposed individuals or in somatic tissues in sporadic cases. Loss of the second allele, which represents the second hit, is seen most commonly as a wholesale loss of a chromosome or a chromosomal recombinational event in somatic tissues. Such large chromosomal losses may be more frequent than the initial point mutation but are only tolerated in the heterozygous state, explaining their prevalence as second rather than first hits. They have proven to be of critical importance in molecular mapping studies of tumor suppressor genes such as those responsible for retinoblastoma and Wilms tumor, since the loss of surrounding restriction fragment length polymorphisms (RFLP) points to the presence of a critical genetic locus.[23]

The epidemiology of Wilms tumor shares a number of features with that of retinoblastoma. Bilateral tumors are noted in 5 to 10

percent of patients, and as predicted by the Knudson model, these present at an earlier age than unilateral cases.[14,24,25] However, familial Wilms tumor is rare, estimated at 1 percent of patients. Based on the number of bilateral tumors, the mathematical model proposed by Knudson and Strong predicts that some 30 percent of children have a genetic predisposition to Wilms tumor. In the majority of cases, this genetic susceptibility appears to represent a *de novo* germ-line mutation rather than a transmitted parental gene. In this context, it is of interest that in most Wilms tumors that show allelic DNA losses involving the 11p13 genetic locus, the lost allele (representing the second hit) is of maternal origin. These observations suggest that the initial mutation is likely to occur in the paternal germ cells during spermatogenesis.

Another distinction between retinoblastoma and Wilms tumor is the presence of a phenotype conferred by a single mutated allele. Individuals with a germ-line mutation in *RB1* who fail to develop a tumor during the first few years of life have no detectable ocular abnormalities as adults, suggesting that hemizygosity for *RB1* is phenotypically silent. In contrast, children with hemizygous deletions involving the 11p13 Wilms tumor locus (WAGR syndrome) have developmental abnormalities of the genitourinary tract as well as nephrogenic rests within both kidneys.[26,27] Since nephrogenic rests consist of a proliferation of primitive blastemal cells, their presence may increase the size of the target cell population, thus enhancing the probability of a second genetic hit. The number of genetic lesions important in the development of Wilms tumor may in fact be greater than two. The Knudson model, based on the statistics of "hit kinetics," has proved to be accurate in predicting the number of genetic events that are rate-limiting. However, genetic events that are necessary for malignant transformation but that are more frequent or that are dependent on these initial "hits" will not be detected by such an analysis. At least three genetic loci have been implicated in the initial events in Wilms tumorigenesis, and tumor specimens have been shown to have a number of additional chromosomal abnormalities that may have a role in tumor progression. The isolation of the first of these genes and the characterization of the genetic lesions that contribute to the development of Wilms tumor have provided an initial appreciation for the genetic complexity of this malignancy.[28]

GENETIC LOCI ASSOCIATED WITH WILMS TUMOR

The identification of the major genetic loci associated with the development of Wilms tumor has resulted from studies of both germ-line and tumor material, using karyotype analysis, genetic linkage and molecular genetic studies, as well as clinical observations on patients with congenital abnormalities. Two distinct genetic loci have been mapped to the short arm of chromosome 11 (Table 24-1), while a third locus on chromosome 17q has been implicated in some familial cases.

Chromosome 11p13 Locus

The first linkage of Wilms tumor susceptibility to a chromosomal locus was derived from a clinical observation. In 1964, Miller and coworkers noted a higher than expected incidence of Wilms tumor in children with aniridia, a rare eye abnormality consisting of malformation or absence of the iris.[29] While Wilms tumor arises in 1 in 10,000 children and aniridia occurs in 1 in 70,000 children, aniridia is noted in 1 in 70 children with Wilms tumor, and this tumor develops in 1 in 3 children with aniridia. As would be expected from the Knudson model, children with aniridia who develop a Wilms tumor have a high incidence of bilateral tumors, consistent with the presence of a predisposing germ-line lesion. This lesion is most clearly evident in children with a constellation of symptoms that includes aniridia, developmental abnormalities of the genitourinary tract (such as hypospadias, undescended testes, renal hypoplasia, or ureteral atresia), and mental retardation.[26,27] Children with this so-called WAGR syndrome (an acronym for *W*ilms, *a*nirida, *g*enitourinary defects, *m*ental

Table 24-1 Summary of the Two Major Congenital Syndromes Associated with Increased Susceptibility to Wilms Tumor*

	WAGR Syndrome	Beckwith-Wiedemann Syndrome
Chromosomal locus	11p13	11p15
Tumor suppressor gene	*WT1*	Unknown
Wilms tumor incidence	<50%	<5%
Associated features	Aniridia	Macroglossia
	Genitourinary defects	Organomegaly/hemihypertrophy
		Umbilical hernia
	Mental retardation	Neonatal hypoglycemia
		Additional tumors
		Adrenocortical carcinoma
		Hepatoblastoma

*The WAGR syndrome results from a hemizygous chromosomal deletion within the chromosome 11p13 locus, affecting the *WT1* and aniridia genes. Beckwith-Wiedemann syndrome results from an abnormality in the 11p15 locus that may involve gene dosage as well as parental imprinting. The gene responsible for this syndrome and for the associated risk of developing Wilms tumor has not been identified.

retardation) were found to have a gross cytogenetic deletion within band 13 of the short arm of chromosome 11[30,31] (Fig. 24-3). This discovery was the first to link a gene conferring susceptibility to Wilms tumor to a genetic locus. The complex congenital abnormalities of children with WAGR syndrome results from a deletion that affects a number of adjacent genes, a so-called contiguous-gene syndrome (Fig. 24-4). The aniridia locus was distinguished from the Wilms tumor locus by the existence of patients with an 11p13 chromosome translocation who suffered from aniridia without developing Wilms tumor.[32,33] Aniridia is now known to result from a hemizygous deletion of a homeobox gene, *Pax6*.[34] The genitourinary defects associated with WAGR syndrome are variable in their severity and appear to result from hemizygosity for the Wilms tumor gene itself (see below). The etiology of the mental retardation is still unclear.

The involvement of the chromosome 11p13 locus in Wilms tumor development also was evidenced by molecular analysis of tumor specimens. Chromosome abnormalities in Wilms tumor specimens are complex but frequently involve the short arm of chromosome 11.[35–38] More precise molecular studies, involving the use of polymorphic DNA markers, were used to demonstrate loss of heterozygosity on chromosome 11p.[39–42] This represents the loss of gross chromosomal fragments or recombinational events resulting in the loss of the second allele of a putative tumor suppressor gene (the second genetic hit). The loss of heterozygosity at chromosome 11p13 that results from such mechanisms

usually extends to the telomere, spanning the 11p15 locus. It therefore can be difficult to distinguish involvement of the two Wilms loci on the short arm of chromosome 11, but cases in which a more limited loss of DNA affects each locus in isolation have confirmed the independence of these two genetic loci.[43,44]

Chromosome 11p15

Like the 11p13 Wilms tumor locus, the 11p15 locus has been implicated both by genetic susceptibility studies and by allelic losses in tumor specimens.[39–46] However, the genetic mechanisms underlying the effects of the 11p15 locus appear to be more complex, involving genomic imprinting and unequal duplication of parental chromosomes. Increased susceptibility to Wilms tumor was noted by Wiedemann and by Beckwith in a syndrome that now bears their name.[47,48] Beckwith-Wiedemann syndrome consists of abnormally enlarged organs, particularly the tongue and abdominal viscera, which can result in an umbilical hernia. Soft tissues also can be enlarged, with one side more affected than the other, resulting in hemihypertrophy of the body. Neonatal hypoglycemia is also evident in more serious cases. Pediatric neoplasms are seen in 7.5 percent of children with Beckwith-Wiedemann syndrome, a far lower incidence than that in patients with WAGR syndrome, and these tumors include adrenocortical carcinoma and hepatoblastoma as well as Wilms tumor. The true penetrance of Beckwith-Wiedemann syndrome is difficult to ascertain, since the different manifestations of the syndrome can be quite variable, often rendering the clinical diagnosis uncertain.[49,50]

The association of Beckwith-Wiedemann syndrome with the chromosome 11p15 locus is based on genetic linkage studies in the rare families in which the condition is inherited,[51,52] as well as

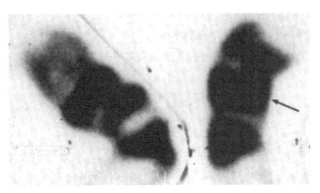

Fig. 24-3 Cytogenetic abnormality in WAGR syndrome. One of the two chromosomes 11 in the germ line of a child with WAGR syndrome contains a deletion within band p13 (arrow). This large hemizygous deletion, encompassing a number of contiguous genes, leads to a 50 percent probability of developing Wilms tumor, abnormal development of the iris (aniridia), abnormalities of genitourinary development, and mental retardation.

chromosome band 11p13:

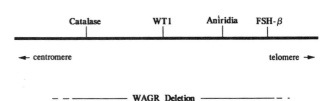

Fig. 24-4 Schematic map of the WAGR region. The 11p13 chromosomal deletion in children with WAGR syndrome is flanked on the centromeric side by the gene encoding catalase and on the telomeric side by the gene for the β subunit of follicle-stimulating hormone. Within the deletion are located the Wilms tumor susceptibility gene *WT1* and the aniridia gene.

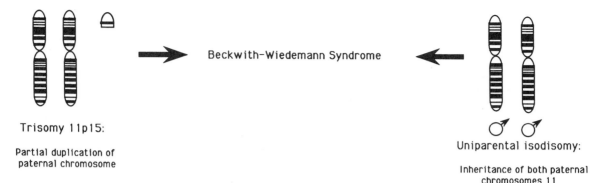

Trisomy 11p15:

Partial duplication of
paternal chromosome

Uniparental isodisomy:

Inheritance of both paternal
chromosomes 11

Fig. 24-5 Genetic mechanisms underlying Beckwith-Wiedemann syndrome. Beckwith-Wiedemann syndrome (hemihypertrophy, organomegaly, neonatal hypoglycemia, and susceptibility to Wilms tumor, adrenocortical carcinoma, and hepatoblastoma) can be inherited and has been linked to chromosome 11p15 by studies of large pedigrees. In sporadic cases, gross chromosome abnormalities in the germ line of affected children also have implicated chromosome 11p15 and have suggested that genomic imprinting may play a role in the syndrome. In some cases, RFLP analysis has shown that affected children have inherited two copies of the paternal chromosomes 11 and neither of the maternal chromosomes 11.[57,58] In other cases, a partial duplication of the paternal 11p15 chromosomal fragment results in trisomy for this genetic locus.[52] These observations are consistent with a mechanism whereby the maternal allele is silent or "imprinted" and the syndrome results from the increased gene dosage caused by the presence of two paternal alleles.

gross cytogenetic abnormalities in the germ line of some sporadically affected individuals.[53,54] Abnormal karyotypes in such patients most frequently consist of a duplication of chromosome band 11p15, although in two cases a ring chromosome has been reported.[55] The role of genetic imprinting in Beckwith-Wiedemann syndrome is suggested by a number of unusual observations. In the familial syndrome, the disease appears to be more severe when the affected chromosome is transmitted by the mother rather than the father.[56] In contrast, in cases where trisomy for 11p15 is present, the duplicated chromosome is invariably of paternal origin.[57] Finally, molecular studies have shown that in some cases of Beckwith-Wiedemann syndrome, affected children are diploid for 11p15 but have inherited two copies of the paternal chromosome and no maternal chromosome—so-called uniparental isodisomy.[58,59] One possible explanation for these unusual genetic abnormalities may be that they can lead to differences in the dosage of a critically regulated gene (Fig. 24-5). If such a gene were imprinted and expressed only from the paternal allele, duplication of the paternal chromosome, either in the form of uniparental isodisomy or partial 11p15 trisomy, would then lead to a twofold overexpression. In familial transmission of Beckwith-Wiedemann syndrome, a mutation resulting in increased expression of this gene would be expected to have a greater impact if it arose on the imprinted maternal allele than in the already expressed paternal allele.

The Wilms tumor gene at the 11p15 locus remains to be identified, but a number of candidate genes are of particular interest. The insulin-like growth factor II (*IGFII*) gene encodes an embryonic growth factor whose expression in most tissues is derived solely from the paternally derived allele. Inactivation of one allele of *IGFII* in the mouse germ line results in small-sized offspring if the disrupted gene is transmitted by the father but has no effect if transmitted by the mother.[60,61] Thus the organomegaly associated with Beckwith-Wiedemann syndrome could be attributed to the doubling of IGFII expression levels caused by duplication of the actively transcribed paternal allele.[62,63] The potential role of *IGFII* in Beckwith-Wiedemann syndrome is supported by the observation that some affected children show constitutional loss of imprinting of this gene (i.e., expression from both alleles), without evidence of gross chromosomal alterations.[64,65] Furthermore, sporadic Wilms tumors have high expression of IGFII,[66,67] and some tumors also show loss or relaxation of imprinting,[68,69] suggesting that this growth factor also may contribute directly to tumorigenesis. However, two other candidate genes at chromosome 11p15 have been reported recently. The cyclin-dependent kinase inhibitor *p57* is also imprinted,[70] and

inactivating mutations in the expressed paternal allele have been detected in the germ line of two children with Beckwith-Wiedemann syndrome.[71] These observations suggest that the overgrowth syndrome may result from loss of growth inhibition by p57, although additional genetic events would presumably be required to explain the chromosomal evidence for increased paternal gene copy number. A third gene at chromosome 11p15, *H19*, also has been implicated in Wilms tumorigenesis. *H19* encodes an abundant transcript lacking an open reading frame, suggesting that it functions as RNA.[72] Transfection studies have shown that it suppresses tumor formation in nude mice without affecting *in vitro* growth properties.[73] Of particular interest is the observation that *H19* and *IGFII* share regulatory sequences, with a reciprocal pattern of imprinting. Thus *H19* is expressed from the maternally derived allele,[72] and expression would be lost in children who inherit two copies of the paternally derived chromosome 11.

The association between the 11p15 chromosomal locus and Wilms tumor is supported by the increased incidence of this tumor in children with Beckwith-Wiedemann syndrome. However, molecular genetic analyses of Wilms tumor specimens have demonstrated allelic losses that affect 11p15 but spare the 11p13 genetic locus.[43,45] These allelic losses are usually indicative of gene deletion or loss-of-function events, which are difficult to reconcile with the apparent increased gene dosage mechanism commonly invoked for Beckwith-Wiedemann syndrome. It is therefore possible that the 11p15 Beckwith-Wiedemann and Wilms tumor locus contains multiple genes, disrupted by different genetic mechanisms. Molecular studies also have suggested that both the 11p13 and 11p15 Wilms tumor genes can contribute to tumorigenesis within the same tumor, based on cases in which distinct allelic losses are seen at both of these loci.[45,74] Unlike the *WT1* gene isolated from the Wilms tumor locus on chromosome 11p13, which appears to be specifically involved in kidney development and tumorigenesis (see below), the putative gene(s) residing at chromosome locus 11p15 has been linked to a number of different tumor types. In addition to adrenocortical carcinoma, Wilms tumor, and hepatoblastoma that are associated with Beckwith-Wiedemann syndrome, somatic allelic losses at 11p15 have been reported in breast cancer, lung cancer, and acute myelogenous leukemia.[75,76]

Familial Wilms Tumor

Familial transmission of susceptibility to Wilms tumor is rare, estimated at less than 1 percent of cases.[14,25] Thus the majority of children with evidence of genetic susceptibility appear to have *de*

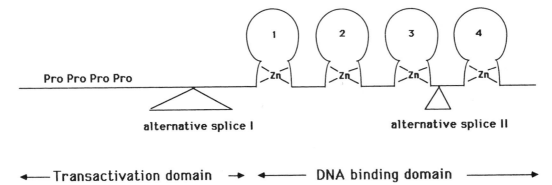

←—— Transactivation domain ——→ ←—— DNA binding domain ——————→

Fig. 24-6 Functional domains of the *WT1* gene product. The predicted polypeptide encoded by *WT1* contains two functional domains: The C-terminus contains four "zinc fingers" of the cysteine-histidine class, which constitute the DNA-binding domain of *WT1*. This domain has a high degree of homology with that of the early growth response gene 1 (EGR1), and it confers a similar DNA-binding specificity. The N-terminus of *WT1* is rich in prolines (Pro) and constitutes the transactivation domain of *WT1*. This domain appears to be capable of suppressing the transcription of genes that are potential targets of WT1. Two alternative splices are variably inserted in the *WT1* transcript, resulting in the presence of four distinct mRNA species. The function of alternative splice I is unknown, while insertion of alternative splice II disrupts the linker between zinc fingers 3 and 4 and alters the DNA-binding specificity of the encoded protein.

novo germ-line mutations. The 11p13 Wilms tumor gene *WT1* has been implicated in a few familial cases of children with bilateral tumors or genitourinary defects.[8,9] However, in three large pedigrees of familial Wilms tumor, genetic linkage analysis has excluded chromosome 11.[77–79] Recently, analysis of a Canadian Wilms tumor kindred, remarkable for the relatively late onset of tumors and the absence of associated genitourinary defects, has indicated genetic linkage to chromosome 17q12-22.[80]

THE *WT1* GENE AT CHROMOSOME 11p13

Identification and Characterization of *WT1*

The isolation of the 11p13 Wilms tumor gene resulted from the analysis of patients with chromosomal deletions and translocations as well as the generation of human-hamster cell hybrids containing defined segments of chromosome 11p13.[81–86] These studies provided detailed maps of the WAGR region within chromosome 11p13, flanked on the centromeric side by the gene encoding catalase[87,88] and on the telomeric side by the gene for the β subunit of follicle-stimulating hormone[89–92] (see Fig. 24-4). The *WT1* gene was isolated within the smallest region of overlap among chromosomal deletions.[93,94]

WT1 encodes a protein migrating at 55 kDa, with two regions of recognizable homology that indicate it functions as a transcription factor (Fig. 24-6). The C-terminus contains four *zinc-finger domains*, loop structures of amino acids that each contain two regularly spaced cysteines and histidines, bind to zinc ions, and mediate recognition of a specific DNA sequence.[95] The N-terminus of *WT1* is rich in prolines and glutamines, a feature shared by the transactivation domains of some transcription factors.[96] Two alternative splices are present within the *WT1* transcript, resulting in four distinct mRNA species that are expressed in constant proportion to each other.[97] Alternative splice I, inserted within the N-terminus of *WT1*, encodes 17 amino acids including five serines and one threonine, potential sites for protein phosphorylation. Alternative splice II encodes three amino acids (lysine, threonine, serine, or KTS) that disrupt the critical spacing between the third and fourth zinc-finger domains. In the absence of alternative splice II, the *WT1* zinc-finger domains share extensive homology with the early growth response gene (*EGR1,* also known as *NGFIA, Krox 24,* or *Zif 268*)[98] and recognize the *EGR1* DNA-binding consensus sequence.[89] WT1 protein also recognizes a GC-rich sequence,[100,101] and binding-site-selection experiments have identified the sequence 5'-GCGTGGGAGT-3' as a potential higher-affinity binding site.[102] In transient transfection experiments using promoter reporter constructs, WT1 functions as a repressor of transcription.[103] This effect, combined with the ability of WT1 to bind the GC-rich sequences present in many promoters, has led to the identification of many potential WT1 target genes.[104] These have included *EGR1,*[99] *IGFII,*[105] platelet-derived growth factor-A (*PDGF-A*),[106,107] IGF receptor,[108,109] epidermal growth factor receptor (*EGFR*),[101] c-*myc, bcl2,*[110] retinoic acid receptor α,[111] *Pax2,*[112] and transforming growth factor β[113] among many others. However, with the possible exception of *EGFR,*[101] *IGFII,*[114] and *IGFR,*[109] none of these WT1-regulated promoters are correlated with regulation of endogenous genes by WT1. Thus a level of target specificity may be evident with native promoters that is not observed in transient transfection assays. Interpretation of transient transfection experiments is further confounded by evidence that WT1 can function as an activator as well as a repressor of transcription, depending on cellular and promoter context and even on the choice of expression vector.[115–117]

The potential physiological significance of transcriptional activation by WT1(−KTS) is supported by a number of observations. In many cell types, ectopic expression of *WT1(−KTS)* leads to a G$_1$ phase arrest of the cell cycle, which is correlated with transcriptional induction of the cyclin-dependent kinase inhibitor p21^{Cip1} [159–162] and dependent upon a direct protein interaction with the transcriptional co-activator CBP[163]. A Wilms tumor-associated point mutation in WT1 abrogates transcriptional activation of the p21^{Cip1} promoter, without disrupting transcriptional repression of GC-rich promoters.[161] Recently, the use of expression profile analysis using high-density microarrays has yielded potentially physiological transcriptional targets of WT1(−KTS), including amphiregulin, a secreted growth factor implicated in epithelial differentiation.[164] Other potential target genes that are induced by WT1(−KTS) include *Dax1, Mullerian inhibiting substance, Bcl2, Syndecan-1, E-cadherin* and *CSF1* (see Ref. 165 for review).

Insertion of alternative splice II (KTS) abolishes binding of WT1 to the GC-rich promoters.[99] An alternative DNA-binding sequence has been proposed,[118] but no potential targets have been identified. The WT1(+KTS) isoform accounts for 80 percent of the cellular WT1 transcript,[97] suggesting that it makes an important contribution to the function of this tumor suppressor. Recently, WT1(+KTS) has been shown to associate with subnuclear clusters, in contrast to WT1(−KTS), which is diffusely localized in the nucleus.[119,120] Colocalization and coimmunoprecipitation studies have suggested that WT1(+KTS) is associated with small nucleoriboproteins (snRNPs), implying a potential role in pre-mRNA splicing.[119] However, the subnuclear clusters containing WT1(+KTS) are distinct from interchromatin granules containing the essential splicing factor SC35, which are thought to

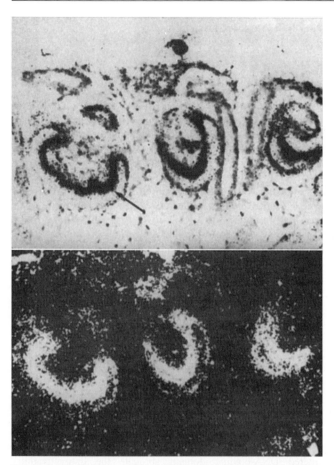

Fig. 24-7 Localization of *WT1* mRNA expression in the developing kidney. Analysis of 20-week human kidney by *in situ* hybridization with the *WT1* probe. Light phase (*upper panel*) and dark phase (*lower panel*) photomicrographs are shown to demonstrate the hybridization signal and the structures within the developing kidney that express *WT1* mRNA. The "S-shaped body" is a precursor of the renal glomerulus, whose inner surface demonstrates high levels of *WT1* mRNA expression (arrow). (*Photomicrograph kindly provided by Dr. Nic Hastie, Medical Research Council, Edinburgh, UK.*)

constitute assembly sites for the cellular splicing machinery.[120] WT1 proteins (+/−KTS) have been shown to physically interact with the essential splicing factor U2AF65 and to be detectable in the poly(A)$^+$ fraction of cellular nuclear extracts.[166,167] Thus the identity of WT1-associated subnuclear clusters is uncertain, and the relationship between WT1 and the pre-mRNA splicing machinery remains to be defined. The importance of the KTS alternative splice is underscored by Frasier Syndrome, characterized by abnormalities of renal and sexual differentiation and associated with a germ-line mutation in the KTS splice donor site.[168] In addition to alternative splicing, WT1 is phosphorylated *in vivo*, although the physiologic consequences of this protein modification are unknown.[121]

Expression of WT1 during Kidney Development

WT1 is normally expressed in a small number of tissues, primarily those of the developing genitourinary tract.[122,123] This expression pattern is in marked contrast to the ubiquitously expressed tumor suppressor genes *RB* and *p53* and may provide insight into the normal role of WT1 in cellular growth and differentiation. In the mouse kidney, WT1 expression is detectable by day 8 of gestation, rising to peak sharply around birth and then rapidly declining to low adult levels by day 17.[123] In humans, WT1 expression has been reported to be high in 20-week kidney and barely detectable in the adult organ.[74] Within the developing kidney, specific structures have been shown by *in situ* RNA hybridization to express WT1, including the condensed mesenchyme, renal vesicle, and glomerular epithelium[122] (Fig. 24-7). The transient expression pattern of WT1 in these early kidney structures is consistent with a gene that is critical during a defined period in normal kidney development (Fig. 24-8). Disruption of this gene by a mutation thus may lead to uncontrolled proliferation of the early renal progenitor cells that are characteristic of Wilms tumor.

WT1 is also expressed in other specific cell types, such as the Sertoli cells of the testis, granulosa cells of the ovary, muscle cells of the uterus, stromal cells of the spleen, and mesothelial cells of the pericardial, pleural, and peritoneal lining.[124–126] The WT1 pattern of expression in these tissues differs from that seen in the kidney, with persistent high levels of expression in adult organs. Expression of WT1 is also noted in acute leukemia cells, although the normal hematopoietic counterparts that express WT1 have not been identified. In addition to Wilms tumors, *WT1* mutations have been reported in mesothelioma and leukemia.[126,127] However, with

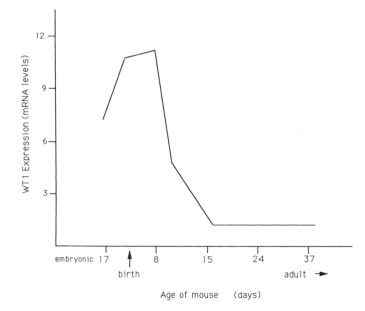

Fig. 24-8 Time course of *WT1* expression in the mouse kidney. Schematic representation of *WT1* mRNA levels in the mouse kidney assayed by Northern blot. *WT1* expression is detectable at the earliest embryonic time point, peaks about the time of birth, and then rapidly declines to adult levels.[95] In human kidney, *WT1* is expressed at high levels at 20 weeks and is no longer detectable in the adult organ.[66,94] Other tissues with high *WT1* mRNA levels, such as the gonads, do not show this dramatic pattern of expression. Instead, *WT1* expression increases during fetal development and remains high in the adult tissue.[96]

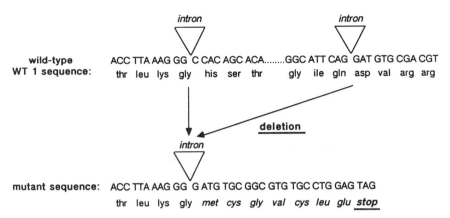

Fig. 24-9 Presence of inactivating mutations within the *WT1* transcript. A subset of Wilms tumors contain inactivated copies of *WT1*, consistent with its characterization as a tumor suppressor gene. Gross deletions of *WT1* appear to be rare, but small internal deletions or mutations can be found by nucleotide sequence analysis using the polymerase chain reaction (PCR). In this example,[7] a fragment of genomic DNA encoding an entire exon (flanked by two introns) has been deleted. The *WT1* transcript in this Wilms tumor is the product of abnormal splicing, joining together the exons on either side of the deletion. The abnormal splice junction results in a frameshift, leading to seven novel amino acids (italics) followed by premature chain termination caused by a stop codon.

the exception of one case of gonadoblastoma,[128] individuals with a germ-line *WT1* mutation do not have an increased incidence of tumors from tissues other than kidney. This suggests that the role played by WT1 in these tissues is not rate-limiting for tumorigenesis, as it appears to be in the kidney.[28]

Inactivation of *WT1* in the Germ Line and in Wilms Tumors

Germ-line mutations in one *WT1* allele have been documented in children with bilateral Wilms tumors, consistent with the predictions of Knudson and Strong.[8,9] The germ-line mutation results either from a *de novo* event or, rarely, from familial transmission. Tumor specimens from these children confirm loss of the remaining wild-type *WT1* allele, evidence of the "second hit." However, unlike retinoblastoma, in which the initial germ-line mutation is phenotypically silent, a heterozygous *WT1* mutation in the germ line may result in dramatic developmental abnormalities. Mutations that result in a premature termination result in a phenotype that is similar to that of WAGR patients, bearing a hemizygous deletion of *WT1*.[9] This consists of variable severity of genitourinary abnormalities (undescended testes, abnormal urethral meatus, malformed kidneys) that are more severe in boys than in girls. This observation suggests that *WT1* itself is the gene responsible for the genitourinary defects seen in children with WAGR syndrome. However, children with specific germ-line mutations that affect the *WT1* DNA-binding domains develop a far more severe constellation of genitourinary abnormalities known as *Denys-Drash syndrome*.[128] These children have gross abnormalities of sexual development, resulting in pseudohermaphroditism and mesangial sclerosis of the kidney, leading to renal failure within the first years of life. These observations suggest that expression of WT1 proteins with altered DNA-binding domains can exert a "dominant negative" effect that disrupts normal genitourinary development to a far greater extent than simple reduction in gene dosage seen in WAGR syndrome.

Most Wilms tumors express high levels of *WT1* mRNA and protein, consistent with their apparent cells of origin in the fetal kidney. By *in situ* RNA hybridization, *WT1* expression has been localized to the epithelial and blastemal histologic components within the tumor.[122] While in most Wilms tumors the *WT1* transcript appears to be grossly intact, in 10 percent of patients deletions and point mutations within the gene have been identified[74,129–133] (Fig. 24-9). These mutations identify *WT1* as the target of gene inactivation events at the chromosome 11p13 locus and confirm its characterization as a tumor-suppressor gene. The majority of *WT1* mutations reported in Wilms tumors are homozygous, resulting from an initial point mutation in one allele

and followed by loss of the second allele through a gross chromosomal event. However, some tumors have been found to express a single mutated *WT1* allele, along with the remaining wild-type allele.[74,131] These observations have suggested that specific types of mutations, particularly those involving the DNA-binding domain of *WT1*, may act as "dominant negative" mutations, in effect suppressing the function of the coexpressed wild-type allele.[134,135] A potential mechanism of action for such dominant negative mutations has been defined *in vitro*. WT1 dimerizes through the N-terminal domain, and mutants with an altered DNA-binding domain abrogate the transactivational properties of wild-type WT1.[120,136,137] These mutants physically associate with subnuclear clusters and recruit transcriptionally active WT1(−KTS), in effect achieving an apparent intranuclear sequestration of the wild-type protein.[120]

In addition to mutational inactivation, unusual mechanisms of disrupting WT1 function contribute to Wilms tumor. An in-frame deletion of *WT1* exon 2, within the transactivation domain, is observed in 10 percent of primary Wilms tumor specimens.[138] This splicing abnormality is not associated with a mutation in flanking exon-intron junctions, but it is observed together with omission of alternative splice II (WT1 exon 5), suggesting a gene-specific abnormality in pre-mRNA processing. The encoded protein, WT1-del2, is a potent transcriptional activator, capable of antagonizing transcriptional repression of promoter reporters by wild-type WT1.[138] Another unusual disruption of *WT1* occurs in a rare pediatric sarcoma, desmoplastic small round cell tumor (DSRT), which is characterized by a chromosomal translocation fusing the potent transactivation domain of the Ewing sarcoma gene *EWS* to zinc fingers 2 to 4 of *WT1*.[139,140] These two transactivating variants of *WT1*, together with Wilms tumor-associated point mutations that modulate the transactivational properties of WT1,[126,141,161] support the link between tumorigenesis and altered expression of transcriptional targets.

In addition to abnormalities in pre-mRNA splicing, RNA editing has been reported in WT1.[142] The altered amino acid, within the transactivation domain of *WT1*, appears to result in a subtle change in transactivational activity. The RNA-edited *WT1* transcripts constitute a fraction of the mRNA in rat kidney, but their role in Wilms tumor development is unknown.

Inactivation of *WT1* in the Mouse and Animal Models of Wilms Tumor

WT1 is highly conserved in the mouse, both in terms of nucleotide conservation and pattern of tissue and developmental expression.[123] However, the genetic consequences of *WT1* inactivation differ between human and mouse, particularly with respect to tumorigenesis. The small eye mouse mutation[143,144] is homologous to the aniridia phenotype in humans and involves the *Pax6* gene on mouse chromosome 2, which is syntenic with human chromosome band 11p13. One variant of the mouse mutation, so-called *Sey/Dey*, includes small eyes, a small body size, and a white belly patch. The *Sey/Dey* mutation results from a hemizygous chromosomal deletion analogous to the WAGR deletion in humans, including hemizygosity for the mouse *WT1* gene.[123,145] Homozygosity for the *Sey/Dey* allele is an embryonic lethal, but heterozygous mice have no detectable abnormalities of genitourinary development, nor do they appear to have an increased risk of renal tumors. These observations have been confirmed in *WT1*-hemizygous mice generated by homologous recombination.[146] This apparent discrepancy between the effect of hemizygosity for *WT1* in mouse and humans raises a number of interesting questions. *WT1* pathways in the mouse may involve greater functional redundancy or genetic safeguards than in humans, conferring protection against malignant transformation in a somatic kidney cell following loss of the remaining wild-type allele. Alternatively, the small number of target cells in the mouse kidney may reduce the probability of the second genetic hit. Finally, an intriguing genetic observation is that the two Wilms tumor loci that share the short arm of human chromosome 11 are separated in the mouse, with 11p13 syntenic with mouse chromosome 2, while 11p15 maps to mouse chromosome 7.[145] Thus, whereas a single chromosomal recombinational event is sufficient to cause loss of both genes in humans, two separate genetic events would be required in the mouse. While the mouse appears to be a reluctant Wilms tumor model, nephroblastomas do arise in the rat. The best studied models are nephroblastomas that arise either spontaneously or following transplacental treatment with the chemical carcinogen *N*-ethylnitrosourea or x-irradiation.[147–149] Point mutations in *WT1* have been observed in some rat nephroblastomas,[150] implying that its inactivation contributes to tumorigenesis.

In contrast to the *WT1*-hemizygous mice, homozygous inactivation of *WT1* has profound developmental consequences. *WT1*-null mice die at embryonic day 11.[146] The precise cause of death is uncertain, but gross cardiac and diaphragmatic defects appear to be implicated. WT1 is expressed in the mesothelial lining of these organs,[125,126] suggesting a potential developmental role. Of particular interest, *WT1*-null mice fail to develop either kidneys or gonads. Developmental arrest in the gonads precedes the sexually undifferentiated stage, implicating WT1 in a very early step in gonadogenesis. The arrest in kidney differentiation precedes the induction of mesoderm by the ureteric bud, and mesenchymal tissue from *WT1*-null mice is resistant to exogenous induction signals.[146] Histologic analysis of nephrogenic tissue from *WT1*-null mice reveals widespread apoptosis of blastemal stem cells. The role of WT1 in kidney development thus appears to involve a survival and potentially a permissive function for differentiating stem cells. The stage of peak WT1 expression that accompanies the differentiation of glomeruli is not reached in *WT1*-null mice, consistent with a developmental arrest at the first developmental stage requiring WT1 expression. Partial rescue of the *WT1*-null phenotype has been accomplished by transgenic expression of a yeast artificial chromosome (YAC) containing the *WT1* locus within 280 kb of genomic sequence.[169] Unidentified regulatory sequences within this large genomic locus appear to be required for the appropriate temporal and spatial expression pattern of *WT1* during kidney development.

Functional Properties of WT1

Reconstitution of WT1 function in models of kidney differentiation remains to be achieved. However, a number of different functional properties are evident in cultured cell lines. Stable transfection of wild-type *WT1* into a Wilms tumor cell line results in growth inhibition.[138] Inducible expression of the WT1($-$KTS) isoform triggers G_1 phase cell cycle arrest, followed by p53-independent apoptosis in osteosarcoma cell lines.[101] More recently, infection of primary hematopoietic progenitors with retroviral constructs encoding *WT1* has been shown to result in the rapid induction of lineage-specific cellular differentiation.[170] This effect is preceded by induction of the cyclin-dependent kinase inhibitor p21[Cip1], but *WT1*-mediated cellular differentiation is not simply the consequence of cell cycle arrest, since ectopic expression of p21[Cip1] is insufficient to reproduce the effect of *WT1*. Together with the specific spatial and temporal expression pattern of *WT1* in the developing kidney, its induction of target genes associated with renal differentiation, and the consequences of its inactivation in human syndromes and in mouse models, these observations point to a functional role for *WT1* in the activation of an organ-specific differentiation program. The precise function of the various WT1 isoforms, and the specific downstream targets that contribute to the effect of *WT1* on survival of renal blastemal cells, gonadal differentiation and tumorigenesis remain to be uncovered.

Concluding Remarks

Wilms tumor is a genetically complex embryonic tumor whose histologic appearance is consistent with arrested differentiation of renal stem cells. The identification of the first Wilms tumor suppressor gene, *WT1*, has revealed a transcriptional regulator that is required for early kidney differentiation but whose inactivation, presumably at a later stage of kidney development, results in Wilms tumor. Further characterization of this gene and isolation of additional Wilms tumor genes will provide greater understanding of the link between normal differentiation in the kidney and malignant transformation.

REFERENCES

1. Bennington J, Beckwith J: Tumors of the kidney, renal pelvis and ureter, in *Atlas of Tumor Pathology,* series 2, fascile 12. Washington, DC, Armed Forces Institute of Pathology, 1975.
2. Breslow N, Churchill F, Nesmith B, Thomas P, Beckwith J, Othersen H, D'Angio G: Clinicopathologic features and prognosis for Wilms' tumor patients with metastases at dignosis. *Cancer* **58**:2501, 1986.
3. Coppes M, Wilson P, Weitzman S: Extrarenal Wilms' tumor: Staging, treatment and prognosis. *J Clin Oncol* **9**:167, 1991.
4. Bove K, McAdams A: The nephroblastomatosis complex and its relationship to Wilms' tumor: a clinicopathologic treatise. *Perspect Pediatr Pathol* **3**:185, 1976.
5. Beckwith J, Kiviat N, Bonadio J: Nephrogenic rests, nephroblastomatosis, and the pathogenesis of Wilms' tumor. *Pediatr Pathol* **10**:1, 1989.
6. Park S, Bernard A, Bove K, Sens D, Hazen-Martin D, Garvin A, Haber D: Inactivation of WT1 in nephrogenic rests, genetic precursors to Wilms' tumour. *Nature Genet* **5**:363, 1993.
7. National Wilms Tumor Study Committee: Wilms' tumor: Status report, 1990. *J Clin Oncol* **9**:877, 1990.
8. Huff V, Miwa H, Haber D, Call K, Housman D, Strong L, Saunders G: Evidence for WT1 as a Wilms tumor (WT) gene: Intragenic germinal deletion in bilateral WT. *Am J Hum Genet* **48**:997, 1991.
9. Pelletier J, Bruening W, Li F, Haber D, Glaser T, Housman D: WT1 mutations contribute to abnormal genital system development and hereditary Wilms' tumour. *Nature* **353**:431, 1991.
10. Grundy P, Breslow N, Green D, Sharples K, Evans A, D'Angio G: Prognostic factors for children with recurrent Wilms' tumor: Results from the second and third National Wilms' Tumor Study. *J Clin Oncol* **7**:638, 1989.
11. Bryd R, Levine A: Late treatment of Wilms' tumor, in Pochedly C, Baum ES (eds): *Clinical and Biological Manifestations,* vol 19. New York, Elsevier, 1984, p 347.
12. Li F, Gimbrere K, Gelber R, Sallan S, Flamant F, Green D, Heyn R, Meadows A: Outcome of pregnancy in survivors of Wilms' tumor. *JAMA* **257**:216, 1987.
13. Knudson A: Mutation and cancer: Statistical study of retinoblastoma. *Proc Natl Acad Sci USA* **68**:820, 1971.
14. Knudson A, Strong L: Mutation and cancer: A model for Wilms tumor of the kidney. *J Natl Cancer Inst* **48**:313, 1972.
15. Knudson A, Strong L: Mutation and cancer: Neuroblastoma and pheochromocytoma. *Am J Hum Genet* **24**:514, 1972.
16. Friend S, Bernards R, Rogelj S, Weinberg R, Rapaport J, Albert D, Dryja T: A human DNA segment with properties of the gene that

predisposes to retinoblastoma and osteosarcoma. *Nature* **323**:643, 1986.

17. Lee W, Bookstein R, Hong F, Young L, Shew J, Lee E: Human retinoblastoma susceptibility gene: Cloning, identification, and sequence. *Science* **235**:1394, 1987.

18. Fung Y, Murphree A, T'Ang A, Ouian J, Hinrichs S, Benedict W: Structural evidence for the authenticity of the retinoblastoma tumor susceptibility gene. *Science* **236**:1657, 1987.

19. Comings D: A general theory of carcinogenesis. *Proc Natl Acad Sci USA* **70**:3324, 1973.

20. Knudson A: Hereditary cancer, oncogenes, and antioncogenes. *Cancer Res* **45**:1437, 1985.

21. Dunn J, Philips R, Becker A, Gallie B: Identification of germline and somatic mutations affecting the retinoblastoma gene. *Science* **241**:1797, 1988.

22. Yandell D, Campbell T, Dayton S, Petersen R, Walton D, Little J, McConkie-Rosell A, Buckley E, Dryja T: Oncogenic point mutations in the human retinoblastoma gene: Their application to genetic counselling. *N Engl J Med* **321**:1689, 1989.

23. Cavenee W, Dryja T, Phillips R, Benedict W, Godbout R, Gallie B, Murphree A, Strong L, White R: Expression of recessive alleles by chromosomal mechanisms in retinoblastoma. *Nature* **305**:779, 1983.

24. Matsunaga E: Genetics of Wilms' tumor. *Hum Genet* **57**:231, 1981.

25. Cochran W, Froggatt P: Bjilateral nephroblastoma in two sisters. *J Urol* **97**:216, 1967.

26. Pendergrass T: Congenital anomalies in children with Wilms' tumor, a new survey. *Cancer* **37**:403, 1976.

27. Breslow N, Beckwith J: Epidemiological features of Wilms' tumor: Results of the National Wilms' Tumor Study. *J Natl Cancer Inst* **68**:429, 1982.

28. Haber D, Housman D: Rate-limiting steps: The genetics of pediatric cancers. *Cell* **64**:5, 1991.

29. Miller R, Fraumeni J, Manning M: Association of Wilms' tumor with aniridia, hemihypertrophy and other congenital malformations. *N Engl J Med* **270**:922, 1964.

30. Riccardi V, Sujansky E, Smith A, Francke U: Chromosomal imbalance in the aniridia-Wilms' tumor association: 11p interstitial deletion. *Pediatrics* **61**:604, 1978.

31. Francke U, Holmes L, Atkins L, Riccardi V: Aniridia-Wilms' tumor association: Evidence for specific deletion of 11p13. *Cytogenet Cell Genet* **24**:185, 1979.

32. Simola K, Knuutila S, Kaitila I, Pirkola A, Pohja P: Familial aniridia and translocation t(4;11)(q22;p13) without Wilms' tumor. *Hum Genet* **63**:158, 1983.

33. Moore J, Hyman S, Antonarakis S, Mules E, Thomas F: Familial isolated aniridia associated with a translocation involving chromosomes 11 and 22 [t(11;22)(p13;q12.20)]. *Hum Genet* **72**:297, 1986.

34. Ton C, Hirronen M, Miwa H, Weil M, Monaghan P, Jordan T, van Heyningen V, Hastie N, Meigers-Heijboer H, Drechsler M, Royer-Pokora B, Collins F, Swaroop A, Strong LC, Saunders GF: Positional cloning and characterization of a paired box- and homeobox-containing gene from the aniridia region. *Cell* **67**:1059, 1991.

35. Kondo K, Chilcote R, Maurer H, Rowley J: Chromosome abnormalities in tumor cells from patients with sporadic Wilms' tumor. *Cancer Res* **44**:5376, 1984.

36. Douglass E, Wilimas J, Green A, Look A: Abnormalities of chromosomes 1 and 11 in Wilms' tumor. *Cancer Genet Cytogenet* **14**:331, 1985.

37. Solis V, Pritchard J, Cowell J: Cytogenetic changes in Wilms' tumors. *Cancer Genet Cytogenet* **34**:223, 1988.

38. Wang-Wuu S, Soukup S, Bove K, Gotwals B, Lampkin B: Chromosome analysis of 31 Wilms tumors. *Cancer Res* **50**:2786, 1990.

39. Fearon E, Vogelstein B, Feinberg A: Somatic deletion and duplication of genes on chromosome 11 in Wilms' tumours. *Nature* **309**:176, 1984.

40. Koufos A, Hansen M, Lampkin B, Workman M, Copeland N, Jenkins N, Cavenee W: Loss of alleles at loci on human chromosome 11 during genesis of Wilms' tumour. *Nature* **309**:170, 1984.

41. Orkin S, Goldman D, Sallan S: Development of homozygosity for chromosome 11p markers in Wilms' tumour. *Nature* **309**:172, 1984.

42. Reeve A, Housiaux P, Gardner R, Chewing W, Grindley R, Millow L: Loss of a Harvey ras allele in sporadic Wilms' tumour. *Nature* **309**:174, 1984.

43. Mannens M, Slater R, Heyting C, Bliek J, Kraker JD, Coad N, Pagter-Holthuizen P, Pearson P: Molecular nature of genetic changes resulting in loss of heterozygosity for chromosome 11 in Wilms' tumor. *Hum Genet* **81**:41, 1988.

44. Glaser T, Jones C, Douglass E, Housman D: Constitutional and somatic mutations of chromosome 11p in Wilms' tumor. Cold Spring Harbor Lab, Cold Spring Harbor, New York, pp. 253–277, 1989.

45. Henry I, Jeanpierre M, Couillin P, Barichard F, Serre J, Journel H, Lamouroux A, Turleau C, Grouchy J, Junien C: Molecular definition of the 11p15.5 region involved in Beckwith-Wiedemann syndrome and probably in predisposition to adrenocortical carcinoma. *Hum Genet* **81**:273, 1989.

46. Reeve A, Sih S, Raizis A, Feinberg A: Loss of allelic heterozygosity at a second locus on chromosome 11 in sporadic Wilms' tumor cells. *Mol Cell Biol* **9**:1799, 1989.

47. Wiedemann H: Complexe malformatif familial avec hernie ombilicale et macroglossie — Un syndrome nouveau? *J Genet Hum* **13**:223, 1964.

48. Beckwith J: Macroglossia, omphalocele, adrenal cytomegaly, gigantism and hyperplastic visceromegaly. *Birth Defects* **5**:188, 1969.

49. Sotelo-Avila C, Gonzalez-Crussi F, Fowler J: Complete and incomplete forms of Beckwith-Wiedemann syndrome: Their oncogenic potential. *J Pediatr* **96**:47, 1980.

50. Wiedemann H: Tumor and hemihypertrophy associated with Wiedemann-Beckwith's syndrome. *Eur J Pediatr* **141**:129, 1983.

51. Koufos A, Grundy P, Morgan K, Aleck K, Hadro T, Lampkin B, Kalbakji A, Cavenee W: Familial Wiedemann-Beckwith syndrome and a second Wilms' tumor locus both map to 11p15.5. *Am J Hum Genet* **44**:711, 1989.

52. Ping J, Reeve A, Law D, Young M, Boehnke M, Feinberg A: Genetic linkage of Beckwith-Wiedemann syndrome to 11p15. *Am J Hum Genet* **23**:165, 1989.

53. Waziri M, Patil S, Hanson J, Bartley S: Abnormality of chromosome 11 in patients with features of Beckwith-Wiedemann syndrome. *J Pediatr* **102**:873, 1983.

54. Turleau C, Grouchy J, Nihoul-Fekete C, Chavin-Colin F, Junien C: Del 11p13/nephroblastoma without aniridia. *Hum Genet* **67**:455, 1984.

55. Romain D, Gebbie O, Parfitt R, Columbano-Green L, Smythe R, Chapman C, Kerr A: Two cases of ring chromosome 11. *J Med Genet* **20**:380, 1983.

56. Niikawa N, Ishikiriyama S, Takahashi S, Inagawa A, Tonoki H, Ohta Y, Hase N, Kamei T, Kajii T: The Wiedemann-Beckwith syndrome: Pedigree studies on five families with evidence for autosomal dominant inheritance with variable expressivity. *Am J Med Genet* **24**:41, 1986.

57. Brown K, Williams J, Maitland N, Mott M: Genomic imprinting and the Beckwith-Wiedemann syndrome. *Am J Hum Genet* **46**:1000, 1990.

58. Henry I, Bonaiti-Pellie C, Chehensse V, Beldjord C, Schwartz C, Utermann G, Junien C: Uniparental paternal disomy in a genetic cancer-predisposing syndrome. *Nature* **351**:665, 1991.

59. Grundy P, Telzerow P, Haber D, Li F, Paterson M, Garber J: Chromosome 11 uniparental isodisomy in a child with hemihypertrophy and embryonal neoplasms. *Lancet* **338**: 1079, 1992.

60. DeChiara T, Efstradiadis A, Robertson E: A growth-deficiency phenotype in heterozygous mice carrying an insulin-like growth factor II gene disrupted by targeting. *Nature* **345**:78, 1990.

61. DeChiara T, Roberson E, Efstradiatis A: Parental imprinting of the mouse insulin-like growth factor II gene. *Cell* **64**:849, 1991.

62. Giannoukakis N, Deal C, Paquette J, Goodyer C, Polychronakos C: Parental genomic imprinting of the human IGF2 gene. *Nature Genet* **4**:98, 1993.

63. Ohlsson R, Nystrom A, Pfeifer-Ohlsson S, Tohonen V, Hedborg F, Schofield P, Flam F, Ekstrom T: IGF2 is parentally imprinted during human embryogenesis and in the Beckwith-Wiedemann syndrome. *Nature Genet* **4**:94, 1993.

64. Weksberg R, Shen D, Fei Y, Song Q, Squire J: Disruption of insulin-like growth factor 2 imprinting in Beckwith-Wiedemann syndrome. *Nature Genet* **5**:143, 1993.

65. Ogawa O, Becroft D, Morison I, Ecles M, Skeen J, Mauger D, Reeve A: Constitutional relaxation of insulin-like growth factor II gene imprinting associated with Wilms' tumour and gigantism. *Nature Genet* **5**:408, 1993.

66. Reeve A, Eccles M, Wilkins R, Bell G, Millow L: Expression of insulin-like growth factor-II transcripts in Wilms' tumour. *Nature* **317**:258, 1985.

67. Scott J, Cowell J, Roberson M, Priestly L, Wadey R, Hopkins B, Pritchard J, Bell G, Rall L, Graham C, Knott T: Insulin like growth factor-II gene expression in Wilms' tumor and embryonic tissues. *Nature* **317**:260, 1985.

68. Rainier S, Johnson L, Dobry C, Ping A, Grundy P, Feinberg A: Relaxation of imprinted genes in human cancer. *Nature* **362**:747, 1993.

69. Ogawa O, Eccles M, Szeto J, McNoe L, Yun K, Maw M, Smith P, Reeve A: Relaxation of insulin-like growth factor II gene imprinting implicated in Wilms' tumour. *Nature* **362**:749, 1993.

70. Matsuoka S, Thompson J, Edwards M, Barletta J, Grundy P, Kalikin L, Harper J, Elledge S, Feinberg A: Imprinting of the gene encoding a human cyclin-dependent kinase inhibitor, p57^{KIP2}, on chromosome 11p15. *Proc Natl Acad Sci USA* **93**:3026, 1996.

71. Hatada I, Ohashi H, Fukushima Y, Kaneko Y, Inoue M, Komoto Y, Okada A, Ohishi S, Nabetani A, Morisaki H, Nakayama M, Niikawa N, Mukai T: An imprinted gene p57^{KP2} is mutated in Beckwith-Wiedemann syndrome. *Nature Genet* **14**:171, 1996.

72. Bartolomei M, Zemel S, Tilghman S: Parental imprinting of the mouse H19 gene. *Nature* **351**:153, 1991.

73. Hao Y, Crenshaw T, Moulton T, Newcomb E, Tycko B: Tumour-suppressor activity of H19 RNA. *Nature* **365**:764, 1993.

74. Haber D, Buckler A, Glaser T, Call K, Pelletier J, Sohn R, Douglass E, Housman D: An internal deletion within an 11p13 zinc finger gene contributes to the development of Wilms' tumor. *Cell* **61**:1257, 1990.

75. Weston A, Willey J, Modali R, Sugimura H, McDowell E, Resau J, Light B, Haugen A, Mann D, Trump B, Harris C: Differential DNA sequence deletions from chromosomes 3, 11, 13, and 17 in squamous-cell carcinoma, large-cell carcinoma and adenocarcinoma of the lung. *Proc Natl Acad Sci USA* **86**:5099, 1989.

76. Ahuja H, Foti A, Zhou D, Cline M: Analysis of proto-oncogenes in acute myeloid leukemia: Loss of heterozygosity for the Ha-ras gene. *Blood* **75**:819, 1990.

77. Huff V, Compton D, Chao L, Strong L, Geiser C, Saunders G: Lack of linkage of familial Wilms' tumour to chromosomal band 11p13. *Nature* **336**:377, 1988.

78. Grundy P, Koufos A, Morgan K, Li F, Meadows A, Cavenee W: Familial predisposition to Wilms' tumour does not map to the short arm of chromosome 11. *Nature* **336**:374, 1988.

79. Schwartz C, Haber D, Stanton V, Strong L, Skolnick M, Housman D: Familial predisposition to Wilms tumor does not segregate with the WT1 gene. *Genomics* **10**:927, 1991.

80. Rahman N, Arbour A, Tonin P, Renshaw J, Pelletier J, Baruchel S, Pritchard-Jones K, Stratton M, Narod S: Evidence for a familial Wilms' tumour gene (FWT1) on chromosome 17q12-21. *Nature Genet* **13**:461, 1996.

81. Glaser T, Jones C, Call K, Lewis W, Bruns G, Junien C, Waziri M, Housman D: Mapping the WAGR region of chromosome 11p: Somatic cell hybrids provide a fine-structure map. *Cytogenet Cell Genet* **46**:620, 1987.

82. Glaser T, Rose E, Morse H, Housman D, Jones C: A panel of irradiation-reduced hybrids selectively retaining human chromosome 11p13: Their structure and use to purify the WAGR gene complex. *Genomics* **6**:48, 1990.

83. Porteous D, Bickmore W, Christie S, Boyd P, Cranston G, Fletcher J, Gosden J, Rout D, Seawright A, Simola K, van Heyningen V, Hastie N: HRAS1 selected chromosome transfer generates markers that colocalize aniridia- and genitourinary dysplasia-associated translocation breakpoints and the Wilms' tumor gene within 11p13. *Proc Natl Acad Sci USA* **84**:5355, 1987.

84. Davis L, Byers M, Fukushima Y, Quin S, Nowak N, Scoggin C, Shows T: Four new DNA markers are assigned to the WAGR region of 11p13: Isolation and regional assignment of 112 chromosome 11 anonymous DNA segments. *Genomics* **3**:264, 1988.

85. Couillin P, Azoulay M, Henry I, Ravise N, Grisard M, Jeanpierre C, Barichard F, Metezeau F, Chandelier J, Lewis W, van Heyningen V, Junien C: Characterization of a panel of somatic cell hybrids for subregional mapping along 11p and within band 11p13. Subdivision of the WAGR complex region. *Hum Genet* **82**:171, 1989.

86. Gessler M, Thomas G, Couillin P, Junien C, McGillvray B, Hayden M, Jaschek G, Bruns G: A deletion map of the WAGR region of chromosome 11. *Am J Hum Genet* **44**:486, 1989.

87. Junien C, Turleau C, Grouchy JD, Said R, Rethore M, Tenconi R, Dufier J: Regional assignment of catalase (CAT) gene to band 11p13: Association with the aniridia-Wilms' tumor-gonadoblastoma (WAGR) complex. *Ann Genet* **23**:165, 1980.

88. van Heyningen V, Boyd P, Seaqright A, Fletcher J, Fantes J, Buckton K, Spowart G, Porteous D, Hill R, Newton M, Hastie N: Molecular analysis of chromosome 11 deletions in aniridia-Wilms' tumor syndrome. *Proc Natl Acad Sci USA* **82**:8592, 1985.

89. Glaser T, Lewis W, Bruns G, Watkins P, Rogler C, Shows T, Powers V, Willard H, Goguen J, Simola K, Housman D: The B-subunit of follicle-stimulating hormone is deleted in patients with aniridia and Wilms'

tumour, allowing a further definition of the WAGR locus. *Nature* **321**:882, 1986.

90. Compton D, Weil M, Jones C, Riccardi V, Strong L, Saunders G: Long range physical map of the Wilms' tumor-aniridia region on human chromosome 11. *Cell* **55**:827, 1988.

91. Gessler M, Bruns G: A physical map around the WAGR complex on the short arm of chromosome 11. *Genomics* **5**:43, 1989.

92. Rose E, Glaser T, Jones C, Smith C, Lewis W, Call C, Minden M, Champagne E, Boncetta L, Yeger H, Housman D: Complete physical map of the WAGR region of 11p13 localizes a candidate Wilms' tumor gene. *Cell* **60**:495, 1990.

93. Call K, Glaser T, Ito C, Buckler A, Pelletier J, Haber D, Rose E, Kral A, Yeger H, Lewis W, Jones C, Housman D: Isolation and characterization of a zinc finger polypeptide gene at the human chromosome 11 Wilms' tumor locus. *Cell* **60**:509, 1990.

94. Gessler M, Poustka A, Cavenee W, Neve R, Orkin S, Bruns G: Homozygous deletion in Wilms tumours of a zinc-finger gene identified by chromosome jumping. *Nature* **343**:774, 1990.

95. Evans R, Hollenberg S: Zinc fingers: Gilt by association. *Cell* **52**:1, 1988.

96. Mitchell P, Tijan R: Transcriptional regulation in mammalian cells by sequence-specific DNA binding proteins. *Science* **245**:371, 1989.

97. Haber D, Sohn R, Buckler A, Pelletier J, Call K, Housman D: Alternative splicing and genomic structure of the Wilms tumor gene WT1. *Proc Natl Acad Sci USA* **88**:9618, 1991.

98. Sukhatme V, Cao X, Chang L, Tsai-Morris C, Stamenkovich D, Ferreira P, Cohen D, Edewards S, Shows T, Curran T, LeBeau M, Adamson E: A zinc finger encoding gene coregulated with c-fos during growth and differentiation and after cellular depolarization. *Cell* **53**:37, 1988.

99. Rauscher F, Morris J, Tournay O, Cook D, Curran T: Binding of the Wilms' tumor locus zinc finger protein to the EGR-1 consensus sequence. *Science* **250**:1259, 1990.

100. Wang Z, Qiu Q, Enger K, Deuel T: A second transcriptionally active DNA-binding site for the Wilms tumor gene product, WT1. *Proc Natl Acad Sci USA* **90**:8896, 1993.

101. Englert C, Hou X, Maheswaran S, Bennett P, Ngwu C, Re G, Garvin A, Rosner M, Haber D: WT1 suppresses synthesis of the epidermal growth factor receptor and induces apoptosis. *EMBO J* **14**:4662, 1995.

102. Nakagama H, Heinrich G, Pelletier J, Housman D: Sequence and structural requirements for high-affinity binding by the WT1 gene product. *Mol Cell Biol* **15**:1489, 1995.

103. Madden S, Cook D, Morris J, Gashler A, Sukhatme V, Rauscher F III: Transcriptional repression mediated by the WT1 Wilms tumor gene product. *Science* **253**:1550, 1991.

104. Rauscher F III: The WT1 Wilms tumor gene product: A developmentally regulated transcription factor in the kidney that functions as a tumor suppressor. *FASEB J* **7**:896, 1993.

105. Drummond I, Badden S, Rohwer-Nutter P, Bell G, Sukhatme V, Rauscher F III: Repression of the insulin-like growth factor II gene by the Wilms tumor suppressor WT1. *Science* **257**:674, 1992.

106. Gashler A, Bonthron D, Madden S, Rauscher F III, Collins T, Sukhatme V: Human platelet-derived growth factor A chain is transcriptionally repressed by the Wilms tumor suppressor WT1. *Proc Natl Acad Sci USA* **89**:10984, 1992.

107. Wang Z, Madden S, Deuel T, Rauscher F III: The Wilms' tumor gene product, WT1, represses transcription of the platelet-derived growth factor A-chain gene. *J Biol Chem* **267**:21999, 1992.

108. Werner H, Re G, Drummond I, Sukhatme V, Rauscher F III, Sens D, Garvin A, LeRoith D, Roberts C Jr: Increased expression of the insulin-like growth factor I receptor gene IGF1R in Wilms tumor is correlated with modulation of IGF1R promoter activity by the WT1 Wilms tumor gene product. *Proc Natl Acad Sci USA* **90**:5828, 1993.

109. Werner H, Shen-Orr Z, Rauscher F III, Morris J, Toberts C, LeRoith D: Inhhibition of cellular proliferation by the Wilms' tumor suppressor WT1 is associated with suppression of insulin-like growth factor I receptor gene expression. *Mol Cell Biol* **15**:3516, 1995.

110. Hewitt S, Hamada S, McDonnell T, Rauscher F III, Saunders G: Regulation of the proto-oncogenes bcl-2 and c-myc by the Wilms' tumor suppressor gene WT1. *Cancer Res* **55**:5386, 1995.

111. Goodyer P, Dehbi M, Torban E, Bruening W, Pelletier J: Repression of the retinoic acid receptor-α gene by the Wilms' tumor suppressor gene product, wt1. *Oncogene* **10**:1125, 1995.

112. Ryan G, Steele-Perkins V, Morris J, Rauscher F III: Repression of Pax-2 by WT1 during normal kidney development. *Development* **121**:867, 1995.

113. Dey B, Sukhatme V, Roberts A, Sporn M, Rauscher F III, Kim S: Repression of the transforming growth factor β1 gene by the Wilms tumor suppressor WT1 gene product. *Mol Endocrinol* **8**:595, 1994.

114. Nichols K, Re G, Yan Y, Garvin A, Haber D: WT1 induces expression of insulin-like growth factor 2 in Wilms' tumor cells. *Cancer Res* **55**:4540, 1995.

115. Wang Z-Y, Qiu Q-Q, Deuel T: The Wilms' tumor gene product WT1 activates or suppresses transcription through separate functional domains. *J Biol Chem* **268**:9172, 1993.

116. Maheswaran S, Park S, Bernard A, Morris J, Rauscher F III, Hill D, Haber D: Physical and functional interction between WT1 and p53 proteins. *Proc Natl Acad Sci USA* **90**:5100, 1993.

117. Reddy J, Hosono S, Licht J: The transcriptional effect of WT1 is modulated by choice of expression vector. *J Biol Chem* **270**:29976, 1995.

118. Bickmore W, Oghene K, Little M, Seawright A, van Heyningen V, Hastie N: Modulation of DNA binding specificity by alternative splicing of the Wilms tumor wt1 gene transcript. *Science* **257**:235, 1992.

119. Larsson S, Charlieu J, Miyagawa K, Engelkamp D, Rassoutzadegan M, Ross A, Cuzin F, van Heyningen V, Hastie N: Subnuclear localization of WT1 in splicing or transcription factor domains is regulated by alternative splicing. *Cell* **81**:391, 1995.

120. Englert C, Vidal M, Maheswaran S, Ge Y, Ezzell R, Isselbacher K, Haber D: Truncated WT1 mutants alter the subnuclear localization of the wild-type protein. *Proc Natl Acad Sci USA* **92**:11960, 1995.

121. Ye Y, Raychaudhuri B, Gurney A, Campbell C, Williams B: Regulation of WT1 by phosphorylation: inhibition of DNA binding, alteration of transcriptional activity and cellular translocation. *EMBO J* **15**:5606, 1996.

122. Pritchard-Jones K, Fleming S, Davidson D, Bickmore W, Porteous D, Gosden C, Bard J, Buckler A, Pelletier J, Housman D, van Heyningen V, Hastie N: The candidate Wilms' tumour gene is involved in genitourinary development. *Nature* **346**:194, 1990.

123. Buckler A, Pelletier J, Haber D, Glaser T, Housman D: Isolation, characterization, and expression of the murine Wilms' tumor gene (WT1) during kidney development. *Mol Cell Biol* **11**:1707, 1991.

124. Pelletier J, Schalling M, Buckler A, Rogers A, Haber D, Housman D: Expression of the Wilms' tumor gene WT1 in the murine urogenital system. *Genes Dev* **5**:1345, 1991.

125. Armstrong J, Pritchard-Jones K, Bickmore W, Hastie N, Bard J: The expression of the Wilms' tumor gene, WT1, in the developing mammalian embryo. *Mech Dev* **40**:85, 1992.

126. Park S, Schalling M, Bernard A, Maheswaran S, Shipley G, Roberts D, Fletcher J, Shipman R, Rheinwald J, Demetri G, Griffin J, Minden M, Housman D, Haber D: The Wilms tumour gene WT1 is expressed in murine mesoderm-derived tissues and mutated in a human mesothelioma. *Nature Genet* **4**:415, 1993.

127. King-Underwood L, Renshaw J, Pritchard-Jones K: Mutations in the Wilms' tumor gene WT1 in leukemias. *Blood* **87**:2171, 1996.

128. Pelletier J, Bruening W, Kashtan C, Mauer S, Manivel J, Striegel J, Houghton D, Junien C, Habib R, Fouser L, Fine R, Silverman B, Haber D, Housman D: Germline mutations in the Wilms' tumor suppressor gene are associated with abnormal urogenital development in Denys-Drash syndrome. *Cell* **67**:437, 1991.

129. Ton C, Huff V, Call K, Cohn S, Strong L, Housman D, Saunders G: Smallest region of overlap in Wilms' tumor deletions uniquely implicates an 11p13 zinc finger gene as the disease locus. *Genomics* **10**:293, 1991.

130. Cowell J, Wadey R, Haber D, Call K, Housman D, Prichard J: Structural rearrangements of the WT1 gene in Wilms' tumor cells. *Oncogene* **6**:595, 1991.

131. Little M, Prosser J, Condie A, Smith P, van Heyningen V, Hastie N: Zinc finger point mutations within the WT1 gene in Wilms tumor patients. *Proc Natl Acad Sci USA* **89**:4791, 1992.

132. Coppes M, Liefers G, Paul P, Yeger H, Williams B: Homozygous somatic WT1 point mutations in sporadic unilateral Wilms tumor. *Proc Natl Acad Sci USA* **90**:1416, 1993.

133. Varanasi R, Bardeesy N, Gharemani M, Petruzzi M-J, Nowak N, Adam M, Grundy P, Shows T, Pelletier J: Fine structure analysis of the WT1 gene in sporadic Wilms tumors. *Proc Natl Acad Sci USA* **91**:3554, 1994.

134. Herskowitz I: Functional inactivation of genes by dominant negative mutations. *Nature* **329**:219, 1987.

135. Haber D, Timmers H, Pelletier J, Sharp P, Housman D: A dominant mutation in the Wilms tumor gene WT1 cooperates with the viral oncogene E1A in transformation of primary kidney cells. *Proc Natl Acad Sci USA* **89**:6010, 1992.

136. Reddy J, Morris J, Wang J, English M, Haber D, Shi Y, Licht J: WT1-mediated transcriptional activation is inhibited by dominant negative mutant proteins. *J Biol Chem* **270**:10878, 1995.

137. Moffett P, Bruening W, Nakagama H, Bardeesy N, Housman D, Housman D, Pelletier J: Antagonism of WT1 activity by protein self-association. *Proc Natl Acad Sci USA* **92**:11105, 1995.

138. Haber D, Park S, Maheswaran S, Englert C, Re G, Hazen-Martin D, Sens D, Garvin A: WT1-mediated growth suppression of Wilms tumor cells expressing a WT1 splicing variant. *Science* **262**:2057, 1993.

139. Ladanyi M, Gerald W: Fusion of the EWS and WT1 genes in the desmoplastic small round cell tumor. *Cancer Res* **54**:2837, 1994.

140. Gerald W, Rosai J, Ladanyi M: Characterization of the genomic breakpoint and chimeric transcripts in the EWS-WT1 gene fusion of desmoplastic small round cell tumor. *Proc Natl Acad Sci USA* **92**:1028, 1995.

141. Park S, Tomlinson G, Nisen P, Haber D: Altered trans-activational properties of a mutated WT1 gene product in a WAGR-associated Wilms' tumor. *Cancer Res* **53**:4757, 1993.

142. Sharma P, Bowman M, Madden S, Rauscher F III, Sukumar S: RNA editing in the Wilms' tumor susceptibility gene, WT1. *Genes Dev* **8**:720, 1994.

143. Theiler K, Varnum D, Stevens L: Development of Dickie's small eye, a mutation in the house mouse. *Anat Embryol* **155**:81, 1978.

144. Hogan B, Horsburgh G, Cohen J, Hetherington C, Fisher G, Lyon M: Small eyes (Sey): A homozygous lethal mutation on chromosome 2 which affects the differentiation of both lens and nasal placodes in the mouse. *J Embryol Exp Morphol* **97**:95, 1986.

145. Glaser T, Lane J, Housman D: A mouse model of the aniridia-Wilms' tumor deletion syndrome. *Science* **250**:823, 1990.

146. Kreidberg J, Sariola H, Loring J, Maeda M, Pelletier J, Housman D, Jaenisch R: WT1 is required for early kidney development. *Cell* **74**:679, 1993.

147. Hasgekar N, Pendse A, Lalitha V: Rat renal mesenchymal tumor as an experimental model for human congenital mesoblastic nephroma. *Pediatr Pathol* **9**:131, 1989.

148. Ohaki Y: Renal tumors induced transplacentally in the rat by N-ethylnitrosourea. *Pediatr Pathol* **9**:19, 1989.

149. Deshpande R, Hasgekar N, Chitale A, Lalitha V: Rat renal mesenchymal tumor as an experimental model for human congenital mesoblastic nephroma: II. Comparative pathology. *Pediatr Pathol* **9**:141, 1989.

150. Sharma P, Bowman M, Yu B, Sukumar S: A rodent model for Wilms tumors: Embryonal kidney neoplasms induced by N-nitros-N9-methylurea. *Proc Natl Acad Sci USA* **91**:9931, 1994.

151. Kudoh T, Ishidate T, Moriyama M, Toyoshima K, Akiyama T: G1 phase arrest induced by Wilms tumor protein WT1 is abrogated by cyclin/CDK complexes. *Proc Natl Acad Sci USA* **92**:4517, 1995.

152. Englert C, Maheswaran S, Garvin AJ, Kreidberg J, Haber DA: Induction of p21 by the Wilms' tumor suppressor gene WT1. *Cancer Res* **57**:1429–1434, 1970.

153. Sherr C, Roberts R: Inhibitors of mammalian G1 cyclin-dependent kinases. *Genes Dev* **9**:1149, 1995.

154. Wang J, Walsh K: Resistance to apoptosis conferred by cdk inhibitors during myocyte differentiation. *Science* **273**:359, 1996.

155. Maheswaran S, Englert C, Bennett P, Heinrich G, Haber D: The WT1 gene product stabilizes p53 and inhibits p53-mediated apoptosis. *Genes Dev* **9**:2143, 1995.

156. Lemoine N, Hughes C, Cowell J: Aberrant expression of the tumour suppressor gene p53 is very frequent in Wilms' tumours. *J Pathol* **168**:237, 1992.

157. Malkin D, Sexsmith E, Yeger H, Williams B, Coppes M: Mutations of the p53 tumor suppressor gene occur infrequently in Wilms' tumor. *Cancer Res* **54**:2077, 1994.

158. Bardeesy N, Falkoff D, Petruzzi M, Nowak N, Zabel B, Adam M, Aguiar M, Grundy P, Shows T, Pelletier J: Anaplastic Wilms' tumour, a subtype displaying poor prognosis, harbours p53 gene mutations. *Nature Genet* **7**:91, 1994.

159. Kudoh T, Ishidate T, Moriyama M, Toyoshima K, Akiyama T: G1 phase arrest induced by Wilms tumor protein WT1 is abrogated by cyclin/CDK complexes. *Proc Natl Acad Sci USA* **92**:4517, 1995.

160. Englert C, Maheswaran S, Garvin AJ, Kreidberg J, Haber DA: Induction of p21 by the Wilms' tumor suppressor gene WT1. *Cancer Res* **57**:1429, 1970.

161. English MA, Licht JD: Tumor associated WT1 missense mutants indicate that transcriptional activation by WT1 is critical for growth control. *J Biol Chem* **274**:13258, 1999.

162. Maheswaran S, Englert C, Zheng G, Lee SB, Wong J, Harkin DP, Bean J, Ezzell R, Garvin AJ, McCluskey RT, DeCaprio J, Haber DA: Inhibition of cellular proliferation by the Wilms tumor suppression WT1 requires association with the inducible chaperone Hsp70. *Genes Dev* **12**:1108, 1998.

163. Wang W, Lee SB, Palmer R, Ellisen LW, Haber DA: A functional interaction with CBP contributes to transcriptional activation by the Wilms tumor suppressor WT1. *J Biol Chem* **276**:16810, 2001.

164. Lee SB, Huang K, Palmer R, Truong VB, Herzlinger D, Kolquist KA, Wong J, Paulding C, Yoon SK, Gerald W, Oliner JD, Haber DA: The Wilms tumor suppressor WT1 encodes a transcriptional activator of amphiregulin. *Cell* **98**:663, 1999.

165. Lee SB, Haber DA. Wilms tumor and the WT1 gene. *Exp Cell Res* **264**:74, 2001.

166. Davies RC, Calvio C, Bratt E, Larsson SH, Lamond AI, Hastie ND: WT1 interacts with the splicing factor U2AF65 in an isoform-dependent manner and can be incorporated into spliceosomes. *Genes Dev* **12**:3217, 1998.

167. Ladomery MR, Slight J, McGhee S, Hastie ND: Presence of WT1, the Wilms tumor suppressor gene product, in nuclear poly(A)(+) ribonucleoprotein. *J Biol Chem* **274**:36520, 1999.

168. Barbaux S, Niaudet P, Gubler MC, Grunfeld JP, Jaubert F, Kuttenn F, Fekete CN, Souleyreau-Therville N, Thibaud E, Fellous M, McElreavey K: Donor splice-site mutations in WT1 are responsible for Frasier syndrome. *Nature Genet* **17**:467, 1997.

169. Moore AW, McInnes L, Kreidberg J, Hastie ND, Schedl A: YAC complementation shows a requirement for WT1 in the development of epicardium, adrenal gland and throughout nephrogenesis. *Development* **126**:1845, 1999.

170. Ellisen L, Carlesso N, Cheng T, Scadden DT, Haber DA: The Wilms tumor suppressor WT1 directs stage-specific quiescence and differentiation of human hematopoietic progenitor cells. *EMBO J* **20**:1897, 2001.

CHAPTER 25

Neurofibromatosis 1

David H. Gutmann ■ *Francis S. Collins*

1. Von Recklinghausen neurofibromatosis, or neurofibromatosis type 1 (NF1), is a common autosomal dominant disorder that affects 1 in 3000 individuals. It is characterized clinically by the finding of two or more of the following: café-au-lait spots, neurofibromas, freckling in non-sun-exposed areas, optic glioma, Lisch nodules, distinctive bony lesions, and a first-degree relative with NF1. Less common manifestations include short stature and macrocephaly. NF1 patients also can have learning disabilities, seizures, scoliosis, hypertension, plexiform neurofibromas, or pheochromocytomas.

2. There is a high spontaneous mutation rate in NF1, with 30 to 50 percent of cases representing new mutations. Although the penetrance of NF1 is essentially 100 percent, NF1 tends to show variable expressivity in that there is a wide range of clinical severity and complications in patients within the same family, who all presumably carry the same mutation.

3. Syndromes related to NF1 include neurofibromatosis type 2 (bilateral vestibular neurofibromatosis), segmental or mosaic NF1, Watson syndrome, and neurofibromatosis 1–Noonan syndrome.

4. The gene for NF1 was identified by positional cloning and resides on chromosome 17q11.2. This gene has an open reading frame of 8454 nucleotides and spans approximately 300,000 nucleotides of genomic DNA. The messenger RNA is 11,000 to 13,000 nucleotides and is detectable at varying levels in all tissues examined. Germ-line mutations in the *NF1* gene have been found in affected patients and range from large (megabase) deletions to missense and nonsense mutations.

5. The protein product of the *NF1* locus (neurofibromin) is 2818 amino acids and is expressed as a 250-kDa protein in brain, spleen, kidney, testis, and thymus. This protein has structural and functional similarity to a family of GTPase-activating proteins (GAPs) that down-regulate a cellular proto-oncogene, p21-*ras. ras* has been implicated in the control of cell growth and differentiation, and the ability of neurofibromin to down-regulate p21-*ras* suggests that the loss of neurofibromin may lead to uncontrolled cell growth or tumor formation. Subcellular localization and biochemical purification experiments have demonstrated that neurofibromin is associated with cytoplasmic microtubules.

6. Somatic mutations in the *NF1* gene that result in an absence of neurofibromin expression have been described for a variety of tumor types. Loss of neurofibromin in neurofibrosarcomas derived from NF1 patients results in increased p21-*ras* activation and presumably tumor formation. Neurofibromin expression is also absent in non-NF1 patients' tumors, including metastatic malignant melanomas and neuroblastomas. The loss of neurofibromin in malignancy supports the notion that neurofibromin is a tumor-suppressor gene product.

7. The diagnosis of neurofibromatosis 1 is based largely on clinical criteria despite progress in defining the molecular genetics of the disorder. Treatment of patients with NF1 is directed at education and genetic counseling, early detection of malignancy, and surveillance for the appearance of complications of NF1.

Von Recklinghausen neurofibromatosis, or neurofibromatosis type 1 (NF1), is one of the most common autosomal dominant disorders in humans, afflicting all ethnic groups, both sexes, and all age groups. It is more common than Duchenne muscular dystrophy and Huntington disease combined and has a greater prevalence in the Western world than does cystic fibrosis. Yet NF1 has received far less attention in the public eye and the medical literature than have these other single-gene disorders. Among the multitude of reasons for this decreased visibility, three seem to stand out: (1) The pleiotropic and variable manifestations of NF1 affect many different organ systems and thus lead to the involvement of a multitude of subspecialists in the care of these patients. However, until recently no single specialist or subspecialist had considered NF1 a disease of major concern. Now this role has been taken on by medical geneticists. (2) Until very recently, NF1 lacked a firm biologic basis, and investigations into its pathogenesis were more descriptive than definitive. In the absence of a biologic hypothesis for the basic defect, very little attention was given to this disorder by basic scientists. (3) It is a tragic reality that many patients with NF1 are at least to some degree disfigured. In a society that often values physical beauty more than strength of character, such individuals have been discriminated against, either overtly or subtly, and often have responded by remaining in the background. There have been few poster children for von Recklinghausen neurofibromatosis, no telethons, and very little public sympathy. The learning disabilities suffered by many individuals with NF1 have further inhibited their ability to achieve positions of power, wealth, and influence.

All these circumstances are undergoing a turnaround. The founding of the National Neurofibromatosis Foundation (NNFF) in America in 1978, LINK (Let's Increase Neurofibromatosis Knowledge) in 1982, and the International Neurofibromatosis Association in 1992 signifies a new determination of NF1 sufferers and their families to increase public awareness of the disease, support research, and reach out to each other in support groups. The clinical care of NF patients, previously fragmented and poorly coordinated, has been greatly improved over the past 15 years by the establishment of a large number of NF specialty clinics, which are now present in most major medical centers. The directors of such clinics are usually pediatricians, internists, neurologists, or geneticists, and the clinics offer diagnosis, counseling, and regular evaluation of affected individuals for complications of the disease and coordinated access to subspecialists when the need arises. Such clinics, initially arising out of the pioneering efforts of Vincent Riccardi at Baylor, have provided a wealth of information about the natural history of the disease and corrected a number of misconceptions.

A list of standard abbreviations is located immediately preceding the index. Nonstandard abbreviations used in this chapter include: NF1 = neurofibromatosis type 1; UBOs = unidentified bright objects; NGF = nerve growth factor; GAPs = GTPase-activating proteins; MAPs = microtubule-associated proteins.

Table 25-1 *Estimates of Prevalence and Mutation Rate of NF1*

Methods of Study (Year)	Ascertainment	Prevalence	Mutation Rate
Crowe et al. (1956)	Surveys of admissions at general hospital and state mental institutions	1/2500–3000	$1.4-2.6 \times 10^{-4}$
Sergeyev (1975)	Population sample of 16-year-old Russian youths	1/7800	$4.4-4.9 \times 10^{-5}$
Samuelsson and Axelson (1981)	Population-based	1/4600	4.3×10.5^{-5}
Huson et al. (1989)	Population-based	1/2500–4950	$3.1-10.5 \times 10^{-5}$

From the scientific point of view, identification of the *NF1* gene by a positional cloning strategy[1–3] and recognition that the protein product is a participant in p21-*ras*-mediated growth control[4–7] have catapulted NF1 into the scientific spotlight, resulting in the recruitment of a significant number of basic scientists into research on this disorder who previously would not have paid it much mind. Thus the complexion of NF1 has changed dramatically over the past 15 years, and it now seems highly appropriate to include a chapter on this disorder in this textbook.

There are three recent excellent books[8–10] on neurofibromatosis, with particular emphasis on the clinical aspects. No attempt will be made here to duplicate those sources and the wealth of clinical detail they provide; the interested reader is referred to those sources as well as to the classic monograph of Crowe, Schull, and Neel.[11] Furthermore, no coverage of neurofibromatosis type 2 (NF2, formerly referred to as *central neurofibromatosis* or *bilateral vestibular neurofibromatosis*) will be attempted.[12,13]

CLINICAL ASPECTS

Historical Perspective

Scattered descriptions of cases that almost certainly represent NF1, sometimes even including drawings, can be found through many centuries of medical writing.[14,15] While other writers previously had focused on the skin tumors and occasionally had noted the familial nature of the disorder, it was von Recklinghausen in 1882 who gave the disease its first full description, including recognition that the tumors arose from the fibrous tissue surrounding small nerves, leading to his designation of these tumors as *neurofibromas*.[16] The autosomal dominant inheritance pattern was defined early in the twentieth century.[17] A crucial diagnostic element, the iris nodule, was defined by the Viennese ophthalmologist Lisch in 1937,[18] although the true significance and usefulness of this observation have come to general attention only in the past decade.[19,20]

The landmark study of Crowe, Schull, and Neel[11] brought together for the first time all the salient clinical features of NF1, including the high incidence, the high spontaneous mutation rate, the usefulness of the café-au-lait spot as a diagnostic feature, and recognition of the wide range of complications that can occur. Other important large-scale studies of the disease include those of Borberg[21] (followed up 35 years later by Sorenson *et al.*[22]), Carey *et al.*,[23] Riccardi,[9,24] and Huson *et al.*[25–27] While none of these studies is completely devoid of bias of ascertainment, together they provide a wealth of information about this pleiotropic disease.

Incidence

Because NF1 often is not diagnosed at birth, especially if the case is a new mutation, true birth incidence rates are difficult to obtain. Population surveys in the United States,[11] Russia,[28] Denmark,[29] and Wales[26] (Table 25-1) have resulted in an estimate of disease prevalence of approximately 1 in 2500 to 1 in 5000. A lower estimate of 1 in 7800 is provided by the Russian study, but this almost certainly represents an underestimate. When underascertainment and increased mortality are considered, the true birth incidence of NF1 is probably about 1 in 3000. There is no evidence that this frequency varies among ethnic groups. This is expected for a disorder with such a high percentage of spontaneous mutations.

Diagnostic Criteria

Despite opinions to the contrary in the medical literature, the diagnosis of NF1 usually is not difficult or controversial when performed by an experienced clinician. In 1987, the National Institutes of Health (NIH) convened a consensus panel to define diagnostic criteria for NF1, and the list that resulted (Table 25-2) reflects extensive clinical experience and only rarely leads to a false-positive diagnosis.[30] The same panel also set out the distinguishing features between NF1 and NF2 (see below), ending many decades of confusion about these two disorders, which are now known to be completely distinct, both genetically and clinically. Recently, these diagnostic criteria were updated based on a decade of improved clinical and basic science insights.[31]

The diagnostic criteria listed in Table 25-2 do not eliminate the occurrence of certain clinical dilemmas, however. A frequent dilemma is the identification of a child under 4 years of age with six or more café-au-lait spots, no family history, and no other manifestations of NF1. According to the NIH criteria, this is insufficient evidence to make a diagnosis of NF1, but such children must be followed for the appearance of other manifestations. Most of these children will eventually turn out to have NF1 as additional features manifest.

Defining Features Present in Most Patients

Café-au-Lait Spots. The café-au-lait spot (Fig. 25-1), a flat, evenly pigmented macule, usually is not apparent at birth but becomes visible during the first year of life. While up to 25 percent of the normal population will have one to three café-au-lait

Table 25-2 *Diagnostic Criteria for NF1*

Two or more of the following:
  Six or more café-au-lait spots
    1.5 cm or larger in postpubertal individuals
    0.5 cm or larger in prepubertal individuals
  Two or more neurofibromas of any type or
    one or more plexiform neurofibromas
  Freckling of armpits or groin
  Optic glioma (tumor of the optic pathway)
  Two or more Lisch nodules (benign iris hamartomas)
  A distinctive bony lesion
  Dysplasia of the sphenoid bone
  Dysplasia or thinning of long bone cortex
  First-degree relative with NF1

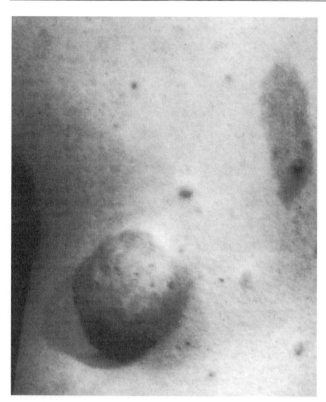

Fig. 25-1 Typical neurofibroma and a café-au-lait spot on the skin of an adult with NF1.

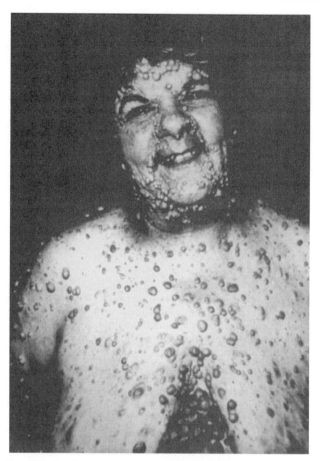

Fig. 25-2 An older individual with NF1, demonstrating extensive involvement on the skin surface with peripheral neurofibromas.

spots,[32] the presence of six or more is highly suspicious for NF1[11] if the size criteria listed in Table 25-2 are closely followed. Melanocytes within a café-au-lait spot have an increased number of macromelanosomes,[33] although this is not diagnostic for NF1. The café-au-lait spots tend to fade in later life and may be difficult or impossible to identify in elderly individuals. Visualization using a Wood's lamp often reveals these macules when they are not discernible on bedside examination.

Peripheral Neurofibromas. Peripheral neurofibromas are soft, fleshy tumors (Figs. 25-1 and 25-2) that are usually not present in childhood but make their appearance slightly before or during adolescence.[9] They tend to increase in size and number with age, although the rate can be extremely variable. Some females affected with NF1 note an increase in the rate of progression during pregnancy, suggesting that these tumors may be hormone-responsive. Pathologically, these lesions arise from cells in the peripheral nerve sheath and are made up of a mixture of cell types, including Schwann cells, fibroblasts, mast cells, and vascular elements.[34]

There are typically two types of neurofibromas: discrete and plexiform. While a discrete neurofibroma arises from a single site along a peripheral nerve as a focal mass with well-defined margins, plexiform neurofibromas usually involve multiple nerve fascicles (see below). A subset of patients can have firmer and sometimes painful neurofibromas along the course of peripheral nerves. These neurofibromas can be quite difficult to manage surgically. Even more challenging are the spinal neurofibromas arising from dorsal nerve roots, which can lead to pain and neurologic compromise. It should be emphasized that dermal neurofibromas are benign tumors without a propensity for malignant transformation.

Freckling. The occurrence of freckles in the axilla, groin, and intertriginous areas was first pointed out by Crowe[35] and is a useful diagnostic feature. Such freckling is not apparent at birth but often appears during childhood. In adults, freckling may be

seen in the neck regions or inframammary areas in women. The occurrence of such freckling in the inframammary areas and other skin folds[36] is a curious observation that suggests that these lesions are modulated by the local environment.

Lisch Nodules. Raised, often pigmented nodules of the iris, pathologically representing hamartomas, are now called *Lisch nodules* (Fig. 25-3) and represent an extremely important diagnostic feature of NF1.[19,20] Like café-au-lait spots and freckling, Lisch nodules never result in significant disease but

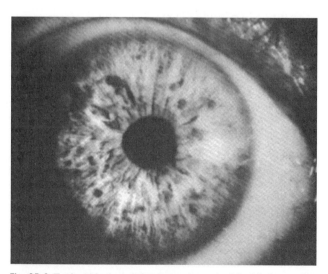

Fig. 25-3 Typical Lisch nodules (hamartomas) of the iris in an adult with NF1.

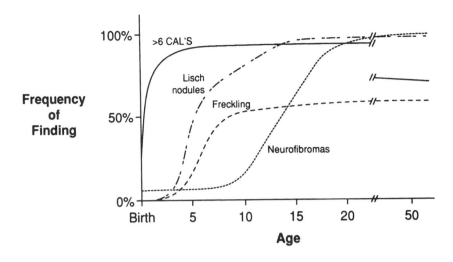

Fig. 25-4 Typical time course of appearance of the major clinical features of NF1. CAL = café-au-lait spots.

can be helpful in establishing the diagnosis. While they can be seen with simple lighting in individuals with light irises, a slit-lamp examination is usually essential to be certain of their presence and to distinguish them from iris nevi. Typically, these lesions are not detected until after 5 years of age.

Time Course

The defining features of NF1 described earlier, while somewhat variable in appearance, tend to follow the pattern shown in Fig. 25-4. As implied by the figure, it is unusual for an individual with NF1 to reach adolescence without having amply satisfied the diagnostic criteria in Table 25-2.

Common but Nondiagnostic and Nonmorbid Features

While not considered specific enough for inclusion in the list of diagnostic criteria, macrocephaly[25] and short stature[24] are common accompaniments of NF1. The macrocephaly reflects concomitant megalencephaly. Careful studies of adult height suggest that individuals with NF1 are on average about 3 inches shorter than predicted by their family backgrounds.[9,25] With both these circumstances, it is important not to overlook other, more significant causes. For instance, aqueductal stenosis leading to hydrocephalus is a known but uncommon complication of NF1 that requires surgical intervention.[37] Similarly, growth failure occasionally can arise as a result of hypothalamic involvement by optic glioma.

Variable but Significant Complications

The defining features of NF1 listed in Table 25-2 are found in most affected patients and, while often associated with significant cosmetic concerns related to neurofibroma growth, usually are not life-threatening. A range of other complications that are quite variable from one patient to the next can be more serious. Approximately one-third of patients with NF1 suffer from one or more of these serious complications during their lifetimes (Fig. 25-5).

Learning Disability. Frank mental retardation (IQ < 70) is uncommon in NF1. Recent molecular information indicates that such patients are much more likely to have the disease because of a large deletion that removes the entire *NF1* gene and considerable flanking DNA.[38] Presumably, other nearby genes are also reduced to hemizygosity by the deletion in these patients and contribute to the retardation.

Although retardation is uncommon, standard IQ testing reveals a downward shift of performance scores by 5 to 10 IQ points in affected individuals.[36] Approximately 40 to 60 percent of all individuals with NF1 have learning disabilities. Analysis of the

specific behavioral phenotype in children with NF1 has demonstrated a higher incidence of minor signs of neurologic impairment (motor abnormalities involving balance and gait), lower IQ scores, and poor performance on tasks involving nonverbal learning. In addition, children with NF1 often exhibit areas of increased T_2 signal intensity on magnetic resonance imaging (MRI) of the brain. It has been suggested that children with such areas (unidentified bright objects, or UBOs) have significantly lower

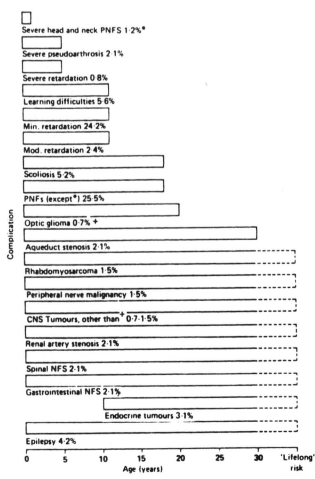

Fig. 25-5 Age range of presentation and frequency of major NF1 complications. PNF = plexiform neurofibroma; NFS = neurofibrosarcoma. (*From Huson et al.[27] Used by permission.*)

IQ and language scores, with impaired visual motor integration and coordination.[39] Although this hypothesis is intriguing, it has not been confirmed in all studies examining this association.[40,41] UBOs are seen most commonly in the basal ganglia, cerebellum, brainstem, and subcortical white matter regions. In one pathologic study, these hyperintense foci corresponded to areas of vacuolar and spongiotic change, with fluid-filled vacuoles surrounded by infiltrating astrocytes.[42] Recent studies have demonstrated increased neurofibromin expression in activated astrocytes both *in vivo* and *in vitro*, suggesting that reduced *NF1* gene expression may alter the normal astrogliotic response in the brain.[43,44] Intervention is highly warranted if the preceding problems emerge, and all children with NF1 should be followed closely for developmental progress and subjected to a thorough educational evaluation at age 3 or 4 if there is any indication of significant delay.

Plexiform Neurofibromas. A plexiform neurofibroma is a much more complex, usually congenital (though often not immediately visible) lesion that may diffusely involve nerve, muscle, connective tissue, vascular elements, and overlying skin.[36] Such lesions, which occur in approximately 20 percent of affected individuals, commonly lead to overgrowth of surrounding tissues during childhood and in their most severe form can lead to massive distortion of the face or an extremity (Fig. 25-6).[36a] When these lesions occur around the orbit, they are often associated with sphenoid wing dysplasia, and the tumor may extend inside the cranial vault, accompanied by pulsating exophthalmos.[9] Severe plexiform lesions are almost invariably apparent by age 4 or 5, so it is possible to reassure older individuals without plexiform lesions that they are not at significant risk for the development of this particularly troubling and disfiguring complication.

Malignancy. The frequency of malignancy in NF1 is difficult to discern accurately, since most series reflect a referral bias and therefore overestimate the occurrence of this complication.[42] Nonetheless, there is clearly an increased risk of specific cancers in NF1, amounting to perhaps 2 to 5 percent of affected individuals.[9,23,25,29,46,46a]

A particularly aggressive and often fatal malignancy is the neurofibrosarcoma, or malignant peripheral nerve sheath tumor (MPNST), which commonly arises in a plexiform neurofibroma in a young adult. Often the first symptom is pain or rapid growth, which should always prompt rapid investigation in an individual with a plexiform lesion. These malignancies are highly aggressive and metastatic cancers that are relatively resistant to chemotherapy and radiation.[47] Survival remains poor when wide excision or amputation is not possible.

A second strongly associated tumor is optic glioma. MRI scanning of affected children with NF1 has revealed radiographic evidence of optic nerve or optic chiasm enlargement in up to 15 to 20 percent of patients,[48–50] but the vast majority of these patients have normal vision and never become symptomatic. Most of these tumors are detected in children younger than 6 years. A small subgroup, however, presents with progressive visual loss associated with an expanding lesion. Occasionally, optic pathway gliomas can lead to precocious puberty when hypothalamic involvement ensues. While this occurs only in a minority of patients with NF1, all children with NF1 should have regular ophthalmologic evaluations.

While the risk of other malignancies of the nervous system is less impressive, there appears to be a moderately increased risk of central nervous system tumors, especially astrocytomas.[34] Pheochromocytoma is commonly quoted as a complication of NF1 but is in fact quite uncommon in this population.[11,45,46]

Seizures. A seizure disorder will develop in approximately 5 percent of patients with NF1, and the onset can occur at any time.[9] While occasionally a definable intracranial tumor will be found to be at fault, usually no cause can be defined. In this regard, the

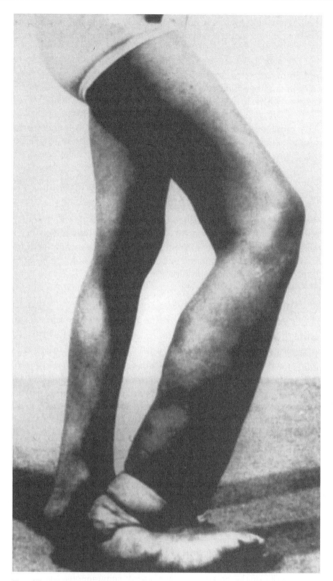

Fig. 25-6 Massive plexiform neurofibroma of the lower extremity in an adolescent with NF1.

recent advent of MRI scanning has uncovered MRI inhomogeneities in the brains of many children with NF1 on T_2-weighted images. These UBOs are of uncertain etiology and generally should not be interpreted as clinically significant.[51] There is some evidence that they tend to disappear with age, and it is not correct, on the basis of current evidence, to refer to them as hamartomas.

Scoliosis. Vertebral defects, including scalloping from dural ectasia,[52] are extremely common in NF1, and approximately 10 percent of affected individuals have scoliosis during late childhood and adolescence.[9] In some instances this can be severe enough to require bracing and/or surgery and may or may not be associated with local neurofibroma formation.

Pseudarthrosis. A peculiar and uncommon complication that defies the classification of NF1 as a disorder purely of the neural crest is the involvement of long bones. This often is noted first as bowing, particularly of the tibia, in young children. This may progress to thinning of the cortex, pathologic fracture, and severe difficulties with nonunion of the fragments. This process may go on to form a pseudarthrosis, or false joint, leaving the limb severely compromised. The pathologic basis of this unusual process is unknown.

Hypertension. Hypertension is extremely common in adults with NF1, affecting perhaps one-third of these patients.[24] In general, this proves to be essential hypertension with no underlying cause, but the new development of hypertension always should raise the possibility of renal artery stenosis, which is particularly common in children,[53] or pheochromocytoma, which occasionally occurs in adults with NF1 (see above).

Miscellaneous Complications. Frequent but less well understood problems associated with neurofibromatosis 1 include headache, which can be bothersome but usually not disabling. The new onset of headache always should trigger evaluation for an intracranial tumor, but many patients experience lifelong stable headache patterns with no identifiable etiology. Generalized itching or itching localized to newly developing neurofibromas is reported by many individuals.[9] Similarly, constipation seems to be a frequent concomitant of the disease, especially in patients who have plexiform neurofibromas in the pelvic area.[54] These complications may interfere with autonomic innervation of the colon and produce both bowel and bladder problems.

GENETIC ASPECTS

Inheritance Pattern

Preiser and Davenport[17] surveyed the literature in 1918 and concluded that approximately 50 percent of the children of individuals affected with NF1 also were afflicted, regardless of sex. They noted numerous examples of male-to-male transmission, concluding that the disease follows an autosomal dominant pattern of inheritance. In 1981, Hall suggested that the sex of the affected parent might have an impact on the severity of the disease,[55,56] a phenomenon we would now ascribe to parental imprinting.[57] In that study, children of affected mothers tended to be slightly more severely affected than did children of affected fathers. Subsequent careful analyses of this issue have failed to confirm this maternal effect,[23,54,55] although a very modest effect would be difficult to exclude with such variability of the disease.[58,59]

Mutation Rate

All large series indicate after careful examination that 30 to 50 percent of patients with NF1 do not have an affected parent.[11,29,59] Such individuals presumably represent spontaneous mutations. With the cloning of the *NF1* gene, several examples have now been documented of *de novo* alterations in the *NF1* gene in such individuals (see below). Given that NF1 is a common disease and that so many of its sufferers have new mutations, one cannot escape the conclusion that the mutation rate for this locus is unusually high. In fact, calculations of this frequency (see Table 25-1) indicate a mutation rate of approximately 10^{-4} per allele per generation. Evidence based on linkage analysis has indicated that the vast majority of new mutations arise from the paternal allele,[60,61] indicating that these mutations apparently occur during spermatogenesis. Whether they are meiotic or mitotic errors has not been determined, although mitotic errors are suggested by the absence of a significant paternal age effect in new mutation cases.

With such a high mutation rate, it would be predicted that the reproductive fitness of individuals with NF1 must be significantly reduced in order for the disease to be present at an equilibrium frequency. The Welsh study[59] found a fitness of 0.31 for affected males and 0.60 for affected females (1.0 is the expected value). A large proportion of the reduced fertility can be attributed to a failure of affected individuals to marry, which presumably reflects the psychosocial consequences of the condition.

Penetrance

The penetrance of NF1 is essentially 100 percent in individuals who have reached adulthood and have been subjected to careful examination by an experienced physician, including a slit-lamp examination. Rare cases of normal parents giving rise to two affected children have been described[62] and could be examples of germ-line mosaicism in one of the parents, although the possibility of independent spontaneous mutations cannot be excluded until molecular studies are carried out in such patients. The importance of careful examination of both parents before giving genetic counseling cannot be overemphasized, however. There are numerous reports of circumstances in which one of the parents was sufficiently mildly affected to be unaware of his or her diagnosis.

Variable Expressivity

NF1 is a classic example of the tendency for autosomal dominant conditions to show variable expressivity, which can at times be dramatic in NF1. Even the more constant defining features of the disease are subject to considerable heterogeneity when considered closely. It has been known for some time that large families with multiple afflicted individuals are likely to demonstrate a wide range of severity and complications, and the variability within a family of significant size is similar to the variability seen in comparisons of different families. This indicates that the specific germ-line mutation at the *NF1* locus does not accurately predict the phenotype in a specific individual, since all affected individuals in the same family carry the same germ-line mutation.

To distinguish between genetic influences and environmental and/or chance influences, Easton and coworkers[63] examined a series of monozygotic twins concordant for NF1 and compared them with other pairs of first-degree affected relatives. There was a significant correlation in the number of café-au-lait spots and neurofibromas between identical twins, with a lower but significant correlation in first-degree relatives and almost no correlation between more distant relatives. This suggests that these features are controlled by other genetic influences but that the specific mutation in the *NF1* gene itself plays a minor role. Optic glioma, scoliosis, epilepsy, and learning disability were concordant in twin pairs, but plexiform neurofibromas were not. Furthermore, there was no indication that the presence of one complication predicted the occurrence of another except for the fact that neurofibrosarcoma has been observed commonly to occur almost exclusively in individuals with plexiform neurofibromas.

Related Syndromes

NF1 has been described in the literature in association with almost every imaginable disorder, but most of these reports appear to represent the coincidental occurrence of two unrelated conditions. A classification scheme proposed by Riccardi and Eichner[9] divides the neurofibromatoses into eight syndromes, but this scheme has not found wide application because of the blurred boundaries between several categories. A full discussion of variant syndromes is beyond the scope of this chapter, but a few of the most relevant conditions will be mentioned.

Neurofibromatosis Type 2. Type 2 neurofibromatosis, formerly designated *central neurofibromatosis* or *bilateral vestibular neurofibromatosis,* is now appreciated to be distinct, both clinically and genetically, from NF1.[64,65] The *NF2* gene has been mapped to chromosome 22 and was identified in 1993.[12,13] Individuals with NF2 often have a small number of café-au-lait spots (rarely more than six) and may have one or two peripheral neurofibromas but usually not more. They occasionally have Lisch nodules.[66] Ophthalmologic evaluation is extremely useful because of the presence of posterior subcapsular cataracts in a sizable proportion of these patients.[67] The hallmark of NF2 is the development of bilateral eighth cranial nerve tumors, properly called *vestibular schwannomas* rather than acoustic neuromas, in 95 percent of these patients by age 30 years.[64] Inheritance is autosomal dominant. Other tumors of cranial and cervical nerve roots are common, and management presents great challenges for neurosurgeons and otolaryngologists. Past statements that acoustic neuroma is a complication of NF1 are almost certainly due to the confusion between these two entities; since more careful definitions of the two disorders have been applied, there has been no indication that individuals with NF1 have an increased risk of eighth cranial nerve tumors compared with the general population. NF2 is much less common than NF1, affecting approximately 1 in 40,000 individuals.

Segmental (Mosaic) NF1. Occasionally individuals are encountered who have features of NF1 limited to one segment of the body.[68] These features may include café-au-lait spots, freckling, and peripheral or plexiform neurofibromas, and Lisch nodules may be seen in an individual who has that segment of the body affected. Such individuals invariably have normal parents but on rare occasions can have a child with classic NF1.[69] There is strong circumstantial evidence that these cases represent somatic mutation of the *NF1* gene early in embryogenesis so that derivatives of that mutant line display the features of NF1. If the mosaicism involves the germ line, the disease can then be transmitted. Recently, germ-line mosaicism for an *NF1* gene mutation was found in a clinically unaffected father of a child with new onset NF1.[70] In addition, somatic mosaicism for an *NF1* gene deletion was detected in an individual with NF1.[71,71a] Analysis of cases of segmental NF1 probably will demonstrate similar somatic mosaicism.

Watson Syndrome. A variant of NF1 that appears to breed true in certain families involves multiple café-au-lait spots, dull intelligence, short stature, pulmonary valvular stenosis, and only a small number of neurofibromas.[72] Reevaluation of these families has indicated that they also have Lisch nodules, further contributing to the blurring of these two phenotypes. In fact, molecular analyses have demonstrated that in at least two families that appear to fall into the category of Watson syndrome, deletions are present in the *NF1* gene. Currently, there appears to be no distinguishing aspect between the deletions causing Watson syndrome and those associated with more classic NF1.

Neurofibromatosis–Noonan Syndrome. The occurrence of features reminiscent of Noonan syndrome in patients with neurofibromatosis 1 has been noted for some time,[73] raising the question of whether these could be overlapping syndromes or even could be due to deletion of adjacent genes. In most of these families, however, individuals with clear-cut Noonan syndrome represent only a proportion of those affected with NF1, and some of the features associated with Noonan syndrome (such as pectus excavatum, mild hypertelorism, and short stature) are frequently observed in NF1.[74] A linkage study of autosomal dominant Noonan syndrome occurring in the absence of NF1 has indicated no linkage to markers in the *NF1* region of chromosome 17, casting into doubt any notion that Noonan syndrome, at least in the aggregate, could be due to a mutation in a gene closely adjacent to *NF1*. At least one family with neurofibromatosis–Noonan syndrome (NFNS) has been found to harbor a deletion in the *NF1* gene, but the fact that very large deletions removing flanking regions on either side of *NF1* do not consistently result in NFNS casts further doubt on the adjacent gene theory. The most appropriate synthesis of the data at the present time indicates that the phenotype of NF1 can include features that overlap with those described in Noonan syndrome, but these disorders are probably genetically distinct.

Spinal Neurofibromatosis. Rare families have been identified with a predominance of spinal tumors and relatively few peripheral neurofibromas. A linkage study has indicated that one such family appears to be linked to NF1, whereas another does not, implying locus heterogeneity for this set of conditions.[75] While this condition underscores the variable expressivity of NF1, spinal neurofibromatosis does not represent a distinct subtype of NF1.

MOLECULAR BIOLOGY OF THE *NF1* GENE

Cloning of the *NF1* Gene

Since no information was available on the structure or function of the *NF1* gene product before the 1980s, the only feasible approach available to identify the gene was positional cloning.[76] The isolation of the gene for von Recklinghausen neurofibromatosis began with an international collaboration to assemble linkage data in families with NF1. By early 1987, this worldwide effort made possible the construction of an exclusion map that narrowed the candidate chromosomes to a handful.[77] Examination of these selected chromosomes with RFLP markers culminated in the establishment of linkage of NF1 to the pericentromeric region of chromosome 17 in the late spring of 1987.[77–80] No linkage disequilibrium was ever found. One of the linked markers was an anonymous probe called pA10-41, and another was the gene for nerve growth factor receptor (17q12-22).[81] The linkage of NF1 with the nerve growth factor (NGF) receptor gene was exciting because of the role of NGF in neural crest tissue development. Further analysis using RFLP markers, however, excluded the NGF receptor gene as a candidate for the *NF1* gene, since numerous crossover events were identified.[82]

An intense genetic mapping effort resulted in the establishment of a multipoint linkage map constructed from data assembled by the NF1 collaborative group (Fig. 25-7). This map represented the outcome of the study of 142 families with over 700 affected individuals and narrowed the distance between flanking probes and the *NF1* gene to 3 cM, or about 3 million bp.[83] Candidate genes in this interval, such as the *erbA1* and *erbB2* proto-oncogenes, were subsequently excluded as candidate genes for NF1 by the identification of recombinants.

The discovery of two patients with NF1 and balanced translocations involving the long arm of chromosome 17 dramatically accelerated the process. These two NF1 patients had reciprocal translocations, one between chromosomes 1p34.3

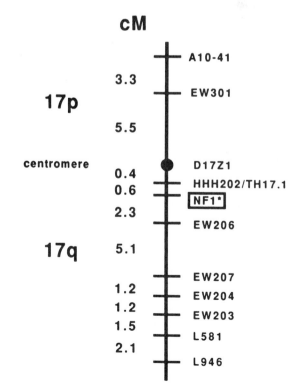

Fig. 25-7 Linkage map for chromosome 17 demonstrating the position of the *NF1* locus relative to other DNA markers linked to the disease. The map distance of the various markers is represented in centimorgans (cM).

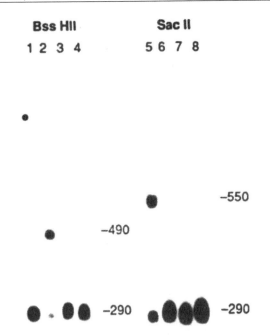

Bss HII

Sac II

1 2 3 4   5 6 7 8

−550

−490

−290   −290

Fig. 25-8 Pulsed-field gel analysis with probe 17L1A in an NF1 patient with [1;17] translocation. Genomic DNA is digested with a rare-cutting restriction enzyme (either BssHII or SacII), separated by pulsed-field gel electrophoresis, and probed with 17L1A. The DNA source in each lane is 1 and 8, patients with NF1; 2 and 5, a patient with a 1;17 translocation has a unique band not seen in the other DNA samples, indicating the presence of a rearrangement of the DNA in the region near the NF1 gene in this patient. (*Adapted from Fountain et al.[84] Used by permission.*)

and 17q11.2 and the other between chromosomes 17q11.2 and 22q11.2.[84–88] Support for the notion that these translocations disrupt the *NF1* gene was provided by the fact that one breakpoint in each of the translocations involved 17q11.2, precisely where the *NF1* gene had been mapped by linkage analysis.

The identification of translocation breakpoints permitted analysis of the genetic region by physical mapping techniques and bridged the gap between linkage mapping and physical mapping.[89] Using restriction enzymes that recognize rare restriction sites in DNA, one could search for an anomalously migrating DNA fragment resulting from the disruption of this region by the translocations. To identify the translocation breakpoints by physical mapping, markers capable of visualizing these areas had to be generated. Using a series of chromosome 17-specific *NotI*-linking clones tested against a somatic cell hybrid mapping panel, a clone termed *17L1A* was identified that detected abnormalities by pulsed-field gel electrophoresis in the 1;17 translocation patient and her affected offspring (Fig. 25-8). The presence of abnormal fragments provided conclusive evidence that the translocation breakpoints map near the 17L1A clone.

The use of cosmid libraries to look for abnormal fragments on pulsed-field gel electrophoresis provided an additional clone, called *1F10*, that detected abnormal fragments in both translocation patients. These two cloned probes were then shown to reside on the same 600-kb DNA fragment and bracketed the two translocations. This narrowed the interval in which the *NF1* gene must reside to 600 kb of DNA.[87] Of interest was the fact that 17L1A represented a CpG island, a hypomethylated region often associated with five regulatory sequences of active genes.

The construction of a physical map of the region around the *NF1* gene laid the groundwork for identifying candidate cDNA transcripts. Using a combination of jump library clones, yeast artificial chromosome probes, and cosmids, candidate cDNA transcripts were identified. Unexpectedly, however, the first candidate gene came from another route: By comparison with a syntenic region on mouse chromosome 11, the mouse *evi2* gene,

which is involved in virally induced murine leukemia, was found to map between these two breakpoints.[90–92] Cloning of the human *EVI2A* gene excluded it as a candidate for the *NF1* gene in that neither translocation actually interrupted the gene and no mutations were found in it in other patients with NF1.[93] A second candidate gene, *EVI2B,* similar to *EVI2A,* was identified but also was excluded as a potential candidate.[92] The third candidate gene, *OMGP* (oligodendrocyte myelin glycoprotein), which was exciting because of its almost exclusive expression in Schwann cells and oligodendrocytes, also failed to satisfy the criteria for an *NF1* gene candidate, since no mutations could be identified in this gene in NF1 patients.[94,95]

The fourth candidate gene was much larger and was cloned and shown to be the *NF1* gene in several ways.[1–3] First, the transcript crossed both translocation breakpoints and would therefore be interrupted in these unique NF1 patients.[1–3] Second, more subtle mutations were identified in patients with NF1 that would alter the coding potential of this candidate transcript.[2] These included a patient with a *de novo* 400-nucleotide insertion that produced an abnormally large fragment on Southern blot analysis using the NF1 cDNA as a probe and another patient with a nonsense mutation.[96] These mutations provided conclusive evidence that the correct gene had been found.

The *NF1* gene has an open reading frame of nearly 9 kb and spans approximately 300 kb of genomic DNA[97] (Fig. 25-9). The messenger RNA has been estimated to be 11 to 13 kb and has been detected in all tissues examined by RT-PCR and northern blot analysis. At least 57 exons have been identified, with three additional alternatively spliced exons (see "Identification of NF1 Gene Product" below). The three previous candidate genes were all found embedded in one large intron and were transcribed from the opposite strand from the *NF1* gene.[93] The predicted protein has 2818 amino acids and a molecular weight of 327 kDa.[98] Analysis of the amino acid sequence failed to reveal any nuclear localization signals or transmembrane domains, suggesting that the gene product resides in the cytoplasm. Comparison of the gene with other previously identified coding sequences revealed unexpected sequence similarity between the *NF1* gene product and a family of GTPase-activating proteins (GAPs) (see "Neurofibromin as a GTPase-Activating Protein" below).[4] Analyses of homologous genes from mouse, chicken, hamster, and *Drosophila* species demonstrate striking species conservation and underscore the fundamental importance of this gene.[99–102]

Further analysis of the genomic organization of the *NF1* gene demonstrated that the promoter of this gene resides within a CpG-rich region; this is consistent with the observation that most active eukaryotic gene promoters are contained within CpG islands.[103] During the construction of a yeast artificial chromosome contig containing the entire *NF1* gene, other homologous loci were found by low-stringency hybridization on Southern blot.[104,105] These loci were determined by a hybrid mapping panel and fluorescent *in situ* hybridization to reside on chromosomes 14, 15, and 22. At least two loci were found on chromosome 14. These homologous loci apparently represent unprocessed pseudogenes in that their coding sequences contain frameshift, nonsense, and missense mutations. However, these loci also may represent mutation reservoirs that can be crossed into the *NF1* locus on chromosome 17 by interchromosomal gene conversion. This phenomenon potentially could contribute to the high rate of mutation in NF1.

Patient Mutations

Analysis of NF1 patients for mutations is still in its infancy and is hampered by the large size of the gene. Approximately 20 mutations have been studied in some detail. Five types of *NF1* gene mutations have been described to date in patients with NF1: (1) Translocations have been described in two patients with NF1 and were described earlier in this chapter. These balanced translocations provided some of the first clues to the precise physical location of the *NF1* gene on chromosome 17. (2) Megabase deletions have been reported in patients with NF1.[38]

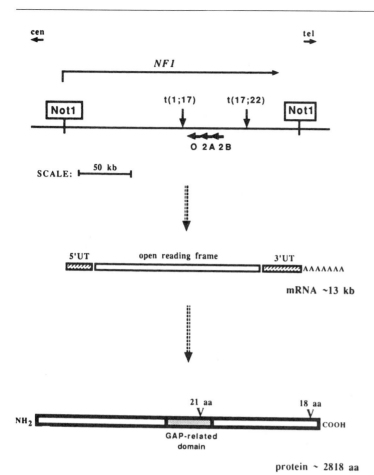

Fig. 25-9 The genetic organization of the *NF1* locus. The genomic structure of the *NF1* locus demonstrates the location of the two NotI restriction sites separated by 1300 kb. The initiation codon is located upstream of the centromeric NotI site and is positioned within a CpG-rich area. The position of the two translocation breakpoints [t(1;17) and t(17;22)] described in two patients with NF1 and their interruption of the *NF1* gene are illustrated. Three genes (O for *OMgP,* 2A for *EVI2A,* and 2B for *EVI2B*) are embedded within one intron on the opposite strand from the *NF1* gene. The mRNA for NF1 is 11 to 13 kb and has an open reading frame of 8454 nucleotides with at least 2 kb of 3′ untranslated sequence. Translation of this open reading frame predicts a protein of 2818 amino acids with an estimated molecular weight of 327 kDa. Sequence similarity between a central 300- to 400-amino-acid region of the *NF1* gene product, neurofibromin, and a family of GTPase-activating proteins (GAPs) is illustrated by the GAP-related domain. The location of the two alternatively spliced isoforms is denoted by the 21-amino-acid insertion into the GAP-related domain and the 18-amino-acid insertion in the C-terminus of neurofibromin.

These deletions extend well beyond the *NF1* gene and may include other genes on chromosome 17q11.2. These patients manifest typical NF1 but also have significant mental retardation. (3) Large internal deletions entirely contained within the *NF1* gene have been reported in patients with NF1. One of these deletions removed 90 kb of DNA encompassing the 5′ portion of the *NF1* gene, while the other deleted 40 kb of NF1 DNA.[106] The phenotypes of these patients were indistinguishable from those of classic NF1 patients. (4) Small rearrangements within the *NF1* gene have been described. One of these rearrangements involved the insertion of a human Alu repeat in the intron between two *NF1* exons, resulting in abnormal mRNA splicing and premature termination of the *NF1* mRNA coding sequence.[96] (5) Many point mutations have been described in patients with NF1.[2] These mutations include the creation of stop codons, missense mutations, and frameshift mutations. One of these missense mutations involves a nonconservative substitution at codon 1423 within the NF1-GAP-related domain (*NF1GRD*).[107] This mutation, when expressed in insect Sf9 cells, results in a reduced ability of the *NF1GRD* to accelerate the hydrolysis of *ras*-GTP and perhaps altered *NF1* gene product, termed *neurofibromin,* function. This mutation also has been observed in anaplastic astrocytomas and colonic adenocarcinomas. Thus far there does not appear to be a hotspot for mutation within the *NF1* gene, since all these mutations are randomly distributed throughout the *NF1* coding sequences.[108] To this end, the phenotypes of patients with all the preceding mutation types (except megabase deletions) are likely to be similar in that they all result in the loss of a functional protein. The fact that mutations all result in a loss of *NF1* protein function is consistent with the notion of *NF1* as a tumor-suppressor gene.

The tumor-suppressor mechanism suggests that loss of both copies of the *NF1* gene would culminate in a transformed or neoplastic phenotype.[109–112] In this hypothesis, affected individuals would inherit one mutated *NF1* gene from their parents (or as

a new mutation), but neurofibromas or neurofibrosarcomas would develop only when the second gene became nonfunctional as a result of somatic mutation. This set of events is termed the *Knudson hypothesis* and was first elegantly demonstrated for retinoblastoma.[113,114] In patients with retinoblastoma, all somatic cells contain the germ-line-inherited mutation in one of the retinoblastoma genes. Retinoblastomas arise as a result of loss of the second copy of the retinoblastoma gene in retinal cells.

Occasionally, the second somatic mutation in the tumor can be detected by Southern blot analysis. In white blood cells from patients with NF1, the DNA may be heterozygous for a particular DNA marker polymorphism on chromosome 17, but when tumor cells develop, the remaining wild-type gene is lost, eliminating that particular allele (Fig. 25-10). This is termed *loss of*

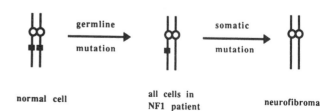

Fig. 25-10 Illustration of loss of heterozygosity in NF1. A given DNA marker polymorphism, denoted by the filled squares, is present in a normal NF1 chromosome 17. A germ-line mutation found in all cells in an NF1 patient would alter the *NF1* gene to result in the loss of one of the DNA markers. Because the patient has one normal chromosome 17 DNA polymorphism and one mutated chromosome 17 DNA polymorphism, the patient is said to be heterozygous with respect to that DNA marker. Mutation of the one remaining normal *NF1* gene in a tumor results in the loss of both copies of the gene and loss of heterozygosity with respect to that DNA marker polymorphism.

heterozygosity and is taken as proof that a second somatic event has occurred that results in the loss of the one remaining functional *NF1* gene. Interpretation of these data for chromosome 17 are confounded by the frequent loss of heterozygosity for markers near the *p53* gene on chromosome 17p as well.[115] Loss of heterozygosity centered at the *NF1* locus has been observed in selected tumors from some patients with NF1, supporting the notion that *NF1* is a tumor-suppressor gene and that the manifestations of the disease result from somatic loss of the second *NF1* gene copy. A tumor in an NF1 patient has been found to display loss of heterozygosity for chromosome 17 markers but in addition demonstrates a large deletion in the *NF1* gene in tumor cell but not white blood cell DNA.[116] This supports the notion that a "second hit" occurs in the *NF1* gene during the development of neurofibrosarcomas in patients with NF1.

Mutations in the *NF1* gene have been described in other tumor types, including malignant melanomas, neuroblastomas, pheochromocytomas, and neurofibrosarcomas.[117,118] Examination of a series of malignant melanoma cell lines derived from metastatic foci demonstrated reduced or absent neurofibromin expression in up to 25 percent of tumors.[119,120] Similar examination of neuroblastomas revealed that *NF1* mRNA and neurofibromin expression is reduced in up to 30 percent of neuroblastomas.[120,121] Similarly, three neurofibrosarcomas derived from NF1 patients demonstrated elevated levels of *ras*-GTP and nearly undetectable levels of neurofibromin, suggesting a relationship between lack of neurofibromin expression and unregulated *ras* activity in these cells (see below).[122,123] Abnormalities at the DNA level have been reported for pheochromocytomas from NF1 patients.[124] Examination of these fresh tumors demonstrated loss of neurofibromin expression in six of six pheochromocytomas as well as one adrenal cortical tumor from patients with NF1.[125] It is likely that examination of other tumors will uncover alterations in neurofibromin expression that are consistent with its proposed role as a tumor-suppressor gene product. Consistent with the proposed role of neurofibromin as a negative growth regulator, tumors from patients with and without NF1 have been examined for alterations in *NF1* gene expression. The hallmark of NF1 is the neurofibroma, a benign tumor composed predominantly of Schwann cells, fibroblasts, and to a lesser extent, mast cells. It has been presumed that the cellular defect in the neurofibroma results from abnormal Schwann cell function secondary to loss of neurofibromin function. Malignancies in NF1 are believed to result from the constitutional inactivation of one *NF1* gene followed by a number of somatic events, including inactivation of the other *NF1* allele. Although loss of the normal allele has been proved for the malignant nerve sheath tumor (neurofibrosarcoma),[116] it had not been evaluated in the etiology of the benign neurofibroma. Recent work has demonstrated loss of heterozygosity in 22 neurofibromas from five unrelated NF1 patients.[126] In eight of these tumors, somatic deletions involving the wild-type *NF1* gene could be demonstrated, indicating that inactivation of the normal *NF1* gene is associated with the development of the neurofibroma. In related studies on Schwann cells derived from the dorsal root ganglia of neurofibromin-deficient mice, abnormalities in Schwann cell proliferation and high levels of activated p21-*ras* were observed, as would be predicted by loss of neurofibromin GAP function.[127] In addition, these neurofibromin-deficient Schwann cells had abnormal proliferative responses to neuronal contact.[128] Additional studies also have demonstrated abnormalities in fibroblasts derived from neurofibromin-deficient mouse embryos.[129] These results collectively suggest that defects in both the Schwann cells and the fibroblasts may contribute to the development of the benign neurofibroma.

Children with NF1 are at increased risk for the development of malignant myeloid disorders. Although myeloid disorders are an uncommon complication of NF1 in childhood, NF1 constitutes as many as 10 percent of the spontaneous cases of myeloid proliferative disorders in children. Examination of bone marrow samples from children with NF1 in whom malignant myeloid disorders developed demonstrated loss of heterozygosity at the *NF1* locus.[130] In each case, the mutant *NF1* allele was inherited from the parent with NF1, and the normal allele was deleted in the myeloid leukemic cells. These results are consistent with the hypothesis that loss of neurofibromin expression predisposes myeloid cells to leukemic transformation. Mice heterozygous for a germ-line *NF1* mutation also develop myeloid leukemias with loss of the wild-type *NF1* allele in the leukemic cells.[131] Analysis of these myeloid leukemic cells with loss of neurofibromin expression demonstrates an exaggerated and prolonged increase in p21-*ras* activation in response to granulocyte macrophage colony stimulating factor (GM-CSF). This increased sensitivity to GM-CSF reflects abnormal p21-*ras* signaling that probably leads to chronic clonal hyperproliferation and malignant transformation. Primary leukemic cells from children with NF1 also show an exaggerated increase in p21-*ras* activity in response to GM-CSF.[132]

Support for the hypothesis that neurofibromin functions to suppress growth by regulating *ras* derives from experiments on the ability of one of these neurofibrosarcoma cell lines (ST88-14) to grow in soft agar.[133] Whereas ST88-14 cells form colonies in soft agar, ST88-14 cells treated with pharmacologic agents that block *ras* function fail to grow in soft agar. In addition, increased ras activity and neurofibromin loss has now been reported in NF1-associated malignant peripheral nerve sheath tumors, benign neurofibromas, and low-grade pilocytic astrocytomas.[133a,133b,133c] These results argue that neurofibromin loss leads to increased *ras* activity, which in turn is partly responsible for the abnormal growth properties of these tumor cells.

Animal Models

The search for spontaneous animal models of NF1 was initially disappointing. Three early models of NF1 were reported. In the bicolor damselfish, spontaneous neurofibromas and hyperpigmented spots develop, but the disorder appears to be transmissible, and these tumors tend to be more invasive and malignant than human neurofibromas.[134] One murine model was reported as resulting from the overexpression of the HTLV-I *tat* gene in mice.[135] Neurofibroma-like tumors developed in the offspring. However, other phenotypic features of NF1 were absent, and the neurofibromas lacked Schwann cells, unlike human NF1 neurofibromas. Similarly, the relationship between HTLV-I and human NF1 is unclear, since there is no increased incidence of HTLV-I exposure or infection in NF1 patients.[136] The third model of NF1 was achieved by injecting *N*-nitroso-*N*-ethylurea into pregnant Syrian golden hamsters.[102,137] The progeny develop neurofibromas histologically identical to those observed in NF1 patients, as well as pigmented lesions similar to café-au-lait spots. However, these hamsters also have Wilms tumors and other malignancies not typically seen in NF1 patients. Recently, point mutations in the *neu* proto-oncogene were identified in these hamster tumors. No mutations have been identified to date in the hamster *NF1* gene by Southern or Western blot analysis.[137]

In an effort to develop a mouse model for neurofibromatosis 1, mice were generated that carried a null mutation at the murine *NF1* locus using gene targeting in embryonic stem cells.[138,139] Heterozygous mutant mice containing one mutant *NF1* and one wild-type allele are phenotypically normal without evidence of neurofibromas, pigmentary abnormalities, or Lisch nodules. However, 75 percent of heterozygous mice succumb to tumors within 27 months compared with 15 percent of wild-type animals.[138] In addition to developing the tumor type seen in older wild-type mice, heterozygote *NF1* mice develop certain tumor types characteristic of human NF1. One animal developed a neurofibrosarcoma at 21 months of age, and 12 developed adrenal tumors at 15 to 28 months. Nine of the adrenal tumors were pheochromocytomas. Examination of these tumors demonstrated loss of the wild-type *NF1* allele and evidence of reduction to homozygosity for the *NF1* gene in the tumor DNA. These data support the hypothesis that the loss of *NF1* gene function contributes to the development of tumors.

The breeding of heterozygous knockout animals to yield mice in which both copies of the *NF1* gene were disrupted by homologous recombination (homozygous knockout mice) produced embryos that died *in utero* from generalized tissue edema.[138,139] Examination of the hearts in these mice at embryonic day 12.5 demonstrates a double-outlet right ventricle defect resulting from a failure of the aorta and pulmonary artery to separate. Double-outlet right ventricles have been observed in developing chicks in which the neural crest cells migrating to form elements of the cardiac vasculature are ablated. These results suggest that neurofibromin may be critical for the function of these neural crest–derived cells, although other mechanisms are possible. In addition to the cardiac vessel defect, the skeletal musculature is hypoplastic relative to normal mouse embryos. The existence of a muscle-specific isoform of the *NF1* gene and the observation that neurofibromin expression is increased in skeletal and cardiac muscle during embryonic development argue that neurofibromin also may be critical for normal muscle differentiation.[140,141] Additionally, examination of the sympathetic ganglia in these homozygous mutant mice demonstrates hyperplasia and an increased mitotic index.[142] These neurons also exhibit a reduced requirement for exogenous survival factors (neurotrophins), arguing that loss of neurofibromin may drive some cells to proliferate even in the absence of survival factors. In addition, there may be some genetic cooperativity between NF1 and p53 such that superior cervical ganglia neurons deficient in both neurofibromin and p53 have longer survival in the absence of neurotrophins.[143]

Mice heterozygous for a targeted mutation in the *Nf1* gene (*Nf1*[+/−]) have been carefully analyzed for features seen in patients with NF1 who also are heterozygous for a mutant *Nf1* allele. *Nf1*[+/−] mice demonstrate learning and memory deficits.[144] As observed in people with NF1, these deficits are restricted to specific types of learning (spatial memory but not associative learning), are not fully penetrant, and can be compensated for with extended training.

Several groups have endeavored to develop more sophisticated models for NF1-associated tumors. Mice that are chimeric for disruption of the *Nf1* gene have been generated such that a small minority of the cells in their bodies has both copies of the *Nf1* gene inactivated.[144a] These chimeric mice are viable and some of these animals develop tumors that are histologically similar to the benign neurofibromas seen in patients affected with NF1. In addition to chimeric mice, mice with conditional tissue-specific disruption of the *Nf1* gene have been developed. Preliminary observations suggest that *Nf1* inactivation has profound tissue specific effects on cell growth and differentiation.

Studies on human malignant peripheral nerve sheath tumors have demonstrated that half of these tumors harbor mutations in another tumor suppressor gene (p53), suggesting that malignant tumor formation requires additional cooperating genetic events. In support of this hypothesis, mice genetically engineered with targeted disruptions of both *Nf1* and *p53* develop high grade MPNSTs.[144a,144b] In addition, some of these mice when maintained on a C57B1/6 genetic background develop high-grade astrocytomas.[144c] Although these high-grade brain tumors are not observed in patients with NF1, these results suggest that modifying genes exist on this strain background that influence the development of brain tumors.

In *Drosophila*, the *NF1* gene may function in the protein kinase A (PKA) signaling pathway.[145] Targeted disruption of both *Drosophila NF1* genes results in reductions in fly size. Whereas homozygous null *NF1*[−/−] mice are embryonic lethal, *Drosophila NF1*-null flies are fertile and viable. Partial rescue of the *Drosophila* mutant phenotype can be obtained with activated PKA. In addition, *Drosophila NF1* is essential for the response to certain polypeptides at the neuromuscular junction in flies.[146]

Identification of the *NF1* Gene Product

The protein product of the *NF1* locus has been identified. Using antibodies generated against fusion proteins and synthetic peptides, a unique 250-kDa protein is identifiable in all cell lines examined.[147–151] This NF1-GAP-related protein was originally termed *NF1GRP* to underscore its relationship to mammalian GAP and the yeast *IRA1* and *IRA2* genes (see below).[4,149] The NNFF consortium agreed to call this protein product *neurofibromin*. This protein was localized to the cytoplasm by differential centrifugation, glycerol gradients, and indirect immunofluorescence.[147,150] The difference between the predicted (327 kDa) and the observed (250 kDa) molecular weights results from anomalous migration in SDS-PAGE, not from posttranslational modifications (DH Gutmann, unpublished results). Expression of the full-length cDNA in insect cells produces a protein that migrates at 250 kDa.[153] Similarly, antibodies directed against both N- and C-terminal epitopes all recognize the same 250-kDa protein.[154]

The tissue distribution of neurofibromin is somewhat controversial in that the mRNA appears to be present at some level in all tissues.[1] Initial examination of whole-cell homogenates from mouse and rat tissues suggested that neurofibromin also was ubiquitously expressed.[149] Subsequent analysis by western blotting, immunoprecipitation, and immunohistochemistry demonstrated that the highest levels of expression are in the brain, spleen, kidney, testis, and thymus[102,148] (DH Gutmann, unpublished data). Immunohistochemical analysis of tissue sections from human and rodent tissues demonstrates prominent nervous system expression of neurofibromin.[102,147,148] Neurofibromin can be detected in the dendritic processes of central nervous system neurons (pyramidal neurons in cortical layers 2 and 5 and cerebellar Purkinje cells), peripheral nervous system neuronal axons, nonmyelinating Schwann cells, oligodendrocytes, and dorsal root ganglia but not astrocytes, microglia, and myelinating Schwann cells.[148,155] Neurofibromin expression is expressed in reactive astrocytes.[156] There does not appear to be abundant expression in adult lung, muscle, intestine, heart, or skin.

The expression of neurofibromin during embryogenesis is being studied in the avian and rodent systems. Preliminary results suggest that neurofibromin is expressed in the developing brain and spinal cord.[100,101] This pattern of expression potentially could account for the described learning disabilities previously unattributable to a purely neural crest–derived tissue disorder. Neurofibromin expression appears to rise dramatically after day 10 of mouse development. In the rat, neurofibromin is ubiquitously expressed from days 10 through 16, after which it becomes increased in spinal cord and brain.[157] At this time, neurofibromin can be found in skeletal muscle, skin, lung, adrenal cortex, and cartilage. By postnatal day 6, the distribution of neurofibromin is identical to that seen in adults. These data, combined with the observation that homozygous mouse *NF1* gene knockouts exhibit developmental arrest and death around embryonic day 13, suggest that events occurring during this time interval depend heavily on the proper expression of neurofibromin. Future studies directed at understanding these events will provide insights into the pathogenesis of NF1.

Neurofibromin as a GTPase-Activating Protein

As mentioned earlier, analysis of the amino acid sequence of the *NF1* gene product revealed sequence similarity between a small portion of the gene and a family of GAPs.[4,158–163] These proteins, both in mammals and in yeast, appear to regulate the GTP state of the cellular p21-*ras* proto-oncogene.[164,165] GAP molecules accelerate the hydrolysis of p21-*ras*-GTP to p21-*ras*-GDP, converting the proto-oncogene from the active form to the inactive form.[162,166] Although the effector of p21-*ras* in mammalian cells is unknown, in yeast, p21-*ras* is important in cAMP regulation.[164,167,168] This sequence similarity was supported by functional studies in mammalian cells and yeast, suggesting that the NF1GRD can act as a GAP molecule *in vitro* and *in vivo*.[5–7,169,170,170a] Recent experiments also have demonstrated that the full-length neurofibromin molecule has GAP-like activity.[122,123,153]

It is exciting to postulate that neurofibromin functions as a tumor-suppressor gene product by down-regulating the normal

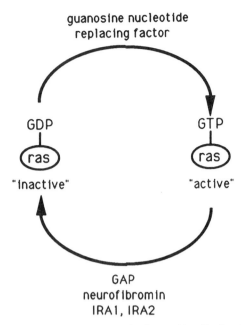

guanosine nucleotide
replacing factor

GDP   GTP
ras   ras
"inactive"   "active"

GAP
neurofibromin
IRA1, IRA2

Fig. 25-11 The p21-*ras* cycle of activation and inactivation by GAP-related proteins. p21-*ras* is inactive in the GDP-bound state and is converted to an active GTP-bound state by guanosine nucleotide-replacing proteins that substitute GTP for GDP. Interaction of GAP-like proteins with p21-*ras* accelerates the conversion of p21-*ras*-GTP to p21-*ras*-GDP by increasing the intrinsic GTPase activity of p21-*ras* and converting p21-*ras* to the inactive GDP-bound form. In resting cells, the majority of p21-*ras* is inactive and in the GDP-bound form.

function of the p21-*ras* proto-oncogene (Fig. 25-11). Previous studies demonstrated that p21-*ras* functions as part of a tyrosine kinase signal transduction pathway involving receptor tyrosine kinases such as epidermal, nerve, and platelet-derived growth factors (EGF, NGF, and PDGF) receptors.[171–173] Support for the involvement of p21-*ras* in such pathways derives from a large number of experiments in a wide variety of signal transduction systems. First, overexpression of the active form of p21-*ras* (v-*ras*) results in neurite extension in a rat pheochromocytoma cell line (PC12) similar to that observed with NGF treatment.[174,175] This effect can be reversed by injecting PC12 cells with antibodies against p21-*ras*.[176] There are conflicting data regarding the existence of a separate p21-*ras*-independent pathway that also culminates in neurite extension.[177] Second, overexpression of activated p21-*ras* can induce morphologic transformation of fibroblast cell lines and unlimited cell proliferation.[178,179] Third, some fibroblast cell lines can be induced to differentiate into adipocytes with overexpression of activated p21-*ras*.[180] Fourth, p21-*ras* is associated with surface immunoglobulin capping as part of a signal transduction (antigen presentation) pathway in B lymphocytes.[181,182]

GAP molecules such as mammalian GAP and the yeast IRA1 and IRA2 proteins may serve to regulate p21-*ras*-mediated growth and differentiation pathways by maintaining p21-*ras* in the inactive GDP-bound state. This model is supported by studies that demonstrate that stimulation of tyrosine kinase receptors such as the EGF and PDGF receptors results in phosphorylation of mammalian GAP on tyrosine residues and inactivation of its GTPase-activating properties.[172,183,184] This inactivation would lead to increased p21-*ras* in the active GTP-bound state and to unregulated cell proliferation in the case of EGF and PDGF. The role of GAP in NGF receptor signal transduction pathways leading to cell differentiation and neurite extension is less well understood. By analogy, it is appealing to suggest that inactivation of neurofibromin as a result of mutation results in higher levels of

p21-*ras*-GTP within affected cells and unlimited cell proliferation, leading to the formation of neurofibromas or neurofibrosarcomas. As was stated previously, examination of three neurofibrosarcomas demonstrated dramatically reduced expression of neurofibromin and elevated p21-*ras*-GTP levels.[122,123] Neurofibromin is phosphorylated on serine and threonine residues in response to EGF and PDGF stimulation but not on tyrosine residues and therefore must involve a pathway distinct from the tyrosine phosphorylation cascade that acts on mammalian GAP.[185,186]

Recent studies have suggested that neurofibromin may suppress cell growth through mechanisms unrelated to *ras* regulation. In NIH3T3 fibroblasts, overexpression of the *NF1* tumor-suppressor gene resulted in a threefold reduction in cell growth without any changes in *ras* activity.[187] Similarly, overexpression of full-length neurofibromin in a human colon carcinoma cell line resulted in reduced tumor growth in nude mice. In these experiments, the growth-suppressor activity of neurofibromin resulted from neurofibromin interfering with *ras* activation of *raf*.[188,189] Finally, *ras* activity can regulate neurofibromin expression.[44] This finding suggests either that neurofibromin is a critical regulator of *ras* in some cells or that neurofibromin may be stimulated by *ras* activation to perform some other function or functions within cells. Further work will be required to distinguish between these nonmutually exclusive possibilities.

Neurofibromin Associates with Cytoplasmic Microtubules

Subcellular localization of neurofibromin demonstrated an association with cytoplasmic microtubules by indirect immunofluorescence and biochemical purification.[150,154,190] Previously described microtubule-associated proteins (MAPs) fall into three classes based on their molecular weights: MAP1 (250 kDa), MAP2 (250 kDa), and tau (35 to 65 kDa).[191–194] Some of these proteins are involved in the stabilization of microtubules through bundling, a process in which the tight association of microtubule filaments is facilitated.[195,196] Other MAP molecules actively promote microtubule movement, and some are involved in microtubule-mediated intracytoplasmic transport.[197] Subpopulations of microtubules are implicated in signal transduction pathways involving neurotransmitters and surface receptors.[198]

Biochemical properties of MAP molecules include GTP and temperature-dependent microtubule association, dissociation from microtubules by ion-exchange chromatography, improved association with taxol treatment, and coimmunoprecipitation with tubulin.[199–204] These properties have been observed with neurofibromin and indicate that there are specific interactions between neurofibromin and microtubules. Studies also have demonstrated that tubulin can partially inhibit the GAP activity of neurofibromin, an effect that is reversed with antitubulin antibodies.[153] In addition, a 20-amino-acid sequence is found in neurofibromin that is shared with two other MAP molecules (MAP2 and tau) and has been reported to be a serine phosphorylation sequence that is important in regulating tau association with microtubules.[150,205] Phosphorylation of tau on that serine residue results in a conformational change and dissociation from the microtubules.

The finding that neurofibromin associates with microtubules does not mean that neurofibromin is a MAP. Intracytoplasmic organelles copurify with microtubules in a manner analogous to MAP molecules, yet these organelles would not be considered MAP molecules because they lack a role in stabilizing or facilitating microtubule-mediated functions. Further examination of the biochemical and physical nature of this association is necessary before neurofibromin can be assigned as a member of the MAP family.

The discovery that neurofibromin is a GAP-like molecule that associates with microtubules suggests several hypotheses to explain its function in cell growth and differentiation (Fig. 25-12). One model, which fits the upstream view of p21-*ras*-GAP interactions, envisions that neurofibromin is regulated by serine/threonine kinases.[206,207] Neurofibromin would be active as a GAP

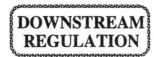

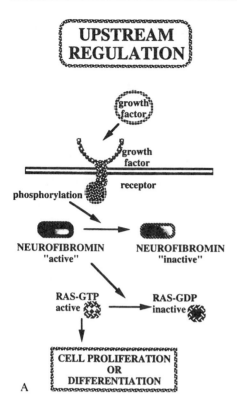

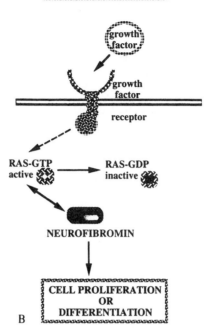

Fig. 25-12 Upstream versus downstream models of p21-*ras*-neurofibromin interactions. *A.* In the upstream model, stimulation of appropriate cells expressing growth factor receptors leads to an inactivation of neurofibromin, perhaps through phosphorylation cascades. Inactivation of neurofibromin releases p21-*ras* from its down-regulation, allowing p21-*ras* to predominate in the active GTP-bound form and signal other intracellular proteins to culminate in cell proliferation or differentiation. *B.* The downstream model on the other hand envisions p21-*ras* as a regulator of neurofibromin and states that it transmits a signal via neurofibromin and p21-*ras* to culminate in cell proliferation or differentiation. For more detail, refer to the text.

while associated with microtubules, keeping p21-*ras* in the inactive form and inhibiting cell division. After phosphorylation, neurofibromin would dissociate from the microtubules, and its GAP activity would be reduced or altered. Alternatively, neurofibromin could be compartmentalized in the microtubule compartment (perhaps performing some other function) until it is required for the control of p21-*ras*. Phosphorylation of neurofibromin on critical serine residues would release it from the microtubules to interact with p21-*ras*. Support for this alternative model is provided by experiments that have failed to demonstrate any alteration of GAP activity after neurofibromin phosphorylation *in vitro*. Similarly, the interaction of neurofibromin with microtubules may actually reduce its GAP activity, as suggested by recent experiments,[153] and its dissociation from the microtubules may allow neurofibromin to associate with and down-regulate p21-*ras*. Of interest is the finding that the same domain of neurofibromin, the GAP-related domain, is the portion of neurofibromin required for microtubule association, suggesting a direct relationship between neurofibromin, p21-*ras* regulation, and microtubule association.[152,153,208] Further studies have demonstrated the involvement of neurofibromin in a B-lymphocyte signal transduction pathway involving microtubules and p21-*ras*. In this system, neurofibromin and p21-*ras* colocalize during immunoglobulin receptor internalization, and neurofibromin is rapidly phosphorylated.[186] A second model, which falls into the category of a downstream hypothesis for p21-*ras*-GAP interaction, is that neurofibromin is induced by the process of p21-*ras*-GTP to p21-*ras*-GDP conversion to transmit a signal through its influence on microtubule organization. Further investigations will be required to refute or support either of these two nonmutually exclusive hypotheses unequivocally.

Neurofibromin Isoforms

Several isoforms of neurofibromin have been identified that arise from alternative splicing.[2,98] The first inserts 21 amino acids within the NF1GRD. This type 2 isoform is expressed in tissues different from those in which type 1 neurofibromin is expressed and may be regulated by brain-specific differentiation events.[209] It

is expressed in many species, including chickens.[210] The type 2 isoform is the predominant mRNA species after week 22 of human fetal development and can be induced in a neuroblastoma cell line by retinoic acid treatment.[209] Similar induction of type 2 neurofibromin expression is observed during Schwann cell differentiations, as reflected by an increase in *NF1* mRNA and neurofibromin levels as well as a switch from type 1 to type 2 *NF1* mRNA in Schwann cells stimulated to differentiate in response to treatments that increase intracellular cAMP.[210,211] In addition, *NF1* isoform expression is altered during mouse embryogenesis, with type 2 *NF1* mRNA expressed before embryonic day 10 and type 1 *NF1* mRNA predominating thereafter.[212] Studies in yeast demonstrate that this isoform also has GAP-like catalytic activity, although moderately reduced from that observed with native type 1 neurofibromin.[210] Whether this isoform can associate with cytoplasmic microtubules is being investigated.

A second, less well-characterized isoform has been identified near the C-terminus of the protein and results from an 18-amino-acid insertion.[2,98] This isoform is detected on the RNA level predominantly in muscle. It is expressed in cardiac muscle (both fetal and adult), skeletal muscle, and some smooth muscle tissues.[213] Little or no expression is found in brain, spleen, or kidney. The expression of an isoform of *NF1* in muscle is intriguing in light of a small number of patients with NF1 and cardiac disease.[214,215] In addition, it was demonstrated recently that neurofibromin expression increases while p21-*ras* activity decreases in myoblasts stimulated to differentiate *in vitro*.[141] Similarly, neurofibromin is transiently expressed in developing myotomes during murine and chick embryonic development.[100,151,157] The relationship between the muscle expression of this isoform and the clinical manifestations of NF1 remains unelucidated.

Recently, an additional isoform of the *NF1* gene was identified that is expressed predominantly in the brain.[216] This alternatively spliced isoform containing exon 9a is enriched in human and rodent cerebral cortex, where its expression correlates with cortical neuron maturation both *in vitro* and *in vivo*.[217] The finding of a brain-specific *NF1* isoform suggests that neurofibromin may play unique roles during central nervous system development.

BIOLOGIC PROPERTIES OF NEUROFIBROMAS

Both plexiform and cutaneous neurofibromas can arise from any nerve throughout the body and at any time, including embryonically. Neurofibromas tend to grow more rapidly during pregnancy and puberty, implying some hormone sensitivity.[218,219] Neurofibromas grow as a mixed population of cells that includes fibroblasts, mast cells, Schwann cells, axons, perineural cells, and endothelial cells.[218–224] The clonal nature of neurofibromas is controversial and has not been resolved conclusively.[225,226]

It has been postulated that the S100+ cells might be primarily responsible for the development of a neurofibroma.[226a] These S100+ cells are believed to be Schwann cells, although they do not always express myelin P0, which is a marker of differentiated Schwann cells. S100+ cells from neurofibroma tumors lack *NF1* mRNA in contrast to the fibroblasts which retain neurofibromin expression. These findings argue that the defective cell type in the neurofibroma is likely the Schwann cell.

Neurofibromas have been found to contain mitogens that stimulate Schwann cell and fibroblast proliferation.[226b,227,228] One study using purified Schwann cells from neurofibromas demonstrated that these NF1 Schwann cells promoted angiogenesis and could invade chick chorioallantoic membranes.[229] These results suggest that neurofibroma Schwann cells are intrinsically different from normal Schwann cells. NF1 fibroblasts also have been examined for evidence of abnormal growth characteristics. Although many of these studies have been difficult to reproduce, it has been suggested that NF1 fibroblasts are more sensitive to ionizing radiation and have an increased rate of transformation by Kirsten murine sarcoma viruses.[230–233]

BIOLOGIC PROPERTIES OF ASTROCYTOMAS

Optic pathway gliomas represent the second most common tumor seen in individuals affected with NF1, suggesting that the *NF1* gene might be a critical growth regulator for astrocytes. In resting astrocytes, neurofibromin expression is low; however, in response to several physiological stimuli, expression can be dramatically increased *in vitro* and *in vivo*.[233a,223b] Support for a role of neurofibromin as a growth regulator for astrocytes derives from several studies. First, increased astrogliosis has been observed in brains from patients with NF1.[223c] Second, mice heterozygous for an *Nf1* targeted mutation demonstrate increased astrocyte proliferation *in vitro* and *in vivo*.[223d,223e] Third, increased ras activity is associated with reduced neurofibromin expression and increased astrocyte growth in *Nf1+/−* astrocytes.[223e]

Loss of neurofibromin expression has been demonstrated in NF1-associated astrocytomas by several complementary methods.[223f] Since only a minority of NF1-associated astrocytomas are clinically progressive, it is possible that other genetic changes cooperate with neurofibromin loss to promote tumor progression.[223g] The identification of these genes will have enormous impact on our understanding of these tumors.

Diagnosis and Treatment

Conventional Treatment of NF1 Patients. The treatment of patients affected with NF1 often requires the expertise of many medical and surgical subspecialists coordinated by one physician or a team of physicians familiar with NF1.[234] For this reason, we advocate the establishment of neurofibromatosis clinics staffed by physicians who regularly see NF1 patients and are familiar with the diagnosis, management, and complications of the disorder. Closely affiliated with the clinic should be a diverse collection of other physicians and health care providers with subspecialties in given areas of medicine or surgery. These persons include ophthalmologists, neurologists, plastic surgeons, neurosurgeons, otolaryngologists, psychiatrists, social workers, child psychologists, orthopedic surgeons, dermatologists, and oncologists. The role of an NF clinic is not only to provide coordinated care from a centralized caregiver familiar with NF1 but also to provide up-to-date information to patients and their families about the disease through regular communication via NNFF-sponsored newsletters and scientific symposia.

The approach to a new patient suspected of having NF1 involves careful history taking and examination. Before the clinic appointment, it is helpful for a genetic counselor to contact the patient to review the patient's clinical features and family history. Often this phone call will precipitate further investigation on the part of the patient and family members in an attempt to determine which other family members have features consistent with NF1. A careful exploration of the family may uncover relatives with subtle features of NF1; this is particularly true in light of its variable expressivity. Hospital records, autopsy reports, and surgical pathology reports also should be requested.

Once the patient arrives in the clinic, he or she should be examined thoroughly by one of the NF1 physicians. A careful cutaneous examination is performed to look for palpable neurofibromas, axillary or inguinal freckling, and café-au-lait spots. The café-au-lait spots can be better visualized under a Wood lamp. The number of pigmented lesions and their greatest diameters are recorded. An ophthalmologic examination with attention to measurement of visual acuity is important to rule out symptomatic optic glioma. In individuals beyond the age of 7 to 8, inspection of the iris should reveal Lisch nodules, especially in patients with light-colored irises. If Lisch nodules are not appreciated and diagnostic criteria for NF1 have not been met, referral to an opthalmologist for a slit-lamp evaluation is made. During a general physical examination, attention is focused on the detection of any curvature of the spine, especially in young children. Severe cases are referred to an orthopedic surgeon. In addition, inspection of the long bones of the upper and lower extremities is warranted in young children to exclude bowing and thinning of the cortices of these bones and prevent the formation of pseudarthroses. Suspicious bones are examined by plain x-rays, and affected patients are referred to an orthopedic surgeon knowledgeable about the bracing and management of this problem. In children, height, weight, and head circumference are noted during each visit and are charted to evaluate the child's growth curve. Inspection of the face and fingers is done to look for facial dysmorphisms or dermatoglyphics suggestive of disorders besides NF1. In addition, blood pressure should be measured during each visit. We recommend routine general medical appointments spaced 6 months after each visit to the NF1 clinic to allow for blood pressure determinations twice a year. Any abnormal rise in blood pressure always warrants further investigation for renal artery stenosis or pheochromocytoma. Patients should be questioned about headache (location, frequency, and character) and bowel or bladder difficulties to screen for deep neurofibromatous involvement of splanchnic nerves.

A screening neurologic examination should be performed during each visit, with special attention to visual acuity, visual fields, and funduscopic evaluation. We strongly advocate the limited and directed use of brain imaging studies and do not obtain them unless there is a change in the symptoms or in the neurologic examination. The limited use of brain imaging studies is based on the low yield of these studies in detecting asymptomatic lesions that require treatment as well as the high likelihood of finding a high-intensity lesion on T_2-weighted MRI. These high-intensity lesions are sometimes referred to as UBOs and can be seen in upward of 60 percent of these children. Their clinical significance is uncertain, and their detection often raises unnecessary concern on the part of both the family and the physician.

During the evaluation, attention is also paid to the social history. In children, school performance is a good reflection of overall learning ability. Formal evaluation of IQ by the school district is recommended early (age 3 to 4) to identify children with learning disabilities. Early detection and aggressive intervention appear to be beneficial in NF1 patients. We encourage families to communicate regularly with the school and to obtain physical, speech, and occupational therapy as appropriate.

Patients with NF1 are seen on a yearly basis in the clinic, during which time they are educated about new information regarding the disease; a forum is provided for a discussion of their concerns and questions. In addition, patients are monitored for the development of new complications, and new family members are evaluated for signs of NF1. The removal of neurofibromas that are particularly large or cosmetically distressing or that rub on clothing straps is coordinated with a plastic surgeon. Otherwise, we encourage patients not to have multiple neurofibromas removed solely for cosmetic reasons, since they can grow back in these areas after surgery.

An integral part of the diagnosis and care of NF1 patients involves the genetic counselor. In our clinic, genetic counselors explain in detail the pattern of inheritance of NF1 (autosomal dominant), its penetrance (essentially 100 percent by 5 years of age), and its variable expressivity. Education is provided, and common misconceptions regarding the disease are dispelled. The emotional impact of NF1 on the patient as well as the other family members is addressed. Families are also given information about support group resources. Explanations of the natural history of the disorder, its behavior during puberty and pregnancy, and its unpredictability are explored. Prenatal counseling is provided for the parents and siblings of affected patients. Prenatal testing, when appropriate, is offered to families in which linkage analysis is informative (see below).

Molecular Genetic Approaches to NF1 Patients. With the entire *NF1* gene cloned and the protein identified, it is now theoretically possible to study gene mutations in patients with NF1. The approaches taken to screen for mutations involve a combination of DNA, RNA, and protein analysis. However, given the large size of the gene and the heterogeneity of the mutations, the search for causative mutations is quite labor-intensive. In the years since cloning of the full-length *NF1* gene, only a handful of mutations have been characterized owing to the arduous task of screening 60 exons for DNA alterations. Therefore, routine clinical application of DNA analysis in the diagnosis of NF1 is not yet a reality. In families in which the clinical diagnosis is certain, multiple members are affected, and closely linked polymorphic markers are informative, linkage analysis using closely spaced markers or microsatellite repeat sequences remains the most practical application of DNA diagnostics.[235]

It is possible that mutations in different regions and/or domains of the *NF1* gene will produce different phenotypes, as has been demonstrated for mutations within the dystrophin gene. As was true with the dystrophin gene, in which other related but distinct disorders were caused by mutations within the same gene, it is important to study neurologic disorders with abnormalities similar to those found in NF1 for alterations in the *NF1* gene.

To date, it has not been possible to provide diagnostic information by surveying for alterations at the protein level. No anomalously migrating protein species have been observed, as was noted for Becker muscular dystrophy. It appears that all the mutations described so far result in a lack of neurofibromin expression as opposed to a smaller or larger protein product. Theoretically, an assay capable of distinguishing 100 percent levels from 50 percent levels of neurofibromin could detect most affected individuals (since most mutations would be null at the protein level). This requires a level of reliable quantification that has not been achieved, however.

NF1 remains a clinical diagnosis. Using the diagnostic criteria established in the NIH consensus statement, the diagnosis of NF1 can be made confidently in the vast majority of individuals. For selected individuals desiring prenatal diagnosis, genetic testing and counseling can be provided. In families with two or more affected individuals with NF1, linkage analysis can be performed.

Recently, a commercial test for *NF1* gene mutations was developed that relies on a protein truncation assay.[236] With this technique, RNA from white blood cells is reverse transcribed and converted into overlapping *NF1* cDNA fragments *in vitro*. Neurofibromin proteins from individuals with NF1 that are larger or smaller than the predicted fragment sizes are then used to direct the search for the underlying *NF1* gene mutation. The advantage of this system is the speed with which mutations potentially can be identified. However, it is unclear at this point whether this test will identify a significant portion of *NF1* gene mutations in individuals with NF1 to warrant more widespread use.

The cloning of the *NF1* gene has opened the door to a more complete understanding of NF1 pathobiology with the eventual goal of designing specific, nonsurgical treatments for affected patients. The finding of elevated p21-*ras*-GTP levels in tumors from NF1 patients suggests that drug therapies directed at up-regulating neurofibromin GAP activity or down-regulating p21-*ras* activity may have a beneficial effect on the growth of neurofibromas. A number of groups have been studying the lipid sensitivity of neurofibromin GAP activity *in vitro* and have found that specific lipids preferentially alter neurofibromin GAP activity as opposed to mammalian p120-GAP catalytic activity.[169,237–239] The discovery of a compound capable of up-regulating or replacing neurofibromin may prove to be a useful therapy in the future.

Similarly, drugs that interfere with p21-*ras* activity, such as pharmaceutical agents that block farnesylation, a reaction necessary for p21-*ras* membrane localization, may have therapeutic potential in NF1.[240–242] Farnesylation-blocking agents have been shown to inhibit the mitogenic effects of growth factors and the tumorigenic properties of neuroblastoma cells. More useful therapies may involve drugs that inhibit farnesyl transferase (the addition of farnesyl groups to the p21-*ras* protein) rather than lovastatin and compactin, which are HMG-CoA reductase inhibitors that block farnesyl synthesis. Further study of these and related drugs may uncover useful therapies for NF1 patients.

ACKNOWLEDGMENTS

We thank the members of our neurofibromatosis research group, past and present. We also thank our collaborators, including Drs. C. Wade Clapp, Abhijit Guha, Tyler Jacks, David Louis, Luis Parada, Arie Perry, Nancy Ratner, J. Lynn Rutkowski, Alcino Silva, Margaret Wallace, and Mark Watson. We also thank numerous members of the NF1 research community for providing preprints of manuscripts and are particularly grateful to Dr. Susan Huson for supplying drafts of several chapters on the clinical manifestations of NF1. Nancy North provided expert assistance in the preparation of this manuscript.

REFERENCES

1. Wallace MR, Marchuk DA, Anderson LB, Letcher R, Odeh HM, Saulino AM, Fountain JW, Brereton A, Nicholson J, Mitchell AL, Brownstein BH, Collins FS: Type 1 neurofibromatosis gene: Identification of a large transcript disrupted in three NF1 patients. *Science* **249**:181, 1990.
2. Cawthon RM, Weiss R, Xu G, Viskochil D, Culver M, Stevens J, Robertson M, Dunn D, Gesteland R, O'Connell P, White R: A major segment of the neurofibromatosis type 1 gene: cDNA sequence, genomic structure, and point mutations. *Cell* **62**:193, 1990.
3. Viskochil D, Buchberg AM, Xu G, Cawthon RM, Stevens J, Wolff RK, Culver M, Carey JC, Copeland NG, Jenkins NA, White R, O'Connell P: Deletions and a translocation interrupt a cloned gene at the neurofibromatosis type 1 locus. *Cell* **62**:187, 1990.
4. Xu G, O'Connell P, Viskochil D, Cawthon R, Robertson M, Culver M, Dunn D, Stevens J, Gesteland R, White R, Weiss R: The neurofibromatosis type 1 gene encodes a protein related to GAP. *Cell* **62**:599, 1990.
5. Xu G, Lin B, Tanaka K, Dunn D, Wood D, Gesteland R, White R, Weiss R, Tamanoi F: The catalytic domain of the neurofibromatosis type 1 gene product stimulates ras GTPase and complements ira mutants of *S. cerevisiae*. *Cell* **63**:835, 1990.

6. Martin GA, Viskochil D, Bollag G, McCabe PC, Crosier WJ, Haubruck H, Conroy L, Clark R, O'Connell P, Cawthon RM, Innis MA, McCormick F: The GAP-related domain of the neurofibromatosis type 1 gene product interacts with ras p21. *Cell* **63**:843, 1990.

7. Ballester R, Marchuk DA, Boguski M, Saulino AM, Letcher R, Wigler M, Collins FS: The *NF1* locus encodes a protein functionally related to mammalian GAP and yeast IRA proteins. *Cell* **63**:851, 1990.

8. Huson SM, Hughes RAC: *The Neurofibromatoses: A Pathogenetic and Clinical Overview.* London, Chapman and Hall, 1994.

9. Friedman J, Gutmann DH, MacCollin M, RiccardiVM: Neurofibromatosis: Phenotype, Natural History and Pathogenesis, 3rd ed. Baltimore, Johns Hopkins University Press, 1999.

10. Korf BR, Carey JC: Molecular genetics of neurofibromatosis, in Rubenstein AE, Korf BR (eds): *Neurofibromatosis: A Handbook for Patients, Families, and Health-Care Professionals.* New York, Thieme, 1990, p 178.

11. Crowe FW, Schull WJ, Neel JV: *A Clinical, Pathological and Genetic Study of Multiple Neurofibromatosis.* Springfield, IL, Charles C Thomas, 1956.

12. Trofatter JA, MacCollin MM, Rutter JL, Murrell JR, Duyao MP, Parry DM, Eldridge R, Kley N, Menon AG, Pulaski K, Haase VH, Ambrose CM, Munroe E, Bove C, Haines JL, Martuzza RL, MacDonald ME, Seizinger DR, Short MP, Buckler AJ, Gusella JF: A novel moesin-, ezrin-, radixin gene is a candidate for the neurofibromatosis 2 tumor suppressor. *Cell* **72**:791, 1993.

13. Rouleau GA, Merel P, Lutchman M, Sanson M, Zucman J, Marineau C, Hoang-Zuan K, Demczuk S, Desmaze C, Plougastel B, Pulst SM, Lenoir G, Bijlsma E, Fashold R, Dumanski J, de Jong P, Parry D, Eldridge R, Aurias A, Delattre O, Thomas G: Alteration in a new gene encoding a putative membrane-organizing protein causes neurofibromatosis type 2. *Nature* **363**:515, 1993.

14. Zanca A: Antique illustrations of neurofibromatosis. *Int J Dermatol* **19**:55, 1980.

15. Hecht F: Recognition of neurofibromatosis before von Recklinghausen. *Neurofibromatosis* **2**:180, 1989.

16. Von Recklinghausen FD: *Ueber die multiplen fibrome der Hautund inhre beziehung zu den multiplen neuromen.* Berlin, Hirschwald, 1882.

17. Preiser SA, Davenport CB: Multiple neurofibromatosis (von Recklinghausen disease) and its inheritance. *Am J Med Sci* **156**:507, 1918.

18. Lisch K: Ueber beteiligung der augen, insbesondere das vorkommen von irisknoten bei der neurofibromatose (Recklinghausen). *Augenheilkde* **93**:137, 1937.

19. Lewis RA, Riccardi VM: Von Recklinghausen neurofibromatosis: Incidence of iris hamartomata. *Ophthalmology* **88**:348, 1981.

20. Lubs M-LE, Bauer MS, Formas ME, Djokic B: Lisch nodules in neurofibromatosis type 1. *N Engl J Med* **324**:1264, 1991.

21. Borberg A: Clinical and genetic investigations into tuberous sclerosis and Recklinghausen's neurofibromatosis. *Acta Psychiatr Neurol Suppl* **71**:1, 1951.

22. Sorenson SA, Mulvhill JT, Nielsen A: Long-term follow up of von Recklinghausen neurofibromatosis: Survival and malignant neoplasms. *N Engl J Med* **314**:1010, 1986.

23. Carey JC, Laub JM, Hall BD: Penetrance and variability in neurofibromatosis: A genetic study of 60 families. *Birth Defects* **15(5B)**:271, 1979.

24. Riccardi VM: Von Recklinghausen neurofibromatosis. *N Engl J Med* **305**:1617, 1981.

25. Huson SM, Harper PS, Compston DAS: Von Recklinghausen neurofibromatosis: A clinical and population study in south east Wales. *Brain* **111**:1535, 1988.

26. Huson SM, Compston DAS, Harper PS, Clark P: A genetic study of von Recklinghausen neurofibromatosis in south east Wales: I. Prevalence, fitness, mutation rate, and effect of parental transmission on severity. *J Med Genet* **26**:704, 1989.

27. Huson SM, Compston DAS, Harper PS: A genetic study of von Recklinghausen neurofibromatosis in south east Wales: II. Guidelines for genetic counselling. *J Med Genet* **26**:712, 1989.

28. Sergeyev AS: On the mutation rate of neurofibromatosis. *Hum Genet* **28**:129, 1975.

29. Samuelsson B, Axelsson R: Neurofibromatosis: A clinical and genetic study of 96 cases in Gothenburg, Sweden. *Acta Dermatol Venereol Suppl (Stockh)* **95**:67, 1981.

30. NIH Consensus Development Conference: Neurofibromatosis statement. *Arch Neurol* **45**:575, 1988.

31. Gutmann DH, Aylsworth A, Carey JC, Korf B, Marks J Pyertiz RE, Rubunstein A, Viskochil D: The diagnostic evaluation and multidisciplinary management of neurofibromatosis 1 and neurofibromatosis 2. *JAMA* **278**:51, 1997.

32. Burwell RG, James NJ, Johnston DI: Café au lait spots in school children. *Arch Dis Child* **57**:631, 1982.

33. Benedict PH, Szabo G, Fitzpatrick TB, Sinesi SJ: Melanotic macules in Albright syndrome and in neurofibromatosis. *JAMA* **205**:72, 1968.

34. Lott IT, Richardson EP Jr: Neuropathological findings and the biology of neurofibromatosis. *Adv Neurol* **28**:23, 1981.

35. Crowe FW: Axillary freckling as a diagnostic aid in neurofibromatosis. *Ann Intern Med* **61**:1142, 1964.

36. Riccardi VM, Eichner JE: *Neurofibromatosis: Phenotype, Natural History, and Pathogenesis.* Baltimore, Johns Hopkins University Press, 1986.

36a. Waggoner DJ, Towbin J, Gottesman G, Gutmann DH: A clinic-based study of plexiform neurofibromas in neurofibromatosis 1. *Am J Med Genetics* **92**:132, 2000.

37. Horwich A, Riccardi VM, Francke V: Brief clinical report: Aqueductal stenosis leading to hydrocephalus, an unusual manifestation of neurofibromatosis. *Am J Med Genet* **14**:577, 1983.

38. Kayes LM, Riccardi VM, Burke W, Bennett RL, Stephens K: Large *de novo* DNA deletion in a patient with sporadic neurofibromatosis, mental retardation and dysmorphism. *J Med Genet* **29**:686, 1992.

39. North K, Joy P, Yuille D, Cocks N, Mobbs E, Hutchiins P, McHugh K, de Silva M: Specific learning disability in children with neurofibromatosis type 1: Significance of MRI abnormalities. *Neurology* **44**:878, 1994.

40. North KK, Riccardi V, Samango-Sprouse C, Ferner R, Moore B, Leguis E, Ratner N, Denckla MG: Cognitive function and academic performance in neurofibromatosis 1: Consensus statement from the NF1 Cognitive Disorders Task Force. *Neurology* **48**:1121, 1997.

41. Moore BD, Slopis JM, Schomer D, Jackson EF, Levy BM: Neuropsychological significance of areas of high signal intensity on brain MRIs of children with neurofibromatosis. *Neurology* **46**:1660, 1996.

42. DiPaolo DP, Zimmerman RA, Rorke LB, Zackai EH, Bilaniuk LT, Yachnis AT: Neurofibromatosis type 1: Pathologic substrate of high signal intensity foci in the brain. *Radiology* **195**:721, 1995.

43. Giordano MJ, Mahadeo DK, He YY, Geist RT, Hsu C, Gutmann DH: Increased expression of the neurofibromatosis 1 (NF1) gene product, neurofibromin, in astrocytes in response to cerebral ischemia. *J Neurosci Res* **43**:246, 1996.

44. Gutmann DH, Giordano MJ, Mahadeo DK, Lau N, Silbergeld D, Guha A: Increased neurofibromatosis 1 gene expression in astrocytic tumors: Positive regulation by p21-*ras*. *Oncogene* **12**:2121, 1996.

45. Brasfield RD, Das Gupta TK: Von Recklinghausen's disease: A clinicopathological study. *Ann Surg* **175**:86, 1972.

46. Hope DG, Mulvhill JJ: Malignancy in neurofibromatosis. *Adv Neurol* **29**:33, 1981.

46a. King AA, DeBaun MR, Riccardi VM, Gutmann DH: Malignant peripheral nerve sheath tumors in neurofibromatosis 1. *Am J Med Genetics* **93**:388, 2000.

47. Thomas JE, Piepgras DG, Scheithauer BW, Onofrio BM, Shives TC: Neurogenic tumors of the sciatic nerve: A clinicopathologic study of 35 cases. *Mayo Clin Proc* **58**:640, 1983.

48. Lewis RA, Gerson LP, Axelsson KA, Riccardi VM, Whitford RP: Von Recklinghausen neurofibromatosis: II. Incidence of optic gliomata. *Ophthalmology* **91**:929, 1984.

49. Listernick R, Charrow J, Greewald MJ, Esterly NA: Optic gliomas in children with neurofibromatosis type 1. *J Pediatr* **114**:788, 1989.

50. Listernick R, Louis DN, Packer PJ, Gutmann DH: Optic pathway gliomas in children with neurofibromatosis 1: Consensus statement from the NF1 Optic Pathway Glioma Taskforce. *Ann Neurol* **41**:143, 1997.

51. Duffner PK, Cohen ME, Seidel FG, Shucard DW: The significance of MRI abnormalities in children with neurofibromatosis. *Neurology* **39**:373, 1989.

52. Holt JF: Neurofibromatosis in children. *AJR* **130**:615, 1978.

53. Daniels SR, Loggie JM, McEnery PT, Towbin RB: Clinical spectrum of intrinsic renovascular hypertension in children. *Pediatrics* **80**:698, 1993.

54. Hochberg FH, Dasilva AB, Galdabini J, Richardson EP Jr: Gastrointestinal involvement in von Recklinghausen's neurofibromatosis. *Neurology* **24**:1144, 1974.

55. Hall JG: Possible maternal and hormonal factors in neurofibromatosis. *Adv Neurol* **29**:125, 1981.

56. Miller M, Hall JG: Possible maternal effect on severity of neurofibromatosis. *Lancet* **2**:1071, 1978.

57. Hall JG: Genomic imprinting: Review and relevance of genetic diseases. *Am J Hum Genet* **46**:857, 1990.

58. Riccardi VM, Wald JS: Discounting an adverse maternal effect on severity of neurofibromatosis. *Pediatrics* **79**:386, 1987.

59. Huson SM, Clark D, Compston DAS, Harper PS: A genetic study of von Recklinghausen's neurofibromatosis in south east Wales: I. Prevalance, fitness, mutation rate and effect of parental transmission on severity. *J Med Genet* **26**:704, 1989.

60. Jadayel D, Fain P, Upadhyaya M, Ponder MA, Huson SM, Carey J, Fryer A, Mathew CGP, Barker DF, Ponder BAJ: Paternal origin of new mutations in von Recklinghausen neurofibromatosis. *Nature* **343**:558, 1990.

61. Stephens K, Kayes L, Riccardi VM, Rising M, Sybert VP, Pagon RA: Preferential mutation of the neurofibromatosis type 1 gene in paternally-derived chromosomes. *Hum Genet* **88**:279, 1992.

62. Riccardi VM, Lewis RA: Penetrance of von Recklinghausen neurofibromatosis: A distinction between predecessors and descendents. *Am J Hum Genet* **42**:284, 1988.

63. Easton DF, Ponder MA, Huson SM, Ponder BAJ: An analysis of variation in expression of neurofibromatosis (NF) type (NF1): Evidence for modifying genes. *Am J Hum Genet* **53**:305, 1993.

64. Eldridge R: Central neurofibromatosis with bilateral acoustic neuroma. *Adv Neurol* **29**:57, 1981.

65. Martuza RL, Eldridge R: Neurofibromatosis 2 (bilateral acoustic neurofibromatosis). *N Engl J Med* **318**:684, 1988.

66. Charles SJ, Moore AT, Yates JRW, Ferguson-Smith MA: Lisch nodules in neurofibromatosis type 2. *Arch Ophthalmol* **107**:1571, 1989.

67. Kaiser-Kupfer MI, Freidlin V, Datiles MB: The association of posterior capsular lens opacity with bilateral acoustic neuromas in patients with neurofibromatosis. *Arch Ophthalmol* **107**:541, 1989.

68. Trattner A, David M, Hodak E, Ben-David E, Sandbank M: Segmental neurofibromatosis. *J Am Acad Dermatol* **23**:866, 1990.

69. Rubenstein AE, Bader JL, Aron AA, Wallace S: Familial transmission of segmental neurofibromatosis. *Neurology* **33(suppl 2)**:76, 1983.

70. Lazaro C, Ravella A, Gaona A, Volpini V, Estivill X: Neurofibromatosis type 1 due to germline mosaicism in a clinically normal father. *N Engl J Med* **33**:1403, 1994.

71. Colman SD, Rasmussen SA, Ho VT, Abernathy CR, Wallace MR: Somatic mosaicism in a patient with neurofibromatosis type 1. *Am J Hum Genet* **58**:484, 1996.

71a. Tinschert S, Naumann I, Stegmann E, Buske A, Kaufmann D, Thiel G, Jenne DE. Segmental neurofibromatosis is caused by somatic mutation of the neurofibromatosis type 1 (NF1) gene. *Eur J Hum Genet* **8**:455, 2000.

72. Allanson JE, Upadhyaya M, Watson GH, Parington M, Mackenzie A, MacLeod A, Safarazi M, Broadhead W, Harper PS: Watson syndrome: Is it a subtype of type 1 NF? *J Med Genet* **28**:752, 1991.

73. Opitz JM, Weaver DD:L The neurofibromatosis-Noonan syndrome. *Am J Med Genet* **21**:477, 1985.

74. Stern HJ, Saal HM, Fain PR, Golgar DE, Rosenbaum KN, Barher DF: Clinical reliability of type 1 neurofibromatosis: Is there a NF-Noonan syndrome? *J Med Genet* **29**:184, 1992.

75. Pulst S-M, Riccardi VM, Fain P, Korenberg JR: Familial spinal neurofibromatosis: Clinical and DNA linkage analysis. *Neurology* **41**:1923, 1991.

76. Collins FS: Positional cloning: Let's not call it reverse anymore. *Nature Genet* **1**:3, 1992.

77. Barker D, Wright E, Nguyen K, Cannon L, Fain P, Goldgar D, Bishop DT, Carey J, Kivlin J, Willard H, Nakamura Y, O'Connell P, Leppert M, White RL, Skolnick M: A genomic search for linkage of neurofibromatosis to RFLPs. *J Med Genet* **24**:536, 1987.

78. Diehl SR, Boehnke M, Erickson RP, Baxter AB, Bruce MA, Lieberman JL, Platt DJ, Ploughman LM, Seiler KA, Sweet AM, Collins FS: Linkage analysis of von Recklinghausen neurofibromatosis to DNA markers on chromosome 17. *Genomics* **1**:361, 1987.

79. Seizinger BR, Rouleau GA, Lane AH, Farmer G, Ozelius LJ, Haines JL, Parry DM, Korf BR, Pericak-Vance MA, Faryniarz AG, Hobbs WJ, Iannazzi JA, Roy JC, Menon A, Bader JL, Spence MA, Chao MV, Mulvihill JJ, Roses AD, Martuza RL, Breakefield XO, Conneally PM, Gusella JF: Linkage analysis in von Recklinghausen neurofibromatosis (NF1) with DNA markers for chromosome 17. *Genomics* **1**:346, 1987.

80. Skolnick MH, Ponder B, Seizinger B: Linkage of NF1 to 12 chromosome 17 markers: A summary of eight concurrent reports. *Genomics* **1**:382, 1987.

81. Seizinger BR, Rouleau GA, Ozelius LJ, Lane AH, Faryniarz AG, Chao MV, Huson S, Korf BR, Parry DM, Pericak-Vance MA, Collins FS, Hobbs WJ, Falcone BG, Iannazzi JA, Roy JC, St. George-Hyslop PH, Tanzi RE, Bothwell MA, Upadhyaya M, Harper P, Goldstein AE, Hoover DL, Bader JL, Spence MA, Mulvihill JJ, Aylsworth AS, Vance JM, Rossenwasser GOD, Gaskell PC, Roses AD, Martuza RL, Breakefield XO, Gusella JF: Genetic linkage of von Recklinghausen neurofibromatosis to the nerve growth factor receptor gene. *Cell* **49**:589, 1987.

82. Darby JK, Feder J, Selby M, Riccardi V, Ferrel R, Siao D, Goslin K, Rutter W, Shooter EM, Cavilli-Sforza LL: A discordant sibship analysis between beta-NGF and neurofibromatosis. *Am J Hum Genet* **37**:52, 1985.

83. Goldgar DE, Green P, Parry DM, Mulvihill JJ: Multipoint linkage analysis in neurofibromatosis type 1: An international collaboration. *Am J Hum Genet* **44**:6, 1989.

84. Fountain JW, Wallace MR, Bruce MA, Seizinger BR, Menon AG, Gusella JF, Michels VV, Schmidt MA, Dewald GW, Collins FS: Physical mapping of a translocation breakpoint in neurofibromatosis. *Science* **244**:1085, 1989.

85. Ledbetter DH, Rich DC, O'Connell P, Leppert M, Carey JC: Precise localization of NF1 to 17q11.2 by balanced translocation. *Am J Hum Genet* **44**:20, 1989.

86. Menon AG, Ledbetter DH, Rich DC, Seizinger BR, Rouleau GA, Michels VV, Schmidt MA, Dewald G, DallaTorre CM, Haines JL, Gusella JF: Characterization of a translocation within the von Recklinghausen neurofibromatosis region of chromosome 17. *Genomics* **5**:245, 1989.

87. O'Connell P, Leach R, Cawthon RM, Culver M, Stevens J, Viskochil D, Fournier REK, Rich DC, Ledbetter DH, White R: Two NF1 translocations map within a 600-kilobase segment of 17q11.2. *Science* **244**:1087, 1989.

88. Schmidt MA, Michels VV, Dewald GW: Cases of neurofibromatosis with rearrangements of chromosome 17 involving band 17q11.2. *Am J Med Genet* **28**:771, 1987.

89. Fountain JW, Wallace MR, Brereton AB, O'Connell P, White RL, Rich DC, Ledbetter DH, Leach RJ, Fournier REK, Menon AG, Gusella JF, Barker D, Stephens K, Collins FS: Physical mapping of the von Recklinghausen neurofibromatosis region on chromosome 17. *Am J Hum Genet* **44**:58, 1989.

90. Buchberg AM, Bedigian HG, Taylor BA, Brownell E, Ihle JN, Nagata S, Jenkins NA, Copeland NG: Localization of *evi-2* to chromosome 11: Linkage to other proto-oncogene and growth factor loci using interspecific backcross mice. *Oncogene Res* **2**:149, 1989.

91. Cawthon RM, Anderson LB, Buchberg AM, Xu G, O'Connell P, Viskochil D, Weiss RB, Wallace MR, Marchuk DA, Culver M, Stevens J, Jenkins NA, Copeland NG, Collins FS, White R: cDNA sequence and genomic structure of *EVI2B*, a gene lying within an intron of the neurofibromatosis type 1 gene. *Genomics* **9**:446, 1991.

92. O'Connell P, Viskochil D, Buchberg AM, Fountain J, Cawthon RM, Culver M, Stevens J, Rich DC, Ledbetter DH, Wallace M, Carey JC, Jenkins NA, Copeland NG, Collins FS, White R: The human homolog of murine evi2 lies between two von Recklinghausen neurofibromatosis translocations. *Genomics* **7**:547, 1990.

93. Cawthon RM, O'Connell P, Buchberg AM, Viskochil D, Weiss RB, Culver M, Stevens J, Jenkins NA, Copeland NG, White R: Identification and characterization of transcripts from the neurofibromatosis 1 region: The sequence and genomic structure of *EVI2* and mapping of other transcripts. *Genomics* **7**:555, 1990.

94. Mikol DD, Gulcher JR, Stefansson K: The oligodendrocyte-myelin glycoprotein belongs to a distinct family of proteins and contains the HNK-1 carbohydrate. *J Cell Biol* **110**:471, 1990.

95. Viskochil D, Cawthon R, O'Connell P, Xu G, Stevens J, Culver M, Carey J, White R: The gene encoding the oligodendrocyte-myelin glycoprotein is embedded within the neurofibromatosis type 1 gene. *Mol Cell Biol* **11**:906, 1991.

96. Wallace MR, Anderson LB, Saulino AM, Gregory P, Glover T, Collins FS: A *de novo* insertion mutation causing neurofibromatosis type 1. *Nature* **353**:864, 1991.

97. Li Y, O'Connell P, Breidenbach HH, Cawthon R, Stevens J, Xu G, Neil S, Robertson M, White R, Viskochil D: Genomic organization of the neurofibromatosis 1 gene (NF1). *Genomics* **25**:9, 1995.

98. Marchuk DA, Saulino AM, Tavakkol R, Swaroop M, Wallace MR, Andersen LB, Mitchell AL, Gutmann DH, Boguski M, Collins FS: cDNA cloning of the type 1 neurofibromatosis gene: Complete sequence of the *NF1* gene product. *Genomics* **11**:931, 1991.

99. Buchberg AM, Cleveland LS, Jenkins NA, Copeland NG: Sequence homology shared by neurofibromatosis type 1 gene and IRA1 and IRA2 negative regulators of the *RAS* cyclic AMP pathway. *Nature* **347**:291, 1990.

100. Kavka AL, Chan SW, Hellen K, Yu H, Gutmann DH, Barabld KF: Expression of avian neurofibromatosis (aNF1) message and protein in neural crest cells (unpublished observation).

101. Stocker KM, Baizer L, Coston T, Sherman L, Ciment G: Regulated expression of neurofibromin in migrating neural crest cells of avian embryos. *J Neurobiol* **27**:535, 1995.

102. Nakamura T, Nemotto T, Arai M, Kasuga T, Gutmann DH, Collins FS, Ishikawa T: Specific expression of the neurofibromatosis type 1 (NF1) gene in hamster Schwann cell. *Am J Pathol* **144**:549, 1994.

103. Bird AP: CpG-rich islands and the function of DNA methylation. *Nature* **321**:209, 1986.

104. Legius E, Marchuk DA, Hall BK, Andersen LB, Wallace MR, Collins FS, Glover TW: NF1-related locus on chromosome 15. *Genomics* **13**:1316, 1993.

105. Marchuk DA, Tavakkol R, Wallace MR, Brownstein BH, Taillon-Miller P, Fong C-T, Legius E, Andersen LB, Glover TW, Collins FS: A yeast artificial chromosome contig encompassing the type 1 neurofibromatosis gene. *Genomics* **13**:372, 1992.

106. Upadhyaya M, Cheryson A, Broadhead W, Fryer A, Shaw DJ, Huson S, Wallace MR, Andersen LB, Marchuk DA, Viskochil D, Black D, O'Connell P, Collins FS, Harper PS: A 90 kb DNA deletion associated with neurofibromatosis type 1. *J Med Genet* **27**:738, 1990.

107. Li Y, Bollag G, Clark R, Stevens J, Conroy L, Fults D, Ward K, Friedman E, Samowitz W, Robertson M, Bradley P, McCormick F, White R, Cawthon R: Somatic mutations in the neurofibromatosis 1 gene in human tumors. *Cell* **69**:275, 1993.

108. Upadhyaya M: Analysis of mutations at the neurofibromatosis 1 (NF1) locus. *Hum Mol Genet* **1**:735, 1992.

109. Marshall CJ: Tumor suppressor genes. *Cell* **64**:313, 1991.

110. Sager R: Tumor suppressor genes: The puzzle and the promise. *Science* **246**:1406, 1989.

111. Weinberg RA: Tumor suppressor genes. *Science* **254**:1138, 1991.

112. Stanbridge EJ: Human tumor suppressor genes. *Annu Rev Genet* **24**:615, 1990.

113. Knudson AG: Mutation and cancer: Statistical study of retinoblastoma. *Proc Natl Acad Sci USA* **68**:820, 1971.

114. Knudson AG: Hereditary cancer, oncogenes, and antioncogenes. *Cancer Res* **45**:1437, 1985.

115. Menon AG, Anderson KM, Riccardi VM, Chung RY, Whaley JM, Yandell DW, Farmer GE, Freiman RM, Lee JK, Li FP, Barker DF, Ledbetter DH, Kleider A, Martuza RL, Gusella JF, Seizinger BR: Chromosome 17p deletions and *p53* gene mutation associated with the formation of malignant neurofibrosarcomas in von Recklinghausen neurofibromatosis. *Proc Natl Acad Sci USA* **87**:5435, 1990.

116. Legius E, Marchuk DA, Collins FS, Glover TW: Somatic depletion of neurofibromatosis type 1 gene in a neurofibrosarcoma supports a tumor suppressor gene hypothesis. *Nature Genet* **3**:122, 1993.

117. Glover TW, Stein CK, Legius E, Andersen LB, Brereton A, Johnson S: Molecular and cytogenetic analysis of tumors in von Recklinghausen neurofibromatosis. *Gene Chrom Cancer* **3**:62, 1991.

118. Seizinger BR: NF1: A prevalent cause of tumorigenesis in human cancers. *Nature Genet* **3**:97, 1993.

119. Andersen LB, Fountain JW, Gutmann DH, Tarle SA, Glover TW, Dracopoli NC, Housman DE, Collins FS: Mutations in the neurofibromatosis 1 gene in sporadic malignant melanomas. *Nature Genet* **3**:118, 1993.

120. Johnson MR, Look AT, DeClue JE, Valentine MB, Lowy DR: Inactivation of the NF1 gene in human melanoma and neuroblastoma cell lines without impaired regulation of GTP-ras. *Proc Natl Acad Sci USA* **90**:5539, 1993.

121. The I, Murthy AE, Hannigan GE, Jacoby LB, Menon AG, Gusella JF, Bernards A: Neurofibromatosis type 1 gene mutations in neuroblastoma. *Nature Genet* **3**:62, 1993.

122. DeClue JE, Papageorge AG, Fletcher J, Diehl SR, Ratner N, Vass WC, Lowy DR: Abnormal regulation of mammalian p21*ras* contributes to malignant tumor growth in von Recklinghausen (type 1) neurofibromatosis. *Cell* **69**:265, 1992.

123. Basu TN, Gutmann DH, Fletcher JA, Glover TW, Collins FS, Downward J: Aberrant regulation of *ras* proteins in tumor cells from type 1 neurofibromatosis patients. *Nature* **356**:713, 1992.

124. Xu W, Mulligan LM, Ponder MA, Liu L, Smith BA, Mathew CGP, Ponder BAJ: Loss of NF1 alleles in phaeochromocytomas from patients with type 1 neurofibromatosis. *Gene Chrom Cancer* **4**:337, 1992.

125. Gutmann DH, Cole JL, Stone WJ, Ponder BAJ, Collins FS: Loss of neurofibromin in adrenal gland tumors from patients with neurofibromatosis type 1. *Gene Chrom Cancer* **10**:55-58, 1994.

126. Colman SD, Williams CA, Wallace MR: Benign neurofibromas in type 1 neurofibromatosis (NF1) show somatic deletions of the *NF1* gene. *Nature Genet* **11**:90, 1995.

127. Kim HA, Rosenbaum T, Marchionni MA, Ratner N, DeClue JE: Schwann cells from neurofibromin-deficient mice exhibit activation of p21-*ras,* inhibition of cell proliferation and morphological changes. *Oncogene* **11**:324, 1995.

128. Kim HA, Ling B, Ratner N: NF1-deficient mouse Schwann cells are angiogenic and invasive and can be induced to hyperproliferate: Reversion of some phenotypes by an inhibitor of farsenyl protein transferase. *Mol Cell Biol* **17**:862, 1997.

129. Rosenbaum T, Boissy YL, Kombrinck K, Brannan CI, Jenkins NA, Copeland NG, Ratner NA: Neurofibromin-deficient fibroblasts fail to form perineurium in vitro. *Development* **121**:3583, 1995.

130. Shannon KM, O'Connell P, Martin GA, Paderanga D, Olson K, Kinndorf P, McCormick F: Loss of normal *NF1* allele from the bone marrow of children with type 1 neurofibromatosis and malignant myeloid disorders. *New Engl J Med* **330**:597, 1994.

131. Largaespada DA, Brannan CI, Jenkins NA, Copeland NG: NF1 deficiency causes ras-mediated granulocyte/macrophage colony stimulating factor hypersensitivity and chronic myeloid leukemia. *Nature Genet* **12**:137, 1996.

132. Bollag G, Clapp DW, Shih S, Adler F, Zhang YY, Thompson P, Lange BJ, Freedman MH, McCormick F, Jacks T, Shannon K: Loss of *NF1* results in activation of the *Ras* signaling pathway and leads to abberant growth in haematopoietic cells. *Nature Genet* **12**:144, 1996.

133. Yan N, Ricca C, Fletcher J, Glover T, Seizinger BR, Manne V: Farnesyltransferase inhibitors block the neurofibromatosis type 1 (NF1) malignant phenotype. *Cancer Res* **55**:3569, 1995.

133a. Guha A, Lau N, Huvar I, Gutmann DH, Provias J, Pawson T, Boss G: Ras-GTP levels are elevated in human NF1 peripheral nerve tumors. *Oncogene* **12**:507, 1996.

133b. Sherman LS, Atit R, Rosenbaum T, Cox AD, Ratner N: Single cell Ras-GTP analysis reveals altered ras activity in a single population of neurofibroma Schwann cells but not fibroblasts. *J Biol Chem* **275**:30740, 2000.

133c. Lau N, Feldkamp MM, Roncari L, Loehr AH, Shannon P, Gutmann DH, Guha A: Loss of neurofibromin is associated with activation of ras/MAPK and PI3K/akt signaling in a neurofibromatosis 1 astrocytoma. *J Neuropath Exp Neurol* **59**:759, 2000.

134. Schmale MC, Hensley GT, Udey LR: Neurofibromatosis in the bicolor damselfish as a model of von Recklinghausen neurofibromatosis. *Ann NY Acad Sci* **486**:386, 1986.

135. Hinrichs SH, Nerenberg M, Reynolds RK, Khoury G, Jay G: A transgenic mouse model for human neurofibromatosis. *Science* **237**:1340, 1987.

136. Nerenberg MI, Minor T, Nagashima K, Takebayashi K, Akai K, Wiley CA, Riccardi VM: Absence of association of HTLV-1 infection with type 1 neurofibromatosis in the United States or Japan. *Neurology* **41**:1687, 1991.

137. Nakamura T, Hara M, Kasuga T: Transplacental induction of peripheral nervous tumor in the Syrian golden hamster by *N*-nitroso-*N*-ethylurea. *Am J Pathol* **135**:251, 1989.

138. Jacks T, Shih TS, Schmitt EM, Bronson RT, Bernards A, Weinberg RA: Tumor predisposition in mice heterozygous for a targeted mutation in *NF1. Nature Genet* **7**:353, 1994.

139. Brannan CI, Perkins AS, Vogel KS, Ratner N, Nordlund ML, Reid SW, Buchberg AM, Jenkins NA, Parada LF, Copeland NG: Targeted disruption of the neurofibromatosis type-1 gene leads to developmental abnormalities in heart and various neural crest-derived tissues. *Gene Dev* **8**:1019, 1994.

140. Gutmann DH, Andersen LB, Cole JL, Swaroop M, Collins FS: An alternatively spliced mRNA in the carboxy terminus of the neurofibromatosis type 1 (NF1) gene is expressed in muscle. *Hum Mol Genet* **2**:989, 1993.

141. Gutmann DH, Cole JL, Collins FS: Modulation of neurofibromatosis type 1 (NF1) gene expression during in vitro myoblast differentiation. *J Neurosci Res* **37**:398, 1994.

142. Vogel KS, Brannan CI, Jenkins NA, Copeland NG, Parada LF: Loss of neurofibromin results in neurotrophin-independent survival of embryonic sensory and sympathetic neurons. *Cell* **82**:733, 1995.

143. Vogel KS, Parada LF: Sympathetic neuron survival and proliferation are prolonged by loss of p53 and neurofibromin. *Mol Cell Neurosci* **11**:19, 1998.

144. Silva AJ, Frankland PW, Marowitz Z, Friedman E, Lazlo G, Cioffi D, Jacks T, Bourtchladze R: A mouse model for the learning and memory deficits associated with neurofibromatosis type 1. *Nature Genet* **15**:281, 1997.

144a. Cichowski K, Shih TS, Schmitt E, Santiago S, Reilly K, McLaughlin ME, Bronson RT, Jacks T: Mouse models of tumor development in neurofibromatosis type 1. *Science* **286**:2172, 1999.

144b. Vogel KS, Kleese LJ, Velasco-Miguel S, Meyers K, Rushing EJ, Parada LF: Mouse tumor model for neurofibromatosis type 1. *Science* **286**:2176, 1999.

144c. Reilly KM, Loisel DA, Bronson RT, McLaughlin ME, Jacks T: *Nf1;Trp53* mutant mice develop glioblastoma with evidence of strain-specific effects. *Nature Genetics* **26**:109, 2000.

145. The I, Hannigan GE, Cowley GS, Reginald S, Zhong Y, Gusella JF, Hariharan IK, Bernards A: Rescue of a *Drosophila NF1* mutant phenotype by protein kinase A. *Science* **276**:791, 1997.

146. Guo H-F, The I, Hannan F, Bernards A, Zhong Y: Requirement of *Drosophila NF1* for activation of adenylyl cyclase by PACAP38-like neuropeptides. *Science* **276**:795, 1997.

147. DeClue JE, Cohen BD, Lowy DR: Identification and characterization of the neurofibromatosis type 1 protein product. *Proc Natl Acad Sci USA* **88**:9914, 1991.

148. Daston MM, Scrable H, Nordlund M, Sturbaum AK, Nissen LM, Ratner N: The protein product of the neurofibromatosis type 1 gene is expressed at highest abundance in neurons, Schwann cells, and oligodendrocytes. *Neuron* **8**:415, 1992.

149. Gutmann DH, Wood DL, Collins FS: Identification of the neurofibromatosis type 1 gene product. *Proc Natl Acad Sci USA* **88**:9658, 1991.

150. Hattori S, Ohmi N, Makawa M, Hoshino M, Kawakita M, Nakamura S: Antibody against neurofibromatosis type 1 gene product reacts with a triton-insoluble GTPase activating protein ras p21. *Biochem Biophys Res Commun* **177**:83, 1991.

151. Golubic M, Roudebush M, Dobrowolski S, Wolfman A, Stacey DW: Catalytic properties, tissue, and intracellular distribution of the native neurofibromatosis type 1 protein. *Oncogene* **7**:2151, 1992.

152. Gregory PE, Gutmann DH, Boguski M, Mitchell AM, Parks S, Jacks T, Wood DL, Jove R, Collins FS: The neurofibromatosis type 1 gene product, neurofibromin, associates with microtubules. *Somat Cell Mol Genet* **19**:265, 1993.

153. Bollag G, McCormick F, Clark R: Characterization of full-length neurofibromin: Tubulin inhibits *RAS* GAP activity. *EMBO J* **12**:1923, 1993.

154. Gutmann DH, Collins FS: Recent progress toward understanding the molecular biology of von Recklinghausen neurofibromatosis. *Ann Neurol* **31**:555, 1992.

155. Nordlund M, Gu X, Shipley MT, Ratner N: Neurofibromin is enriched in the endoplasmic reticulum of CNS neurons. *Neuroscience* **13**:1588, 1993.

156. Hewett SJ, Choi DW, Gutmann DH: Expression of the neurofibromatosis 1 (NF1) gene in reactive astrocytes in vitro. *Neuroreport* **6**:1565, 1995.

157. Daston MM, Ratner N: Neurofibromin, a predominantly neuronal GTPase activating protein in the adult, is ubiquitously expressed during development. *Dec Dyn* **19**:216, 1993.

158. Tanaka K, Nakafuku M, Satoh T, Marshall MS, Gibbs JB, Matsumoto K, Kaziro Y, Toh-e A: *S. cerevisiae* genes IRA1 and IRA2 encode proteins that may be functionally equivalent to mammalian ras GTPase activating protein. *Cell* **60**:803, 1990.

159. Tanaka K, Matsumoto K, Toh-e A: IRA1, an inhibitory regulator of the *RAS*-cyclic AMP pathway in *Saccharomyces cerevisiae*. *Mol Cell Biol* **9**:757, 1989.

160. Tanaka K, Nakafuku M, Tamanoi F, Kaziro Y, Matsumoto K, Toh-e A: *IRA2*, a second gene of *Saccharomyces cerevisiae* that encodes a protein with a domain homologous to mammalian *ras* GTPase-activating protein. *Mol Cell Biol* **10**:4303, 1990.

161. Tanaka K, Lin BK, Wood DR, Tamanoi F: *IRA2*, an upstream negative regulator of *RAS* in yeast, is a *RAS* GTPase-activating protein. *Proc Natl Acad Sci USA* **88**:468, 1991.

162. Trahey M, Wong G, Halenbeck R, Rubinfeld B, Martin GA, Ladner M, Long CM, Crosier WJ, Watt K, Koths K, McCormick F: Molecular cloning of two types of GAP complementary DNA from human placenta. *Science* **242**:1697, 1988.

163. Wang Y, Boguski M, Riggs M, Rodgers L, Wigler M: *Sar1*, a gene from *Schizosaccharomyces pombe* encoding a GAP-like protein that regulates *ras1*. *Cell Regul* **2**:253, 1992.

164. Wigler MH: GAPs is understanding *ras*. *Nature* **346**:696, 1990.

165. Marshall CJ: How does p21 *ras* transform cells? *Trends Genet* **7**:91, 1991.

166. Adari H, Lowy DR, Willumsen BM, Der CJ, McCormick F: Guanosine triphosphatase activating protein (GAP) interacts with the p21 *ras* effector binding domain. *Science* **240**:518, 1988.

167. Mitts MR, Bradshaw-Rouse J, Heideman W: Interactions between adenylate cyclase and the yeast GTPase-activating protein IRA1. *Mol Cell Biol* **11**:4591, 1991.

168. Broach JR: *RAS* genes in *Saccharomyces cerevisiae:* Signal transduction in search of a pathway. *Trends Genet* **7**:28, 1991.

169. Golubic M, Tanaka K, Dobrowolski S, Wood D, Tsai MH, Marshall M, Tamanoi F, Stacey DW: The GTPase stimulatory activity of the neurofibromatosis type 1 and yeast IRA2 proteins are inhibited by arachidonic acid. *EMBO J* **10**:2897, 1991.

170. Weismuller L, Wittinghofer A: Expression of the GTPase activating domain of the neurofibromatosis type 1 (NF1) gene in *Escherichia coli* and the role of the conserved lysine residue. *J Biol Chem* **267**:10207, 1992.

170a. Hiatt KK, Ingram DA, Zhang Y, Bollag G, Clapp CW: Neurofibromin GAP related domains (GRDs) restore normal growth in *Nf1* −/− cells. *J Biol Chem* **276**:7240, 2001.

171. Kamata T, Feramisco JR: Epidermal growth factor stimulates guanine nucleotide binding activity and phosphorylation of ras oncogene proteins. *Nature* **310**:147, 1984.

172. Moran MF, Polakis P, McCormick F, Pawson T, Ellis C: Protein-tyrosine kinases regulate the phosphorylation, protein interactions, subcellular distribution, and activity of p21*ras* GTPase-activating protein. *Mol Cell Biol* **11**:1804, 1991.

173. Satoh T, Endo M, Nakafuku M, Akiyama T, Yamamoto T, Kaziro Y: Accumulation of p21 *ras*-GTP in response to stimulation with epidermal growth factor and oncogene products with tyrosine kinase activity. *Proc Natl Acad Sci USA* **87**:7926, 1990.

174. Bar-Sagi D, Feramisco JR: Microinjection of the *ras* oncogene protein into PC12 cells induces morphological differentiation. *Cell* **42**:841, 1985.

175. Noda M, Ko M, Ogura A, Liu D-G, Amano T, Takano T, Ikawa Y: Sarcoma viruses carrying *ras* oncogenes induce differentiation-associated properties in a neuronal cell line. *Nature* **318**:73, 1985.

176. Hagag N, Halegoua S, Viola M: Inhibition of growth factor-induced differentiation of PC12 cells by microinjection of antibody to *ras* p21. *Nature* **319**:680, 1986.

177. Zhang K, Papageorge AG, Lowy DR: Mechanistic aspect of signalling through *ras* in NIH3T3 cells. *Science* **257**:671, 1992.

178. Feramisco JR, Clark R, Wong G, Arnheim N, Milley R, McCormick F: Transient reversion of *ras* oncogene-induced cell transformation by antibodies specific for amino acid 12 of *ras* protein. *Nature* **314**:639, 1985.

179. Feramisco JR, Gross M, Kamata T, Rosenberg M, Sweet RW: Microinjection of the oncogene form of the human H-*ras* (T-24) protein results in rapid proliferation of quiecent cells. *Cell* **38**:109, 1984.

180. Benito M, Porras A, Nebreda AR, Santos E: Differentiation of 3T3-L1 fibroblasts to adipocytes induces by transfection of *ras* oncogenes. *Science* **253**:565, 1991.

181. Graziadei L, Raibowol K, Bar-Sagi D: Co-capping of *ras* proteins with surface immunoglobulins in B lymphocytes. *Nature* **347**:396, 1990.

182. Kaplan S, Bar-Sagi D: Association of p21 *ras* with cellular polypeptides. *J Biol Chem* **266**:18934, 1991.

183. Downward J, Graves JD, Warne PH, Rayter S, Cantrell DA: Stimulation of p21*ras* upon T-cell activation. *Nature* **346**:719, 1990.

184. Ellis C, Moran M, McCormick F, Pawson T: Phosphorylation of GAP and GAP-associated proteins by transforming and mitogenic tyrosine kinases. *Nature* **343**:377, 1990.

185. Gutmann DH, Basu TN, Gregory PE, Wood DL, Downward J, Collins FS: The role of the neurofibromatosis type 1 (NF1) gene product in growth factor-mediated signal transduction. *Neurology* **42**:A183, 1992.

186. Boyer M, Gutmann DH, Collins F, Bar-Sagi D: Co-capping of neurofibromin, but not GAP, with surface immunoglobulins in B lymphocytes. *Oncogene* **9**:349, 1994.

187. Johnson MR, DeClue JE, Felzmann S, Vass WC, Xu G, White R, Lowy DR: Neurofibromin can inhibit *ras*-dependent growth by a mechanism independent of its GTPase-accelerating function. *Mol Cell Biol* **14**:641, 1994.

188. Li Y, White R: Suppression of a human colon cancer cell line by introduction of an exogenous *NF1* gene. *Cancer Res* **56**:2872, 1996.

189. Clark GJ, Drugan JK, Terrell RS, Bradham C, Der CJ, Bell RM, Campbell S: Peptides containing a consensus *Ras* binding sequence from Raf-1 and the GTPase activating protein NF1 inhibit *Ras* function. *Proc Natl Acad Sci USA* **93**:1577, 1996.

190. Gutmann DH, Gregory PE, Wood DL, Collins FS: The neurofibromatosis type 1 gene product encodes a signal transduction protein which associates with microtubules. *J Cell Biochem* **16B**:A143, 1992.

191. Cleveland DW: Microtubule mapping. *Cell* **60**:701, 1990.

192. Matus A: Microtubule-associated proteins. *Curr Opin Cell Biol* **2**:10, 1990.

193. Olmsted JB: Microtubule-associated proteins. *Annu Rev Cell Biol* **2**:421, 1986.

194. Wiche G: High-MW microtubule-associated proteins: Properties and functions. *Biochem J* **259**:1, 1989.

195. Obar RA, Collins CA, Hammarback JA, Shpetner HS, Vallee RB: Molecular cloning of the microtubule-associated mechanochemical enzyme dynamin reveals homology with a new family of GTP-binding proteins. *Nature* **347**:256, 1990.

196. Shpetner HS, Vallee RB: Identification of dynamin, a novel mechanochemical enzyme that mediates interactions between microtubules. *Cell* **59**:421, 1989.

197. Van der Bliek AM, Meyerowitz EM: Dynamin-like protein encoded by the *Drosophila* shibire gene associated with vesicular traffic. *Nature* **351**:411, 1991.

198. Jasmin BJ, Changeux J-P, Cartaud J: Compartmentalization of cold-stable and acetylated microtubules in the subsynaptic domain of chick skeletal muscle fibre. *Nature* **344**:673, 1990.

199. Vallee RB: A taxol-dependent procedure for the isolation of microtubules and microtubule-associated proteins (MAPs). *J Cell Biol* **92**:435, 1982.

200. Vallee RB: Reversible assembly purification of microtubules without assembly-promoting agents and further purification of tubulin, microtubule-associated proteins, and MAP fragments. *Methods Enzymol* **134**:89, 1986.

201. Vallee RB: Molecular characterization of high molecular weight microtubule-associated proteins: Some answers, many questions. *Cell Motil Cytoskel* **15**:204, 1990.

202. Vallee RB, Bloom GS, Theurkauf WE: Microtubule-associated proteins: Subunits of the cytomatrix. *Cell Biol* **99**:38, 1984.

203. Vallee RB, Collins CA: Purification of microtubules and microtubule-associated proteins from sea urchin eggs and cultured mammalian cells using taxol, and use of exogenous taxol-stabilized brain microtubules for purifying microtubule-associated proteins. *Methods Enzymol* **134**:116, 1986.

204. Collins CA: Reversible assembly purification of taxol-treated microtubules. *Methods Enzymol* **196**:246, 1991.

205. Steiner B, Mandelkow E-M, Biernat J, Gustke N, Meyer HE, Schmidt B, Mieskes G, Soauling HD, Drechsel D, Kirschner MW, Goedert M, Mandelkow E: Phosphorylation of microtubule-associated protein tau: Identification of the site for calcium-calmodulin dependent kinase and relationship with tau phosphorylation in Alzheimer tangles. *EMBO J* **9**:3539, 1990.

206. Hall A: ras and GAP: Who's controlling whom? *Cell* **61**:921, 1990.

207. McCormick F: *ras* GTPase activating protein: Signal transmitter and signal terminator. *Cell* **56**:5, 1989.

208. Mitchell AL, Gutmann DH, Gregory PE, Cole J, Park S, Jove R, Collins FS: Localization of the domain in the neurofibromatosis type 1 protein (neurofibromin) that interacts with microtubules. *Am J Hum Genet* **43**:A62, 1993.

209. Nishi T, Lee PSY, Oka K, Levin VA, Tanase S, Morino Y, Saya H: Differential expression of two types of the neurofibromatosis type 1 (NF1) gene transcripts related to neuronal differentiation. *Oncogene* **6**:1555, 1991.

210. Anderson LB, Ballester R, Marchuk DA, Chang E, Gutmann DH, Saulino AM, Camonis J, Wigner M, Collins FS: A conserved alternative splice in the von Recklinghausen neurofibromatosis (NF1) gene produces two neurofibromin isoforms, both of which have GTPase activating protein ability. *Mol Cell Biol* **13**:487, 1993.

211. Gutmann DH, Tennekoon GI, Cole JL, Collins FS, Rutkowski JL: Modulation of the neurofibromatosis type 1 gene product, neurofi-

212. Gutmann DH, Cole JL, Collins FS: Expression of the neurofibromatosis type 1 (NF1) gene during mouse embryonic development. *Prog Brain Res* **105**:327, 1995.

213. Gutmann DH, Geist RT, Rose K, Wright DE: Expression of two new protein isoforms of the neurofibromatosis type 1 (NF1) gene product, neurofibromin, in muscle tissues. *Dev Dyn* **202**:302, 1995.

214. Neiman HL, Mena E, Holt JF, Stern AM, Perry BL: Neurofibromatosis and congenital heart disease. *AJR* **122**:146, 1974.

215. Kaufman RL, Hartmann AF, McAlister WH: Congenital heart disease associated with neurofibromatosis. *Birth Defects* **8**:92, 1972.

216. Danglot G, Regnier V, Fauvet D, Vassal G, Kujas M, Bernheim A: Neurofibromatosis 1 (NF1) mRNAs expressed in the central nervous system are differentially spliced in the 59 part of the gene. *Hum Mol Gen* **34**:915, 1995.

217. Geist RT, Gutmann DH: Expression of a developmentally-regulated neuron-specific isoform of the neurofibromatosis 1 (NF1) gene. *Neurosci Lett* **211**:85, 1996.

218. Martuza RL, MacLaughlin DT, Ojemann RG: Specific estradiol binding in schwannomas, meningiomas, and neurofibromas. *Neurosurgery* **9**:665, 1981.

219. Riccardi VM: Growth-promoting factors in neurofibroma crude extracts. *Ann NY Acad Sci* **486**:66, 1986.

220. Peltonen J, Aho H, Rinne UK, Penttinen R: Neurofibromatosis tumor and skin cells in culture. *Acta Neuropathol (Berl)* **61**:275, 1983.

221. Peltonen J, Jaakkola S, Lebwohl M, Renvall S, Risteli L, Virtanen I, Uitto J: Cellular differentiation and expression of matrix genes in type 1 neurofibromatosis. *Lab Invest* **59**:760, 1988.

222. Pintar JE, Sonnenfeld KH, Fisher J, Klein RS, Kreider B: Molecular and immunocytochemical studies of neurofibromas and related cell types. *Ann NY Acad Sci* **486**:96, 1986.

223. Krone W, Jirikowski G, Muhleck O, Kling H, Gall H: Cell culture studies on neurofibromatosis (von Recklinghausen): II. Occurrence of glial cells in primary cultures of peripheral neurofibromas. *Hum Genet* **63**:247, 1983.

224. Krone W, Mao R, Muhleck S, Kling H, Fink T: Cell culture studies on neurofibromatosis (von Recklinghausen): Characterization of cells growing from neurofibromas. *Ann NY Acad Sci* **486**:354, 1986.

225. Fialkow PJ, Sagebiel RW, Gartler SM, Rimoin DL: Multiple cell origin of hereditary neurofibromatosis. *N Engl J Med* **284**:298, 1971.

226. Skuse GR, Kosciolek BA, Rowley PT: The neurofibroma in von Recklinghausen neurofibromatosis has a unicellular origin. *Am J Hum Genet* **49**:600, 1991.

226a. Rutkowski JL, Wu K, Gutmann DH, Boyer P, Legius E: Multiple mechanisms of benign tumor formation in neurofibromatosis type 1. *Human Mol Genetics* **9**:1059, 2000.

226b. Mashour GA, Ratner N, Khan GA, Wang H-L, Martuza RL, Kurtz A: The angiogenic factor midkine is aberrantly expressed in NF1-deficient Schwann cells and is a mitogen for neurofibroma-derived cells. *Oncogene* **20**:97, 2001.

227. Pleasure D, Kreider B, Sobue G, Ross AH, Koprowski H, Sonnenfeld KH, Rubenstein AE: Schwann-like cells cultured from human dermal neurofibromas: Immunohistological identification and response to Schwann cell mitogens. *Ann NY Acad Sci* **486**:227, 1986.

228. Ratner N, Lieberman MA, Riccardi VM, Hong D: Mitogen accumulation in von Recklinghausen neurofibromatosis. *Ann Neurol* **27**:298, 1990.

229. Sheela S, Riccardi VM, Ratner N: Angiogenic and invasive properties of neurofibroma Schwann cells. *J Cell Biol* **111**:645, 1990.

230. Bidot-Lopez P, Frankel JW: Enhanced viral transformation of skin fibroblasts from neurofibromatosis patients. *Ann Clin Lab Sci* **13**:27, 1983.

231. Frankel JW, Bidot P, Kopelovich L: Enhanced sensitivity of skin fibroblasts from neurofibromatosis patients to transformation by the Kirsten murine sarcoma virus. *Ann NY Acad Sci* **486**:403, 1986.

232. Kopelovich L, Rich RF: Enhanced radiotolerance to ionizing radiation is correlated with increased cancer proneness of cultured fibroblasts from precursor states in neurofibromatosis patients. *Cancer Genet Cytogenet* **22**:203, 1986.

233. Woods WG, McKenzie B, Letourneau MA, Byrne TD: Sensitivity of cultured skin fibroblasts from patients with neurofibromatosis to DNA-damaging agents. *Ann NY Acad Sci* **486**:336, 1986.

233a. Giordano MJ, Mahadeo DK, He YY, Geist RT, Hsu C, Gutmann DH: Increased expression of the neurofibromatosis 1 (NF1) gene product, neurofibromin, in astrocytes in response to cerebral ischemia. *J Neuroscience Res* **43**:246, 1996.

bromin, during Schwann cell differentiation. *J Neurosci Res* **36**:216, 1993.

233b. Hewett SJ, Choi DW, Gutmann DH: Increased expression of the neurofibromatosis 1 (NF1) tumor suppressor gene protein, neurofibromin, in reactive astrocytes in vitro. *Neuroreport* **6**:1505, 1995.

233c. Nordlund ML, Rizvi TA, Brannan CI, Ratner N: Neurofibromin expression and astrogliosis in neurofibromatosis (type 1) brains. *J Neuropath Exp Neurol* **54**:588, 1995.

233d. Gutmann DH, Loehr A, Zhang Y, Kim J, Henkemeyer M, Cashen A: Haploinsufficiency for the neurofibromatosis 1 (NF1) tumor suppressor results in increased astrocyte proliferation. *Oncogene* **18**:4450, 1999.

233e. Bajenaru ML, Donahoe J, Corral T, Reilly KM, Brophy S, Pellicer A, Gutmann DH: Neurofibromatosis 1 (NF1) heterozygosity results in a cell-autonomous growth advantage for astrocytes. *Glia* **33**:314, 2001.

233f. Gutmann DH, Donahoe J, Brown T, James CD, Perry A: Loss of neurofibromatosis 1 (NF1) gene expression in NF1-associated pilocytic astrocytomas. *Neuropath Exp Neurobiol* **26**:361, 2000.

233g. Li J, Perry A, James CD, Gutmann DH: Cancer-related gene expression in neurofibromatosis 1 (NF1)-associated pilocytic astrocytomas. *Neurology* **56**:885, 2001.

234. Huson SM: Recent developments in the diagnosis and management of neurofibromatosis. *Arch Dis Child* **64**:745, 1989.

235. Andersen LB, Tarle SA, Marchuk DA, Leguis E, Collins FS: A compound nucleotide repeat in the neurofibromatosis (NF1) gene. *Hum Mol Genet* **2**:1083, 1993.

236. Heim RA, Silvermna LM, Farber RA, Kam-Morgan LNW, Luce MC: Screening for truncated NF1 proteins. *Nature Genet* **8**:218, 1994.

237. Tsai M-H, Yu C-L, Stacey DW: A cytoplasmic protein inhibits the GTPase activity of H-*Ras* in a phospholipid-dependent manner. *Science* **250**:982, 1990.

238. Gibbs JB: *Ras* C-terminal processing enzymes: New drug targets? *Cell* **65**:1, 1991.

239. Bollag G, McCormick F: Differential regulation of *ras*GAP and neurofibromatosis gene product activities. *Nature* **351**:576, 1991.

240. Chen W-J, Andres DA, Goldstein JL, Brown MS: Cloning and expression of a cDNA encoding the alpha subunit of rat p21ras protein farnesyltransferase. *Proc Natl Acad Sci USA* **88**:11368, 1991.

241. Kinsella BT, Erdman RA, Maltese WA: Posttranslational modification of Ha-*ras* p21 by farnesyl versus geranylgeranyl isoprenoids is determined by the COOH-terminal amino acid. *Proc Natl Acad Sci USA* **88**:8934, 1991.

242. Pitts AF, Winters TR, Green SH: Ras isoprenylation is required for ras-induced but not for NGF-induced neuronal differentiation of PC12 cells. *J Cell Biol* **115**:795, 1991.

Neurofibromatosis 2

Mia MacCollin ■ James Gusella

1. **Neurofibromatosis 2 (NF2) is an autosomal dominant disorder that affects approximately 1 in 40,000 individuals. It is characterized by the development of bilateral vestibular schwannomas and other histologically benign intracranial, spinal, and peripheral nerve tumors. The only nontumorous manifestations of NF2 are cataract and retinal hamartoma. NF2 is fully penetrant by age 60 years, and half of all cases represent new mutations.**

2. **Syndromes related to NF2 include sporadic unilateral vestibular schwannoma, mosaic inactivation of the NF2 gene, schwannomatosis, and multiple meningiomas. NF2 is genetically and clinically distinct from von Recklinghausen disease or neurofibromatosis 1.**

3. **Positional cloning identified the gene for NF2 on chromosome 22q. It spans 110 kb with 16 constitutive exons and 1 alternatively spliced exon. The NF2 protein product is a member of the protein 4.1 family of cytoskeleton-associated proteins. These proteins play a critical role in maintaining membrane stability and cell shape by connecting integral membrane proteins to the spectrin–actin lattice of the cytoskeleton.**

4. **A large number of germ-line mutations have been detected in NF2 patients, with the majority predicted to result in gross protein truncation. Detection of somatic alterations in NF2-related tumors has supported the hypothesis that the *NF2* gene acts as a true tumor suppressor in both schwannomas and meningiomas. NF2 also appears to play a role in the development of mesothelioma, although this tumor is not seen in patients with NF2.**

5. **Diagnosis of NF2 is currently dependent on clinical criteria, although genetic diagnosis may soon be feasible. Treatment of NF2-related tumors remains largely surgical. Advances in hearing augmentation, such as auditory brainstem implants, may improve the quality of life for many patients.**

CLINICAL ASPECTS

Historical Notes and Nomenclature

In 1822, J.H. Wishart made a case report of an unfortunate 21-year-old man who was found at autopsy to have multiple dural-based tumors, hydrocephalus, and multiple tumors at the skull base, a classic description of what is now recognized as neurofibromatosis 2 (NF2).[1] Seventy years after Wishart's observations, Fredrich Daniel von Recklinghausen published his famous monograph on neurofibromatosis 1 (NF1),[2] and in several subsequent publications the presence of skin and spinal cord tumors in both NF1 and NF2 blurred the distinctions between the disorders. In 1902, Henneberg and Koch recognized a clinically distinct form of NF, which lacked skin alterations typical of von Recklinghausen disease and included "acoustic neuromas."[3]

They referred to this distinct disorder as "central neurofibromatosis" in contrast to the peripheral features of von Recklinghausen disease. In 1915, Bassoe and Nuzum described a patient with bilateral cerebellopontine angle tumors and other central nervous system tumors.[4] In 1930, a family with 38 members who had bilateral cerebellopontine angle tumors transmitted in an autosomal dominant fashion was reported, emphasizing the genetic nature of this disorder.[5] Several subsequent works confirmed that the form of NF characterized by bilateral cerebellopontine angle tumors is a disorder distinct from the more common or peripheral NF.[6–8] Overlapping clinical features, such as multiple spinal and skin tumors, continue to cause confusion between these two diseases.[9]

In 1987, a Consensus Development Conference was held at the National Institutes of Health (NIH) to clarify the various clinical types of NF, and 4 years later a second NIH conference was held to evaluate the clinical aspects of acoustic neuroma.[10,11] As a result of these efforts, formal diagnostic criteria were proposed that have improved diagnostic certainty and allowed clinical and molecular genetic studies of phenotypically homogenous groups of patients. The conferees recommended the adoption of the term neurofibromatosis type 2 (NF2) instead of central, bilateral vestibular, or bilateral acoustic neurofibromatosis. In addition, the term "vestibular schwannoma" was preferred to the previously used "acoustic neuroma," based on the observation that the tumors originate from the vestibular rather than the acoustic branch of the eighth cranial nerve. Finally, the older term "neurilemmoma" has been replaced by "schwannoma," based on work implicating the Schwann cell as the cell of origin in these tumors.

Incidence of Inherited and Sporadic Disease

NF2 is a rare disorder, and because of the wide variety of specialists who manage these patients and because of frequent misdiagnoses, its prevalence is difficult to ascertain. Antinheimo et al, found the incidence at birth to be 1 in 87, 410[12] while Evans et al. found the incidence at birth to be approximately 1 in 40,000.[13] This makes NF2 an order of magnitude less common than neurofibromatosis type 1 (NF1), which has an incidence of 1 in 3000.[10] Half of all persons with NF2 are sporadic with unaffected parents.[13,14] This may reflect a relatively high mutation rate at the *NF2* locus and low reproductive fitness, especially in severely affected patients. Unilateral vestibular schwannoma, unlike NF2, is a very common disorder, with an incidence of about 1 per 100,000 per year.[11] In two large autopsy series, the incidence of occult vestibular schwannoma was even higher (0.82 to 0.87 percent).[15,16] Less than 5 percent of individuals with unilateral vestibular schwannoma eventually develop bilateral disease and NF2.[11,17] Both unilateral vestibular schwannoma and NF2 show no racial, ethnic, or gender predilection.

Diagnostic Criteria

Diagnostic criteria for both NF1 and NF2 have been proposed by the NIH (Table 26-1).[10] Several workers have suggested expansion of these criteria in the hope that diagnosis may be made earlier in patients with multiple features of the disorder but without bilateral vestibular schwannoma.[18,19] Caution must be used in counseling patients on their reproductive and health risks when they do not

---

A list of standard abbreviations is located immediately preceding the index. Additional abbreviations used in this chapter include: ERM = ezrin, radixin, moesin; BAER = brain stem auditory evoked response; NF = neurofibromatosis; NIH = National Institutes of Health.

Table 26-1 Diagnostic Criteria for NF2

Bilateral eighth-nerve masses seen with appropriate imaging
  techniques
  or
A first-degree relative with NF2 and unilateral eighth nerve mass or
  two of the following:
    Neurofibroma
    Meningioma
    Glioma
    Schwannoma
    Juvenile posterior subcapsular lenticular opacity

SOURCE: Adapted from Mulvihill JJ, Parry DM, Sherman JL, Pikus A, Kaiser-Kupfer MI, Eldridge R: NIH conference: Neurofibromatosis 1 (Recklinghausen disease) and neurofibromatosis 2 (bilateral acoustic neurofibromatosis): An update. *Ann Intern Med* 113:39, 1990.

meet the NIH criteria because the more liberal criteria have not been validated clinically. When the NIH criteria are applied strictly, it is rare to find an overlap between NF1 and NF2 in a single patient. Nearly all individuals with NF2 eventually develop bilateral vestibular schwannoma, and this alone is enough to diagnose the disorder. In the presence of other cardinal features of NF2, such as a positive family history, or other NF2-related tumors, the diagnosis may be considered in an individual with unilateral vestibular schwannoma on the presumption that bilateral tumors will appear in time. Because the appearance of all NF2-related tumors increases with age, the diagnosis should be strongly suspected in a child of an affected individual who has any manifestation, including a skin tumor alone.[20]

Major Clinical Features of NF2

Vestibular Schwannoma. The occurrence of bilateral vestibular schwannoma is a nearly universal feature of individuals with NF2, and so the diagnosis of NF2 should be reconsidered in any individual without a positive family history who does not have these tumors. Vestibular tumors originate within the internal auditory canal, where the eighth nerve lies in close proximity to the facial nerve (Fig. 26-1). Initial symptoms include tinnitus, hearing loss, and balance dysfunction. Significant facial palsy is rare even in large tumors and if present should suggest a facial nerve tumor. Disability is often insidious in onset, although occasionally sudden hearing loss may occur, presumably owing to

vascular compromise by the tumor. Patients often report difficulty in using the telephone in one ear, or unsteadiness when walking at night or on uneven ground. With time, vestibular tumors extend medially into the cerebellopontine angle and, if left untreated, cause compression of the brain stem and hydrocephalus. Schwannomas also may develop on other cranial nerves, with sensory nerves more frequently affected than motor nerves.[7,14]

Meningioma. Approximately half of individuals with NF2 develop meningioma (Fig. 26-2).[14,18] Most of these tumors are intracranial; spinal meningioma is not uncommon, and there is a single report of a cutaneous meningioma.[9] There is no site of predilection for meningioma as there is for schwannoma, although meningioma intermixed with schwannoma is a common and incidental finding when the cerebral pontine angle is explored surgically.[21] Because of the multiplicity and slow growth patterns of these tumors, it is often neither possible nor advisable to remove all meningiomas from an NF2 patient. Therapy should be considered when a tumor causes symptoms resulting from compression or development of edema in the adjacent brain. Special attention is needed for meningiomas in the orbit that may compress the optic nerve and result in visual loss, and meningiomas at the skull base that may cause symptoms of cranial neuropathy, brain stem compression, and hydrocephalus.

Spinal Tumors. Two-thirds or more of NF2 patients develop spinal tumors. This can be one of the most devastating and difficult to manage aspects of this disease (Fig. 26-3).[14,22] The most common spinal tumor is a schwannoma, which often originates within the intravertebral canal on the dorsal root and extends both medially and laterally to form a dumbbell shape. This configuration is identical to that of spinal neurofibromas in NF1, and occasionally may cause diagnostic confusion between the two disorders. Less commonly, patients develop meningiomas of the spinal coverings. Intramedullary tumors, such as astrocytoma and ependymoma, are reported to occur in 5 to 10 percent of all NF2 patients,[14,18] although 33 percent of severely affected individuals who underwent complete spinal imaging had evidence of intramedullary cord tumors.[22] Most individuals with spinal cord tumors have multiple tumors (50 percent in the study of Mautner et al.[22]), and there is no site of predilection for either intra- or extramedullary tumor formation. Although ependymoma in patients without NF2 is optimally treated with complete resection and occasionally with radiotherapy and chemotherapy,[23] it is unclear whether ependymoma in NF2 patients warrants aggressive management.

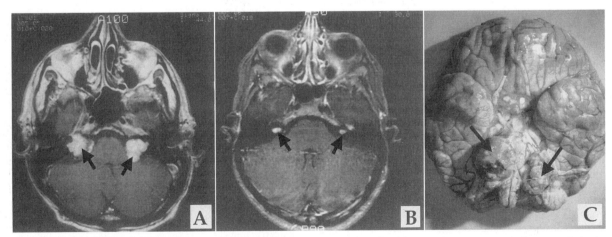

Fig. 26-1. Bilateral vestibular schwannoma. *A,* Axial T1-weighted contrast-enhanced image of the skull base in a 45-year-old man with NF2. Very large multilobulated tumors with extracannicular extension are seen (arrows). *B,* Similar MRI of the patient's presymptomatic adolescent nephew. Small enhancing masses are seen in both internal auditory canals (arrows). *C,* Gross pathologic view of the skull base in an NF2 patient; arrows point to tumors in the cerebellar pontine angles (Photo courtesy of Dr. David Louis, Neuropathology Department, Massachusetts General Hospital.)

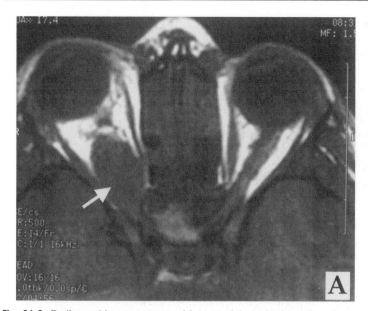

Fig. 26-2. Radiographic appearance of intracranial meningioma in NF2. *A*, Orbital mass in a child with NF2. Orbital tumors in NF2 affected children may be confused with optic glioma; the latter tumor is seen in NF1 but not NF2. T1-weighted MRI. *B*, Multiple discrete lesions (arrows) and diffuse enhancement (arrowheads) suggestive of meningiomatosis in an adult with NF2.

Other Features of NF2. In addition to vestibular schwannoma and spinal schwannoma, NF2 patients are prone to the development of schwannomas along other cranial nerves, in the brachial and lumbar plexuses, and along peripheral nerves. Two-thirds of these patients will develop skin tumors, primarily schwannomas.[14,18,24] Unlike NF1 patients, it is rare for a single patient to develop more than 10 skin tumors.[14,24] There have been several reports of peripheral neuropathy or monomelic atrophy occurring in the context of NF2, although the pathophysiology of this process is unknown.[14,18,25,26]

The ophthalmologic consequences of NF2 are an underrecognized and important aspect of the disease.[27–29] For example, Bouzas et al. studied 54 NF2 patients and found that one-third had decreased visual acuity in one or both eyes, which was directly or indirectly related to the diagnosis.[28] Posterior subcapsular lens opacity progressing to actual cataract is the most common ocular finding (Fig. 26-4). Lens opacities may appear before vestibular schwannoma in at-risk children.[20] Retinal hamartoma and epiretinal membrane are seen in up to one-third of these patients, making indirect ophthalmoscopy mandatory in the evaluation of NF2 patients. Finally, the neuro-ophthalmologic consequences of intracranial and intraorbital tumors may result in decreased visual acuity and diplopia. Because all NF2 patients are also at risk for hearing loss, early recognition of visual impairment from any of these causes is extremely important.

Features not Associated with NF2. Because NF2 is uncommon and because diagnostic confusion continues to exist, it is worth noting several features associated with NF1 that are not increased in the NF2 population. NF2 patients do not have the associated

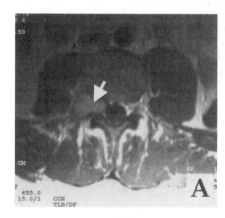

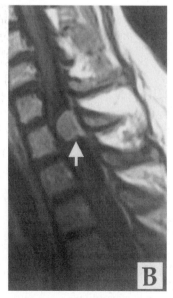

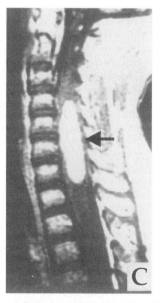

Fig. 26-3. Spinal cord tumors associated with NF2. *A*, Dorsal root schwannoma that has assumed a "dumbbell" configuration (arrow). *B*, Meningioma lying posterior to and displacing the thoracic spinal cord of a child with NF2 (arrow). *C*, Intramedullary cervical spine tumor. Biopsy revealed ependymoma, although the radiographic appearance also is consistent with astrocytoma. T1-weighted contrast enhanced MRIs.

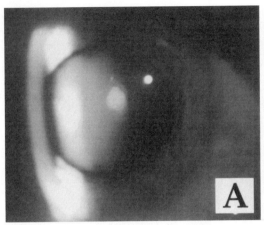
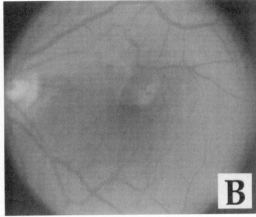

Fig. 26-4. Ocular findings in NF2. *A,* Slit-lamp photograph revealing posterior capsular cataract. *B,* Fundus photograph revealing an epiretinal membrane near the macula. (Courtesy of Dr. Muriel Kaiser, National Eye Institute.)

cognitive problems, including mental retardation and learning disability, that NF1 patients have, nor do they have significant numbers of Lisch nodules. The schwannomas of NF2 rarely, if ever, transform to malignant peripheral nerve sheath tumors, and the overall incidence of malignant tumors in the NF2 population is probably not increased over that in the general population. Approximately half of NF2-affected individuals have small numbers of café-au-lait macules.[14,18] Because 10 percent of the general population also has one or two of these macules, this finding has limited diagnostic value.[30,31] NF2 patients do not have significant numbers of café-au-lait macules (six or more over 15 mm in greatest diameter in postpubertal persons), although their skin is more frequently scrutinized, perhaps leading to this misconception.

Clinical Course

In a large population-based study, the average age of the onset of symptoms among NF2 patients was 21 years, with a range of 2 to 52 years.[18] Similar findings were reported by Parry et al., who reported an average age at onset of symptoms of 20 years and a range of 7 to 70 years.[14] Most patients present with symptoms referable to compression of the eighth cranial nerve, including deafness, tinnitus, and balance dysfunction. Other presenting problems may include facial weakness, visual impairment, and painful skin tumors. Headache and seizure are distinctly uncommon modes of presentation. In the case of deafness, the inability to use a phone in one ear is often an important clue, as it is the only test of unilateral hearing that normally occurs in everyday life. Unfortunately, the study of Parry et al. documented an 8-year lag between age at first symptom and diagnosis, underscoring the need for increased clinical recognition of this disorder.[14] Recognition of NF2 in the pediatric population is an especially critical area, as NF2 is classically thought of as an adult disease. Skin tumors and ocular findings, which often are not prominent in an older patient, may be important clues in the pediatric age range.[20]

The clinical course of NF2 is extremely variable and depends on tumor burden, surgical management, and complications. A small number of NF2 patients develop only vestibular schwannoma with disability primarily related to the seventh and eighth cranial nerves. More commonly, patients exhibit a progressive deterioration with loss of hearing, ambulation, and sight along with chronic pain caused by the tumor burden. Although the spectrum of NF2 among affected individuals is quite wide, there is some intrafamilial homogeneity that may be helpful in the counseling and management of patients with a positive family history. The course of NF2 is most likely minimally affected by gender or pregnancy.[32,33]

The average age at death in the NF2 population has been reported to be 36 years; in the same study, actuarial survival after

diagnosis was 15 years.[18] It is important to realize that several factors may affect this figure in the near future. Early recognition of the disease, both clinically and by presymptomatic diagnosis of at-risk offspring, allows diagnosis of tumors at an earlier and presumably more surgically approachable stage.[34] Improvements in imaging techniques have allowed the detection of smaller tumors and better preoperative assessment of anatomy. Finally, the advances in surgical techniques described below certainly will improve outcome.[35,36]

Related Syndromes

Unilateral Vestibular Schwannoma. Sporadic unilateral vestibular schwannoma is a common tumor in the general population, accounting for 5 to 10 percent of all intracranial tumors and the vast majority of cerebellopontine angle tumors.[37] Less than 5 percent of individuals with vestibular schwannoma develop bilateral tumors, and the probability of doing so is critically dependent on the age at which the tumor is detected (Fig. 26-5).[17] For those under age 25, the development of a unilateral vestibular schwannoma should prompt a careful evaluation for other features of the disease. Conversely, there is little rationale for screening persons 55 and over with unilateral vestibular schwannoma for NF2. The offspring of persons with unilateral vestibular schwannoma alone do not have an increased incidence of either NF2 or unilateral vestibular schwannoma.

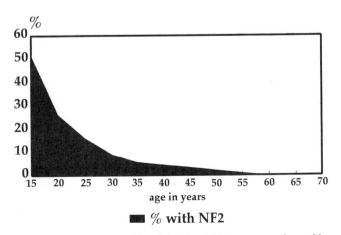

Fig. 26-5. Age-specific risk of having NF2 on presenting with vestibular schwannoma. (From Evans et al.[17] by permission of the author and *The Journal of Laryngology and Otology.*)

Mosaicism in the NF2 Gene. Somatic mosaicism of frameshifting and nonsense mutation has been reported to cause a mild form of sporadic NF2.[38] Other reports of clinically suspected mosaicism have been made in individuals with unilateral vestibular schwannoma and multiple other ipsilateral tumors.[39] A single case of isolated germ-line mosaicism has been reported, resulting in affected sibs carrying identical *NF2* gene mutations with clinically normal parents in whom the mutation could not be detected in lymphoblast DNA.[40] It remains unclear to what extent persons with somatic mosaicism carry genetic risk for bearing affected offspring (i.e., to what extent somatic mosaicism may coexist with germ-line mosaicism).

Recognition of mosaic individuals may be problematic, as they may not have bilateral vestibular schwannomas and genetic analysis in peripheral tissues such as lymphocytes may not reveal the underlying mutation. Mosaicism should be considered in any individual with unilateral vestibular schwannoma and other NF2-related tumors, especially if the tumors are anatomically localized. Molecular genetic analysis of resected tumor material may be a viable alternative to analysis of peripheral tissues for a definitive diagnosis of mosaicism. Germ-line mosaicism for *NF2* mutations appears to be sufficiently rare to make screening of the sibs of an affected individual with normal parents unnecessary.

Schwannomatosis. Schwannomatosis is defined as multiple pathologically proven schwannomas without vestibular schwannoma diagnostic of NF2.[41] Previous terms for this condition have included multiple neurilemmomas, agminated neurilemmomas, multiple schwannomas, and neurilemmomatosis. Schwannomatosis appears to be a clinically distinct entity from NF1 and NF2. Persons with schwannomatosis may develop intracranial, spinal nerve root, or peripheral tumors; like persons with NF2, they do not develop malignancy. In one-third of all reported cases, schwannomatosis patients have had anatomically localized tumors suggestive of segmental disease.[41–43] There are few cases of familial involvement with schwannomatosis; in these rare kindreds autosomal dominant inheritance with highly variable expressivity and incomplete penetrance is seen.[41] Although schwannomatosis appears to be a tumor-suppressor gene syndrome, it is unclear if it is due to an aberration in *NF1*, *NF2*, or an unknown transcript.

Multiple Meningiomas. Although many patients with NF2 develop multiple meningiomas, the appearance of meningiomas rarely predates that of vestibular schwannoma in a single patient. Rare instances of families with multiple meningiomas without vestibular schwannoma segregating as an autosomal dominant trait have been reported.[44] Genetic linkage analysis of one such family showed that the trait segregates separately from the *NF2* gene, implicating a second genetic locus.[45] This result is supported by the data presented below, which implicate a non-NF2 gene in approximately half of all sporadic meningiomas. Multiple meningiomas in a patient without a family history are more commonly due to noncontiguous spread of a single tumor.[46] Presumably, the latter condition carries no genetic risk to offspring. Because sporadic meningioma is classically a tumor of older adults, the finding of a single meningioma in an individual under age 25 years should prompt an evaluation for an underlying genetic condition.[17]

Histopathology

The tumors of NF2 are derived from Schwann cells, meningeal cells, and glial cells, and are histologically benign. Vestibular schwannomas from NF2 patients have several pathologic differences from those that occur sporadically. About 40 percent of vestibular tumors from NF2 patients have a lobular pattern that is uncommon in sporadic tumors.[21] Intermixture of meningioma with vestibular schwannoma in NF2 patients is not uncommon.[21] NF2-associated vestibular schwannomas have been reported to be more invasive of the eighth cranial nerve and to have a higher proportion

of dividing cells.[47,48] Less is known about histologic distinctions between nonvestibular tumors in their sporadic and NF2-associated forms. Some workers have reported a predominance of fibroblastic meningioma, although others have found equal numbers of fibroblastic and meningothelial tumors in NF2 patients.[49] No histologic differences between glial tumors in NF2 and those in sporadic cases have been reported.[49]

GENETIC ASPECTS OF NF2

Historical Aspects

Early studies on the pathogenetic mechanisms underlying NF2 revealed that NF2-related tumors often lost large stretches of chromosome 22.[50–52] This finding not only suggested that the *NF2* gene is on chromosome 22, but also supported the hypothesis that it is a classic tumor suppressor.[53] In conjunction with these initial investigations on tumors, studies were made of a large NF2-affected kindred by the method of linkage analysis.[54] This genetic linkage approach confirmed the position of *NF2* on chromosome 22 and refined its localization to band 22q12. Further work with tumor material and other affected kindreds narrowed the critical region on chromosome 22 to approximately 6 Mb.[55]

In 1992, a single, affected individual was identified, who, along with her affected daughter, carried a 30-kb deletion recognizable with the probe neurofilament heavy chain and the rare cutting enzyme *NotI*. Taking this patient's deleted region as a target, the transcribed sequences within this area were isolated by using the method of exon trapping. Subsequent identification of cDNA using these exons as probes revealed that the predicted protein carried especially high homology to the 4.1 family of cytoskeletal-associated proteins. Because of this homology, the putative protein product has been named *merlin* (for moezin-ezrin-radixin-like protein); alternatively, schwannomin has been suggested to reflect the role of this protein in the prevention of the development of schwannomas.[56]

Clinical Genetics

NF2 shows autosomal-dominant transmission with full penetrance by age 60.[14,18] In two studies, a parent of origin effect on severity was observed, with the mean age in paternally inherited cases being 24 years, and that in maternally inherited cases being 18 years.[6,18] Subsequent work has not confirmed this disparity, which may reflect a difference in the reproductive fitness of severely affected males versus females.[14] There is a marked degree of heterogeneity in NF2, and several authors have divided the disease into clinical subtypes. The mild, or Gardner, subtype is characterized by the onset of symptoms in the third decade or later, few associated brain or spinal tumors, and survival into the sixth decade. The severe, or Wishart, subtype involves onset before age 25, rapid clinical progression, multiple intracranial and spinal tumors, and death in the third or fourth decade. The existence of a third subtype (Lee-Abbott) with variable age at hearing loss, cataract, and early age at death has not been confirmed.[14,18,57] The manifestations and clinical subtype of NF2 usually are similar within members of a family.[14,18,40] All series have shown that half of affected individuals are sporadic with unaffected parents. *De novo* alteration in the *NF2* gene has been documented in several sporadic cases, with most arising on the paternal allele.[40,58,59] In these sporadic cases, mutations arising on the paternal allele resulted in a more severe phenotype then those arising on the maternal allele.[59]

The *NF2* Gene and Protein Product

The *NF2* gene spans 110 kilobases and includes 16 constitutive exons and 1 alternatively spliced exon.[55,56] *NF2* is widely expressed, producing mRNAs in three different size ranges of approximately 7, 4.4, and 2.6 kb.[55,60] Two major alternative forms of the NF2 protein product exist. Isoform 1 is a protein of 595 amino acids produced from exons 1 through 15 and exon 17. The

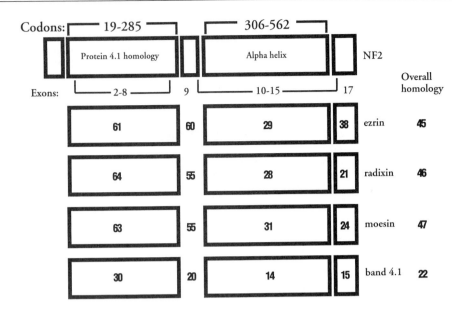

Fig. 26-6. ERM proteins related to NF2. The NF2 protein product is a member of the band 4.1 family of cytoskeletal-associated proteins. This diagram depicts the domain of the NF2 protein, which includes a region of homology in the amino terminal half that defines membership in the protein 4.1 family, an α-helical domain, and a terminus affected by alternative splicing. The percentage amino acid identity with the three most closely related family members ezrin, radixin, and moesin, and with band 4.1 itself is shown within each region. The C-terminus of the ERM proteins contains an actin-binding region not found in the NF2 protein.

presence of the alternatively spliced exon 16 alters the C-terminus of the protein, replacing 16 amino acids with 11 novel residues in isoform 2. Additional alternative splices predicting other minor species have also been described.[61,62] The *NF2* gene is highly conserved through evolution, as the mouse protein is 98 percent identical to human *NF2*, and the mouse *NF2* gene, which maps to chromosome 11 in a region of synteny conservation with 22q, is similarly alternatively spliced.[63,64]

The NF2 protein product is a member of the protein 4.1 family of cytoskeleton-associated proteins (Fig. 26-6). The proteins of this family include protein 4.1 itself, talin, ezrin, radixin, moesin, and several protein tyrosine phosphatases. All family members have a homologous domain of approximately 270 amino acids at the N-terminus.[65] In the NF2 protein and its close relatives, this domain is followed by a long α-helical segment and a charged C-terminal domain. Protein 4.1, the best-studied member of the family, plays a critical role in maintaining membrane stability and cell shape in the erythrocyte by connecting integral membrane proteins, glycophorin, and the anion channel to be spectrin-actin lattice of the cytoskeleton. Protein 4.1 is the only other family member in which disease-causing mutation is known (hereditary elliptocytosis).

The ERM proteins, to which the NF2 protein is most closely related, share 70 to 75 percent amino acid identity with each other and are located in actin-rich surface projections such as microvilli, filopodia, membrane ruffles, lamellipodia in migrating cells, neuronal growth cones, and mitotic cleavage furrows. The NF2 protein is 45 to 46 percent identical to the ERMs with a common structural pattern except for the two different charged C-termini produced by alternative splicing. Both isoforms localize preferentially to the motile regions of cultured cells, such as the leading or ruffling edges, where they colocalize with F-actin. Where it has been tested, the NF2 protein does not colocalize with ezrin or moesin, suggesting a membrane-cytoskeleton linker function that is distinguishable from the ERM proteins.[66] A function of the NF2 protein in the motile regions of the cell suggests that schwannomas and meningiomas may form when the appropriate cell loses the ability to accurately regulate cell movement, shape, or communication, leading to a loss of growth control.

Germ-Line Mutations

Several studies aimed at identifying germ-line mutations in typical NF2 patients have been reported.[38,67–69] In at least two studies, exon scanning was shown to detect mutation in two-thirds of patients.[40,59] Smaller numbers of patients have been reported to have gene deletions.[55,70–72] A wide variety of mutations have been

identified in all *NF2* exons except for exons 16 and 17. The vast majority of the alterations predict truncation of the protein product as a result of the introduction of a stop codon, a frameshift with premature termination, or a splicing alteration, supporting the view that loss of the protein's normal function is crucial to the development of tumors. C to T transitions in CGA codons causing nonsense mutations are an especially common occurrence.[73] Less than 10 percent of detected mutations involve in-frame deletions and missense mutations, which indicates that alteration of particular functional domains can abolish the *NF2* tumor-suppressor activity.[74] No frequent polymorphisms, even in codon wobble positions, have been reported in the *NF2* gene.

A strong effect of the genotype on the resulting phenotype in NF2 is suggested by the clinical observations that intrafamilial homogeneity is marked in NF2. Several studies have supported the hypothesis that the underlying *NF2* gene mutation is predictive of the resulting phenotype when the gross variables of mild versus severe disease is examined.[40,55,56,59,67–69,73,75–77] In these studies, a total of 110 independently occurring nonsense and frameshift mutations produced severe disease in 95 cases studied (86 percent), while splice-site mutation produced severe disease in 49 percent of cases and rare nontruncating changes produced severe disease in only 33 percent of cases. Despite studies in other tumor-suppressor genes that have linked position within the gene to specific manifestations, no effect of the position of the mutation has been determined in NF2.

Several studies that present a more detailed analysis of the effects of genotype on phenotype have been reported.[38,40,67,75] Overall, patients with nonsense or frameshift mutations have earlier ages at onset and diagnosis and greater numbers of tumors then any other group of patients. At the other end of the spectrum, families in whom mutations cannot be identified by exon scanning have late ages of onset and diagnosis and a low frequency of nonvestibular tumors.[40] Such families may harbor larger deletions or insertions not identified by the methodologies used in these studies, mutations in introns and untranslated regulatory elements, or mosaicism not detectable in the tissue analyzed. Also of importance to the clinician is that families with splice-site mutation display far more intrafamilial variability than other families,[77] so that caution should be exercised when giving anticipatory guidance to these families. These studies also point out an irony in current *NF2* screening protocols, because patients with mild phenotypes may be more likely to seek molecular diagnostic services than those with severe manifestations, and are the least likely to have identifiable *NF2* gene changes by current techniques.

Somatic Mutations

A number of studies have looked at somatic mutations in the *NF2* gene in resected tumor tissues from both NF2-affected and NF2-unaffected individuals. Mutations found in tumor material but not in normal tissue from the same individual are essential in confirming that *NF2* behaves like other well-documented tumor-suppressor genes.[53] In a study of 38 sporadic and NF2-derived schwannomas, Jacoby et al. found 25 somatic mutations affecting expression of the *merlin* protein.[78] All 25 mutations involved gross truncation with nonsense, frameshift, or splice-site alteration. Deletion was an especially common mechanism of mutation, with over half the mutations (14 of 25) involving the removal of 1 to 34 base pairs. As would be expected, many of these tumors (16 of 38) also showed loss of polymorphic markers on chromosome 22, indicating large deletions of that chromosome. Similar results have been reported in a follow-up study by the same group and by several other groups.[79–85] No differences have been reported between mutations detected in vestibular and nonvestibular tumors, or between tumors derived from NF2 patients and sporadic tumors. These studies support the hypothesis that the *NF2* gene is the major tumor suppressor for schwannoma.

Analysis of meningiomas, the second most common tumor type in NF2, has revealed slightly different results. Wellenreuther et al., in a comprehensive analysis of 70 sporadic meningiomas, identified 43 mutations in 41 tumors.[86] Similar to the results in schwannoma, only 1 of the 43 involved a nontruncating event. Mutational events were much more common in tumors that had lost heterozygosity for chromosome 22, supporting the hypothesis that *NF2* is the meningioma locus on chromosome 22. These authors found that *NF2* mutations occurred much more frequently in specific pathologic subtypes of meningiomas. These and other studies suggest that *NF2* is a tumor suppressor for meningioma but that another protein or proteins not on chromosome 22 may also fill this role.[83,84,87,88]

Analysis of glial tumors has shown conflicting results. A comprehensive study of 62 sporadic ependymomas revealed loss of heterozygosity of 22q markers in 12 and *NF2* mutation in 6.[89] All tumors carrying *NF2* mutation were WHO grade II and spinal in location, suggesting a different pathogenetic mechanism for this subset of tumors. No mutations have been found in astrocytic tumors, even those with loss of heterozygosity of chromosome 22 markers.[90] Further work is needed to determine if pathologic or anatomic subgroups of astrocytomas exist in which the *NF2* gene is more important as a tumor suppressor.

Loss of heterozygosity has also been observed for chromosome 22q markers in many different types of tumors that are not characteristic of NF2. Screening for mutations that affect the *NF2* gene in such tumors has yielded mixed results. Only a handful of putative mutations of the *NF2* gene have been found in malignant melanoma, breast adenocarcinoma, and colon cancer, and none have been seen in ovarian carcinoma or hepatocellular carcinoma.[91–93] A high rate of *NF2* mutation has been detected in malignant mesothelioma, suggesting that loss of *NF2* may be important in the progression of this aggressive mesodermal tumor type.[94,95] Further work is needed to determine what role *NF2* plays in the proliferation of cells beyond those giving rise to the nervous system tumors of NF2.

DIAGNOSIS AND TREATMENT

Diagnosis of NF2 is based on the NIH clinical criteria (Table 26-1). A careful clinical examination with special attention to a dermatologic evaluation, the neurologic symptomatology, and a slit-lamp examination to evaluate possible retinal or lenticular manifestations are mandatory. Initial radiographic evaluation of a patient known or suspected to have NF2 should include a cranial MRI scan with and without gadolinium enhancement. Small intracanalicular tumors may not be seen on standard 5-mm slice thickness through the posterior fossa. Optimal evaluation includes

3-mm cuts overlapping by 1.5 mm on both axial and coronal post-contrast enhancement views through the internal auditory canals.[35] Large vestibular schwannomas (those greater than 2 cm) and meningiomas may be visualized by computer tomography (CT). In general, however, CT is obscured by bony artifact in the region of the internal auditory canal and skull base and cannot substitute for MRI. Audiologic evaluation including brain stem auditory evoked response (BAER) may rarely reveal a functional deficit in a nerve in which no enhancement is visible. BAER also may be useful in defining the baseline functional impact of an otherwise presymptomatic tumor. Spinal MRI may be helpful in defining asymptomatic tumors; it is mandatory in individuals with unexplained neurologic symptoms or signs.

Increasingly, presymptomatic genetic testing may supplant clinical testing for individuals at risk for NF2.[34,96,97] Because NF2 is a fully penetrant disease and because the age of onset shows homogeneity within families, such testing probably is useful only for the children of an at-risk individual. The age at testing depends on the family's attitude toward presymptomatic surgery and the severity of disease in the family. Genetic testing may be done on the basis of linkage when there is more than one affected family member, or on the basis of mutational analysis of a known affected individual. Caution must be exercised when using a founder to phase chromosomes for linkage because of the high incidence of mosaicism in this disorder.[98] Because no mutation can be detected in at least one-third of individuals with typical NF2, mutational analysis is not useful for confirming or excluding a suspected diagnosis in a proband.

Therapy for vestibular schwannoma remains primarily surgical.[35,36,99,100] Close neurologic monitoring is mandatory for determining the timing of surgical intervention. Small vestibular tumors (less than 1.5 cm) that are completely intracanalicular can often be completely resected with preservation of both hearing and facial function.[35,36] Larger tumors probably are best managed expectantly, with debulking or decompression carried out when brain stem compression, or increasing facial and/or hearing function ensues.[36] Special consideration should be given when considering intervention on a small or large tumor in an only hearing ear. Other cranial and spinal tumors, including meningiomas, other cranial nerve schwannomas, and ependymomas, should be monitored for symptomatology. These tumors are very slow growing, and intervention on a minimally functionally active tumor may produce disability years before it would occur otherwise. Facial nerve reconstruction may be very important for patients who find facial palsy more debilitating than hearing loss.[36,101]

Stereotactic radiosurgery, most commonly with the gamma knife, has been offered as an alternative to surgery in selected patients with vestibular schwannomas.[102–104] Radiation therapy for other NF2-associated tumors should be carefully considered because radiation exposure may induce, accelerate, or transform tumors in a patient with an inactivated tumor-suppressor gene. There is currently no medical therapy available for NF2 patients. Various agents, including quinidine, and antiangiogenesis factors have shown promising results in cell culture and animal models.[105–107] Management of patients with vestibular tumors should include counseling on the often insidious problems with balance they may encounter. Drowning or near-drowning owing to underwater disorientation is an especially important consideration.[6]

Hearing and speech augmentation and preservation play an important role in the management of NF2 patients. All patients and their families should be referred to audiologists to receive training in optimization of hearing and speech production. Teaching may enhance lip-reading skills, and sign language often may be more effectively acquired before the patient loses hearing. Hearing aids may be helpful early in the course of the disease. Rarely, patients who have had a vascular insult to the cochlea, but who are otherwise without nerve damage, may benefit from a cochlear implant.[108] An alternative technology has been developed for placement of a cochlear implant-type electrode proximal to the nerve in the lateral recess of the fourth ventricle.[109,110] Initial results with the auditory brainstem implant or ABI in 24 adult-deafened NF2 patients have been extremely promising.[111]

Resources for Patients with NF2

Diagnosis, evaluation, and treatment of complex patients with NF2 is best done in a neurofibromatosis center that is experienced in the multiple complications and delicate management of this disease.[17,32] Such multidisciplinary clinics are now available in most major medical centers and are accredited by the National Neurofibromatosis Foundation (New York, NY) and Neurofibromatosis, Inc. (Lanthan, MD). Both organizations publish newsletters and maintain a network of local support chapters that are invaluable resources for patient and family education and support.

REFERENCES

1. Wishart JH: Case of tumours in the skull, dura mater, and brain. *Edinburgh Med Surg J* **18**:393, 1822.
2. Crump TT: Translation of case reports in Ueber die multiplen Fibrome der Haut und ihre Beziehung zu den multiplen Neuromen by F.V. Recklinghausen. *Adv Neurol* **29**:259, 1981.
3. Henneberg R, Koch M: Ueber centrale Neurofibromatose und die Geschwulste des Kleinhirnbruckenwinkels (Acusticus-neurome). *Arch Psychiatrie* **36**:251, 1902.
4. Bassoe P, Nuzum F: Report of a case of central and peripheral neurofibromatosis. *J Nerv Ment Dis* **42**:785, 1915.
5. Gardner WJ, Frazier CH: Bilateral acoustic neurofibromas: A clinical study and field survey of a family of five generations with bilateral deafness in thirty-eight members. *Arch Neurol Psychiatr* **23**:266, 1929.
6. Kanter WR, Eldridge R, Fabricant R, Allen JC, Koerber T: Central neurofibromatosis with bilateral acoustic neuroma: Genetic, clinical and biochemical distinctions from peripheral neurofibromatosis. *Neurology* **30**:851, 1980.
7. Martuza RL, Eldridge R: Neurofibromatosis 2 (bilateral acoustic neurofibromatosis). *N Engl J Med* **318**:684, 1988.
8. Friedman JM, Gutmann DH, MacCollin M, Riccardi VM: *Neurofibromatosis: Phenotype, Natural History, and Pathogenesis*, 3rd ed. Baltimore: Johns Hopkins University Press, 1999, pp 299–365.
9. Argenyi ZB, Thieberg MD, Hayes CM, Whitaker DC: Primary cutaneous meningioma associated with von Recklinghausen's disease. *J Cutan Pathol* **21**:549, 1994.
10. Mulvihill JJ, Parry DM, Sherman JL, Pikus A, Kaiser-Kupfer MI, Eldridge R: NIH conference: Neurofibromatosis 1 (Recklinghausen disease) and neurofibromatosis 2 (bilateral acoustic neurofibromatosis): An update. *Ann Intern Med* **113**:39, 1990.
11. Eldridge R, Parry DM: Summary: Vestibular schwannoma (acoustic neuroma): Consensus development conference. *Neurosurgery* **30**:961, 1992.
12. Antinheimo J, Sankila R, Carpen O, Pukkala E, Sainio M, Jaaskelainen J: Population-based analysis of sporadic and type 2 neurofibromatosis-associated meningiomas and schwannomas. *Neurology* **54**:71, 2000.
13. Evans DG, Huson SM, Donnai D, Neary W, Blair V, Teare D, Newton V, Strachan T, Ramsden R, Harris R: A genetic study of type 2 neurofibromatosis in the United Kingdom: I. Prevalence, mutation rate, fitness and confirmation of maternal transmission effect on severity. *J Med Genet* **29**:841, 1992.
14. Parry DM, Eldridge R, Kaiser-Kupfer MI, Bouzas E, Pikus A, Patronas N: Neurofibromatosis 2 (NF2): Clinical characteristics of 63 affected individuals and clinical evidence for heterogeneity. *Am J Med Genet* **52**:450, 1994.
15. Leonard J, Talbot M: Asymptomatic acoustic neurilemoma. *Arch Otolaryngol* **91**:117, 1970.
16. Stewart T, Liland J, Schuknecht H: Occult schwannomas of the vestibular nerve. *Arch Otolaryngol* **101**:91, 1975.
17. Evans DGR, Ramsden R, Huson SM, Harris R, Lye R, King T: Type 2 neurofibromatosis: The need for supraregional care? *J Laryngol Otol* **107**:401, 1993.
18. Evans DGR, Huson SM, Donnai D, Neary W, Blair V, Newton V, Harris R: A clinical study of type 2 neurofibromatosis. *QJM* **304**:603, 1992.
19. Gutmann, DH, Aylsworth, A, Carey, JC, Korf, B, Marks, J, Pyeritz, RE, Rubenstein, A, Viskochil, D. The diagnostic evaluation and multi-disciplinary management of neurofibromatosis 1 and neurofibromatosis 2. *JAMA* **278**:51, 1997.
20. MacCollin M, Mautner VF: The diagnosis and management of neurofibromatosis 2 in childhood. *Semin Pediatr Neurol* **5**:243, 1998.
21. Sobel R, Wang Y: Vestibular (acoustic) schwannomas: Histological features in neurofibromatosis 2 and in unilateral cases. *J Neuropathol Exp Neurol* **52**:106, 1993.
22. Mautner VF, Tatagiba M, Lindenau M, Funsterer C, Pulst SM, Kluwe L, Zanella F: Spinal tumors in patients with neurofibromatosis type 2: MR imaging study of frequency, multiplicity, and variety. *AJR Am J Roentgenol* **165**:951, 1995.
23. McCormick P, Torres R, Post K, Stein B: Intramedullary ependymoma of the spinal cord. *J Neurosurg* **72**:523, 1990.
24. Mautner VF, Lindenau M, Baser M, Kluwe L, Gottschalk J: Skin abnormalities in neurofibromatosis 2. *Arch Dermatol* **133**:1539, 1997.
25. Thomas PK, King RHM, Chiang TR, Scaravilli F, Sharma AK, Downie AW: Neurofibromatosis neuropathy. *Muscle Nerve* **13**:93, 1990.
26. Trivedi R, Byrne J, Huson SM, Donaghy M: Focal amyotrophy in neurofibromatosis 2. *J Neurol Neurosurg Psychiatry* **69**:257, 2000.
27. Kaiser-Kupfer M, Freidlin V, Datiles M, Edwards P, Sherman J, Parry D, McCain L, Eldridge R: The association of posterior capsular lens opacities with bilateral acoustic neuromas in patients with neurofibromatosis type 2. *Arch Ophthalmol* **107**:541, 1989.
28. Bouzas E, Parry D, Eldridge R, Kaiser-Kupfer M: Visual impairment in patients with neurofibromatosis 2. *Neurology* **43**:622, 1993.
29. Ragge N, Baser M, Klein J, Nechiporuk A, Sainz J, Pulst SM, Riccardi V: Ocular abnormalities in neurofibromatosis 2. *Am J Ophthalmol* **20**:634, 1995.
30. Crowe FW, Schull WJ: Diagnostic importance of the cafe au lait spot in neurofibromatosis. *Arch Intern Med* **91**:758, 1953.
31. Kopf AW, Levine LJ, Rigel DS, Friedman RJ, Levenstein M: Prevalence of congenital-nevus-like nevi, nevi spili and café au lait spots. *Arch Dermatol* **121**:766, 1985.
32. Short MP, Martuza RL, Huson SM: Neurofibromatosis 2: Clinical features, genetic counselling and management issues, in Huson SM, Hughes RAC (eds): *The Neurofibromatoses: A Pathogenetic and Clinical Overview*. London: Chapman and Hall, 1994, p 414.
33. Evans DG, Blair V, Strachan T, Lye RH, Ramsden RT: Variation of expression of the gene for type 2 neurofibromatosis: Absence of a gender effect on vestibular schwannomas, but confirmation of a preponderance of meningiomas in females. *J Laryng Oto* **109**:830, 1995.
34. Harsh G, MacCollin M, McKenna M, Nadol J, Ojemann R, Short MP: Molecular genetic screening for children at risk of neurofibromatosis 2. *Arch Otolaryngol Head Neck Surg* **121**:590, 1995.
35. Slattery WH, Brackmann DE, Hiteselberger W: Hearing preservation in neurofibromatosis type 2. *Am J Otol* **19**:638, 1998.
36. Samii M, Matthies C, Tatagiba M: Management of vestibular schwannomas (acoustic neuromas): Auditory and facial nerve function after resection of 120 vestibular schwannomas in patients with neurofibromatosis 2. *Neurosurgery* **40**:696, 1997.
37. Bruce J, Fetell M: Tumors of the skull and cranial nerves, in Rowland LP (ed): *Merritt's Textbook of Neurology*, 9th ed. Baltimore: Williams & Wilkins, 1995, p 320.
38. Evans DGR, Wallace AJ, Wu CL, Trueman L, Ramsden RT, Strachan T: Somatic mosaicism: a common cause of classic disease in tumor prone syndromes? Lessons from type 2 neurofibromatosis. *Am J Hum Genet* **63**:727, 1998
39. MacCollin MM, Jacoby LB, Jones D, Ojemann R, Feit H, Gusella J: Somatic mosaicism of the neurofibromatosis 2 tumor suppresser gene. *Neurology* **48**:A29, 1997.
40. Parry DM, MacCollin M, Kaiser-Kupfer M, Pulaski K, Nicholson HS, Bolesta M, Eldridge R, Gusella J: Germ line mutations in the neurofibromatosis 2 (NF2) gene: Correlations with disease severity and retinal abnormalities. *Am J Hum Genet* **59**:529, 1996.
41. Jacoby LB, Jones D, Davis K, Kronn D, Short MP, Gusella J, MacCollin M: Molecular analysis of the NF2 tumor-suppressor gene in schwannomatosis. *Am J Hum Genet* **61**:1293, 1997.
42. MacCollin M, Woodfin W, Kronn D, Short MP: Schwannomatosis: A clinical and pathologic study. *Neurology* **46**:1072, 1996.
43. Buenger K, Porter N, Dozier S, Wagner R: Localized multiple neurilemmoma of the lower extremity. *Cutis* **51**:36, 1993.
44. Sieb JP, Pulst SM, Buch A: Familial CNS tumors. *J Neurol* **239**:343, 1992.
45. Pulst SM, Rouleau G, Marineau C, Fain P, Sieb J: Familial meningioma is not allelic to neurofibromatosis 2. *Neurology* **43**:2096, 1993.

46. Von Deimling A, Kraus JA, Stangl AP, Wellenreuther R, Lenartz D, Schramm J, Louis DN, Ramesh V, Gusella JF, Wiestler OD: Evidence of subarachnoid spread in the development of multiple meningiomas. *Brain Pathol* 5:11, 1995.

47. Jaaskelainin J, Paetau A, Pyykko I, Blomstedt G, Palva T, Troupp H: Interface between the facial nerve and large acoustic neurinomas: Immunohistochemical study of the cleavage plane in NF2 and non-NF2 cases. *J Neurosurg* 870:541, 1993.

48. Aguiar P, Tatagiba M, Samii M, Dankoweit-Timpe E, Ostertag H: The comparison between the growth fraction of bilateral vestibular schwannomas in neurofibromatosis 2 (NF2) and unilateral vestibular schwannomas using the monoclonal antibody MIB 1. *Acta Neurochir (Wien)* 134:40, 1995.

49. Louis D, Ramesh V, Gusella J: Neuropathology and molecular genetics of neurofibromatosis 2 and related tumors. *Brain Pathol* 5:163, 1995.

50. Seizinger B, Martuza R, Gusella J: Loss of genes on chromosome 22 in tumorigenesis of human acoustic neuroma. *Nature* 322:644, 1986.

51. Seizinger B, de la Monte S, Atkins L, Gusella J, Martuza R: Molecular genetic approach to human meningioma: Loss of genes on chromosome 22. *Proc Natl Acad Sci U S A* 68:820, 1971.

52. Seizinger B, Rouleau G, Ozelius L, Lane LJ, St. George-Hyslop P, Huson S, Gusella J, Martuza R: Common pathogenetic mechanism for three tumor types in bilateral acoustic neurofibromatosis. *Science* 236:317, 1987.

53. Knudson AG: Mutation and cancer: A statistical study. *Proc Natl Acad Sci U S A* 68:820, 1971.

54. Rouleau GA, Wertelecki W, Haines JL, Hobbs WJ, Trofatter JA, Seizinger BR, Martuza RL, Superneau DW, Connealy PM, Gusella JF: Genetic linkage of bilateral acoustic neurofibromatosis to a DNA marker on chromosome 22. *Nature* 329:246, 1987.

55. Trofatter J, MacCollin M, Rutter J, Murrell J, Duyao M, Parry D, Eldridge R, Kley N, Menon A, Pulaski K, Haase V, Ambrose C, Munroe D, Bove C, Haines J, Martuza R, MacDonald M, Seizinger B, Short MP, Buckler A, Gusella J: A novel moesin-, ezrin-, radixin-like gene is a candidate for the neurofibromatosis 2 tumor suppressor. *Cell* 72:791, 1993.

56. Rouleau G, Merel P, Lutchman M, Sanson M, Zucman J, Marineau C, Hoang-Xuan K, Demczuk S, Desmaze C, Plougastel B, Pulst S, Lenoir G, Bijlsma E, Rashold R, Dumanski J, de Jong P, Parry D, Eldridge R, Aurias A, Delattre O, Thomas G: Alteration in a new gene encoding a positive membrane-organizing protein causes neuro-fibromatosis type 2. *Nature* 363:515, 1993.

57. Lee DK, Abbott ML: Familial central nervous system neoplasia: Case report of a family with von Recklinghausen's neurofibromatosis. *Arch Neurol* 20:154, 1969.

58. Kluwe L, Mautner V, Parry DM, Jacoby LB, Baser M, Gusella J, Davis K, Stavrou D, MacCollin M: The parental origin of new mutations in neurofibromatosis 2. *Neurogenetics* 3:17, 2000.

59. MacCollin M, Ramesh V, Jacoby LB, Louis D, Rubio M, Pulaski K, Trofatter J, Short MP, Bove C, Eldridge R, Parry D, Gusella J: Mutational analysis of patients with neurofibromatosis 2. *Am J Hum Genet* 55:314, 1994.

60. Gutmann DH, Wright DE, Geist R, Snider W: Expression of the neurofibromatosis 2 (NF2) gene isoforms during rat embryonic development. *Hum Mol Genet* 4:471, 1995.

61. Pykett M, Murphy M, Harnish P, George D: The neurofibromatosis 2 (NF2) tumor suppressor gene encodes multiple alternatively spliced transcripts. *Hum Mol Genet* 3:559, 1994.

62. Hitotsumatsu T, Kitamoto T, Iwaki T, Fukui M, Tateishi J: An exon 8 spliced out transcript of the neurofibromatosis 2 gene is constitutively expressed in various human tissues. *J Biochem (Tokyo)* 116:1205, 1994.

63. Haase V, Trofatter J, MacCollin M, Tarttelin E, Gusella J, Ramesh V: The murine NF2 homologue encodes a highly conserved merlin protein with alternative forms. *Hum Mol Genet* 3:407, 1994.

64. Hara T, Bianchi A, Seizinger B, Kley N: Molecular cloning and characterization of alternatively spliced transcripts of the mouse neurofibromatosis 2 gene. *Cancer Res* 54:330, 1994.

65. Arpin M, Algrain M, Louvard D: Membrane-actin microfilament connections: An increasing diversity of players related to band 4.1. *Curr Opin Cell Biol* 6:136, 1994.

66. Gonzalez-Agosti C, Xu L, Pinney D, Beauchamp R, Hobbs W, Gusella J, Ramesh V: The merlin tumor suppressor localizes preferentially in membrane ruffles. *Oncogene* 13:1239, 1996.

67. Kluwe L, Bayer S, Baser M, Hazim W, Wolfgang H, Funsterer C, Mautner VF: Identification of NF2 germ-line mutations and comparison with neurofibromatosis 2 phenotypes. *Hum Genet* 98:534, 1996.

68. Merel P, Hoang-Xuan K, Sanson M, Bijlsma E, Rouleu G, Laurent-Puig P, Pulst S, Baser M, Lenoir G, Sterkers JM, Philippon J, Resche F, Mautner V, Fischer G, Hulsebos T, Aurias A, Delattre O, Thomas G: Screening for germ-line mutations in the NF2 gene. *Genes Chrom Cancer* 12:117, 1995.

69. Bourn D, Carter S, Mason S, Evans DGR, Strachan T: Germline mutations in the neurofibromatosis type 2 tumour suppressor gene. *Hum Mol Genet* 3:813, 1994.

70. Watson C, Gaunt L, Evans G, Patel K, Harris R, Strachan T: A disease-associated germline deletion maps the type 2 neurofibromatosis (NF2) gene between the Ewing sarcoma region and the leukaemia inhibitory factor locus. *Hum Mol Genet* 2:701, 1993.

71. Kluwe L, Pulst S, Koppen J, Matner VP: A 163-bp deletion at the C-terminus of the schwannomin gene associated with variable phenotypes of neurofibromatosis type 2. *Hum Genet* 95:443, 1995.

72. Bruder CE, Hirvela C, Tapia-Paez I, Fransson I, Segraves R, et al: High resolution deletion analysis of constitutional DNA from neurofibromatosis type 2 (NF2) patients using microarray-CGH. *Hum Mol Genet* 10:271, 2001.

73. Sainz J, Figueroa K, Baser M, Mautner VF, Pulst SM: High frequency of nonsense mutations in the NF2 gene caused by C to T transitions in five CGA codons. *Hum Mol Genet* 4:137, 1995.

74. Stokowski RP, Cox DR: Functional analysis of the neurofibromatosis type 2 protein by means of disease-causing point mutations. *Am J Hum Genet* 66:873, 2000.

75. Ruttledge M, Andermann A, Phelan C, Claudio J, Han F, Chretien N, Rangaratnam S, MacCollin M, Short MP, Parry D, Michels V, Riccardi V, Weksberg R, Kitamura K, Bradburn J, Hall B, Propping P, Rouleau G: Type of mutation in the neurofibromatosis type 2 gene (NF2) frequently determines severity of disease. *Am J Hum Genet* 59:331, 1996.

76. MacCollin M, Braverman N, Viskochil D, Ruttledge M, Davis K, Ojemann R, Gusella J, Parry D: A point mutation associated with a severe phenotype of neurofibromatosis 2. *Ann Neurol* 40:440, 1996.

77. Kluwe L, MacCollin M, Tatagiba M, Thomas S, Hazim W, Haase W, Mautner VF: Phenotypic variability associated with 14 splice-site mutations in the NF2 gene. *Am J Med Genet* 18:228, 1998.

78. Jacoby LB, MacCollin M, Louis DN, Mohney T, Rubio MP, Pulaski K, Trofatter J, Kley N, Seizinger B, Ramesh V, Gusella J: Exon scanning for mutation of the NF2 gene in schwannomas. *Hum Mol Genet* 3:413, 1994.

79. Jacoby L, MacCollin M, Barone R, Ramesh V, Gusella J: Frequency and distribution of NF2 mutations in schwannomas. *Genes Chromosomes Cancer* 17:45, 1996.

80. Biljlsma E, Merel P, Bosch A, Westerveld A, Delatre O, Thomas G, Hulsebos T: Analysis of mutations in the SCh gene in schwannomas. *Genes Chromosomes Cancer* 11:7, 1994.

81. Twist E, Ruttledge M, Rousseau M, Sanson M, Papi L, Merel P, Delattre O, Thomas G, Rouleau G: The neurofibromatosis type 2 gene is inactivated in schwannomas. *Hum Mol Genet* 3:147, 1994.

82. Sainz J, Huynh D, Figueroa K, Ragge N, Baser M, Pulst SM: Mutations of the neurofibromatosis type 2 gene and lack of the gene product in vestibular schwannomas. *Hum Mol Genet* 3:885, 1994.

83. Deprez R, Bianchi A, Groen N, Seizinger B, Hagemeijer A, van Drunen E, Bootsma D, Koper J, Avezaat C, Kley N, Zwarthoff E: Frequent NF2 gene transcript mutations in sporadic meningiomas and vestibular schwannomas. *Am J Hum Genet* 54:1022, 1994.

84. Merel P, Hoang-Xuan K, Sanson M, Moreau-Aubry A, Bijlsma EK, Lazaro C, Moisan JP, Resche F, Nishisho J, Estivill X, Delattre JY, Poisson M, Theillet C, Hulsebos T, Delattre O, Thomas G: Predominant occurrence of somatic mutations of the NF2 gene in meningiomas and schwannomas. *Genes Chromosomes Cancer* 13:211, 1995.

85. Welling DB, Guida M, Goll F, Pearl DK, Glasscock ME, Pappas DG, Linthicum FH, Rogers D, Prior TW: Mutational spectrum in the neurofibromatosis type 2 gene in sporadic and familial schwannomas. *Hum Genet* 98:189, 1996.

86. Wellenreuther R, Kraus JA, Lenartz D, Menon AG, Schramm J, Louis DN, Ramesh V, Guesella JF, Wiestler OD, von Deimling A: Analysis of the neurofibromatosis 2 gene reveals molecular variants of meningioma. *Am J Pathol* 146:827, 1995.

87. Ruttledge M, Sarrazin J, Rangaratnam S, Phelan C, Twist E, Merel P, Delattre O, Thomas G, Nordenskjold M, Collins VP, Dumanski J, Rouleau G: Evidence for the complete inactivation of the NF2 gene in the majority of sporadic meningiomas. *Nat Genet* 6:180, 1994.

88. Evans JJ, Jeun SS, Lee JH, Harwalkar JA, Shoshan Y, Cowell JK, Golubic M: Molecular alterations in the neurofibromatosis type 2 gene

and its protein rarely occurring in meningothelial meningiomas. *J Neurosurg* **94**:111, 2001.

89. Ebert C, von Haken M, Meyer-Puttliz B, Wiestler OD, Reifenberger G, Pietsch T, von Deimling A: Molecular genetic analysis of ependymal tumors. NF2 mutations and chromosome 22q loss occur preferentially in intramedulalary spinal ependymomas *Am J Pathol* **155**:627, 1999.

90. Hoang-Xuan K, Merel P, Vega F, Hugot JP, Cornu P, Delattre JY, Poisson M, Thomas G, Delattre O: Analysis of the NF2 tumor-suppressor gene and of chromosome 22 deletions in gliomas. *Int J Cancer* **60**:478, 1995.

91. Bianchi A, Hara T, Ramesh V, Gao J, Klein-Szanto AJP, Morin F, Menon A, Trofatter J, Gusella J, Seizinger B, Kley N: Mutations in transcript isoforms of the neurofibromatosis 2 gene in multiple human tumour types. *Nat Genet* **6**:185, 1994.

92. Englefield P, Foulkes W, Campbell I: Loss of heterozygosity on chromosome 22 in ovarian carcinoma is distal to and is not accompanied by mutations in NF2 at 22112. *Br J Cancer* **70**:905, 1994.

93. Kanai Y, Tsuda H, Oda T, Sakamoto M, Hirohashi S: Analysis of the neurofibromatosis 2 gene in human breast and hepatocellular carcinomas. *Jpn J Clin Oncol* **25**:1, 1995.

94. Sekido Y, Pass H, Bader S, Mew D, Christman M, Gazdar A, Minna J: Neurofibromatosis type 2 (NF2) gene is somatically mutated in mesothelioma but not in lung cancer. *Cancer Res* **55**:1227, 1995.

95. Cheng JQ, Lee WC, Klein MA, Cheng GZ, Jhanwar SC, Testa JR: Frequent mutations of NF2 and allelic loss from chromosome band 22q12 in malignant mesothelioma: evidence for a two-hit mechanism of NF2 inactivation *Genes Chromosomes Cancer.* **24**:238, 1999.

96. Sainio M, Strachan T, Blomstedt G, Salonen O, Setala K, Palotie A, Palo J, Pyykoo I, Peltonen L, Jaaskelainen J: Presymptomatic DNA and MRI diagnosis of neurofibromatosis 2 with mild clinical course in an extended pedigree. *Neurology* **45**:1314, 1995.

97. Bijlsma EK, Merel P, Fleury P, van Asperen C, Westerveld A, Delattre O, Thomas G, Hulsebos T: Family with neurofibromatosis type 2 and autosomal dominant hearing loss: Identification of carriers of the mutated NF2 gene. *Hum Genet* **96**:1, 1995.

98. Bijlsma EK, Wallace AJ, Evans DG: Misleading linkage results in an NF2 presymptomatic test owing to mosaicism. *J Med Genet* **34**:934, 1997.

99. Nadol JB Jr, Chiong CM, Ojemann RG, McKenna MJ, Martuza RL, Montgomery WW, Levine RA, Ronner SF, Glynn RJ: Preservation of hearing and facial nerve function in resection of acoustic neuroma. *Laryngoscope* **102**:1153, 1992.

100. Samii M, Matthies C, Tatagiba M: Management of vestibular schwannomas (acoustic neuromas): Auditory and facial nerve function after resection of 120 vestibular schwannomas in patients with neurofibromatosis 2. *Neurosurgery* **40**:696, 1997.

101. Tatagiba M, Matthies C, Samii M: Facial nerve reconstruction in neurofibromatosis 2. *Acta Neurochir (Wien)* **126**:72, 1994.

102. Kondziolka D, Lunsford LD, MacLaughlin MR, Flickinger JC: Long-term outcomes after radiosurgery for acoustic neuromas *N Engl J Med* **339**:1426, 1998.

103. Kida Y, Kobayashi T, Tanaka T, Mori Y: Radiosurgery for bilateral neurinomas associated with neurofibromatosis type 2 *Surg Neurol* **53**:383, 2000.

104. Subach BR, Kondziolka D, Lunsford LD, Bissonette DJ, Flickinger JC, Maitz AH: Sterotactic radiosurgery in the management of acoustic neuromas associated with neurofibromatosis type 2 *J Neurosurg* **90**:815, 1999.

105. Rosenbaum C, Kamleiter M, Grafe P, Kluwe L, Mautner V, Muller HW, Hanemann CO: Enhanced proliferation and potassium conductance of Schwann cells isolated from NF2 schwannomas can be reduced by quinidine *Neurobiol Dis* **7**:483, 2000.

106. Takamiya Y, Friedlander R, Brem H, Malick A, Martuza R: Inhibition of angiogenesis and growth of human nerve-sheath tumors by AGM-1470. *J Neurosurg* **78**:470, 1993.

107. Schrell UM, Rittig MG, Anders M, Koch UH, Marschalek R, Kiewewetter F, Fahlbusch, R: Hydroxyurea for treatment of unresectable and recurrent meningiomas. II. Decrease in the size of meningiomas in patients treated with hydroxyurea. *J Neurosurg* **86**:840, 1997.

108. Temple RH, Axon PR, Ramsden RT, Keles N, Deger K, Yucel E: Auditory rehabilitation in neurofibromatosis type 2: A case for cochlear implantation *J Laryngol Otol* **113**:161, 1999.

109. Brackmann D, Hitselberger W, Nelson R, Moore J, Waring M, Portillo F, Shannon R, Telischi F: Auditory brainstem implant: I. Issues in surgical implantation. *Otolaryngol Head Neck Surg* **108**:624, 1993.

110. Shannon R, Fayad J, Moore J, Lo W, Otto S, Nelson R, O'Leary M: Auditory brainstem implant: II. Postsurgical issues and performance. *Otolaryngol Head Neck Surg* **108**:634, 1993.

111. Otto SR, Shannon RV, Brackmann DE, Hitselberger WE, Staller S, Menapace C: The multichannel auditory brain stem implant: performance in twenty patients. *Otolaryngol Head Neck Surg* **118(3 Pt 1)**:291, 1998.

Renal Carcinoma

W. Marston Linehan ▪ *Berton Zbar* ▪ *Richard D. Klausner*

1. Renal carcinoma appears in both a sporadic and a hereditary form. Eighty-five percent of sporadic renal carcinomas are of the clear-cell histologic type; 5 to 10 percent are papillary renal carcinoma and the remainder are less-common histologic types such as chromophobe and collecting-duct renal carcinomas.

2. The best characterized form of hereditary renal carcinoma is von Hippel-Lindau (VHL). VHL is a hereditary cancer syndrome in which affected individuals are at risk to develop tumors in a number of organs, including the kidneys, cerebellum, spine, eye, inner ear, adrenal gland, and pancreas. VHL families are categorized as VHL Type I (without pheochromocytoma) or VHL Type II (with pheochromocytoma).

3. The VHL gene, which has the characteristics of a tumor-suppressor gene, has been identified on the short-arm of chromosome 3. The VHL gene has 3 exons and encodes a protein of 213 amino acids. Both copies of the VHL gene are inactivated in tumors in VHL patients. There is mutation in the inherited allele and loss of the wild-type allele. VHL gene mutation analysis provides a method for early diagnosis of VHL in asymptomatic individuals, or in clinical situations such as hereditary pheochromocytoma when the diagnosis is in doubt. Because VHL manifestations often occur in childhood, testing early in life is recommended so that appropriate intervention can be instituted. There is a marked genotype/phenotype correlation with VHL gene mutation and the manifestation of the VHL; VHL Type II families are characterized by missense mutations of the VHL gene. There is a hot spot for VHL Type II at a single codon in the 5' end of exon 3 of the VHL gene.

4. Inactivation of both copies of the VHL gene is an early event in clear-cell renal carcinoma, where a high percentage of VHL gene mutations and loss-of-heterozygosity (LOH) have been detected. VHL gene mutations, including nucleotide insertions, deletions, substitutions, and nonsense mutations, have been found in each of the three exons. Neither VHL gene mutation nor VHL LOH is found in papillary renal carcinoma. A molecular genetic classification of renal carcinoma, clear-cell versus papillary, has been proposed, with clear-cell renal carcinoma characterized by VHL gene mutation. VHL gene mutations have been detected in DNA extracted from formalin-fixed material and tissue aspirates, providing a potentially useful diagnostic tool. Somatic VHL gene mutations have been detected in sporadic tumors from other organs affected in VHL, including cerebellar hemangioblastoma and epididymal cystadenoma. With the exception of rare reports, VHL is not mutated or implicated in other sporadic cancers.

5. pVHL forms a complex with elongin C, elongin B, Cul2, and the RINGH2 protein Rbx1. This complex is referred to as the VCB-Cul2 complex. Portions of the complex are homologous to components of the SCF family of ubiquitin-ligase complexes (Skp1/Cul1-Cdc53/F-box protein). The complex targets ubiquitin-mediated degradation of the oxygen-dependent domain of the α subunit of the transcription factor, HIF-1α. HIF-1α is a transcription factor that regulates a number of hypoxia-inducible genes, including vascular endothelial growth factor (VEGF), paltelet-derived growth factor (PDGF), and the glucose transporter GLUT-1. Studies of the crystal structure of the VCB-Cul2 complex reveal an α-domain of pVHL, which is the binding site for elongin C, and a β-domain, which is the binding site for HIF. Inactivation of pVHL is associated with increased levels of HIFα and VEGF, PDGF, and Glut 1. Although there are likely other targets for the VCB-Cul2 complex, this provides a potential explanation for the high degree of vascularity observed in VHL and sporadic renal carcinoma.

6. Sporadic clear cell renal carcinomas are characterized by a high degree of neoangiogenesis; angiogenesis is also a striking feature in the clinical manifestations of VHL. Both clear-cell renal carcinoma and cerebellar hemangioblastoma are characterized by a marked elevation in expression of VEGF. The increased expression of VEGF is reversed in renal carcinoma cells by reintroduction of the wild-type VHL gene. This reversal is blocked by either anoxia or by low serum conditions, suggesting that VHL may play a role in the normal regulated induction of angiogenesis. This critical gene is one of the first identified targets of VHL function.

7. Hereditary papillary renal-cell carcinoma (HPRC) is a hereditary cancer syndrome in which affected individuals are at risk to develop bilateral, multifocal papillary renal cell carcinoma. This syndrome, which has an autosomal dominant inheritance pattern, is caused by missense mutations in the tyrosine kinase domain of the MET protooncogene. Patients with germ line or somatic mutations in the MET protooncogene develop a specific subtype of papillary renal carcinoma—papillary renal carcinoma type 1. The mutations in the tyrosine kinase domain of the MET protooncogene can be readily detected by denaturing high-performance liquid chromatography (DHPLC).

8. Familial renal oncocytoma is characterized by a predisposition to develop bilateral, multiple renal oncocytomas in affected family members.

9. The Birt-Hogg-Dubé syndrome (BHD), a rare inherited cutaneous disorder characterized by hamartomas of the hair follicle, may be associated with an increased risk for development of renal cancer. BHD was found in two families with familial renal oncocytoma, and in one family with members affected with papillary renal carcinoma.

Renal carcinoma, the most common cancer in the kidney, affects nearly 28,000 Americans annually and is associated with over 12,000 deaths per year.[1] Renal carcinoma, which accounts for approximately 3 percent of adult cancers, most commonly occurs in adults between the ages of 50 and 70 years; however, it has been reported in children as young as 3 years of age.[2] Clear-cell type (or a variant of clear-cell) makes up 80 to 85 percent of renal carcinoma. Little is known about the etiology of renal cancer, although a number of environmental, hormonal, and cellular

Table 27-1 Hereditary Forms of Renal Carcinoma

1. Hereditary clear-cell renal carcinoma	(HCRC)
2. Von Hippel-Lindau	(VHL)
3. Hereditary papillary renal carcinoma	(HPRC)

factors have been studied. Renal carcinoma has been increasing at a rate of approximately 2 percent per year and affects males twice as frequently as females.[3] There is a strong correlation with cigarette smoking and an increased incidence of renal cancer among leather workers and workers exposed to asbestos.[4–7] There is an increased incidence of renal carcinoma in patients with end-stage renal disease, which is particularly notable in patients who have acquired cystic disease.[8,9] The risk of developing renal-cell carcinoma for end-stage renal patients with cystic changes on dialysis is estimated to be 30 times higher than that in the general population.[10] Five to 10 percent of renal carcinoma is of the papillary histologic type.[11,12] The remaining tumors are made up of rare histologic types such as chromophobe and collecting-duct renal carcinoma.

Renal carcinoma occurs in hereditary, as well as nonhereditary, sporadic forms. Estimates from case-control studies suggest that up to 4 percent of renal carcinoma may be hereditary on the basis of family history.[3] There are three forms of hereditary renal-cell carcinoma (Table 27-1). One is hereditary clear-cell renal carcinoma (HCRC) in which 50 percent of offspring of an affected individual are likely to develop renal carcinoma.[13,14] A second form of hereditary renal carcinoma is that associated with VHL, in which affected individuals develop tumors in a number of organs, including the kidneys.[3,15] A third form of inherited renal carcinoma is HPRC.[16,17] While patients with sporadic renal carcinoma are likely to develop a solitary renal tumor between the ages of 50 and 70 years, patients with hereditary renal cell carcinoma tend to develop multifocal, early onset renal carcinoma.[3]

LOCATION OF THE CLEAR-CELL RENAL CARCINOMA GENE: CHROMOSOME 3

An initial indication of the location of renal carcinoma gene came from the studies of Cohen et al., who, in 1979, reported a family with an autosomal dominant inheritance pattern of bilateral, multifocal renal carcinoma.[13] Affected individuals in this kindred were characterized by a balanced germ line translocation from chromosome 3 to chromosome 8. Subsequently, Pathak reported a renal cell carcinoma family with a chromosome 3 to chromosome 11 translocation.[18] In 1989, Kovaks et al. described a family carrying a constitutional translocation (3;6)(p13;q25.1) in which affected individuals developed multiple, bilateral, early onset renal carcinoma.[19]

These and other findings led to genetic studies of chromosome 3 in nonhereditary renal cell carcinoma. When renal carcinoma was evaluated for loss of heterozygosity on chromosome 3 by restriction fragment length polymorphism (RFLP) analysis (Fig. 27-1), consistent loss of a segment of the short-arm of chromosome 3 was detected in tumor tissue from patients with sporadic, nonhereditary clear-cell renal carcinoma.[20–28] Cytogenetic analysis of sporadic renal cell carcinoma confirmed these findings.[23,28–30] Loss of a segment of chromosome 3 was found to be a consistent feature of clear-cell renal carcinoma, the common form of renal carcinoma, but not in papillary renal carcinoma.[21,32,33] In a detailed analysis of 60 tumors, Anglard et al. detected LOH in nearly 90% of clear-cell renal carcinomas, and defined by deletion analysis (Fig. 27-2) an area of minimal deletion in the 3p21-26 region of chromosome 3.[21] As this region was too large to study by conventional cloning methods available at the time, investigators turned to the hereditary form of renal-cell

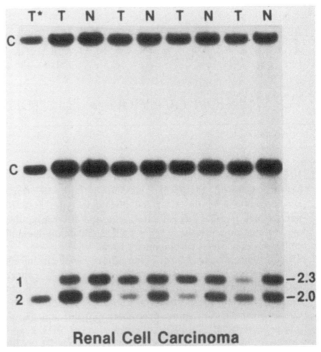

Fig. 27-1 RFLP analysis of sporadic renal-cell carcinoma tumors (T) and corresponding normal tissue (N) with a probe for the chromosome 3p DNF 15S2 locus. One and 2 indicate the two polymorphic chromosome 3p alleles; C indicates a constant band. The bands on the lower part of the figure represent the 2.3- and 2.0-kb alleles, one of which is lost in the tumors indicated. The residual bands represent the presence of normal lymphocytes; the lane marked T* indicates a renal tumor grown in an immunodeficient mouse. (*From Zbar et al.[20] Used with permission.*)

carcinoma associated with von Hippel-Lindau to search for the kidney cancer gene.

VON HIPPEL-LINDAU

VHL is a hereditary cancer syndrome, in which affected individuals are at risk to develop tumors in a number of organs, including the kidneys. In the early 1860s, reports by ophthalmologists began to appear that described angiomatous lesions of the retina that were associated with blindness, and that were occasionally associated with similar cerebellar lesions.[34] In 1894, Collins described angiomas which appeared in the retinas of two siblings.[35] Von Hippel, a German ophthalmologist, first recognized that there was a hereditary component to the retinal angiomas.[36] The Swedish ophthalmologist, Arvid Lindau determined that the retinal angiomas and cerebellar hemangioblastomas together were part of the familial syndrome that bears his name.[37] Although subsequent clinical reports of small families confirmed the association of the retinal angiomas, central nervous system (CNS) hemangioblastomas, renal tumors and cysts, epididymal cystadenomas, pancreatic cysts and tumors, and pheochromocytomas,[34] it was in 1964, that Melmon and Rosen codified the term *von Hippel-Lindau* with the definitive article in which a large family with these diverse manifestations was characterized (Table 27-2).[38]

VHL is estimated to occur in 1/36,000 live births; inheritance of the gene follows an autosomal dominant pattern with a penetrance from 80 to 90 percent, but with highly varied expressivity.[15] The age of onset of VHL is variable and depends on (a) which asymptomatic lesions are sought and (b) the expression within the family. The retinal angiomas are generally the earliest lesions detected, followed by CNS and spinal hemangiomas. The mean age at diagnosis of retinal hemangiomas is 25 years (range, 1 to 67 years); for CNS hemangioblastoma, it is

CHROMOSOME 3 DELETION MAP: SPORADIC RENAL CELL CARCINOMA

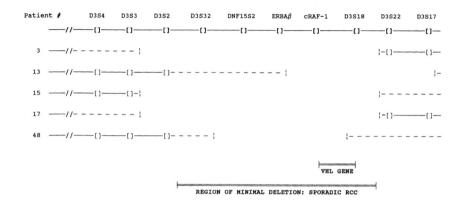

Fig. 27-2 Deletion map showing the area of minimal deletion on chromosome 3p in sporadic renal-cell carcinoma. Analysis of the genotypes identified the locus in the telomeric portion of chromosome 3p bounded by the markers D3S2 and D3S22 as the region of a potential renal-cell carcinoma disease gene. (*From Anglard et al.*[21] *Used with permission.*)

30 years (range, 11 to 78 years); and for renal-cell carcinoma, the mean age is 37 years (range, 16 to 67 years).[34] In kindreds with pheochromocytoma (VHL Type II), pheochromocytoma is often detected before other manifestations and can appear before the age of 10 years.

Renal Manifestations of VHL

Renal-cell carcinoma occurs in 28 to 45 percent of individuals affected with VHL. Affected individuals may develop renal cysts, renal cysts lined with renal-cell carcinomas, or solid renal-cell carcinomas. Although the renal tumors are often detected when they are small and confined to the kidney, these tumors are malignant and can metastasize (Fig. 27-3). Poston et al. characterized the findings after renal surgery in 161 lesions from 12 patients with von Hippel-Lindau and renal-cell carcinoma. Pathologic evaluation revealed 45 solid lesions, 41 of which were renal-cell carcinoma, and 116 cystic lesions, 25 of which were malignant. Of 66 malignant lesions, 35 (53%) contained cells with only clear-cell cytologic features; 30 (46%) were comprised of predominantly clear cells with scattered granular cells. A single malignant lesion (1.5%) was found to have sarcomatoid renal cell carcinoma with clear and granular cells. This study established the clear-cell cytologic feature as the primary finding in renal lesions of VHL patients.[39] When Walther et al. examined in detail grossly normal renal parenchyma from 16 VHL patients, microscopic renal cystic and solid neoplasms containing only clear-cell cytologic features were found (Fig. 27-4). The extrapolated number of lesions in the average kidney, represented at the mean age of 37 years, was estimated as 1100 nonmalignant cysts with a clear-cell lining and 600 clear-cell neoplasms.[40]

For detection of even small renal lesions in VHL, computerized tomography (CT) scan and ultrasound are the preferred techniques.[34,41,42] Treatment of renal-cell carcinoma involves parenchymal sparing surgery whenever possible.[43–47] Intraoperative ultrasound may be used to identify both solid and cystic lesions to be removed surgically.[48,49] The prevalence of microscopic renal carcinoma makes it likely that tumors will reappear; the goal of surgery is to maintain renal function as long as possible while reducing the risk of metastases. A serial CT study of the natural history of renal lesions in VHL patients revealed that there is a wide variation in the growth rates of the renal lesions.[50] Although

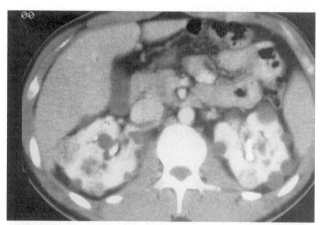

A

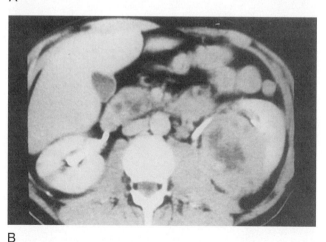

B

Fig. 27-3 *A*, Abdominal CT scan of a VHL patient reveals bilateral multifocal renal carcinomas and cysts. *B*, Abdominal CT scan of a VHL patient reveals a large renal mass, which had spread to the lungs. (*From Linehan et al.*[145] *Used with permission.*)

Table 27-2 Von Hippel-Lindau Manifestations

Bilateral, multifocal clear-cell renal carcinoma
Bilateral, multifocal renal cysts
Cerebellar and spinal hemangioblastoma
Endolymphatic sac tumors (ELSTs)
Retinal angioma
Pancreatic cysts, microcystic adenomas, islet-cell tumors
Pheochromocytoma
Epididymal cystadenoma

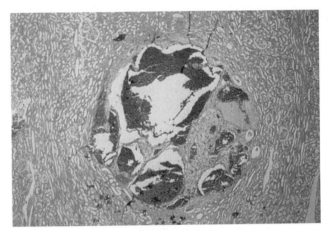

Fig. 27-4 A microscopic focus of renal cell carcinoma detected in grossly "normal" renal tissue from a VHL patient. (*From Linehan et al.*[145] *Used with permission.*)

clinicians often recommend surgery when the solid renal lesions reach the 2.5- to 3-cm size, the role of surgical resection in the management of VHL-associated renal carcinoma, i.e., whether survival can be extended or quality of life enhanced by aggressive screening and early detection programs, remains to be determined.

RETINAL ANGIOMA

Retinal angiomas are often the first manifestation of VHL (Fig. 27-5). Fifty-eight to 60 percent of affected VHL patients develop these benign vascular tumors of the retina. The histologic pattern of the ocular manifestation is strikingly similar to that of clear-cell renal-cell carcinoma and cerebellar hemangioblastoma. These tumors can be multifocal, bilateral, and recurrent. Although the mean age of diagnosis is reported to be 25 years, these tumors can occur in infants. Although the retinal angiomas are nonmalignant, these tumors can cause glaucoma, cataracts, retinal detachment, and blindness. It is critical that at-risk individuals

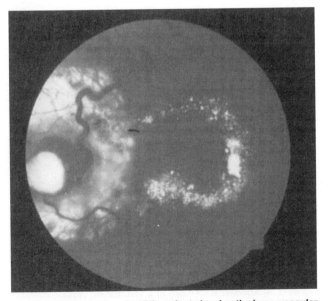

Fig. 27-5 Retinal lesion of a VHL patient showing the hypervascular retinal angioma that characterize VHL. (*From Linehan et al.*[145] *Used with permission.*)

have a thorough ophthalmologic examination. Ophthalmologic examination often includes tonometry, fluorescein angioscopy and indirect ophthalmoscopy. Periodic ophthalmologic evaluation is a part of the management of VHL patients. Treatment of retinal angiomas is often by laser therapy. An aggressive approach to screening and treatment of eye lesions in VHL patients can often result in successful, long-term preservation of vision. Many clinicians recommend initiation of ophthalmologic screening at an early age (1 year of age) so that preservation of vision can be maintained.[15]

CNS HEMANGIOBLASTOMA

CNS hemangioblastomas occur in 60 to 65 percent of affected VHL individuals and can cause increased intracranial pressure, obstructive hydrocephalus, hemorrhage or death. The hemangioblastomas are characterized by three cell types: endothelial cells, stromal cells, and pericytes. These vascular tumors form channels and caverns, and can organize into a vascular mural nodule within a fluid-filled cyst. The cells in the CNS tumors are remarkably similar to those seen in the clear-cell renal carcinoma, as well as in the epididymal cystadenoma. There is marked hypertrophy of the afferent and efferent vessels in the cerebellar and spinal tumors; the gross appearance of these tumors can be one of a mass of blood vessels. The VHL-associated CNS hemangioblastomas occur most often in the spine and cerebellum, as well as in the brainstem at the craniocervical junction. These tumors occasionally occur above the tentorium.[15,51] Hemangioblastoma can occur in the pituitary, although this is an infrequent occurrence. The number of CNS lesions, as well as the number of renal and pancreatic lesions, is often underestimated by radiographic imaging studies.

Although the mean age of diagnosis of CNS hemangioblastoma in VHL patients is 29 years, these tumors can occur in children. Symptoms can include headache, nausea, broad-based gait, and vertigo. Signs include papilledema, dysmetria, ataxia, slurred speech, nystagmus; focal weakness may be an indication of a spinal lesion. Diagnosis of CNS hemangioblastoma is by T_1-weighted MRI of both the head and spine (Fig. 27-6).[15,51] Treatment is most often by surgical removal. Surgical selection is often complicated in VHL patients. The decision to recommend surgery relates to the size, number, locations of tumors, and the presence of associated findings, such as syringomyelia or hydrocephalus. More studies are needed to determine whether quality of life can be enhanced, or survival extended, by early CNS tumor detection and aggressive genetic and clinical screening programs.[51] Focused radiation therapy with the "gamma knife" is sometimes utilized, although its role in the management of CNS hemangioblastoma remains to be determined.

THE CELL OF ORIGIN IN HEMANGIOBLASTOMA

Hemangioblastomas are a mixture of stromal cells and immature vascular cells. The neoplastic cell that forms these tumors is not known. Two advances provide further understanding of VHL hemangioblastomas. First, Lee and Vortmeyer used microdissection to identify which cell type showed loss of heterozygosity in sporadic hemangioblastomas.[52,53] Microdissected stromal cells from hemangioblastomas showed loss of heterozygosity with markers on chromosome 3p, suggesting that stromal cells had one of the two hits (molecular events) required to produce tumors. It was not possible to isolate the immature vascular cells by microdissection. These results suggest that the stromal cell is the neoplastic cell in hemangioblastomas. By using cultures of mouse embryonic stem cells, a common progenitor that gives rise to both blood cells and vascular endothelial cells was identified.[54,55] Because this progenitor cell can be grown in culture, it now can be studied in detail. It is possible that the hemangioblast described by Choi, et al. may be related to the cell of origin of VHL hemangioblastomas.

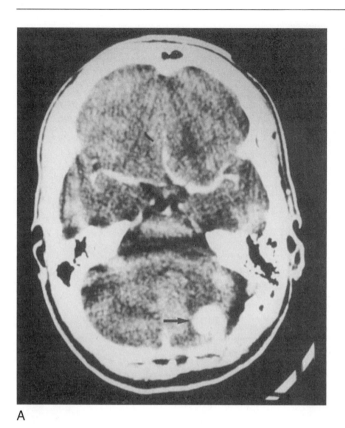

A

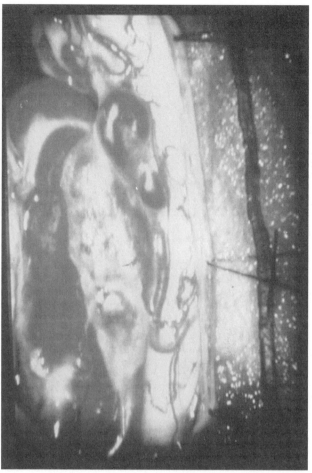

B

Fig. 27-6 *A*, Cerebellar hemangioblastoma detected by an MRI examination. *B*, Spinal hemangioblastoma revealing the intense hypervascularity of these lesions. (*From Linehan et al.*[145] *Used with permission.*)

PHEOCHROMOCYTOMA

Pheochromocytoma has been reported to occur in 18 percent of affected individuals.[15] There is a marked clustering of pheochromocytoma in certain families and this is now known as a distinct subtype of VHL — VHL Type II. Pheochromocytomas can be bilateral, multifocal, extraadrenal, and can become malignant. Symptoms of pheochromocytoma in VHL patients include paroxysmal or sustained hypertension, episodic sweating, palpitations, headaches, and anxiety attacks, and are caused by the release of the catecholamines epinephrine and norepinephrine. Blood pressure can increase to levels that cause fatal cerebral hemorrhage or acute myocardial infarction. Unsuspected pheochromocytoma can be particularly ominous in a patient who has a cerebellar hemangioblastoma, who is pregnant, or who is undergoing surgical resection of a CNS, renal, or pancreatic lesion.

Abdominal CT scanning, which is often performed in the initial screening of VHL patients, frequently provides the initial detection of VHL-associated pheochromocytoma (Fig. 27-7). MRI scanning is a particularly useful method for making the diagnosis. If there is a suspicion that a patient may have an extra-adrenal pheochromocytoma, I[131]-MIBG (metaiodobenzylguanidine) scintigraphy may be recommended (Fig. 27-8).[56] The diagnosis of pheochromocytoma is made by demonstration of elevated levels of catecholamines and/or their metabolites in the urine or blood. Evaluation of VHL patients includes measurement of serum and blood catecholamines, most often epinephrine, norepinephrine, and metanephrine. The clonidine suppression and/or glucagon

stimulation tests may aid in making the diagnosis of an indeterminate or potentially nonfunctioning adrenal mass lesion.[57,58] The treatment of pheochromocytoma is surgical resection of tumors that are functioning or larger than 5 cm. Treatment of bilateral pheochromocytoma may require surgical removal of both glands. Because removal of both adrenal glands requires that the patient be on a lifetime of replacement therapy, some physicians perform partial adrenalectomies to preserve functioning adrenal tissue. Although this has the potential advantage of preserving adrenal function, such patients need careful monitoring for recurrent pheochromocytoma. The addition of laparoscopic adrenalectomy has added another potentially less invasive method for management of VHL-associated tumors.[57,59] Detection and treatment of functioning pheochromocytomas is important. Undetected pheochromocytomas are life-threatening and have lead to the deaths of VHL patients. The role of treatment of occult, nonfunctioning pheochromocytomas is currently under study.

PANCREATIC MANIFESTATIONS OF VHL

VHL-associated pancreatic lesions include pancreatic cysts, serous microcystic adenomas and islet cell tumors (Fig. 27-9). Pancreatic cysts are the most common manifestations; however, the frequency depends on the individual family being studied. The reported frequency of pancreatic cysts in VHL patients varies from 0 percent in two large families[60,61] to 93 percent in other families.[62]

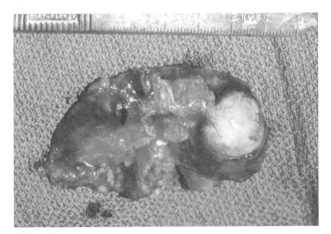

A

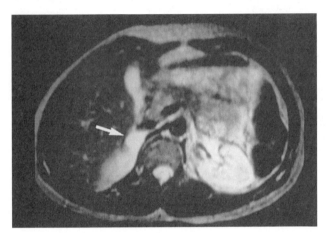

B

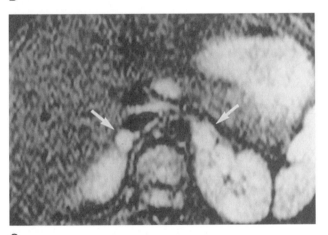

C

Fig. 27-7 *A,* **Adrenal gland removed at surgery with a large pheochromocytoma on the left side of the gland.** *B* **and** *C* **Abdominal CT imaging reveals a solitary, right-sided pheochromocytoma (***B,* **middle panel). In another patient abdominal MRI scan reveals the presence of bilateral pheochromocytomas in a 12-year-old boy (***C,* **right panel). (***From Linehan et al.*[145] *Used with permission.*)

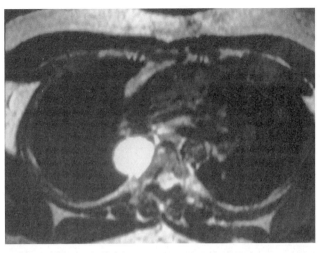

Fig. 27-8 MRI scan showing an extra-adrenal pheochromocytoma. (*From Linehan et al.*[145] *Used with permission.*)

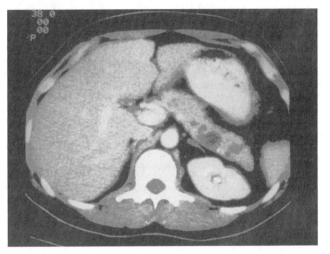

Fig. 27-9 Abdominal imaging reveals pancreatic cysts and islet cell tumors in a VHL patient. (*From Linehan et al.*[145] *Used with permission.*)

Pancreatic cysts usually appear in the 20- to 40-year-old age group, however, they have been detected in patients as young as 15 years of age. The cysts appear throughout the body of the pancreas with no localization to a particular site. Epithelium-lined collections of serous fluid produce the cysts, which vary in size from 7 mm to larger than 10 cm. Serous cystadenoma (or micro-

cystic adenoma) contains multiple macroscopic and microscopic cysts that are separated by thickened walls of stroma arranged in a stellate pattern with a central nidus, which can be scar-like or calcified.[34] Pancreatic cysts are most often asymptomatic. Symptoms can be caused by biliary obstruction or associated with such diffuse disease that pancreatic insufficiency results and steatorrhea and diarrhea occur. Obstruction is managed by the placement of biliary stents; pancreatic insufficiency by enzyme replacement. Rarely, cystic enlargement is associated with such local pain or early satiety that percutaneous drainage is required.[34]

Pancreatic islet cell tumors occur in VHL patients, apparently independently of pancreatic cystic disease. These tumors, of neural origin, are comprised of nests of polygonal cells with vesicular nuclei. Like VHL-associated renal tumors and CNS and retinal tumors, the pancreatic islet cell tumors are markedly vascular. While most are slow growing and asymptomatic, pancreatic islet cell tumors can grow rapidly or metastasize. Diagnosis of islet cell tumors is by CT scan, where the tumor appears as a characteristically intensely enhancing lesion. Although the standard treatment of growing islet cell tumors is surgical resection, the decision to recommend surgery for the management of VHL-associated islet cell tumors is complicated. While advanced islet cell tumors are life-threatening, they can invade locally and metastasize, and the role of surgical resection in prolonging survival and quality of life remains to be determined.

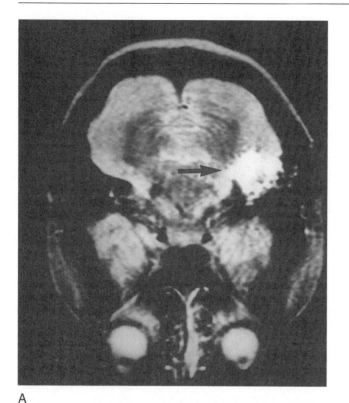

A

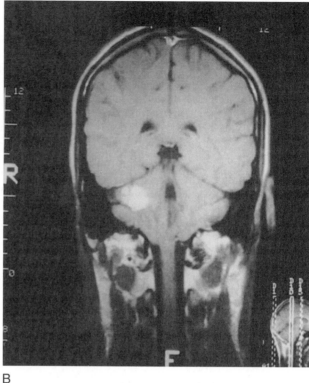

B

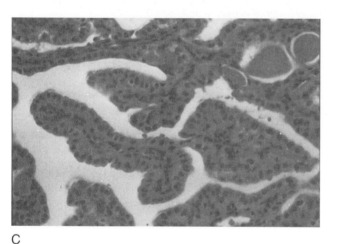

C

Fig. 27-10 *A* and *B*, Imaging studies reveal endolymphatic sac tumors (ELST) in VHL patients. *C*, Histologically this tumor is a low grade, papillary neoplasm which invades locally but which has low potential to metastasize. (*From Linehan et al.*[145] *Used with permission.*)

PAPILLARY CYSTADENOMA OF THE EPIDIDYMIS AND BROAD LIGAMENT

Papillary cystadenomas of the epididymis can be unilateral or bilateral and are present in 10 to 26 percent of affected VHL males. These benign tumors, which can involve the spermatic cord, are most often found in the globus major of the epididymis. The lesions, which are typically 2 to 3 cm in size, can reach 5 cm. The histology of these tumors resembles that of renal and pancreatic cysts and endolymphatic sac tumors. The epididymal cysts are lined by clear cells that contain glycogen and fat with papillary and tubular structures and a surrounding collagenous pseudocapsule.[34] These tumors do not have malignant potential and treatment is most often conservative. Rarely, a symptomatic epididymal cystadenoma requires surgery. Papillary cystadenomas may also occur in women, in tissue associated with the mesonephric tubules near the ovaries and uterine tubes, and in

remanants of the longer mesonephric duct, close to the lateral walls of the uterus and vagina.[34,63]

ENDOLYMPHATIC SAC TUMORS

A more recently appreciated manifestation of VHL is the presence of a tumor in the inner ear, an endolymphatic sac tumor (ELST) (Fig. 27-10). Lying between the dura of the posterior fossa, the endolymphatic sac is located at the end of the endolymphatic sac canal.[34] Although the prevalence and clinical characteristics of endolymphatic sac tumors in VHL patients are only recently being characterized,[64] it has been estimated that as many as 10 percent of VHL patients may have ELST. ELST is a low-grade malignancy with a papillary histologic growth pattern. Although a metastatic ELST has not been reported, this tumor can invade locally and can be associated with hearing damage or facial paresis. Evaluation of

VHL patients for ELST involves imaging with high-resolution CT and MRI imaging through the inner ear. Audiologic evaluation is used for assessment of hearing and cochlear function. Significant audiologic abnormalities may be detected in up to 50 percent of VHL patients. The possibility exists that there are two components, one neoplastic and the other neurologic, to the otologic manifestations of VHL. It is unknown whether these two aspects of VHL are related. Early detection of the endolymphatic sac tumors is possible with MRI and CT scanning of the internal auditory canal (IAC). The role of early surgical intervention to preserve hearing remains to be determined.[34]

THE VHL GENE: CHARACTERISTICS OF A TUMOR-SUPPRESSOR GENE

To determine whether the genetics of VHL fit Knudson's two-hit hypothesis of a tumor-suppressor gene, Tory et al. evaluated renal cell carcinomas, pheochromocytoma, spinal hemangioblastoma, and cerebellar hemangioblastoma from von Hippel-Lindau patients. Multiple renal-cell carcinomas, pheochromocytomas, and spinal and cerebellar hemangioblastomas from VHL patients showed loss of the wild-type chromosome 3p allele, demonstrating that both copies of the VHL gene were inactivated in VHL tumor tissue.[65] To assess for the earliest abnormalities in renal manifestations of VHL, Lubensky et al. performed detailed analysis of chromosome 3p LOH in microdissected renal lesions from VHL

patients by polymerase chain reaction-single-strand conformation polymorphism (PCR-SSCP) analysis (Fig. 27-11). Two benign cysts, five atypical cysts, five microscopic renal cell carcinoma *in situ*, five single-cell-lined cysts, two microscopic and seven macroscopic renal-cell carcinomas were evaluated. Twenty-five of 26 of the renal lesions had (a) nonrandom allelic loss at the VHL gene locus with loss of the wild-type allele, and (b) retention of the inherited, mutated VHL allele.[66] Although clinical, radiologic, and pathologic data suggest that benign and atypical renal lesions may represent the precursors of renal-cell carcinoma in VHL patients, the finding of LOH of the VHL gene as an early event suggests that atypical and benign clear cell cysts may represent early stages in the development and progression of renal-cell carcinoma in VHL patients.[66]

THE VHL GENE IS LOCALIZED TO CHROMOSOME 3

In 1988, Seizinger et al. localized the VHL gene to a locus in the telomeric region of the short-arm of chromosome 3, in the region of the cRAF1 oncogene at 3p25.[67] To further characterize the VHL gene locus, Lerman et al. isolated a collection of 2000 lambda phage-carrying single-copy DNA fragments which were ordered as RFLP markers for construction of a fine linkage map spanning the distal portion of chromosome 3p encompassing the VHL locus.[68] These markers made the localization and subsequent identification of the VHL gene possible. When Hosoe et al., and Richards et al. performed multipoint linkage analysis (Fig. 27-12) with chromosome 3p markers in VHL families, the gene locus was determined to be in a 4-cM interval between cRAF1 and D3S18, an anonymous marker at 3p25.5.[69,70]

PRESYMPTOMATIC DIAGNOSIS OF VON HIPPEL LINDAU BY DNA POLYMORPHISM ANALYSIS

With flanking DNA markers available, Glenn et al. compared the results of DNA linkage analysis with a comprehensive clinical screening examination. Forty-three individuals at risk for developing VHL were informative with polymorphic markers. In 42 of 43 at-risk individuals, polymorphism analysis accurately identified individuals carrying the VHL gene among asymptomatic family members.[71] All 9 of the at-risk individuals predicted to carry the VHL gene were found on clinical examination to have evidence of occult manifestations; no clinical evidence of VHL was detected in 32 of 33 of the at-risk individuals predicted to carry the wild-type

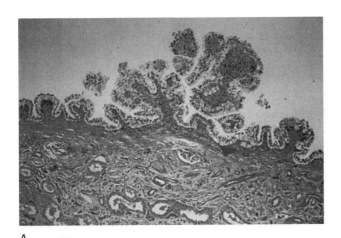

A

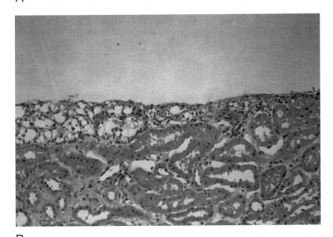

B

Fig. 27-11 *A* and *B*, Histology of early renal lesions in a VHL patient. Lubensky et al. detected VHL gene LOH in microdissected material from 25/26 renal lesions, including lesions such as renal cell carcinoma (*A*) and atypical cysts lined by 2 to 3 layers of clear epithelial cells. (*From Lubensky et al.*[66] *Used with permission.*)

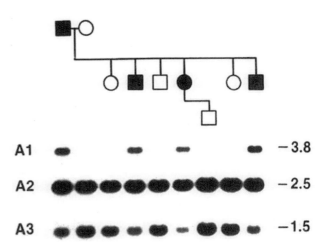

Fig. 27-12 Linkage analysis demonstrating cosegregation of the A1 allele of the chromosome 3p marker D3S18 with VHL. The darkened boxes represent individuals affected with VHL. (*From Hosoe et al.*[69] *Used with permission.*)

Table 27-3 Classification of VHL

Type I	VHL without pheochromocytoma
Type II	VHL with pheochromocytoma
Type IIA	Pheochromocytoma, CNS hemangioblastomas, and retinal angiomas
Type IIB	VHL IIA plus pancreatic involvement and renal manifestations (tumors, cysts)

allele of the VHL gene.[71] The single patient who was classified clinically as having VHL and who was not predicted by linkage analysis to carry the VHL gene was a 42-year-old at-risk female who had a solid renal mass. When the mass was surgically removed, a small focus of clear-cell renal-cell carcinoma was found. When the VHL gene was later identified and the mutation in this kindred was determined, this patient was found not to carry a germ line VHL mutation. A somatic VHL gene mutation was, however, subsequently found in her tumor,[72] which, as would be predicted, was different from that identified in her affected siblings. She was an example of a "phenocopy"; i.e., an individual who is found to have a tumor in a target organ in a hereditary cancer syndrome who does not carry the VHL gene.[71]

VHL: GENOTYPIC HOMOGENEITY/PHENOTYPIC HETEROGENEITY

To further localize the VHL gene, more than 100 VHL families from North America were evaluated. Different patterns of VHL manifestation appeared among the VHL families. In the initial genetic studies, one large family was identified whose VHL phenotype was markedly distinct from typical VHL. Whereas pheochromocytoma is normally identified in 18 percent of affected VHL individuals, in this kindred, 57 percent (27 of 47) of affected family members were found to have pheochromocytoma. Four of 47 affected family members had spinal or cerebellar hemangioblastomas; none of the affected family members had renal-cell carcinoma (0 of 47) or pancreatic cysts (0 of 24).[71,73] The clinical findings were confirmed by genetic analysis. The family linked to RAF1 and D3S18, markers shown to be linked to typical VHL. Subsequently a number of families have been characterized with this pattern of VHL, that is with pheochromocytomas. These

findings formed the initial basis for the classification of VHL kindreds (Table 27-3) as VHL Type I (VHL without pheochromocytomas) or VHL Type II (with pheochromocytomas).

IDENTIFICATION OF THE VHL GENE

After the VHL gene was localized to the 3p25 locus, the area was covered with overlapping yeast artificial chromosomes (YACs) and cosmid-phage contigs.[74] A critical step in the identification of the gene occurred when Yao et al. identified overlapping germ line deletions in three unrelated VHL patients during the construction of a long-range (2.5 megabase) restriction map of the regions surrounding the VHL gene. A cosmid (cosmid 11) was identified that mapped to the smallest nested deletion. Two candidate cDNAs, denoted g7 and g6, were isolated from a λGT11 terato-carcinoma library screened by conserved sequences in cosmid 11. As previous studies had determined that there was genotypic homogeneity in VHL, the VHL gene was considered to be at a single locus; g6 was an unlikely candidate because no mutations were detected in 120 unrelated VHL patients. When inactivating mutations were searched for in constitutional DNA derived from 221 unrelated VHL patients by Southern blot analysis, aberrant bands ranging in size from 4 to 25 kb were detected in 28 of the 221 VHL kindreds. SSCP analysis revealing inactivating mutations that segregated with VHL were identified in three families. These findings (Fig. 27-13) indicated that g7 is the VHL tumor-suppressor gene.[74] VHL gene expression has been detected in all human tissues tested; the 6- and 6.5-kb transcripts likely represent alternatively spliced forms of g7 mRNA. The human VHL gene, which has three exons, encodes a protein of 213 amino acids.

GENETIC DIAGNOSIS OF VHL

The gold standard for diagnosis of von Hippel-Lindau disease is the identification of germ line mutations in patients suspected of having the illness. Previously, the best available diagnostic test in at-risk asymptomatic VHL family members was the use of linkage analysis.[71] Now that the VHL gene has been identified, germ line mutation detection can be used to establish the diagnosis of VHL in individuals with clinical pictures suggestive of von Hippel-Lindau disease, to identify mutation carriers in at-risk members of VHL families, and to identify the germ line mutation that characterizes each family. The detection of germ line mutation

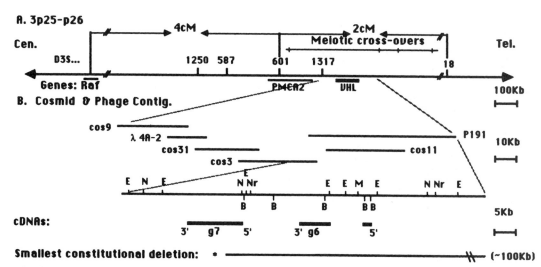

Fig. 27-13 Physical and genetic map encompassing the VHL gene locus on chromosome 3p. The VHL locus was determined by meiotic mapping and by multipoint linkage analysis. The nested deletions identified in the germ line DNA of the three unrelated VHL patients[146] are shown under the map. (*From Latif et al.[74] Used with permission.*)

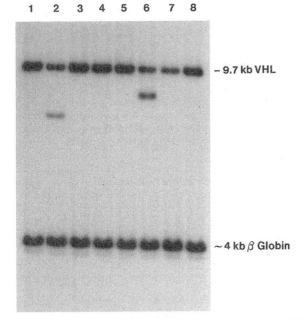

Fig. 27-14 Stolle et al. Analyzed in detail the characteristics of the germ line VHL gene in 93 families seen at the National Cancer Institute. A new method for detection of deletion (or partial deletion) of the VHL gene was developed. In normal individuals, a single 22-kb *Eco*RI or 9.7-kb *Eco*RI/*Ase*I fragment was detected by hybridization with the g7 cDNA probe. In individuals with partial deletions of the VHL gene, a slower or faster migrating fragment was detected in addition to the normal-sized fragment. A germ line deletion of the entire VHL gene was suspected when there was a reduction of signal intensity of the fragment hybridized to the g7 cDNA. Lane 7 VHL is deleted, lanes 2 and 6 represent partial deletion (*From Stolle et al.[75] Used with permission.*)

initially varied from 39 to 75 percent. Now, with improved methodology, it should be possible to identify germ line mutations in virtually all families with VHL (Fig. 27-14).[75]

The National Cancer Institute and University of Pennsylvania groups reported detection of germ line mutations in 100 percent (93/93) of VHL families. Improved mutation detection in VHL required the use of panel mutation detection methods to detect all the types of mutations that produce VHL disease (Fig. 27-15). The methods used included quantitative Southern blotting to detect deletions of the entire VHL gene, Southern blotting to detect gene

Improved Detection of Germline VHL Mutations
Cathe Stolle/U of P

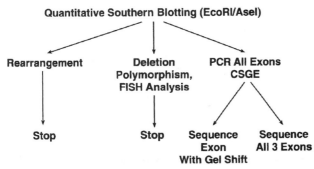

Fig. 27-15 Flow sheet of methods used sequentially by Cathy Stolle at the University of Pennsylvania to detect germ line VHL mutations in 100 percent (93/93) of VHL families.

rearrangements, fluorescence *in situ* hybridization to confirm deletions, and complete sequencing of the gene.

GENOTYPE/PHENOTYPE CORRELATIONS

Clinical heterogeneity is a feature of VHL. To determine the relationship between VHL gene mutations and the clinical manifestation of the VHL, Chen et al. searched for VHL gene mutations in 114 families (Fig. 27-16). Mutations, including microdeletions/insertions, nonsense mutations, deletions, or missense mutations, were detected in 85/114 (75 percent) families. Mutations were detected in each of the three exons, clustering in the 3' end of exon 1 and the 5' end of exon 3. There were a small number of mutations in exon 2. While 56 percent of the mutations associated with VHL Type I mutations were deletions, nonsense mutations, or microdeletions/insertions, 96 percent of mutations in VHL Type II (VHL with pheochromocytoma) kindreds were found to be missense mutations. There was also a clustering of VHL Type II mutations in a small region in the 5' end of exon 3 of the VHL gene; mutation in codon 238 accounted for 43 percent of the VHL Type II mutations.[76] Subsequent studies confirm the association of missense mutations with VHL Type II families. Brauch et al. identified a missense mutation at nucleotide 505 (T to C) in 14 VHL Type II families from the Black Forest region of Germany. This mutation had been previously identified in two VHL Type II families living in Pennsylvania (the kindred previously described in "VHL: Genotypic Homogeneity/Phenotypic Heterogeneity"). Haplotype analysis among the 100 patients with the 505 mutation indicated a founder effect.[77] A nucleotide 547 missense mutation has also been described in a large VHL family with pheochromocytoma, with no members affected with renal cell carcinoma.[78] Similar mutation patterns have been detected in families from Europe[79,80] and Japan.[81–83]

Hereditary forms of pheochromocytoma are associated with VHL, multiple endocrine neoplasia type II (MEN II), or neurofibromatosis type 1. Families with multiple pheochromocytomas in which there is uncertainty about the diagnosis are candidates for VHL gene mutation analysis.[77,79,80,82–85] For example, the abdominal imaging studies in Fig. 27-17 are from an 11-year-old boy with pheochromocytoma whose mother had had a pheochromocytoma removed when she was 11 years of age and whose uncle had died at age 9 years with severe hypertension. The clinical impression had previously been that this family was affected with either MENII or "familial pheochromocytoma."

When the child's mother underwent abdominal imaging (Fig. 27-18), she was found to have a pancreatic mass, which was removed surgically and found to be an islet cell tumor. Germ line VHL gene mutation analysis was performed and a nucleotide 595 (leucine-phenylalanine) missense mutation was detected, confirming the diagnosis of von Hippel Lindau Type II.

When a 25-year-old female from a pheochromocytoma family (6 other members were diagnosed with pheochromocytoma) was evaluated, a retroperitoneal mass was detected (Fig. 27-19). She was found to have malignant pheochromocytoma with pulmonary metastases. Germ line VHL mutation analysis revealing a missense mutation in exon 2 confirmed the diagnosis of VHL, Type II.

Penetrance of Different Mutations

There is evidence that the penetrance of the VHL gene depends on the particular germ line mutation. About 60 percent of people with the 505 mutation develop clinical or radiologic evidence of VHL during their lifetimes (Neumann; unpublished work).

Modifier Genes and VHL

Individuals with identical germ line VHL mutations differ in the degree of disease severity. In a search for evidence of genes modifying the expression of VHL mutant genes, Webster et al. examined 183 individuals with germ line VHL mutations for the

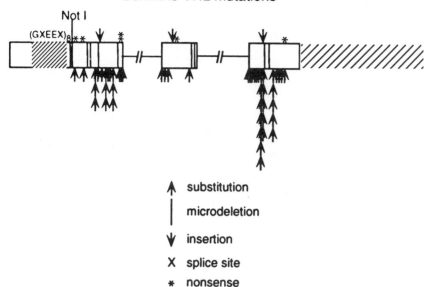

Fig. 27-16 VHL gene germ line mutation distribution in VHL kindreds. The boxes indicate cloned exons. The 3′ UTR and the exon 1 pentameric acidic repeat are indicated by cross hatching. (*From Chen et al.*[76] *Used with permission.*)

presence and number of retinal angiomas.[86] The number of ocular tumors was significantly correlated in closely related individuals, but not in more distantly related individuals. The findings suggested that the development of ocular tumors was determined at an early age and was influenced by genetic or environmental modifier effects that act at multiple sites.

MUTATIONS OF THE VHL TUMOR-SUPPRESSOR GENE IN RENAL CARCINOMA

To evaluate the role of VHL in the origin of sporadic, non-hereditary renal-cell carcinoma, Gnarra et al.[87] searched for VHL gene mutation in tumors from 108 patients with both localized and advanced renal-cell carcinoma (Fig. 27-20). LOH of the VHL gene was detected in 98 percent of clear-cell renal carcinomas; VHL mutations were identified in 57 percent of the samples (Fig. 27-21A). Mutations, including nucleotide deletions, substitutions, insertions, and nonsense mutations, were found in each of the three exons. The presence of splice-site mutations that would eliminate the translation of exon 2 and the high percentage of mutations (45 percent) involving exon 2, indicated that exon 2 may have an importatn function of the protein.[3,72] The detection of somatic VHL mutation in small, clinically localized renal cell carcinomas (<2 cm) suggests that inactivation of this gene is an early event in renal carcinogenesis.[88] When 119 tumors from 11 different tissues were evaluated, no additional somatic VHL gene mutations were detected. Neither chromosome 3 LOH nor VHL gene mutations were detected in tumor tissue from patients with papillary renal carcinoma (Fig. 27-21B). VHL gene mutations have been identified in clear-cell renal carcinomas in Japan,[89] Europe,[90–92] and North America.[84]

When tumor tissues from patients with hereditary renal carcinoma characterized by 3;8 translocation[13] were analyzed for VHL mutations,[72,93] two of four tumors were found to have mutations of the wild-type VHL gene. In this kindred, it is the inherited derivative chromosome 8 carrying the portion of chromosome 3 distal to the breakpoint that is deleted in the kidney tumors and the normal chromosome 3 that is retained.[14] The wild-type VHL allele was found to be mutated in the tumors, demonstrating a mechanism of clear-cell renal carcinoma tumorigenesis in the chromosome (3;8) translocation family that involves the loss of both copies of the VHL gene.[72,93] The association of

VHL gene mutation and clear-cell renal carcinoma in three independent clinical entities [(a) sporadic clear-cell renal carcinoma, (b) clear-cell renal carcinoma associated with von Hippel Lindau, and (c) clear-cell renal carcinoma associated with the 3;8 translocation hereditary clear-cell renal carcinoma], demonstrates that inactivation of the VHL gene is a critical event in clear-cell renal carcinoma. Detection of VHL gene inactivation in clear-cell renal carcinoma but not in papillary renal carcinoma, supports the proposal of a molecular genetic classification of renal carcinoma, papillary versus clear-cell renal carcinoma, with clear-cell renal carcinoma being characterized by inactivation of the VHL gene.

The microdissection techniques for archival DNA[94] provide a method for detection of VHL gene mutations in paraffin-embedded material,[95] which may furnish clinicians with improved strategies for both diagnosis[96] and classification of renal tumors. Similar methods applied to aspirate cytology may enable improved clarification of whether or not an indeterminate mass in a kidney or other organ is a clear-cell renal carcinoma.

VHL gene mutations were detected when the sporadic form of other tumors that appear in VHL patients were analyzed. Kanno et al. detected abnormal VHL gene SSCP patterns in 7 of 13 sporadic hemangioblastomas, 3 of which were characterized by direct sequencing. Somatic mutations in the three tumors included two missense mutations and one microdeletion; one in exon 1 and two in exon 2.[97] Gilcrease et al. detected a somatic VHL gene mutation in 1 of 2 sporadic cystadenomas of the epididymis.[98] VHL gene mutations appear to play a role in tumorigenesis in a subset of sporadic epididymal cystadenomas and CNS hemangioblastomas.

SILENCING THE VHL GENE BY DNA METHYLATION

Herman et al. demonstrated another potential mechanism for inactivation of the VHL gene in clear-cell renal carcinoma by showing hypermethylation of the normally unmethylated CpG island in the 5′ region of the gene. The hypermethylation was observed in 5 of 26 (19 percent) clear-cell renal carcinomas evaluated. In four of the tumors, one copy of the VHL gene was lost; the fifth retained two heavily methylated VHL alleles. One of the five tumors had a missense mutation in addition to hypermethylation of the single remaining allele. The other four

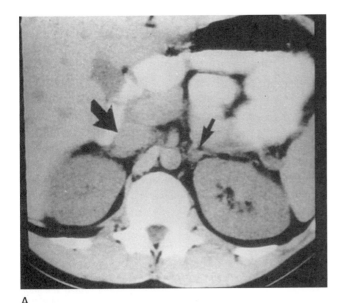

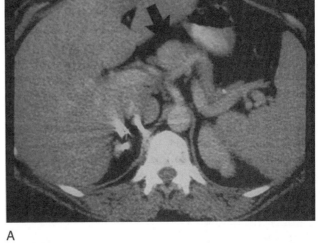

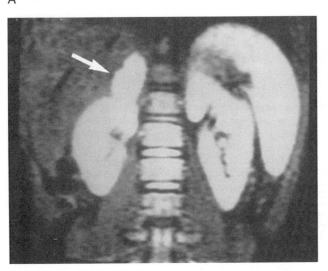

A

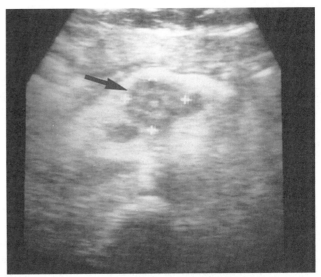

B

Fig. 27-17 Abdominal CT scan (*A*) and abdominal MRI examination (*B*) reveal the presence of pheochromocytoma in an 11-year-old child found to have a mutation of the VHL gene. (*From Linehan et al.*[145] *Used with permission.*)

Fig. 27-18 Abdominal CT scan (*A*) revealed a pancreatic lesion in a woman whose 11-year-old child was found to have a pheochromocytoma. Abdominal ultrasound (*B*) confirmed that the pancreatic lesion is solid. The mass was removed surgically and found to be an islet cell tumor. (*From Linehan et al.*[145] *Used with permission.*)

tumors with VHL hypermethylation had no detectable mutations. None of the five tumors expressed the VHL gene. When one of the renal cell carcinoma cell lines with a hypermethylated (and silent) VHL gene was treated with 5-aza-2′-deoxycytidine, the VHL gene was reexpressed. Although the extent of hypermethylation of the VHL gene in a larger series of tumors and the potential role of agents such as 5-aza-2′-deoxycytidine remain to be determined, this study does provide an additional mechanism for inactivation of the VHL gene in clear-cell renal carcinoma.[99]

FUNCTION OF VHL

Recently, the function of VHL has begun to be elucidated. The VHL tumor-suppressor gene forms a complex with homology to components of the SCF family of E3 ubiquitin-ligase complex and targets HIF for degradation. VHL exists as part of a multisubunit complex containing four other characterized subunits. The complex is now recognized to be one of several SCF complexes, which represent one class of ubiquitin ligases (Fig. 27-22*A*). Based on protein sequence homologies, the VHL complex was proposed to be one of several FCS complexes, which represent one class of ubiquitin ligases. The VHL complex has been isolated and shown to be capable of mediating the transfer of ubiquitin to at least one critical intracellular substrate, thereby targeting it for proteosome-mediated degradation. The substrate, the α subunit of the hypoxia-inducible transcription factor HIF-1, is bound to the VHL complex, but is only ubiquinated and degraded in the presence of oxygen (Fig. 27-22*B*). The absence of VHL-dependent ubiquitination under hypoxic conditions results in the accumulation of HIF-1 and its ability to control the transcription of hypoxia-induced genes. Structural studies demonstrate that VHL is most likely the homologue of the F-box proteins found in all SCF complexes. These proteins represent the substrate recognition subunits of the ubiquitin ligases.

The recently solved structure of VHL bound to elongin C[100] reveals three classes of missense mutations that are found in families with germ-line mutations of the VHL gene as well as in tumors from patients with clear-cell renal carcinoma.[72,101] (a) Those that affect complex formation: The structure of the ternary VCB complex reveals an interface between VHL and elongin C

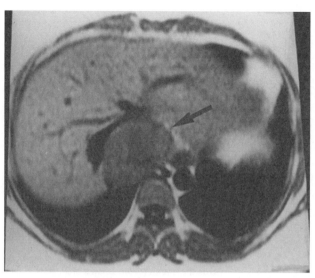

A

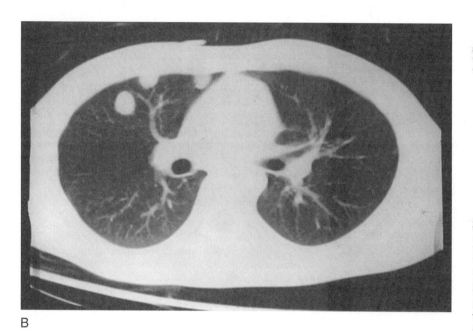

B

Fig. 27-19 Abdominal CT scan (*A*) revealed a retroperitoneal mass in a 25-year-old female who had had two previous surgical resections of pheochromocytoma. Lung CT (*B*) revealed the presence of metastatic foci in the chest. VHL gene analysis revealed a mutation in exon 2 of the VHL gene, confirming the diagnosis of VHL. (*From Linehan et al.*[145] *Used with permission.*)

and suggests similarity between a 35-residue domain of VHL that binds elongin C (the α domain) and the F box that binds Skp1 (Fig. 27-22*C*).[100] (b) Those that affect substrate binding: The structural analysis revealed the presence of a β domain, which has been shown to bind directly to the HIF, targeting HIF for ubiquitin-mediated degradation[102] (Fig. 27-22*C*). (c) Overall structural stability: Mutations of residues buried in the structure outside of the α or β domain are predicted to affect overall structural stability of the VCB-Cul2 complex.

The oxygen-controlled ubiquitination of HIF via the VHL complex explains several biochemical phenotypes associated with the inactivation of VHL. Most striking are the highly vascular tumors associated with homozygous loss of VHL function. Tumor development in von Hippel-Lindau (as well as clear-cell renal-cell carcinoma) is associated with inactivation of both copies of the VHL gene. The highly vascular nature of the VHL-associated renal, adrenal, pancreatic, ocular, and CNS tumors can be understood in the setting of the regulation of HIF stability by the VCB-Cul2 complex. A hallmark of these tumors is their high degree of vascularity and expression of hypoxia-inducible genes, including VEGF.[103] Cells lacking functional pVHL fail to degrade

HIF under normoxic conditions[104] (see Fig. 27-22*C*). Naturally occurring, disease-causing VHL mutations can be found in either the α domain or the β domain. β-Domain mutants fail to bind to HIF,[104] whereas α-domain mutants (elongin C/B binding box) retain HIF-1α binding activity, but will not ubiquinate HIF.[102,105,106] Given the many manifestations of the VHL −/− phenotype, it is likely that the VCB-Cul2 complex targets other substrates.[103] Pause et al. demonstrated that VHL is required for cell-cycle exit upon serum withdrawal, and a VHL target is thus implicated in the regulation of cell-cycle exit.[107] Whether the ubiquitin ligase activity of the VCB-Cul2 complex will explain the full spectrum of the VHL −/− phenotype remains to be determined.

Carbonic Anhydrases and VHL

Ivanov et al. reported that carbonic anhydrases 9 and 12 are downregulated by the VHL gene.[108] The authors used RNA differential display to compare genes expressed in a VHL null renal carcinoma cell line with the same cell line expressing wild-type VHL. Increased expression of CA9 and CA12 was found in two VHL

Sporadic renal carcinoma *VHL* mutations

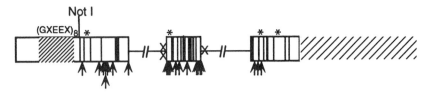

↑ substitution

| microdeletion

↓ insertion

X splice site

* nonsense

Fig. 27-20 VHL gene mutation distribution in sporadic, clear cell renal carcinoma. The boxes indicate cloned exons. The 3′ UTR and the exon 1 pentameric acidic repeat are indicated by crosshatching. (*From Gnarra et al.*[72] *Used with permission.*)

null renal carcinoma cell lines. Carbonic anhydrases 9 and 12 are single-pass cell membrane-spanning proteins that catalyze the reversal hydration of CO_2. Of particular interest, CA9 is identical to the MN antigen, and is the target of the G250 antibody.[109,110] The MN antigen is reported to be characteristic of clear-cell renal carcinomas; one antigen that is characteristic of clear-cell renal carcinomas is a protein under the control of the VHL gene.

Constitutional Translocation of Chromosome 3p and Clear-Cell Renal Carcinoma

Several families have been described with an inherited predisposition to develop clear-cell renal carcinoma associated with constitutional balanced translocations involving chromosome 3p and either chromosome 2, 6, or 8.[13,19,111] Studies of the renal tumors from these families have provided insight into mechanisms of formation of clear-cell renal carcinomas. Clear-cell renal carcinomas from members of the t(3;8) family, and from members of the t(3;2) family showed a loss of the derivative chromosome (the chromosome to which the distal portion of chromosome 3p had been translocated).[14,111] Clear-cell renal carcinomas from members of these families also showed somatic mutation of the VHL remaining gene in 2 of 4 tumors studied in the t(3,8) family and in 4 of 5 tumors studied in the t(3,2) family.[93,111] The VHL mutation found in each renal tumor was different.

These results suggest that clear-cell renal carcinomas develop in members of chromosome t(3;8) and t(3;2) translocation families by a series of steps: (a) inheritance of the balanced chromosome 3p translocation; (b) loss of the derivative chromosome bearing the distal portion of chromosome 3p (a somatic event leading to the loss of one copy of the VHL gene); and (c) somatic mutation of the VHL gene located on the normal chromosome 3. These three events occur within a single renal epithelial cell and initiate malignant transformation. The process of formation of clear cell renal carcinomas in individuals with the chromosome t(3;8) and t(3;2) translocations appears to be a variation of the events leading to sporadic clear-cell renal carcinomas.[88] The initiating event in both situations appears to be a loss or inactivation of both copies of the VHL gene. See Fig. 27-23.

PAPILLARY RENAL CARCINOMA

Five to 10 percent of sporadic renal carcinoma is the papillary histologic type.[3,11,72] Papillary renal carcinoma is significantly less hypervascular and tends to be of lower grade than clear-cell renal carcinoma. The clinical course of papillary renal carcinoma may be more indolent than that of clear-cell renal carcinoma.[112,113] Sporadic papillary renal carcinoma frequently appears as bilateral, multifocal disease; multiple tumor nodules and areas of atypical hyperplastic growth may appear throughout the kidney.[114,115] Whether the presence of multifocal, bilateral papillary renal

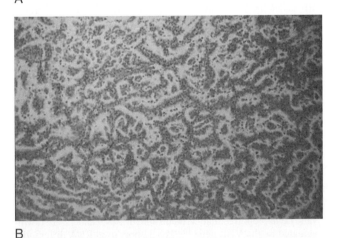

A

B

Fig. 27-21 Somatic VHL gene mutations and LOH are characteristic of clear-cell renal carcinoma (*A*) but are not found in papillary renal carcinoma (*B*). (*From Linehan et al.*[145] *Used with permission.*)

carcinoma is primarily a result of genetic events, is secondary to an agent such as a renotrophic virus, or is the result of exposure to environmental factors, is not known.

Most common among the cytogenetic changes that have been described in tumor tissue from patients with papillary renal carcinoma are those involving trisomy of chromosomes 7, 10, and 17.[32,114,116] More recently, a consistent t(X;1)(p11.2;q21) translocation in papillary renal cell carcinoma was described as a feature of at least some papillary renal carcinomas.[117–119] Whether or not the t(X;1) translocation represents a distinct subtype of papillary renal cell carcinoma is currently under study.

HEREDITARY PAPILLARY RENAL CELL CARCINOMA

Multigenerational kindreds in which members develop papillary renal cell carcinoma have been described by Zbar et al (Fig. 27-24).[16,17,120] Affected family members develop multiple tumors of varying size in both kidneys (Fig. 27-25). In this disorder, which has an autosomal dominant inheritance pattern, the renal tumors are the uniformly papillary histologic type.[16]

Germ Line and Somatic Mutations in the Tyrosine Kinase Domain of the MET Protooncogene in Papillary Renal Carcinomas

Malignant papillary renal carcinomas are characterized by trisomy of chromosomes 7, 16, and 17, and in men, by loss of the Y

chromosome. The HPRC was localized to chromosome 7q31.1-34 in a 24 cM interval between D7S496 and D7S1837. Among the genes located in the nonrecombinant interval was the MET protooncogene. Emphasis was placed on the MET protooncogene because cytogenetic and fluorescent *in situ* hybridization (FISH) studies showed chromosome 7 duplication rather than loss, suggesting that the gene responsible for HPRC was a protooncogene rather than a tumor-suppressor gene. Also, the MET gene was in the same supergene family (receptor tyrosine kinase) as RET, a protooncogene mutated in another inherited cancer syndrome (MEN II).

Genome Structure of the MET Protooncogene

Although discovered in 1984, the MET protooncogene's genomic structure was not determined until later, as a first step toward mutation analysis.[121] The MET gene contains 21 exons. These exons encode a receptor tyrosine kinase that contains extracellular, transmembrane, juxtamembrane, and tyrosine kinase domains. Primers were designed for the polymerase chain reaction to test for mutations in MET in affected members of HPRC families. Germ line missense mutations located in the tyrosine kinase domain of the MET protooncogene were detected in the germ line of affected members of HPRC families and in a subset of sporadic papillary renal carcinomas. Two large North American families with HPRC were identified with identical mutations in the MET protooncogene.[122] Affected members of the two families shared the same haplotype within and immediately distal to the MET gene,

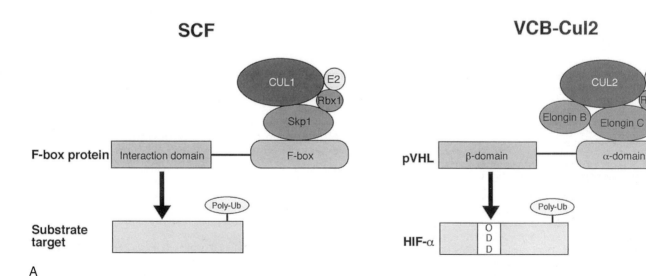

A

Fig. 27-22 *A*, A model of the interaction between pVHL and ElonginC–ElonginB, CUL2, Rbx1 and hypoxia-inducible factor (modified from Krek et al.[105]) Structural analogies exist between the recently described class of ubiquitin ligases, termed Skp1-Cdc53/CUL1-F-box protein (SCF) and the pVHL ElonginC–ElonginB CUL2 Rbx1 complex.[103] *B*, Under hypoxic conditions, HIF accumulates, leading to increased VEGF, Glut 1, and PDGF. *C*, Mutations in the α-domain affect VCB complex formation; mutations in the β-domain of pVHL affect substrate specificity.[102,105,147]

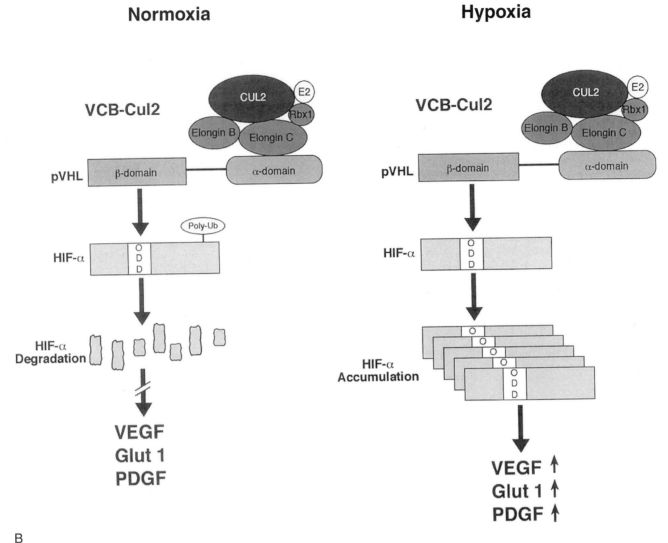

B

Fig. 27-22 (Continued)

suggesting a founder effect. That is, both families had a common ancestor. The age-dependent penetrance of the H1112R mutation was determined (Fig. 27-26). The H1112R mutation produced a late-onset malignancy of low penetrance. The estimated risk at 40 years of age among carriers was 19 percent (95 percent confidence interval, 5 to 34 percent).

Duplication of the Chromosome Carrying the Mutant MET Allele in HPRC Tumors

Although trisomy of chromosome 7 was demonstrated in HPRC renal tumors, it was not known whether the process of chromosome duplication in HPRC tumors was random or nonrandom. Sixteen renal tumors from two patients with the MET H1112R mutation were studied by FISH and by quantitative PCR to identify which chromosome 7 was duplicated in the tumors.[123] FISH showed trisomy 7 in all renal tumors. In all 16 tumors, there was an increased signal intensity of the microsatellite allele from the chromosome bearing the mutant MET allele, as compared with the chromosome bearing the wild-type MET.[123] Similar work was independently performed by the Kovacs laboratory with identical results.[124] The study demon-

strates nonrandom duplication of the chromosome bearing the mutated MET in hereditary papillary renal carcinomas.

Mutations in the MET Protooncogene Produce a Gain of Function

The MET receptor tyrosine kinase transduces motility, proliferation, and morphogenic signals of hepatocyte growth factor/scatter factor in epithelial cells.[125–127] During embryogenesis, the MET receptor HGF/SF pathway is required for normal muscle and liver development. The effect of each MET mutation was examined in biological and biochemical assays.[128]

MET mutants exhibited increased levels of tyrosine phosphorylation and enhanced kinase activity toward an exogenous substrate when compared to wild-type MET. NIH3T3 cells expressing mutant MET molecules formed foci *in vitro* and were tumorigenic in nude mice versus wild-type MET. A strong correlation was observed between the enzymatic and biological activity of the MET mutants, indicating that the tumorigenesis is quantitatively related to its level of activation.

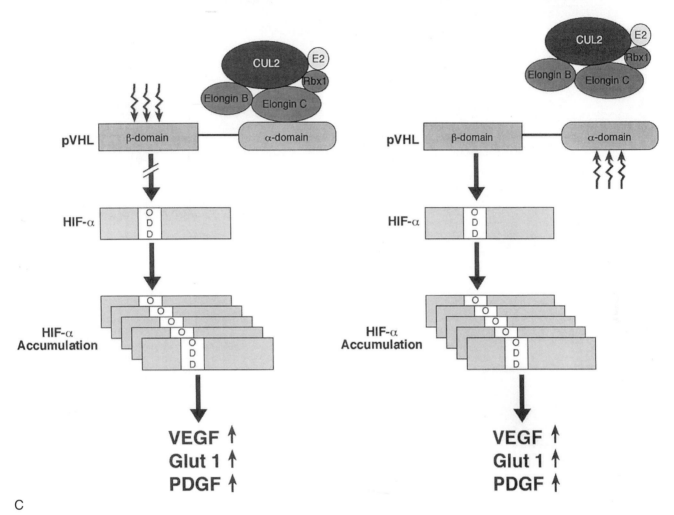

VHL mutation, β-domain

VHL mutation, α-domain

C

Fig. 27-22 (Continued)

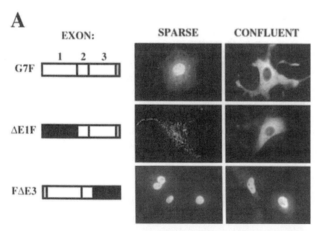

Fig. 27-23 Localization of the VHL gene. The wild-type VHL protein is found predominantly in the cytoplasm when transiently transfected COS-7 cells are grown under confluent conditions and in the nucleus under sparse conditions (*top* panel). When an exon 1 deletion mutant is analyzed, immunofluorescence localizes the protein to the cytoplasm in both sparse as well as confluent cells. When an exon 3 deletion mutant is introduced into the COS-7 cells, there is striking localization predominantly to the nucleus in the sparse, as well as the confluent, conditions. (*From Lee et al.[148] Used with permission.*)

Similarities Between Mutations in MET, RET, c-KIT, and c-erbB Protooncogenes

There are striking homologies in the location of the mutations observed in the MET, RET, c-KIT, and c-erbB protooncogenes.[122,129] c-KIT is a receptor tyrosine kinase that is expressed on stem cells in the bone marrow. Activating c-KIT mutations have been detected in mastocytosis and can be associated with malignant hematologic disorders.[130] RET, also a receptor tyrosine kinase expressed in thyroid cells, is the receptor for glial-derived growth factor. Germ line mutations in RET are found in the hereditary cancer syndrome MEN II. The c-erbB protooncogene is an avian protooncogene.[131]

All four transmembrane tyrosine kinase receptors have mutation in the tyrosine kinase domains. In four instances, the mutations in MET were located in codons homologous to mutation in RET, c-KIT, or c-erbB. The results indicate that there are hot spots for mutation within the tyrosine kinase domain that are common to several receptor tyrosine kinases (Fig. 27-27).[131]

Hereditary Papillary Renal Carcinoma: Morphologic Correlations

Studies by Delahunt and Eble indicated that papillary renal carcinoma could be subdivided into types 1 and 2 based on

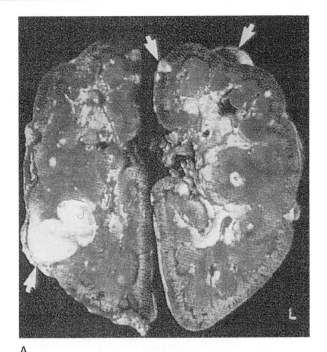

A

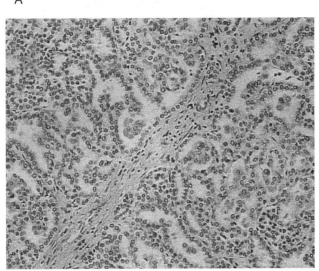

B

Fig. 27-24 *A,* Photograph of renal tumor from patient IV-8 (family 160) with HPRC, a 35-year-old woman treated by bilateral nephrectomy. Arrows point to renal tumors. *B,* Photomicrograph of renal tumor from patient IV-8. Note papillary histology. (*From Schmidt et al.*[131] *Used with permission.*)

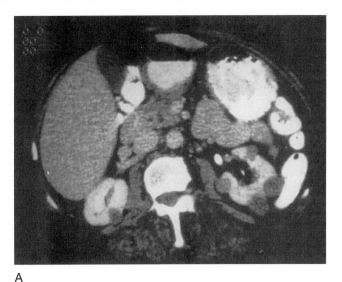

A

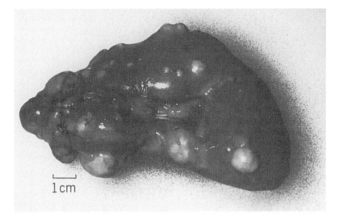

B

Fig. 27-25 A kidney from an affected individual in a HPRC kindred showing multifocal papillary renal carcinomas. (*From Zbar et al.*[16] *Used with permission.*)

morphologic criteria.[132] Studies by Moch et al. indicate that papillary renal carcinoma type 1 and type 2 had a different prognosis.[133] Careful morphologic studies show that patients with HPRC had type 1 papillary renal carcinomas.[134] Patients with sporadic papillary renal carcinomas associated with somatic MET mutations also had type 1 papillary renal carcinomas.

Denaturing high-performance liquid chromatorgraphy (DHPLC) is a recently developed sensitive mutation detection method. Nickerson et al.[135] demonstrated that the mutations in the tyrosine kinase domain of the MET protooncogene could be readily detected by DHPLC; each MET mutation had a characteristic elution profile, a molecular signature.

Familial Renal Oncocytomas

At the National Cancer Institute, five families were seen in which individuals were affected with bilateral, multiple, renal oncocytomas.[136] One identical twin pair was affected with bilateral multiple renal oncocytomas. Because renal oncocytomas were in most cases asymptomatic, occurred at a late age, and required imaging studies for detection, it was initially difficult to detect the hereditary pattern of this disorder. Further studies are in progress to identify the genetic factor that predisposes individuals to the development of renal oncocytomas.

The Birt-Hogg-Dubé Syndrome

The Birt-Hogg-Dubá syndrome (BHD) is a rare disorder, inherited as an autosomal dominant trait (Fig. 27-28*A*), characterized by the presence of multiple, smooth, skin-colored papules located on the head and neck (Fig. 27-28*B*).[137] Histologic examination of these skin papules show disorganization of hair follicle structure, increased amounts of mucin, and thin, elongated, anastomosing epithelial strands (Fig. 27-28*C*);[138] these hamartomas of the hair follicle are called fibrofolliculomas. In 1993, Roth et al. described a single patient with BHD and bilateral renal carcinoma.[139] In 2000, Toro et al. revisited the renal tumor families described by

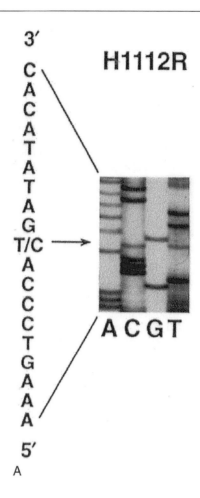

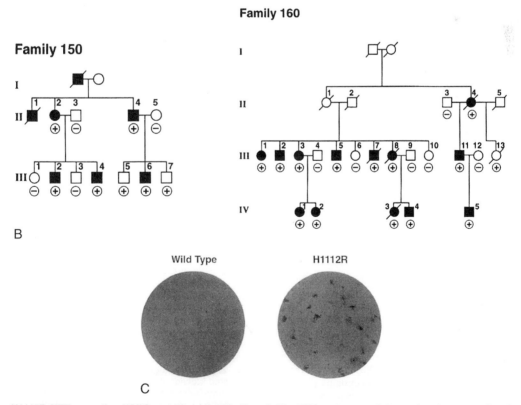

Fig. 27-26 The H1112R MET germ line HPRC mutation identification *A*, The DNA sequence of the region demonstrating the mutation. *B*, Segregation of the germ line mutation with the phenotype in pedigrees of two HPRC families, 150 and 160. Individuals predicted not to be carriers of the HPRC gene,—; individuals predicted to be carriers of the HPRC gene,+. The solid symbols represent those found to be affected. *C*, The NIH3T3 growth focus induced by wild-type and mutant MET. (*From Schmidt et al.*[131] *Used with permission.*)

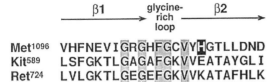

Fig. 27-27 The amino acid sequence of the homologous regions of Hir, Ret and Kit shown in comparison with MET in the region of the H1112R mutation. The site of the H1112R mutation is outlined in black. The codons conserved in the four proteins are outlined in gray. (*From Schmidt et al.*[131] *Used with permission.*)

Weirich et al.[136] In renal oncocytoma families 166 and 168, multiple members were affected with BHD. To evaluate these findings, Toro et al. studied 152 members of families with inherited renal cancer.

The signs of BHD were found in renal oncocytoma families 166 and 168, and also in family 171, a family with papillary renal carcinoma type 2. The signs of BHD were not found in families with members affected with von Hippel-Lindau disease or with hereditary papillary renal carcinoma type 1. Families with BHD did not display mutations in the VHL gene or the tyrosine kinase domain of the MET protooncogene.[138] These results suggest BHD may be a novel marker of kidney neoplasia, and that BHD patients and their relatives should be screened for renal tumors.

GENETICS OF HEREDITARY RENAL CARCINOMA

There are three forms of hereditary renal carcinoma: von Hippel-Lindau; hereditary clear cell renal carcinoma; and hereditary papillary renal carcinoma. VHL is characterized by mutation of the VHL gene. Currently VHL gene mutation can be detected in 75 to 99 percent of VHL families. As advanced mutation detection methods are used (FISH-based deletion analysis, analysis of the 3′UTR, promoter, etc.), the mutation detection percentage increases. VHL has been categorized as Type I and Type II, with Type II families being characterized by the presence of pheochromocytoma. Nearly all of the Type II families carry a missense mutation, and there is a VHL Type II hot spot in exon 3 of the VHL gene. Further studies in progress will determine whether there are genotype/phenotype correlations with other VHL-associated tumors, such as CNS hemangioblastoma, pancreatic tumors, and endolymphatic sac tumors.

The role of genetic and clinical screening programs in the management of individuals at risk for a multisystem hereditary cancer syndrome such as VHL is complex. Unlike some syndromes in which testing is not routinely performed in at-risk individuals under the age of 18 because medical intervention is not required, in individuals at risk for VHL germ line mutation, testing is recommended by most clinicians at an early age. Early intervention may be of significant benefit to affected VHL patients, particularly those with retinal, adrenal, and CNS lesions. Retinal angiomas, which can occur in very young children, are bilateral and multifocal and can cause early loss of vision, which eventually may lead to blindness. Treatment with laser therapy is performed with the goal of preservation of vision and with the intent of decreasing the morbidity of VHL-associated retinal angiomas.

Pheochromocytoma and CNS hemangioblastomas can appear before the age of 10. Occult pheochromocytoma can be lethal, and early detection of functioning pheochromocytomas is critical. While the benefit of detection of an occult functioning pheochromocytoma is clear, the benefit of detection and treatment of occult, nonfunctioning pheochromocytomas is not yet determined. In some patients, occult CNS hemangioblastomas also can have significant morbidity, including stroke, paralysis, and death. However, longitudinal studies will be needed to determine whether

aggressive screening for CNS lesions, as well as other manifestations of VHL, will enhance quality of life or increase survival.

The role of early diagnosis of VHL-associated renal, pancreatic, and endolymphatic sac tumors is less well defined. Greater understanding of the natural history of these VHL manifestations is required for determining the most appropriate management of patients with these malignancies. At present, there is no consensus for which patients with VHL-associated renal carcinomas are best treated with surgical resection. Renal-cell carcinoma can spread in asymptomatic individuals, and advanced renal carcinoma has been reported as the direct cause of death in one-third of VHL patients.[15,140] As such, physicians managing these patients often recommend removal of the tumors when they have reached a certain size, such as 2.5 to 3 cm. The clinical rationale is that removal of tumors of this size may reduce the incidence of metastasis, while preserving quality of life. VHL-associated pancreatic islet cell tumors are malignant lesions that can become metastatic. Surgical resection is often recommended with the intent to prevent metastasis, however, prospective trials are

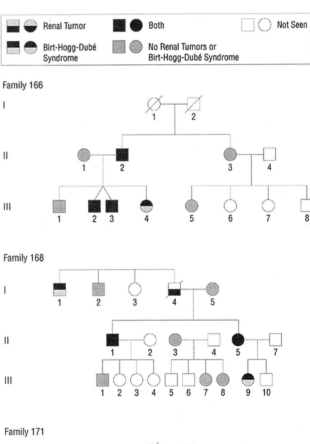

Fig. 27-28 A, Pedigrees from Birt-Hogg-Dubé (BHD) kindreds. Indicated individuals are affected with cutaneous manifestations of Birt-Hogg-Dubé syndrome and renal tumors. B, Cutaneous manifestations of BHD (A,B,C,D) most often appear in the facial area, neck, and upper trunk. C, The microscopic features of the cutaneous manifestations of BHD (A,B,C,D) reveal fibrofolliculoma with multiple anastomosing strands of epithelial cells extending from the central follicle. (*From Toro et al.*[138] *Used with permission.*)

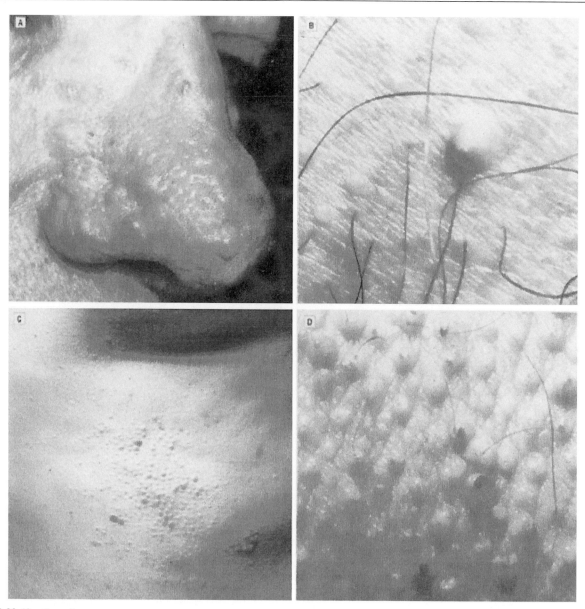

Fig. 27-28 (Continued)

required to define the role of surgery in the management of these tumors. The endolymphatic sac tumors represent a similar clinical challenge. These tumors can have profound manifestations in VHL patients. Patients with ELST may lose total hearing in an ear within a matter of 3 to 4 days. Trials are in progress to determine whether early surgical intervention will preserve hearing in VHL patients with ELST.

When tumors which had formed in other organs affected by VHL (such as sporadic cerebellar hemangioblastoma and epididymal cystadenoma) were analyzed, mutations were found. Further studies of these tumors, as well as of other sporadic tumors from organs affected by VHL (such as pancreatic tumors, ELST, retinal angiomas, and pheochromocytoma), are required to determine the role of the VHL gene inactivation in these neoplasms.

Papillary Renal Carcinoma

Much remains to be learned about the genetics and the subtypes of papillary renal carcinoma. Little is known about the factors associated with the development of multifocal, bilateral sporadic papillary renal carcinoma. The genetic or environmental features that characterize individuals with bilateral, multifocal papillary renal carcinoma with no apparent hereditary feature (no parents, siblings, or offspring involved) remain to be determined. A number of kindreds have been evaluated in which multiple members (two to six) have clear-cell renal carcinoma. Whether these findings are coincidental, the result of an undetermined combination of genetic and environmental factors, or an example of complex genetics, is not yet known.

VHL gene mutation analysis is now an integral aspect in the diagnosis of VHL and of screening of at-risk, asymptomatic individuals. Predictions about which types of tumors will appear are possible in some instances, particularly in VHL Type II kindreds. Germ line VHL gene mutation analysis is likely to be useful in kindreds with "familial pheochromocytoma," or in those with clinical manifestations of MEN II in whom the diagnosis is in doubt. VHL gene mutation analysis may be useful for assisting in

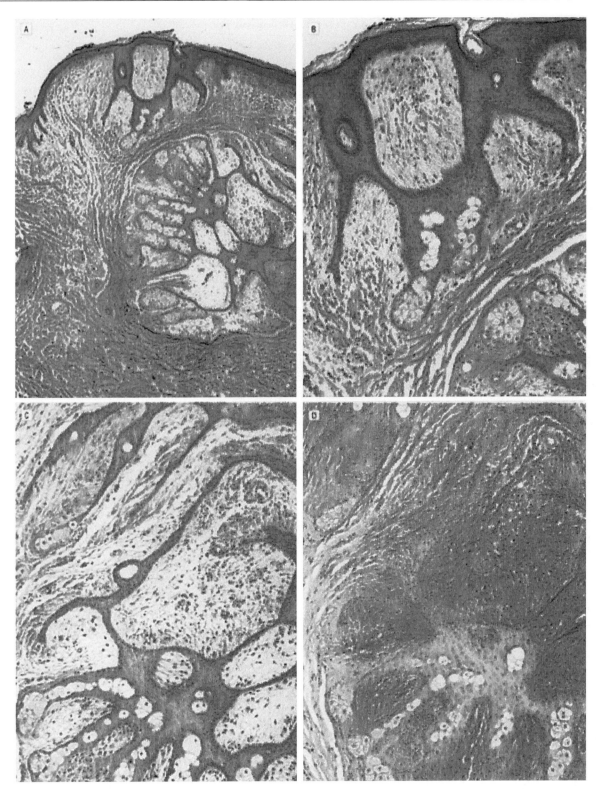

Fig. 27-28 (Continued)

the diagnosis of an indeterminate renal mass or in an extrarenal mass in a patient with clear-cell kidney cancer.

Patients who present with advanced renal carcinoma have an 8 to 15 percent 2-year survival. Those who are diagnosed with Stage I renal carcinoma have a 95 percent 5-year survival. It is possible that detection of an inactivated VHL gene will aid in the early diagnosis of clear-cell renal carcinoma. Cancer cells, including renal carcinoma cells, may circulate years in advance of the clinical detection of metastasis.[141-144] It is possible that detection of a mutated VHL gene in the urine or in circulating cells may provide a method for early diagnosis of this disease.

Ultimately, it is hoped that knowledge of the mechanism of the VHL gene and other genes involved in renal carcinoma will lead to the development of targeted methods for early diagnosis, prevention, and treatment of diseases such as sporadic and hereditary renal carcinoma.

ACKNOWLEDGMENT

We greatly acknowledge the work of our many collaborators and colleagues whose studies are discussed here.

REFERENCES

1. Boring CC, Squires TS, Tong T: Cancer statistics. *CA Cancer J Clin* **44**:7, 1994.
2. Linehan WM, Shipley W, Parkinson D: Cancer of the kidney and ureter, in DeVita VT, Hellman S, Rosenberg SA (eds): *Cancer: Principles and Practice of Oncology*, vol. 2, 4th ed. Philadelphia, JB Lippincott, 1996, pp. 19–46.
3. Linehan WM, Lerman MI, Zbar B: Identification of the VHL gene: its role in renal carcinoma. *JAMA* **273**:564, 1995.
4. Malker HR, Malker BK, McLaughlin JK, Blot WJ: Kidney cancer among leather workers. *Lancet* **1**:56, 1984.
5. Maclure M: Asbestos and renal adenocarcinoma: A case-control study. *Environ Res* **42**:353, 1987.
6. Maclure M, Willett W: A case-control study of diet and risk of renal adenocarcinoma. *Epidemiology* **1**:430, 1990.
7. Yu MC, Mack TM, Hanisch R, Cicioni C, Henderson BE: Cigarette smoking, obesity, diuretic use, and coffee consumption as risk factors for renal cell carcinoma. *J Natl Cancer Inst* **77**:351, 1986.
8. Chung-Park M, Parveen T, Lam M: Acquired cystic disease of the kidneys and renal cell carcinoma in chronic renal insufficiency without dialysis treatment. *Nephron* **53**:157, 1989.
9. Matson MA, Cohen EP: Acquired cystic kidney disease: occurrence, prevalence, and renal cancers. *Medicine (Baltimore)* **69**:217, 1990.
10. Brennan JF, Stilmant MM, Babayan RK, Siroky MB: Acquired renal cystic disease: Implications for the urologist. *Br J Urol* **67**:342, 1991.
11. Kovacs G, Ishikawa I: High incidence of papillary renal cell tumours in patients on chronic haemodialysis. *Histopathology* **22**:135, 1993.
12. Bard RH, Lord B, Fromowitz F: Papillary adenocarcinoma of kidney. *Urol.* **19**:16, 1982.
13. Cohen AJ, Li FP, Berg S, Marchetto DJ, Tsai S, Jacobs SC, Brown RS: Hereditary renal-cell carcinoma associated with a chromosomal translocation. *N Engl J Med* **301**:592, 1979.
14. Li FP, Decker H-JH, Zbar B, Stanton VP, Kovacs G, Seizinger BR, Aburantani H, Sandberg AA, Berg S, Hosoe S, Brown RS: Clinical and genetic studies of renal cell carcinomas in a family with a constitutional chromosome 3;8 translocation: Genetics of familial renal carcinoma. *Ann Intern Med* **118**:106, 1993.
15. Glenn GM, Choyke PL, Zbar B, Linehan WM: Von Hippel-Lindau disease: clinical review and molecular genetics, in Anderson EE (ed.): *Problems in Urologic Surgery: Benign and Malignant Tumors of the Kidney*, Philadelphia, JB Lippincott, 1990, pp. 312–330.
16. Zbar B, Tory K, Merino M, Schmidt L, Glenn G, Choyke P, Walther MM, Lerman M, Linehan WM: Hereditary papillary renal cell carcinoma. *J Urol* **151**:561, 1994.
17. Zbar B, Glenn G, Lubensky IA, Choyke P, Magnusson G, Bergerheim U, Pettersson S, Amin M, Hurley K, Linehan WM, Walther MM: Hereditary papillary renal cell carcinoma: Clinical studies in 10 families. *J Urol* **153**:907, 1995.
18. Pathak S, Strong LC, Ferrell RE, Trindade A: Familial renal cell carcinoma with a 3:11 chromosome translocation limited to tumor cells. *Science* **217**:939, 1982.
19. Kovacs G, Brusa P, de Riese W: Tissue-specific expression of a constitutional 3;6 translocation: Development of multiple bilateral renal-cell carcinomas. *Int J Cancer* **43**:422, 1989.
20. Zbar B, Brauch H, Talmadge C, Linehan WM: Loss of alleles of loci on the short arm of chromosome 3 in renal cell carcinoma. *Nature* **327**:721, 1987.
21. Anglard P, Brauch TH, Weiss GH, Latif F, Merino MJ, Lerman MI, Zbar B, Linehan WM: Molecular analysis of genetic changes in the origin and development of renal cell carcinoma. *Cancer Res* **51**:1071, 1991.
22. Szucs S, Muller-Brechlin R, DeRiese W, Kovacs G: Deletion 3p: The only chromosome loss in a primary renal cell carcinoma. *Cancer Genet Cytogenet* **26**:369, 1987.
23. Kovacs G, Erlandsson R, Boldog F, Ingvarsson S, Muller-Brechlin R, Klein G, Sumegi J: Consistent chromosome 3p deletion and loss of heterozygosity in renal cell carcinoma. *Proc Natl Acad Sci U S A* **85**:1571, 1988.
24. Linehan WM, Miller E, Anglard P, Merino M, Zbar B: Improved detection of allele loss in renal cell carcinomas after removal of leukocytes by immunologic selection. *J Natl Cancer Inst* **81**:287, 1989.
25. Boldog F, Arheden K, Imreh S, Strombeck B, Szekely L, Erlandsson R, Marcsek Z, Sumegi J, Mitelman F, Klein G: Involvement of 3p deletions in sporadic and hereditary forms of renal cell carcinoma. *Genes Chromosomes Cancer* **3**:403, 1991.
26. Morita R, Ishikawa J, Tsutsumi M, Hikiji K, Tsukada Y, Kamidono S, Maeda S, Nakamura Y: Allelotype of renal cell carcinoma. *Cancer Res* **51**:820, 1991.
27. Ogawa O, Kakehi Y, Ogawa K, Koshiba M, Sugiyama T, Yoshida O: Allelic loss at chromosome 3p characterizes clear cell phenotype of renal cell carcinoma. *Cancer Res* **51**:949, 1991.
28. Presti JC, Rao PH, Chen Q, Reuter VE, Li FP, Fair WR, Jhanwar SC: Histopathological, cytogenetic, and molecular characterization of renal cortical tumors. *Cancer Res* **51**:1544, 1991.
29. Yoshida HA, Ohyashiki K, Ochi H, Gibas Z, Pontes JE, Prout GR, Huben R, Sandberg AA: Cytogenetic studies of tumor tissue from patients with nonfamilial renal cell carcinoma. *Cancer Res* **46**:2139, 1986.
30. Carroll PR, Murty VVS, Reuter V, Jhanwar S, Fair WR, Whitemore WF, Chaganti RSK: Abnormalities of chromosome region 3p12-14 characterize clear cell renal carcinoma. *Cancer Genet Cytogenet* **26**:253, 1987.
31. Kovacs G, Wilkens L, Papp T, de Riese W: Differentiation between papillary and nonpapillary renal cell carcinomas by DNA analysis. *J Natl Cancer Inst* **81**:527, 1989.
32. Kovacs G, Fuzesi L, Emanual A, Kung HF: Cytogenetics of papillary renal cell tumors. *Genes Chromosomes Cancer* **3**:249, 1991.
33. Anglard P, Trahan E, Liu S, Latif F, Merino M, Lerman M, Zbar B, Linehan WM: Molecular and cellular characterization of human renal cell carcinoma cell lines. *Cancer Res* **52**:348, 1992.
34. Choyke PL, Glenn GM, Walther MM, Patronas NJ, Linehan WM, Zbar B: Von Hippel Lindau disease: Genetic, clinical and imaging features. *Radiology* **194**:629, 1995.
35. Collins ET: Two cases, brother and sister, with peculiar vascular new growth, probably primarily retinal, affecting both eyes. *Trans Ophth Soc UK* **14**:141, 1894.
36. von Hippel E: Uber eine sehr seltene erkrankung der netzhaut. *Klinische Boebachtungen Arch Ophthalmol* **59**:83, 1904.
37. Lindau A: Studien uber kleinhirncysten bau: pathogenese und beziehungen zur angiomatous retinae. *Acta Pathol Microbiol Scand* (Supp) **1**:1, 1926.
38. Melmon KL, Rosen SW, Lindau's disease: Review of the literature and study of a large kindred. *Am J Med* **36**:595, 1964.
39. Poston CD, Jaffe GS, Lubensky IA, Solomon D, Zbar B, Linehan WM, Walther MM: Characterization of the renal pathology of a familial form of renal cell carcinoma associated with von Hippel-Lindau disease: Clinical and molecular genetic implications. *J Urol* **153**:22, 1995.
40. Walther MM, Lubensky IA, Venzon D, Zbar B, Linehan WM: Prevalence of microscopic lesions in grossly normal renal parenchyma from patients with von Hippel-Lindau disease, sporadic renal cell carcinoma and no renal disease: Clinical implications. *J Urol* **154**:2010, 1995.
41. Choyke PL, Filling-Katz MR, Shawker TH, Gorin MB, Travis WD, Chang R, Seizinger BR, Dwyer AJ, Linehan WM: Von hippel-lindau disease: Radiologic screening for visceral manifestations. *Radiology* **174**:815, 1990.
42. Jamis-Dow CA, Choyke PL, Jennings SB, Linehan WM, Thakore KN, Walther MM: Small (<3-cm) Renal masses: Detection with CT versus US and pathologic correlation. *Radiology* **198**:785, 1996.
43. Pearson JC, Weiss J, Tanagho EA: A plea for conservation of kidney in renal adenocarcinoma associated with von Hippel-Lindau disease. *J Urol* **124**:910, 1980.
44. Palmer JM, Swanson DA: Conservative surgery in solitary and bilateral renal carcinoma: Indications and technical considerations. *J Urol* **120**:113, 1987.
45. Frydenberg M, Malek RS, Zincke H: Conservative renal surgery for renal cell carcinoma in von Hippel-Lindau's disease. *J Urol* **194**:461, 1993.
46. Walther MM, Choyke PL, Weiss G, Manolatos C, Long J, Reiter R, Alexander RB, Linehan WM: Parenchymal sparing surgery in patients with hereditary renal cell carcinoma. *J Urol* **153**:913, 1995.
47. Walther MM, Thompson N, Linehan WM: Enucleation procedures in patients with multiple hereditary renal tumors. *World J Urol* **13**:248, 1995.
48. Walther MM, Choyke PL, Hayes W, Shawker TH, Thakore K, Alexander RB, Linehan WM: Evaluation of color doppler intraoperative ultrasound in parenchymal sparing renal surgery. *J Urol* **152**:1984, 1995.

49. Marshall FF, Holdford SS, Hamper UM: Intraoperative sonography of renal tumors. *J Urol* **148**:1393, 1992.

50. Choyke PL, Glenn G, Walther MM, Zbar B, Weiss GH, Alexander RB, Hayes WS, Long JP, Thakore KN, Linehan WM: The natural history of renal lesions in von Hippel-Lindau disease: A serial CT study in 28 patients. *AJR Am J Roentgenol* **159**:1229, 1992.

51. Filling-Katz MR, Choyke PL, Oldfield E, Charnas L, Patronas NJ, Glenn GM, Gorin MB, Morgan JK, Linehan WM, Seizinger BR, Zbar B: Central nervous system involvement in von Hippel Lindau disease. *Neurology* **41**:41, 1991.

52. Lee J, Dong S, Park WS, Yoo N, Kim S, Kim C, Jang J, Zbar B, Lubensky IA, Linehan WM, Vortmeyer AO, Zhuang Z: Loss of heterozygosity and somatic mutations of the VHL tumor suppressor gene in sporadic cerebellar hemangioblastomas. *Cancer Res* **58**:504, 1998.

53. Vortmeyer AO, Gnarra JR, Emmert-Buck MR, Katz D, Linehan WM, Oldfield EH, Zhuang Z: von Hippel-Lindau gene deletion detected in the stromal cell component of a cerebellar hemangioblastoma associated with von Hippel-Lindau disease. *Hum Pathol* **28**:540, 1997.

54. Robb L, Elefanty AG: The hemangioblast an elusive cell captured in culture. *Bioessays* **20**:611, 1998.

55. Choi K, Kennedy M, Kazarov A, Papadimitriou JC, Keller G: A common precursor for hematopoietic and endothelial cells. *Development* **125**:725, 1998.

56. Maurea S, Cuocolo A, Reynolds JC, Tumeh SS, Begley MG, Linehan WM, Norton JA, Walther MM, Keiser HR, Neumann RD: Iodine-313-metaiodobenzylguanidine scintigraphy in preoperative and postoperative evaluation of paragangliomas: Comparison with CT and MRI. *J Nucl Med* **34**:173, 1993.

57. Keiser HR, Doppman JL, Robertson CN, Linehan WM, Averbuch SD: Diagnosis, localization and management of pheochromocytoma, in EE Lack (ed.). *Pathology of the Adrenal Gland, 14th ed.*, New York: Churchill-Livingston, 1990, pp. 237–255.

58. Bouck NP, Polverini PJ: Identification of a new inhibitor of neovascularization controlled by a tumor suppressor gene. *J Northwestern Univ Cancer Center* **1**:4, 1990.

59. Perry RR, Keiser HJ, Norton JA, Wall RT, Robertson CN, Travis W, Pass HI, Walther MM, Linehan WM: Surgical management of pheochromocytoma with the use of metyrosine. *Ann Surg* **212**:621, 1990.

60. Green JS, Bowmer MI, Johnson GJ: Von Hippel-Lindau disease in a Newfoundland kindred. *CMAJ* **134**:133, 1986.

61. Seizinger BR: Von Hippel-Lindau disease: A model system for the isolation of tumor suppressor genes associated with the primary genetic mechanisms of cancer. *Adv Nephrol Necker Hosp* **23**:29, 1994.

62. Neumann HPH: Basic criteria for clinical diagnosis and genetic counselling in von Hippel-Lindau syndrome. *Vasa* **16** 220, 1987.

63. Karsdorp N, Elderson A, Wittebol-Post D: Von Hippel-Lindau disease: new strategies in early detetion and treatment. *Am J Med* **97**:158, 1994.

64. Vortmeyer AO, Choo D, Pack SD, Oldfield E, Zhuang Z: von Hippel-Lindau disease gene alterations associated with endolymphatic sac tumor. *J Natl Cancer Inist* **89**:970, 1997.

65. Tory K, Brauch H, Linehan WM, Barba D, Oldfield E, Filling-Katz M, Seizinger B, Nakamura Y, White R, Marshall FF, Lerman MI, Zbar B: Specific genetic change in tumors associated with von Hippel-Lindau disease. *J Natl Cancer Inst* **81**:1097, 1989.

66. Lubensky IA, Gnarra JR, Bertheau P, Walther MM, Linehan WM, Zhuang Z: Allelic deletions of the VHL gene detected in multiple microscopic clear cell renal lesions in von Hippel-Lindau disease patients. *Am J Pathol* **149**:2089, 1996.

67. Seizinger BR, Rouleau GA, Ozelius LJ, Lane AH, Farmer GE, Lamiell JM, Haines J, Yuen JW, Collins D, Majoor-Krakauer D, et al: Von Hippel-Lindau disease maps to the region of chromosome 3 associated with renal cell carcinoma. *Nature* **332**:268, 1988.

68. Lerman MI, Latif F, Glenn GM, Daniel LN, Brauch H, Hosoe S, Hampsch K, Delisio J, Orcutt M.-L, McBride OW, Grzeschik K.-H, Takahashi T, Minna J, Anglard P, Linehan WM, Zbar B: Isolation and regional localization of a large collection (2,000) of single copy DNA fragments on human chromosome 3 for mapping and cloning tumor suppressor genes. *Hum Genet* **86**:567, 1991.

69. Hosoe S, Brauch H, Latif F, Glenn G, Daniel L, Bale S, Choyke P, Gorin M, Oldfield E, Berman A, Goodman J, Orcutt ML, Hampsch K, Delisio J, Modi W, McBride W, Anglard P, Weiss G, Walther MM, Linehan WM, Lerman MI, Zbar B: Localization of the von Hippel-Lindau disease gene to a small region of chromosome 3. *Genomics*, **8**:634, 1990.

70. Richards FM, Maher ER, Latif F, Phipps ME, Tory K, Lush M, Croosey PA, Oostra B, Gustavson KH, Green J, Turner G, Yates JRW, Linehan WM, Affara NA, Lerman M, Zbar B, Ferguson-Smith MA: Detailed genetic mapping of the von Hippel-Lindau disease tumour suppressor gene. *J Med Genet* **30**:104, 1993.

71. Glenn GM, Linehan WM, Hosoe S, Latif F, Yao M, Choyke P, Gorin MB, Chew E, Oldfield E, Manolatos C, Orcutt ML, Walther MM, Weiss GH, Tory K, Jensson O, Lerman MI, Zbar B: Screening for von Hippel-Lindau disease by DNA-polymorphism analysis. *JAMA* **267**:1226, 1992.

72. Gnarra JR, Tory K, Weng Y, Schmidt L, Wei MH, Li H, Latif F, Liu S, Chen F, Duh F.-M, Lubensky IA, Duan R, Florence C, Pozzatti R, Walther MM, Bander NH, Grossman HB, Brauch H, Pomer S, Brooks JD, Issacs WB, Lerman MI, Zbar B, Linehan WM: Mutation of the VHL tumour Suppressor Gene in Renal Carcinoma. *Nat Genet* **7**:85, 1994.

73. Glenn GM, Daniel LN, Choyke P, Linehan WM, Oldfield E, Gorin M, Hosoe S, Latif F, Weiss G, Walther MM, Lerman MI, Zbar B: Von Hippel-Lindau disease: Distinct phenotypes suggest more than one mutant allele at the VHL locus. *Hum Genet* **87**:207, 1991.

74. Latif F, Tory K, Gnarra JR, Yao M, Duh F.-M, Orcutt ML, Stackhouse T, Kuzmin I, Modi W, Geil L, Schmidt L, Zhou F, Li H, Wei MH, Chen F, Glenn G, Choyke P, Walther MM, Weng Y, Duan D-SR, Dean M, Glavac D, Richards FM, Crossey PA, Ferguson-Smith MA, Le Paslier D, Chumakov I, Cohen D, Chinault CA, Maher ER, Linehan WM, Zbar B, Lerman MI: Identification of the von Hippel-Lindau disease tumor suppressor gene. *Science* **260**:1317, 1993.

75. Stolle CA, Glenn G, Zbar B, Humphrey JS, Choyke P, Walther MM, Pack S, Hurley K, Ondrey C, Klausner RD, Linehan WM: Improved detection of germline mutations in the von Hippel-Lindau disease tumor suppressor gene. *Hum Mutat* **12**:417, 1998.

76. Chen F, Kishida T, Yao M, Hustad T, Glavac D, Dean M, Gnarra JR, Orcutt ML, Duh FM, Glenn G, Green J, Hsia YE, Lamiell J, Li H, Wei MH, Schmidt L, Tory K, Kuzmin I, Stackhouse T, Latif F, Linehan WM, Lerman M, Zbar B: Germline mutations in the von Hippel-Lindau disease tumor suppressor gene: Correlation with phenotype. *Hum Mutat* **5**:66, 1995.

77. Brauch H, Kishida T, Glavac D, Chen F, Pausch F, Hofler H, Latif F, Lerman MI, Zbar B, Neumann HPH: Von Hippel Lindau (VHL) disease with pheochromocytoma in the Black forest region of Germany: Evidence for a founder effect. *Hum Genet* **95**:551, 1995.

78. Tisherman SE, Tisherman BG, Tisherman SA, Dunmire S, Levey GS, Mulvihill JJ: Three-decade investigation of familial pheochromocytoma. *Arch Intern Med* **153**:2550, 1993.

79. Crossey PA, Eng C, Ginalska-Malinowska M, Lennard TW, Wheeler DC, Ponder BA, Maher ER: Molecular genetic diagnosis of von Hippel-Lindau disease in familial phaeochromocytoma. *J Med Genet* **32** 885, 1995.

80. Neumann HP, Eng C, Mulligan LM, Glavac D, Zauner I, Ponder BA, Crossey PA, Maher ER, Brauch H: Consequences of direct genetic testing for germline mutations in the clinical management of families with multiple endocrine neoplasia, type II [see comments]. *JAMA* **274**: 1149, 1995.

81. Kanno H, Shuin T, Kondo K, Ito S, Hosaka M, Torigoe S, Fujii S, Tanaka Y, Yamamoto I, Kim I, Yao M: Molecular genetic diagnosis of von Hippel-Lindau disease: Analysis of five Japanese families. *Jpn J Cancer Res* **87**:423, 1996.

82. Shuin T, Kondo K, Kaneko S, Sakai N, Yao M, Hosaka M, Kanno H, Ito S, Yamamoto I: Results of mutation analyses of von Hippel-Lindau disease gene in Japanese patients: Comparison with results in United States and United Kingdom. *Hinyokika Kiyo* **41**:703, 1995.

83. Clinical Research Group for VHL in Japan Germline mutations in the von Hippel-Lindau disease (VHL) gene in Japanese VHL: *Hum Mol Genet* **4**:2233, 1995.

84. Whaley JM, Naglich J, Gelbert L, Hsia YE, Lamiell JM, Green JS, Collins D, Neumann PH, Laidlaw J, Li FP, Klein-Szanto AJP, Seizinger BR, Kley N: Germ-line mutations in the von Hippel-Lindau tumor-suppressor gene are similar to von Hippel-Lindau aberrations in sporadic renal cell carcinoma. *Am J Hum Genet* **55**:1092, 1994.

85. Gross DJ, Avishai N, Meiner V, Filon D, Zbar B, Abeliovich D: Familial pheochromocytoma associated with a novel mutation in the von Hippel-Lindau gene. *J Clin Endocrinol Metab* **81**:147, 1996.

86. Webster AR, Maher ER, Moore AT: Clinical characteristics of ocular angiomatosis in von Hippel-Lindau disease and correlation with germline mutation. *Arch Ophthalmol* **117**:371, 1999.

87. Gnarra JR, Tory K, Weng Y, Schmidt L, Wei MH, Li H, Latif F, Liu S, Chen F, Duh F-M, Lubensky IA, Duan R, Florence C, Pozzatti R,

Walther MM, Bander NH, Grossman HB, Brauch H, Pomer S, Brooks JD, Issacs WB, Lerman MI, Zbar B, Linehan WM: Mutation of the VHL tumour suppressor gene in renal carcinoma. *Nat Genet* **7**:85, 1994.

88. Knudson AG: VHL gene mutation and clear-cell renal carcinomas. *Cancer J* **1**:180, 1995.

89. Shuin T, Kondo K, Torigoe S, Kishida T, Kubota Y, Hosaka M, Nagashima Y, Kitamura H, Latif F, Zbar B, Lerman MI, Yao M: Frequent somantic mutations and loss of heterozygosity of the von Hippel-Lindau tumor suppressor gene in primary human renal cell carcinomas. *Cancer Res* **54**:2852, 1994.

90. Crossey PA, Richards FM, Foster K, Green JS, Prowse A, Latif F, Lerman MI, Zbar B, Affara NA, Ferguson-Smith MA, Maher ER: Identification of intragenic mutations in the von Hippel-Lindau disease tumor suppressor gene and correlation with disease phenotype. *Hum Mol Genet* **3**:1303, 1994.

91. Foster K, Prowse A, van den Berg A, Fleming S, Hulsbeek MMF, Crossey PA, Richards FM, Cairns P, Affara NA, Ferguson-Smith MA, Buys CHCM, Maher ER: Somatic mutations of the von Hippel-Lindau disease tumour suppressor gene in nonfamilial clear cell renal carcinoma. *Hum Mol Genet* 2169, 1994.

92. Bailly M, Bain C, Favrot MC, Ozturk M: Somatic mutations of von Hippel-Lindau (VHL) tumor-suppressor gene in European kidney cancers. *Int J Cancer* **63**:660, 1995.

93. Schmidt L, Li F, Brown RS, Berg S, Chen F, Wei MH, Tory K, Lerman MI, Zbar B: Mechanism of tumorigenesis of renal carcinomas associated with the constitutional chromosome 3; 8 translocation. *Cancer J Sci Am* **1**:191, 1995.

94. Zhuang Z, Bertheau P, Emmert-Buck MR, Liotta LA, Gnarra JR, Linehan WM, Lubensky IA: A microdissection technique for archival DNA analysis of specific cell populations in lesions <1 mm in size. *Am J Pathol* **146**:620, 1995.

95. Zhuang Z, Gnarra JR, Dudley CF, Zbar B, Linehan WM, Lubensky IA: Detection of von Hippel-Lindau disease gene mutations in paraffin-embedded sporadic renal cell carcinoma specimens. *Mod Pathol* **9**:838, 1996.

96. Long JP, Anglard P, Gnarra JR, Walther MM, Merino MJ, Liu S, Lerman MI, Zbar B, Linehan WM: The use of molecular genetic analysis in the diagnosis of renal cell carcinoma. *World J Urol* **12**:69, 1994.

97. Kanno H, Kondo K, Ito S, Yamamoto I, Fujii S, Torigoe S, Sakai N, Masahiko H, Shuin T, Yao M: Somatic mutations of the von Hippel-Lindau tumor suppressor gene in sporadic central nervous system hemangioblastomas. *Cancer Res* **54**:4845, 1994.

98. Gilcrease MZ, Schmidt L, Zbar B, Truong L, Rutledge M, Wheeler TM: Somatic von Hippel-Lindau mutation in clear cell papillary cystadenoma of the epididymis. *Hum Pathol* **26**:1341, 1995.

99. Herman JG, Latif F, Weng Y, Lerman MI, Zbar B, Liu S, Samid D, Duan D.-SR, Gnarra JR, Linehan WM, Baylin SB: Silencing of the VHL tumor suppressor gene by DNA methylation in renal carcinoma. *Proc Natl Acad Sci U S A* **91**:9700, 1994.

100. Stebbins CE, Kaelin WGJ, Pavletich NP: Structure of the VHL-ElonginC–ElonginB complex: Implications for VHL tumor suppressor function. *Science* **284**:455, 1999.

101. Chen F, Kishida T, Yao M, Hustad T, Glavac D, Dean M, Gnarra JR, Orcutt ML, Duh FM, Glenn G, Green J, Hsia YE, Lamiell J, Li H, Wei MH, Schmidt L, Tory K, Kuzmin I, Stackhouse T, Latif F, Linehan WM, Lerman M, Zbar B: Germline mutations in the von hippel-lindau disease tumor suppressor gene: Correlation with phenotype. *Hum Mutat* **5**:66, 1995.

102. Ohh M, Park CW, Ivan M, Hoffman MA, Kim TY, Huang LE, Pavletich N, Chau V, Kaelin WG: Ubiquitination of hypoxia-inducible factor requires direct binding to the beta-domain of the von Hippel-Lindau protein. *Nat Cell Biol.* **2**:423, 2000.

103. Tyers M, Rottapel R, VHL: A very hip ligase. *Proc Natl Acad Sci U S A* **96**:12230, 1999.

104. Maxwell PH, Wiesener MS, Chang GW, Clifford SC, Vaux EC, Cockman ME, Wykoff CC, Pugh CW, Maher ER, Ratcliffe PJ: The tumour suppressor protein VHL targets hypoxia-inducible factors for oxygen-dependent proteolysis. *Nature* **399**:271, 1999.

105. Krek W: VHL takes HIF's breath away. *Nat Cell Biol* **2**:E1, 2000.

106. Krieg M, Haas R, Brauch H, Acker T, Flamme I, Plate KH: Up-regulation of hypoxia-inducible factors HIF-1alpha and HIF-2alpha under normoxic conditions in renal carcinoma cells by von Hippel-Lindau tumor suppressor gene loss of function. *Oncogene* **19**:5435, 2000.

107. Pause A, Lee S, Lonergan KM, Klausner RD: The von Hippel-Lindau tumor suppressor gene is required for cell cycle exit upon serum withdrawal. *Proc Natl Acad Sci U S A* **95**:993, 1998.

108. Ivanov SV, Kuzmin I, Wei MH, Pack S, Geil L, Johnson BE, Stanbridge EJ, Lerman MI: Down-regulation of transmembrane carbonic anhydrases in renal cell carcinoma cell lines by wild-type von Hippel-Lindau transgenes. *Proc Natl Acad Sci U S A* **95**:12596, 1998.

109. Oosterwijk E, Ruiter DJ, Hoedemaeker PJ, Pauwels EK, Jonas U, Zwartendijk J, Warnaar SO: Monoclonal antibody G 250 recognizes a determinant present in renal-cell carcinoma and absent from normal kidney. *Int J Cancer* **38**:489, 1986.

110. McKiernan JM, Buttyan R, Bander NH, Stifelman MD, Katz AE, Chen MW, Olsson CA, Sawczuk IS: Expression of the tumor-associated gene MN: A potential biomarker for human renal cell carcinoma. *Cancer Res.* **57**:2362, 1997.

111. Koolen MI, van der Meyden AP, Bodmer D, Eleveld M, van der Looij E, Brunner H, Smits A, van den Berg E, Smeets D, Geurts VK: A familial case of renal cell carcinoma and a t(2;3) chromosome translocation. *Kidney Int* **53**:273, 1998.

112. Mydlo JH, Bard RH: Analysis of papillary renal adenocarcinoma. *Urology* **30**:529, 1987.

113. Boczko S, Fromowitz FB, Bard RH: Papillary adenocarcinoma of kidney. *Urology* **14**:491, 1979.

114. Kovacs G: Papillary renal cell carcinoma. A morphologic and cytogenetic study of 11 cases. *Am J Pathol* **134**:27, 1989.

115. Kovacs G, Hoene E: Multifocal renal cell carcinoma: A cytogenetic study. *Virchows Arch A Pathol Anat Histopathol* **412**:79, 1987.

116. Hughson MD, Johnson LD, Silva FG, Kovacs G: Nonpapillary and papillary renal cell carcinoma: a cytogenetic and phenotypic study. *Mod Pathol.* **6**:449, 1993.

117. Shipley JM, Birdsall S, Clark J, Crew J, Gill S, Linehan WM, Gnarra JR, Fisher S, Craig IW, Cooper CS: Mapping the X chromosome breakpoint in two papillary renal cell carcinoma cell lines with a t(X;1)(p11.2;q21.2) and the first report of a female case. *Cytogenet Cell Genet* **71**:280, 1995.

118. Suijkerbuijk RF, Meloni AM, Sinke RJ, de Leeuw B, Wilbrink M, Janssen HA, Geraghty MT, Monaco AP, Sandberg AA, Geurts van Kessel A: Identification of a yeast artificial chromosome that spans the human papillary renal cell carcinoma-associated t(X;1) breakpoint in Xp 11.2. *Cancer Genet Cytogenet* **71**:164, 1993.

119. Meloni AM, Dobbs RM, Pontes JE, Sandberg AA: Translocation (X;1) in papillary renal cell carcinoma. A new cytogenetic subtype. *Cancer Genet Cytogenet* **65**:1, 1993.

120. Zbar B, Lerman M: Inherited Carcinomas of the Kidney. *Adv Cancer Res* **75**:163, 1998.

121. Duh F-M, Scherer SW, Tsui LC, Lerman M, Zbar B, Schmidt L: Gene structure of the human MET proto-oncogene. *Oncogene* **15**:1583, 1997.

122. Schmidt L, Duh F-M, Chen F, Kishida T, Glenn G, Choyke P, Scherer SW, Zhuang Z, Lubensky IA, Dean M, Allikmets R, Chidambaram A, Bergerheim UR, Feltis TJ, Casadevall C, Zamarron A, Bernues M, Richard S, Lips CJM, Walther MM, Tsui L, Geil L, Orcutt ML, Stackhouse T, Lipan J, Slife L, Brauch H, Decker J, Niehans G, Hughson MD, Moch H, Storkel S, Lerman MI, Linehan WM, Zbar B: Germline and somatic mutations in the tyrosine kinase domain of the MET proto-oncogene in papillary renal carcinomas. *Nat Genet* **16**:68, 1997.

123. Zhuang Z, Park WS, Pack S, Schmidt L, Pak E, Pham T, Weil RJ, Candidus S, Lubensky IA, Linehan WM, Zbar B, Weirich G: Trisomy 7 harboring non-random duplication of the mutant MET allele in hereditary papillary renal carcinomas. *Nat Genet* **20**:66, 1998.

124. Fischer J, Palmedo G, von Knobloch R, Bugert P, Prayer-Galetti T, Pagano F, Kovacs G: Duplication and overexpression of the mutant allele of the MET protooncogene in multiple hereditary papillary renal cell tumours. *Oncogene* **17**:733, 1998.

125. Park M, Dean M, Kaul K, Braun MJ, Gonda MA, Vande WG: Sequence of MET protooncogene cDNA has features characteristic of the tyrosine kinase family of growth-factor receptors. *Proc Natl Acad Sci U S A* **84**:6379, 1987.

126. Weidner KM, Sachs M, Birchmeier W: The Met receptor tyrosine kinase transduces motility, proliferation, and morphogenic signals of scatter factor/hepatocyte growth factor in epithelial cells. *J Cell Biol.* **121**:145, 1993.

127. Bladt F, Riethmacher D, Isenmann S, Aguzzi A, Birchmeier C: Essential role for the c-met receptor in the migration of myogenic

precursor cells into the limb bud [see comments]. *Nature* **376**:768, 1995.

128. Jeffers M, Schmidt L, Nakaigawa N, Webb CP, Weirich G, Kishida T, Zbar B, Vande WG: Activating mutations for the MET tyrosine kinase receptor in human cancer. *Proc Natl Acad Sci U S A* **94**:11445, 1997.

129. Schmidt L, Junker K, Weirich G, Glenn G, Choyke P, Lubensky IA, Zhuang Z, Jeffers M, Woude GV, Neumann H, Walther MM, Linehan WM, Zbar B: Two North American families with hereditary papillary renal carcinoma and identical novel mutations in the MET proto-oncogene. *Cancer Res* **58**:1719, 1998.

130. Buttner C, Henz BM, Welker P, Sepp NT, Grabbe J: Identification of activating c-KIT mutations in adult-, but not in childhood-onset indolent mastocytosis: A possible explanation for divergent clinical behavior. *Journal of Investigative Dermatology* **111**:1227, 1998.

131. Schmidt L, Junker K, Kinjerski T, Weirich G, Neumann H, Brauch H, Decker J, Storkel S, Miller M, Moch H, Jenkins W, Linehan WM, Zbar B: Novel mutations of the MET proto-oncogene in papillary renal carcinomas. *Oncogene* **18**:2343, 1999.

132. Delahunt B, Eble JN: Papillary renal cell carcinoma: A clinicopathologic and immunohistochemical study of 105 tumors. *Mod Pathol* **10**:537, 1997.

133. Moch H, Gasser T, Amin MB, Torhorst J, Sauter G, Mihatsch MJ: Prognostic utility of the recently recommended histologic classification and revised TNM staging system of renal cell carcinoma: A Swiss experience with 588 tumors. *Cancer* **89**:604, 2000.

134. Lubensky IA, Schmidt L, Zhuang Z, Weirich G, Pack S, Zambrano N, Walther MM, Choyke P, Linehan WM, Zbar B: Hereditary and sporadic papillary renal carcinomas with c-MET mutations share a distinct morphological phenotype. *Am J Pathol.* **155**:517, 1999.

135. Nickerson ML, Weirich G, Zbar B, Schmidt LS: Signature-based analysis of MET proto-oncogene mutations using DHPLC. *Hum Mutat* **16**:68, 2002.

136. Weirich G, Glenn G, Junker K, Merino M, Storkel S, Lubensky IA, Choyke P, Pack S, Amin M, Walther MM, Linehan WM, Zbar B: Familial renal oncocytoma: Clinicopathologic study of 5 families. *Urol* **160**:335, 1998.

137. Birt AR, Hogg GR, Dube WJ: Hereditary multiple fibrofolliculomas with trichodiscomas and acrochordons. *Arch Dermatol.* **113**:1674, 1977.

138. Toro J, Duray PH, Glenn GM, Darling T, Zbar B, Linehan WM, Turner M: Birt-Hogg-Dube syndrome: A novel marker of kidney neoplasia. *Arch Dermatol* **135**:1195, 1999.

139. Roth JS, Rabinowitz AD, Benson M, Grossman ME: Bilateral renal cell carcinoma in the Birt-Hogg-Dube syndrome. *J Am Acad Dermatol.* **29**:1055, 1993.

140. Horton WA, Wong V, Eldridge R: Von Hippel-Lindau disease: Clinical and pathological manifestations in nine families with 50 affected members. *Arch Intern Med* **136**:769, 1976.

141. Pontes JE, Pescatori E, Connelly R, Hashimura T, Tubbs R: Circulating cancer cells in renal-cell carcinoma. *Prog Clin Biol Res* **348**:1, 1990.

142. Liotta LA, Kleinerman J, Seidel GM: Quantitative relationships of intravascular tumor cells, tumor vessels and pulmonary metastasis following tumor implantation. *Cancer Res* **34**:997, 1974.

143. Buttler TP, Gullino PM: Quantitation of cell shedding into efferent blood of mammary adenocarcinoma. *Cancer Res* **35**:512, 1975.

144. Moreno JG, Croce CM, Fischer R, Monne M, Vihko P, Mulholland SG, Gomella LG: Detection of hematogenous micrometastasis in patients with prostate cancer. *Cancer Res* **52**:6110, 1992.

145. Linehan WM, Klausner RD: Renal carcinoma, in Vogelstein B, Kinzler K, (eds): *The Genetic Basis of Human Cancer*, New York, McGraw-Hill, 1998, pp. 455–473.

146. Yao M, Latif F, Kuzmin I, Stackhouse T, Zhou FW, Tory K, Orcutt ML, Duh FM, Richards F, Maher E, La Forgia S, Huebner K, Le Pasilier D, Linehan WM, Lerman M, Zbar B: Von Hippel-Lindau disease: Identification of deletion mutations by pulsed field gel electrophoresis. *Hum Genet* **92**:605, 1993.

147. Tyers M, Rottapel R, VHL: A very hip ligase. *Proc Natl Acad Sci U S A* **96**:12230, 1999.

148. Lee S, Chen DYT, Humphrey JS, Gnarra JR, Linehan WM, Klausner RD: Nuclear/cytoplasmic localization of the VHL tumor suppressor gene product is determined by cell density. *Proc Natl Acad Sci U S A* **93**:1770, 1996.

Multiple Endocrine Neoplasia Type 1

Stephen J. Marx

1. **Multiple endocrine neoplasia type 1 (MEN1) is an autosomal dominant disorder with endocrine tumors of the parathyroids, the enteropancreatic neuroendocrine tissues, the anterior pituitary, and foregut carcinoid. Associated nonendocrine tumors include facial angiofibromas, skin collagenomas, lipomas and leiomyomas.**
2. **Most of the tumors are benign and produce symptoms and signs by oversecreting hormones (parathyroid hormone, gastrin, prolactin, etc.). Associated gastrinomas and foregut carcinoid tumors have a substantial malignant potential.**
3. **The most common endocrinopathy is primary hyperparathyroidism with several features different from features in sporadic parathyroid adenoma. Hyperparathyroidism in MEN1 is expressed earlier than in sporadic adenoma; 50 percent of mutation carriers express it by ages 18 to 30. Most MEN1 patients have multiple parathyroid tumors and, after successful subtotal parathyroidectomy, have a high likelihood of late recurrence. Hyperparathyroidism can exacerbate the simultaneous Zollinger-Ellison syndrome in MEN1.**
4. **The *MEN1* gene was identified by positional cloning in 1997. Its sequence predicted a novel protein termed *menin*.**
5. ***MEN1* germ-line mutations have been found in about 80 percent of MEN1 families and in a similar fraction of patients with sporadic MEN1. Clinical use of germ-line *MEN1* mutation testing can give valuable information. Because it does not mandate an intervention, it does not have the urgency of germ-line *RET* mutation testing for MEN2a or MEN2b.**
6. **Certain sporadic endocrine and nonendocrine tumors often show somatic *MEN1* mutation. In fact, *MEN1* is the known gene most commonly mutated in sporadic parathyroid adenoma, gastrinoma, insulinoma, and bronchial carcinoid tumor.**
7. ***MEN1* is likely a tumor-suppressor gene, since most MEN1 tumors and many sporadic endocrine tumors with *MEN1* mutation also show inactivation (recognized as loss of heterozygosity) of the normal allele at 11q13, the *MEN1* locus.**
8. **The *MEN1*-encoded protein, menin, is mainly located in the nucleus. It shows no protein homologies. It binds to and inhibits junD, an AP1 transcription factor. It also binds closely to several other proteins. Most germ-line or somatic *MEN1* mutations predict truncation of the menin protein and are thus likely to cause inactivation of menin function. Inactivation-type mutation further supports menin's predicted role as a tumor suppressor.**

A list of standard abbreviations is located immediately preceding the index. Nonstandard abbreviations used in this chapter include: MEN1 = multiple endocrine neoplasia type 1; MEN2 = multiple endocrine neoplasia type 2; Z-E = Zollinger-Ellison; BAO = basal acid output; MAO = maximal acid output; LOH = loss of heterozygosity.

INTRODUCTION AND HISTORY

Multiple endocrine neoplasia is a broad term that encompasses many distinct disorders. Literally interpreted, it includes all patients and families with endocrine neoplasia in more than one tissue type. Thus it includes patients with two coincidental endocrine neoplasms such as parathyroid adenoma and pituitary microadenoma, and it can include patients with a neoplasm that stimulates another tumor, such as pancreatic islet tumor secreting growth hormone-releasing hormone, which causes pituitary hyperplasia.

Within this broad definition, multiple endocrine neoplasia type 1 (MEN1) and multiple endocrine neoplasia type 2 (MEN2) stand out as occurring repeatedly in sporadic cases and also within families. The main endocrine expressions of MEN1 are parathyroid tumor, enteropancreatic neuroendocrine tumor, anterior pituitary tumor, and foregut carcinoid tumor. Nonendocrine expressions include lipoma, facial angiofibroma, skin collagenoma and leiomyoma (Table 28-1).

The first description of a patient with MEN1 is generally attributed to Erdheim.[1] He reported in 1903 the autopsy of a patient with acromegaly, pituitary adenoma, and four enlarged parathyroids. Familial transmission of MEN1 was established in 1953–1954 by Moldawar[2,3] and Wermer.[4] Subsequently, *Wermer's syndrome* has been an eponym for MEN1. With delineation of sporadic gastrinoma[5–7] and prolactinoma[8,9] as clinical entities in 1955 and 1971, respectively, they were almost simultaneously recognized as possible components of MEN1. In the 1970s and 1980s, knowledge about MEN1 advanced with the development of new and improved radioimmunoassays for hormones and other peptides. During this time, the clinical spectrum of MEN1 also changed with advances in pharmacology, such as acid secretion-blocking drugs for Zollinger-Ellison syndrome[10–13] and dopamine agonists for prolactinoma.[14] Important surgical advances also were made, beginning with total gastrectomy for Zollinger-Ellison syndrome through improved pituitary microsurgery and use of new pre- and intraoperative tumor imaging methods.[15–17,17b,17c]

The genetic etiology of MEN1 has been clarified only recently. Larsson *et al.*[18] showed in 1988 that the *MEN1* gene was likely a tumor-suppressor gene, based on MEN1 tumors showing loss of the normal allele from chromosome 11. At the same time, these authors reported tight genetic linkage of the MEN1 trait to the *PYGM* locus at 11q13. The *MEN1* gene was identified in 1997.[19]

CLINICAL ASPECTS

Prevalence

There are no population-based studies of the prevalence of MEN1. Autopsy series have estimated a prevalence of 2.5 per 1000.[20,21] However, biochemical tests have suggested a prevalence of 0.01 to 0.175 per 1000.[22–25]

An alternate estimate can be derived from the fraction of MEN1 among patients with evaluation for single-tissue endocrine tumor. Primary hyperparathyroidism is likely to be one main

Table 28-1 Summary Features of Multiple Endocrine Neoplasia Type 1 with Estimated Average Penetrance (in Parentheses) among Patients Expressing *MEN1* Mutation

Endocrine Features	Nonendocrine Features
Parathyroid adenomas (90%)	Facial angiofibromas (85%)
Enteropancreatic tumor	Collagenomas (70%)
Gastrinoma (40%)	Lipomas (30%)
Insulinoma (10%)	Leiomyoma (1%)
Pancreatic polypeptide or	Ependymoma ($<$ 1%)
nonfunctioning (20%)*	
Other—glucagonoma, VIPoma,	
somatostatinoma, etc. (2%)	
Anterior pituitary tumor	
Prolactinoma (25%)	
Other—growth hormone/prolactin,	
growth hormone, ACTH, etc. (5%)	
Nonsecreting (10%)	
Foregut carcinoid tumor	
Thymic carcinoid (2%)	
Bronchial carcinoid (4%)	
Gastric enterochromaffin-like	
tumor (10%)	
Other tumor: adrenal cortex (5%),	
pheochromocytoma ($<$ 1%)	

* Does not include near 100% prevalence of nonfunctioning and clinically silent tumors, which are detected incidental to pancreaticoduodenal surgery in MEN1.

source of MEN1 case ascertainment; the fraction of MEN1 among patients with primary hyperparathyroidism has been estimated at 1 to 18 percent.[26] The cause for this variable fraction is not known, but selection bias is likely. The true fraction is probably 2 to 3 percent[26b] this, combined with a population annual incidence of 0.5 per 1000 for primary hyperparathyroidism,[27] gives an estimate of MEN1 annual incidence of 0.015 per 1000.

Among patients with Zollinger-Ellison syndrome, the prevalence of MEN1 has been 16 to 38 percent, much higher than that of MEN1 among sporadic primary hyperparathyroidism.[25,28,29] Among patients with pituitary tumor, the prevalence of MEN1 has been 2.7 to 5 percent[30–32] but as high as 14 percent among prolactinoma patients.[32]

Familial versus Sporadic Cases

The majority of cases of MEN1 are familial. In a British series, there were 36 sporadic cases versus 220 familial cases among 62 families.[33] In our series (Marx et al., unpublished), there are 30 sporadic cases versus approximately 500 familial cases in 80 families. Two reports from Japan indicated an inverted sporadic/familial ratio with 61 sporadic cases and 45 affected cases from 15 families[33b] and similarly 20 sporadic cases plus 41 *MEN1* mutation carriers from 16 families.[33c,33d] This high frequency of apparently sporadic MEN1 cases in Japan may arise from a reluctance to discuss illness in a patient or a relative in that society. Sporadic cases, of course, may have unrecognized familial MEN1.

Diagnostic Criteria

Similar broad diagnostic criteria have been used informally by most groups.[19,33] MEN1 is usually defined as a patient with an endocrine tumor in two (not necessarily simultaneously) of the three major tissue systems (parathyroid, enteropancreatic neuroendocrine, and anterior pituitary). This is to say, carcinoid tumor, lipoma, facial angiofibroma, and certain other features (see Table 28-1) have not been used traditionally for ascertainment. *Familial* MEN1 is defined as a family that includes at least one patient with MEN1 and at least one first-degree relative with an endocrine tumor in one of the three principal MEN1-associated tissues. It is understood that these operational criteria will

encompass, occasionally, several disorders that are not caused by *MEN1* mutation. Similarly, some, presumably small, kindreds with *MEN1* mutation will not meet these clinical criteria.

Expressions of MEN1 by Tissue System

Benign and Malignant Neoplasia. An important feature of MEN1 is that most of its main expressions are determined by the hormone(s) that are oversecreted. Thus MEN1 is expressed mainly as hyperparathyroidism, Zollinger-Ellison (Z-E) syndrome, and hyperprolactinemia. The neoplasms in general are small and benign. Only the pituitary tumor, and much less commonly a pancreatic islet tumor, can produce clinical signs through a local mass effect. At the same time, MEN1 is a genuine familial cancer syndrome. Gastrinomas, thymic carcinoid, and bronchial carcinoid all are common expressions of MEN1 with a substantial malignant potential. Some less common expressions (see below) also have substantial malignant potential. The hormonal expressions of MEN1 generally have excellent treatment options; the malignant expressions usually do not. Malignant enteropancreatic neuroendocrine tumor and malignant carcinoid account for one-third of deaths among MEN1 patients.[34] This is a similar or even higher syndrome-related cancer mortality than with MEN2a.

Parathyroid Gland

Primary Hyperparathyroidism as the Most Common Endocrinopathy in MEN1. Primary hyperparathyroidism is the most common endocrine expression of MEN1,[35–41] with 87 to 100 percent prevalence among carriers expressing any endocrinopathy (see Table 28-1). Among obligate carriers of the mutated *MEN1* gene, approximately 50 percent will express hyperparathyroidism by ages 18 to 25 and 90 percent by age 50.[33,39–41] Rare carriers do not express the trait at any age.[42] The prevalences for other endocrinopathies vary widely, depending largely on the methods to test the tissue.

Primary Hyperparathyroidism in MEN1 Differs from Sporadic Occurrences. Most features of primary hyperparathyroidism in MEN1 are similar to those in sporadic primary hyperparathyroidism.[24,33,43,44] These include a long early asymptomatic stage, generally low morbidity, and rapid amelioration after parathyroidectomy. Typical symptoms and signs include weakness, kidney stones, and back pain. Hypercalcemic crisis[45] or parathyroid cancer[46,47,47b,47c] is extremely rare, and one of three reported cancer cases[46] has been reinterpreted as not parathyroid cancer (JJ Shepherd, personal communication).

However, the hyperparathyroidism in MEN1 also has important differences from that in sporadic cases (Table 28-2). Primary hyperparathyroidism begins earlier in MEN1, with 50 percent of carriers expressing this by ages 18 to 25,[33,39–41] and with recognition as early as age 8.[33] Clinically important primary hyperparathyroidism in MEN1 is rare before age 15. The female-to-male ratio is 1.0 in MEN1 versus 3.0 in sporadic hyperparathyroidism. Early onset brings potential for osteopenia in young adults.[47d] Primary hyperparathyroidism can exacerbate Z-E syndrome (see below) in MEN1 (Fig. 28-1). This can influence a decision toward parathyroid surgery for this criterion, which is not relevant in sporadic hyperparathyroidism. On the other hand, because of excellent stomach acid control by antisecretory drugs, concomitant Z-E syndrome is usually not a sole indication for parathyroid surgery in MEN1.

Parathyroid gland clinical biology differs in MEN1 and sporadic cases. In sporadic cases there is usually a single benign parathyroid tumor (adenoma). In MEN1, multiple parathyroid glands are usually enlarged, and the enlargement is highly asymmetric.[48,49] These are multiple mono- or oligoclonal adenomas, not a diffuse polyclonal process.[49b] Surgical outcomes differ in MEN1 from outcomes in sporadic cases. Because of the multiplicity of tumors and the associated occurrence of occasional tumor in unusual locations, postoperative persistence of hyperparathyroidism in MEN1 can be 40 to 60 percent with inexperienced

Table 28-2 Distinguishing Features Among Three Categories of Primary Hyperparathyroidism

Feature	Sporadic Adenoma(s)	Multiple Endocrine Neoplasia Type 1	Familial Hypocalciuric Hypercalcemia
Percent of all hyperparathyroids	94	2	2
Heredity	Sporadic	Autos. dom.	Autos. dom.
Hypercalcemia onset age (year)	50–60	15–25	0 (at birth)
Sex ratio (F:M)	3:1	1:1	1:1
Calcium in urine	High	High	Normal to low
Parathyroid hormone in serum	High	High	Normal (15% high)
Endocrine tumors outside parathyroid	No	Often	No
Parathyroid gland pathology	Adenoma, often one	Adenoma, multiple	Hyperplasia, mild
Parathyroidectomy result*			
Immediate cure (%)	95%	92%	Below 5%
Persistence (%)	5%	10%	Above 95%
Hypoparathyroidism (%)	2%	5%	2%
Late recurrence (%)	2%	Above 50%	NA†

*Surgical results are for patients with appropriate preoperative evaluation and with an experienced parathyroid surgeon. Hypoparathyroidism is not considered a "cure."

†NA = Not applicable, since virtually no operations lead to stable normocalcemia in familial hypocalciuric hypercalcemia.

surgeons[50] and as high as 10 percent with experienced surgeons.[49–52] The desire, in MEN1, to identify all four parathyroid glands and to remove all but part of one results in an increased rate of postoperative hypoparathyroidism, as high as 30 percent.[49,52,53] While rare in sporadic cases,[54] in MEN1, postoperative late recurrent primary hyperparathyroidism reaches very high rates with time, 50 percent after 8 to 12 years.[50,51]

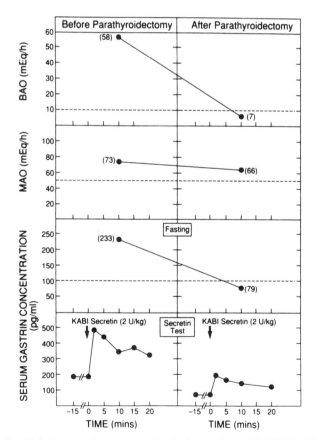

Fig. 28-1 The gastrin-gastric acid axis in a patient with MEN1 with Zollinger-Ellison syndrome, before and after normalization of serum calcium through parathyroidectomy. Successful parathyroidectomy caused remission in typical expressions of gastrinoma. Panels show basal acid output (BAO) or maximal acid output (MAO), and gastrin fasting or after intravenous secretin. Dashed lines are upper limits of normal. (*From Metz et al.*[60] Used with permission.)

Enteropancreatic Neuroendocrine Tissues

Overview. Like parathyroid tumors, enteropancreatic neuroendocrine tumors develop at younger ages and in more sites (multiplicity) in MEN1 than in sporadic cases.[33,41] The enteropancreatic neuroendocrine tumors in MEN1 are virtually always multiple at the time of surgery.[55] Although primary hyperparathyroidism is usually present when the enteropancreatic neuroendocrine tumor expresses itself, in a small fraction of prolactinoma cases, Z-E syndrome or insulinoma can be expressed first.[56b]

The enteropancreatic neuroendocrine tumors in MEN1 usually present with symptoms of hormone release rather than symptoms of tumor expansion or metastasis.[56,57] In fact, some hormone-oversecreting tumors may be too small to be imaged.[57]

Hormone Oversecretion and Storage in Tumors. Among the enteropancreatic neuroendocrine tumors in MEN1, gastrinoma is expressed most commonly at up to 54 percent.[45,57–59] Insulinoma is expressed second most commonly in MEN1, as often as 21 percent.[45,57] Glucagonoma, VIPoma, growth hormone-releasing factor-secreting tumor, intestinal carcinoid, and somatostatinoma each have been much less frequent (Table 28-1). Furthermore, MEN1 patients can express more than one enteropancreatic neuroendocrine tumor. Conversely, MEN1 occurs in approximately 20 percent of all patients with Z-E syndrome, 4 percent with insulinoma, and 33 percent with GRFoma.[60]

Nonfunctional endocrine tumors are a major component of MEN1. Although only one tumor may hypersecrete a hormone and cause symptoms and signs, typically there are many associated pancreatic islet tumors. While these may synthesize hormonal peptides, they do not oversecrete them. Still they have the potential to progress and cause subsequent oversecretion and/or cancer.[61]

Histologic evaluations of the MEN1 pancreas from surgical specimens have shown multiple tumors in about 50 percent,[55,62,63] but diffuse micronodules (diameter 0.5 cm) have been found in all.[55,62] The rates of positivity of immunostaining in 201 macro- or micronodules were pancreatic polypeptide (26 percent), glucagon (24 percent), insulin (23 percent), gastrin (4 percent), and no hormone (18 percent);[54,62] this study was done without evaluation for the frequent extrapancreatic locations of gastrinomas in MEN1.[64–66] There do not appear to be important components of diffuse islet hyperplasia or nesidioblastosis (islets budding from ducts) in the MEN1 pancreas. This differs from the histology in a mouse MEN1 model (see below).

Gastrinoma. Z-E syndrome is a symptom complex resulting from gastrinomas. Gastrinomas originate in the pancreatic islets or proximal duodenum.[6,64–66] The initial syndrome was the triad of

(1) non-beta islet cell tumor of the pancreas, (2) gastric acid hypersecretion, and (3) severe peptic ulcers of the stomach and small intestine. With increasing awareness of the disease, and with ready availability of acid-blocking drugs, the disease is now seen in milder and different forms (see below).[58,59,67] All the usual features of Z-E syndrome result from gastrin's ability to stimulate secretion of acid from the stomach.

Gastrinomas in sporadic and familial MEN1 are mostly in the "gastrinoma triangle," the duodenum or pacreatic head.[57–59,64,68–71] The specific distribution (concentrated in the duodenum) of MEN1 gastrinomas within this zone may differ from that of sporadic gastrinomas, of which 40 to 80 percent occur in the pancreas.[59,65,69,70,72] Furthermore, while most sporadic gastrinomas are solitary and large, those in MEN1 are often multiple, small, and submucosal.[64] Gastrinoma in MEN1 versus sporadic has been suggested to have lesser[59,65,73] or similar malignant propensity.[59,65,74,75] "Milder" malignancy can be an artefact from earlier ascertainment age; however, it is clear that metastases can occur,[58,64,75] and they can dominate the clinical picture in MEN1.[76–78]

Many gastrinomas in MEN1 occur after age 40.[33,57,59,65] Abdominal pain is the most common symptom, and symptoms of gastrointestinal (GI) reflux occur in up to two-thirds of patients. Some patients do not show these symptoms despite high acid output.[60] Diarrhea can be associated; in 10 to 30 percent of patients it is the sole symptom or sign. The diarrhea is a direct consequence of acid oversecretion with associated (1) high fluid secretion into bowel, (2) inactivation of pancreatic enzymes, and (3) mucosal ulceration.[58,59,76,79,80] Whereas atypical ulcer location was once common in Z-E syndrome, current practices recognize most ulcers in locations similar to locations with idiopathic peptic disease.[58,59]

Gastrinoma should be evaluated in any MEN1 patient with any of the symptoms listed above. Furthermore, fasting gastrin should be measured periodically in asymptomatic MEN1 patients older than age 20. The most useful tests for diagnosis are acid output, fasting gastrin, and secretin-stimulated gastrin. Endoscopy, because of widespread availability, is often used as a substitute for acid measurements. This is not optimal.

The upper limit for basal acid output (BAO) in the absence of acid-reducing surgery is 15 meq/h for both genders.[58,59,81] This criterion alone is insufficient for diagnosis of Z-E syndrome. There are many false positives (such as some cases of idiopathic peptic disease, a much more common disorder)[58,59] and some false negatives (exemplified by the postparathyroidectomy state)[82] (see Fig. 28-1). Maximal acid output (MAO) after subcutaneous pentagastrin (6 mg/kg) correlates with parietal cell mass.[57,58,68] However, the variability of this response and of the BAO/MAO ratio give them little diagnostic use.[58,59,76,79] Documentation of fasting gastric pH above 3.0 in a patient not taking acid-blocking medications can exclude Z-E syndrome. In a patient with hypergastrinemia, this can establish hypo- or achlorhydria (Table 28-3).

The clinical diagnosis of gastrinoma depends on documentation of dysregulated hypersecretion of gastrin. Virtually all cases have high fasting gastrin levels.[76,77] With the widespread use of acid-blocking drugs, drug-induced hypergastrinemia has become the most common condition to exclude[85] (see Table 28-3). Another consideration is hypochlorhydria, which is very common among patients with sporadic primary hyperparathyroidism (both states are concentrated among women beyond age 50). Another consideration specific to MEN1 is the interaction of gastrinoma and hyperparathyroidism. Z-E syndrome can diminish or even enter remission after successful parathyroidectomy[85] (see Fig. 28-1). It is not known if parathyroidectomy slows the growth of the gastrinomas.

Two separate gastrin measurements should be made because values can fluctuate. Most cases of Z-E syndrome show a gastrin level more than 10-fold above the upper limit of normal. With gastric acid pH below 3.0, the diagnosis is established. When the diagnosis is uncertain, provocative testing for hypergastrinemia should be done. Stimulants have included secretin, calcium infusion, and a standardized meal. The most effective stimulus is secretin. The criterion for an abnormal response to secretin is a positive change of serum gastrin greater than 200 pg/ml.[58,59,86] Unfortunately secretin became unavailable in 2000.

Once the diagnosis has been established, management must combine acid control, which may be accomplished pharmacologically, and tumor evaluation. The mainstay of tumor evaluation is imaging with radioactive octreotide. This agent is usually effective in distinguishing local from metastatic gastrinoma.[87–89]

Insulinoma. Insulinoma is expressed in 10 to 20 percent of patients with familial MEN1.[37,90] Onset has been as early as age 6 years.[56b] Mean age of onset is younger in MEN1 than in sporadic cases (age 30 versus 45 years).[33,41] Although they are associated with multiple islet tumors, their high surgical cure rate suggests that (1) the insulinoma syndrome in MEN1 usually results from one hypersecreting adenoma, and (2) the adenoma is usually 1–3 cm and often the largest islet tumor in that patient.[91–93]

The most common expression of insulinoma is neuroglycopenia, often worst on fasting and relieved by eating sweets. Once suspected, hypoglycemia should be documented during symptoms and during fasting. Other possible etiologies should be excluded, including prescribed medications, surreptitious use of hypoglycemic agents, wasting, hypoadrenalism, and growth hormone deficiency (in children). The most reliable test is a supervised fast. Most patients show hypoglycemia (sugar below 40 mg/dl) and neuroglycopenic symptoms by 48 h, but apparently negative tests should be carried to 72 h. Glucose, insulin, C-peptide, and proinsulin fraction should be measured at the time of hypoglycemia.[94] The single most useful indicator is an insulin concentration above 6 mU/ml at the time of hypoglycemia. This establishes insulin mediation of hypoglycemia; however, it does not exclude surreptitious use of insulin or sulfonylureas or hypoglycemia caused by antibodies against the insulin receptor.

Treatment of insulinoma in MEN1 is surgery. Insulinoma in MEN1 is usually benign. Failed initial operation was common in the past.[95] Because of the frequent association with multiple nonfunctioning islet tumors, it is desirable to identify the approximate location of insulin hypersecretion before resection. This can be done most effectively by selective arteriography with calcium infusion.[96] Transhepatic venous sampling has high yield, but it is not widely available, and it has substantial potential for

Table 28-3 Causes of Fasting Hypergastrinemia

With Deficient Gastric Acid Production	With Gastric Acid Production
Medications	Retained gastric antrum syndrome
Histamine H$_2$-receptor antagonists	Small bowel resection
Blockers of stomach acid pump	Chronic gastric outlet obstruction
Atrophic gastritis (includes pernicious anemia)	Antral G-cell hyperplasia or hyperfunction
Chronic renal failure	Gastrinoma
Postvagotomy/gastric resection	Laboratory error

morbidity.[97] Individual tumors are often small and are best localized with intraoperative ultrasound.[15,98] Noninvasive imaging methods, including octreotide radionuclide scanning, have low sensitivity for insulinoma, based on experience with sporadic insulinoma.[97] Approximately 15 percent of MEN1 insulinomas recur late after surgery; this could reflect insulinoma malignancy, benign insulinoma resected incompletely, or most likely a second and independently arising insulinoma.

Glucagonoma. Glucagonomas are islet tumors causing a syndrome of a specific dermatitis, weight loss, glucose intolerance, and anemia.[99–101] The specific skin rash is termed *migratory necrolytic erythema*.[102,103] Glucagonoma is rare in MEN1 (1 percent), and glucagonoma patients rarely have MEN1. Most tumours occur after age 40. They are usually in the pancreatic body or tail and large at presentation,[98,103] with 50 to 80 percent showing metastases at presentation.[100,101] Glucose intolerance characteristically predates recognition of glucagonoma by 5 years.[101] Glucose intolerance in MEN1 is more often idiopathic or secondary to Cushing syndrome.

VIPoma. VIPomas are enteropancreatic neuroendocrine tumors that oversecrete vasoactive intestinal protein (VIP). They cause severe watery diarrhea ("pancreatic cholera," a misnomer), hypokalemia, and hypochlorhydria.[105–109] This is sometimes called *Verner-Morrison syndrome* and sometimes called *WDHA syndrome*, for watery diarrhea, hypokalemia, and achlorhydria. Over 80 percent are in the pancreas,[110,111] but several occur in intestinal carcinoid or pheochromocytoma.[112] In children (age 2–4 years), the tumor is usually an extrapancreatic ganglioneuroma or ganglioneuroblastoma[111] and is not associated with MEN1. Just as glucagonomas, VIPomas in adults present usually after age 40 and are usually large and metastatic. Associated hypercalcemia in up to 50 percent of patients may be caused by tumor secretion of parathyroid hormone-related peptide,[112b] but in MEN1 this must be distinguished from associated primary hyperparathyroidism.

GRFoma. Growth hormone-releasing factor (GRF or GHRH) can be oversecreted by a tumor, a GRFoma. This is a rare tumor that stimulates the pituitary to release excessive growth hormone.[113,114] Approximately one-third of GRFomas are associated with MEN1.[115–117] GRFomas occur in the lung (53 percent), pancreas (30 percent), or small intestine (10 percent). They are often large and metastatic at presentation.[115,118] GRF is a 44-amino-acid peptide. Its oversecretion results in pituitary somatotroph hyperplasia and growth hormone excess. Most cases of growth hormone excess (with or without MEN1) are caused by primary tumor of the pituitary. GRFoma is diagnosed by finding growth hormone excess and high blood levels of GRF.

Somatostatinoma. Somatostatin-secreting tumor causes a syndrome of mild diabetes mellitus, gall bladder disease, weight loss, and anemia.[119,120] There is a frequent association of this rare tumor with MEN1 or with MEN2, but its prevalence in an MEN1 population seems very low. Most somatostatinomas are in the pancreatic head.[121,122] Fewer are in the proximal duodenum or ampulla of Vater. At presentation, most are large and metastatic. Commonly, somatostatin is the "second" hormone secreted by the tumor.[122] Somatostatin is a 14-amino-acid peptide with multiple inhibitory effects on the GI tract. It inhibits release of many hormones, including insulin, gastrin, and growth hormone. It decreases stomach acid secretion; decreases bile flow and gall bladder contractility; decreases pancreatic enzyme and fluid secretion; and decreases absorption of lipid, D-xylose, vitamin B$_{12}$, and folate.[123] All these actions contribute to somatostatinoma presentations.

PPomas and Nonfunctional Pancreatic Endocrine Tumors. P-Pomas are pancreatic tumors that oversecrete pancreatic polypeptide but do not cause a recognizable syndrome.[55,124–128] Nonfunctional tumors may or may not produce a hormonal peptide, but they do not secrete enough to cause a recognizable syndrome.[57,121,126] Nonfunctional tumors or PPomas, if they cause symptoms, do so by local or metastatic growth. They are among the most common tumors in MEN1,[45,55,61,127] but because they do not cause endocrine symptoms, they have received limited attention.[61] The finding of multiple pancreatic islet tumors is a strong predictor of MEN1.[61–63] If these tumors cause symptoms through growth, they are usually in the pancreatic head, large, and malignant.

Carcinoid Tumor of Bronchus or Thymus. Carcinoid tumors occur in derivatives of foregut, midgut, or hindgut. Carcinoid tumor in MEN1 is in foregut derivatives (bronchi, thymus, stomach, pancreas, duodenum).[129] This contrasts with sporadic carcinoid, which is predominantly hindgut in origin.[130] Unlike the equal sex distribution of sporadic bronchial carcinoid, female sex predominates by 4:1 in MEN1. Thymic carcinoids are 90 percent male in sporadic cases as well as in MEN1.[129]

Common presentations of mediastinal carcinoid in MEN1 are through mass effect, incidental to chest imaging, or incidental to prophylactic thymectomy (for primary hyperparathyroidism in MEN1). Carcinoid tumors of the bronchus or thymus in MEN1 rarely cause the carcinoid syndrome or secrete serotonin. They occasionally oversecrete histamine, which is converted to 5-hydroxyindoleacetic acid and measurable in urine. Occasionally, they cause an atypical carcinoid syndrome with facial flushing, lacrimation, headache, and bronchoconstriction; the biochemical cause is not known. Bronchial and thymic carcinoid can oversecrete endocrine peptides including ACTH,[132,133] GHRH,[134] calcitonin, and others, but this has been rare in MEN1. Sporadic carcinoid tumors are often malignant, and this also has been even more aggressive in thymic carcinoid in MEN1.[131]

Gastric ECLomas. Histamine-secreting enterochromaffin-like cells (ECL cells) are prominent among the endocrine cells of the human gastric oxyntic mucosa. In sporadic cases they produce tumors unrelated to hypergastrinemia. In MEN1, these ECLomas (also termed *gastric carcinoids*) are associated with hypergastrinemia.[135–137] It is thought that hypergastrinemia is associated with ECL cell stimulation. This has been seen in animal models and in pernicious anemia. ECLoma in MEN1 can remit following treatment with a somatostatin receptor blocker (octreotide), perhaps secondary to its lowering of gastrin secretion.[137b] Despite a presumed relation to hypergastrinemia, ECLomas are uncommon in association with sporadic gastrinoma.[65,135,136] Gastric ECLomas have no associated hormonal syndrome, and their natural history is unknown. They have been recognized in up to 15 percent of MEN1 patients incidental to endoscopies for gastrinoma.[138] Their malignant potential in MEN1 may be substantial.[139]

GI Tract Carcinoid Tumor. Carcinoid tumors are structurally indistinguishable from other peptide hormone non-secreting, enteropancreatic neuroendocrine tumors; thus the term *carcinoid tumor* has sometimes been applied to all these tumors.[57,65] Carcinoid of the midgut or hindgut is somewhat common in the general population, but there seems to be no real association of these latter carcinoids with MEN1. The non-MEN1 carcinoid of the terminal ileum often metastasizes to the liver, secretes serotonin, and can cause the carcinoid syndrome.[58,130,140]

Carcinoid Tumor Syndrome. Carcinoid tumors can secrete a variety of bioactive peptides and small molecules.[58,130,140] Carcinoid tumor syndrome is a complex thought to result from these products. It includes episodes of flushing, diarrhea, abdominal cramping, wheezing, dyspnea, and palpitations. Blood pressure falls rather than rises. It usually arises when a midgut carcinoid tumor metastasizes to the liver. It can arise from

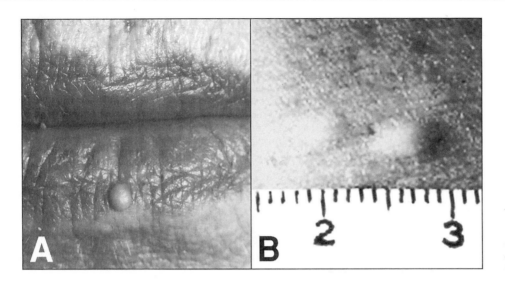

Fig. 28-2 Angiofibroma and collagenoma of the skin in MEN1. *A.* Facial angiofibroma. The papular, telangiectatic lesion, often multiple in MEN1, is mainly on the nose and cheeks. *B.* Collagenoma. This papular whitish lesion can be multiple. It appears on the upper torso, neck, and shoulders.

bronchial carcinoid without metastases. Most foregut carcinoids in MEN1 do not produce this syndrome.

Anterior Pituitary Tumor

Symptoms and signs of pituitary tumor are evident in 10 to 40 percent of symptomatic MEN1 patients. The symptoms and signs of pituitary tumor have age, sex, and hormone distributions (MEN1 shows some enrichment for prolactin[32]) similar to those in tumors not associated with MEN1.[33,38,41] The sex ratio favors women because the majority of tumors are prolactinomas (40–75 percent), with approximately 10 percent secreting prolactin and growth hormone, 10 percent growth hormone only, and 5 percent ACTH.[140,140b] Oversecretion of luteinizing hormone/follicle-stimulating hormone (LH/FSH) or thyroid-stimulating hormone (TSH) are even less common. Five percent are hormone nonsecreting and important because they present by mass effect (hypopituitarism, pituitary apoplexy, visual compromise).

Aside from mass effect, prolactinoma is recognized as galactorrhea, amenorrhea, and/or infertility in women. Hypogonadism may occur in men. Biochemical diagnosis depends mainly on a fasting prolactin level above 300 ng/ml (upper normal about 12 ng/ml). Milder elevations occur too but are hard to distinguish from loss of inhibition through stalk compression. Imaging is a useful supplement for diagnosis and management. Excellent images can be obtained with gadolinium-enhanced magnetic resonance imaging (MRI). As for prolactinoma, the features of other hormone-secreting pituitary tumors are similar in MEN1 and sporadic cases.

Other Tissue Features of MEN1

Thyroid Neoplasms. Thyroid follicular adenoma has long been recognized as an occasional association in MEN1,[36] but no detailed analysis has established other than a random association.

Primary Adrenocortical Neoplasms. Rare patients with MEN1 have shown hypercortisolism or hyperaldosteronism.[36,95,142] Analyses of adrenal cortical enlargement in MEN1 indicated frequent silent enlargement in 30 to 40 percent.[142] Adrenocortical cancer has been reported.[143]

Pheochromocytoma. Unilateral pheochromocytoma has been encountered in 8 cases of familial MEN1.[144b,144c] However, tumor documentation has so far been incomplete in each. All the same, it seems likely that this is a true but uncommon feature of MEN1.

Lipoma. While a common neoplasm, lipoma is especially common in MEN1, at 20 to 30 percent of patients.[36,145] Lipomas may occur anywhere, single or multiple. Large visceral lipomas can be noted by imaging or at laparotomy.

Skin Lesions. Surveys of MEN1 patients showed facial angiofibromas in 40–90 percent.[145] These were clinically and histologically identical to the lesions in tuberous sclerosis. Another highly specific finding was collagenomas in 72 percent. (Fig. 28-2) Confetti-like hypopigmented macules (6 percent) and multiple gingival papules (6 percent) were other findings that previously had been associated with tuberous sclerosis. Malignant melanoma has been noted in one member of seven different MEN1 kindreds,[145c] but separate MEN1 mutational studies have suggested that this is a coincidental, not an etiologic, association (see below).

Leiomyoma. Leiomyoma has been reported in the esophagus, uterus, or rectum in MEN1;[36,145d–145f] its frequency in MEN1 has not been analyzed.

Intrafamilial Homogeneity of MEN1

Prolactinoma Variant. One or two unusual expressions of MEN1 sometimes occur in a small kindred, such as a kindred with hyperparathyoridism, two cases of Cushing's disease, and no enteropancreatic tumor.[146] Such associations may be rare and random events. Ideally, large kindreds are preferred for efforts to recognize an unusual phenotype. Three large MEN1 kindreds (9–83 affected members) have shown a high frequency of prolactinoma (35–65 percent) but a low frequency of gastrinoma (2.5–11 percent).[147–151] The largest family also showed 14 percent carcinoid tumors.[151] The trait in these families has been termed the *prolactinoma variant* of MEN1, with MEN1$_{Burin}$ applied to the similar subfamilies about the Burin peninsula of Newfoundland.

In an extraordinarily large MEN1 pedigree from Tasmania, prolactinoma was found commonly (50 percent) in two branches but uncommonly in others. Although gastrinoma was not included in the analysis, the observations were used to suggest that the "prolactinoma phenotype" required a second mutation other than that causing MEN1.[152]

Other Possible Variants of MEN1

Hyperparathyroidism Variant. Several kindreds, reported initially as familial isolated hyperparathyroidism, subsequently expressed features of MEN1.[37] One large kindred showed only minimal features of MEN1 on follow-up.[37,153] Another large kindred showed likely linkage to 11q13 with a LOD (Logarithm of the odds) score of 2.1 and no other features of MEN1.[154] There are types of familial primary hyperparathyroidism not caused by the

Table 28-4 Syndromes of Hereditary Endocrine Neoplasia with Proven or Presumed Clonal Basis for Tumors*

Multiple Endocrine Neoplasia	Single Endocrine Neoplasia in Syndrome of Multiple Neoplasia	Isolated Endocrine Neoplasia
Multiple endocrine neoplasia type1	Hyperparathyroidism–jaw tumor syndrome	Hyperparathyroidism
Multiple endocrine neoplasia type 2a and type 2b	Cowden syndrome	Pituitary tumor
Von Hippel-Lindau syndrome	Neurofibromatosis type 1	Insulinoma
Carney complex	Li-Fraumeni syndrome	Carcinoid
McCune-Albright syndrome*	Tuberous sclerosis	Thyroid oxyphil

* Fibrous dysplasia in McCune-Albright syndrome is likely a post-zygotic mosaic proliferation that includes the clonal mutation.[197] This lesion may not be neoplastic and clonality or other criteria for neoplasia have not been tested in other pathologic tissues in this syndrome.

MEN1 gene (see below). It is not yet known if *MEN1* mutation can cause a stable phenotype of isolated hyperparathyroidism.

Insulinoma Variant. Several MEN1 kindreds showed disproportional prevalence of insulinoma with little gastrinoma.[37,39]

Cancer Variant. Most gastrinomas are multiple in MEN1.[64] A high, though undetermined, fraction have metastasized by the time they cause symptoms. In some kindreds, gastrinomas have seemed particularly aggressive.[39] In one large kindred, there was clustering of enteropancreatic malignancy cases, suggesting that modifiers determined penetrance of this *MEN1* expression.[155] This question requires additional study.

Earliest Penetrance by Organ

In general, expression of MEN1 begins with slowly developing hyperparathyroidism between the ages of 15 and 30 years. In planning biochemical and genetic screening programs, it is helpful to know about frequency and severity of very early expressions. There is little information on these points. The earliest reported expressions in MEN1 have been as follows: primary hyperparathyroidism at age 8,[33] prolactinoma at age 5,[156,157] and insulinoma at age 6.[44,56b]

TREATMENT OF MEN1

Treatment of the multiple expressions of MEN1 is not covered here. Suffice it to say that treatment can be complex and expensive. In general, each hormone-oversecreting tumor must be handled as an independent disorder requiring pharmacologic or surgical management.[158] Mild expressions (such as mild hyperparathyroidism) may only require periodic monitoring, whereas malignant expressions may prove refractory to most measures.

DIFFERENTIAL DIAGNOSIS

As pleiomorphic as it is, MEN1 has a potentially long list of conditions from which it must be distinguished. Conditions to be covered here are those which are the most relevant clinically and also those which may have special relevance with regard to understanding the metabolic pathway disturbed in MEN1.

Sporadic Multiple Endocrine Neoplasia

Any combination of endocrine neoplasia in more than one tissue is multiple endocrine neoplasia. Some such cases are expressions of *MEN1* germ-line mutation. Some others could be termed *MEN1 phenocopies*.

Pancreatic islet tumors can cause secondary endocrine tumors when the primary pancreatic tumor secretes "ectopically" ACTH[159,160] or growth hormone-releasing hormone.[161]

Some reports, based on single cases, are probably random coincidences.[162] There has been an association between primary hyperparathyroidism and nonmedullary thyroid cancer,[163,164] perhaps independent of the association attributable to radiation (see below). There have been other endocrine tumors with prolactinoma[165–168] or with acromegaly.[169,170] Some of the more intriguing cases have combined components of MEN1 and MEN2 within a single patient.[170–182]

A relation between radiation and thyroid neoplasia has been long recognized.[183,184] More recently, a relation between radiation and parathyroid neoplasia also has been recognized. Parathyroid and thyroid neoplasia, when they coexist, are often a consequence of prior radiation exposure.[184–193] The thyroid neoplasms may be uni- or multifocal and benign or malignant; the parathyroid tumors are almost always benign and sometimes multiple.

Hereditary Endocrine Neoplasia

There is a spectrum of hereditary endocrine neoplasias (Table 28-4). However, MEN1 is the only one for which endocrine/metabolic hyperfunctions are the principal manifestation.

Disorders with Hyperfunction in Multiple Endocrine Organs

McCune-Albright Syndrome. The McCune-Albright syndrome combines features of sporadic and hereditary neoplasia. The McCune-Albright syndrome is a complex of polyostotic fibrous dysplasia, café-au-lait skin pigmentation, and any among the following endocrine disorders: sexual precocity, hyperthyroidism, growth hormone oversecretion, and adrenal cortical hyperfunction.[194] This is usually caused by an activating mutation in Gs-α, a subunit of the stimulatory G-protein involved in signal transduction.[195] The mutation is apparently lethal in the germ line, but it can occur early in ontogeny so that the carrier is a mosaic. The mutation appears to cause tumor in tissues where overproduction of cyclic AMP leads to cell proliferation.[196] Fibrous dysplasia of bone, which is not clearly neoplastic, is composed of a mixture of cells with mutated $Gs\alpha$ and cells without mutated $Gs\alpha$.[197,197b]

Multiple Endocrine Neoplasia Type 2. MEN2[198] consists of neoplasms of thyroid C-cells, adrenal medulla, and parathyroid. A distinct, more morbid variant, MEN2b, has low penetrance for parathyroid tumors but has ganglioneuromas, submucosal neuromas, and a marfanoid habitus. MEN2 is caused usually or always by mutation of the *RET* gene on chromosome 10. It encodes the catalytic subunit of a membrane-bound tyrosine kinase whose normal extracellular ligands include glial cell-derived growth factor and nurturin. The mutations in MEN2 are in focused regions of the *RET* gene, and all are believed to be activating mutations. Because MEN2 rarely presents as hyperparathyroidism alone,[199] MEN2 is not difficult to distinguish from MEN1.

Carney Complex. Carney complex is a rare autosomal dominant complex of myxomas (cardiac, cutaneous, and breast), pigmented skin lesions, and endocrine tumors.[200,201] The endocrinopathies include pigmented bilateral adrenal lesions (often cortisol hypersecreting), acromegaly, Sertoli or Leydig cell tumor of testis, and thyroid neoplasms.[202] The disorder is usually linked to chromosome 2p or to 17q.[203,204] One of the two causative genes is at 17q and encodes a regulatory subunit of protein kinase-A (cyclic AMP dependent protein kinase).[204b]

Von Hippel-Lindau Syndrome. This disorder is characterized by hemangioblastoma of the central nervous system (CNS), retinal angiomatosis, renal clear cell carcinoma, visceral cysts, and pheochromocytoma.[205] Pancreatic cysts and pancreatic islet cell tumors are associated. The islet cell tumors occur in 10 percent, are usually nonfunctional, and can be benign or malignant.[206] Patients with this disease also rarely show other endocrine tumor such as carcinoid, prolactinoma, and medullary thyroid cancer.[207] The *VHL* gene functions by a tumor-suppressor mechanism, is at chromosome 3p, and has been cloned.[208] It encodes a protein that may interact with several other proteins important in the cell cycle.[209]

Hereditary Disorders with Hyperfunction in One Endocrine Organ (Likely Clonal)

Cloned Tumor-Suppressor Genes with Endocrine Tumor as a Minor Feature. Li-Fraumeni syndrome (*p53* inactivating mutations) can be expressed as many types of cancer. Adrenal cortical cancer occurs in about 1 percent of patients with the Li-Fraumeni syndrome.[210]

Cowden syndrome (*PTEN* inactivating mutations) is expressed most often as breast cancer and hamartomas. Thyroid neoplasia is seen in some 50 percent of patients with Cowden syndrome (about 20 percent of the thyroid neoplasms are malignant).[211]

Neurofibromatosis type 1 causes neural disturbances including café-au-lait spots, neurofibromas, benign and malignant tumors of the nervous system, Lisch nodules of the iris, and mental retardation.[212] Pheochromocytoma occurs in about 1 percent. Hyperparathyroidism, usually a single adenoma, has been associated at least 11 times.[213] It is unclear if this is a random association; 17q loss of heterozygosity (LOH) analysis in associated parathyroid tumors could clarify this question. Rare associations include duodenal somatostatinoma[214] and adrenocortical adenoma.[215,216] The *NF1* gene is on 17q, functions as a tumor suppressor, and has been cloned.[217] It encodes a protein, neurofibromin, with a GTPase activating protein-like domain that down-regulates GTP-bound ras.

Familial Hyperparathyroidism and Jaw Tumors. About 20 families have been described with parathyroid tumors and fibroosseus jaw tumors.[218] The parathyroid tumors sometimes have a micro- or macrocystic appearance.[219] Parathyroid cancer also has occurred in 10% of these cases. Other features clearly associated in one large family are kidney cysts, Wilms tumor, and nephroblastoma.[220] The trait in most of these families has been linked to chromosome 1q21-32, and there was LOH about this locus in renal hamartomas and in parathyroid tumors, suggesting cause by a tumor-suppressor gene at this locus.[220–222] Two large families with autosomal dominant hyperparathyroidism plus parathyroid cancer[223,223b,224] may express this disorder but were not originally tested for linkage to chromosome 1q.

Isolated Hyperparathyroidism. Familial isolated hyperparathyroidism has been described in many, mostly small kindreds. Some undoubtedly have MEN1,[37] others have familial hypocalciuric hypercalcemia (see below), few likely have the hyperparathyroidism–jaw tumor syndrome, while others probably have still different disorders.[224b] Most transmission patterns have been consistent with autosomal dominant transmission, with one suggesting a recessive mode.[225] Unusual features in some families have been early age of onset, severe hypercalcemia, and occasionally tumor of one parathyroid gland.[226,227] In one report, three or four tumors representing different kindreds showed LOH at chromosome 13q,

raising the possibility of germ-line mutation in a tumor-suppressor gene in that region.[228]

Isolated Pancreatic Islet Tumors. There are two reports of familial insulinoma without other endocrinopathy.[229,230] In each kindred, this was seen in a father and a daughter.

Isolated Pituitary Tumors. Acromegaly alone has been seen in several families.[231–235] Haplotype and tumor LOH studies in two families suggested that the tumor might be an expression of *MEN1* germ-line mutation.[237,237b] Four small families have had prolactinomas in first-degree relatives.[238]

Isolated Carcinoid Tumors. Occasionally, carcinoid tumors show familial clustering independent of MEN1.[239–243] The tumors have been in the terminal ileum or appendix (five families) or in the duodenum (one family).

Hereditary Disorders with Non-Neoplastic Hyperfunction of One Hormone-Secreting Tissue (Likely Polyclonal or Hyperplastic)

Hypocalciuric Hypercalcemia and Neonatal Severe Primary Hyperparathyroidism. The hereditary disorder most often requiring differentiation from MEN1 is familial hypocalciuric hypercalcemia (FHH), also termed *familial benign hypercalcemia*.[244] This is an autosomal dominant form of hypercalcemia with a prevalence similar to that of MEN1. Features that distinguish it from MEN1 are highlighted (see Table 28-2). In FHH, serum calcium level (if tested) is high near birth, and its degree of elevation remains stable throughout life. In FHH, urine calcium level is usually in the normal range; as a result, the hypercalcemia does not raise the incidence of calcium urolithiasis. A useful diagnostic index in hypercalcemic patients is the ratio of calcium clearance over creatinine clearance. Values in FHH are usually below 0.01, whereas those in typical primary hyperparathyroidism are usually above. Parathyroid hormone (PTH) levels are typically normal in FHH.[245] The parathyroid glands are normal to minimally enlarged,[246] and subtotal parathyroidectomy is followed by persistent hypercalcemia in FHH. FHH is usually or always a disturbance in calcium recognition by the parathyroid cells and perhaps by the renal tubular cells.[247] Most familial cases are linked to chromosome 3q and can be attributed to mutations in a parathyroid cell surface calcium-sensing receptor (*CaS-R*).[248] Cases in rare kindreds are linked to chromosome 19p, 19q, (Table 28-5).[249,250]

FHH patients with homozygous inactivating mutation of the *CaS-R* express extremely severe neonatal primary hyperparathyroidism with impressive enlargement of all parathyroid glands and with serum total calcium generally above 4 mM.[248,251,252]

Non-Neoplastic Hyperfunction in Endocrine Tissue Other than Parathyroid. Mutation in one of several genes has been identified as a cause of endocrine polyclonal hyperfunction limited to one, presumed hyperplastic hormone-secreting tissue and not associated with a multiple neoplasia syndrome (Table 28-5). The resulting syndromes all begin in the neonatal period and vary from hyperparathyroidism,[248] to hyperthyroidism,[253] to testotoxicosis (isosexual male precocious puberty),[254] or to hyperinsulinism.[255–258,258b]

The causative genes generally show a relatively organ-specific expression pattern. Their encoded proteins include three serpentine G-protein-coupled membrane receptors (the calcium ion-sensing receptor of the parathyroid gland, the TSH receptor of the thyroid follicular cell, and the LH/HCG receptor of Leydig cells) and four proteins involved in glucose recognition by the pancreatic beta cell (two nonhomologous membrane subunits of the ATP-sensitive potassium channel and two cytoplasmic enzymes that determine the islet beta cell ATP concentration). Each functions in recognition by a hormone-secreting cell of a major extracellular factor that regulates hormone secretion by that cell (Table 28-5).

Table 28-5 Cloned Genes Whose Mutation Can Cause Hereditary Hyperfunction of One Non-Neoplastic (Presumably Hyperplastic or Polyclonal) Hormone-Secreting Tissue

Syndrome	Oversecreted Hormone	Gene Mutation(s)*	Extracellular Sensor Pathway Disturbed
Hypocalciuric hypercalcemia	PTH	CaS-R⁻ †	Parathyroid cell response to serum ionized calcium
Neonatal severe primary hyperparathyroidism	PTH	CaS-R⁻ × CaS-R⁻	Parathyroid cell response to serum ionized calcium
Juvenile thyrotoxicosis	T_3/T_4	TSH-R⁺	Thyrocyte response to serum TSH
Testotoxicosis	Testosterone	LH/CG-R⁺	Leydig cell response to serum LH
Persistent hyperinsulinemic hypoglycemia of infancy	Insulin	SUR⁻ × SUR1⁻	Pancreatic islet beta cell response to blood glucose
Persistent hyperinsulinemic hypoglycemia of infancy	Insulin	Kir6.2⁻ × Kir6.2⁻	Pancreatic islet beta cell response to blood glucose
Persistent hyperinsulinemic hypoglycemia of infancy	Insulin	GK⁺	Pancreatic islet beta cell response to blood glucose
Persistent hyperinsulinemic hypoglycemia of infancy	Insulin	GLUD1⁺	Pancreatic islet beta cell response to blood glucose

* Gene abbreviations: *Ca-SR* = calcium ion-sensing receptor (mainly on plasma membrane of parathyroid cell); *TSH-R* = receptor for thyroid stimulating hormone (mainly on plasma membrane of thyrocyte); *LH/CG-R* = receptor for luteinizing hormone or chorionic gonadotropin (in males, mainly on plasma membrane of Leydig cells); *SUR1* = sulfonylurea receptor (part of ATP-sensitive K⁺ channel of pancreatic beta cells); *Kir6.2* = inward rectifying K⁺ channel subunit (part of ATP-sensitive K⁺ channel of pancreatic beta cells); *GK* = glucokinase; *GLUD1*=glutamate dehydrogenase.
† Mutation momenclature: − = inactivating mutation; + = activating mutation; × = accompanied by a second, in these cases mutated, allele (i.e., homozygous mutation).

The neonatal onset or lack of postnatal latency interval seems to reflect one-hit expression and this disturbance in hormone secretory regulation, independent of a period for clonal cell accumulation.

The underlying endocrine gland histology often suggests a diffuse or polyclonal process[246,259,260,260a]; endocrine malignancy is not an expression of these hereditary syndromes. However, mutation of the *TSH-R* or of the *LH/CG-R* also has been implicated in sporadic, clonal neoplasm of the thyrocyte and Leydig cell, respectively, and thus could even contribute to malignancy in these tissues.[261,262] Most of the preceding features (excepting involvement in sporadic neoplasia) and mechanisms contrast in important ways with features of the genes for MEN1 and other multiple neoplasia syndromes.[258b]

CELLULAR EXPRESSIONS OF MEN1

MEN1 Growth Factor

An early phase in MEN1 angiofibroma may be clonal proliferation of perivascular cells.[262b]

A growth promoting activity was detected in MEN1 plasma when incubated with cultured parathyroid cells.[263–266] High levels were independent of age among adults.[267] Preliminary data pointed to high levels even in young, asymptomatic *MEN1* gene carriers.[268] This growth factor shared many features with FGF-2 or basic fibroblast growth factor, including size, immunologic epitopes, and reactivity toward endothelium.[269,270] The FGF family is small, but all members are potent mitogens.[271] The growth activity in MEN1 plasma could be tumor-derived. However, parathyroid tumors apparently have been excluded as the source.[266] Pituitary tumor is a possible source because the circulating growth activity fell after treatment of pituitary tumors by surgery or medication.[272]

Any role for a circulating growth factor in MEN1 remains unknown. It could be an unimportant by-product of the neoplastic process. It could be an autocrine or paracrine factor that escapes into the circulation. It could be a circulating factor that acts on one or more target tissues to help initiate the neoplastic process. Since the *MEN1* gene is a tumor suppressor, the MEN1 growth factor is not likely to be a product of the *MEN1* gene. However, it

remains possible that overexpression of the MEN1 growth factor is an early, albeit downstream, consequence of inactivation of one or both copies of the *MEN1* gene.

Chromosomal Instability

Several studies have suggested increased frequency of chromosomal breakage in MEN1. Cultured lymphocytes in familial MEN1 showed increased frequency of gaps and chromatid-type abnormalities[273] Lymphocytes also showed increased chromosomal breakage[274] and a subtle defect in DNA repair.[274b,274c] Cultured lymphocytes and cultured fibroblasts from MEN1 patients showed increased chromosomal instability.[275]

GENETIC LOCI

Hereditary Patterns

Genetic Linkage

Near Homogeneity. In 1988, Larsson first reported, in three Swedish kindreds, genetic linkage of MEN1 trait to *PYGM* (muscle phosphorylase locus) at chromosome 11q13.[18] This was confirmed in a single large American kindred, with MEN1 linked to *INT-2* at 11q13.[276] Subsequently, many MEN1 kindreds showed similar linkage to several probes at 11q13. The kindreds have been in Japan,[277] Asia,[278] Finland,[279] and North America,[280] plus England, France, Tasmania, and Sweden.[281] A workshop-based survey of 87 families (including many of those cited above) suggested that the trait was linked to 11q13 in all kindreds evaluated to that point.[282]

Prolactinoma Variant. The largest kindreds with the prolactinoma variant of MEN1 are located almost solely in Newfoundland, Canada. This variant has been termed *MEN1*ₐ, after the Burin Peninsula where most patients live.[148] Linkage of MEN1 to 11q13 was demonstrated in those kindreds.[283] Furthermore, a common founder for the four apparently separate families with MEN1ᴮᵘʳⁱⁿ was suggested by finding linkage to the same allele of *PYGM* in each Newfoundland family[283] and strongly supported by a detailed demonstration of a shared 11q13 haplotype and a shared *MEN1* mutation.[284]

Locus Heterogeneity. Subsequently, one large kindred almost meeting the criteria of MEN1 (but no member showed two major MEN1 features) raised the possibility of locus heterogeneity, since their MEN1 trait was not linked to 11q13.[285] This kindred had several features that would be unusual for MEN1. In generation 1 there was a patient with primary hyperparathyroidism. In generation 2 there were (1) a patient with acromegaly, (2) a patient with acromegaly and possible hyperparathyroidism, and (3) an asymptomatic carrier. In generation 3 there was a patient with prolactinoma. Screening suggested that other members may express the trait in mild forms. Linkage analysis of affected patients excluded 11q13. This kindred could be categorized, alternately, as showing familial pituitary tumors (see also above and below).

Rare Situations

Twins. MEN1 was described in a pair of identical twins. Their disease expressions differed, though not strikingly.[286] At age 25, both had hyperparathyroidism and prolactinoma. One also had gastrinoma and Cushing disease. Few other twin pairs have been reported in the accumulated experience.[286a] The stochastic nature of the tumors makes interindividual variability likely.

Possible Homozygotes. A sibship was reported in which apparently unrelated parents each were likely heterozygotes for MEN1.[287] Haplotype analysis suggested that two of three siblings were homozygotes (double heterozygotes) for MEN1. Their features of MEN1 were not unusually severe or early in onset, although both (a male and a female) had unexplained infertility. *MEN1* mutation has been identified in only one side of the family,[287b] so compound heterozygosity is not proven. Another sibship includes two remotely related parents with MEN1_Burin, the prolactinoma variant of MEN1.[148,284] They had two children. One seemed unaffected, and a daughter expressed galactorrhea at age 23 (presumed prolactinoma) and died at age 30 of an invasive thymic carcinoid without expressing hyperparathyroidism. Her *MEN1* allele status or *MEN1* mutation status was not known.

Sporadic MEN1

There have been many reports of sporadic MEN1 cases.[36] These cases have two, three, or more features of MEN1. Some such cases represent coincidental occurrence of common plus uncommon diseases. Many others, however, are likely expressions of the *MEN1* gene (see below, *MEN1* germ-line mutations among sporadic cases).

Endocrine tumor in a single tissue system is also a predictable expression of the *MEN1* gene. This had not been possible to test rigorously until the *MEN1* gene was isolated.[288] In the near future, *MEN1* germ-line mutation will be explored in apparently sporadic primary hyperparathyroidism (particularly that caused by multiple parathyroid tumors and that in younger patients),[26b] sporadic Z-E syndrome, and sporadic pituitary tumor.

11q13 LOSS OF HETEROZYGOSITY

MEN1 Tumors and Tissues

Endocrine Tumors. Larsson reported in 1988 that two MEN1 insulinomas had loss of alleles from the chromosome 11 copy, inherited from the unaffected parent.[18] This led to their prediction that the *MEN1* gene would be a tumor-suppressor gene; i.e., it would cause tumors by a sequential gene inactivation mechanism in the tumor precursor cell(s) ("two hit" hypothesis).[289,290] Subsequently, depending on the probes and on variable normal DNA contamination of tumor DNA, 11q13 LOH has been shown to be frequent in MEN1 tumors of the parathyroids[49b,292–296] and pituitary,[297] approaching 100 percent of tumors following microdissection.[297–301b] 11q13 LOH also has been found in 85 percent of nongastrinoma pancreatic islet tumors,[302] in 40 percent of gastrinomas,[302] and in 75 percent of gastric carcinoids.[303] Fewer

MEN1 bronchial carcinoids and lipomas have been tested, but approximately 50 percent of each type show 11q13 LOH.[304] It is likely that the 11q13 LOH rate in MEN1 tumors would be near 100 percent if near-in probes were used with noncontaminated tumor DNA specimens. Adrenal cortex shows generally silent bilateral enlargement in about a third of MEN1 patients; 11q13 LOH was not found.[142] 11q13 LOH was also not found in any thymic carcinoids of MEN1 cases.[131]

Studies of MEN1 tumors have suggested involvement of other tumor-suppressor genes in addition to *MEN1*. In particular there was 1p LOH in 21 percent of MEN1 parathyroids.[305] And comparative genomic hybridization studies of multiple tumors from one patient showed losses from large regions of seven chromosomes, including chromosome 11.[144c,306] There has been no extensive survey in MEN1 to determine the full spectrum of other genes that may cooperate in development of these neoplasms.

Nonendocrine Tumors. Initially, three MEN1 angiofibromas did not show 11q13 LOH.[304] It is notable that two angiofibromas in tuberous sclerosis also did not show LOH at either of the two tuberous sclerosis disease loci.[307] Both diseases are associated with other tumors that show LOH at the locus of the germ-line mutation; however, it was uncertain if the syndrome-associated angiofibromas were neoplasms or other dysplasias. If they were neoplasms, they might have a large stromal/fibrous component, and the neoplastic component may not have been sufficiently cleared from normal tissue admixture to allow LOH to be recognized. Single-cell analysis (FISH or fluorescent *in situ* hybridization) of angiofibroma, collagenoma, lipoma, and leiomyoma in MEN1 subsequently showed loss of one *MEN1* allele, establishing that these are neoplasms and "two hit" in development.[145e,145f,309] 11q13 LOH was identified in two esophageal leiomyomata of one MEN1 case.[145c]

Sporadic Tumors

Endocrine Tumors. In general, sporadic endocrine tumors have shown frequent 11q13 LOH, though not as frequent as in MEN1-associated tumors. This suggests that mutation of the *MEN1* gene often contributes to these sporadic tumors and also that other oncogenes and tumor-suppressor genes play an even more important role in these sporadic tumors than in MEN1.[309] Twenty to 60 percent of sporadic parathyroid tumors show 11q13 LOH.[49b,228,293,295] 11q13 LOH has been found in 19 percent of sporadic insulinomas[302] and in 45 percent of sporadic gastrinomas, this latter being a similar incidence to that in MEN1 gastrinoma in the same study.[302] Analyses on smaller numbers of sporadic islet tumors have found similar frequencies of 11q13 LOH.[293,311] Sporadic pituitary tumors have shown variable frequency of 11q13 LOH, perhaps relating to contamination by normal tissue and to variable informativeness of the probes used: 3 percent (selectively high LOH for prolactinoma?),[293] 33 percent in somatotropinomas,[311] and 15 to 30 percent similarly distributed among 88 nonfunctioning growth hormone-secreting, prolactin-secreting, and ACTH-secreting.[312] One large analysis found approximately 30 percent 11q13 LOH in invasive pituitary tumors versus 3 percent in noninvasive.[313] The highest rate of 11q13 LOH among sporadic tumors has been reported at 78 percent among carcinoids.[314] In this series, 11q13 LOH had similar frequency in carcinoids of the foregut, midgut, and hindgut. However, a more recent report did not find 11q13 LOH in intestinal or rectal carcinoids.[303] One report found 15 percent 11q13 LOH in benign follicular tumors of the thyroid but not in papillary tumors or malignant follicular tumors of the thyroid.[315] Thirty-five percent of aldosteronomas showed 11q13 LOH.[316] A separate analysis found 11q13 LOH in most adrenocortical cancers but in few adrenocortical benign tumors.[317] Not surprisingly, 11q13 LOH also has been found in some endocrine tumors in familial settings different from MEN1: in particular, familial hyperparathyroidism[318] and familial acromegaly.[237,319]

Uremic Parathyroids. Renal failure causes a multifactorial enlargement of the parathyroid glands (secondary hyperparathyroidism). Occasionally, the process becomes sufficiently dysregulated as to resist suppression and occasionally to cause PTH-mediated hypercalcemia (tertiary hyperparathyroidism). In either secondary or tertiary hyperparathyroidism, occasionally surgical removal of portions of the parathyroids is the best treatment. Four studies of these abnormal tissues have found that they usually contain monoclonal components.[228,320–322] 11q13 LOH was found in 0 to 16 percent.

Nonendocrine tumors. 11q13 LOH has been found in several tumors without known relation to MEN1. This includes *in situ* and invasive breast cancer[323,324] and cervical cancer.[325,326]

MEN1 GENE

Methods of Discovery

Positional Candidates. The search for the *MEN1* gene was accelerated by findings in 1988 that it was linked to 11q13 and that, since MEN1 tumors showed LOH about this locus, it was likely to be a tumor-suppressor gene.[18] In the ensuing years, the candidate interval was gradually narrowed by identifying kindred members with important meiotic recombinations between *MEN1* and nearby loci.[280,281,327] In addition, several "positional candidate" genes,[328] which had been mapped to this interval, did not show mutation in MEN1 and thus seemed unlikely to be the *MEN1* gene, including *FAU*,[329] *phospholipase C beta*,[330] and *REL A*.[331] In retrospect, it is evident that testing of the few available positional candidates could not have uncovered the *MEN1* gene at that time.

Positional Cloning. Identification of the *MEN1* gene was achieved by positional cloning, a strategy that used a combination of methods.[19] In short, these methods were (1) assemble a large set of overlapping DNA clones including development of new polymorphic markers therein, (2) narrow the candidate interval using recombinant cases in kindreds and using 11q13 LOH in tumors, (3) identify candidate genes, all possible (near 100%) from genomic sequence in the narrowest candidate interval, and (4) search for mutations in candidate genes by dideoxy fingerprinting

for mutation screening and then selective sequencing analysis of MEN1 probands (Fig. 28-2).

A contig (overlapping DNA, cloned in YACs, bacterial artificial clones (BACs), PACs, P1s, and cosmids) was assembled to ensure uninterrupted coverage of 2.8 million bases encompassing the *MEN1* gene.[332] Thirty-three candidate genes were identified in this interval.[333] New polymorphic probes were developed[334] to help narrow the interval through linkage and 11q13 LOH analyses.[301,327]

The candidate interval was narrowed with analysis of recombinants in families (genetic linkage) and with 11q13 LOH in tumors using the newly developed polymorphic probes. Almost 200 tumors were analyzed, mostly from familial MEN1 but some from sporadic cases.[298,301,302] Because PCR reactions with tumor DNA sometimes gave confusing results (unexpected retention of two alleles within a larger zone of allelic loss) attributable to admixture with nontumor DNA, most tumors were microdissected with customized pipettes or with laser capture.[299,300]

The minimal candidate interval from meiotic recombinations was between *D11S1883* and *D11S449*[281,302] (Fig. 28-3). However 11q13 LOH in four tumors allowed an inward shift of the centromeric border to *PYGM,* and one tumor moved the telomeric border centromerically to *DS11S4936.* Thus the size of the candidate interval had been narrowed from 3000 kb, based on meiotic recombination, down to only 300 kb based on 11q13 LOH.[301]

Genomic sequence for most of the 300-kb interval in the final steps of the search was obtained by "shotgun" sequencing of two BACs and by obtaining additional cosmid sequences available publicly. This sequence was used to identify eight genes in the minimal interval. Segments of seven genes were matched initially through computer software to publicly available ESTs (expressed sequence tags), and one gene was identified from a computer software prediction of introns and exons.

Mutation Testing of Candidate Genes with a DNA Panel from MEN1 Probands. Full-length cDNA of a candidate transcript was isolated and sequenced. The intron/exon boundaries were determined from comparing the cDNAs and genomic sequences. Candidate genes were tested for mutations, using a DNA panel from probands representing 15 MEN1 kindreds. Mutations were screened by dideoxy fingerprinting, a method that combines

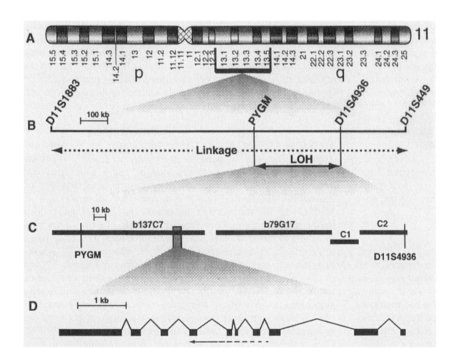

Fig. 28-3 Steps in positional cloning of the *MEN1* gene. Initial genetic linkage to chromosome 11q13 (*A*) was followed by finer mapping by meiotic recombination (an extension of genetic linkage) (*B*) and yet finer mapping by loss of heterozygosity (LOH) analyses in tumors (*B*). Nearly complete bacterial clone coverage was achieved across the most likely interval (*C*). Shotgun DNA sequencing revealed eight new candidate genes. One of these candidates had 10 exons (*D*). revealing mutations in 14 MEN1 probands among a testing panel of 15 probands. (*From Chandrasekharappa et al.*[19] *Used with permission.*)

features of dideoxy chain termination sequencing and single-strand conformation polymorphism.[335]

Most genes showed occasional polymorphisms (present in normal individuals and MEN1 probands). Only one anonymous gene (*Mu*) showed mutations in many MEN1 probands. Mutations of this anonymous gene were identified in 14 of the 15 probands. The mutations were present in other MEN1-affected family members and not in 142 normal chromosomes. Most mutations were nonsense/stop codons or frameshifts; a few were missense mutations or inframe deletions. These mutations, thereby specific for MEN1 and likely deleterious for function of the encoded protein, established the identification of the *MEN1* gene.

Germ-Line *MEN1* Mutations

In MEN1 Families. Germ-line mutations in the open reading frame of the *MEN1* gene were found initially in members of 47 of 50 MEN1 kindreds from North America.[336] Germ-line mutation was not evaluated in most of the noncoding 5′, 3′, or intronic portions of the *MEN1* gene. Thus it is apparent that all or most families with typical MEN1 do have germ-line mutations in the open reading frame of this gene. Similar mutation rates also were found in other centers.[33c,56b,287b,319,337–340]

Among Sporadic Cases. Sporadic MEN1, defined as endocrine tumor in two or more of the main MEN1-related tissues, has shown high *MEN1* mutation prevalence, similar to that in familial cases.[33d,336,340,340b] Several of these cases were proven to have new mutations, with 10 percent of all mutations being new in an extensive survey.[340]

Repeating *MEN1* Germ-Line Mutations. Eight mutations occurred more than one time among 50 North American MEN1 kindreds.[336] The six mutations occurring twice each did not reflect founder effects but rather mini-hot spots of mutation.[341] The most frequent mutations occurred six (512delC) and five (416delC) times. Haplotype analysis indicated that, like the Newfoundland cluster with R460X and with the prolactinoma variant of MEN1,[283,284] all kindreds in the two large clusters must share a common ancestor.[341] A similar conclusion was possible for a cluster of six Finnish families with 1466del12.[342] The Newfoundland and Finland MEN1 clusters in particular are typical of the founder effects that characterize hereditary diseases in geographically or socially constrained populations.

Genotype/Phenotype Correlations. Three kindreds with the prolactinoma variant of MEN1 were tested to explore possible genotype/phenotype correlations.[147–151,283,284] Two kindreds had germ-line *MEN1* mutations (R460X and Y312X). The third did not have a mutation identified but showed MEN1 linkage to 11q13 (LOD score 3.25), suggesting that it has an unrecognized *MEN1* mutation. The three presumed different *MEN1* mutations showed no recognizable difference from other *MEN1* mutations.[336] Thus no explanation for the prolactinoma variant could be recognized from the type of *MEN1* mutation. Other explanations for such a phenotype could include other associated polymorphisms in *MEN1*, linked feature in a neighboring gene, *MEN1* mutation occurring in a modifying background, and unrecognized ascertainment bias. *MEN1* mutation has been found in more than ten families with isolated hyperparathyroidism, also with no specific genotype (see below).[224b,342a,342b,342c]

Possible *MEN1* Phenocopies

Familial Isolated Hyperparathyroidism. Familial isolated hyperparathyroidism can be an early or incomplete expression of MEN1,[37,342a,342b,342c] but most such families have other causes. In an analysis of 36 kindreds with familial isolated hyperparathyroidism, none had *MEN1* mutation.[224b] However, five had mutation of the *calcium-sensing receptor* gene as in familial hypocalciuric hypercalcemia, and three had the hyperparathyroidism-jaw tumor syndrome. The remaining 28 families did not have an etiology

proven, but occult hyperparathyroidism-jaw tumor syndrome could not be tested as that gene had not been identified yet, and the families were too small for analysis of genetic linkage to that locus.

Familial Pituitary Tumors. None among 13 small families with hereditary pituitary tumor, mainly acromegaly, have shown germ-line *MEN1* mutation.[319,342,342c] One of these families (see above) with three members with pituitary tumor also had a member with hyperparathyroidism; the MEN1-like trait in this family was not linked to 11q13.[285,342]

Sporadic Endocrine Tumor as a Possible *MEN1* Phenocopy. As part of evaluations of tumors for somatic *MEN1* mutation (see below), tumor-bearing patients also were evaluated for germ-line *MEN1* mutation. As a result, *MEN1* germ-line mutation was excluded in the following 119 cases of sporadic endocrine tumor: 31 with hyperparathyroidism,[318] 38 with pituitary tumor,[156] 27 with gastrinoma,[345] 12 with insulinoma[345] and 11 with bronchial carcinoid.[347] In Japan, germline *MEN1* mutation was found in 3 of 64 cases of sporadic hyperparathyroidism;[26b] there, familial involvement with MEN1 may be particularly difficult to determine by routine questioning (see above).

Somatic *MEN1* Mutations

A somatic *MEN1* mutation, by definition, arises in a somatic tissue and is not in the germ line of the patient. In fact, germ-line mosaicism is sometimes impossible to exclude. 11q13 LOH indicates, in sporadic or hereditary tumor, a large somatic mutation, reflecting a chromosomal or subchromosomal rearrangement. Small somatic mutation, generally L-3 bases of the *MEN1* gene has been found in 12 to 21 percent of sporadic parathyroid adenomas,[318,343,344] 33 percent of sporadic gastrinomas,[345,346] 17 percent of sporadic insulinomas,[345] and 36 percent of sporadic bronchial carcinoids.[347] For each of those four tumors, *MEN1* is the known gene most frequently found to be mutated. *MEN1* mutation did not correlate with any clinical feature, such as invasivness in a large series of gastrinomas.[347b] The *MEN1* mutation frequency has been lower (0–5 percent) in sporadic pituitary tumors, in parathyroid cancer, or in uremic hyperparathyroidism.[156,348,349,349b,349c] In the prior analyses, *MEN1* mutation was almost always associated with 11q13 LOH if this was evaluated.[349d] Furthermore, for all but bronchial carcinoid, 11q13 LOH also was found in a similar fraction of tumors with and without *MEN1* mutation. Most likely, this excess of 11q13 LOH without *MEN1* mutation reflects other mechanisms (such as promoter methylation)[350] for inactivation of the first *MEN1* allele. Additional possibilities include undiscovered *MEN1* mutations and inactivation of other, unknown 11q13 tumor-suppressor gene(s).[351] Despite frequent LOH at 11q13, thyroid tumors or adrenocortical cancer have not had somatic *MEN1* mutation.[317,351b]

Somatic *MEN1* mutation also has been implicated in certain nonendocrine tumors: angiofibroma (2 of 19)[352] and lipoma (1 of 6).[353]

MEN1 as One of Many Genes Implicated in Parathyroid Tumors. The *MEN1* gene is frequently mutated in certain endocrine tumors, but it is just one of many genes that can contribute by mutation to endocrine tumorigenesis. By way of illustration, parathyroid tumor is notable for its importance in MEN1 and for the number of genes that have already been implicated in tumor development (Table 28-6). Activating mutation in either of two genes, *RET* or *Cyclin D1*, contributes to parathyroid tumorigenesis.[198,199,354,355] However, *RET* activation has not been found in sporadic parathyroid tumor,[356] and *Cyclin D1* activating mutation has been found in only 4 percent of sporadic parathyroid tumors.[354,355] Other loci of possible gene amplification have been suggested with comparative genome hybridization, but there was insufficient agreement between the two studies to conclude that any one locus was important.[355b,355c] Gene inactivation has been recognized more frequently than gene

Table 28-6 Genes Contributing by Mutation to Hereditary and/or Sporadic Parathyroid Tumor, Including Parathyroid Cancer*

	Parathyroid Tumorigenesis from Gain of Gene Function	Parathyroid Tumorigenesis from Loss of Gene Function
Cloned genes	Cyclin D1 (S) RET(H)	MEN1 (S & H) CaS-R(H) RB1(S) P53(S)
Loci of noncloned genes		1q21-32 (hyperpara–jaw tumor) (H) LOH evidence (1p, 6q, 15q, X) (S)

* Abbreviations: S = sporadic; H = hereditary.

activation in parathyroid tumors. Heterozygous or homozygous mutation of the calcium-sensing receptor is implicated in hereditary variants of hyperparathyroidism (see Table 28-5), but these have not been identified in sporadic parathyroid tumor.[357–359] Inactivation of *RB1* or *p53* is common in sporadic parathyroid cancer but rare in common-variety parathyroid adenoma.[360–363] As yet unidentified genes are also likely to be implicated. The gene for hyperparathyroidism–jaw tumor is probably a tumor suppressor[219] but LOH at this 1q24 locus has not been implicated in sporadic parathyroid tumors. LOH has been identified in several loci in parathyroid tumors;[309] in particular, 1p34 LOH seems about as frequent as 11q13 LOH. Additional loci have been implicated by recognizing chromosomal or subchromosomal DNA loss with comparative genome hybridization.[355b,355c]

Functions of the *MEN1* Gene

The function of the *MEN1* gene is not known.[19] The gene is approximately 9000 bases long with a message of 2800 bases. Across exons 2–10, it encodes a predicted protein, named *menin*, that is 610 amino acids long. The protein is highly homologous to mouse, fish, and fly menin,[364,365] but it is absent in *S. cerevisiae* and *C. elegans*. The encoded menin protein resides all or mainly in the nucleus, and it has two nuclear localization domains near its C-terminus.[366] Human menin binds to junD, a jun/fos transcription factor, and it inhibits transcription stimulated by junD. Tumor

suppression might arise from a cooperative role of menin and junD.[366b,366c] Other possibly close-interacting proteins include SMAD3, PEM, NFKB, and NM23.

Limited information can be derived from the identified mutations (Fig. 28-4). Tumors in different organs show similar *MEN1* mutations. The somatic mutations in tumors are similar to germ-line mutations. Two-thirds of germ-line and somatic mutations predict protein truncation. Thus they are likely inactivating mutations. This is made more likely because each truncating mutation would remove one or both of the C-terminal nuclear localization signals.[366] The inactivating mutations, together with loss of the remaining normal allele in tumors, thus indicate that both alleles had been inactivated in the tumor clone precursor(s). Most genes that cause tumors through inactivation of both alleles are classified as tumor-suppressor genes. This is supported further by overexpression of menin in ras-transformed cells, causing partial suppression of the the tumor phenotype.[366c] The predicted normal function of menin still could be in a pathway of cell birth, cell death, or DNA repair. Or to state this differently, the proof of an *MEN1* gene inactivation mechanism in tumorigenesis does not narrow the choices among the possible critical molecular pathways.

The missense *MEN1* mutations are not clustered and thus do not highlight a particularly critical menin region. The related interpretation is that missense mutation at various loci can compromise the molecule.

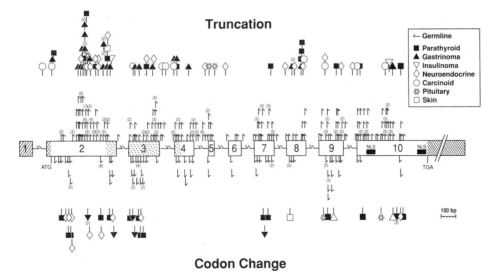

Truncation

←	Germline
■	Parathyroid
▲	Gastrinoma
▽	Insulinoma
◇	Neuroendocrine
○	Carcinoid
✸	Pituitary
□	Skin

Codon Change

Fig. 28-4 Unique germ-line *MEN1* mutations in families and in sporadic cases. Somatic *MEN1* mutations in diverse non-hereditary tumors are shown separately along the top and bottom of the figure. *MEN1* message is diagrammed with exons numbered; untranslated regions are cross-hatched. The critical junD-binding domain is dotted. Truncating mutations [frameshift mutations, splice error, and nonsense (stop codons) mutations] are shown above the mRNA diagram. Codon shift mutations (missense mutations or in-frame deletions) are shown below. Repeating mutations within germline or somatic category are shown only once with a number nearby to count repeats. NLS = nuclear localization sequence. One large deletion, likely of the entire *MEN1* gene, is not shown.[367]

Only one large deletion, likely eliminating the entire *MEN1* open reading frame, has been reported to date.[367] A large deletion excludes menin function as a dominant negative in that kindred and thus in all others. No unusual phenotype was commented on in this kindred.[367]

Animal Models of MEN1

Homozygous inactivation of the *MEN1* gene in the mouse gives a phenotype of lethality during late gestation.[367b] Heterozygous *Men1* inactivation in the mouse gives a phenotype with striking resemblance to human MEN1.[367b] The mice develop multiple tumors, particularly parathyroid tumors, insulinomas, and prolactinoma. These are associated with inactivation of the second allele at the *Men1* locus. Interesting differences from human MEN1 include a milder degree of parathyroid hyperfunction, no gastrinomas up to adulthood, and a striking insulinoma precursor lesion in the form of hyperplastic and probably polyclonal pancreatic islets; the mice also develop bilateral pheochromocytoma and adrenocortical cancer.

A second mouse model of MEN1 was discovered from inactivation of two types of cyclin-dependent kinase inhibitor, specifically $p18^{INK4c}$ and $p27^{KIP1}$. Mice with knockouts of both genes develop various combinations of tumors in the parathyroid, anterior pituitary, pancreatic islets, and duodenum (similar to MEN1).[367c] They also develop C-cell cancers and pheochromocytoma (like MEN2). Since both inactivated genes are in the G1 phase of the cell cycling pathway, this model raises the possibility that MEN1 and/or MEN2 have otherwise unsuspected disruption in this pathway.

Mice have been developed with homozygous inactivation of junD. Though there is evidence that menin and junD interact directly with each other in a pathway critical for endocrine tumorigenesis,[366b] the only phenotype from junD inactivation was male infertility, decreased body size, and decreased growth hormone in serum.[367d] Furthermore, the effects of junD knockout in cultured fibroblasts from the mice were highly context dependent; there was inhibition of cell accumulation in primary cultures but stimulation of accumulation in immortalized cells.[367e]

IMPLICATIONS FOR DIAGNOSIS

Periodic Biochemical Testing

For Diagnosis of MEN1. The standard of care has been that members of MEN1 kindreds undergo periodic biochemical testing. Recent recommendations have been to begin this testing at age 15[40] or as early as age 5.[157] The latter is based on the projected age when important signs may begin. Parameters for testing such as chromogranin A[367b] must be dictated by clinical importance, cost, and local availability. A cost-effective panel could consist of ionized calcium, parathyroid hormone, and prolactin. Such a panel should be repeated approximately every 2 years. Any patient who does not convert to a positive test by age 30 has far reduced (about 10 percent) likelihood of being a gene carrier. But testing should be continued at longer intervals indefinitely, since no maximal age for conversion to a positive test has been determined.[42] Because the screened tumor is not totally specific for MEN1, occasionally a sporadic tumor will predispose to a false positive diagnosis of MEN1.[367f]

For Monitoring of MEN1. Patients with established MEN1 should undergo periodic testing for expression of new endocrinopathies and for recurrence of treated endocrinopathies.[367g,367h] Monitoring and treatment of recognized hormone excess states are beyond this chapter. Even more so than for diagnostic testing, testing of known carriers should be more extensive and must depend on cost and availability (Table 28-7). Sometimes symptoms, such as those from ulcer or hypoglycemia, will present before an abnormality is found by biochemical testing.

Table 28-7 A Typical Panel of Tests for Periodic Monitoring of a Patient with MEN1 or with *MEN1* Mutation

Parathyroids	Enteropancreatic Neuroendocrine
Ionized calcium (annually)	Fasting sugar chromogranin-A and gastrin (annually)
PTH (annually)	CT scan and Octreoscan (every 5 years; needs more evaluation)

Pituitary	Carcinoid
Prolactin (annually) Sella MRI (every 5 years)	CT scan and Octreoscan (every 5 years)

Genetic Linkage Testing

Until the isolation of the *MEN1* gene, genetic linkage or haplotype was the only method to establish that the trait in a family was linked to 11q13 and similarly to make a confident genetic diagnosis in an asymptomatic member of an MEN1 family.[282] After *MEN1* gene discovery, genetic linkage analysis has had less frequent applications. The main use is in the MEN1 family with no *MEN1* mutation identified. There, linkage analysis may establish if the disease is linked to 11q13 or not. Of course, when positive, it also can be used for ascertainment within a family. Where 11q13 linkage testing has been possible in "mutation negative" MEN1 families, it has confirmed linkage to 11q13 in 3 of 4 families.[42,336]

Detection Rates with Mutation Testing

By dideoxy fingerprinting and cycle sequencing, germ-line mutation was recognizable in 47 of 50 families.[336] This implies that virtually every MEN1 family has a mutation in the open reading frame of the *MEN1* gene. The implication is that robust *MEN1* germ-line mutation testing is possible, and this can be applied to families and sporadic cases. Detection rates in academic centers, reporting more than 30 tested MEN1 families and using various detection methods, range from 51 to 94 percent.[56b,144b,336,340,342,342c,367i] Thus the false negative rate in a new MEN1 family will be 10–30%.

Difficulty of *MEN1* Germ-Line Mutation Testing

Approximately 200 different germ-line *MEN1* mutations are spread over nine coding exons (see Fig. 28-4). Many familial and sporadic MEN1 patients continue to reveal a previously undescribed mutation. There is only limited clustering of mutations in the 3′ two-thirds of exon 2. Thus there is little prospect for test shortcuts directed at several bases or several exons. Furthermore, the relatively high fraction with missense mutations predicts that even if most truncated messages are expressed, a protein truncation type assay would fail to recognize at least one-third of mutations. Of course, within a family or in a population with a founder effect,[19,284,342] simplified tests directed at the known mutation should be used.

Currently available methods (cycle sequencing alone or with dideoxy fingerprinting, with single-strand conformer polymorphism or with heteroduplex analysis) are likely to have similarly high diagnostic yield under carefully controlled conditions.

Cases for Possible *MEN1* Germ-Line Mutation Testing

Several categories of clinical presentation have rather clear justification for *MEN1* germ-line mutation testing at presentation or after a delay (see 5):

1. An affected member in an MEN1 or MEN1 phenocopy family that has not previously had a member tested. Testing can

Table 28-8 Major Differences Between MEN1 and MEN2a/MEN2b. Some Can Affect Decisions About Gene Testing

The Concerns	MEN1	MEN2a/MEN2b
Gene and locus	*MEN1*, 11q13	*RET*, 10 cen
Encoded protein location and action	Nucleus, unknown action Binds junD	Plasma membrane, tyrosine kinase
How mutation promotes tumor	Gene inactivation	Gene activation
Mutation distribution	Throughout open reading frame	Few exons, few codons
Main clinical expressions	Hormone excess effects	Cancer of C-cells
Gene-testing benefits	Information to MD and patient	Information to MD and patient Cancer prevention or cure
Age to offer mutation test	5 years	5 years in MEN2a; 0.5 year in MEN2b
False negative rate	10–30%	1–2%

confirm the diagnosis and also assist in possible development of an inexpensive mutation test for other members, such as based on a specific restriction digest or based on hybridization to allele specific oligonucleotides.

2. A likely affected member of an MEN1 or MEN1 phenocopy family with known familial mutation, concerned for confirmation of mutational status.

3. An unaffected adult in an MEN1 family. This is mainly dependent upon a known family mutation or 11q13 haplotype. Any without mutation would be freed from the recommendation to undergo regular biochemical screening (Table 28-8). Any with mutation would be given opposite recommendations with more confidence.

4. A sporadic case with MEN1 or an MEN1 phenocopy. Certain phenocopies (such as combined hyperparathyroidism and bronchial carcinoid) will have a high likelihood of mutation, while others (such as sporadic hyperparathyroidism) will have low likelihood.

5. An unaffected child in an MEN1 family. The consensus of the U.S. genetics community is that children in the United States generally should not be offered genetic testing that will not have a major effect on their immediate care.[368] Since aggressive prolactinoma in familial MEN1 has been noted before age 5,[157] testing of children for MEN1 ascertainment can begin by age 5. As this guideline is based on only one case, many physicians might begin testing at a later age.

Issues for Genetic Counseling

The issues to consider for counseling are, in general, covered in detail in the body of this chapter. Several additional points can be made. The similarity in names leads to confusion among some patients and among some physicians between MEN1 and MEN2, but the differences are more important than their similarities (see Table 28-8). Above all, *RET* gene testing in MEN2a or MEN2b carries major therapeutic implications (possible prevention or cure of cancer)[198]; major therapeutic implications are uncommon from *MEN1* gene testing in MEN1. Unlike in MEN2, in MEN1 there is no tumor host organ that is readily dispensable to prevent or cure a major malignancy. A patient education manual, which has been updated regularly, is available on the international communications Web at *http://www.niddk.nih.gov/health/endo/pubs/fmen1/fmen1.htm*.[369]

MEN1 generally does not have major effects on fertility. Primary hyperparathyroidism in a mother is considered a risk factor for pregnancy complications.[370] However, the mild hyperparathyroidism that is common in MEN1 rarely leads to complications for mother or child. MEN1 carrier state in a fetus is not a pregnancy risk factor for fetus or mother. Prolactinoma can clearly impair fertility in women or men, and it should be monitored for enlargement during pregnancy. Most women (and men) with prolactinoma are able to conceive when treated with a dopamine agonist.[371]

ACKNOWLEDGMENTS

I wish to thank many collaborators who contributed to our work on MEN1, particularly those in the NIH intramural programs, including Sunita K. Agarwal, MaryBeth Kester, Christina Heppner, Young S. Kim, Paul K. Goldsmith, Monica C. Skarulis, Allen M. Spiegel, and A. Lee Burns (All National Institute of Diabetes and Digestive and Kidney Diseases), Sirandanahalli C. Guru, Judith S. Crabtree, Pachiapan Manickam, Francis S. Collins, and Settara C. Chandrasekharappa (All National Human Genome Research Institute), Michael R. Emmert-Buck, Larissa V. Debelenko, Zhengping Zhuang, Irina A. Lubensky, and Lance A. Liotta (National Cancer Institute). I am also indebeted for many contributions from John L. Doppman, H. Richard Alexander, Mark S. Boguski, Thomas L. Darling, Lee S. Weinstein, William F. Simonds, and many members of the NIH Interinstitute Endocrine Program. Many persons outside NIH also made important contributions, particularly Bruce A. Roe, Jane S. Green, Joseph E. Green III, and also many patients and their families.

REFERENCES

1. Erdheim J: Zur normalen und pathologischen histologie der glandula throidea, parathyroidea, und hypophysis. *Beitr Z Pathol Anat* **33**:158, 1903.
2. Moldawer MP: Case records of the Massachusetts General Hospital, case 39501. *N Engl J Med* **249**:990, 1953.
3. Moldawer MP, Nardi GL, Raker JW: Concomitance of multiple adenomas of the parathyroids and pancreatic islet cells with tumor of the pituitary a syndrome with familial incidence. *Am J Med Sci* **228**:190, 1954.
4. Wermer P: Genetic aspects of adenomatosis of endocrine glands. *Am J Med* **16**:363, 1954.
5. Schmid JR, Labhart A, Rossier PH: Relationship of multiple endocrine adenomas to the syndrome of ulcerogenic islet cell adenomas (Zollinger-Ellison): Occurrence of both syndromes in one family. *Am J Med* **31**:343, 1961.
6. Zollinger RM, Ellison EH: Primary peptic ulceration of the jejunum associated with islet cell tumors of the pancreas. *Ann Surg* **142**:709, 1955.
7. Gregory RH, Tracy HJ, French JM, Sircus W: Extraction of a gastrin-like substance from a pancreatic tumor in a case of Zollinger-Ellison syndrome. *Lancet* **1**:1040, 1960.
8. Lewis UJ, Singh RN, Seavey BK: Human prolactin: Isolation and some properties. *Biochem Biophys Res Commun* **44**:1169, 1971.
9. Malarkey WB: Prolactin and the diagnosis of pituitary tumors. *Annu Rev Med* **30**:249, 1979.
10. Howard JM, Chremos AN, Collen MJ: Famotidine, a new potent long acting histamine H$_2$-receptor antagonist: comparison with cimetidine and ranitidine in the treatment of Zollinger-Ellison syndrome. *Gastroenterology* **188**:1026, 1985.
11. Metz DC, Pisegna JR, Fishbeyn VA, Benya RV, Jensen RT: Control of gastric acid hypersecretion in the management of patients with Zollinger-Ellison syndrome. *World J Surg* **17**:468, 1993.
12. Frucht H, Maton PN, Jensen RT: Use of omeprazole in patients with Zollinger-Ellison syndrome. *Dig Dis Sci* **36**:394, 1991.

13. Maton PN, Vinayek R, Frucht H: Long term efficacy and safety of omeprazole in patients with Zollinger-Ellison syndrome. *Gastroenterology* **97**:827, 1989.

14. Bevan JS, Webster J, Burke CW, Scanlon MF: Dopamine agonists and pituitary tumor shrinkage. *Endocr Rev* **13**:220, 1992.

15. Norton JA, Cromack DT, Shawker TH: Intraoperative ultrasonographic localization of islet cell tumors: A prospective comparison to palpation. *Ann Surg* **207**:160, 1988.

16. Norton JA, Shawker TH, Jones BL, Spiegel AM, Marx SJ, Fitzpatrick L, Aurbach GD, Doppman JL: Intraoperative ultrasound and reoperative parathyroid surgery: an initial evaluation. *World J Surg* **10**:631, 1986.

17. Doppman JL: Tumor localization in multiple endocrine neoplasia type 1. *Ann Intern Med* **129**:484, 1998.

17b. Norton JA: Intraoperative methods to stage and localize pancreeatic and duodenal tumors. *Ann Oncol* **10**(Suppl 4):182, 1999.

17c. Tonelli F, Spini S, Tommasi M et al: Intraoperative PTH measurement in patients with MEN1 syndrome and hyperparathyroidism. *World J Surg* **24**:556, 2000.

18. Larsson C, Skogseid B, Oberg K, Nakamura Y, Nordenskjold M: Multiple endocrine neoplasia type 1 gene maps to chromosome 11 and is lost in insulinoma. *Nature* **332**:85, 1988.

19. Chandrasekharappa SC, Guru SC, Manickam P, Olufemi S-E, Collins FS, Emmert-Buck MR, Debelenko LV, Zhuang Z, Lubensky IA, Liotta LA, Crabtree JS, Wang Y, Roe BA, Weiseman J, Bogusky MS, Agarwal SK, Kester MB, Kim YS, Heppner C, Dong Q, Spiegel AM, Burns AL, Marx SJ: Positional cloning of the gene for multiple endocrine neoplasia type 1. *Science* **276**:404, 1997.

20. Lips CJM, Vasen HFA, Lamers CBHW, Berdjis CC: Polyglandular syndrome: II. Multiple endocrine adenomas in man: A report of 5 cases and a review of the literature. *Oncologia* **15**:288, 1962.

21. Lips CJM, Vasen HFA, Lamers CBHW: Multiple endocrine neoplasia syndromes. *CRC Crit Rev* **2**:117, 1984.

22. Eberle F, Grun R: Multiple endocrine neoplasia, type I (MEN1). *Ergeb Inn Med* **46**:76, 1981.

23. Oberg K, Skogseid B, Eriksson B: Multiple endocrine neoplasia type 1 (MEN-1): Clinical, biochemical and genetical investigations. *Acta Oncologia* **28**:383, 1989.

24. Betts JB, O'Malley BP, Rosenthal FD: Hyperparathyroidism: A prerequisite for Zollinger-Ellison syndrome in multiple endocrine adenomatosis type 1. *Q J Med* **193**:69, 1980.

25. Watson RGP, Johnston CF, O'Hare MMT, Anderson JR, Wilson BG, Collins JS, Sloan JM, Buchanan KD: The frequency of gastrointestinal endocrine tumors in a well defined population — Northern Ireland. *Q J Med* **72**:647, 1985.

26. Brandi ML, Marx SJ, Aurbach GD, Fitzpatrick LA: Familial multiple endocrine neoplasia type I: A new look at pathophysiology. *Endocr Rev* **8**:391, 1987.

26b. Uchino S, Noguchi S, Sato M, Yamashita H, Watanabe S, et al: Screening of the MEN1 gene and discovery of germ-line and somatic mutations in apparently sporadic parathyroid tumors. *Cancer Res* **60**:5553, 2000.

27. Heath H III, Hodgson S, Kennedy MA: Primary hyperparathyroidism: Incidence, morbidity, and potential economic impact in a community. *N Engl J Med* **302**:189, 1980.

28. Bardram L, Stage JG: Frequency of endocrine disorders in patients with the Zollinger-Ellison syndrome: A collective surgical experience. *Scand J Gastroenterol* **20**:233, 1985.

29. Farley DR, van Heerden JA, Grant CS, Miller LJ, Ilstrup DM: The Zollinger-Ellison syndrome: A collective surgical experience. *Ann Surg* **215**:561, 1992.

30. Schaaf L, Gerschner M, Geissler W, Eckert B, Seif FJ, Usadel KH: The importance of multiple endocrine neoplasia syndromes in differential diagnosis. *Klin Wochenschr* **68**:669, 1990.

31. Scheithauer BW, Laws ER Jr, Kovacs K, Horvath E, Randall RV, Carney JA: Pituitary adenomas of the multiple endocrine neoplasia type I syndrome. *Semin Diagn Pathol* **4**:205, 1987.

32. Corbetta S, Pizzocaro A, Peracchi M, Beck-Peccoz P, Faglia G, Spada A: Multiple endocrine neoplasia type 1 in patients with recognized pituitary tumors of different types. *Clin Endocrinol* **47**:507, 1997.

33. Trump D, Farren B, Wooding C, Pang JT, Besser GM, Buchanan KD, Edwards CR, Heath DA, Jackson CE, Jansen S, Lips K, Monson JP, O'Halloran D, Sampson J, Shalet SM, Wheeler MH, Zink A, Thakker RV: Clinical studies of multiple endocrine neoplasia type 1 (MEN1). *Q J Med* **89**:563, 1996.

33b. Yoshimoto K, Saito S: Clinical characteristics in multiple endocrine neoplasia type 1 in Japan: a review of 106 patients. *Folia Endocrinol* **67**:764, 1991.

33c. Hai N, Aoki N, Matsuda A, Mori T, Kosugi S: Germline MEN1 mutations in sixteen Japanese families with multiple endocrine neoplasia type 1 (MEN1). *Eur J Endocrinol* **141**:475, 1999.

33d. Hai N, Aoki N, Shimatsu A, Mori T, Kosugi S: Clinical features of multiple endocrine neoplasia type 1 (MEN1) phenocopy without germline MEN1 gene mutations: analysis of 20 Japanese sporadic cases without MEN1. *Clin Endocrinol* **52**:509, 2000.

34. Doherty GM, Olson JA, Frisella MM, Lairmore TC, Wells SA Jr, Norton JA: Lethality of multiple endocrine neoplasia type 1. *World J Surg* **22**:581, 1998.

35. Majewski JT, Wilson SD: The MEA-I syndrome: An all or none phenomenon? *Surgery* **86**:475, 1979.

36. Ballard HS, Frame B, Hartsock RJ: Familial multiple endocrine adenoma-peptic ulcer complex. *Medicine* **43**:481, 1964.

37. Marx SJ, Spiegel AM, Levine MA, Rizzoli RE, Lasker RD, Santora AC II, Downs RW, Aurbach GD: Familial hypocalciuric hypercalcemia: The relation to primary parathyroid hyperplasia. *N Engl J Med* **307**:416, 1982.

38. Vasen HFA, Lamers CBHW, Lips CJM: Screening for multiple endocrine neoplasia syndrome type I. *Arch Intern Med* **149**:2717, 1989.

39. Skogseid B, Eriksson B, Lundqvist G: Multiple endocrine neoplasia type 1: A 10-year prospective screening study in four kindreds. *J Clin Endocrinol Metab* **73**:281, 1991.

40. Marx SJ, Vinik AI, Santen RJ, Floyd JC Jr, Mills JL, Green JE III: Multiple endocrine neoplasia type I: Assessment of laboratory tests to screen for the gene in a large kindred. *Medicine* **65**:226, 1986.

41. Skarulis MC: Clinical expressions of MEN1 at NIH. *Ann Intern Med* **129**:484, 1998.

42. Giraud S, Choplin H, Teh B, Lespinasse J, Jouvet A, Labat-Moleur F, Lenoir G, Hamon B, Hamon P, Calender A: A large multiple endocrine neoplasia type 1 family with clinical expression suggestive of anticipation. *J Clin Endocrinol Metab* **82**:3487, 1997.

43. Samaan NA, Ovais S, Ordonez NG, Choksi UA, Selvin RV, Hickey RC: Multiple endocrine syndrome type 1: Clinical laboratory findings, and management in five families. *Cancer* **64**:741, 1989.

44. Lamers CBHW, Froeling PGAM: Clinical significance of hyperparathyroidism in familial multiple endocrine adenomatosis type I (MEA I). *Am J Med* **66**:422, 1979.

45. Eberle F, Grun R: Multiple endocrine neoplasia, type I (MEN I), in Frick P, Harnack G-A, Kochsiek K, Martini GA, Prade A (eds): *Advances in Internal Medicine and Pediatrics*. Berlin, Springer-Verlag, 1981, p 77.

46. Shepherd JJ: Latent familial multiple endocrine neoplasia in Tasmania. *Med J Aust* **142**:395, 1985.

47. Wu CW, Huang CI, Tsai ST, Chiang H, Liu W-Y, P'eng F-K: Parathyroid carcinoma in a patient with non-secretory pituitary tumor: A variant of multiple endocrine neoplasia type-I? *Eur J Surg Oncol* **18**:517, 1992.

47b. Knee TS, Yohihashi AK, Aprill BS, et al: Parathyroid carcinoma associated with MEN type 1. Program and Abstracts 80th Annual Meeting of the Endocrine Society, 494 (Abstract), 1998.

47c. Sato M, Miyauchi A, Namihira H, Bhuiyan MMR, Imachi H, Murao K, Takahara J: A newly recognized germline mutation of MEN1 gene identified in a patient with parathyroid adenoma and carcinoma. *Endocrine* **12**:223, 2000.

47d. Burgess JR, David R, Greenaway TM, Parameswaran V, Shepherd JJ: Osteoporosis in multiple endocrineoplasia type 1. *Arch Surg* **134**:1119, 1999.

48. Marx SJ, Menczel J, Campbell G, Aurbach GD, Spiegel AM, Norton JA: Heterogeneous size of the parathyroid glands in familial multiple endocrine neoplasia type 1. *Clin Endocrinol* **35**:521, 1991.

49. Hellman P, Skogseid B, Juhlin C, Akerstrom G, Rastad J: Findings and long-term result of parathyroid surgery in multiple endocrine neoplasia type 1. *World J Surg* **16**:718, 1992.

49b. Friedman E, Sakaguchi K, Bale AE, Falchetti A, Streeten A, Zimering MB, Weinstein LS, McBride WO, Nakamura Y, Brandi ML, Norton JA, Aurbach GD, Spiegel AM, Marx SJ: Clonality of parathyroid tumors in familial multiple endocrine neoplasia type 1. *N Engl J Med* **321**:213, 1989.

50. Rizzoli R, Green J III, Marx SJ: Primary hyperparathyroidism in familial multiple endocrine neoplasia type I. *Am J Med* **78**:468, 1985.

51. Burgess JR, David R, Parameswaran V, Greenaway TM, Shepherd JJ: The outcome of subtotal parathyroidectomy for the treatment of hyperparathyroidism in multiple endocrine neoplasia type 1. *Arch Surg* **133**:126, 1998.

52. Prinz RA, Gamvros OI, Sellu D, Lynn JA: Subtotal parathyroidectomy for primary chief cell hyperplasia of the multiple endocrine neoplasia type I syndrome. *Ann Surg* **193**:26, 1981.

53. van Heerden JA, Kent RB III, Sizemore GW, Grant CS, ReMine WH: Primary hyperparathyroidism in patients with multiple endocrine neoplasia syndromes. *Arch Surg* **118**:533, 1983.

54. Rudberg C, Akerstrom G, Palmer M, Ljunghall S, Adami HO, Johansson H, Grimelius L, Thoren L, Bergstrom R: Later results of operation for primary hyperparathyroidism in 441 patients. *Surgery* **99**:643, 1986.

55. Le Bodic M-F, Heymann M-F, Lecompte M, Berger N, Berger F, Louvel A, De Micco C, Patey M, De Mascarel A, Burtin F, Saint-Andre J-P: Immunohistochemical study of 100 pancreatic tumors in 28 patients with multiple endocrine neoplasia, type 1. *Am J Surg Pathol* **20**:1378, 1996.

56. Benya RV, Metz DC, Venzon DJ, Fishbeyn VA, Strader DB, Orbuch M, Jensen RT: Zollinger-Ellison syndrome can be the initial endocrine manifestation in patients with multiple endocrine neoplasia-type I. *Am J Med* **5**:436, 1994.

56b. Giraud S, Zhang CX, Serova-Sinilnikova O, Wautot V, Salandre J, Buisson N, Waterlot C, Bauters C, Porchet N, Aubert J-P, Emy P, Cadiot G, Delemer B, Chabre O, and 27 additional coauthors: Germline mutation analysis in patients with multiple endocrine neoplasia type 1 and related disorders. *Am J Hum Genet* **63**:455, 1998.

57. Norton JA, Levin B, Jensen RT: Cancer of the endocrine system, in DeVita VT Jr, Hellman S, Rosenberg SA (eds): *Cancer: Principles and Practice of Oncology.* Philadelphia, Lippincott, 1993, p 1335.

58. Metz DC, Jensen RT: Endocrine tumors of the pancreas, in Haubrich WB, Berk JE, Schaffner F (eds): *Bockus Gastroenterology.* Philadelphia, Saunders, 1994, p 3002.

59. Jensen RT, Gardner JD: Gastrinoma, in Go VLW, Brooks FP, DiMagno EP (eds): *The Exocrine Pancreas.* New York, Raven Press, 1993.

60. Metz DC, Jensen RT, Bale A, Skarulis MC, Eastman RC, Nieman L, Norton JA, Friedman E, Larsson C, Amorosi A, Brandi ML, Marx SJ: Multiple endocrine neoplasia type 1: Clinical features and management, in Bilezekian JP, Levine MA, Marcus R (eds): *The Parathyroids.* New York, Raven Press, 1994, p 591.

61. Skogseid B, Oberg K, Eriksson B, Juhlin C, Grandberg D, Akerstrom G, Rastad J: Surgery for asymptomatic pancreatic lesion in multiple endocrine neoplasia type I. *World J Surg* **7**:872, 1996.

62. Kloppel G, Sillemar S, Stamm B, Hacki WH, Heitz PN: Pancreatic lesions and hormonal profile in pancreatic tumors in multiple endocrine neoplasia type I. *Cancer* **57**:1824, 1986.

63. Thompson NW, Lloyd RU, Nishiyama RH: MEN-1 pancreas: A histological and immunohistochemical study. *World J Surg* **8**:561, 1984.

64. Pipeleers-Marichial M, Somers G, Willems G: Gastrinomas in the duodenum of patients with multiple endocrine neoplasia type 1 and the Zollinger-Ellison syndrome. *N Engl J Med* **322**:723, 1990.

65. Jensen RT, Gardner JD: Zollinger-Ellison syndrome: Clinical presentation, pathology, diagnosis and treatment, in Dannenberg A, Zakim D (eds): *Peptic Ulcer and Other Acid-Related Diseases.* New York, Academic Research Association, 1991, p 117.

66. Norton JA, Doppman JL, Jensen RT: Curative resection in Zollinger-Ellison syndrome: Results of a 10 year prospective study. *Ann Surg* **215**:8, 1992.

67. Ruszniewski P, Podevin P, Cadiot G, Marmuse JP, Mignon M, Vissuzaine C, Bonfils S, Lehy T: Clinical anatomical, and evolutive features of patients with the Zollinger-Ellison syndrome combined with type I multiple endocrine neoplasia. *Pancreas* **8**:295, 1993.

68. Neuburger P, Lewin M, Bonfils S: Parietal and chief cell population in four cases of the Zollinger-Ellison syndrome. *Gastroenterology* **63**:937, 1972.

69. Norton JA, Doppman JL, Collen MJ: Prospective study of gastrinoma localization and resection in patients with Zollinger-Ellison syndrome. *Ann Surg* **204**:468, 1986.

70. Stabile BE, Morrow DJ, Passaro E Jr: The gastrinoma triangle: Operative implications. *Am J Surg* **147**:25, 1984.

71. Norton JA, Jensen RT: Unresolved issues in the management of patients with Zollinger-Ellison syndrome. *World J Surg* **15**:151, 1991.

72. Zollinger RM, Ellison EH, Fabri PJ, Johnson J, Sparks J, Carey LC: Primary peptic ulceration of the jejunum associated with islet cell tumors: Twenty-five year appraisal. *Ann Surg* **192**:422, 1980.

73. Oberg K, Skogseid B, Eriksson B: Multiple endocrine neoplasia type 1 (MEN-1). *Acta Oncol* **28**:383, 1989.

74. Zollinger RM: Gastrinoma factors influencing prognosis. *Surgery* **97**:49, 1985.

75. Podevin P, Ruszniewski P, Mignon M: Management of multiple endocrine neoplasia type 1 (MEN1) in Zollinger-Ellison syndrome. *Gastrenterology* **98**:A230, 1990.

76. Jensen RT, Gardner JD, Raufman J-P: Zollinger-Ellison syndrome: Current concepts and management. *Ann Intern Med* **98**:59, 1983.

77. Weber HC, Venzon DJ, Lin JT, Fishbein VA, Orbuch M, Strader DB, Gibril F, Metz DC, Fraker DL, Norton JA, Jensen RT: Determinants of metastatic rate and survival in patients with Zollinger-Ellison syndrome: A prospective long-term study. *Gastroenterology* **108**:1637, 1995.

78. Jensen RT: Management of the Zollinger-Ellison syndrome in patients with multiple endocrine neoplasia type 1. *Ann Intern Med* **243**:477, 1998.

79. Isenberg JI, Walsh JH, Grossman MI: Zollinger-Ellison syndrome. *Gastroenterology* **65**:140, 1973.

80. Shimoda SS, Saunders DR, Rubin C: The Zollinger-Ellison syndrome with steatorrhea: Mechanisms of fat and vitamin B_{12} malabsorption. *Gastroenterology* **55**:705, 1968.

81. Feldman M: Gastric secretion, in Sleisenger MH, Fordtran JS (eds): *Gastrointestinal Disease.* Philadelphia, Saunders, 1983, p 541.

82. Norton JA, Cornelius MJ, Doppman JL: Effect of parathyroidectomy in patients with hyperparathyroidism and multiple endocrine neoplasia type I. *Surgery* **102**:958, 1987.

83. Yonda RJ, Ostroff JW, Ashbaugh CD, Guis MS, Goldberg HI: Zollinger-Ellison syndrome with a normal screening gastrin level. *Dig Dis Sci* **34**:1929, 1989.

84. Wolfe MM, Jensen RT: Zollinger-Ellison syndrome. *N Engl J Med* **317**:1200, 1987.

85. Metz DC, Pisegna JR, Fishbeyn VA, Benya RV, Jensen RT: Current maintenance doses of omeprazole in Zollinger-Ellison syndrome are too high. *Gastroenterology* **103**:1498, 1992.

86. Frucht H, Howard JM, Slaff JE: Secretin and calcium provocative tests in patients with Zollinger-Ellison syndrome: A prospective study. *Ann Intern Med* **111**:713, 1989.

87. Krenning EP, Kwekkeboom DJ, Oei HY, de Jong RJB, Dop FJ, Reubi JC, Lambers SWJ: Somatostatin-receptor scintigraphy in gastroenteropancreatic tumors. *Ann NY Acad Sci* **733**:416, 1994.

88. Gibril F, Reynolds JC, Doppman JL, Chen CC, Venzon DJ, Termanini B, Weber HC, Stewart CA, Jensen RT: Somatostatin receptor scientigraphy: A prospective study of its sensitivity compared to other imaging modalities in detecting primary and metastatic gastrinomas. *Ann Intern Med* **125**:26, 1996.

89. Termanini B, Gibril F, Reynolds JC, Doppman JL, Chen CC, Sutliffe VE, Jensen RT: Value of somatostatin receptor scintigraphy: A prospective study in gastrinoma of its effect on clinical management. *Gastroenterology* **112**:335, 1997.

90. Galbut DL, Markowitz AM: Insulinoma: Diagnosis, surgical management and long term followup. Review of 41 cases. *Am J Surg* **139**:682, 1980.

91. Rasbach DA, van Heerden JA, Telander RL, Grant CS, Carney A: Surgical management of hyperinsulinism in the multiple endocrine neoplasia type 1 syndrome. *Arch Surg* **123**:584, 1985.

92. Pasieka JL, McLoed MK, Thompson NW, Burney RE: Surgical approach to insulinomas. Assessing the need for preoperative localization. *Arch Surg* **127**:442, 1992.

93. van Heerden JA, Edis AJ, Service FJ: Surgical aspects of insulinomas. *Ann Surg* **189**:677, 1992.

94. Eastman RC, Kahn CR: Hypoglycemia, in Moore WT, Eastman EC (eds): *Diagnostic Endrocrinology.* Toronto, BC Decker, 1990, p 183.

95. Boukhman MP, Karam JH, Shaver J, Siperstein AE, Duh Q-Y, Clark OH: Insulinoma: Experience from 1950 to 1995. *West J Med* **169**:98, 1998.

96. Doppman JL, Miller DL, Chang R: Insulinomas: Localization with selective intrarterial injection of calcium. *Radiology* **178**:237, 1991.

97. Doherty GM, Doppman JL, Shawker TH, Miller DL, Eastman RC, Gorden P, Norton JA: Results of a propective strategy to diagnose, localize and resect insulinomas. *Surgery* **110**:989, 1991.

98. Grant CS, van Heerden JA, Charboneau JW, James EM, Reading CC: Insulinoma: The value of intraoperative ultrasonography. *Arch Surg* **123**:843, 1988.

99. Boden G: Glucagonomas and insulinomas. *Gastroenterol Clin North Am* **18**:831, 1989.

100. Leichter SB: Clinical and metabolic aspects of glucagonoma. *Medicine* **59**:100, 1980.

101. Guillausseau PJ, Guillausseau C, Villet R: Les glucagonomas. Aspect Cliniques biologiques, Anatomo-pathologiques et therapeutiques (Revue général de 130 cas). *Gastroenterol Clin Biol* **6**:1029, 1982.

102. Wilkinson DS: Necrolytic migratory erythema with carcinoma of the pancreas. *Trans St Johns Hosp Dermatol Soc* **59**:244, 1973.

103. Mallison CN, Bloom SR, Warin AP: A glucagonoma syndrome. *Lancet* **2**:1, 1974.

104. Holst JJ: Hormone producing tumors of the gastrointestinal tract, in Cohen S, Soloway RD (eds): *Glucagon-Producing Tumors*. New York, Churchill-Livingstone, 1985, p 57.

105. Verner JV, Morrison AB: Endocrine pancreatic ilset disease with diarrhea: Report of a case due to diffuse hyperplasia of non beta islet tissue with a review of 54 additional cases. *Arch Intern Med* **133**:492, 1974.

106. Matsumoto KK, Peter JB, Schultze RG: Watery diarrhea and hypokalemia associated with pancreatic islet cell adenoma. *Gastroenterology* **50**:231, 1966.

107. Mekhjian H, O'Dorisio TM: VIPoma syndrome. *Semin Oncol* **14**:282, 1987.

108. Kane MG, D'Dorisio TM, Krejs GJ: Production of secretory diarrhea by intravenous infusion of vasoactive intestinal peptide. *N Engl J Med* **309**:1482, 1983.

109. Namihara Y, Achord JL, Subramony C: Multiple endocrine neoplasia, type 1, with pancreatic cholera. *Am J Gastroenterol* **82**:794, 1987.

110. Welbourn RB, Wood SM, Polak JM, Bloom SR: Pancreatic endocrine tumors, in Bloom SR, Polak JM (eds): *Gut Hormones*. New York, Churchill-Livingstone, 1981, p 547.

111. Long RG, Bryant MG, Mitchell SJ, Adrian TE, Polak JM, Bloom SR: Clinicopathological study of pancreatic and ganglioneuroblastoma tumors secreting vasoactive intestinal polyeptide (Vipomas). *Br Med J* **282**:1767, 1981.

112. Capella C, Polak JM, Butta R: Morphologic patterns and diagnostic criteria of VIP-producing endocrine tumors: A histologic, histochemical, ultrastructural and biochemical study of 32 cases. *Cancer* **52**:1860, 1983.

112b. Wu TJ, Lin CL, Taylor RL, Kvols LK, Kao PC: Increased parathyroid hormone-related peptide in patients with hypercalcemia associated with islet cell carcinoma. *Mayo Clin Proc* **72**:1111, 1997.

113. Rivier J, Spress J, Thorner M, Vale W: Characterization of a growth-hormone releasing factor from a human pancreatic islet cell tumor. *Nature* **300**:276, 1982.

114. Thorner M, Perryman RI, Cronin MJ: Somatotroph hyperplasia. *J Clin Invest* **70**:965, 1982.

115. Sano T, Asa SL, Kovacs K: Growth hormone releasing-producing tumors: Clinical, biochemical and morphological manifestations. *Endocr Rev* **9**:357, 1988.

116. Asa SL, Singer W, Kovacs K, Horvath E, Murray D, Colapinto N, Thorner MO: Pancreatic endocrine tumour producing growth hormone-releasing hormone associated with multiple endocrine neoplasia type I syndrome. *Acta Endocrinol* **115**:331, 1987.

117. Barkan AL, Shenker Y, Grekin RJ: Acromeglay from ectopic GHRH secretion by malignant carcinoid tumor: Successful treatment with long-acting somatostain analogue SMS. *Cancer* **61**:221, 1986.

118. Sano T, Yamasaki R, Saito H: Growth hormone releasing hormone (GHRH)-secreting pancreatic tumor in a patient with multiple endocrine neoplasia type 1. *Am J Surg Pathol* **11**:810, 1987.

119. Larsson LI, Hirsch MA, Holst JJ: Pancreatic somatostatinoma: Clinical features and physiologic implications. *Lancet* **1**:666, 1977.

120. Ganda OP, Weir GC, Soeldner JS: Somatostatinoma: A somatostatin-containing tumor of the endocrine pancreas. *N Engl J Med* **296**:963, 1977.

121. Vinik AI, Strodel WE, Eckhauser FE, Moattari AR, Lloyd R: Somatostatinomas, Ppomas and neurotensinomas. *Semin Oncol* **14**:263, 1987.

122. Boden G, Shimoyama R: Hormone-producing tumors of the gastrointestinal tract, in Cohen S, Soloway RD (eds): *Somatostatinoma*. New York, Churchill-Livingstone, 1985, p 85.

123. Yamada T, Chiha T: The gastrointestinal system, in Makhlouf GM (ed): *Handbook of Physiology,* sec 6: *Somatostatin*. Bethesda, MD, American Physiological Society, 1979, p 431.

124. Eckhauser FE, Cheung PS, Vinik A, Strodel WE, Lloyd R, Thompson NW: Nonfunctioning malignant neuroendocrine tumors of the pancreas. *Surgery* **100**:978, 1986.

125. Kent RB, van Heerden JA, Weiland LH: Nonfunctioning islet cell tumors. *Ann Surg* **193**:185, 1981.

126. O'Dorisio TM, Vinik AI: Pancreatic polypeptide and mixed peptide-producing tumors of the gastrointestinal tract, in Cohen S, Soloway RD (eds): *Contemporary Issues in Gastroenterology.* Edinburgh, Churchill-Livingstone, 1984, p 117.

127. Takahashi H, Nakano K, Adachi Y: Multiple nonfunctional pancreatic islet cell tumor in multiple endocrine neoplasia type 1: A case report. *Acta Pathol Jpn* **38**:667, 1988.

128. Heitz PU, Kasper M, Polak JM, Kloppel G: Pancreatic endocrine tumors: immunocytochemical analysis of 125 tumors. *Hum Pathol* **13**:163, 1982.

129. Duh Q-Y: Carcinoids associated with multiple endocrine neoplasia syndromes. *Am J Surg* **154**:142, 1987.

130. Godwin JD: Carcinoid tumors. An analysis of 2837 cases. *Cancer* **36**:560, 1975.

131. Teh BT, McArdle J, Chan SP, Menon J, Hartley L, Pullan P, Ho J, Khir A, Wilkinson S, Larsson C, Cameron D, Shepherd J: Clinicopathologic studies of thymic carcinoids in multiple endocrine neoplasia type 1. *Medicine* **76**:21, 1997.

132. Pass HI, Doppman JL, Nieman L: Management of the ectopic ACTH syndrome due to thoracic carcinoids. *Ann Thorac Surg* **50**:52, 1990.

133. Doppman JL, Pass HI, Nieman LK: Detection of ACTH-producing bronchial carcinoid tumors: MR imaging vs CT. *AJR* **156**:39, 1991.

134. Glikson M, Gil-Ad I, Calun E, Dresner R: Acromegaly due to ectopic growth hormone-releasing hormone secretion by a bronchial carcinoid tumour: Dynamic hormonal responses to various stimuli. *Acta Endocrinol (Copenh)* **125**:366, 1991.

135. Maton PN, Dayal Y: Clinical implication of hypergastrinemia, in Dannenberg A, Zakim D (eds): *Peptic Ulcer and Other Acid-Related Diseases.* New York, Academic Research Association, 1993, p 213.

136. Frucht H, Maton PN, Jensen RT: Use of omeprazole in patients with Zollinger-Ellison syndrome. *N Engl J Med* **322**:723, 1990.

137. Jensen RT: Gastrinoma as a model for prolonged hypergastrinemia, in Walsh JH (ed): *Gastrin.* New York, Raven Press, 1993.

137b. Tomassetti P, Migliori M, Caletti GC, Fusaroli P, Corinaldesi R, Gullo L: Treatment of type II gastric carcinoid tumors with somatostatin analogues. *N Engl J Med* **343**:551, 2000.

138. Benya RV, Metz DC, Hijazi YM, Fishbeyn VA, Pisegna JR, Jensen RT: Fine needle aspiration cytology for the evaluation of submucosal nodules in patients with Zollinger-Ellison sndrome. *Am J Gastroenterol* **88**:258, 1993.

139. Bordi C, Falchetti A, Azzoni C, D'Adda T, Canavese G, Guariglia A, Santini D, Tomasetti P, Brandi ML: Aggressive forms of gastric neuroendocrine tumors in multiple endocrine neoplasia type 1. *Am J Surg Pathol* **21**:1075, 1997.

140. Thompson GB, van Heerden JA, Martin JK, Scutt AJ, Ilstrup DM, Carney JA: Carcinoma of the gastrointestinal tract: Presentation, management, and prognosis. *Surgery* **98**:1054, 1985.

140b. O'Brien T, O'Riordan DS, Gharib H, Scheithauer BW, Ebersold MJ, van Heerden JA: Results of treatment of pituitary disease in multiple endocrine neoplasia type 1. *Neurosurg* **39**:273, 1996.

141. Scheithauer BW, Laws ER Jr, Kovacs K, Horvath E, Randall RV, Carney JA: Pituitary adenomas of the multiple endocrine neoplasia type I syndrome. *Semin Diagn Pathol* **4**:205, 1987.

142. Skogseid B, Larsson C, Lindgren PG, Kvanta E, Rastad J, Theodorsson E, Wide L, Wilander E, Oberg K: Clinical and genetic features of adrenocortical lesions in multiple endocrine neoplasia type 1. *J Clin Endorcrinol Metab* **75**:76, 1992.

143. Houdelette P, Chagnon A, Dumotier J, Marthan E: Corticosurrenalome malin dans le cadre d'un syndrome de Wermer. *J Chir (Paris)* **126**:385, 1989.

144. Marx SJ, Agarwal SK, Kester MB, Heppner C, Kim YS, Skarulis MC, James LA, Goldsmith PK, Saggar SK, Park SY, Spiegel AM, Burns AL, Debelenko LV, Zhuang Z, Lubensky IA, Liotta LA, Emmert-Buck MR, Guru SC, Manickam P, Crabtree J, Erdos MR, Collins FS, Chandrasekharappa SC: Multiple endocrine neoplasia type 1: Clinical

and genetic features of the hereditary endocrine neoplasias. *Rec Prog Horm Res* **54**:397, 1999.

144b. Dackiw APB, Cote GJ, Fleming JB, Schultz PN, Stanford P, Vassilopoulous-Sellin R, Evans DB, Gagel RF, Lee JE: Screening for MEN1 mutations in patients with atypical endocrine neoplasia.. *Surgery* **126**:1097, 104 1999.

144c. Sigl E, Behmel A, Henn T, Wirnsberger G, Weinhausel A, Kaserer K, Neiderle B, Pfranger R: Cytogenetic and CGH studies of four neuroendocrine tumors and tumor-derived cell lines of a patient with multiple endocrine neoplasia type 1. *Int J Oncol* **15**:41, 1999.

145. Darling TN, Skarulis MC, Steinberg SM, Marx SJ, Spiegel AM, Turner M: Multiple facial angiofibromas and collagenomas in patients with multiple endocrine neoplasia type 1. *Arch Dermatol* **133**:853, 1997.

145c. Nord B, Platz A, Smoczynski K, Kytola S, Robertson G, Calender A, Murat A, Weintraub D, Burgess J, Edwards M, Skogseid B, Owen D, Lassam N, Hogg D, Larsson C, Teh BT: Malignant melanoma in patients with multiple endocrine neoplasia type 1 and involvement of the MEN1 gene in sporadic melanoma. *Int J Cancer* **87**:463, 2000.

145d. Sakurai A, Matsummoto K, Ikeo Y, et al. Frequency of facial angiofibromas in Japanese patients with multiple endocrine neoplasia type 1. *Endoc J* **47**:569, 2000.

145e. Vortmeyer AO, Lubensky IA, Skarulis M, Li G, Moon YW, Park WS, Weil R, Barlow C, Spiegel AM, Marx SJ, Zhuang Z: Multiple endocrine neoplasia type 1: atypical presentation, clinical course, and genetic analysis of multiple tumors. *Mod Pathol* **12**:919, 1999.

145f. McKeeby JL, Li X, Zhuang Z, Vortmeyer AO, Huang S, Pirner M, Skarulis MC, James-Newton L, Marx SJ, Lubensky IA: Multiple leiomyomas of the esophagus and uterus in multiple endocrine neoplasia type 1. *Am J Pathol* **159**:1121, 2001.

146. Gaitan D, Loosen PT, Orth DN: Two patients with Cushing's disease in a kindred with multiple endocrine neoplasia type 1. *J Clin Endocrinol Metab* **76**:1580, 1993.

147. Hershon KS, Kelly WA, Shaw CM, Schwartz R, Bierman EL: Prolactinomas as part of the multiple endocrine neoplastic syndrome type 1. *Am J Med* **74**:713, 1983.

148. Farid NR, Buehler S, Russell NA, Maroun FB, Allerdice P, Smyth HS: Prolactinomas in familial multiple endocrine neoplasia syndrome type 1. *Am J Med* **69**:874, 1980.

149. Bear JC, Urbina RB, Fahey JF, Farid NR: Variant multiple endocrine neoplasia I (MEN I-Burin): Further studies and non-linkage to HLA-1. *Hum Hered* **35**:15, 1985.

150. Marx SJ, Powell D, Shimkin PM, Wells SA, Ketcham AS, McGuigan JE, Bilezikian JP, Aurbach GD: Familial hyperparathyroidism: Mild hypercalcemia in at least nine members of a kindred. *Ann Intern Med* **78**:371, 1973.

151. Green JS: Development implementation and evaluation of clinical and genetic screening programs for hereditary tumor syndromes. Ph.D. thesis, Memorial University, Newfoundland, Canada, 1995.

152. Burgess JR, Shepherd JJ, Parameswaran V, Hoffman L, Greenaway TM: Prolactinomas in a large kindred with multiple endocrine neoplasia type 1: Clinical features and inheritance pattern. *J Clin Endocrinol Metab* **81**:1841, 1996.

153. Goldsmith RE, Sizemore GW, Chen I, Zalme E, Altemeier WA: Familial hyperparathyroidism description of a large kindred with physiologic observations and a review of the literature. *Ann Intern Med* **842**:36, 1976.

154. Kassem M, Zhang X, Brask S, Ericksen EF, Mosekilde L, Kruse TA: Familial isolated primary hyperparathyroidism. *Clin Endocrinol* **41**:415, 1994.

155. Burgess JR, Greenaway TM, Parameswaran V, Challis DR, David R, Shepherd JJ: Enteropancreatic malignancy associated with multiple endocrine neoplasia type 1: Risk factors and pathogenesis. *Cancer* **83**:428, 1998.

156. Zhuang Z, Ezzat SZ, Vortmeyer AS, Weil R, Oldfield EH, Park WS, Pack S, Huang S, Agarwal SK, Guru SC, Manickam P, Debelenko LV, Kester MB, Olufemi SE, Heppner C, Burns AL, Spiegel AM, Marx SJ, Chandrasekharappa SC, Collins FS, Emmert-Buck MR, Liotta L, Asa SL, Lubensky IA: Mutations of the MEN1 tumor suppressor gene in pituitary tumors. *Cancer Res* **57**:5446, 1997.

157. Stratakis CA, Schussheim DH, Freedman SM, Keil MF, Pack SD, Agarwal SK, Skarulis MC, Weil RJ, Zhuang Z, Oldfield EH, Marx SJ: Pituitary macroadenoma in a 5-year old: an early expression of MEN1. *J Clin Endocrinol Metab* **85**:4776, 2000.

158. Arnold A (ed): *Endocrine Neoplasms*. Boston, Kluwer Academic Publishers, 1997.

159. Maton PN, Gardner JD, Jensen RT: Cushing's syndrome in patients with Zollinger-Ellison syndrome. *N Engl J Med* **315**:1, 1986.

160. Kloppel G, Heitz PU: Pancreatic endocrine tumors. *Pathol Res Pract* **183**:155, 1988.

161. Melmed S, Ezrin C, Kovacs K, Goodman RS, Frohman LA: Acromegaly due to secretion of growth hormone by an ectopic pancreatic islet-cell tumor. *N Engl J Med* **312**:9, 1986.

162. Schimke RN: Multiple endocrine adenomatosis syndrome. *Adv Intern Med* **21**:249, 1976.

163. Calcatera TC, Paglia D: The coexistence of parathyroid adenoma and thyroid carcinoma. *Laryngoscope* **89**:1166, 1979.

164. Simpson RJ, Moss J Jr: Parathyroid adenoma and nonmedullary thyroid carcinoma association. *Otolaryngol Head Neck Surg* **101**:584, 1989.

165. Doumith R, Gennes JL, Cabane JP, Zygelman N: Pituitary prolactinoma, adrenal aldosterone producing adenoma, gastric schwannoma and clonic polyadenomas: A possible variant of multiple endocrine neoplasia (MEN) type 1. *Acta Endocrinol* **100**:189, 1982.

166. Holland OB, Gomez-Sanchez CE, Kem DC, Weiberger MH, Kramer NJ, Higgins JR: Evidence against prolactin stimulation of aldosterone in normal subjects and in patients with primary hyperaldosteronism, including a patient with primary hyperaldosteronismn and prolactin producing pituitary macroadenoma. *J Clin Endocrinol Metab* **45**:1064, 1977.

167. Blumenkopf B, Boekelheide K: Neck paraganglinoma with a pituitary adenoma: Case report. *J Neurosurg* **57**:426, 1982.

168. Nelson DR, Stachura ME, Dunlap DB: Case report: Ileal carcinoid tumor complicated by retroperitoneal fibrosis and prolactinoma. *Am J Med Sci* **296**:129, 1988.

169. Barzilay J, Heatley GJ, Cushing GW: Benign and malignant tumors in patients with acromegaly. *Arch Intern Med* **151**:1629, 1991.

170. Anderson RJ, Lufkin EG, Sizemore GW, Carney JA, Sheps SG, Silliman YE: Acromegaly and pituitary adenoma with pheochromocytoma: A variant of multiple endocrine neoplasia. *Clin Endocrinol* **14**:605, 1981.

171. Morris JA, Tymms DJ: Oat cell carcinoma, pheochromocytoma and carcinoid tumors—Multiple APUD neoplasia. A case report. *J Pathol* **131**:107, 1980.

172. Farhi F, Dikman SH, Lawson W, Cobin RH, Zak FG: Paragangliomatosis associated with multiple endocrine adenomas. *Arch Pathol Lab Med* **100**:495, 1976.

173. Hansen OP, Hansen M, Hansen HH, Rose B: Multiple endocrine adenomatosis of the mixed type. *Acta Med Scand* **200**:327, 1976.

174. Cameron D, Spiro HM, Lansberg L: Zollinger-Ellison syndrome with multiple endocrine adenomatosis type II. *N Engl J Med* **299**:152, 1978.

175. Janson KL, Roberts JA, Varela M: Multiple endocrine adenomatosis: In support of the common origin theories. *J Urol* **119**:161, 1978.

176. Alberts MW, Mcmeekin JO, George JM: Mixed multiple endocrine neoplasia syndromes. *JAMA* **244**:1236, 1980.

177. Cusick JF, Ho KC, Hagen TC, Kun LE: Granular-cell pituicytoma associated with multiple endocrine neoplasia type 2. *J Neurosurg* **56**:594, 1982.

178. Manning GS, Stevens KA, Stock JL: Multiple endocrine neoplasia type 1: Association with marfanoid habitus, optic atrophy, and other abnormalities. *Arch Intern Med* **143**:2315, 1983.

179. Bertnard JH, Ritz P, Reznik Y, Grollier G, Potier JC, Evrad C, Mahoudeau JA: Sipple's syndrome associated with a large prolactinoma. *Clin Endocrinol* **27**:607, 1987.

180. Jerkins TW, Sacks HS, O'Dorisio TM, Tuttle S, Solomon SS: Medullary carcinoma of the thyroid, pancreatic nesidioblastosis and microadenosis, and pancreatic polypeptide hypersecretion: A new association and clinical and hormonal response to a long-acting somatostatin analog. *J Clin Endocrinol Metab* **64**:1313, 1987.

181. Maton PN, Norton JA, Nieman LK, Doppman JL, Jensen RT: Multiple endocrine neoplasia type II with Zollinger-Ellison syndrome caused by a solitary pancreatic gastrinoma. *JAMA* **262**:535, 1989.

182. Reschini E, Catania A, Airaghi L, Manfredi MG, Crosignani PG: Scintigraphic study of extra-adrenal ganglioneuroma in a patient with overlap between multiple endocrine neoplasia types 1 and 2. *Clin Nucl Med* **17**:573, 1992.

183. Modan B, Baidatz D, Mart H, Steinitz R, Levin SG: Radiation-induced head and neck tumors. *Lancet* I 277, 1975.

184. Schneider AB, Shore-Freedman E, Weinstein RA: Radiation-induced thyroid and other head and neck tumors: Occurrence of multiple tumors and analysis of risk factors. *J Clin Endocrinol Metab* **63**:107, 1986.

185. Rosen IB, Strawbridge HG, Bain J: A case hyperparathyroidism associated with radiation of the head and neck area. *Cancer* **36**:1111, 1975.

186. Tisell LE, Carlsson S, Lindberg S, Ragnhult I: Autonomous hyperparathyroidism: A possible late complication of neck radiotherapy. *Acta Chir Scand* **142**:889, 1976.

187. Hedman I, Hansson G, Lundberg LM, Tisell LE: A clinical evaluation of radiation-induced hyperparathyroidism based on 148 surgically treated patients. *World J Surg* **8**:96, 1984.

188. Christmas TJ, Chapple CR, Noble JG, Milroy EJG, Cowie AGA: Hyperparathyroidism after neck irradiation. *Br J Surg* **75**:873, 1988.

189. Fujiwara S, Spoto R, Ezaki HAB, Akiba S, Neriishi K, Kodama K, Hosada Y, Shimaoka K: Hyperparathyroidism among atomic bomb survivors in Hiroshima. *Radiat Res* **130**:372, 1992.

190. Printz RA, Paloyan E, Lawrence AM, Pickleman JR, Braithwaite S, Brooks MH: Radiation-associated hyperparathyroidism: A new syndrome? *Surgery* **822**:276, 1977.

191. Tisell LE, Hansson G, Lindberg S, Ragnhult I: Hyperparathyroidism in persons treated with X-rays for tuberculous cervical adenitis. *Cancer* **40**:846, 1977.

192. Cohen J, Gierlowski TC, Schneider AB: A prospective study of hyperparathyroidism in individuals exposed to radiation in childhood. *JAMA* **264**:581, 1990.

193. Katz A, Braunstein GD: Clinical, biochemical and pathologic features of radiation-associated hyperparathyroidism. *Arch Intern Med* **143**:79, 1983.

194. Weinstein LS: Other skeletal diseases of G proteins — McCune-Albright syndrome, in Bilezikian J, Raisz L, Rodan G (eds): *Principles of Bone Biology*. New York, Academic Press, 1996, p 877.

195. Weinstein LS, Shenker A, Gejman PV, Merino MJ, Friedman E, Spiegel AM: Activating mutations of the stimulatory G protein in the McCune-Albright syndrome. *N Engl J Med* **325**:1688, 1991.

196. Landis CA, Masters SB, Spada A, Pace AM, Bourne HR, Vallar L: GTPase inhibiting mutations activate the subunit of Gs and stimulate adenylyl cyclase in human pituitary tumors. *Nature* **340**:692, 1989.

197. Bianco P, Kuznetsov SA, Riminucci M, Fisher LW, Spiegel AM, Robey PG: Reproduction of human fibrous dysplasia of bone in immunocompromised mice by transplanted mosaics of normal and Gsalpha-mutated skeletal progenitor cells. *J Clin Invest* **101**:1737, 1998.

197b. Bianco P, Riminucci M, Majolagbe A, Kuznetsov SA, Collins MT, Mankani MH, Corsi A, Bone HG, Wientroub S, Spiegel AM, Fisher LW, Robey PG: Mutations of the GNAS1 gene, stromal cell dysfunction, and osteomalacic changes in non-McCune-Albright fibrous dysplasia of bone. *J Bone Min Res* **15**:120, 2000.

198. Ponder B: Multiple endocrine neoplasia type 2, in Scriver CR, Beaudet A, Sly WS, Valle D, Vogelstein B (eds): *Metabolic and Molecular Bases of Inherited Disease*, 8th ed. New York, McGraw-Hill, 2000.

199. Schuffenecker I, Virally-Monod M, Brohet R, Goldgar D, Conte-Devolx B, Leclerc L, Chabre O, Boneu A, Caron J, Houdent C and the Groupe D'Etude des Tumeurs a Calcitonine: Risk and penetrance of primary hyperparathyroidism in multiple endocrine neoplasia type 2A families with mutations at codon 634 of the RET proto-oncogene. *J Clin Endocrinol Metab* **83**:487, 1998.

200. Schweitzer-Cagianut M, Froesch ER, Hedinger C: Familial Cushing's syndrome with primary adrenocortical microadenomatosis (primary adrenocortical nodular dysplasia). *Acta Endocrinol (Copenh)* **94**:529, 1980.

201. Carney JA, Gordon H, Carpenter PC, Shenoy BV, Go VLW: The complex of myxomas, spotty pigmentation and endocrine over-activity. *Medicine* **64**:270, 1985.

202. Stratakis CA, Courcoutsakis NA, Abati A, Filie A, Doppman JL, Carney JA, Shawker T: Thyroid gland abnormalities in patients with the syndrome of spotty skin pigmentation, myxomas, endocrine overactivity, and schwannomas (Carney complex). *J Clin Endocrinol Metab* **82**:2037, 1997.

203. Stratakis CA, Carney JA, Lin JP, Papaniccolaou DA, Karl M, Kastner DL, Pras E, Chrousos GP: Carney complex, a familial multiple neoplasia and lentiginosis syndrome: Analysis of 11 kindreds and linkage to the short arm of chromosome 2. *J Clin Invest* **97**:699, 1996.

204. Basson CT, MacRae CA, Korf B, Merliss A: Genetic heterogeneity of familial atrial myxoma syndromes (Carney complex). *Am J Cardiol* **79**:994, 1997.

204b. Kirschner LS, Carney JA, Pack SD, Taymans SE, Giatzakis C, Cho YS, Cho-Chung YS, Stratakis CA: Mutations of the gene encoding the protein kinase A type I-alpha regulatory subunit in patients with the Carney complex. *Nature Genet* **26**:89, 2000.

205. Linehan WM, Klausner R: Renal carcinoma, in Scriver CR, Beaudet A, Sly WS, Valle D, Vogelstein B (eds): *Metabolic and Molecular Bases of Inherited Disease*, 8th ed. New York, McGraw-Hill, 2000.

206. Lubensky IA, Pack S, Ault D, Vortmeyer AO, Libutti SK, Choyke PL, Walther MM, Linehan WM, Zhuang ZP: Multiple neuroendocrine tumors of the pancreas in von Hipple-Lindau disease patients. *Am J Pathol* **153**:1, 1998.

207. Neumann HPH: Basic criteria for clinical diagnosis and genetic counseling in von Hippel-Lindau syndrome. *J Vasc Dis* **16**:220, 1987.

208. Latif F, Tory K, Gnara J, Yao M, Duh FM, Orcutt S, Stackhouse T, Kuzmin I, Modi W, Geil L: Identification of the von Hipple-Lindau disease tumor suppressor gene. *Science* **260**:1317, 1993.

209. Pause A, Lee S, Worrell RA, Chen DY, Burgess WH, Linehan WM, Klausner RD: The von Hippel-Landau tumor-suppressor gene product forms a stable complex with human CUL-2, a member of the Cdc53 family of proteins. *Proc Natl Acad Sci USA* **94**:2156, 1997.

210. Malkin D: Li-Fraumeni syndrome, in Scriver CR, Beaudet A, Sly WS, Valle D, Vogelstein B (eds): *Metabolic and Molecular Bases of Inherited Disease*, 8th ed. New York, McGraw-Hill, 2000.

211. Eng C, Parsons R: Cowden syndrome, in Scriver CR, Beaudet A, Sly WS, Valle D, Vogelstein B (eds): *Metabolic and Molecular Bases of Inherited Disease*, 8th ed. New York, McGraw-Hill, 2000.

212. Guttman GH, Collins FS: Neurofibromatosis, in Scriver CR, Beaudet A, Sly WS, Valle D, Vogelstein B (eds): *Metabolic and Molecular Bases of Inherited Disease*, 8th ed. New York: McGraw-Hill, 2000.

213. Weinstein RS, Harris RL: Hypercalcemic hyperparathyroidism and hypophosphatemic osteomalacia complicating neurofibromatosis. *Calcif Tissue Int* **46**:261, 1990.

214. Swinburn BA, Yeong ML, Lane MR, Nicholson GI, Holdaway IM: Neurofibromatosis associated with somatostatinoma: A report of two patients. *Clin Endocrinol* **28**:353, 1988.

215. Sartori P, Symons JC, Taylor NF, Grant OB: Adrenal cortical adenoma in a 13 year old girl with neurofibromatosis. *Acta Paediatr Scand* **78**:476, 1989.

216. DeAngelis LM, Kelleher MB, Kalmon DP, Fetell MR: Multiple paragangliomatosis in neurofibromatosis: A new neuroendocrine neoplasia. *Neurology* **37**:129, 1987.

217. Cawthon RM, Weiss R, Xu C, Viskochill D, Culver M, Stevens J, Robertson M, Dunn D, Gesteland R, O'Connel P, White R: A major segment of the neurofibromatosis type 1 gene: cDNA sequence, genomic structure, and point mutations. *Cell* **62**:193, 1990.

218. Jackson CE, Norum RA, Boyd SB, Talpos GB, Wilson SD, Taggart T, Mallette LE: Hereditary hyperparathyroidism and multiple ossifying jaw fibromas: A clinically and genetically distinct syndrome. *Surgery* **108**:1006, 1990.

219. Mallette LE, Malini S, Rappaport MP, Kirkland JL: Familial cystic parathyroid adenomatosis. *Ann Intern Med* **107**:54, 1987.

220. Teh BT, Farnebo F, Kristoffersson U, Sundelin B, Cardinal J, Axelson R, Yap A, Epstein M, Heath H III, Cameron D, Larsson C: Autosomal dominant primary hyperparathyroidism and jaw tumor syndrome associated with renal hamartomas and cystic kidney disease: Linkage to 1q21-q32 and loss of the wild type allele in renal hamartomas. *J Clin Endocrinol Metab* **81**:4204, 1996.

221. Szabo J, Heath B, Hill VM, Jackson CE, Zarbo RJ, Mallette LE, Chew SL, Besser GM, Thakker RV, Huff V, Leppert MF, Heath H III: Hereditary hyperparathyroidism-jaw tumor syndrome: The endocrine tumor gene HRPT2 maps to chromosome 1q21-q31. *Am J Hum Genet* **56**:944, 1995.

222. Teh BT, Farnebo F, Twigg S, Kristoffersson U, Sundelin B, Cardinal J, Axelson R, Yap A, Epstein M, Heath H III, Camerson D, Larsson C: Familial isolated hyperparathyroidism maps to the hyperparathyroidism-jaw tumor locus in 1q21-q32 in a subset of families. *J Clin Endocrinol Metab* **83**: 2114, 1998.

223. Wassif WS, Moniz CF, Friedman E, Wong S, Weber G, Nordenskjold M, Peters TJ, Larsson C: Familial isolated hyperparathyroidism: A distinct genetic entity with an increased risk of parathyroid cancer. *J Clin Endocrinol Metab* **77**:1485, 1993.

223b. Kassem M, Kruse TA, Wong FK, Larsson C, Teh BT: Familial isolated hyperparathyroidism as a variant of multiple endocrine neoplasia type 1 in a large Danish pedigree. *J Clin Endocrinol Metab* **85**:165, 2000.

224. Streeten E, Weinstein LS, Norton JA, Mulvihill JJ, White B, Friedman E, Jaffe G, Brandi ML, Stewart K, Zimering MB, Spiegel AM, Aurbach GD, Marx SJ: Studies in a kindred with parathyroid carcinoma. *J Clin Endocrinol Metab* **75**:362, 1992.

224b. Simonds WF, James-Newton LA, Agarwal SK, Yang B, Skarulis MC, Hendy GN, Marx SJ: Familial isolated hyperparathyroidism: Clinical and genetic characteristics of 36 kindreds. *Medicine*. In press.

225. Law WM Jr, Hodgson S, Heath H III: Autosomal recessive inheritance of familial hyperparathyroidism. *N Engl J Med* **309**:650, 1983.

226. Allo M, Thompson NW: Familial hyperparathyroidism caused by solitary adenomas. *Surgery* **92**:486, 1982.

227. Huang SM, Duh O-Y, Shaver J, Siperstein AE, Kraimp JL, Clark OH: Familial hyperparathyroidism without multiple endocrine neoplasia. *World J Surg* **21**:22, 1997.

228. Farnebo F, Teh B, Dotzenrath C, Wassif WS, Svensson A, White I, Betz R, Goretzki P, Sandelin K, Farnebo LO, Larsson C: Differential loss of heterozygosity in familial, sporadic, and uremic hyperparathyroidism. *Hum Genet* **99**:342, 1997.

229. Tragl KH, Mayr WR: Familial islet cell adenomatosis. *Lancet* **1**:426, 1977.

230. Maioli M, Cicarese M, Pacifico A, Tonolo G, Ganau A, Cossu S, Tanda F, Realdi G: Familial insulinoma: Description of two cases. *Acta Diabetol* **29**:38, 1992.

231. Kinnamon JEC: Heredity and symptoms in acromegaly. *Acta Otolaryngol* **82**:230, 1976.

232. Kurisaka M, Takei Y, Tsubokawa T, Motiyasu N: Growth hormone-secreting pituitary adenoma in uniovular twin brothers: Case report. *Neurosurgery* **8**:226, 1981.

233. Jones MK, Evans PJ, Jopnes IR, Thomas JP: Familial acromegaly. *Clin Endocrinol (Oxf)* **20**:355, 1984.

234. Abbassioun K, Fatourechi V, Amirjamshidi A, Meibodi NA: Familial acromegaly with pituitary adenoma: Report of three affected siblings. *J Neurosurg* **64**:510, 1986.

235. Gadelha MR, Kineman RD, Frohman LA: Familial somatotropinomas: Clinical and genetic aspects. *Endocrinologist* **9**:277, 1999.

236. Benlian P, Giraud S, Lahlou N, Roger M, Blin C, Holler C, Lenoir G, Sallandre J, Calender A, Turpin G: Familial acromegaly: A specific clinical entity. Further evidence from the genetic study of a three-generation family. *Eur J Endocrinol* **133**:451, 1995.

237. Yamada S, Yoshimoto K, Sano T, Takada K, Itakura M, Usui M, Teramoto A: Inactivation of the tumor suppressor gene on 11q13 in brothers with familial acrogigantism without multiple endocrine neoplasia type 1. *Clin Endocrinol Metab* **82**:239, 1997.

237b. Gadelha MR, Une KN, Rohde K, Vaisman M, Kineman RD, Frohman LA. Isolated familial somatotropinomas: Establishment of linkage to chromosome 11q13.1-11q13.3 and evidence for a potential second locus at chromosome 2p16-12. *J Clin Endocrinol Metab* **85**:707, 2000.

238. Berezin M, Karasik A: Familial prolactinoma. *Clin Endocrinol* **42**:483, 1995.

239. Eschbach JW, Rinaldo JA: Metastatic carcinoid: A familial occurrence. *Ann Intern Med* **57**:647, 1962.

240. Anderson RE: A familial instance of appendiceal carcinoid tumors. *Am J Surg* **111**:738, 1966.

241. Wale RJ, William JA, Veeley AH: Familial occurrence in carcinoid tumors. *Aust NZ J Surg* **53**:325, 1983.

242. Moertel CG, Dockerty MB: Familial occurrence of metastasizing carcinoid tumors. *Ann Intern Med* **78**:389, 1973.

243. Yeatman TJ, Sharp JV, Kimura AK: Can susceptibility to carcinoid tumors be inherited? *Cancer* **63**:390, 1989.

244. Marx SJ, Attie M, Levine MA, Spiegel AM, Downs RW Jr, Lasker RD: The hypocalciuric or benign variant of familial hypercalcemia: Clinical and biochemical features in fifteen kindreds. *Medicine* **60**:397, 1981.

245. Firek AF, Kao PC, Heath H III: Plasma intact parathyroid hormone (PTH) and PTH-related peptide in familial benign hypercalcemia: Greater responsiveness to endogenous PTH than in primary hyperparathyroidism. *J Clin Endocrinol Metab* **72**:541, 1991.

246. Thorgeirsson U, Costa J, Marx SJ: The parathyroid glands in familial hypocalciuric hypercalcemia. *Hum Pathol* **12**:229, 1981.

247. Attie MF, Gill JR Jr, Stock JL, Spiegel AM, Downs RW Jr, Levine MA, Marx SJ: Urinary calcium excretion in familial hypocalciuric hypercalcemia: Persistence of relative hypocalciuria after induction of hypoparathyroidism. *J Clin Invest* **72**:667, 1983.

248. Brown EM, Pollak M, Hebert SC: The extracellular calcium-sensing receptor: its role in health and disease. *Annu Rev Med* **49**:15, 1998.

249. Heath H III, Jackson CE, Otterud B, Leppert MF: Genetic linkage analysis in familial benign (hypocalciuric) hypercalcemia: Evidence for locus heterogeneity. *Am J Hum Genet* **53**:193, 1993.

250. Trump D, Whyte MP, Wooding C, Pang JT, Pearce SHS, Kocher DV, Thakker RV: Linkage studies in a kindred from Oklahoma, with familial benign (hypocalciuric) hypercalcaemia (FBH) and developmental elevations in serum parathyroid hormone levels, indicate a third locus for FBH. *Hum Genet* **96**:183, 1995.

251. Pollack MR, Chou YHW, Marx SJ, Steinman B, Cole DEC, Brandi ML, Papopoulos SE, Menko F, Hendy GN, Brown EM, Seidman CE, Seidman JG: Familial hypocalciuric hypercalcemia and neonatal severe hyperparathyroidism: Effects of mutant gene dosage on phenotype. *J Clin Invest* **93**:1108, 1994.

252. Pearse SHR, Trump D, Wooding C, Besser GM, Hew SL, Grant DB, Heath DA, Hughes IA, Paterson CR, Whyte MP, Thakker RV: Calcium-sensing receptor mutations in familial benign hypercalcemia and neonatal hyperparathyroidism. *J Clin Invest* **96**:2683, 1995.

253. Tonacchera M, Van Sande J, Cetani F, Swillens S, Schvartz C, Winiszewski L, Portmann L, Dumont JE, Vassart G, Parma J: Functional characteristics of three new germline mutations of the thyrotropin receptor gene causing autosomal dominant toxic thyroid hyperplasia. *J Clin Endocrinol Metab* **81**:547, 1996.

254. Shenker A, Laue L, Kosugi S, Merendino JJ, Menegishi T, Cutler GB Jr: A constitutively activating mutation of the luteinizing-hormone receptor in familial male precocious puberty. *Nature* **365**:652, 1993.

255. Thomas PM, Cote GJ, Wohlik N, Haddad B, Mathew PM, Rabel W, Aguilar-Bryan L, Gagel RF, Bryan J: Mutations in the sulfonylurea receptor gene in familial persistent hyperinsulinemic hypoglycemia of infancy. *Science* **268**:426, 1995.

256. Thomas PM, Ye Y, Lightner E: Mutation of the pancreatic islet inward rectifier Kir6.2 also leads to familial persistent hyperinsulinemic hypoglycemia of infancy. *Hum Mol Genet* **11**:1809, 1996.

257. Glaser B, Kesavan P, Heyman M, Davis E, Cuesta A, Buchs A, Stanley CA, Thornton PS, Permutt MA, Matschinsky FM, Herold KC: Familial hyperinsulinism caused by an activating glucokinase mutation. *N Engl J Med* **338**:226, 1998.

258. Stanley CA, Lieu YK, Hsu BY, Burlina AB, Greenberg CR, Hopwood NJ, Perlman K, Rich BH, Zammarchi E, Poncz M: Hyperinsulinism and hyperammonemia in infants with regulatory mutations of the glutamate dehydrogenase gene. *N Engl J Med* **338**:1352, 1998.

258b. Marx SJ: Contrasting paradigms for hereditary hyperfunction of endocrine cells. *J Clin Endocrinol Metab* **84**:3001, 1999.

259. Ho C, Conner DA, Pollak MR, Ladd DJ, Kifor O, Warren HB, Brown EM, Seidman JG, Seidman CE: A mouse model of human familial hypocalciuric hypercalcemia and neonatal severe hyperparathyroidism. *Nature Genet* **11**:389, 1995.

260. Vassart G: New pathophysiological mechanisms in hyperthyroidism. *Horm Res* **48(suppl 4)**:47, 1997.

260a. Verkarre V, Fournet J-C, de Lonlay P, Gross-Morand M-S, Devillers M, Rahier J, Brunelle F, Robert J-J, Nihoul-Fekete C, Saudubray J-M, Junien C: Paternal mutation of the sulfonylurea receptor (SUR1) gene and maternal loss of 11p15 imprinted genes lead to persistent hyperinsulinism in focal adenomatous hyperplasia. *J Clin Invest* **102**:1286, 1998.

261. Parma J, Duprez L, Van Sande J, Hermans J, Roomans P, Van Vliet G, Costagliola S, Rodien P, Dumont JE, Vassart G: Diversity and prevalence of somatic mutations in the thyrotrophin receptor and Gs alpha genes as a cause of toxic thyroid adenomas. *J Clin Endocrinol Metab* **82**:2695, 1997.

262. Liu G, Duranteau L, Carel J, Monroe J, Doyle DA, Shenker A: Leydig-cell tumors caused by an activating mutation of the gene encoding the luteinizing hormone receptor. *N Eng J Med* **341**:1731, 1999.

262b. Vortmeyer AO, Boni R, Pack SD, Darling TN, Zhuang Z: Perivascular cells harboring multiple endocrine neoplasia type 1 alteration are neoplastic cells in angiofibromas. *Cancer Res* **59**:274, 1999.

263. Brandi ML, Fitzpatrick LA, Coon HG, Aurbach GD: Bovine parathyroid cells: Cultures maintained for more than 140 population doublings. *Proc Natl Acad Sci USA* **83**:1709, 1986.

264. Sakaguchi K, Santora A, Zimering M, Curcio F, Aurbach GD, Brandi ML: Functional epithelial cell line cloned from rat parathyroid glands. *Proc Natl Acad Sci USA* **84**:3269, 1987.

265. Brandi ML, Ornberg R, Sakaguchi K, Curcio F, Fattorossi A, Lelkes P, Matsui T, Zimering M, Aurbach GD: Establishment and characterization of a clonal line of parathyroid endothelial cells. *FASEB J* **4**:3152, 1990.

266. Brandi ML, Aurbach GD, Fitzpatrick LA: Parathyroid mitogenic activity in plasma from patients with familial multiple endocrine neoplasia type 1. *N Engl J Med* **314**:1287, 1985.

267. Marx SJ, Sakagucki K, Green JE III, Aurbach GD, Brandi ML: Mitogenic activity on parathyroid cells in plasma from members of a large kindred with multiple endocrine neoplasia type 1. *J Clin Endocrinol Metab* **67**:149, 1988.

268. Friedman E, Larsson C, Amorosi A, Brandi ML, Bale A, Metz D, Jensen RT, Skarulis M, Eastman RC, Nieman L, Norton JA, Marx SJ: Multiple endocrine neoplasia type 1: Pathology pathophysiology, and differential diagnosis, in Bilezekian JP, Levine MA, Marcus R (eds): *The Parathyroids*. New York, Raven Press, 1994, p 647.

269. Zimering MB, Brandi ML, DeGrange DA, Marx SJ, Streeten E, Katsumata N, Murphy PR, Sato Y, Friesen HG, Arubach GD: Circulating fibroblast growth factor-like substance in familial multiple endocrine neoplasia type 1. *J Clin Endocrinol Metab* **70**:149, 1990.

270. Bikealvi A, Klein S, Pintucci G, Rifkin DB: Biological roles of fibroblast growth factor-2. *Endocr Rev* **18**:26, 1997.

271. Brem H, Klagsbrun M: The role of fibroblast growth factors and related oncogenes in tumor growth. *Cancer Treat Res* **63**:211, 1992.

272. Zimering MB, Katsumata N, Sato Y, Brandi ML, Aurbach GD, Marx SJ, Friesen HG: Increased basic fibroblast growth factor in plasma from multiple endocrine neoplasia type 1: Relation to pituitary tumor. *J Clin Endocrinol Metab* **76**:1182, 1993.

273. Gustavsson KH, Jansson R, Oberg K: Chromosomal breakage in multiple endocrine adenomatosis (type 1 and II). *Clin Genet* **23**:143, 1983.

274. Benson L, Gustavson KH, Rastad J, Akerstrom G, Oberg K, Ljunghall S: Cytogenetical investigations in patient with primary hyperparathyroidism and multiple endocrine neoplasia type 1. *Hereditas* **108**:227, 1988.

274b. Ikeo Y, Sakurai A, Suzuki R, Zhang MX, Koizumi S, Takeuchi Y, Yumita W, Nakayama J, Hashizume K: Proliferation-associated expression of the MEN1 gene as revealed by in situ hybridization: possible role of the menin as a negative regulator of cell proliferation under DNA damage. *Lab Invest* **80**:797, 2000.

274c. Itakura Y, Sakurai A, Katai M, Ikeo Y, Hashizume K: Enhanced sensitivity to alkylating agent in lymphocytes from patients with multiple endocrine neoplasia type 1. *Biomed & Pharmacother* **54** (**Suppl**):187S, 2000.

275. Scappaticci S, Maraschio P, Del Ciotto N, Fossati GS, Zonta A, Fraccarp M: Chromosome abnormalities in lymphocytes and fibroblasts of subjects with multiple endocrine neoplasia type 1. *Cancer Genet Cytogenet* **52**:85, 1991.

276. Bale SJ, Bale AE, Stewart K, Dachowski L, McBride OW, Glaser T, Green JE III, Mulvihill JJ, Brandi ML, Sakaguchi K, Aurbach GD, Marx SJ: Linkage analysis of multiple endocrine neoplasia type 1 with int-2 and other markers on chromosome 11. *Genomics* **4**:320, 1989.

277. Sakurai A, Katai M, Itakura Y, Nakajima K, Baba K, Hashizume K: Genetic screening in hereditary multiple endocrine neoplasia type 1: Absence of a founder effect among Japanese families. *Jpn J Cancer Res* **87**:985, 1996.

278. Teh BT, Hii SI, David R, Parameswaran V, Grimmond S, Walters MK, Tan TT, Nancarrow DJ, Chan SP, Mennon J, Larsson C, Zaini A, Khalid AK, Shepherd JJ, Cameron DP, Hayward NK: Multiple endocrine neoplasia type (MEN1) in two Asian families. *Hum Genet* **94**:468, 1994.

279. Kytola S, Leisti J, Winqvist R, Salmela P: Improved carrier testing for multiple endocrine neoplasia, type 1, using new microsatellite-type DNA markers. *Hum Genet* **96**:449, 1995.

280. Smith CM, Wells SA, Gerhard DS: Mapping eight new polymorphisms in 11q13 in the vicinity of multiple endocrine neoplasia type 1: Identification of a new distal recombinant. *Hum Genet* **96**:377, 1995.

281. Courseaux A, Grosgeorge J, Gaudray P, Pannett AAJ, Forbes SA, Williamson C, Bassett D, Thakker RV, Teh BT, Farnebo F, Shepherd J, Skogseid B, Larsson C, Giraud S, Zhang CX, Salandre J, Calender A: The European Consortium on MEN1: Definition of the minimal MEN1 candidate area based on a 5-Mb integrated map of proximal 11q13. *Genomics* **37**:354, 1996.

282. Larsson C, Calender A, Grimmond S, Giraud S, Hayward NK, Teh BT, Farnebo F: Molecular tools for presymptomatic testing in multiple endocrine neoplasia type 1. *J Intern Med* **2328**:239, 1995.

283. Petty EM, Green JS, Marx SJ, Taggart RT, Farid N, Bale AE: Mapping the gene for hereditary hyperparathyroidism and prolactinoma (MEN1-Burin) to chromosome 11q: Evidence for a founder effect in patients from Newfoundland. *Am J Hum Genet* **54**:1060, 1994.

284. Olufemi SE, Green JS, Manickam P, Guru SC, Agarwal SK, Kester MB, Dong Q, Burns AL, Spiegel AM, Marx SJ, Coillins FS, Chandrasekharappa SC: A common ancestral mutation in the MEN1 gene is likely responsible for the prolactinoma variant (MEN1-Burin) in four kindreds from Newfoundland. *Hum Mutat* **11**:264, 1998.

285. Stock JL, Warth MR, Teh BT, Coderre JA, Overdorf JH, Baumann G, Hintz RL, Hartman ML, Seizinger BR, Larsson C, Aronin N: A kindred with a variant of multiple endocrine neoplasia type 1 demonstrating frequent expression of pituitary tumors but not linked to the multiple endocrine neoplasia type 1 locus at chromosome region 11q13. *J Clin Endocrinol Metab* **82**:486, 1997.

286. Bahn RS, Scheithauer BW, van Heerden JA, Laws ER Jr, Horvath E, Gharib H: Nonidentical expressions of multiple endocrine neoplasia type 1 in identical twins. *Mayo Clin Proc* **61**:689, 1986.

286a. Flanagan DE, Armitage M, Clein GP, Thakker RV: Prolactinoma presenting in identical twins with multiple endocrine neoplasia type 1. *Clin Endocrinol* **45**:117, 1996.

287. Brandi ML, Weber G, Svensson A, Falchetti A, Tonelli F, Castello R, Furlani L, Scappaticci S, Fraccaro M, Larsson C: Homozygotes for the autosomal dominant neoplasia syndrome (MEN1). *Am J Hum Genet* **53**:1167, 1993.

287b. Morelli A, Falchetti A, Martineti V, Becherini L, Mark W, Friedman E, Brandi ML: MEN1 gene mutation analysis in Italian patients with multiple endocrine neoplasia type 1. *Eur J Endocrinol* **142**:131, 2000.

288. Muhr C, Ljunghall S, Akerstrom G, Palmer M, Bergstrom K, Enoksson P, Lundqvist G, Wide L: Screening for multiple endocrine neoplasia syndrome (type 1) in patients with primary hyperparathyroidism. *Clin Endocrinol* **20**:153, 1984.

289. de Mars R: Published discussion, *23rd Annual Symposium of Fundamental Cancer Research*. Baltimore, Williams & Wilkins, 1969, p 105 (abstract).

290. Knudson AG: Mutation and cancer: Statistical study of retinoblastoma. *Proc Natl Acad Sci USA* **68**:820, 1971.

292. Thakker RV, Bouloux P, Wooding C, Chotai K, Broad PM, Spurr NK, Besser GM, O'Riordan JLH: Association of parathyroid tumors in multiple endocrine neoplasia type 1 with loss of alleles on chromosome 11. *N Engl J Med* **321**:218, 1989.

293. Bystrom C, Larsson C, Blomberg C, Sandelin K, Falkermern U, Skogseid B, Oberg K, Werner S, Nordenskhold M: Localization of the MEN 1 gene to a small region within chromosome 11q13 by deletion mapping in tumors. *Proc Natl Acad Sci USA* **87**:1968, 1990.

294. Radford DM, Ashley SM, Wells SA, Gerhard DS: Loss of hetrozygosity of markers on chromosome 11 in tumors from patients with multiple endocrine neoplasia syndrome type 1. *Cancer Res* **50**:6529, 1990.

295. Friedman E, DeMarco L, Gejman PV, Norton JS, Bale AE, Aurbach GD, Spiegel AM, Marx SJ: Allelic loss from chromosome 11 in parathyroid tumors. *Cancer Res* **525**:6804, 1992.

296. Morelli A, Falchetti A, Amorosi A, Tonelli F, Bearzi I, Ranaldi R, Tomassetti P, Brandi ML: Clonal analysis by chromsome 11 microsatellite-PCR of microdissected parathyroid tumors from MEN1 patients. *Biochem Biophys Res Commun* **227**:736, 1996.

297. Weil RJ, Vortmeyer AO, Huang S, Huang S, Boni R, Lubensky IA, Pack S, Marx SJ, Zhuang Z, Oldfield EH: 11q13 Allelic loss in pituitary tumors in patients with multiple endocrine neoplasia type 1. *Clin Cancer Res* **4**:1673, 1998.

298. Lubensky IA, Debelenko LV, Zhuang Z, Emmet-Buck MR, Dong Q, Chandrasekharappa SC, Guru SC, Manickam P, Olufemi SE, Marx SJ, Spiegel AM, Collins FS, Liotta LA: Allelic deletions in chromosome 11q13 in multiple tumors from individual MEN1 patients. *Cancer Res* **56**:5272, 1996.

299. Zhuang Z, Bertheau P, Emmert-Buck MR, Liotta LA, Gnarra J, Linehan WM, Lubensky IA: A microdissection technique for archival DNA analysis of specific cell populations in lesions, 1 mm in size. *Am J Pathol* **146**:620, 1995.

300. Emmert-Buck MR, Bonner RF, Smith PD, Chuaqui RF, Zhuang Z, Goldstein SR, Weiss RA, Liotta LA: Laser capture microdissection. *Science* **274**:998, 1996.

301. Emmert-Buck MR, Lubensky IA, Dong Q, Manickam P, Guru SC, Kester MB, Olufemi S-E, Agarwal SK, Burns AL, Spiegel AM, Collins FS, Marx SJ, Zhuang Z, Liotta LA, Chandrasekharappa SC, Debelenko LV: Localization of the MEN1 gene based on tumor LOH analysis. *Cancer Res* **57**:1855, 1997.

301b. Pannett AAJ, Wooding C, Bassett JHD, Forbes SA, Thakker RV: Somatic mutations in multiple endocrine neoplasia type 1 (MEN1) tumours, consistent with the Knudson hypothesis. *Bone* **23 Suppl**:S187 (abstract), 1998.

302. Debelenko LV, Zhuang Z, Emmert-Buck MR, Chandrasekharappa SC, Manickam P, Guru SC, Marx SJ, Spiegel AM, Collins FS, Jensen RT, Liotta LA, Lubensky IA: Allelic deletions on chromosome 11q13 in MEN1-associated and sporadic duodenal gastrinomas and pancreatic endocrine tumors. *Cancer Res* **157**:2238, 1997.

303. Debelenko LV, Emmert-Buck MR, Zhuang Z, Epshteyn E, Moskaluk CA, Jensen RT, Liotta LA, Lubensky IA: The multiple endocrine neoplasia type 1 gene locus is involved in the pathogenesis of type II gastric carcinoids. *Gastroenterology* **113**:773, 1997.

304. Dong Q, Debelenko L, Chandrasekharappa S, Emmert-Buck MR, Zhuang Z, Guru SC, Manickam P, Skarulis M, Lubensky IA, Liotta LA, Collins FS, Marx SJ, Spiegel AM: Loss of heterozygosity at 11q13: Analysis of pituitary tumors, lung carcinoids, lipomas, and other uncommon tumors in familial multiple endocrine neoplasia type 1. *J Clin Endocrinol Metab* **82**:1416, 1997.

305. Williamson C, Pannett A, Pang JT, McCarthy M, Sherppard MN, Monson JP, Clayton RN, Thakker RV: Localisation of a tumour suppressor gene causing endocrine tumours to a four centimorgan region on chromosome 1, in *Program and Abstracts of the Endocrinology Society*, 1996, p 961 (abstract).

306. Kytola S, Makinen MJ, Kahkonen M, Teh BT, Leisti J, Salmela P: Comparative genomic hybridization studies in tumors from a patient with multiple endocrine neoplasia type 1. *Eur J Endocrinol* **139**:202, 1998.

307. Henske EP, Scheithauer BW, Short MP, Wollmann R, Nahmias J, Hornigold N, Slegtenhorst M, Welsh CT, Kwiatkowski DJ: Allelic loss is frequent in tuberous sclerosis kidney lesions but rare in brain lesions. *Am J Hum Genet* **59**:400, 1996.

308. Pack S, Turner ML, Zhuang Z, Vortmeyer AO, Boni R, Skarulis M, Marx SJ, Darling TN: Cutaneous tumors in patients with multiple endocrine neoplasia type 1 show allelic deletions of the MEN1 gene. *J Invest Dermatol* **11**:438, 1998.

309. Tahara H, Smith AP, Gaz RD, Cryns VL, Arnold A: Genomic localization of novel candidate tumor suppressor gene loci in human parathyroid adenomas. *Cancer Res* **56**:599, 1996.

310. Eubanks PJ, Sawicki MP, Samara GJ, Gratti R, Nakamura Y, Tsao D, Johnson C, Hurwitz M, Wan YJ, Passaro E: Putative tumor-suppressor gene on chromosome 11 is important in sporadic endocrine tumor formation. *Am J Surg* **167**:180, 1994.

311. Thakker RV, Pook MA, Wooding C, Boscaro M, Scanarini M, Clayton RN: Association of somatotrophinomas with loss of alleles on chromsome 11 and with gsp mutations. *J Clin Invest* **91**:2815, 1993.

312. Boggild MD, Jenkinson S, Pistorello M, Boscaro M, Scanarini M, McTernan P, Perrett CW, Thakker RV, Clayton RN: Molecular genetic studies of sporadic pituitary tumors. *J Clin Endocrinol Metab* **78**:387, 1994.

313. Bates AS, Farrell WE, Bicknell EJ, McNicol AM, Talbots AJ, Broome JC, Perrett CW, Thakker RV, Clayton RN: Allelic deletion in pituitary adenomas reflects aggressive biological activity and has potential value as a prognostic marker. *J Clin Endocrinol Metab* **82**:818, 1997.

314. Jakobovitz O, Devora N, DeMarco L, Barbosa AJA, Simoni FB, Rechavi G, Friedman E: Carcinoid tumors frequently display genetic abnormalities involving chromosome 11. *J Clin Endocrinol Metab* **81**:3164, 1996.

315. Matsuo K, Tang SH, Fagin JA: Allelotype of human thyroid tumors: Loss of chromosome 11q13 sequences in follicular neoplasms. *Mol Endocrinol* **5**:1873, 1991.

316. Iida A, Blake K, Tunny T, Klemm S, Stowasser M, Hayward N, Gordon R, Nakamura Y, Imai TK: Allelic losses on chromosome band 11q13 in aldosterone-producing adrenal tumors. *Genes Chromosom Cancer* **12**:73, 1995.

317. Heppner C, Reincke M, Agarwal SK, Mora P, Allolio B, Burns AL, Spiegel AM, Marx SJ: MEN1 gene analysis in sporadic adrenocortical neoplasms. *J Clin Endocrinol Metab* **84**:216, 1999.

318. Heppner C, Kester MB, Agarwal SK, Debelenko LV, Emmert-Buck MR, Guru SC, Manickam P, Olufemi SE, Skarulis MC, Doppman JL, Alexander RH, Kim YS, Saggar SK, Lubensky IA, Zhuang Z, Liotta LA, Chandrasekharappa SC, Collins FS, Spiegel AM, Burns AL, Marx SJ: Somatic mutation of the MEN1 gene in parathyroid tumors. *Nature Genet* **16**:375, 1997.

319. Tanaka C, Yoshimoto K, Yamada S, Lnishioka H, Moritani M, Yamaoka T, Itakura M: Absence of germ-line mutations of the

multiple endocrine neoplasia type 1 (MEN1) gene in familial pituitary adenoma in contrast to MEN1 in Japanese. *J Clin Endocrinol Metab* **83**:960, 1998.

320. Falchetti A, Bale AE, Amorosi A, Bordi C, Cicci P, Bandini S, Marx SJ, Brandi ML: Progression of uremic hyperparathyroidism involves allelic loss on chromosome 11. *J Clin Endocrinol Metab* **76**:139, 1993.

321. Arnold A, Brown MF, Urena P, Gaz RD, Sarfati E, Drueke TB: Monoclonality of parathyroid tumors in chronic renal failure and in primary parathyroid hyperplasia. *J Clin Invest* **95**:2047, 1995.

322. Farnebo F, Farnebo L-O, Nordenstrom J, Larsson C: Allelic loss on chromosome 11 is uncommon in parathyroid glands of patients with hypercalcemic secondary hyperparathyroidism. *Eur J Surg* **163**:331, 1997.

323. Zhuang Z, Merino MJ, Chuaqui R, Liotta LA, Emmert-Buck MR: Identical allelic loss on chromosome 11q13 in microdissected *in situ* and invasive human breast cancer. *Cancer Res* **55**:467, 1995.

324. Chuaqui RF, Zhuang Z, Emmert-Buck MR, Liotta LA, Merino MJ: Analysis of loss of heterozygosity on chromosome 11q13 in atypical ductal hyperplasia and *in situ* carcinoma of the breast. *Am J Pathol* **150**:297, 1997.

325. Srivatsan ES, Misra BC, Venugopalan M, Wilczynski SP: Loss of heterozygosity for alleles on chromosome 11 in cervical carcinoma. *Am J Hum Genet* **49**:868, 1991.

326. Popescu NC, Zimonjic DB: Alterations of chromosome 11q13 in cervical carcinoma cell lines. *Am J Hum Genet* **58**:422, 1996.

327. Debelenko LV, Emmert-Buck MR, Manickam P, Kester MB, Guru SC, DiFranco EM, Olufemi SE, Agarwal SK, Lubensky IA, Zhuang Z, Burns AL, Spiegel AM, Liotta LA, Collins FS, Marx SJ, Chandrasekharappa SC: Haplotype analysis defines a minimal interval for the multiple endocrine neoplasia type 1 (MEN1) gene. *Cancer Res* **57**:1039, 1997.

328. Collins FS: Positional cloning moves from perditional to traditional. *Nature Genet* **9**:347, 1995.

329. Kas K, Weber G, Merregaert J, Michiels L. Sandelin K, Skogseid B, Thompson N, Nordenskjold M, Larsson C, Friedman E: Exclusion of FAU as the multiple endocrine neoplasia type 1 (MEN1) gene. *Hum Mol Genet* **2**:349, 1993.

330. DeWit MJ, Landsvater RM, Sinke RJ, van Kessel A, Lips CJ, Hoppener JW: Exclusion of the phosphatidylinositol-specific phospholipase C beta 3 (PLC beta 3) gene as candidate for the multiple endocrine neoplasia type 1 (MEN1) gene. *Hum Genet* **99**:133, 1997.

331. Landsvater RM, DeWit MJ, Peterson LF, Sinke RJ, van Kessel AD, Lips CJM, Hoppener JWM: Exclusion of the nuclear factor-kB3 (REL A) gene as candidate for the multiple endocrine neoplasia type 1 (MEN1) gene. *Biochem Mol Med* **60**:76, 1997.

332. Guru SC, Olufemi S-E, Manickam P, Cummings C, Gieser LM, Pike BM, Bittner ML, Jiang Y, Chinnault AC, Nowack NJ, Brzozowska A, Crabtree JS, Wang Y, Roe BA, Weisemann J, Boguski MS, Agarwal SK, Burns AL, Spiegel AM, Marx SJ, Flejter WL, de Jong PJ, Collins FS, Chandrasekharappa SC: A 2.8 Mb clone contig of the multiple endocrine neoplasia type 1 (MEN1) region at 11q13. *Genomics* **42**:436, 1997.

333. Guru SC, Agarwal SK, Manickam P, Olufemi S-E, Crabtree JS, Weisemann J, Kester MB, Kim YS, Wang Y, Emmert-Buck MR, Liotta LA, Spiegel AM, Boguski MS, Roe BA, Collins FS, Marx SJ, Burns AL, Chandrasekharappa SC: A transcript map for the 2.8 Mb region containing the multiple endocrine neoplasia type 1 (MEN1) locus. *Genome Res* **7**:725, 1997.

334. Manickam P, Guru SC, Debelenko LV, Agarwal SK, Olufemi S-E, Weisemann JM, Boguski M, Crabtree JS, Wang Y, Roe BA, Lubensky IA, Zhuang Z, Kester MB, Burns AL, Spiegel AM, Marx SJ, Liotta LA, Emmert-Buck MR, Collins FS, Chandrasekharappa SC: Eighteen new polymorphic markers in the multiple endocrine neoplasia type 1 (MEN1) region. *Hum Genet* **101**:102, 1997.

335. Sarkar G, Yoon HS, Sommer SS: Dideoxy fingerprinting (ddF): A rapid and efficient screen for the presence of mutations. *Genomics* **13**:441, 1992.

336. Agarwal SK, Kester MB, Debelenko LV, Heppner C, Emmert-Buck MR, Skarulis MC, Doppman JL, Kim YS, Lubensky IA, Zhuang Z, Green JS, Guru SC, Manickam P, Olufemi SE, Liotta LA, Chandrasekharappa SC, Collins FS, Spiegel AM, Burns AL, Marx SJ: Germline mutations of the MEN1 gene in familial multiple endocrine neoplasia type 1 and related states. *Hum Mol Genet* **7**:1177, 1997.

337. Lemmens I, Van de Ven WJM, Kas K, Zhang CX, Giraud S, Wautot V, Buisson N, De Witte K, Salandre J, Lenoir G, Pugeat M, Calender

A, Parente F, Quincey D, Gaudray P, De Wit MJ, Lips CJM, Hoppener JWM, Khodaei S, Grant AL, Weber G, Kytola S, Teh BT, Farnebo F, Phelan C, Hayward N, Larsson C, Pannett AJ, Forbes SA, Bassett JHD, Thakker RV: The European Consortium on MEN1: Identification of the multiple endocrine neoplasia type 1 (MEN1) gene. *Hum Mol Genet* **6**:1177, 1997.

338. Mayr B, Apenberg S, Rothamel T, von zur Muhlen A, Brabant G.: Menin mutations in patients with multiple endocrine neoplasia type 1. *Eur J Endocrinol* **137**:684, 1997.

339. Shimizu S, Tsukada T, Futami H, Ui K, Kameya T, Kawanaka M, Uchiyama S, Aoki A, Yasuda H, Kawano S, Ito Y, Kanbe M, Obara T, Yamaguchi K: Germline mutations of the MEN1 gene in Japanese kindred with multiple endocrine neoplasia type 1. *Jpn J Cancer Res* **88**:1029, 1997.

340. Bassett JHD, Forbes SA, Pannett AAJ, Lloyd SE, Christie PT, Wooding C, Harding B, Besser GM, Edwards CR, Monson JP, Sampson J, Wass JAH, Wheeler MH, Thakker RV: Characterization of the mutations in patients with multiple endocrine neoplasia type 1. *Am J Hum Genet* **62**:232, 1998.

340b. Roijers JFM, de Wit MJ, van der Luijt RB, van Amstel HKP, Hoppener JWM, Lips CJM: Criteria for mutation analysis in MEN 1-suspected patients: MEN1 case-finding. *Eur J Clin Invest* **30**:487, 2000.

341. Agarwal SK, Debelenko LV, Kester MB, Guru SC, Manickam P, Olufemi SE, Skarulis MC, Heppner C, Crabtree JS, Lubensky IA, Zhuang Z, Kim YS, Chandrasekharappa SC, Collins FS, Liotta LA, Spiegel AM, Burns AL, Emmert-Buck MR, Marx SJ: Analysis of recurrent germline mutations in the MEN1 gene encountered in apparently unrelated families. *Hum Mutat* **12**:75, 1998.

342. Teh BT, Kytola S, Farnebo F, Bergman L, Wong FK, Weberf G, Hayward N, Larsson C, and a Clinical Diagnosis Group: Mutation analysis of the MEN1 gene in multiple endocrine neoplasia type 1, familial acromegaly and familial isolated hyperparathyroidism. *J Clin Endocrinol Metab* **83**:2621, 1998.

342a. Takami H, Shirahama S, Ikeda Y, et al. Familial hyperparathyroidism. *Biomed & Pharmacother* **54 (Suppl 1)**:21, 2000.

342b. Kassem M, Kruse TA, Wong FK, Larsson C, Teh BT: Familial isolated hyperparathyroidism as a variant of multiple endocrine neoplasia type 1 in a large Danish pedigree. *J Clin Endocrinol Metab* **85**:165, 2000.

342c. Poncin J, Abs R, Velkeniers B, Bonduelle M, Abramawicz M, Legros JJ, et al: Mutation analysis of the *MEN1* gene in Belgian patients with multiple endocrine neoplasia type 1 and related diseases. *Hum Mut* **13**:54, 1999.

343. Farnebo F, Teh BT, Kytola S, Svensson A, Phelan C, Sandelinm K, Thompson NW, Hoog A, Weber G, Farnebo L-O, Larsson C: Alterations of the MEN1 gene in sporadic parathyroid tumors. *J Clin Endocrinol Metab* **83**:2627, 1998.

344. Carling T, Correa P, Hessman O, Hedberg J, Skogseid B, Lindberg D, Rastad J, Westin G, Akerstrom G: Parathyroid MEN1 gene mutations in relation to clinical characteristics of nonfamilial primary hyperparathyroidism. *J Clin Endocrinol Metab* **83**:2960, 1998.

345. Zhuang Z, Vortmeyer AO, Pack S, Huang S, Pham TA, Wang C, Park WS, Agarwal SK, Debelenko LV, Kester MB, Guru SC, Manickam P, Olufemi SE, Yu F, Heppner C, Skarulis MC, Venzon DJ, Emmert-Buck MR, Spiegel AM, Chandrasekharappa SC, Collins FS, Burns AL, Marx SJ, Jensen RT, Liotta LA, Lubensky IA: Somatic mutations of the MEN1 tumor suppressor gene in sporadic gastrinomas and insulinomas. *Cancer Res* **57**:4682, 1997.

346. Wang EH, Ebrahimi SA, Wu AY, Kashefi C, Passaro E Jr, Sawicki MP: Mutation of the menin gene in sporadic pancreatic endocrine tumors. *Cancer Res* **58**:4417, 1998.

347. Debelenko LV, Brambilla E, Agarwal SK, Swalwell JI, Kester MB, Lubensky IA, Zhuang Z, Guru SC, Manickam P, Olufemi S-E, Chandrasekharappa SC, Crabtree JS, Kim YS, Heppner C, Burns AL, Spiegel AM, Marx SJ, Collins FS, Travis WB, Emmert-Buck MR: Identification of MEN1 gene mutations in sporadic carcinoid tumors of the lung. *Hum Mol Genet* **6**:2285, 1997.

347b. Goebel SU, Heppner C, Burns AL, Marx SJ, Spiegel AM, Zhuang Z, et al: Genotype/phenotype correlation of *MEN1* gene mutations in sporadic gastrinomas. *J Clin Endocrinol Metab* **85**:116–123, 2000.

348. Prezant TR, Levine J, Melmed S: Molecular characterization of the MEN1 tumor suppressor gene in sporadic pituitary tumors. *J Clin Endocrinol Metab* **83**:1388, 1998.

349. Tanaka C, Kimura T, Yang P, Moritani M, Yamaoka T, Yamada S, Sano T, Yoshimoto K, Itakura M: Analysis of loss of heterozygosity

on chromosome 11 and infrequent inactivation of the MEN1 gene in sporadic pituitary adenomas. *J Clin Endocrinol Metab* **83**:2631, 1998.

349b. Imanishi Y, Palanisamy N, Tahara H, Vickery A, Cryns VL, Gaz RD, et al: Molecular pathogenetic analysis of parathyroid carcinoma. *J Bone Min Res* **14**(Suppl 1):S421 (abstract), 1999.

349c. Tahara H, Imanishi Y, Yamada T, Tsujimota Y, Taabata T, Inoue T, Inaba M, Morii H, Nishizawa Y: Rare somatic inactivation of the multiple endocrine neoplasia type 1 gene in secondary hyperparathyroidism of uremia. *J Clin Endocrinol Metab* **85**:4113, 2000.

349d. Pannett, AAJ, Thakker RV: Somatic mutations in MEN type 1 tumors, consistent with the Knudson "two-hit" hypothesis. *J Clin Endocrinol Metab* **86**:4371, 2001.

350. Herman, JG, Latif F, Weng Y, Lerman MI, Zbar B, Liu S, Samid D, Duan DS, Gnarra JR, Linehan WM: Silencing of the VHL tumor-suppressor gene by DNA methylation in renal carcinoma. *Proc Natl Acad Sci USA* **91**:9700, 1994.

351. Chakrabarti R, Srivatsan ES, Wood TF, Eubanks PJ, Ebrahimi SA, Gatti RA, Passaro E, Sawicki MP: Deletion mapping of endocrine tumors localizes a second tumor supressor gene on chromosome band 11q13. *Genes Chromosom Cancer* **22**:130, 1998.

351b. Nord B, Larsson C, Wong FK, Wallin G, Teh BT, Zedenius J: Sporadic follicular thyroid tumors of a 200-kb region in 11q13 without evidence for mutations in the *MEN1* gene. *Genes Chromosomes* **35**, 1999.

352. Boni R, Vortmeyer AO, Pack S, Park WS, Burg G, Hofbauer G, Darling T, Liotta L, Zhuang Z: Somatic mutations of the *MEN1* tumor suppressor gene detected in sporadic angiofibromas. *J Invest Derm* **111**:539, 1998.

353. Vortmeyer AO, Boni R, Pak E, Pack S, Zhuang Z: Multiple endocrine neoplasia 1 gene alterations in MEN1-associated and sporadic lipomas. *J Natl Cancer Inst* **90**:398, 1998.

354. Motokura T, Bloom T, Kim HG, Juppner H, Ruderman JV, Kronenberg HM, Arnold A: A novel cyclin encoded by a bcl-1 linked candidate oncogene. *Nature* **350**:512, 1991.

355. Hsi ED, Zukerberg LF, Yang WI, Arnold A: Cyclin D1/PRAD1 expression in parathyroid adenomas: An immunohistochemical study. *J Clin Endocrinol Metab* **81**:1736, 1996.

355b. Palanisamy N, Imanishy Y, Rao PH, Tahara H, Chaganti RSK, Arnold A: Novel chromosomal abnormalities identified by comparative genomic hybridization in parathyroid adenomas. *J Clin Endocrinol Metab* **83**:1766, 1998.

355c. Agarwal SK, Schrock E, Kester MB, Burns AL, Heffess CS, Reid T, Marx SJ: Comparative genome hybridization analysis of human parathyroid tumors. *Cancer Genet Cytogenet* **106**:30, 1998.

356. Pausova Z, Soliman E, Amizuka N, Janicic N, Konrad EM, Arnold A, Goltzman D, Hendy GN: Role of the RET proto-oncogene in sporadic hyperparathyroidism and in hyperparathyroidism of multiple endocrine neoplasia type 2. *J Clin Endocrinol Metab* **81**:2711, 1996.

357. Hosokawa Y, Pollak MR, Brown EM, Arnold A: Mutational analysis of the extracellular Ca(2+)-sensing receptor gene in human parathyroid tumors. *J Clin Endocrinol Metab* **80**:3107, 1995.

358. Thompson DB, Samowitz WS, Odelberg S, Davis RK, Szabo J, Heath H III: Genetic abnormalities in sporadic parathyroid adenomas: Loss of heterozygosity for chromosome 3q markers flanking the calcium receptor locus. *J Clin Endocrinol Metab* **80**:3377, 1995.

359. Kifor O, Moore FD Jr, Wang P, Goldstein M, Vassilev P, Kifor I, Hebert SC, Brown EM: Reduced immunostaining for the extracellular Ca^{2+}-sensing receptor in primary and uremic secondary hyperparathyroidism. *J Clin Endocrinol Metab* **81**:1598, 1996.

360. Cryns VL, Rubio MP, Thor AD, Louis DL, Arnold A: P53 abnormalities in human parathyroid carcinoma. *J Clin Endocrinol Metab* **78**:1320, 1994.

361. Cryns VL, Thor AD, Xu HJ, Hu SH, Wierman ME, Vickery AL Jr, Benedict WF, Arnold A: Loss of the retinoblastoma tumor-suppressor gene in parathyroid carcinoma. *N Engl J Med* **330**:757, 1994.

362. Dotzenrath C, Teh BT, Farnebo T, Cupisti K, Svensson A, Toell A, Goretzki P, Larsson C: Allelic loss of the retinoblastoma tumor suppressor gene: A marker for aggressive parathyroid tumors? *J Clin Endocrinol Metab* **81**:3194, 1996.

363. Pearce SH, Trump D, Woodling C, Sheppard MN, Clayton RN, Thakker RV: Loss of heterozygosity studies at the retinoblastoma and breast cancer susceptibility (BRCA2) loci in pituitary, parathyroid, pancreatic and carcinoid tumors. *Clin Endocrinol* **45**:195. 1996.

364. Guru SC, Crabtree JS, Brown KD, Dunn KJ, Manickam P, Prasad BN, Wangsa D, Burns AL, Spiegel AM, Marx SJ, Pavan WJ, Collins FS,

Chandrasekharappa SC: Isolation, genomic organization and expression analysis of *Men1*, the murine homolog of the MEN1 gene. *Mammalian Genome* **10**:592–596, 1999.

365. Guru S, Prasad NB, Shin EJ, Hemavathy K, Lu J, Ip YT, Agarwal SK, Marx SJ, Spiegel AM, Collins FS, Oliver B, Chandrasekharappa SC: Characterization of a *MEN1* ortholog from Drosophila melanogaster. *Gene* **263**:31, 2001.

366. Guru SC, Goldsmith PK, Burns AL, Marx SJ, Spiegel AM, Collins FS, Chandrasekharappa SC: Menin, the product of the MEN1 gene, is a nuclear protein. *Proc Natl Acad Sci USA* **95**:1630, 1998.

366b. Agarwal SK, Guru SC, Heppner C, Erdos MR, Collins M, Park SY, Saggar S, Chandrasekharappa SC, Collins FS, Spiegel AM, Marx SJ, Burns AL: Menin interacts with the AP1 transcrition factor JunD and represses JunD activated transcription. *Cell* **96**:143, 1999.

366c. Knapp JL, Heppner C, Hickman AB, Burns AL, Chandrasekharappa SC, Collins FS, Marx SJ, Spiegel AM, Agarwal SK: Identification and characterization of junD missense mutants that lack menin binding. *Oncogene* **19**:4706, 2000.

366d. Kim YS, Burns AL, Goldsmith PK, Heppner C, Park SY, Chandrasekharappa SC, Collins FS, Spiegel AM, Marx SJ: Stable overexpression of *MEN1* suppresses tumorigenictiy of *RAS*. *Oncogene* **18**:5936, 1999.

367. Kishi M, Tsukada T, Shimizu S, Futami H, Ito Y, Kanbe M, Obara T, Yamaguchi K: A large germline deletion of the MEN1 gene in a family with multiple endocrine neoplasia type 1. *Jpn J Cancer Res* **81**:1, 1998.

367b. Crabtree JS, Scacheri PC, Ward JM, Garrett-Beal L, Emmert-Buck MR, Edgemon KA, Lorang D, Libutti SK, Chandrasekharappa SC, Marx SJ, Spiegel AM, Collins FS: A mouse model of MEN1 develops multiple endocrine tumors. *Proc Natl Acad Sci USA* **98**:1118, 2001.

367c. Franklin DS, Godfrey VL, O'Brien DA, Deng C, Xiong Y: Functional collaboration between different cyclin-dependent kinase inhibitors suppresses tumor growth with distinct tissue specificity. *Mol Cell Biol* **20**:6147, 2000.

367d. Thepot D, Weitzman JB, Barra J, Segretain D, Stinnakre MG, Babinet C, Yaniv M: Targeted disruption of the murine junD gene results in multiple defects in male reproductive function. *Development* **127**:143, 2000.

367e. Weitzman JB, Fiette L, Matsuo K, Yaniv M: JunD protects cells from p53-dependent senescence and apoptosis. *Molec Cell* **6**:1109, 2000.

367f. Burgess JR, Nord B, David R, Greenaway TM, Parameswaran V, Larsson C, Shepherd JJ, Teh BT: Phenotype and phenocopy: the relationship between genotype and clinical phenotype in a single large family with multiple endocrine neoplasia type 1 (MEN 1). *Clin Endocrinol* **53**:205, 2000.

367g. Granberg D, Stridsberg M, Seensalu R, Eriksson B, Lundqvist G, Oberg K, Skogseid B: Plasma chromogranin A in patients with multiple endocrin neoplasia type 1. *J Clin Endocrinol Metab* **84**:2712, 1999.

367h. Brandi ML, Gagel RF, Angeli A, Bilezekian JP, Beck-Peccoz P, Bordi C, Conte-Delvox B, Falchetti A, Gheri RG, Libroia A, Lips CJM, Lombardi G, Mannelli M, Pacini F, Ponder BAJ, Raue F, Skogseid B, Tamburrano G, Thakker RV, Thompson NW, Tomassetti P, Tonelli F, Wells SA Jr, Marx SJ: Guidelines for diagnosis and therapy of multiple endocrine neoplasia type I and type 2. *J Clin Endocrinol Metab*. In press.

367i. Mutch MG, Dilley WG, Sanjurjo F, DeBenedetti MK, Doherty G, Wells SA Jr, et al: Germline mutations in the multiple endocrine neoplasia type 1 gene: Evidence for frequent splicing defects. *Hum Mutat* **13**:175, 1999.

368. American Society of Human Genetics Board of Directors and the American College of Medical Genetics Board of Directors: Points to consider: Ethical, legal, and psychosocial implications of genetic testing in children and adolescents. *Am J Hum Genet* **57**:1233, 1995.

369. Marx SJ: Familial multiple endocrine neoplasia type 1. NIH publication no 96-3048, 1997.

370. Kohlmeier L, Marcus R: Calcium disorders of pregnancy. *Endocrinol Metab Clin North Am* **1**:15, 1995.

371. Ciccarelli E, Camanni F: Diagnosis and drug therapy of prolactinoma. *Drugs* **51**:954, 1996.

Multiple Endocrine Neoplasia Type 2

B. A. J. Ponder

1. Multiple endocrine neoplasia type 2 (MEN 2) is an uncommon autosomal disorder of tumor formation and developmental abnormalities which affects about 1 in 30,000 individuals. It is characterized by the occurrence of C-cell tumors of the thyroid (medullary thyroid carcinoma), often in association with tumors of the adrenal medulla (pheochromocytoma) and parathyroid hyperplasia or adenoma. Developmental abnormalities, which occur in a minority of cases, principally affect the autonomic nerve plexuses of the intestine. The thyroid C cells, adrenal medulla, and intestinal autonomic plexuses but not the parathyroid glands are derived from neural ectoderm.

2. Distinct clinical subtypes of MEN 2 are defined by the combination of tissues affected and the presence or absence of developmental abnormalities. In MEN 2A, thyroid C cells, adrenal medulla, and parathyroids may all be involved, but developmental abnormalities are rare. In familial MTC (FMTC), only thyroid C-cell tumors are seen; there are no developmental abnormalities. In MEN 2B, thyroid C cells and adrenal medullary tumors are common, but parathyroid abnormality is uncommon; there are constant developmental abnormalities involving hyperplasia of the intestinal autonomic nerve plexuses and disorganized growth of peripheral nerve axons in the lips, oral mucosa, and conjunctiva, giving rise to a characteristic facies. The onset of thyroid and adrenal tumors in MEN 2B tends to occur early, and their behavior may be more aggressive.

3. The gene for MEN 2 was identified by positional cloning. It lies on chromosome 10q11.2. This gene, *ret*, is a previously known receptor tyrosine kinase. Mutations in *ret* in MEN 2A and FMTC result in constitutive activation of the receptor; in MEN 2B, the extent of activation is unclear, but the substrate specificity of the tyrosine kinase may be altered. There are clear correlations between specific mutations in *ret* and the phenotypes that result. Loss-of-activity mutations in *ret* result in Hirschsprung disease of the colon and rectum (HSCR), in which there is an absence of intestinal autonomic nerve plexuses, in distinction to the hyperplasia in MEN 2B. In a few families, MEN 2A and HSCR coexist, apparently as a result of the same *ret* mutation; the mechanism for this is not understood. *ret* is unusual among tumor-predisposing genes in that MEN 2 mutations result in gain of function; it is not a tumor-suppressor gene.

4. The tumors characteristic of MEN 2 also occur in a nonhereditary form. Somatic mutations of *ret* are found in these tumors, but almost all are of the same type as the germ-line mutations characteristic of MEN 2B, which alter the substrate specificity of the tyrosine kinase. This may imply that *ret* mutations of the type seen in MEN 2A and FMTC, which result in activation of a normal tyrosine kinase domain, are for the most part effective in tumorigenesis only during a restricted period in development.

5. MEN 2 is a good example of an inherited cancer syndrome in which screening of family members leads to early diagnosis and effective treatment by thyroidectomy and adrenalectomy. Since each of the tissues involved in tumor formation secretes a characteristic product (calcitonin, epinephrine, parathyroid hormone), biochemical monitoring of family members at risk provides a sensitive means of early detection. This can now be refined by predictive genetic testing for the characteristic *ret* mutations.

Multiple endocrine neoplasia (MEN) is characterized by the occurrence of tumors that involve two or more endocrine glands in a single patient or in close relatives. There are two types of MEN syndrome,[1] with distinct patterns of tissue involvement (Table 29-1). Multiple endocrine neoplasia type 1 (MEN 1), sometimes called *Wermer syndrome*,[1–3] includes tumors of parathyroid, pituitary, and pancreatic islet cells and less frequently adrenocortical, carcinoid, and multiple lipomatous tumors.[4–6] MEN 1 is dominantly inherited; the predisposing locus has been mapped by linkage to chromosome 11q13,[7] and the gene has been identified recently.[7a] There is no evidence to suggest genetic heterogeneity. Multiple endocrine neoplasia type 2 (MEN 2), sometimes called *Sipple syndrome* and previously called *MEA II* or *MEN II,* although MEN 2 is now preferred, includes tumors of the thyroid C cells and adrenal medulla and hyperplasia or adenoma of the parathyroids.[8–10] There also may be various developmental abnormalities, which are described below. The predisposing gene for MEN 2 is *ret,* a receptor tyrosine kinase that maps to chromosome 10q11.2. The great majority of MEN 2 families have detectable mutations in *ret,* but a few are unaccounted for,[11] and genetic heterogeneity remains a possibility.[12]

Patients occasionally have been described as having tumors that are a combination of those associated with MEN 1 and MEN 2, e.g., pituitary tumors and pheochromocytoma. It is unclear whether these are more than chance occurrences[13] and whether there is an additional MEN "overlap" syndrome. A spectrum of endocrine tumors that overlaps that of MEN 1 and MEN 2 is seen in some inbred strains of rats[14,15] and in transgenic mice homozygous for loss of activity of the retinoblastoma gene, which have been reported to develop thyroid C-cell and pituitary tumors. The human MEN 1 and MEN 2 syndromes are genetically and almost always clinically distinct. Familial pheochromocytomas occur in two other human inherited cancer syndromes: von

A list of standard abbreviations is located immediately preceding the index. Nonstandard abbreviations used in this chapter include: MEN 1 = multiple endocrine neoplasia type 1; MEN 2 = multiple endocrine neoplasia type 2; FMTC = familial medullary thyroid carcinoma; MTC = medullary thyroid carcinoma; HSCR = Hirschsprung disease of the colon and rectum.

Table 29-1 Endocrine Involvement in the MEN Syndromes

MEN 1	MEN 2
Parathyroid	Thyroid C cells
Anterior pituitary	Adrenal medulla
Pancreatic islets	Parathyroid
Adrenal cortex	

Hippel-Lindau (VHL) syndrome (see Chap. 27) and neurofibromatosis type 1 (see Chap. 25).

CLINICAL ASPECTS OF MEN 2

Three clinical types of MEN 2 [MEN 2A, MEN 2B, and familial medullary thyroid carcinoma (FMTC)] are distinguished by the combination of tissues involved[16-18] (Table 29-2).

The Component Tumors of MEN 2

As in the other inherited cancer syndromes, each of the component tumors of MEN 2 also has a nonhereditary counterpart.

Medullary Thyroid Carcinoma. The characteristic tumor of MEN 2 is the medullary thyroid carcinoma (MTC), which is derived from the C cells of the thyroid. These are malignant tumors, metastasizing usually at a stage when the primary tumor is 5 to 10 mm in diameter, at first locally within the neck and then to distant sites.[19,20] The C cells and the tumors derived from them secrete the hormone calcitonin. This provides a valuable marker for early diagnosis and for following the later course of disease.[21] There is no obvious syndrome of calcitonin overproduction.

Pheochromocytoma. The tumor derived from the adrenal medulla is the pheochromocytoma. Generally these tumors are nonmalignant, at least until they are of large size.[22] They commonly secrete epinephrine and norepinephrine, which, if undetected, can lead to fatal hypertensive episodes, especially in situations such as general anesthesia and childbirth.

Parathyroid. The parathyroid abnormalities in MEN 2 are benign, either hyperplasia or the formation of true benign adenomas.[23] Parathyroid involvement is often clinically silent but may present with symptomatic hypercalcemia or renal stones.

THE CLINICAL TYPES OF MEN 2 SYNDROMES

MEN 2A

Clinical Features. MEN 2A is the most common type, accounting for about 65 percent of families that could be classified in an

Table 29-2 Patterns of Tissue Involvement in the MEN 2 Syndromes

	MEN 2A	MEN 2B	FMTC
Thyroid C cells	Tumor	Tumor	Tumor
Adrenal medulla	Tumor	Tumor	Not involved
Parathyroid	Hyperplasia/ benign tumor	Not involved	Not involved
Enteric ganglia	Normal*	Hyperplasia	Normal
Other developmental abnormalities	None	Various†	None

*Usually there is no abnormality of enteric ganglia in MEN 2A, but a few families have been described in which there is absence of ganglia from a variable length of the intestine in some individuals.
†Includes musculoskeletal abnormalities and others; see text.

international survey of *ret* mutations in MEN 2 families.[11] The penetrance of *ret* mutations in MEN 2A is incomplete.[24] About 70 percent of gene carriers develop symptomatic disease within their lifetimes, with MTC as the usual first manifestation. Almost all gene carriers can, however, be detected by biochemical screening for MTC by age 40 (Fig. 29-1; see below). On average, about 50 percent of gene carriers will develop pheochromocytoma, and perhaps 5 to 10 percent will develop symptomatic parathyroid disease, but the pattern varies considerably both between and within families.[24] Some of the variation between families can be attributed to different mutant *ret* alleles (see below); the contribution of genetic background, environment, and chance to within-family variation has not been elucidated.

Incidence. The incidence of MEN 2A has not been documented accurately. An attempt to identify all new cases of MTC (hereditary and nonhereditary) in a 2-year period in the United Kingdom, using ascertainment from cancer registries and requests for calcitonin estimations from regional assay laboratories, suggested an overall incidence of about 1 per 1 million per year.[25] Wide variations in the number of registrations between different registries suggested, however, that the data may not be very accurate. It generally is assumed that 20 to 25 percent of MTCs are heritable. This figure is not based on a systematic population-based study but derives largely from two observations: In early clinical studies, about 15 percent of consecutive cases of MTC had an evident family history[19,20,26]; in later series in which families of apparently isolated cases were investigated further by more careful history taking or by genetic or biochemical screening, up to 10 percent showed familial involvement.[27,28] Together, these figures add up to about 20 to 25 new cases of MEN 2 (all types) per year in the United Kingdom (population 55 million).

New Mutations. Some apparently sporadic cases of MTC are new mutations to the hereditary disease. The frequency is not known precisely. There are a few documented cases,[29] and MEN 2 mutations occur on many different haplotypes, indicating separate origins.[30] However, many MEN 2A families have been traced back through several generations, suggesting that founder mutations are not uncommon. This contrasts with MEN 2B, where new mutations are more usual.[31]

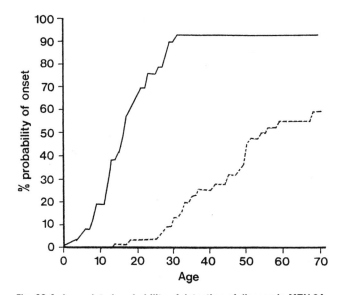

Fig. 29-1 Age-related probability of detection of disease in MEN 2A. Shown is the probability that an individual with the gene for MEN 2A will have presented to medical attention (dotted line) or be detectable by a pentagastrin stimulation test (solid line) by a given age. (*Reproduced with permission from Easton et al: Am J Hum Genet 44:208, 1989. Published by University of Chicago Press.*)

Clinical Variants. No developmental abnormalities are known to be consistently associated with MEN 2A. There are, however, two clinical variants. A small number of families have been described in which several individuals have an itchy skin lesion in the interscapular area with histologic features of lichen amyloidosis.[32,33] A dermatomal distribution in one family[33] suggested a neurologic basis for the lesion, but this remains unsubstantiated. Several families have been described in which there is cosegregation of MEN 2A (or FMTC) and Hirschsprung disease of the colon and rectum (HSCR), with individuals having both phenotypes.[34–37] This is a surprising and intriguing observation, because the *ret* mutations in MEN 2 are thought to result in activation of the gene, whereas those typical of HSCR are associated with loss of activity. It is almost certainly significant that each of the MEN 2/HSCR families described to date has one of two specific *ret* mutations (see below).

Familial MTC

Clinical Features and Definition. The term *familial MTC* denotes families in which MTC is the only abnormality. The original evidence for a separate category of site-specific MTC came from two large kindreds in the United States in which there were multiple cases of MTC but no evidence, either clinically or on biochemical screening, of adrenal or parathyroid involvement.[18] A particular feature of these families was the late onset and low mortality of the tumors. There were no developmental abnormalities. The categorization of FMTC as a distinct variety of MEN 2 was justifiable in these extensive kindreds and subsequently has received support from mutational analysis of the *ret* gene that indicates that the spectrum of mutations in families designated as having FMTC is indeed different from (although overlapping) that described in MEN 2A.[11] Nevertheless, the inconstant occurrence of adrenal or parathyroid involvement in MEN 2A families clearly leads to a difficulty in the classification of small families in which MTC is the only feature: Is the family truly FMTC or a MEN 2A family in which by chance the adrenal or parathyroid components have not yet manifested? As more data are collected, it may be possible to classify families with respect to risks of different tumors on the basis of the *ret* mutation that is present (see below). For the present, however, an arbitrary definition has been generally adopted: To qualify as FMTC, a family should have at least four individuals with proven MTC and no clinical or biochemical evidence of an adrenal or parathyroid abnormality either in the affected members or in available first-degree relatives.[38] Families that fail to meet these criteria either because there are fewer affected cases or because clinical or biochemical data are not available are assigned to an "MEN 2—other" or "undefined" category. Clinical impressions as well as the results of *ret* mutation analysis indicate that FMTC is less common than MEN 2A.

MEN 2B

Clinical Features. MEN 2B is probably the least common variety of MEN 2 but is the most clearly distinct. MTC and pheochromocytoma are common, as in MEN 2A, but tend to present at a younger age (18 and 24 years for MTC and pheochromocytoma in MEN 2B compared with 38 years for MTC in MEN 2A (EuroMEN collaboration, unpublished data).[39] Parathyroid involvement in MEN 2B is rare or absent.[22] The main distinguishing features of MEN 2B are the consistent developmental abnormalities.[17,40–46] A characteristic facies (Fig. 29-2) with thick blubbery lips, nodules on the anterior tongue and the conjunctivae, and thickening of the corneal nerves visible on ophthalmologic examination results from disorganized growth of axons, leading to thickening and irregularity of peripheral nerves.[40,41] (Note, however, that the corneal nerve thickening may be difficult to score.[42]) Hyperplasia of the intrinsic autonomic ganglia in the wall of the intestine leads to disordered gut motility,[43] which commonly presents in infancy or childhood as failure to thrive or alternating episodes of constipation and diarrhea. These abnormalities can be

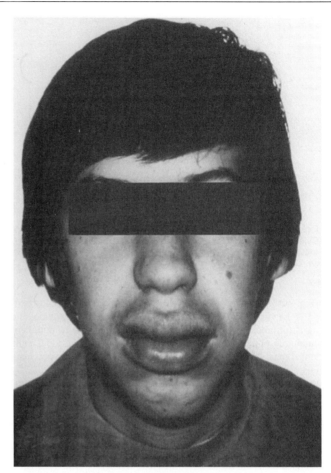

Fig. 29-2 Typical facies of MEN 2B showing the prominent "blubbery" lips caused by neuroma tissue.

recognized on rectal biopsy. A generalized hypotonia ("floppy baby") has been described in newborn infants.[44] There may be a variety of skeletal abnormalities, including pes cavus, slipped femoral epiphyses, pectus excavatum, and bifid ribs,[45] and a general abnormality of body shape with features resembling those of Marfan syndrome but without the aortic, palatal, or lens abnormalities. Delayed puberty has been noted in a few girls with MEN 2B; the mechanism is unclear. Impotence in men is neurologic in origin.

New Mutations. The earlier onset of tumors and the developmental abnormalities presumably confer a reproductive disadvantage. As a result, perhaps one-half of all MEN 2B cases result from new mutations.[31] As in retinoblastoma and neurofibromatosis type 1, new mutations occur predominantly on the chromosome from the male parent.[46] It has been suggested that the sex of the transmitting parent also may affect the probability that the disease will manifest in a male or a female child, with an excess of affected female children among the offspring of transmitting males.[46] An interesting commentary on these findings was written by Sapienza.[47]

Differences Between Hereditary and Nonhereditary Tumors: Multifocal Hyperplasia

The histologic appearances of the fully developed MTC, pheochromocytoma, or parathyroid adenomas of MEN 2 patients are indistinguishable from those of nonhereditary cases. However, just as familial cancers at any site are commonly multiple and associated with multiple preneoplastic changes in the target tissue, in the MEN 2 syndromes there are multiple foci of hyperplasia in the target tissues before the development of overt tumors[48,49]

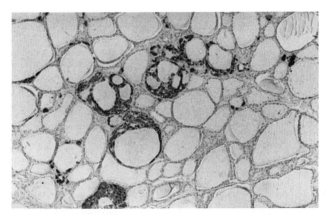

Fig. 29-3 C-cell hyperplasia in MEN 2A thyroid. Prominent groups of C cells are demonstrated by immunochemistry for calcitonin among the thyroid follicles which are unstained. (*Photograph courtesy of Dr. G. Thomas.*)

(Fig. 29-3). This may provide a histologic basis for recognition of an isolated case as being of the hereditary type and provides the basis for biochemical screening to detect the increased amounts of calcitonin or catecholamines produced by the hyperplastic C cells and adrenal medulla.[21] The biochemical test for C-cell hyperplasia (see "Biochemical Screening" below) is made more sensitive by the use of a stimulus (usually intravenous pentagastrin or calcium) that causes the C cells to release stored calcitonin into the circulation. Measurement of calcitonin levels before and after the stimulus provides an indication of C-cell mass. The test is sufficiently sensitive to detect C-cell hyperplasia before the stage of progression to invasive tumor, and surgery based on presymptomatic calcitonin screening is likely to be curative.[21]

Other Causes of C-Cell Hyperplasia. It is important to note that although it is a useful indication of hereditary disease, C-cell hyperplasia may not be completely specific for MEN 2. Increased C-cell numbers (although possibly in a different histologic pattern) have been described in autopsy samples from the general population,[50–52] and there are several well-documented instances in which members of MEN 2 families have had thyroidectomy on the basis of increased calcitonin levels on screening and the thyroid histology has been reported as C-cell hyperplasia but subsequent genetic testing has shown them not to have inherited the familial MEN 2 mutation.[53,54] There may be genetic or nongenetic influences on C-cell mass independent of the MEN 2 mutation that complicate the assessment of C-cell hyperplasia.

Diagnostic Criteria for MEN 2

Failure to Recognize Hereditary Disease. A recent survey for the Royal College of Physicians in the United Kingdom[25] showed that the diagnosis of MEN 2 often is missed. The possibility of hereditary disease in an apparently isolated case of MTC is discounted or not pursued with sufficient vigor.

Part of the problem may stem from terminology. An isolated case of MTC is often referred to as *sporadic*. *Sporadic* in turn is often incorrectly used to signify *nonhereditary,* and so clinicians may come to regard any isolated case as nonhereditary. In fact, of course, a sporadic case may be hereditary, lacking a family history because the phenotype was not manifest in immediate relatives (MEN 2 is incompletely penetrant; see Fig. 29-1), because the history has been poorly taken, or because the case is a new mutation (particularly common in MEN 2B, and in such cases, the diagnosis should be signaled by the associated phenotype) (see Fig. 29-2).

Evaluation of an Apparently Sporadic Case. Guidelines for estimating the probability that an apparently isolated patient presenting with MTC at a given age is in fact hereditary are given by Ponder et al.[55] An apparently sporadic case of MTC, pheochromocytoma, or parathyroid disease should be evaluated carefully for the possibility of MEN 2 first by taking a detailed family history (with special attention to possible indications of the MEN 2 syndrome — goiter, possible hypertensive sudden death, renal stones) and second by evaluation of the surgical specimen for evidence of multifocal hyperplasia.

GENETIC LOCI

Genetic Loci Involved in Germ-Line Mutations in MEN 2

The great majority of MEN 2 families show linkage to chromosome 10q11.2 and have demonstrable mutations in *ret*[11] (Table 29-3). Most published reports suggest that around 10 to 15 percent of FMTC families and families with fewer than four cases of MTC (in the "MEN 2 — other" category) have not been found to have *ret* mutations,[11] even though in some of these families the known coding region of *ret* has been examined carefully. Probably some mutations are missed, even on careful analysis. Evidence in support of this comes from the report of a German group who describe a previously undetected "hot spot" for mutations in codons 790 and 791 of *ret* (exon 13) in families with FMTC and a single family with MEN 2A. This group claims to be able to detect *ret* mutation in 100 percent of their MEN 2 families.[55a] A further possibility, not completely excluded, is that another locus also predisposes primarily to MTC, possibly with low penetrance.[12] There have been occasional reports of "MTC-only" families in which there is evidence against linkage on chromosome 10q, but the linkage results have relied on C-cell hyperplasia as the MEN 2 phenotype. Because C-cell hyperplasia can be a difficult phenotype to define,[50–54] it is uncertain how these results should be interpreted.

Genetic Loci Involved in Somatic Mutations

Loss of heterozygosity (LOH) studies show a low level of chromosomal instability in MTC and pheochromocytomas. Mulligan et al.,[56] in a systematic search, identified six chromosomal regions that showed a frequency of LOH of 10 percent or more in a combined series of MTC and pheochromocytoma: 1p, 3p, 3q, 11p, 13, and 22. There were no clear differences between sporadic and familial tumors. Losses are rarely seen at the *ret* locus on chromosome 10q. Chromosome 1p is the most frequently involved in both MTC and pheochromocytoma.[56,57] In almost all cases, the entire chromosome arm is lost. This is not associated with isochromosome 1q formation.[56] A localized region of loss at 1p32 was reported[57] but appears not to be a consistent finding in

Table 29-3 Percentages of MEN 2 Families with Different Phenotypes in Which *ret* Mutations Have Been Detected

Phenotype	No. of Families	Mutation +ve(%)	Mutation −ve (%)
MEN 2A			
MTC, pheochromocytoma, PTH	94	91 (97)	3 (3)
MTC, pheochromocytoma, no PTH	96	95 (99)	1 (1)
MTC, PTH, no pheochromocytoma	13	13 (100)	0 (0)
MEN 2B	79	75 (95)	4 (5)
FMTC*	34	30 (88)	4 (12)
Other MTC*	161	136 (85)	25 (15)
Total	477	440 (92)	37 (8)

*See text.

SOURCE: Data from the International Mutation Consortium.[11]

other studies. No mutations have been identified in candidate genes lying within the regions of LOH.

SPECIFIC GENES

ret is the only gene known to be involved in the inherited predisposition to MEN 2 and the only gene known to cause a predisposition to MTC. Germ-line mutations in other genes may predispose to pheochromocytoma in VHL syndrome (see Chap. 27) neurofibromatosis type 1 (see Chap. 7). It has not been clear whether there is an additional syndrome of site-specific pheochromocytoma or whether these families fall within VHL. However, germline mutations in the mitochondrial complex II subunit SDHB have recently been reported in familial and sporadic phaeochromocytoma and in familial paraganglioma.[57a,57b] Germline mutations in the Menin gene in MEN 1 predispose to parathyroid tumors.[4-6]

Mutations of *ret* in MEN 2

Identification of *ret* as a Proto-Oncogene. The *ret* proto-oncogene is a cell-surface glycoprotein that is a member of the receptor tyrosine kinase (RTK) family.[58] The name *ret* is an acronym for "*re*arranged during *t*ransfection," reflecting the original identification of *ret* as a chimeric oncogene formed by rearrangement during transfection assays using DNA from human lymphomas and gastric tumors.[59] Three different rearranged versions of *ret* have since been described *in vivo*, specifically in papillary thyroid carcinomas (which arise from thyroid follicular epithelial cells and are therefore distinct from the C-cell-derived MTC).[60-62] These rearranged versions are termed *ret PTC-1, -2,* and -3. In each case, the effect of the rearrangement, which occurs as a somatic event, is to fuse the tyrosine kinase region of *ret* with different activating sequences that are expressed in thyroid epithelial cells. The fused activating genes contribute a new N-terminal portion to the ret protein that is capable of dimerization, leading to activation of the tyrosine kinase domain independent of any ligand. Mutations of the *ret-PTC* type are not seen in MEN 2-related tumors.

Identification of *ret* in MEN 2. *ret* lies in the region of the MEN 2 locus defined by linkage analysis and was therefore a candidate gene.[63,64] At that time, *ret* was known as a proto-oncogene, whereas all the tumor-predisposing genes identified to that point acted as suppressor genes. The plausibility of *ret* as a candidate was, however, strengthened by the first reports that the *ret* knockout mouse had a phenotype that resembled HSCR[65] and the known association of MEN 2 and HSCR in some families. Mutation analysis of *ret* in MEN 2 families revealed mutations in the extracellular domain of the gene in MEN 2A and FMTC[66-68] and subsequently in the tyrosine kinase domain in MEN 2B.[69-71]

ret Structure. The coding sequence consists of 21 exons in a genomic sequence of approximately 55 kb.[72,73] The protein exists in three main 39 alternatively spliced forms of 1072 to 1114 amino acids.[74] There is a cleavable signal sequence of 28 amino acids; an extracellular domain, which is glycosylated and has a conserved[75,76] cysteine-rich region close to the cell membrane and a region of cadherin homology further out[77]; a transmembrane domain; and a tyrosine kinase domain with a short interkinase region of 27 amino acids (Fig. 29-4). Further details of the structure are given in references 72–74 and 78–80.

Ligands for the _ret_ Receptor. Four ligands have so far been identified: glial cell line-derived neurotrophic factor (GDNF),[81] neurturin,[81a] persephin[81b] and artemin.[81i] These are structurally related secreted proteins that are widely expressed in the nervous system and in other tissues and promote the survival of neurons during development.[81c,81d] Each signals through a multicomponent receptor consisting of *ret* and one of the GFRα family of glycosylphosphatidylinositol (GP1)-linked proteins.[81e,81f,81g,81h,81i,84,85] GFRα1 is the preferred ligand-binding protein for GDNF; GFRα2, for neurturin; and GFRα4, for persephin.[81e,81f,81h] Mouse knockouts of the *GDNF* gene have a phenotype similar to that of *ret* knockouts.[82,83] The distinct and overlapping roles of the different *ret*-ligand combinations in development are currently under study.

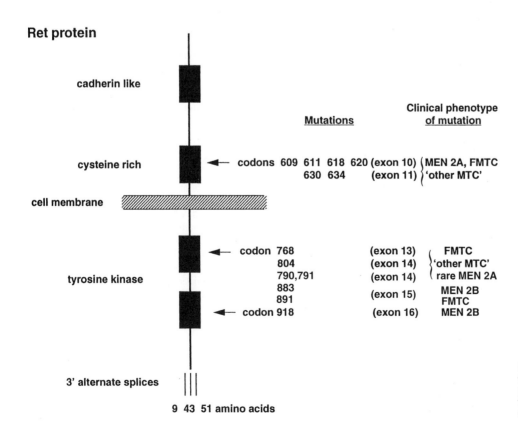

Ret protein

Fig. 29-4 The main features of the protein encoded by the *ret* proto-oncogene and the sites of the mutations in the different clinical varieties of MEN 2.

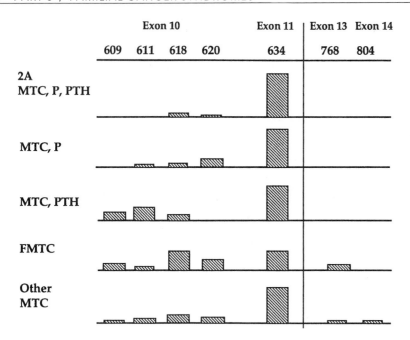

Fig. 29-5 Proportion of mutations in different codons of *ret* in different phenotypic subtypes of MEN 2A, FMTC, and other MTC families. Based on data from the International *ret* Mutation Consortium summarized in Table 29-3.

Germ-Line *ret* Mutations in MEN 2. A summary of the mutations is given in Table 29-3 and Fig. 29-4. With the exception of rare in-frame insertions in the cysteine-rich domain,[85a] all MEN 2 germ-line mutations so far identified are point mutations that lead to amino acid substitution.

Mutations in MEN 2A and FMTC. The majority of mutations in MEN 2A and FMTC lie in one of five cysteine codons in the cysteine-rich region of the extracellular domain[11,38] and result in substitution of the cysteine by another amino acid. A few mutations in families with MTC have been found in exons 13, 14, and 15 of the intracellular domain,[86,87] and a single MEN 2A family has been reported with mutation in codon 790 (exon 13)[55a] (see Figs. 29-4 and 29-5). Figure 29-5 shows clearly that there is a correlation between the codon involved in the mutation and the MEN 2 phenotype.[11] In families with MEN 2A with both pheochromocytoma and parathyroid involvement, almost all the mutations are in codon 634; in MEN 2A families lacking pheochromocytoma and in FMTC, codons 609, 611, 618, and 620 are more frequently involved. This correlation is highly significant; 160 of 186 families with at least one proven case of pheochromocytoma have mutations in codon 634, compared with 18 of 43 families with no evidence of pheochromocytoma ($p <$ 0.0001).[11,11a] There also may be an effect not only of the position of the cysteine codon but of the particular amino acid substitution involved. Mutations at codon 634 seen in MEN 2 include all the possible amino acid substitutions allowed by the coding sequence. The most common changes are cysteine to arginine (C634R; TGC → CGC) and cysteine to tyrosine (C634Y; TGC → TAC), which may reflect the known frequency of T → C and G → A changes rather than the particular biologic significance of these substitutions. Nevertheless, it is intriguing that while C634R was present in 88 of 169 MEN 2A families with a codon 634 mutation, none of 9 FMTC families with a codon 634 mutation had this change.[11] Furthermore, Mulligan et al.[38] found a highly significant association between the C634R mutation, compared with all other 634 mutations, and the presence in the family of parathyroid disease. This, however, has not so far been replicated in an independent study.[11a] Four families (three meeting the criteria for FMTC and one "other") have been identified with a glu → asp mutation in codon 768 (exon 13),[86,87] and two families with MTC have been placed in the "other" category with a leu → val mutation in codon 804 (exon 14).[86] Mutations in codons 790 and 791 have been reported in several small families with MTC and one with MEN 2A.[55a] Thus mutations in this region of the intracellular domain seem mostly to be specifically associated with MTC rather than with pheochromocytoma or parathyroid disease, although the MEN 2A family with codon 790 mutation indicates that this correlation may not be absolute.

Mutations in MEN 2B. Some 95 percent of MEN 2B families reported to date have an identical mutation: methionine → threonine in codon 918 of exon 16.[11,69–71,88] Each of four families lacking this mutation had typical and well-documented phenotypic features.[89] In four families without M918T mutation, a mutation of A883F recently has been reported.[89a,89b] One case has been reported of MEN 2B phenotype in a patient with a mutation in codon 804 and a further base substitution in codon 806.[89c]

Mutations in Families with MEN 2 and HSCR. Each of the 17 or so families reported has a mutation in either cys 609, cys 618, or cys 620.[33,37,90,90a,90b,90c] No other mutation has been found after careful examination of the remainder of the gene in these families, and so the conclusion must be that the same mutation can result in apparently contrasting phenotypes in the same individual. Families with HSCR alone with no evidence of MEN 2 also have been reported to have missense mutations in cysteine codons 609 and 620.[35,36]

Expression of *ret* in Development. Three of the tissues principally involved in MEN 2 — thyroid C cells, adrenal medulla, and intestinal autonomic ganglia — are derived from neural ectoderm.[91] The parathyroids are derived from the endoderm of the third and fourth pharyngeal pouches. The lineage relationships between C cells and other cells of neuroectodermal origin are still unclear, but the origin of C cells from vagal neural crest and the biochemical similarities with enteric neurons[92] suggest that they share a common precursor with enteric neurons and ultimately with the sympathoadrenal progenitor that is the precursor of chromaffin cells and sympathetic neurons.[93]

In situ hybridization studies during mouse and rat development show that *ret* is expressed in the neural crest-derived cells that migrate from the region of the hindbrain into the posterior pharyngeal arches and from there to form the thyroid C cells and the vagal neural crest that gives rise to the intestinal autonomic nerves.[94,95] *ret* is also expressed in migrating cells derived from the trunk neural crest as they coalesce alongside the aorta to form the sympathetic ganglia and the chromaffin cells that will form the adrenal medulla and in the endoderm of the pharyngeal pouches that give rise to the parathyroids.[94,96] The expression of *ret* is therefore consistent with a role in the development and differentiation of the tissues that are involved in MEN 2. It is perhaps surprising that *ret* homozygous knockout mice appear at birth to have absent intestinal autonomic ganglia but normal C cells and adrenal medulla.[65] The mice die at this stage, probably of respiratory or kidney failure resulting from other developmental defects, and so the possible role of *ret* expression in postnatal development cannot be assessed. However, the tentative conclusion must be that while disordered *ret* expression can lead to tumor formation, normal *ret* expression is not necessary for C-cell or adrenal medullary development up to the time of birth. A caveat is that while the C cells and adrenal medulla may appear grossly normal, the development of the cells may have been perturbed in some way that is not readily apparent. There is a further possibility, with some evidence to support it, that the C-cell population is heterogeneous, with only some C cells expressing *ret*.[95,97] It may be, therefore, that the C cells that are seen in the knockout mice are only one component of the population, with the other component being absent.

In the later stages of embryogenesis in the mouse and in rodent and human thyroid and adrenal medullas after birth, there appears to be only weak and patchy expression of *ret* by the criteria of *in situ* hybridization and immunohistochemistry.[95,97] In most MTCs and pheochromocytomas, by contrast, *ret* is expressed at high levels.[98,99] At present, nothing is known about the role of *ret* in C-cell or adrenal medullary development or in the adult glands. The mechanism and significance of the apparent increase in the expression in tumors are uncertain but may in part have a trivial explanation in terms of stabilization of the *ret* mRNA or protein as a result of the mutation.[100]

Function of *ret* at the Cellular Level. *ret* is a receptor tyrosine kinase (RTK). Binding of ligand results in dimerization of the receptor, activation of the tyrosine kinase, and initiation of onward signaling pathways.[101] Evidence is slowly accumulating,[102–106,106a,106b] but there is no coherent picture of the signaling events that follow *ret* activation. Analysis is complicated by the three 39 alternative splice forms of *ret,* which might be predicted from the sequence context of their tyrosines to differ in the affinity with which they bind different signaling molecules and may therefore signal through different pathways, and by the likelihood (supported by some evidence[106]) that the pathways of signaling are specific for different cell types, which implies that studies should be done in cells that resemble as closely as possible those involved in MEN 2.

Consequences of *ret* Mutations. Transfection experiments[101,104] have shown that both the MEN 2A (cys 634 arg) and the MEN 2B (met 918 thr) mutations lead to activation of *ret* tyrosine kinase. The evidence is of two types: (1) biologic, in which transfection of mutant but not wild-type *ret* induces transformation of NIH 3T3 cells and differentiation of rat PC12 (pheochromocytoma) cells, and (2) biochemical, in which the *ret* protein becomes phosphorylated on tyrosine and acquires tyrosine kinase activity against added substrates.

Extracellular Domain Cysteine Mutations. The cysteine mutations activate *ret* by inducing covalent dimerization[101,104,107,108] (Fig. 29-6). The genotype-phenotype correlation observed with different cysteine mutations is probably explained by quantitative differences in signaling. The different cysteine mutants have been shown to differ both in their efficiency of dimerization and in their maturation to the fully glycosylated form, which is necessary for insertion into the plasma membrane. Either or both of these differences may be responsible for differences in the level of *ret* activation.[108a,108b]

The Met 918 Thr MEN 2B Mutation. This mutation has proved to be of great interest because one effect of the mutation is to convert the substrate specificity of the *ret* tyrosine kinase from that typical of a receptor tyrosine kinase (RTK) to that typical of a

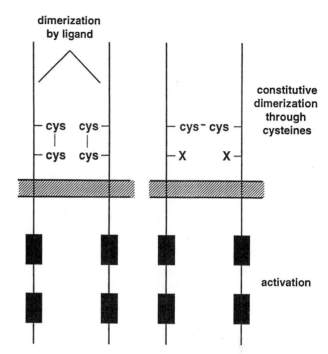

Fig. 29-6 Constitutive activation of *ret* as a result of mutation of a cysteine in the extracellular domain.

cytoplasmic tyrosine kinase. It also confers some activity on the receptor, independent of dimerization (see below).

Residue 918 is predicted from modeling studies to lie at the base of a pocket in the protein that is involved in substrate binding.[58,69] The substitution of threonine for methionine is predicted to alter the dimensions of the pocket and thus the substrate specificity. Tyrosine kinases fall into two classes: RTKs and cytoplasmic tyrosine kinases. Almost all RTKs have methionine at the equivalent position to codon 918, whereas almost all cytoplasmic tyrosine kinases have threonine (Fig. 29-7).[58] Songyang et al.[109] used degenerate peptide libraries to demonstrate that whereas RTKs prefer hydrophobic amino acids at positions 11 and 13 downstream of the target tyrosine in their substrate, cytoplasmic tyrosine kinases prefer a hydrophilic residue at 11 and a hydrophobic residue at 13. These different amino acid contexts flanking the tyrosine provide different preferred substrates for different groups of SH2 domains on signaling molecules and hence the possibility of different pathways of downstream signaling.

When wild-type (equivalent to MEN 2A) and MEN 2B *ret* tyrosine kinases were compared for their ability to phosphorylate model substrates, a clear shift toward the specificity characteristic of a cytoplasmic tyrosine kinase was seen with the MEN 2B mutation.[109] The inference that the MEN 2B mutation has altered the pathway of downstream signaling is supported by the observation that activated MEN 2B *ret* differs from activated wild-type *ret* both in the pattern of tyrosine phosphorylation of the *ret* protein itself[110] and in the patterns of tyrosine phosphorylations seen in cell extracts.[104]

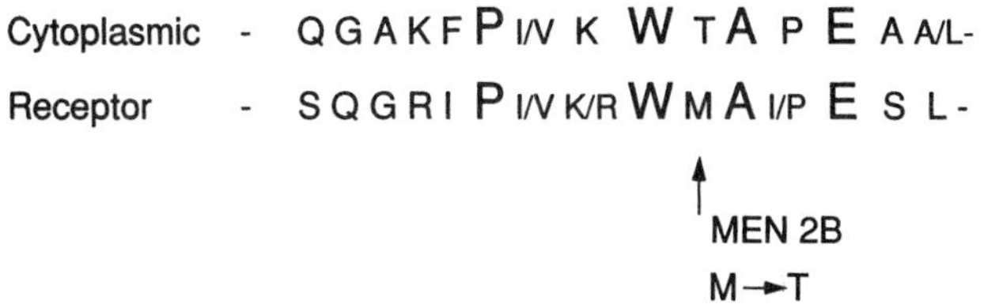

Cytoplasmic - Q G A K F P I/V K W T A P E A A/L-

Receptor - S Q G R I P I/V K/R W M A I/P E S L -

↑
MEN 2B

M → T

Fig. 29-7 Amino acid sequence of consensus receptor and cytoplasmic tyrosine kinases in the substrate binding region of Hanks domain VIII, showing the mutation characteristic of MEN 2B.

The MEN 2B mutation does not lead to covalent dimerization of *ret*.[104] However, there is *in vitro* evidence that it does lead to activation of the receptor through an intramolecular mechanism.[101,104,105] Activation by this mechanism may be further enhanced by ligand binding, and the combined result may be a higher activity than is conferred by the cysteine MEN 2A mutations. It is unclear whether this increased activity, or the altered substrate specificity, is responsible for the characteristic features of the MEN 2B phenotype.

The 768 and 804 Mutations. The glu 768 asp mutation[86,87] involves a residue that is highly conserved in different receptor tyrosine kinases (RTKs). Modeling suggests a possible effect both on ATP binding and on substrate specificity, each of which is being tested experimentally. The val 804 leu mutation[86] also affects a conserved residue, but no modeling studies have been reported.

Genes Involved in Somatic Mutations

The genetic events in the progression of MEN 2 tumors and in the initiation and progression of the related nonhereditary tumors are largely unknown. Baylin et al.[111] showed that the tumors are clonal. Several candidate oncogenes have been screened for mutations or altered expression (N-*ras*, Ha-*ras*, N-*myc*, c-*myc*, 1-*myc*, c-*mos*, β nerve growth factor, and the low-affinity nerve growth factor receptor).[112,113] Apart from one report of overexpression of N-*myc* in 6 of 21 MTCs analyzed by *in situ* hybridization,[114] all the studies were negative.

The role of mutations of *ret* in sporadic tumors is of some interest. In the inherited cancer syndromes, nonhereditary tumors often have mutations in the same gene that shows germ-line mutations in hereditary cases. In MEN 2 this is partly true, with an interesting twist. Among 157 apparently sporadic MTCs in the literature, 39 percent are reported to have a somatic mutation in *ret* codon 918 (the MEN 2B mutation), but mutations of the cysteine codons characteristic of MEN 2A and FMTC are uncommon, probably on the order of 1 to 3 percent.[28,67,115,115a,115b] Somatic mutations in the intracellular domain are seen a little more frequently, e.g., codon 768 in 4 of 72 sporadic MTCs[87,87a,116] and codons 790 and 791 in 11 tumors[55] and codon 883 in exon 15 in 4 of 111 MTCs[116,117] (Eng et al., unpublished data). In pheochromocytomas, the picture is slightly different. Six of 112 (5 percent) sporadic pheochromocytomas had a mutation in the *ret* codon 918,[118,119] 2 of 112 had proven somatic mutations of codon 634,[119,120] and a further 3 tumors have been reported with novel somatic mutations affecting the 39 splice acceptor site of exon 9, codons 632 through 633, and codon 925.[118,121] None of 32 non-MEN 2–associated parathyroid lesions was found to have *ret* mutations.[122] No *ret* mutations have been found in sporadic or hereditary neuroblastoma.[122a]

Detailed study of codon 918 mutations in sporadic MTCs by PCR analysis of microdissected portions of primary tumors and metastases has shown that the tumors are most often mosaic for the mutation; i.e., there are mutant and nonmutant clones, implying that the 918 mutation is not the initiating event in formation of sporadic MTC.[123] One tumor was found to have different areas with codon 918 and codon 883 mutations. Mosaicism for codon 918 mutation also was found in two of three MEN 2A tumors studied, in which a germ-line codon 634 also was present.

Synthesis: Speculation on How *ret* Mutations Result in Tumor Formation

Carlson et al.[124] showed that induction of raf-1 signaling in TT cells (an MTC cell line bearing a codon 634 mutation)[125] results in both differentiation and silencing of *ret* expression. Possibly, during development, C cells move from a ''predetermined'' to a terminally differentiated state in which *ret* expression is reduced and the potential for proliferation is lost.[124] Inappropriate continued activation of *ret* by a cysteine mutation may override the differentiation program, allowing continued proliferation and

the hyperplasias seen in MEN 2. In this scheme, the effects of mutations in the different cysteine codons may depend on the degree of activation that resulted. The combined HSCR/MEN 2 phenotype occasionally seen with mutations of cys 609, cys 618, and cys 620 may (speculatively) be a result of these mutations causing inappropriate activation of *ret* sufficient to result in tumor formation but insufficient to sustain the development of enteric neurons. If these mutations also impaired ligand binding, any reinforcement of *ret* activation by that means would be reduced. The lack of developmental abnormalities in MEN 2A and FMTC compared with MEN 2B may be the case because although the timing of *ret* signaling is inappropriate, the pathways of signaling are normal and the degree of activation of *ret* signaling is probably less. Similarly, the preponderance of MEN 2B-type somatic mutations in tumors could occur because once they are past a certain stage of differentiation and development, thyroid C cells and adrenal medullary cells are no longer susceptible to transformation by increased *ret* activity alone but are susceptible to the altered pathways of signaling induced by the MEN 2B mutation, or because MEN 2B mutations are associated with a higher level of activation. The lack of parathyroid involvement in MEN 2B may be the case either because the MEN 2B-specific signaling pathways are not present in parathyroid cells or because the MEN 2B mutations, unlike MEN 2A, still retain partial dependence on ligand binding for activity and the ligand may not be present in parathyroid tissue. Evidence is not currently available to distinguish any of these alternatives but may become available through studies of transgenic models in which the design of both mutant *ret* and ligand can be modulated.

Implications for Diagnosis

Biochemical Screening. Regular screening by biochemical testing and imaging, followed by surgery where necessary, has been shown to be effective in preventing mortality and morbidity in MEN 2 families.[21,126–128]

In families with MEN 2A or FMTC, it is generally recommended that screening be started at about 4 to 5 years of age, continued annually until about age 20, and then possibly (this is controversial) continued at rather wider intervals until age 35. Screening should consist of measurement of plasma calcitonin after stimulation with intravenous pentagastrin, calcium, or both combined[21,127,128]; blood pressure measurement; urinary or plasma catecholamines; possibly imaging of the adrenals; and serum calcium levels. Thyroid surgery should consist of total thyroidectomy and central node dissection with conservation of normal parathyroid *in situ* or autotransplantation to the forearm.[129] It is controversial whether after the detection of a unilateral adrenal abnormality one or both adrenals should be removed.[130] The risks of serious problems from pheochromocytoma developing subsequently in the remaining adrenal must be balanced against the inconvenience and possible dangers of life after adrenalectomy and hormone replacement. Current opinion generally favors bilateral adrenalectomy. There is no consensus about screening for MEN 2B. Because of the sometimes early development and aggressive nature of the thyroid tumor, screening for MTC in a *ret* mutation-positive child of a known MEN 2B patient probably should start by age 1 year.[131,132] Normal calcitonin levels may be high in infants, and screening results may be difficult to interpret. In this situation, some clinicians have advocated thyroidectomy on the basis of the MEN 2B phenotype alone. Greater certainty can now be provided by DNA testing for the MEN 2B mutation.

Although generally effective, biochemical screening has several problems. The stimulated calcitonin tests are somewhat unpleasant, and compliance is not always good. Occasional false-positive results have been obtained, and results on successive tests that fluctuate at and just above the normal level are common and a frequent cause of anxiety to physicians and family members. Finally, there is the problem of whether to initiate a program of screening for the families of apparently sporadic cases of one of the MEN 2 component tumors. Although many physicians are reluctant to burden a family with these tests, not following such a screening program will inevitably lead to missing some opportunities for early diagnosis.

DNA Testing. The number of distinct *ret* mutations that occur in MEN 2 is small. One of these mutations can be detected in over 90 percent of patients. DNA testing is therefore relatively simple and is now in routine clinical use.[53]

In a family known to have MEN 2 in which the causative mutation can be identified, DNA testing of unaffected family members at risk will eliminate those who do not have the mutation from the need for biochemical screening and simplify the decision to have surgery in those whose screening results are equivocal. Increasingly, opinion is moving toward a recommendation for thyroidectomy in childhood on the basis of DNA testing alone, without waiting for biochemical testing to show abnormalities indicative of C-cell hyperplasia. This may seem surprising given that the chances of presentation with symptomatic disease in MEN 2A are only on the order of 50 percent by age 50[24] and that a good biochemical screen for early disease is available. It probably reflects a mixture of concern about continued compliance with the biochemical screening and the possibility that equivocation over borderline results may lead to surgery being carried out too late; there is also the view that thyroidectomy even in young children has low morbidity and that the best thing for the child and family is to deal with the problem and put it behind them. Because of the lower probability of adrenal disease and the much greater morbidity of adrenalectomy, prophylactic removal of the adrenals is not advised except when there is evidence of abnormality.

The genotype-phenotype correlations outlined above[11] may provide some indication of the probability of adrenal or parathyroid involvement, but at present the data are too few and the overlaps too great to recommend that mutation data be used to exclude families from adrenal or parathyroid screening.

DNA Testing in an Apparently Sporadic Case. DNA testing plays an important role in determining which apparently sporadic cases have heritable disease. All apparently sporadic cases of MTC should be offered DNA testing. If the patient is dead, normal or tumor tissues from pathology specimens may be tested. The limited range of mutations makes this technically feasible in most cases, and since MEN 2A-type mutations are uncommon as somatic events, they can be interpreted as probably germ line in origin even if they are found in tumor (the same does not, of course, apply to MEN 2B mutations). If there is no family history on careful review and no evidence of C-cell hyperplasia on the thyroidectomy specimen, the probability of hereditary disease will vary according to the age at diagnosis of the index case but is almost certainly well below 10 percent.[27,55] In this case, failure to find a mutation in exons 10, 11, 13, 14, and 16 of *ret* excludes MEN 2A with 99 percent probability[11] and, if there is no abnormal phenotype, MEN 2B as well. The residual probability of FMTC or "MTC only" familial disease is a little higher, since up to 10 percent of such families have no detectable *ret* mutation, but it is still probably below 2 percent. It remains a matter of clinical judgment, according to the circumstances and perceptions of each family, whether to pursue biochemical screening of family members at these levels of risk. On the one hand, one does not wish to lose any possibility of early diagnosis and treatment of a potentially lethal and unpleasant cancer (but possibly the FMTC, which is most likely to be missed, could be treated satisfactorily at clinical presentation); on the other hand, one does not want to run the risk of unnecessarily "medicalizing" a family over a period of many years.

Direct mutation testing of unselected cases of apparently sporadic pheochromocytomas suggests that roughly 5 percent may carry a *ret* mutation and that another 5 percent will have a VHL mutation.[119] A few may have mutations in the mitochondrial complex II subunit SDHB, also associated with familial

paraganglioma[57b,119a] (see Chap. 27). Mutation screening of apparently sporadic cases of pheochromocytoma for MEN 2A and VHL mutations is probably worthwhile. The incidence of occult MEN 2 among apparently sporadic cases of parathyroid hyperplasia and adenoma appears to be low,[122] and unless there are other suggestive features, DNA screening probably is not justified. Children presenting with Hirschsprung disease should be tested for *ret* mutation and, if a mutation is found in exons 10 or 11, for thyroid C-cell tumor.

ACKNOWLEDGMENTS

B. A. J. Ponder is a Gibb Fellow of The Cancer Research Campaign [CRC].

REFERENCES

1. Thakker RV, Ponder BAJ: Multiple endocrine neoplasia. *Clin Endocrinol Metab* **2**:1031, 1988.
2. Thakker RV: Multiple endocrine neoplasia type 1, in Grossman A (ed): *Clinical Endocrinology*. Oxford, Blackwell, 1992, p 597.
3. Wermer P: Multiple endocrine adenomatosis: Multiple hormone producing tumours: A familial syndrome. *Clin Gastroenterol* **3**:671, 1974.
4. Marx SJ, Vinik AI, Santen RJ, Floyd JC, Mills JL, Green J: Multiple endocrine neoplasia type 1: Assessment of laboratory tests to screen for the gene in a large kindred. *Medicine* **65**:226, 1986.
5. Vasen HFA, Lamers CBHW, Lips CJM: Screening for multiple endocrine neoplasia syndrome type 1: A study of 11 kindreds in the Netherlands. *Arch Intern Med* **149**:2717, 1989.
6. Trump D, Farren B, Wooding C, Pang JT, Besser GM, Buchanan KD, Edwards CR, et al: Clinical studies of multiple endocrine neoplasia type 1 (MEN 1). *Q J Med* **89**:653, 1996.
7. Larsson C, Skogseld B, Oberg K. Nakamura Y, Nordenskjold M: Multiple endocrine neoplasia type 1 gene maps to chromosome 11 and is lost in insulinoma. *Nature* **332**:85, 1988.
7a. Chandrasekharappa SC, et al: Positional cloning of the gene for multiple endocrine neoplasia type 1. *Science* **276**:404, 1997.
8. Smith DP, Ponder BAJ: The MEN 2 syndromes and the role of the *ret* protooncogene. *Adv Cancer Res* **70**:199, 1996.
9. Schimke RN: Genetic aspects of multiple endocrine neoplasia. *Annu Rev Med* **35**:25, 1984.
10. Cancer WG, Wells SA: Multiple endocrine neoplasia type 2A. *Curr Probl Surg* **22**:7, 1985.
11. Eng C, Clayton D, Schuffenecker I, et al: The relationship between specific *ret* protooncogene mutations and disease phenotype in multiple endocrine neoplasia type 2: International RET Mutation Consortium. *JAMA* **276**:1575, 1996.
11a. Schuffenecker I, Virally Monod M, Brohet R, Goldgar D, Conte Devolx C, Leclerc L, Chabre O, et al: Risk and penetrance of primary hyperparathyroidism in multiple endocrine neoplasia type 2A families with mutations at codon 634 of the *ret* protooncogene. *J Clin Endocrinol Metab* **83**:487, 1998.
12. Nelkin BD, De Bustros AC, Mabrey M, Baylin SB: The molecular biology of medullary thyroid carcinoma. *JAMA* **261**:3130, 1989.
13. Schimke RN: Multiple endocrine neoplasia: How many syndromes? *Am J Med Genet* **37**:375, 1990.
14. DeLellis RA, Nunnemacher G, Bitman WR, Gagel RF, Tashjian AH, Blount M, Wolfe HJ: C-cell hyperplasia and medullary thyroid carcinoma in the rat. *Lab Invest* **40**:140, 1979.
15. Sass B, Rabstein LS, Madison R, Nims AM, Peters RL, Kelloff GJ: Evidence of spontaneous neoplasms in F344 rats throughout the natural life-span. *J Natl Cancer Inst* **54**:1449, 1975.
16. Schimke KN, Hartmann WH, Prout TE, Rimoin DL: Syndrome of bilateral pheochromocytoma, medullary thyroid carcinoma and multiple neuromas. *N Engl J Med* **279**:1, 1968.
17. Khairi MRA, Dexter RN, Burzynoki NJ, Johnson CC Jr: Mucosal neuroma, pheochromocytoma and medullary thyroid carcinoma: Multiple endocrine neoplasia type 3. *Medicine* **54**:89, 1975.
18. Farndon JR, Leight GS, Dilley WG, Baylin SB, Smallridge RC, Harrison TC, Wells SA Jr: Familial medullary thyroid carcinoma without associated endocrinopathies: A distinct clinical entity. *Br J Surg* **73**:278, 1986.
19. Chong GC, Beaths OH, Sizemore GW, Woolmer LH: Medullary carcinoma of the thyroid gland. *Cancer* **35**:695, 1975.

20. Saad MF, Ordonez NG, Rashid RK, Guido JJ, Hill CS Jr, Hickey RC, Samaan NA: Medullary carcinoma of the thyroid: A study of the clinical features and prognostic factors in 161 patients. *Medicine* **63**:319, 1984.

21. Gagel RF, Tashjian AH, Cummings T, Papathanasopoulos N, Kaplan MM, Delellis RA, Wolfe HJ, et al: The clinical outcome of prospective screening for multiple endocrine neoplasia type 2A. *N Engl J Med* **318**:478, 1988.

22. Dralle H, Schurmeyer TH, Kotzerke TH, Kemnitz J, Crosse H, von zur Muhlen A: Surgical aspects of familial phaeochromocytoma. *Hormone Metab Res Suppl Series* **21**:34, 1989.

23. Van Heerden JA, Kent RB, Sizeman GW, Grant CS, ReMine WH: Primary hyperparathyroidism in patients with multiple endocrine neoplasia syndromes. *Arch Surg* **118**:533, 1983.

24. Easton DF, Ponder MA, Cummings T, Gagel RF, Hansen HH, Reichlin S, Tashjian AH Jr, et al: The clinical and age-at-onset distribution for the MEN 2 syndrome. *Am J Hum Genet* **44**:208, 1989.

25. Harris R, Williamson P: Confidential enquiry into counselling for genetic disorders. *J R Coll Phys Lond* **30**:316, 1991.

26. Sizemore GW, Carney JA, Hunter H II: Epidemiology of medullary carcinoma of the thyroid gland: A 5-year experience (1971–1976). *Surg Clin North Am* **57**:633, 1977.

27. Ponder BAJ, Finer M, Coffey R, Harmer CL, Maisey M, Ormerod MG, Pembrey ME, et al: Family screening in medullary thyroid carcinoma presenting without a family history. *Q J Med* **252**:299, 1986.

28. Eng C, Mulligan LM, Smith DP, Healey CS, Frilling A, Raue F, Neumann HPH, et al: Mutation of the *RET* pro-oncogene in sporadic medullary thyroid carcinoma. *Genes Chromosom Cancer* **12**:209, 1995.

29. Mulligan LM, Eng C, Healey CS, Ponder MA, Feldman CL, Li P, Jackson CE, et al: A *de novo* mutation of the *RET* proto-oncogene in a patient with MEN 2A. *Hum Mol Genet* **3**:1007, 1994.

30. Narod SA, Lavone MF, Morgan K, Calmettes C, Solbol H, Goodfellow PJ, Lenoir GM: Genetic analysis of 24 French families with multiple endocrine neoplasia type 2A. *Am J Hum Genet* **51**:469, 1992.

31. Norum RA, Lafreniere RC, O'Neal LW, Nikolai TF, Delaney JP, Sisson JC, Sobol H: Linkage of the multiple endocrine neoplasia type 2B gene (MEN 2B) to chromosome 10 markers linked to MEN 2A. *Genomics* **8**:313, 1990.

32. Gagel RF, Levy ML, Donovan DT, Alford BR, Wheeler T, Tschen JA: Multiple endocrine neoplasia type 2A associated with cutaneous lichen amyloidosis. *Ann Intern Med* **111**:802, 1989.

33. Chabre O, Labat F, Berthod F, Jarel V, Bachelot Y: Cutaneous lesions associated with multiple endocrine neoplasia type 2A: Lichen amyloidosis or notalgia paresthetica? *Henry Ford Hosp Med J* **40**:245, 1992.

34. Verdy M, Weber AM, Roy CC, Morin CL, Cadotte M, Brochu P: Hirschsprung's disease in a family with multiple endocrine neoplasia type 2. *J Paediatr Gastroenterol Nutr* **1**:603, 1982.

35. Mulligan LM, Eng C, Attie T, Lyonnet S, Marsh DJ, Hyland VJ, Robinson BG, et al: Diverse phenotypes associated with exon 10 mutations of the *RET* proto-oncogene. *Hum Mol Genet* **3**:2163, 1994.

36. Angrist M, Bolk S, Thiel B, Puffenberger EG, Hofstra RM, Buys CHCM, Cass DT, et al: Mutation analysis of the *RET* receptor tyrosine kinase in Hirschsprung's disease. *Hum Mol Genet* **4**:821, 1995.

37. Borst MJ, van Camp JM, Peacock ML, Decker RA: Mutation analysis of multiple endocrine neoplasia type 2A associated with Hirschsprung disease. *Surgery* **117**:386, 1995.

38. Mulligan LM, Eng C, Healey CS, Clayton D, Kwok JBJ, Gardner E, Ponder MA, et al: Specific mutations of the *RET* proto-oncogene are related to disease phenotype in MEN 2A and FMTC. *Nature Genet* **6**:70, 1994.

39. Vasen HFA, Kruseman ACN, Berkel H: Multiple endocrine neoplasia syndrome type 2: the value of screening and central registration: A study of 15 kindreds in the Netherlands. *Am J Med* **83**:487, 1987.

40. Dyck PJ, Carney JA, Sizemore GW: Multiple endocrine neoplasia type 2B: Phenotype recognition. *Ann Neurol* **6**:302, 1979.

41. Khalil MK, Lorenzetti DWC: Eye manifestations in medullary carcinoma of the thyroid. *Br J Ophthalmol* **64**:789, 1980.

42. Kinoshita S, Tanaki F, Ohasi Y, Ikeda M, Takai S: Incidence of prominent corneal nerves in multiple endocrine neoplasia type 2A. *Am J Ophthalmol* **111**:307, 1991.

43. Carney JA, Go VLW, Sizemore GW, Hayles AB: Alimentary-tract ganglioneuromatosis: A major component of the syndrome of multiple endocrine neoplasia, type 2B. *N Engl J Med* **295**:1287, 1976.

44. Fryns JP, Chrzanowska K: Mucosal neuromata syndrome [MEN type IIb (III)]. *J Med Genet* **25**:703, 1988.

45. Carney JA, Bianco AJ, Sizeman GW, Hayles AB: Multiple endocrine neoplasia with skeletal manifestations. *J Bone Joint Surg* **63A**:405, 1981.

46. Carlson KM, Bracamontes J, Jackson CE, Clark R, Lacroix A, Wells SA Jr, Goodfellow PJ: Parent of origin effects in multiple endocrine neoplasia type 2B. *Am J Hum Genet* **55**:1076, 1994.

47. Sapienza C: Parental origin effects, genomic imprinting and sex-ratio distortion: Double or nothing? *Am J Hum Genet* **55**:1073, 1994.

48. Wolfe HJ, Melvin KEW, Cervi-Skinner SJ: C cell hyperplasia preceding medullary thyroid carcinoma. *New Engl J Med* **289**:437, 1973.

49. Block MA, Jackson CE, Greenawald KA, Yott JB, Tashjian AH: Clinical characteristics distinguishing hereditary from medullary thyroid carcinoma. *Arch Surg* **115**:142, 1980.

50. O'Toole K, Genoglio-Prieser C, Pushparag N: Endocrine changes associated with the aging process: III. Effect of age on the number of calcitonin immunoreactive cells in the thyroid gland. *Hum Pathol* **16**:991, 1985.

51. Gibson WGH, Peng TC, Croker BP: C cell nodules in adult human thyroid: A common autopsy finding. *Am J Clin Pathol* **75**:347, 1981.

52. Gibson WGH, Peng TC, Croker BP: Age-associated C-cell hyperplasia in the human thyroid. *Am J Pathol* **106**:388, 1982.

53. Lips CJM, Landsvater RM, Hoppener JWM, Geerdink RA, Blijham G, Jansen-Schillhorn van Veen JM, van Gils APG, et al: Clinical screening as compared with DNA analysis in families with multiple endocrine neoplasia type 2A. *N Engl J Med* **331**:828, 1994.

54. Wolfe HJ, Kaplan M, Cummings T, Ponder BAJ, Ponder M, Gardner G, Papi L, et al: Re-evaluation of histologic ceriteria for C cell hyperplasia in MEN 2A using genetic recombinant markers. *Henry Ford Hosp J Med* **40**:312, 1992.

55. Ponder BAJ, Ponder MA, Coffey R, Pembrey ME, Gagel RP, Telenius-Berg M, Semple P, et al: Risk estimation and screening in families of patients with medullary thyroid carcinoma. *Lancet* **1**:397, 1988.

55a. Berndt I, Reuter M, Saller B, Frank-Raue K, Groth P, Grussendorf M, Raue F, et al: A new hot spot for mutations in the *ret* protooncogene causing familial medullary thyroid carcinoma and multiple endocrine neoplasia. *J Clin Endocrinol Metab* **83**:770, 1998.

56. Mulligan LM, Gardner E, Smith BA, Mathew CGP, Ponder BAJ: Genetic events in tumor initiation and progression in multiple endocrine neoplasia. *Genes Chrom Cancer* **6**:166, 1993.

57. Moley JF, Brother MB, Fong CT, White PS, Baylin SB, Nelkin B, Wells SA, et al: Consistent association of 1p loss of heterozygosity with phaeochromocytomas from patients with multiple endocrine neoplasia type 2 syndromes. *Cancer Res* **52**:770, 1992.

57a. Astuti D, Douglas F, Lennard TWJ, Agaliaganis I, Woodward ER, Evans DGR, Eng C, et al: Germline SDHD mutation in familial phaeochromocytoma. *Lancet* **357**:1181, 2001.

57b. Astuti D, Latif F, Dallol A, Dahia PLM, Douglas F, George E, Skoldberg F, et al: Mutations in the mitochondrial complex II subunit gene SDHD cause susceptibility to familial paraganglioma and phaeochromocytoma. *Am J Hum Genet* (in press).

58. Hanks SK, Quinn AM, Hunter T: The protein kinase family: Conserved features and deduced phylogeny of the catalytic domain. *Science* **241**:42, 1988.

59. Takahashi M, Cooper GM: *RET* fusion protein encodes a fusion protein homologous to tyrosine kinases. *Mol Cell Biol* **7**:1378, 1987.

60. Grieco M, Santoro M, Berlingieri MT, Melillo RM, Donghi R, Bonzagzone I, Pierotti MA, et al: PTC is a novel rearranged form of the *RET* proto-oncogene and is frequently expressed in vivo in human papillary thyroid carcinomas. *Cell* **60**:557, 1990.

61. Bongarzone I, Monzini N, Borrello MG, Carcano C, Ferraresi G, Arighi E, Mondellini P, et al: Molecular characterisation of a thyroid fusion-sapecific transforming sequence formed by the fusion of *ret* tyrosine kinase and the regulatory subunit R1 of cyclic AMP-dependent protein kinase A. *Mol Cell Biol* **13**:358, 1993.

62. Santoro M, Dathan NA, Berlingieri MT, Bongarzone I, Paulin C, Grieco M, Pierotti MA, Vecchio G, Fusco A: Molecular characterisation of RET/PTC3, a novel rearranged version of the *RET* protooncogene in a human papillary thyroid carcinoma. *Oncogene* **9**:509, 1994.

63. Gardner E, Mullian LM, Eng C, Healey CS, Kwok JAJ, Ponder MA, Ponder BAJ: Haplotype analysis of MEN 2 mutations. *Hum Mol Genet* **3**:1771, 1994.

64. Mole SE, Mulligan LM, Healey CS, Ponder BAJ, Tunnacliffe A: Localisation of the gene for multiple endocrine neoplasia type 2A to a

480 kb region in chromosome band 10q11.2. *Hum Mol Genet* **2**:247, 1993.

65. Schuchardt A, D'Agati V, Larrson-Blomberg L, Constantini F, Pachnis V: The c-*ret* receptor tyrosine kinase gene is required for the development of the kidney and the enteric nervous systrem. *Nature* **367**:380, 1994.

66. Mulligan LM, Kwok JBJ, Healey CS, Elsdon M, Eng C, Gardner E, Love DR, et al: Germ-line mutations of the *RET* proto-oncogene in multiple endocrine neoplasia type 2A. *Nature* **363**:458, 1993.

67. Donis-Keller H, Dou S, Chi D, Carlson KM, Toshima K, Lairmore TC, Howe JR, et al: Mutations in the *RET* proto-oncogene are associated with MEN 2A and FMTC. *Hum Mol Genet* **2**:851, 1993.

68. Schuffenecker I, Billaud M, Calender A, Chambe B, Ginet N, Calmettes C, Modigliani E, et al: *RET* proto-oncogene mutations in French MEN 2A and FMTC families. *Hum Mol Genet* **3**:1939, 1994.

69. Carlson KM, Dou S, Chi D, Scavarda N, Toshima K, Jackson CE, Wells SA, et al: Single missense mutation in the tyrosine kinase catalytic domain of the *RET* protoncogene is associated with multiple endocrine neoplasia type 2B. *Proc Natl Acad Sci USA* **91**:1579, 1994.

70. Eng C, Smith DP, Mulligan LM, Nagai MA, Healey CS, Ponder MA, Gardner E, et al: Point mutation within the tyrosine kinase domain of the *RET* proto-oncogene in multiple endocrine neoplasia type 2B and related sporadic tumours. *Hum Mol Genet* **3**:237, 1994.

71. Hofstra RMW, Landsvater RM, Ceccherini I, Stulp RP, Stelwagen T, Luo Y, Pasini B, et al: A mutation in the *RET* proto-oncogene associated with multiple endocrine neoplasia type 2B and sporadic medullary thyroid carcinoma. *Nature* **367**:375, 1994.

72. Ceccherini I, Hofstra RMW, Luo Y, Stulp RP, Barone V, Stelwagen T, Bocciardi R, et al: DNA polymorphisms and conditions for SSCP analysis of the 20 exons of the *ret* proto-oncogene. *Oncogene* **9**:3025, 1994.

73. Kwok JBJ, Gardner E, Warner JP, Ponder BAJ, Mulligan LM: Structural analysis of the human *ret* proto-oncogene using exon trapping. *Oncogene* **8**:2575, 1993.

74. Myers SM, Eng C, Ponder BAJ, Mulligan LM: Characterisation of *ret* protooncogene 39 splicing variants and polyadenylation sites: A novel C terminus for *ret*. *Oncogene* **11**:2039, 1995.

75. Iwamoto I, Taniguchi M, Asai N, Ohkusu K, Nakashima I, Takahashi M: cDNA cloning of mouse *ret* proto-oncogene and its sequence similarity to the cadherin superfamily. *Oncogene* **8**:1087, 1993.

76. Sugaya R, Ishimaru S, Hosoya T, Saigo K, Emori Y: A *Drosophila* homology of human protooncogene *ret* transiently expressed in embryonic neuronal precursor cells including neuroblast and CNS cells. *Mech Dev* **45**:139, 1994.

77. Schneider R: The human protooncogene *ret*: A communicative cadherin? *Trends Biochem Sci* **17**:468, 1992.

78. Lorenzo MJ, Eng C, Mulligan LM, Stonehouse TJ, Healey CS, Ponder BAJ, Smith DP: Multiple mRNA isoforms of the human ret protooncogene generated by alternate splicing. *Oncogene* **10**:1377, 1995.

79. Takahashi M, Buma Y, Iwamoto T, Iwaguma Y, Ikeda H, Hiai H: Cloning and expression of the *ret* protooncogene encoding a tyrosine kinase with two potential transmembrane domains. *Oncogene* **3**:571, 1988.

80. Asai N, Iwashita T, Matsumama M, Takahashi M: Mechanism of activation of the *ret* protooncogene by multiple endocrine neoplasia type 2A mutations. *Mol Cell Biol* **15**:1613, 1995.

81. Liu LF-H, Doherty DH, Uke JD, Behtash S, Collins F: GDNF: A glial cell line-derived neurotrophic factor for mid-brain dopaminergic neurons. *Science* **260**:1130, 1993.

81a. Kotzbauer PT, Lampe PA, Heuckeroth RO, Golden JP, Creedon DJ, Johnson EMJ, et al: Neurturin, a relative of glial-cell-line-derived neurotrophic factor. *Nature* **384**:467, 1996.

81b. Milbrandt J, de Sauvage FJ, Fahrner TJ, Baloh RH, Leitner ML, Tansey MG: Persephin, a novel neurotrophic factor related to GDNF and neurturin. *Neuron* **20**:245, 1998.

81c. Buj-Bello A, Buchman VL, Horton A, Rosenthal A, Davies AM: GDNF is an age-specific survival factor for sensory and autonomic neurons. *Neuron* **15**:821, 1995.

81d. Trupp M, Ryden M, Jornvall H, Funakoshi H, Timmusk T, Arenas E, Ibanez CF: Peripheral expression and biological activities of GDNF, a new neurotrophic factor for avian and mammalian peripheral neurons. *J Cell Biol* **130**:137, 1995.

81e. Klein RD, Sherman D, Ho WH, Stone D, Bennett GL, Moffat B, Vandlen R, et al: A GPI-linked protein that interacts with *Ret* to form a candidate neurturin receptor. *Nature* **387**:717, 1997.

81f. Buj-Bello A, Adu J, Pinon LGP, Horton A, Thompson J, Rosenthal A, Chinchetru M, et al: Neurturin responsiveness requires a GPI-linked receptor plus the *Ret* receptor tyrosine kinase. *Nature* **387**:721, 1997.

81g. Trupp M, Raynoschek C, Belluardo N, Ibanez CF: Multiple GPI-anchored receptors control GDNF-dependent and independent activation of the c-*ret* receptor tyrosine kinase. *Mol Cell Neurosci* **11**:47, 1998.

81h. Enokido Y, de Sauvage F, Hongo J-A, Ninkina N, Rosenthal A, Buchman VL, Davies AM: GFRa-4 and the tyrosine kinase *Ret* form a functional receptor complex for persephin. *Curr Biol* **8**:1019, 1998.

81i. Baloh RH, Tansey MG, Lampe PA, Fahrner TJ, Enomoto H, Simburger KS, Leitner ML, et al: Artemin: a novel member of the GDNF ligand family. Supports peripheral and central neurons and signals through the GFR alpha-3-RET receptor complex. *Neuron* **21**:1291, 1998.

82. Sanchez MP, Silos-Santiago I, Frisen J, He B, Lira SA, Barbacid M: Renal agenesis and the absence of enteric neurons in mice lacking GDNF. *Nature* **382**:70, 1996.

83. Pichel JG, Shen L, Sheng HZ, Granholm A-C, Drago J, Grinberg A, Lee EJ, et al: Defects in enteric innervation and kidney development in mice lacking GDNF. *Nature* **382**:73, 1996.

84. Treanor JS, Goodman L, de Sauvage F, Stone DM, Poulsen KT, Beck CD, Gray C, et al: Characterisation of a multicomponent receptor for GDNF. *Nature* **382**:80, 1996.

85. Jing S, Wen D, Yu Y, Holst PL, Luo Y, Fang M, Tamir R, et al: GDNF-induced activation of the *ret* protein tyrosine kinase is mediated by GDNF-α, a novel receptor for GDNF. *Cell* **85**:1113, 1996.

85a. Hoppner W, Ritter MM: A duplication of 12bp in the critical cysteine rich domain of the *ret* protooncogene results in a distinct phenotype of multiple endocrine neoplasia type 2A. *Hum Mol Genet* **6**:587, 1997.

86. Bolino A, Schuffenecker I, Luo Y, Seri M, Silengo M, Tocco T, Chabrier G, et al: RET mutations in exons 13 and 14 of FMTC patients. *Oncogene* **10**:2415, 1995.

87. Eng C, Smith DP, Mulligan LM, Healey CS, Zvelebil MJ, Stonehouse TJ, Ponder MA, et al: A novel point mutation in the tyrosine kinase domain of the *RET* proto-oncogene in sporadic medullary thyroid carcinoma and in a family with FMTC. *Oncogene* **10**:509, 1995.

87a. Eng C, Mulligan LM, Smith DP, Healey CS, Frilling A, Raue F, Neumann HPH, et al: Low frequency of germline mutations in the *ret* protooncogene in patients with apparently sporadic medullary thyroid carcinoma. *Clin Endocrinol* **43**:123, 1995.

88. Rossel M, Schuffenecker I, Schlumberger M, Bonnardel C, Modigliani E, Gardet P, Navarro J, et al: Detection of a germ line mutation at codon-918 of the *ret* protooncogene in French MEN 2B families. *Hum Genet* **95**:403, 1995.

89. Toogood AA, Eng C, Smith DP, Ponder BAJ, Shalet SM: No mutation at codon 918 of the *ret* gene in a family with multiple endocrine neoplasia type 2B. *Clin Endocrinol* **43**:759, 1995.

89a. Smith DP, Houghton C, Ponder BAJ: Germline mutation of RET codon 883 in two cases of de novo MEN 2B. *Oncogene* **15**:1213, 1997.

89b. Gimm O, Marsh DJ, Andrew SD, Frilling A, Dahia PLM, Mulligan LM, Zajac JD, et al: Germline dinucleotide mutation in codon 883 of the *RET* protooncogene in multiple endocrine neoplasia type 2B without codon 918 mutation. *J Clin Endocrinol Metab* **82**:3902, 1997.

89c. Miyauchi A, Futami H, Hai N, Yokozawa T, Kuma K, Aoki N, Kosugi S, et al: Two germline missense mutations at codons 804 and 806 of the *RET* proto-oncogene in the same allele in a patient with multiple endocrine neoplasia type 2B without codon 918 mutation. *Jpn J Cancer Res* **90**:1, 1999.

90. Landsvater RM, Jansen RPM, Hofstra RMW, Buys CHCM, Lips CJM, Ploos van Amstel HK: Mutation analysis of the *ret* protooncogene in Dutch families with MEN 2 and FMTC. *Hum Genet* **97**:11, 1996.

90a. Decker RA, Peacock ML, Watson P: Hirschsprung disease in MEN 2A: Increased spectrum of *RET* exon genotypes and strong genotype-phenotype correlation. *Hum Mol Genet* **7**:129, 1998.

90b. Peretz H, Luboshitsky R, Baron E, Biton A, Gershoni R, Usher S, Grynberg E, et al: Cys 618 Arg mutation in the *RET* protooncogene associated with familial medullary thyroid carcinoma and maternally transmitted Hirschsprung disease suggesting a role for imprinting. *Hum Mutat* **10**:155, 1997.

90c. Romeo G, Ceccherini I, Celli J, Priolo M, Betsos N, Bonardi G, Seri M, Yin L, et al: Association of multiple endocrine neoplasia type 2A and Hirschsprung disease. *J Intern Med* **243**:515, 1998.

91. Le Douarin N: *The Neural Crest.* Cambridge, UK, Cambridge University Press, 1982.

92. Tamir H, Liu K-P, Playette RF, Hsuing S-C, Adlersberg M, Nurez EA, Gershon MD: *J Neurosci* **9**:1199, 1989.

93. Anderson DJ: Molecular control of cell fate in the neural crest: The sympathoadrenal lineage. *Annu Rev Neurosci* **16**:129, 1993.

94. Pachnis V, Maukoo B, Constantini F: Expression of the *c-ret* proto-oncogene during mouse embryogenesis. *Development* **119**:1005, 1993.

95. Tsuzuki T, Takahashi M, Asai N, Iwashita T, Matsuyene M, Asai J: Spatial and temporal expressio of the *ret* proto-oncogene product in embryonic, infant and adult rat tissues. *Oncogene* **10**:191, 1995.

96. Van der Geer P, Wiley S, Lai VK-M, Olivier JP, Gish GD, Stephens R, Kaplan D, et al: A conserved amino terminal shc domain binds to glycophosphotyrosine motifs in activated receptors and phosphopeptides. *Curr Biol* **5**:404, 1995.

97. Durbec PL, Larsson-Blomberg WB, Schuchardt A, Constantini P, Pachnis V: Common origin and developmental dependence on *c-ret* of subsets of enteric and sympathetic neuroblasts. *Development* **122**:349, 1996.

98. Fabien N, Paulin C, Santoro M, Berger B, Grieco M: The *ret* protooncogene is expressed in normal human parafollicular thyroid cells. *Int J Oncol* **4**:623, 1994.

99. Santoro M, Rosati R, Grieco M, Berlinger M, D'Amato GLC, de Franciscis V, Fusco A: The *ret* proto-oncogene is consistently expressed in human pheochromocytoma and thyroid medullary carcinomas. *Oncogene* **5**:1595, 1990.

100. Miya A, Yamamoto M, Morimoto H, Tanaka N, Shin E, Karakawa K, Toyoshima K, et al: Expression of the *ret* proto-oncogene in human medullary thyroid carcinomas and pheochromocytomas of MEN 2A. *Henry Ford Hosp Med J* **40**:215, 1992.

101. Pawson T, Schlessinger J: SH2 and SH3 domains. *Curr Biol* **3**:434, 1993.

102. Borrello MG, Pelicci G, Arighi E, De Filippis L, Greco A, Bongarzone I, Rizzetti MG, et al: The oncogenic versions of the *Ret* and *Trk* tyrosine kinases bind Shc and Grb2 adaptor proteins. *Oncogene* **9**:1661, 1994.

103. Santoro M, Wong WT, Aroca P, Santos E, Matoskova B, Grieco M, Fusco A, Di Fiore PP: An epidermal growth factor receptor/ret chimera generates mitogenic and transforming signals: Evidence for a *ret*-specific signalling pathway. *Mol Cell Biol* **14**:663, 1994.

104. Pandey A, Duan H, Di Fiore PP, Dixit VM: The *ret* receptor protein tyrosine kinase associates with the SH2-containing adapter protein Grb10. *J Biol Chem* **270**:21461, 1995.

105. Santoro M, Carlomagno F, Romanova A, Bottaro DP, Dathan NA, Grieco M, Fusco A, et al: Activation of *RET* as a dominant transforming gene by germ line mutations of MEN 2A and MEN 2B. *Science* **267**:381, 1995.

106. Iwashita T, Asai N, Murakami H, Matsuyama M, Takahashi M: Identification of tyrosine residues that are essential for transforming activity of the *ret* proto-oncogene with MEN 2A or MEN 2B mutation. *Oncogene* **12**:481, 1996.

106a. Xing S, Furminger TL, Tong Q, Jhiang SM: Signal transduction pathways activated by *ret* oncoproteins in phaeochromocytoma cells. *J Biol Chem* **273**:4909, 1997.

106b. Durick K, Gill GN, Taylor S: Shc and Enigma are both required for mitogenic signalling by *ret/ptc2. Mol Cell Biol* **18**:2298,1998.

107. Van Weering DHJ, Medema JP, van Puijenbroek A, Burgering BMT, Baas PD, Bos JL: Ret receptor tyrosine kinase activates extracellular signal regulated kinase Z in SK-N-Mc cells. *Oncogene* **11**:2207, 1995.

108. Wada M, Asai N, Tsuzuki T, Maruyama S, Ohiwa M, Imai T, Funahashi H, et al: Detection of *ret* homodimers in MEN 2A associated phaeochromocytomas. *Biochem Biophys Res Commun* **218**:606, 1996.

108a. Carlomagno F, Salvatore G, Cirafici AM, DeVita G, Mellillo RM, de Franciscus V, Billaud M, et al: The different *ret* activating capability of mutations of cysteine 620 or cysteine 634 correlates with multiple endocrine neoplasia type 2 phenotype. *Cancer Res* **57**:391, 1997.

108b. Ito S, Iwashita T, Asai N, Mutakami H, Iwata Y, Sobue G, Takahashi M: Biological properties of *ret* with cysteine mutations correlate with multiple endocrine neoplasia type 2A, familial medullary thyroid carcinoma and Hirschsprungs disease phenotype. *Cancer Res* **57**:2870, 1997.

109. Songyang Z, Carraway KL III, Eck MJ, Harrison SC, Feldman RA, Mohammadi M, Schlessinger J, et al: Catalytic specificity of protein-

110. Liu X, Vega QC, Decker RA, Plandey A, Worby CA, Dixon JE: Oncogenic *RET* receptors display different autophosphorylation sites and substrate binding specificities. *J Biol Chem* **271**:5309, 1996.

111. Baylin SB, Gann DS, Hsu SH: Clonal origin of inherited medullary thyroid carcinoma and phaeochromocytoma. *Science* **193**:321, 1976.

112. Moley JF, Brother MB, Wells SA, Spengler BA, Bredler JL, Brodeur GM: Low frequency of ras gene mutations in neuroblastomas, phaeochromocytomas and medullary thyroid cancers. *Cancer Res* **51**:1596, 1991.

113. Moley JF, Wallin GK, Brother MB, Kim M, Wells SA Jr, Brodeur GM: Oncogene and growth factor expression in MEN 2 and related tumours. *Henry Ford Hosp Med J* **40**:284, 1992.

114. Boultwood J, Wyllie FS, Williams GD, Wynford Thomas D: N-*myc* expression in neoplasia of human thyroid C cells. *Cancer Res* **48**:4073, 1988.

115. Zedenius J, Wallin G, Hamberger B, Nordenskjold M, Weber G, Larsson C: Somatic and MEN2A de novo mutations identified in the *ret* protooncogene by screening of sporadic MTCs. *Hum Mol Genet* **3**:1259, 1994.

115a. Shirahama S, Ogura K, Takami H, Itoh K, Tohsen T, Miyauchi A, Nakamura Y: Mutational analysis of the *RET* protooncogene in 71 Japanese patients with medullary thyroid carcinoma. *J Hum Genet* **43**:101, 1998.

115b. Jhiang SM, Fithian L, Weghorst CM, Clark OH, Falko JM, Odorisio TM, Mazzaferri EL: *Ret* mutation screening in MEN 2 patients and discovery of a novel mutation in a sporadic medullary thyroid carcinoma. *Thyroid* **6**:115, 1996.

115c. Ixalinin V, Frilling A: 27bp deletion in the ret protooncogene as a somatic mutation associated with medullary thyroid carcinoma. *J Mol Med* **76**:365, 1998.

115d. Romei C, Elisei R, Pinchera A, Ceccherini I, Molinari E, Mancusi F, Martino E, et al: Somatic mutations of the *ret* protooncogene in sporadic medullary thyroid carcinoma are not restricted to exon 16 and are associated with tumour recurrence. *J Clin Endocrinol Metab* **81**:1619, 1996.

116. Marsh DJ, Andrew SD, Learoyd DL, Pojer R, Eng C, Robinson BG: Deletion-insertion mutation encompassing *RET* codon 634 is associated with medullary thyroid carcinoma. *Hum Mutat* Suppl **1**:3, 1998.

117. Dou S, Chi D, Carlson KM, Moley JA, Wells SA Jr, Donis-Keller H: *RET* proto-oncogene mutations associated with sporadic cases of medullary thyroid carcinoma. *Fifth International Workshop on Multiple Endocrine Neoplasia, Karolinska Inst*, Stockholm, Sweden, 1994, p 3.

118. Beldjord C, Desclaux-Arramond F, Raffin-Sanson M, Corvol J-C, De Keyzer Y, Luton J-P, Plouin P-F, et al: The ret proto-oncogene in sporadic phaeochromocytomas: Frequent MEN 2-like mutations and new molecular defects. *J Clin Endocrinol Metab* **80**:2063, 1995.

119. Eng C, Crossey PA, Mulligan LM, Healey CS, Houghton C, Prowse A, Chew SL, et al: Mutations of the *ret* protooncogene and the Von Hippel-Lindau disease tumour suppressor gene in sporadic and syndromic phaeochromocytoma. *J Med Genet* **32**:934, 1995.

119a. Gimm O, Armanios M, Dziema H, Neumann HPH, Eng C: Somatic and occult germline mutations in SDHD, a mitochondrial complex II gene, in non-familial phaeochromocytomas. *Cancer Res* **60**:6822, 2000.

120. Komminoth P, Kunz EK, Matias-Guiu X, Hiort O, Christensen G, Colomer A, Rother J, et al: Analysis of *ret* protooncogene point mutations distinguishes heritable from non-heritable thyroid carcinomas. *Cancer* **76**:479, 1995.

121. Lindor NM, Honchel R, Khosla S, Thibodeau SN: Mutations in the *ret* plrotooncogene in sporadic phaeochromocytomas. *J Clin Endocrinol Metab* **80**:627, 1995.

122. Padberg BC, Schroder S, Jochum W, Kastendieck H, Roth J, Heitz PU, Komminoth P: Absence of *ret* protooncogene point mutations in sporadic hyperplastic and neoplastic lesions of the parathyroid gland. *Am J Pathol* **147**:1600, 1995.

122a. Hofstra RMW, Cheng NC, Hausen C, Stulp RP, Stelwagen T, Clausen N, Tommerup N, et al: No mutations found by *ret* screening in sporadic and hereditary neuroblastoma. *Hum Genet* **97**:362, 1996.

123. Eng C, Mulligan LM, Healey CS, Houghton C, Frilling A, Raue F, Thomas GA, et al: Heterogeneous mutation of the *RET* proto-oncogene

in subpopulations of medullary thyroid carcinoma. *Cancer Res* **56**:2167, 1996.

124. Carson EB, McMahon M, Baylin SB, Nelkin BD: *Ret* gene silencing is associated with Raf-1-induced medullary thyroid carcinoma cell differentiation. *Cancer Res* **55**:2048, 1995.

125. Carlomagno F, Salvatore D, Santoro M, de Franciscis V, Quadro L, Panariello L, Colantuoni V, et al: Point mutation of the *RET* proto-oncogene in the TT human medullary thyroid carcinoma cell line. *Biochem Biophys Res Commun* **207**:1022, 1995.

126. Ponder BAJ: Medullary carcinoma of the thyroid, in Peckham M, Pinedo, Veronesi U (eds): *Oxford Textbook of Oncology*, vol 2. Oxford, UK, Oxford Medical Publications, 1996, p 2110.

127. Telenius-Berg M, Berg B, Hamberger B: Impact of screening on prognosis in the multiple endocrine neoplasia type 2 syndromes: Natural history and treatment results in 105 patients. *Henry Ford Hosp Med J* **32**:225, 1984.

128. Wells SA, Baylin SB, Leight GS, Dale JK, Dilley WG, Farndon JR: The importance of early diagnosis in patients with hereditary medullary thyroid carcinoma. *Ann Surg* **195**:595, 1982.

129. Malletta LE, Blewins T, Jordan PM, Noon GP: Autogenous parathyroid grafts for generalized primary parathyroid hyperplasia: Contrasting outcome in sporadic hyperplasia versus multiple endocrine neoplasia type 1. *Surgery* **101**:738, 1987.

130. Jansson S, Tisell LE, Fjalling M, Lindberg S, Jacobson L, Zacharison BF: Early diagnosis of and surgical strategy for adrenal medullary disease in MEN II gene carriers. *Surgery* **103**:11, 1988.

131. Vasen HFA, van der Feltz M, Raue F, Kruseman AN, Koppeschaar HPF, Pieters G, Seif FJ, et al: The natural course of multiple endocrine neoplasia type IIb. *Arch Intern Med* **251**:1250, 1992.

132. Samaan NA, Draznin MB, Halpin RE, Bloss RS, Hawkins E, Lewis RA: Multiple endocrine syndrome type IIb in early childhood. *Cancer* **68**:1832, 1991.

Malignant Melanoma

Alexander Kamb ■ *Meenhard Herlyn*

1. Melanoma is one of the more common cancers in the United States and is increasing rapidly in occurrence. Environmental factors, particularly sun exposure, have been strongly implicated in melanoma risk.

2. An accumulation of evidence points to a set of genetic changes that underlie the evolution from melanocyte to metastatic melanoma. In addition, a significant fraction of the disease is familial, suggesting that specific genes regulate susceptibility. Study of familial melanoma provides one route to identification of genes that contribute to all melanomas, including the more common sporadic form.

3. The investigation of somatic lesions in melanoma tumors and cell lines has permitted clinicians and molecular geneticists to focus on defined regions in the genome. Several chromosomal areas have been delineated based on various types of analyses. These regions exhibit loss of heterozygosity (LOH) and, in some cases, homozygous deletions. The most commonly observed abnormality in melanoma is LOH and homozygous deletion at 9p21. Chromosomal aberrations at 9p21 may occur early in tumor development, although certain results suggest that their ultimate effect may be manifested later.

4. Linkage analysis of melanoma-prone kindreds also identified 9p21 as the site of a potential tumor-suppressor gene involved in melanoma susceptibility. Interestingly, initial linkage studies were hindered by use of dysplastic nevi as the phenotypic trait rather than melanoma itself, emphasizing the importance of phenotype definition in linkage analysis. The melanoma susceptibility locus discovered at 9p21, called *MLM*, is inherited as a dominant allele with penetrance that ranges upward from 50 percent. Its expressivity is highly variable.

5. The identity of *MLM* has been determined largely through deletion mapping in melanoma cell lines. It encodes a negative growth regulator called p16, the expression of which causes cell cycle arrest. p16 is part of a growth-control pathway that involves cyclin-dependent kinases, cyclins, and the retinoblastoma gene product Rb. An impressive list of experiments supports a role for p16 not only in melanoma formation but also in the genesis of many other tumors. p16 inactivation may occur in nearly half of all advanced human cancers.

6. Genes other than *p16* also play a part in melanoma formation. One of these is cyclin-dependent kinase 4 (cdk4), a target of *p16's* biochemical inhibitory activity. *CDK4* is mutated in some tumors and in the germ line of rare familial melanoma cases. It is only the second germ-line oncogene to be described. Through cdk4 and Rb, *p16* is tied into the basic cell cycle control apparatus.

7. The identification of genes involved in familial and sporadic melanoma raises the possibility of gene-based tests for cancer predisposition and for the classification of tumors.

p16, as the primary genetic element in familial melanoma, is an interesting case study for genetic testing. Technical and economic issues are especially important in this realm. With respect to somatic gene testing, technical concerns are superseded by the pressing need to demonstrate clinical utility of information about *p16* status in tumors. Therapeutic implications of genetic discoveries are not insignificant but remain largely speculative and long term.

Melanoma is a malignancy that originates from melanocytes, the pigment-producing cells in skin. Melanocytes generate a light-absorbing shield of melanin that protects the skin from damage caused by ultraviolet (UV) radiation. They transfer much of this pigment to keratinocytes in the suprabasal skin layers via dendritic connections. It is ironic that melanocytes themselves are among the targets of UV, spurred into malignant growth by the agent they are intended to counter. Melanocytes arise from neural crest-derived progenitors that migrate from the developing central nervous system into the skin and are homogeneously distributed at the junction between the epidermal and dermal layers. Born of colonists themselves, it is perhaps not surprising that melanocytes, when fully transformed, are as aggressive and migratory as any tumor cells. Melanocytes are present in the skin at roughly equal densities in all the races.[1] Dark-skinned people do not have more melanocytes; rather, each melanocyte produces, on average, more melanin pigment than melanocytes from light-skinned people. Consequently, individuals differ little in the numbers of precursor cells that can give rise to melanomas.

Several factors have contributed recently to a heightened awareness of melanoma. People are more conscious of the dangers imposed by sun exposure. Melanoma, like lung cancer, is gaining a reputation as a neoplasm on the rise, a cancer whose incidence is profoundly affected by controllable environmental influences. In addition, genetic principles that underlie the disease are beginning to emerge.[2]

Melanoma responds poorly to chemical and radiation therapy, and the most effective treatment is surgical excision before the tumor is well advanced.[3] Early detection thus is of paramount importance. Because the skin lesions are relatively easy to spot, frequent examination and prompt treatment are highly successful medical strategies. On the other hand, clinical and histologic diagnosis of early lesions remains difficult and controversial. For individuals who have hundreds of moles, diagnosis is especially problematic. Partly because of the efficacy of early detection, genetic analysis of melanoma offers hope in a comprehensive plan to limit the morbidity of the disease. Genetic tests may provide the means to assess risk and recognize individuals who require more intensive observation. Although genetic studies in melanoma have lagged somewhat behind other neoplasias such as colon cancer, the future appears bright in the effort to understand the biology of melanoma, predict its clinical behavior, and eventually discern how to defeat it.[4]

INCIDENCE OF MELANOMA

The overall melanoma incidence in the United States currently is nearly 40,000 cases per year, placing it significantly below only prostate, breast, lung, and colon cancers in occurrence.[5] The

---

A list of standard abbreviations is located immediately preceding the index. Nonstandard abbreviations used in this chapter include: LOH = loss of heterozygosity; DNS = dysplastic nevus syndrome.

population-averaged lifetime risk of developing melanoma can be as high as 1 in 60 in particular groups; more typically, it is 1 in 90.[6,7] This rate of occurrence is increasing rapidly, more so than for any other cancer site except lung. Since the 1930s, the incidence of melanoma has jumped nearly 20-fold.[7] The reason is likely related to the fashion for tanning and outdoor activities. The development of melanoma is strongly influenced by genetic as well as environmental factors—especially exposure to UV.[8] This is dramatically illustrated by epidemiologic studies that relate melanoma incidence to ethnographic and geographic factors. Melanoma is nearly three times more common in southern latitudes of the United States than in the northern United States.[3] The highest incidence of melanoma occurs in Queensland, Australia, whereas one of the lowest occurs in South India. Both these regions have a high degree of sun exposure. The difference is that Australians are largely light-skinned, whereas South Indians are dark-skinned. Thus, the genetics of skin color interact with sunlight exposure to determine the overall rate of melanoma.

DEVELOPMENT OF MELANOMA

Clinical Features

Melanoma presents in a variety of clinically distinct forms: superficial spreading melanoma, lentigo maligna melanoma, acral lentigious melanoma, and nodular melanoma.[3] At least two of these types, lentigo maligna melanoma and superficial spreading melanoma, may exist for several years in a preinvasive state, providing a long window of opportunity for removal. Once the lesion thickens and begins to invade, the prognosis worsens considerably. The survival of melanoma patients correlates strongly with the thickness of the primary lesion and its degree of invasion into the dermis. If the lesion is clinically localized, the 5-year survival rate is 85 percent.[3]

Specific genetic components are presumed to account for the morphologic features that distinguish the various clinical forms of melanoma. One important goal of melanoma research is to identify genes that influence the phenotype of the tumor. Thus it is helpful to develop a tractable experimental system in which to study tumor progression. Fortunately, some of the features of melanoma *in situ* can be reproduced in tissue culture.[9]

Often it is useful to classify cells in culture based not on the clinical criteria described earlier but on a scheme with a more chronologic emphasis. The transition from normal melanocyte to metastatic melanoma occurs in a series of defined stages. Each stage is characterized broadly by changes in morphology and growth properties (Fig. 30-1). The first abnormal state that is recognizably different from the melanocyte is the nevus cell. This cell type differs little in microscopic appearance from a normal melanocyte, yet it can contain random chromosomal abnormalities. The next stage is the premalignant melanoma, discernible often as a raised mole that has acquired atypical architectural and cytologic features. This premalignant lesion can evolve further into a primary melanoma that is capable of breaking through the dermal layer into the underlying blood vessels. Finally, the most insidious form, metastatic melanoma, arises from the primary lesion. This end stage is invasive, migratory, and ultimately, if unchecked, kills the patient. The secondary sites of metastasis include brain, bone, lung, and liver.

Models of Melanoma in Tissue Culture

Much has been learned about the properties of the different melanoma stages by study of cells in culture. The overall pattern of melanoma, as of other cancer types, involves progressive loss of dependence on exogenous growth signals as melanocytes evolve toward malignancy (Table 30-1). For example, normal melanocytes placed in culture require phorbol ester, basic fibroblast

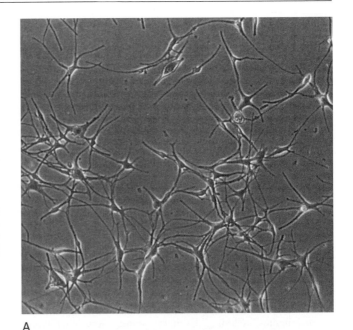

A

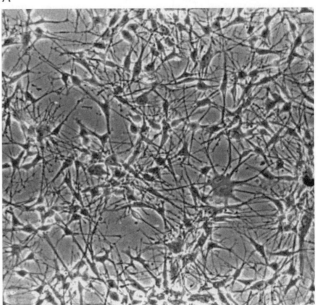

B

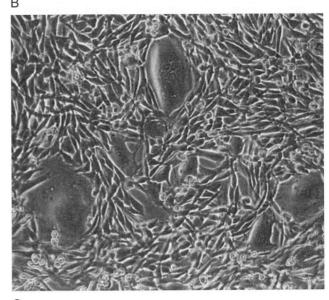

C

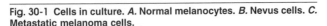

Fig. 30-1 Cells in culture. *A.* Normal melanocytes. *B.* Nevus cells. *C.* Metastatic melanoma cells.

Table 30-1 Culture Characteristics of Normal Melanocytes and Cells from Nonmalignant Primary and Metastatic Melanocytic Lesions

| Parameter | Melanocytes | Nevus | Primary Melanoma | | Metastatic Melanoma |
			Early	Late	
Chromosomal abnormalities	None	None (few random)	(#1, 6, 7, 9) Nonrandom	(#1, 6, 7, 9) Nonrandom	(#1, 6, 7, 9, 11) Nonrandom
Life span (doublings)	Finite ($<$60)	Finite ($<$50)	Infinite ($>$100)	Infinite ($>$100)	Infinite ($>$100)
Response to phorbol ester	Stimulation	Stimulation	Inhibition	Inhibition	Inhibition
Growth factor requirements	I, FGF, aMSH, TPA*	Same as melanocytes†	I only	None	None
Growth in soft agar (percent)	$<$0.001	0.001–3 (average 0.9)	5–10 (average 8)	5–20	5–70 (average 25)
Growth in nude mice (percent)	None	None	80	100	100

*I = insulin; FGF = basic fibroblast growth factor; αMSH = α-melanocyte stimulating hormone. †Cultures are often independent of FGF and/or TPA.

growth factor, α-melanocyte-stimulating factor, and insulin-like growth factor 1. However, most lines derived from early melanomas no longer require phorbol ester. By the time metastases appear, the cells have lost their dependence on any of these factors. They grow rapidly in culture dishes without special serum factors. Behavior of cells in culture that have been established from clinically defined stages of melanoma is presumed relevant to the transitions that occur as melanocytes evolve in the body toward metastatic melanoma. Thus thorough characterization of such cell lines is likely to be of great value in understanding the biology of melanoma.

GENETICS OF MELANOMA

Genetic analysis of melanoma has two aspects: the study of predisposition in melanoma-prone kindreds and the study of somatic genetic alterations that occur as tumors evolve in the body. Both approaches have considerable appeal and, as described in the following, may converge on the same set of genes important in melanoma development.

Somatic Genetics of Melanoma Tumors

Melanomas, like practically all tumors, progressively accumulate abnormalities in their DNA as they evolve more malignant traits.[10,11] These abnormalites include chromosomal losses, duplications, translocations, and deletions. In addition to cytogenetically detectable aberrations, melanomas incorporate more subtle somatic changes such as microsatellite variability and point mutations.[12–15] Which of these changes are causal in tumorigenesis and which are merely the effect of the transformed state are difficult questions to answer in many cases.

9p21 Loss of Heterozygosity

One of the most consistent somatic changes in melanomas is the loss of chromosomal material from the short arm of chromosome 9 (9p).[11,16,17] This cytogenetic abnormality is observed in over half of malignant melanomas. Some studies suggest that the initial change involving loss of heterozygosity (LOH) on 9p is a relatively early event in melanoma development, occurring before the primary lesion matures.[11] More recent work has demonstrated that a large fraction of the 9p abnormalities ultimately are detected as homozygous deletions of 9p21 in advanced malignancies.[18] Whether or not the homozygous deletions are present at an earlier stage in tumor development remains an open question, although some studies suggest that they may be a later phenomenon.[19] If so, the role of the early LOH lesions in melanoma is unclear. In a subsequent section, the molecular identity of the 9p21 tumor suppressor is discussed.

Other LOH Sites

Chromosomal abnormalities other than 9p LOH also have been observed as common features in primary melanoma tumors[11]

(Table 30-2). These include LOH regions on 3p, 6q, 10q, 11q, and 17p. 3p and 10q losses are detected in tumors less than 1.5 mm in thickness, suggesting that hypothetical tumor-suppressor loci located on these chromosomal arms may be important at earlier stages of melanoma formation. 6q, 11q, and 17p LOH is detected only in more invasive tumors. Homozygous deletions at a specific site on 3p have been described recently.[20] These deletions frequently remove a gene termed *FHIT*, suggesting that it may be the relevant tumor-suppressor locus in the region. However, the *FHIT* location on 3p is a fragile site, prone to rearrangement, and further studies are necessary to establish a causal relationship between *FHIT* inactivation and tumor growth. 17p contains the *p53* tumor-suppressor gene, and although point mutations in *p53* are relatively uncommon in melanomas, *p53* may account for a fraction of 17p LOH.[21,22] Additional regions of abnormality on 1p, 3q, and 17q have been described in melanoma cell lines and metastases.[23–27] 17q contains the metastasis-suppressor gene *NM23* and the *NF1* tumor-suppressor gene, a gene found to be mutated in some melanoma cell lines.[27–29] The *PTEN* tumor-suppressor gene located on 10q is likely the underlying cause of 10q LOH because the gene is altered in a significant percentage of melanoma tumors and cells lines.[30]

Kindred Analysis

Apart from skin tone, predisposition to melanoma may be strongly influenced by heredity. As early as 1952, the familial nature of nonocular melanoma was described, and current estimates indicate that 5 to 10 percent of all melanoma cases may have a genetic basis.[30,31] This heritable component is inferred from melanoma cases that cluster in specific families. The definition of familiality varies, but typically, melanoma patients who have at least one

Table 30-2 Loss of Heterozygosity in Primary Melanoma Specimens

Chromosome Arm	Percent LOH
1p	5
3p	19
3q	14
6q	31
9p	47
9q	19
10q	31
11q	17
13q	9
17p	16
17q	4
22q	6

SOURCE: Data are taken from Ref. 11. Experiments on each chromosome arm involved 21 to 41 informative samples.

first-degree relative with melanoma are classified as familial cases. For first-degree relatives of melanoma patients, the increased risk is calculated to be 2.0; with a relative under age 50 affected, the risk is 6.5.[32,33]

Based on the commonly accepted figures, over 90 percent of melanomas are predicted to be of a nongenetic, or sporadic, origin, percentages similar to those reported for other cancer sites such as breast and colon the Sporadic melanoma truly may be independent of heredity, arising solely from random wear and tear that occur during a lifetime. Alternatively, it may be caused by multiple genes or weakly penetrant alleles that modify an individual's risk modestly but, in aggregate, strongly affect the overall incidence of disease in a population.

Dysplastic Nevus Syndrome

During the past few decades, numerous families with multiple cases of melanoma have been identified.[34–36] Individuals in many of these kindreds were reported to have unusual numbers of large nevi, and the nevus count on the skin was shown to be a risk factor for melanoma.[37] A variety of pathologic studies suggested that certain nevi could be classified as dysplastic and, therefore, more likely to produce melanomas.[38,39] These nevi resemble the clinically miniature early superficial spreading melanomas.[3] Such observations gave rise to the notion of a disease, dysplastic nevus syndrome (DNS), characterized by frequent occurrence of atypical moles and increased risk of melanoma.

MLM

Some DNS/melanoma kindreds served as the basis for genetic linkage analysis in which molecular genetic markers positioned at various places throughout the genome were tested for linkage to DNS and to melanoma. Because dysplastic nevi are believed to be precursors to melanomas, initial attempts to determine a genetic basis for melanoma focused on DNS. However, these attempts were hindered by the difficulties of diagnosis and classification of moles. A reported linkage assignment on 1p36 was not reproduced in other families.[40–46] When the phenotype was restricted to melanoma itself, definitive linkage was obtained with markers in 9p21[47] (Fig. 30-2). This linkage study produced a cumulative Lod score (base 10 logarithm of the odds of linkage) of nearly 13, suggesting a probability of linkage in excess of 1 trillion to 1; one large kindred had a Lod score of nearly 6. The genetic locus identified by linkage analysis was designated *MLM*.

The history of the discovery of *MLM* is an ideal example of the importance of phenotypic definition to linkage analysis.[48] DNS proved to be an unreliable phenotype, difficult to diagnose objectively. The use of melanoma itself as the primary phenotypic trait reduced the number of affecteds in the analysis but placed the phenotypic definition on a firm, objective foundation. This definition provided the key to identification of *MLM*.

MLM is inherited in a dominant Mendelian fashion; a single defective germ-line copy of the gene predisposes to melanoma. The penetrance of the disease gene, the likelihood that an individual carrier will develop melanoma by age 80, has been estimated at 53 percent using three 9p21-linked kindreds.[49] More recent studies suggest that the penetrance may vary depending on the particular allele and/or the kindreds under consideration. In some kindreds, the penetrance appears to approach 100 percent.[50] However, in general, as with many other cancer-predisposition genes, inheritance of a defective *MLM* allele increases the *probability* of melanoma; it does not guarantee illness. For melanoma, the increased lifetime risk caused by inheritance of predisposing *MLM* alleles is roughly 50-fold. This risk depends on the level of sun exposure.[49]

MLM behaves as a classic tumor-suppressor locus. Although the increased risk is dominantly inherited, the mutant locus acts in cells as a recessive. Tumors that arise in *MLM* gene carriers invariably lose the wild-type chromosome by deletion or nondisjunction.[51] This feature accords with the proposal of Knudson based originally on studies of the retinoblastoma (*RB1*)

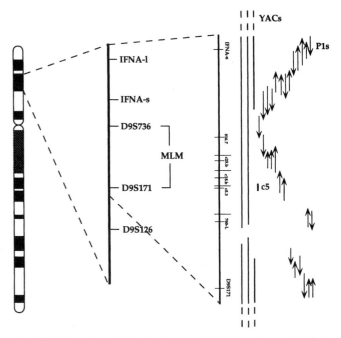

Fig. 30-2 Genetic and physical maps of 9p21 region containing *MLM*. A cartoon of human chromosome 9 is shown with the 9p21 region expanded. Shown are 5 microsatellite markers; *MLM* maps between *D9S736* and *D9S171* by recombinant analysis. This region was aligned to a physical map of P1, yeast artificial chromosome (YAC), and cosmid clones. Several new markers were generated, some of which are shown (e.g., c5.3). In addition, the location of cosmid c5 is shown. This cosmid contains sequences from *p15* and *p16*.

tumor-suppressor gene.[52] In the general case of a tumor-suppressor gene, two "hits" are required to inactivate the locus, one for the maternal copy and one for the paternal copy. In familial cancers, one hit occurs through inheritance of a defective allele. Thus a single somatic event is necessary to complete the functional inactivation of the locus.

The relationship between nevi and melanoma remains unclear. The role of nevi as melanoma precursors has not been disputed, but the genetic underpinnings of mole incidence and size are unresolved. No simple genetic basis for nevi has been discovered. Nevertheless, *MLM* may influence mole size and number. A comparison of *MLM* carriers and noncarriers revealed that carriers had roughly 50 percent more nevi.[49] If real, the phenotypic effect is dominant or codominant, involving inheritance of a single defective *MLM* copy. This deduction has implications for the role of *MLM* in melanocyte biology.

GENES THAT INFLUENCE MELANOMA

p16

Following the establishment of melanoma linkage to 9p21 markers, an effort to isolate *MLM* was undertaken. However, isolation of the gene proceeded largely without recourse to the 9p21-linked kindreds (see Fig. 30-2). Instead, cell lines were used as the primary tools for gene localization. Previous work had revealed the presence of melanoma cell lines with large homozygous deletions in 9p21.[16,17] This implied that the genetic locus *MLM* and a tumor-suppressor locus presumed to underlie the 9p21 deletions might be one and the same. Under this assumption, standard positional cloning methods of recombinant chromosome analysis were bypassed in favor of the simpler strategy of deletion breakpoint localization in cell lines.

In one study, a collection of nearly 100 melanoma cell lines was assembled to identify and map deletion breakpoints in 9p21.[18] Roughly 60 percent of these lines proved to have detectable

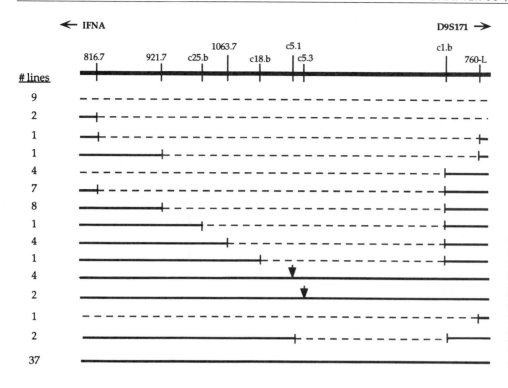

Fig. 30-3 Homozygous deletions in melanoma cell lines. Markers used to detect homozygous deletions are shown above. Melanoma cell lines are grouped into families based on which markers are missing, indicated by dashed lines. The two arrows show homozygous deletions that remove a single marker. The number of cell lines per family is listed on the left.

homozygous deletions, and the deletions clustered around a single site in 9p21 (Fig. 30-3). This site contained two genes, one that encoded the previously identified cyclin-dependent kinase (CDK) inhibitor p16, and the second subsequently shown to encode the related CDK inhibitor p15.[53–57] A variety of deletional and DNA sequence-based studies soon pointed to *p16* (also designated *P16INK4A, MTS1, CDKN2*) as the relevant locus. Inactivating point mutations were found in the *p16* coding sequence but not in *p15* in cell lines and tumors.[54,58,59] In addition, no homozygous

deletions were found that removed *p15* but left *p16* intact.[60] In contrast, there were several examples of deletions that left *p15* intact but selectively removed *p16*.

Clinching evidence for the role of *p16* in tumorigenesis was obtained through study of the gene in 9p21-linked families. Linked *p16* sequence variants were found in many, although not all, of these kindreds[61–66] (Table 30-3). Several of the sequence variants obviously were disruptive to the protein causing truncation of the predicted product, and several other missense changes subse-

Table 30-3 Parameters Associated with Melanoma-Prone Kindreds and Mutations

Kindred	Lod Score	Cases	Cases with Haplotype or Mutation	Mutation	Effect
3346	5.97	21	21	—	—
1771	3.57	12	12	Val126Asp	Missense
3137	1.90	17	16	—	—
1764	1.04	4	4	—	—
3012	0.64	4	4	Gly101Trp	Missense
3006	0.19	6	3	—	—
D4	1.22	6	6	Del(218-237)	Frameshift
2482	1.65	—	—	—	—
377	1.64	—	—	—	—
1016	1.41	6	6	Val126Asp	Missense
1017	1.24	4	4	Gly101Trp	Missense
567	1.08	4	4	Arg58Ter	Stop
479	1.03	5	5	Val126Asp	Missense
2884	0.52	2	2	IVS2+1	Splice
909	0.47	—	—	—	—
2209	0.24	—	—	—	—
928	0.12	4	6	Gly101Trp	Missense
481	0.00	3	3	Gly101Trp	Missense
873	−0.03	2	3	Arg87Pro	Missense
373	−0.34	3	3	Asn71Ser	Missense

NOTE: Lod scores for the first five kindreds were calculated for markers between IFNA and D9S171.[63] The Lod score for D4 was computed using D9S171.[66] Note that this mutation was misreported in the original work. Lod scores for the last 12 kindreds were calculated for IFNA.[62] A number of other studies have reported germ-line p16 mutations that are not listed here.[51,64,67]

quently were shown to encode defective p16 molecules.[67-69] *p16* germ-line mutations are found rarely in sporadic cases and in familial cases that do not manifest strong signs of 9p21 linkage. For instance, in 38 patients who meet the typical definition of familiality but who were not part of extended 9p21-linked kindreds, no *p16* mutations were detected.[62] Based on such studies, it is likely that *p16* accounts for a fraction of the total melanoma incidence that is generally considered to be familial. To date, there are no firm estimates for the population frequency of predisposing *MLM* alleles. Extrapolation from some of the work previously cited suggests a frequency in the U.S. population of no more than 1 in a few thousand.[60,64]

Through remarkable serendipity, two individuals homozygous for a predisposing *MLM* allele have been identified.[65] Both homozygous persons carried two copies of the same mutant *p16* allele that contains a deletion of 19 base pairs, an allele that is prevalent especially in melanoma-prone families in Holland. The chance intermarriage of two gene carriers from relatively isolated Dutch villages produced the homozygous individuals. Interestingly, the homozygous gene carriers were normal, except that one of them developed two primary melanomas by age 15. The other individual, however, lived to the age of 55 with no melanomas, although she died of an internal adenocarcinoma. It is worth noting that the melanoma patient had numerous nevi, whereas the other carrier was relatively mole-free. The latter individual, however, had offspring, some of whom were classified as DNS cases. These facts demonstrate two important aspects of *p16* function. First, *p16* is not essential for normal development or viability, a conclusion confirmed by the recent demonstration of viable *p16* knockout mice.[70] Second, *p16* mutations have variable expressivity; phenotypic effects may depend on unknown genetic factors as well as environmental factors, including but perhaps not restricted to sun exposure.

The weight of the evidence strongly supports the view that *p16* is *MLM*. As is the case with many familial tumor suppressors, *p16* germ-line mutations increase cancer risk, whereas *p16* somatic mutations also occur in sporadic tumors during the transition toward malignancy.

p15

A continuing mystery is the existence of kindreds that are definitely 9p21-linked but for whom mutations cannot be found in *p16*[60,61] (see Table 30-3). These kindreds served as the initial impetus to explore *p15* as a candidate for a second melanoma-susceptibility gene on 9p21. *p15* has considerable sequence similarity to *p16* (77 percent at the protein level in humans) and encodes a protein with biochemical behavior nearly identical to p16.[56,57] It is located within 20 kb of *p16* on chromosome 9 and likely was derived from *p16* by gene duplication, divergence, and in the human lineage, a gene conversion event.[71] Both proteins cause growth arrest when overexpressed in certain cell lines and in normal cells.[59,67,72,73] *p15* regulation, however, is markedly different from *p16*. *p15* is induced by transforming growth factor beta (TGF-β); *p16* is not.[56] This adds further interest to the possible role of p15 in cancer, since TGF-β is an important regulator of cell growth. Despite the obvious appeal of *p15* as an alternative *MLM*-like gene, no germ-line mutations have been reported so far in *p15*.[59]

E1β/p19^ARF

Another potential tumor suppressor is encoded at the *p16* locus, although its role in cancer is obscure (Fig. 30-4). The gene, termed *p19^ARF* or *p16^E1β*, actually overlaps the *p16* coding sequence.[74-76] The *p16^E1β* transcript originates from a promotor distinct from the normal *p16* promotor. This second upstream promotor produces a transcript that contains the second and third coding exons of *p16* (E2 and E3) but incorporates an alternative first exon (*E1β*) in place of the normal first exon of *p16* (see Fig. 30-3). The reading frame used to encode *p16* is closed immediately upstream of the *E1β-E2* junction, suggesting that if this frame were used for

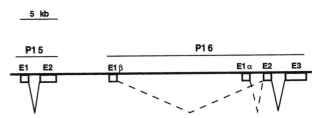

Fig. 30-4 The *p16* locus is complex. The relative position of *p16* coding exons (1 and 2) and *p16* exons are shown. Dashed lines indicate an alternative splice that distinguishes the *E1β* transcript from the *p16* transcript.

translation, a truncated *p16* molecule missing the first third of the protein would result. No such protein has been detected *in vivo*. An alternative reading frame (*ORF2*), however, potentially encodes a protein of 19 kDa; hence the name p19^ARF. This protein bears no homology to any known protein sequence. However, it is conserved between mouse and human.[71,77]

The *E1β* exon is deleted selectively in several melanoma cell lines, leaving the *p16* transcript and protein intact. This implies an important role for *p16^E1β* in the tumor-suppressor function of the *p16* locus. No *E1β* mutations have been observed in the germ lines of familial cases. Moreover, no *E1β*-specific point mutations have been detected in cell lines or tumors.[74]

Antibodies raised against p19^ARF detect a 19-kDa protein *in vivo*, and overexpression of p19^ARF causes cessation of cell growth.[77] However, unlike p16 and other CDK inhibitors, p19^ARF does not inhibit cdk4 *in vitro*. Paradoxically, the level of the *E1β* transcript increases as quiescent T cells enter the cell cycle.[74] In addition, comparison of human and mouse sequences reveals that the reading frame predicted to encode p19^ARF is no more conserved than the other alternative to the *p16* reading frame (*ORF3*).[71,74] Thus there is little evidence for evolutionary selective pressure on the p19^ARF protein. The p19^ARF protein binds to mdm2, which in turn interacts with p53, thus potentially tying the p53 and p16 pathways together.[79-81] *E1β/p19^ARF* may represent one of the more bizarre genes in the mammalian genome: a member of a complex locus; transcribed from a separate, independently regulated promotor; overlapping a gene that is translated in a different reading frame; and both genes participating in the cell cycle regulatory apparatus.

CDK4

On the heels of the discovery that *p16* germ-line mutations predispose to melanoma, a second melanoma-predisposition gene was uncovered. A fraction of melanoma-prone families that are not linked to 9p21 segregate mutations in a gene that encodes one of the targets of p16's inhibitory activity, cdk4.[79] These mutations affect a single site in the *CDK4* coding sequence that renders the molecule resistant to p16 binding and inhibition. The identical lesion also has been observed as a somatic mutation in a sporadic melanoma.[80] Thus *CDK4* behaves as a proto-oncogene; the mutant form is converted into an overactive growth promotor, an oncogene. This is only the second example of germ-line mutations in a proto-oncogene. The other example is the *RET* proto-oncogene, germ-line mutations in which predispose to the cancer-susceptibility syndrome multiple endocrine neoplasia 2A.[81] Based on the observed frequency of mutations, kindreds that segregate *CDK4* mutations may be tenfold less frequent than *p16* kindreds.

A Growth-Control Pathway in Melanocytes

The identification of *CDK4* germ-line mutations in melanoma-prone kindreds is exciting for another reason. cdk4, p16, Rb, and D cyclins comprise part of a growth-control pathway that operates in a variety, perhaps all, tissues[82] (Fig. 30-5). Several lines of evidence suggest that p16 inhibits cdk4, which has the consequence of preventing phosphorylation of Rb protein. Hypophos-

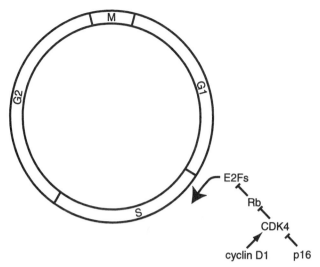

Fig. 30-5 The cell cycle and the p16 growth-control pathway. Eukaryotic cell division is broken up into four phases: G1, during which the cell prepares to synthesize DNA; S, the phase of DNA replication; G2 during which the cell prepares for mitosis; and M, the mitotic period. The transition between G1 and S is monitored carefully by the cell. p16, acting through cdk4 and Rb, exercises its control over cell division at this point. Arrows indicate a positive effect; blunt-ended lines an inhibitory effect.

phorylated Rb binds transcription factors such as members of the *E2F* family, interfering with their ability to activate transcription of genes involved in DNA synthesis.[83] Sporadic tumors seldom contain mutations in more than one component of this pathway, an observation that supports the mutually dependent function of the genes.[84–87] In contrast, mutations in *p53,* although rare in melanoma, occur as frequently in *p16*-positive tumors as in *p16*-negative tumors, an indication that p53 and p16 function in separate pathways of growth control.[13] It should be emphasized, however, that p19[ARF] may link the two pathways in some functional sense. p16, cdk4, and Rb thus play a central part in the regulation of the cell cycle. They may comprise a primary circuit that integrates information relevant in the decision to proceed through the first stage of cell division and DNA replication.

To date, three of the four known components of the pathway have been implicated in hereditary cancer syndromes: *CDK4, p16,* and *RB1.* Curiously, *RB1* mutant gene carriers do not suffer from excessive melanoma but rather from a specific childhood tumor of the eye.[88] Why the phenotype of *CDK4* and *p16* mutations differs from the *RB1* mutant phenotype is unclear, but it emphasizes the complexity of the growth-control pathways that operate in cells.

The evidence that *p16* is an important cancer gene is compelling. Germ-line mutations in *p16* increase melanoma risk. Deletions in *p16,* as well as a smaller number of point mutations, are found in a large percentage of melanomas and many other cancer types.[89] In melanoma tumors and cell lines, the large majority of point mutations that are detected have the hallmarks of UV-induced changes, signs of the link between UV and *p16* inactivation in tumors.[58,90,91] Loss of *p16* expression owing to methylation has been reported in a variety of cell lines.[92–94] Overexpression of p16 in a range of cell types causes arrest at the G1/S checkpoint in the cell cycle.[67,70,73] Mice in which the *p16* gene has been inactivated by homologous recombination are cancer-prone.[70] p16 functions *in vitro* as a biochemical inhibitor of cdk4, a protein known to promote passage through the G1/S checkpoint. Taken together, this body of data leaves little doubt that *p16* plays a key role in a variety of human cancers but does not delineate the precise nature of the role.

p16 and Other CDK Inhibitors

Many other CDK inhibitors have been identified including p15, p18, p21, p27, and p57.[56,95–102] All, including p16, are expressed in a wide variety of tissues.[74] The biochemical behavior of p16 protein differs little from, for example, p15.[56] All CDK inhibitors, when overexpressed in particular cell types, induce cell cycle arrest. Yet *p16* appears to be a special case. None of the other genes is mutated at appreciable frequencies in tumors or cell lines.[59,103–105] The physiologic function of p16 that may distinguish it from other CDK inhibitors, rendering it more vulnerable to mutational inactivation, is not obvious.

Attempts to define the physiologic function of p16 *in vivo* have focused on two general areas: its role in programmed cell death, or apoptosis, and its role in cellular senescence. In one model system, p16 expression correlated with protection from apoptosis, a finding that does not explain why tumor cells would dispense with *p16*.[106] More germane, perhaps, *p16*-deficient mouse cells are highly sensitive to oncogenic transformation and readily form colonies in culture.[70] This result suggests that loss of p16 expression may contribute to immortalization. Other studies have reported an increase in p16 levels as cells approach senescence, followed by a fall as cells become immortalized.[107–109] Based on this correlation, it seems reasonable to propose a role for p16 in suppressing immortalization. To achieve this effect, p16 must work through Rb. Consequently, Rb and the other components of the p16 pathway are implicated as accessory molecules in the control of cellular life span. This proposed role for p16 leaves unexplained the early 9p LOH events in melanoma development.

p16 Mutations and Predisposition to Nonmelanoma Cancers

It is perplexing given the widespread involvement of *p16* in sporadic cancer that *p16* mutant gene carriers are predisposed only to melanoma. Some studies have suggested an association between pancreatic cancer and melanoma in certain families, but a clear role for *MLM* in cancers besides melanoma has been difficult to prove.[51,110] A simple explanation may lie in considerations about rate-limiting steps in tumorigenesis. If, as the data begin to suggest, p16 inactivation is a relatively late step in tumor development, its removal may not be rate-limiting in most tumor types. For reasons that are obscure, p16 inactivation may be important at an earlier stage in melanoma formation, or it may be the final brake that is released in cells that suffer an environmental insult in the form of UV exposure and consequent high rates of mutation. It is more complicated, although not impossible, to hypothesize a role for *p16* mutations both early during melanoma formation in nevi and later in the escape from senescence.

GENETICS AND MELANOMA DIAGNOSIS

Germ-Line Testing for Melanoma Susceptibility

With identification of the major genetic factors underlying hereditary melanoma, *p16* and, to a lesser extent, *CDK4,* the possibility of germ-line testing for melanoma risk has arrived. Contrary to many other types of genetic testing, a melanoma-predisposition screen has certain clear advantages. First, in principle, the results of such a test provide valuable information to guide behavior. If an individual tests positive (i.e., carries a high-risk allele), steps can be taken to avoid sun exposure and to maintain vigilance for abnormal growths on the skin. Such behavior not only would diminish the chance of melanoma but also would facilitate early detection and removal of the lesion, by far the most successful approach to combating the disease. Second, although many independent sequence changes have been described, the *p16* gene is small, consisting of only 158 codons. By contrast, coding sequences of the breast cancer-susceptibility genes *BRCA1* and *BRCA2* are huge, roughly 12 and 25 times the size of *p16*, respectively.[111,112] The relatively small size of *p16* should reduce dramatically the technical difficulties and cost associated with a genetic screen. In the case of *CDK4*, a screen that targets a single codon may be sufficient.[79]

Excitement about the value of a melanoma-susceptibility screen is blunted somewhat by other considerations, especially the economic realities of such a test. The combined gene frequency of *p16* and *CDK4* predisposing alleles is low. Thus, for random, population-based screening, the *a priori* probability of getting a positive result is very small, a disincentive to pay for such a test. In addition, the possibility of missing *MLM* mutations that fall outside the coding sequence must be considered. Several kindreds that show a strong indication of 9p21 linkage appear to have wild-type *p16* coding regions.[61,62] This suggests that a percentage of *p16* mutations fall outside the coding sequences or that a second *MLM* gene resides in 9p21. Either a test must be devised to detect such mutations, or the test may have limited informativeness.

The greatest value of a melanoma-susceptibility test may apply to individuals at higher risk of melanoma than the majority of the population. These include people with many moles and people with affected relatives. With roughly 40,000 melanoma cases per year in the United States, such a test might be relevant to over 100,000 people every year. If the criterion of numerous nevi also is used, the number of higher-risk individuals may exceed 1 million. This is a potential market size that may drive development of a commercial test, but whether a specialized melanoma genetic test could be economically self-sustaining in the short term remains debatable. It may make more sense to provide an *MLM* test when the costs of such gene-based diagnostic screens are lower or when it becomes part of a larger panel of susceptibility gene tests.

Somatic Gene Testing

An alternative to germ-line *p16* and *CDK4* testing is afforded by the potential for somatic gene testing in tumors. *p16* is one of the most frequently altered genes in human cancer, inactivated in perhaps half of all advanced tumors.[54] Here, economic considerations contribute a strong impulse for test development, providing certain criteria can be met. First, there is a slew of technical issues that involve detection of *p16* alterations in cancer cells: homozygous deletions, the most common form of *p16* inactivation, methylated DNA, and other somatic changes. Detection of such disparate lesions is a particularly significant problem in tumors that are invariably adulterated by normal somatic cells.[60] Second, the clinical relevance of such a somatic *p16* gene test must be demonstrated firmly. The test must prove useful in the diagnosis or prognosis of cancer. Most desirable would be test results that aid in customization of cancer therapy. Clinical studies that address these issues are critically important. At least one report so far details the significance of *p16* gene status as a prognostic indicator in childhood acute lymphocytic leukemia.[113] Thus there is the exciting possibility that *p16* gene tests, as well as tests for multiple other cancer genes, ultimately may supplement or replace traditional modes of subjective histologic analysis in the classification and treatment of tumors.

GENETICS AND MELANOMA THERAPY

Advances in understanding the genetics of melanoma so far have had little impact on treatment, nor are they likely to have a rapid effect in the future. The difficulties of translating genetic knowledge into practical therapeutic advances are immense. Here, as in the traditional approach to cancer therapy, the challenge is to achieve specificity. An effective therapeutic agent must target cancer cells and leave normal cells relatively unharmed. With some of the molecules that regulate melanoma development now in hand, it is at least possible to formulate potential strategies.

Targeting cdk4

Immunotherapy tailored to abnormal cdk4 molecules offers a route to novel melanoma therapy. Indeed, T cells have been identified that recognize tumor cells that harbor mutant cdk4 proteins.[80] One of the weaknesses of this approach, however, is the small number of tumors likely to have sustained cdk4 alterations. Thus a treatment that targets mutant cdk4 is unlikely to have general success in combating the vast majority of melanomas.

Complementation of Defective *p16* Genes in Tumors

An alternative approach is to devise treatments that rely on *p16*. Because *p16* mutations occur in many tumors besides melanoma, the investment in such a treatment likely would have benefits that extend well beyond melanoma. Once again, however, specificity and delivery are key factors. Simple reintroduction of functional *p16* sequences into tumor cells causes growth arrest.[114,115] However, the sequences also arrest normal cells.[73] Therefore, a strategy that depends on restored expression of p16 in tumor cells must include either a means for selective delivery of *p16* into tumor cells or a mechanism for regulated expression that permits normal cell growth.

Manipulating the Cell Cycle

Small-molecule drugs that mimic p16 may find some use in cancer treatment and are currently under development by certain pharmaceutical companies. However, the issue of selectivity remains problematic here as with gene therapy.

Finally, it may be possible to use cell cycle regulators such as p16 to protect normal cells from the ravages of conventional chemo- or radiotherapy. If a method for specific induction of growth arrest in normal cells could be found, a state of temporary arrest could be induced in normal cells that would endow them with resistance to subsequent cytotoxic treatments. This general concept has been explored in the past.[116–119] *p16* provides a new molecular tool to study the value of such an approach. At least in one model system, p16 expression causes reversible cell cycle arrest that protects cells from chemotherapeutics.[120] The challenge in this approach is to achieve a general protection of normal tissues by reversible induction of p16 or other regulators. The strategy is attractive because the induction does not need to be selective. Many tumors have lost the function of the p16 growth-control pathway, either by mutation of *p16* itself or by alteration of downstream components such as cdk4 or Rb. Thus most tumors would not respond to an agent that induces p16 expression by entering a state of arrest. Only normal cells, which maintain the integrity of the p16 pathway, would arrest and be rendered resistant to cytotoxic treatments.

REFERENCES

1. Clark WH: The skin, in Rubin E, Farber JL (eds): *Pathology.* Philadelphia, Lippincott, 1988.
2. Kamb A: Human melanoma genetics. *J Invest Dermatol Symp Proc* **1**:177, 1996.
3. Fitzpatrick TB, Sober AJ, Mihm MC Jr: Malignant melanoma of the skin, in Braunwald E, Isselbacher KJ, Petersdorf RG, Wilson JD, Martin JB, Fauci AS (eds): *Principles of Internal Medicine.* New York, McGraw-Hill, 1987.
4. Fearon ER, Vogelstein B: A genetic model for colorectal tumorigenesis. *Cell* **61**:759, 1990.
5. National Cancer Institute: *1987 Annual Cancer Statistics Review.* NIH publication no 88-2789, 1988.
6. Sober AJ, Lew RA, Koh HK, Barnhill RL: Epidemiology of cutaneous melanoma. *Dermatol Clin* **9**:617, 1991.
7. Nigel DS, Fridman RJ, Kopf AW: The incidence of malignant melanoma in the United States: Issues as we approach the 21st century. *J Am Acad Dermatol* **34**:839, 1996.
8. Green A, Swerdlow AJ: Epidemiology of melanocytic nevi. *Epidemiol Rev* **11**:204, 1989.

9. Herlyn M: *Molecular and Cellular Biology of Melanoma.* Austin, TX, RG Landes, 1993.

10. Fountain JW, Bale SJ, Housman DE, Dracopoli NC: Genetics of melanoma. *Cancer Surv* **9**:645, 1990.

11. Healy E, Rehman I, Angus B, Rees JL: Loss of heterozygosity in sporadic primary cutaneous melanoma. *Genes Chromosom Cancer* **12**:152, 1995.

12. Walker GJ, Palmer JM, Walters MK, Nancarrow DJ, Hayward NK: Microsatellite instability in melanoma. *Melanoma Res* **4**:267, 1994.

13. Gruis NA, Weaver-Feldhaus J, Liu Q, Frye C, Ecles R, Orlow I, Lacombe L, Ponce-Castoneda V, Lianes E, et al: Genetic evidence in melanoma and bladder cancers that p16 and p53 function in separate pathways of tumor suppression. *Am J Pathol* **146**:1199, 1995.

14. Peris K, Keller G, Chimenti S, Amantea A, Derl H, Hofler H: Microsatellite instability and loss of heterozygosity in melanoma. *J Invest Dermatol* **105**:625, 1995.

15. Quinn AG, Healy E, Rehman I, Sikkink S, Rees JL: Microsatellite instability in human non-melanoma and melanoma skin cancer. *J Invest Dermatol* **104**:309, 1995.

16. Olopade OI, Jenkins R, Linnenbach AJ, et al: Molecular analysis of chromosome 9p deletion in human solid tumors. *Proc Am Assoc Cancer Res* **21**:318, 1990.

17. Fountain JW, Karayiorgou M, Ernstoff MS, Kirkwood JM, Vlock DR, Titus-Ernstoff L, Bouchard B, Vijayasaradhi S, Houghton AN, Lahti J, et al: Homozygous deletions within human chromosome band 9p21 in melanoma. *Proc Natl Acad Sci USA* **89**:10557, 1992.

18. Weaver-Feldhaus J, Gruis NA, Neuhausen S, Le Paslier D, Stockert E, Skolnick MH, Kamb A: Localization of a putative tumor suppressor gene by using homozygous deletions in melanomas. *Proc Natl Acad Sci USA* **91**:7563, 1994.

19. Reed JA, Loganzo F Jr, Shea CR, Walker GJ, Flores JF, Glending JM, Bogdany JK, Shiel MJ, Haluska FG, Fountain JW, Albino AP: Loss of expression of the p16/cyclin-dependent kinase inhibitor 2 tumor suppresser gene in melanocytic lesions correlates with invasive stage of tumor progression. *Cancer Res* **55**:2713, 1995.

20. Sozzi G, Veronese ML, Negrini M, Baffa R, Cotticelli MG, Inoue H, Tornielli S, Pilotti S, De Gregorio L, Pastorino U, Pierotti MA, Ohta M, Huebner K, Croce CM: The *FHIT* gene 3p14.2 is abnormal in lung cancer. *Cell* **85**:17, 1996.

21. Volkenandt M, Schlegel U, Nanus DM, Albino AP: Mutational analysis of the human *p53* gene in malignant melanoma cell lines. *Pigment Cell Res* **4**:35, 1991.

22. Levin DB, Wilson K, Valadares de Amorim G, Webber J, Kenny P, Kusser W: Detection of *p53* mutations in benign and dysplastic nevi. *Cancer Res* **55**:4278, 1995.

23. Balaban GB, Herlyn M, Clark WH Jr, Nowell PC: Karyotypic evolution in human malignant melanoma. *Cancer Genet Cytogenet* **19**:113, 1986.

24. Dracopoli ND, Alhadeff B, Houghton AN, Old LJ: Loss of heterozygosity at autosomal and X-linked loci during tumor progression in a patient with melanoma. *Cancer Res* **47**:3995, 1987.

25. Cowan JM, Halaban R, Francke U: Cytogenetic analysis of melanocytes from premalignant nevi and melanomas. *J Natl Cancer Inst* **80**:1159, 1988.

26. Horsman DE, White VA: Cytogenetic analysis of uveal melanoma: Consistent occurrence of monosomy 3 and trisomy 8q. *Cancer* **71**:811, 1993.

27. Andersen LB, Fountain JW, Gutmann DH, Tarle SA, Glover TW, Dracopoli NC, Housman DE, Collins FS: Mutations in the neurofibromatosis 1 gene in sporadic melanoma cell lines. *Nature Genet* **3**:118, 1993.

28. Johnson MR, Look AT, DeClue JE, Valentine MB, Lowy DR: Inactivation of the *NF1* gene in human melanoma and neuroblastoma cell lines without impaired regulation of *GRP.ras. Proc Natl Acad Sci USA* **90**:5539, 1993.

29. Welch DR, Chen P, Miele ME, McGary CT, Bower JM, Stanbridge EJ, Weissman BE: Microcell-mediated transfer of chromosome 6 into metastatic human C8161 melanoma cells suppresses metastasis but does not inhibit tumorigenicity. *Oncogene* **9**:255, 1994.

30. Teng DH, Hu R, Lin H, Davis T, Iliev D, Frye C, Swedlund B, Hansen KL, Vinson VL, Gumpper KL, Ellis L, El-Nagger A, Frazier M, Jasser S, Langford LA, Lee J, Mills GB, Pershouse MA, Pollack RE, Tornos C, Troncoso P, Yung WK, Fujii G, Berson A, Steck PA, et al: MMAC1/PTEN mutations in primary tumor specimens and tu cell lines *Cancer Res* **57**:5221, 1997.

31. Cawley EP: Genetic aspects of malignant melanoma. *Arch Dermatol* **65**:440, 1952.

32. Greene MH, Fraumeni JF Jr: The hereditary variant of malignant melanoma, in Clark WH Jr, Goldman LI, Mastrangelo MJ (eds): *Human Malignant Melanoma.* New York, Grune and Stratton, 1979.

33. Wallace DC, Exton LA, McLeod GR: Genetic factor in malignant melanoma. *Cancer* **27**:1262, 1971.

34. Goldgar DE, Easton DF, Cannon-Albright LA, Skolnick MH: A systematic population-based assessment of cancer risk in first degree relatives of cancer probands. *J Natl Cancer Inst* **86**:1600, 1994.

35. Turkington RW: Familial factors in malignant melanoma. *JAMA* **192**:77, 1965.

36. Smith EE, Henley WS, Knox JM, Lane M: Familial melanoma. *Arch Intern Med* **117**:820, 1966.

37. Anderson DE, Smith JL Jr, McBride CM: Hereditary aspects of malignant melanoma. *JAMA* **200**:741, 1967.

38. Swerdlow AJ, English J, Mackie RM, O'Doherty CJ, Hunter JAA, Clark J: Benign nevi associated with high risk of melanoma. *Lancet* **2**:168, 1984.

39. Clark WH, Reimer RR, Greene M, Ainsworth AM, Mastrangelo M: Origin of familial malignant melanomas from heritable melanocyte lesions. *Arch Dermatol* **114**:732, 1978.

40. Lynch HT, Frichot BC, Lynch J: Familial atypical multiple mole melanoma syndrome. *J Med Genet* **15**:352, 1978.

41. Greene MH, Goldin LR, Clark WH, et al: Familial malignant melanoma: Autosomal dominant trait possibly linked to the Rhesus locus. *Proc Natl Acad Sci USA* **80**:6071, 1983.

42. Bale SJ, Dracopoli NC, Tucker, MA, Clark WH Jr, Fraser MC, Stanger BZ, Green P, Donis-Keller H, Housman DE, Green MH: Mapping the gene for hereditary cutaneous malignant melanoma-dysplastic nevus to chromosome 1p. *N Engl J Med* **320**:1367, 1986.

43. van Haeringen A, Bergman W, Nolen MR, van der Kooij-Meijs E, Hendrikse I, Wijnen JT, Khan PM, Klasen EC, Frants RR: Exclusion of the dysplastic nevus syndrome (DNS) locus from the short arm of chromsome 1 by linkage studies in Dutch families. *Genomics* **5**:61, 1989.

44. Cannon-Albright LA, Goldgar DE, Wright EC, et al: Evidence against the reported linkage to the cutaneous melanoma-dysplastic nevus syndrome locus to chromosome 1p36. *Am J Human Genet* **46**:912, 1990.

45. Kefford RF, Salmon J, Shaw HM, Donald JA, McCarthy WH: Hereditary melanoma in Australia: Variable association with dysplastic nevi and absence of genetic linkage to chromosome 1p. *Cancer Genet Cytogenet* **51**:45, 1991.

46. Nancarrow DJ, Palmer JM, Walters MK, Kerr BM, Hofner GJ, Garske L, McLeod GR, Hayward NK: Exclusion of the familial melanoma locus (*MLM*) from the *PND/DIS47* and *MYCL1* regions of chromosome arm 1p in 7 Australian pedigrees. *Genomics* **12**:18, 1992.

47. Goldstein AM, Dracopoli NC, Engelstein M, Fraser MC, Clark WH Jr, Tucker MA: Linkage of cutaneous malignant melanoma/dysplastic nevi to chromosome 9p, and evidence for genetic heterogeneity. *Am J Hum Genet* **54**:489, 1994.

48. Cannon-Albright LA, Goldgar DE, Meyer LJ, Lewis CM, Anderson DE, Fountain JW, Hegi ME, Wiseman RW, Petty EM, Bale AE, Olopade OI, Diaz MO, Kwiatkowski DJ, Piepkorn MW, Zone JJ, Skolnick MH: Assignment of a locus for familial melanoma, *MLM*, to chromosome 9p 13-p22. *Science* **258**:1148, 1992.

49. Skolnick MH, Cannon-Albright LA, Kamb A: Genetic predisposition to melanoma. *Eur J Cancer* **30**:1991, 1994.

50. Cannon-Albright LA, Meyer LJ, Goldgar DE, Lewis CM, McWhorter WP, Jost M, Harrison D, Anderson DE, Zone JJ, Skolnick MH: Penetrance and expressivity of the chromosome 9p melanoma susceptibility locus (*MLM*). *Cancer Res* **54**:6041, 1994.

51. Walker GJ, Hussussian CJ, Flores JF, Glendening JM, Haluska FG, Drocopoli NC, Hayward NK, Fountain JW: Mutations of the *CDKN2/p16INK4* gene in Australian melanoma kindreds. *Hum Mol Genet* **4**:1845, 1995.

52. Gruis NA, Sandkuijl LA, van der Velden PA, Bergman W, Frants RR: CDKN2 explains part of the clinical phenotype in Dutch familial atypical multiple-mole melanoma (FAMMM) syndrome families. *Melanoma Res* **5**:169, 1995b.

53. Knudson AG: Mutation and cancer: Statistical study of retinoblastoma. *Proc Natl Acad Sci USA* **68**:820, 1971.

54. Serrano M, Hannon GJ, Beach D: A new regulatory motif in cell-cycle control causing specific inhibition of cyclin D/CDK4. *Nature* **366**:704, 1993.

55. Kamb A, Gruis NA, Weaver-Feldhaus J, Liu Q, Harshman K, Tavtigian SV, Stockert E, Day RS, Johnson BE, Skolnick MH: A cell cycle regulator potentially involved in genesis of many tumor types. *Science* **264**:436, 1994.

56. Nobori T, Miura K, Wu DJ, Lois A, Takabayashi K, Carson DA: Deletions of the cyclin-dependent kinase-4 inhibitor gene in multiple human cancers. *Nature* **368**:753, 1994.

57. Hannon GJ, Beach D: p15INK4B is a potential effector of TFG-β–induced cell cycle arrest. *Nature* **371**:257, 1994.

58. Jen J, Harper JW, Bigner SH, Bigner DD, Papadopoulos N, Markowitz S, Wilson JKV, Kinzler KW, Vogelstein B: Deletion of *p16* and *p15* genes in brain tumors. *Cancer Res* **54**:6353, 1994.

59. Liu Q, Neuhausen S, McClure M, Frye C, Weaver-Feldhaus J, Gruis NA, Eddington K, Allalunis-Turner MJ, Skolnick MH, Fujimura FK, Kamb A: *CDKN2* (*MTS1*) tumor suppressor gene mutations in human tumor cell lines. *Oncogene* **10**:1061, 1995.

60. Stone S, Dayananth P, Jiang P, Weaver-Feldhaus JM, Tavtigian SV, Skolnick MH, Kamb A: Genomic structure, expression, and mutational analysis of the *P15* (*MTS2*) gene. *Oncogene* **11**:987, 1995.

61. Kamb A, Liu Q, Harshman K, Tavtigian SV: Response to rate of *p16* (*MTS1*) mutations in primary tumors with 9p loss. *Science* **265**:416, 1994.

62. Hussussian CJ, Struewing JP, Goldstein AM, Higgins PAT, Ally DS, Sheahan MD, Clark WHJ, Tucker MA, Dracopoli NC: Germline *p16* mutations in familial melanoma. *Nature Genet* **8**:15, 1994.

63. Kamb A, Shattuck-Eidens D, Eeles R, Liu Q, Gruis NA, Ding W, Hussey C, Tran T, Miki Y, Weaver-Feldhaus J, McClure M, Aitken JF, Anderson DE, Bergman W, Frants R, Goldgar DE, Green A, MacLennan R, Martin NG, Meyer LJ, Youl P, Zone JJ, Skolnick MH, Cannon-Albright LA: Analysis of the *p16* gene (*CDKN2*) as a candidate for the chromosome 9p melanoma susceptibility locus. *Nature Genet* **8**:22, 1994.

64. Borg A, Johannsson U, Johannsson O, Hakansson S, Westerdahl J, Masback A, Olsson H, Ingvar C: Novel germline *p16* mutation in familial malignant melanoma in southern Sweden. *Cancer Res* **56**:2497, 1996.

65. Holland EA, Beaton SC, Becker TM, Grulet OM, Peters BA, Rizos H, Kefford RF, Mann GJ: Analysis of the *p16* gene, *CDKN2*, in 17 Australian melanoma kindreds. *Oncogene* **11**:2289, 1995.

66. Gruis NA, van der Velden PA, Sandkuijl LA, Prins DE, Weaver-Feldhaus J, Kamb A, Bergman W, Frants RR: Homozygotes for *CDKN2* (*p16*) germline mutation in Dutch familial melanoma kindreds. *Nature Genet* **10**:351, 1995.

67. Liu L, Lassam NJ, Slingerland JM, Bailey D, Cole D, Jenkins R, Hogg D: Germline *p16INK4A* mutation and protein dysfunction in a family with inherited melanoma. *Oncogene* **11**:405, 1995.

68. Koh J, Enders GH, Cynlacht BD, Harlow E: Tumor-derived p16 alleles encoding proteins defective in cell-cycle inhibition. *Nature* **375**:506, 1995.

69. Ranade K, Hussussian CJ, Sikorski RS, Varmus HE, Goldstein AM, Tucker MA, Serrano M, Hannon GJ, Beach D, Dracopoli NC: Mutations associated with familial melanoma impair *p16INK4* function. *Nature Genet* **10**:114, 1995.

70. Yang R, Gombart AF, Serrano M, Koeffler P: Mutational effects on the *p16INK4a*. *Cancer Res* **55**:2503, 1995.

71. Serrano M, Lee H, Chin L, Cordon-Cardo C, Beach D, DePinho RA: Role of the *INK4a* locus in tumor suppression and cell mortality. *Cell* **85**:27, 1996.

72. Jiang P, Stone S, Wagner R, Wang S, Dayananth P, Kozak CA, Wold B, Kamb A: Comparative analysis of *Homo sapiens* and *Mus musculus* cyclin-dependent kinase (CDK) inhibitor genes *p16* (*MTS1*) and *p15* (*MTS2*). *J Mol Evol* **41**:795, 1995.

73. Serrano M, Gomez-Lahoz E, DePinho RA, Beach D, Bar-Sagi D: Inhibition of ras-induced proliferation and cellular transformation by *p16INK4*. *Science* **267**:249, 1995.

74. Lukas J, Parry D, Aagaard L, Mann DJ, Bartkova J, Strauss M, Peters G, Bartek J: Retino-blastoma-protein-dependent cell-cycle inhibition by the tumor suppressor p16. *Nature* **375**:503, 1995.

75. Stone S, Jiang P, Dayannanth P, Tavtigian SV, Katcher H, Parry D, Peters G, Kamb A: Complex structure and regulation of the *P16* (*MTS1*) locus. *Cancer Res* **55**:2988, 1995.

76. Mao L, Merlo A, Bedi G, Shapiro GI, Edwards CD, Rollins BJ, Sidransky DA: A novel *p16INK4A* transcript. *Cancer Res* **55**:2995, 1995.

77. Duro D, Bernard O, Della Valle V, Berger R, Larsen CJ: A new type of p161INK4/MTS1 gene transcript expressed in B-cell malignancies. *Oncogene* **11**:212, 1995.

78. Quelle D, Zindy F, Ashmun RA, Sherr CJ: Alternative reading frames of the *INKa* tumor suppressor gene encode two unrelated proteins capable of inducing cell cycle arrest. *Cell* **83**:993, 1995.

79. Pomerantz J, Schreiber-Agus N, Liegeois NJ, et al: The Ink4a tumor suppressor gene product, p19Arf, interacts with MDM2 and neutralizes MDM2's inhibition of p53. *Cell* **92**:713, 1998.

80. Zhang Y, Xiong Y, Yarbrough WG: ARF promotes MDM2 degradation and stabilizes p53: ARF-INK4a locus deletion impairs both the Rb and p53 tumor suppression pathways. *Cell* **92**:725, 1998.

81. Kamijo T, Weber JD, Zambetti G, et al: Functional and physical interactions of the ARF tumor suppressor with p53 and Mdm2. *Proc Natl Acad Sci USA* **95**:8292, 1998

82. Glendening JM, Flores JF, Wlaker GJ, Stone S, Albino AP, Fountain JW: Homozygous loss of the *p15INK4B* gene (and not the *p16INK4* gene) during tumor progression in a sporadic melanoma patient. *Cancer Res* **55**:5531, 1995.

83. Zuo L, Weger J, Yang Q, Goldstein AM, Tucker MA, Walker GJ, Hayward N, Dracopoli NC: Germline mutations in the *p16INK4a* binding domain of CDK4 in familial melanoma. *Nature Genet* **12**:97, 1996.

84. Wolfel T, Hauer M, Schneider J, Serrano M, Wolfel C, Klehmann-Hieb E, De Plaen E, Hankeln T, Meyer zum Buschenfelde KH, Beach D: A *p16INK4a*-insensitive CDK4 mutant targeted by cytolytic T lymphocytes in human melanoma. *Science* **269**:1281, 1995.

85. Mulligan LM, Kwok JBJ, Healey CS, Elsdon MJ, Gardner E, Love DR, Moore JK, Papi L, Ponder MA, Telenius H, Tunnacliffe A, Ponder BAJ: Germ-line mutations of the *RET* proto-oncogene in multiple endocrine neoplasia type 2A. *Nature* **363**:774, 1993.

86. Sherr CJ: G1 phase progression: Cycling on cue. *Cell* **79**:551, 1994.

87. Lukas J, Petersen BO, Holm K, Bartek J, Helin K: Deregulated expression of E2F family members induces S-phase entry and overcomes *p16INK4A*-mediated growth suppression. *Mol Cell Biol* **16**:1047, 1996.

88. He J, Allen JR, Collins VP, Allalunis-Turner MJ, Godbout R, Day RS 3d, James CD: CDK4 amplification is an alternative mechanism to *p16* gene homozygous deletion in glioma cell lines. *Cancer Res* **54**:5804, 1994.

89. Okamoto A, Demetrick DJ, Spillare EA, Hagiwara K, Hussain SP, Bennett WP, Forrester K, Gerwin B, Serrano M, Beach DH, et al: Mutations and altered expression of *P16INK4* in human cancer. *Proc Natl Acad Sci USA* **91**:11045, 1994.

90. Otterson GA, Dkatzke RA, Coxon A, Kin YW, Kaye FJ: Absence of p16INK4 protein is restricted to the subset of lung cancer lines that retains wildtype RB. *Oncogene* **9**:3375, 1994.

91. Aagaard L, Lukas J, Bartkova J, Kjerulff AA, Strauss M, Bartek J: Aberrations of p16Ink4 and retinoblastoma tumor-suppressor genes occur in distinct sub-sets of human cancer cell lines. *Int J Cancer* **61**:115, 1995.

92. DeVita VT, Hellman S, Rosenberg SA: *Cancer: Principles and Practice of Oncology.* Philadelphia, Lippincott, 1989.

93. Kamb A: Cell-cycle regulators and cancer. *Trends Genet* **11**:136, 1995.

94. Maestro R, Boiocchi M: Sunlight and melanoma: An answer from MTS1 (p16). *Science* **267**:15, 1995.

95. Pollock PM, Yu F, Qiu L, Parsons PG, Hayward NK: Evidence for UV induction of *CDKN2* mutations in melanoma cell lines. *Oncogene* **11**:663, 1995.

96. Herman JG, Merlo A, Mao L, Issa JJ-P, Davidson NE, Sidransky D, Baylin SB: Inactivation of the *CDKN2/p16/MTS1* gene is frequently associated with aberrant DNA methylation in all common human cancers. *Cancer Res* **55**:4525, 1995.

97. Merlo A, Herman JG, Mao L, Lee DJ, Gabrielson E, Burger PC, Baylin SB, Sidransky D: 5′ CpG island methylation is associated with transcriptional silencing of the tumour suppressor *p16/CDKN2/MTS1* in human cancers. *Nature Med* **1**:686, 1995.

98. Gonzalez-Zulueta M, Bender CM, Yang AS, Nguyen T, Beart RW, Van Tornout JM, Jones PA: Methylation of the 5′ CpG island of the *p16/CDKN2* tumor suppressor gene in normal and transformed human tissues correlates with gene silencing. *Cancer Res* **55**:4531, 1995.

99. El-Deiry WF, Tokino T, Velculescu VE, Levy DB, Parsons R, Trent JM, Lin D, Mercer WE, Kinzler KW, Vogelstein B: WAF1, a potential mediator of p53 tumor suppression. *Cell* **75**:817, 1993.

100. Gu W, Turck CW, Morgan DO: Inhibition of CDK2 activity *in vivo* by an associated 20K regulatory subunit. *Nature* **366**:707, 1993.

101. Harper JW, Adami GR, Wei N, Keyomarsi K, Elledge KK: The p21 Cdk-interacting protein Cip1 is a potent inhibitor of G1 cyclin-dependent kinases. *Cell* **75**:805, 1993.

102. Xiong Y, Hannon GJ, Zhang H, Casso D, Kobayashi R, Beach D: p21 is a universal inhibitor of cyclin kinases. *Nature* **366**:701, 1993.

103. Polyak K, Lee M-H, Bromage HE, Koff A, Roberts JM, Tempst P, Massague J: Cloning of p27Kip1, a cyclin-dependent kinase inhibitor

and a potential mediator of extracellular antimitogenic signals. *Cell* **78**:59, 1994.

104. Toyoshima H, Hunter T: p27, a novel inhibitor of G1 cyclin-Cdk protein kinase activity, is related to p21. *Cell* **78**:67, 1994.

105. Guan K-L, Jenkins CW, Li Y, Nichols MA, Wu X, O'Keefe CL, Matera AG, Xiong Y: Growth suppression by p18, a p16INK4/MTS1 and p14INK4B/MTS2-related CDK6 inhibitor, correlates with wild-type pRb function. *Genes Dev* **8**:2939, 1994.

106. Lee MH, Reynisdottir I, Massague J: Cloning of p57KIP2, a cyclin-dependent kinase inhibitor with unique domain structure and tissue distribution. *Genes Dev* **9**:639, 1995.

107. Kawamata N, Seriu T, Koeffler HP, Bartram CR: Molecular analysis of the cyclin-dependent kinase inhibitor family: *p16(CDKN2/MTS1/INK4A), p18(INK4C)* and *p27(Kip1)* genes in neuroblastomas. *Cancer* **77**:570, 1996.

108. Orlow I, Iavorone A, Crider-Miller SJ, Bonilla F, Latres E, Lee MH, Gerald WL, Massague J, Weissman BE, Cordon-Cardo C: Cyclin-dependent kinase inhibitor p57/KIP2 in soft tissue sarcomas and Wilms tumors. *Cancer Res* **56**:1219, 1996.

109. Rusin MR, Okamoto A, Chorazy M, Czyzewski K, Harasim J, Spillare EA, Hagiwara K, Hussain SP, Xiong Y, Demetrick DJ, Harris CC: Intragenic mutation of the *p16(INK4), p15(INK4B)* and *p18* genes in primary non-small-cell lung cancers. *Int J Cancer* **65**:734, 1996.

110. Wang J, Walsh K: Resistance to apoptosis conferred by Cdk inhibitors during myocyte differentiation. *Science* **273**:359, 1996.

111. Reznikoff CA, Yeager TR, Belair CD, Savelieva E, Puthenveettil JA, Stadler WM: Elevated p16 at senescence and loss of p16 at immortalization in human papillomavirus 16 E6, but not E7, transformed human uroepithelial cells. *Cancer Res* **56**:2886, 1996.

112. Hara E, Smith R, Parry D, Tahara H, Stone S, Peters G: Regulation of p16/CDKN2 expression and its implications for cell immortalization and senescence. *Mol Cell Biol* **16**:859 1986.

113. Rogan EM, Bryan TM, Hukku B, Maclean K, Chang AC, Moy EL, Englezou A, Warneford SG, Dalla-Pozza L, Reddel RR: Alterations in p53 and p16INK4 expression and telomere length during spontaneous immortalization of Li-Fraumeni syndrome fibroblasts. *Mol Cell Biol* **15**:475, 1986.

114. Bergman W, Watson P, de Jong J, Lunch HT, Fusaro RM: Systemic cancer and the FAMMM syndrome. *Br J Cancer* **61**:932, 1990.

115. Miki Y, Swensen J, Shattuck-Eidens D, et al: A strong candidate for the breast and ovarian cancer susceptibility gene *BRCA1*. *Science* **266**:66, 1994.

116. Tavtigian SV, Simard J, Rommens J: The complete *BRCA2* gene and mutations in chromosome 13Q-linked kindreds. *Nature Genet* **12**:1, 1996.

117. Heyman M, Rasool O, Borgonovo Brandter L, et al: Prognostic importance of *p15INK4B* and *p16INK4* gene inactivation in childhood acute lymphocytic leukemia. *J Clin Oncol* **14**:1512, 1996.

118. Jin X, Nguyen D, Zhang WW, Kyritsis AP, Roth JA: Cell cycle arrest and inhibition of tumor cell proliferation by the *p16INK4* gene mediated by an adenovirus vector. *Cancer Res* **55**:3250, 1995.

119. Fueyo J, Gomez-Manzano C, Yung WK, Clayman GL, Liu TJ, Bruner J, Levin VA, Kyritsis AP: Adenovirus-mediated *p16/CDKN2* gene transfer induces growth arrest and modifies the transformed phenotype of glioma cells. *Oncogene* **12**:103, 1996.

120. Pardee AB, James LJ: Selective killing of transformed baby hamster kidney (BHK) cells. *Cell Biol* **72**:4994, 1975.

121. Hartwell LH, Kastan MB: Cell cycle control and cancer. *Science* **266**:1821, 1994.

122. Kohn KW, Jackman J, O'Connor PM: Cell cycle control and cancer chemotherapy. *J Cell Biochem* **54**:440, 1994.

123. Darzynkiewicz Z: Apoptosis in anticancer strategies: Modulation of cell cycle or differen-tiation. *J Cell Biochem* **58**:151, 1995.

124. Stone S, Dayananth P, Kamb A: Reversible, p16-mediated cell cycle arrest as protection from chemotherapy. *Cancer Res* **56**:3199, 1996.

Cowden Syndrome

Charis Eng ■ *Ramon Parsons*

1. Cowden syndrome (CS) is an autosomal dominant disorder characterized by multiple hamartomas and a risk of breast and thyroid cancers.
2. The great majority of tumors, including those of the thyroid and breast, are benign. Up to 10 percent of affected individuals develop nonmedullary thyroid carcinoma and up to 50 percent of affected females develop breast cancer. Preliminary data suggest that endometrial cancer is a component of CS.
3. The pathognomonic hamartoma is the trichilemmoma, a benign tumor of the infundibulum of the hair follicle.
4. The susceptibility gene for CS is a tumor suppressor gene, as evidenced by loss of heterozygosity in the *PTEN* region of 10q23 in various tumors and by transfection assays. Overexpression of *PTEN* results in G1 cell cycle arrest and/or apoptosis.
5. The *CS* gene, *PTEN*, was isolated by a combination of genetic mapping analyses, somatic genetics, and a candidate gene approach. *PTEN* located on 10q23.3 encodes a 403-amino acid protein that contains a phosphatase signature motif and has sequences homologous to tensin.
6. PTEN is a dual-specificity lipid phosphatase. PTEN is the 3-phosphatase for phosphatidylinositol-3,4,5-triphosphate and hence, coordinately regulates the cell survival factor PKB/Akt via the PI3 kinase-signaling pathway. However, it is becoming clear that PTEN can mediate growth arrest via PI3K-dependent and -independent pathways.
7. Germ-line mutations in *PTEN* have been found in CS families, as well as in the related, but distinct, hamartoma disorder Bannayan-Ruvalcaba-Riley syndrome. A subset of Proteus-like patients also has germ line *PTEN* mutations. These mutations result in predicted protein truncation or loss of function, hence supporting its predicted function as a tumor suppressor.
8. Somatic mutations of *PTEN* occur to a variable extent in several cancer types. However, alternate mechanisms of PTEN inactivation does occur.

Cowden syndrome or multiple hamartoma syndrome (CS, MIM 158350) can be a great imitator of many inherited cancer syndromes, and therefore, should be in many differential diagnoses. Named after Rachel Cowden who died of bilateral breast cancer in her early thirties, CS is characterized by multiple hamartomas, which are benign, hyperplastic, disorganized growths, involving organ systems derived from all three germ cell layers and a risk of breast and thyroid cancers.[1,2] Females with CS are reported to have as high as a 67 percent risk of fibrocystic disease of the breasts and a 25 to 50 percent lifetime risk of developing invasive adenocarcinoma of the breast.[2,3] This maximum lifetime risk exceeds that of the general population in the United States (11 percent). Furthermore, affected individuals are said to have a 3 to 10 percent lifetime risk of developing epithelial thyroid carcinoma;[3–5] this, too, exceeds that of the general population (1 percent). Recent preliminary observations subsequent to the identification of the susceptibility gene suggest

that endometrial carcinoma is also a true component tumor of this syndrome.[6–8] The precise lifetime risk for endometrial cancer is as yet unknown.

The CS susceptibility gene, *PTEN*, is located on chromosome sub-band 10q23.3, and accounts for the great majority of classic CS cases.[9–11] Apart from CS, a subset of Bannayan-Riley-Ruvalcaba syndrome (BRR, MIM 153480) and a previously unclassified Proteus-like syndrome, both previously not suspected of having an increased risk of cancer, have also been found to be caused by germ line *PTEN* mutations.[12,13]

CLINICAL ASPECTS

Epidemiology

Because the diagnosis of CS is difficult, the true incidence is unknown. From an informal population-based study, the estimated gene frequency is one in one million.[9] However, after identification of the susceptibility gene, the same population base yielded an incidence of 1 in 200,000,[14,15] although the latter is likely still an underestimate. Because of frequencies such as these, this syndrome is often listed as rare, but exponents of the field suspect that it is much more common than believed. Because of the variable, protean, and often subtle external manifestations of CS, many cases remain undiagnosed[16,17] (Eng, unpublished). Indeed, between two centers in the US dedicated to the study of Cowden syndrome, more than 150 cases have been ascertained (Eng and Peacocke, unpublished). Furthermore, each of the features of CS could occur in the general population as well, thus confounding recognition of this disease. Nonetheless, CS has been reported from many countries from around the world, including those in North America, Europe, and Asia. Despite the apparent rarity of CS, the syndrome is worthy of note from both scientific and clinical viewpoints.

Because CS is likely underdiagnosed, a true count of the fraction of isolated cases (defined as no obvious family history) and familial cases (defined as two or more related affected individuals) cannot be performed. From the literature and the experience of both major US CS centers, the majority of CS cases are isolated. As a broad estimate, perhaps 10 to 50 percent of CS cases are familial.[18]

Diagnostic Criteria

CS usually presents by the time the individual is in her late twenties. It is believed that >90 percent of affected individuals should manifest a phenotype by the twenties.[8,9] By the third decade, 99 percent of affected individuals would have developed the mucocutaneous stigmata, although any of the features could be present already (Tables 31-1 and 31-2). Because the clinical literature on CS consists mostly of reports of the most obvious or most unusual families, or of case reports by subspecialists interested in their respective organ systems, the true spectrum of component signs is unknown. Despite this, the most commonly reported manifestations are mucocutaneous lesions; thyroid abnormalities; fibrocystic disease and carcinoma of the breast; gastrointestinal hamartomas; multiple, early onset uterine leiomyoma; macrocephaly (specifically, megencephaly); and mental

Table 31-1 Common Manifestations of Cowden Syndrome

Mucocutaneous Lesions (90–100%)
  Trichilemmomas
  Acral keratoses
  Verucoid or papillomatous papules
Thyroid Abnormalities (50–67%)
  Goiter
  Adenoma
  Cancer (3–10%)
Breast Lesions
  Fibroadenomas/fibrocystic disease (76% of affected females)
  Adenocarcinoma (25–50% of affected females)
Gastrointestinal Lesions (40%)
  Hamartomatous polyps
Macrocephaly (38%)
Gentiourinary Abnormalities (44% of females)
  Uterine leiomyoma (multiple, early onset)

Table 31-2 International Cowden Syndrome Consortium Operational Criteria for the Diagnosis of Cowden Syndrome (Ver. 2000)*

Pathognomonic Criteria
  Mucocutanous lesions:
    Trichilemmomas, facial
    Acral keratoses
    Papillomatous papules
    Mucosal lesions
Major Criteria
  Breast carcinoma
  Thyroid carcinoma (nonmedullary), especially follicular thyroid carcinoma
  Macrocephaly (Megalencephaly) (say, ≥97%ile)
  Lhermitte-Duclos disease (LDD)
  Endometrial carcinoma
Minor Criteria
  Other thyroid lesions (e.g., adenoma or multinodular goiter)
  Mental retardation (say, IQ ≤ 75)
  GI hamartomas
  Fibrocystic disease of the breast
  Lipomas
  Fibromas
  GU tumors (e.g., renal cell carcinoma, uterine fibroids) or malformation
Operational Diagnosis in an Individual:
1. Mucocutanous lesions alone if:
  (a) there are 6 or more facial papules, of which 3 or more must be trichilemmoma, or
  (b) cutaneous facial papules and oral mucosal papillomatosis, or
  (c) oral mucosal papillomatosis and acral keratoses, or
  (d) palmoplantar keratoses, 6 or more
2. 2 Major criteria but one must include macrocephaly or LDD
3. 1 Major and 3 minor criteria
4. 4 Minor criteria
Operational Diagnosis in a Family Where One Individual Is Diagnostic for Cowden
1. The pathognomonic criterion/ia
2. Any one major criterion with or without minor criteria
3. Two minor criteria

*Operational diagnostic criteria are reviewed and revised on a continuous basis as new clinical and genetic information becomes available. The 1995 version and the 2000 version have been accepted by the US-based National Comprehensive Cancer Network High Risk/Genetics Panel.

retardation (Table 31-1).[3–5,8,19] Pathognomonic mucocutaneous lesions are trichilemmomas and papillomatous papules (Table 31-2, Fig. 31-1). Because of the lack of uniform diagnostic criteria for CS prior to 1995, a group of individuals, the International Cowden Consortium, interested in systematically studying this syndrome to localize the susceptibility gene, arrived at a set of consensus operational diagnostic criteria.[9,20] These criteria were revised recently in the context of new data and are reflected in the practice guidelines of the US-based National Comprehensive Cancer Network Genetics/High Risk Panel (Table 31-2).[8,21]

The two documented component cancers in CS are carcinoma of the breast and thyroid[3] (illustrated by pedigree shown in Fig. 31-2). By contrast, in the general population, lifetime risks for breast and thyroid cancers are approximately 11 percent (in women), and 1 percent, respectively. In women with CS, lifetime risk estimates for the development of breast cancer range from 25 to 50 percent.[3–5,22] The mean age at diagnosis is likely 10 years earlier than breast cancer occurring in the general population.[3,5] Although Rachel Cowden died of breast cancer at the age of 31,[1,2] and the earliest recorded age of diagnosis of breast cancer is 14,[3] the majority of CS breast cancers are diagnosed after the age of 30 to 35 years (range, 14 to 65).[5] Until genotype-phenotype analyses were performed with the discovery of the susceptibility gene, it was thought that male breast cancer was not a component of CS. However, male breast cancer does occur in *PTEN* mutation-positive CS, but with unknown frequency.[11,23]

The lifetime risk for nonmedullary thyroid cancer can be as high as 10 percent in males and females with CS. Because of small numbers, it is unclear whether the age of onset is truly earlier than that of the general population. Histologically, the thyroid cancer is predominantly follicular carcinoma although papillary histology has also been rarely observed[3–5] (Eng, unpublished observations). After identification of *PTEN* as the susceptibility gene, preliminary data suggest that endometrial carcinoma is a component cancer of CS.[6–8] What its frequency is in mutation carriers is as yet unknown.

Benign tumors are also common in CS (Tables 31-1 and 31-3). Apart from those of the skin, benign tumors or disorders of breast and thyroid are the most frequently noted and likely represent true component features of this syndrome (Table 31-1). Fibroadenomas and fibrocystic disease of the breast are common signs in CS, as are follicular adenomas and multinodular goiter of the thyroid. An unusual central nervous system tumor, cerebellar dysplastic gangliocytoma or Lhermitte-Duclos disease, was only recently associated with CS[24,25] (illustrated in pedigree in Fig. 31-2).

Other malignancies and benign tumors have been reported in patients or families with CS (Tables 31-3 and 31-4). Whether malignant tumors other than those in the breast, thyroid, and endometrium, are true components of CS, or whether some are coincidental findings, is as yet unknown.

Histology

Like other inherited cancer syndromes, multifocality and bilateral involvement is the rule. Hamartomas are the hallmark of CS. These are classic hamartomas in general. They are benign tumors that comprise all the elements of a particular organ but in a disorganized fashion. Of note, the hamartomatous polyps found in this syndrome are different in histomorphology from Peutz-Jeghers polyps, which have a distinct appearance. A preliminary report examining the gastrointestinal manifestations of nine patients from six unrelated CS kindreds found that all patients examined had colonic nonadenomatous hamartomatous polyps.[26] Additionally, a majority had acanthosis of the esophagus.[26]

With regard to the individual cancers, even of the breast and thyroid, as of mid 1997, there has yet to be a systematic study published. Recently, however, one study has attempted to look at benign and malignant breast pathology in CS patients. Although these are preliminary studies, without true matched controls, it is, to date, the only study that examines breast pathology in a series of CS cases. Breast histopathology from 59 cases belonging to 19 CS women was systematically analyzed.[17] Thirty-five specimens had some form of malignant pathology. Of these, 31 (90 percent) had ductal adenocarcinoma, 1 had tubular carcinoma, and 1 had lobular

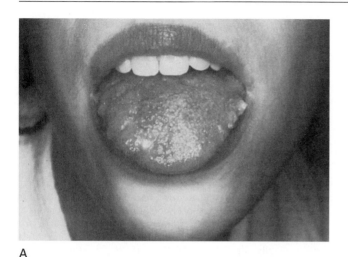

A

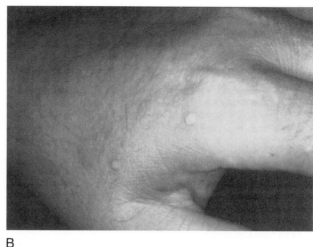

B

Figure 31-1 Characteristic mucocutaneous features of Cowden syndrome. *A*, Scrotal tongue comprising papillomatous papules. *B*, Papillomatous papules of the skin.

carcinoma-*in-situ*. Sixteen of the 31 specimens had both invasive and *in situ* (DCIS) components of ductal carcinoma, while 12 specimens had DCIS only, and 2 had only invasive adenocarcinoma. Interestingly, it was noted that 19 of these carcinomas appeared to have arisen in the midst of densely fibrotic hamartomatous tissue.

Benign thyroid pathology is more common in CS than is malignant thyroid pathology. Multinodular goiter and thyroid adenomas are often noted. Follicular thyroid carcinomas are much more common than papillary histology.[3,19,22] No systematic studies on thyroid or endometrial pathology in CS have been performed.

GENETICS

CS is an autosomal dominant disorder with age-related penetrance. It is believed that the penetrance is 90 percent after the age of 20 years.[9] Not much was known about the genetics of CS prior to 1996. The International Cowden Consortium examined 12 classic CS families and found that the then putative susceptibility locus was on 10q22-24, without genetic heterogeneity,[9] although it has also been suggested that rare locus heterogeneity might occur.[27] Subsequently, germ-line mutations of *PTEN*, which encodes a dual

specificity phosphatase, were found in CS.[10] That *PTEN* is the CS gene has been confirmed by other groups.[14,27,28]

Germline *PTEN* mutations in families with Bannayan-Riley-Ruvalcaba syndrome (BRR) have also been found.[12] Thus, at least a subset of BRR and CS may be considered allelic. Recently, an individual with an unclassified Proteus-like syndrome, who did not meet the criteria for diagnosis of either BRR or Proteus syndrome, was found to harbor a germ line *PTEN* mutation, as well as a germ-line mosaic *PTEN* mutation.[13] What proportion of Proteus-like or even classic Proteus patients actually have *PTEN* mutations is currently unknown and the topic of ongoing investigation.

Table 31-3 Noncutaneous Benign Lesions Reported in Cowden Syndrome

Nervous System	Genitourinary
Lhermitte-Duclos disease	Female
Megencephaly	Leiomyomas
Glioma	Ovarian cysts
Meningioma	Vaginal and vulvar cysts
Neuroma	Various developmental
Neurofibroma	anomalies (e.g., duplicated
Bridged sella turcica	collecting system)
Mental retardation	Male
Breast	Hydrocele
Fibrocystic disease	Varicocele
Fibroadenoma	Hypoplastic testes
Hamartoma	Skeletal
Gynecomastia of male breast	Craniomegaly
Thyroid	Adenoid facies
Goiter	High arched palate
Adenoma	Hypoplastic zygoma
Thyroiditis	Kyphoscoliosis
Thyroglossal duct cyst	Pectus excavatum
Rudimentary sixth digit	Bone cysts
Hyperthyroidism	Other
Hypothyroidism	Hypoplastic vulva
Gastrointestinal	Atrial septal defect
Hamartomatous polyposis	Arteriovenous
of entire tract	malformations
Diverticuli of colon and sigmoid	Eye cataracts
Ganglioneuroma	Retinal angioid streaks
Leiomyoma	
Hepatic hamartoma	

LDD 60

Meg Birth
MNG 26
Trich 15
PP 12

FTC 27
BR 36
PP 15
Trich 15

Trich 10
PP 10
MNG 15

Figure 31-2 Hypothetical CS family pedigree. *LDD*, Lhermitte-Duclos disease; *Meg*, megencephaly; *MNG*, multinodular goiter; *Trich*, trichilemmoma; *PP*, papillomatous papules; *FTC*, follicular thyroid carcinoma; *BR*, breast adenocarcinoma.

Table 31-4 Reported Malignancies in Patients with Cowden Syndrome

Central Nervous System
  Glioblastoma multiforme
Mucocutaneous
  Squamous cell carcinoma
  Basal cell carcinoma
  Malignant melanoma
  Merkel cell carcinoma
Breast
  Adenocarcinoma
Endocrine
  Nonmedullary thyroid carcinoma (classically of follicular histology)
Pulmonary
  Nonsmall-cell carcinoma
Gastrointestinal
  Colorectal carcinoma
  Hepatocellular carcinoma
  Pancreatic carcinoma
Genitourinary
  Uterine carcinoma
  Ovarian carcinoma
  Transitional cell carcinoma of the bladder
  Renal cell carcinoma
Other
  Liposarcoma

Genotype-Phenotype Associations in CS

For purposes of genotype-phenotype analyses, a series of 37 unrelated CS probands were ascertained by the operational diagnostic criteria of the International Cowden Consortium (Ver. 1995).[8,9] Thirty of the 37 (81 percent) probands were found to harbor germ line *PTEN* mutations.[11] Approximately two-thirds of all mutations were found in exons 5, 7, or 8. Forty percent of mutations were found within exon 5 alone, which encodes the phosphatase core motif, although this exon represents only 20 percent of the PTEN coding sequence. In the worldwide experience as of January 2000,[29] approximately one-third of all *CS* mutations were noted to be in exon 5 and 65 percent were noted to be in exons 5, 7, or 8 (Fig. 31-3). Of anecdotal note, there were two male probands with germ line *PTEN* mutations and breast cancer.[23] Association analyses revealed that CS families with germ line *PTEN* mutations are more likely to develop malignant breast disease, as compared to *PTEN* mutation-negative families.[11] In addition, missense mutations and those within the phosphatase core motif and 5' of it appeared to be associated with involvement of 5 or more organs, a surrogate phenotype for severity of disease.[11] Another group examined families for germ line *PTEN* mutations and found mutations in only 13 probands.[15] They could not find any clear genotype-phenotype associations, most likely because of their small sample size.

Genotype-Phenotype Associations in BRR

Because CS and a subset of BRR are allelic, 43 unrelated BRR cases were ascertained by standard clinical criteria for purposes of examining their *PTEN* mutation spectrum in the context of that of CS and to analyze genotype-phenotype associations. In contrast to CS, 60 percent of BRR were found to have germ line *PTEN* mutations.[18] In addition, two of these mutations were one with a cytogenetically detectable deletion of 10q23, encompassing *PTEN*, and another with a translocation involving 10q23.[18,30,31] The mutational spectra of BRR and CS seemed to overlap, thus lending formal proof that CS and BRR are allelic.[18] In the published literature as of January 2000,[18,29] approximately 17 percent of BRR probands with *PTEN* mutations have mutations located in exon 5, in contrast to 33 percent for CS. There was no difference in mutation frequencies between isolated BRR and familial BRR.[18] Of note, >90 percent of CS-BRR overlap families had germ line *PTEN* mutations. The presence of *PTEN* mutations in BRR was associated with the development of any cancer, tumors of the breast, and lipomas.[18] Therefore, the presence of *PTEN* mutations in BRR may have implications for cancer surveillance in this syndrome, which was previously not believed to be associated with malignancy. In view of the genetic and molecular epidemiologic data to date, clinical cancer geneticists have found it more useful to consider, and thus to medically manage, individuals with germ line *PTEN* mutations not by clinical syndromic names but under the rubric of *PTEN* Hamartoma Tumor syndrome (PHTS).[18]

Occult Germ Line *PTEN* Mutations and Cryptic PHTS

The true range of the clinical PHTS spectrum is unknown. This spectrum is important to delineate for purposes of understanding the biology and for the practical purpose of practicing evidence-based clinical cancer genetics. When CS is ascertained by the strict Consortium criteria (Table 31-2), a full 80 percent of patients carry germ line *PTEN* mutations.[11] Because CS is difficult to diagnose

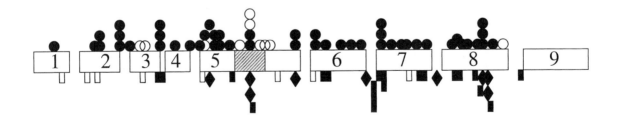

      ▨ Phosphatase core motif

      ● Cowden syndrome, truncating mutation

      ○ Cowden syndrome, missense mutation

■ BRR, truncating mutation

□ BRR, missense mutation

◆ CS-BRR overlap family

Figure 31-3 Representation of *PTEN* and its mutations found in CS, BRR, and CS-BRR probands in the published literature.[11,18,29] Spaces between exons (boxes) represent introns. Nonsense, frameshift, and splice mutations are considered truncating mutations for purposes of this figure.

clinically, ascertainment of CS varies from center to center; thus, the frequency of germ line *PTEN* mutations also varies greatly. Mutation frequencies as low as 10 percent have been described.[27] For purposes of examining the clinical spectrum of PHTS and to test the robustness of the Consortium clinical criteria, probands and families were ascertained with the minimal features of breast cancer and thyroid disease in a single individual or two first-degree relatives, but must not meet the 1995 version of the Consortium criteria.[6] Of the 64 families in this initial series, approximately 2 percent were found to harbor occult germ line *PTEN* mutations.[6] This study concluded that the presence of endometrial carcinoma might increase the probability of finding the presence of occult germ line *PTEN* mutation in such CS-like families.[6] It also demonstrated that even at a molecular level, the Consortium criteria for clinical diagnosis of CS are robust. That endometrial carcinoma might be an important component of CS may be corroborated by another study that sought to examine the frequency of occult germ line *PTEN* mutation in women with multiple primary cancers.[7] In this nested cohort of 103 eligible women from the Nurses Health Study, 5 women had germ line *PTEN* missense mutations. Of these five women, two had endometrial cancer. This study, therefore, suggests that occult germ line mutations of *PTEN* and, by extrapolation, of CS, occur with a higher frequency than previously believed. These two studies together, as well as increasing clinical experience with CS and PHTS, suggested that endometrial cancer might be a true component of CS, and thus, has been added to the revised diagnostic criteria of the Consortium (Table 31-2).[8]

What is the frequency of occult germ line *PTEN* mutations when individuals present with a single CS-component tumor? This is germane as it addresses the issue of penetrance and has implications for medical and surgical oncology practices. When 62 unrelated women under the age of 40 years with diagnosed breast cancer were examined for the occult presence of germ line *PTEN* mutations, two (3.2 percent) were found to have missense mutations.[32] Despite all these studies, site-specific breast cancer families without CS features not linked to *BRCA1* or *BRCA2* were found not to be linked to 10q23[33] and were not found to have germ line *PTEN* mutations.[34] There have been no formal studies ascertaining the frequency of occult germ line *PTEN* mutations in presentations of nonmedullary thyroid cancer or endometrial cancer. Such information, nonetheless, can be extrapolated from studies primarily examining for somatic *PTEN* mutations in these sporadic cancers. Amongst these series, there have been no cases of occult germ line *PTEN* mutations in presentations of nonfamilial nonmedullary thyroid cancer cases or sporadic endometrial cancer cases.[35–40]

CLINICAL CANCER GENETICS

Differential Diagnosis

Because CS has variable expression, several differential diagnoses have to be considered. BRR could be considered in the differential diagnosis although with the identification of *PTEN* mutations in patients and families with BRR, it is believed that CS and at least one subset of BRR should be considered a single genetic entity, with the proposed name of PTEN Hamartoma Tumor Syndrome.[18] The PHTS entity is of practical importance because there are currently at least 14 families with an overlap of both CS and BRR features[18] (Eng, unpublished observations). To date, at least one Proteus-like individual has been found to have germ line *PTEN* mutation.[13]

Other differential diagnoses to consider are encompassed by other hamartoma syndromes, including juvenile polyposis (JPS, MIM 174900) and Peutz-Jeghers syndrome (PJS, MIM 174900). JPS is an autosomal dominant disorder that is characterized by hamartomatous polyps in the gastrointestinal tract and a high risk of colorectal cancer, and may be viewed as a clinical diagnosis of exclusion. A single report claimed that germ line *PTEN* mutations

can occur in JPS.[41] However, closer inspection of these probands revealed that one likely had CS and the other was too young to clinically exclude CS, given that the penetrance under the age of 20 for classic CS is <10 percent. When Kurose and colleagues ascertained a series of patients with the diagnosis of juvenile polyposis, he found one with germ line *PTEN* mutation, and unlike the previous series, these investigators were able to recall that patient for reexamination, and discovered clinical stigmata of CS.[42] Recently, a report described a 55-year-old father and two young children, the latter of whom presented with hamartomatous polyps and was given the presumptive clinical diagnosis of JPS, were found to have germ line *PTEN* mutation.[43] Although it was stated that these individuals had no other signs of CS/BRR, little detail on the physical examination was noted in the report. It is suspected that examination of the father by clinical cancer geneticists facile with the manifestations of CS would reveal some physical findings consistent with CS/BRR. Nonetheless, the discovery of occult germ line mutations in this "JPS" family should initiate management of this family as a PHTS. Thus, finding a germ line *PTEN* mutation in a presumed JPS case alters the diagnosis to CS, i.e., to PHTS.[44] After all, a major *JPS* locus was identified on 18q, and germ line mutations in *SMAD4* have been found in a subset of JPS.[45–47] PJS, which carries a high risk of intestinal carcinomas and breast cancers, should be clinically quite distinct. The pigmentation of the peroral region in this autosomal dominant hamartoma syndrome is pathognomonic.[48,49] The hamartomatous polyp in PJS has a diagnostic appearance as well, and is referred to as the Peutz-Jeghers polyp. They are unlike the hamartomatous polyps seen in CS and JPS. Clinically, although Peutz-Jeghers polyps are often symptomatic (intersusception, rectal bleeding), CS polyps are rarely so. Germ line mutations in *LKB1/STK11*, on 19p, have been found in isolated and familial PJS cases,[50–52] although some believe that there is a minor susceptibility gene on 19q as well.[53]

Proteus syndrome (MIM176920) might be considered in the differential diagnosis of CS because of the common theme of overgrowth, e.g., hemihypertrophy, macrocephaly, and lipomatosis.[54] Like CS, Proteus syndrome can have a broad spectrum of phenotypic expression and so, its diagnosis is also made by consensus operational criteria.[55] Mandatory diagnostic criteria include mosaic distribution of lesions, progressive course, and sporadic occurrence.[55] In a small pilot study to determine if Proteus syndrome is part of PHTS, an apparently isolated case of a Proteus-like syndrome comprising hemihypertrophy, macrocephaly, lipomas, connective tissue nevi, and multiple arteriovenous malformations was found to have a germ line *PTEN* mutation R335X.[13] Interestingly, a nevus, a lipomatous region and arteriovenous malformation tissue were found to harbor a second hit nongerm line *PTEN* mutation R130X, possibly representing a germ line mosaic. Both these mutations have been previously described in classic CS and BRR. Thus, this Proteus-like case may be classified as PHTS at the molecular level, with implications for the development of malignancies characteristic of CS/BRR. What proportion of clinical Proteus syndrome or Proteus-like cases will be reclassified as PHTS at the molecular level is unknown and currently under study by several centers.

Other, less likely, differential diagnoses to consider are neurofibromatosis type 1 (NF-1), and basal cell nevus (Gorlin) syndrome, although the latter should not be confused clinically with CS or BRR. In NF-1, the only two consistent features seen in both NF-1 and CS/BRR are café-au-lait macules and fibromatous tumors of the skin. Plexiform neuromas are highly suggestive of NF-1. The susceptibility gene for this syndrome has been isolated as *NF1* on 17q.[56,57] Because of the large size of the gene, direct mutation analysis is still impractical. In informative families, linkage analysis is feasible for predictive testing purposes and is 98 percent accurate.[58] Basal cell nevus syndrome is an autosomal dominant condition characterized by basal cell nevi, basal cell carcinoma, and diverse developmental abnormalities. In addition, affected individuals can develop other tumors and cancers, such as fibromas, hamartomatous gastric polyps, and medulloblastomas. However, the dermatologic findings and developmental features in CS and basal cell nevus syndrome are quite different. For instance, the palmar pits together with the characteristic facies of the latter are never seen in CS. The (A major?) susceptibility gene for basal cell nevus syndrome is also distinct from CS/BRR, and is the human homologue of the Drosophila *patched* gene, *PTC* on 9q22-31.[59] Linkage analysis and mutation analysis are technically possible. However, because it is not known what proportion of patients with this syndrome will actually turn out to have mutations in *PTC*, predictive testing based on mutation analysis alone should be deferred until more data become available.

Clinical Cancer Genetic Management

The key to proper clinical cancer genetic consultation in CS is recognition of the syndrome. Families with CS should be advised as for any autosomal dominant trait with high penetrance. What is unclear, however, is the variability of expression between and within families. We suspect that there are CS families who have nothing but trichilemmomas and, therefore, never come to medical attention. Based on the current data, it might also be prudent to treat all patients with PHTS, no matter what their apparent clinical syndrome is, as if it were CS.

The two most serious, and established, component tumors in CS are breast cancer and nonmedullary thyroid cancer for both affected females and males. Endometrial cancer is now believed to be a component of CS, at least for medical management purposes (see above).[8] Patients with CS or those who are at risk for CS should undergo surveillance for these three cancers. Beginning in their teens, these individuals should undergo annual physical examinations paying particular attention to the thyroid. Beginning in their mid twenties, women with CS or those at risk for it, should be encouraged to perform monthly breast self-examinations and to have careful breast examinations during their annual physicals. The value of annual imaging studies is unclear because there are no objective data available. Nonetheless, we usually recommend annual mammography and/or breast ultrasounds performed by skilled individuals in women-at-risk beginning at age 30 years, or 5 years earlier than the earliest breast cancer case in the family, whichever is younger. Some women with CS develop severe, sometimes disfiguring, fibroadenomas of the breasts well before age 30 years. This situation should be treated individually. For example, if the fibroadenomas cause pain, or if they make breast cancer surveillance impossible, then some have advocated prophylactic mastectomies.[2] Careful annual physical examination of the thyroid and neck region beginning at age 18 years, or 5 years younger than the earliest diagnosis of thyroid cancer in the family (whichever is earlier), should be sufficient, although a single baseline thyroid ultrasound in the early twenties might be considered as well. Surveillance for endometrial carcinoma is recommended, perhaps beginning at the age of 35 to 40 years (no data for age at onset), or at 5 years younger than the earliest onset case in the family (whichever is earlier). For premenopausal women, annual blind repel (suction) biopsies of the endometrium should be performed. In the postmenopausal years, transabdominal uterine ultrasound examinations should suffice.

Whether other tumors are true components of CS is unknown. It is believed, however, that skin cancers, for instance, might be features of CS. For now, however, surveillance for other organs should follow the American Cancer Society guidelines, although proponents of CS will advise routine skin surveillance also. Some clinical cancer geneticists recommend surveillance for the development of renal cell carcinoma as well, including urinalysis for occult blood and perhaps renal ultrasound.

A preliminary study demonstrated that the presence of germ line *PTEN* mutation in BRR is associated with cancer development.[18] Until additional data become available, it might be conservative to manage all BRR individuals and families, especially those harboring germ line *PTEN* mutations, as if it were CS with respect to cancer formation and surveillance. Given the data that

have accumulated regarding *PTEN* mutations and PHTS, it seems that routine clinical laboratory testing for *PTEN* mutations both as a molecular diagnostic tool and as a predictive tool might become commonplace. In the United States, at least one academic center offers clinical *PTEN* testing, with the molecular diagnostics laboratory working very closely with the Clinical Cancer Genetics Program.

The key to successful management of CS and all PHTS patients and their families is a multidisciplinary team. There should always be a primary care provider, usually a general internist, who orchestrates the care of such patients, many of whom may need the care of surgeons, gynecologists, dermatologists, oncologists, and clinical cancer geneticists.

SOMATIC GENOMIC AND EPIGENETIC *PTEN* ALTERATIONS IN SPORADIC NEOPLASIA

Somatic *PTEN* mutations and/or deletions occur with variable frequency depending on neoplasia type. When *PTEN* was initially isolated, a wide variety of neoplastic cell line models yielded apparently high frequencies of homozygous *PTEN* mutations and deletions,[60,61] and were somewhat misleading indicators for predicting the frequency of "two-hit" genetic alterations in noncultured primary malignancies.

PTEN Alterations in Sporadic Counterparts of CS-Component Cancers

The sporadic CS-component cancers illustrating somatic mutation and PTEN silencing are those of the breast, thyroid, and endometrium. Interestingly, among the three types of sporadic component tumors, only endometrial carcinoma had any frequency of somatic intragenic *PTEN* mutations. In noncultured primary breast carcinomas, the high mutation and deletion frequency observed in breast cancer cell lines has not been borne out.[62-65] In one study of 54 unselected primary breast carcinomas, only 1 true somatic mutation was noted.[62] Even when selected for 10q23 hemizygous deletion, only 1 of 14 samples had a somatic intragenic mutation.[64] Consistently, deletions in the region of *PTEN*, 10q22-24, occur in 30 to 40 percent of primary breast carcinomas.[63-65] In one study, hemizygous deletion of *PTEN* and the 10q23 region occurred with any frequency only in invasive carcinomas of the breast but not in *in situ* cancers, and appeared to be associated with loss of estrogen receptor expression.[64] In order to examine mechanisms of PTEN inactivation other than genetic, 33 well-characterized primary invasive breast adenocarcinomas without intragenic *PTEN* mutations[66] were analyzed for *PTEN* deletion and PTEN expression by immunohistochemistry.[67] Of these cancers, 11 had hemizygous deletion of *PTEN*. Five of these 11 cancers with hemizygous deletion had complete PTEN silencing, while the remainder had decreased PTEN expression. These observations argue that the second hit in breast cancers might be epigenetic.

Shortly after the identification of *PTEN* as the *CS* gene, three studies have revealed somatic *PTEN* mutation in 34 to 50 percent of apparently sporadic endometrial carcinoma.[37-39] From these three early series, it was noted that the frequency of intragenic mutation was much higher (86 percent) in those of endometrioid histology with microsatellite instability.[38] Recently, however, 83 percent of endometrioid endometrial carcinomas belonging to a single institutional series were shown to have somatic intragenic mutations, and the frequency was equivalently high irrespective of microsatellite stability status.[40] This observation regarding microsatellite status was corroborated independently.[68] Interestingly, in the single institutional series, only 33 percent had deletions or mutations involving both *PTEN* alleles, yet 61 percent expressed no protein.[40] In matched precancers, 55 percent had intragenic mutation, while 75 percent had no expression. Hence, *PTEN* mutation is an early event initiating endometrial precancers[40,69] and epigenetic PTEN silencing can precede genetic alteration in the earliest precancers.[40]

Deletions, represented by loss of heterozygosity (LOH) of anonymous polymorphic markers residing on chromosome 10, have been well documented in both benign and malignant epithelial thyroid neoplasia over the course of the last 10 years.[70] Three series, based mainly on thyroid tumors of European origin, demonstrated that hemizygous deletion of *PTEN* occurs with a higher frequency in follicular adenomas (20 to 25 percent) as compared to follicular carcinomas (5 to 10 percent).[35,71,72] The apparent higher LOH frequency in adenomas, as compared to carcinomas, was not observed in a single US-based series.[36] The only intragenic point mutation amongst all series to date was a somatic frameshift mutation in a single papillary thyroid carcinoma.[35] These observations suggest that the pathogenesis of adenomas and carcinomas may proceed along two different pathways, and that the adenoma-carcinoma sequence is not the rule in epithelial thyroid neoplasia.[72] The data were at-first surprising in that epithelial thyroid malignancies do occur in 3 to 10 percent of CS patients,[3,22] and one would expect that a larger proportion of sporadic thyroid carcinomas are associated with somatic *PTEN* alteration. It was rationalized that benign thyroid disease occurs in 50 to 67 percent of CS individuals, far outnumbering the frequency of thyroid carcinomas. However, a recent expression and genetic analysis of 139 benign and malignant nonmedullary thyroid tumors yielded some interesting data that may begin to address this apparent paradox.[73] In this series, follicular adenomas, follicular carcinomas, and papillary thyroid carcinomas all had a 20 to 30 percent frequency of hemizygous deletion, while almost 60 percent of undifferentiated (anaplastic) carcinomas had hemizygous *PTEN* deletion. Of note, hemizygous deletion and decreased PTEN expression were associated. Decreasing PTEN expression was observed with declining degree of differentiation. Decreasing nuclear PTEN expression seemed to precede that in the cytoplasm. The thyroid data suggest that in addition to structural deletion, inappropriate subcellular compartmentalization might also contribute to PTEN inactivation.[73]

Somatic *PTEN* Alterations in Sporadic Noncomponent Neoplasias

Of several types of sporadic non-CS-component neoplasias, glioblastoma multiforme has been consistently found to harbor the highest frequency of somatic intragenic *PTEN* mutations and deletions, as well as "second-hit" intragenic mutations or deletions.[74-77] However, lower grade gliomas were not found to be associated with *PTEN* mutations, nor were meningiomas.[74,78] Similar to glioblastoma multiforme, it would appear that up to a quarter of sporadic primary squamous cell carcinomas of the cervix, at least of Japanese origin, carry two somatic genetic hits comprising an intragenic mutation together with deletion of the wild-type allele or homozygous deletion.[79] Somatic *PTEN* alterations have not been previously noted in noncultured cervical cancers,[80] which may be explained by technical issues or country of origin.

In a series of 44 sporadic ovarian carcinomas, approximately 75 percent have no or decreased PTEN expression, of which half are a result of epigenetic means.[81] Again, intragenic somatic mutation occurred rarely, <5 percent of tumors. Many tumors with altered PTEN expression have increased levels of P-Akt, a known proapoptotic factor (see Mechanism of PTEN Tumor Suppression below), but there were carcinomas which had decreased/no PTEN expression and decreased levels of P-Akt as well. The latter suggests that PTEN might signal down the Akt pathway, as well as down an Akt-independent pathway, a postulate that has been corroborated by *in vitro* biochemical studies as well.[82]

LOH of markers along chromosome arm 10q in malignant melanomas is not a new finding.[83,84] Although melanoma cell lines carry a high frequency of intragenic *PTEN* mutations and "two-hit" genetic alterations, the frequencies of intragenic *PTEN* mutations in noncultured melanomas are variable.[61,85-87] A recent study using unselected, uncultured primary and metastatic malignant melanomas clearly demonstrated that somatic intragenic *PTEN* mutations are rare, occurring in <10 percent of melanomas.[88] Confirming previous studies, about a third of these tumors had hemizygous deletion in the *PTEN* region. What was surprising, however, was the high frequency of complete abrogation of PTEN expression (15 percent) and depressed levels of PTEN expression (50 percent).[88] Thus, epigenetic monoallelic and biallelic *PTEN* silencing might be a major mechanism of PTEN inactivation in uncultured melanomas.

It is now obvious, with accumulating knowledge of somatic *PTEN* genetics in sporadic tumors, that several different mechanisms, and not just somatic intragenic mutations, may inactivate PTEN. Several mechanisms of inactivation can occur in a single tumor type, like in primary ovarian carcinomas,[81] although the sense is that one particular mechanism predominates in any one tissue type. For example, in the endometrial neoplasia system, either two genetic hits or one genetic hit and one epigenetic silencing hit can occur, although the latter predominates.[40] In malignant melanoma, both inactivating hits for PTEN are epigenetic.[88] In contrast, PTEN might also be inactivated by differential subcellular compartmentalization as illustrated by thyroid neoplasia and endocrine pancreatic tumours.[73,89] This mechanism is puzzling, as PTEN has no obvious nuclear localization signal. The precise mechanisms of nongenetic inactivation need further exploration.

MECHANISM OF PTEN TUMOR SUPPRESSION

The initial identification of PTEN's tyrosine phosphatase domain, and the germ line and somatic missense mutations within it, stimulated the search for substrates. Initial experiments identified that PTEN could remove phosphates from proteins and peptides containing phosphotyrosines, phosphoserines, and phosphothreonines.[90,91] Moreover, phosphatase activity correlated with tumor suppressor function because most of the germ line missense mutations lacked phosphatase activity *in vitro*. However, a few CS phosphatase domain mutations remained fully functional in these assays suggesting that the protein substrates were not physiologic.[90]

One potential candidate substrate was the oncogenic phospholipid phosphatidylinositol-3,4,5-triphosphate (PI3,4,5P). No known phosphatase was able to remove the D-3 phosphate from PI3,4,5P. PI3,4,5P is generated when phosphatidylinositol-3 (PI3) kinase phosphorylates the D-3 position of phosphatidylinositol-4,5-diphosphate on the inner leaflet of the plasma membrane.[92] Increased enzymatic activity of PI3 kinase (PI3K) is associated with the oncogenic transformation of cells. The polyoma middle-T-antigen oncogene binds and activates PI3K.[93] Moreover, the catalytic subunit of PI3K is a retroviral oncogene and is amplified in ovarian cancer.[94,95] In normal cells, PI3K activity is tightly regulated. Ligands for a variety of receptors elicit the association of the activated receptor complex with the p85 regulatory subunit of PI3K. The association of the receptor complex with PI3K stimulates the enzyme for several minutes following ligand binding. The PI3,4,5P level rises as a result but is rapidly metabolized.

Mahaema and Dixon tested the hypothesis that PI3,4,5P is a substrate for PTEN.[96] They demonstrated that PTEN could remove the D-3 phosphate from PI3,4,5P and thereby directly opposed the effect of PI-3 kinase. Moreover, they found that PTEN could metabolize the PI3,4,5P generated *in vivo* in response to insulin. Soon thereafter *pten* −/− cells were found to have elevated levels of PI3,4,5P.[97,98] CS-type *PTEN* mutations that were able to dephosphorylate protein substrates were then tested for their ability to remove the D-3 phosphate from PI3,4,5P. Interestingly, all of the mutations that were enzymatically active on protein substrates were unable to dephosphorylate PIP3,4,5.[99,100] These data strongly support the conclusion that the lipid phosphatase activity of PTEN is its major mechanism of tumor suppression.

Cells express a variety of proteins that are regulated by PI3,4,5P. These proteins contain a form of pleckstrin homology

(PH) domain that binds PI3,4,5P with high affinity. One such protein that has attracted a great deal of attention is AKT/protein kinase B.[101] The gene for this protein was first isolated from a mouse retroviral oncogene, and AKT1 and AKT2 are amplified in different forms of human cancer. AKT has an impact on many signaling pathways through the phosphorylation of substrates. In particular, AKT is able to inhibit apoptosis and stimulate the cell cycle. After binding PI3,4,5P at the membrane, AKT is phosphorylated at amino acids 308 and 473, which activates its kinase. Increased phosphorylation of these amino acids and increased kinase activity was observed in *PTEN* −/− tumors and mouse embryo fibroblasts.[97,102–105] In addition, the transient expression of PTEN reduced AKT phosphorylation and activation. Expression of exogenous PTEN led to G1 arrest of the cell cycle and/or apoptosis depending upon the cell system. In several systems, AKT was able to rescue cells from PTEN-mediated apoptosis.[97,104] Moreover, *pten* −/− mouse embryo fibroblasts and +/− B lymphocytes were resistant to apoptosis.[97,106,107] On the other hand, *pten* −/− embryos exhibited increased proliferation prior to lethality, as did *pten* −/− embryonic stem cells in soft agar and under serum-deprived conditions. Therefore, it appears that loss of PTEN affects both the cell cycle and apoptosis.

The relationship of PTEN to PI3K and AKT has been reproducibly confirmed in the lower organisms *Caenorhabditis elegans* and *Drosophila melanogaster*.[108–114] In both systems, a single homologue has been mapped by epistasis analysis to be downstream of an insulin-like receptor and PI3K and upstream of AKT. The role of PTEN in insulin signaling might also hold true in a human tumor model, whereby PTEN, in the presence of insulin, depresses phosphorylation of insulin receptor substrate-1 (IRS-1) with consequent failure to recruit Grb-2 and Sos to IRS-1.[115] Interestingly, PTEN also induces the expression of IRS-2 and the latter's association with the p85 subunit of PI3K.[116] In *Drosophila*, *Pten* −/− cells reduce apoptosis and increase proliferation and cell size in a PI3K/AKT-dependent and independent manner,[109] an observation that holds true in humans as well.[82] The domain structure of Pten also supports its function as a PI3,4,5P phosphatase. The crystal structure of Pten contains two globular domains, the phosphatase and C2 domains.[117] The catalytic pocket of PTEN is wider than the pocket of tyrosine phosphatases, which allows for the binding of inositol head groups. The C2 domain binds to phosphatidyl serine, positions the protein at the membrane and is necessary for productive interaction with the PI3,4,5P substrate.

The introduction of germline mutations of *pten* in mice has validated the tumor suppressor function of pten.[106,107,118,119] Mice develop spontaneous tumors of the uterus, thyroid (papillary histology), prostate, mammaries, lymphocytes, liver, intestine, and adrenal medulla. Tumors frequently demonstrate loss of the wild-type *pten* allele, elevated proliferation, and increased AKT activity. Interestingly, the mice do not develop hamartomas, the hallmark of human CS and BRR, and the types of tumors that they do develop are not reminiscent of human CS or BRR. Recently, a single knock-out mouse model was found to develop endometrial carcinoma relatively late; although this occurred with some frequency in the mouse, this has only recently been recognized as a secondary component tumor of CS.[8] Although the murine tumors affecting the lymphoid system, liver, and adrenal medulla are never seen in human CS or BRR, these are organs in which *PTEN* is highly expressed in both human and murine development.[120,121]

REFERENCES

1. Lloyd KM, Denis M: Cowden's disease: A possible new symptom complex with multiple system involvement. *Ann Intern Med* **58**:136, 1963.
2. Brownstein MH, Wolf M, Bilowski JB: Cowden's disease. *Cancer* **41**:2393, 1978.
3. Starink TM, van der Veen JPW, Arwert F, de Waal LP, de Lange GG, Gille JJP, Eriksson AW: The Cowden syndrome: A clinical and genetic study in 21 patients. *Clin Genet* **29**:222, 1986.
4. Hanssen AMN, Fryns JP: Cowden syndrome. *J Med Genet* **32**:117, 1995.
5. Longy M, Lacombe D: Cowden disease. Report of a family and review. *Ann Genet* **39**:35, 1996.
6. Marsh DJ, Caron S, Dahia PLM, Kum JB, Frayling IM, Tomlinson IPM, Hughes KS, Hodgson SV, Murday VA, Houlston R, Eng C: Germline *PTEN* mutations in Cowden syndrome-like families. *J Med Genet* **35**:881, 1998.
7. De Vivo I, Gertig D, Nagase S, Hankinson SE, OBrien R, Speizer FE, Parsons R, Hunter DJ: Novel germline mutations in the *PTEN* tumour suppressor gene found in women with multiple cancers. *J Med Genet* **37**:336, 2000.
8. Eng C: Will the real Cowden syndrome please stand up: Revised diagnostic criteria. *J Med Genet* **37**:828, 2000.
9. Nelen MR, Padberg GW, Peeters EAJ, Lin AY, van den Helm B, Frants RR, Coulon V, Goldstein AM, van Reen MMM, Easton DF, Eeles RA, Hodgson S, Mulvihill JJ, Murday VA, Tucker MA, Mariman ECM, Starink TM, Ponder BAJ, Ropers HH, Kremer H, Longy M, Eng C: Localization of the gene for Cowden disease to 10q22-23. *Nature Genet* **13**:114, 1996.
10. Liaw D, Marsh DJ, Li J, Dahia PLM, Wang SI, Zheng Z, Bose S, Call KM, Tsou HC, Peacocke M, Eng C, Parsons R: Germline mutations of the *PTEN* gene in Cowden disease, an inherited breast and thyroid cancer syndrome. *Nat Genet* **16**:64, 1997.
11. Marsh DJ, Coulon V, Lunetta KL, Rocca-Serra P, Dahia PLM, Zheng Z, Liaw D, Caron S, Duboué B, Lin AY, Richardson A-L, Bonnetblanc J-M, Bressieux J-M, Cabarrot-Moreau A, Chompret A, Demange L, Eeles RA, Yahanda AM, Fearon ER, Fricker J-P, Gorlin RJ, Hodgson SV, Huson S, Lacombe D, LePrat F, Odent S, Toulouse C, Olopade OI, Sobol H, Tishler S, Woods CG, Robinson BG, Weber HC, Parsons R, Peacocke M, Longy M, Eng C: Mutation spectrum and genotype-phenotype analyses in Cowden disease and Bannayan-Zonana syndrome, two hamartoma syndromes with germline *PTEN* mutation. *Hum Mol Genet* **7**:507, 1998.
12. Marsh DJ, Dahia PLM, Zheng Z, Liaw D, Parsons R, Gorlin RJ, Eng C: Germline mutations in *PTEN* are present in Bannayan-Zonana syndrome. *Nat Genet* **16**:333, 1997.
13. Zhou XP, Marsh DJ, Hampel H, Mulliken JB, Gimm O, Eng C: Germline and germline mosaic mutations associated with a Proteus-like syndrome of hemihypertrophy, lower limb asymmetry, arteriovenous malformations and lipomatosis. *Hum Mol Genet* **9**:765, 2000.
14. Nelen MR, van Staveren CG, Peeters EAJ, Ben Hassel M, Gorlin RJ, Hamm H, Lindboe CF, Fryns J-P, Sijmons RH, Woods DG, Mariman ECM, Padberg GW, Kremer H: Germline mutations in the *PTEN/MMAC1* gene in patients with Cowden disease. *Hum Mol Genet* **6**:1383, 1997.
15. Nelen MR, Kremer H, Konings IBM, Schoute F, van Essen AJ, Koch R, Woods CG, Fryns J-P, Hamel B, Hoefsloot LH, Peeters EAJ, Padberg GW: Novel *PTEN* mutations in patients with Cowden disease: Absence of clear genotype-phenotype correlations. *Eur J Hum Genet* **7**:267, 1999.
16. Haibach H, Burns TW, Carlson HE, Burman KD, Deftos LJ: Multiple hamartoma syndrome (Cowden's disease) associated with renal cell carcinoma and primary neuroendocrine carcinoma of the skin (Merkel cell carcinoma). *Am J Clin Pathol* **97**:705, 1992.
17. Schrager CA, Schneider D, Gruener AC, Tsou HC, Peacocke M: Clinical and pathological features of breast disease in Cowden's syndrome: An underrecognised syndrome with an increased risk of breast cancer. *Hum Pathol* **29**:47, 1997.
18. Marsh DJ, Kum JB, Lunetta KL, Bennett MJ, Gorlin RJ, Ahmed SF, Bodurtha J, Crowe C, Curtis MA, Dazouki M, Dunn T, Feit H, Geraghty MT, Graham JM, Hodgson SV, Hunter A, Korf BR, Manchester D, Miesfeldt S, Murday VA, Nathanson KA, Parisi M, Pober B, Romano C, Tolmie JL, Trembath R, Winter RM, Zackai EH, Zori RT, Weng LP, Dahia PLM, Eng C: *PTEN* mutation spectrum and genotype-phenotype correlations in Bannayan-Riley-Ruvalcaba syndrome suggest a single entity with Cowden syndrome. *Hum Mol Genet* **8**:1461, 1999.
19. Mallory SB: Cowden syndrome (multiple hamartoma syndrome). *Dermatol Clin* **13**:27, 1995.
20. Eng C: Genetics of Cowden syndrome—through the looking glass of oncology. *Int J Oncol* **12**:701, 1998.
21. NCCN: NCCN Practice Guidelines: Genetics/Familial High Risk Cancer. *Oncology* **13**:161, 1999.

22. Eng C: Cowden syndrome. *J Genet Counsel* **6**:181, 1997.
23. Fackenthal J, Marsh DJ, Richardson AL, Cummings SC, Eng C, Robinson BG, Olopade OI: Male breast cancer in Cowden syndrome patients with germline *PTEN* mutations. *J Med Genet* **38**:159, 2001.
24. Padberg GW, Schot JDL, Vielvoye GJ, Bots GTAM, de Beer FC: Lhermitte-Duclos disease and Cowden syndrome: A single phakomatosis. *Ann Neurol* **29**:517, 1991.
25. Eng C, Murday V, Seal S, Mohammed S, Hodgson SV, Chaudary MA, Fentiman IS, Ponder BAJ, Eeles RA: Cowden syndrome and Lhermitte-Duclos disease in a family: A single genetic syndrome with pleiotropy? *J Med Genet* **31**:458, 1994.
26. Weber HC, Marsh D, Lubensky I, Lin A, Eng C: Germline *PTEN/ MMAC1/TEP1* mutations and association with gastrointestinal manifestations in Cowden disease. *Gastroenterology* **114S:**G2902, 1998.
27. Tsou HC, Teng D, Ping XL, Broncolini V, Davis T, Hu R, Xie X-X, Gruener AC, Schrager CA, Christiano AM, Eng C, Steck P, Ott J, Tavtigian SV, Peacocke M: Role of *MMAC1* mutations in early onset breast cancer: Causative in association with Cowden's syndrome and excluded in *BRCA1*-negative cases. *Am J Hum Genet* **61**:1036, 1997.
28. Lynch ED, Ostermeyer EA, Lee MK, Arena JF, Ji H, Dann J, Swisshelm K, Suchard D, MacLeod PM, Kvinnsland S, Gjertsen BT, Heimdal K, Lubs H, Moller P, King M-C: Inherited mutations in *PTEN* that are associated with breast cancer, Cowden syndrome and juvenile polyposis. *Am J Hum Genet* **61**:1254, 1997.
29. Bonneau D, Longy M: Mutations of the human *PTEN* gene. *J Med Genet* **16**:109, 2000.
30. Arch EM, Goodman BK, van Wesep RA, Liaw D, Clarke K, Parsons R, McKusick VA, Geraghty MT: Deletion of *PTEN* in a patient with Bannayan-Riley-Ruvalcaba syndrome suggests allelism with Cowden disease. *Am J Med Genet* **71**:489, 1997.
31. Ahmed SF, Marsh DJ, Weremowicz S, Morton CC, Williams DM, Eng C: Balanced translocation of 10q and 13q, including the *PTEN* gene, in a boy with an HCG-secreting tumor and the Bannayan-Riley-Ruvalcaba syndrome. *J Clin Endocrinol Metab* **84**:4665, 1999.
32. FitzGerald MG, Marsh DJ, Wahrer D, Caron S, Bell S, Shannon KEM, Ishioka C, Isselbacher KJ, Garber JE, Eng C, Haber DA: Germline mutations in *PTEN* are an infrequent cause of genetic predisposition to breast cancer. *Oncogene* **17**:727, 1998.
33. Shugart YY, Cour C, Renard H, Lenoir G, Goldgar D, Teare D, Easton D, Rahman N, Gusterton R, Seal S, Barfoot R, Stratton M, Mangion J, Peelen T, van den Ouweland A, Meijers H, Devilee P, Eccles D, Lynch H, Weber B, Stoppa-Lyonnet D, Bignon Y-J, Chang-Claude J: Linkage analysis of 56 multiplex families excludes the Cowden disease gene PTEN as a major contributor to familial breast cancer. *J Med Genet* **36**:720, 1999.
34. Chen J, Lindblom P, Lindblom A: A study of the *PTEN/MMAC1* gene in 136 breast cancer families. *Hum Genet* **102**:124, 1998.
35. Dahia PLM, Marsh DJ, Zheng Z, Zedenius J, Komminoth P, Frisk T, Wallin G, Parsons R, Longy M, Larsson C, Eng C: Somatic deletions and mutations in the Cowden disease gene, *PTEN*, in sporadic thyroid tumors. *Cancer Res* **57**:4710, 1997.
36. Halachmi N, Halachmi S, Evron E, Parsons R, Sidransky D: Somatic mutations of the *PTEN* tumor suppressor gene in sporadic follicular thyroid tumors. *Gene Chrom Cancer* **23**:239, 1998.
37. Risinger JI, Hayes AK, Berchuck A, Barrett JC: *PTEN/MMAC1* mutations in endometrial cancers. *Cancer Res* **57**:4736, 1997.
38. Tashiro H, Blazes MS, Wu R, Cho KR, Bose S, Wang SI, Li J, Parsons R, Ellenson LH: Mutations in *PTEN* are frequent in endometrial carcinoma but rare in other common gynecological malignancies. *Cancer Res* **57**:3935, 1997.
39. Kong D, Suzuki A, Zou T-T, Sakurada A, Kemp LW, Wakatsuki S, Yokohama T, Yamakawa H, Furukawa T, Sato M, Ohuchi N, Sato S, Yin J, Want S, Abraham JM, Souza RF, Smolinksi KN, Meltzer SJ, Horii A: *PTEN1* is frequently mutated in primary endometrial carcinomas. *Nat Genet* **17**:143, 1997.
40. Mutter GL, Lin M-C, Fitzgerald JT, Kum JB, Baak JPA, Lees JA, Weng L-P, Eng C: Altered PTEN expression as a diagnostic marker for the earliest endometrial precancers. *J Natl Cancer Inst* **92**:924, 2000.
41. Olschwang S, Serova-Sinilnikova OM, Lenoir GM, Thomas G: *PTEN* germline mutations in juvenile polyposis coli. *Nat Genet* **18**:12, 1998.
42. Kurose K, Araki T, Matsunaka T, Takada Y, Emi M: Variant manifestation of Cowden disease in Japan: Hamartomatous polyposis of the digestive tract with mutation of the *PTEN* gene. *Am J Hum Genet* **64**:308, 1999.
43. Huang SC, Chen CR, Lavine JE, Taylor SF, Newbury RO, Pham TT, Ricciardiello L, Carethers JM: Genetic heterogeneity in familial juvenile polyposis. *Cancer Res* **60**:6882, 2000.
44. Eng C, Ji H: Molecular classification of the inherited hamartoma polyposis syndromes: Clearing the muddied waters. *Am J Hum Genet* **62**:1020, 1998.
45. Howe JR, Ringold JC, Summers RW, Mitros FA, Nishimura DY, Stone EM: A gene for familial juvenile polyposis maps to chromosome 18q21.1. *Am J Hum Genet* **62**:1129, 1998.
46. Howe JR, Roth S, Ringold JC, Summers RW, Jarvinen HJ, Sistonen P, Tomlinson IPM, Houlston RS, Bevan S, Mitros FA, Stone EM, Aaltonen LA: Mutations in the *SMAD4/DPC4* gene in juvenile polyposis. *Science* **280**:1086, 1998.
47. Houlston R, Bevan S, Williams A, Young J, Dunlop M, Rozen P, Eng C, Markie D, Woodford-Richens K, Rodriguez-Bigas M, Leggett B, Neale K, Phillips R, Sheridan E, Hodgson D, Iwama T, Eccles D, Fagan K, Bodmer W, Tomlinson I: Mutations in *DPC4* (*SMAD4*) cause juvenile polyposis syndrome, but only account for a minority of cases. *Hum Mol Genet* **7**:1907, 1998.
48. Eng C, Blackstone MO: Peutz-Jeghers syndrome. *Med Rounds* **1**:165, 1988.
49. Rustgi AK: Medical progress—hereditary gastrointestinal polyposis and nonpolyposis syndromes. *N Engl J Med* **331**:1694, 1994.
50. Hemminki A, Tomlinson I, Markie D, Järvinen H, Sistonen P, Björkqvist A-M, Knuutila S, Salovaara R, Bodmer W, Shibata D, de la Chapelle A, Aaltonen LA: Localisation of a susceptibility locus for Peutz-Jeghers syndrome to 19p using comparative genomic hybridization and targeted linkage analysis. *Nat Genet* **15**:87, 1997.
51. Hemminki A, Markie D, Tomlinson I, Avizienyte E, Roth S, Loukola A, Bignell G, Aminoff WM, Högland P, Järvinen H, Kristo P, Pelin K, Ridanpää M, Salovaara R, Toro T, Bodmer W, Olschwang S, Olsen AS, Stratton MR, de la Chapelle A, Aaltonen LA: A serine/threonine kinase gene defective in Peutz-Jeghers syndrome. *Nature* **391**:184, 1998.
52. Jenne DE, Reimann H, Nezu J-I, Friedel W, Loff S, Jeschke R, Müller O, Back W, Zimmer M: Peutz-Jeghers syndrome is caused by mutations in a novel serine threonine kinase. *Nat Genet* **18**:38, 1998.
53. Mehenni H, Blouin JL, Radhakrishna U, Baradwaj S, Baradwaj K, Dixit VB, Richards KF, Fenoll BA, Leaf AS, Raval RC, Antonarakis SE: Peutz-Jeghers syndrome: confirmation of linkage to chromosome 19p13.3 and identification of a potential second locus on 19q13.4. *Am J Hum Genet* **61**:1327, 1997.
54. Gorlin RJ: Proteus syndrome. *J Dysmorphol* **2**:8, 1984.
55. Biesecker LG, Happle R, Mulliken JB, Weksberg R, Graham JM, Viljoen DL, Cohen MM: Proteus syndrome: Diagnostic criteria, differential diagnosis and patient evaluation. *Am J Med Genet* **84**:389, 1999.
56. Viskochil D, Buchberg AM, Xu G, Cawthon RM, Stevens J, Wolff RK, Culver M, Carey JC, Copeland NG, Jenkins NA, White R, O'Connell P: Deletions and translocation interrupt a cloned gene at the neurofibromatosis type 1 locus. *Cell* **62**:187, 1990.
57. Wallace MR, Marchuk DA, Anderson LB, Letcher R, Oden HM, Saulino AM, Fountain JW, Bereton A, Nicholson J, Mitcehll AL, Brownstein BH, Collins FS: Type 1 neurofibromatosis gene: Identification of a large transcript disrupted in three NF-1 patients. *Science* **249**:181, 1990.
58. Ward K, O'Connell P, Carey J, Leppert M, Jolley S, Plaetke R, Ogden B, White R: Diagnosis of neurofibromatosis 1 by using tightly linked, flanking DNA markers. *Am J Hum Genet* **46**:943, 1990.
59. Johnson RL, Rothman AL, Xie J, Goodrich LV, Bare JW, Bonifas JM, Quinn AG, Myers RM, Cox DR, Epstein EH, Scott MP: Human homolog of *patched*, a candidate gene for the basal cell nevus syndrome. *Science* **272**:1668, 1996.
60. Li J, Yen C, Liaw D, Podsypanina K, Bose S, Wang S, Puc J, Miliaresis C, Rodgers L, McCombie R, Bigner SH, Giovanella BC, Ittman M, Tycko B, Hibshoosh H, Wigler MH, Parsons R: *PTEN*, a putative protein tyrosine phosphatase gene mutated in human brain, breast and prostate cancer. *Science* **275**:1943, 1997.
61. Teng DH-F, Hu R, Lin H, David T, Iliev D, Frye C, Swedlund B, Hansen KL, Vinson VL, Grumpper KL, Ellis L, El-Naggar A, Frazier M, Jasser S, Langford LA, Lee J, Mills GB, Pershouse MA, Pollack RE, Tornos C, Troncoso P, Yung WKA, Fujii G, Berson A, Bookstein R, Bolen JB, Tavtigian SV, Steck PA: *MMAC1/PTEN* mutations in primary tumor specimens and tumor cell lines. *Cancer Res* **57**:5221, 1997.
62. Rhei E, Kang L, Bogomoliniy F, Federici MG, Borgen PI, Boyd J: Mutation analysis of the putative tumor suppressor gene *PTEN/ MMAC1* in primary breast carcinomas. *Cancer Res* **57**:3657, 1997.

63. Singh B, Ittman MM, Krolewski JJ: Sporadic breast cancers exhibit loss of heterozygosity on chromosome segment 10q23 close to the Cowden disease locus. *Genes Chromosomes Cancer* **21**:166, 1998.

64. Bose S, Wang SI, Terry MB, Hibshoosh H, Parsons R: Allelic loss of chromosome 10q23 is associated with tumor progression in breast carcinomas. *Oncogene* **17**:123, 1998.

65. Feilotter HE, Nagai MA, Boag AH, Eng C, Mulligan LM: Analysis of *PTEN* and the 10q23 region in primary prostate carcinomas. *Oncogene* **16**:1743, 1998.

66. Feilotter HE, Coulon V, McVeigh JL, Boag AH, Dorion-Bonnet F, Duboué B, Latham WCW, Eng C, Mulligan LM, Longy M: Analysis of the 10q23 chromosomal region and the *PTEN* gene in human sporadic breast carcinoma. *Br J Cancer* **79**:718, 1999.

67. Perren A, Weng LP, Boag AH, Ziebold U, Thakore K, Dahia PLM, Komminoth P, Less JA, Mulligan LM, Mutter GL, Eng C: Immunohistochemical evidence of loss of PTEN expression in primary ductal adenocarcinomas of the breast. *Am J Pathol* **155**:1253, 1999.

68. Cohn DE, Basil JB, Venegoni AR, Mutch DG, Rader JS, Herzog TJ, Gersell DJ, Goodfellow PJ: Absence of *PTEN* repeat tract mutation in endometrial cancers with microsatellite instability. *Gynecol Oncol* **79**:101, 2000.

69. Levine RL, Cargile CB, Blazes MS, van Rees B, Kurman RJ, Ellenson LH: *PTEN* mutations and microsatellite instability in complex atypical hyperplasia, a precursor lesion to uterine endometrioid carcinoma. *Cancer Res* **58**:3254, 1998.

70. Zedenius J, Wallin G, Svensson A, Grimelius L, Hoog A, Lundell G, Backdahl M, Larsson C: Allelotyping of follicular thyroid tumors. *Hum Genet* **96**:27, 1995.

71. Marsh DJ, Zheng Z, Zedenius J, Kremer H, Padberg GW, Larsson C, Longy M, Eng C: Differential loss of heterozygosity in the region of the Cowden locus within 10q22-23 in follicular thyroid adenomas and carcinomas. *Cancer Res* **57**:500, 1997.

72. Yeh JJ, Marsh DJ, Zedenius J, Dwight T, Delbridge L, Robinson BG, Eng C: Fine structure deletion analysis of 10q22-24 demonstrates novel regions of loss and suggests that sporadic follicular thyroid adenomas and follicular thyroid carcinomas develop along distinct parallel neoplastic pathways. *Genes Chromosomes Cancer* **26**:322, 1999.

73. Gimm O, Perren A, Weng LP, Marsh DJ, Yeh JJ, Ziebold U, Gil E, Hinze R, Delbridge L, Lees JA, Robinson BG, Komminoth P, Dralle H, Eng C: Differential nuclear and cytoplasmic expression of PTEN in normal thyroid tissue, and benign and malignant epithelial thyroid tumors. *Am J Pathol* **156**:1693, 2000.

74. Dürr E-M, Rollbrocker B, Hayashi Y, Peters N, Meyer-Puttlitz B, Louis DN, Schramm J, Wiestler OD, Parsons R, Eng C, von Deimling A: *PTEN* mutations in gliomas and glioneuronal tumours. *Oncogene* **16**:2259, 1998.

75. Wang SI, Puc J, Li J, Bruce JN, Cairns P, Sidransky D, Parsons R: Somatic mutations of *PTEN* in glioblastoma multiforme. *Cancer Res* **57**:4183, 1997.

76. Rasheed BKA, Stenzel TT, McLendon RE, Parsons R, Friedman AH, Friedman HS, Bigner DD, Bigner SH: *PTEN* gene mutations are seen in high-grade but not in low-grade gliomas. *Cancer Res* **37**:4187, 1997.

77. Maier D, Zhang ZW, Taylor E, Hamou MF, Gratzl O, van Meir EG, Scott RJ, Merlo A: Somatic deletion mapping on chromosome 10 and sequence analysis of *PTEN/MMAC1* point to the 10q25-26 region as the primary target in low-grade and high-grade gliomas. *Oncogene* **16**:3331, 1998.

78. Peters N, Wellenreuther R, Rollbrocker B, Hayashi Y, Meyer-Puttlitz B, Dürr E-M, Lenartz D, Marsh DJ, Schramm J, Wiestler OD, Parsons R, Eng C, von Deimling A: Analysis of the *PTEN* gene in human meningiomas. *Neuropathol Appl Neurobiol* **24**:3, 1998.

79. Kurose K, Zhou XP, Araki T, Eng C: Biallelic inactivating mutations and an occult germline mutation of *PTEN* in primary cervical carcinomas. *Genes Chromosomes Cancer* **29**:166, 2000.

80. Su TH, Chang JG, Perng LI, Chang CP, Wei HJ, Wang NM, Tsai CH: Mutation analysis of the putative tumor suppressor gene *PTEN/MMAC1* in cervical cancer. *Gynecol Oncol* **76**:193, 2000.

81. Kurose K, Zhou X-P, Araki T, Cannistra SA, Maher ER, Eng C: Frequent loss of PTEN expression is linked to elevated phosphorylated Akt levels, but not associated with p27 and cyclin D1 expression, in primary epithelial ovarian carcinomas. *Am J Pathol* **158**:2097, 2001.

82. Weng LP, Brown JL, Eng C: PTEN induces apoptosis and cell cycle arrest through phosphoinositol-3-kinase/Akt-dependent and independent pathways. *Hum Mol Genet* **10**:237, 2001.

83. Herbst RA, Weiss J, Ehnis A, Cavanee WK, Arden KC: Loss of heterozygosity for 10q22-10qter in malignant melanoma progression. *Cancer Res* **54**:3111, 1994.

84. Healy E, Belgaid C, Takata M, Harrison D, Zhu NW, Burd DA, Rigby HS, Matthews JN, Rees JL: Prognostic significance of allelic losses in primary melanomas. *Oncogene* **16**:2213, 1998.

85. Guldberg P, thorStraten P, Birck A, Ahrenkiel V, Kirkin AF, Zeuthen J: Disruption of the *MMAC1/PTEN* gene by deletion or mutation is a frequent event in malignant melanoma. *Cancer Res* **57**:3660, 1997.

86. Robertson GP, Furnari FB, Miele ME, Glendening MJ, Welch DR, Fountain JW, Lugo TG, Huang HJ, Cavanee WK: In vitro loss of heterozygosity targets the PTEN/MMAC1 gene in melanoma. *Proc Natl Acad Sci U S A* **95**:9418, 1998.

87. Tsao H, Zhang X, Benoit E, Haluska FG: Identification of *PTEN/MMAC1* mutations in uncultured melanomas and melanoma cell lines. *Oncogene* **16**:3397, 1998.

88. Zhou XP, Gimm O, Hampel H, Niemann T, Walker MJ, Eng C: Epigenetic PTEN silencing in malignant melanomas without *PTEN* mutation. *Am J Pathol* **157**:1123, 2000.

89. Perren A, Komminoth P, Saremaslani P, Matter C, Feurer S, Lees JA, Heitz PU, Eng C: Mutation and expression analyses reveal differential subcellular compartmentalization of PTEN in endocrine pancreatic tumors compared to normal islet cells. *Am J Pathol* **157**:1097, 2000.

90. Myers MP, Stolarov J, Eng C, Li J, Wang SI, Wigler MH, Parsons R, Tonks NK: PTEN, the tumor suppressor from human chromosome 10q23, is a dual specificity phosphatase. *Proc Natl Acad Sci U S A* **94**:9052, 1997.

91. Li D-M, Sun H: TEP1, encoded by a candidate tumor suppressor locus, is a novel protein tyrosine phosphatase regulated by transforming growth factor B. *Cancer Res* **57**:2124, 1997.

92. Carpenter CL, Cantley LC: Phosphoinositide 3-kinase and the regulation of cell growth. *Biochim Biophys Acta* **1288**:M11, 1996.

93. Whitman M, Kaplan DR, Schaffhausen B, Cantley L, Roberts TM: Association of phosphoinositol kinase activity with polyoma middle-T competent for transformation. *Nature* **315**:239, 1985.

94. Chang HW, Aoki M, Fruman D, Auger KR, Bellacosa A, Tsichlis PN, Cantley LC, Roberts TM, Vogt PK: Transformation of chicken cells by the gene encoding the catalytic subunit of PI3-kinase. *Science* **276**:1848, 1997.

95. Shayesteh L, Lu Y, Kuo WL, Baldocci R, Godfrey T, Collins C, Pinkel D, Powell B, Mills GB, Gray JW: PIK3CA is implicated as an oncogene in ovarian cancer. *Nat Genet* **21**:99, 1999.

96. Maehama T, Dixon JE: The tumor suppressor, PTEN/MMAC1, dephosphorylates the lipid second messenger phosphoinositol 3,4,5-triphosphate. *J Biol Chem* **273**:13375, 1998.

97. Stambolic V, Suzuki A, de la Pompa JL, Brothers GM, Mirtsos C, Sasaki T, Rulland J, Penninger JM, Siderovski DP, Mak TW: Negative regulation of PKB/Akt-dependent cell survival by the tumor suppressor PTEN. *Cell* **95**:1, 1998.

98. Sun H, Lesche R, Li DM, et. al.: PTEN modulates cell cycle progression and cell survival by regulating phosphatidylinositol-3,4,5-triphosphate and Akt/protein kinase B signaling pathway. *Proc Natl Acad Sci U S A* **96**:6199, 1999.

99. Myers MP, Pass I, Batty IH, van der Kaay J, Storalov JP, Hemmings BA, Wigler MH, Downes CP, Tonks NK: The lipid phosphatase activity of PTEN is critical for its tumor suppressor function. *Proc Natl Acad Sci U S A* **95**:13513, 1998.

100. Furnari FB, SuHuang H-J, Cavanee WK: The phosphoinositol phosphatase activity of *PTEN* mediates a serum-sensitive G1 growth arrest in glioma cells. *Cancer Res* **58**:5002, 1998.

101. Datta SR, Brunet A, Greenberg ME: Cellular survival: A play in three Akts. *Genes Dev* **13**:2905, 1999.

102. Weng L-P, Smith WM, Dahia PLM, Ziebold U, Gil E, Lees JA, Eng C: PTEN suppresses breast cancer cell growth by phosphatase function-dependent G1 arrest followed by apoptosis. *Cancer Res* **59**:5808, 1999.

103. Wu X, Senechal K, Neshat MS, Whang YE, Sawyers CL: The PTEN/MMAC1 tumor suppressor phosphatase functions as a negative regulator of the phosphoinositide 3-kinase/Akt pathway. *Proc Natl Acad Sci U S A* **95**:15587, 1998.

104. Li J, Simpson L, Takahashi M, Miliaresis C, Myers MP, Tonks N, Parsons R: The *PTEN/MMAC1* tumor suppressor induces cell death that is rescued by the AKT/protein kinase B oncogene. *Cancer Res* **58**:56–67, 1998.

105. Dahia PLM, Aguiar RCT, Alberta J, Kum J, Caron S, Sills H, Marsh DJ, Freedman A, Ritz J, Stiles C, Eng C: PTEN is inversely correlated with the cell survival factor PKB/Akt and is inactivated by diverse mechanisms in haematologic malignancies. *Hum Mol Genet* **8**:185, 1999.

106. Podsypanina K, Ellenson LH, Nemes A, Gu J, Tamura M, Yamada KM, Cordon-Cardo C, Catoretti G, Fisher PE, Parsons R: Mutation of Pten/Mmac1 in mice causes neoplasia in multiple organ systems. *Proc Natl Acad Sci U S A* **96**:1563, 1999.
107. Di Cristofano A, Pesce B, Cordon-Cardo C, Pandolfi PP: *Pten* is essential for embryonic development and tumour suppression. *Nat Genet* **19**:348, 1998.
108. Gil EB, MaloneLink E, Liu LX, Johnson CD, Lees JA: Regulation of the insulin-like developmental pathway of Caenorhabditis elegans by a homolog of the PTEN tumor suppressor gene. *Proc Natl Acad Sci* **96**:2925, 1999.
109. Mihaylova VT, Borland CZ, Manjarrez L, Stern MJ, Sun H: The PTEN tumor suppressor homolog in *Caenorhabditis elegans* regulates longevity and dauer formation in an insulin receptor-like signaling pathway. *Proc Natl Acad Sci U S A* **96**:7427, 1999.
110. Ogg S, Ruvkun G: The C. elegans PTEN homolog, DAF-18, acts in the insulin receptor-like metabolic signaling pathway. *Mol Cell* **2**:887, 1998.
111. Rouault JP, Kuwabara PE, Sinilnikova OM, Duret L, Thierry-Mieg D, Billaud M: Regulation of dauer larva development in *Caenorhabditis elegans* by daf-18, a homologue of the tumour suppressor PTEN. *Curr Biol* **9**:329, 1999.
112. Scanga SE, Ruel L, Binari RC, Snow B, Stambolic V, Bouchard D, Peters M, Calvieri B, Mak TW, Woodgett JR, Manoukian AS: The conserved PI3'K/PTEN/Akt signaling pathway regulates both cell size and survival in Drosophila. *Oncogene* **19**:3971, 2000.
113. Gao X, Neufeld TP, Pan D: PTEN regulates cell growth and proliferation through PI3K-dependent and -independent pathways. *Devel Biol* **221**:404, 2000.
114. Huang H, Potter CJ, Tao W, Li DM, Brogiolo W, Hafen E, Sun H, Xu T: PTEN affects cell size, cell proliferation and apoptosis during Drosophila eye development. *Development* **126**:5365, 1999.
115. Weng LP, Smith WM, Brown JL, Eng C: PTEN inhibits insulin-stimulated MEK/MAPK activation and cell growth by blocking IRS-1 phosphorylation and IRS-1/Grb-2/Sos complex formation in a breast cancer model. *Hum Mol Genet* **10**:605, 2001.
116. Simpson L, Li J, Liaw D, Hennessey I, Oliner J, Christians F, Parsons R: PTEN expression causes a feedback upregulation of IRS-2 signaling. *Mol Cell Biol* **21**:3947, 2001.
117. Lee J, Yang H, Georgescu M-M, Di Cristafano A, Maehama T, Shi Y, Dixon JE, Pandolfi P, Pavletich NP: Crystal structure of the PTEN tumor suppressor: Implications for its phosphoinositide phosphatase activity and membrane association. *Cell* **99**:323, 1999.
118. Suzuki A, de la Pompa JL, Stambolic V, Elia AJ, Sasaki T, del Barco Barrantes I, Ho A, Wakeham A, Itie A, Khoo W, Fukumoto M, Mak TW: High cancer susceptibility and embryonic lethality associated with mutation of the *PTEN* tumor suppressor gene in mice. *Curr Biol* **8**:1169, 1998.
119. Stambolic V, Tsao MS, MacPherson D, Suzuki A, Chapman WB, Mak TW: High incidence of breast and endometrial neoplasia resembling human Cowden syndrome in pten +/− mice. *Cancer Res* **60**:3605, 2000.
120. Gimm O, Attié-Bitach T, Lees JA, Vekemens M, Eng C: Expression of PTEN protein in human embryonic development. *Hum Mol Genet* **9**:1633, 2000.
121. Luukko K, Ylikorkala A, Tiainen M, Mäkelä TP: Expression of LKB1 and PTEN tumor suppressor genes during mouse and embryonic development. *Mech Devel* **83**:187, 1999.

Skin Cancer (Including Nevoid Basal Cell Carcinoma Syndrome)

Jonathan L. Rees

1. Nonmelanoma skin cancer is the most common malignancy in many Caucasian populations. Approximately 80 percent of the tumors are basal cell carcinomas (BCCs), the majority of the remaining 20 percent being squamous cell carcinomas (SCCs). Putative precursor lesions, such as actinic keratoses, are even more common. Basal cell carcinomas and squamous cell carcinomas are readily diagnosed on the basis of clinical and histopathologic appearance. Basal cell carcinomas rarely metastasize, and although squamous cell carcinomas have a low rate of metastasis, overall case fatality is low. Surgical therapy or radiotherapy is highly effective.

2. The main environmental cause is ultraviolet radiation, and the major genetic influence is through the major physiologic adaptation to ultraviolet radiation, namely, pigmentation. Studies of coat color in the mouse suggest that over 100 loci are involved in determining pigmentation, and to date, the loci important in accounting for differences in pigmentary characteristics between different human populations are largely unknown. Recently, mutations in the melanocortin 1 receptor (MC1R), a receptor for melanocyte-stimulating hormone, have been shown to be strongly associated with red hair and fair skin.

3. Familial disorders characterized by a simple Mendelian inheritance pattern probably account for fewer than 1 percent of all cases of skin cancer. The most common disorder is the nevoid basal cell carcinoma syndrome (NBCCS, Gorlin syndrome), an autosomal dominant disorder with an estimated minimum prevalence of 1 in 56,000 in a U.K. population. Nevoid basal cell carcinoma syndrome is characterized by multiple BCCS, a high incidence of other neoplasms including medulloblastomas, ocular abnormalities, and a variety of developmental abnormalities including odontogenic keratocysts. The gene for nevoid basal cell carcinoma syndrome was mapped by several groups to 9q22-31 and has been identified as the human homologue (PTC) of the *Drosophila* gene *patched* (*ptc*). Mutations of *PTC* have been found in NBCCS probands and in sporadic BCC as well as in a range of central nervous system (CNS) tumors including medulloblastomas, which are a feature of the NBCCS syndrome. Loss of heterozygosity data is compatible with its role as a tumor suppressor, and some developmental anomalies, such as the odontogenic keratocysts, also may fit the two-hit model. The other developmental anomalies suggest a dosage effect. The pattern of expression in the mouse is compatible with its putative role in developmental abnormalities in the human. *PTC* acts in the Hedgehog signaling pathway so as to inhibit the action of *smoothened* (*SMO*); mutations of *patched* therefore may exert similar effects to activating mutations of *smoothened*, a model supported by the recent identification of activating mutations of *SMO* in sporadic BCCs.

4. There is no inherited syndrome principally characterized by an elevated risk of squamous cell carcinoma (increased rates of SCC and BCC are seen in xeroderma pigmentosum). The Ferguson Smith syndrome (self-healing epitheliomata of Ferguson Smith) is characterized by lesions that clinically and pathologically resemble squamous cell carcinomas but are distinct because they involute spontaneously. On a worldwide basis, the syndrome is extremely rare. The Ferguson Smith syndrome maps to the same locus as the nevoid basal cell carcinoma syndrome. It is not known at present whether the two conditions are allelic or caused by separate genes.

5. *p53* mutations are common in both BCC and SCC. Nonmelanoma skin cancers, however, are not a feature of the Li-Fraumeni syndrome. The mutational spectrum in nonmelanoma skin cancer with frequent $C \rightarrow T$ and $CC \rightarrow TT$ transitions strongly supports ultraviolet radiation as the relevant mutagen.

6. Although BCCs and SCCs show frequent *p53* mutations and *ras* mutations have been described in both tumor types, loss of heterozygosity studies show clear differences between the two tumor types. In BCCs, which usually are diploid, allelic loss is uncommon and is almost entirely confined to the Gorlin locus on 9q. By contrast, in SCC, the fractional allelic loss is 25 to 30 percent, with loss of heterozygosity being common on chromosomes 3, 9, 13, and 17. Loss of heterozygosity studies clearly distinguish SCC from BCC, keratoacanthoma (a regressing form of nonmelanoma skin cancer), and other rarer tumor types, including appendageal tumors.

Based on their underlying biology and clinical behavior, skin cancers are usefully classified according to their cell of origin: melanoma from melanocytes or melanocyte precursors (melanoma skin cancer) and nonmelanoma skin cancer (NMSC), the majority of which are derived from the major cell type of the epidermis, the keratinocyte. There are two common types of NMSC, basal cell

---

A list of standard abbreviations is located immediately preceding the index. Nonstandard abbreviations used in this chapter include: NMSC = nonmelanoma skin cancer; BCC = basal cell carcinoma; SCC = squamous cell carcinoma; NBCCS = nevoid basal cell carcinoma syndrome; LOH = loss of heterozygosity; KA = keratoacanthoma.

carcinoma (BCC) and (cutaneous) squamous cell carcinoma (SCC). A small number of tumors arise from other cell types of the epidermis or dermis including Merkel cells and endothelial cells, and although they are technically nonmelanoma skin cancers, they have little in common with the keratinocyte-derived tumors and will not be discussed further. Melanoma skin cancer is discussed in Chap. 30. Xeroderma pigmentosum is associated with dramatically increased rates of both NMSC and melanoma skin cancer and is dealt with in Chap. 14.

Because NMSC has a low case-fatality rate and often is treated outside the hospital setting, and because some lesions may be treated without histologic confirmation, incidence data for NMSC are notoriously unreliable.[1] Nevertheless, for predominantly Caucasian populations in many parts of the world, NMSC is the most common human malignancy.[2–5] It is estimated that in the United States over three-quarters of a million individuals present with NMSC every year, accounting for over one-third of all incident cancers. Approximately 80 percent of NMSCs are BCCs, with most of the remaining 20 percent being SCCs. In areas with high ambient ultraviolet radiation and a predominantly Caucasian population, such as Australia, over half the population over the age of 40 have NMSCs or cognate lesions.[1,6–8] The relative neglect of serious study of NMSC probably reflects a number of facts, most notably the relative ease and success of surgical or other destructive therapy.[9–12] Although in part this may be attributed to the ease of their detection, their visibility, is not a complete explanation because melanomas are equally, if not more, visible and yet show a significant mortality. Recent work has shown that even when keratinocytes have accumulated multiple genetic abnormalities and when by conventional histopathologic criteria they show considerable dedifferentiation, their clinical behavior is relatively benign in comparison with other epithelial malignancies.[13,14] Given the frequency of NMSC and that ultraviolet radiation, the main cause of NMSC, is the most ubiquitous human carcinogen, it is tempting to speculate that evolutionary constraints on keratinocytes make them relatively resistant to the adoption of an aggressive malignant phenotype.

ETIOLOGY

The population contribution of single-gene disorders to NMSC is dwarfed by the influence of ultraviolet radiation. Clinically characterized single-gene disorders such as the nevoid basal cell carcinoma syndrome (Gorlin syndrome) and the Ferguson Smith syndrome (self-healing epitheliomata of Ferguson Smith) and other rarer syndromes account for fewer than 1 percent of incident cases of NMSC. Even in these disorders, expressivity is influenced by the biology of the response to ambient ultraviolet radiation. In black skin BCC may be entirely absent in the nevoid BCC syndrome (highlighting the inadequacy of the syndrome name), whereas in countries with high ambient ultraviolet radiation such as Australia, the age of presentation is markedly younger than in countries in more temperate latitudes.[15–18] Despite the small contribution from these characterized Mendelian syndromes, the genetic contribution to NMSC is considerable, as can be appreciated by considering the relation between pigmentary status, cancer risk, and ultraviolet exposure.[19,20]

Proof of the importance of ultraviolet radiation in the causation of NMSC comes from several sources.[1,19–21] First, both SCC and BCC are most common on sun-exposed body sites (although there are differences in body-site distribution between the two tumors, suggesting that other factors may be important or that the quantitative relation with ultraviolet radiation differs between BCC and SCC). Second, the results of forced or voluntary population migrations, most notably of individuals of Anglo-Saxon origin to Australia, support a role for sun exposure.[1,20] Within genetically homogeneous populations, tumor rates are inversely proportional to distance from the equator, with rates, for instance, being higher in Brisbane than in Melbourne. Third, the mutational spectra of target genes such as *p53* directly implicate a

role for ultraviolet radiation mutagenesis in NMSC.[22,23] Fourth, NMSC rates are orders of magnitude different between human populations with different pigmentary characteristics.[24–26] Finally, some, but possibly not all, forms of iatrogenically administered ultraviolet radiation cause NMSC.[27,28] It is salutary to remember that the color of one's skin and the ability to tan in response to ultraviolet radiation are largely the result of an evolutionary tradeoff between the need to protect against solar damage in areas of high ambient ultraviolet radiation and the need to ensure that adequate ultraviolet B radiation reaches the spinous and basal layers of skin to ensure adequate vitamin D synthesis to avoid metabolic bone disease.[20,29–31] The genetic basis of these pigmentary differences is likely to be complex. In the mouse, over a hundred loci are known to be important in determining coat color, although recent candidate approaches based on the melanocortin 1 receptor (MC1R) may explain the predisposition of those with red hair and/or pale skin to NMSC.[32–35] Although ultraviolet radiation is the major cause of NMSC, other etiologic factors with smaller attributable risks include ionizing radiation, chemical carcinogens, and some forms of iatrogenic immunosuppression.[10,11,36]

BASAL CELL CARCINOMA

Basal cell carcinomas are characteristically indolent, small, pearly edged lesions with accompanying telangiectasia and an ulcerated center occurring most commonly on the face or less commonly on the upper trunk or elsewhere.[11,12,37–39] They are the most common tumor in the United States, with over 750,000 incident cases per year.[40] Histologically, the tumors show downgrowths of keratinocytes from the epidermis lined by palisades of cells resembling basal cells. There are a number of clinicopathologic variants with differences in clinical behavior, although the molecular basis for these differences is unknown, and different tumor subtypes may be seen in the same individual. Differentiation with features of eccrine or hair epithelia may occur. Although BCCs are invasive and can track down nerves or invade underlying tissues such as bone, metastasis is extremely uncommon (< 1 in 4000) and calls into question the diagnosis.[11,12,41] Destruction of the tumor using a variety of modalities including surgical excision, curetting, and cautery, cryotherapy, or radiotherapy is usually curative. BCCs are a central feature of the nevoid basal cell carcinoma syndrome and the Bazex-Dupre-Christol syndrome.

Nevoid Basal Cell Carcinoma Syndrome (Gorlin Syndrome) (OMIM 109400)

Nevoid basal cell carcinoma syndrome (NBCCS) is inherited as an autosomal dominant fashion with a high rate (40 percent) of new mutations and an estimated minimum incidence in a U.K. population of 1 in 56,000.[42] Fewer than 0.5 percent of patients presenting with a BBC will have NBCCS, although the proportion will be higher in patients presenting with a BCC at an early age or with multiple tumors. Patients show a characteristic facial appearance, an increased frequency of a number of neoplasms, most notably BCCs, odontogenic keratocysts, and a variety of other developmental abnormalities.[42–44] Gorlin recently has reviewed the clinical features.[18] Cutaneous signs include the development of multiple (up to several hundred or more) BCCs and palmar-plantar pits. BCCs occur most commonly on the face, neck, or upper trunk and histologically are identical to sporadic BCCs. Tumors commonly appear at or after puberty, but presentation appears to be influenced by the amount of ambient ultraviolet radiation and other cutaneous characteristics. In blacks, BCCs may be uncommon or not seen at all, whereas among whites in Australia, the average age of BCC presentation is relatively young.[15,16] Tumors have been reported as early as 2 years of age. BCCs do not occur in about 10 percent of documented cases of NBCCS. The clinical appearance of the lesions is said to be distinctive and may resemble benign cutaneous lesions, including skin tags or seborrhoeic warts or melanocytic nevi.[18] Gorlin reports that before puberty these lesions are harmless and that only a minority change and become aggressive.[18] Palmar or plantar pits occur in over half the cases, more commonly on the hands than feet, and are more common in adults than in children. Typically, they are several millimeters across, have a telangiectatic base, and are clinically distinct from the pits seen in Darier disease. BCC may develop in the bases of the pits.

Patients with NBCCS are at increased risk of a number of other neoplasms, benign or malignant, including medulloblastoma (approximately 5 percent), meningioma, cardiac fibromas, and ovarian sarcomas and fibromas (15 percent). Patients also show a variety of other developmental defects: multiple odontogenic keratocysts that are often asymptomatic and peak during the second or third decade and occur in up to 85 percent of subjects; a characteristic facial appearance with frontal and biparietal bulging, prominent supraorbital ridges, and a low occiput and a long mandible (such patients are often tall, with some showing a marfanoid build); and a variety of skeletal manifestations including bifid ribs, short fourth metacarpals, and cortical defects of the long bones. Ophthalmic abnormalities such as squint or cataract are also seen in 25 percent of patients.[17] Patients with unilateral cutaneous signs have been described.[45] It seems likely that some of the many patients who present with multiple BCCs may be forme frustes of the NBCCS syndrome.

Genetic Loci Involved in BCC

Mapping of NBCCS by several groups to 9q22-31 and the finding of loss of heterozygosity (LOH) in up to 70 percent of sporadic BCCs suggests an underlying tumor-suppressor gene important in both familial and sporadic BCC.[46,47] Loss of the same wild-type allele in multiple BCCs from the same individual with NBCCS is in keeping with this.[48] There is no evidence of genetic heterogeneity.

The gene underlying NBCCS was identified recently using positional cloning strategies by two groups and has been found to be the human homologue (PTC) of the *Drosophila* gene *ptc*.[49,50] PTC is a 23-exon gene spanning 34 kb and consists of an open reading frame of 4242 nucleotides encoding a putative protein of 1296 amino acids, which shows 39 percent identity and 60 percent similarity to its *Drosophila* counterpart.[49–51] Over 15 different mutations of PTC have been identified in approximately one-third of individuals with NBCCS, as well as in variable numbers (20–50 percent) of sporadic BCCs and in other tumors, including medulloblastomas characteristic of the NBCCS syndrome, and sporadic medulloblastomas.[52–57] Why a higher proportion of PTC mutations has not been found in sporadic or familial cases is not yet clear. There is no evidence of locus heterogeneity, but because PTC is a large gene, mutations may have been missed for technical reasons, or alternatively, other mechanisms of inactivation may occur. Whereas some of the abnormalities such as the odontogenic keratocysts may, like BCC, be explained by a two-hit mechanism, the widespread developmental abnormalities suggest a dosage effect and, of course, fall outside the strict Knudson paradigm for the recessive nature at the cellular level of tumor-suppressor genes.[58] Little genotype-phenotype correlation between the various mutations and clinical phenotype has been reported so far.[59] Most mutations of PTC in BCC are truncations leading to presumed loss of function, and about 40 percent have the hallmark of ultraviolet radiation-induced damage.[49,50,57]

Work in *Drosophila* and other model organisms has facilitated understanding the oncogenic role of the patched signaling pathway. PTC encodes a transmembrane receptor for the secreted ligand Sonic Hedgehog (SHH). In the absence of SHH, PTC inhibits Smoothened (SMO), an adjacent transmembrane receptor. SMO in humans is believed to activate a family of genes including Gli1 and, through this pathway, activates transcription of a number of genes, including PTC itself, TGFβ, and the Wnt class of genes. From this model it would be predicted that activating mutations of SMO may produce similar effects to loss of function of PTC and that Gli expression would increase with either loss of PTC function

or activation of *Smoothened*. Recent experiments have provided support for this model. First, activation mutations of *Smoothened* have been described recently in sporadic BCCs, and transgenic mice with mutated *Smoothened* under a basal keratin promoter develop changes consistent with those seen in human BCC.[60,61] Second, transgenic mice for SHH under the control of the K14 promoter developed many of the cutaneous features of NBCCS with multiple BCCs like epidermal proliferations.[62,63] Interestingly, transplantation of the skin from these mice to SCID mice resulted in a normalization of the phenotype, suggesting the importance of mesenchymal interaction in these tumours (as is believed to be the case in humans). Third, following the transgenic SHH experiments, mutations of SHH have been found in sporadic BCC.[64] Finally, as would be expected, PTC and Gli1 are overexpressed in human BCC and, in keeping with the presumed hair follicle origin of BCC, are normally expressed in the developing follicle.[63,65] It seems likely that mutations of other components of these pathways may be involved in sporadic BCC.

Other Genetic Targets in BCC

Unusually for an epithelial malignancy LOH studies on sporadic BCC show a low frequency of allele loss (at loci other than the NBCCS locus that is lost in up to 70 percent of BCCs), a result in keeping with the usual diploid nature of these tumors.[47,66,67] LOH of 14 to 33 percent for chromosome arm 1q has been reported, but otherwise, LOH appears uncommon, unless it is confined to small areas that have not been examined. Interestingly, despite the presence of p53 mutation, LOH of 17p is uncommon, but a second inactivating p53 mutation on the remaining allele is relatively common.[47,68,69]

Mutations of p53, ras, and a GTPase-activating protein have been described in BCC. Abnormal expression of p53 is common in BCC and, depending on the antibody and exact immunocyto-chemical method employed, is increased compared with normal skin in upward of 50 percent of tumors.[69–74] In many instances this increased expression represents overexpression of wild-type sequence.[69] Various studies have reported the presence of p53 mutations in BCC. As with SCC, the mutation spectrum reflects in large part the particular characteristics of ultraviolet radiation mutagenesis with frequent C → T transitions at (dipyrimidine sites) and double CC → TT transitions, with the result that the mutation "hot spots" differ from those seen in many internal malignancies.[22,23,75,76] The absolute rate of p53 mutation in BCC varies considerably between different studies, ranging from 20 to 60 percent.[68,69,77,78] These differences may be accounted for by small statistical sample sizes and technical factors, particularly relating to the difficulties in separating stromal or inflammatory elements in small tumors, but also could conceivably represent genuine differences in molecular epidemiology. The presence of more than one p53 point mutation, one on each allele, perhaps reflects the high ultraviolet radiation mutagenic load skin is exposed to.[68,69]

Ras mutations are common in the murine chemical carcinogenesis model of skin cancer, and investigators early on examined human NMCS including BCC for the presence of such changes.[79,80] Activating mutations of *ras* could be expected based on the known properties and base specificity of ultraviolet radiation-induced mutations. As for p53, and possibly for similar reasons, ras mutation rates show a wide scatter between 0 and 30 percent.[77,80–82] There is one report of mutations of the GTPase-activating protein (which is involved in down-regulating ras proteins and in signal transduction) in 3 of 21 BCCs.[83] To date, there are no studies showing a relation between the presence of specific genetic change and clinical behavior or histologic subtype of BCC, nor has a definite precursor lesion been identified, although some authors have identified p53 immunopositive clones harboring p53 mutations close to clinically obvious BCC.[78,81,84] It remains possible, perhaps likely, that these lesions are precursors of other types of NMSCs.[72]

Bazex-Dupre-Christol Syndrome (OMIM 301845)

This is an extremely uncommon X-linked dominant condition characterized by multiple BCCs developing in the second and third decades and follicular atrophoderma present from birth or early childhood.[85–88] Hypotrichosis and other abnormalities may be present. The BCCs may resemble those seen in the NBCCS. It has been mapped to Xq24-27.[89]

Rombo Syndrome (MIM 180730)

There is one report of this syndrome that was transmitted through four generations consistent with an autosomal dominant trait. BCCs were described together with vermiculate atrophoderma, abnormal eyelashes and eyebrows, and in one case, trichoepitheliomas.

SQUAMOUS CELL CARCINOMA

SCCs are invasive tumors with the ability to metastasize that have a histologic resemblance to differentiated suprabasal keratinocytes.[4,10,39,90,91] They usually arise on sun-exposed skin, grow quicker than BCCs, and produce a more indurated, untidy keratotic lesion with ulceration. There may be associated signs of ultraviolet radiation damage to skin, including actinic keratoses. Histology shows aberrant differentiation, frequent mitoses, and variable degrees of dysplasia. Metastasis rates are between 0.1 and 4 percent, but the overall mortality is low.[4,10,91,92] Cutaneous SCCs are less aggressive in their biologic behavior than other keratinocyte-derived tumors such as those of the oral cavity or cervix and SCC of the lip, which are also caused by ultraviolet radiation exposure.[10,91] There is some evidence that SCC arising in the sites of thermal burns or in sites of chronic inflammation may behave more aggressively.[10] Most cutaneous SCCs are readily amenable to surgery or radiotherapy.

Whereas there are no clinically identified precursor lesions for BCC, some SCCs are thought to arise from actinic keratoses or areas of Bowen disease (*in situ* carcinoma).[10,93] Actinic keratoses are focal areas of cutaneous dysplasia characterized clinically by redness and scaling that are usually only minimally indurated or show no induration.[93,94] They are usually multiple, and their body-site distribution mirrors cumulative ultraviolet radiation exposure, being high on the scalps of balding men, face, and backs of hands and lower arms.[94] Epidemiologic studies in Australia report a prevalence for actinic keratoses of around 50 percent over age 40 and that the risk of progression from a single actinic keratosis to a SCC is less than 1:1000 per year.[1,95] One-quarter of actinic keratoses may resolve spontaneously over a 1-year period, whereas approximately half of SCCs arise in a preexisting actinic keratosis, with the other half apparently arising *de novo*.[95,96] Actinic keratoses are at least 15 times more common than SCC.[1] Sporadic SCCs, unlike keratoacanthomas or the epitheliomata of Ferguson Smith, show no significant propensity to clinical regression.[10] There are no single-gene disorders that specifically feature SCCs. (Ferguson Smith tumors, although showing certain similarities, are distinct.)

Genetic Change in SCC

Aneuploidy is common in SCC (unlike BCC), occurring in between 20 and 80 percent of patients. SCCs show distinct patterns of LOH compared with other noncutaneous squamous cell cancers and other skin tumors such as BCCs or keratoacanthomas.[67,97,98] LOH in SCC is especially common on chromosomes 3 (25 percent), 9 (40 percent), and 17 (40 percent), with an overall fractional allelic loss of 30 percent.[14,47] With the exception of chromosome 17 and *p53,* the identity of the underlying putative tumor-suppressor genes for cutaneous SCC are unknown. Loss of 3p is common in other keratinocyte squamous malignancies including oral carcinoma, but the target gene is at present unknown: *FHIT* mutations were not found in one study of cutaneous SCC.[99,100] The target gene(s) underlying LOH on

chromosome 9 also is unknown. Current data suggest that the NBCCS or the Ferguson Smith locus is not a primary target in SCC; rather, deletion mapping studies suggest an area of 9p that includes *p16* and *p15*.[101,102] Studies examining these genes for mutation have not been reported, nor have other areas of 9p been excluded.[103]

Brash first showed that *p53* mutations were common in SCC but, perhaps more important, showed that the pattern of mutation involving frequent $C \rightarrow T$ and $CC \rightarrow TT$ transitions bore the molecular footprint of ultraviolet radiation-induced mutagenesis.[22] Ultraviolet radiation can influence the carcinogenic process in a number of ways.[20] Ultraviolet radiation is mutagenic, in animal systems can act as a tumor promoter, and there is evidence in animals, if not in humans, that local and systemic immunosuppression induced by ultraviolet radiation may be important in skin carcinogenesis. The finding of ultraviolet radiation-induced mutations was therefore important direct proof of the mutagenic role of ultraviolet radiation in human skin cancer (the increased incidence of SCC in patients with xeroderma pigmentosum could, although perhaps not very convincingly, be attributed to the ultraviolet radiation-induced abnormalities of immune function or to effects on tumor promotion). Subsequent studies have in large part confirmed the earlier findings, although not unfamiliarly for studies of genetic change in NMSC, the absolute rates of *p53* mutation in SCC vary considerably from 10 to over 60 percent.[22,76,77,82,104,105] These differences may reflect genuine epidemiologic differences, technical factors, or statistical sampling errors, since most studies were relatively small. There is a suggestion that the type of mutations may vary in different studies. Studies of premalignant lesions such as Bowen disease and actinic keratoses also show a high rate of *p53* mutation.[106,107] It is not known whether preinvasive lesions harboring *p53* mutations are more likely to progress to SCC than those without mutation, although given the frequency of nonprogression, even with *p53* mutations, the majority of actinic keratoses would be expected to regress or at least not progress. In contrast with BCC, where allelic loss is uncommon, as with many other malignancies, loss of the remaining wild-type allele is common in SCC. It remains possible that there are targets other than *p53* on chromosome 17.[14]

The timing of *p53* mutation during SCC development and the role *p53* plays in keratinocyte physiology also have been examined.[23,107] Wild-type p53 protein expression is increased in human skin following exposure to doses of ultraviolet radiation too small to induce erythema.[108–110] Increased expression is seen with ultraviolet A, B, and C, although when normalized so that equal amounts of erythema are produced, the largest increase is seen for ultraviolet B.[108] The pattern of induction throughout the epidermis is not easily explained on the basis of the known penetration characteristics of the various wavebands of ultraviolet radiation.[108] It is widely assumed that the up-regulation of *p53* expression in response to ultraviolet radiation is a direct result of DNA damage, although more modest increases are seen following a range of stimuli that are not known to cause DNA damage.[109] The functional significance of the increased expression is not clear. For instance, individuals with the Li-Fraumeni syndrome harboring *p53* mutations do not show an excess of NMSC, nor has photosensitivity been reported in this group of patients (although I have seen one such patient). In an attempt to assess the function of *p53*, Brash and colleagues irradiated mice null for *p53* and showed that the number of sunburn cells formed in response to ultraviolet radiation was diminished.[107] (Sunburn cells are defined morphologically and are thought to represent apoptotic—probably basal—keratinocytes.[111,112]) They argued that wild-type *p53* plays an important role in facilitating apoptosis in response to DNA damage and that loss of this function would allow clonal expansion of mutated clones, thus implicating a role for ultraviolet radiation in mutagenesis and tumor promotion.[107,113] It remains unclear why the increase in *p53* expression following ultraviolet B radiation is seen throughout both the proliferative and terminally differentiated compartment.[108] No increase in sunburn cell formation following irradiation was reported in mice carrying a mutant *p53* transgene.[114]

The timing of *p53* mutations in the development of SCC also has been studied. Sensitive techniques such as the ligase-mediated PCR that do not rely on the presence of a clonally expanded group of cells have shown that *p53* mutations can be identified in normal sun-exposed skin and in irradiated cultured keratinocytes.[115] Clusters of *p53* immunopositive cells harboring *p53* mutation also have been described close to BCC and in sun-exposed skin in the absence of any clinical tumor, and although these could represent BCC precursors, perhaps it is more likely that they are related to SCC development.[72,81,113,116,117] It has been suggested that because dissection of different regions of actinic keratoses shows no heterogeneity for *p53* mutation, then *p53* mutation may be the initiating event in SCC development.[107] Given the high proliferative rate of many actinic keratoses, this argument is not decisive, since other changes may have occurred already. In keeping with this, recent work has shown that in many actinic keratoses, increased proliferation, elevated wild-type *p53* expression, changes in p21[waf/cip1] expression, and chromosomal loss all occur without or before *p53* mutation.[14] There may be many pathways to SCC development, and within certain limits, the order of genetic change may not be critical. The high rate of regression and the low rate of progression to SCC raise the possibility that actinic keratoses and SCC are cognate phenomena, both responses to ultraviolet radiation-induced genetic damage, and that the rare apparent progression from an actinic keratosis to an SCC is the result of misdiagnosis of early *in situ* SCC as actinic keratosis.[118,119] The finding of higher rates of genetic change in actinic keratosis than in SCC, although compatible with this, does not prove it, and the hypothesis remains speculative.[14,120]

As with BCC, a number of studies have looked for *ras* mutations in SCC. Although some early studies reported a high frequency of *ras* mutations (principally of H-*ras* at codon 12), as has been found in studies of other human cancers, later results have qualified earlier work, with lower mutation rates being reported. Rates therefore vary from 0 to 46 percent in different studies.[77,80,121–123] There is some evidence that *ras* mutation rates are higher in some risk groups such as patients with xeroderma pigmentosum than in control tumors.[124–126] Definitive studies conducted simultaneously on samples from different populations are required. In addition to studies of point mutations of *ras,* there are reports of alteration in *ras* expression, gene amplification, or gene deletion that appear particularly common in tumors occurring on the basis of xeroderma pigmentosum.[124,125]

Keratoacanthoma

Keratoacanthomas (KAs) are interesting tumors that, although sharing histologic and clinical overlap with SCC, are defined by their history of spontaneous regression.[39,127,128] Characteristically, KAs develop over the course of a few months and show rapid growth resulting in lesions a few centimeters across, with a keratin plug and a cellular shoulder, before regressing leaving a scar. KAs show many similarities to SCCs, and because the defining feature of a KA is natural regression, in clinical practice where lesions are excised or biopsied, differentiation from SCC is often problematic. KAs are distinct from the self-healing epitheliomata of Ferguson Smith.[129]

Even in the face of their interesting natural history, KAs have received little serious attention. Various theories have been proposed to account for their regressing course: that they have a viral pathogenesis, that they are follicular tumors and that their growth pattern mimics the hair follicle's anagen and telogen, and that they are SCCs that are immunologically rejected by the host.[127,128,130] There are particular diagnostic problems with any analysis of these tumors because the "gold standard" of distinction between a KA and an SCC relies on natural history, which is compromised by removal or biopsy.

Studies conflict as to the frequency of aneuploidy in KA and whether it is possible to clearly distinguish KA from SCC on the basis of ploidy[67,97,131] (although subsequent allelotyping of KA and SCC suggest that differences are likely[98]). Increases in *p53* expression have been described, although definitive studies of mutation rates have not been reported.[77,80,121–123] *Ras* mutations have been described in a small number of tumors, and an attempt has been made to link the presence of mutation with regression rather than progression.[136,137] A recent study of LOH in KAs showed a low fractional allelic loss based on examination of 26 autosomes of only 1.3 percent, with only sporadic loss seen.[98] This suggests clear differences from SCC (score of 30 percent) and makes it likely that KAs and SCCs are different *de novo* rather than KAs being the result of a successful immunologic attack on an SCC.[14,47,130] LOH at the Ferguson Smith locus was uncommon.[98]

Ferguson Smith Syndrome (OMIM 132800)

This syndrome was described originally in a single individual, and the familial nature of the disorder was recognized only later.[129,132,133] It is inherited as an autosomal dominant fashion, has been reported to skip generations, and the largest series all originate from Scotland, with the possibility that they all derive from a single mutation in the late eighteenth century.[132] The incidence is unknown, but worldwide the tumors appear exceptionally rare. Clinically, the condition is characterized by the presence of recurrent lesions identical to SCCs that develop over a few months and then resolve spontaneously, leaving a depressed scar. More than one lesion may be present at the same time. Histologically, the lesions are well-differentiated SCCs rather than KAs[127] (although many workers still refer to them as KAs or argue that they are indeed a form of familial KA). Tumors may present in the second decade but occur more commonly later in life. Tumors on the face and scalp are common, and although most tumors occur on sun-exposed areas, tumors have been reported on the anus and the perineum.[134] There are no associated extracutaneous features, and while disabling and destructive with tumors capable of underlying infiltration, they do not usually affect mortality. There are reports of genuine SCC with metastases developing in individuals with the Ferguson Smith syndrome.[129] The disorder may be unilateral.[134]

In studies of 13 British families, linkage has been shown to 9q22-31, the same locus as for the NBCCS.[135] Whether the two disorders are allelic or reflect mutations of two different genes is not known.[136] Studies of LOH in Ferguson Smith tumors have not been published, and it remains possible that the target gene is not a tumor suppressor.

Muir Torre Syndrome (OMIM 158320)

This is best considered part of the Lynch type 2 family cancer syndrome secondary to an underlying defect in mismatch repair.[137–139] The cutaneous manifestations are characterised by sebaceous gland tumors, including sebaceous adenomas, sebaceous epitheliomas, and sebaceous carcinomas, and less commonly KAs.[140] The syndrome is inherited as an autosomal dominant trait, but expressivity is variable.[141] The true incidence is unknown, but I suspect that the cutaneous aspects are widely underdiagnosed or misdiagnosed. Replication errors have been demonstrated in the cutaneous tumors, including tumors such as actinic keratoses not considered part of the syndrome (replication errors are otherwise uncommon in NMSC).[142,143]

Epidermodysplasia Verruciformis (OMIM 226400)

This disorder is characterized by the onset in childhood of a combination of plane wart, red plaque, and pityriasis versicolor-like lesions in which a range of human papillomavirus types may be identified, with the development of SCCs on sun-exposed areas later, and depressed cell-mediated immunity.[144,145] The mode of inheritance is unclear, although the majority of reports favor an autosomal recessive inheritance.[144] The condition is extremely rare, and apart from identification of new papillomaviruses, it has received little genetic attention.[145]

Dyskeratosis Congenita (OMIM 305000)

SCCs of the skin and other epithelia have been reported in this condition, which is characterized by leukoplakia, nail dystrophy, and cutaneous atrophy and pigmentation.[146,147] It is usually an X-linked recessive syndrome, although other patterns of inheritance have been described.[146,152] The X-linked form has been mapped to Xq28 and is the result of mutations in the gene coding for dyskerin (*DKC1*).[148,149]

APPENDAGEAL TUMORS

BCC and SCC aside, there are a large number of different types of epidermal tumors of varying degrees of aggressiveness that on a clinicopathologic basis are believed to relate to the pilosebaceous unit or eccrine or apocrine sweat glands.[150,151] They are uncommon in comparison with BCC or SCC and often are only correctly diagnosed after histologic examination. The vast majority of tumors are solitary and occur without any family history. Examination of a range of appendageal tumors for LOH showed a low frequency of LOH at selected loci and failed to find any consistent pattern, a finding perhaps not surprising given their pathologic heterogeneity and relatively benign clinical course.[84] Particular familial syndromes that usually are characterized by multiple tumors include Cowden syndrome (multiple hamartoma syndrome, OMIM 158350), an autosomal dominant trait comprising multiple hair follicle tumors, oral papillomas, and breast cancer, which maps to 10q22-23 and is due to mutations in the *PTEN* gene; familial trichoepithelioma (OMIM 132700), which recently has been mapped tentatively to 9p (see below); and familial cyclindromatosis (turban tumors, OMIM 132700), which maps to 16q12-q13 and that shows LOH for this locus in the tumors.[129,152–154] Mutations of *PTC* also have been described in sporadic trichoepitheliomas, a benign hair follicle-related tumor with many similarities to BCCs, although no *PTC* mutations were seen in two familial cases.[155] Clinical and pathologic diagnosis in appendageal tumors is often difficult, and some individuals suffer from more than one type of tumor. It is likely that genetic strategies may assist in understanding the nosology and relation of the different tumors.

COMPLEX TRAITS AND SKIN CANCER SUSCEPTIBILITY

In numerical terms, the contribution of the highly penetrant single-gene disorders described earlier to NMSC is small, accounting for perhaps fewer than 1 percent of cases. Nevertheless, the genetic influence on skin cancer development is considerable. Although ultraviolet radiation is viewed as the major environmental cause of NMSC, this is true in large part only because populations adapted to areas of low ambient ultraviolet radiation have in the relatively recent evolutionary past migrated to areas of high exposure.[20,156] The major genetic determinant of NMSC worldwide therefore is pigmentation (and any other genetic determinants of the cutaneous response to ultraviolet radiation). Blacks have rates of NMSC greater than 50-fold lower than whites, and Japanese who have migrated to areas of higher ultraviolet radiation still show rates 4 to 12 times lower than those seen in Caucasians (although differences in sun-exposure habits cannot be excluded entirely).[24,157–159] Even within Caucasian populations, rates vary perhaps fivefold between those with red hair or who tend to burn rather than tan (and who are often red-haired or of Irish, or Welsh, or Scottish—so-called Celtic—ancestry) and those who tan rather than burn from southern Europe.[160,161] Although the genetics of pigmentation appear complex with, in the mouse, upward of a 100 loci involved in determining coat color, there are in humans single loci effecting pigmentation that exert considerable effects on skin cancer rates.[33,162] For instance, oculocutaneous albinos living in areas of high ambient ultraviolet radiation

show dramatically increased risks of NMSC, and without appropriate care and sun avoidance, they may die from complications of their tumors in early adult life.[157,163–165]

Recently, associations between variants of the melanocortin 1 receptor and the inability to tan and red hair have been described.[34,166,167] The melanocortin 1 receptor is a receptor for melanocyte-stimulating hormone and is present on a range of cells including melanocytes and keratinocytes. Genetic analyses in the mouse (and other mammals) have shown that melanocyte-stimulating hormone controls the switch from the production of pheomelanin (red/yellow melanin) to eumelanin (black/brown melanin), an action antagonized by agouti.[32,168] Although eumelanin is photoprotective, pheomelanin has poor sunscreen activities and actually may generate free radicals in response to ultraviolet radiation.[169–171] Over 75 percent of the population of the United Kingdom has been shown to harbor coding region variants of the MC1R, with three alleles in particular (Arg151Cys, Arg160Trp, and Asp294His) looking as though they are functionally important. Evidence for loss of function in transient transfection assays for the Arg151Cys variant has been published recently.[172] The majority of individuals with bright red hair are compound heterozygotes for these alleles, and family studies suggest that as operationally defined, the trait often approximates to a recessive model. That other loci are important in determining the red hair phenotype, however, came from twin studies in which different (hair color) phenotypes in discordant twins concordant for the MC1R locus were seen.[167] An overrepresentation of particular MC1R putative mutant alleles has been reported in melanoma and non-melanoma skin cancer.[166,173] It is likely that there are a number of other genetic influences on NMSC development of unknown magnitude, including the relation between immunologic aspects of cutaneous function and tumor risk.[174,175] Associations have been reported between NMSC and glutathione *S*-transferase GSTM1 polymorphisms, between HLA haplotypes and NMSC, and between NMSC and genetic determinants of susceptibility to the immunosuppressive actions of ultraviolet radiation.[176–179] The influence of differences in DNA repair rates on NMSC is discussed in Chap. 14 and references 180 and 181.

REFERENCES

1. Marks R: An overview of skin cancers: Incidence and causation. *Cancer* **75**(suppl):607, 1995.
2. Gallagher RP, Ma B, McLean DI, Yang CP, Ho V, Carruthers JA, Warshawski LM: Trends in basal cell carcinoma, squamous cell carcinoma, and melanoma of the skin from 1973 through 1987. *J Am Acad Dermatol* **23**:413, 1990.
3. Glass AG, Hoover RN: The emerging epidemic of melanoma and squamous cell skin cancer. *JAMA* **262**:2097, 1989.
4. Preston DS, Stern RS: Nonmelanoma cancers of the skin. *N Engl J Med* **327**:1649, 1992.
5. Green A: Changing patterns in incidence of non-melanoma skin cancer (review). *Epithel Cell Biol* **1**(1):47, 1992.
6. Marks R, Jolley D, Dorevitch AP, Selwood TS: The incidence of non-melanocytic skin cancers in an Australian population: Results of a five-year prospective study. *Med J Aust* **150**(9):475, 1989.
7. Kricker A, English DR, Randell PL, Heenan PJ, Clay CD, Delaney TA, Armstrong BK: Skin cancer in Geraldton, Western Australia: A survey of incidence and prevalence. *Med J Aust* **152**:399, 1990.
8. Marks R, Staples M, Giles GG: Trends in non-melanocytic skin cancer treated in Australia: The second national survey. *Int J Cancer* **53**(4):585, 1993.
9. Fleming ID, Amonette R, Monaghan T, Fleming MD: Principles of management of basal and squamous cell carcinoma of the skin. *Cancer* **75**(suppl):699, 1995.
10. Kwa RE, Campana K, Moy RL: Biology of cutaneous squamous cell carcinoma. *J Am Acad Dermatol* **26**:1, 1992.
11. Miller SJ: Biology of basal cell carcinoma, part 1. *J Am Acad Dermatol* **24**:1, 1991.
12. Miller SJ: Biology of basal cell carcinoma, part 2. *J Am Acad Dermatol* **24**:161, 1991.

13. Rehman I, Quinn AG, Healy E, Rees JL: High frequency of loss of heterozygosity in actinic keratoses, a usually benign disease. *Lancet* **344**:788, 1994.

14. Rehman I, Takata M, Wu YY, Rees JL: Genetic change in actinic keratoses. *Oncogene* **122**:483, 1996.

15. Goldstein AM, Pastakia B, DiGiovanna JJ, Poliak S, Santucci S, Kase R, Bale AE, Bale SJ: Clinical findings in two African-American families with the nevoid basal cell carcinoma syndrome (NBCC) (review). *Am J Med Genet* **50**(3):272, 1994.

16. Shanley S, Ratcliffe J, Hockey A, Haan E, Oley C, Ravine D, Martin N, Wicking C, Chenevix-Trench G: Nevoid basal cell carcinoma syndrome: Review of 118 affected individuals (review). *Am J Med Genet* **50**(3):282, 1994.

17. Evans DG, Ladusans EJ, Rimmer S, Burnell LD, Thakker N, Farndon PA: Complications of the naevoid basal cell carcinoma syndrome: Results of a population based study. *J Med Genet* **30**(6):460, 1993.

18. Gorlin RJ: Nevoid basal-cell carcinoma syndrome. *Medicine* **66**(2):98, 1987.

19. IARC: IARC *Monographs on the Evaluation of Carcinogenic Risks to Humans: Solar and Ultraviolet Radiation.* Lyon, France: IARC, World Health Organization, 1992, p 55.

20. Report of an advisory group on non-ionising radiation: Board statement on effects of ultraviolet radiation on human health and health effects from ultraviolet radiation.Chilton, Didcot, Oxon: National Radiation Protection Board, 1995, p 6(2). Documents of the NRPB.

21. Urbach F, Rose DB, Bonnem RDH, Urbach F, Rose DB, Bonnem RDH, Bonnem M, eds: *Genetic and Environmental Carcinogenesis.* Baltimore: Williams & Wilkins; 1972, pp 355–371.

22. Brash DE, Rudolph JA, Simon JA, Lin A, McKenna GJ, Baden HP, Halperin AJ, Ponten J: A role for sunlight in skin cancer: UV-induced *p53* mutations in squamous cell carcinoma. *Proc Natl Acad Sci* USA **88**:10124, 1991.

23. Brash DE, Ziegler A, Jonason AS, Simon JA, Kunula S, Leffel DJ: Sunlight and sunburn in human skin cancer: *p53,* apoptosis, and tumour promotion. *J Invest Dermatol Symp* **1**(suppl):136S, 1996.

24. Scotto J, Fears TR, Fraumeni JF: *Incidence of Non-Melanoma Skin Cancer in the United States.* Washington, National Institutes of Health, 1983.

25. Fleming ID, Barnawell JR, Burlison PE, Rankin JS: Skin cancer in black patients. *Cancer* **35**(3):600, 1975.

26. Weinstock MA: Epidemiology of nonmelanoma skin cancer: Clinical issues, definitions, and classification. *J Invest Dermatol* **102**(suppl):4S, 1994.

27. Stern RS: Risks of cancer associated with long-term exposure to PUVA in humans: Current status — 1991. *Blood Cells* **18**:91, 1992.

28. Bhate SM, Sharpe GR, Marks JM, Shuster S, Ross WM: Prevalence of skin and other cancers in patients with psoriasis. *Clin Exp Dermatol* **18**(5):401, 1993.

29. Bodmer WF, Cavalli-Sforza LL: *Genetics, Evolution and Man.* San Fransisco, WH Freeman, 1976.

30. Freemon FR, Loomis WF: Vitamin D and skin pigments. *Science* **158**(801):579, 1967.

31. Loomis WF: Skin-pigment regulation of vitamin-D biosynthesis in man. *Science* **157**(788):501, 1967.

32. Jackson IJ: Molecular and developmental genetics of mouse coat color. *Annu Rev Genet* **28**:189, 1994.

33. Jackson IJ: Mouse coat colour mutations: A molecular genetic resource which spans the centuries. *Bioessays* **13**(9):439, 1991.

34. Valverde P, Healy E, Jackson I, Rees JL, Thody AJ: Variants of the mealnocyte-stimulating hormone receptor gene are associated with red hair and fair skin in humans. *Nature Genet* **11**:328, 1995.

35. Smith R, Healy E, Siddiqui S, Flanagan N, Steijlen PM, Rosdahl I, Jacques JP, Rogers R, Turner R, Jackson IJ, Birch-Machi MA, Rees JL: Melanocortin 1 receptor variants in an Irish population. *J Invest Dermatol* **111**(1):119, 1998.

36. Bouwes Bavinck JM, Vermeer BJ, Claas FHJ, Schegget JT, Van Der Woude FJ: Skin cancer and renal transplantation. *J Nephrol* **7**(5):261, 1994.

37. Lang PJJ, Maize JC, Friedman RJ, Rigel DS, Kopf AW, Harris MN, Baker D, eds: *Cancer of the Skin.* Philadelphia, Saunders, 1991, pp 35–73.

38. Mackie RM: *Skin Cancer,* 2d ed. London, Martin Dunitz, Ltd, 1996, pp 112–132.

39. Mackie RM, Champion RH, Burton JL, Ebling FJG, eds: *Textbook of Dermatology,* 5th ed. London, Blackwell Scientific, 1992, pp 1505–1524.

40. Miller DL, Weinstock MA: Nonmelanoma skin cancer in the United States: Incidence. *J Am Acad Dermatol* **30**:774, 1994.

41. Lo JS, Snow SN, Reizner GT, Mohs FE, Larson PO, Hruza GJ: Metastatic basal cell carcinoma: Report of twelve cases with a review of the literature (see comments) (review). *J Am Acad Dermatol* **24**(5:pt 1):715, 1991.

42. Evans DG, Ladusans EJ, Rimmer S, Burnell LD, Thakker N, Farndon PA: Complications of the naevoid basal cell carcinoma syndrome: Results of a population based study. *J Med Genet* **30**(6):460, 1993.

43. Gorlin RJ, Goltz RW: Multiple nevoid basal-cell epithelioma, jaw cysts and bifid rib. *N Engl J Med* **262**(18):908, 1960.

44. Bale AE, Gailani MR, Leffell DJ: Nevoid basal cell carcinoma syndrome. *J Invest Dermatol* **103**(suppl):126S, 1994.

45. Sharpe GR, Cox NH: Unilateral naevoid basal cell carcinoma syndrome: An individually controlled study of fibroblast sensitivity to radiation. *Clin Exp Dermatol* **15**:352, 1990.

46. Farndon PA, Mastro RGD, Evans DGR, Kilpatrick MW: Location of gene for Gorlin syndrome. *Lancet* **339**:581, 1992.

47. Quinn AG, Sikkink S, Rees JL: Basal cell carcinomas and squamous cell carcinomas of human skin show distinct patterns of chromosome loss. *Cancer Res* **54**(17):4756, 1994.

48. Bonifas JM, Bare JW, Kerschmann RL, Epstein EH: Parental origin of chromosome 9q22.3-q31 lost in basal cell carcinomas from basal cell nevus syndrome patients. *Hum Mol Genet* **3**:447, 1994.

49. Hahn H, Wicking C, Zaphiropoulos PG, Gailani MR, Shanley S, Chidambaram A, Vorechovsky I, Holmberg E, Unden AB, Gillies S, Negus K, Smyth I, Pressman C, Leffell DJ, Gerrard B, Goldstein AM, Dean M, Toftgard R, Chenevix-Trench G, Wainwright B, Bale AE: Mutations of the human homologue of *Drosophila patched* in the nevoid basal cell carcinoma syndrome. *Cell* **85**(6):841, 1996.

50. Johnson RL, Rothman AL, Xie JW, Goodrich LV, Bare JW, Bonifas JM, Quinn AG, Myers RM, Cox DR, Epstein EH Jr, Scott MP: Human homologue of *patched,* a candidate gene for the basal cell nevus syndrome. *Science* **272**(5268):1668, 1996.

51. Hahn H, Christiansen J, Wicking C, Zaphiropoulos PG, Chidambaram A, Gerrard B, Vorechovsky I, Bale AE, Toftgard R, Dean M, Wainwright B: A mammalian *patched* homolog is expressed in target tissues of *sonic hedgehog* and maps to a region associated with developmental abnormalities. *J Biol Chem* **271**(21):12125, 1996.

52. Chidambaram A, Goldstein AM, Gailani MR, Gerrard B, Bale SJ, DiGiovanna JJ, Bale AE, Dean M: Mutations in the human homologue of the *Drosophila patched* gene in Caucasian and African-American nevoid basal cell carcinoma syndrome patients. *Cancer Res* **56**(20):4599, 1996.

53. Lench NJ, Telford EA, High AS, Markham AF, Wicking C, Wainwright BJ: Characterisation of human patched germ line mutations in naevoid basal cell carcinoma syndrome. *Hum Genet* **100**(5-6):497, 1997.

54. Raffel C, Jenkins RB, Frederick L, Hebrink D, Alderete B, Fults DW, James CD: Sporadic medulloblastomas contain *PTCH* mutations. *Cancer Res* **57**(5):842, 1997.

55. Wolter M, Reifenberger J, Sommer C, Ruzicka T, Reifenberger G: Mutations in the human homologue of the *Drosophila* segment polarity gene patched (*PTCH*) in sporadic basal cell carcinomas of the skin and primitive neuroectodermal tumors of the central nervous system. *Cancer Res* **57**(13):2581, 1997.

56. Xie J, Johnson RL, Zhang X, Bare JW, Waldman FM, Cogen PH, Menon AG, Warren RS, Chen LC, Scott MP, Epstein EH Jr: Mutations of the *patched* gene in several types of sporadic extracutaneous tumors. *Cancer Res* **57**(12):2369, 1997.

57. Aszterbaum M, Rothman A, Johnson RL, Fisher M, Xie JW, Bonifas JM, Zhang XL, Scott MP, Epstein EH Jr: Identification of mutations in the human *patched* gene in sporadic basal cell carcinomas and in patients with the basal cell nevus syndrome. *J Invest Dermatol* **110**(6):885, 1998.

58. Levanat S, Gorlin RJ, Fallet S, Johnson DR, Fantasia JE, Bale AE: A two-hit model for developmental defects in Gorlin syndrome. *Nature Genet* **12**(1):85, 1996.

59. Wicking C, Shanley S, Smyth I, Gillies S, Negus K, Graham S, Suthers, Haites N, Edwards M, Wainwright B, Chenevix-Trench G: Most germ-line mutations in the nevoid basal cell carcinoma syndrome lead to a premature termination of the *patched* protein, and no genotype-phenotype correlations are evident. *Am J Hum Genet* **60**(1):21, 1997.

60. Xie J, Murone M, Luoh SM, Ryan A, Gu Q, Zhang C, Bonifas JM, Lam CW, Hynes M, Goddard A, Rosenthal A, Epstein EHJ,

de Sanvage FJ: Activating Smoothened mutations in sporadic basal-cell carcinoma. *Nature* **391**(6662):90, 1998.

61. Reifenberger J, Wolter M, Weber RG, Megahed M, Ruzicka T, Lichter P, Reifenberger G: Missense mutations in *SMOH* in sporadic basal cell carcinomas of the skin and primitive neuroectodermal tumors of the central nervous system. *Cancer Res* **58**(9):1798, 1998.

62. Fan H, Oro AE, Scott MP, Khavari PA: Induction of basal cell carcinoma features in transgenic human skin expressing sonic hedgehog. *Nature Med* **3**(7):788, 1997.

63. Dahmane N, Lee J, Robins P, Heller P, Ruiz: Activation of the transcription factor Gli1 and the sonic hedgehog signalling pathway in skin tumours. *Nature* **389**(6653):876, 1997.

64. Oro AE, Higgins KM, Hu Z, Bonifas JM, Epstein EHJ, Scott MP: Basal cell carcinomas in mice overexpressing sonic hedgehog. *Science* **276**(5313):817, 1997.

65. Unden AB, Zaphiropoulos PG, Bruce K, Toftgard R, Stahle-Backdahl M: Human patched (PTCH) mRNA is overexpressed consistently in tumor cells of both familial and sporadic basal cell carcinoma. *Cancer Res* **57**(12):2336, 1997.

66. Bare JW, Lelbo RV, Epstein EH: Loss of heterozygosity at chromosome 1q22 in basal cell carcinomas and exclusion of the basal cell nevus syndrome gene from this site. *Cancer Res* **52**:1494, 1992.

67. Newton JA, Camplejohn RS, McGibbon DH: A flow cytometric study of the significance of DNA aneuploidy in cutaneous lesions. *Br J Dermatol* **117**:169, 1987.

68. Ziegler A, Leffell DJ, Kunala S, Sharma HW, Gailani M, Simon JA, Halperin AJ, Baden HP, Shapiro PE, Bale AE, et al: Mutation hotspots due to sunlight in the *p53* gene of nonmelanoma skin cancers. *Proc Natl Acad Sci USA* **90**(9):4216, 1993.

69. Campbell C, Quinn AG, Angus B, Rees JL: The relation between *p53* mutation and p53 immunostaining in non-melanoma skin cancer. *Br J Dermatol* **129**:235, 1993.

70. McGregor JM, Yu CC, Dublin EA, Levison DA, Macdonald DM: Aberrant expression of p53 tumour-suppressor protein in non-melanoma skin cancer. *Br J Dermatol* **127**:463, 1992.

71. McNutt NS, Saenz-Santamaria C, Volkenandt M, Shea CR, Albino AP: Abnormalities of p53 protein expression in cutaneous disorders (editorial, review). *Arch Dermatol* **130**:225, 1994.

72. Rees JL: *p53* and the origins of skin cancer (editorial, comment). *J Invest Dermatol* **104**(6):883, 1995.

73. Ro YS, Cooper PN, Lee JA, Quinn AG, Harrison D, Lane D, Horne CH, Rees JL, Angus B: p53 protein expression in benign and malignant skin tumours. *Br J Dermatol* **128**:237, 1993.

74. Rees J: Genetic alterations in non-melanoma skin cancer (review). *J Invest Dermatol* **103**(6):747, 1994.

75. Hollstein M, Sidransky D, Vogelstein B, Harris CC: *p53* mutations in human cancers. *Science* **253**:49, 1991.

76. Dumaz N, Stary A, Soussi T, Daya-Grosjean L, Sarasin A: Can we predict solar ultraviolet radiation as the causal event in human tumours by analysing the mutation spectra of the *p53* gene? (review). *Mutat Res* **307**(1):375, 1994.

77. Moles JP, Moyret C, Guillot B, Jeanteur P, Guihou J, Theillet C, Basset-Seguin N: *p53* gene mutations in human epithelial skin cancers. *Oncogene* **8**:583, 1993.

78. Gailani MR, Leffell DJ, Ziegler A, Gross EG, Brash DE, Bale AE: Relationship between sunlight exposure and a key genetic alteration in basal cell carcinoma. *J Natl Cancer Inst* **88**(6):349, 1996.

79. Burns PA, Bremner R, Balmain A: Genetic changes during mouse skin tumorigenesis (review). *Environ Health Perspect* **93**:41, 1991.

80. Campbell C, Rees JL: The role of ras gene mutations in murine and human skin carcinogenesis. *Skin Cancer* **8**:245, 1993.

81. Urano Y, Asano T, Yoshimoto K, Iwahana H, Kubo Y, Kato S, Sasaki S, et al: Frequent p53 accumulation in the chronically sun-exposed epidermis and clonal expansion of p53 mutant cells in the epidermis adjacent to basal cell carcinoma. *J Invest Dermatol* **104**:928, 1995.

82. Kubo Y, Urano Y, Yoshimoto K, Iwahana H, Fukuhara K, Arase S, Itakura M: *p53* gene mutations in human skin cancers and precancerous lesions: comparison with immunohistochemical analysis. *J Invest Dermatol* **102**(4):440, 1994.

83. Friedman E, Gejman PV, Martin GA, McCormick F: Nonsense mutations in the C-terminal SH2 region of the GTPase activating protein (*GAP*) gene in human tumours. *Nature Genet* **5**:242, 1993.

84. Takata M, Quinn AG, Hashimoto K, Rees JL: Low frequency of loss of heterozygosity at the nevoid basal cell carcinoma locus and other selected loci in appendageal tumors. *J Invest Dermatol* **106**(5):1141, 1996.

85. Bazex A, Dupre A, Christol B: Atrophodermaie folliculaire, proliferations basocellulaires et hypothichose. *Ann Dermatol Syphiol* **93**:241, 1966.

86. Viksnins P, Berlin A: Follicular atrophoderma and basal cell carcinomas: The Bazex syndrome. *Arch Dermatol* **113**(7):948, 1977.

87. Goeteyn M, Geerts ML, Kint A, De Weert J: The Bazex-Dupre-Christol syndrome. *Arch Dermatol* **130**:337, 1994.

88. Kidd A, Carson L, Gregory DW, De Silva D, Holmes J, Dean JCS, Haites N: A Scottish family with Bazex-Dupre-Christol syndrome: Follicular atrophoderma, congenital hypotrichosis, and basal cell carcinoma. *J Med Genet* **33**(6):493, 1996.

89. Vabres P, Lacombe D, Rabinowitz LG, Aubert G, Anderson CE, Taieb A, Bonafe JL, Hors-Cayla MC: The gene for Bazex-Dupre-Christol syndrome maps to chromosome Xq. *J Invest Dermatol* **105**(1):87, 1995.

90. Mackie RM: *Skin Cancer*, 2d ed. London, Martin Dunitz, Ltd, 1996, pp 133–156.

91. Rowe DE, Carroll RJ, Day CL: Prognostic factors for local recurrence, metastasis, and survival rates in squamous cell carcinoma of the skin, ear, and lip. *J Am Acad Dermatol* **26**:976, 1992.

92. Lund HZ: How often does squamous cell carcinoma of the skin metastasize. *Arch Dermatol* **92**:635, 1965.

93. Callen JP, Friedman RJ, Rigel DS, Kopf AW, Harris MN, Baker D, eds: *Cancer of the Skin*. Philadelphia, Saunders, 1991, pp 27–34.

94. Sober AJ, Burstein JM: Precursors to skin cancer. *Cancer* **75**(suppl):645, 1995.

95. Marks R, Rennie G, Selwood TS: Malignant transformation of solar keratoses to squamous cell carcinoma. *Lancet* **1**:795, 1988.

96. Marks R, Foley P, Goodman G, Hage BH, Selwood TS: Spontaneous remission of solar keratoses: the case for conservative management. *Br J Dermatol* **115**:649, 1986.

97. Stephenson TJ, Cotton DW: Flow cytometric comparison of keratoacanthoma and squamous cell carcinoma (letter). *Br J Dermatol* **118**(4):582, 1988.

98. Waring AJ, Takata M, Rehman I, Rees JL: Loss of heterozygosity analysis of keratoacanthoma reveals multiple differences from cutaneous squamous cell carcinoma. *Br J Cancer* **73**(5):649, 1996.

99. Roz L, Wu CL, Porter S, Scully C, Speight P, Read A, Sloan P, et al: Allelic imbalance on chromosome 3p in oral dysplastic lesions: An early event in oral carcinogenesis. *Cancer Res* **56**(6):1228, 1996.

100. Sikkink SK, Rehman I, Rees JL: Deletion mapping of chromosome 3p and 13q and preliminary analysis of the *FHIT* gene in human nonmelanoma skin cancer. *J Invest Dermatol* **109**(6):801, 1997.

101. Quinn AG, Sikkink S, Rees JL: Delineation of two distinct deleted regions on chromosome 9 in human non-melanoma skin cancers. *Genes Chromosome Cancer* **11**:222, 1994.

102. Quinn AG, Campbell C, Healy E, Rees JL: Chromosome 9 allele loss occurs in both basal and squamous cell carcinomas of the skin. *J Invest Dermatol* **102**:300, 1994.

103. Puig S, Ruiz A, Lázaro C, Castel T, Lynch M, Palou J, Vilalta A, Weissenbach J, Mascaro J-M, Estivill X: Chromosome 9p deletions in cutaneous malignant melanoma tumors: The minimal deleted region involves markers outside the *p16* (*CDKN2*) gene. *Am J Hum Genet* **57**(2):395, 1995.

104. Sato M, Nishigori C, Zghal M, Yagi T, Takebe H: Ultraviolet-specific mutations in *p53* gene in skin tumors in xeroderma pigmentosumpatients. *Cancer Res* **53**:2944, 1993.

105. Pierceall WE, Mukhopadhyay T, Goldberg LH, Ananthaswamy HN: Mutations in the *p53* tumor suppressor gene in human cutaneous squamous cell carcinomas. *Mol Carcinog* **4**(6):445, 1991.

106. Campbell C, Quinn AG, Ro YS, Angus B, Rees JL: *p53* mutations are common and early events that precede tumor invasion in squamous cell neoplasia of the skin. *J Invest Dermatol* **100**:746, 1993.

107. Ziegler A, Jonason AS, Leffell DJ, Simon JA, Sharma HW, Kimmelman J, Remington L, Jacks T, Brash DE: Sunburn and *p53* in the onset of skin cancer. *Nature* **372**:773, 1994.

108. Campbell C, Quinn AG, Angus B, Farr PM, Rees JL: Wavelength specific patterns of *p53* induction in human skin following exposure to UV radiation. *Cancer Res* **53**:2697, 1993.

109. Healy E, Reynolds NJ, Smith M, Campbell C, Farr PM, Rees JL: Dissociation between erythema and *p53* expression in human skin: Effects of UVB irradiation and skin irritants. *J Invest Dermatol* **103**:493, 1994.

110. Hall PA, McKee PH, Menage HD, Dover R, Lane DP: High levels of *p53* protein in UV-irradiated normal human skin. *Oncogene* **8**:203, 1993.

111. Young AR: The sunburn cell. *Photodermatology* **4**:127, 1987.

112. Danno K, Horio T: Sunburn cell: Factors involved in its formation. *Photochem Photobiol* **45**:683, 1987.

113. Jonason AS, Kunala S, Price GJ, Restifo RJ, Spinelli HM, Persing JA, Leffell DJ, Tarone RE, Brash DE: Frequent clones of p53-mutated keratinocytes in normal human skin. *Proc Natl Acad Sci USA* **93**(24):14025, 1996.

114. Li G, Mitchell DL, Ho VC, Reed JC, Tron VA: Decreased DNA repair but normal apoptosis in ultraviolet-irradiated skin of p53-transgenic mice. *Am J Pathol* **148**(4):1113, 1996.

115. Nakazawa H, English D, Randell PL, Nakazawa K, Martel N, Armstrong BK, Yamasaki H: UV and skin cancer: Specific p53 gene mutation in normal skin as a biologically relevant exposure measurement. *Proc Natl Acad Sci USA* **91**:360, 1994.

116. Ren ZP, Hedrum A, Ponten F, Nister M, Ahmadian A, Lundeberg J, Uhlen M, Ponten J: Human epidermal cancer and accompanying precursors have identical p53 mutations different from p53 mutations in adjacent areas of clonally expanded non-neoplastic keratinocytes. *Oncogene* **12**(4):765, 1996.

117. Ren ZP, Ahmadian A, Ponten F, Nister M, Berg C, Lundeberg J, Uhlen M, Ponten J: Benign clonal keratinocyte patches with p53 mutations show no genetic link to synchronous squamous cell precancer or cancer in human skin. *Am J Pathol* **150**(5):1791, 1997.

118. Marks R: Premalignant disease of the epidermis: The Parkes Weber lecture 1985. *J R Coll Phys Lond* **20**(2):116, 1986.

119. Harvey I, Shalom D, Marks RM, Frankel SJ: Non-melanoma skin cancer (review). *Br Med J* **299**(6708):1118, 1989.

120. Rees JL, Altmeyer P, Hoffman K, Stücker M, eds: *Skin Cancer and UV Radiation.* Berlin, Spriner-Verlag, 1997, pp 700–708.

121. Anathaswamy HN, Pierceall WE: Molecular alterations in human skin tumors. Klein-Szanto AJP, Anderson MW, Barrett JC, Slaga TJ, eds *Comparative Molecular Carcinogenesis* New York, Wiley, 1992, pp 61–84.

122. Van der Schroeff J, Evers LM, Boot AJM, Bos JL: *ras* oncogene mutations in basal cell carcinomas and squamous cell carcinomas of human skin. *J Invest Dermatol* **94**:423, 1990.

123. Spencer JM, Kakhn SM, Jiang W, DeLeo VA, Weinstein IB: Activated *ras* genes occur in human actinic keratoses, premalignant precursors to squamous cell carcinomas. *Arch Dermatol* **131**:796, 1995.

124. Suarez HG, Daya-Grosjean L, Schlaifer D, Nardeux P, Renault G, Bos JL, Sarasin A: Activated oncogenes in human skin tumors from a repair-deficient syndrome, xeroderma pigmentosum. *Cancer Res* **49**(5):1223, 1989.

125. Daya-Grosjean L, Robert C, Drougard C, Suarez H, Sarasin A: High mutation frequency in *ras* genes of skin tumors isolated from DNA repair deficient xeroderma pigmentosum patients. *Cancer Res* **53**:1625, 1993.

126. Ishizaki K, Tsujimura T, Nakai M, Nishigori C, Sato K, Katayama S, Kurimura O, Yoshikawa K, Imamura S, Ikenaga M: Infrequent mutation of the *ras* genes in skin tumors of xeroderma pigmentosum patients in Japan. *Int J Cancer* **50**:382, 1992.

127. Straka BF, Grant-Kels JM, Friedman RJ, Rigel DS, Kopf AW, Harris MN, Baker D, eds: *Cancer of the Skin.* Philadelphia, Saunders, 1991, pp 390–407.

128. Schwartz RA: Keratoacanthoma (review). *J Am Acad Dermatol* **30**(1):1, 1994.

129. Mackie RM: *Skin Cancer,* 2d ed. London, Martin Dunitz, Ltd, 1996, pp 30–51.

130. Patel A, Halliday GM, Cooke BE, Barneston RS: Evidence that regression in keratoacanthoma is immunologically mediated: A comparison with squamous cell carcinoma. *Br J Dermatol* **131**:789, 1994.

131. Herzberg AJ, Kerns BJ, Pollack V, Kinney RB: DNA image cytometry of keratoacanthoma and squamous cell carcinoma. *J Invest Dermatol* **97**:495, 1991.

132. Ferguson-Smith MA, Wallace DC, James ZH, Renwick JH: Multiple self-healing squamous epithelioma. *Birth Defects* **7**(8):157, 1971.

133. Ferguson-Smith J: Multiple primary, self-healing epitheliomata of the skin. *Br J Dermatol* **60**:315, 1948.

134. Rook A, Moffatt JL: Multiple self-healing epitheliomata of Ferguson Smith type: Report of a case of ulilateral distribution. *Arch Dermatol* **74**:525, 1956.

135. Goudie DR, Yuille MAR, Leversha MA, Furlong RA, Carter NP, Lush MJ, Affara NA, Ferguson-Smith MA: Multiple self healing squamous epitheliomata (*ESS1*) mapped to chromosome 9q22-q31 in families with common ancestry. *Nature Genet* **3**:165, 1993.

136. Richards FM, Goudie DR, Cooper WN, Jene Q, Barroso I, Wicking C, Wainwright BJ, Ferguson-Smith MA: Mapping the multiple self-healing squamous epithelioma (*MSSE*) gene and investigation of xeroderma pigmentosum group A (*XPA*) and *PATCHED* (*PTCH*) as candidate genes. *Hum Genet* **101**(3):317, 1997.

137. Lynch HT, Fusaro RM, Roberts L, Voorhees GJ, Lynch JF: Muir-Torre syndrome in several members of a family with a variant of the cancer family syndrome. *Br J Dermatol* **113**:295, 1985.

138. Papadopoulos N, Nicolaides NC, Wei Y-F, Ruben SM, Carter KC, Rosen CA, Haseltine WA, Fleischmann RD, Fraser CM, Adams MD, Venter JC, Hamilton SR, Petersen GM, Watson P, Lynch HT, Peltomakl P, Mecklin J-P, de la Chapelle A, Kinzler KW, Vogelstein B: Mutation of a *mut*L homolog in hereditary colon cancer. *Science* **263**:1625, 1994.

139. Nyström-Lahti M, Parsons R, Sistonen P, Pylkkänen L, Aaltonen LA, Leach FS, Hamilton SR, Watson P, Bronson E, Fusaro R, Cavalieri J, Lynch J, Lanspa S, Smyrk T, Lynch P, Drouhard T, Kinzler KW, Vogelstein B, Lync HT, de la Chapelle A, Peltomäkl P: Mismatch repair genes on chromosomes 2p and 3p account for a major share of hereditary nonpolyposis colorectal cancer families evaluable by linkage. *Am J Hum Genet* **55**:659, 1994.

140. Schwartz RA, Torre DP: The Muir-Torre syndrome: A 25-year retrospect. *J Am Acad Dermatol* **33**(1):90, 1995.

141. Hall NR, Murday VA, Chapman P, Williams MA, Burn J, Finan PJ, Bishop DT: Genetic linkage in Muir-Torre syndrome to the same chromosomal region as cancer family syndrome. *Eur J Cancer* **30A**(2):180, 1994.

142. Honchel R, Halling KC, Schaid DJ, Pittelkow M, Thibodeau SN: Microsatellite instability in Muir-Torre syndrome. *Cancer Res* **54**:1159, 1994.

143. Quinn AG, Healy E, Rehman I, Sikkink S, Rees JL: Microsatellite instability in human non-melanoma and melanoma skin cancer. *J Invest Dermatol* **104**:309, 1995.

144. Jablonska S, Friedman RJ, Rigel DS, Kopf AW, Harris MN, Baker D, eds: *Cancer of the Skin.* Philadelphia, Saunders, 1991, pp 101–116.

145. Majewski S, Jablonska S: Epidermodysplasia verruciformis as a model of human papillomavirus-induced genetic cancer of the skin. *Arch Dermatol* **107**(11):1312, 1996.

146. Davidson HR, Connor JM: Dyskeratosis congenita. *J Med Genet* **25**(12):843, 1988.

147. Connor JM, Teague RH: Dyskeratosis congenita: Report of a large kindred. *Br J Dermatol* **105**(3):321, 1981.

148. Arngrimsson R, Dokal I, Luzzatto L, Connor JM: Dyskeratosis congenita: Three additional families show linkage to a locus in Xq28. *J Med Genet* **30**(7):618, 1993.

149. Heiss NS, Knight SW, Vullimany TJ, Klauck SM, Wiemann S, Mason PJ, Poustk A, Dokal I: X-linked dyskeratosis congenita is caused by mutations in a highly conserved gene with putative nucleolar functions. *Nature Genet* **19**:32, 1998.

150. Hashimoto K, Friedman RJ, Rigel DS, Kopf AW, Harris MN, Baker D, eds: *Cancer of the Skin.* Philadelphia, Saunders, 1991, pp 209–218.

151. Mackie RM: *Skin Cancer,* 2d ed. London, Martin Dunitz, Ltd, 1996, pp 242–277.

152. Nelen MR, van Staveren WC, Peeters EA, Hassel MB, Gorlin RJ, Hamm H, Lindboe CF, Fryns JP, Sijmons RH, Woods DG, Mariman EC, Padberg GW, Kremer H: Germline mutations in the PTEN/ MMAC1 gene in patients with Cowden disease. *Hum Mol Genet* **6**:1383, 1997.

153. Biggs PJ, Wooster R, Ford D, Chapman P, Mangion J, Quirk Y, Easton DF, Burn J, Atratton MR: Familial cylindromatosis (turban tumour syndrome) gene localised to chromosome 16q12-q13: Evidence for its role as a tumour suppressor gene. *Nature Genet* **11**(4):441, 1995.

154. Harada H, Hashimoto K, Ko MSH: The gene for multiple familial trichoepithelioma maps to chromosome 9p21. *J Invest Dermatol* **107**(1):41, 1996.

155. Vorechovsky I, Unden AB, Sandstedt B, Toftgard R, Stahle-Backdahl M: Trichoepitheliomas contain somatic mutations in the overexpressed *PTCH* gene: Support for a gatekeeper mechanism in skin tumorigenesis. *Cancer Res* **57**(21):4677, 1997.

156. Kricker A, Armstrong BK, English DR: Sun exposure and non-melanocytic skin cancer (review). *Cancer Causes Control* **5**(4):367, 1994.

157. Halder RM, Bridgeman-Shah S: Skin cancer in African Americans (review). *Cancer* **75**(suppl):667, 1995.

158. Chuang TY, Reizner GT, Elpern DJ, Stone JL, Farmer ER: Nonmelanoma skin cancer in Japanese ethnic Hawaiians in Kauai, Hawaii: An incidence report. *J Am Acad Dermatol* **33**(3):422, 1995.

159. Weinstock MA, Grob JJ, Stern RS, MacKie RM, Weinstock MA, eds: *Epidemiology, Causes and Prevention of Skin Diseases.* London, Blackwell Scientific, 1998, pp 121–128.

160. Kricker A, Armstrong BK, English DR, Heenan PJ: Pigmentary and cutaneous risk factors for non-melanocytic skin cancer: A case-control study. *Int J Cancer* **48**:650, 1991.

161. Urbach F, Rose DB, Bonnem RDH, Urbach F, Rose DB, Bonnem RDH, Bonnem M, eds: *Genetic and Environmental Carcinogenesis.* Baltimore, Williams & Wilkins, 1971, pp 355–371.

162. Barsh GS: The genetics of pigmentation: From fancy genes to complex traits. *Trends Genet* **12**(8):299, 1996.

163. Spritz RA: Molecular genetics of oculocutaneous albinism (review). *Hum Mol Genet* **3**(spec no):1469, 1994.

164. Lookingbill DP, Lookingbill GL, Leppard B: Actinic damage and skin cancer in albinos in northern Tanzania: Findings in 164 patients enrolled in an outreach skin care program. *J Am Acad Dermatol* **32**(4):653, 1995.

165. Luande J, Henschke CI, Mohammed N: The Tanzanian human albino skin: Natural history. *Cancer* **55**(8):1823, 1985.

166. Valverde P, Healy E, Sikkink S, Haldane F, Thody AJ, Carothers A, Jackson IJ, Rees JL: The ASP84GLU variant of the melanocortin 1 receptor (*MC1R*) is associated with melanoma. *Hum Mol Genet* **5**:1663, 1996.

167. Box NF, Wyeth JR, O'Gorman LE, Martin NG, Sturm RA: Characterization of melanocyte stimulating hormone receptor variant alleles in twins with red hair. *Hum Mol Genet* **6**(11):1891, 1997.

168. Cone RD, Lu D, Koppula S, Vage DI, Klungland H, Boston B, Chen W, Orth DN, Pouton C, Kesterson RA: The melanocortin receptors: Agonists, antagonists, and the hormonal control of pigmentation (review). *Recent Prog Horm Res* **51**:287, 1996.

169. Hill HZ: The function of melanin or six blind people examine an elephant. *Bioessays* **14**(1):49, 1992.

170. Thody AJ, Priestly GC, eds: *Molecular Aspects of Dermatology.* New York, Wiley, 1993, pp 55–73.

171. Persad S, Menon IA, Haberman HF: Comparison of the effects of UV-visible irradiation of melanins and melanin-hematoporphyrin complexes from human black and red hair. *Photochem Photobiol* **37**(1):63, 1983.

172. Frändberg PA, Doufexis M, Kapas S, Chhajlani V: Human pigmentation phenotype: A point mutation generates nonfunctional MSH receptor. *Biochem Biophys Res Commun* **245**(2):490, 1998.

173. Rees JL, Birch-Machin M, Flanagan N, Healy E, Philipp S, Todd C: Melanocortin 1 receptor (MCR1). *Ann NY Acad Sci* 1999, in press.

174. Streilein JW, Taylor JR, Vincek V, Kurimoto I, Shimizu T, Tie C, Golomb C: Immune surveillance and sunlight-induced skin cancer. *Immunol Today* **15**(4):174, 1994.

175. de Berker D, Ibbotson S, Simpson NB, Matthew JNS, Idle JR, Rees JL: Reduced experimental contact sensitivity in squamous cell but not basal cell carcinomas of the skin. *Lancet* **345**:425, 1995.

176. Heagerty AH, Fitzgerald D, Smith A, Bowers B, Jones P, Fryer AA, Zhao L, Alldersea J, Strange RC: Glutathione *S*-transferase GSTM1 phenotypes and protection against cutaneous tumours. *Lancet* **343**:266, 1994.

177. Bouwes Bavinck JN, Claas FHJ: The role of HLA molecules in the development of skin cancer. *Hum Immunol* **41**:173, 1994.

178. Czarnecki D, Tait B, Nicholson I, Lewis A: Multiple non-melanoma skin cancer: Evidence that different *MHC* genes are associated with different cancers. *Dermatology* **188**:88, 1994.

179. Streilein JW, Taylor JR, Vincek V, Kurimoto I, Richardson J, Tie C, Medema J-P, Golomb C: Relationship between ultraviolet radiation-induced immunosuppression and carcinogenesis. *J Invest Dermatol* **103**(suppl):107S, 1994.

180. Wei Q, Matanoski GM, Farmer ER, Hedayati MA, Grossman L: DNA repair and aging in basal cell carcinoma: A molecular epidemiology study. *Proc Natl Acad Sci USA* **90**:1614, 1993.

181. Hall J, English DR, Artuso M, Armstrong BK, Winter M: DNA repair capacity as a risk factor for non-melanocytic skin cancer: A molecular epidemiological study. *Int J Cancer* **58**:179, 1994.

Breast Cancer

Fergus J. Couch ∎ *Barbara L. Weber*

1. **Breast cancer is the most frequently diagnosed cancer in Western women and the leading cause of death in U.S. women aged 40 to 55. Breast cancer is heterogeneous in its clinical, genetic, and biochemical profile. The large majority of affected women present with a breast mass or mammographic abnormality as the only clinically detectable manifestation of disease, yet approximately 30 percent of women diagnosed with breast cancer go on to develop metastatic disease that ultimately is fatal.**

2. **Numerous risk factors for the development of breast cancer have been identified. Family history suggesting an inherited component in the development of some breast cancers is one of the strongest known risk factors. It is estimated that 15 to 20 percent of women with breast cancer have a family history of the disease, with approximately 5 percent of all breast cancers attributable to dominant susceptibility alleles. Two major breast cancer susceptibility genes (*BRCA1* and *BRCA2*) have been identified; others are being actively sought.**

3. **Breast cancer may present in a preinvasive form or an invasive form. Treatment depends on the stage at diagnosis, patient age at the time of diagnosis, and the presence or absence of the estrogen receptor in tumor cells. The prognosis is largely dependent on the stage at diagnosis.**

4. ***BRCA1* is a highly penetrant breast cancer susceptibility gene on chromosome 17q21 that is thought to account for 20 to 30 percent of inherited breast cancers. Families with germ-line mutations in *BRCA1* have an autosomal dominant inheritance pattern of breast cancer as well as an increased incidence of ovarian cancer. The mutation spectrum of *BRCA1* is well defined, and functional links to transcription regulation, cellular response to DNA damage, and development are becoming evident.**

5. ***BRCA2* is a highly penetrant breast cancer susceptibility gene on chromosome 13q12-13 that is thought to account for 10 to 20 percent of inherited breast cancers. Families with germ-line mutations in *BRCA2* also have an autosomal dominant inheritance pattern of breast cancer, an increased incidence of ovarian cancer that is less striking than that with *BRCA1*, and an increased incidence of male breast cancer. The mutation spectrum of *BRCA2* is well defined, and functional links also have been made to transcription regulation, cellular response to DNA damage, and development.**

6. **Sporadic breast cancers have been studied extensively for molecular changes that may provide clues to etiology, prognosis, and improved treatment approaches. Growth factors and their receptors, intracellular signaling molecules, regulators of cell cycling, adhesion molecules, and**
proteases have all been shown to be altered in sporadic breast cancer.

Breast cancer is among the most common human cancers, representing 32 percent of all incident cancers in the United States. Currently, more than 180,000 women in the United States and almost 1 million women worldwide are diagnosed with breast cancer every year.[1] Because of the magnitude of the public health problem, the desire to reduce the impact of this disease on American women, and the suitability of breast cancer as a model for the study of the molecular basis of cancer, an increasing number of investigators have focused on this disease in recent years. As a result, tremendous strides have been made in identifying susceptibility genes for breast cancer, defining regions of the human genome that harbor unidentified breast cancer-related genes, and characterizing a number of genes that are somatically altered in sporadic breast cancers. In turn, advances in these areas provide the reagents necessary to translate scientific discoveries into clinical practice as a means of improving the detection, treatment, and ultimately, prevention of breast cancer. In an effort to catalogue this large body of knowledge, this chapter provides (1) an overview of the clinical aspects of breast cancer, (2) a detailed description of the two recently isolated breast cancer susceptibility genes, *BRCA1* and *BRCA2*, (3) information on genes that contribute to less common inherited breast cancer susceptibility syndromes, (4) a summary of the genomic regions thought to harbor unidentified breast cancer-related genes, (5) a synopsis of genes that have been implicated in the development and progression of sporadic breast cancer, and (6) a review of the clinical uses of these genes for predisposition testing, disease detection, prognostication, and therapy selection.

CLINICAL ASPECTS OF BREAST CANCER

Incidence and Mortality

Breast cancer is the leading cause of death for American women between the ages of 50 and 55.[2] The most recent data suggest that 12 percent of all American women (1 in 8) will be diagnosed with breast cancer, and approximately 30 percent of the women diagnosed with breast cancer will die of the disease. Overall, there are more than 50,000 deaths from breast cancer every year in the United States alone. Adding to this concern is the fact that breast cancer incidence in the United States has been rising steadily since 1930, with an average increase of 1.2 percent per year, as reported by the Connecticut Tumor Registry.[3] The incidence in all age groups has increased, with the greatest increase occurring in older women.[4] Many investigators have attempted to explain these data, and while it appears that the advent of screening mammography and the aging of the population play a role in the increasing incidence of breast cancer, the increase reflects a real trend, suggesting that environmental or lifestyle changes may be effecting an increase in the number of breast cancers that develop. However, it is important to evaluate the age-adjusted risk for breast cancer because breast cancer risk rises steeply with age. Data from the National Cancer Institute Surveillance Program indicate that a 35-year-old woman has a risk

---

A list of standard abbreviations is located immediately preceding the index. Nonstandard abbreviations used in this chapter include: DCIS = ductal carcinoma *in situ*; LCIS = lobular carcinoma *in situ*; LFS = Li-Fraumeni syndrome; PJS = Peutz-Jeghers syndrome; LOH = loss of heterozygosity.

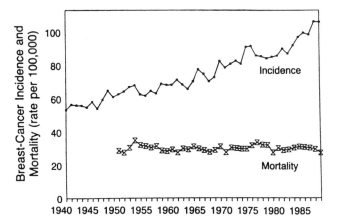

Fig. 33-1 Breast cancer incidence and mortality trends. Incidence of breast cancer in the United States from 1940 to 1985 is indicated by closed circles. Mortality rates, indicated by Xs, have remained fairly constant despite the rising incidence. (*Used with permission from Holford et al.[5]*)

of 1 in 2500, a 50-year-old woman has a risk of 1 in 50, and it is not until age 85 that risk reaches 1 in 8. Interestingly, while incidence rates have been increasing steadily, mortality rates have remained relatively constant[5] (Fig. 33-1). This constancy in the face of increasing incidence may be explained by better reporting, increases in less aggressive forms of the disease, improved detection strategies, and/or improvements in treatment.

Risk Factors

The search for breast cancer risk factors is based on a desire to explain the rising incidence of breast cancer and an obvious interest in identifying modifiable lifestyle or environmental factors that will reduce the likelihood of developing breast cancer in individual women. The best-studied and most significant risk factor is a family history of breast cancer. While shared exposure to another risk factor cannot be excluded, this most commonly represents heritable factors that increase the likelihood of developing breast cancer. The breast cancer susceptibility genes *BRCA1* and *BRCA2* represent the most dramatic examples, but since they probably account for only 15 to 20 percent of the breast cancer that clusters in families,[6] it is clear that other, less penetrant, but more common heritable factors remain to be identified. Relative risk for breast cancer with respect to family history ranges from 1.4 for a woman whose mother was diagnosed with breast cancer after age 60[7,8] to 150 for a 40-year-old woman with an inherited *BRCA1* alteration.[9] Weaker risk factors for breast cancer include early age at menarche (relative risk 1.2),[10] nulliparity (relative risk 2.0),[11] and late age at menopause (relative risk 2.0).[12] Pike and colleagues postulated that these factors all

reflect an increased number of menstrual cycles compared with multiparous women and that this is the underlying risk factor; work on this hypothesis is ongoing.[13] Additionally, terminal differentiation of breast epithelial cells does not occur until the onset of lactation after the completion of a full-term pregnancy. This final stage of differentiation may confer increased resistance to carcinogens. Radiation exposure is clearly a risk factor, with significant increases in breast cancer observed among atomic bomb survivors (maximum relative risk 13),[14,15] and in women who received mantle radiation for Hodgkin disease as children (incidence ratio 75.3).[16] Additional factors that have appeared as risk factors in some but not all studies include bottle feeding as opposed to breast feeding, alcohol intake greater than two drinks per day, a high-fat diet, prolonged oral contraceptive use, and estrogen replacement therapy.[17,18] Risk factor data are summarized in Table 33-1.

Histology of Breast Cancer

Breast carcinoma arises from the epithelium of the mammary gland, which includes the milk-producing lobules and the ducts that carry milk to the nipple (Fig. 33-2). Malignant transformation of the stromal, vascular, or fatty components of the breast is not included in this definition and is extremely rare. These facts may largely explain why breast size is not a risk factor for breast cancer, since all women have a similar amount of breast epithelium, whereas breast size is determined largely by the amount of stromal and fatty tissue. The transition from normal to malignant breast epithelium has not been as well studied as the parallel changes in colonic epithelium; however, there is increasing evidence that the breast epithelium undergoes a transformation from normal to hyperplasic, followed by the appearance of atypia in association with the hyperplasia, ultimately becoming malignant. Malignant cells continue to evolve from noninvasive carcinoma, typified by ductal carcinoma *in situ* (DCIS), to invasive carcinoma, and ultimately, to cells with metastatic potential.

Lobular Carcinoma *in Situ*. Lending confusion to the progression from normal to malignant epithelium is the entity of lobular carcinoma *in situ* (LCIS), which is not a preinvasive lesion but appears to be a marker of increased risk for the development of invasive cancer. LCIS was not identified as a clinical entity until 1941 and originally was believed to be the precursor lesion of invasive lobular carcinoma. Since its original description, LCIS has been recognized as a purely histologic diagnosis. Clinical diagnosis is not possible because LCIS does not form a palpable lesion and therefore cannot be identified on physical examination, and because it is not visible on mammography. Thus the diagnosis of LCIS always is made as an incidental finding on a breast biopsy obtained for diagnosis of an adjacent lesion. In addition, the incidence of LCIS in the general population is unknown because the nature of the diagnosis precludes studies based on mammographic screening. Evidence that LCIS is a marker lesion and not a

Table 33-1 Risk Factors for Breast Cancer

Risk Factor	Risk Category	Relative Risk	References
Family history	Mother > 60	1.4	7
	Two first-degree relatives	4–6	8
BRCA1/BRCA2 mutations	Carriers	150 (at age 40)	9
Age at menarche	< 14	1.3	10
Age at menopause	> 55	1.5	12
Parity	No full-term birth	1.9	11
Benign breast disease	Atypical hyperplasia	4.0	18
Radiation	Atomic bomb survivors	13	14,15
	Mantle radiation for Hodgkin disease	75	16

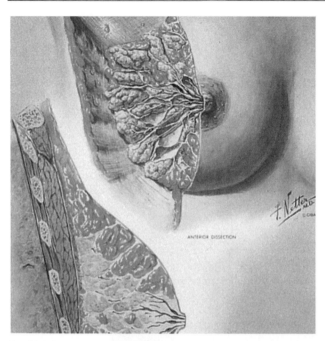

Fig. 33-2 Normal breast architecture. The breast is shown partially dissected from an anterior view (above) and in a sagittal section. Mammary ducts are seen radiating out from the nipple and terminating in milk-producing lobules. Fat and stoma surround and interdigitate with the ductal and lobular structure.

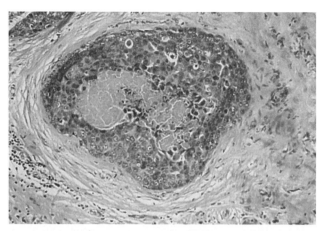

Fig. 33-3 Ductal carcinoma *in situ*. A focus of comedo-type DCIS is shown stained with hematoxylin and eosin. The malignant cells are wholly contained within the duct and do not invade the surrounding stroma. The central region is filled with necrotic cellular debris.

true malignant lesion comes from studies demonstrating that it is frequently multicentric and/or bilateral and that the invasive cancer that may develop subsequently is likely to occur distant from the known focus of LCIS and is more often of ductal rather than lobular histology.[19] The risk of invasive breast cancer after a diagnosis of LCIS has been the subject of many studies; the series with the longest follow-up was reported by Rosen and colleagues at the Memorial Sloan-Kettering Cancer Institute.[20] In this cohort, followed for a mean of 24 years, 37 percent of the women with LCIS who were not lost to follow-up developed invasive breast cancer; more than half these women developed an invasive lesion within at least 15 years following the initial diagnosis of LCIS. When the data were analyzed with the assumption that all the women lost to follow-up remained cancer-free, the percentage of patients developing invasive disease dropped to 31 percent.[20] Because of the substantial risk of invasive carcinoma and the inability to predict where it will occur in the breasts of a woman with LCIS, the treatment of LCIS presents a conundrum. Currently, patients are offered a choice between frequent mammographic surveillance and bilateral mastectomies. This widely discrepant choice is, for obvious reasons, a difficult one and seems particularly harsh when considering the emphasis on breast conservation for the treatment of invasive disease.

Although there has been considerable speculation that LCIS represents a histologic marker of genetic predisposition to breast cancer, recent work suggests that this may not be the case. In a study of 436 women with familial breast cancer and an equal number of age-matched controls selected randomly from a general hospital, Lakhani and colleagues provided evidence that LCIS was underrepresented in the familial cohort, including the subset of known *BRCA1* and *BRCA2* mutation carriers, compared with the controls (3 versus 6 percent, $p < 0.013$).[21] Data suggest that women with LCIS and a family history of breast cancer may be more likely to develop invasive cancer than those with LCIS alone[22]; however, no studies that compare invasive cancer risk in women with a family history of LCIS with that of women with no family history have been reported. Thus the question of whether family history and LCIS represent compounding risk factors remains unanswered.

Ductal Carcinoma *in Situ*. Unlike LCIS, DCIS is considered a true precursor lesion of invasive ductal carcinoma (Fig. 33-3). Historically, patients presented with a palpable breast mass, a nipple discharge, or both. Before the use of mammography, pure DCIS lesions without an invasive component were uncommon, constituting only 1 to 5 percent of all breast cancer cases.[23] Patients were treated with total mastectomy. However, after the widespread dissemination of screening mammography, the clinical picture of DCIS changed radically, with 50 to 60 percent of DCIS being diagnosed solely as a mammographic abnormality and pure DCIS representing more than 30 percent of breast cancers diagnosed by screening mammography.[24] The most common mammographic manifestation of DCIS is clustered microcalcifications. Information on the risk of progression from DCIS to invasive cancer is limited because until recently patients were treated with total mastectomy. While this is essentially 100 percent effective in preventing disease progression and death, the natural history of the lesion was obscured by the procedure. Estimates from small series of patients inadvertently treated with biopsy alone suggest that 30 to 50 percent of DCIS lesions evolve into invasive cancer within 6 to 10 years of diagnosis.[25,26] In nearly all these patients, the invasive cancer occurred at or near the original biopsy site and was of ductal histology.

As noted earlier, historically treatment of DCIS consisted of mastectomy, and in women with multifocal lesions, this is still the treatment of choice. However, recent data suggest that when the lesion is localized, lumpectomy followed by radiation does not compromise survival, allowing breast conservation for women who choose this approach.[27] A large, randomized clinical trial designed to confirm this observation and validate this treatment is being conducted by the National Surgical Adjuvant Breast and Bowel Project (NSABP).

It is clear that DCIS alone or in association with an invasive lesion may be found in women with breast cancer caused by germline mutations in the breast cancer susceptibility genes *BRCA1* or *BRCA2*. However, recent data suggest that the frequency of DCIS may be lower in inherited breast cancers than in age-matched unselected controls.[21] The biologic meaning of this finding is unclear but could reflect an early transition from noninvasive to invasive breast cancer and/or an invasive tumor with a rapid growth rate. This would result in a lesion where the noninvasive component may be too small to be clinically recognizable or where the ratio of invasive to noninvasive cancer in a given lesion makes the detection of the noninvasive component difficult.

Invasive Breast Cancer. Invasive breast cancer may be ductal or lobular in histologic type, and while there are a few distinguishing clinical features, the natural history and treatment of the two

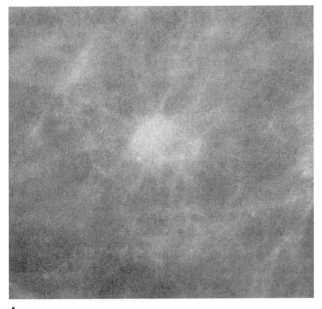

A

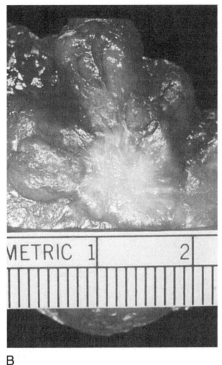

B

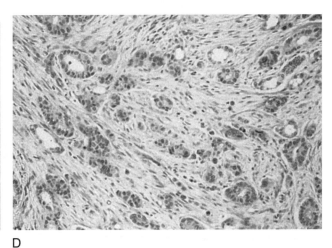

C

D

Fig. 33-4 Invasive breast cancer. *A.* Mammogram showing a spiculated mass with poorly defined borders that is characteristic of an invasive breast cancer. *B.* Invasive ductal carcinoma gross pathology. An unfixed biopsy specimen illustrates the gross pathologic correlates of the mammogram. The hard white invasive cancer extends into the breast in all directions with no defined border and numerous stellate extensions. *C.* Normal breast histopathology. The ducts are shown cut in cross section lined with a single layer of ductal epithelium. The surrounding stroma stains pink in this preparation (hematoxylin and eosin). *D.* Invasive ductal carcinoma histopathology. Malignant epithelial cells are characterized by large pleomorphic nuclei invading the breast stroma individually and in clusters and forming ductlike structures in some cases.

lesions are virtually identical. About 80 percent of invasive breast cancers are ductal carcinomas. Infiltrating lobular carcinoma is less common, representing only 5 to 10 percent of breast cancers. The remainder of invasive breast cancer consists of a variety of "special types," including tubular cancer, characterized by prominent tubule formation; medullary carcinoma, a lesion that appears poorly differentiated under the microscope but is thought to have a more favorable prognosis than other breast cancers[28]; and mucinous (or colloid) carcinoma, characterized by the abundant accumulation of extracellular mucin, bulky tumors, and a good prognosis.[17] Of particular note is the fact that approximately 15 percent of invasive carcinomas are not detectable mammographically, particularly invasive lobular carcinomas. The clinical implication of this false-negative rate is that mammography alone is not sufficient for the evaluation of a breast

mass. In the presence of a palpable breast mass, a negative mammogram should be followed by ultrasound and/or biopsy. A cystic lesion on ultrasound may be presumed benign and aspirated or followed. A solid or complex lesion should be subjected to excisional biopsy. The mammographic and histopathologic appearance of invasive breast cancer is illustrated in Fig. 33-4.

The treatment and prognosis of a woman with breast cancer are strongly influenced by the stage at the time of diagnosis. Multiple staging systems have been proposed, but the most commonly used system is the one adopted by both the American Joint Committee (AJC) and the International Union against Cancer (UICC).[29] This staging system is a detailed TNM (tumor, nodes, metastasis) system but can be summarized as in Table 33-2. Data compiled from several studies with extensive follow-up suggest that 10-year disease-free survival rates for women with invasive breast cancer

Table 33-2 AJC and IUCC Staging System for Breast Cancer

State 0	Carcinoma *in situ*
Stage I	Tumor ≤ 2 cm, negative axillary nodes
State II	Tumor from 2–5 cm and/or mobile positive axillary nodes
Stage III	Tumor > 5 cm and/or fixed axillary nodes; inflammatory breast cancer
Stage IV	Distant metastases beyond ipsilateral axillary nodes

Table 33-3 Adjuvant Treatment Options for Women with Breast Cancer

Patient Characteristics	Standard Treatment
Premenopausal	
Tumor <1 cm, node negative	None
Tumor ≥1 cm, node negative	Chemotherapy with tamoxifen if ER+
Tumor ≥1 cm, node positive	Chemotherapy with tamoxifen if ER+
Postmenopausal	
Tumor <1 cm, node negative	None
Tumor ≥1 cm, node negative, ER+	Tamoxifen or observation
Tumor ≥1 cm, node negative, ER −	Chemotherapy or observation
Tumor ≥1 cm, node negative, ER+	Tamoxifen ± chemotherapy
Tumor ≥1 cm, node negative, ER −	Chemotherapy

are approximately 80 percent for women diagnosed with stage I disease, decreasing to 55 percent (stage II), 40 percent (stage III), and 10 percent (stage IV) as the stage at diagnosis increases[30,31] (Fig. 33-5).

Since breast cancer is considered a systemic disease at the time of detection, treatment is designed to achieve two distinct goals: (1) local control of the tumor in the breast and the ipsilateral axillary lymph nodes and (2) eradication of clinically occult systemic micrometastases. Local control may be obtained in most cases by mastectomy alone or by lumpectomy (removal of the tumor with histologically negative margins) followed by radiation therapy to the affected breast. Lumpectomy without radiation is associated with a 35 percent local recurrence rate and thus is considered unacceptable[32] and is rarely used. Since multiple randomized studies have shown that the breast-conserving approach of lumpectomy and radiation does not compromise survival compared with mastectomy, this therapeutic choice is often left to the individual patient. Relative contraindications to the use of breast conservation are related to the presence of a multicentric or multifocal tumor, extensive DCIS in association with an invasive tumor, or a large tumor (> 5 cm). Large tumors are particularly problematic in a small breast, where the cosmetic result associated with a complete excision may be compromised by the relative amount of tissue that must be removed to obtain clear margins around the tumor. However, the choice of procedure generally is dictated only by personal preference (some patients feel more comfortable with removal of the entire breast despite data supporting the safety of lumpectomy) and convenience (some patients choose mastectomy to avoid 6 to 7 weeks of daily radiotherapy treatments).

Once local control has been achieved by one of the two surgical options just discussed, adjuvant therapy may be used to reduce the likelihood of a systemic recurrence. Often confusing to patients, the decision to use adjuvant chemotherapy is not dictated by the choice of local therapy but by the stage of disease and the menopausal status of the patient. The adjuvant regimens most commonly used include a 3- to 6-month course of chemotherapy and/or a prolonged course of the partial estrogen antagonist tamoxifen. Surgical oophorectomy (removal of both ovaries) performed after local therapy also has been shown to reduce the risk of systemic recurrence in premenopausal patients. While the needs of each patient must be addressed individually, generalizations can be made about the choice of therapy (Table 33-3). First, there is increasing evidence that women with tumors less than 1 cm in diameter without involved axillary nodes do not require adjuvant therapy. The 10-year survival rates for women in this category exceed 90 percent, and the relative benefit derived from adjuvant treatment adds little to this excellent prognosis. In contrast, numerous studies support the use of adjuvant therapy in premenopausal women with tumors greater than 1 cm in diameter regardless of nodal status. In this setting, chemotherapy is associated with the greatest increase in overall survival, with tamoxifen generally being added for women with tumors that appear to be hormonally responsive by virtue of expressing the estrogen receptor (ER). More controversial is the treatment of postmenopausal women because tamoxifen alone may be of benefit equivalent to that of chemotherapy, obviating the need for chemotherapy in postmenopausal women with ER-positive tumors. Postmenopausal women with ER-negative tumors without involved axillary nodes may receive no adjuvant therapy or be given a course of chemotherapy depending on a number of variables, including the size and grade of the tumor as well as the general health status of the patient. Postmenopausal women with involved axillary nodes may receive chemotherapy and/or tamoxifen depending on their ER status. Chemotherapy may be administered for 3 to 6 months, is given in the outpatient setting, and generally is well tolerated. The most commonly employed regimens include cyclophosphamide and doxorubicin or cyclophosphamide, methotrexate, and 5-fluorouracil. A taxane increasingly is becoming an important part of this regimen. Tamoxifen is self-administered orally and is taken daily for a minimum of 5 years after the diagnosis.

Finally, autologous bone marrow transplantation is an experimental adjuvant therapy approach that may be an option for women with a high risk of systemic relapse. These women generally are defined by the presence of 10 or more involved axillary lymph nodes or by the presence of inflammatory breast cancer, a particularly aggressive form of invasive carcinoma that presents clinically with diffuse breast pain, swelling, and redness.

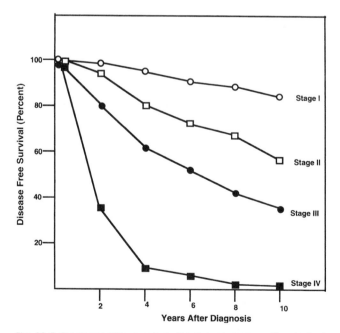

Fig. 33-5 Stage-specific survival for breast cancer. Survival at 2-year intervals is indicated by stage (IUCC). Stage I: open circles; stage II: open squares; stage III: shaded circles; stage IV: shaded squares.

Ten-year survival rates for patients with both these clinical entities are only 15 to 20 percent in the absence of systemic therapy. Conventional-dose chemotherapy, which may improve survival by 10 to 15 percent, is still associated with 10-year recurrence rates of 60 to 65 percent.[33]

Autologous bone marrow transplantation for breast cancer was designed as a means of delivering very high doses of chemotherapy that would be fatal in the absence of a method for protecting bone marrow stem cells from the toxic effects of treatment. In this setting, bone marrow cells may be harvested directly from the iliac crest or by pheresis of stem cells from peripheral blood. Stem cells are stored (by freezing) during intensive chemotherapy and reinfused into the patient when the drugs have been cleared. While this approach is promising, the long-term results are not available.

The interventions just described are of clear benefit in reducing the risk of recurrence; nonetheless, overall, at least 30 percent of patients with breast cancer will relapse and die of the disease. Metastatic disease (stage IV) may be extremely variable in course. Ten-year survival rates are dismal at 5 to 10 percent,[33] with the median survival for patients with metastatic disease being approximately 18 months. However, while some patients with metastatic breast cancer may succumb within months of a recurrence, others, particularly those with metastases to bone as the only site of disease, may do well with minimally progressive disease for years. Time to recurrence is also extremely variable, since some patients will relapse with aggressive drug-resistant tumors within weeks of the completion of adjuvant therapy and some patients will have disease-free intervals of up to 30 years before ultimate disease recurrence.

Treatment for metastatic disease must be individualized but may include chemotherapy, hormonal therapy, and palliative radiation therapy. Surgical resection of chest wall recurrences after mastectomy may be indicated in some patients. Unfortunately, treatment of metastatic breast cancer is uniformly considered palliative. The only exception at present may be a subset of patients who achieve complete remission of all clinically detectable tumors with standard chemotherapy and then undergo autologous bone marrow transplantation. While early studies suggested that 10 to 15 percent of these patients may attain durable complete remissions[34], recent studies have failed to show a benefit of this approach.[34b]

THE GENETICS OF BREAST CANCER

Breast cancer is a complex and heterogeneous disease caused by interactions of both genetic and nongenetic factors; however, a family history of breast cancer has long been recognized as a significant risk factor, as evidenced by the fact that familial clustering of breast cancer was first described by physicians in ancient Rome.[35] The first modern documentation of familial clustering of breast cancer was published in 1866 by a French surgeon who reported 10 cases of breast cancer in four generations of his wife's family; four other women in this family died as a result of hepatic tumors that may well have been metastatic breast cancer.[36] In 1984, Williams and Anderson were the first to provide statistical evidence for an autosomal dominant breast cancer susceptibility gene with age-related penetrance, using segregation analysis to compare various models that might explain the pattern of aggregation of breast cancer in families.[37] This model was supported in 1988 by Newman and colleagues,[38] and the hypothesis was proven correct in 1994 with isolation of the susceptibility gene BRCA1.[39]

Two high-penetrance breast cancer susceptibility genes have been identified (BRCA1 and BRCA2),[39–41] and others are being actively sought. Breast cancer in families with germ-line mutations in these genes appears as an autosomal dominant trait, as predicted by previous work. In addition, mutations in several other genes such as TP53, MSH2, and PTEN have been identified as rare causes of hereditary breast cancer. Finally, it is very likely

that other lower-penetrance genes are responsible for inherited susceptibility to breast cancer in families in which the incidence of breast cancer is higher than that in the general population, but the susceptibility inheritance pattern does not fit the classic model of Mendelian inheritance.

Given the strong influence of molecular genetics in medicine in recent years, there is a tendency to assume that familial clustering of disease results from a genetically inherited predisposition. However, other explanations for familial clustering of breast cancer are possible, including (1) geographically limited environmental exposure to carcinogens that might affect an extended family living in close proximity, (2) culturally motivated behavior that alters the risk factor profile such as age at first live birth and contraceptive choice, and (3) socioeconomic influences that, for example, may result in differing dietary exposures. In addition, multiple, complex inherited genetic factors are likely to influence the extent to which a risk factor for breast cancer plays a role in any single individual; such modifying effects are likely to be shared among genetically similar members of an extended family. Nonetheless, while noninherited factors certainly play a role in familial clustering of breast cancer, recent advances have provided unequivocal evidence for the presence of breast cancer susceptibility genes that are directly responsible for 5 to 10 percent of all breast cancers.

Breast cancer due to inherited susceptibility has several distinctive clinical features: Age at diagnosis is considerably lower than in sporadic cases, the prevalence of bilateral breast cancer is higher, and the presence of associated tumors in affected individuals is noted in some families. Associated tumors may include ovarian, colon, prostate, and endometrial cancers and sarcomas.[42] However, breast cancer due to inherited susceptibility does not appear to be distinguished by histologic type, metastatic pattern, or survival characteristics. The study of BRCA1 and BRCA2[39,40] has greatly expanded our knowledge of inherited susceptibility breast cancer, and the study of these and other genes continues at a rapid pace.

BRCA1

Clinical Features of Affected Families. In 1990, chromosome 17q21 was identified as the location of a susceptibility gene for early-onset breast cancer now termed BRCA1.[39] Linkage between the genetic marker D17S74 on 17q21 and the appearance of ovarian cancer in several large kindreds was subsequently demonstrated.[43] A collaborative study of more than 200 families suggested that breast/ovarian cancer was linked to markers in this region in more than 90 percent of families with apparent autosomal dominant transmission of breast cancer and at least one case of ovarian cancer. Linkage between breast cancer and genetic markers on 17q12-q21 was observed in just 45 percent of families with breast cancer only. However, the percentage of site-specific breast cancer families in this study attributed to BRCA1 mutations rose to almost 70 percent when the median age of onset of breast cancer in the families was less than 45 years.[9] As greater numbers of breast cancer families have been screened for mutations in BRCA1, it has become apparent that the role of BRCA1 in familial breast and/or ovarian cancer may have been overestimated. These data were collected from the largest, most severely affected families that were suitable for linkage analysis, thereby introducing substantial ascertainment bias. Recent studies of the complete spectrum of families (from 3 to 12 affected members) that present at high-risk breast cancer clinics suggest that BRCA1 mutations are responsible for 20 to 30 percent of familial breast cancer and 10 to 20 percent of familial ovarian cancer.[44–47] While the families used in these studies most likely include cancer clusters not associated with a dominant susceptibility gene, it is clear that BRCA1 is responsible for far less familial breast cancer than the widely quoted estimate of 45 percent.[9]

As described earlier, breast cancer in highly penetrant families appears as a classic Mendelian trait of autosomal dominant

Breast Cancer Penetrance

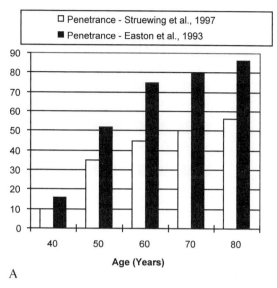

A

Ovarian Cancer Penetrance

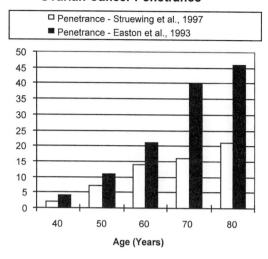

B

Fig. 33-6 Breast and ovarian cancer risks associated with *BRCA1* and *BRCA2* mutations. *A.* Age-adjusted penetrance for breast cancer in *BRCA1* and *BRCA2* mutation carriers comparing data from Easton et al.[48] **and Struewing et al.**[49] ***B.* Age-adjusted penetrance for ovarian cancer in *BRCA1* and *BRCA2* mutation carriers comparing data from Easton et al.**[48] **and Struewing et al.**[49]

transmission with high penetrance, with almost 50 percent of the children of carriers developing breast and/or ovarian cancer by age 85. Female mutation carriers are estimated to have an 87 percent lifetime risk of developing breast cancer[9] and a 40 to 60 percent lifetime risk of developing ovarian cancer[48] (Fig. 33-6). Approximately 20 percent of female *BRCA1* mutation carriers will develop breast cancer by age 40 years, 51 percent by age 50 years, and 87 percent by age 70. *BRCA1* mutation carriers also have an increased incidence of bilateral breast cancer. In a study of 33 families with evidence of germ-line mutations in *BRCA1* conducted by the Breast Cancer Linkage Consortium, the cumulative risk of developing a second breast cancer was estimated to be 65 percent for mutations carriers who live to age 70.[48] However, ascertainment bias again affects these risk estimates.

However, studies of families segregating *BRCA1* mutations have shown that in many cases the mutations are nonpenetrant. By focusing on founder mutations in the Ashkenazi population, Struewing and colleagues estimated the penetrance of *BRCA1* and *BRCA2* mutations in this population at 56 and 16 percent, respectively[49] (Fig. 33-6). Results from three additional population-based studies using estimates of *BRCA1* and *BRCA2* prevalence suggest that the risk for breast and ovarian cancer by age 80 years in mutation carriers is 73.5 and 27.8 percent, respectively.[50] Thus it is likely that different mutations, variable genetic background, and differential exposure to certain risk factors result in a great variation in penetrance. Currently, penetrance for breast cancer is thought to range between 56 and 86 percent.[51]

Risk for other cancers also may be increased in the presence of an inherited *BRCA1* mutation. Data published in 1993 from a study of a large Icelandic breast/ovarian cancer family suggested that prostate cancer may be a component of the *BRCA1* syndrome.[52] Subsequently, the Breast Cancer Linkage Consortium estimated a relative risk of 3.33 for prostate cancer in males thought to carry *BRCA1* germ-line mutations and a relative risk of 4.11 for colon cancer.[53] It is important to note that the excess colon cancer risk reflects the experience of only a few families, suggesting either very low penetrance with regard to colon cancer or a limited number of specific mutations that increase colon cancer risk. No significant excesses were observed for cancers originating from other anatomic sites.[53] Male breast cancer is also associated with *BRCA1* germ-line mutations.

To determine whether tumors that arise as a result of *BRCA1* mutations have clinical and pathologic characteristics that differ from those of sporadic tumors, Lynch and colleagues analyzed 180 tumors from hereditary breast/ovarian or site-specific breast cancer families.[54] Ninety-eight of the 180 tumors were considered as a subset more likely than the remainder to result from *BRCA1* mutations on the basis of linkage analysis or the presence of ovarian cancer in the family. Patients in both subgroups were significantly younger than the population average for women with breast cancer. In addition, the "*BRCA1* group" was found to have more aneuploid and more high S-phase tumors, but surprisingly, disease-free survival was longer in this group than in the group thought less likely to have *BRCA1* mutations. Tubular and lobular cancers were less common in the group where the presence of *BRCA1* mutations was suspected. These investigators suggested that *BRCA1* mutations may result in tumors with adverse pathologic indicators but a paradoxically better survival than expected. Unfortunately, this study was performed before it was possible to determine which tumors were actually attributable to *BRCA1* mutations. Subsequent studies of the pathobiology of breast tumors associated with *BRCA1* verified that these tumors are often high grade and tend to be estrogen and progesterone receptor negative[20,55–59] (Fig. 33-7). One further study suggested a correlation between the absence of *BRCA1* in the nucleus of cells from *BRCA1* tumors and high proliferative rate.[60] However, the possibility that these tumors are associated with a paradoxically better survival has not been substantiated.

Several more recent studies have shown that survival for carriers of *BRCA1* mutations may be similar to that of sporadic breast cancer patients when controlling for stage of diagnosis,[61,62] and a study of Ashkenazi Jewish *BRCA1* mutation carriers suggested that *BRCA1* mutation is an adverse prognostic factor.[63] Genetic studies of *BRCA1*-related breast and ovarian tumors by comparative genome hybridization indicate that these tumors have high levels of amplification and deletion, suggesting that the tumors are genetically unstable and highly proliferative.[64,65] Several regions of amplification and deletion were identified in familial breast tumors, but not in sporadic breast tumors, whereas amplification of 2q24-q32 accounted for the only apparent difference between familial and sporadic ovarian tumors.[65]

Several environmental factors have been identified that modify the risk of breast and ovarian cancer in *BRCA1* mutation carriers.

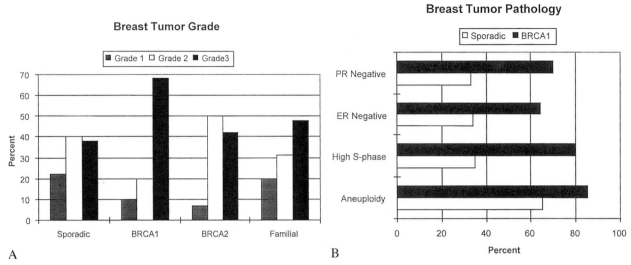

Fig. 33-7 Pathologic features of *BRCA1* and *BRCA2* breast cancers. **A.** Grade distribution of sporadic *BRCA1*, *BRCA2*, and combined familial breast tumors. (*Used with permission from MR Stratton.*[21]) *B.* Frequency of pathobiologic characteristics of sporadic and *BRCA1*-related breast tumors. PR refers to the progesterone receptor, and ER refers to the estrogen receptor. (Data from refs. 21,30,56, and 62.)

A recent study reported that women who smoke and have *BRCA1* or *BRCA2* mutations have a lower risk of breast cancer.[66] Subjects who smoked more than 4 pack-years had a lower breast cancer risk (odds ratio of 0.46, 95% CI = 0.27–0.80) than nonsmokers. One explanation for this observation is based on the relationship of estrogen to breast cancer and on the fact that women smokers are found to have lower levels of estrogen on average. This study is preliminary and needs to be repeated, taking into account the clustering of cases within specific families and adjusting for other effectors of circulating estrogen levels in the subjects.

Another recent study also reported that oral contraceptives may reduce the risk of ovarian cancer in *BRCA1* or *BRCA2* mutation carriers.[67] The odds ratio for ovarian cancer associated with any use of oral contraceptives was 0.5 (95% CI = 0.3–0.8). Oral contraceptive use for greater than 6 years was associated with a 60 percent risk reduction. While this result supports previous observations that oral contraceptives are protective for ovarian cancer, no consideration was given to the possible increased risk of breast cancer in this study. The study also contained a possible source of bias in the control group. First, many of the controls did not have a defined *BRCA1* or *BRCA2* mutation. Second, many of the controls who were assessed for ovarian cancer development had previously undergone prophylactic oophorectomy. And third, the controls contained a significantly lower proportion of Ashkenazi Jewish individuals than the study population. These findings await further confirmation.

It also is becoming clear that modifying genes affect the penetrance of *BRCA1* mutations.[68] In the first study to assess the role of potential modifiers of *BRCA1* penetrance, rare alleles at the *HRAS1* (*Harvey ras* proto-oncogene) VNTR were associated with an increased risk of ovarian cancer in individuals with a *BRCA1* mutation.[69] Recently, it has been reported that the common *APC I1307K* variant that occurs in 6 percent of the Ashkenazi Jewish population and has been associated with colorectal neoplasia is also associated with an increased risk of developing breast cancer in the Ashkenazi population.[70] In this study, 10.4 percent of individuals with breast cancer (unselected for family history of breast cancer) carried the variant in comparison with 6.8 percent of unaffected Ashkenazi controls. The frequency of the variant in carriers of *BRCA1* and *BRCA2* mutations was significantly greater than in controls (OR = 1.9, 95% CI = 1.2–3.0), suggesting an association between *BRCA1/2* mutations and the *APC* variant. However, no association between breast cancer risk and the *APC* variant was seen in patients without *BRCA1* or *BRCA2* mutations

(OR = 1.4, 95% CI = 1.0–1.8),[70] nor was age at onset of breast cancer afffected by the presence of *I1307K* mutation.

Isolation of *BRCA1*. No information was available on the structure and function of the *BRCA1* gene before its identification in 1994; thus positional cloning was used by several groups in an attempt to isolate the gene. These efforts began in 1990 with identification of chromosome 17q21 as the location of *BRCA1*. Initial linkage analysis was performed on seven families and yielded a maximum cumulative Lod score of 5.98.[71] Several groups adopted linkage analysis and positional cloning strategies in an attempt to locate the *BRCA1* gene. In late 1994, this effort culminated in identification of the *BRCA1* gene by Miki and colleagues.[39]

BRCA1 is a novel gene composed of 24 exons, with an mRNA that is 7.8 kb in length, and 22 coding exons translating into a protein of 1863 amino acids (Fig. 33-8). The entire gene covers approximately 80 kb of genomic sequence. The structure of *BRCA1* is unusual, with most exons in the expected 100- to 500-bp size, but with exon 11 (approximately 3500 bp) constituting approximately 60 percent of the coding region of the gene (see Fig. 33-8). The functional or evolutionary significance of this unusual structure is unknown. Exon 4 is thought to be an artifact of the isolation method and is omitted from the gene sequence. The BRCA1 protein contains a zinc-binding RING finger motif near the N-terminus and two BRCT (*BRCA1* C-terminal) domains in tandem (motif 1: amino acids 1653–1736; motif 2: amino acids 1760–1855). The RING finger motif has been identified in numerous transcription factors and cofactors involved in both DNA and protein binding, suggesting a role for *BRCA1* in transcription regulation, while the BRCT motifs have been found in a number of proteins involved in cell cycle control and DNA repair.[72]

The murine homologue of *BRCA1* has been characterized by several groups.[73–75] The mouse cDNA sequence predicts a protein of 1812 amino acids, 51 residues shorter than the human cDNA. The human and mouse proteins display 58 percent identity and 73 percent similarity, with perfect conservation in the RING finger domain near the N-terminus and high homology in a putative acidic transactivation domain at the C-terminus.[73] The canine form of *BRCA1* also has been identified and sequenced and, similar to the murine form, displays greater than 80 percent identity in both the RING domain and in 80 amino acids at the C-terminus containing the acidic transactivation domain.[76] Finally, a fragment of the rat *BRCA1* gene containing the RING domain has been

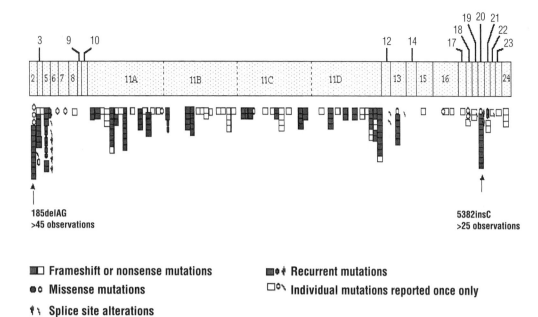

Frameshift or nonsense mutations

Missense mutations

Splice site alterations

Recurrent mutations

Individual mutations reported once only

Fig. 33-8 Structure and mutation spectrum of *BRCA1*. Diagram demonstrating even distribution of mutations across the *BRCA1* coding sequence. The 24 exons of *BRCA1* are represented by vertical lines within the gene. Mutations are depicted beneath the *BRCA1* exon where the mutation occurrs. Mutations are categorized according to recurrance and mutation type, as shown in the accompanying key. The idiogram was copied from the Breast Cancer Information Core (BIC) Web site and was generated by Simon Gayther, Cambridge, U.K. in 1997. Updated data is available on the BIC Web site.

sequenced and shown to have high homology with the human form.[77]

Mutational Spectrum. Since the identification of *BRCA1*, more than 500 sequence variations have been detected (see Fig. 33-8). Initial reports described eight disease-associated mutations within the gene,[39,78] followed shortly afterward by an increasing number of novel mutations.[79–81] Surprisingly, almost all described mutations are germ-line mutations, with *BRCA1* mutations being extremely rare in sporadic breast and ovarian tumors,[82–85] suggesting that *BRCA1* coding-region mutations play a limited role in the development of sporadic breast cancer. A single individual has been reported to be homozygous for a *BRCA1* mutation, inheriting the same mutation from each parent.[86] This apparently homozygous individual is developmentally normal but was diagnosed with breast cancer at age 32. It has recently been suggested that PCR error led to erroneous classification of this individual as a homozygote for a *BRCA1* mutation.

A variety of mutation-detection techniques have been used to identify *BRCA1* mutations, including SSCP,[79,80,87] protein truncation assays,[88,89] multiplex heteroduplex analysis,[90] conformation-sensitive gel electrophoresis,[44,91] and most commonly, direct sequencing. Details of these techniques are available on the Breast Cancer Information Core (BIC) Web site: *http://www.nhgri.nih.gov/Intramural_research/Lab_transfer/Bic/.* A report from 1996 describing the first 254 sequence variants in the *BRCA1* gene showed that 55 percent of the mutations were located in exon 11 (which contains 62 percent of the gene-coding sequence), suggesting that sequence alterations are scattered evenly throughout *BRCA1*.[92] In this early summary, the great majority of mutations resulted in truncation or absence of the protein product. This number included frameshift and nonsense mutations, splice variants that also create frameshifts and stop codons in the gene, and ill-defined noncoding region mutations. The remaining sequence variants were nontruncating missense mutations within the *BRCA1* coding sequence. The four noncoding region mutations were inferred from inactivation of transcription of one allele of *BRCA1*.[39,93,94] The specific DNA alterations that result in inactivation of transcription in these samples have not been determined. Serova and colleagues also identified various

regions of the *BRCA1* cDNA that when mutated led to complete loss of the allele-specific transcript, presumably as a result of destabilization and degradation of mRNA.[94]

Analysis of more than 500 *BRCA1* mutations in the BIC database suggests that the data for the earlier study were biased toward truncating mutations. It is now believed that approximately 30 percent of all *BRCA1* mutations are missense alterations. This group of sequence alterations includes defined disease-associated mutations, polymorphisms, and unclassified variants. Several *BRCA1* missense mutations are thought to inactivate *BRCA1* function. The C61G variant is thought to alter the structure of the RING finger domain,[95] which is known to bind both the BARD[96] and BAP[97] proteins. The C64G variant originally was reported as a RING finger missense mutation; however, this variant could also result in altered splicing and a frameshift within *BRCA1* due to the formation of a cryptic slice site. In addition, a G → C transversion at nucleotide 117 in the Kozak site of the *BRCA1* gene recently has been postulated to alter translation of the BRCA1 protein.[98] Several missense mutations from the exon 17–21 region of *BRCA1,* which is now known to encode a transcription activation domain, also have been shown to ablate *BRCA1* function by a yeast growth assay.[99] The assay also was successful in identifying several nonfunctional polymorphisms. In the absence of functional assays, frequency data currently are being used to predict the role of missense mutation in disease. However, conclusive evidence awaits the establishment of a robust *BRCA1* functional assay.

Two studies have determined that large genomic deletions form part of the constellation of *BRCA1* mutations. Mazoyer and colleagues identified a 1.7-kb deletion within *BRCA1* that was postulated to result from inter-Alu recombination.[100] Three genomic deletions within the *BRCA1* gene have been shown to account for 30 percent of *BRCA1* mutations in the Dutch-Belgian high-risk breast cancer population.[101] The high frequency of Alu-related repetitive sequences in the intronic regions of *BRCA1* is thought to facilitate the formation of these deletions by homologous recombination.

Two studies have identified a genotype-phenotype correlation,[93,102] suggesting that mutations in the 5′ half of *BRCA1* predispose to both breast and ovarian cancer, whereas mutations closer to the 3′ portion of the gene are predominantly associated with site-specific breast cancer. This correlation is rarely seen in the *BRCA1* populations from the United States but holds up well in the majority of European studies. Mutations occurring in two terminal regions of *BRCA1* may be associated with a more severe phenotype, as defined by high tumor grade,[103] suggesting that these two regions may be important in the control of mammary cell growth.

The two most common mutations in *BRCA1* are 185delAG and 5382insC.[92] These mutations have been shown to occur at a frequency of 8 and 1.2 per 1000 individuals in the Ashkenazi Jewish population,[49,104] as compared with the overall frequency of *BRCA1* mutations in an unselected Caucasian population of about 1 in 1500, suggesting the presence of a founder effect in the Ashkenazi Jewish population. This observation has been expanded to include the Moroccan Iraqi and Yemenite Jewish populations.[105] Analysis of germ-line *BRCA1* mutations in Jewish and non-Jewish women with early onset breast cancer indicated that approximately 21 percent of Jewish women who develop breast cancer before age 40 may carry the 185delAG mutation.[106,107] Preliminary screening of unselected Ashkenazi Jewish patients showed that 20 to 60 percent with ovarian cancer and 30 percent with early onset breast cancer carried either the 185delAG *BRCA1* mutation or the 6174delT *BRCA2* mutation.[108–110]

Haplotype analysis of 185delAG *BRCA1* mutation carriers has identified two common haplotypes within the Ashkenazi Jewish population.[111] These studies suggest that although these are ancestral mutations, several founder populations may have arisen independently. The location of the mutation in a tandem AG repeat suggests that this may be a hypermutable region. Other haplotype studies have identified three common haplotypes in a large series of breast and ovarian cancer cases using four common polymorphisms.[112] No association was found between the presence of the common haplotypes and breast or ovarian cancer, suggesting that common polymorphisms in *BRCA1* do not make a significant contribution to development of breast or ovarian cancer. However, the same study suggested that the Gln356Arg polymorphism may be associated with a protective effect against breast cancer and thus actually may be a gain-of-function mutation.

A number of studies have investigated the frequency of *BRCA1* mutations in subpopulations. Founder mutations identified thus far include the G5193A mutation in three Icelandic families,[113] the 3745delT and IVS1-2A→G mutations in the Finnish population,[114] and the185delAG and 5382insC mutations in the Ashkenazi Jewish,[49] Hungarian,[115] and Russian[116] populations. Common genomic deletions have been found in the Dutch-Belgian population,[101] along with the 1675delA mutation in the Norwegian population.[117] King and Szabo recently presented a comprehensive review of many of these studies.[118]

A number of large mutation screening studies of women with breast and/or ovarian cancer with and without a family history of breast and/or ovarian cancer also have been completed in an effort to define the prevalence of *BRCA1* mutations in certain subsets of the population and to determine risk estimates for women conforming to the selection criteria. Studies of *BRCA1* mutations in women with early onset breast cancer have shown that approximately 10 percent of unselected breast cancer patients under 40 years of age carry *BRCA1* mutations. Similarly, only 7 percent of site-specific breast cancer families carry mutations. In comparison, 17 to 20 percent of all breast cancer families including those with breast and ovarian cancer possess *BRCA1* mutations. This indicates that ovarian cancer within a family is a strong predictor of the presence of a *BRCA1* mutation.[44] The data also suggest that other, as yet unidentified genes exist that predispose to early onset breast cancer and site-specific breast cancer. A number of other studies have validated these results and have extended the studies to show that only 7 percent of breast cancer patients under 45 years of age with an affected first-degree relative carried *BRCA1* mutations.[119] In a similar study and the first to consider *BRCA1* mutation prevalence in the African-American population, it was reported that 3 percent of Caucasians

Table 33-4 Germ-line BRACA1 and BRCA2 Mutations in Select Populations

Population	No. of Cases	Percent with Germ-line Mutations
BRCA1		
High-risk families*		
Britain	339	21%
France	160	24%
Sweden	106	23%
USA	238	26.5%
High-risk Ashkenazi Jewish		
Israel	42	38%
Early onset breast cancer, non-Ashkenazi Jewish		
USA, <40 y	94	13%
USA, <32 y	73	12.3%
Japan, <35, bilateral	103	4%
Early onset breast cancer, Ashkenazi		
USA, <40 y	39	21%
Population based		
USA, Jewish	5318	1.15%
US Breast cancer cases (North Carolina)		
White	120	3.3%
Black	88	8%
US breast cancer cases (Seattle)		
<35 y	193	6.2%
<45 y, 1st degree affected	208	7.2%
BRCA2		
High-risk families		
Finland	100	11%
Sweden	106	11.3%
Europe	22	27%
USA	238	13%
High-risk Ashkenazi Jewish		
Israel	42	21%
Early onset breast cancer, non-Ashkenazi Jewish		
USA, <32	73	2.7%
Early onset breast cancer, Ashkenazi Jewish		
Israel, <40 y	43	7%
Population based		
Washington, D.C., Jewish	5318	1.11%
Male breast cancer (USA)		
Family history	50	14%
Unselected	54	3.7%

*High-risk families have three or more cases of female breast and/or any cases of ovarian cancer.

NOTE: All cases represent individuals affected with breast cancer.[118] Visit the BIC Web site at for a comprehensive listing at: http://ruly70.medfac.leidenuniv.nl/~devilee/screen.htm.

and less than 1 percent of African-Americans with breast cancer unselected for family history possessed *BRCA1* mutations.[120] Cumulatively, these data suggest that *BRCA1* mutations are rare in those individuals who do not have a significant family history of breast and/or ovarian cancer. Similar studies have not yet been reported for Hispanics, Asians, Native Americans, and other ethnic populations. A summary of these studies is presented in Table 33-4.[44,45,47,49,92,94,108,110,119–123]

Clinical Utility of Mutation Testing. Testing for *BRCA1* and *BRCA2* mutations is now widely available both commercially and in research studies. One problem associated with mutation screening is the identification of missense mutations that cannot be classified as either benign variants or disease-associated mutations. Approximately 20 percent of all identified variants reported in the BIC database excluding common polymorphisms are missense mutations. Improvement in the identification of disease-associated variants awaits the development of functional assays for the *BRCA1* and *BRCA2* genes. A second difficulty is the recent realization that current mutation screening technology may fail to identify as many as 20 to 30 percent of mutations in families linked to the *BRCA1* and *BRCA2* genes. A third problem associated with testing is the observation that perhaps only 40 percent of high-risk breast cancer families are associated with *BRCA1* and *BRCA2* mutations. Thus a high percentage of mutation tests will produce negative results.

In an attempt to improve the selection of patients for mutation testing, several laboratories have generated frequency tables and models based on screening of high-risk women that predict the presence of a *BRCA1* mutation. The first study of this kind identified *BRCA1* mutations in 169 women with breast cancer from high-risk families containing from 1 to 11 cases of breast cancer. A probability model was developed that predicts the presence of a *BRCA1* mutation by considering family characteristics, including (1) average age of onset of breast cancer in the family, (2) Ashkenazi Jewish ancestry, (3) presence of ovarian cancer, and (4) presence of breast and ovarian cancer in a single individual.[44] A second *BRCA1* predictive model used frequency data from mutation studies of several hundred individuals to provide probabilities for the presence of a *BRCA1* mutation. Probability tables were provided for (1) number of breast cancers, (2) number of ovarian cancers, and (3) age of onset of the individual.[46] A third group generated a mathematical model for predicting the presence of *BRCA1* or *BRCA2* mutations. Estimates of *BRCA1* and *BRCA2* mutation frequencies and age-specific incidence rates for breast and ovarian cancer were used to predict the presence of a mutation. The model is based on the cancer status of all first- and second-degree relatives and the age of onset of affected individuals.[124] Thus the probability that an individual from a high-risk family has a *BRCA1* or *BRCA2* mutation can be estimated using one or more of the models described earlier.

Molecular Biology of *BRCA1*. *BRCA1* does not appear to be a member of a known gene family on the basis of sequence analysis, other than as a member of a widespread group of cell cycle control and DNA repair genes that contain BRCT domains. Southern blotting of human genomic DNA detects a single band, suggesting that only one copy is present in the human genome. Northern blotting of human and mouse tissue with a *BRCA1* probe has been performed by a number of laboratories. Initial reports using a *BRCA1* fragment as a probe described a 7.8-kb RNA and several splice variants formed as a result of alternate splicing at the 5′ end of the transcript.[39,125,126] Subsequent work with a probe representing the complete coding region of *BRCA1* identified several additional transcripts. Three of these variants have been identified as (1) an in-frame deletion of exon 11, (2) a deletion of exon 11 117 bp from the 5′ splice acceptor, and (3) an in-frame deletion of exon 10.[127,128] Of greatest significance is the observation that deletion of exon 11 results in removal of the nuclear localization signal of *BRCA1*. Thus the proteins encoded by the exon 11-deleted forms of *BRCA1* may be localized in the cytoplasm of the cell. The functional significance of these isoforms is under investigation.

The two regions of near 100 percent homology between human and murine *BRCA1* have been studied in detail by several groups. The N-terminal RING finger domain has been screened extensively for a DNA-binding function with no success reported. Studies of protein-protein interaction by yeast twin-hybrid analysis has resulted in the identification of a BRCA1-binding protein termed *BRCA1 activator protein-1* (BAP)[97] that is thought to function as a ubiquitin hydrolase that enhances BRCA1-mediated cell growth suppression. BAP and BRCA1 co-localize in the cell

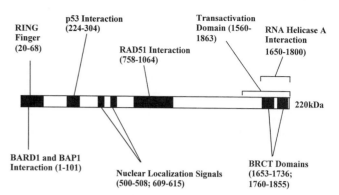

BRCA1

Fig. 33-9 Functional domains of *BRCA1*. Idiogram of the 220-kDa BRCA1 protein depicting known functional domains. Domains are shown as filled areas within the diagram.

nucleus. A second protein shown to bind the RING finger of BRCA1 has been termed *BARD1*.[129] This protein contains a zinc finger domain and two BRCT domains that are commonly found in proteins involved in DNA repair. BARD1 colocalizes with BRCA1 in the cell nucleus during S phase but not G phase of the cell cycle.[130] It has recently been suggested that the BRCA1-BARD1 complex facilitates ubiquitination of other proteins. BRCA1 also complexes with Rad51[131] and BRCA2.[132] Since both these proteins have been associated with cellular response to double-strand DNA breaks, this further suggests a role for BRCA1 in DNA damage repair.

Studies of the C-terminal acidic activation domain by yeast two-hybrid and mammalian two-hybrid assays have shown that this region of BRCA1, as well as the complete BRCA1 protein, can function as a coactivator of transcription, as detailed below[133–135] (Fig. 33-9). BRCA1 also has been shown to bind to the oligomerization domain of p53.[136] The interaction between BRCA1 and p53 has been associated with activation of p21 expression, leading to a cell cycle pause.[137] These data suggest that BRCA1 functions as a coactivator of p53-regulated transcription. Finally, BRCA1 has been shown to bind to the RNA polymerase II holoenzyme through RNA helicase A[138,139] and to the transcription coactivator and histone acetylase CREB-binding protein (CBP).[140] The association of BRCA1 with these proteins also suggests that BRCA1 functions as a transcriptional coactivator and forms a key component of the bridge between DNA-binding transcription factors and RNA polymerase II.

In addition, a novel kinase activity has been copurified with amino acids 329–435 of BRCA1.[141] This activity does not involve protein kinase A (PKA), protein kinase C (PKC), or casein kinase II (CKII). However, the purification of a kinase activity supports the observation that BRCA1 is a phosphoprotein and suggests that this kinase may play a role in regulation of BRCA1 function.

***BRCA1* Gene Regulation.** Shortly after identification of *BRCA1*, the sequence of 1345 bp of genomic DNA proximal to the putative transcription start site was identified.[125] This 1345-bp region was notable for the inclusion of the putative promoters of both the *BRCA1* gene and the *1A1.3B* gene, a homologue of CA-125 encoding a protein of unknown function that is overexpressed in some ovarian tumors. These genes are located head to head with transcription start sites located 295 bp apart, raising the possibility that sharing of promoters between the two genes acts as a regulatory mechanism. Physical mapping of the *BRCA1* region identified a large duplicated region containing the 5′ end of the *BRCA1* gene; a partial pseudogene of *BRCA1* containing exons 1A, 1B, and 2; the functional *1A1.3B* gene; and a *1A1.3B* pseudogene containing exons 1A, 1B, and 3.[125] A second transcription start site for *BRCA1* also was identified that initiates transcription in an alternative exon 1 located in intron 1. Thus two promoters for *BRCA1* have been located separated by approximately 2 kb of genomic DNA. These *BRCA1* promoters contain consensus binding elements for multiple transcription factors including p53 and AP2, although no data are available concerning the functionality of these sites. Recent data suggest that external agents such as adriamycin downregulate BRCA1 transcription in a p53 dependent manner. Studies of the *BRCA1* promoter detected CpG methylation of a CREB (cAMP-responsive element-binding) site in breast tumors but not in normal tissues, suggesting that methylation of regulatory sequences in the *BRCA1* promoter may be a method of inactivation of *BRCA1* in breast tumors.[142] A further report of hypermethylation of two of seven sporadic breast carcinomas with no methylation of normal tissues supports this hypothesis.[143]

BRCA1 and Estrogen Response. Little is known about the transcriptional regulation of the *BRCA1* gene, although BRCA1 mRNA and protein levels have been shown to be altered by some steroid hormones in an indirect manner.[144–147] In these studies, estrogen, as well as a mixture of estrogen and progesterone, has been shown to increase BRCA1 mRNA and protein levels in human cell line[144,145] and mRNA levels in animal models; however, protein levels were not analyzed in this system.[147] This induction appears to result indirectly in association with the increased cellular proliferation and DNA synthesis following estrogen exposure and not from direct activity of the estrogen receptor on the *BRCA1* promoter.[148,149] This is evidenced by the fact that putative estrogen response elements in the *BRCA1* promoter fails to respond to 17-β-estradiol,[148] and application of cyclohexamide to block protein synthesis inhibits the induction of *BRCA1* expression.[150]

Subcellular Localization of BRCA1. The subcellular localization of BRCA1 was studied initially by cell fractionation and immunofluorescence of breast cancer cell lines, "normal" breast epithelial cell lines, and breast tumor tissue. BRCA1 was detected in the nucleus of the normal cells and in the cytoplasm or in both the cytoplasm and the nucleus of almost all breast cancer cell lines through the use of three polyclonal BRCA1 antibodies.[151] Staining of primary cells from pleural effusions and cells in tissue sections also provided evidence that BRCA1 was located predominantly in the cytoplasm of malignant cells, suggesting that subcellular mislocalization of BRCA1 may be a mechanism by which BRCA1 plays a role in the pathogenesis of sporadic breast tumors. However, a similar study performed by Scully and colleagues using fixed tissue sections and BRCA1 monoclonal antibodies demonstrated localization of BRCA1 to the nucleus in every section analyzed. This group also tested a variety of methods of tissue fixation and determined that technical variation may lead to apparent cytoplasmic localization of BRCA1.[152] To add to this confusion, BRCA1 was noted to have homology to a granin consensus sequence. Granins are proteins that are secreted and modified to form bioactive peptides that act on the cell surface. In studies by Jensen and colleagues, polyclonal antibodies against the last 20 C-terminal amino acids identified a 190-kDa protein localized to the cytoplasm, Golgi network, and secretory vesicles.[153] Fractionation studies and confocal imaging supported these results, the latter purportedly identifying the protein they believed to be BRCA1 being released from a secretory body on the extracellular surface. Subsequent experiments indicate that the two polyclonal antibodies used by Jensen and colleagues detect BRCA1 as well as EGF-R and HER-2/*neu* and that it is the latter two proteins that are detected on the extracellular surface and in the Golgi network.[154] Immunofluorescence studies of BRCA1 using a variety of BRCA1 polyclonal and monoclonal antibodies have demonstrated that BRCA1 transfected into cell lines is localized in the nucleus, whereas BRCA1 splice forms or mutants deleted for the consensus nuclear localization signal in exon 11 are located in the cytoplasm.[127] The current consensus is that BRCA1 is localized to the nucleus in normal cells; however, no consensus

has been reached concerning the location of BRCA1 in cells from breast cancer lines or tumors. Therefore, it is unknown whether aberrant localization of BRCA1 is a mechanism by which BRCA1 plays a role in the development of sporadic breast cancer. A functional consensus nuclear localization signal in BRCA1 exon 11 has been identified[127] (see Fig. 33-9), multiple laboratories have replicated the initial observation that BRCA1 is a nuclear protein, and the controversy is largely resolved.

BRCA1 and Tumor Suppression. Before its isolation, *BRCA1* was predicted to function as a tumor-suppressor gene based on frequent loss of heterozygosity in *BRCA1*-associated tumors, where the deleted region invariably included the wild-type allele.[155,156] These data suggested that malignant transformation occurs when both functional copies of *BRCA1* are lost, a pattern indicative of a tumor-suppressor gene. After isolation of the gene, Thompson and colleagues demonstrated that the presence of antisense oligonucleotides complementary to BRCA1 RNA significantly increased the growth rate of MCF-7 cells in comparison with untreated cells, indicating that reduction of BRCA1 RNA levels was associated with an increased growth rate in these cells.[157] Analysis of BRCA1 RNA levels in tumors also suggested that *BRCA1* was down-regulated in sporadic tumors compared with normal breast epithelium. Subsequent studies using NIH-3T3 fibroblasts indicated that BRCA1 antisense RNA could reduce native BRCA1 RNA levels and result in a transformed phenotype in these cells. This group also demonstrated that nontumorigenic NIH-3T3 cells formed tumors in nude mice when treated with antisense BRCA1 RNA.[102] The growth-inhibitory properties of BRCA1 were then tested in animal models and cell lines. Retroviral transfer of wild-type BRCA1 inhibited the growth of two breast cancer cell lines and three ovarian cancer cell lines. Finally, it was demonstrated that the development of MCF-7 tumors in nude mice was inhibited in the presence of wild-type BRCA1 and unaffected by the presence of mutant BRCA1, adding further support to the hypothesis that *BRCA1* functions as a tumor suppressor.[102]

Further study of the role of BRCA1 in cell growth control has proved difficult because of consistent problems with the development of cell lines stably transfected with wild-type BRCA1, since transfected cells die rapidly in culture. Shao and colleagues analyzed this phenomenon and determined that constitutive expression of an exon 11-deleted form of BRCA1 results in induction of apoptosis, especially notable in conjunction with serum starvation or calcium ionophore treatment.[158] However, the use of the deleted form of BRCA1 complicates the interpretation of this study and suggests that further evidence is required in order to associate BRCA1 with apoptosis.

Of note, a recent report described the characterization of a novel breast cancer cell line derived from the breast carcinoma of a germ-line *BRCA1* mutation carrier. The patient carried a 5382insC mutation in *BRCA1*, and the tumor demonstrated loss of the wild-type *BRCA1* allele. Thus the cell line only contains a truncated form of the *BRCA1* gene that may or may not retain some level of function. While a number of additional genetic alterations have been identified in this cell line (a *p53* mutation, a *PTEN* deletion, and others), further cellular studies of *BRCA1* function will be greatly enhanced by the availability of this breast epithelial *BRCA1* mutant cell line.[159]

BRCA1 and the Cell Cycle. A connection between *BRCA1* and the cell cycle was suggested originally by studies of breast cancer cell lines treated with estrogen, which demonstrated that BRCA1 and cyclin A RNA levels increased in parallel in response to the hormone treatment.[144] It is now known that BRCA1 is a nuclear phosphoprotein that is phosphorylated in a cell cycle-dependent manner.[160] The greatest expression and phosphorylation of BRCA1 are observed in the S and M phases of the cell cycle. Cyclin-dependent kinase 2 and cyclin D- and A-associated kinases bind to and phosphorylate BRCA1, suggesting that BRCA1 function may be regulated by cyclin-dependent kinase phosphorylation. Subsequent studies showed that BRCA1 RNA levels were highest in rapidly growing cells, decreased after growth factor withdrawal, and increased at the G1/S phase boundary in synchronized cells.[145] BRCA1 RNA levels also were reduced in senescent cells and cells treated with transforming growth factor beta (TGFβ), indicating that BRCA1 expression is sensitive to *in vitro* growth conditions and may play a role in G1/S phase checkpoint control or merely be up-regulated at this point in the cell cycle in response to cellular messages. Vaughan and colleagues described similar findings and extended their analysis to include BRCA1 protein levels. In this study, induction of BRCA1 occurred before the initiation of DNA synthesis at the G1/S boundary.[146] Finally, overexpression of the BRCT transactivation domain led to increased growth rate through loss of a colchicine-induced G2/M block.[161] The cumulative data suggest that BRCA1 plays a role in cell cycle checkpoint control and is regulated by kinases and phosphatases that are known to play a role in the regulation of the cell cycle.

BRCA1 and Development. The first studies of the role of BRCA1 in development were performed by *in situ* hybridization of mouse embryos. Whole-mount embryos hybridized with mouse BRCA1 probe indicated that BRCA1 was widely expressed in many developing tissues, suggesting that BRCA1 may play a role in tissue development, possibly as a ubiquitous transcription factor.[147] Northern blots of mouse mammary gland RNAs also were used to demonstrate that BRCA1 was highly expressed in the mouse gland during pregnancy, remaining above pregestational levels at least 4 weeks after postlactational regression of the mammary epithelium. These results suggest that BRCA1 is involved in cell proliferation in breast epithelial cells and is regulated at least secondarily by ovarian hormone changes during pregnancy.

Further studies have supported the observation that BRCA1 is expressed in proliferating cells of embryos in the mammary gland during morphogenesis and in most adult tissues. BRCA1 exhibited a hormone-independent expression pattern in the oocytes, granulosa cells, and thecal cells of developing ovarian follicles and in the mitotic spermatogenia and meiotic spermatocytes of the testes.[162]

Gowen and colleagues produced the first *BRCA1* nullizyous mice. The disrupted allele was generated by the complete deletion of *BRCA1* exon 11 and flanking intron sequences, resulting in embryonic lethality 10 to 13 days after conception.[163] Abnormalities were most evident in the neural tube, with 40 percent of the embryos exhibiting spina bifida and anencephaly. In all homozygous null mice, the neuroepithelium appeared disorganized, with excessive cell growth as well as increased cell death. This report substantiated the work of Marquis and colleagues,[147] suggesting that *BRCA1* plays an important role in early murine development.

Hakem and colleagues also reported on the development of homozygous null *BRCA1* mice. The construct used for the generation of these mice was made by targeted deletion of exons 5 and 6, introducing stop codon in all three reading frames. The early truncation of the protein, coupled with deletion of a portion of the RING finger domain, was expected to yield a severely affected phenotype. These homozygous null mice have a phenotype slightly different from that of mice produced by Koller and colleagues and die before day 7.5 of embryogenesis.[164] The death of mutant embryos before gastrulation was postulated to result from failure of the proliferative burst necessary for the development of early germ layers. No increase in apoptosis was detected in these mice, but cell proliferation was reduced. These results again suggest a role for BRCA1 as a growth activator in early development. Further analysis demonstrated that the absence of BRCA1 was associated with reduced expression of mdm-2 and cyclin E, whereas expression of the cyclin-dependent kinase (cdk) inhibitor p21 was dramatically increased.

Liu and colleagues also generated a mouse with homozygous disruptions in *BRCA1* by replacing 186 bp of exon 11 with a neomycin resistance gene, resulting in protein truncation. These animals die at 4.5 to 8.5 days of embrogenesis.[165] The embryos fail to form egg cylinders and are unable to complete gastrulation. The difference between the Koller mice and the Liu mice may be accounted for by mouse strain differences and by stability differences in the mutant transcripts of *BRCA1*. Finally, Ludwig and colleagues reported that loss of p53 in association with loss of BRCA1 by deletion of exon 2 in a $BRCA1^{-/-}, p53^{-/-}$ embryo resulted in a less severe phenotype than that observed in the $BRCA1^{-/-}$ embryo. The *BRCA1/p53* double nullizygous mutants were significantly more advanced developmentally than the $BRCA1^{-/-}$ mice and survived to 9.5 days of embryogenesis.[166] These data support the data described above that suggest that p53 and BRCA1 are functionally associated. The accumulating data increasingly suggest that BRCA1 plays a role in cell cycle regulation, but how this function is associated with tumor suppression and early embryonic development is not yet understood.

BRCA1 and Transcription. As noted earlier, *BRCA1* contains a C-terminal transactivation domain,[133,134] as first defined by the yeast two-hybrid system. The transactivation domain was mapped to the region of the protein encoded by exons 21–24 using deletion constructs of *BRCA1* fused to the Gal4 DNA binding domain in both the yeast and mammalian systems. The ability of the transactivation domain to activate a Gal4 promoter was ablated by the addition of specific missense mutations in both hosts.[99,134] It also was shown that expression of human BRCA1 in *Saccharomyces cereviseae* resulted in a small-colony or slow-growth phenotype. Expression of mutant *BRCA1* failed to produce the small-colony effect, leading to the suggestion that the yeast growth assay could be used as a functional assay for C-terminal *BRCA1* mutations.[99] The transactivation domain of *BRCA1* coincides with the position of the second BRCT domain, suggesting that the BRCT domain can, but does not always, function as an activation domain.[167] Thus different proteins may use this domain for diverse functions.

The association between BRCA1 and transcription was further strengthened when Somasundaram and colleagues demonstrated that BRCA1 was capable of activating the p21 promoter.[137] This activation was reported initially as p53-independent and resulted in a partial S phase block and a reduction of DNA synthesis in SW480 p53 null cells. Missense mutations in the *BRCA1* transactivation domain resulted in decreases in p21 induction. Subsequent studies determined that the p21, mdm2, and bax promoters could all be activated by BRCA1 in a p53-dependent manner and that amino acids 261–314 of BRCA1 physically interacted with the oligomerization domain of p53[135,136] (see Fig. 33-9). Hanafusa and colleagues were unable to validate the p53-independent transactivating potential of BRCA1[135] but provided supporting data for the role of BRCA1 as a coactivator of p53-dependent transcription.

In support of this role, Scully and colleagues demonstrated that BRCA1 interacts with the RNA polymerase II holoenzyme[168] (see Fig. 33-9). Other investigators have shown that BRCA1 colocalizes with PCNA at DNA replication forks and transcription sites and interacts specifically with RNA helicase A.[138] Finally, it has been suggested that BRCA1 associates with CBP and modulates histone transacetylase activity[140] during the S phase of the cell cycle and in response to DNA damage. The amalgamation of these studies strongly suggests that one of the primary roles of BRCA1 in the cell is to function as a coactivator of transcription.

BRCA1 and Cellular Response to DNA Damage. A substantial amount of evidence implicating BRCA1 in the response to DNA damage has been generated. BRCA1 nullizygous embryos present with the same phenotype at 6.5 days of embryogenesis as seen in Rad51 nullizygous embryos.[169] BRCA1 also colocalizes with

Rad51 and BARD1 to nuclear foci during S phase of the cell cycle in mitotic cells and coimmunoprecipitates.[130,131] Rad51 is a RecA homologue and has been implicated in double-strand DNA break repair and recombination in yeast.[170] In meiotic cells, the BRCA1 and Rad51 proteins colocalize to axial filaments of the synaptonemal complex. The S phase foci disperse in response to hydroxyurea, ultraviolet radiation, mitomycin C, or gamma irradiation[168] and are not associated with altered phosphorylation states of BRCA1. Following dispersal, BRCA1, BARD1, and Rad51 accumulate at PCNA replication structures. A similar study demonstrated that hydrogen peroxide also induces BRCA1 phosphorylation and nuclear focus dispersal and suggests that BRCA1 undergoes cyclic hyperphosphorylation in the cell cycle and in response to DNA damage.[171] These studies implicate BRCA1 in several different DNA damage-associated pathways. Further attempts to identify damaging agents and response pathways involving BRCA1 showed that adriamycin and ultraviolet irradiation was associated with down-regulated BRCA1 expression in a mutant p53 ovarian cancer cell line,[172] suggesting that BRCA1-associated DNA damage response may be dependent on p53 function. However, in a separate study, overexpression of wild-type BRCA1 increased prostate cancer cell line sensitivity to adriamycin and drug-induced apoptosis and reduced efficiency of single-strand DNA break repair.[173] Resistance to *cis*-diamine dichloroplatinum (CDDP) also has been associated with induction of BRCA1 expression, and antisense BRCA1 expression has been associated with CDDP sensitivity.[174]

Finally, *BRCA1* nullizygous mouse embryonic stem cells have been shown to be hypersensitive to ionizing radiation and hydrogen peroxide and are unable to perform preferential transcription-coupled repair of oxidative DNA damage, as measured by thymine glycol removal.[175] Ultraviolet radiation damage of the transcribed strand was unaffected by the absence of BRCA1. Taken together, these data suggest that BRCA associates with Rad51 and plays a role in transcription-coupled double-strand DNA damage repair. However, it is possible that BRCA1 is also involved in other mechanisms of DNA damage repair that are uncoupled from transcription.

A recent commentary introduced the concept of gatekeeper and caretaker genes in cancer initiation and progression. In this model, caretaker genes including *BRCA1* and *BRCA2* do not promote tumor initiation directly but function to regulate genome stability. Elimination of the caretaker function leads to eventual mutation of gatekeeper genes that directly initiate tumorigenesis.[176] The discovery that cells without functional BRCA1 are hypersensitive to DNA damage supports this hypothesis. Further evidence comes from the observation that *p53* mutations are significantly more common in *BRCA1*-associated breast tumors than in sporadic tumor controls.[177] In addition, an increased frequency of *p53* mutations was found in association with loss of heterozygosity at the *BRCA1* and *BRCA2* loci in breast carcinomas.[178] Mutations in *p53* also were found in 80 percent of *BRCA1*-associated ovarian tumors, suggesting that *p53* mutations are important in but perhaps not essential for *BRCA1*-associated tumorigenesis.[179] In this case, mutation of *BRCA1* may lead to increased genome instability, resulting in mutation of the gatekeeper *p53* gene and subsequent tumor formation.

BRCA2

Clinical Features of Affected Families. Initial progress toward the identification of a second breast cancer susceptibility gene came from a linkage analysis of 22 families with multiple cases of early onset female breast cancer and at least one case of male breast cancer. Twelve of these families also had at least one individual diagnosed with ovarian cancer.[180] All 22 families were analyzed for linkage between breast cancer and genetic markers flanking the *BRCA1* candidate region on chromosome 17. A maximum Lod score of −6.63 was obtained, providing strong evidence against linkage to *BRCA1* in these families. This study demonstrated that only a small proportion of breast cancer families

with at least one case of male breast cancer were likely to be associated with germ-line mutations in *BRCA1*, arguing strongly for the existence of at least one additional breast cancer susceptibility gene, now known to be *BRCA2*. Shortly after the appearance of this report, a large collaborative group succeeded in identifying linkage in large female and male breast cancer families between polymorphic genetic markers on chromosome 13q12-13 and the disease phenotype.[181] A genomewide linkage search, using 15 large breast cancer families, located a familial early onset breast cancer susceptibility gene (*BRCA2*) in a 6-cM region between the markers D13S289 and D13S267, with a maximum total multipoint Lod score of 9.58, 5 cM proximal to D13S260. *BRCA2*, which was identified in late 1995, has a cancer risk profile similar but not identical to that of *BRCA1*.

A number of studies have been carried out in an attempt to define lifetime risk for breast and ovarian cancer in carriers of *BRCA2* mutations. The first studies of this type focused only on *BRCA1* mutation carriers, and only recently have estimates become available for *BRCA2* carriers. Initial reports from families used for linkage analysis estimated that lifetime breast cancer risk for *BRCA2* mutation carriers is 86 percent, and lifetime ovarian cancer risk is 27 percent.[182] While significantly above the general population risk of 1 percent, the *BRCA2*-associated ovarian cancer risk is lower than the 40 to 60 percent lifetime risk of ovarian cancer associated with *BRCA1* mutations found in the same type of heavily affected families (see Fig. 33-6). Predictably, when using a more population-based ascertainment strategy, more recent analyses of the Ashkenazi Jewish population estimated that a lower lifetime *BRCA2*-associated risk of breast cancer is 56 percent, whereas the lifetime risk for ovarian cancer is 10 to 20 percent.[49] Thus these risks are often presented as ranging between 56 and 86 percent for breast cancer and between 10 and 27 percent for ovarian cancer.

BRCA2 mutations are also associated with a 6 percent lifetime risk of male breast cancer. Although in absolute terms this represents significantly less cancer risk to men than to women, the relative risk represents a similar 100-fold increase over the general population risk. Elevated risks for the development of prostate, pancreatic, non-Hodgkin lymphoma, basal cell carcinoma, and other cancers may be associated with *BRCA2* mutations but remain poorly defined.

Like *BRCA1* tumors, *BRCA2* tumors have been reported as highly proliferative and may be of either ductal or lobular origin. A significant increase in tubule formation was identified in these tumors, along with aneuploidy and high S phase fraction.[21] These tumors are often high grade (see Fig. 33-7),[21,56,57] and in a recent study of tumors from Icelandic 999del5 mutation carriers, many were shown to be estrogen and progesterone receptor positive.[183] This is in contrast to *BRCA1*-associated tumors, which are often ER negative.

Isolation of *BRCA2*. After demonstration of the linkage of familial breast cancer to chromosome 13q12-13, several laboratories began evaluating families not linked to *BRCA1* for linkage to this region, particularly those with male breast cancer cases. Icelandic pedigrees with male breast cancer cases were shown to be linked to chromosome 13q12-13, and a common haplotype was identified, suggesting a common founder.[184] An unexpected addition to the fine mapping of the *BRCA2* region was provided by the identification of a homozygous somatic deletion in a single pancreatic cancer[185] that spanned a region estimated at 250 kb.

Sequence data from a 900-kb region thought to contain *BRCA2* were completed by DNA sequencing groups at the Sanger Center and Washington University, and the assembled sequence was released over the Internet, greatly facilitating this effort. The culmination of this effort was the identification of a partial sequence of the *BRCA2* gene[40] and six mutations that truncated the putative BRCA2 protein. Shortly afterward, the complete cDNA sequence of *BRCA2* was published by another collaborative group.[41]

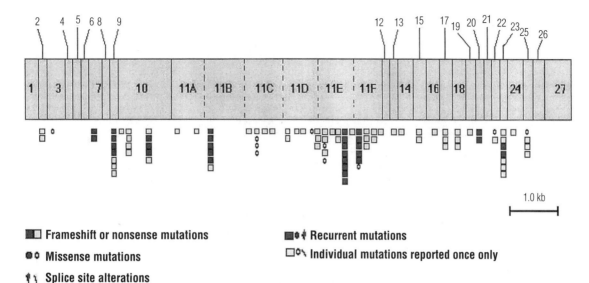

Frameshift or nonsense mutations

Missense mutations

Splice site alterations

Recurrent mutations

Individual mutations reported once only

Fig. 33-10 Structure and mutation spectrum of *BRCA2*. The 27 exons of the *BRCA2* cDNA are shown as sections within the *BRCA2* gene structure. Mutations are drawn as boxes beneath the exons of the gene in which they were detected and are categorized by frequency and mutation type. The idiogram was copied from the Breast Cancer Information Core (BIC) Web site and was generated by Simon Gayther, Cambridge, U.K. in 1997. Updated information is available on the BIC Web site.

The *BRCA2* cDNA is approximately 11.5 kb in length and is contained within 70 kb of genomic DNA. The coding region is 10.4 kb in length and is composed of 26 exons, with exon 1 forming part of the 5′ untranslated region. Like *BRCA1*, *BRCA2* has a large exon 11 (4.8 kb) and has no significant homology to any previously described gene (Fig. 33-10). *BRCA2* does not appear to be a member of a known gene family on the basis of sequence analysis and Southern blotting of human genomic DNA. Northern blotting using a *BRCA2* fragment as a probe described an 11.4-kb RNA with no predominant splice variants. The BRCA2 protein is composed of 3418 amino acids and has an estimated molecular mass of 384 kDa.[41]

Neither *BRCA2* cDNA nor protein contain previously defined functional domains (Fig. 33-11). However, eight copies of a 30- to 80-amino-acid repeat (BRC repeats) are encoded by exon 11. Comparison of sequences from several species demonstrates that the repeats are conserved but that exon 11 in general is poorly conserved.[186,187] The functional significance of the conserved repeats remains controversial, but at least some of the repeats form the binding site for the interaction between BRCA2 and Rad51 (discussed below).

BRCA2 is expressed in most human tissues at very low levels, with higher expression in testes.[41] The murine *BRCA2* gene has been identified and sequenced, and a similar pattern exists in the mouse.[188,189] The murine cDNA encodes a protein of 3329 amino acids that shares 59 percent identity with human BRCA2. However, identity is higher in certain regions, including the putative transactivation domain encoded by exon 3, the BRC repeats encoded by exon 11, and the C-terminus of the protein between amino acids 2414 and 3092 with 77 percent identity. The complete rat *BRCA2* sequence also is available and displays 58 percent identity with human *BRCA2* over 3343 amino acids. The mouse and rat genes are 73 and 72 percent identical, respectively, to the human gene.

Mutational Spectrum. More than 500 *BRCA2* mutations have been defined to date[40,41,190–196] (see Fig. 33-10), with a tabulated list available on the BIC Web site (*http://www.nhgri.nih.gov/ Intramural_research/Lab_transfer/Bic/.*). Interestingly, several similarities with *BRCA1* are apparent. First, *BRCA2* mutations span the entire coding region of the gene, adding little information on important functional regions and making mutation screening in this very large gene difficult. No mutation hotspots have been detected. Second, 80 percent of mutations reported to date are truncating mutations created mainly by small insertions and deletions, again adding little in the way of clues for defining functional regions. Missense mutations in the *BRCA2* gene account for approximately 20 percent of all variants detected in this gene (see Fig. 33-10). As with *BRCA1*, a number of these variants have not been classified as either polymorphisms, benign rare variants, or disease-causing mutations. One example, however, is likely to be the G2901N mutation, which recently was detected in three siblings with ovarian cancer. Evidence supporting the disease association of this mutation is that the glycine residue and the surrounding amino acids are conserved in human, mouse, and chicken, and the mutation was not present in 220 controls and was found only in affected members of the family. Definitive evidence awaits a functional assay.

Several mutations have been identified in *BRCA2*, which have helped to delimit specific functional domains. One variant of particular importance is the Lys3326ter alteration, which truncates the BRCA2 protein close to the C-terminus. Analysis of families

BRCA2

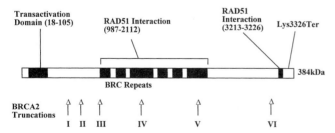

Fig. 33-11 Functional domains of *BRCA2*. The known functional domains of the BRCA2 protein including the N-terminal transactivation domain, the C-terminal Rad51 binding site, and the central Rad51-binding BRC repeats are depicted as black boxes within the diagram. The position of mutations leading to truncations in several *BRCA2* homozygous mutant mice are depicted as arrows beneath the gene.

with this variant showed that the putative mutation did not segregate with breast cancer in the family.[198] Furthermore, families were identified that carried other truncating BRCA2 mutations along with the Lys3326ter variant. This observation indicates that the discrete C-terminus of BRCA2 is not important for normal protein function and that Lys3326ter is a nonfunctional polymorphism. Another potentially useful mutation is a 126-bp deletion in exon 23 that does not create a frameshift, suggesting that the protein encoded by exon 23 may be important for BRCA2 function.[190] In addition, a large 5068-bp genomic deletion in BRCA2 spanning from intron 2 to intron 3 removes the exon 3 transactivation domain and is expected to alter the putative transcription-associated function of BRCA2,[199] whereas two missense mutations, V1283G and T1302N, in the BRC repeats have been shown to ablate the ability of BRCA2 to repair methylmethane sulfonate-induced DNA damage.[200] Thus the analysis of mutations within the gene has partially validated the role of BRCA2 in transcription regulation and DNA repair.

Several founder mutations have been identified in the BRCA2 gene in specific populations. The 6174delT mutation has been found in the Ashkenazi Jewish population at a prevalence of 1.2 percent, with a total of 2.5 percent of the entire Ashkenazi Jewish population now thought to carry one of three specific BRCA1 and BRCA2 mutations.[201] No human homozygotes of any of the three founder mutations have been reported, suggesting that the null phenotype involving any of these three mutations is an embryonic lethal. However, double mutants with one BRCA1 mutation and one BRCA2 mutation have been noted by numerous groups. Studies of the BRCA2 gene in the Icelandic population have determined that a founder effect also exists in that population, with the majority of high-risk breast and ovarian cancer patients sharing a common haplotype flanking BRCA2,[184] which is associated with a 999del5 mutation.[202] It also has been shown that 8.5 percent of breast cancer patients, 7.9 percent of ovarian cancer patients, and 2.7 percent of prostate cancer patients under 65 years of age in Iceland carry the 999del5 mutation. Finally, founder mutations have been identified in Finland. These include the IVS23-2A → G mutation and the 999del5 mutation, which suggests that individuals from Finland may have introduced this mutation into Iceland.[114] Analysis of haplotypes associated with nine recurrent mutations in BRCA2 provides evidence of common origins of each founder BRCA2 mutation.[111]

Mutations in the BRCA2 gene have been identified in individuals with apparently sporadic ovarian cancer at a prevalence of less than 1 percent, in comparison with a prevalence of 10 percent for BRCA1.[203] Mutations also have been detected in 7.3 percent of germ-line pancreatic carcinomas.[204] No mutations have been reported in sporadic meningiomas[205] or in sporadic breast cancer. Few studies have been performed on BRCA2 because of the difficulty in screening the entire coding sequence for mutations. However, one study has shown that BRCA2 mutations account for only 2.7 percent of breast cancer in women under 32 years of age,[122] suggesting that BRCA2 contributes to fewer cases of early onset breast cancer than does BRCA1. In a large study of Ashkenazi Jewish breast cancer patients, 7 percent of women with breast cancer diagnosed under age 40 years and 5 percent of those diagnosed over age 50 years carried the 6174delT mutation. In those with breast cancer and no family history, 4.5 percent were accounted for by 6174delT.[110] The same study determined that cumulatively the common BRCA1 and BRCA2 mutations failed to account for 79 percent of high-incidence breast cancer families and 35 percent of high-risk breast and ovarian cancer families in the Ashkenazi Jewish population. This suggests that other BRCA1 and BRCA2 mutations may have been overlooked because of the focus on the founder mutations and also that other breast cancer predisposition genes remain to be identified. This observation is supported by recent studies suggesting that the prevalence of BRCA2 mutations in high-risk breast cancer families appears to have been overestimated. These studies found BRCA2 mutations in 10 to 20 percent of

high-risk breast and/or ovarian cancer families (Table 33-4), whereas earlier studies suggested that BRCA2 mutations accounted for up to 35 percent of familial breast and/or ovarian cancer.[45,47,49,108,110,118,121,122,190,206–208]

Molecular Biology of BRCA2. The regions of high homology between human and murine BRCA2 have been studied by several groups; however, little functional data are available to date. Of note, exon 3 has been shown to encode a transactivation domain,[197] using a mammalian one-hybrid system, and the BRC repeats have been shown to bind the Rad51 a DNA repair protein, as does a C-terminal domain,[188,189] suggesting a role for BRCA2 in DNA repair. Most recently, BRCA2 has been shown to interact with BRCA1 (as discussed earlier), suggesting that the two proteins function in the same pathway.[132] This hypothesis makes sense teleologically, since mutations in each of the two genes produce an almost identical phenotype.

The sequence of the single BRCA2 promoter has been available since the entire BRCA2 region was sequenced by groups at Washington University in St. Louis and at the Sanger Center. Interestingly, the promoter does not appear to contain either a CCAAT box or a TATA box. The BRCA2 promoter contains consensus binding elements for multiple transcription factors, including the arylhydrocarbon receptor, AP2, and SP1; however, no data are available concerning the functionality of these sites. Basal transcription of the BRCA2 gene appears to be regulated by the USF1 and USF2 transcription factors. BRCA2 transcription can also be induced by NFKB and ETS factors, and repressed by certain DNA damaging agents such as adriamycin.

BRCA2 has been detected in the nucleus of MCF7 breast cancer cells. Cells were fractionated into nuclear and cytoplasmic fractions and probed on western blots with TFIIH, p89, and β-tubulin as controls for nuclear and cytoplasmic proteins. BRCA2 was detected predominantly in the nucleus.[208] BRCA2 also has been localized to the nucleus by transfection of cells with a GFP-tagged BRCA2 construct.[132] A series of basic amino acids including the sequence KKRR beginning at amino acid 3382 of the human BRCA2 protein has been suggested as a consensus nuclear binding site.[189]

BRCA2 and the Cell Cycle. Shortly after the identification of BRCA2, the gene was shown to be regulated in a cell cycle-dependent manner and in association with cellular proliferation. Levels of BRCA2 are low in G1 but increase as the cell approaches the G1/S boundary. Highest levels of BRCA2 are detected in S phase. Expression of BRCA2 also was shown to be independent of bulk DNA synthesis.[209] A second study reported that BRCA2 RNA levels were maintained through the S and G2/M phases of the cell cycle.[210] The cell cycle kinetics of BRCA2 are similar to the kinetics of BRCA1 and suggest that these proteins are coordinately regulated.

BRCA2 and Development. The first studies of the role of BRCA2 in development were performed by in situ hybridization of mouse embryos similarly to BRCA1. BRCA2 hybridization to whole-mount embryos showed widespread expression in many developing tissues, suggesting that BRCA2 may play a role in tissue development, possibly as a ubiquitous transcription factor.[211] Further studies have supported the observation that BRCA2 is expressed in proliferating cells of embryos in the mammary gland during morphogenesis and in most adult tissues. Similar to BRCA1, BRCA2 exhibited a hormone-independent expression pattern in the oocytes, granulosa cells, and thecal cells of developing ovarian follicles and in the mitotic spermatogenia and meiotic spermatocytes of the testes.[162] However, the time course of BRCA2 expression in spermatogonia was delayed relative to BRCA1, possibly suggesting distinct roles for BRCA1 and BRCA2 in meiosis.

Sharan and colleagues produced the first BRCA2 nullizygous mice. The null allele was generated by the deletion of BRCA2 exon

11 encoding amino acids 626–1437 and resulted in embryonic lethality at day 8.5 of embryogenesis at the same time that BRCA2 expression levels were detected in the normal animals.[212] However, unlike *BRCA1* nullizygous animals, mesoderm formation had begun prior to developmental arrest. Heterozygous mice were healthy and fertile. Suzuki and colleagues also demonstrated that embryos nullizygous for *BRCA2* due to deletion of exons 10 and 11 die before day 9.5 of development.[213] Cellular proliferation was shown to be inhibited, and p21 levels were increased. The death of the *BRCA2* nullizygous mice during early postimplantation suggests a role for BRCA2 in cellular proliferation and development. Embryos nullizygous for both *BRCA1* and *BRCA2* exhibited a *BRCA1* nullizygous phenotype.[166] In this case, the *BRCA2* mutation involved a large deletion of exon 11. *BRCA2/ p53* nullizygous embryos had a partially rescued phenotype, surviving to 11.5 days of embryogenesis. These data suggest that p53 and BRCA2 are functionally associated similar to BRCA1 and p53.

Each of the three nullizygous embryos just described involved mutations that truncated the BRCA2 protein in the region encoded by exon 10 or early exon 11 and eliminated the BRC repeats. However, viable nullizygous *BRCA2* mice also have been generated by two groups.[214,215] In these animals, truncation of BRCA2 occurred in regions encoded by the central and 3′ sections of exon 11 and by exon 27. Each of these alleles removes the C-terminal *Rad51* interaction domain of *BRCA2*. The allele described by Connor and colleagues contains seven of the eight BRC repeats,[215] whereas the Friedman *et al.*[214] mice retain three of the four BRC repeats. These animals are sickly and growth-retarded but survive to adulthood. Levels of p21 and p53 were elevated in mouse embryo fibroblasts derived from these animals. The data suggest that the presence of at least three BRC repeats is essential for regulation of embryonic development and cellular proliferation by BRCA2.

BRCA2 **and Transcription.** BRCA2 contains an N-terminal transactivation domain,[197] as defined by the yeast two-hybrid system and the mammalian one-hybrid system (Fig. 33-11). This BRCA2 transactivation domain was segregated into repression and activation domains. The ability of the domain to transactivate a Gal4 promoter was ablated by the addition of a Y42C missense mutation located in exon 3 of the *BRCA2* gene. BRCA2 has not been shown to interact with the RNA polymerase II holoenzyme; however, studies have demonstrated that BRCA2 complexes with BRCA1 and with RAD51.[132,210] The association with BRCA1 has not been shown to be a direct interaction, but the formation of a protein complex does support the hypothesis that BRCA2 may function as a coactivator or corepressor of transcription similarly to BRCA1. RAD51 has been shown to bind to both p53 and the RNA polymerase II holoenzyme, suggesting a role for this protein in regulation of transcription, perhaps through transcription-coupled double-strand DNA break repair.[169] Evidence that BRCA2 can bind DNA directly has yet to be presented.

BRCA2 **and Cellular Response to DNA Damage.** Several experiments have supported the hypothesis that BRCA2 plays a role in double-strand break repair. Hasty and colleagues successfully identified a C-terminal portion of mouse BRCA2 as a RAD51-binding protein in a two-hybrid screen in yeast (see Fig. 33-11). Further analysis by this group and others demonstrated that Rad51 binds to a 36-amino-acid domain (residues 3196–3232).[212,216] These amino acids are 95 percent conserved between mouse and human BRCA2, suggesting that the domain is important for BRCA2 function. As mentioned previously, Rad51 is a human homologue of *Escherchia coli* RecA and of yeast ScRad51, a member of the RAD52 epistasis group. ScRad51 is involved in mitotic and meiotic recombination and double-strand DNA break repair in yeast,[170] the human form of which associates with BRCA1 in S phase of the cell cycle.[168] Several other studies expanded on this discovery, showing that RAD51 also binds to the

BRC repeats of BRCA2. Wong and colleagues reported that residues 98 to 339 of human RAD51 interact with a 59-amino-acid region within each of the eight BRC repeats[210] (see Fig. 33-11). Katagiri found that RAD51 bound to at least two regions of BRCA2 involving residues 982 to 1066 and 1139 to 1266.[217] More recently, RAD51 was shown to bind directly to the four 5′ BRC repeats and was shown to form complexes in vivo by coimmunoprecipitation. In contrast to previous studies, RAD51 was shown not to bind the four 3′ BRC repeats or at the C-terminus of BRCA2.[200] While it is unclear which BRC repeats bind RAD51, it is now well established that BRCA2 binds RAD51 at several positions and thus likely plays a role in response to double-strand breaks and in both mitotic and meiotic recombination.

Further evidence supporting this role for BRCA2 has been provided by studies of *BRCA2* mutant embryos. The first such evidence was provided by the homozygous mutant embryos generated by Sharan and colleagues that display hypersensitivity to ionizing radiation.[189] Following exposure of these mutant embryos to 400 rads of γ-irradiation at day 3.5 of development, the inner cell mass outgrowth of these embryos was completely ablated, and this effect not seen in heterozygous or normal embryos. The number of trophoblast cells also was greatly reduced in the homozygous mutant embryos. Mouse embryo fibroblasts (MEF) from viable *BRCA2* homozygous mutant animals with mutations 3′ of the BRC repeats are also hypersensitive to agents that create double-strand DNA breaks.[215,218,219] This suggests that the BRC repeats may be necessary for development of the embryo but may not be essential for radiation resistance because even in the presence of these repeats the MEF cells are hypersensitive to radiation damage in comparison with controls. Thus the C-terminal Rad51 interaction domain or other as yet unidentified C-terminal domains may regulate the DNA damage response function of BRCA2.

Studies of a pancreatic cell line (CAPAN-1) expressing truncated BRCA2 have shown these cells to be hypersensitive to methyl methanesulfonate (MMS) treatment.[200] CAPAN-1 cells carry the 6174delT common Ashkenazi Jewish *BRCA2* mutation of one allele and a deletion of the wild-type allele. Introduction of wild-type BRCA2 into these cells conferred resistance to MMS, whereas introduction of BRCA2 with BRC repeat deletions or missense mutations in the BRC repeats had no effect. This suggests that the BRC repeats and the interaction between RAD51 and BRCA2 is essential for repair of MMS-induced DNA damage. Further studies by Abbott and colleagues showed that CAPAN-1 cells are highly sensitive to double-strand DNA break-inducing drugs such as etoposide and to ionizing radiation.[220] Thus it is likely that binding of RAD51 to both the BRC repeats and the C-terminal interaction domain is important for the DNA damage-repair function of BRCA2. Tumors in mice derived from CAPAN-1 injection also demonstrated hypersensitivity to radiation and mitoxantrone, suggesting that irradiation or treatment with DNA-damaging agents may be a useful method for elimination of BRCA2 null cells.[220]

The discovery that cells without functional BRCA2 are sensitive to DNA damage supports the hypothesis that *BRCA2* is a caretaker of the genome. Further evidence comes from the observation that *p53* mutations are significantly more common in *BRCA2*-associated breast tumors[221] and ovarian tumors[179] than in sporadic tumor controls.

Rare Causes of Inherited Breast Cancer Syndromes

Li-Fraumeni Syndrome. Li-Fraumeni syndrome (LFS), now known to be associated with germ-line mutations in *TP53*, was first identified as a syndrome in 1969 in a description of four kindreds in which cousins or sibs had childhood soft tissue sarcomas and other relatives had excessive cancer occurrence.[222] Subsequent epidemiologic efforts resulted in enumeration of the major component neoplasms, including breast cancer, soft tissue sarcomas and ostersarcomas, brain tumors, leukemias, and adrenocortical carcinomas, with several additional tumor types likely to merit inclusion.[223,224] Segregation analysis of families identified through a family member with sarcoma confirmed the autosomal dominant pattern of transmission of cancer susceptibility, with age-specific penetrance functions estimated to reach 90 percent by age 70. Nearly 30 percent of tumors in reported families occur before age 15 years.[224]

The pattern of breast cancer in LFS families is remarkable. Among 24 LFS families currently under study, 44 women have been diagnosed with breast cancer, of whom 77 percent were between the ages of 22 and 45 years.[225] Bilateral disease was documented in 25 percent of these women; 11 percent had additional primary tumors. It has been suggested that males may have later onset tumors in LFS families because they tend not to get breast cancer, which is so dramatic among female LFS family members.

As noted previously, in 1990, germ-line mutations were identified in the *p53* tumor-suppressor gene (*TP53*) in affected members of LFS families.[226,227] Mutations were clustered in the conserved sequences of the gene (exons 5 through 9), an observation that was thought to increase the significance of these findings. Additional families meeting the classic criteria for the clinical syndrome of LFS have been evaluated for the presence of germ-line alterations in *p53*. Approximately 50 percent of such carefully defined families have had alterations identified in the *p53* gene. While mutations are more frequently identified in hotspots within the conserved sequences, they have been seen throughout the gene.[228–232] *p53* genes ostensibly normal by sequencing but abnormal in a functional assay or with regard to expression also have been observed.[233,234] The prevalence of germ-line *TP53* alterations among women diagnosed with breast cancer before age 40 has been estimated at less than 1 percent.[235,236] It is therefore a rare explanation for breast cancer occurrence in the population; nonetheless, *p53* mutation screening formed the basis for the first predisposition testing programs for breast cancer susceptibility. Recently, mutations in the Chk2 gene have been implicated as the cause of Li-Fraumenilike syndrome.

Cowden Disease. Cowden disease, also known as the *multiple hamartoma syndrome,* is a rare autosomal dominant familial cancer syndrome that is characterized by an increased risk of breast cancer, genodermatosis, and multiple, more variable clinical features. The most consistent and characteristic findings are mucocutaneous lesions, including multiple facial trichilemmomas, papillomatosis of the lips and oral mucosa, and acral keratoses. Vitiligo and angiomas also have been reported. The syndrome is inherited in an autosomal dominant mode with variable expressivity and complete penetrance of the dermatologic lesions by age 20.[237]

Benign proliferations in other organ systems are common in patients with Cowden disease, including thyroid goiter, thyroid adenomas, gastrointestinal polyps, uterine leiomyomas, and lipomas. Nonmalignant abnormalities of the breast similarly are noted in these patients and include fibroadenomas, fibrocystic lesions, areolar and nipple malformations, and ductal epithelial hyperplasia.[237–239] Central nervous system involvement was recognized only recently and includes megaencephaly, epilepsy, and gangliocytomas of the cerebellum.[240,241]

A marked increase in breast cancer incidence compared with the general population was observed in a series of recently published cases of Cowden disease.[239] Breast neoplasms occurred in 10 of the 21 female patients; the lesions were bilateral in 4 of these women. Lesions were said to be exclusively intraductal in 2 of the 10 women; however, given the fact that these are true precursor lesions, these intraductal carcinomas are likely to represent a manifestation of the underlying genetic defect. Additional cases of Cowden disease have been published, bringing the number of reported patients to 83, of whom 51 are female.[237] Thus the total number of women with breast cancer and Cowden disease totals 15 (29 percent), with bilateral invasive tumors in 4 women. Since many of the women in these families are still alive

and at risk of developing breast cancer, the number of these women with breast cancer is likely to increase, increasing current estimates for the lifetime risk of developing breast cancer in women with this syndrome. However, increased recognition of Cowden disease could continue to disproportionately increase the number of Cowden patients without breast cancer and ultimately reduce estimates of the breast cancer rate. The gene for Cowden disease recently was mapped to chromosome 10q22-23 by linkage analysis of 12 families from four different countries.[242] Haplotype analysis demonstrated that all 12 families were linked to this locus, indicating that Cowden disease is a single-gene disorder.

A candidate tumor-suppressor gene *PTEN/MMAC1/TEP1* (phosphatase and tensin homologue/mutated in multiple advanced cancers 1/TGFβ-regulated and epithelial cell–enriched phophatase 1) was recently identified on chromosome 10q23.[242–245] Somatic mutations in the gene were identified in cancer cell lines and in 70 percent of primary glioblastomas and 60 percent of advanced prostate, breast, and kidney tumors.[244] Subsequently, mutations were identified in the *PTEN* gene in the germ line of Cowden disease patients.[246,247] Several more mutations identified in Cowden disease patients demonstrated that *PTEN* mutations are causative of Cowden disease and associated breast cancer.[248] In the same study, certain Cowden disease families were shown to have no *PTEN* coding-region mutations, suggesting that the mutations in these families are not readily detectable by PCR-based strategies or that other Cowden disease genes remain to be identified. Germ-line and somatic *PTEN* mutations have not been detected in sporadic breast cancers or in early onset breast cancers, suggesting that only breast cancer in association with the Cowden disease phenotype is caused by *PTEN* mutations. A *PTEN* pseudogene also has been identified.[249] The presence of the pseudogene may result in coamplification of pseudogene and functional gene fragments when using PCR-based mutation screening strategies. Thus accumulated variants in the pseudogene may be mistaken for mutations within the functional *PTEN* gene.

The PTEN protein has dual-specificity tyrosine phosphatase activity[245] and can dephosphorylate serine, threonine, or tyrosine residues. PTEN has homology to tensin, an SH2 domain actin-binding cytoskeletal protein localized to focal adhesions.[246] PTEN also contains a PDZ-binding domain at the C-terminus.[247] Thus PTEN also may function as an assembly factor for protein signaling complexes.

Peutz-Jeghers Syndrome. Peutz-Jeghers syndrome (PJS) is a rare autosomal dominant disorder characterized by gastrointestinal hamartomas and macular melanotic pigmentation of the mucosa, lips, fingers, and toes.[250] Pigmented lesions often appear at 1 to 2 years of age and accumulate with age. PJS predisposes to cancers of the gastrointestinal tract,[251] respiratory tract,[252] urinary tract,[253] female genital tract,[254] breast,[255] and ovary.[256] The female genital tract tumors are rare and not well recognized and include Sertoli cell tumors,[257] sex cord tumors with annular tubules (SCTAT),[258] and adenoma malignum of the cervix.[259] A recent follow-up study of 34 PJS patients identified a relative risk for cancer in females of 20 and of 7 in males.[260] A total of 6 cases of breast cancer were reported in the 34 individuals, and 50 percent of women with PJS developed a gynecologic or breast malignancy.

A PJS locus was recently mapped to chromosome 19p13.3 by a combination of comparative genome hybridization and loss of heterozygosity (LOH) studies in tumors, followed by linkage studies of PJS families.[261] Subsequently, the PJS gene, *LKB1* (*STK11*), was identified as a serine-threonine kinase.[262] Mutation screening in 12 patients determined that most mutations result in truncation of the STK11 protein product by creating a premature stop codon or by intragenic deletion.[262] Thus *STK11* is the first kinase gene associated with hereditary cancer that is inactivated by mutations. A series of mutation studies of *STK11* in sporadic breast,[263] colon,[264] and testicular[265] tumors has failed to identify any variants, suggesting that the involvement of *STK11* in these cancers is limited to those associated with an inherited predis-

Table 33-5 Causes of Inherited Breast Cancer Syndromes

	Clinical Manifestations	Mutation	Inheritance
Li-Fraumeni syndrome	Breast cancer, sarcoma, brain tumors, leukemia, adrenocortical carcinoma	*TP53*	Autosomal dominant
Cowden disease	Mucocutaneous lesions, angiomas, hamartomatous polyps of the colon, breast, and thyroid cancer	*PTEN*	Autosomal dominant
Muir-Torre syndrome	Gastrointestinal and genitourinary tumors, skin and breast tumors	*MLH1, MSH2*	Autosomal dominant
Peutz-Jeghers syndrome	Melanin deposits, hamartomatous polyps of the colon, breast, ovary, cervical, uterine, and testicular tumors	*LKB1/STK11*	Autosomal dominant
Ataxia-telangiectasia	Cerebellar ataxia, oculocutaneous telangiectasias, radiation hypersensitivity, lymphoma, leukemia, and breast tumors	*ATM*	Autosomal recessive

position. Further studies have determined that a small number of PJS families are not linked to the *STK11* locus, suggesting the presence of another PJS gene elsewhere in the genome.[266]

Muir-Torre Syndrome. Muir-Torre syndrome, a variant of Lynch syndrome type II, is the eponym given to the association between multiple skin tumors and multiple benign and malignant tumors of the upper and lower gastrointestinal and genitourinary tracts.[267,268] Many of the manifestations are common lesions (basal cell carcinomas, keratoacanthomas, colonic diverticula) that occur at younger ages but in a distribution similar to that in the general population. Inheritance of this syndrome is autosomal dominant with high penetrance.[268] Females with the syndrome reportedly have an increased risk of breast cancer, particularly after menopause, although lifetime risk has not been calculated.[269] Five genes responsible for inherited forms of colon cancer not associated with polyposis recently were described, including *MLH1* and *MSH2, PMS1, PMS2,* and *MSH6*.[270–274] Mutations in these genes are thought to lead to the development of hereditary nonpolyposis colorectal cancer (HNPCC) through loss of the ability to repair damaged DNA, accumulation of replication errors, and genome instability. Since various malignancies in Muir-Torre syndrome display microsatellite instability similar to that seen in colon cancer patients with HNPCC, it was postulated that mutations in one or more HNPCC-related genes may be the underlying defect in Muir-Torre syndrome. This observation was verified recently by linkage and mutation analysis demonstrating that mutations in *MSH2* predispose to Muir-Torre syndrome.[275] A truncating mutation in *MLH1* also has been detected in a Muir-Torre syndrome family.[276] Further discussion of the role of *MLH1* and *MSH2* in carcinogenesis is presented in Chap. 18.

Ataxia-Telangiectasia. Ataxia-telangiectasia (AT) is an autosomal recessive disorder that is characterized by cerebellar ataxia, oculocutaneous telangiectasias, radiation hypersensitivity, and an increased incidence of malignancy. Chromosomal fragility and resulting DNA rearrangements are thought to result from the genetic defect that underlies the clinical syndrome of AT. AT is characterized by an autosomal recessive pattern of inheritance, with the complete clinical syndrome occurring only in homozygous individuals. Of note, AT homozygotes, accounting for 3 to 11 live births per million,[277] are estimated to have a risk of cancer that is 60 to 180 times greater than that of the general population.[278] Cancers observed in association with AT include non-Hodgkin lymphoma (nearly 100 percent lifetime risk) and a significant but lower risk of developing breast cancer, ovarian cancer, lymphocytic leukemia, and malignancies of the oral cavity, stomach, pancreas, and bladder. However, breast cancer risk in AT mutation carriers does not approach the risk observed in women with inherited mutations in *p53, BRCA1,* or *BRCA2.* Initially, reports of increased susceptibility to cancer were limited to

homozygous AT mutation carriers, who represent approximately 0.2 to 0.7 percent of the general population in the United States.[278] However, a study published in 1987 suggested that AT heterozygotes who do not display the typical neurologic findings seen in homozygotes have a fivefold increased incidence of breast cancer.[279] This finding was particularly significant given that AT heterozygotes represent up to 7 percent of the general population[277] and that screening mammography, a source of ionizing radiation, could possibly contribute to the increased breast cancer incidence seen in this population. However, this study has been criticized for methodologic flaws, including small sample size, inappropriateness of the control group, and lack of quantitation of radiation exposure. In addition, two groups have analyzed a total of 80 families with evidence for an inherited form of breast cancer for linkage between breast cancer and genetic markers flanking the AT locus on chromosome 11, finding strong evidence against this association.[280,281] Both groups concluded that the contribution of AT mutations to familial breast cancer is likely to be minimal. Nonetheless, since AT results from an alteration in the ability to repair DNA damage, the hypothesis that AT heterozygotes may have a decreased capacity to repair DNA could explain an increased susceptibility to cancer in such individuals. The AT gene (*ATM*) on human chromosome 11q22 has been identified[282] and is described in detail in Chap. 15. A summary of the clinical and genetic characteristics of the rare genetic syndromes associated with increased breast cancer risk is presented in Table 33-5.

Other Breast Cancer Susceptibility Loci

A large number of genes have been implicated in breast cancer tumorigenesis through identification of mutations in tumors, and several of these genes are discussed later in this chapter. Two genes in addition to those described earlier have been implicated in familial breast cancer susceptibility by identification of mutations that segregate with the disease in families or by linkage analysis. First, the estrogen receptor (ER) has been suggested as a candidate locus for familial late onset breast cancer susceptibility.[283] One extended family with eight women with late onset breast cancer was identified with a single haplotype flanking the ER locus that consistently segregated with the disease, yielding a maximum Lod score of 1.85. The frequent expression of the ER in breast cancer is associated with responsiveness to hormonal treatment and a favorable prognosis. Therefore, mutations in the ER may modify the hormonal response in breast epithelium and potentially result in inherited susceptibility to breast cancer. However, no mutations associated with inherited cancer have been identified in the ER, although several somatic mutations have been identified in breast cancer biopsies and established breast cancer cell lines.[284]

Another breast cancer susceptibility locus has been proposed on chromosome 8p12-22[285] based on linkage analysis of several breast cancer families with polymorphic genetic markers on chromosome 8p. This analysis yielded a maximum Lod score of

2.51 using the polymorphic markers NEFL and D8S259. Several groups have attempted to reproduce this result with little success. However, the region is thought to harbor tumor-suppressor genes involved in sporadic prostate cancer[286] and sporadic breast tumors,[285] as defined by LOH studies. Studies of male breast tumors identified 83 percent LOH at one marker on chromosome 8p and two distinct regions of loss on chromosome 8p12-21.3 and 8p22.[287] These data suggest that a tumor-suppressor gene functioning as an inherited susceptibility gene may be involved in breast cancer pathogenesis in a small subset of families, especially those with cases of male breast cancer. As whole-genome linkage studies commence in an effort to identify other familial breast cancer susceptibility genes, the 8p12-22 region will be at the forefront as a strong candidate locus.

Somatic Alterations in Breast Cancer

Another approach to understanding the pathogenesis of breast cancer is the study of noninherited (sporadic) breast cancers. This is an important complementary approach to the study of germ-line alterations for several reasons. First, the large majority of breast cancers do not arise as a result of inherited mutations in single breast cancer susceptibility genes, and sporadic tumors may have fundamental molecular genetic differences. Second, genes that are frequently dysregulated or mutated in sporadic breast cancer are candidate genes for susceptibility loci, as was demonstrated with *p53* and LFS. Third, the study of genetic alterations per se, such as mutations, deletions, and amplifications, provides clues to the mechanisms that result in the genomic instability that is inherent in cancer cells. This section provides a summary of chromosomal regions commonly deleted in breast cancer (resulting in LOH), as well as an overview of genes that are mutated or dysregulated in sporadic breast cancers. Some of these genetic alterations have been identified as markers of particularly aggressive tumor behavior, whereas a few have become potential therapeutic targets. A summary of the genes altered in sporadic breast cancers is given in Table 33-6.

Table 33-6 Somatic Alterations in Breast Cancer

Gene/Region	Modification	Frequency
Growth factors and receptors		
EGFR	Overexpression	20–40%
HER-2/neu	Overexpression	20–40%
FGF1/FGF4	Overexpression	20–30%
TGFα	Overexpression	Not reported
Intracellular signaling molecules		
Ha-ras	Mutation	5–10%
c-src	Overexpression	50–70%
Regulators of cell cycle		
TP53	Mutation/inactivation	30–40%
RB1	Inactivation	20%
Cyclin D	Overexpression	35–45%
TGFβ	Dysregulation	Not reported
Adhesion molecules and proteases		
E-cadherin	Reduced/absent	60–70%
P-cadherin	Reduced/absent	30%
Cathepsin D	Overexpression	20–24%
MMPs	Increased expression	20–80%
Other genes		
bcl-2	Overexpression	30–45%
c-myc	Amplification	5–20%
nm23 (NME1)	Decreased expression	Not reported

Loss of Heterozygosity. Loss of heterozygosity has long been associated with the presence of tumor-suppressor genes in DNA because the analysis of many tumors has demonstrated that the wild-type allele of a mutated tumor-suppressor gene is often lost during tumorigenesis. In the case of germ-line mutations in tumor-suppressor genes, as suggested by Knudsen's "two hit" hypothesis,[288] individuals from "cancer families" inherit an inactivating mutation in one allele of the implicated tumor-suppressor gene in all cells. Therefore, only one somatic event is required to inactivate the remaining copy, making the development of cancer a much more common event than it is in individuals born without the "first hit." The mechanism by which LOH occurs is not known, but the end result is physical deletion of large regions of chromosomes. LOH has been studied in detail in sporadic and familial breast tumors, resulting in identification of many putative tumor-suppressor loci. A subset of these loci is likely to function as inherited breast cancer susceptibility loci.

The most common regions of LOH in breast cancer are located on chromosomes 17p, 17q, 16q, 13q, 11p, 1p, 3p, 6q, 7q, 18q, and 22q.[289–293] Many other loci have been identified. The 17q LOH region originally was thought to harbor the *BRCA1* gene, but more complete analysis has identified at least three and as many as six independent regions on chromosome 17q, only one of which contains *BRCA1*.[294–297] LOH also has been associated with the *BRCA2* gene on chromosome 13q12-13. These data demonstrate that the known inherited susceptibility genes are associated with LOH in tumors and that other susceptibility genes may be isolated from other LOH regions.

The 17p LOH region can be divided into two separate loci, one containing *TP53* on 17p13.1 and a second, more distal region on 17p13.3.[298] Two candidate tumor-suppressor genes have been isolated from the 17p13.3 region.[299] Studies of chromosome 1 also have identified multiple regions of loss on 1p13, 1p31, and 1p32-p34 and 1p36.2 in the same region as the neuroblastoma gene.[300,301] Three regions of LOH have been identified on chromosome 11 at 11p15.5, 11q13, and 11q22-qter, with 19, 23, and 37 to 43 percent LOH, respectively, demonstrated in a group of breast tumors. More detailed mapping has suggested that as many as five different LOH regions exist on chromosome 11q22-q24.[302] Significant association between LOH on chromosomes 11p15, 17q21, and 3p also has been detected, suggesting that the putative tumor-suppressor genes at these loci may function together in a tumorigenic pathway.[291] LOH has been detected on chromosomes 16q22.1 and 16q22.4-qter in a large number of breast tumors[303]; this is of interest because chromosome 16q is the location of the E-cadherin gene, which has been implicated in metastasis of sporadic breast cancers. Further discussion of the role of E-cadherin in breast cancer can be found below. Finally, an association has been seen between LOH on chromosomes 9p, 3p, and 6q,[304] suggesting the existence of a tumorigenic pathway involving all these loci. Another example of cooperativety between distant loci was reported by Smith and colleagues,[305] who analyzed 133 breast cancers for *TP53* mutations and LOH on 13 chromosome arms. In this series, *TP53* mutations were strongly associated with LOH at two specific loci: 3p24-26 ($p < 0.001$) and 7q31 ($p < 0.05$). Surprisingly, there was no association between *TP53* mutations and LOH at 17p, the site of the *p53* gene, suggesting that breast cancers frequently have only one defective *TP53* allele.

Many sites of LOH correspond with the location of known tumor-suppressor genes. Examples include the *DCC* gene on chromosome 18q, with 52 percent LOH in breast tumors, and the *APC* gene on chromosome 5q21.[306] These genes have been screened for mutations in familial breast cancer samples, and none has been identified, seemingly eliminating these LOH regions as candidate loci for inherited susceptibility genes. However, it is possible that tumor-suppressor genes other than *DCC* and *APC* exist in these locations. The previously described *I1307K* variant may account for the association of LOH with the *APC* gene.

Recently, investigators began analyzing atypical ductal hyperplasia, a precancerous lesion of the breast, for LOH, which has been demonstrated on chromosomes 16q and 17p in these lesions.[307] Analysis of DCIS, a malignant but noninvasive lesion of the breast, resulted in the identification of LOH on chromosomes 8p, 13q, 16q, 17p, and 17q.[308] These results suggest that known genes such as *BRCA1*, *BRCA2*, and *p53* or unknown tumor-suppressor genes in these chromosomal regions are altered as the first steps in breast tumorigenesis and may provide clues to the location of additional breast cancer susceptibility genes. LOH in breast cancer also has been tracked in stages from primary tumors to the onset of metastasis, demonstrating LOH on chromosome 7q31 at all stages[309] and suggesting that LOH of chromosome 7q31 is another early event in breast tumorigenesis.

Growth Factor Receptors. An important class of genes frequently altered in sporadic breast cancer are members of the epidermal growth factor receptor (EGFR) family of growth factor receptors. The members of this family of proto-oncogenes (*EGFR*, *erbB-2* or *HER-2/neu*, *erbB-3*, and *erbB-4*) all share extensive homology and encode transmembrane glycoproteins with tyrosine kinase activity. They become oncogenic through gene amplification or overexpression at the mRNA and protein levels, leading to aberrations in signal transduction pathways and deregulation of cellular proliferation.[310] All the members of this family have been described as overexpressed in breast carcinoma; the most extensively studied receptors, EGFR and erbB-2, are known to be overexpressed in 20 to 40 percent of breast cancers.[311–316]

Recent work has revealed a complex system of interaction between the various members of the EGFR family, as well as cross-regulation between growth factor-activated signal transduction pathways and estrogen-responsive pathways. For example, estrogen receptor-positive breast cancer cell lines that overexpress erbB-2 demonstrate decreased erbB-2 protein expression in response to treatment with estradiol or EGF.[317] The erbB-2 pathway also has been linked to the *ras* oncogene signal transduction pathway and activation of mitogen-activated protein kinase (MAPK),[318,319] suggesting that cooperation between various oncogenes may be important in breast tumorigenesis. Overexpression of erbB-2 has been associated with a less favorable prognosis in patients with breast cancer, particularly in tumors with involvement of axillary lymph nodes.[315,320,321] It also has been reported that overexpression of erbB-2 identifies a subgroup of patients who are more resistant to chemotherapy, and a recent study suggested that higher doses of chemotherapy with regimens containing doxorubicin can in part overcome this effect.[322] In fact, overexpression of p185/c-erbB2 renders cells resistant to tamoxifen.[323] In addition, ER-positive patients who overexpress erbB-2 are less likely to have a clinically significant response to the estrogen antagonist tamoxifen and have overall shorter survival than do patients with ER-positive, erbB-2-negative tumors.[324] Finally, evidence is accumulating that down-regulation of erbB-2 protein levels with monoclonal antibodies or antisense oligonucleotides may be useful therapeutically. p185HER2/neu monoclonal antibodies have antiproliferative effects *in vitro* on cells that overexpress erbB-2 and sensitize human breast cancer cells to tumor necrosis factor.[325] In addition, erbB-2 antisense oligonucleotides[326] can inhibit the proliferation of breast cancer cells. Down-regulation of EGFR using antisense oligonucleotides also has been shown to result in down-regulation of protein kinase A and reduced growth potential in breast cancer cells.[327] Furthermore, neutralizing antibodies against EGFR and HER2/neu result in down-regulation of vascular endothelial growth factor and reduced angiogenesis.[328]

Of note, the well-described growth factor transforming growth factor alpha (TGFα) is a member of the EGF family and is a ligand for EGFR. Elevated expression of TGFα consistently has been associated with neoplastic transformation, with transgenic mouse models providing direct evidence for the role of TGFα in malignant transformation of breast epithelium. In this regard, metallothionein-directed expression of TGFα in transgenic mice and constitutive TGFα expression promote uniform epithelial hyperplasia of several organs and induce postlactational secretory mammary adenocarcinomas.[329]

The fibroblast growth factors (FGFs) and their receptors (FGFRs) also are thought to play a role in breast cancer. However, since specific genetic alterations in FGFs or FGFRs have not been reported in breast tumors, their causal role in breast tumorigenesis is less clear than that of EGFR or HER-2/neu. This large group of proteins may be involved in cell transformation by deregulated activation of a receptor tyrosine kinase through an autocrine mechanism. FGF signaling activates the STAT1 and p21 pathways and inhibits the estrogen response and cell proliferation in breast cancer cells.[330] Acidic FGF (FGF1) and basic FGF (FGF2) initially were identified as heparin-binding growth factors that stimulate the proliferation of vascular endothelium. They are expressed in a number of tumors and have strong angiogenic properties.[331,332] Basic FGF also is known to down-regulate Bcl-2 and induce apoptosis.[333] Acidic FGF plays a role in estrogen-independent cell growth regulation and anti-estrogen-resistant growth of MCF-7 cells.[330] FGF3, initially identified as int-2 because it is activated by the insertion of murine mammary tumor provirus, is associated with the transformation of murine mammary epithelium. At least nine FGFs and four FGFRs have been identified. A recent study of seven of the nine known family members and all four known receptors in a panel of 10 tumor cell lines and 103 breast tumor samples provided evidence for FGF1 and FGF2 expression in almost all samples, as well as limited expression of FGF5, FGF6, FGF7, and FGF9. FGF3 was not expressed in any sample, and FGF4 and FGF8 were not assayed. FGF8 recently has been shown to be expressed at high frequency in breast tissues.[334]

Intracellular Signaling Molecules. While it is clear that overexpression and/or mutation of mediators of intracellular signaling play a key role in malignant transformation, relatively little work has focused on the specific role of these molecules in the development of breast cancer. However, recent work suggests that dysregulation of several signaling pathways intersects directly with many breast cancer-related proteins such as the receptor tyrosine kinases. The proto-oncogene *Ha-ras* is the most extensively studied example of the involvement of signaling pathways in breast cancer development. Additionally, work in the past few years has produced evidence that rare *Ha-ras* alleles are associated with inherited susceptibility to breast cancer.[335] More recent work suggests that these rare alleles may be associated with altered penetrance of the major breast cancer susceptibility gene *BRCA1*.[69] However, the mechanism underlying this association remains unclear. Some investigators have suggested that the presence of the rare alleles is a marker of genomic instability that predisposes to cancer, whereas others have suggested that function may be altered by changes in *ras* regulatory regions or that mutations in genes in close physical proximity to the *Ha-ras* locus that are therefore genetically linked may be the underlying cause of the increase in cancer susceptibility associated with these alleles.

Experimental models have been used to determine whether chemically induced breast neoplasia is associated with *Ha-ras* changes. Using the spontaneously immortalized but nontransformed breast line MCF10A, loss of one *Ha-ras* allele and induction of a mutation in the remaining allele at the first position of codon 12 have been observed after carcinogen exposure.[336] These changes were associated with the ability of these cells to form colonies in soft agar, but not with the emergence of tumorigenesis in animals.

There is evidence that while *ras* coding region mutations occur in less than 10 percent of breast cancers, the pathway *ras* services may be deregulated in breast cancer more frequently. Bland and colleagues examined 85 breast cancer specimens with immuno-histochemical staining for the presence of multiple oncogene products, including *Ha-ras,* and correlated the results with the clinical outcome.[337] The oncogenes with the strongest prognostic correlation to survival were *Ha-ras* and c-*fos.* Coexpression of c-*myc* and *Ha-ras* with c-*fos* also correlated with an increased likelihood of recurrence and decreased survival. Other studies also suggested cooperativity between *Ha-ras* and both rat c-erbB-2 and human TGFα in transformation but similarly demonstrated that additional genetic changes are required for a fully tumorigenic phenotype.[338] Finally, a link has been established between the expression of *Ha-ras* and the appearance of the multidrug resistance phenotype. Transfection of the breast cell line MCF-10A with c-*Ha-ras* and c-erbB-2 results in up-regulation of the *mdr-1* gene (multidrug resistance-1), appearance of the protein product on the cell surface, and the multidrug resistance phenotype.[339] Transfection with either proto-oncogene alone has no effect, strongly suggesting cooperativity. As noted earlier, the association between c-erbB-2 expression and breast cancer prognosis has been investigated extensively, and recent work suggests that erbB-2 expression may correlate with Ha-ras expression.[340] Interestingly, in this study, if chemotherapy is included in the model, tumors coexpressing Ha-ras and c-erbB-2 are less responsive to both chemotherapy and the partial estrogen antagonist tamoxifen.

The signaling pathway involving the proto-oncogene c-*src* also has been linked to genetic alterations in breast cancer. Specifically, the phosphotyrosine residues of receptor tyrosine kinases serve as binding sites for proteins that contain SRC homology 2 (SH2) domains. Using glutathione-*S*-transferase fusion proteins containing the SH2 region, it has been demonstrated that in human breast carcinoma cell lines the SH2 domain binds to activated EGFR and to p185her2/neu. These investigators also have shown that endogenous pp60c-src is tightly associated with tyrosine-phosphorylated EGFR, raising the possibility that this association may be an integral part of malignant transformation of breast epithelium.[341] In a related study, protein tyrosine kinase activity was assayed in 72 primary breast cancer specimens; increased activity compared with normal breast tissue was identified in all 72 samples. In this study, at least 70 percent of the cytosolic protein tyrosine kinase activity originated from the presence of the c-*src* oncogene product.[342] Since cytosolic protein tyrosine kinase activity parallels malignancy in breast tumors,[343] and since most of this activity is precipitated by anti-src antibodies, it appears likely c-*src* plays a significant role in the manifestation of breast cancer.[342]

Regulators of the Cell Cycle. Accumulating evidence indicates that derangements in the protein machinery that normally regulates passage through the cell cycle are critical contributors to uncontrolled cell growth and cancer.[344,345] *TP53* (encoding p53) initially was regarded as a tumor-suppressor gene that is deleted or mutated in a large number of human tumors from a variety of tissue types. p53 was known to have DNA-binding and transcriptional activation domains, and more recent work has established that p53 plays a central role in regulating progression through the cell cycle. The strongest link between *TP53* mutations and breast cancer comes from the increased incidence of early onset breast cancer seen in LFS, the family cancer syndrome caused by germline alterations in *TP53.*[226] Additional evidence for the involvement of *TP53* in breast cancer comes from studies demonstrating decreased ability to form tumors in nude mice and reduced capacity for growth in soft agar when wild-type *TP53* in a retroviral vector is introduced into breast cancer cell lines with mutated *TP53.* Alterations in *TP53* in breast cancer may be detected by analyzing the coding region for mutations[236,346] or in some cases by using antibody demonstrating aberrant localization or altered levels of p53. *TP53* mutations have been detected in 15 to 45 percent of human breast cancer specimens in several studies.[347–350] Of note, several groups have investigated racial differences in the *TP53* mutations found in breast cancer. While striking differences between Caucasian and African-American

patients in the type and/or frequency of *TP53* mutations have not been reported, significantly lower survival rates have been reported in association with *TP53* mutations in black patients compared with white patients (four- to fivefold excess death rate, $p < 0.012$).[351]

Interestingly, *TP53* mutations do not appear to be evenly distributed among the various histologic types of breast cancer. In one series, 148 human breast cancers were surveyed for *TP53* mutations, with mutations identified in 39 percent of medullary cancers and 26 percent of invasive ductal lesions but only 12 percent of invasive lobular cancers. No *TP53* mutations were detected in the 19 mucinous and 8 papillary carcinomas examined.[352] In all studies where survival data were available, *TP53* mutations were associated with a significantly poorer prognosis. Finally, *TP53* mutations have been reported in approximately 15 percent of DCIS lesions.[349]

In addition to mutations, alterations in the subcellular location of p53 have been noted in breast cancer specimens compared with normal breast epithelium. In an analysis of 27 breast cancers, sequestration of p53 in the cytoplasm was demonstrated in 37 percent of the breast cancers analyzed, overexpression of nuclear p53 in another 30 percent of tumors, and complete lack of staining in the remaining 33 percent.[353] While other studies have not found p53 alterations in all samples studied, these data suggest that p53 alterations are among the most common genetic changes found in breast carcinoma.

The relationship between *TP53* mutations and the chemoresistance of breast cancer cells was suggested initially by a report hinting that specific mutations in the DNA-binding domain of p53 lead to primary resistance to doxorubicin, one of the most widely used and most effective chemotherapeutic agents for breast cancer.[354] In this study, 11 of 63 tumors had mutations in this region. Four of these 11 patients progressed on doxorubicin, as opposed to only 2 of 52 patients without p53 DNA-binding region mutations. Among the patients with p53 DNA-binding-domain mutations who did respond to doxorubicin, most relapsed within 3 months of treatment. Similar data were reported in a second study reporting a smaller benefit from chemotherapy, hormonal therapy, and radiation in patients with tumors harboring *TP53* mutations.[355]

The retinoblastoma tumor-suppressor gene (*RB1*) appears to play a role in breast tumorigenesis in at least a proportion of cases; however, *RB1* has not been as well characterized in breast cancer as *TP53.* Like p53, RB regulates cell cycle progression, with dephosphorylated RB acting to halt cell cycle progression in G1. The link between *RB1* and breast cancer was first suggested by studies demonstrating structural rearrangements and inactivation of *RB1* in breast cancer.[356,357] This observation was followed by work demonstrating that estradiol decreases expression of RB, fueling speculation that estogen may act as a tumor promoter by decreasing expression of critical tumor-suppressor genes.[358] Further evidence for the role of *RB1* in breast cancer was provided by demonstration that using retroviral-mediated gene transfer, wild-type *RB1* introduced into breast cancer cells with a known *RB1* mutation results in decreased tumorgenicity in nude mice and a reduction in anchorage-independent growth.[359]

Current estimates suggest that *RB1* may be inactivated in approximately 20 percent of breast cancers.[360] One group of investigators described the incidence of RB1 alterations in 96 primary breast cancers and related their findings to patient and tumor characteristics, as well as oncogene amplifications and *TP53* mutations.[361] In this series, RB1 alterations were found to occur more frequently in ER-positive tumors and less frequently in tumors with HER2/neu or c-myc amplification. RB1 alterations were associated with small (< 2 cm) tumors without axillary node involvement. In contrast, a study of 197 breast cancer specimens using immunohistochemistry to evaluate the expression of RB1[362] suggested that loss of RB1 expression was correlated with the presence of axillary nodal metastasis; however, neither group of investigators was able to demonstrate a correlation with relapse-free or overall survival.

Various cyclins accumulate at cell cycle checkpoints and complex with cdks. Binding of a cdk to a specific cyclin partner activates the kinase activity of the cdk, which in turn phosphorylates and activates downstream target proteins that are necessary to propel the cell into the next phase of the cell cycle.[363,364] Overproduction of cyclins and cdks or their presence at an inappropriate time would be expected to cause unregulated cell division. Consequently, these molecules are candidate proto-oncogenes. In one of the first studies of the role of cyclins in breast carcinoma, 20 breast cancer cell lines were assayed for expression of cyclin A, B1, C, D1, D2, D3, and E; increased expression of one or more cyclins was demonstrated in 7 of 20 lines (35 percent). Five of the seven displayed increased expression of cyclin D1. This group also noted cyclin D1 overexpression in 45 percent of 124 primary breast cancers.[363] Cyclin D1, which regulates the G1/S transition, recently was identified as the *PRAD1* oncogene located at chromosome 11q13.[364] Cyclin D1 overexpression appears to be a relatively early event in tumor development.[365,366] Evidence for the early involvement of cyclin D in breast cancer was provided by Steeg and colleagues, who demonstrated cyclin D1 overexpression in 18 percent of benign breast lesions but in 76 percent of low-grade DCIS, 87 percent of high-grade DCIS, and 83 percent of infiltrating ductal cancers.[367] Significantly lower frequencies of overexpression were seen in a recent study, where 39 percent of atypical ductal hyperplasia, 43 percent of DCIS, and 48 percent of invasive carcinoma demonstrated overexpression of cyclin D1.[368] Cyclin D1 overexpression also has been identified in up to 80 percent of invasive lobular carcinomas of the breast.[369] Induced expression of cyclin D1 in breast cancer cells leads to an increase in the proportion of cells progressing through G1 and removes the requirement for growth factor stimulation normally necessary for completion of the cell cycle.[370] Overexpression of cyclin D1 in 30 to 50 percent of breast tumors does not correlate with observations of cyclin D1 gene amplification in 15 percent of tumors. Thus a mechanism other than amplification leads to overexpression and oncogenesis. A more recent analysis of cyclin D1-null mice provides an interesting and not unexpected link with mammary development as these mice do not undergo the massive mammary epithelial proliferation associated with pregnancy despite a normal ovarian hormone response.[371] Finally, Cyclin D1 is capable of activating the estrogen receptor in the absence of estrogen and independently of cdk4 activation.[372,373] This suggests that overexpression of cyclin D1 may exhibit some of its oncogenic effect through regulation of ER-responsive genes. However, one group found that this activation can be inhibited by tamoxifen,[373] while the other group states that antiestrogens do not inhibit ER activation.[372]

Tumor-specific mutations are rare in the p27Kip1 and cyclin E cell cycle regulators. However, levels of expression of these genes can be altered by posttranscriptional mechanisms. Thus, by observing protein levels, Porter and colleagues demonstrated that p27 and cyclin E correlate with survival in early onset breast cancer patients.[374]

The growth inhibitory protein of transforming growth factor beta (TGFβ) is thought to exert its effect on cell growth through inhibition of cell cycle progression. Because a number of tumorigenic cell lines have lost responsiveness to TGFβ, it is believed to play a role in tumor suppression, with malignant transformation being partially dependent on the loss of TGFβ expression or function. The growth-inhibitory effects of TGFβ are initiated by binding to cell surface TGFβ receptors. After ligand-receptor binding, multiple molecular targets have been suggested, including down-regulation of c-myc and cyclin expression, accumulation of hypophosphorylated RB, and inactivation of cdk2 and cdk4.[375] Work in this area is ongoing, but any one of these effects potentially could result in G1 arrest. Of particular interest in regard to breast cancer, TGFβ is hormonally regulated. Jeng and colleagues demonstrated that TGFβ isoforms are differentially regulated,[376] with TGFβ2 and TGFβ3 levels being suppressed by estrogen with little effect on TGFβ1 levels. While early work suggested that TGFβ (isoforms not specified) is induced to high levels by the growth inhibitory estrogen antagonist tamoxifen,[377] later work demonstrated that short exposure (6 h) to tamoxifen resulted in a slight decrease in TGFβ1 protein, whereas longer exposure had no effect. Thus the increase in unfractionated TGFβ in response to tamoxifen probably is due to increases in TGFβ2 and/or TGFβ3.[378] Paradoxically, while TGFβ is a strong growth inhibitor of normal mammary tissue, recent evidence suggests that enhanced TGFβ secretion correlates with aggressive malignant behavior. This was first demonstrated with the growth-stimulatory effect of TGFβ1 on the breast cancer cell lines T47D and MCF-7.[379] In support of these studies, the breast cancer cell line MCF-7, transfected with TGFβ1 cDNA, formed tumors in ovariectomized mice in the absence of estrogen supplementation, whereas the parental MCF-7 cells did not.[380] Prominent TGFβ1 expression also has been associated with axillary lymph node metastases ($p < 0.015$), but this association was not found in tumors that expressed both TGFβ1 and TGFβ2.[381] In a study of 50 breast cancers, one group reported that 90 percent expressed TGFβ1, 78 percent expressed TGFβ2, and 94 percent expressed TGFβ3, with 74 percent of the tumors expressing all three isoforms. Expression of all three isoforms was more likely to be associated with lymph node metastases than with the expression of one or two isoforms ($p < 0.025$).[382] However, other studies have not confirmed the usefulness of TGFβ expression as a prognostic factor in breast cancer.[383]

Regulators of Apoptosis. Apoptosis, the genetically programmed process of active (energy-requiring) cell death, is clearly important in understanding both neoplastic transformation and resistance to cytotoxic chemotherapy in breast cancer. Apoptosis can be induced by a variety of stimuli, including withdrawal of growth factors, DNA damage, viral infection, and expression of p53.[384] Since emerging evidence suggests that cytotoxic chemotherapy may exert a major effect on cancer cells by inducing apoptosis in response to chemotherapy-induced DNA damage, resistance to chemotherapy in some cases may result from inhibition of the apoptotic response.[385]

The proto-oncogene *bcl*-2, which normally functions to suppress apoptosis in a variety of cell types, has been studied extensively in several human cancers, including breast carcinoma, where it is overexpressed in 30 to 45 percent of cases.[386,387] Bcl-2 expression in human breast tissue varies dramatically throughout the menstrual cycle, suggesting that bcl-2 regulation is hormone-dependent.[388] Consistent with this hypothesis is the finding that bcl-2 expression is increased in ER-positive tumors and further increases after treatment with tamoxifen.[386] Conversely, bcl-2 expression is down-regulated in tumors expressing aberrant p53.[389] However, no genetic alterations that would increase bcl-2 levels have been reported in breast cancers.

c-myc. Numerous investigators have examined the role of the c-*myc* proto-oncogene in breast cancer with variable results. c-*myc* amplification was examined in 89 Norwegian breast cancer patients without axillary node involvement; amplification was noted in only one tumor.[390] However, another group used immunohistochemical methods to study 206 breast carcinomas and reported nuclear staining in 12 percent and cytoplasmic staining in 95 percent of these tumors. The presence of cytoplasmic staining was associated with increased disease-free survival compared with patients with tumors where c-myc was detected in the nucleus.[391] Finally, a study of 42 invasive breast cancers and 11 normal breast tissues suggested that while c-myc as detected by immunohistochemistry was present in both normal and malignant tissues, the level of expression in tumors was higher than it was in normal breast tissue.[392]

Cell Adhesion Molecules. Normal mammary epithelial cells are arranged in two layers: (1) a luminal epithelium and (2) a basal layer composed of myoepithelial cells and a small number of basal or stem cells. The basal layer is highly proliferative and is in direct contact with the basement membrane. During mammary carcinogenesis, tumor cells must escape normal adhesion mechanisms and traverse the basement membrane to invade surrounding structures. In this setting, interactions between breast carcinoma cells and their microenvironment are important determinants of the growth, invasion, and metastatic potential of tumor cells. In an effort to elucidate these interactions, researchers have investigated cell adhesion mechanisms, proteolytic enzymes, and the paracrine stimulation of growth factor receptors.[393]

Several factors participate in the maintenance of normal cell-cell and cell-matrix interactions. Cell-cell interactions are mediated via desmosomes and cadherin-containing junctions. In adult breast tissue, E-cadherin is expressed in normal ductal epithelial cells, and a reduction in E-cadherin expression is being investigated as a possible marker of invasive and metastatic potential. P-cadherin normally is expressed only in embryonal cells and in the basal layer of the adult epithelium. In examining cell-cell interactions, one study of 11 cases of invasive breast carcinoma suggested that in histologically normal areas, myoepithelial cells contain higher levels of cell-matrix adhesion molecules than do luminal epithelial cells.[394] In these normal areas, both myoepithelial and luminal cells have cadherin-containing junctions necessary for cell-cell interactions. In regions containing invasive carcinoma, normal E-cadherin staining was maintained in 10 of 11 cases, but β-catenin, the cytoplasmic component of E-cadherin-mediated junctions, was down-regulated or was distributed in an irregular punctate pattern. Similar findings were reported in a study of 26 primary breast carcinomas in which E-cadherin expression was decreased or lost in 63 percent of cases and α-catenin was reduced or absent in 81 percent of cases.[395] In this study, all patients with known metastatic disease at the time of biopsy had abnormal β-catenin staining, suggesting a role for β-catenin in maintaining normal cell-cell interactions. In keeping with other studies, expression of both E- and P-cadherin in 57 invasive breast carcinomas was noted to be altered, with reduced E-cadherin expression in 67 percent of tumors and abnormal P-cadherin in the luminal cells of 30 percent of invasive carcinomas.[396] All specimens with abnormal P-cadherin staining were histologic grade III and also revealed decreased E-cadherin expression. Of note, while an earlier study observed P-cadherin expression in lobular carcinomas of all grades,[397] P-cadherin expression in ductal carcinomas has been limited to high-grade lesions. These findings suggest that in some aggressive breast carcinomas, decreased or absent E-cadherin may be replaced by P-cadherin. This association between reduced E-cadherin staining and an aggressive histologic appearance also was noted in 109 patients with invasive ductal carcinomas, with an association between reduced E-cadherin expression and reduced disease-free survival in univariate analysis (5-year DFS = 70 percent in the E-cadherin positive group; DFS = 38 percent in the reduced E-cadherin group; $p = 0.027$).[398] However, longer follow-up and further validation will be required to determine whether E-cadherin is an independent predictor of disease prognosis.

Matrix Metalloproteinases. Extracellular proteinases are believed to be important in modulating both cell-matrix interactions and the degradation of the basement membrane necessary for invasion and metastasis. The matrix metalloproteinases (MMPs) include the gelatinases MMP-2 (gelatinase A) and MMP-9 (gelatinase B). The gelatinases, which are secreted as zymogens and are activated by cell membrane-associated proteins, have specific activity against type IV collagen, a component of the basement membrane.[399] This collagenase activity, the results of specific inhibition studies, and higher levels of immunostaining in invasive breast cancers (relative to preinvasive cancers) implicate these MMPs in tumor invasiveness.[393,400] Membrane-type metalloproteinase (MT-MMP), another member of the MMP family, has been postulated to be the membrane-associated activator of

MMP-2. The inhibitory component of this pathway consists of tissue inhibitors of metalloproteinase (TIMP-1 and -2). TIMPs are believed to exert their inhibitory activity by direct binding with the activated MMPs.

In an analysis of MMP-8, MMP-9, and TIMP-1 expression in breast cancer cells, protein levels were measured in the tumor tissue of 53 breast cancer patients.[401] MMP-8 and MMP-9 appeared to be coordinately regulated, and both were elevated in invasive tumors. However, increased levels of the MMP inhibitor TIMP-1 also were found in association with increased levels of the MMPs. These findings do not support earlier data suggesting that metastatic potential is associated with decreased TIMP-1 expression.

Of great interest is whether these proteases are produced by tumor cells or surrounding "normal" stromal cells, and if they are produced by stromal cells, whether the tumor cells are able to induce the expression of proteases. In an attempt to address this question, *in situ* hybridization was used to demonstrate that MT-MMP mRNA was expressed exclusively in the stromal cells in 83 of 83 human tumor specimens (including breast) analyzed.[402] In contrast, using an antibody directed against MT-MMP, protein was detected on the surface of invasive carcinoma cells.[403] This apparent discrepancy also has been described for MMP-2, with MMP-2 mRNA detected in tumor fibroblasts but MMP-2 protein detected in carcinoma cells.[404] Taken together with earlier studies suggesting that conditioned medium or the membrane fraction from breast carcinoma lines up-regulates the expression of MMP-2 in fibroblasts,[405,406] these findings suggest close interaction between tumor and stromal cells. A unifying hypothesis is that both MT-MMP and MMP-2 are produced in peritumor fibroblasts in response to the paracrine stimulation of carcinoma cells, that MT-MMP may activate MMP-2 on the stromal cell membrane, that the enzymes are secreted into the extracellular matrix, that each binds to the surface of malignant cells, and that one or both enzymes subsequently may be internalized by tumor cells.

Cathepsins. The cathepsins are another class of proteases that may affect the invasive and metastatic potential of malignant cells. These proteins are expressed at low levels in all cells, and once they are auto-activated, they have enzymatic activity against several matrix proteins, including those in the basement membrane. Levels of cathepsin expression in breast cancer have been studied as possible prognostic markers. Cathepsin D expression has been examined by immunostaining of 151 breast carcinomas, with "strong" cathepsin D expression detected in 22 percent of cases correlating with the nonductal histologic type ($p = 0.0243$) and metastases at the time of diagnosis ($p = 0.0068$) but not with tumor size, histologic grade, lymph node metastases, or ER/PR status. On univariate analysis, "strong" cathepsin D staining appeared to predict a significantly worse prognosis (median survival < 40 months in the high-cathepsin D group, median survival not yet reached at 140 months of follow-up in the low-cathepsin D group; $p = 0.047$). In multivariate analysis, however, no significant correlation between "strong" cathepsin D staining and prognosis persisted after adjusting for other known prognostic markers.[407] The relationship between cathepsin D and other pathologic features has been investigated in a large series of 1752 primary breast cancer patients. In this study, cathepsin D was associated with tumor size and grade and the presence or absence of nodal metastasis. On multivariate analysis performed on 489 patients from this series, cathepsin D independently predicted relapse-free survival and overall survival.[408] While the reason for the discrepancy between the findings of these two studies is not clear; it may be that the scoring of the intensity of cathepsin D staining as a continuous variable and the larger sample size of later study allowed detection of the prognostic significance of this marker.

Mediators of Metastasis. In addition to the well-characterized cell adhesion molecules and matrix metalloproteases that are thought to play a role in the development of metastatic breast cancer, *NME1* (encoding nm23) is a gene that is difficult to characterize with regard to its normal function and as result of decreased expression.[409] *NME1* was isolated initially as a gene that is differentially expressed in melanoma cells with discrepant metastatic potential.[410] The highest level of nm23 expression is seen in cells with low metastatic potential. Shortly after the isolation of *NME1*, data were presented suggesting that NME1 is differentially expressed in human breast cancers, with low NME1 mRNA levels found in association with histopathologic indicators of high metastatic potential.[411] These data are supported by studies demonstrating that transfection of NME1 into human MDA-MB-435 breast carcinoma cells reduces the metastatic potential of these cells when injected into the mammary fat pad of mice. Reduction in metastatic potential was associated with decreased ability of cells to form colonies in soft agar and an altered response to TGFβ.[412] Murine developmental studies also demonstrated a role for nm23 in the functional differentiation of the mammary gland. In this study, NME1 expression increased with functional differentiation of the mammary gland in nulliparous and pregnant animals.[413] Howlett and colleagues subsequently demonstrated a link between nm23 and human breast epithelial differentiation by using a culture system designed to mimic breast stroma. In this system, transfected breast cancer cell lines that overexpressed nm23 regained several aspects of the normal phenotype, including acinar formation, basement membrane production, and eventual growth arrest.[414] In investigations of the biologic function of NME1, it became clear that this gene is identical to PUF, a factor known to alter myc transcription *in vitro*.[415] However, data suggesting that nm23 can function as a growth inhibitor[414] led to confusion about how nm23 can be both a tumor suppressor and an activator of the proto-oncogene c-*myc*. It is possible that this is due to a tissue-specific effect, since NME1 expression is increased in aggressive neuroblastomas but is reduced in aggressive breast cancers.[416]

CLINICAL IMPLICATIONS OF BREAST CANCER SUSCEPTIBILITY

As was discussed in this chapter, advances in molecular genetics have provided data that allow risk estimation for women with inherited mutations in dominant cancer susceptibility genes and prognostic determinations for women with sporadic breast cancer. Unfortunately, our ability to make clinically useful interventions on the basis of these data remains limited. Prospective studies that allow an estimation of risk reduction from prophylactic surgical intervention are unavailable, and the science of chemoprevention is in its infancy. There are limited data available to assess the efficacy of enhanced surveillance programs for individuals at high risk of developing breast cancer. Finally, there is little information available about the interaction of multiple risk factors, so recommendations regarding modification of exposure to hormonal agents or dietary changes in the face of increased breast cancer risk caused by family history may be premature. Thus, in counseling women at increased risk of breast cancer, clinicians rely almost entirely on clinical judgment and the wishes of the women being counseled. Women at increased risk of breast cancer are offered the options of increased surveillance and prophylactic surgery and may be eligible for chemoprevention as part of an approved research protocol.

For women diagnosed with breast cancer, whether inherited or sporadic, prognostic information is most useful when coupled with targeted therapeutic approaches, very few of which exist. Identification of highly aggressive tumors is of little benefit if we have only the standard treatment to offer. The challenge for the future is to learn to use data on the molecular characteristics of an individual tumor to benefit patients and, ultimately, to prevent the development of breast cancer.

RECOMMENDATIONS FOR WOMEN WITH INHERITED SUSCEPTIBILITY TO BREAST CANCER

As noted earlier, it is not known whether increased surveillance will reduce breast cancer-related mortality in high-risk women. Furthermore, women from high-risk breast cancer families are well aware that mammography and clinical breast examination may not detect premalignant lesions. In the face of a striking family history and close personal losses, these women may be unconvinced that mammography and clinical breast examination offer the protection they seek. Such women often inquire about prophylactic mastectomy in the absence of other preventive options. There are few prospective data demonstrating the efficacy of prophylactic mastectomy in this setting. Furthermore, there are theoretical considerations that call into question the rationale for prophylactic surgery. Current surgical technique does not allow the complete removal of all breast tissue in a prophylactic total mastectomy. Since a germ-line mutation will be present in all residual breast tissue, individuals may remain at increased risk after surgery. Similarly, prophylactic oophorectomy does not guarantee protection from ovarian carcinoma, since tumors may arise spontaneously in the peritoneal reflection. These uncertainties make it difficult to counsel individuals about the potential benefits of these procedures. Nonetheless, the anxiety faced by women who harbor mutations in a breast cancer susceptibility gene can be overwhelming. Women must be presented with available data and allowed to make decisions that reflect their needs but do not offer a false sense of security.

Current recommendations include breast examination and mammography every 6 to 12 months beginning between the ages of 25 and 35 for women at increased risk of breast cancer resulting from direct or indirect molecular demonstration of a breast cancer-related genetic mutation.[417,418] Although no data exist to determine whether an increased frequency of clinical examination and screening mammography in this population reduces mortality, there are preliminary data that *BRCA1*-related tumors may have a faster growth rate than do sporadic tumors.[419] In addition, patient anxiety may be allayed somewhat by offering the option of two mammograms per year. Prophylactic mastectomy may be an option for interested women, who should be provided with information regarding the limited evidence for or against risk reduction by this procedure.

In women with a documented *BRCA1* or *BRCA2* mutation, pelvic examinations with transvaginal ultrasound every 6 to 12 months for those under age 40 and/or those still interested in childbearing may be of benefit. Prophylactic oophorectomy at the completion of childbearing or at the time of menopause is recommended by the American College of Obstetrics and Gynecology; however, there is a low but measurable incidence of peritoneal malignancies after oophorectomy that may derive from peritoneal cells, which are at similar risk for malignant transformation and are not removed by oophorectomy. It may be prudent for women at increased risk of breast cancer to avoid the use of exogenous estrogens when possible, since no data exist regarding the effect of estrogens on the penetrance of susceptibility genes in breast cancer. However, a dilemma arises in that there may be some benefit to taking oral contraceptives to reduce ovarian cancer risk and in that heart disease and osteoporosis are more prevalent in women who do not use estrogen replacement therapy after menopause.

ACKNOWLEDGMENTS

We are extremely grateful to Mary Jo Marchionni for assistance with the preparation of this chapter.

REFERENCES

1. Kelsey JL, Horn-Ross PL: Breast cancer: Magnitude of the problem and descriptive epidemiology. *Epidemiol Rev* **15**:7, 1993.

2. Miller BA: Causes of breast cancer and high risk groups, incidence and demographics, in Harris JR, Hellman S, Henderson IC, Kinne DW (eds): *Breast Diseases*. Philadelphia, Lippincott, 1991, p 119.

3. Miller BA, Feuer EJ, Hankey BF: The increasing incidence of breast cancer since 1982: Relevance of early detection. *Cancer Causes Control* **2**:67, 1991.

4. Glass A, Hoover RN: Changing incidence of breast cancer (letter). *J Natl Cancer Inst* **80**:1076, 1988.

5. Holford TR, Roush GC, McKay LA: Trends in female breast cancer in Connecticut and the United States. *J Clin Epidemiol* **44**:29, 1991.

6. Slattery ML, Kerber RA: A comprehensive evaluation of family history and breast cancer risk: The Utah Population Database (see comments). *JAMA* **270**:1563, 1993.

7. Colditz GA, et al: Family history, age, and risk of breast cancer: Prospective data from the Nurses' Health Study (see comments) [published erratum appears in *JAMA* **270**:1548, 1993]. *JAMA* **270**:338, 1993.

8. Gail MH, et al: Projecting individualized probabilities of developing breast cancer for white females who are being examined annually (see comments). *J Natl Cancer Inst* **81**:1879, 1989.

9. Easton DF, Bishop DT, Ford D, Crockford GP: Genetic linkage analysis in familial breast and ovarian cancer: Results from 214 families. The Breast Cancer Linkage Consortium. *Am J Hum Genet* **52**:678, 1993.

10. Kampert JB, Whittemore AS, Paffenbarger RS Jr: Combined effect of childbearing, menstrual events, and body size on age-specific breast cancer risk. *Am J Epidemiol* **128**:962, 1988.

11. White E: Projected changes in breast cancer incidence due to the trend toward delayed childbearing. *Am J Public Health* **77**:495, 1987.

12. Trichopoulos D, MacMahon B, Cole P: Menopause and breast cancer risk. *J Natl Cancer Inst* **48**:605, 1972.

13. Pike MC, Spicer DV, Dahmoush L, Press MF: Estrogens, progestogens, normal breast cell proliferation, and breast cancer risk. *Epidemiol Rev* **15**:17, 1993.

14. Tokunaga M, et al: Incidence of female breast cancer among atomic bomb survivors, 1950–1985. *Radiat Res* **138**:209, 1994.

15. McGregor H, et al: Breast cancer incidence among atomic bomb survivors, Hiroshima and Nagasaki, 1950–69. *J Natl Cancer Inst* **59**:799, 1977.

16. Bhatia S, et al: Breast cancer and other second neoplasms after childhood Hodgkin's disease (see comments]. *N Engl J Med* **334**:745, 1996.

17. Harris JR, Lippman ME, Veronesi U, Willett W: Breast cancer (1) (see comments). *N Engl J Med* **327**:319, 1992.

18. Dupont WD, Page DL: Risk factors for breast cancer in women with proliferative breast disease. *N Engl J Med* **312**:146, 1985.

19. Kinne DW: Clinical measurement of lobular carcinoma in situ, in Harris JR, Hellman S, Henderson IC, Kinne DW (eds): *Breast Diseases*. Philadelphia, Lippincott, 1985, pp 239–244.

20. Rosen PP, Kosloff C, Lieberman PH, Adair F, Braun DW Jr: Lobular carcinoma *in situ* of the breast: Detailed analysis of 99 patients with average follow-up of 24 years. *Am J Surg Pathol* **2**:225, 1978.

21. Consortium BCL: Pathology of familial breast cancer: Differences between breast cancers in carriers of *BRCA1* or *BRCA2* mutations and sporadic cases. Breast Cancer Linkage Consortium (see comments). *Lancet* **349**:1505, 1997.

22. Haagensen CD, Bodian C, Haagensen DE Jr: *Breast Carcinoma, Risk and Detection*. Philadelphia, Saunders, 1981, p. 238.

23. Rosner D, Bedwani RN, Vana J, Baker HW, Murphy GP: Noninvasive breast carcinoma: Results of a national survey by the American College of Surgeons. *Ann Surg* **192**:139, 1980.

24. Baker LH: Breast Cancer Detection Demonstration Project: Five-year summary report. *Cancer J Clin* **32**:194, 1982.

25. Page DL, Dupont WD, Rogers LW, Landenberger M: Intraductal carcinoma of the breast: Follow-up after biopsy only. *Cancer* **49**:751, 1982.

26. Rosen PP, Braun DW Jr, Kinne DE: The clinical significance of pre-invasive breast carcinoma. *Cancer* **46**:919, 1980.

27. Solin LJ, et al: Ten-year results of breast-conserving surgery and definitive irradiation for intraductal carcinoma (ductal carcinoma *in situ*) of the breast. *Cancer* **68**:2337, 1991.

28. Fisher ER, et al: Medullary cancer of the breast revisited. *Breast Cancer Res Treat* **16**:215, 1990.

29. American Joint Committee on Cancer: *Manual for Staging for Breast Carcinoma*. Philadelphia, Lippincott, 1989.

30. Harris JR: Staging of breast carcinoma, in Harris JR, Hellman S, Henderson IC, Kinne DW (eds): *Breast Diseases*. Philadelphia, Lippincott, 1991, p 330.

31. Clark GM, Sledge GW Jr, Osborne CK, McGuire WL: Survival from first recurrence: Relative importance of prognostic factors in 1015 breast cancer patients. *J Clin Oncol* **5**:55, 1987.

32. Fisher B, Anderson S, Redmond C: Reanalysis and results after 12 years follow-up in a randomized clinical trial comparing total mastectomy with lumpectomy with or without irradiation in the treatment of breast cancer. *N Engl J Med* **333**:1456, 1995.

33. Valero V, Buzdar AU, Hortobagyi GN: Locally advanced breast cancer. *Oncologist* **1**:8, 1996.

34. Peters WP: High-dose chemotherapy with autologous bone marrow transplantation for the treatment of breast cancer: Yes. *Import Adv Oncol* 215, 1995.

34b. Stadtmauer EA, O'Neill A, Goldstein LJ, Crilley PA, Mangan KF, Ingle JN, Brodsky I, et al: Conventional-does chemotherapy compared with high-dose chemotherapy plus autologous hematopoietic stem-cell transplatation for metastatic breast cancer. *N Engl J Med* **342**:1069, 2000.

35. Lynch HT, et al: Genetic heterogeneity and familial carcinoma of the breast. *Surg Gynecol Obstet* **142**:693, 1976.

36. Broca: *Taite de tumerus*. Asselin, 1866.

37. Williams WR, Anderson DE: Genetic epidemiology of breast cancer: Segregation analysis of 200 Danish pedigrees. *Genet Epidemiol* **1**:7, 1984.

38. Newman B, Austin MA, Lee M, King MC: Inheritance of human breast cancer: Evidence for autosomal dominant transmission in high-risk families. *Proc Natl Acad Sci USA* **85**:3044, 1988.

39. Miki Y, et al: A strong candidate for the breast and ovarian cancer susceptibility gene *BRCA1*. *Science* **266**:66, 1994.

40. Wooster R, et al: Identification of the breast cancer susceptibility gene *BRCA2* (see comments) [published erratum appears in *Nature* **379(6567)**:749, 1996]. *Nature* **378**:789, 1995.

41. Tavtigian SV, et al: The complete *BRCA2* gene and mutations in chromosome 13q-linked kindreds (see comments). *Nature Genet* **12**:333, 1996.

42. Nelson CL, et al: Familial clustering of colon, breast, uterine, and ovarian cancers as assessed by family history. *Genet Epidemiol* **10**:235, 1993.

43. Narod SA, et al: Familial breast-ovarian cancer locus on chromosome 17q12-q23 (see comments). *Lancet* **338**:82, 1991.

44. Couch FJ, et al: *BRCA1* mutations in women attending clinics that evaluate the risk of breast cancer (see comments). *N Engl J Med* **336**:1409, 1997.

45. Stoppa-Lyonnet D, et al: *BRCA1* sequence variations in 160 individuals referred to a breast/ovarian family cancer clinic: Institut Curie Breast Cancer Group (see comments). *Am J Hum Genet* **60**:1021, 1997.

46. Shattuck-Eidens D, et al: *BRCA1* sequence analysis in women at high risk for susceptibility mutations: Risk factor analysis and implications for genetic testing (see comments). *JAMA* **278**:1242, 1997.

47. Frank TS, et al: Sequence analysis of *BRCA1* and *BRCA2*: Correlation of mutations with family history and ovarian cancer risk. *J Clin Oncol* **16**:2417, 1998.

48. Easton DF, Bishop DT, Ford D, Crockford GP, Consortium BCL: Breast and ovarian cancer incidence in *BRCA1* mutation carriers. *Lancet* **343**:962, 1994.

49. Struewing JP, et al: The risk of cancer associated with specific mutations of *BRCA1* and *BRCA2* among Ashkenazi Jews (see comments). *N Engl J Med* **336**:1401, 1997.

50. Whittemore AS, Gong G, Itnyre J: Prevalence and contribution of *BRCA1* mutations in breast cancer and ovarian cancer: Results from three U.S. population-based case-control studies of ovarian cancer. *Am J Hum Genet* **60**:496, 1997.

51. Brody LC, Biesecker BB: Breast cancer susceptibility genes: *BRCA1* and *BRCA2*. *Medicine* **77**:208, 1998.

52. Arason A, Barkardottir RB, Egilsson V: Linkage analysis of chromosome 17q markers and breast-ovarian cancer in Icelandic families and possible relationship to prostatic cancer. *Am J Hum Genet* **52**:711, 1993.

53. Ford D, Easton DF, Bishop DT, Narod SA, Goldgar DE: Risks of cancer in *BRCA1*-mutation carriers: Breast Cancer Linkage Consortium. *Lancet* **343**:692, 1994.

54. Lynch HT, Marcus J, Watson P, Page D: Distinctive clinicopathologic features of *BRCA1*-linked hereditary breast cancer. *Proc ASCO* **13**:56, 1994.

55. Marcus JN, et al: Hereditary breast cancer: Pathobiology prognosis and *BRCA1* and *BRCA2* gene linkage (see comments). *Cancer* **77**:697, 1996.

56. Karp SE, et al: Influence of *BRCA1* mutations on nuclear grade and estrogen receptor status of breast carcinoma in Ashkenazi Jewish women. *Cancer* **80**:435, 1997.

57. Robson M, et al: *BRCA*-associated breast cancer: Absence of a characteristic immunophenotype. *Cancer Res* **58**:1839, 1998.

58. Wagner TM, et al: *BRCA1*-related breast cancer in Austrian breast and ovarian cancer families: Specific *BRCA1* mutations and pathological characteristics. *Int J Cancer* **77**:354, 1998.

59. Eisinger F, et al: Germ line mutation at *BRCA1* affects the histoprognostic grade in hereditary breast cancer. *Cancer Res* **56**:471, 1996.

60. Jarvis EM, Kirk JA, Clarke CL: Loss of nuclear *BRCA1* expression in breast cancers is associated with a highly proliferative tumor phenotype. *Cancer Genet Cytogenet* **101**:109, 1998.

61. Johannsson OT, Ranstam J, Borg A, Olsson H: Survival of *BRCA1* breast and ovarian cancer patients: A population-based study from southern Sweden (see comments). *J Clin Oncol* **16**:397, 1998.

62. Verhoog LC, et al: Survival and tumour characteristics of breast-cancer patients with germline mutations of *BRCA1*. *Lancet* **351**:316, 1998.

63. Foulkes WD, Wong N, Rozen F, Brunet JS, Narod SA: Survival of patients with breast cancer and *BRCA1* mutations (letter). *Lancet* **351**:1359, 1998.

64. Tirkkonen M, et al: Distinct somatic genetic changes associated with tumor progression in carriers of *BRCA1* and *BRCA2* germ-line mutations. *Cancer Res* **57**:1222, 1997.

65. Tapper J, et al: Genetic changes in inherited and sporadic ovarian carcinomas by comparative genomic hybridization: Extensive similarity except for a difference at chromosome 2q24-q32. *Cancer Res* **58**:2715, 1998.

66. Brunet JS, et al: Effect of smoking on breast cancer in carriers of mutant *BRCA1* or *BRCA2* genes (see comments). *J Natl Cancer Inst* **90**:761, 1998.

67. Narod SA, et al: Oral contraceptives and the risk of hereditary ovarian cancer: Hereditary Ovarian Cancer Clinical Study Group (see comments). *N Engl J Med* **339**:424, 1998.

68. Easton D: Breast cancer genes: What are the real risks? (news). *Nature Genet* **16**:210, 1997.

69. Phelan CM, et al: Ovarian cancer risk in *BRCA1* carriers is modified by the HRAS1 variable number of tandem repeat (VNTR) locus. *Nature Genet* **12**:309, 1996.

70. Redston M, Nathanson K, Yuan ZQ: The APC I1307K allele and cancer risk in a community-based study of Ashkenazi Jews. *Nature Genet* **20**:62, 1998.

71. Hall JM, et al: Linkage of early-onset familial breast cancer to chromosome 17q21. *Science* **250**:1684, 1990.

72. Bork P, et al: A superfamily of conserved domains in DNA damage-responsive cell cycle checkpoint proteins. *FASEB J* **11**:68, 1997.

73. Abel KJ, et al: Mouse *Brca1*: Localization sequence analysis and identification of evolutionarily conserved domains. *Hum Mol Genet* **4**:2265, 1995.

74. Bennett LM, et al: Isolation of the mouse homologue of *BRCA1* and genetic mapping to mouse chromosome 11. *Genomics* **29**:576, 1995.

75. Sharan SK, Wims M, Bradley A: Murine *Brca1*: Sequence and significance for human missense mutations. *Hum Mol Genet* **4**:2275, 1995.

76. Szabo CI, et al: Human, canine and murine *BRCA1* genes: Sequence comparison among species. *Hum Mol Genet* **5**:1289, 1996.

77. Chen KS, Shepel LA, Haag JD, Heil GM, Gould MN: Cloning genetic mapping and expression studies of the rat *Brca1* gene. *Carcinogenesis* **17**:1561, 1996.

78. Futreal PA, et al: *BRCA1* mutations in primary breast and ovarian carcinomas. *Science* **266**:120, 1994.

79. Castilla LH, et al: Mutations in the *BRCA1* gene in families with early-onset breast and ovarian cancer. *Nature Genet* **8**:387, 1994.

80. Friedman LS, et al: Confirmation of *BRCA1* by analysis of germline mutations linked to breast and ovarian cancer in ten families. *Nature Genet* **8**:399, 1994.

81. Simard J, et al: Common origins of *BRCA1* mutations in Canadian breast and ovarian cancer families. *Nature Genet* **8**:392, 1994.

82. Merajver SD, et al: Somatic mutations in the *BRCA1* gene in sporadic ovarian tumours. *Nature Genet* **9**:439, 1995.

83. Hosking L, et al: A somatic *BRCA1* mutation in an ovarian tumour (letter). *Nature Genet* **9**:343, 1995.

84. Takahashi H, et al: Mutation analysis of the *BRCA1* gene in ovarian cancers. *Cancer Res* **55**:2998, 1995.

85. Matsushima M, et al: Mutation analysis of the *BRCA1* gene in 76 Japanese ovarian cancer patients: Four germline mutations but no evidence of somatic mutation. *Hum Mol Genet* **4**:1953, 1995.

86. Boyd M, Harris F, McFarlane R, Davidson HR, Black DM: A human *BRCA1* gene knockout (letter). *Nature* **375**:541, 1995.

87. Inoue R, et al: Germline mutation of *BRCA1* in Japanese breast cancer families. *Cancer Res* **55**:3521, 1995.

88. Hogervorst FB, et al: Rapid detection of *BRCA1* mutations by the protein truncation test. *Nature Genet* **10**:208, 1995.

89. Plummer SJ, et al: Detection of *BRCA1* mutations by the protein truncation test. *Hum Mol Genet* **4**:1989, 1995.

90. Gayther SA, et al: Rapid detection of regionally clustered germ-line *BRCA1* mutations by multiplex heteroduplex analysis: UKCCCR Familial Ovarian Cancer Study Group. *Am J Hum Genet* **58**:451, 1996.

91. Ganguly T, Dhulipala R, Godmilow L, Ganguly A: High throughput fluorescence-based conformation-sensitive gel electrophoresis (F-CSGE) identifies six unique *BRCA2* mutations and an overall low incidence of *BRCA2* mutations in high-risk *BRCA1*-negative breast cancer families. *Hum Genet* **102**:549, 1998.

92. Couch FJ, Weber BL: Mutations and polymorphisms in the familial early-onset breast cancer (*BRCA1*) gene: Breast Cancer Information Core. *Hum Mutat* **8**:8, 1996.

93. Gayther SA, et al: Germline mutations of the *BRCA1* gene in breast and ovarian cancer families provide evidence for a genotype-phenotype correlation. *Nature Genet* **11**:428, 1995.

94. Serova O, et al: A high incidence of *BRCA1* mutations in 20 breast-ovarian cancer families. *Am J Hum Genet* **58**:42, 1996.

95. Brzovic PS, Meza J, King MC, Klevit RE: The cancer-predisposing mutation *C61G* disrupts homodimer formation in the NH$_2$-terminal *BRCA1* RING finger domain. *J Biol Chem* **273**:7795, 1998.

96. Wu GS, et al: KILLER/DR5 is a DNA damage-inducible p53-regulated death receptor gene (letter). *Nature Genet* **17**:141, 1997.

97. Jensen DE, et al: *BAP1*: A novel ubiquitin hydrolase which binds to the *BRCA1* RING finger and enhances *BRCA1*-mediated cell growth suppression. *Oncogene* **16**:1097, 1998.

98. Papa S, et al: Identification of a possible somatic *BRCA1* mutation affecting translation efficiency in an early-onset sporadic breast cancer patient (letter). *J Natl Cancer Inst* **90**:1011, 1998.

99. Humphrey JS, et al: Human *BRCA1* inhibits growth in yeast: Potential use in diagnostic testing. *Proc Natl Acad Sci USA* **94**:5820, 1997.

100. Puget N, et al: A 1-kb Alu-mediated germ-line deletion removing *BRCA1* exon 17. *Cancer Res* **57**:828, 1997.

101. Petrij-Bosch A, et al: *BRCA1* genomic deletions are major founder mutations in Dutch breast cancer patients [published erratum appears in *Nature Genet* **17**(4):503, 1997]. *Nature Genet* **17**:341, 1997.

102. Holt JT, et al: Growth retardation and tumour inhibition by *BRCA1* (see comments). *Nature Genet* **12**:298, 1996.

103. Sobol H, et al: Truncation at conserved terminal regions of BRCA1 protein is associated with highly proliferating hereditary breast cancers. *Cancer Res* **56**:3216, 1996.

104. Tonin P, et al: *BRCA1* mutations in Ashkenazi Jewish women (letter). *Am J Hum Genet* **57**:189, 1995.

105. Bar-Sade RB, et al: The 185delAG *BRCA1* mutation originated before the dispersion of Jews in the diaspora and is not limited to Ashkenazim. *Hum Mol Genet* **7**:801, 1998.

106. FitzGerald MG, et al: Germ-line *BRCA1* mutations in Jewish and non-Jewish women with early-onset breast cancer (see comments). *N Engl J Med* **334**:143, 1996.

107. Offit K, et al: Germline *BRCA1* 185delAG mutations in Jewish women with breast cancer (see comments). *Lancet* **347**:1643, 1996.

108. Levy-Lahad E, et al: Founder *BRCA1* and *BRCA2* mutations in Ashkenazi Jews in Israel: Frequency and differential penetrance in ovarian cancer and in breast-ovarian cancer families (see comments). *Am J Hum Genet* **60**:1059, 1997.

109. Muto MG, Cramer DW, Tangir J, Berkowitz R, Mok S: Frequency of the *BRCA1* 185delAG mutation among Jewish women with ovarian cancer and matched population controls. *Cancer Res* **56**:1250, 1996.

110. Abeliovich D, et al: The founder mutations 185delAG and 5382insC in *BRCA1* and 6174delT in *BRCA2* appear in 60% of ovarian cancer and 30% of early-onset breast cancer patients among Ashkenazi women. *Am J Hum Genet* **60**:505, 1997.

111. Neuhausen SL, et al: Haplotype and phenotype analysis of nine recurrent *BRCA2* mutations in 111 families: Results of an international study. *Am J Hum Genet* **62**:1381, 1998.

112. Dunning AM, et al: Common *BRCA1* variants and susceptibility to breast and ovarian cancer in the general population. *Hum Mol Genet* **6**:285, 1997.

113. Bergthorsson JT, et al: Chromosome imbalance at the 3p14 region in human breast tumours: High frequency in patients with inherited predisposition due to BRCA2. *Eur J Cancer* **34**:142, 1998.

114. Huusko P, et al: Evidence of founder mutations in Finnish *BRCA1* and *BRCA2* families (letter). *Am J Hum Genet* **62**:1544, 1998.

115. Ramus SJ, et al: Analysis of *BRCA1* and *BRCA2* mutations in Hungarian families with breast or breast-ovarian cancer (letter). *Am J Hum Genet* **60**:1242, 1997.

116. Gayther SA, et al: Variation of risks of breast and ovarian cancer associated with different germline mutations of the *BRCA2* gene. *Nature Genet* **15**:103, 1997.

117. Dorum A, et al: A *BRCA1* founder mutation, identified with haplotype analysis, allowing genotype/phenotype determination and predictive testing. *Eur J Cancer* **33**:2390, 1997.

118. Szabo CI, King MC: Population genetics of *BRCA1* and *BRCA2* (editorial; comment). *Am J Hum Genet* **60**:1013, 1997.

119. Malone KE, et al: *BRCA1* mutations and breast cancer in the general population: Analyses in women before age 35 years and in women before age 45 years with first-degree family history (see comments). *JAMA* **279**:922, 1998.

120. Newman B, et al: Frequency of breast cancer attributable to *BRCA1* in a population-based series of American women (see comments). *JAMA* **279**:915, 1998.

121. Hakansson S, et al: Moderate frequency of *BRCA1* and *BRCA2* germ-line mutations in Scandinavian familial breast cancer (see comments). *Am J Hum Genet* **60**:1068, 1997.

122. Krainer M, et al: Differential contributions of *BRCA1* and *BRCA2* to early-onset breast cancer (see comments). *N Engl J Med* **336**:1416, 1997.

123. Katagiri T, et al: Mutations in the *BRCA1* gene in Japanese breast cancer patients. *Hum Mutat* **7**:334, 1996.

124. Berry DA, Parmigiani G, Sanchez J, Schildkraut J, Winer E: Probability of carrying a mutation of breast-ovarian cancer gene *BRCA1* based on family history (see comments). *J Natl Cancer Inst* **89**:227, 1997.

125. Brown MA, Xu C, Nicolai H: The 59 end of the *BRCA1* gene lies within a duplicated region of human chromosome 17q21. *Cancer Res* **12**:2507, 1996.

126. Fetzer S, Tworek HA, Piver MS, Dicioccio RA: An alternative splice site junction in exon 1a of the *BRCA1* gene (letter). *Cancer Genet Cytogenet* **105**:90, 1998.

127. Thakur S, et al: Localization of *BRCA1* and a splice variant identifies the nuclear localization signal. *Mol Cell Biol* **17**:444, 1997.

128. Wilson CA, et al: Differential subcellular localization expression and biological toxicity of *BRCA1* and the splice variant *BRCA1-delta11b*. *Oncogene* **14**:1, 1997.

129. Wu LC, et al: Identification of a RING protein that can interact in vivo with the *BRCA1* gene product. *Nature Genet* **14**:430, 1996.

130. Jin Y, et al: Cell cycle-dependent colocalization of BARD1 and BRCA1 proteins in discrete nuclear domains. *Proc Natl Acad Sci USA* **94**:12075, 1997.

131. Scully R, et al: Association of BRCA1 with Rad51 in mitotic and meiotic cells. *Cell* **88**:265, 1997.

132. Chen J, Silver DP, Walpita D, Cantor SB, Gazdar AF, Tomlinson G, Couch FJ, Weber BL, Ashley T, Livingston DM, Scully R: Stable interaction between the products of the BRCA1 and BRCA2 tumor suppressor genes in mitotic and meiotic cells. *Mol Cell* **2**:317, 1998.

133. Chapman MS, Verma IM: Transcriptional activation by *BRCA1* (letter; comment). *Nature* **382**:678, 1996.

134. Monteiro AN, August A, Hanafusa H: Evidence for a transcriptional activation function of *BRCA1* C-terminal region. *Proc Natl Acad Sci USA* **93**:13595, 1996.

135. Ouchi T, Monteiro AN, August A, Aaronson SA, Hanafusa H: *BRCA1* regulates p53-dependent gene expression. *Proc Natl Acad Sci USA* **95**:2302, 1998.

136. Zhang H, et al: *BRCA1* physically associates with *p53* and stimulates its transcriptional activity. *Oncogene* **16**:1713, 1998.

137. Somasundaram K, et al: Arrest of the cell cycle by the tumour-suppressor *BRCA1* requires the CDK-inhibitor p21WAF1/CiP1. *Nature* **389**:187, 1997.

138. Anderson SF, Schlegel BP, Nakajima T, Wolpin ES, Parvin JD: *BRCA1* protein is linked to the RNA polymerase II holoenzyme complex via RNA helicase A. *Nature Genet* **19**:254, 1998.

139. Scully R, et al: *BRCA1* is a component of the RNA polymerase II holoenzyme. *Proc Natl Acad Sci USA* **94**:5605, 1997.

140. Cui JQ, et al: *BRCA1* splice variants *BRCA1a* and *BRCA1b* associate with CBP co-activator. *Oncol Rep* **5**:591, 1998.

141. Burke TF, et al: Identification of a *BRCA1*-associated kinase with potential biological relevance. *Oncogene* **16**:1031, 1998.

142. Mancini DN, et al: CpG methylation within the 5′ regulatory region of the *BRCA1* gene is tumor specific and includes a putative CREB binding site. *Oncogene* **16**:1161, 1998.

143. Dobrovic A, Simpfendorfer D: Methylation of the *BRCA1* gene in sporadic breast cancer. *Cancer Res* **57**:3347, 1997.

144. Gudas JM, Nguyen H, Li T, Cowan KH: Hormone-dependent regulation of *BRCA1* in human breast cancer cells. *Cancer Res* **55**:4561, 1995.

145. Gudas JM, et al: Cell cycle regulation of *BRCA1* messenger RNA in human breast epithelial cells. *Cell Growth Diff* **7**:717, 1996.

146. Vaughn JP, et al: *BRCA1* expression is induced before DNA synthesis in both normal and tumor-derived breast cells. *Cell Growth Diff* **7**:711, 1996.

147. Marquis ST, et al: The developmental pattern of *Brca1* expression implies a role in differentiation of the breast and other tissues. *Nature Genet* **11**:17, 1995.

148. Marks JR, et al: *BRCA1* expression is not directly responsive to estrogen. *Oncogene* **14**:115, 1997.

149. Romagnolo D, et al: Estrogen upregulation of *BRCA1* expression with no effect on localization. *Mol Carcinogen* **22**:102, 1998.

150. Spillman MA, Bowcock AM: *BRCA1* and *BRCA2* mRNA levels are coordinately elevated in human breast cancer cells in response to estrogen. *Oncogene* **13**:1639, 1996.

151. Chen Y, et al: Aberrant subcellular localization of *BRCA1* in breast cancer (see comments) [published erratum appears in *Science* **270**:5241, 1995]. *Science* **270**:789, 1995.

152. Scully R, Ganesan S, Brown M: Localization of *BRCA1* in human breast and ovarian cancer cells. *Science* **272**:122, 1996.

153. Jensen RA, et al: *BRCA1* is secreted and exhibits properties of a granin (see comments). *Nature Genet* **12**:303, 1996.

154. Wilson CA, et al: *BRCA1* protein products: Antibody specificity. *Nature Genet* **13**:264, 1996.

155. Chamberlain JS, et al: *BRCA1* maps proximal to D17S579 on chromosome 17q21 by genetic analysis. *Am J Hum Genet* **52**:792, 1993.

156. Smith SA, Easton DF, Evans DG, Ponder BA: Allele losses in the region 17q12-21 in familial breast and ovarian cancer involve the wild-type chromosome. *Nature Genet* **2**:128, 1992.

157. Thompson ME, Jensen RA, Obermiller PS, Page DL, Holt JT: Decreased expression of *BRCA1* accelerates growth and is often present during sporadic breast cancer progression. *Nature Genet* **9**:444, 1995.

158. Shao N, Chai YL, Shyam E, Reddy P, Rao VN: Induction of apoptosis by the tumor suppressor protein *BRCA1*. *Oncogene* **13**:1, 1996.

159. Tomlinson GE, et al: Characterization of a breast cancer cell line derived from a germ-line *BRCA1* mutation carrier. *Cancer Res* **58**:3237, 1998.

160. Chen Y, et al: *BRCA1* is a 220-kDa nuclear phosphoprotein that is expressed and phosphorylated in a cell cycle-dependent manner [published erratum appears in *Cancer Res* **56**:17, 1996]. *Cancer Res* **56**:3168, 1996.

161. Larson JS, Tonkinson JL, Lai MT: A *BRCA1* mutant alters G2-M cell cycle control in human mammary epithelial cells. *Cancer Res* **57**:3351, 1997.

162. Blackshear PE, et al: *Brca1* and *Brca2* expression patterns in mitotic and meiotic cells of mice. *Oncogene* **16**:61, 1998.

163. Gowen LC, Johnson BL, Latour AM, Sulik KK, Koller BH: *Brca1* deficiency results in early embryonic lethality characterized by neuroepithelial abnormalities. *Nature Genet* **12**:191, 1996.

164. Hakem R, et al: The tumor suppressor gene *Brca1* is required for embryonic cellular proliferation in the mouse. *Cell* **85**:1009, 1996.

165. Liu CY, Flesken-Nikitin A, Li S, Zeng Y, Lee WH: Inactivation of the mouse *Brca1* gene leads to failure in the morphogenesis of the egg cylinder in early postimplantation development. *Genes Dev* **10**:1835, 1996.

166. Ludwig T, Chapman DL, Papaioannou VE, Efstratiadis A: Targeted mutations of breast cancer susceptibility gene homologs in mice: Lethal phenotypes of *Brca1*, *Brca2*, *Brca1/Brca2*, *Brca1/p53*, and *Brca2/p53* nullizygous embryos. *Genes Dev* **11**:1226, 1997.

167. Shore D: *RAP1*: A protean regulator in yeast. *Trends Genet* **10**:408, 1994.

168. Scully R, et al: Dynamic changes of *BRCA1* subnuclear location and phosphorylation state are initiated by DNA damage. *Cell* **90**:425, 1997.

169. Lim DS, Hasty P: A mutation in mouse *rad51* results in an early embryonic lethal that is suppressed by a mutation in *p53*. *Mol Cell Biol* **16**:7133, 1996.

170. Shinohara A, Ogawa H, Ogawa T: Rad51 protein involved in repair and recombination in *S. cerevisiae* is a RecA-like protein [published erratum appears in *Cell* **71**:180, 1992]. *Cell* **69**:457, 1992.

171. Thomas JE, Smith M, Tonkinson JL, Rubinfeld B, Polakis P: Induction of phosphorylation on *BRCA1* during the cell cycle and after DNA damage. *Cell Growth Diff* **8**:801, 1997.

172. Fan S, et al: Down-regulation of *BRCA1* and *BRCA2* in human ovarian cancer cells exposed to adriamycin and ultraviolet radiation. *Int J Cancer* **77**:600, 1998.

173. Fan S, et al: *BRCA1* as a potential human prostate tumor suppressor: Modulation of proliferation damage responses and expression of cell regulatory proteins. *Oncogene* **16**:3069, 1998.

174. Husain A, He G, Venkatraman ES, Spriggs DR: *BRCA1* up-regulation is associated with repair-mediated resistance to cis-diamminedichloroplatinum(II). *Cancer Res* **58**:1120, 1998.

175. Gowen LC, Avrutskaya AV, Latour AM, Koller BH, Leadon SA: *BRCA1* required for transcription-coupled repair of oxidative DNA damage. *Science* **281**:1009, 1998.

176. Kinzler KW, Vogelstein B: Cancer-susceptibility genes: Gatekeepers and caretakers (news; comment). *Nature* **386**:761, 1997.

177. Crook T, Crossland S, Crompton MR, Osin P, Gusterson BA: *p53* mutations in *BRCA1*-associated familial breast cancer (letter). *Lancet* **350**:638, 1997.

178. Tseng SL, et al: Allelic loss at *BRCA1*, *BRCA2*, and adjacent loci in relation to *TP53* abnormality in breast cancer. *Genes Chromosom Cancer* **20**:377, 1997.

179. Rhei E, et al: Molecular genetic characterization of *BRCA1*- and *BRCA2*-linked hereditary ovarian cancers. *Cancer Res* **58**:3193, 1998.

180. Stratton MR, et al: Familial male breast cancer is not linked to the *BRCA1* locus on chromosome 17q. *Nature Genet* **7**:103, 1994.

181. Wooster R, et al: Localization of a breast cancer susceptibility gene *BRCA2* to chromosome 13q12-13. *Science* **265**:2088, 1994.

182. Ford D, et al: Genetic heterogeneity and penetrance analysis of the *BRCA1* and *BRCA2* genes in breast cancer families: The Breast Cancer Linkage Consortium. *Am J Hum Genet* **62**:676, 1998.

183. Agnarsson BA, et al: Inherited *BRCA2* mutation associated with high grade breast cancer. *Breast Cancer Res Treat* **47**:121, 1998.

184. Gudmundsson J, et al: Frequent occurrence of *BRCA2* linkage in Icelandic breast cancer families and segregation of a common *BRCA2* haplotype. *Am J Hum Genet* **58**:749, 1996.

185. Schutte M, et al: An integrated high-resolution physical map of the DPC/BRCA2 region at chromosome 13q12. *Cancer Res* **55**:4570, 1995.

186. Bignell G, Micklem G, Stratton MR, Ashworth A, Wooster R: The BRC repeats are conserved in mammalian BRCA2 proteins. *Hum Mol Genet* **6**:53, 1997.

187. Bork P, Blomberg N, Nilges M: Internal repeats in the BRCA2 protein sequence (letter). *Nature Genet* **13**:22, 1996.

188. Sharan SK, Bradley A: Murine *Brca2*: Sequence map position and expression pattern. *Genomics* **40**:234, 1997.

189. McAllister KA, et al: Characterization of the rat and mouse homologues of the *BRCA2* breast cancer susceptibility gene. *Cancer Res* **57**:3121, 1997.

190. Couch FJ, et al: *BRCA2* germline mutations in male breast cancer cases and breast cancer families. *Nature Genet* **13**:123, 1996.

191. Neuhausen S, et al: Recurrent *BRCA2* 6174delT mutations in Ashkenazi Jewish women affected by breast cancer. *Nature Genet* **13**:126, 1996.

192. Phelan CM, et al: Mutation analysis of the *BRCA2* gene in 49 site-specific breast cancer families (see comments) [published erratum appears in *Nature Genet* **13(3)**:374, 1996]. *Nature Genet* **13**:120, 1996.

193. Lancaster JM, et al: *BRCA2* mutations in primary breast and ovarian cancers. *Nature Genet* **13**:238, 1996.

194. Miki Y, Katagiri T, Kasumi F, Yoshimoto T, Nakamura Y: Mutation analysis in the *BRCA2* gene in primary breast cancers. *Nature Genet* **13**:245, 1996.

195. Teng DH, et al: Low incidence of *BRCA2* mutations in breast carcinoma and other cancers. *Nature Genet* **13**:241, 1996.

196. Takahashi H, et al: Mutations of the *BRCA2* gene in ovarian carcinomas. *Cancer Res* **56**:2738, 1996.

197. Milner J, Ponder B, Hughes-Davies L, Seltmann M, Kouzarides T: Transcriptional activation functions in *BRCA2* (letter; see comments). *Nature* **386**:772, 1997.

198. Mazoyer S, et al: A polymorphic stop codon in *BRCA2* (letter). *Nature Genet* **14**:253, 1996.

199. Nordling M, et al: A large deletion disrupts the exon 3 transcription activation domain of the *BRCA2* gene in a breast/ovarian cancer family. *Cancer Res* **58**:1372, 1998.

200. Chen PL, et al: The BRC repeats in *BRCA2* are critical for *RAD51* binding and resistance to methyl methanesulfonate treatment. *Proc Natl Acad Sci USA* **95**:5287, 1998.

201. Tonin P, et al: Frequency of recurrent *BRCA1* and *BRCA2* mutations in Ashkenazi Jewish breast cancer families (see comments). *Nature Med* **2**:1179, 1996.

202. Thorlacius S, et al: A single *BRCA2* mutation in male and female breast cancer families from Iceland with varied cancer phenotypes (see comments). *Nature Genet* **13**:117, 1996.

203. Rubin SC, et al: Clinical and pathological features of ovarian cancer in women with germ-line mutations of *BRCA1* (see comments). *N Engl J Med* **335**:1413, 1996.

204. Goggins M, et al: Germline *BRCA2* gene mutations in patients with apparently sporadic pancreatic carcinomas. *Cancer Res* **56**:5360, 1996.

205. Kirsch M, Zhu JJ, Black PM: Analysis of the *BRCA1* and *BRCA2* genes in sporadic meningiomas. *Genes Chromosom Cancer* **20**:53, 1997.

206. Schubert EL, et al: *BRCA2* in American families with four or more cases of breast or ovarian cancer: Recurrent and novel mutations variable expression penetrance and the possibility of families whose cancer is not attributable to *BRCA1* or *BRCA2* (see comments). *Am J Hum Genet* **60**:1031, 1997.

207. Friedman LS, et al: Mutation analysis of *BRCA1* and *BRCA2* in a male breast cancer population. *Am J Hum Genet* **60**:313, 1997.

208. Bertwistle D, et al: Nuclear location and cell cycle regulation of the BRCA2 protein. *Cancer Res* **57**:5485, 1997.

209. Vaughn JP, et al: Cell cycle control of *BRCA2*. *Cancer Res* **56**:4590, 1996.

210. Wong AKC, Pero R, Ormonde PA, Tavtigian SV, Bartel PL: *RAD51* interacts with the evolutionarily conserved BRC motifs in the human breast cancer susceptibility gene brca2. *J Biol Chem* **272**:31941, 1997.

211. Rajan JV, Marquis ST, Gardner HP, Chodosh LA: Developmental expression of *Brca2* colocalizes with *Brca1* and is associated with proliferation and differentiation in multiple tissues. *Dev Biol* **184**:385, 1997.

212. Sharan SK, et al: Embryonic lethality and radiation hypersensitivity mediated by *Rad51* in mice lacking *Brca2* (see comments). *Nature* **386**:804, 1997.

213. Suzuki A, et al: *Brca2* is required for embryonic cellular proliferation in the mouse. *Genes Dev* **11**:1242, 1997.

214. Friedman LS, et al: Thymic lymphomas in mice with a truncating mutation in *Brca2*. *Cancer Res* **58**:1338, 1998.

215. Connor F, et al: Tumorigenesis and a DNA repair defect in mice with a truncating *Brca2* mutation. *Nature Genet* **17**:423, 1997.

216. Mizuta R, et al: RAB22 and RAB163/mouse BRCA2: Proteins that specifically interact with the RAD51 protein. *Proc Natl Acad Sci USA* **94**:6927, 1997.

217. Katagiri T, et al: Multiple possible sites of BRCA2 interacting with DNA repair protein RAD51. *Genes Chromosom Cancer* **21**:217, 1998.

218. Patel KJ, et al: Involvement of *Brca2* in DNA repair. *J Clin Monit Comput* **1**:347, 1998.

219. Morimatsu M, Donoho G, Hasty P: Cells deleted for *Brca2* COOH terminus exhibit hypersensitivity to gamma-radiation and premature senescence. *Cancer Res* **58**:3441, 1998.

220. Abbott DW, Freeman ML, Holt JT: Double-strand break repair deficiency and radiation sensitivity in *BRCA2* mutant cancer cells (see comments). *J Natl Cancer Inst* **90**:978, 1998.

221. Gretarsdottir S, et al: *BRCA2* and *p53* mutations in primary breast cancer in relation to genetic instability. *Cancer Res* **58**:859, 1998.

222. Li FP, Fraumeni JF: Soft-tissue sarcomas breast cancer and other neoplasms: Familial syndrome? *Ann Intern Med* **71**:747, 1969.

223. Li FP, Fraumeni JF, Mulvihill JJ: A cancer family syndrome in 24 kindreds. *Cancer Res* **48**:5358, 1988.

224. Strong LC, Williams WR, Tainsky MA: The Li-Fraumeni syndrome: From clinical epidemiology to molecular genetics. *Am J Epidemiol* **135**:190, 1992.

225. Li FP: Unpublished data, 1997.

226. Malkin D, et al: Germ line *p53* mutations in a familial syndrome of breast cancer sarcomas and other neoplasms (see comments). *Science* **250**:1233, 1990.

227. Srivastava S, Zou ZQ, Pirollo K, Blattner W, Chang EH: Germ-line transmission of a mutated *p53* gene in a cancer-prone family with Li-Fraumeni syndrome (see comments). *Nature* **348**:747, 1990.

228. Law JC, Strong LC, Chidambaram A, Ferrell RE: A germ line mutation in exon 5 of the *p53* gene in an extended cancer family. *Cancer Res* **51**:6385, 1991.

229. Santibanez-Koref MF, et al: *p53* germline mutations in Li-Fraumeni syndrome. *Lancet* **338**:1490, 1991.

230. Srivastava S, et al: Detection of both mutant and wild-type p53 protein in normal skin fibroblasts and demonstration of a shared "second hit" on *p53* in diverse tumors from a cancer-prone family with Li-Fraumeni syndrome. *Oncogene* **7**:987, 1992.

231. Brugieres L, et al: Screening for germ line *p53* mutations in children with malignant tumors and a family history of cancer. *Cancer Res* **53**:452, 1993.

232. Sameshima Y, et al: Detection of novel germ-line *p53* mutations in diverse-cancer-prone families identified by selecting patients with childhood adrenocortical carcinoma. *J Natl Cancer Inst* **84**:703, 1992.

233. Frebourg T, et al: Germ-line mutations of the *p53* tumor suppressor gene in patients with high risk for cancer inactivate the p53 protein. *Proc Natl Acad Sci USA* **89**:6413, 1992.

234. Barnes DM, et al: Abnormal expression of wild type p53 protein in normal cells of a cancer family patient. *Lancet* **340**:259, 1992.

235. Sidransky D, et al: Inherited *p53* gene mutations in breast cancer. *Cancer Res* **52**:2984, 1992.

236. Borresen AL, et al: Screening for germ line *TP53* mutations in breast cancer patients. *Cancer Res* **52**:3234, 1992.

237. Starink TM: Cowden's disease: Analysis of fourteen new cases. *J Am Acad Dermatol* **11**:1127, 1984.

238. Wood DA, Darling HH: A cancer family manifesting multiple occurrences of bilateral carcinoma of the breast. *Cancer Res* **3**:509, 1943.

239. Brownstein MH, Wolf M, Bikowski JB: Cowden's disease: A cutaneous marker of breast cancer. *Cancer* **41**:2393, 1978.

240. Padberg GW, Schot JD, Vielvoye GJ, Bots GT, de Beer FC: Lhermitte-Duclos disease and Cowden disease: A single phakomatosis (see comments). *Ann Neurol* **29**:517, 1991.

241. Eng C, et al: Cowden syndrome and Lhermitte-Duclos disease in a family: A single genetic syndrome with pleiotropy? *J Med Genet* **31**:458, 1994.

242. Nelen MR, et al: Localization of the gene for Cowden disease to chromosome 10q22-23. *Nature Genet* **13**:114, 1996.

243. Steck PA, et al: Identification of a candidate tumour suppressor gene *MMAC1* at chromosome 10q23.3 that is mutated in multiple advanced cancers. *Nature Genet* **15**:356, 1997.

244. Li J, et al: *PTEN:* A putative protein tyrosine phosphatase gene mutated in human brain breast and prostate cancer (see comments). *Science* **275**:1943, 1997.

245. Li DM, Sun H: TEP1, encoded by a candidate tumor suppressor locus, is a novel protein tyrosine phosphatase regulated by transforming growth factor beta. *Cancer Res* **57**:2124, 1997.

246. Liaw D, et al: Germline mutations of the *PTEN* gene in Cowden disease, an inherited breast and thyroid cancer syndrome. *Nature Genet* **16**:64, 1997.

247. Nelen MR, et al: Germline mutations in the *PTEN/MMAC1* gene in patients with Cowden disease. *Hum Mol Genet* **6**:1383, 1997.

248. Tsou HC, et al: The role of *MMAC1* mutations in early-onset breast cancer: Causative in association with Cowden syndrome and excluded in *BRCA1*-negative cases. *Am J Hum Genet* **61**:1036, 1997.

249. Chiariello E, Roz L, Albarosa R, Magnani I, Finocchiaro G: *PTEN/MMAC1* mutations in primary glioblastomas and short-term cultures of malignant gliomas. *Oncogene* **16**:541, 1998.

250. Jeghers H, McKusick VA, Katz KH: Generalized intestinal polyposis and melanin spots of the oral mucosa lips and digits: A syndrome of diagnostic significance. *N Engl J Med* **241**:993, 1949.

251. Utsunomiya J, Gocho H, Miyanaga T: Peutz-Jeghers syndrome: Its natural course and management. *Johns Hopkins Med J* **136**:71, 1975.

252. Jancu J: Peutz-Jeghers syndrome: Involvement of the gastrointestinal and upper respiratory tracts. *Am J Gastroenterol* **56**:545, 1971.

253. Sommerhaug RG, Mason T: Peutz-Jeghers syndrome and ureteral polyposis. *JAMA* **211**:120, 1970.

254. Chen KT: Female genital tract tumors in Peutz-Jeghers syndrome. *Hum Pathol* **17**:858, 1986.

255. Riley E, Swift M: A family with Peutz-Jeghers syndrome and bilateral breast cancer. *Cancer* **46**:815, 1980.

256. Young RH, Scully RE: Mucinous ovarian tumors associated with mucinous adenocarcinomas of the cervix: A clinicopathological analysis of 16 cases. *Int J Gynecol Pathol* **7**:99, 1988.

257. Cantu JM, Rivera H, Ocampo-Campos R: Peutz-Jeghers syndrome with feminizing Sertoli cell tumor. *Cancer* **46**:223, 1980.

258. Scully RE: Sex cord tumor with annular tubules: A distinctive ovarian tumor of the Peutz-Jeghers syndrome. *Cancer* **25**:1107, 1970.

259. Sristava PJ, Keeney GL, Podratz KC: Disseminated cervical adenoma malignum and bilateral ovarian sex cord tumors with annular tubules associated with Peutz-Jeghers syndrome. *Gynecol Oncol* **53**:256, 1994.

260. Boardman LA: Unpublished data, 1998.

261. Hemminki A, Tomlinson I, Markie D: Localization of a susceptibility locus for PJS to 19p using comparative genomic hybridization and targeted linkage analysis. *Nature Genet* **15**:87, 1997.

262. Hemminki A, et al: A serine/threonine kinase gene defective in Peutz-Jeghers syndrome. *Nature* **391**:184, 1998.

263. Bignell GR, et al: Low frequency of somatic mutations in the LKB1/Peutz-Jeghers syndrome gene in sporadic breast cancer. *Cancer Res* **58**:1384, 1998.

264. Wang ZJ, Taylor F, Curchman M: Genetic pathways of colorectal carcinogenesis rarely involve the *PTEN* and *LKB1* genes outside the inherited hamartoma syndromes. *Am J Pathol* **153**:363, 1998.

265. Avizienyte E: Somatic mutations in *LKB1* are rare in sporadic colorectal and testicular tumors. *Cancer Res* **58**:2087, 1998.

266. Olschwang S, Markie D: Peutz-Jeghers disease: Most but not all families are compatible with linkage to 19p13.3. *J Med Genet* **35**:42, 1998.

267. Muir EG, Bell AJ, Barlow KA: Multiple primary carcinomata of the colon duodenum and larynx associated with kerato-acanthomata of the face. *Br J Surg* **54**:191, 1967.

268. Hall NR, Williams MA, Murday VA, Newton JA, Bishop DT: Muir-Torre syndrome: A variant of the cancer family syndrome. *J Med Genet* **31**:627, 1994.

269. Anderson DE: An inherited form of large bowel cancer: Muir's syndrome. *Cancer* **45**:1103, 1980.

270. Papadopoulos N, et al: Mutation of a *mutL* homolog in hereditary colon cancer (see comments). *Science* **263**:1625, 1994.

271. Bronner CE, et al: Mutation in the DNA mismatch repair gene homologue *hMLH1* is associated with hereditary nonpolyposis colon cancer. *Nature* **368**:258, 1994.

272. Fishel R, et al: The human mutator gene homolog *MSH2* and its association with hereditary nonpolyposis colon cancer [published erratum appears in *Cell* **77**:167, 1994]. *Cell* **75**:1027, 1993.

273. Leach FS, et al: Mutations of a *mutS* homolog in hereditary nonpolyposis colorectal cancer. *Cell* **75**:1215, 1993.

274. Nicolaides NC, et al: Genomic organization of the human *PMS2* gene family. *Genomics* **30**:195, 1995.

275. Kolodner RD, et al: Structure of the human *MSH2* locus and analysis of two Muir-Torre kindreds for *msh2* mutations [published erratum appears in *Genomics* **28(3)**:613, 1995]. *Genomics* **24**:516, 1994.

276. Bapat B, et al: The genetic basis of Muir-Torre syndrome includes the *hMLH1* locus (letter). *Am J Hum Genet* **59**:736, 1996.

277. Swift M, et al: The incidence and gene frequency of ataxia-telangiectasia in the United States. *Am J Hum Genet* **39**:573, 1986.

278. Morrell D, Cromartie E, Swift M: Mortality and cancer incidence in 263 patients with ataxia-telangiectasia. *J Natl Cancer Inst* **77**:89, 1986.

279. Swift M, Morrell D, Massey RB, Chase CL: Incidence of cancer in 161 families affected by ataxia-telangiectasia (see comments). *N Engl J Med* **325**:1831, 1991.

280. Cortessis V, et al: Linkage analysis of DRD2, a marker linked to the ataxia-telangiectasia gene in 64 families with premenopausal bilateral breast cancer. *Cancer Res* **53**:5083, 1993.

281. Wooster R, et al: Absence of linkage to the ataxia telangiectasia locus in familial breast cancer. *Hum Genet* **92**:91, 1993.

282. Savitsky K, et al: A single ataxia telangiectasia gene with a product similar to PI-3 kinase (see comments). *Science* **268**:1749, 1995.

283. Zuppan P, Hall JM, Lee MK, Ponglikitmongkol M, King MC: Possible linkage of the estrogen receptor gene to breast cancer in a family with late-onset disease. *Am J Hum Genet* **48**:1065, 1991.

284. Sluyser M: Mutations in the estrogen receptor gene. *Hum Mutat* **6**:97, 1995.

285. Kerangueven F, Essioux L, Dib A: Loss of heterozygosity and linkage analysis in breast carcinoma: Indication for a putative third susceptibility gene on the short arm of chromosome 8. *Oncogene* **10**:1023, 1995.

286. Latil A, et al: Genetic alterations in localized prostate cancer: Identification of a common region of deletion on chromosome arm 18q. *Genes Chromosom Cancer* **11**:119, 1994.

287. Chuaqui RF, et al: Loss of heterozygosity on the short arm of chromosome 8 in male breast carcinomas. *Cancer Res* **55**:4995, 1995.

288. Knudson AG Jr: Mutation and cancer: Statistical study of retinoblastoma. *Proc Natl Acad Sci USA* **68**:820, 1971.

289. Callahan R, et al: Genetic and molecular heterogeneity of breast cancer cells. *Clin Chim Acta* **217**:63, 1993.

290. Cleton-Jansen AM, et al: At least two different regions are involved in allelic imbalance on chromosome arm 16q in breast cancer. *Genes Chromosom Cancer* **9**:101, 1994.

291. Gudmundsson J, et al: Loss of heterozygosity at chromosome 11 in breast cancer: Association of prognostic factors with genetic alterations. *Br J Cancer* **72**:696, 1995.

292. Morelli C, et al: Characterization of a 4-Mb region at chromosome 6q21 harboring a replicative senescence gene. *Cancer Res* **57**:4153, 1997.

293. Huang H, Qian C, Jenkins RB, Smith DI: Fish mapping of YAC clones at human chromosomal band 7q31.2: Identification of YACS spanning FRA7G within the common region of LOH in breast and prostate cancer. *Genes Chromosom Cancer* **21**:152, 1998.

294. Cropp CS, Champeme MH, Lidereau R, Callahan R: Identification of three regions on chromosome 17q in primary human breast carcinomas which are frequently deleted. *Cancer Res* **53**:5617, 1993.

295. Kirchweger R, et al: Patterns of allele losses suggest the existence of five distinct regions of LOH on chromosome 17 in breast cancer. *Int J Cancer* **56**:193, 1994.

296. Nagai MA, et al: Five distinct deleted regions on chromosome 17 defining different subsets of human primary breast tumors. *Oncology* **52**:448, 1995.

297. Phelan CM, et al: Consortium study on 1280 breast carcinomas: Allelic loss on chromosome 17 targets subregions associated with family history and clinical parameters. *Cancer Res* **58**:1004, 1998.

298. Cornelis RS, et al: Evidence for a gene on 17p13.3 distal to *TP53* as a target for allele loss in breast tumors without *p53* mutations. *Cancer Res* **54**:4200, 1994.

299. Schultz DC, et al: Identification of two candidate tumor suppressor genes on chromosome 17p13.3. *Cancer Res* **56**:1997, 1996.

300. Mathew S, Murty VV, Bosl GJ, Chaganti RS: Loss of heterozygosity identifies multiple sites of allelic deletions on chromosome 1 in human male germ cell tumors. *Cancer Res* **54**:6265, 1994.

301. Bieche I, Khodja A, Lidereau R: Deletion mapping in breast tumor cell lines points to two distinct tumor-suppressor genes in the 1p32-pter region, one of deleted regions (1p36.2) being located within the consensus region of LOH in neuroblastoma. *Oncol Rep* **5**:267, 1998.

302. Kerangueven F, et al: Loss of heterozygosity in human breast carcinomas in the ataxia telangiectasia Cowden disease and *BRCA1* gene regions. *Oncogene* **14**:339, 1997.

303. Dorion-Bonnet F, Mautalen S, Hostein I, Longy M: Allelic imbalance study of 16q in human primary breast carcinomas using microsatellite markers. *Genes Chromosom Cancer* **14**:171, 1995.

304. Eiriksdottir G. et al: Loss of heterozygosity on chromosome 9 in human breast cancer: Association with clinical variables and genetic changes at other chromosome regions. *Int J Cancer* **64**:378, 1995.

305. Smith HS, et al: Molecular aspects of early stages of breast cancer progression. *J Cell Biochem Suppl* **17G**:144, 1993.

306. Medeiros AC, Nagai MA, Neto MM, Brentani RR: Loss of heterozygosity affecting the *APC* and *MCC* genetic loci in patients with primary breast carcinomas. *Cancer Epidemiol Biomark Prevent* **3**:331, 1994.

307. Lakhani SR, Collins N, Stratton MR, Sloane JP: Atypical ductal hyperplasia of the breast: Clonal proliferation with loss of heterozygosity on chromosomes 16q and 17p. *J Clin Pathol* **48**:611, 1995.

308. Radford DM, et al: Allelotyping of ductal carcinoma in situ of the breast: deletion of loci on 8p, 13q, 16q, 17p, and 17q. *Cancer Res* **55**:3399, 1995.

309. Champeme MH, Bieche I, Beuzelin M, Lidereau R: Loss of heterozygosity on 7q31 occurs early during breast tumorigenesis. *Genes Chromosom Cancer* **12**:304, 1995.

310. Bacus SS, Zelnick CR, Plowman G, Yarden Y: Expression of the erbB-2 family of growth factor receptors and their ligands in breast cancers: Implication for tumor biology and clinical behavior. *Am J Clin Pathol* **102**:S13, 1994.

311. Slamon DJ, Godolphin W, Jones LA: Studies of the *Her-2/neu* proto-oncogene in human breast and ovarian cancer. *Science* **244**:707, 1989.

312. Kraus MH, Issing W, Miki T, Popescu NC, Aaronson SA: Isolation and characterization of ERBB3, a third member of the ERBB/epidermal growth factor receptor family: Evidence for overexpression in a subset of human mammary tumors. *Proc Natl Acad Sci USA* **86**:9193, 1989.

313. Lewis S, et al: Expression of epidermal growth factor receptor in breast carcinoma. *J Clin Pathol* **43**:385, 1990.

314. Hawkins RA, et al: Epidermal growth factor receptors in intracranial and breast tumours: Their clinical significance. *Br J Cancer* **63**:553, 1991.

315. Paik S, et al: Pathologic findings from the National Surgical Adjuvant Breast and Bowel Project: Prognostic significance of erbB-2 protein overexpression in primary breast cancer. *J Clin Oncol* **8**:103, 1990.

316. Clark GM, McGuire WL: Follow-up study of *HER-2/neu* amplification in primary breast cancer. *Cancer Res* **51**:944, 1991.

317. Antoniotti S, et al: Oestrogen and epidermal growth factor down-regulate erbB-2 oncogene protein expression in breast cancer cells by different mechanisms. *Br J Cancer* **70**:1095, 1994.

318. Janes PW, Daly RJ, deFazio A, Sutherland RL: Activation of the *Ras* signalling pathway in human breast cancer cells overexpressing *erbB-2*. *Oncogene* **9**:3601, 1994.

319. Nowak F, Jacquemin-Sablon A, Pierre J: Expression of the activated p185erbB2 tyrosine kinase in human epithelial cells leads to MAP kinase activation but does not confer oncogenicity. *Exp Cell Res* **231**:251, 1997.

320. Toikkanen S, Helin H, Isola J, Joensuu H: Prognostic significance of *HER-2* oncoprotein expression in breast cancer: A 30-year follow-up (see comments). *J Clin Oncol* **10**:1044, 1992.

321. Gusterson BA, et al: Prognostic importance of c-*erbB*-2 expression in breast cancer: International (Ludwig) Breast Cancer Study Group (see comments). *J Clin Oncol* **10**:1049, 1992.

322. Thor AD, et al: *erbB*-2, *p53,* and efficacy of adjuvant therapy in lymph node-positive breast cancer (see comments). *J Natl Cancer Inst* **90**:1346, 1998.

323. Yu D, et al: Overexpression of both *p185c-erbB2* and *p170mdr-1* renders breast cancer cells highly resistant to Taxol. *Oncogene* **16**:2087, 1998.

324. Leitzel K, et al: Elevated serum c-erbB-2 antigen levels and decreased response to hormone therapy of breast cancer. *J Clin Oncol* **13**:1129, 1995.

325. Sleijfer S, Asschert JG, Timmer-Bosscha H, Mulder NH: Enhanced sensitivity to tumor necrosis factor-alpha in doxorubicin-resistant tumor cell lines due to down-regulated c-*erbB2*. *Int J Cancer* **77**:101, 1998.

326. Colomer R, Lupu R, Bacus SS, Gelmann EP: erbB-2 antisense oligonucleotides inhibit the proliferation of breast carcinoma cells with *erbB*-2 oncogene amplification. *Br J Cancer* **70**:819, 1994.

327. Ciardiello F, et al: Down-regulation of type I protein kinase A by transfection of human breast cancer cells with an epidermal growth factor receptor antisense expression vector. *Breast Cancer Res Treat* **47**:57, 1998.

328. Petit AM, et al: Neutralizing antibodies against epidermal growth factor and ErbB-2/neu receptor tyrosine kinases down-regulate vascular endothelial growth factor production by tumor cells in vitro and in vivo: Angiogenic implications for signal transduction therapy of solid tumors. *Am J Pathol* **151**:1523, 1997.

329. Sandgren EP, Luetteke NC, Palmiter RD, Brinster RL, Lee DC: Overexpression of TGF alpha in transgenic mice: Induction of epithelial hyperplasia pancreatic metaplasia and carcinoma of the breast. *Cell* **61**:1121, 1990.

330. Johnson MR, Valentine C, Basilico C, Mansukhani A: FGF signaling activates STAT1 and p21 and inhibits the estrogen response and proliferation of MCF-7 cells. *Oncogene* **16**:2647, 1998.

331. Burgess WH, Maciag T: The heparin-binding (fibroblast) growth factor family of proteins. *Annu Rev Biochem* **58**:575, 1989.

332. Penault-Llorca F, et al: Expression of FGF and FGF receptor genes in human breast cancer. *Int J Cancer* **61**:170, 1995.

333. Wang Q, et al: Basic fibroblast growth factor downregulates *Bcl-2* and promotes apoptosis in MCF-7 human breast cancer cells. *Exp Cell Res* **238**:177, 1998.

334. Tanaka A, et al: High frequency of fibroblast growth factor (FGF) 8 expression in clinical prostate cancers and breast tissues immunohistochemically demonstrated by a newly established neutralizing monoclonal antibody against FGF 8. *Cancer Res* **58**:2053, 1998.

335. Conway K, et al: Ha-ras rare alleles in breast cancer susceptibility. *Breast Cancer Res Treat* **35**:97, 1995.

336. Zhang PL, Calaf G, Russo J: Allele loss and point mutation in codons 12 and 61 of the c-*Ha-ras* oncogene in carcinogen-transformed human breast epithelial cells. *Mol Carcinogen* **9**:46, 1994.

337. Bland KI, Konstadoulakis MM, Vezeridis MP, Wanebo HJ: Oncogene protein co-expression: Value of *Ha-ras*, c-*myc*, c-*fos*, and *p53* as prognostic discriminants for breast carcinoma (see comments). *Ann Surg* **221**:706, 1995.

338. Ciardiello F, et al: Additive effects of c-erbB-2, c-Ha-ras, and transforming growth factor-alpha genes on in vitro transformation of human mammary epithelial cells. *Mol Carcinogen* **6**:43, 1992.

339. Sabbatini AR, et al: Induction of multidrug resistance (MDR) by transfection of MCF-10A cell line with c-Ha-ras and c-erbB-2 oncogenes. *Int J Cancer* **59**:208, 1994.

340. Giai M, Roagna R, Ponzone R: Prognostic and predictive relevance of c-erB-2 and ras expression in node-positive and negative breast cancer. *Anticancer Res* **14**:1441, 1994.

341. Luttrell DK, et al: Involvement of pp60c-src with two major signaling pathways in human breast cancer. *Proc Natl Acad Sci USA* **91**:83, 1994.

342. Ottenhoff-Kalff AE, et al: Characterization of protein tyrosine kinases from human breast cancer: Involvement of the c-src oncogene product. *Cancer Res* **52**:4773, 1992.

343. Hennipman A, van Oirschot BA, Smits J, Rijksen G, Staal GE: Tyrosine kinase activity in breast cancer benign breast disease and normal breast tissue. *Cancer Res* **49**:516, 1989.

344. Hunter T, Pines J: Cyclins and cancer. II: Cyclin D and CDK inhibitors come of age (see comments). *Cell* **79**:573, 1994.

345. Marx J: How cells cycle toward cancer (news). *Science* **263**:319, 1994.

346. Hollstein M, Sidransky D, Vogelstein B, Harris CC: p53 mutations in human cancers. *Science* **253**:49, 1991.

347. Deng G, et al: Loss of heterozygosity and p53 gene mutations in breast cancer. *Cancer Res* **54**:499, 1994.

348. Andersen TI, et al: Prognostic significance of TP53 alterations in breast carcinoma. *Br J Cancer* **68**:540, 1993.

349. Elledge RM, Fuqua SA, Clark GM, Pujol P, Allred DC: William L. McGuire Memorial Symposium: The role and prognostic significance of p53 gene alterations in breast cancer. *Breast Cancer Res Treat* **27**:95, 1993.

350. Saitoh S, et al: p53 gene mutations in breast cancers in midwestern U.S. women: Null as well as missense-type mutations are associated with poor prognosis. *Oncogene* **9**:2869, 1994.

351. Shiao YH, Chen VW, Scheer VW, Wu XC, Correa P: Racial disparity in the association of p53 gene alterations with breast cancer survival. *Cancer Res* **55**:1485, 1995.

352. Marchetti A, et al: p53 mutations and histological type of invasive breast carcinoma. *Cancer Res* **53**:4665, 1993.

353. Moll UM, Riou G, Levine AJ: Two distinct mechanisms alter p53 in breast cancer: Mutation and nuclear exclusion. *Proc Natl Acad Sci USA* **89**:7262, 1992.

354. Aas T, et al: Specific p53 mutations are associated with de novo resistance to doxorubicin in breast cancer patients. *Nature Med* **2**:811, 1996.

355. Bergh J, Norberg T, Sjogren S, Lindgren A, Holmberg L: Complete sequencing of the p53 gene provides prognostic information in breast cancer patients, particularly in relation to adjuvant systemic therapy and radiotherapy. *Nature Med* **1**:1029, 1995.

356. T'Ang A, Varley JM, Chakraborty S, Murphree AL, Fung YK: Structural rearrangement of the retinoblastoma gene in human breast carcinoma. *Science* **242**:263, 1988.

357. Lee EY, et al: Inactivation of the retinoblastoma susceptibility gene in human breast cancers. *Science* **241**:218, 1988.

358. Gottardis MM, et al: Regulation of retinoblastoma gene expression in hormone-dependent breast cancer. *Endocrinology* **136**:5659, 1995.

359. Wang NP, To H, Lee WH, Lee EY: Tumor suppressor activity of RB and p53 genes in human breast carcinoma cells. *Oncogene* **8**:279, 1993.

360. Fung YK, T'Ang A: The role of the retinoblastoma gene in breast cancer development. *Cancer Treat Res* **61**:59, 1992.

361. Berns EM, et al: Association between RB-1 gene alterations and factors of favourable prognosis in human breast cancer without effect on survival. *Int J Cancer* **64**:140, 1995.

362. Sawan A, et al: Retinoblastoma and p53 gene expression related to relapse and survival in human breast cancer: An immunohistochemical study. *J Pathol* **168**:23, 1992.

363. Buckley MF, et al: Expression and amplification of cyclin genes in human breast cancer. *Oncogene* **8**:2127, 1993.

364. Motokura T, Bloom T, Kim HG: A BCL1-linked candidate oncogene, which is rearranged in parathyroid tumors, encodes a novel cyclin. *Nature* **350**:512, 1991.

365. Bartokova J, Lukas J, Muller H: Cyclin D1 protein expression and function in human breast cancer. *Int J Cancer* **57**:353, 1994.

366. Zhang SY, Caamano J, Cooper F, Guo X, Klein-Szanto AJ: Immunohistochemistry of cyclin D1 in human breast cancer. *Am J Clin Pathol* **102**:695, 1994.

367. Weinstat-Saslow D, et al: Overexpression of cyclin D mRNA distinguishes invasive and in situ breast carcinomas from non-malignant lesions (see comments). *Nature Med* **1**:1257, 1995.

368. Alle KM, Henshall SM, Field AS, Sutherland RL: Cyclin D1 protein is overexpressed in hyperplasia and intraductal carcinoma of the breast. *Clin Cancer Res* **4**:847, 1998.

369. Oyama T, Kashiwabara K, Yoshimoto K, Arnold A, Koerner F: Frequent overexpression of the cyclin D1 oncogene in invasive lobular carcinoma of the breast. *Cancer Res* **58**:2876, 1998.

370. Musgrove EA, Lee CS, Buckley MF, Sutherland RL: Cyclin D1 induction in breast cancer cells shortens G1 and is sufficient for cells arrested in G1 to complete the cell cycle. *Proc Natl Acad Sci USA* **91**:8022, 1994.

371. Sicinski P, et al: Cyclin D1 provides a link between development and oncogenesis in the retina and breast. *Cell* **82**:621, 1995.

372. Zwijsen RM, et al: CDK-independent activation of estrogen receptor by cyclin D1. *Cell* **88**:405, 1997.

373. Neuman E, et al: Cyclin D1 stimulation of estrogen receptor transcriptional activity independent of cdk4. *Mol Cell Biol* **17**:5338, 1997.

374. Porter PL, et al: Expression of cell-cycle regulators p27Kip1 and cyclin E alone and in combination correlate with survival in young breast cancer patients (see comments). *Nature Med* **3**:222, 1997.

375. Alexandrow MG, Moses HL: Transforming growth factor beta and cell cycle regulation. *Cancer Res* **55**:1452, 1995.

376. Jeng MH, ten Dijke P, Iwata KK, Jordan VC: Regulation of the levels of three transforming growth factor beta mRNAs by estrogen and their effects on the proliferation of human breast cancer cells. *Mol Cell Endocrinol* **97**:115, 1993.

377. Knabbe C, et al: Evidence that transforming growth factor-beta is a hormonally regulated negative growth factor in human breast cancer cells. *Cell* **48**:417, 1987.

378. Perry RR, Kang Y, Greaves BR: Relationship between tamoxifen-induced transforming growth factor beta 1 expression cytostasis and apoptosis in human breast cancer cells (see comments). *Br J Cancer* **72**:1441, 1995.

379. Croxtall JD, Jamil A, Ayub M, Colletta AA, White JO: TGF-beta stimulation of endometrial and breast-cancer cell growth. *Int J Cancer* **50**:822, 1992.

380. Arteaga CL, Dugger TC, Winnier AR, Forbes JT: Evidence for a positive role of transforming growth factor-beta in human breast cancer cell tumorigenesis. *J Cell Biochem Suppl* **17G**:187, 1993.

381. Walker RA, Dearing SJ, Gallacher B: Relationship of transforming growth factor beta 1 to extracellular matrix and stromal infiltrates in invasive breast carcinoma. *Br J Cancer* **69**:1160, 1994.

382. MacCallum J, et al: Expression of transforming growth factor beta mRNA isoforms in human breast cancer (see comments). *Br J Cancer* **69**:1006, 1994.

383. Dublin EA, Barnes DM, Wang DY, King RJ, Levison DA: TGF alpha and TGF beta expression in mammary carcinoma. *J Pathol* **170**:15, 1993.

384. Thompson CB: Apoptosis in the pathogenesis and treatment of disease. *Science* **267**:1456, 1995.

385. Fisher DE: Apoptosis in cancer therapy: Crossing the threshold. *Cell* **78**:539, 1994.

386. Johnston SR, et al: Modulation of Bcl-2 and Ki-67 expression in oestrogen receptor-positive human breast cancer by tamoxifen. *Eur J Cancer* **30A**:1663, 1994.

387. Joensuu H, Pylkkanen L, Toikkanen S: Bcl-2 protein expression and long-term survival in breast cancer. *Am J Pathol* **145**:1191, 1994.

388. Sabourin JC, et al: bcl-2 expression in normal breast tissue during the menstrual cycle. *Int J Cancer* **59**:1, 1994.

389. Haldar S, Negrini M, Monne M, Sabbioni S, Croce CM: Down-regulation of bcl-2 by p53 in breast cancer cells. *Cancer Res* **54**:2095, 1994.

390. Ottestad L, et al: Amplification of c-erbB-2, int-2, and c-myc genes in node-negative breast carcinomas: Relationship to prognosis. *Acta Oncol* **32**:289, 1993.

391. Pietilainen T, et al: Expression of c-myc proteins in breast cancer as related to established prognostic factors and survival. *Anticancer Res* **15**:959, 1995.

392. Pavelic ZP, et al: c-myc, c-erbB-2, and Ki-67 expression in normal breast tissue and in invasive and noninvasive breast carcinoma. *Cancer Res* **52**:2597, 1992.

393. Porter-Jordan K, Lippman ME: Overview of the biologic markers of breast cancer. *Hematol Oncol Clin North Am* **8**:73, 1994.

394. Glukhova M, Koteliansky V, Sastre X, Thiery JP: Adhesion systems in normal breast and in invasive breast carcinoma. *Am J Pathol* **146**:706, 1995.

395. Rimm DL, Sinard JH, Morrow JS: Reduced alpha-catenin and E-cadherin expression in breast cancer (see comments). *Lab Invest* **72**:506, 1995.

396. Palacios J, et al: Anomalous expression of P-cadherin in breast carcinoma: Correlation with E-cadherin expression and pathological features. *Am J Pathol* **146**:605, 1995.

397. Rasbridge SA, Gillett CE, Sampson SA, Walsh FS, Millis RR: Epithelial (E-) and placental (P-) cadherin cell adhesion molecule expression in breast carcinoma. *J Pathol* **169**:245, 1993.

398. Siitonen SM, et al: Reduced E-cadherin expression is associated with invasiveness and unfavorable prognosis in breast cancer. *Am J Clin Pathol* **105**:394, 1996.

399. Stetler-Stevenson WG: Type IV collagenases in tumor invasion and metastasis. *Cancer Metastas Rev* **9**:289, 1990.

400. Yu M, Sato H, Seiki M, Thompson EW: Complex regulation of membrane-type matrix metalloproteinase expression and matrix metalloproteinase-2 activation by concanavalin A in MDA-MB-231 human breast cancer cells. *Cancer Res* **55**:3272, 1995.

401. Duffy MJ, et al: Assay of matrix metalloproteases types 8 and 9 by ELISA in human breast cancer. *Br J Cancer* **71**:1025, 1995.

402. Okada A, et al: Membrane-type matrix metalloproteinase (*MT-MMP*) gene is expressed in stromal cells of human colon breast and head and neck carcinomas. *Proc Natl Acad Sci USA* **92**:2730, 1995.

403. Sato H, et al: A matrix metalloproteinase expressed on the surface of invasive tumour cells (see comments). *Nature* **370**:61, 1994.

404. Polette M, et al: Gelatinase A expression and localization in human breast cancers: An *in situ* hybridization study and immunohistochemical detection using confocal microscopy. *Virchows Arch* **424**:641, 1994.

405. Ito A, Nakajima S, Sasaguri Y, Nagase H, Mori Y: Co-culture of human breast adenocarcinoma MCF-7 cells and human dermal fibroblasts enhances the production of matrix metalloproteinases 1, 2, and 3 in fibroblasts. *Br J Cancer* **71**:1039, 1995.

406. Noel AC, et al: Coordinate enhancement of gelatinase A mRNA and activity levels in human fibroblasts in response to breast-adenocarcinoma cells. *Int J Cancer* **56**:331, 1994.

407. Aaltonen M, Lipponen P, Kosma VM, Aaltomaa S, Syrjanen K: Prognostic value of cathepsin-D expression in female breast cancer. *Anticancer Res* **15**:1033, 1995.

408. Gion M, et al: Relationship between cathepsin D and other pathological and biological parameters in 1752 patients with primary breast cancer. *Eur J Cancer* **31A**:671, 1995.

409. Steeg PS, et al: Evidence for a novel gene associated with low tumor metastatic potential. *J Natl Cancer Inst* **80**:200, 1988.

410. Rosengard AM, et al: Reduced Nm23/Awd protein in tumour metastasis and aberrant *Drosophila* development. *Nature* **342**:177, 1989.

411. Bevilacqua G, Sobel ME, Liotta LA, Steeg PS: Association of low nm23 RNA levels in human primary infiltrating ductal breast carcinomas with lymph node involvement and other histopathological indicators of high metastatic potential. *Cancer Res* **49**:5185, 1989.

412. Leone A, Flatow U, VanHoutte K, Steeg PS: Transfection of human *nm23-H1* into the human MDA-MB-435 breast carcinoma cell line: Effects on tumor metastatic potential colonization and enzymatic activity. *Oncogene* **8**:2325, 1993.

413. Steeg PS, et al: *Nm23* and breast cancer metastasis. *Breast Cancer Res Treat* **25**:175, 1993.

414. Howlett AR, Petersen OW, Steeg PS, Bissell MJ: A novel function for the *nm23-H1* gene: Overexpression in human breast carcinoma cells leads to the formation of basement membrane and growth arrest (see comments). *J Natl Cancer Inst* **86**:1838, 1994.

415. Postel EH, Berberich SJ, Flint SJ, Ferrone CA: Human c-*myc* transcription factor PuF identified as nm23-H2 nucleoside diphosphate kinase, a candidate suppressor of tumor metastasis (see comments). *Science* **261**:478, 1993.

416. Chang CL, et al: *Nm23-H1* mutation in neuroblastoma (letter). *Nature* **370**:335, 1994.

417. Hoskins KF, et al: Assessment and counseling for women with a family history of breast cancer: A guide for clinicians. *JAMA* **273**:577, 1995.

418. Burke W, et al: Recommendations for follow-up care of individuals with an inherited predisposition to cancer: II. *BRCA1* and *BRCA2*. Cancer Genetic Studies Consortium (see comments). *JAMA* **277**:997, 1997.

419. Lakhani SR, Sloane JP, Gusterson BA: Pathology of familial breast cancer: Differences between breast cancers in carriers of *BRCA1* or *BRCA2* mutations and sporadic cases. *Lancet* **349**:1505, 1997.

Colorectal Tumors

Kenneth W. Kinzler ▪ *Bert Vogelstein*

1. Colorectal tumors progress through a series of clinical and histopathologic stages ranging from single crypt lesions (aberrant crypt foci) through small benign tumors (adenomatous polyps) to malignant cancers (carcinomas). This progression is the result of a series of genetic changes that involve activation of oncogenes and inactivation of tumor-suppressor genes.

2. There are several inherited predispositions to colorectal cancer. The two best characterized and most pronounced are hereditary nonpolyposis colorectal cancer (HNPCC) and familial adenomatous polyposis (FAP). Patients with HNPCC inherit defective DNA mismatch repair genes (see Chap. 18). Although HNPCC and FAP are both associated with a marked predisposition to colorectal cancer, they only account for a small fraction of colorectal cancers. Most colorectal cancers occur in the absence of a recognized inherited factor and are considered sporadic.

3. The majority of mutations contributing to colorectal tumorigenesis are acquired in the tumor cell (i.e., somatic). To date, over a dozen genes have been found to be somatically mutated in colorectal cancer. Four genetic events are particularly common in colorectal cancers and have been described at the molecular level. These include activation of *RAS* oncogenes and inactivation of tumor-suppressor genes on chromosomes 5q, 17p, and 18q.

4. Activating mutations of one of the *RAS* oncogenes occur in about 50 percent of colorectal cancers and in a similar percentage of adenomas larger than 1.0 cm in diameter. The majority of these mutations affect the *c-Ki-RAS* gene, with the rest affecting the *N-RAS* gene. The RAS proteins are homologous to G proteins and are believed to play a role in signal transduction.

5. The tumor-suppressor gene on chromosome 17p has been identified as the *p53* gene. The *p53* gene is inactivated in at least 85 percent of colorectal cancers but rarely in benign tumors. Inactivation of *p53* is most often due to a missense mutation combined with a loss of the other allele. Biochemical studies of the p53 protein suggest that it functions through transcriptional activation of genes controlling cell birth and cell death, such as the cyclin-dependent kinase inhibitor p21WAF1/CIP1. The p53 protein has been shown to bind to specific recognition elements within the promoters of these genes. Mutant p53 is defective in these activities.

6. Three candidate tumor-suppressor genes, *DCC, SAMD4/ DPC4,* and *SMAD2,* have been isolated from chromosome 18q. At least one copy of these genes is lost in 70 percent of colorectal cancers and in over 40 percent of large adenomas with foci of carcinomatous transformation. Somatic alterations, including homozygous deletions, point mutations, or insertions, have been detected in all three candidate genes, with mutations of *SMAD4* being most frequent. However, mutations of these genes cannot account for the majority of 18q chromosome loss events, suggesting that additional mechanism of inactivation or other undefined tumor-suppressor genes are playing a role. Additional studies will be necessary to fully understand the role of 18q losses in colorectal tumorigenesis.

7. The tumor-suppressor gene on chromosome 5q has been identified as the *APC* gene. In addition to causing FAP through germ-line transmission, mutations of the *APC* gene occur somatically in over 80 percent of sporadic colorectal tumors, whether benign or malignant. Almost all these mutations, like the inherited mutations causing FAP, are predicted to result in truncation of the APC protein. Mutation of the *APC* gene is the earliest genetic event yet identified in colorectal tumorigenesis, with mutations being identified in lesions as small as a few crypts. At the biochemical level, one critical function of APC is inhibition of β-catenin/Tcf–mediated transcription. Mutation of *APC* leads to increased β-catenin/Tcf–mediated transcription of growth-promoting genes including the *c-MYC* oncogene. In rare tumors with wild-type APC, increased β-catenin/ Tcf–mediated transcription results from mutations of β-catenin that render it resistant to the inhibitory effects of APC.

8. Despite the requirement for multiple somatic mutations to drive the neoplastic process, several inherited predispositions can result from inheritance of a single defective gene, as noted earlier. The genes responsible for cancer predispositions can be grouped broadly into three categories of defects: *caretakers, gatekeepers,* and *landscapers.* Examples of all three defects exist for colon cancer. Caretaker defects are typified by the DNA mismatch repair alterations observed in HNPCC. While these defects do not act directly to affect cellular growth, they act as caretakers, reducing the accumulation of mutations that arise during the normal replication of DNA. Defects in DNA mismatch repair lead to a genetic instability that accelerates the progression of cancer. In contrast, patients with FAP inherit truncating mutations of the *APC* tumor-suppressor gene. *APC* functions as a gatekeeper, directly regulating the growth of colorectal epithelial cells. As a result of inheriting a mutant gatekeeper gene, patients with FAP develop hundreds of benign colorectal tumors, some of which progress to carcinomas. The third category of predispositions results from landscaper defects. Landscaper defects do not directly affect cancer cell growth but contribute to abnormal stromal environment that contributes to the neoplastic transformation of the overlying epithelium. The increased risk of colorectal cancer observed in juvenile polyposis syndrome and Peutz-Jeghers syndrome may be the result of landscaper defects.

9. The analysis of mutations in colorectal tumors at various stages of their development allows definition of a model for

---

A list of standard abbreviations is located immediately preceding the index. Nonstandard abbreviations used in this chapter include: ACF = aberrant crypt foci; FAP = familial adenomatous polyposis coli; GS = Gardner syndrome; HNPCC = hereditary nonpolyposis colorectal cancer; JPS = juvenile polyposis syndrome.

colorectal tumor development. Mutations in the *APC* gene appear to initiate this process, resulting in small tumors representing the clonal growth of a single cell. One of the cells in this small tumor may acquire an additional mutation (often in the *K-RAS* gene), allowing it to overgrow surrounding cells and resulting in a larger tumor. Subsequent waves of clonal expansion are driven by sequential mutations in the 18q suppressor and *p53* genes. Along with this expansion comes further cellular disorganization and eventually the ability to invade and metastasize. While this accumulation of multiple genetic changes is driven by growth advantages, it also can be facilitated by an innate genetic instability. In a small but significant fraction of cancers, this genetic instability is due to a defect in DNA mismatch repair. In the majority of cancers, accumulation of genetic changes is facilitated by a chromosomal instability, perhaps associated with defects in mitotic spindle checkpoints.

CLINICAL FEATURES

Incidence and Scope

Colorectal cancer is the second leading cause of cancer death in the United States. In 1998, there were an estimated 131,000 new cases of colorectal cancers and 56,000 deaths from this disease.[1] The cases are roughly equally distributed between the sexes. The average age of incidence of colon cancer in the United States is 67 years,[2] and over 90 percent of colon cancer deaths occur in individuals over the age of 55.[3] Approximately 5 percent of the population develop colorectal cancer, and this figure is expected to rise as life expectancy increases.[3] Furthermore, when nonmalignant colorectal tumors are considered, up to half the population is affected.[4–6]

Histopathology

A single layer of epithelial cells lines the invaginations (crypts) of the colon and rectum (Fig. 34-1). As is true throughout the digestive tract, these crypts substantially increase the surface area occupied by the epithelium. Four to six stem cells at the base of each crypt give rise to the three major epithelial cell types (absorptive cells, mucus-secreting goblet cells, and neuroepithelial cells). The cells multiply in the lower third of the crypt and differentiate in the upper two-thirds. The journey from the base of the crypt to its apex, where the epithelial cells are extruded, takes 3 to 6 days.[7,8]

Normally, the birth rate of the colonic epithelial cells precisely equals the rate of loss from the crypt apex to the lumen of the bowel. If the birth/loss ratio increases, a neoplasm results (a *neoplasm* is here defined as any abnormal accumulation of cells originating from a single progenitor cell). A tumor of the colon is often first observed clinically as a polyp, a mass of cells protruding from the bowel wall (Fig. 34-2). There are predominantly two types of polyps, which can be distinguished histologically but not

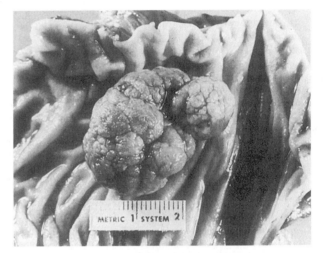

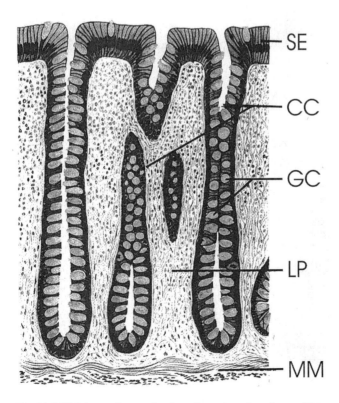

Fig. 34-1 Histology of normal colon. Examples of surface epithelium (SE), colonic crypts (CC), goblet cells (GC), lamina propria (LP), and muscularis mucosa (MM) are marked. (*Used with permission from Clara et al.*[417])

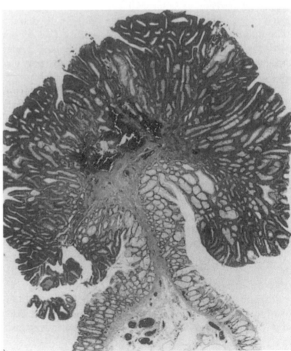

Fig. 34-2 Morphology of a colonic polyp showing its pedunculated nature. (*A*) A macroscopic view of a large tubular adenoma. (*B*) A cross section of a tubular adenoma with a clearly visible stalk. (*Used with permission from Kent and Mitros.*[9])

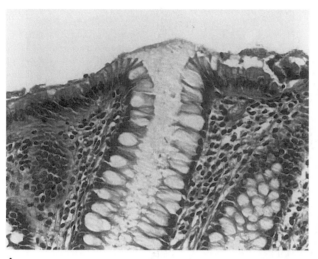

A

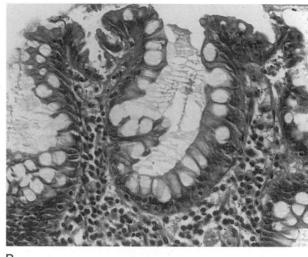

B

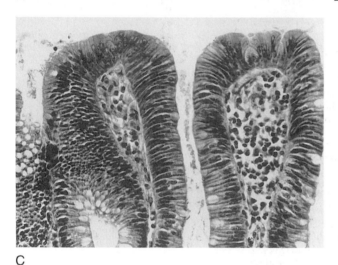

C

Fig. 34-3 Histopathology of colonic polyps. Panels show high-power views of hematoxylin and eosin–stained sections of normal colonic mucosa, (A) a hyperplastic polyp (nondysplastic), and an adenomatous polyp (dysplastic) (B), respectively. Note (C) the increased disruption of normal architecture present in the adenomatous polyp compared with the hyperplastic polyp. (From Dr. Stanley R. Hamilton, Johns Hopkins University School of Medicine, Baltimore MD.)

by their external appearance.[9] The nondysplastic or hyperplastic type consists of large numbers of cells that have a normal morphology (Fig. 34-3B). The cells are lined up in a single row along the basement membrane, and these polyps apparently have little tendency to become neoplastic. The other polyp type (adenomatous) is dysplastic, i.e., has an abnormal intracellular and intercellular organization (see Fig. 34-3C). Several layers of epithelial cells, in addition to the one adjacent to the basement membrane, are evident; the nuclei of the epithelial cells are larger than normal; and their position within the cell is often aberrant. Crypts crowd together in a kaleidoscopic pattern. As adenomas grow in size, they become more dysplastic. They also are more likely to contain "villous" components, i.e., fingerlike projections of dysplastic crypts that can be distinguished from the smooth contour of the less advanced "tubular" adenomas. As adenomas progress, they are more likely to become malignant, defined as the ability to invade surrounding tissues and travel to distant organs through direct spread or transport by blood vessels and lymphatics (metastasis). Malignant tumors are not necessarily larger or more dysplastic than benign tumors; their sole determining feature is invasiveness. Adenocarcinomas are the most common malignant tumor of the colon, although other cancers (e.g., lymphomas, sarcomas) that arise from nonepithelial cells occur occasionally.[10] As noted earlier, polyps are the earliest clinical manifestation of colorectal neoplasia, but methylene blue staining or microscopic examination of the colonic mucosa also can detect lesions affecting one or a small number of crypts (Fig. 34-4). These lesions are termed *aberrant crypt foci* (ACF) and, like their larger

counterparts, can be either dysplastic (microadenomas) or nondysplastic.

Colorectal neoplasia is not a rare condition. About 5 percent of individuals 40 to 50 years of age have adenomatous polyps, as do about half of those over 70 years old.[4–6] These figures are even higher when ACF are considered. Adenomas less than 10 mm in diameter have a very low probability of developing a focus of malignancy, whereas tumors larger than 10 mm have a 15 percent chance of becoming malignant over a 10-year period.[11] Benign tumors are easily removed by colonoscopy or surgery. Malignant tumors are usually excisable by surgery, but if they have already metastized, additional therapy is necessary. The most common site of metastasis is the mesenteric lymph nodes.[2] These lymph nodes are usually excised at the time of the initial surgery for the cancer. If distant metastasis has occurred (to the peritoneal surface or liver), surgery will not be curative. Patients with metastatic disease are usually treated with radiation and/or chemotherapeutic agents (adjuvant therapy). Although such treatments can induce remissions of many months, they are usually not curative, as evidenced by the fact that about 40 percent of patients with colorectal cancer die from their disease within 5 years of diagnosis despite adjuvant treatment.[1]

Inherited Predispositions

Familial colorectal cancers can be divided broadly into two groups: those characterized by the presence of multiple benign colorectal polyps (polyposis) and those characterized by the absence of polyposis. Several types of polyposis syndromes have

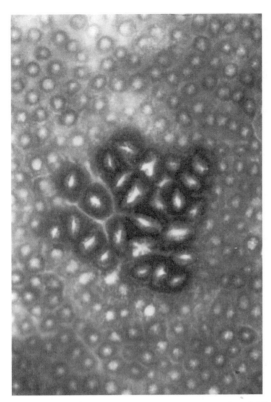

Fig. 34-4 Morphology of an ACF. Macroscopic view of an ACF after staining with methylene blue. (*From Dr. Stanley R. Hamilton, Johns Hopkins University School of Medicine, Baltimore, MD.*)

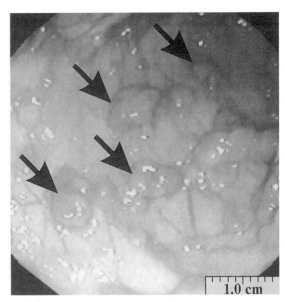

Fig. 34-5 Polyposis in an FAP patient. Colonoscopic view of polyps in a patient with FAP. (*Used with permission from Kinzler and Vogelstein.*[418])

been described, including familial adenomatous polyposis coli (FAP), Peutz-Jegher syndrome (see Chap. 20), familial juvenile polyposis (see Chap. 21), Cowden syndrome (see Chap. 31), Cronkhite-Canada syndrome, and hyperplastic polyposis. We will limit our discussion of the polyposis syndromes to FAP and its variants because its pathogenesis has been proven to be especially relevant to sporadic colorectal tumorigenesis.

FAP is inherited in autosomal dominant fashion, and affected individuals develop hundreds to thousands of adenomatous polyps during their lifetime (Fig. 34-5). The polyps are first observed during the second decade of life and increase in number over the next two decades. The histologic and biologic features of these polyps are indistinguishable from those of sporadic adenomatous polyps that develop in the general population. Although an individual polyp in an FAP patient is no more likely to progress to cancer than a sporadic polyp with the same degree of dysplasia, their large numbers in FAP patients essentially guarantee that some will progress to cancer. Indeed, the median age for colorectal cancer in untreated FAP patients is about 40.[12] Thus prophylactic colectomies are performed routinely on FAP patients to reduce their risk of cancer. Although about 1 in 5000 to 10,000 individuals is affected with FAP in the United States,[13] less than 1 percent of all colon cancers occur in FAP patients. Patients with FAP are also at increased risk for cancers of the thyroid, small intestine, stomach, and brain.[12,14] Variants of FAP have been described that include all the colonic manifestations of FAP plus varied extracolonic manifestations.[15,16] The most common variant is Gardner syndrome (GS), which is characterized by soft tissue tumors, osteomas, dental abnormalities, and congenital hypertrophy of the retinal pigment epithelium (CHRPE).[15] Still other attenuated variants of FAP are characterized by a reduced number of intestinal polyps (10 to 100).[17,18] Finally, many cases of Turcot syndrome, which is characterized by the presence of central nervous system (CNS) tumors in combination with familial predisposition to colorectal cancer, are variants of FAP.[14] As detailed below, FAP and its variants can now be traced to germline mutations of the *APC* gene. Molecular, physiologic, and epidemiologic studies all suggest that FAP represents a defect in the control of tumor initiation.

It is estimated that hereditary nonpolyposis colorectal cancer (HNPCC) accounts for about 2 to 4 percent of colorectal cancer in the Western world.[19] Like FAP patients, HNPCC patients develop colorectal cancer at a median age of approximately 42 years (see Chap. 18 for a detailed review).[20] However, unlike FAP patients, HNPCC patients do not have a marked increase in the number of precursor adenomas. Thus, until recently, HNPCC kindred have had to be defined operationally. The standard clinical criterion for HNPCC included the identification of at least three first-degree relatives in at least two different generations with colorectal cancer, with at least one individual affected at less than 50 years of age. The identification of the underlying genetic defect now allows a genetic definition.[21] It is now known that the majority of HNPCC patients inherit a defect in DNA mismatch repair (*MMR*) genes. Tumors arising in these patients are DNA mismatch repair deficient and as a result are genetically unstable and progress rapidly to cancer. Thus, in contrast to FAP, the defect in HNPCC primarily affects tumor progression. In addition to colorectal cancer, HNPCC patients are at increased risk for other cancers, including those of the uterus, ovary, and brain.[21] Indeed, those cases of Turcot syndrome which are not due to germ-line defects in *APC* usually have germ-line defects in an *MMR* gene.[14]

Other Genetic Factors

The majority of patients with colorectal cancer do not have first-degree relatives with colorectal cancer, and therefore, the cancers are considered sporadic. Only about 3 to 5 percent of all colorectal cancers occur in individuals with well-characterized inherited predispositions such as those described earlier. However, several studies suggest a broader role for inheritance.[22–24] For example, the relatives of patients with sporadic colon cancers also have an increased risk for colon cancer; detailed studies of this phenomenon have suggested a dominant inheritance of susceptibility to adenomatous polyps and associated cancers.[23,24] Furthermore, it has been estimated that such inherited susceptibility could account for 15 to more than 50 percent of the total colorectal cancers in the population at large. Although these studies await to be confirmed through identification of the specific genetic factors involved, it is reasonable to assume that hereditary factors, when combined with environmental factors (see below), determine the aggregate risk for colorectal cancer. Whether the hereditary factors turn out to be embodied in a few major genes, rather than in a synergistic combination of multiple genes, remains to be determined.

Environmental Factors

While inherited genetic factors can clearly play an important role in the development of colon cancers, they are by no means the sole determinant.[25] This point is well illustrated by classic studies of Japanese immigrants to the United States. Historically, the incidence of colon cancer has been low in Japan, whereas the incidence of gastric cancer has been high. Japanese populations that moved to the United States show a progressive increase in colorectal cancer.[26] Today, this change in cancer incidence is being repeated on a larger scale in Japan, where the incidence of gastric cancer is declining, while the incidence of colon cancer is increasing.[27] These changes have been hypothesized to be due to the westernization of the Japanese diet. Epidemiologic studies indicate that certain diets[28–32] are associated with increased risk for colorectal cancer. The components of these diets that are responsible for the effects on risk and the mechanisms underlying such effects have not yet been fully elucidated. Presumably, they affect either the incidence of mutations or the ability of mutated cells to expand clonally.

MOLECULAR GENETICS OF COLORECTAL CANCER

Clonal Nature of Colorectal Cancers

The clonal nature of tumors is a critical feature of the somatic mutation/clonal evolution model of carcinogenesis.[33] In this model, a single cell acquires a mutation providing a selective growth advantage that allows its progeny to outnumber those of neighboring cells (Fig. 34-6). From within this clonal population, a single cell may acquire a second mutation, providing an additional growth advantage that allows further clonal expansion. Repeated cycles of mutation followed by clonal expansion eventually lead to a fully developed malignant tumor.

The clonal nature of human colorectal tumors was first demonstrated using techniques based on X chromosome inactivation in females. Only a single X chromosome is active in any somatic cell of a female. This inactivation occurs early during embryogenesis and is random with regard to which copy of the X chromosome (maternal or paternal) is inactivated in any given cell. The pattern of X inactivation is transmitted in a highly stable manner to progeny cells. The inactivation is also accompanied by changes in methylation of cytosine residues on the inactivated X

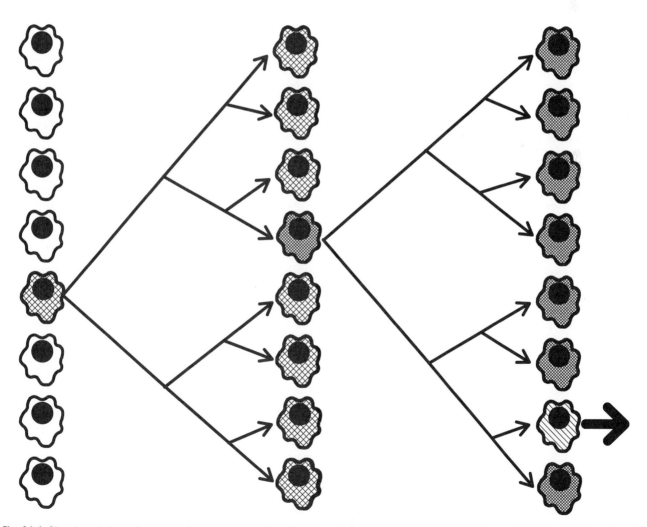

Fig. 34-6 Clonal evolution of tumor cells. A normal cell suffers a mutation that gives it a slight growth advantage. With time, this clone expands, and one of the progeny cell acquires another mutation providing an additional growth advantage. After several rounds of mutation followed by expansion, a malignant tumor results. The expansion phase is important because it provides additional targets for subsequent mutation. Without this expansion, mutations would be so infrequent that multiple genetic changes would be unlikely to occur, and tumors would be very rare.

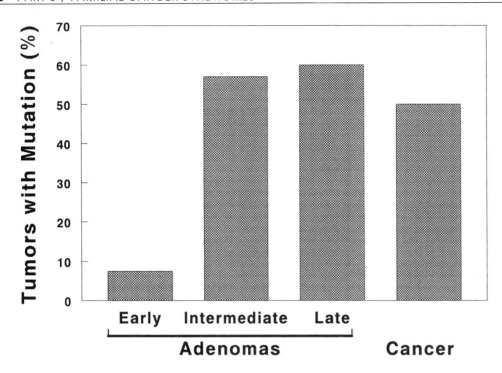

Fig. 34-7 Frequency of *RAS* mutations in colorectal tumors. Early adenomas were defined as less than 1.0 cm; intermediate adenomas were larger than 1.0 cm but without foci of carcinomatous transformation; late adenomas were larger than 1.0 cm and contained at least one focus of carcinomatous transformation; the cancers were adenocarcinomas of the colon. Tumors were assessed for *RAS* mutations as described.[45]

chromosome. Thus methylation-sensitive restriction enzymes in combination with restriction fragment length polymorphism can be used to distinguish which copy of the X chromosome is inactivated.[34] When this type of analysis is performed on small portions of normal colonic mucosa, the inactivation of X is equally distributed between the maternal and paternal copies. In contrast, when benign or malignant colorectal tumors are analyzed, they are found to display a monoclonal pattern of X inactivation.[35,36] The monoclonal nature of these tumors was further demonstrated using autosomal polymorphic markers that demonstrated clonal chromosomal losses.[36] These observations were consistent with cytogenetic studies that had demonstrated clonal chromosomal abnormalities in many carcinomas[37–39] and a major fraction of adenomas.[40–42] Subsequently, the identification of somatic point mutations in specific growth-controlling genes provided conclusive proof of the monoclonal nature of human colorectal tumors.

The *RAS* Oncogenes

The first breakthrough in the molecular genetics of colorectal tumors was the identification of *RAS* gene mutations.[43–45] The first *RAS* genes were identified as the transforming components of the Kirsten and Harvey rat sarcoma virus genomes (see Chap. 11). Three cellular *RAS* genes, *K-RAS, H-RAS,* and *N-RAS,* were later identified and shown to transform cells in tissue culture when mutated.[46,47] Specific point mutations of *K-RAS* or *N-RAS* are found in approximately 50 percent of colorectal adenomas larger than 1.0 cm and in 50 percent of carcinomas; *RAS* mutations are seen rarely in adenomas less than 1.0 cm in size[45] (Fig. 34-7). The lack of mutations in smaller adenomas suggests that *RAS* mutations are acquired during adenoma progression. Direct evidence for this premise comes from microdissection studies demonstrating subpopulations of adenoma cells that have acquired *RAS* mutations.[48] *RAS* mutations are not limited to dysplastic colorectal lesions; 100 percent of nondysplastic ACF and 25 percent of hyperplastic polyps have *RAS* mutations.[49,50] However, these nondysplastic lesions appear to be largely self-limited with respect to their potential for neoplastic progression. Regardless of the lesion's histology, most of the mutations identified (85 percent) are in codons 12 and 13 of *K-RAS,* with the rest affecting codon 61 of *K-RAS* or *N-RAS.* These studies clearly indicate that *RAS* oncogene mutations play a role during the development of a significant fraction of colorectal tumors. However, they also

suggest that many tumors can develop in the absence of *RAS* mutations or fail to progress in the presence of one. The importance of *RAS* in colorectal tumorigenesis also has been emphasized by the finding that colorectal tumor cells in which the mutated *RAS* gene has been removed by homologous recombination still grow indefinitely *in vitro* but lose their ability to form tumors in nude mice.[51]

The *RAS* oncogenes encode 21-kDa monomeric proteins with homology to G proteins.[52] Like G proteins, RAS can bind GTP and catalyze its hydrolysis to GDP. RAS is active only when bound to GTP, with the hydrolysis to GDP leading to inactivation. The ratio of GTP-RAS to GDP-RAS is higher in cells containing mutant *RAS* genes than in cells with only wild-type *RAS* gene products. The altered ratio is due to decreased hydrolysis of GTP to GDP. However, the intrinsic GTPase activities of wild-type and mutant RAS do not usually account for this difference. The interaction of RAS with a cellular GTPase-activating protein (GAP) is apparently responsible for the difference. The GTPase activity of wild-type RAS is stimulated by GAP, whereas mutant RAS fails to respond to GAP.[53] Interestingly, the gene responsible for neurofibromatosis type 1 (NF1) has been found to have GAP activity (see Chap. 25).[54–57] This is interesting in light of the fact that many colon cancers do not contain *RAS* gene mutations. Accordingly, a mutation of NF1 has been reported to occur in a colon tumor that did not have a *RAS* mutation.[58]

Tumor-Suppressor Genes in Colorectal Cancers

The first molecular evidence for the role of tumor-suppressor genes in colorectal tumorigenesis came from the study of allelic losses.[36,45,59–63] Tumor-suppressor genes can be inactivated in a variety of ways, including point mutations, rearrangements, and deletions. Many of the deletions include entire chromosomal arms or even whole chromosomes. These large deletions can be detected using polymorphic markers that distinguish the two alleles present in the germ line.[64] Comparison of the alleles present in the tumor tissue with those in normal tissue allows the identification of deletions as loss of heterozygosity (LOH). When colorectal cancers were examined using at least one polymorphic marker for each nonacrocentric autosomal arm, certain arms were found to be frequently lost[63] (Fig. 34-8). Most frequently implicated were chromosomes 5q, 8p, 17p, and 18q, which were lost in 36, 50, 73, and 75 percent of the cases, respectively. This frequent loss of

A

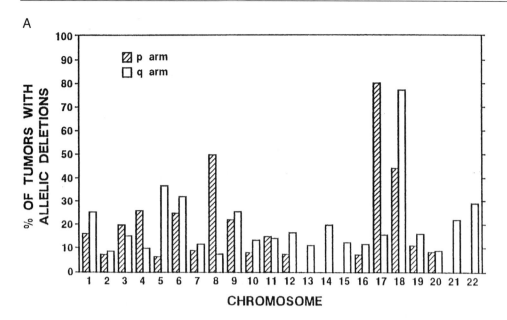

B

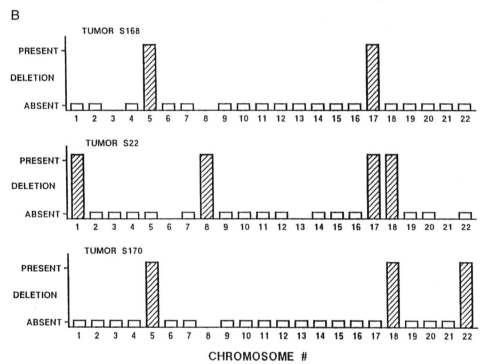

Fig. 34-8 Chromosomal losses in colorectal cancers. (*A*) Frequency of allelic deletions for individual chromosome arms in colorectal carcinomas. Allelic losses were scored in 56 colorectal carcinomas using polymorphic marker for all nonacrocentric autosomal arms.[63] Values for loss are expressed as a percentage of informative cases showing allelic loss. (*Used with permission from Fearon and Vogelstein.[381]*) (B) Allelic losses in three individual tumors (S168, S22, and S170) are shown. Long bars indicate a deletion; short bars indicate no deletion; the lack of an informative marker is indicated by the absence of a bar. Note that although there is a significant trend for loss of chromosomes 5, 8, 17, and 18, the exact pattern in individual tumors varies.

specific chromosomes has been taken to represent one step in the inactivation of a tumor-suppressor gene residing on the lost chromosome. The LOH analyses generally were consistent with karyotypic studies that had shown frequent losses of the same chromosomes.[37–39] To date, presumptive tumor-suppressor genes located on chromosomes 5q, 17p, and 18q have been identified. Chromosome losses, analyzed by LOH or karyotype, obviously underestimate the prevalence of suppressor gene alterations in colorectal tumors because small deletions, rearrangements, or point mutations are not detected in such analyses.

Chromosome 17p: The *p53* Gene

The first tumor-suppressor gene implicated in the development of colorectal tumors was the *p53* gene on chromosome 17p. The existence of a tumor-suppressor gene on 17p was suggested by the aforementioned allelic loss,[36,45,60,62,63] as well as by cytogenetic studies.[38,39] Loss of 17p sequences was detected in 75 percent of cancers, whereas 17p sequences were rarely lost in adenomas,

suggesting that inactivation of the 17p tumor-suppressor gene was a relatively late event in colorectal tumorigenesis[45] (Fig. 34-9).

The *p53* gene was identified originally in 1979 by virtue of its expression in cells infected with tumor viruses.[65–67] During the first 10 years of its study, the cellular *p53* gene was considered to be a proto-oncogene. This was in part because of its increased expression in tumors and also because *p53* was apparently able to transform rat embryo fibroblasts in collaboration with *RAS* oncogenes.[68–70] However, subsequent studies have indicated that the wild-type *p53* gene is a tumor-suppressor gene, not a proto-oncogene. Studies on colorectal tumors were critical to this realization.[71] As mentioned earlier, chromosome 17p losses were noted frequently in colorectal tumors. To further localize the position of the putative tumor-suppressor gene on this chromosome, a large panel of polymorphic markers was used to analyze numerous colorectal cancer cases. The common region of deletion (i.e., the chromosomal region consistently lost in tumors containing any loss of chromosome 17p) was mapped to a region centered

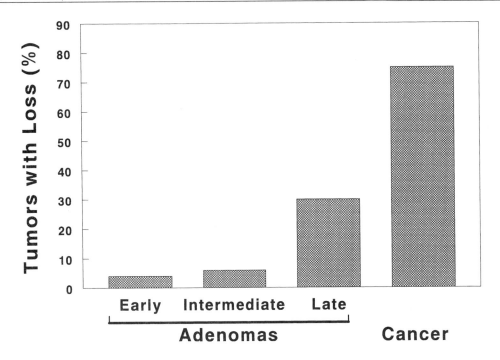

Fig. 34-9 Frequency of 17p losses in colorectal tumors. Tumor classes are defined as in Fig. 34-7. Values for chromosome 17p losses are expressed as a percentage of informative cases showing allelic loss.

at 17p13.1. Based on Knudson's hypothesis,[72] it was hypothesized that the loss of 17p13 removed one copy of a putative suppressor gene from the cell, while the remaining copy was mutant. Because *p53* was known to reside at 17p13 and had been implicated previously in neoplasia (albeit as an oncogene), it was tested to see if it fit Knudson's hypothesis. The remaining *p53* gene from a colorectal tumor that had lost one *p53* allele was sequenced. It was found to harbor a missense mutation at codon 143, changing alanine to valine. The mutation was somatic; i.e., it was not present in the normal colon of the same patient. Further analysis identified somatic mutations in the remaining *p53* gene in 24 of 28 colorectal tumors that had undergone allelic loss of 17p.[73] The majority of these mutations were missense and clustered into four regions that are conserved among mammals, amphibians, birds, and fish (Figs. 34-10 and 34-11).

The frequent allelic loss of 17p, coupled with mutation of the remaining copy of *p53,* strongly suggested that *p53* was a tumor-suppressor gene. Several other observations reinforced this idea. It was found that the wild-type *p53* gene, but not the mutant *p53* gene, could inhibit the growth of transformed cells in culture. This was first demonstrated in rodent cell fibroblasts[74,75] and later in human cancers of the colon[76] and other tissues.[77–79] Conversely, it was found that mutant, but not wild-type, *p53* genes could transform rat embryo fibroblasts in cooperation with *RAS* oncogenes (the presumably normal *p53* genes used for the initial studies on transformation by *p53* turned out to contain a mutation).[80,81] In Friend virus−induced erythroleukemias, the *p53* gene was found to be inactivated by proviral integration.[82–84] The p53 protein appears to be inactivated by viruses in some human cancers as well. In cervical cancers, the human papilloma virus E6 protein binds to the *p53* gene product[85] and inhibits its functional properties.[86] Finally, studies of other human tumor types, including lung, breast, brain, bladder and liver, show that *p53* is frequently mutated, just as in the colon.[87] In fact, the mutations observed in some of these tumors have provided clues as to the responsible mutagen.[88] For example, a specific mutation at codon 249 in liver tumors suggests a role for aflatoxins,[89–91] pyrimidine dimer mutations in skin tumors are consistent with a role for ultraviolet light,[92] and the pattern of mutations in lung cancers suggests mutagens in tobacco smoke as the culprits.[93] It has been estimated that over half the total malignancies in the world involve inactivation of *p53*.

How does *p53* exert its tumor-suppressor effect? The biochemical properties of p53 protein provide some answers to this question. The *p53* gene encodes a 393-amino-acid phospho-protein (Fig. 34-11). Biophysical studies of the p53 protein indicate that it exists as a tetramer.[94,95] The region responsible for this tetramerization has been mapped to the carboxyl terminus,[96] between amino acids 344 to 393, and this tetramerization appears to be critical for defining the biochemical properties of p53.[97] The most compelling property is the ability of wild-type p53 to bind DNA in a sequence-specific manner.[98] Analysis of numerous human and artificially constructed sequences that bind p53 *in vitro* allowed definition of a consensus binding site composed of two copies of the 10-bp motif 5′-PuPuPuC(A/T)(A/T)GPyPyPy-3′.[99–101] One copy of this binding site is insufficient for binding, but binding is preserved even when the two copies are separated by as much as 13 bp. The complete p53 binding site is thus composed of four copies of the 5-bp half site 5′-PuPuPuC(A/T) (A/T)-3′ arranged in opposing directions. The ability of p53 to form tetramers could account for the fourfold symmetry of the binding site.

The fact that tumor-derived mutant p53 proteins nearly always have a reduced ability to bind DNA in a sequence-specific manner accentuates the importance of this activity.[98–100,102,103] The three-dimensional structure of a p53-DNA complex provides a biochemical understanding of the effects of these mutations.[104] Indeed, the Arg 248 and Arg 273 residues, which are the most frequently targeted residues for somatic mutations, were observed to directly contact DNA (Fig. 34-12).

What does this DNA binding accomplish in the cell? The amino terminus of p53 (codons 20−42) has an acidic domain that is similar to those in other transcription factors[81,105–107] (see Fig. 34-11). When this domain is fused to a DNA-binding protein, it conveys the ability to activate transcription.[81,105,106] Additional evidence for the role of p53 as a transcription factor comes from the studies of artificial genes containing a p53 binding site upstream of a reporter gene.[100,108] Expression of wild-type p53 in the presence of these reporter constructs results in strong transcriptional activation of the reporter molecule. The activation of transcription is proportional to the strength of p53 binding, and no transactivation is seen with constructs containing mutated binding sites that no longer bind p53. Additionally, p53 can mediate transactivation of genes containing p53 binding sites in

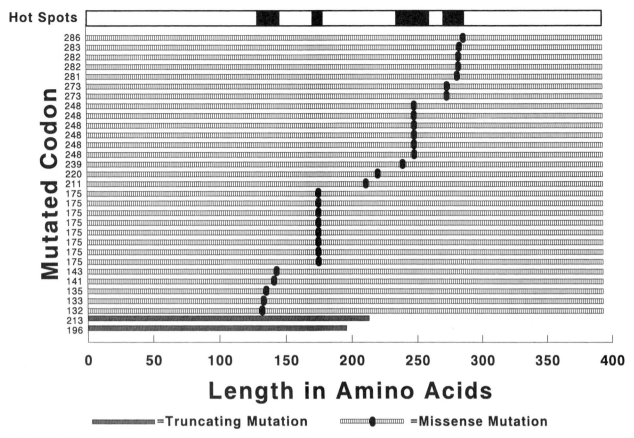

Fig. 34-10 Mutation of *p53* in colorectal tumors. Thirty-one *p53* mutations are illustrated.[73] Length of bar indicates region of *p53* translation terminated normally or by a somatic nonsense mutation. Cross bars indicate the locations of somatic missense mutations.

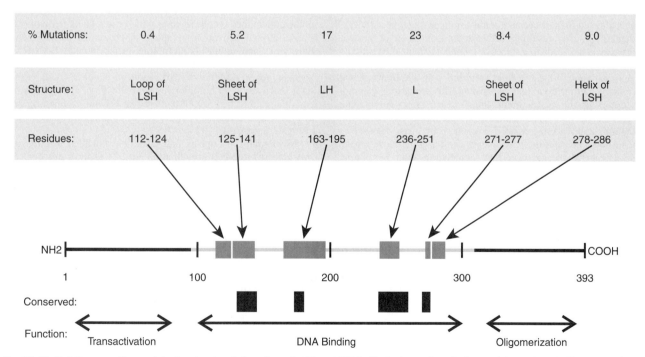

Fig. 34-11 Mutations as they relate to structural domains of p53. Mutations within the indicated region are taken from compiled data (from Greenblatt et al.[419]). Structural domains were determined by x-ray crystallography of the region indicated in yellow.[104] L, LH, and LSH indicate loop, loop-helix, and loop-sheet-helix, respectively. Function domains are indicated and conserved domains are indicated at the bottom. (*Modified with permission from Vogelstein and Kinzler.*[420])

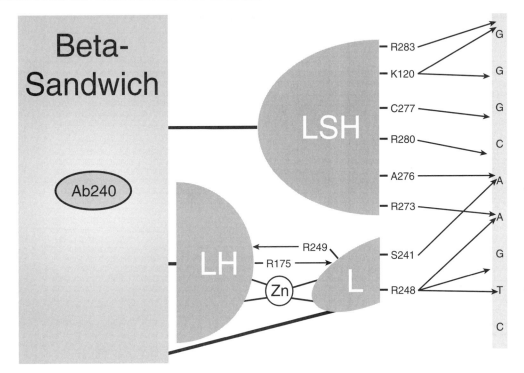

Fig. 34-12 Key structural elements of p53-DNA binding. Based on the crystal structure in Cho et al.[104] L, LH, and LSH indicate loop, loop-helix, and loop-sheet-helix, respectively. Residues are indicated in single-letter code, and DNA contacts are indicated by arrows. For simplicity, only one strand is shown with arrows pointing to bases indicating a base contact and arrows pointing between bases indicating contacts to sugar or phosphate groups. (*Used with permission from Vogelstein and Kinzler.[420]*)

yeast.[108,109] As expected due to the lack of specific DNA binding, mutant p53 proteins are devoid of transactivation activity. Moreover, mutant p53 is able to suppress transactivation by wild-type p53 in a dominant negative manner.[108] This suppression was found to be due to the ability of mutant p53 to inhibit wild-type p53 binding to DNA, likely through the formation of inactive hetero-oligomers between wild-type and mutant p53 molecules.

Taken together, these studies suggest the following model for p53 function[110]: Wild-type p53 is hypothesized to bind to specific sequences within the promoters of growth-inhibitory genes and activate their transcription. If a tumor acquires an inactivating missense mutation in one copy of the *p53* gene, p53 activity in the cell is reduced (in part because of the dominant negative activity of mutant p53). The resulting decrease in expression of growth-inhibitory genes leads to a selective growth advantage. Eventually, the residual wild-type activity is completely eliminated by loss of the normal copy of the *p53* gene, resulting in an additional growth advantage and further clonal expansion. This scenario is common in tumors of the colon, brain, lung, breast, skin, and bladder. Occasionally, *p53* is inactivated by nonsense or splice-site mutations that lead to truncated proteins or by gross deletions of one or both copies of the *p53* gene. In cervical cancers, it appears that p53 is often inactivated by association with the human papilloma virus–produced E6 protein.[85,86] Similarly, p53 appears to be inactivated in some tumors by the product of the *MDM2* gene.[111–113] The *MDM2* gene was identified originally by virtue of its amplification in transformed mouse cells[114] and is often amplified in human sarcomas, particularly the malignant fibrous histiocytoma subclass.[112]

Direct evidence for this model has come from the identification of genes transcriptionally regulated by p53. To date, at least 20 genes have been identified that are regulated by p53.[115–133] These genes appear to affect a variety of cellular processes including apoptosis,[117,118,126] cell cycle arrest,[116,127] and negative regulation of the p53 pathway itself.[115] One of the first to be characterized and best understood of these downstream pathways is that containing p21^{WAF1/CIP1}.[116,134–136] p53 directly induces the expression of p21^{WAF1/CIP1} via binding to three consensus binding sites located within 2.3 kb of the transcription start site.[116,137] p21^{WAF1/CIP1} in turn inhibits growth by inducing a G1 cell cycle arrest.[116,134] This arrest is due to the ability of p21^{WAF1/CIP1} to bind to and inhibit cyclin-dependent kinases.[135,138] Consistent with this, disruption of the p21^{WAF1/CIP1} genes by homologous recombination eliminates the ability of p53 to induce a G1 arrest in colorectal cancer cells[139,140] and (to a lesser extent) in mouse fibroblasts.[141,142]

As indicated above, p53 induces a variety of genes, and accordingly, the growth-inhibitory effects of p53 on the cell are not limited to a G1 arrest. p53 also can produce a sustained G2 arrest that requires p21^{WAF1/CIP1}[143] and the p53-inducible gene *14-3-3σ*.[127,144] In a subset of colon cancers, restoration of p53 function can result in apoptosis rather than cell cycle arrest.[145] Although the specific mechanism for p53-induced apoptosis in colorectal epithelial cells remains unclear, it is likely to involve the transcriptional activation of apoptosis-promoting genes. Candidates for such apoptosis-promoting genes include BAX,[117,118] PIGs,[145] and PUMA.[145a,145b] The definitive identification of the specific genes essential for p53-induced apoptosis will require their inactivation by homologous recombination; analogously, the essential role of p21 in cell cycle arrest became compelling only after its inactivation by homologous recombination was shown to abrogate this arrest.

In summary, it appears that when p53 is called to duty, it is instructed to stop cell growth at all cost. To achieve this goal, the p53 commando has been granted a large arsenal of growth-inhibitory weapons that allow it to function in diverse cellular environments. If all attempts at growth control fail, p53 induces cellular suicide (the "doomsday" weapon of last resort).

Although p53 function is beginning to be understood at the cellular and biochemical levels, its strategic role at the organism level still remains elusive. Mice with both copies of *p53* inactivated by homologous recombination are viable and develop normally, albeit with a predisposition to lymphomas and, to a lesser extent, other tumors.[146–148] Furthermore, individuals with Li-Fraumeni syndrome inherit a mutated *p53* gene and are normal except for an increased risk of leukemia, breast carcinoma, soft tissue sarcoma, brain tumor, and osteosarcoma.[149,150] These results suggest that p53 function is not essential to the normal cell under most circumstances. However, p53 may be critical to normal cells when stressed. Normal cells arrest their growth in response to x-ray- or drug-induced DNA damage, whereas cells with mutant p53 are only partially blocked and continue to divide.[151–153] This has prompted the suggestion that p53 in part protects the integrity of the genome by preventing propagation of cells with DNA damage.[154] Other forms of stress in addition to DNA damage can induce p53 function. For example, hypoxia, such as that found in poorly vascularized tumors, can induce p53 expression and p53-dependent apoptosis in mouse cells.[155,156] Moreover, cells lacking p53 were shown to have a selective advantage in such an environment.[156] Likewise, excess mitogenic signals from overexpression of Myc,[157,158] E1A,[159] or E2F-1[160–162] can induce p53-mediated apoptosis. This induction is dependent on p19[ARF] and is distinct from induction by hypoxia and DNA damage.[163–168] In addition to DNA damage, hypoxia, and mitogenic stimulation, changes in adhesion, redox, or rNTP levels status can modulate p53 activity (reviewed in Giaccia and Kastan[169]). Many of these pathways ultimately lead to activation of p53 by post-translational modification of p53 or by

interference with the negative regulatory protein Mdm2 (reviewed in Giaccia and Kastan[169]). The physiologic importance of appropriate regulation of p53 has been elegantly illustrated by the ability of deletion of *p53* to rescue the lethality of Mdm2 null mice.[170]

Further information about the regulation and function of p53 is provided in Chap. 23. While a great deal has been learned about the function of p53 and models for its role in tumorigenesis can be proposed (Fig. 34-13), several fundamental questions remain unanswered. For example, it is not understood why patients with Li-Fraumeni syndrome do not have a higher incidence of colon cancer. Nor are the intracellular mediators that determine the expression levels of p53 in normal and tumor cells fully elucidated. Finally, while some insight into the ability of p53 to induce growth arrest have been made, our understanding of its ability to induce apoptosis is less developed. These answers have

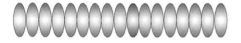

Normal Cells

↓ **Mutation in Tumor Initiating Gene**

Small Tumor

↓ **Additional Mutations**

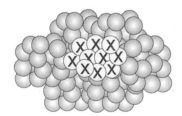

Large Tumor, Central Hypoxia Induces p53, Resulting in Growth Arrest/Apoptosis

↓ **p53 Mutation**

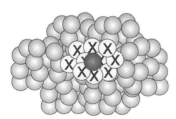

p53 Mutant Cell Resists Growth Arrest/Apoptosis

↓ **Clonal Expansion**

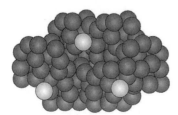

p53 Mutant Cells Become the Predominant Cells in the Tumor

Fig. 34-13 Function of p53 in tumor development. Model of why *p53* mutations occur late in tumorigenesis and lead to selective survival in the adverse environment of a tumor. In this example, hypoxia is the selecting factor, although other adverse conditions also may operate in tumors. (*Used with permission from Kinzler and Vogelstein.*[421])

Ⓧ **= Growth Arrest/Apoptosis**   ⬤ **= p53 Mutant Cell**

been amplified recently with identification of structural and functional homologues to *p53* on chromosomes 1p (p73)[171] and 3q (p63, p51, and p40).[172–174] Although products from both loci share p53's ability to inhibit growth, these genes do not appear to play the same central role in human cancers as does *p53*.

Chromosome 18q: The *DCC, SMAD4,* and *SMAD2* Genes

As with *p53,* the first evidence for a tumor-suppressor gene on chromosome 18q came from the study of chromosomal losses in colorectal cancers.[36,45,62,63] One copy of chromosome 18q is lost in 73 percent of sporadic colorectal cancers and in 47 percent of large adenomas with foci of carcinomatous growth, but the loss occurs infrequently in less advanced adenomas[45] (Fig. 34-14). In the clinical arena, three studies have demonstrated that 18q loss is associated with an unfavorable outcome in stage II colorectal cancers,[175–177] although another has not.[178] On the molecular side, several candidate tumor-suppressor genes have been identified in this region, but efforts to positively pinpoint the culprit genes have been complicated by the inability to identify a candidate gene displaying intragenic mutations in the majority of cases.

The first candidate tumor-suppressor gene was isolated during attempts to map the chromosome 18q losses in human colorectal cancer with molecular techniques.[179] Analysis of 60 cancers with a series of polymorphic markers along 18q localized the most common region of deletion to 18q21. One marker from this region identified one carcinoma with a somatic point mutation that could create a novel splice acceptor site and a second with a complete (homozygous) loss of sequences from this region. Thorough analysis of a 370-kb region flanking this marker, using a variety of techniques, revealed a single expressed gene termed *DCC* for *deleted in colorectal cancer.* The *DCC* gene encodes a 10-kb transcript with a 4347-bp open reading frame.[179,180] The coding portion of the transcript is distributed within 29 exons occupying 1350 kb.[181]

The primary structure of DCC provides important clues to how DCC might function. If initiation occurs at the first methionine of the open reading frame, it would encode a 1447-amino-acid protein. DCC protein has several structural features, indicating that it is a membrane protein.[179,180] The amino-terminal end has a 25-amino-acid hydrophobic leader sequence, and an apparent membrane-spanning region divides the protein into an 1100-

amino-acid extracellular domain and a 324-amino-acid intracytoplasmic domain. The intracytoplasmic domain shows no obvious homologies to previously sequenced proteins. The extracellular domain shows extensive homology to the cell adhesion molecule N-CAM and to other related cell surface glycoproteins. Specifically, the extracellular domain contains four immunoglobulin-like C2 domains and six fibronectin type III repeats. Some of the suspected properties of DCC derived from the primary sequence have been confirmed by direct analysis of the DCC protein. Cell surface labeling studies documented a cell surface localization for the DCC protein. Immunocytochemical analysis of cells expressing high levels of DCC revealed membrane staining concentrated at points of cell-cell contact.[180] Immunohistochemical studies of human tissues indicate that DCC protein is expressed in differentiating cells, particularly in the intestinal epithelium and brain.[182] Consistent with the preceding observations, the DCC protein was shown to be a receptor for netrin, a laminin-related protein involved in guidance of developing axons.[183–185]

The precise role of *DCC* in colorectal cancer has been difficult to define, in part due to its large size and its lack of expression in colorectal cancers. While the *DCC* transcript is expressed in many tissues, including the colonic mucosa, most colorectal cancers fail to express an intact *DCC* transcript, consistent with its potential role as a tumor suppressor.[179,186] Unfortunately, this lack of expression complicates mutational analysis in that mutations leading to such loss of expression need not be limited to the coding portions of *DCC*. Despite this, a small number of somatic mutations of *DCC,* including small insertions and point mutations, have been identified in human tumors.[179,181] Southern blot analysis of DCC has revealed two intronic point mutations by chance, and detailed analysis of 7 of *DCC*'s 29 coding exons in 30 colorectal cancers identified one somatic missense mutation.[179,181] In addition, three homozygous mutations affecting DCC have been described in colorectal cancer cells.[179,186] Homozygous deletions of *DCC* also were observed in 2 of 91 human germ cell cancers screened by Southern blot analysis.[187] Moreover, the lack of expression of DCC in a subset of tumors with mismatch repair deficiency may be due to an unusually large expansion of a repeat in a DCC intron.[179,181] Loss of DCC protein expression has prognostic value and is associated with an unfavorable outcome in stage II and III colorectal cancers.[188–191] These immunohistochemical studies support the previous observations that

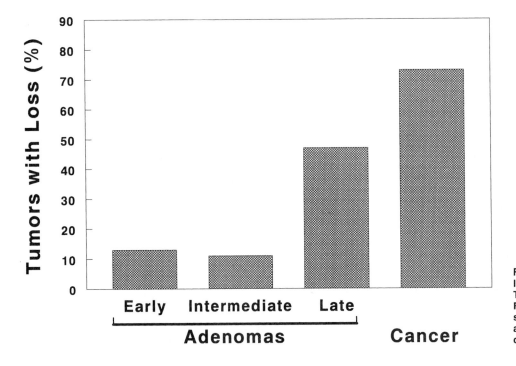

Fig. 34-14 Frequency of 18q losses in colorectal tumors. Tumor classes are defined as in Fig. 34-7. Values for chromosome 18q losses are expressed as a percentage of informative cases showing allelic loss.

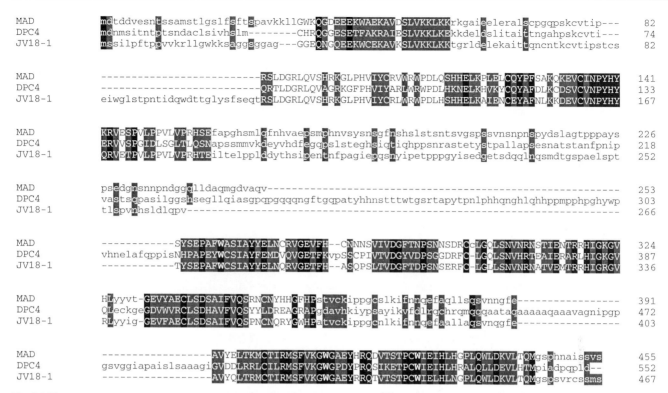

Fig. 34-15 Homology between *SMAD4*, *SMAD2*, and *Drosophila* Mad. The amino acid sequences of *Mad*,[196] *SMAD4* (DPC4),[193] and *SMAD2* (JV18-1)[207] were aligned and shaded by the means of their pairwise score using the MACAW multiple alignment software.[422]

chromosome 18q loss carries an unfavorable prognosis and suggest that the target of such losses is DCC. However, because the mechanisms underlying the loss of DCC expression are not yet known, it is not possible to conclusively implicate DCC as this target from these data. To date, no germ-line mutations of *DCC* have been found. A small fraction of mice with targeted inactivation of one copy of *DCC* showed multiple intestinal tumors or lethal brain tumors that are not observed in normal mice, but the number of mice with these neoplastic phenotypes was not high enough to draw statistically significant conclusions supporting a role for DCC in murine tumorigenesis.[192]

A second tumor-suppressor gene was identified on chromosome 18q21 during the course of investigation of chromosome 18q losses in pancreatic cancers.[193] Chromosome 18q losses occur in nearly 90 percent of pancreatic cancer.[194] Detailed analysis of pancreatic tumors losses identified a marker that revealed homozygous deletions that did not overlap with *DCC*. Characterization of this minimally deleted region identified a single expressed gene, termed *deleted in pancreatic cancer 4 (DPC4)*.[193] Further analysis of *DPC4* revealed that it was homozygously deleted in 25 of 84 pancreatic carcinomas (30 percent). Sequencing analysis of *DPC4* in 27 pancreatic cancers without homozygous mutations identified six intragenic mutations including one splice site, one missense, and four truncating mutations. Together these findings suggest a critical role for *DPC4* inactivation in pancreatic cancers.

DPC4 encodes a 552-residue protein with significant homology to the *Drosophila* mothers against Dpp (Mad) protein as well as *Caenorhabditis elegans* Mad homologues (Fig. 34-15). These proteins have been implicated in the signaling pathway of the transforming growth factor-beta (TGFβ) superfamily of signaling polypeptides.[195–197] This is of particular interest in light of the fact that TGFβ suppresses the growth of most normal cells and many cancer cells are resistant to the growth-suppressing affects of TGFβ (reviewed in Fynan and Reiss[198] and Brattain *et al.*[199]). Indeed, mutations of the TGFβ receptor have been identified in a subset of human colorectal cancers.[200–202] In colorectal cancer cells, DPC4 was shown to be required for TGFβ and activin

signaling by specific disruption of the *DPC4* loci through homologous recombination.[203] At the biochemical level, DPC4 functions in this pathway as a sequence-specific transcription activator.[204–206] To date, over a half dozen human Mad homologues (*SMAD*s) have been identified,[193,197,207–211] and *DPC4* has been redesignated *SMAD4*. Interestingly, *SMAD2*[207,208] and *SMAD7*,[210–212] in addition to *DPC4/SMAD4*, also map to chromosome 18q21, providing additional candidate tumor-suppressor genes. In contrast to SMAD2 and DPC4/SMAD4, SMAD7 appears to function antagonistically in TGFβ signaling, making it less appealing as a candidate tumor-suppressor gene.[210,211]

Mutational analysis of *DPC4/SMAD4* in 18 human colorectal cancers with 18q losses identified one homozygous deletion, one nonsense mutation, and three somatic missense mutations.[186] Analysis of *SMAD2* in the same 18 tumors identified one homozygous deletion that did not affect *DPC4/SMAD4* or *DCC* and a 42-bp deletion.[207] Intact *SMAD4/DPC4* and *SMAD2* transcripts were detected in the remaining tumors. In a separate study, analysis of *SMAD2* in 66 colorectal cancers identified four missense mutations.[208] Three of these mutations were shown to be functionally defective, as assessed by their abnormal TGFβ-induced phosphorylation and *Xenopus* mesoderm induction.[208] Other studies have found somatic mutations of *DPC4/SMAD4* or *SMAD2* in colorectal,[213] lung,[214] and stomach[215] cancers. However, in each case, mutations of *DPC4/SMAD4* could only account for the minority of 18q losses, suggesting that mutations remained undetected or that another chromosome 18q gene is the primary target of the 18q losses in these tumors. These genetic observations have been confirmed at the protein level using immunohistochemistry to detect DPC4 in human cancers with 18q loss.[215a] Germ-line mutations of *DPC4/SMAD4* are observed in a subset of individuals with juvenile polyposis syndrome (JPS). Individuals with JPS develop multiple juvenile polyps (distinct from adenomas) and are at an increased risk for colorectal cancer. The *SMAD4* mutations in JPS may lead to colorectal neoplasia only indirectly, since the mutations appear to initially affect stromal cells rather than the epithelial precursors of cancers

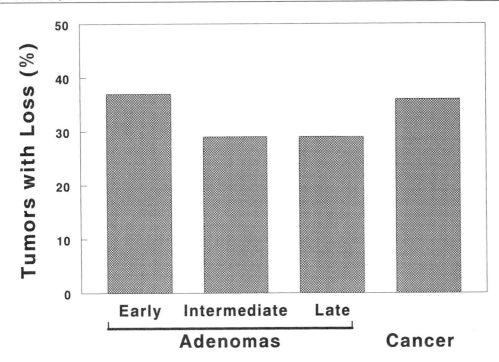

Fig. 34-16 Frequency of 5q losses in colorectal tumors. Tumor classes are defined as in Fig. 34-7. Values for chromosome 5q losses are expressed as a percentage of informative cases showing allelic loss.

(see Chap. 21).[216] In mice, inactivation of one copy of *Dpc4/Smad4* does not lead to increased rate of spontaneous tumors.[217,218] However, inactivation of both copies of *Dpc4/Smad4* did accelerate the progression of tumors arising in mice with a concurrent inactivation of *Apc*.[219] Interestingly, whereas homozygous inactivation of *Smad2*[220,221] or *Smad4*[217,218] is embryonically lethal, certain mouse strains with homozygous inactivation of *Smad3* are viable and develop metastatic colorectal cancer.[222]

Studies employing chromosome transfer demonstrated the ability of chromosome 18q to eliminate or reduce the growth of human colon cancer cells in nude mice.[223,224] In both colorectal cancer and squamous carcinoma cell lines, suppression by chromosome 18 is associated with restoration of TGFβ sensitivity.[224,225] In the squamous carcinoma cell lines, loss of this suppression is associated with loss of *DPC4/SMAD4* but not *DCC*.[225] Evidence for the growth-suppressive effect of DCC has come from antisense studies. When DCC expression in rat cells is inhibited by *DCC* antisense sequences, the cells become anchorage-independent *in vitro* and form tumors in nude mice.[226,227] Conversely, when DCC expression vectors are used to express DCC in human keratinocytes lacking DCC expression, tumorigenicity in nude mice is suppressed.[228] A molecular basis for these observations was provided recently when it was found that DCC induces apoptosis through a novel mechanism requiring receptor proteolysis.[229]

A variety of data point to the existence of a tumor-suppressor gene(s) on chromosome 18q in a number of human cancers. In some cancers, the inactivation of *DPC4/SMAD4* is clearly the target of these loss events. However, mutations of *DPC4/SMAD4* do not appear to account for most cases of chromosome 18q loss, so other known or yet-to-be-discovered candidate tumor-suppressor genes are likely to be the culprit(s) in the majority of cases.

Chromosome 5q: The *APC* Gene

Two lines of evidence suggested that a putative tumor-suppressor gene located on chromosome 5q was of particular interest. The first line of evidence came from the study of FAP, an inherited predisposition to colorectal cancer. The seminal clue to the location of the gene causing FAP came from a patient with polyposis and a constitutional interstitial deletion of 5q that was visible on cytogenetic analysis.[230] This observation suggested that a suppressor gene on chromosome 5q was responsible for the

patient's condition. This suggestion was confirmed and extended by linkage analysis, which established linkage of FAP to chromosome 5q21 markers in all kindreds analyzed.[231–233]

The second line of evidence came from the study of allelic losses in sporadic colorectal tumors. Chromosome 5q losses were reported to occur in 20 to 50 percent of colorectal cancers, depending on the region of chromosome 5q assessed.[45,59,62,63,234–237] Even more important, the loss of chromosome 5 sequences occurred as frequently in small benign colorectal tumors as in larger malignant tumors[45] (Fig. 34-16). These observations suggested that inactivation of a tumor-suppressor gene on chromosome 5q occurs frequently and early during tumor formation.

These two lines of evidence converged with the identification of a small region of chromosome 5q21 that was altered in the germ line of FAP patients and in sporadic colorectal cancers. Four genes were mapped to this region [*MCC, TB2 (DP1), SRP19*, and *APC*].[238,239] One of these genes (*APC*, for *adenomatous polyposis coli*) was found to be mutated in the germ line of FAP patients[240,241] and in sporadic colorectal tumors.[240] The *APC* gene contains an open reading frame of 8538 bp that would encode a 2843-amino-acid protein if translation initiated at the first methionine. This coding sequence is distributed over 15 exons and is remarkable in that the last exon contains a 6579-bp uninterrupted open reading frame. Several alternatively spliced forms of *APC* are known to exist, including variants that affect the coding region.[239,241–243]

The *APC* gene has been examined in over 500 FAP kindreds.[244,245] The most successful of these analyses have identified intragenic mutations in roughly 80 percent of the kindreds examined.[246] The majority of the remaining kindreds also have mutations of the *APC* gene that result in deletion of large portions of the gene or reduce its expression.[247] These latter mutations are difficult to detect because they can be masked by the normal allele.[248] The nature of the intragenic mutations so far documented is quite striking, with more than 95 percent predicted to result in truncation of the APC protein (based on 176 mutations compiled in Nagase and Su[244]). The truncating mutations are largely the result of nonsense point mutations (33 percent) or small insertions (6 percent) and deletions (55 percent) that lead to frameshifts.[244] The majority of mutations occur in the first half of the last exon (Fig. 34-17). A few missense changes have been identified, but it is currently not known whether

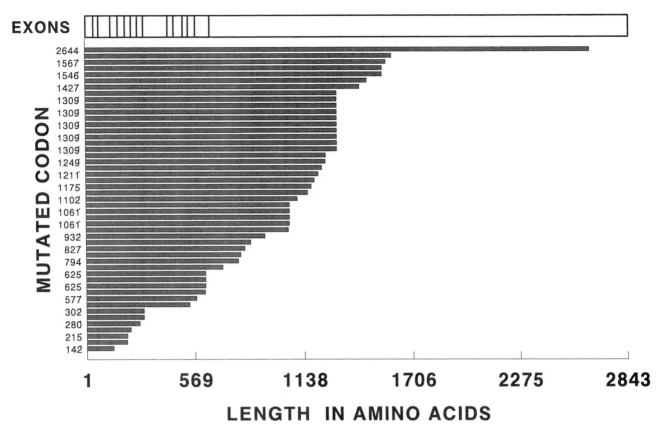

EXONS

MUTATED CODON

2644
1567
1546
1427
1309
1309
1309
1309
1309
1249
1211
1175
1102
1061
1061
932
827
794
625
625
577
302
280
215
142

LENGTH IN AMINO ACIDS

1   569   1138   1706   2275   2843

Fig. 34-17 Mutation of the *APC* gene in the germ line of FAP patients. Truncating *APC* mutations from 49 independent FAP kindreds are illustrated (Miyoshi et al.[423]). Four missense changes are not shown because it is not known whether they represent rare variants or true (functional) mutations. Lengths of bars indicate the region of *APC* translated until terminated by either a nonsense or frameshift mutation.

these missense changes are functional or merely represent rare variants; at least one has been shown not to segregate with the disease.[249]

The phenotypic manifestations of FAP vary considerably and in some cases can be correlated with a specific *APC* mutation (Fig. 34-18). For example, congenital hypertrophy of the retinal pigment epithelium (CHRPE) is associated with truncating mutations between codons 463 and 1387.[250-252] Truncating mutations between codon 1403 and 1578 are associated with increased extracolonic disease, particularly desmoid tumors and mandibular lesions, but patients with such mutations do not exhibit CHRPE.[252-254] Similarly, colonic manifestations have been shown to vary with the position of the mutation. Truncating mutations amino-terminal to codon 157[18] or at the extreme carboxyl-terminal end[255-259] are associated with an attenuated form of FAP in which patients develop a relatively small number of polyps (0–100). Some studies have suggested that mutations between codons 1250 and 1464 are associated with an increased number of colorectal tumors.[260,261] In contrast, patients with identical mutations can develop dissimilar clinical features. For example, some patients with identical truncating mutations develop features of GS (mandibular osteomas and desmoid tumors), whereas others do not.[240,262] Likewise, only a small number of patients within any kindred develop brain tumors, hepatoblastomas, or thyroid cancers, even though there is a clear predisposition to these tumors associated with germ-line *APC* mutations.[12,14]

APC's role in colorectal tumorigenesis is not limited to FAP; it also plays a critical role in the development of sporadic colorectal tumors.[263-265] It is estimated that at least 80 percent of colorectal tumors have somatic mutations of the *APC* gene.[263-265] The nature and distribution of somatic mutations identified in sporadic tumors resemble those observed in FAP patients (Fig. 34-19). Over 95 percent of the mutations are predicted to result in truncations of

the APC protein, due to either splice-site mutations (7 percent), nonsense mutations (40 percent), or insertions (12 percent) or deletions (41 percent) that lead to frameshifts (based on 75 mutations from Miyoshi et al.[263] and Powell et al.[264]). Two observations suggest that mutation of *APC* is an early, perhaps initiating event in sporadic colorectal tumorigenesis. First, the frequency of *APC* mutations is just as high in small benign tumors as in cancers.[50,263,264] This is in marked contrast to mutations of other genes (such as those in *RAS* or *p53*), which appear only as tumors progress. Second, mutations of *APC* have been found in the earliest sporadic lesions analyzed, including those as small as a few crypts (ACF).[50,266]

In addition to FAP and sporadic colorectal cancers, studies of *APC* in individuals with a modest predisposition to colorectal cancer revealed a novel mechanism for cancer predisposition. Genetic testing of an individual with multiple polyps and a family history of late-onset colorectal cancer revealed a missense substitution in codon 1307 (I1307K).[267] This change was present in approximately 6 percent of Ashkenazi Jews but rarely in the general population.[267-269] Among Ashkenazim, the I1307K allele was found to be more common in colorectal cancer patients and in individuals with a family history of colorectal cancer than in the Ashkenazi population at large.[267] In the families of I1307K colorectal cancer survivors, the I1307K allele was found to be associated with individuals with polyps or cancer in a highly nonrandom manner.[267,270] Together the preceding data suggested an increased risk (1.8-fold) for colorectal cancer for I1307K carriers. However, the mechanistic basis for this increased risk was unclear because previously only truncating mutations of *APC* had been shown to be disease-causing. This mechanism became clear, however, on analysis of the codon 1307 region in tumors. Sequencing of the *APC* gene in tumors from individuals with the I1307K variant revealed the presence of somatic truncating

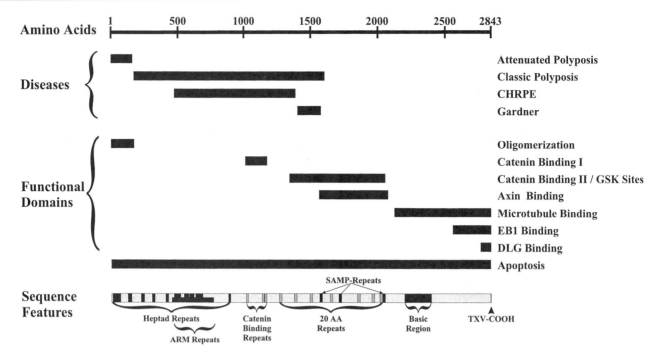

Fig. 34-18 Functional and disease-related domains of *APC*. Disease map: The location of truncating *APC* mutations has been shown to correlate with the extent of colonic and extracolonic manifestations. Truncating mutations prior to codon 157[18] or at the extreme C-terminal end[255–259] are associated with a reduced number of colorectal polyps, whereas the majority of mutations are associated with more pronounced polyposis and occur between codon 169 and 1600.[244] Mutations in codons 463 to 1387 are associated with congenital hypertrophy of the retinal pigment epithelium (CHRPE).[250–252] Mutations in codons 1403 to 1578 have been associated with an increased incidence of extracolonic manifestations.[252–254] Functional domains and sequence features: N-terminal residues 1 to 171 are sufficient for oligomerization.[287,288] This oligomerization is thought to be mediated by the heptad repeats.[238,241,287] APC binds to β-catenin through two motifs, the first comprising three 15-amino-acid repeats located between residues 1020 and 1169.[289,290] A second region, comprising seven 20-amino-acid repeats between residues 1324 and 2075,[241] binds to β-catenin and also acts as substrate for GSK phosphorylation.[293,310] Phosphorylation is thought to occur at SXXXS sites within the 20-amino-acid repeats.[293] Axin homologues bind to three SAMP repeats located between residues 1561 and 2057 of *APC*.[295] When transiently overexpressed, full-length APC decorates the microtubule cytoskeleton. The C-terminus of APC is required for this association, and residues 2130 to 2843 are sufficient.[265,301] Two proteins have been shown to associate with the C-terminus of APC. Residues 2560 to 2843 are sufficient to bind EB-1, a highly conserved 30-kDa protein of unknown function.[300] Residues 2771 to 2843 are sufficient to bind DLG, a human homologue of the *Drosophila* disk large tumor-suppressor gene[303]; the three C-terminal residues of APC (TXV) probably mediate this binding. Expression of full-length APC in colorectal cancer cell lines results in apoptosis, but the regions required for this activity have not been precisely defined.[285] Residues 453 to 767 contain 7 copies of a repeat consensus found in the *Drosophila* segment polarity gene product armadillo,[424] and residues 2200 to 2400 correspond to a basic region.[241] (*Modified with permission from Kinzler and Vogelstein.*[418])

mutations in the immediate vicinity of the codon 1307 change in 48 percent of the tumors.[267] Each of these somatic changes was found to affect the K allele of *APC* rather than the I allele. Taken together, these data suggest that the I1307K change predisposes to colorectal polyps and cancer by creating a premutation, i.e., a genomic region that is predisposed to subsequent somatic mutation. As expected with a mutation that causes only a 1.8-fold increase in risk, such risk increases are difficult to detect using standard epidemiologic methods in small samples of patients. However, several studies have documented an association with colorectal cancer consistent with a 1.5- to 2-fold increase.[267,268,271,272] Other studies could exclude a markedly increased risk but did not have the power to exclude or implicate a modest increase.[273–275] Given the difficulties associated with population studies, examination of the aforementioned somatic mutations may provide a better estimate of the increased risk associated with I1307K. Two studies of somatic mutations suggest that approximately 43 percent of the colorectal cancers that arise in I1307K carriers are attributed to the I1307 change.[267,276] If it is assumed that I1307K patients with colorectal cancer are representative of all I1307K individuals, this would translate to a relative risk of 1.7, in excellent agreement with the epidemiologic studies. The larger implications of the Ashkenazi work are that classic mutations in tumor-suppressor genes can lead to severe disease (like polyposis), while less obvious mutations in the same genes also can lead to milder predispositions to the same tumor types. Indeed,

other missense mutations of *APC* have been suggested to lead to colorectal cancer predisposition in the absence of polyposis.[271]

Evidence for an important role of *APC* in tumorigenesis has been supported by the study of mice with germ-line inactivation of the murine homologue of *APC* (*mAPC*). Three such mouse lineages have been reported, and all three have an increased risk for intestinal tumors.[277–279] The first and best described of these is the multiple intestinal neoplasia (Min) strain of mice.[280] The Min mouse was established from a C57BL/6J male mouse treated with ethylnitrosurea and bred for inherited traits. Min mice exhibit an autosomal dominantly inherited predisposition to multiple intestinal neoplasia and on a susceptible background develop an average of 30 to 50 intestinal tumors by the age of 90 days.[280,281] This phenotype is not exactly like that of FAP patients, since the mouse adenomas are largely found in the small intestine rather than in the colon, whereas the reverse is true in FAP patients. The Min phenotype was traced to a single nonsense mutation resulting in the truncation of mApc protein at codon 850.[277] Similar phenotypes to Min are observed in mouse lineages derived by homologous recombination to specifically inactivate *mAPC*.[278,279] The nature of the mutations in all these mice is similar to those observed in the germ line of FAP patients, making these mice good models of FAP at both the phenotypic and genotypic levels. Furthermore, because these mouse models share at least one important genetic defect with sporadic human colorectal tumors, they may prove to be a good model for colorectal tumorigenesis in general.

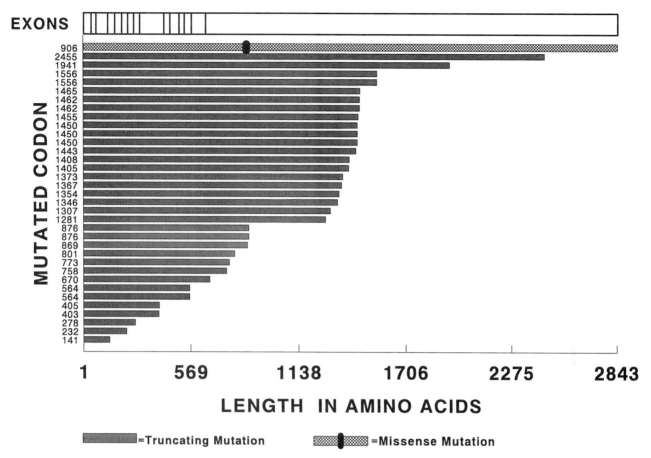

Fig. 34-19 Somatic *APC* mutations in sporadic colorectal tumors. Thirty-five *APC* mutations from 16 adenomas and 26 carcinomas are illustrated (Powell et al.[264]). Lengths of bars indicate the region of *APC* translated until terminated by either a nonsense or frameshift mutation. Cross bar indicates the location of the single somatic missense mutation identified.

Do both copies of the *APC* gene need to be inactivated for it to exert its affect on tumor development, as Knudson's tumor-suppressor gene model would suggest? Studies of *APC* mutations in primary sporadic colorectal tumors suggest that at least a third of both benign and malignant tumors have no normally functioning *APC* gene.[263,264] Studies of primary tumors from FAP patients identify a second inactivating mutation in about 80 percent of the tumors. Both these studies undoubtedly represent underestimates of the true extent of inactivation of both alleles due to the difficulties in analyzing primary human tumors. However, studies of APC protein in colorectal cancer cell lines indicate that most (26 of 32) were totally devoid of full-length APC protein.[265] Similarly, inactivation of both alleles of the *mAPC* gene occurs almost without exception in Min tumors and can be detected in lesions so small that they can only be observed at the microscopic level.[282,283] Together these data strongly suggest that both copies of *APC* must be inactivated during tumorigenesis. This notion is further supported by the rapid development of adenomas after disruption the *Apc* gene in mice with conditional targeting of the *Apc* locus.[284]

What is APC's normal function that is so critical to prevention of intestinal tumor development? Expression of wild-type APC in colorectal epithelial cells with *APC* mutations results in apoptosis, suggesting that APC may control the cell death process.[285] Immunohistochemical analysis indicates that APC protein is apparently located at the basolateral membrane in colorectal epithelial cells, with expression increasing as cells migrate to the top of the crypt.[265,286] Since loss of cells from the top of crypts is an important homeostatic process in the colon, it is easy to imagine how disruption of such a "death signal" could lead to neoplasia.

The primary structure of APC provides few clues as to how it might mediate such functions (see Fig. 34-18). Residues 453 to 767 contain seven copies of repeat consensus found in the *Drosophila* segment polarity gene *armadillo*. The amino-terminal third of *APC* contains several heptad repeats of the type that mediate oligomerization by a coiled-coil structure.[287,288] These regions may mediate homo-oligomerization between mutant and wild-type proteins and could theoretically cause a dominant negative effect, although no such effect has been demonstrated biologically. In addition, seven 20-amino-acid repeats have been identified between residues 1324 and 2075.[241]

Although the preceding sequence features have provided some insights into the function of APC, the identification of proteins that interact with APC has yielded even more tantalizing clues. To date, over a half dozen APC protein interactions have been described, including β-catenin,[289,290] γ-catenin,[291,292] GSK-3β,[293] AXIN family proteins,[294–299] EB-1,[300] microtubules,[301,302] and hDLG.[303] Two of these proteins, EB-1 and hDLG, bind to the C-terminus of APC. *EB-1* encodes a highly conserved 30-kDa protein[300] that is associated with cytoplasmic and spindle microtubules.[304] In yeast, an *EB-1* homologue is required for a cytokinesis checkpoint.[305] The second C-terminal interacting gene product is the human homologue of the *Drosophila* tumor-suppressor gene disks large (*DLG*).[303] Since virtually all *APC* mutations result in loss of the C-terminus of the APC protein (see Figs. 34-17 and 34-19), these data suggest that hDLG and/or EB-1 may be essential for APC's growth-controlling function.

The most penetrating insights into APC function have come from studies of the interaction between β-catenin and APC.[289,290] The central third of APC contains two classes of β-catenin–binding repeats, one of which is modulated by phosphorylation[293]

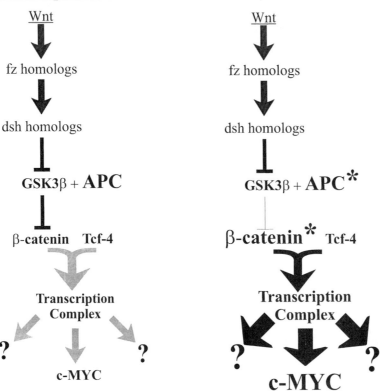

Fig. 34-20 The Wg/Wnt pathway ultimately results in β-catenin/Tcf–mediated transcription. APC cooperates with GSK-3β to degrade β-catenin and inhibit β-catenin/Tcf–mediated transcription. Inactivating mutations of APC or activating mutations of β-catenin can alleviate this inhibition resulting in increased transcription of growth promoting genes. One of these growth-promoting genes is *c-MYC*. See the text for additional detail.

(see Fig. 34-18). Although many mutant APC proteins retain some β-catenin binding, virtually all mutant APC proteins lack at least one type of β-catenin–binding repeat.

The β-catenin association links APC to two apparently diverse cellular processes. The first process is related to cellular adhesion. The catenins originally were identified as cytoplasmic proteins that bind to cadherins, a family of calcium-dependent homophilic cell adhesion molecules. Several studies have indicated that β-catenin is necessary for cadherin-mediated cell adhesion.[306] Given that binding of β-catenin to cadherins or to APC is mutually exclusive, it is possible that APC could modulate such adhesion as part of its tumor-suppressing function. APC additionally could act as a downstream communicator of adhesion status, linking cadherin-catenin complexes to other cellular components.

The second process involving APC has been elucidated by studies of the wingless (Wg) and Wnt signaling pathways in *Drosophila, Xenopus,* and mouse. β-*Catenin* and *armadillo* (the *Drosophila* homologue of β-*catenin*) have been firmly implicated as signal transducers in these pathways.[307–309] This link was fortified by the observation that the APC-β-catenin complex is physically associated with a second member of this pathway, the ZW3/GSK3β protein kinase.[293] Moreover, this kinase was found to promote β-catenin binding to APC, presumably by phosphorylation of APC class II binding sites[293] (see Fig. 34-18). The functional consequence of this binding is the ubiquitin-dependent proteosomal degradation of β-catenin.[310–312] Consistent with this, epistasis evaluations in *Drosophila* suggest that Wg signaling inhibits ZW3 function and that active ZW3 can inhibit β-catenin signaling. Finally, studies in *Xenopus* and mouse suggest that Wnt signaling ultimately results in formation of a heteromeric complex containing β-catenin and members of the Tcf/Lef family of HMG box transcription factors.[313,314] Taken together, these observations suggest that APC works in concert with ZW3/GSK3β to inhibit β-catenin–induced transcription. Given that this pathway had been implicated previously in neoplasia by the ability of truncated β-catenin to transform cells in culture[315] and the involvement of Wnt signaling in breast tumorigenesis in mice,[16] it was plausible

that the β-catenin–APC interaction contributed to the tumor-suppressive function of APC. Further analysis of this pathway in colorectal cancers provided strong support for this notion.[317,318] Constitutive activity of this pathway as measured by β-catenin/Tcf–mediated transcription was elevated in colorectal cancer cell lines but not in cancer cell lines from other organs, and wild-type APC could specifically down-regulate this activity when transfected into appropriate reporter cells. Furthermore, APC mutants derived from colon cancers and FAP patients were deficient in this down-regulating activity. Compelling evidence for the importance of β-catenin came from the study of the rare tumors that lacked APC mutations. Approximately half these tumors possessed β-catenin mutations in the N-terminal regulatory domain.[318–321,322] These mutations render β-catenin superactive and relatively resistant to the effects of APC.[318] These findings strongly suggest that excess β-catenin/Tcf signaling contributes to colorectal tumorigenesis (Fig. 34-20). In the majority of cancers, this is achieved by mutations of the *APC* gene that prevent its inhibition of β-catenin. In a significant fraction of the remaining tumors, this is achieved by dominant activating β-catenin mutations that render the protein insensitive to APC/GSK-3β–mediated degradation. Similar oncogenic mutations of β-catenin have been observed in other human[323–328] and rodent[324,329,330] cancers. These observations led to the prediction that the increased β-catenin/Tcf–mediated transcription ultimately results in expression of genes that promote cell growth or inhibit cell death (see Fig. 34-20). This expectation was confirmed recently by identification of the *c-MYC* oncogene as a direct downstream target of β-catenin/Tcf–mediated transcription.[331] Interestingly, this observation is consistent with previous studies that indicated that restoration of chromosome 5 to colorectal cancer cells was associated with a decrease in c-MYC expression.[332] Other β-catenin/Tcf downstream targets have also been identified.[332a,332b,332c,332d,332e] Whether all of APC tumor-suppressive effects are related to inhibition of β-catenin/Tcf–mediated transcription remains to be determined. In this regard, it is interesting to note that mice with transgenic expression of activated β-catenin in their intestinal epithelial cells did not develop intestinal tumors but did show abnormal intestinal cell homeostasis.[333] More strikingly, mice engineered to allow Cre-mediated deletion of β-catenin exon 3 did develop adenomatous intestinal polyps resembling those observed in Apc (Δ716) knock out mouse when crossed with mice expressing Cre recombinase.[333a] Likewise, mice with transgenic expression of an activated β-catenin in their keratinocytes underwent *de novo* hair follicle morphogenesis but also developed hair follicle tumors.[334] Mice engineered to lack Tcf-4 by homologous recombination showed depletion of intestinal epithelial stem cell compartment.[335] Thus β-catenin/Tcf signaling plays a critical role in regulation of epithelial cell homeostasis, and loss of regulation of this pathway by APC contributes to neoplastic transformation of several cell types. Why germ-line *APC* mutations lead largely to colorectal neoplasia, rather than to more widespread tumorigenesis, remains a mystery. An APC homologue (APCL) that shares APC's ability to interact with β-catenin has been described recently.[336,337] It will be interesting to determine whether APCL functions like APC in noncolonic tissues, with the resulting redundancy perhaps explaining the cell type specificity of APC tumorigenesis.

Other Genetic Changes

MCC. During the search for the gene responsible for FAP, a second gene from chromosome 5q21 was identified that was somatically mutated in sporadic colorectal cancers.[338] The *MCC* gene, for *mutated in colorectal cancer,* is located less than 250 kb away from the *APC* gene[238,239,339] and was chosen for further study because Southern blot analysis revealed a colon carcinoma with a somatic rearrangement. The *MCC* gene transcript contains a 2511-bp open reading frame that is distributed over 17 exons. Detailed analysis of all 17 coding exons identified specific point mutations in 6 of 90 colorectal carcinomas examined. All 6 mutations were predicted to alter the MCC protein either by amino acid substitution or by altered splicing. However, it is unlikely that mutations of *MCC* play a major role in the development of colorectal cancer.[338,340] Comparison of *MCC* with *APC* reveals some interesting similarities in addition to their proximity in the genome. Although the significance of *MCC* mutations in colorectal tumors is not clear, these similarities raise the possibility that *MCC* and *APC* may function along the same pathway.

Gene Amplification. The specific amplification of a small region of the genome (gene amplification) frequently activates oncogenes in some tumor types. One indication of gene amplification is the cytogenetic observation of double-minute chromosomes. These chromosomes are known to harbor amplified sequences. Although double-minute chromosomes have been reported in a significant fraction of primary colorectal cancers,[341] amplification of specific, well-characterized genes has been described rarely in colon cancers. Isolated cases of *c-MYB*,[342] *c-MYC*,[343–346] *NEU*,[345,347,348] and *cyclin*[349] gene amplification have been reported. It is notable that those few colorectal cancers with demonstrable gene amplification are indistinguishable from other colorectal cancers in histology and behavior. It is likely that amplification of these genes, as well as additional (as yet unidentified) oncogenes, contributes to tumor progression, especially at late stages. More recently, it has been reported that *aurora*[350,351] and *Fas decoy*[352] genes are amplified in a subset of colorectal tumors. Although these reports are certainly intriguing, it is often difficult to distinguish true amplification from chromosome imbalance by the techniques used in these studies. Confirmation of the specific amplification of these genes with other techniques and documentation of the importance of these amplifications in colorectal tumorigenesis are eagerly awaited.

Modifying Loci. The existence of genetic loci that modify the risk for colorectal cancer has long been suspected but has been difficult to prove in humans. However, the Min model provides a clear-cut example of a modifying locus in mice. Depending on the inbred mouse strain harboring this mutation, the number of polyps varies significantly.[281] Linkage analysis has demonstrated that a single locus (*MOM1,* for *modifier of Min*) on mouse chromosome 4 accounts for much of this difference between strains.[353] Recently, the *MOM1* gene has been identified as that encoding secreted phospholipase A2 (sPLA2).[354,355] Unfortunately, studies of sPLA2 in humans suggest that it is not a major modifier of colorectal cancer risk.[356]

Gene Expression

One of the most difficult issues in cancer research involves the evaluation of gene expression. Although the expression of numerous genes is different in tumor cells than in normal cells, the significance of these differences is uncertain. For example, the expression of various oncogenes, particularly *c-MYC*,[346,357] a variety of mucins,[358] growth factors and their receptors,[347,359,360] carcinoembryonic antigens,[361] cell surface glycoproteins,[362,363] and enzymes involved in DNA replication and cell division[364] are increased in neoplastic colon cells. Whether these increases in expression drive the process of tumorigenesis or are simply the *result* of the abnormal growth or microenvironment of cancer is impossible to determine at present. Some of the abnormally expressed gene products are likely to play an important role in mediating the biologic effects of the mutant genes discussed in this chapter. Recent results linking *c-MYC* expression to *APC* mutation provide an excellent example of this principle.[331] Other changes in gene expression are likely to be insignificant with regard to pathogenesis. The advent of several new technologies for the analysis of gene expression hopefully will lead to advances in this important area.[365–368] Indeed, using just one of these new approaches,[367] it was possible to analyze over 300,000 transcripts from human cancer cells and identify hundreds of genes that were differentially expressed between normal and tumor tissue.[369] While a complete understanding of the behavior of a neoplastic cell will require a full knowledge of these differentially expressed genes, their large numbers and inherent complexity illustrate why the study of genetic alterations has been so useful.

Methylation

The only known covalent modification of DNA in normal mammalian cells occurs at the fifth position of cytosine at 5′-CG-3′ dinucleotides. In most somatic cells, 80 percent of these dinucleotides are methylated, and such methylation has been implicated in the control of gene expression and chromosome condensation.[370] In cancer cells, a generalized hypomethylation of the genome occurs relatively early during colorectal tumorigenesis and can be observed even in small adenomas.[371,372] Hypermethylation of specific 5′-CG-3′–rich sites also occurs.[373] The causes and effects of these methylation differences are not understood. Hypomethylation is not likely due to the underexpression of methylase activity, because such activity is not decreased in tumors.[374] Changes in methylation of genes, unlike the mutations of genes noted earlier, are not clonal changes in that any specific 5′-CG-3′dinucleotide is methylated differently in only a fraction of the tumor cell population. Nevertheless, these changes could have significant effects on tumor cell biology. For example, decreased methylation could in part allow expression of genes that normally should be silent, such as those required for cellular invasion (proteinases) or growth at metastatic sites (cell surface receptors for growth factors or extracellular matrices). Additionally, it has been demonstrated experimentally that reduced methylation of DNA can lead to aberrant chromosome condensation and adherence of the decondensed regions to one another.[375] This, in turn, could result in abnormal chromosome segregation, particularly chromosome loss, which, as noted earlier, is one of the most common mechanisms for inactivating tumor-suppressor genes. Conversely, increased methylation could lead to silencing of genes important for growth suppression. Indeed, methylation changes have been implicated in the silencing of the *hMLH1* DNA mismatch repair gene in tumors with mismatch repair deficiency[376] and in silencing of the *p16* tumor-suppressor gene in colorectal cancers in general.[377,378] The evidence implicating methylation in colorectal tumorigenesis is not limited to the methylation changes observed in tumors but also includes direct experimental evidence. For example, the hypermethylation of *hMLH1* can be reversed with the demethylating agent 5-aza-cytidine, leading to expression of *hMLH1* and reconstitution of mismatch repair activity.[376] Treatment of cells with 5-aza-cytidine has been shown to be oncogenic *in vitro* and *in vivo*, suggesting a proneoplastic role of decreased methylation *in vivo*.[379] On the other hand, mice with a genetic deficiency for methyltransferase are resistant to intestinal tumors resulting from *mAPC* mutations, and this resistance is potentiated by 5-aza-cytidine.[380] While the evidence implicating methylation changes in tumorigenesis continues to mount, additional studies will be necessary to clarify the significance of these changes and the mechanisms responsible for the differences between methylation in normal and neoplastic cells.

A Genetic Model for Colorectal Tumorigenesis

In molecular terms, the process of colorectal tumor evolution represents the acquisition of sequential mutations[381,382] (Fig. 34-21). Mutations in *APC* seem to be required to initiate the adenomatous process, resulting in the clonal growth of a single cell. In most cases, it appears that inactivation of both alleles of *APC* is both necessary and sufficient for tumor initiation. In rare cases, mutations of β-catenin can substitute for *APC* mutations.[381,382] A small polyp that results from these initial mutations may remain dormant for decades. Eventually, however, one of the cells of this small tumor acquires an additional mutation (often in the *K-RAS* gene), allowing it to overgrow its sister cells and resulting in a larger tumor. Subsequent waves of clonal expansion are driven by further mutations in other genes [particularly the 18q tumor suppressor(s) and *p53*], and along with this expansion comes further dysplasia. When a cell has acquired sufficient mutations (generally affecting at least four genes), it acquires the ability to invade and metastasize and is observed clinically as a malignancy.

There are several points worth noting about the preceding model. First, not every tumor needs to acquire each of the mutations indicated. For example, only half of all colorectal cancers have *RAS* mutations. It is likely that other yet unidentified mutated genes can substitute for *RAS* mutations. Second, it is likely that other genetic events are required for cancer development. Even so, this model predicts that at least seven genetic events (i.e., one oncogene mutation and six mutations to inactivate three tumor-suppressor genes) typically are required for a cancer to develop. Finally, the order of mutations can have a significant impact on tumorigenic process. For example, as noted earlier, nondysplastic ACF with *RAS* gene mutations are remarkably common.[49,50] However, these cells, unlike their dysplastic *APC*

mutant counterparts, appear to have little or no potential to form clinically important tumors. Similarly, patients with germ-line mutations of *p53* do not develop polyposis[383] despite that fact that *p53* mutations occur in over 80 percent of colorectal cancers.[73] Therefore, although it is clear that *p53* can play a role in colorectal tumorigenesis, it is equally clear that it cannot initiate the process in a fashion similar to *APC*. Thus it appears that it is not simply the accumulation of mutations but rather also their order that determines the propensity for neoplasia and that only a subset of the genes that can affect cell growth actually can initiate the neoplastic process. This subset of tumor-suppressor genes has been deemed *gatekeepers*.[384]

It is notable that the genes identified in colorectal tumors affect almost all the cellular compartments (i.e., *RAS* at the inner surface of the cell membrane, *APC* in the cytoplasm, and *p53* in the nucleus). This suggests that human cells have evolved several levels of cellular protection against neoplasia and that many of these protective mechanisms must be disassembled before cancer can fully develop. Even at the malignant stage, however, the tumor continues to evolve, developing subclones with varying degrees of aneuploidy, drug or radiation resistance, and metastatic capability. This whole process, from appearance of a tiny adenomatous tumor to invasion by a carcinoma, takes 20 to 40 years, perhaps reflecting the time required to sequentially mutate the relevant genes and generate clonal expansions.

It has long been suspected that this accumulation of genetic changes may be facilitated by genetic instability.[385–387] In the case of colorectal cancer, tangible proof of this premise came with the identification of defects in DNA mismatch repair in HNPCC patients (see Chap. 18) and in a subset of sporadic colorectal cancers.[388–390] These tumors display an increased rate of small intragenic mutations[391] that can drive the neoplastic process. However, defects in DNA mismatch repair occur in only about 13 percent of all colorectal cancers.[388–390] Recently, there has been growing evidence of a genetic instability that operates in the remaining colorectal cancers. *Aneuploidy,* defined as an abnormal complement of chromosomes, is a classic characteristic of most solid tumors. Until recently, it was not clear whether an abnormal karyotype was the result of a true genetic instability. In this regard, it is interesting to note that cancers with instability due to a defect in DNA mismatch repair generally have a normal karyotype, whereas the remaining cancers are generally aneuploid. Careful measurement of chromosomal losses in colorectal cancer cell lines revealed that aneuploid lines had a persistent and marked increase in chromosomal gains and losses compared with diploid lines.[392] This instability was termed a *chromosomal instability* (CIN) and could be transferred in a dominant manner in cell fusion experiments.[392] Subsequent studies showed that the CIN phenotype was associated with functional defects of mitotic checkpoints.[393] In a small fraction of colorectal cancers, somatic mutations of the mitotic checkpoint gene *BUB1* probably account

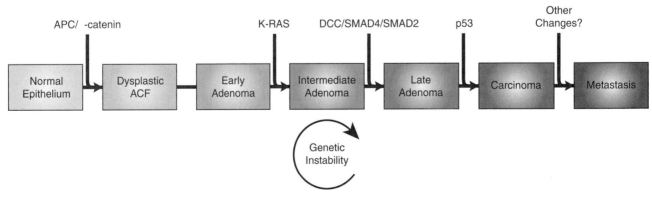

Fig. 34-21 T > A genetic model for colorectal tumorigenesis. See text for explanation. (*Modified with permission from Fearon and Vogelstein.*[381])

for the mitotic checkpoint defect and resulting CIN.[393] Thus it appears that most colorectal cancers possess some form of genetic instability that drives the neoplastic process (see Fig. 34-21). In a minority of cancers, this instability is due to a defect in DNA mismatch repair and results in an increased rate of small intragenic mutations. In the majority of cancers, a chromosomal instability exists that manifests as losses and gains of whole chromosomes or large chromosomal regions. The subset of tumor-suppressor genes that prevents such genetic instabilities has been deemed *caretakers*.[384] Although in a few cases CIN can be traced to defects in a specific gene, the genetic basis of CIN is unknown in the great majority of cases, providing a significant challenge for future research.[394]

This chapter has focused on gene alterations that contribute to the neoplastic process in a direct and cell autonomous manner. Mutations of *APC* (gatekeeper) or DNA mismatch repair genes (caretakers) are examples of such alterations that can result in highly penetrant predispositions to colorectal cancer. The third category of predispositions results from *landscaper* defects. Landscaper defects do not directly affect cancer cell growth but contribute to an abnormal stromal environment that contributes to the neoplastic transformation of the overlying epithelium. The cancer predispositions associated with such landscapers would be expected to be weaker than that observed with a gatekeeper such as *APC*. The increased risk of colorectal cancer observed in JPS and perhaps also inPeutz-Jeghers syndrome, characterized by the intestinal hamartomatous polyps, may be the result of landscaper defects. In the lesions associated with these syndromes, the epithelium does not initially show any neoplastic changes, but rather it is the underlying mesenchymal tissue that appears to be affected. This abnormal mesenchymal growth may create a microenvironment that facilitates that neoplastic transformation of the overlying epithelium. However, because both genes (*PTEN*[395,396] and *SMAD4*[193]) that have been implicated in this pathway can directly affect growth of epithelial cells as well, additional studies will be necessary to distinguish a weak gatekeeper effect from a landscaper effect.

PROSPECTUS

Despite the advances made in understanding the genetics of colorectal tumorigenesis, many questions remain unanswered. First, other chromosomes besides 5q, 17p, and 18q are lost in subsets of colorectal cancers. The identification of the culprit genes on these chromosomes has not been accomplished. It is unclear whether these other genes are simply responsible for the evolution of tumor heterogeneity at late stages of the process or play a more fundamental role in tumorigenesis. Second, about one-half of all colorectal tumors develop without a *RAS* mutation, and a small fraction of tumors apparently do not have abnormalities of *p53* or *APC/β-catenin*. The mechanism that allows such alterations to be bypassed could prove to be very important. Perhaps such tumors develop mutations of other genes in the same pathway that have the same physiologic effects. Third, the biochemical and physiologic functions of oncogenes and tumor-suppressor genes have yet to be fully worked out in cells *in vitro*, much less in the complex environment that exists in tissues *in vivo*. Finally, inherited genetic factors affecting colon cancer risk in the general population have yet to be defined.

Diagnosis

One of the first benefits derived from the study of colorectal cancer genetics is improved diagnosis. Already, knowledge of the genetic bases for FAP and HNPCC is allowing presymptomatic diagnosis in affected families (see Chap. 39). Demonstration that an individual member of such a family has not inherited the disease can have significant impact, reducing the discomfort and expense of repeated medial examinations as well as the anxiety associated with disease expectation. Genetic diagnosis also could be performed *in utero*, although substantial ethical questions are inherent in

such diagnoses when the relevant disease is not necessarily lethal and when mortality, if it occurs at all, is delayed until adulthood. Presymptomatic testing also will have significant clinical implications with the advent of pharmacologic intervention for the possible prevention of polyposis in FAP patients (see below).

Specific gene mutations also may be used as the basis of a very specific test for presymptomatic diagnosis of colorectal tumors in the general population. Tumor cells shed into the stool can be identified by the presence of their mutant *RAS* genes in DNA isolated from stool samples.[397–401] Mutant genes were detected in stool from patients with benign as well as malignant tumors and could be observed in relatively small tumors as well as large ones. Application of this strategy to other mutations known to occur in colorectal tumors could significantly improve the applicability of this test. Numerous additional studies of course will be required to determine whether such assays will lead to improved detection of colorectal neoplasia in a cost-effective manner.

The analysis of genetic changes in colorectal cancers also has been shown to have prognostic value.[175] While *RAS* oncogene mutations and chromosome 5q losses do not show any prognostic utility, chromosome 17p and 18q losses each provide independent prognostic information. Chromosome 17p and 18q losses are associated with distant metastases and poorer prognosis.[175–177,188–191] This analysis represents the first step in the application of molecular genetics to the management of colorectal cancer patients. In the future, one can imagine that the choice of chemotherapeutic regimen will depend on the specific genetic changes present in the patient's tumor.

PREVENTION AND TREATMENT

One of the most important purposes of studying colorectal tumorigenesis lies in the hope that this will lead to better treatment and/or prevention of the disease. The notion that more effective drugs to treat colorectal tumors can be developed is furthered by the apparent success of some conventional drug treatments. Several studies have indicated that the nonsteroidal anti-inflammatory drug (NSAID) sulindac can cause tumor regression in FAP patients.[402–409] Hope that such treatment may prove useful for the general public comes from epidemiologic studies of colon cancer in aspirin users.[410–412] Many of these studies have shown that the use of aspirin, another NSAID, is associated with a reduced colon cancer death risk. Evaluation of these and other drugs may be greatly facilitated by testing in Min mice. Indeed, several studies have already demonstrated the ability of NSAIDs to reduce the incidence of intestinal tumors in the Min mouse.[413–415] Ultimately, it is hoped that the study of cancer genes and their biologic consequences will lead to the knowledge-based development of much more specific and effective chemopreventive and chemotherapeutic agents. In this regard, the identification of specific genetic alterations that commonly underlie human cancers has yielded considerable excitement because it is clear that such changes provide targets that are unique to the cancer cell. However, most of these mutations result in loss of function of a tumor-suppressor gene. Restoration of such function represents a formidable therapeutic challenge because most commonly used drugs are designed to inhibit an activity rather than replace the function of a protein. Fortunately, detailed studies of the tumor-suppressive pathway often reveal consequences of mutations that are more readily targeted. For example, while it is hard to imagine a small drug replacing the function of the 300-kDa APC protein, it is easy to conceive of a drug that inhibits the elevated β-catenin/ Tcf–mediated transcription that results from inactivation of APC. Likewise, it is also simple to imagine the development of agents that exploit the checkpoint defects that arise from mutations in *p53* or are associated with the CIN phenotype.[140,394,416] Future and ongoing studies undoubtedly will provide additional targets for therapeutic intervention.

REFERENCES

1. *Cancer Facts & Figures 1998.* Atlanta, American Cancer Society, 1998.
2. Beart RW: Colorectal cancer, in Holleb AI, Fink DJ, Murphy GP (eds): *American Cancer Society Textbook of Clinical Oncology.* Atlanta, American Cancer Society, 1991, pp 213-218.
3. Cohen AM, Shank B, Friedman MA: Colorectal cancer, in De Vita V, Hellman S, Rosenberg S (eds): *Cancer: Principles and Practice of Oncology.* Philadelphia, Lippincott, 1989, p 895.
4. Ransohoff D, Lang C: Screening for colorectal cancer. *N Engl J Med* **325**:37, 1991.
5. Jass JR, Stewart SM: Evolution of hereditary non-polyposis colorectal cancer. *Gut* **33**:783, 1992.
6. Lieberman D: Cost-effectiveness of colon cancer screening. *Am J Gastroenterol* **86**:1789, 1991.
7. Lipkin M, Bell B, Shelrock P: Cell proliferation kinetics in the gastrointestinal tract of man. *J Clin Invest* **42**:767, 1963.
8. Shorter RG, Moertel CG, Titus JL, Reitemeier RJ: Cell kinetics of in the jejunum and rectum of man. *Am J Dig Dis* **9**:760, 1964.
9. Kent TH, Mitros FA: Polyps of the colon and small bowel, polyp syndromes, and the polyp-carcinoma sequence, in Norris HT (eds): *Pathology of the Colon, Small Intestine, and Anus,* Vol 2. New York, Churchill-Livingstone, 1983, p 167.
10. Cooper HS: Carcinoma of the colon and rectum, in Norris HT (eds): *Pathology of the Colon, Small Intestine and Anus,* Vol 2. New York, Churchill-Livingstone, 1983, p 201.
11. Stryker SJ, Wolff BG, Culp CE, Libbe SD, Ilstrup DM, MacCarty RL: Natural history of untreated colonic polyps. *Gastroenterology* **93**:1009, 1987.
12. Giardiello FM: Gastrointestinal polyposis sydromes and hereditary nonpolyposis colorectal cancer, in Rustgi AK (eds) *Gastrointestinal Cancers: Biology, Diagnosis, and Therapy.* Philadelphia, Lippincott-Raven, 1995, pp 367–377.
13. Bussey HJ, Veale AM, Morson BC: Genetics of gastrointestinal polyposis. *Gastroenterology* **74**:1325, 1978.
14. Hamilton SR, Liu B, Parsons RE, et al: The molecular basis of Turcot's syndrome. *N Engl J Med* **332**:839, 1995.
15. Gardner E, Richards R: Multiple cutaneous and subcutaneous lesions occurring simultaneously with hereditary polyposis and osteomatosis. *Am J Hum Genet* **5**:139, 1953.
16. Bulow S: Extracolonic manifestations of familial adenomatous polyposis, in Herrera L (eds): *Familial Adenomatous Polyposis.* New York, Alan R Liss, 1990, p 109.
17. Spirio L, Otterud B, Stauffer D, et al: Linkage of a variant or attenuated form of adenomatous polyposis coli to the adenomatous polyposis coli (*APC*) locus. *Am J Hum Genet* **51**:92, 1992.
18. Spirio L, Olschwang S, Groden J, et al: Alleles of the *APC* gene: An attenuated form of familial polyposis. *Cell* **75**:951, 1993.
19. Ponz de Leon M, Sassatelli R, Benatti P, Roncucci L: Identification of hereditary nonpolyposis colorectal cancer in the general population: The 6-year experience of a population-based registry. *Cancer* **71**:3493, 1993.
20. Lynch HT, Smyrk T, Jass JR: Hereditary nonpolyposis colorectal cancer and colonic adenomas: Aggressive adenomas? *Semin Surg Oncol* **11**:406, 1995.
21. Lynch HT, Smyrk T, Lynch JF: Overview of natural history, pathology, molecular genetics and management of HNPCC (Lynch syndrome). *Int J Cancer* **69**:38, 1996.
22. Burt RW, Bishop DT, Cannon LA, Dowdle MA, Lee RG, Skolnick MH: Dominant inheritance of adenomatous colonic polyps and colorectal cancer. *N Engl J Med* **312**:1540, 1985.
23. Cannon-Albright LA, Skolnick MH, Bishop DT, Lee RG, Burt RW: Common inheritance of susceptibility to colonic adenomatous polyps and associated colorectal cancers. *N Engl J Med* **319**:533, 1988.
24. Houlston RS, Collins A, Slack J, Morton NE: Dominant genes for colorectal cancer are not rare. *Ann Hum Genet* **56**:99, 1992.
25. Willett W: The search for the causes of breast and colon cancer. *Nature* **338**:389, 1989.
26. Haenszel W, Kurihara M: Studies of Japanese migrants: I. Mortality from cancer and other diseases among Japanese in the United States. *J Natl Cancer Inst* **40**:43, 1968.
27. Lee JA: Recent trends of large bowel cancer in Japan compared to United States and England and Wales. *Int J Epidemiol* **5**:187, 1976.
28. Armstrong B, Doll R: Environmental factors and cancer incidence and mortality in different countries, with special reference to dietary practices. *Int J Cancer* **15**:617, 1975.
29. Pickle LW, Greene MH, Ziegler RG, et al: Colorectal cancer in rural Nebraska. *Cancer Res* **44**:363, 1984.
30. Willett WC, Stampfer MJ, Colditz GA, Rosner BA, Speizer FE: Relation of meat, fat, and fiber intake to the risk of colon cancer in a prospective study among women. *N Engl J Med* **323**:1664, 1990.
31. Burkitt DP: Epidemiology of cancer of the colon and rectum. *Cancer* **28**:3, 1971.
32. Bingham S, Williams DR, Cole TJ, James WP: Dietary fibre and regional large-bowel cancer mortality in Britain. *Br J Cancer* **40**:456, 1979.
33. Nowell PC: The clonal evolution of tumor cell populations. *Science* **194**:23, 1976.
34. Vogelstein B, Fearon ER, Hamilton SR, Feinberg AP: Use of restriction fragment length polymorphisms to determine the clonal origin of human tumors. *Science* **227**:642, 1985.
35. Vogelstein B, Fearon ER, Hamilton SR, et al: Clonal analysis using recombinant DNA probes from the X-chromosome. *Cancer Res* **47**:4806, 1987.
36. Fearon ER, Hamilton SR, Vogelstein B: Clonal analysis of human colorectal tumors. *Science* **238**:193, 1987.
37. Martin P, Levin B, Golomb HM, Riddell RH: Chromosome analysis of primary large bowel tumors: A new method for improving the yield of analyzable metaphases. *Cancer* **44**:1656, 1979.
38. Reichmann A, Martin P, Levin B: Chromosomal banding patterns in human large bowel cancer. *Int J Cancer* **28**:431, 1981.
39. Muleris M, Salmon RJ, Zafrani B, Girodet J, Dutrillaux B: Consistent deficiencies of chromosome 18 and of the short arm of chromosome 17 in eleven cases of human large bowel cancer: A possible recessive determinism. *Ann Genet* **28**:206, 1985.
40. Mark J, Mitelman F, Dencker H, Norryd C, Tranberg KG: The specificity of the chromosomal abnormalities in human colonic polyps: A cytogenetic study of multiple polyps in a case of Gardner's syndrome. *Acta Pathol Microbiol Scand [A]* **81**:85, 1973.
41. Mitelman F, Mark J, Nilsson PG, Dencker H, Norryd C, Tranberg KG: Chromosome banding pattern in human colonic polyps. *Hereditas* **78**:63, 1974.
42. Reichmann A, Martin P, Levin B: Chromosomal banding patterns in human large bowel adenomas. *Hum Genet* **70**:28, 1985.
43. Bos JL, Fearon ER, Hamilton SR, et al: Prevalence of ras gene mutations in human colorectal cancers. *Nature* **327**:293, 1987.
44. Forrester K, Almoguera C, Han K, Grizzle WE, Perucho M: Detection of high incidence of *K-ras* oncogenes during human colon tumorigenesis. *Nature* **327**:298, 1987.
45. Vogelstein B, Fearon ER, Hamilton SR, et al: Genetic alterations during colorectal-tumor development. *N Engl J Med* **319**:525, 1988.
46. Bishop JM: Molecular themes in oncogenesis. *Cell* **64**:235, 1991.
47. Weinberg RA: Oncogenes and tumor suppressor genes. *CA Cancer J Clin* **44**:160, 1994.
48. Shibata D, Schaeffer J, Li ZH, Capella G, Perucho M: Genetic heterogeneity of the c-K-ras locus in colorectal adenomas but not in adenocarcinomas. *J Natl Cancer Inst* **85**:1058, 1993.
49. Pretlow TP, Brasitus TA, Fulton NC, Cheyer C, Kaplan EL: K-ras mutations in putative preneoplastic lesions in human colon. *J Natl Cancer Inst* **85**:2004, 1993.
50. Jen J, Powell SM, Papadopoulos N, et al: Molecular determinants of dysplasia in colorectal lesions. *Cancer Res* **54**:5523, 1994.
51. Shirasawa S, Furuse M, Yokoyama N, Sasazuki T: Altered growth of human colon cancer cell lines disrupted at activated *Ki-ras*. *Science* **260**:85, 1993.
52. Bourne HR, Sanders DA, McCormick F: The GTPase superfamily: Conserved structure and molecular mechanism. *Nature* **349**:117, 1991.
53. Haubruck H, McCormick F: *Ras* p21: Effects and regulation. *Biochim Biophys Acta* **1072**:215, 1991.
54. Xu GF, Lin B, Tanaka K, et al: The catalytic domain of the neurofibromatosis type 1 gene product stimulates *ras* GTPase and complements *ira* mutants of *S. cerevisiae*. *Cell* **63**:835, 1990.
55. Martin GA, Viskochil D, Bollag G, et al: The GAP-related domain of the neurofibromatosis type 1 gene product interacts with *ras* p21. *Cell* **63**:843, 1990.
56. Ballester R, Marchuk D, Boguski M, et al: The *NF1* locus encodes a protein functionally related to mammalian GAP and yeast IRA proteins. *Cell* **63**:851, 1990.
57. Bollag G, McCormick F: Differential regulation of rasGAP and neurofibromatosis gene product activities. *Nature* **351**:576, 1991.
58. Li Y, Bollag G, Clark R, et al: Somatic mutations in the neurofibromatosis 1 gene in human tumors. *Cell* **69**:275, 1992.

59. Solomon E, Voss R, Hall V, et al: Chromosome 5 allele loss in human colorectal carcinomas. *Nature* **328**:616, 1987.

60. Monpezat JP, Delattre O, Bernard A, et al: Loss of alleles on chromosome 18 and on the short arm of chromosome 17 in polyploid colorectal carcinomas. *Int J Cancer* **41**:404, 1988.

61. Okamoto M, Sasaki M, Sugio K, et al: Loss of constitutional heterozygosity in colon carcinoma from patients with familial polyposis coli. *Nature* **331**:273, 1988.

62. Law DJ, Olschwang S, Monpezat JP, et al: Concerted nonsyntenic allelic loss in human colorectal carcinoma. *Science* **241**:961, 1988.

63. Vogelstein B, Fearon ER, Kern SE, et al: Allelotype of colorectal carcinomas. *Science* **244**:207, 1989.

64. Cavenee WK, Dryja TP, Phillips RA, et al: Expression of recessive alleles by chromosomal mechanisms in retinoblastoma. *Nature* **305**:779, 1983.

65. DeLeo AB, Jay G, Appella E, Dubois GC, Law LW, Old LJ: Detection of a transformation-related antigen in chemically induced sarcomas and other transformed cells of the mouse. *Proc Natl Acad Sci USA* **76**:2420, 1979.

66. Linzer DI, Levine AJ: Characterization of a 54-kilodalton cellular SV40 tumor antigen present in SV40-transformed cells and uninfected embryonal carcinoma cells. *Cell* **17**:43, 1979.

67. Lane DP, Crawford LV: T antigen is bound to a host protein in SV40-transformed cells. *Nature* **278**:261, 1979.

68. Eliyahu D, Raz A, Gruss P, Givol D, Oren M: Participation of p53 cellular tumour antigen in transformation of normal embryonic cells. *Nature* **312**:646, 1984.

69. Parada LF, Land H, Weinberg RA, Wolf D, Rotter V: Cooperation between gene encoding p53 tumour antigen and *ras* in cellular transformation. *Nature* **312**:649, 1984.

70. Jenkins JR, Rudge K, Currie GA: Cellular immortalization by a cDNA clone encoding the transformation-associated phosphoprotein p53. *Nature* **312**:651, 1984.

71. Baker SJ, Fearon ER, Nigro JM, et al: Chromosome 17 deletions and *p53* gene mutations in colorectal carcinomas. *Science* **244**:217, 1989.

72. Hethcote HW, Knudson AG Jr: Model for the incidence of embryonal cancers: Application to retinoblastoma. *Proc Natl Acad Sci USA* **75**:2453, 1978.

73. Baker SJ, Preisinger AC, Jessup JM, et al: *p53* gene mutations occur in combination with 17p allelic deletions as late events in colorectal tumorigenesis. *Cancer Res* **50**:7717, 1990.

74. Finlay CA, Hinds PW, Levine AJ: The *p53* proto-oncogene can act as a suppressor of transformation. *Cell* **57**:1083, 1989.

75. Eliyahu D, Michalovitz D, Eliyahu S, Pinhasi-Kimhi O, Oren M: Wild-type p53 can inhibit oncogene-mediated focus formation. *Proc Natl Acad Sci USA* **86**:8763, 1989.

76. Baker SJ, Markowitz S, Fearon ER, Willson JK, Vogelstein B: Suppression of human colorectal carcinoma cell growth by wild-type p53. *Science* **249**:912, 1990.

77. Diller L, Kassel J, Nelson CE, et al: p53 functions as a cell cycle control protein in osteosarcomas. *Mol Cell Biol* **10**:5772, 1990.

78. Mercer WE, Shields MT, Amin M, et al: Negative growth regulation in a glioblastoma tumor cell line that conditionally expresses human wild-type p53. *Proc Natl Acad Sci USA* **87**:6166, 1990.

79. Chen PL, Chen YM, Bookstein R, Lee WH: Genetic mechanisms of tumor suppression by the human *p53* gene. *Science* **250**:1576, 1990.

80. Hinds PW, Finlay CA, Quartin RS, et al: Mutant p53 DNA clones from human colon carcinomas cooperate with ras in transforming primary rat cells: A comparison of the "hot spot" mutant phenotypes. *Cell Growth Diff* **1**:571, 1990.

81. Raycroft L, Wu HY, Lozano G: Transcriptional activation by wild-type but not transforming mutants of the *p53* anti-oncogene. *Science* **249**:1049, 1990.

82. Mowat M, Cheng A, Kimura N, Bernstein A, Benchimol S: Rearrangements of the cellular *p53* gene in erythroleukaemic cells transformed by Friend virus. *Nature* **314**:633, 1985.

83. Hicks GG, Mowat M: Integration of Friend murine leukemia virus into both alleles of the *p53* oncogene in an erythroleukemic cell line. *J Virol* **62**:4752, 1988.

84. Ben David Y, Prideaux VR, Chow V, Benchimol S, Bernstein A: Inactivation of the *p53* oncogene by internal deletion or retroviral integration in erythroleukemic cell lines induced by Friend leukemia virus. *Oncogene* **3**:179, 1988.

85. Werness BA, Levine AJ, Howley PM: Association of human papillomavirus types 16 and 18 E6 proteins with p53. *Science* **248**:76, 1990.

86. Scheffner M, Werness BA, Huibregtse JM, Levine AJ, Howley PM: The E6 oncoprotein encoded by human papillomavirus types 16 and 18 promotes the degradation of p53. *Cell* **63**:1129, 1990.

87. Hollstein M, Shomer B, Greenblatt M, et al: Somatic point mutations in the *p53* gene of human tumors and cell lines: Updated compilation. *Nucl Acids Res* **24**:141, 1996.

88. Vogelstein B, Kinzler KW: Carcinogens leave fingerprints. *Nature* **355**:209, 1992.

89. Hsu IC, Metcalf RA, Sun T, Welsh JA, Wang NJ, Harris CC: Mutational hotspot in the *p53* gene in human hepatocellular carcinomas. *Nature* **350**:427, 1991.

90. Bressac B, Kew M, Wands J, Ozturk M: Selective G to T mutations of *p53* gene in hepatocellular carcinoma from southern Africa. *Nature* **350**:429, 1991.

91. Ozturk M: *p53* mutation in hepatocellular carcinoma after aflatoxin exposure. *Lancet* **338**:1356, 1991.

92. Brash DE, Rudolph JA, Simon JA, et al: A role for sunlight in skin cancer: UV-induced *p53* mutations in squamous cell carcinoma. *Proc Natl Acad Sci USA* **88**:10124, 1991.

93. Hollstein M, Sidransky D, Vogelstein B, Harris CC: *p53* mutations in human cancers. *Science* **253**:49, 1991.

94. Stenger JE, Mayr GA, Mann K, Tegtmeyer P: Formation of stable p53 homotetramers and multiples of tetramers. *Mol Carcinogen* **5**:102, 1992.

95. Jeffrey PD, Gorina S, Pavletich NP: Crystal structure of the tetramerization domain of the *p53* tumor suppressor at 1.7 angstroms. *Science* **267**:1498, 1995.

96. Milner J, Medcalf EA: Cotranslation of activated mutant *p53* with wild type drives the wild-type p53 protein into the mutant conformation. *Cell* **65**:765, 1991.

97. Hupp TR, Meek DW, Midgley CA, Lane DP: Regulation of the specific DNA binding function of p53. *Cell* **71**:875, 1992.

98. Kern SE, Kinzler KW, Bruskin A, et al: Identification of p53 as a sequence-specific DNA-binding protein. *Science* **252**:1708, 1991.

99. El-Deiry WS, Kern SE, Pietenpol JA, Kinzler KW, Vogelstein B: Definition of a consensus binding site for p53. *Nature Genet* **1**:45, 1992.

100. Funk WD, Pak DT, Karas RH, Wright WE, Shay JW: A transcriptionally active DNA-binding site for human p53 protein complexes. *Mol Cell Biol* **12**:2866, 1992.

101. Tokino T, Thiagalingam S, El-Deiry WS, Waldman T, Kinzler KW, Vogelstein B: p53 tagged sites from human genomic DNA. *Hum Mol Genet* **3**:1537, 1994.

102. Bargonetti J, Friedman PN, Kern SE, Vogelstein B, Prives C: Wild-type but not mutant p53 immunopurified proteins bind to sequences adjacent to the SV40 origin of replication. *Cell* **65**:1083, 1991.

103. Kern SE, Kinzler KW, Baker SJ, et al: Mutant p53 proteins bind DNA abnormally in vitro. *Oncogene* **6**:131, 1991.

104. Cho Y, Gorina S, Jeffrey PD, Pavletich NP: Crystal structure of a p53 tumor suppressor-DNA complex: Understanding tumorigenic mutations. *Science* **265**:346, 1994.

105. Fields S, Jang SK: Presence of a potent transcription activating sequence in the p53 protein. *Science* **249**:1046, 1990.

106. O'Rourke RW, Miller CW, Kato GJ, et al: A potential transcriptional activation element in the p53 protein. *Oncogene* **5**:1829, 1990.

107. Unger T, Nau MM, Segal S, Minna JD: *p53:* A transdominant regulator of transcription whose function is ablated by mutations occurring in human cancer. *EMBO J* **11**:1383, 1992.

108. Kern SE, Pietenpol JA, Thiagalingam S, Seymour A, Kinzler KW, Vogelstein B: Oncogenic forms of *p53* inhibit p53-regulated gene expression. *Science* **256**:827, 1992.

109. Scharer E, Iggo R: Mammalian p53 can function as a transcription factor in yeast. *Nucl Acids Res* **20**:1539, 1992.

110. Vogelstein B, Kinzler KW: p53 function and dysfunction. *Cell* **70**:523, 1992.

111. Momand J, Zambetti GP, Olson DC, George D, Levine AJ: The *mdm-2* oncogene product forms a complex with the p53 protein and inhibits p53-mediated transactivation. *Cell* **69**:1237, 1992.

112. Oliner JD, Kinzler KW, Meltzer PS, George DL, Vogelstein B: Amplification of a gene encoding a p53-associated protein in human sarcomas. *Nature* **358**:80, 1992.

113. Oliner JD, Pietenpol JA, Thiagalingam S, Gyuris J, Kinzler KW, Vogelstein B: Oncoprotein MDM2 conceals the activation domain of tumour suppressor p53. *Nature* **362**:857, 1993.

114. Fakharzadeh SS, Trusko SP, George DL: Tumorigenic potential associated with enhanced expression of a gene that is amplified in a mouse tumor cell line. *EMBO J* **10**:1565, 1991.

115. Wu X, Bayle JH, Olson D, Levine AJ: The *p53-mdm-2* autoregulatory feedback loop. *Genes Dev* **7**:1126, 1993.

116. El-Deiry WS, Tokino T, Velculescu VE, et al: *WAF1*, a potential mediator of *p53* tumor suppression. *Cell* **75**:817, 1993.

117. Miyashita T, Krajewski S, Krajewska M, et al: Tumor suppressor *p53* is a regulator of *bcl-2* and *bax* gene expression in vitro and in vivo. *Oncogene* **9**:1799, 1994.

118. Miyashita T, Reed JC: Tumor suppressor *p53* is a direct transcriptional activator of the human *bax* gene. *Cell* **80**:293, 1995.

119. Madden SL, Galella EA, Riley D, Bertelsen AH, Beaudry GA: Induction of cell growth regulatory genes by p53. *Cancer Res* **56**:5384, 1996.

120. Lehar SM, Nacht M, Jacks T, Vater CA, Chittenden T, Guild BC: Identification and cloning of *EI24*, a gene induced by p53 in etoposide-treated cells. *Oncogene* **12**:1181, 1996.

121. Amson RB, Nemani M, Roperch JP, et al: Isolation of 10 differentially expressed cDNAs in p53-induced apoptosis: Activation of the vertebrate homologue of the *Drosophila* seven in absentia gene. *Proc Natl Acad Sci USA* **93**:3953, 1996.

122. Rouault JP, Falette N, Guehenneux F, et al: Identification of BTG2, an antiproliferative p53-dependent component of the DNA damage cellular response pathway. *Nature Genet* **14**:482, 1996.

123. Fiscella M, Zhang H, Fan S, et al: Wip1, a novel human protein phosphatase that is induced in response to ionizing radiation in a p53-dependent manner. *Proc Natl Acad Sci USA* **94**:6048, 1997.

124. Nishimori H, Shiratsuchi T, Urano T, et al: A novel brain-specific p53-target gene, *BAI1*, containing thrombospondin type 1 repeats inhibits experimental angiogenesis. *Oncogene* **15**:2145, 1997.

125. Varmeh-Ziaie S, Okan I, Wang Y, et al: *Wig-1*, a new p53-induced gene encoding a zinc finger protein. *Oncogene* **15**:2699, 1997.

126. Polyak K, Xia Y, Zweier JL, Kinzler KW, Vogelstein B: A model for p53 induced apoptosis. *Nature* **389**:300, 1997.

127. Hermeking H, Lengauer C, Polyak K, et al: 14-3-3s is a p53-regulated inhibitor of G2/M progression. *Mol Cell* **1**:3, 1997.

128. Urano T, Nishimori H, Han H, et al: Cloning of *P2XM*, a novel human P2X receptor gene regulated by p53. *Cancer Res* **57**:3281, 1997.

129. Kimura Y, Furuhata T, Urano T, Hirata K, Nakamura Y, Tokino T: Genomic structure and chromosomal localization of *GML* (GPI-anchored molecule-like protein), a gene induced by p53. *Genomics* **41**:477, 1997.

130. Sheikh MS, Burns TF, Huang Y, et al: p53-dependent and -independent regulation of the death receptor *KILLER/DR5* gene expression in response to genotoxic stress and tumor necrosis factor alpha. *Cancer Res* **58**:1593, 1998.

131. Takei Y, Ishikawa S, Tokino T, Muto T, Nakamura Y: Isolation of a novel *TP53* target gene from a colon cancer cell line carrying a highly regulated wild-type *TP53* expression system. *Genes Chromosom Cancer* **23**:1, 1998.

132. Mashimo T, Watabe M, Hirota S, et al: The expression of the *KAI1* gene, a tumor metastasis suppressor, is directly activated by p53. *Proc Natl Acad Sci USA* **95**:11307, 1998.

133. Utrera R, Collavin L, Lazarevic D, Delia D, Schneider C: A novel p53-inducible gene coding for a microtubule-localized protein with G2-phase-specific expression. *EMBO J* **17**:5015, 1998.

134. Harper JW, Adami GR, Wei N, Keyomarsi K, Elledge SJ: The p21 Cdk-interacting protein Cip1 is a potent inhibitor of G1 cyclin-dependent kinases. *Cell* **75**:805, 1993.

135. Xiong Y, Hannon GJ, Zhang H, Casso D, Kobayashi R, Beach D: p21 is a universal inhibitor of cyclin kinases. *Nature* **366**:701, 1993.

136. Noda A, Ning Y, Venable SF, Pereira-Smith OM, Smith JR: Cloning of senescent cell-derived inhibitors of DNA synthesis using an expression screen. *Exp Cell Res* **211**:90, 1994.

137. El-Deiry WS, Tokino T, Waldman T, et al: Topological control of p21(Waf1/Cip1) expression in normal and neoplastic tissues. *Cancer Res* **55**:2910, 1995.

138. Elledge SJ, Harper JW: Cdk inhibitors: On the threshold of checkpoints and development. *Curr Opin Cell Biol* **6**:847, 1994.

139. Waldman T, Kinzler KW, Vogelstein B: P21 is necessary for the p53-mediated G(1) arrest in human cancer cells. *Cancer Res* **55**:5187, 1995.

140. Waldman T, Lengauer C, Kinzler KW, Vogelstein B: Uncoupling of S phase and mitosis induced by anticancer agents in cells lacking p21. *Nature* **381**:713, 1996.

141. Deng C, Zhang P, Harper JW, Elledge SJ, Leder P: Mice lacking p21CIP1/WAF1 undergo normal development, but are defective in G1 checkpoint control. *Cell* **82**:675, 1995.

142. Brugarolas J, Chandrasekaran C, Gordon JI, Beach D, Jacks T, Hannon GJ: Radiation-induced cell cycle arrest compromised by p21 deficiency. *Nature* **377**:552, 1995.

143. Bunz F, Dutriaux A, Lengauer C, et al: Requirement for p53 and p21 to sustain G2 arrest after DNA damage. *Science* **282**:1497, 1998.

144. Chan T, Hermeking H, Kinzler K, Vogelstein B: Unpublished observation, 1998.

145. Polyak K, Waldman T, He T-C, Kinzler KW, Vogelstein B: Genetic determinants of p53 induced apoptosis and growth arrest. *Genes Dev* **10**:1945, 1996.

145a. Yu J, Zhang L, Hwang PM, Kinzler KW, Vogelstein B: PUMA induces the rapid apoptosis of colorectal cancer cells. *Molecular Cell* **7**:673, 2001.

145b. Nakano K, Vousden KH: PUMA, a novel proapoptotic gene, is induced by p53, *Molecular Cell* **7**:683, 2001.

146. Lowe SW, Schmitt EM, Smith SW, Osborne BA, Jacks T: p53 is required for radiation-induced apoptosis in mouse thymocytes. *Nature* **362**:847, 1993.

147. Clarke AR, Purdie CA, Harrison DJ, et al: Thymocyte apoptosis induced by p53-dependent and independent pathways. *Nature* **362**:849, 1993.

148. Donehower LA, Harvey M, Slagle BL, et al: Mice deficient for p53 are developmentally normal but susceptible to spontaneous tumours. *Nature* **356**:215, 1992.

149. Malkin D, Li FP, Strong LC, et al: Germ line *p53* mutations in a familial syndrome of breast cancer, sarcomas, and other neoplasms. *Science* **250**:1233, 1990.

150. Srivastava S, Zou ZQ, Pirollo K, Blattner W, Chang EH: Germ-line transmission of a mutated *p53* gene in a cancer-prone family with Li-Fraumeni syndrome. *Nature* **348**:747, 1990.

151. Kastan MB, Onyekwere O, Sidransky D, Vogelstein B, Craig RW: Participation of p53 protein in the cellular response to DNA damage. *Cancer Res* **51**:6304, 1991.

152. Kuerbitz SJ, Plunkett BS, Walsh WV, Kastan MB: Wild-type p53 is a cell cycle checkpoint determinant following irradiation. *Proc Natl Acad Sci USA* **89**:7491, 1992.

153. Kastan MB, Zhan Q, el-Deiry WS, et al: A mammalian cell cycle checkpoint pathway utilizing p53 and GADD45 is defective in ataxia-telangiectasia. *Cell* **71**:587, 1992.

154. Lane DP: Cancer: *p53*, guardian of the genome. *Nature* **358**:15, 1992.

155. Graeber TG, Peterson JF, Tsai M, Monica K, Fornace AJ Jr, Giaccia AJ: Hypoxia induces accumulation of p53 protein, but activation of a G1-phase checkpoint by low-oxygen conditions is independent of p53 status. *Mol Cell Biol* **14**:6264, 1994.

156. Graeber TG, Osmanian C, Jacks T, et al: Hypoxia-mediated selection of cells with diminished apoptotic potential in solid tumours. *Nature* **379**:88, 1996.

157. Hermeking H, Eick D: Mediation of c-Myc-induced apoptosis by p53. *Science* **265**:2091, 1994.

158. Wagner AJ, Kokontis JM, Hay N: *Myc*-mediated apoptosis requires wild-type p53 in a manner independent of cell cycle arrest and the ability of p53 to induce p21waf1/cip1. *Genes Dev* **8**:2817, 1994.

159. Lowe SW, Ruley HE: Stabilization of the *p53* tumor suppressor is induced by adenovirus 5 E1A and accompanies apoptosis. *Genes Dev* **7**:535, 1993.

160. Qin XQ, Livingston DM, Kaelin WG Jr, Adams PD: Deregulated transcription factor E2F-1 expression leads to S-phase entry and p53-mediated apoptosis. *Proc Natl Acad Sci USA* **91**:10918, 1994.

161. Shan B, Lee WH: Deregulated expression of E2F-1 induces S-phase entry and leads to apoptosis. *Mol Cell Biol* **14**:8166, 1994.

162. Wu X, Levine AJ: p53 and E2F-1 cooperate to mediate apoptosis. *Proc Natl Acad Sci USA* **91**:3602, 1994.

163. Bates S, Phillips AC, Clark PA, et al: p14ARF links the tumour suppressors *RB* and *p53*. *Nature* **395**:124, 1998.

164. Kamijo T, Weber JD, Zambetti G, Zindy F, Roussel MF, Sherr CJ: Functional and physical interactions of the *ARF* tumor suppressor with *p53* and *Mdm2*. *Proc Natl Acad Sci USA* **95**:8292, 1998.

165. Pomerantz J, Schreiber-Agus N, Liegeois NJ, et al: The *Ink4a* tumor suppressor gene product, p19Arf, interacts with MDM2 and neutralizes MDM2's inhibition of p53. *Cell* **92**:713, 1998.

166. de Stanchina E, McCurrach ME, Zindy F, et al: E1A signaling to p53 involves the p19 (*ARF*) tumor suppressor. *Genes Dev* **12**:2434, 1998.

167. Zhang Y, Xiong Y, Yarbrough WG: *ARF* promotes MDM2 degradation and stabilizes p53: ARF-INK4a locus deletion impairs both the *Rb* and *p53* tumor suppression pathways. *Cell* **92**:725, 1998.

168. Zindy F, Eischen CM, Randle DH, et al: *Myc* signaling via the *ARF* tumor suppressor regulates p53-dependent apoptosis and immortalization. *Genes Dev* **12**:2424, 1998.

169. Giaccia AJ, Kastan MB: The complexity of p53 modulation: Emerging patterns from divergent signals. *Genes Dev* **12**:2973, 1998.

170. Montes de Oca Luna R, Wagner DS, Lozano G: Rescue of early embryonic lethality in *mdm2*-deficient mice by deletion of *p53*. *Nature* **378**:203, 1995.

171. Kaghad M, Bonnet H, Yang A, et al: Monoallelically expressed gene related to p53 at 1p36, a region frequently deleted in neuroblastoma and other human cancers. *Cell* **90**:809, 1997.

172. Osada M, Ohba M, Kawahara C, et al: Cloning and functional analysis of human p51, which structurally and functionally resembles p53. *Nature Med* **4**:839, 1998.

173. Trink B, Okami K, Wu L, Sriuranpong V, Jen J, Sidransky D: A new human *p53* homologue. *Nature Med* **4**:747, 1998.

174. Yang A, Kaghad M, Wang Y, et al: *p63*, a *p53* homolog at 3q27-29, encodes multiple products with transactivating, death-inducing, and dominant-negative activities. *Mol Cell* **2**:305, 1998.

175. Jen J, Kim H, Piantadosi S, et al: Allelic loss of chromosome 18q and prognosis in colorectal cancer. *N Engl J Med* **331**:213, 1994.

176. Martinez-Lopez E, Abad A, Font A, et al: Allelic loss on chromosome 18q as a prognostic marker in stage II colorectal cancer. *Gastroenterology* **114**:1180, 1998.

177. Ogunbiyi OA, Goodfellow PJ, Herfarth K, et al: Confirmation that chromosome 18q allelic loss in colon cancer is a prognostic indicator. *J Clin Oncol* **16**:427, 1998.

178. Carethers JM, Hawn MT, Greenson JK, Hitchcock CL, Boland CR: Prognostic significance of allelic lost at chromosome 18q21 for stage II colorectal cancer. *Gastroenterology* **114**:1188, 1998.

179. Fearon ER, Cho KR, Nigro JM, et al: Identification of a chromosome 18q gene that is altered in colorectal cancers. *Science* **247**:49, 1990.

180. Hedrick L, Cho KR, Fearon ER, Wu TC, Kinzler KW, Vogelstein B: The *DCC* gene product in cellular differentiation and colorectal tumorigenesis. *Genes Dev* **8**:1174, 1994.

181. Cho KR, Oliner JD, Simons JW, et al: The *DCC* gene: Structural analysis and mutations in colorectal carcinomas. *Genomics* **19**:525, 1994.

182. Hedrick L, Cho KR, Boyd J, Risinger J, Vogelstein B: *DCC:* A tumor suppressor gene expressed on the cell surface. *Cold Spring Harb Symp Quant Biol* **57**:345, 1992.

183. Keino-Masu K, Masu M, Hinck L, et al: Deleted in colorectal cancer (*DCC*) encodes a netrin receptor. *Cell* **87**:175, 1996.

184. Chan SS, Zheng H, Su MW, et al: *UNC-40*, a *C. elegans* homologue of *DCC* (deleted in colorectal cancer), is required in motile cells responding to UNC-6 netrin cues. *Cell* **87**:187, 1996.

185. Kolodziej PA, Timpe LC, Mitchell KJ, et al: Frazzled encodes a *Drosophila* member of the DCC immunoglobulin subfamily and is required for CNS and motor axon guidance. *Cell* **87**:197, 1996.

186. Thiagalingam S: Evaluation of chromosome 18q in colorectal cancers. *Nature Genet* **13**:343, 1996.

187. Murty VV, Li RG, Houldsworth J, et al: Frequent allelic deletions and loss of expression characterize the *DCC* gene in male germ cell tumors. *Oncogene* **9**:3227, 1994.

188. Shibata D, Reale MA, Lavin P, et al: The DCC protein and prognosis in colorectal cancer. *N Engl J Med* **335**:1727, 1996.

189. Reymond MA, Dworak O, Remke S, Hohenberger W, Kirchner T, Kockerling F: DCC protein as a predictor of distant metastases after curative surgery for rectal cancer. *Dis Colon Rectum* **41**:755, 1998.

190. Goi T, Yamaguchi A, Nakagawara G, Urano T, Shiku H, Furukawa K: Reduced expression of deleted colorectal carcinoma (DCC) protein in established colon cancers. *Br J Cancer* **77**:466, 1998.

191. Yamamoto H, Itoh F, Kusano M, Yoshida Y, Hinoda Y, Imai K: Infrequent inactivation of *DCC* gene in replication error-positive colorectal cancers. *Biochem Biophys Res Commun* **244**:204, 1998.

192. Fazeli A, Dickinson SL, Hermiston ML, et al: Phenotype of mice lacking functional deleted in colorectal cancer (*DCC*) gene. *Nature* **386**:796, 1997.

193. Hahn SA, Schutte M, Hoque ATMS, et al: *Dpc4*, a candidate tumor suppressor gene at human chromosome 18q21.1. *Science* **271**:350, 1996.

194. Hahn SA, Seymour AB, Hoque AT, et al: Allelotype of pancreatic adenocarcinoma using xenograft enrichment. *Cancer Res* **55**:4670, 1995.

195. Hursh DA, Padgett RW, Gelbart WM: Cross regulation of decapentaplegic and ultrabithorax transcription in the embryonic visceral mesoderm of *Drosophila*. *Development* **117**:1211, 1993.

196. Sekelsky JJ, Newfeld SJ, Raftery LA, Chartoff EH, Gelbart WM: Genetic characterization and cloning of mothers against *dpp*, a gene required for decapentaplegic function in *Drosophila melanogaster*. *Genetics* **139**:1347, 1995.

197. Savage C, Das P, Finelli AL, et al: *Caenorhabditis elegans* genes *Sma2*, *Sma-3*, and *Sma-4* define a conserved family of transforming growth factor beta pathway components. *Proc Natl Acad Sci USA* **93**:790, 1996.

198. Fynan TM, Reiss M: Resistance to inhibition of cell growth by transforming growth factor-beta and its role in oncogenesis. *Crit Rev Oncogen* **4**:493, 1993.

199. Brattain MG, Howell G, Sun LZ, Willson JK: Growth factor balance and tumor progression. *Curr Opin Oncol* **6**:77, 1994.

200. Markowitz S, Wang J, Myeroff L, et al: Inactivation of the type II TGF-beta receptor in colon cancer cells with microsatellite instability. *Science* **268**:1336, 1995.

201. Parsons R, Myeroff LL, Liu B, et al: Microsatellite instability and mutations of the transforming growth factor beta type II receptor gene in colorectal cancer. *Cancer Res* **55**:5548, 1995.

202. Grady WM, Rajput A, Myeroff L, et al: Mutation of the type II transforming growth factor-beta receptor is coincident with the transformation of human colon adenomas to malignant carcinomas. *Cancer Res* **58**:3101, 1998.

203. Zhou S, Buckhaults P, Zawel L, et al: Targeted deletion of Smad4 shows it is required for TGF-β and activin signalin in colorectal cancer cells. *Proc Natl Acad Sci USA* **95**:2412, 1998.

204. Yingling JM, Datto MB, Wong C, Frederick JP, Liberati NT, Wang XF: Tumor suppressor *Smad4* is a transforming growth factor–inducible DNA binding protein. *Mol Cell Biol* **17**:7019, 1997.

205. Zawel L, Dai JL, Buckhaults P, et al: Human *Smad3* and *Smad4* are sequence-specific transcription activators. *Mol Cell* **1**:611, 1998.

206. Dennler S, Itoh S, Vivien D, ten Dijke P, Huet S, Gauthier JM: Direct binding of Smad3 and Smad4 to critical TGF beta–inducible elements in the promoter of human plasminogen activator inhibitor-type 1 gene. *EMBO J* **17**:3091, 1998.

207. Riggins GJ, Kinzler KW, Vogelstein B, Thiagalingam S: *Mad*-related genes in the human. *Nature Genet* **13**:347, 1996.

208. Eppert K, Scherer SW, Ozcelik H, et al: *MADR2* maps to 18q21 and encodes a TGF-beta-regulated MAD-related protein that is mutated in colorectal carcinoma. *Cell* **86**:543, 1996.

209. Riggins GJ, Kinzler KW, Vogelstein B, Thiagalingam S: Frequency of *Smad* gene mutations in human cancers. *Cancer Res* **57**:2578, 1997.

210. Hayashi H, Abdollah S, Qiu Y, et al: The MAD-related protein Smad7 associates with the TGF-beta receptor and functions as an antagonist of TGF-beta signaling. *Cell* **89**:1165, 1997.

211. Nakao A, Afrakhte M, Moren A, et al: Identification of *Smad7*, a TGF-beta–inducible antagonist of TGF-beta signalling. *Nature* **389**:631, 1997.

212. Roijer E, Moren A, ten Dijke P, Stenman G: Assignment of the *Smad7* gene (*MADH7*) to human chromosome 18q21.1 by fluorescence in situ hybridization. *Cytogenet Cell Genet* **81**:189, 1998.

213. MacGrogan D, Pegram M, Slamon D, Bookstein R: Comparative mutational analysis of *DPC4* (*Smad4*) in prostatic and colorectal carcinomas. *Oncogene* **15**:1111, 1997.

214. Uchida K, Nagatake M, Osada H, et al: Somatic in vivo alterations of the *JV18-1* gene at 18q21 in human lung cancers. *Cancer Res* **56**:5583, 1996.

215. Powell SM, Harper JC, Hamilton SR, Robinson CR, Cummings OW: Inactivation of *Smad4* in gastric carcinomas. *Cancer Res* **57**:4221, 1997.

215a. Montgomery E, Goggins M, Zhou S, Argani P, Wilentz R, Kaushal M, Booker S, Romans K, Bhargava P, Hruban R, Kern S: Nuclear localization of Dpc4 (Madh4, Smad4) in colorectal carcinomas and relation to mismatch repair/transforming growth factor-beta receptor defects, *Am J Pathol* **158**:537, 2001.

216. Howe JR, Roth S, Rigold JC, et al: Mutations in the *SMAD4/DPC4* gene in juvenile polyposis. *Science* **280**:1086, 1998.

217. Yang X, Li C, Xu X, Deng C: The tumor suppressor *SMAD4/DPC4* is essential for epiblast proliferation and mesoderm induction in mice. *Proc Natl Acad Sci USA* **95**:3667, 1998.

218. Sirard C, de la Pompa JL, Elia A, et al: The tumor suppressor gene *Smad4/Dpc4* is required for gastrulation and later for anterior development of the mouse embryo. *Genes Dev* **12**:107, 1998.

219. Takaku K, Oshima M, Miyoshi H, Matsui M, Seldin MF, Taketo MM: Intestinal tumorigenesis in compound mutant mice of both *Dpc4* (*Smad4*) and *Apc* genes. *Cell* **92**:645, 1998.

220. Nomura M, Li E: *Smad2* role in mesoderm formation, left-right patterning and craniofacial development. *Nature* **393**:786, 1998.

221. Waldrip WR, Bikoff EK, Hoodless PA, Wrana JL, Robertson EJ: *Smad2* signaling in extraembryonic tissues determines anterior-posterior polarity of the early mouse embryo. *Cell* **92**:797, 1998.

222. Zhu Y, Richardson JA, Parada LF, Graff JM: *Smad3* mutant mice develop metastatic colorectal cancer. *Cell* **94**:703, 1998.

223. Tanaka K, Oshimura M, Kikuchi R, Seki M, Hayashi T, Miyaki M: Suppression of tumorigenicity in human colon carcinoma cells by introduction of normal chromosome 5 or 18. *Nature* **349**:340, 1991.

224. Goyette MC, Cho K, Fasching CL, et al: Progression of colorectal cancer is associated with multiple tumor suppressor gene defects but inhibition of tumorigenicity is accomplished by correction of any single defect via chromosome transfer. *Mol Cell Biol* **12**:1387, 1992.

225. Reiss M, Santoro V, de Jonge RR, Vellucci VF: Transfer of chromosome 18 into human head and neck squamous carcinoma cells: Evidence for tumor suppression by *Smad4/DPC4*. *Cell Growth Diff* **8**:407, 1997.

226. Narayanan R, Lawlor KG, Schaapveld RQ, et al: Antisense RNA to the putative tumor-suppressor gene *DCC* transforms Rat-1 fibroblasts. *Oncogene* **7**:553, 1992.

227. Lawlor KG, Telang NT, Osborne MP, et al: Antisense RNA to the putative tumor suppressor gene "deleted in colorectal cancer" transforms fibroblasts. *Ann NY Acad Sci* **660**:283, 1992.

228. Klingelhutz AJ, Hedrick L, Cho KR, McDougall JK: The *DCC* gene suppresses the malignant phenotype of transformed human epithelial cells. *Oncogene* **10**:1581, 1995.

229. Mehlen P, Rabizadeh S, Snipas SJ, Assa-Munt N, Salvesen GS, Bredesen DE: The *DCC* gene product induces apoptosis by a mechanism requiring receptor proteolysis. *Nature* **395**:801, 1998.

230. Herrera L, Kakati S, Gibas L, Pietrzak E, Sandberg A: Gardner syndrome in a man with an interstitial deletion of 5q. *Am J Med Genet* **25**:473, 1986.

231. Leppert M, Dobbs M, Scambler P, et al: The gene for familial polyposis coli maps to the long arm of chromosome 5. *Science* **238**:1411, 1987.

232. Bodmer W, Bailey C, Bodmer J, et al: Localization of the gene for familial adenomatous polyposis on chromosome 5. *Nature* **328**:614, 1987.

233. Nakamura Y, Lathrop M, Leppert M, et al: Localization of the genetic defect in familial adenomatous polyposis within a small region of chromosome 5. *Am J Hum Genet* **43**:638, 1988.

234. Ashton Rickardt PG, Dunlop MG, Nakamura Y, et al: High frequency of *APC* loss in sporadic colorectal carcinoma due to breaks clustered in 5q21-22. *Oncogene* **4**:1169, 1989.

235. Delattre O, Olschwang S, Law DJ, et al: Multiple genetic alterations in distal and proximal colorectal cancer. *Lancet* **2**:353, 1989.

236. Sasaki M, Okamoto M, Sato C, et al: Loss of constitutional heterozygosity in colorectal tumors from patients with familial polyposis coli and those with nonpolyposis colorectal carcinoma. *Cancer Res* **49**:4402, 1989.

237. Ashton Rickardt PG, Wyllie AH, Bird CC, et al: *MCC,* a candidate familial polyposis gene in 5q.21, shows frequent allele loss in colorectal and lung cancer. *Oncogene* **6**:1881, 1991.

238. Kinzler KW, Nilbert MC, Su LK, et al: Identification of *FAP* locus genes from chromosome 5q21. *Science* **253**:661, 1991.

239. Joslyn G, Carlson M, Thliveris A, et al: Identification of deletion mutations and three new genes at the familial polyposis locus. *Cell* **66**:601, 1991.

240. Nishisho I, Nakamura Y, Miyoshi Y, et al: Mutations of chromosome 5q21 genes in *FAP* and colorectal cancer patients. *Science* **253**:665, 1991.

241. Groden J, Thliveris A, Samowitz W, et al: Identification and characterization of the familial adenomatous polyposis coli gene. *Cell* **66**:589, 1991.

242. Horii A, Nakatsuru S, Ichii S, Nagase H, Nakamura Y: Multiple forms of the *APC* gene transcripts and their tissue-specific expression. *Hum Mol Genet* **2**:283, 1993.

243. Thliveris A, Samowitz W, Matsunami N, Groden J, White R: Demonstration of promoter activity and alternative splicing in the region 5′ to exon 1 of the *APC* gene. *Cancer Res* **54**:2991, 1994.

244. Nagase H, Su Y: Mutations of the *APC* (adenomatous polyposis coli) gene. *Hum Mutat* **2**:425, 1993.

245. Laurent-Puig P, Beroud C, Soussi T: *APC* gene: Database of germline and somatic mutations in human tumors and cell lines. *Nucl Acids Res* **26**:269, 1998.

246. Powell SM, Petersen GM, Krush AJ, et al: Molecular diagnosis of familial adenomatous polyposis. *N Engl J Med* **329**:1982, 1993.

247. Laken SJ, Papadopoulous N, Petersen GM, et al: Analysis of masked mutations in familial adenomatous polyposis. *Proc Natl Acad Sci USA* **96**:2322, 1999.

248. Papadopoulos N, Leach FS, Kinzler KW, Vogelstein B: Monoallelic mutation analysis (MAMA) for identifying germline mutations. *Nature Genet* **11**:99, 1995.

249. Groden J, Gelbert L, Thliveris A, et al: Mutational analysis of patients with adenomatous polyposis: Identical inactivating mutations in unrelated individuals. *Am J Hum Genet* **52**:263, 1993.

250. Olschwang S, Tiret A, Laurent-Puig P, Muleris M, Parc R, Thomas G: Restriction of ocular fundus lesions to a specific subgroup of *APC* mutations in adenomatous polyposis coli patients. *Cell* **75**:959, 1993.

251. Wallis YL, Macdonald F, Hulten M, et al: Genotype-phenotype correlation between position of constitutional *APC* gene mutation and CHRPE expression in familial adenomatous polyposis. *Hum Genet* **94**:543, 1994.

252. Caspari R, Olschwang S, Friedl W, et al: Familial adenomatous polyposis: Desmoid tumours and lack of ophthalmic lesions (CHRPE) associated with *APC* mutations beyond codon 1444. *Hum Mol Genet* **4**:337, 1995.

253. Davies D, Armstrong J, Thakker N, et al: Severe Gardner syndrome in families with mutations restricted to a specific region of the *APC* gene. *Am J Hum Genet* **57**:1151, 1995.

254. Dobbie Z, Spycher M, Mary J-L, et al: Correlation between the development of extracolonic manifestations in FAP patients and mutations beyond codon 1403 of the *APC* gene. *J Med Genet* **33**:274, 1996.

255. Friedl W, Meuschel S, Caspari R, et al: Attenuated familial adenomatous polyposis due to a mutation in the 3′ part of the *APC* gene: A clue for understanding the function of the APC protein. *Hum Genet* **97**:579, 1996.

256. Walon C, Kartheuser A, Michils G, et al: Novel germline mutations in the *APC* gene and their phenotypic spectrum in familial adenomatous polyposis kindreds. *Hum Genet* **100**:601, 1997.

257. Soravia C, Berk T, Madlensky L, et al: Genotype-phenotype correlations in attenuated adenomatous polyposis coli. *Am J Hum Genet* **62**:1290, 1998.

258. Pedemonte S, Sciallero S, Gismondi V, et al: Novel germline *APC* variants in patients with multiple adenomas. *Genes Chromosom Cancer* **22**:257, 1998.

259. Brensinger JD, Laken SJ, Luce MC, et al: Variable phenotype of familial adenomatous polyposis in pedigrees with 3′mutation in the *APC* gene. *Gut* **43**:548, 1998.

260. Gayther S, Wells D, SenGupta S, et al: Regionally clustered *APC* mutations are associated with a severe phenotype and occur at a high frequency in new mutation cases of adenomatous polyposis coli. *Hum Mol Genet* **3**:53, 1994.

261. Nagase H, Miyoshi Y, Horii A, et al: Correlation between the location of germ-line mutations in the *APC* gene and the number of colorectal polyps in familial adenomatous polyposis patients. *Cancer Res* **52**:4055, 1992.

262. Giardiello FM, Krush AJ, Petersen GM, et al: Phenotypic variability of familial adenomatous polyposis in 11 unrelated families with identical *APC* gene mutation. *Gastroenterology* **106**:1542, 1994.

263. Miyoshi Y, Nagase H, Ando H, et al: Somatic mutations of the *APC* gene in colorectal tumors: Mutation cluster region in the *APC* gene. *Hum Mol Genet* **1**:229, 1992.

264. Powell SM, Zilz N, Beazer-Barclay Y, et al: *APC* mutations occur early during colorectal tumorigenesis. *Nature* **359**:235, 1992.

265. Smith KJ, Johnson KA, Bryan TM, et al: The *APC* gene product in normal and tumor cells. *Proc Natl Acad Sci USA* **90**:2846, 1993.

266. Smith AJ, Stern HS, Penner M, et al: Somatic *APC* and *K-ras* codon 12 mutations in aberrant crypt foci from human colons. *Cancer Res* **54**:5527, 1994.

267. Laken SJ, Petersen GM, Gruber SB, et al: Familial colorectal cancer in Ashkenazim due to a hypermutable tract in *APC*. *Nature Genet* **17**:79, 1997.

268. Woodage T, King SM, Wacholder S, et al: The *APCI1307K* allele and cancer risk in a community-based study of Ashkenazi Jews. *Nature Genet* **20**:62, 1998.

269. Lothe RA, Hektoen M, Johnsen H, et al: The *APC* gene I1307K variant is rare in Norwegian patients with familial and sporadic colorectal or breast cancer. *Cancer Res* **58**:2923, 1998.

270. Petersen GM, Parmigiani G, Thomas D: Missense mutations in disease genes: A Bayesian approach to evaluate causality. *Am J Hum Genet* **62**:1516, 1998.

271. Frayling IM, Beck NE, Ilyas M, et al: The *APC* variants I1307K and E1317Q are associated with colorectal tumors, but not always with a family history. *Proc Natl Acad Sci USA* **95**:10722, 1998.

272. Rozen P, Shomrat R, Strul H, et al: Prevalence of the I1307K *APC* gene variant in Israel Jews of differing ethnic origin and risk for cancer. *Gastroenterology* **16**:54, 1999.

273. Petrukhin L, Dangel J, Vanderveer L, et al: The I1307K *APC* mutation does not predispose to colorectal cancer in Jewish Ashkenazi breast and breast-ovarian cancer kindreds. *Cancer Res* **57**:5480, 1997.

274. Abrahamson J, Moslehi R, Vesprini D, et al: No association of the I1307K *APC* allele with ovarian cancer risk in Ashkenazi Jews. *Cancer Res* **58**:2919, 1998.

275. Yuan ZQ, Kasprzak L, Gordon PH, Pinsky L, Foulkes WD: I1307K *APC* and *hMLH1* mutations in a non-Jewish family with hereditary non-polyposis colorectal cancer. *Clin Genet* **54**:368, 1998.

276. Gryfe R, Di Nicola N, Gallinger S, Redston M: Somatic instability of the *APC* I1307K allele in colorectal neoplasia. *Cancer Res* **58**:4040, 1998.

277. Su LK, Kinzler KW, Vogelstein B, et al: Multiple intestinal neoplasia caused by a mutation in the murine homolog of the *APC* gene. *Science* **256**:668, 1992.

278. Fodde R, Edelmann W, Yang K, et al: A targeted chain-termination mutation in the mouse *Apc* gene results in multiple intestinal tumors. *Proc Natl Acad Sci USA* **91**:8969, 1994.

279. Oshima M, Oshima H, Kitagawa K, Kobayashi M, Itakura C, Taketo M: Loss of *Apc* heterozygosity and abnormal tissue building in nascent intestinal polyps in mice carrying a truncated *Apc* gene. *Proc Natl Acad Sci USA* **92**:4482, 1995.

280. Moser AR, Pitot HC, Dove WF: A dominant mutation that predisposes to multiple intestinal neoplasia in the mouse. *Science* **247**:322, 1990.

281. Moser AR, Dove WF, Roth KA, Gordon JI: The *Min* (multiple intestinal neoplasia) mutation: Its effect on gut epithelial cell differentiation and interaction with a modifier system. *J Cell Biol* **116**:1517, 1992.

282. Luongo C, Moser AR, Gledhill S, Dove WF: Loss of *Apc+* in intestinal adenomas from *Min* mice. *Cancer Res* **54**:5947, 1994.

283. Levy DB, Smith KJ, Beazer-Barclay Y, Hamilton SR, Vogelstein B, Kinzler KW: Inactivation of both *APC* alleles in human and mouse tumors. *Cancer Res* **54**:5953, 1994.

284. Shibata H, Toyama K, Shioya H, et al: Rapid colorectal adenoma formation initiated by conditional targeting of the *Apc* gene. *Science* **278**:120, 1997.

285. Morin PJ, Vogelstein B, Kinzler KW: Apoptosis and *APC* in colorectal tumorigenesis. *Proc Natl Acad Sci USA* **93**:7950, 1996.

286. Miyashiro I, Senda T, Matsumine A, et al: Subcellular localization of the APC protein: Immunoelectron microscopic study of the association of the APC protein with catenin. *Oncogene* **11**:89, 1995.

287. Joslyn G, Richardson DS, White R, Alber T: Dimer formation by an N-terminal coiled coil in the APC protein. *Proc Natl Acad Sci USA* **90**:11109, 1993.

288. Su LK, Johnson KA, Smith KJ, Hill DE, Vogelstein B, Kinzler KW: Association between wild type and mutant *APC* gene products. *Cancer Res* **53**:2728, 1993.

289. Rubinfeld B, Souza B, Albert I, et al: Association of the *APC* gene product with beta-catenin. *Science* **262**:1731, 1993.

290. Su LK, Vogelstein B, Kinzler KW: Association of the APC tumor suppressor protein with catenins. *Science* **262**:1734, 1993.

291. Hulsken J, Birchmeier W, Behrens J: E-cadherin and APC compete for the interaction with beta-catenin and the cytoskeleton. *J Cell Biol* **127**:2061, 1994.

292. Rubinfeld B, Souza B, Albert I, Munemitsu S, Polakis P: The APC protein and E-cadherin form similar but independent complexes with alpha-catenin, beta-catenin, and plakoglobin. *J Biol Chem* **270**:5549, 1995.

293. Rubinfeld B, Albert I, Porfiri E, Fiol C, Munemitsu S, Polakis P: Binding of GSK3-beta to the APC-beta-catenin complex and regulation of complex assembly. *Science* **272**:1023, 1996.

294. Ikeda S, Kishida S, Yamamoto H, Murai H, Koyama S, Kikuchi A: Axin, a negative regulator of the Wnt signaling pathway, forms a complex with GSK-3beta and beta-catenin and promotes GSK-3beta-dependent phosphorylation of beta-catenin. *EMBO J* **17**:1371, 1998.

295. Behrens J, Jerchow BA, Wurtele M, et al: Functional interaction of an axin homolog, conductin, with beta-catenin, APC, and GSK3beta. *Science* **280**:596, 1998.

296. Yamamoto H, Kishida S, Uochi T, et al: Axil, a member of the Axin family, interacts with both glycogen synthase kinase 3beta and beta-catenin and inhibits axis formation of *Xenopus* embryos. *Mol Cell Biol* **18**:2867, 1998.

297. Kishida S, Yamamoto H, Ikeda S, et al: Axin, a negative regulator of the wnt signaling pathway, directly interacts with adenomatous polyposis coli and regulates the stabilization of beta-catenin. *J Biol Chem* **273**:10823, 1998.

298. Hart MJ, de los Santos R, Albert IN, Rubinfeld B, Polakis P: Downregulation of beta-catenin by human Axin and its association with the APC tumor suppressor, beta-catenin and GSK3 beta. *Curr Biol* **8**:573, 1998.

299. Nakamura T, Hamada F, Ishidate T, et al: Axin, an inhibitor of the Wnt signalling pathway, interacts with beta-catenin, GSK-3beta and APC and reduces the beta-catenin level. *Genes Cells* **3**:395, 1998.

300. Su LK, Burrell M, Hill DE, et al: APC binds to the novel protein EB1. *Cancer Res* **55**:2972, 1995.

301. Munemitsu S, Souza B, Muller O, Albert I, Rubinfeld B, Polakis P: The *APC* gene product associates with microtubules in vivo and promotes their assembly in vitro. *Cancer Res* **54**:3676, 1994.

302. Smith KJ, Levy DB, Maupin P, Pollard TD, Vogelstein B, Kinzler KW: Wild-type but not mutant *APC* associates with the microtubule cytoskeleton. *Cancer Res* **54**:3672, 1994.

303. Matsumine A, Ogai A, Senda T, et al: Binding of *APC* to the human homolog of the *Drosophila* discs large tumor suppressor protein. *Science* **272**:1020, 1996.

304. Berrueta L, Kraeft SK, Tirnauer JS, et al: The adenomatous polyposis coli-binding protein EB1 is associated with cytoplasmic and spindle microtubules. *Proc Natl Acad Sci USA* **95**:10596, 1998.

305. Muhua L, Adames NR, Murphy MD, Shields CR, Cooper JA: A cytokinesis checkpoint requiring the yeast homologue of an APC-binding protein. *Nature* **393**:487, 1998.

306. Kemler R: From cadherins to catenins: Cytoplasmic protein interactions and regulation of cell adhesion. *Trends Genet* **9**:317, 1993.

307. Perrimon N: The genetic basis of patterned baldness in *Drosophila*. *Cell* **76**:781, 1994.

308. Gumbiner BM: Signal transduction of beta-catenin. *Curr Opin Cell Biol* **7**:634, 1995.

309. Peifer M: Regulating cell proliferation: As easy as APC. *Science* **272**:974, 1996.

310. Munemitsu S, Albert I, Souza B, Rubinfeld B, Polakis P: Regulation of intracellular beta-catenin levels by the adenomatous polyposis coli (APC) tumor-suppressor protein. *Proc Natl Acad Sci USA* **92**:3046, 1995.

311. Aberle H, Bauer A, Stappert J, Kispert A, Kemler R: Beta-catenin is a target for the ubiquitin-proteasome pathway. *EMBO J* **16**:3797, 1997.

312. Orford K, Crockett C, Jensen JP, Weissman AM, Byers SW: Serine phosphorylation-regulated ubiquitination and degradation of beta-catenin. *J Biol Chem* **272**:24735, 1997.

313. Behrens J, von Kries JP, Kuhl M, et al: Functional interaction of beta-catenin with the transcription factor LEF-1. *Nature* **382**:638, 1996.

314. Molenaar M, van de Wetering M, Oosterwegel M, et al: XTcf-3 transcription factor mediates beta-catenin-induced axis formation in *Xenopus* embryos. *Cell* **86**:391, 1996.

315. Whitehead I, Kirk H, Kay R: Expression cloning of oncogenes by retroviral transfer of cDNA libraries. *Mol Cell Biol* **15**:704, 1995.

316. Nusse R, Varmus HE: *Wnt* genes. *Cell* **69**:1073, 1992.

317. Korinek V, Barker N, Morin PJ, et al: Constitutive transcriptional activation by a beta-catenin-Tcf complex in *APC-/-* colon carcinoma. *Science* **275**:1784, 1997.

318. Morin PJ, Sparks AB, Korinek V, et al: Activation of beta-catenin-Tcf signaling in colon cancer by mutations in beta-catenin or APC. *Science* **275**:1787, 1997.

319. Iwao K, Nakamori S, Kameyama M, et al: Activation of the beta-catenin gene by interstitial deletions involving exon 3 in primary colorectal carcinomas without adenomatous polyposis coli mutations. *Cancer Res* **58**:1021, 1998.

320. Ilyas M, Tomlinson IP, Rowan A, Pignatelli M, Bodmer WF: Beta-catenin mutations in cell lines established from human colorectal cancers. *Proc Natl Acad Sci USA* **94**:10330, 1997.

321. Kitaeva MN, Grogan L, Williams JP, et al: Mutations in beta-catenin are uncommon in colorectal cancer occurring in occasional replication error-positive tumors. *Cancer Res* **57**:4478, 1997.

322. Sparks AB, Morin PJ, Vogelstein B, Kinzler KW: Mutational analysis of the APC/b-catenin/Tcf pathway in colorectal cancer. *Cancer Res* **58**:1130, 1998.

323. Rubinfeld B, Robbins P, El-Gamil M, Albert I, Porfiri E, Polakis P: Stabilization of beta-catenin by genetic defects in melanoma cell lines. *Science* **275**:1790, 1997.

324. de la Coste A, Romagnolo B, Billuart P, et al: Somatic mutations of the beta-catenin gene are frequent in mouse and human hepatocellular carcinomas. *Proc Natl Acad Sci USA* **95**:8847, 1998.

325. Voeller HJ, Truica CI, Gelmann EP: Beta-catenin mutations in human prostate cancer. *Cancer Res* **58**:2520, 1998.

326. Miyoshi Y, Iwao K, Nagasawa Y, et al: Activation of the beta-catenin gene in primary hepatocellular carcinomas by somatic alterations involving exon 3. *Cancer Res* **58**:2524, 1998.

327. Palacios J, Gamallo C: Mutations in the beta-catenin gene (*CTNNB1*) in endometrioid ovarian carcinomas. *Cancer Res* **58**:1344, 1998.

328. Zurawel RH, Chiappa SA, Allen C, Raffel C: Sporadic medulloblastomas contain oncogenic beta-catenin mutations. *Cancer Res* **58**:896, 1998.

329. Dashwood RH, Suzui M, Nakagama H, Sugimura T, Nagao M: High frequency of beta-catenin (*ctnnb1*) mutations in the colon tumors induced by two heterocyclic amines in the F344 rat. *Cancer Res* **58**:1127, 1998.

330. Takahashi M, Fukuda K, Sugimura T, Wakabayashi K: Beta-catenin is frequently mutated and demonstrates altered cellular location in azoxymethane-induced rat colon tumors. *Cancer Res* **58**:42, 1998.

331. He TC, Sparks AB, Rago C, et al: Identification of c-MYC as a target of the APC pathway. *Science* **281**:1509, 1998.

332. Rodriguez-Alfageme C, Stanbridge EJ, Astrin SM: Suppression of deregulated c-MYC expression in human colon carcinoma cells by chromosome 5 transfer. *Proc Natl Acad Sci USA* **89**:1482, 1992.

332a. Tetsu O, McCormick F: Beta-catenin regulates expression of cyclin D1 in colon carcinoma cells. *Nature* **398**:422, 1999.

332b. Shtutman M, Zhurinsky J, Simcha I, Albanese C, D'Amico M, Pestell R, Ben-Ze'ev A: The cyclin D1 gene is a target of the beta-catenin/LEF-1 pathway. *Proc Natl Acad Sci USA* **96**:5522, 1999.

332c. Mann B, Gelos M, Siedow A, Hanski ML, Gratche A, Ilyas M, Bodmer WF, Moyer MP, Riecken EO, Buhr HJ, Hanski C: Target genes of beta-catenin-T cell-factor/lymphoid-enhancer-factor signaling in human colorectal carcinomas. *Proc Natl Acad Sci USA* **96**:1603, 1999.

332d. Roose J, Huls G, van Beest M, Moerer P, van der Horn K, Goldschmeding R, Logtenberg T, Clevers H: Synergy between tumor suppressor APC and the beta-catenin-Tcf4 target Tcf1. *Science* **285**:1923, 1999.

332e. He TC, Chan TA, Vogelstein B, Kinzler KW: PPARdelta is an APC-regulated target of nonsteroidal anti-inflammatory drugs. *Cell* **99**:335, 1999.

333. Wong MH, Rubinfeld B, Gordon JI: Effects of forced expression of an NH2-terminal truncated beta-catenin on mouse intestinal epithelial homeostasis. *J Cell Biol* **141**:765, 1998.

333a. Harada N, Tamai Y, Ishikawa T, Sauer B, Takaku K, Oshima M, Taketo MM: Intestinal polyposis in mice with a dominant stable mutation of the beta-catenin gene, *Embo J* **18**:5931, 1999.

334. Gat U, DasGupta R, Degenstein L, Fuchs E: *De novo* hair follicle morphogenesis and hair tumors in mice expressing a truncated beta-catenin in skin. *Cell* **95**:605, 1998.

335. Korinek V, Barker N, Moerer P, et al: Depletion of epithelial stem-cell compartments in the small intestine of mice lacking Tcf-4. *Nature Genet* **19**:379, 1998.

336. Nakagawa H, Murata Y, Koyama K, et al: Identification of a brain-specific APC homologue, APCL, and its interaction with beta-catenin. *Cancer Res* **58**:5176, 1998.

337. van Es J, Kirkpatrick C, van de Wetering M, et al: A homologue of the adenomatous polyposis coli tumor suppressor gene. *Curr Biol* **9**:105, 1999.

338. Kinzler KW, Nilbert MC, Vogelstein B, et al: Identification of a gene located at chromosome 5q21 that is mutated in colorectal cancers. *Science* **251**:1366, 1991.

339. Hampton GM, Ward JR, Cottrell S, et al: Yeast artificial chromosomes for the molecular analysis of the familial polyposis APC gene region. *Proc Natl Acad Sci USA* **89**:8249, 1992.

340. Curtis LJ, Bubb VJ, Gledhill S, Morris RG, Bird CC, Wyllie AH: Loss of heterozygosity of *MCC* is not associated with mutation of the retained allele in sporadic colorectal cancer. *Hum Mol Genet* **3**:443, 1994.

341. Barker PE: Double minutes in human tumor cells. *Cancer Genet Cytogenet* **5**:81, 1982.

342. Alitalo K, Winqvist R, Lin CC, de la Chapelle A, Schwab M, Bishop JM: Aberrant expression of an amplified *c-myb* oncogene in two cell lines from a colon carcinoma. *Proc Natl Acad Sci USA* **81**:4534, 1984.

343. Alitalo K, Schwab M, Lin CC, Varmus HE, Bishop JM: Homogeneously staining chromosomal regions contain amplified copies of an abundantly expressed cellular oncogene (*c-myc*) in malignant neuroendocrine cells from a human colon carcinoma. *Proc Natl Acad Sci USA* **80**:1707, 1983.

344. Alexander RJ, Buxbaum JN, Raicht RF: Oncogene alterations in primary human colon tumors. *Gastroenterology* **91**:1503, 1986.

345. Meltzer SJ, Ahnen DJ, Battifora H, Yokota J, Cline MJ: Proto-oncogene abnormalities in colon cancers and adenomatous polyps. *Gastroenterology* **92**:1174, 1987.

346. Finley GG, Schulz NT, Hill SA, Geiser JR, Pipas JM, Meisler AI: Expression of the *myc* gene family in different stages of human colorectal cancer. *Oncogene* **4**:963, 1989.

347. Tal M, Wetzler M, Josefberg Z, et al: Sporadic amplification of the *HER2/neu* protooncogene in adenocarcinomas of various tissues. *Cancer Res* **48**:1517, 1988.

348. D'Emilia J, Bulovas K, D'Ercole K, Wolf B, Steele G Jr, Summerhayes IC: Expression of the *c-erbB-2* gene product (p185) at different stages of neoplastic progression in the colon. *Oncogene* **4**:1233, 1989.

349. Leach FS, Elledge SJ, Sherr CJ, et al: Amplification of cyclin genes in colorectal carcinomas. *Cancer Res* **53**:1986, 1993.

350. Zhou H, Kuang J, Zhong L, et al: Tumour amplified kinase STK15/BTAK induces centrosome amplification, aneuploidy and transformation. *Nature Genet* **20**:189, 1998.

351. Bischoff JR, Anderson L, Zhu Y, et al: A homologue of *Drosophila aurora* kinase is oncogenic and amplified in human colorectal cancers. *EMBO J* **17**:3052, 1998.

352. Pitti RM, Marsters SA, Lawrence DA, et al: Genomic amplification of a decoy receptor for Fas ligand in lung and colon cancer. *Nature* **396**:699, 1998.

353. Dietrich WF, Lander ES, Smith JS, et al: Genetic identification of *Mom-1,* a major modifier locus affecting Min-induced intestinal neoplasia in the mouse. *Cell* **75**:631, 1993.

354. MacPhee M, Chepenik K, Liddell R, Nelson K, Siracusa L, Buchberg A: The secretory phospholipase A2 gene is a candidate for the *Mom1* locus, a major modifier of ApcMin-induced intestinal neoplasia. *Cell* **81**:957, 1995.

355. Cormier RT, Hong KH, Halberg RB, et al: Secretory phospholipase Pla2g2a confers resistance to intestinal tumorigenesis. *Nature Genet* **17**:88, 1997.

356. Riggins GJ, Markowitz S, Wilson JK, Vogelstein B, Kinzler KW: Absence of secretory phospholipase a(2) gene alterations in human colorectal cancer. *Cancer Res* **55**:5184, 1995.

357. Melhem MF, Meisler AI, Finley GG, et al: Distribution of cells expressing myc proteins in human colorectal epithelium, polyps, and malignant tumors. *Cancer Res* **52**:5853, 1992.

358. Ogata S, Uehara H, Chen A, Itzkowitz SH: Mucin gene expression in colonic tissues and cell lines. *Cancer Res* **52**:5971, 1992.

359. Ciardiello F, Kim N, Saeki T, et al: Differential expression of epidermal growth factor-related proteins in human colorectal tumors. *Proc Natl Acad Sci USA* **88**:7792, 1991.

360. Koenders PG, Peters WH, Wobbes T, Beex LV, Nagengast FM, Benraad TJ: Epidermal growth factor receptor levels are lower in carcinomatous than in normal colorectal tissue. *Br J Cancer* **65**:189, 1992.

361. Gold P, Freedman SO: Demonstration of tumor-specific antigens in human colonic carcinomata by immunological tolerance and absorption techniques. *J Exp Med* **121**:439, 1965.

362. Ransom JH, Pelle B, Hanna MG Jr: Expression of class II major histocompatibility complex molecules correlates with human colon tumor vaccine efficacy. *Cancer Res* **52**:3460, 1992.

363. Tsioulias G, Godwin TA, Goldstein MF, et al: Loss of colonic HLA antigens in familial adenomatous polyposis. *Cancer Res* **52**:3449, 1992.

364. Calabretta B, Kaczmarek L, Ming PM, Au F, Ming SC: Expression of *c-myc* and other cell cycle-dependent genes in human colon neoplasia. *Cancer Res* **45**:6000, 1985.

365. Adams MD, Kerlavage AR, Fleischmann RD, et al: Initial assessment of human gene diversity and expression patterns based upon 83 million nucleotides of Cdna sequence. *Nature* **377**:3, 1995.

366. Liang P, Pardee AB: Differential display of eukaryotic messenger RNA by means of the polymerase chain reaction. *Science* **257**:967, 1992.

367. Velculescu VE, Zhang L, Vogelstein B, Kinzler KW: Serial analysis of gene expression. *Science* **270**:484, 1995.

368. Schena M, Shalon D, Davis RW, Brown PO: Quantitative monitoring of gene expression patterns with a complementary DNA microarray. *Science* **270**:467, 1995.

369. Zhang L, Zhou W, Velculescu VE, Kern SE, Hruban RH, Hamilton SR, Vogelstein B, Kinzler KW: Gene expression profiles in normal and cancer cells. *Science* **276**:1268 1997.

370. Bird A: The essentials of DNA methylation. *Cell* **70**:5, 1992.

371. Goelz SE, Vogelstein B, Hamilton SR, Feinberg AP: Hypomethylation of DNA from benign and malignant human colon neoplasms. *Science* **228**:187, 1985.

372. Feinberg AP, Gehrke CW, Kuo KC, Ehrlich M: Reduced genomic 5-methylcytosine content in human colonic neoplasia. *Cancer Res* **48**:1159, 1988.

373. Silverman AL, Park JG, Hamilton SR, Gazdar AF, Luk GD, Baylin SB: Abnormal methylation of the calcitonin gene in human colonic neoplasms. *Cancer Res* **49**:3468, 1989.

374. El-Deiry WS, Nelkin BD, Celano P, et al: High expression of the DNA methyltransferase gene characterizes human neoplastic cells and progression stages of colon cancer. *Proc Natl Acad Sci USA* **88**:3470, 1991.

375. Schmid M, Haaf T, Grunert D: 5-Azacytidine-induced undercondensations in human chromosomes. *Hum Genet* **67**:257, 1984.

376. Herman JG, Umar A, Polyak K, et al: Incidence and functional consequences of *hMLH1* promoter hypermethylation in colorectal carcinoma. *Proc Natl Acad Sci USA* **95**:6870, 1998.

377. Baylin SB, Makos M, Wu JJ, et al: Abnormal patterns of DNA methylation in human neoplasia: Potential consequences for tumor progression. *Cancer Cells* **3**:383, 1991.

378. Herman JG, Merlo A, Mao L, et al: Inactivation of the *CDKN2/p16/MTS1* gene is frequently associated with aberrant DNA methylation in all common human cancers. *Cancer Res* **55**:4525, 1995.

379. Landolph JR, Jones PA: Mutagenicity of 5-azacytidine and related nucleosides in C3H/10T 1/2 clone 8 and V79 cells. *Cancer Res* **42**:817, 1982.

380. Laird P, Jackson-Grusby L, Fazeli A, et al: Suppression of intestinal neoplasia by DNA hypomethylation. *Cell* **81**:197, 1995.

381. Fearon ER, Vogelstein B: A genetic model for colorectal tumorigenesis. *Cell* **61**:759, 1990.

382. Vogelstein B, Kinzler KW: The multistep nature of cancer. *Trends Genet* **9**:138, 1993.

383. Garber JE, Goldstein AM, Kantor AF, Dreyfus MG, Fraumeni JF Jr, Li FP: Follow-up study of twenty-four families with Li-Fraumeni syndrome. *Cancer Res* **51**:6094, 1991.

384. Kinzler KW, Vogelstein B: Cancer-susceptibility genes: Gatekeepers and caretakers. *Nature* **386**:761, 1997.

385. Loeb LA: Mutator phenotype may be required for multistage carcinogenesis. *Cancer Res* **51**:3075, 1991.

386. Hartwell L: Defects in a cell cycle checkpoint may be responsible for the genomic instability of cancer cells. *Cell* **71**:543, 1992.

387. Heim S, Mitelman F: Cytogenetic analysis in the diagnosis of acute leukemia. *Cancer* **70**:1701, 1992.

388. Ionov Y, Peinado MA, Malkhosyan S, Shibata D, Perucho M: Ubiquitous somatic mutations in simple repeated sequences reveal a new mechanism for colonic carcinogenesis. *Nature* **363**:558, 1993.

389. Thibodeau SN, Bren G, Schaid D: Microsatellite instability in cancer of the proximal colon. *Science* **260**:816, 1993.

390. Aaltonen LA, Peltomaki P, Leach FS, et al: Clues to the pathogenesis of familial colorectal cancer. *Science* **260**:812, 1993.

391. Eshleman JR, Lang EZ, Bowerfind GK, et al: Increased mutation rate at the hprt locus accompanies microsatellite instability in colon cancer. *Oncogene* **10**:33, 1995.

392. Lengauer C, Kinzler KW, Vogelstein B: Genetic instability in colorectal cancers. *Nature* **386**:623, 1997.

393. Cahill DP, Lengauer C, Yu J, et al: Mutations of mitotic checkpoint genes in human cancers. *Nature* **392**:300, 1998.

394. Lengauer C, Kinzler KW, Vogelstein B: Genetic instabilities in human cancers. *Nature* **396**:643, 1998.

395. Li J, Yen C, Liaw D, et al: *PTEN,* a putative protein tyrosine phosphatase gene mutated in human brain, breast, and prostate cancer. *Science* **275**:1943, 1997.

396. Steck PA, Pershouse MA, Jasser SA, et al: Identification of a candidate tumour suppressor gene, *MMAC1,* at chromosome 10q23.3 that is mutated in multiple advanced cancers. *Nature Genet* **15**:356, 1997.

397. Sidransky D, Tokino T, Hamilton SR, et al: Identification of *ras* oncogene mutations in the stool of patients with curable colorectal tumors. *Science* **256**:102, 1992.

398. Smith-Ravin J, England J, Talbot IC, Bodmer W: Detection of *c-Ki-ras* mutations in faecal samples from sporadic colorectal cancer patients. *Gut* **36**:81, 1995.

399. Hasegawa Y, Takeda S, Ichii S, et al: Detection of *K-ras* mutations in DNAs isolated from feces of patients with colorectal tumors by mutant-allele-specific amplification (MASA). *Oncogene* **10**:1441, 1995.

400. Villa E, Dugani A, Rebecchi AM, et al: Identification of subjects at risk for colorectal carcinoma through a test based on K-ras determination in the stool. *Gastroenterology* **110**:1346, 1996.

401. Nollau P, Moser C, Weinland G, Wagener C: Detection of *K-ras* mutations in stools of patients with colorectal cancer by mutant-enriched PCR. *Int J Cancer* **66**:332, 1996.

402. Waddell WR, Ganser GF, Cerise EJ, Loughry RW: Sulindac for polyposis of the colon. *Am J Surg* **157**:175, 1989.

403. Rigau J, Pique JM, Rubio E, Planas R, Tarrech JM, Bordas JM: Effects of long-term sulindac therapy on colonic polyposis. *Ann Intern Med* **115**:952, 1991.

404. Labayle D, Fischer D, Vielh P, et al: Sulindac causes regression of rectal polyps in familial adenomatous polyposis. *Gastroenterology* **101**:635, 1991.

405. Giardiello FM, Hamilton SR, Krush AJ, et al: Treatment of colonic and rectal adenomas with sulindac in familial adenomatous polyposis. *N Engl J Med* **328**:1313, 1993.

406. Nugent K, Farmer K, Spigelman A, Williams C, Phillips R: Randomized controlled trial of the effect of sulindac on duodenal and rectal polyposis and cell proliferation in patients with familial adenomatous polyposis. *Br J Surg* **80**:1618, 1993.

407. Winde G, Gumbinger HG, Osswald H, Kemper F, Bunte H: The NSAID sulindac reverses rectal adenomas in colectomized patients with familial adenomatous polyposis: Clinical results of a dose-finding study on rectal sulindac administration. *Int J Colorectal Dis* **8**:13, 1993.

408. Debinski H, Trojan J, Nugent K, Spigelman A, Phillips R: Effect of sulindac on small polyps in familial adenomatous polyposis. *Lancet* **345**:855, 1995.

409. Winde G, Schmid K, Schlegel W, Fischer R, Osswald H, Bunte H: Complete reversion and prevention of rectal adenomas in colectomized patients with familial adenomatous polyposis by rectal low-dose sulindac maintenance treatment: Advantages of a low-dose nonsteroidal anti-inflammatory drug regimen in reversing adenomas exceeding 33 months. *Dis Colon Rectum* **38**:813, 1995.

410. Kune GA, Kune S, Watson LF: Colorectal cancer risk, chronic illnesses, operations, and medications: Case control results from the Melbourne Colorectal Cancer Study. *Cancer Res* **48**:4399, 1988.

411. Rosenberg L, Palmer JR, Zauber AG, Warshauer ME, Stolley PD, Shapiro S: A hypothesis: Nonsteroidal anti-inflammatory drugs reduce the incidence of large-bowel cancer. *J Natl Cancer Inst* **83**:355, 1991.

412. Thun MJ, Namboodiri MM, Heath CW Jr: Aspirin use and reduced risk of fatal colon cancer. *N Engl J Med* **325**:1593, 1991.

413. Beazer-Barclay Y, Levy DB, Moser AM, et al: Sulindac suppresses tumorigenesis in the Min mouse. *Carcinogenesis* **17**:1757, 1996.

414. Jacoby RF, Marshall DJ, Newton MA, et al: Chemoprevention of spontaneous intestinal adenomas in the APC-Min mouse by the nonsteroidal anti-inflammatory drug piroxicam. *Cancer Res* **56**:710, 1996.

415. Boolbol SK, Dannenberg AJ, Chadurn A, et al: Cyclooxygenase-2 overexpression and tumor formation are blocked by sulindac in a murine model of familial adenomatous polyposis. *Cancer Res* **56**:2556, 1996.

416. Waldman T, Zhang Y, Dillehay L, et al: Cell-cycle arrest versus cell death in cancer therapy. *Nature Med* **3**:1034, 1997.

417. Clara M, Herschel K, Ferner H: *Atlas of Normal Microscopic Anatomy of Man.* New York, Urban & Schwarzenberg, 1974.

418. Kinzler KW, Vogelstein B: Lessons from hereditary colon cancer. *Cell* **87**:159, 1996.

419. Greenblatt MS, Bennett WP, Hollstein M, Harris CC: Mutations in the *p53* tumor suppressor gene: Clues to cancer etiology and molecular pathogenesis. *Cancer Res* **54**:4855, 1994.

420. Vogelstein B, Kinzler K: Tumour-suppressor genes: X-rays strike p53 again. *Nature* **370**:174, 1994.

421. Kinzler KW, Vogelstein B: Life (and death) in a malignant tumour. *Nature* **379**:19, 1996.

422. Altschul SF, Gish W, Miller W, Myers EW, Lipman DJ: Basic local alignment search tool. *J Mol Biol* **215**:403, 1990.

423. Miyoshi Y, Ando H, Nagase H, et al: Germ-line mutations of the *APC* gene in 53 familial adenomatous polyposis patients. *Proc Natl Acad Sci USA* **89**:4452, 1992.

424. Peifer M, Berg S, Reynolds AB: A repeating amino acid motif shared by proteins with diverse cellular roles. *Cell* **76**:789, 1994.

Pilomatricoma and Pilomatrix Carcinoma

Edward F. Chan ▪ *Uri Gat*
Ramanuj Dasgupta ▪ *Elaine Fuchs*

1. Pilomatricoma is a benign hair follicle tumor that is thought to be the most common solid cutaneous tumor in patients 20 years of age or younger. It demonstrates differentiation toward the compartment of cells in the matrix of the hair bulb that forms the hair shaft. These tumors typically present as solitary, firm nodules on the head, neck, and upper extremities. Multiple pilomatricomas are found in 4 percent of cases. There is a bimodal age of presentation, with most cases occurring in the first and sixth decades. In patients younger than 20 years of age, there is a male:female ratio of 1:2.5.

2. Pilomatrix carcinoma is relatively rare; there have been approximately 70 reports in the literature. Unlike pilomatricomas, pilomatrix carcinomas have a male:female ratio of 2:1 and occur at a later age, with a mean age of 48. This tumor may have an invasive growth pattern, with spread into the underlying bone. Local recurrence occurs in 60 percent of cases and metastatic disease occurs in 10 percent of cases.

3. The histologic appearance of a pilomatricoma is of a well-circumscribed tumor in the lower dermis to subcutis comprised of coalescing, irregularly shaped islands of epithelial cells. Two basic cell types form these epithelial islands: basophilic cells and eosinophilic shadow cells. The basophilic cells tend to be at the periphery or sides of the tumor islands and possess scant cytoplasm, indistinct cell borders, basophilic and hyperchromatic nuclei, and numerous mitoses. The eosinophilic shadow cells are at the center of the tumor and show distinct cell borders, faintly eosinophilic cytoplasm, and a central oval clear area which is a shadow of the lost nucleus. These shadow cells form from the basophilic cells and there may be a transition zone where the basophilic cells become more eosinophilic with development of pyknotic nuclei. There are often foci of calcification and ossification associated with the shadow cells.

4. In pilomatrix carcinoma, there are large, anaplastic, hyperchromatic basophilic cells with numerous mitoses, some of which may be atypical. The basophilic cells show variation in nuclear size, with coarse chromatin, and prominent nucleoli. There are cystic areas with central necrosis and shadow cells. Vascular and perineural invasion may also be present.

5. Some syndromes involve pilomatricomas as one of several complex traits. These disorders include myotonic dystrophy, Gardner syndrome, and the Rubinstein-Taybi syndrome. In addition, there are reported cases of familial pilomatricomas without other systemic manifestations. In contrast to the sporadic cases of pilomatricoma in which a solitary lesion is typical, in the case of familial pilomatricomas, the tumors are often multiple.

6. A high percentage of pilomatricomas possess β-catenin missense mutations clustered in the amino-terminal segment, normally involved in phosphorylation-dependent, ubiquitin-mediated degradation of the protein. The initial work that led to this finding developed from the observation that similar tumors develop in transgenic mice expressing a keratin promoter-driven, stable form of β-catenin truncated at its amino terminus. In addition, nuclear LEF-1 is present in the basophilic cells of the tumor, thus providing further biochemical evidence that pilomatricomas are derived from hair matrix cells. These findings point to β-catenin/LEF misregulation as a major cause of tumorigenesis in pilomatricomas.

Pilomatricoma, also known as calcifying epithelioma or pilomatrixoma, is a benign tumor that was first described in 1880 by Malherbe,[1] and is thought to be the most common solid cutaneous tumor in patients 20 years of age or younger.[2,3] It demonstrates hair follicle differentiation toward the compartment of cells in the matrix of the hair bulb that form the cortex of the hair shaft. Evidence for this comes from morphologic, ultrastructural,[4,5] and biochemical data.[6-8] The transitional cells within pilomatricomas express hair keratin basic 1,[9] a hair keratin that is found in the normal hair cortex from the keratogenous zone to the isthmus.[10] Malignant transformation of pilomatricoma into pilomatrix carcinoma is characterized by cytologic atypia and aggressive behavior and occurs infrequently.

CLINICAL ASPECTS OF PILOMATRICOMA AND PILOMATRIX CARCINOMA

Clinical Presentation and Incidence

Pilomatricomas typically present as solitary, firm nodules. A review of cutaneous adnexal tumors in the first two decades of life showed that pilomatric lesions accounted for approximately three-fourths of cases.[2] Most are found on the head and neck (40 to 60 percent), upper extremities (25 to 30 percent), or trunk (13 to 35 percent).[3] The overlying epidermis can be normal appearing, have a red-blue hue, or show atrophy and anetoderma. There may be hard areas of calcification and ossification, and stretching of the overlying skin may show the "tent sign" with multiple facets or angles. In most cases, there is slow growth of the tumor, although hemorrhage can cause sudden, rapid growth. Perforation through the epidermis has been reported.[11] Multiple pilomatricomas are found in 4 percent of cases.[12] Although most cases are sporadic tumors, there are reports of familial pilomatricomas, typically in the setting of myotonic dystrophy.[13]

In a retrospective review of 209 cases of pilomatricomas over 20 years, there was a bimodal age of presentation with tumors found primarily in the first and sixth decades. The age range was between 18 months to 86 years, with peak ages between 5 and 15 years for females and up to 5 years for males. In adults, it occurred mostly between 50 and 65 years of age. In patients younger than 20 years of age, there was a female predilection with a male:female ratio of 1:2.5. The tumors ranged in size from less than 0.5 cm to 6.0 cm, with most between 1.0 and 1.5 cm. Approximately 50 percent were located on the head, with 10 percent on the scalp. None were found on the palms, soles, or genitalia.[14]

Pilomatrix carcinoma is relatively rare, and there have been approximately 70 reports in the literature. Unlike pilomatricomas, pilomatrix carcinomas have a male:female ratio of 2:1 and occur at a later age, with a mean age of 48.[15] This tumor may have an invasive growth pattern, with spread into the underlying bone.[16] Local recurrence occurs in 60 percent of cases. Metastatic disease occurs in 10 percent of cases and has been documented to the lung, bone, and lymphatics. Widespread metastatic disease with multi-organ involvement can also occur; four deaths have been attributed to metastatic disease. Patients have also developed secondary hypercalcemia[6] and angioimmunoblastic lymphadenopathy.[17] In eight cases, the initial biopsy was consistent with a benign lesion, with the recurrent tumor showing malignant transformation.[15]

Diagnostic Criteria and Pathology

The gross appearance of a pilomatricoma is of a variegated tumor with gray, white, and brown areas, often with calcification and bone formation. The histologic appearance of pilomatricomas on low power is of a well-circumscribed tumor in the lower dermis to subcutis comprised of coalescing, irregularly shaped islands of epithelial cells (Fig. 35-1A). There is often a connective tissue capsule and a surrounding foreign body giant cell reaction. Occasionally, the pilomatricoma may be connected to one or several hair follicles.[18] There are two basic cell types which form these epithelial islands: basophilic cells and eosinophilic shadow cells. The basophilic cells tend to be at the periphery or sides of the tumor islands and possess scant cytoplasm, indistinct cell borders, basophilic and hyperchromatic nuclei, and numerous mitoses (Fig. 35-1B). These features on a fine-needle aspirate may result in a false positive diagnosis of malignancy.[19] The basophilic cells express the proliferation associated antigen, Ki-67, and the apoptosis-inhibiting protein, bcl-2, particularly in the basal layer.[20,21] The eosinophilic shadow cells are at the center of the tumor and show distinct cell borders, faintly eosinophilic cytoplasm, and a central oval clear area which is a shadow of the lost nucleus (Fig. 35-1C). These shadow cells show differentiation toward the hair shaft cortex. These shadow cells form from the basophilic cells and there may be a transition zone where the basophilic cells become more eosinophilic with development of pyknotic nuclei (Fig. 35-1D). The nuclei of these transitional cells stain with *in situ* end-labeling techniques such as the TUNEL (transferase-mediated dUTP-biotin nick-end labeling) technique, and thus show DNA fragmentation.[20,22,23] However, nuclear

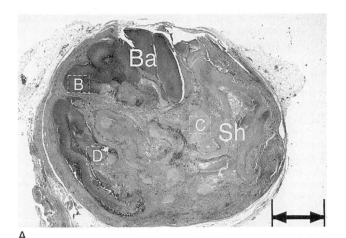

A

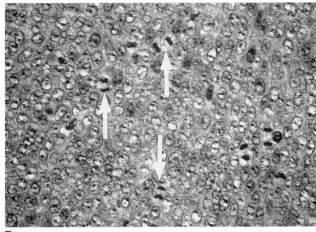

B

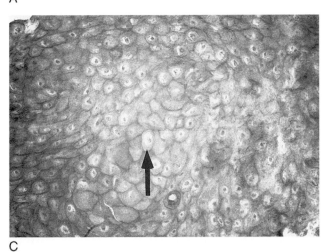

C

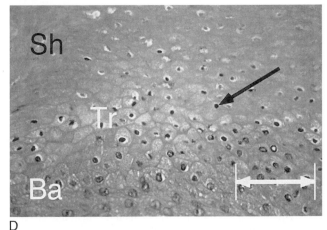

D

Figure 35-1 *A,* Low-power view of a pilomatricoma with basophilic cells labeled Ba and shadow cells labeled Sh. Dotted boxes indicate areas chosen for *B, C,* and *D,* respectively. Magnification bar corresponds to 1.3 mm. *B,* The basophilic cells possess scant cytoplasm, indistinct cell borders, basophilic and hyperchromatic nuclei, and numerous mitoses (*arrows*). *C,* The eosinophilic shadow cells show distinct cell borders, faintly eosinophilic cytoplasm, and a central oval clear area, which is a shadow of the lost nucleus (*arrow*). *D,* The transition zone (Tr) is where the basophilic cells (Ba) become more eosinophilic with development of pyknotic nuclei (*arrow*). Shadow cells are labeled Sh. Magnification bar corresponds to 80 μm in *B, C,* and *D.*

fragmentation does not occur, and it has been hypothesized that these cells are not undergoing conventional apoptosis but some form of terminal differentiation toward the hair cortex.[22]

The histologic appearance of pilomatricomas varies with the age of the lesion, with early lesions containing more basaloid cells and later lesions containing more shadow cells. This continuum has been subdivided into four stages.[24] In the early stage, there are smaller cystic structures lined by basaloid epithelium with a central area containing shadow cells. In the fully developed stage there are larger neoplasms comprised of basaloid epithelium at the periphery surrounding zones of shadow cells. The early regressive stage also has basophilic and shadow cells, but has a surrounding stromal reaction and no epithelial lining. The late regressive stage shows masses of shadow cells without basophilic cells and little or no inflammatory infiltrate.

Calcification is present in more than two-thirds of these tumors, and occurs mainly in the shadow cells. Ossification occurs in 15 to 20 percent, and also occurs mainly in shadow cells, which have been shown to express bone morphogenetic protein-2 by immunohistochemical staining.[25] Bone formation may be accompanied by extramedullary hematopoiesis.[26] Melanin is present in 20 percent of cases and may be found in the shadow cells, the surrounding stroma, or within the islands of basophilic cells.

In pilomatrix carcinoma, there are large, anaplastic, hyperchromatic basophilic cells with numerous mitoses and an infiltrative border.[16] The basophilic cells show variation in nuclear size, with coarse chromatin, and prominent nucleoli. Atypical mitotic figures, cystic areas with central necrosis, vascular invasion, and perineural invasion may also be present. No specific markers to distinguish between pilomatricoma and pilomatrix carcinoma have been identified, and DNA flow cytometry of pilomatrix carcinoma shows no abnormalities.[27,28] Although the average size of these tumors is slightly larger than benign pilomatricomas, this was not predictive of malignancy because of the significant overlap in size.[16]

GENETIC LOCI IN HEREDITARY CASES OF PILOMATRICOMA

There are several syndromes associated with the development of pilomatricomas, including myotonic dystrophy, Gardner syndrome, and the Rubinstein-Taybi syndrome. In addition, there have been rare reported cases of familial pilomatricomas without other systemic manifestations.[29] In the case of pilomatricomas associated with an inherited syndrome, the tumors are often multiple, in contrast to the sporadic cases where a solitary lesion is more typical.

Myotonic dystrophy (Steinert disease) is a hereditary neuromuscular disorder that is the most common cause of muscular dystrophy in adult life. It is characterized by myotonia (hyperexcitability of the skeletal muscle causing inability to relax after contraction), myopathy, cardiac disease, cataracts, testicular atrophy, and frontal baldness. The disease is inherited in an autosomal dominant fashion and is caused by a trinucleotide CTG expansion of the 3' untranslated region of the myotonin protein kinase gene (DMPK) on chromosome 19q13.3.[30,31] The number of triplet repeats can increase with subsequent generations and disease severity correlates with the size of the expansion. Approximately 4 percent of patients with myotonic dystrophy have pilomatricomas.[32] There are 25 reported cases of pilomatrixoma with myotonic dystrophy and of these patients, 84 percent had multiple tumors (from 2 to 41), and 80 percent had tumors located on the scalp.[13] In 11 cases, pilomatricomas were also found in other family members with myotonic dystrophy.[32,33] These tumors have the clinical and histologic appearance of typical sporadic pilomatricomas.

Various other tumors have also been associated with myotonic dystrophy, including neural crest-derived tumors, parathyroid adenomas, and small-bowel carcinomas. The Drosophila *warts* gene is a homologue of DMPK, and homozygous loss of this gene

is associated with abnormal growth of epithelial cells, thus providing evidence that it may function as a tumor suppressor gene.[34] One hypothesis for the occurrence of these tumors in myotonic dystrophy patients is function of DMPK as a tumor-suppressor gene.[35]

Gardner syndrome is a form of familial adenomatous polyposis (FAP) with characteristic extracolonic manifestations. These patients develop intestinal polyposis and colorectal adenocarcinoma with a high degree of penetrance.[36] Other neoplasms associated with this syndrome include follicular or papillary thyroid carcinoma, adrenal adenomas and adenocarcinomas, hepatoblastoma, and duodenal carcinomas. In addition, they develop characteristic pigmented lesions of the ocular fundus, cutaneous cysts, desmoid tumors, and lipomas.

Fifty to 60 percent of patients with Gardner syndrome develop cutaneous cysts.[37] Although initially these cysts were felt to be infundibular or epidermoid cysts, it is now recognized that pilomatricoma-like changes in the walls of these cysts are quite characteristic for Gardner syndrome.[38–40] In addition to these features, there are reports of sebaceous gland differentiation and focal epithelial proliferations of the basal layer that express cytokeratin 19 and that are associated with cytokeratin 20-reactive Merkel cells—both characteristics of bulge cells, the putative stem cell population of the hair follicle.[41] The more typical solid-tumor form of pilomatricoma has also been reported in Gardner syndrome patients.[42]

Patients with familial adenomatous polyposis harbor mutations in the adenomatous polyposis coli (APC) gene,[43] a tumor-suppressor gene that is also mutated in approximately 80 percent of sporadic colon cancers.[44] In addition, patients with the extracolonic manifestations of Gardner syndrome in its severe form tend to have mutations in a specific region of the APC gene.[45] The APC gene codes for a large 2843-amino acid protein that interacts with many other molecules, including β-catenin. The interaction of APC with β-catenin causes the downregulation of β-catenin *in vivo* (see below for a more detailed explanation of this process).[46]

Rubinstein-Taybi syndrome is an autosomal dominant, multisystem, inherited disorder characterized by mental retardation, broad thumbs and great toes, characteristic facial abnormalities, and short stature. Approximately 5 percent of patients develop neoplasms, including those affecting the nervous system, such as medulloblastoma, neuroblastoma, and oligodendroglioma.[47] Pilomatricomas have been reported in six patients with this syndrome, with four of these cases developing multiple pilomatricomas.[48,49] Rubinstein-Taybi may be caused by gross rearrangements or deletions of chromosome 16p13.3 and is associated with point mutations in a gene located in this region coding for CREB binding protein (CBP).[50]

CBP (also known as p300) is a transcriptional coactivator that is recruited to DNA by several different transcription factors, including CREB (cyclic AMP response element-binding protein),[51] the p65 subunit of NFκB,[52] and Dorsal.[53] In vertebrates, CBP is a transcriptional coactivator for β-catenin,[54] whereas in *Drosophila*, dCBP acetylates dTCF in the absence of β-catenin and represses transcription.[55] Of note, if the pilomatricomas in patients with Rubinstein-Taybi syndrome are the result of loss of function mutations, then the overall effect of CBP would be as a repressor.

SPECIFIC GENES

Sporadic Cases

A high percentage of pilomatricomas possess β-catenin missense mutations clustered in the amino-terminal segment.[56,56a] The initial work that led to this finding developed from the observation that similar tumors develop in transgenic mice expressing a keratin promoter-driven, stable form of β-catenin truncated at its amino terminus (NΔ87 βcat).[57] β-Catenin, the vertebrate homologue of

Drosophila armadillo, can perform two separate functions: it has a role in cell-cell adhesion and a role in the Wnt signaling pathway. There are two cellular pools of β-catenin corresponding to these roles. In one pool, β-catenin is part of a cytoskeletal-associated complex with E-cadherin, a protein involved in intercellular adhesion. In another pool, seen only upon transduction of a Wnt signal, β-catenin exists in a monomeric soluble form and can potentially interact with a specific class of DNA binding proteins.[58]

Wnt signaling pathways play critical roles in both development and carcinogenesis.[59] In the absence of most Wnt signals, APC interacts with any β-catenin not used for cell-cell junctions and promotes its phosphorylation, subsequent ubiquitination, and degradation. APC contains a nuclear export sequence, and through its association with β-catenin, can keep β-catenin cytoplasmic.[60–62] APC and β-catenin also bind to the scaffold protein axin/conductin, which also binds the GSK-3β kinase that phosphorylates β-catenin.

In the presence of most extracellular Wnt ligands, there is an activation of Wnt receptors, known as Frizzleds. A low-density lipoprotein receptor-related-protein (LRP) has been shown to be a potential Frizzled coreceptor and LRP's intracellular domain binds to axin.[63] One possible mechanism is that upon activation, LRP alters the conformation of axin in a way that prevents binding of β-catenin but maintains association with APC and GSK-3β. This could involve another protein, Disheveled, which is also implicated at this step.

Once stabilized, β-catenin forms a complex with a member of the TCF/LEF transcription factor family and results in activation of new gene expression patterns.[64] A variety of additional proteins are known to associate with these transcription factor complexes to influence whether the complexes will be repressors or activators of transcription. Such factors include dCBP[55] and Groucho proteins.[58,65,66]

Besides the Wnt/Frizzled ligand receptor genes, three genes in this pathway are known to be mutated in primary human cancers: β-catenin,[67–75] axin,[76,77] and APC.[44] In all three cases, there is accumulation of β-catenin and aberrant activation of downstream genes. Normally, the β-catenin that is not assembled into adherens junctions becomes phosphorylated in its N-terminal segment, thereby targeting the protein for ubiquitin-mediated degrada-

tion.[78,79] Most human cancers that involve β-catenin mutations possess changes in a few specific amino acid residues within the N-terminal segment.[67–75] These affect specific serine and threonine amino acid residues and their adjacent amino acids that play a role in targeting the molecule for degradation. These mutations are clustered within and close to the GSK-3β phosphorylation sites. They inhibit the phosphorylation dependent interaction of the amino-terminal end of β-catenin with a component of E3 ubiquitin ligase, β-TRCP.[80]

Given the predisposition of keratin promoter-driven NΔ87 βcat mice to develop pilomatricoma-like tumors,[57] Chan et al.[56] searched for mutations in the N-terminal segment of the β-catenin gene in human sporadic pilomatricomas. Sixteen human pilomatricomas were screened and single nucleotide substitutions were found in the DNAs from 12 of the samples examined.[56] Sequencing of the DNA fragments amplified from the microdissected normal tissue surrounding the tumor revealed the wild-type β-catenin sequence, thus indicating the somatic nature of these mutations. The 12 nucleotide alterations found all encode putative missense mutations in the amino terminal segment of β-catenin: D32Y (GAC → TAC), D32G (GAC → GGC), 2 X S33F (TCT → TTT), 2 X S33Y (TCT → TAT), 3 X G34E (GGA → GAA), S37C (TCT → TGT), S37F (TCT → TTT) and T41I (ACC → ATC) (Fig. 35-2). Each of these mutations had been previously associated with a variety of nonskin human carcinomas and cell lines (Fig. 35-2). Seven of the 12 mutations represent alterations in serine 33, serine 37, and/or threonine 41 amino acid residues essential for GSK-3β-dependent phosphorylation.[81,82] Five mutations are in the aspartic acid or glycine residues flanking serine 33. This DSG sequence, along with serine 37 (underlined residues in Fig. 35-2), have been characterized as a ubiquitination targeting motif based upon its conservation with IκBα, another protein that is phosphorylated and subsequently degraded by ubiquitin ligases.[82,83] Therefore, mutations in these adjoining residues may interfere with ubiquitination, possibly through altering the GSK-3β kinase-recognition sites. These findings have recently been independently confirmed, with seven out of seven human sporadic pilomatricomas showing β-catenin mutations affecting these same amino acid residues.[56a]

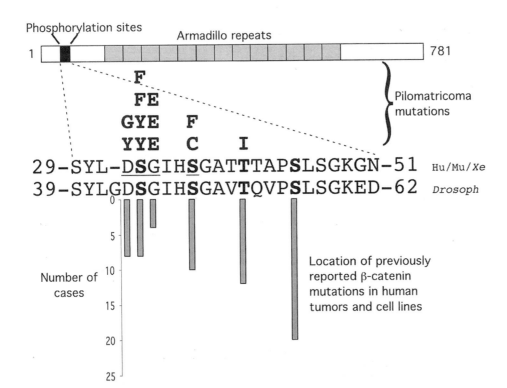

Figure 35-2 Schematic of β-catenin, depicting the location of the GSK3 β-dependent phosphorylation sites in the amino-terminal segment and the *Armadillo* repeats, characteristic of this family of proteins. Shown are the sequences of the wild-type, conserved amino-terminal segment from human (Hu), murine (Mu), *Xenopus* (Xe), and *Drosophila* (*Drosoph*) and the corresponding location of pilomatricoma mutations and previously described mutations from other types of human tumors and cell lines. (*Reprinted with permission from Chan et al.*[56])

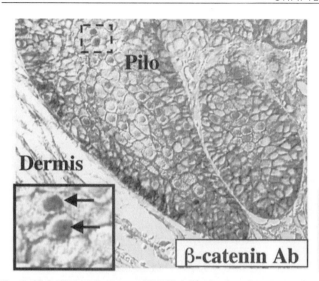

Figure 35-3 Pilomatricomas exhibit high levels of nuclear β-catenin and cyclin D1. Sections of pilomatricoma from a K14-ΔN-βcat transgenic mouse underwent immunohistochemistry. *Left*, a section was stained with anti-β-catenin antibodies at conditions in which nuclear β-catenin can be detected. High levels of nuclear β-catenin (see arrows in inset, dotted box indicates area of magnification) were found in peripheral as well as the more differentiated (inner) layers of the tumor. *Right*, Cyclin D1, a target gene of activated β-catenin is also highly expressed in the tumors (see arrows in inset, dotted box indicates area of magnification) as detected by anti-Cyclin D1-specific antibodies.

The frequency of β-catenin mutations in pilomatricomas is higher than what had previously been described for other tumors; however, recent papers have also revealed a high percentage of β-catenin mutations in some other tumors including hepatoblastomas[84–86] and anaplastic thyroid carcinomas.[87] The findings of Chan et al.[56] suggest that acquisition of a stabilizing mutation in β-catenin plays an important role in the pathogenesis of pilomatricomas. In addition, two genetic syndromes associated with pilomatricomas, Gardner syndrome and Rubinstein-Taybi syndrome, are associated with mutations in a gene that is involved in the β-catenin/LEF signaling pathway—APC in Gardner syndrome and CBP in Rubinstein-Taybi syndrome. Taken together, these findings suggest that β-catenin/LEF misregulation is a major component of tumorigenesis in pilomatricomas.

The exact mechanism whereby aberrant activation of the Wnt/APC/β-catenin signaling pathway causes tumorigenesis is, at this point, unclear. Downstream transcriptional targets of β-catenin include c-myc[88] and cyclin D1,[89,90] which both contain TCF-binding sites in their promoters. In addition, these genes appear to be constitutively activated in several colon cancer cell lines.

To better characterize the differentiation of pilomatricomas, sporadic human tumor sections have been stained with anti-LEF-1 antibodies.[56] Although Lef-1 mRNAs have also been detected in cultured epidermal keratinocytes,[91] and in some melanoma cell lines,[92] hair matrix cells can be distinguished from other epidermal cells by their high level of these mRNAs and by the presence of nuclear LEF-1.[7,91,93] Moreover, recent studies in transgenic mice harboring TOPGAL, a β-galactosidase gene under control of a LEF/TCF and β-catenin inducible promoter, show expression of the gene in the differentiating hair shaft precursor cells of the matrix.[94] This suggests that these cells assemble functional LEF-1/β-catenin complexes that can activate downstream target genes. In the studies of Chan et al.,[56] LEF-1 antibody stained the nuclei of the proliferating cells of pilomatricomas, but was not detected in the transitional or shadow cells of the tumor.[56] These findings, along with data showing expression of hair precortex keratins by pilomatricomas,[9,10] provide further biochemical data in support of morphologic evidence that pilomatricomas are derived from the hair matrix cells that give rise to the cortex of the hair shaft.

Animal Models

Mice Expressing a Truncated β-Catenin in the Skin. To study the effect of LEF/TCF signaling on hair follicle morphogenesis, mice were engineered to express a stabilized, N-terminally truncated, form of β-catenin controlled by an epidermal keratin promoter.[57] During initiation of the first postnatal hair cycle, these mice demonstrate de novo hair follicle morphogenesis. As these mice age, they develop skin tumors, which are histologically indistinguishable from human pilomatricomas. They possess a zone of mitotically active basophilic cells that are separated from an area of shadow cells by a transitional zone of more eosinophilic cells with pyknotic nuclei. The basophilic cells of the pilomatricoma show nuclear localization of β-catenin and cyclin D1 using immunohistochemical methods (Fig. 35-3). Cyclin D1 contains a TCF binding site in its promoter and has recently been shown to be a downstream transcriptional target of β-catenin.[89,90] Furthermore, the basophilic cells of the pilomatricomas in these mice express nuclear LEF-1 and type I, hair-specific keratins in cortical and precortical cells (Fig. 35-4). These findings are further evidence that these tumors are derived from the hair matrix cells that give rise to the cortex of the hair shaft.

In several related studies examining the roles of β-catenin in epidermal and follicular development, mice were engineered to either conditionally ablate the β-catenin gene[95] or to interfere with β-catenin/LEF/TCF function through overexpression of ΔNLEF1, lacking the β-catenin interacting domain of LEF-1.[96] Interestingly, the follicular-derived cysts which are subsequently formed show evidence of epidermal[95] or sebaceous[96] differentiation, rather than follicular differentiation. These findings further illustrate the role of β-catenin in tumorigenesis, in hair follicle development, and possibly in stem cell differentiation.

Mice Carrying a Targeted Mutation in APC. A mouse model for Gardner syndrome has been developed by targeted mutation of the 1639 codon in the APC gene to produce a truncated protein with undetectable levels. The heterozygous mice Apc+/Apc1638N develop attenuated polyposis of the upper gastrointestinal tract, along with cutaneous cysts and desmoid tumors. The cysts show combinations of pilomatricoma-like changes and infundibular differentiation,[97] features that are identical to the cysts found in patients with Gardner syndrome.

IMPLICATIONS FOR DIAGNOSIS

Although the need for the development of genetic screening for pilomatricoma is not necessary because of the benign nature of this

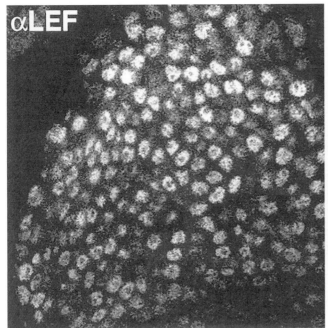

Figure 35-4 Pilomatricomas express nuclear LEF-1 and type I, hair-specific keratins. Sections of pilomatricoma from a K14-ΔN-βcat transgenic mouse underwent immunohistochemistry. *Left,* a section was stained with anti-LEF1 antibodies. High levels of nuclear LEF-1 were found in the basophilic cells of the tumor. *Right,* Hair-specific keratins expressed in cortical and precortical cells are also highly expressed in the same cells exhibiting nuclear LEF-1, as detected by the monoclonal antibody AE13.

tumor, there are several reported cases of pilomatrix carcinoma. The best candidate gene is β-catenin, which is mutated in approximately 75 percent of sporadic pilomatricomas. Moreover, activating mutations in this gene are essentially limited to a series of serine and threonine residues in the amino-terminal region of this molecule, thereby simplifying the analysis. Further studies are needed to determine the prevalence of these genetic changes in pilomatrix carcinoma and the other molecules involved in the formation of pilomatricomas and pilomatrix carcinomas.

REFERENCES

1. Malherbe A, Chenantais J: Note sur l'épithelioma calcifié des glandes sébacés. *Progrés Médical (Paris)* **8**:826, 1880.
2. Marrogi AJ, Wick MR, Dehner LP: Benign cutaneous adnexal tumors in childhood and young adults, excluding pilomatrixoma: Review of 28 cases and literature. *J Cutan Pathol* **18**:20, 1991.
3. Marrogi AJ, Wick MR, Dehner LP: Pilomatrical neoplasms in children and young adults. *Am J Dermatopathol* **14**:87, 1992.
4. McGavron MH: Ultrastructure of pilomatrixoma (calcifying epithelioma). *Cancer* **18**:1445, 1965.
5. Hashimoto K, Lever WF: Histogenesis of skin appendage tumors. *Arch Dermatol* **100**:356, 1969.
6. Manivel C, Wick MR, Mukai K: Pilomatrix carcinoma: An immunohistochemical comparison with benign pilomatrixoma and other benign cutaneous lesions of pilar origin. *J Cutan Pathol* **13**:22, 1986.
7. Moll I, Heid H, Moll R: Cytokeratin analysis of pilomatrixoma: Changes in cytokeratin-type expression during differentiation. *J Invest Dermatol* **91**:251, 1988.
8. Watanabe S, Wagatsuma K, Takahashi H: Immunohistochemical localization of cytokeratins and involucrin in calcifying epithelioma: Comparative studies with normal skin. *Br J Dermatol* **131**:506, 1994.
9. Cribier B, Asch PH, Regnier C, Rio MC, Grosshans E: Expression of human hair keratin basic 1 in pilomatrixoma. A study of 128 cases. *Br J Dermatol* **140**:600, 1999.
10. Regnier CH, Asch PH, Grosshans E, Rio MC: Expression pattern of human hair keratin basic 1 (hHb1) in hair follicle and pilomatricoma. *Exp Dermatol* **6**:87, 1997.
11. Alli N, Gungor E, Artuz F: Perforating pilomatricoma. *J Am Acad Dermatol* **35**:116, 1996.
12. Moehlenbeck FW: Pilomatrixoma (calcifying epithelioma). A statistical study. *Arch Dermatol* **108**:532, 1973.
13. Geh JL, Moss AL: Multiple pilomatrixomata and myotonic dystrophy: A familial association. *Br J Plast Surg* **52**:143, 1999.
14. Julian CG, Bowers PW: A clinical review of 209 pilomatricomas. *J Am Acad Dermatol* **39**:191, 1998.
15. Sassmannshausen J, Chaffins M: Pilomatrix carcinoma: A report of a case arising from a previously excised pilomatrixoma and a review of the literature. *J Am Acad Dermatol* **44**:358, 2001.
16. Sau P, Lupton GP, Graham JH: Pilomatrix carcinoma. *Cancer* **71**:2491, 1993.
17. Zagarella SS, Kneale KL, Stern HS: Pilomatrix carcinoma of the scalp [published erratum appears in *Australas J Dermatol* **33**(2):86, 1992]. *Australas J Dermatol* **33**:39, 1992.
18. Noguchi H, Kayashima K, Ono T: Pilomatricoma associated with several hair follicles. *Am J Dermatopathol* **21**:458, 1999.
19. Viero RM, Tani E, Skoog L: Fine-needle aspiration (FNA) cytology of pilomatrixoma: Report of 14 cases and review of the literature. *Cytopathology* **10**:263, 1999.
20. Fayyazi A, Soruri A, Radzun HJ, Peters JH, Berger H: Cell renewal, cell differentiation and programmed cell death (apoptosis) in pilomatrixoma. *Br J Dermatol* **137**:714, 1997.
21. Farrier S, Morgan M: bcl-2 expression in pilomatricoma. *Am J Dermatopathol* **19**:254, 1997.
22. Nakamura T: A reappraisal on the modes of cell death in pilomatricoma. *J Cutan Pathol* **26**:125, 1999.
23. Kishimoto S, Nagata M, Takenaka H, Yasuno H: Detection of apoptosis by in situ labeling in pilomatricoma. *Am J Dermatopathol* **18**:339, 1996.
24. Kaddu S, Soyer HP, Hodl S, Kerl H: Morphological stages of pilomatricoma. *Am J Dermatopathol* **18**:333, 1996.
25. Kurokawa I, Kusumoto K, Bessho K, Okubo Y, Senzaki H, Tsubura A: Immunohistochemical expression of bone morphogenetic protein-2 in pilomatricoma. *Br J Dermatol* **143**:754, 2000.
26. Kaddu S, Beham-Schmid C, Soyer HP, Hodl S, Beham A, Kerl H: Extramedullary hematopoiesis in pilomatricomas [see comments]. *Am J Dermatopathol* **17**:126, 1995.
27. Panico L, Manivel JC, Pettinato G, De Rosa N, Ruggiero A, De Rosa G: Pilomatrix carcinoma. A case report with immunohistochemical findings, flow cytometric comparison with benign pilomatrixoma and review of the literature. *Tumori* **80**:309, 1994.
28. Rabkin MS, Wittwer CT, Soong VY: Flow cytometric DNA content analysis of a case of pilomatrix carcinoma showing multiple

recurrences and invasion of the cranial vault. *J Am Acad Dermatol* **23**:104, 1990.

29. Hills RJ, Ive FA: Familial multiple pilomatrixomas [letter]. *Br J Dermatol* **127**:194, 1992.

30. Brook JD, McCurrach ME, Harley HG, Buckler AJ, Church D, Aburatani H, Hunter K, et al: Molecular basis of myotonic dystrophy: Expansion of a trinucleotide (CTG) repeat at the 3′ end of a transcript encoding a protein kinase family member [published erratum appears in *Cell* **69**(2):385, 1992]. *Cell* **68**:799, 1992.

31. Mahadevan M, Tsilfidis C, Sabourin L, Shutler G, Amemiya C, Jansen G, Neville C, et al: Myotonic dystrophy mutation: an unstable CTG repeat in the 3′ untranslated region of the gene. *Science* **255**:1253, 1992.

32. Harper PS: Calcifying epithelioma of Malherbe. Association with myotonic muscular dystrophy. *Arch Dermatol* **106**:41, 1972.

33. Delfino M, Monfrecola G, Ayala F, Suppa F, Piccirillo A: Multiple familial pilomatricomas: A cutaneous marker for myotonic dystrophy. *Dermatologica* **170**:128, 1985.

34. Justice RW, Zilian O, Woods DF, Noll M, Bryant PJ: The *Drosophila* tumor-suppressor gene warts encodes a homolog of human myotonic dystrophy kinase and is required for the control of cell shape and proliferation. *Genes Dev* **9**:534, 1995.

35. Jinnai K, Sugio T, Mitani M, Hashimoto K, Takahashi K: Elongation of (CTG)n repeats in myotonic dystrophy protein kinase gene in tumors associated with myotonic dystrophy patients. *Muscle Nerve* **22**:1271, 1999.

36. Naylor EW, Gardner EJ: Penetrance and expressivity of the gene responsible for the Gardner syndrome. *Clin Genet* **11**:381, 1977.

37. Leppard B, Bussey HJ: Epidermoid cysts, polyposis coli and Gardner's syndrome. *Br J Surg* **62**:387, 1975.

38. Leppard BJ, Bussey HJ: Gardner's syndrome with epidermoid cysts showing features of pilomatrixomas. *Clinl Exp Dermatol* **1**:75, 1976.

39. Cooper PH, Fechner RE: Pilomatricoma-like changes in the epidermal cysts of Gardner's syndrome. *J Am Acad Dermatol* **8**:639, 1983.

40. Rutten A, Wenzel P, Goos M: Gardner-Syndrom mit pilomatrixomartigen Haarfollikelzysten. *Hautarzt* **41**:326, 1990.

41. Narisawa Y, Kohda H: Cutaneous cysts of Gardner's syndrome are similar to follicular stem cells. *J Cutan Pathol* **22**:115, 1995.

42. Pujol RM, Casanova JM, Egido R, Pujol J, de Moragas JM: Multiple familial pilomatricomas: a cutaneous marker for Gardner syndrome? *Pediatr Dermatol* **12**:331, 1995.

43. Groden J, Thliveris A, Samowitz W, Carlson M, Gelbert L, Albertsen H, Joslyn G, et al: Identification and characterization of the familial adenomatous polyposis coli gene. *Cell* **66**:589, 1991.

44. Kinzler KW, Vogelstein B: Lessons from hereditary colorectal cancer. *Cell* **87**:159, 1996.

45. Davies DR, Armstrong JG, Thakker N, Horner K, Guy SP, Clancy T, Sloan P, et al: Severe Gardner syndrome in families with mutations restricted to a specific region of the APC gene. *Am J Hum Genet* **57**:1151, 1995.

46. Munemitsu S, Albert I, Souza B, Rubinfeld B, Polakis P: Regulation of intracellular beta-catenin levels by the adenomatous polyposis coli (APC) tumor-suppressor protein. *Proc Natl Acad Sci U S A* **92**:3046, 1995.

47. Miller RW, Rubinstein JH: Tumors in Rubinstein-Taybi syndrome [see comments]. *Am J Med Genet* **56**:112, 1995.

48. Cambiaghi S, Ermacora E, Brusasco A, Canzi L, Caputo R: Multiple pilomatricomas in Rubinstein-Taybi syndrome: A case report. *Pediatr Dermatol* **11**:21, 1994.

49. Masuno M, Imaizumi K, Ishii T, Kuroki Y, Baba N, Tanaka Y: Pilomatrixomas in Rubinstein-Taybi syndrome [letter; comment]. *Am J Med Genet* **77**:81, 1998.

50. Petrij F, Giles RH, Dauwerse HG, Saris JJ, Hennekam RC, Masuno M, Tommerup N, et al: Rubinstein-Taybi syndrome caused by mutations in the transcriptional co-activator CBP [see comments]. *Nature* **376**:348, 1995.

51. Chrivia JC, Kwok RP, Lamb N, Hagiwara M, Montminy MR, Goodman RH: Phosphorylated CREB binds specifically to the nuclear protein CBP. *Nature* **365**:855, 1993.

52. Perkins ND, Felzien LK, Betts JC, Leung K, Beach DH, Nabel GJ: Regulation of NF-kappaB by cyclin-dependent kinases associated with the p300 coactivator. *Science* **275**:523, 1997.

53. Akimaru H, Hou DX, Ishii S: *Drosophila* CBP is required for dorsal-dependent twist gene expression. *Nat Genet* **17**:211, 1997.

54. Takemaru KI, Moon RT: The transcriptional coactivator CBP interacts with beta-catenin to activate gene expression. *J Cell Biol* **149**:249, 2000.

55. Waltzer L, Bienz M: *Drosophila* CBP represses the transcription factor TCF to antagonize Wingless signaling. *Nature* **395**:521, 1998.

56. Chan EF, Gat U, McNiff JM, Fuchs E: A common human skin tumour is caused by activating mutations in beta-catenin. *Nat Genet* **21**:410, 1999.

56a. Kajind Y, Yamaguchi A, Hashimoto N, Matsuura A, Sato N, Kikuchi K: β-Catenin gene mutation in human hair-follicle related tumors. *Pathol Int* **51**:543, 2001.

57. Gat U, DasGupta R, Degenstein L, Fuchs E: De Novo hair follicle morphogenesis and hair tumors in mice expressing a truncated beta-catenin in skin. *Cell* **95**:605, 1998.

58. Morin PJ: Beta-catenin signaling and cancer. *Bioessays* **21**:1021, 1999.

59. Miller JR, Hocking AM, Brown JD, Moon RT: Mechanism and function of signal transduction by the Wnt/beta-catenin and Wnt/Ca2+ pathways. *Oncogene* **18**:7860, 1999.

60. Neufeld KL, Zhang F, Cullen BR, White RL: APC-mediated down-regulation of beta-catenin activity involves nuclear sequestration and nuclear export. *EMBO Reports* **1**:519, 2000.

61. Henderson BR: Nuclear-cytoplasmic shuttling of APC regulates beta-catenin subcellular localization and turnover. *Nat Cell Biol* **2**:653, 2000.

62. Rosin-Arbesfeld R, Townsley F, Bienz M: The APC tumour suppressor has a nuclear export function. *Nature* **406**:1009, 2000.

63. Mao J, Wang J, Liu B, Pan W, Farr GH 3rd, Flynn C, Yuan H, et al: Low-density lipoprotein receptor-related protein-5 binds to Axin and regulates the canonical Wnt signaling pathway. *Mol Cell* **7**:801, 2001.

64. Behrens J, von Kries JP, Kuhl M, Bruhn L, Wedlich D, Grosschedl R, Birchmeier W: Functional interaction of beta-catenin with the transcription factor LEF-1. *Nature* **382**:638, 1996.

65. Roose J, Molenaar M, Peterson J, Hurenkamp J, Brantjes H, Moerer P, van de Wetering M, et al: The Xenopus Wnt effector XTcf-3 interacts with Groucho-related transcriptional repressors. *Nature* **395**:608, 1998.

66. Brantjes H, Roose J, van De Wetering M, Clevers H: All Tcf HMG box transcription factors interact with Groucho-related co-repressors. *Nucleic Acids Res* **29**:1410, 2001.

67. Morin PJ, Sparks AB, Korinek V, Barker N, Clevers H, Vogelstein B, Kinzler KW: Activation of beta-catenin-Tcf signaling in colon cancer by mutations in beta-catenin or APC [see comments]. *Science* **275**:1787, 1997.

68. Palacios J, Gamallo C: Mutations in the beta-catenin gene (CTNNB1) in endometrioid ovarian carcinomas. *Cancer Res* **58**:1344, 1998.

69. Muller O, Nimmrich I, Finke U, Friedl W, Hoffmann I: A beta-catenin mutation in a sporadic colorectal tumor of the RER phenotype and absence of beta-catenin germline mutations in FAP patients. *Genes Chromosomes Cancer* **22**:37, 1998.

70. Zurawel RH, Chiappa SA, Allen C, Raffel C: Sporadic medulloblastomas contain oncogenic beta-catenin mutations. *Cancer Res* **58**:896, 1998.

71. Miyoshi Y, Iwao K, Nagasawa Y, Aihara T, Sasaki Y, Imaoka S, Murata M, et al: Activation of the beta-catenin gene in primary hepatocellular carcinomas by somatic alterations involving exon 3. *Cancer Res* **58**:2524, 1998.

72. Voeller HJ, Truica CI, Gelmann EP: Beta-catenin mutations in human prostate cancer. *Cancer Res* **58**:2520, 1998.

73. Fukuchi T, Sakamoto M, Tsuda H, Maruyama K, Nozawa S, Hirohashi S: Beta-catenin mutation in carcinoma of the uterine endometrium. *Cancer Res* **58**:3526, 1998.

74. Sparks AB, Morin PJ, Vogelstein B, Kinzler KW: Mutational analysis of the APC/beta-catenin/Tcf pathway in colorectal cancer. *Cancer Res* **58**:1130, 1998.

75. de La Coste A, Romagnolo B, Billuart P, Renard CA, Buendia MA, Soubrane O, Fabre M, et al: Somatic mutations of the beta-catenin gene are frequent in mouse and human hepatocellular carcinomas. *Proc Natl Acad Sci U S A* **95**:8847, 1998.

76. Satoh S, Daigo Y, Furukawa Y, Kato T, Miwa N, Nishiwaki T, Kawasoe T, et al: AXIN1 mutations in hepatocellular carcinomas, and growth suppression in cancer cells by virus-mediated transfer of AXIN1. *Nat Genet* **24**:245, 2000.

77. Liu W, Dong X, Mai M, Seelan R, Taniguchi K, Krishnadath KK, Halling KC, et al: Mutations in AXIN2 cause colorectal cancer with defective mismatch repair by activating beat-catenin/TCF signaling. *Nat Genet* **26**:146, 2000.

78. Munemitsu S, Albert I, Rubinfeld B, Polakis P: Deletion of an amino-terminal sequence beta-catenin in vivo and promotes hyperphosphorylation of the adenomatous polyposis coli tumor suppressor protein. *Mol Cell Biol* **16**:4088, 1996.

79. Aberle H, Bauer A, Stappert J, Kispert A, Kemler R: Beta-catenin is a target for the ubiquitin-proteasome pathway. *EMBO J* **16**:3797, 1997.

80. Hart M, Concordet JP, Lassot I, Albert I, del los Santos R, Durand H, Perret C, et al: The F-box protein beta-TrCP associates with phosphorylated beta-catenin and regulates its activity in the cell. *Curr Biol* **9**:207, 1999.

81. Yost C, Torres M, Miller JR, Huang E, Kimelman D, Moon RT: The axis-inducing activity, stability, and subcellular distribution of beta-catenin is regulated in *Xenopus* embryos by glycogen synthase kinase 3. *Genes Dev* **10**:1443, 1996.

82. Orford K, Crockett C, Jensen JP, Weissman AM, Byers SW: Serine phosphorylation-regulated ubiquitination and degradation of beta-catenin. *J Biol Chem* **272**:24735, 1997.

83. Chen ZJ, Parent L, Maniatis T: Site-specific phosphorylation of IκBα by a novel ubiquitination-dependent protein kinase activity. *Cell* **84**:853, 1996.

84. Koch A, Denkhaus D, Albrecht S, Leuschner I, von Schweinitz D, Pietsch T: Childhood hepatoblastomas frequently carry a mutated degradation targeting box of the beta-catenin gene. *Cancer Res* **59**:269, 1999.

85. Wei Y, Fabre M, Branchereau S, Gauthier F, Perilongo G, Buendia MA: Activation of beta-catenin in epithelial and mesenchymal hepatoblastomas. *Oncogene* **19**:498, 2000.

86. Jeng YM, Wu MZ, Mao TL, Chang MH, Hsu HC: Somatic mutations of beta-catenin play a crucial role in the tumorigenesis of sporadic hepatoblastoma. *Cancer Lett* **152**:45, 2000.

87. Garcia-Rostan G, Tallini G, Herrero A, D'Aquila TG, Carcangiu ML, Rimm DL: Frequent mutation and nuclear localization of beta-catenin in anaplastic thyroid carcinoma. *Cancer Res* **59**:1811, 1999.

88. He TC, Sparks AB, Rago C, Hermeking H, Zawel L, da Costa LT, Morin PJ, et al: Identification of c-MYC as a target of the APC pathway [see comments]. *Science* **281**:1509, 1998.

89. Shtutman M, Zhurinsky J, Simcha I, Albanese C, D'Amico M, Pestell R, Ben-Ze'ev A: The cyclin D1 gene is a target of the beta-catenin/LEF-1 pathway. *Proc Natl Acad Sci U S A* **96**:5522, 1999.

90. Tetsu O, McCormick F: Beta-catenin regulates expression of cyclin D1 in colon carcinoma cells. *Nature* **398**:422, 1999.

91. Zhou P, Byrne C, Jacobs J, Fuchs E: Lymphoid enhancer factor 1 directs hair follicle patterning and epithelial cell fate. *Genes Develop* **9**:700, 1995.

92. Rubinfeld B, Robbins P, El-Gamil M, Albert I, Porfiri E, Polakis P: Stabilization of beta-catenin by genetic defects in melanoma cell lines [see comments]. *Science* **275**:1790, 1997.

93. van Genderen C, Okamura RM, Farinas I, Quo RG, Parslow TG, Bruhn L, Grosschedl R: Development of several organs that require inductive epithelial-mesenchymal interactions is impaired in LEF-1-deficient mice. *Genes Dev* **8**:2691, 1994.

94. DasGupta R, Fuchs E: Multiple roles for activated LEF/TCF transcription complexes during hair follicle development and differentiation. *Development* **126**:4557, 1999.

95. Huelsken J, Vogel R, Erdmann B, Cotsarelis G, Birchmeier W: Beta-catenin controls hair follicle morphogenesis and stem cell differentiation in the skin. *Cell* **105**:533, 2001.

96. Merrill BJ, Gat U, DasGupta R, Fuchs E: Tcf3 and Lef1 regulate lineage differentiation of multipotent stem cells in skin. *Genes Dev* **15**:1688, 2001.

97. Smits R, van der Houven van Oordt W, Luz A, Zurcher C, Jagmohan-Changur S, Breukel C, Khan PM, et al: Apc1638N: a mouse model for familial adenomatous polyposis-associated desmoid tumors and cutaneous cysts. *Gastroenterology* **114**:275, 1998.

CHAPTER 36

Hereditary Paragangliomas of the Head and Neck

Peter Devilee ■ *Andel G.L. van der Mey* ■ *Cees J. Cornelisse*

1. Paragangliomas are mostly benign, slow growing tumors in the head and neck region originating from the parasympathetic paraganglion system.
2. Between 10 and 50 percent of the cases are caused by an inherited gene-defect. The inheritance pattern seen in most families displays a parent-of-origin effect. In these families, children of affected mothers never develop the disease; only paternal transmission of the gene-defect confers susceptibility.
3. Mutations in SDHD gene are the major cause of this inherited tumor. SDHD is a subunit of the mitochondrial respiratory chain complex II. Two families have been identified in which the disease mutation resides in other genes, namely in SDHC in a family of German origin, and in an as yet unidentified gene (PGL2) in a Dutch family. Mutations in SDHB have been found in a small number of families with adrenal pheochromocytoma, with or without head and neck paraganglioma. SDHB and SDHC are two other subunits of the mitochondrial complex II.
4. Tumors developing in carriers of an SDHC or SDHD mutation have invariably lost the wild-type allele, suggesting that both genes function as a tumor-suppressor gene in parasympathetic paraganglion tissues.
5. SDHC and SDHD are the first tumor suppressor genes whose normal cellular function are exerted in the mitochondria.

Head and neck (HN-) paragangliomas are rare, predominantly benign tumors that arise from extra-adrenal paraganglion tissue associated with the parasympathetic nervous system. Most frequently, these hypervascular tumors originate from the carotid body at the carotid bifurcation.[1] Less common are paragangliomas originating from the glomus bodies of the jugular bulb, the tympanic plexus of Jacobson's nerve, and the vagal nerve. The average age at which a tumor is diagnosed is approximately 45 years in most studies, and the tumors characteristically progress extremely slowly. Histories spanning several decades are not uncommon. At present, surgery is considered to be the optimal method of treatment.

CLINICAL ASPECTS

Diagnostic Criteria and Site of Origin

The clinical symptoms associated with paragangliomas depend on their site of origin. Jugulotympanic paragangliomas are confined to the middle ear cavity and usually cause pulsatile tinnitus and hearing loss. Local extension may lead to palsies of cranial nerves VII to XII. Eventually, intracranial growth can lead to compression of the brainstem and death. Carotid and vagal body tumors usually present as a firm, painless, lateral neck mass (Fig. 36-1A) and may lead to impairment of cranial nerves X and XII. In a very small proportion of patients (~1 percent), the tumors are vasoactive in

that they produce large amounts of catecholamines.[2] For this reason, and to distinguish them from the excreting phaeochromocytomas originating from the sympathetic paraganglion system, HN paragangliomas are sometimes also referred to as nonchromaffin paragangliomas. Yet the normal function of carotid bodies, i.e., chemo- and oxygen-sensing, is exerted by excretion of physiological levels of a neurotransmitter (most probably catecholamines).[3] Negation of the excretory potential of carotid body tumors may cause fatal complications during surgery.

In 5 to 10 percent of cases, the tumor progresses into malignancy, metastasizing to regional lymph nodes, lungs, or bone.[4] The gold standard for their diagnosis is magnetic resonance (MR) imaging. Open biopsies are dangerous because of their extreme vascularity. MR angiography (MRA) usually reveals the number of HN-paragangliomas and their extension. At high resolution, MRA may also reveal the smallest, clinically occult, tumors.[5]

Incidence

The overall incidence of HN-paragangliomas has been estimated to be 1 in 100,000 to 1,000,000 annually.[6–8] An unknown proportion has an inherited origin (MIM 168000). Because the disease is so rare, any patient with at least one first-, second-, or third-degree relative with HN-paragangliomas can already be considered to be genetic. On this basis, about 10 to 15 percent of all patients are estimated to be familial.[4,9–11] Patients with a positive family history more often present with bilateral or multicentric tumors than do sporadic patients (30 percent versus 10 percent), which holds for both synchronous and metachronous lesions. The bilateral carotid body tumor is the most common occurrence among these cases. Yet the exact proportion of familial disease is difficult to estimate because the tumors often occur in adult life, grow slowly, and initially cause a few mild nonspecific symptoms. Thus, a number of relatives of an index case may be incorrectly ascertained as unaffected, and the heritability aspect may be missed. Another factor contributing to this is the typical inheritance pattern (see below). Repeated transmission of the gene-defect by females will mask the familiality of the disease. Extensive genealogical analysis of a large number of HN-paraganglioma patients in the Netherlands, combined with detailed clinical ascertainment in the relatives, indicated that more than 50 percent of the cases may have a genetic basis.[8,12,13]

Developmental Aspects

The paraganglion system of the head and neck belongs to the extra-adrenal parasympathetic system, which functions as a series of afferent receptor organs. The carotid bodies are sensitive to fluctuations in arterial oxygen and pH, and as such are the most probable regulators of the cardiorespiratory system under certain hypoxic conditions.[3,14] A current model of carotid body chemotransduction postulates that transmitter-laden glomus cells initiate the neural activity by being depolarized by hypoxemia and releasing an excitatory neurotransmitter, which binds to postsynaptic receptors of the adjacent sensory afferent fibers. However,

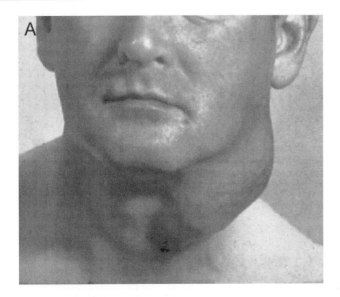

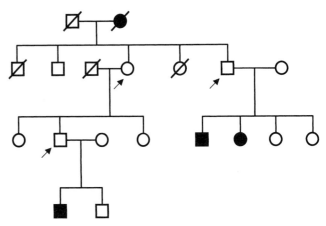

Figure 36-2 Demonstration of the typical inheritance pattern of HN-paragangliomas, linked to PGL1 (SDHD). Genomic imprinting is seen after maternal transmission. Filled symbols represent affected individuals. Arrows indicate obligate, imprinted carriers of the gene.

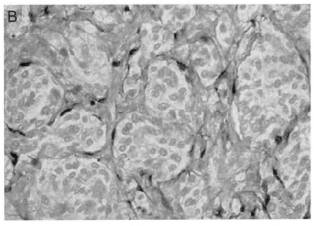

Figure 36-1 *A*, Example of the clinical presentation of a carotid body tumor. A firm lateral neck mass is clearly visible. *B*, Histologic picture of a typical carotid body tumor (hematoxylin and eosin-stained section). Note the clustered arrangement of chief cells (type I cells) in so-called Zellballen, surrounded by fibrovascular stroma and sustentacular cells (type II cells, immunostained with an antibody against the S-100 antigen).

the molecular and neural details of this mechanism are unresolved at present, certainly in humans.

The paraganglion system is of neurectodermal origin and its most prominent organ is the adrenal medulla. On the basis of anatomic distribution, paraganglia are subdivided into parasympathetic and sympathetic paraganglia.[15] Tumors of the latter group, which include pheochromocytomas, are often chromaffin-positive and secrete catecholamines, while the parasympathetic tumors do not secrete catecholamines.[1] The parasympathetic paraganglia appear to arise from the neural crest, and neuroectodermal cells are the forerunners of the glomus tissue. In the human fetus and newborn infant, the distribution of extra-adrenal parasympathetic paraganglion cells is considerably wider than in the adult.[16] Carotid bodies and jugulotympanic bodies, however, develop postnatally and attain their largest size at the age of 20, after which they become sclerotic and progressively smaller.[17–19]

Histology

Whereas the carotid body is macroscopically visible (rice grain-sized), the other parasympathetic paraganglia are frequently composed of aggregates comprising only a few cells. The histologic appearance of the parasympathetic paraganglia characteristically consists of two types of cells: the chief cell and the sustentacular cell.[15,20] The chief cell (type I) has a copious

cytoplasm with poorly defined margins and a large round or oval nucleus. The sustentacular cell (type II) is elongated and ensheathes a nerve axon. The cells are arranged in clusters, each cluster composed by a central core of chief cells surrounded by a shell of sustentacular cells (Fig. 36-1B). There is no clear histologic difference between a carotid body tumor, glomus jugulare tumor, or vagal body tumor.[15] There is also no satisfactory separation into benign, locally invasive, and malignant metastasizing tumors on histologic grounds. As such they resemble the tissue from which they arise and are, in fact, a caricature of that tissue. There is thus no evident correlation between the histologic appearance of these tumors and their biological behavior, even though the incidence of malignant transformation does vary somewhat with the site of origin of the tumor.

Inheritance Pattern

The pattern of inheritance in families with multiple cases of paraganglioma was initially determined to be autosomal dominant with reduced penetrance.[10] In-depth analyses of clinical data of 15 extended Dutch pedigrees, in conjunction with case reports by others, revealed the absence of mother-to-offspring transmission of the phenotype.[5,21] Affected individuals were observed only upon paternal transmission (Fig. 36-2). These observations were subsequently confirmed in paraganglioma families of US origin,[6,22,23] and very strongly suggested the involvement of genomic imprinting. When the gene-defect underlying the disease is passed through the female germ line, its expression is somehow "inactivated" by an epigenetic mechanism. This cannot be achieved by a change in the primary DNA sequence, because subsequent transmission of a female-derived gene-defect by a male "reactivates" the mutation, so that his offspring is again at risk. Generation skipping upon maternal transmission is likely to have led to a severe underestimation of the proportion of inherited cases. Parasympathetic paragangliomas have been observed in the context of other tumor syndromes, such as multiple endocrine neoplasia type 2,[24] neurofibromatosis,[25] von Hippel-Lindau,[26] and adrenal pheochromocytoma,[27,28] but these combinations are very rare. The familial association with pheochromocytoma, their shared ultrastructural similarities, and their common neuroectodermal paraganglionic origin suggests a possible etiological link between these two tumor types.

GENETIC LOCI

Linkage Analysis

A genome-wide linkage-search in a single large Dutch pedigree led to the mapping of the gene defect to 11q22.3-q23.[29] This locus was named PGL1. Independently, another Dutch team found linkage to a 5-cM interval on 11q13.1 in another family identified in another geographical locale.[30,31] Both families appear mutually exclusive for the other locus, suggesting that there are at least two loci for this trait. Linkage to PGL1 was significantly confirmed in 11 North American families,[22,23] whereas linkage to PGL2 was excluded in 8 of these families. HN-paraganglioma is caused by PGL2 in only a single kindred thus far. Initially, only paternally derived patients were ascertained in this family,[9,30] but a recent extension of the genealogy revealed evidence for generation skipping upon maternal transmission.[31,32] This indicates that the expression of PGL2, like that of PGL1, is modified in a parent-of-origin–dependent way. The existence of yet another gene (PGL3) was suggested by linkage analysis in a family of German origin, by which both PGL1 and PGL2 were excluded.[33] Remarkably, in this family, the trait is transmitted maternally, indicating that PGL3 is not subject to the same imprinting effect as is PGL1 and PGL2.

By comparing carrier status of family members, as defined by haplotype analysis, with tumor diagnoses as ascertained by clinical examination and MRI, it has been possible to estimate cumulative risks conferred by PGL1 in the large Dutch pedigree. By clinical symptoms alone, the penetrance of the gene was estimated to be 53 percent by age 40 years, and leveled off at 66 percent by age 53 years (Jansen JC, Van der Mey AGL, manuscript submitted for publication). Including MRI data, which detected nonsymptomatic paragangliomas in 6 carrier individuals older than age 45 years, the penetrance was estimated to be 53 percent by age 40 years, 84 percent by age 60 years, and 100 percent by age 70 years. Hence all carriers of a paternally inherited PGL1 mutation will eventually develop head and neck paragangliomas, but the slow growth rate of these tumors[13] delays the onset of symptoms in a considerable proportion of the cases.

Genealogy analysis on all families known to be of Dutch origin and known to derive from the same small geographical area led to the identification of a common ancestor, born in 1776, for three families. Disease-linked haplotypes of 25 patients in the lowest 2 generations were determined. Because all patients descend from the same ancestral female, they all carry the same gene-defect. Alleles of markers closely bordering this gene were expected to be identical by descent. This was indeed found for several closely linked markers. Surprisingly, this haplotype was also seen in several other Dutch families that were not yet linked by genealogy, strongly suggesting that all these families descended from a common ancestor and shared the same genetic defect.[34] This finding, together with a few critical recombinants in other families, finally led to the identification of a small segment on 11q22.3 where PGL1 had to reside.[35]

Somatic Genetics

At least one-third of HN-paragangliomas show clear aneuploid DNA stem lines in flow cytometry.[36] This suggests the presence of numerical chromosome aberrations, and indicates that these tumors contain true clonal proliferations. Loss of heterozygosity (LOH) was found mainly on the long arm of chromosome 11 in 60–80 percent of the tumors.[37,38] Although complex LOH-patterns were seen, LOH seemed to focus around the PGL1 locus. Intriguingly, the lost allele always derived from the mother in the eight cases in which its parental origin could be determined.[37]

Many cases with LOH at 11q often display only weak losses of allele-signal intensity.[37] This suggests that either not all cells carry the LOH-event, or that the tumor is not clonally derived. An aneuploid DNA stem line is, by definition, clonally derived, and so in these tumors the most likely explanation for the partial LOH is cellular heterogeneity for the LOH events. This was confirmed by a study in which complete allele loss was seen in flow-sorted aneuploid cells, as well as in the microdissected chief cells.[39] These results strongly suggest that the chief cells represent the clonal aneuploid DNA stem line seen in flow cytometry, and are therefore the true neoplastic cells in these tumors. The stromal component, and possibly also the sustentacular cells, does not

sustain LOH at 11q. This remains to be proven for diploid tumors. In fact, in two diploid tumors, the X-inactivation assay suggested that the majority of cells were polyclonally derived.[37] Possibly, the development of clonally derived (aneuploid) tumor foci in HN-paragangliomas is a late event in tumor progression.

SPECIFIC GENES

SDHD: A Mitochondrial Respiratory Chain Defect that Causes PGL

Recently, PGL1 was identified to be the SDHD gene by using positional cloning methods.[40] The SDHD gene encodes the small subunit D of cytochrome b558 of the mitochondrial respiratory chain complex II (succinate: ubiquinone oxidoreductase). SDHD was found to map in the chromosomal segment defined by haplotype and recombinant analyses in families and was an immediate candidate, given the role of the carotid body as a sensory organ for arterial oxygen levels. The 103 amino acids of the mature SDHD-protein (without the leader signal-peptide) are encoded by 4 exons, which cover about 10 kb genomic DNA.[41] Germ-line mutations were found in all families that were previously linked to PGL1. The mutations found to date include nonsense and frameshifting mutations, some occurring in the mitochondrial signal peptide, or missense mutations replacing evolutionary conserved amino acids (Fig. 36-3). In the Dutch population, in which a strong founder effect had already been noted, over 90 percent of all hereditary cases were found to be caused by either of two missense mutations.[42] Germ-line SDHD mutations have also been detected in sporadic and familial nonsyndromic pheochromocytomas.[40,43]

In four HN-paraganglioma patients with a germ-line mutation, DNA from flow-sorted diploid and aneuploid tumor cell fractions could be examined. In the aneuploid fraction, only the mutation could be demonstrated to be present. The maternally derived wild-type allele was lost. These results are in agreement with Knudson's two-hit hypothesis for the inactivation of a tumor-suppressor gene. Accordingly, SDHD is the first tumor suppressor gene to exert its normal cellular function in the mitochondria. Knudson's hypothesis also predicts that acquired (or ''somatic'') mutations would occur in SDHD, in truly sporadic HN-paragangliomas. One such mutation has been reported in 42 analyzed pheochromocytomas,[40,43] but not yet in HN-paragangliomas.

Other Complex II Proteins

The mitochondrial complex II is composed of four peptides: the flavoprotein and iron-sulfur protein of the succinate dehydrogenase (SDHA and SDHB, respectively), and two integral membrane proteins (SDHC and SDHD) that anchor the enzymatic subunits to the inner-mitochondrial membrane. The link between complex II dysfunction and tumorigenesis was further supported by two findings. First, the HN-paragangliomas in the German family linked to PGL3 were found to be due to a mutation in SDHC.[44] This mutation destroys the start-codon ATG of the gene, which leads to a rapid degradation of the mutant transcript. Second, SDHB mutations were detected in two of five kindreds with familial pheochromocytoma, in two of three kindreds with pheochromocytoma and paraganglioma, and in one of 24 sporadic pheochromocytomas.[45] Further work is now required to establish the proportions of HN-paraganglioma families carrying mutations in SDHB, SDHC, or SDHD.

Function

At the moment, it is not clear how a defect in a protein that is part of complex II of the respiratory chain can cause tumor growth specifically in HN-paraganglia. It is possible that complex II dysfunction in paraganglia cells interferes with their physiological function as chemoreceptors for blood oxygen pressure. In rats, the rise in partial pressure of oxygen in arterial blood around the time of birth is critical for normal maturation and function of the type I

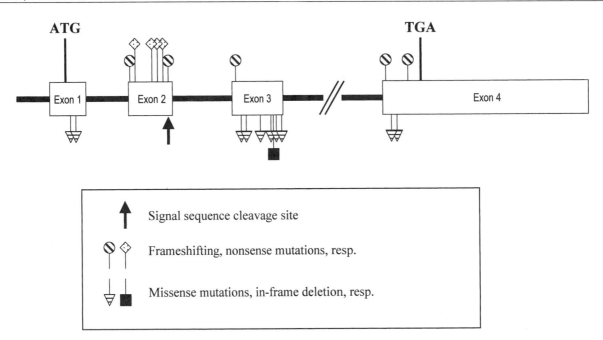

Figure 36-3 Gene organization of SDHD and position of disease-related mutations in HN-paraganglioma families. ATG and TGA represent the start and stop codons for protein-translation, respectively. Exons 1–4 are 62, 117, 145, and 989 bp, respectively. Mutation data compiled from refs 40, 42, 43, and 58–60.

carotid body cells. This is accompanied by a concomitant rise in hypoxia sensitivity (reviewed in Ref. 3). Chronic hypoxia after birth (imposed by maintaining the rats in a low-oxygen environment) inhibits this maturation and results in glomus cell hypertrophy. On this basis, it is tempting to speculate that in humans, the loss of SDHD mimics the chronic hypoxic state, despite the actual normoxia conditions in the blood. As a result, the carotid body paraganglia become persistently hyperplastic,[2,46] which increases the chance of acquiring further gene mutations and eventual genuine monoclonal tumor growth (Fig. 36-4). Hyperplasia of glomus bodies has been noted in patients with chronic hypoxemia.[47] Increased hyperplasia, as well as increased incidence of HN-paragangliomas, has been noted in individuals living for prolonged time at very high altitudes in the Andes of Peru.[48] Finally, two-thirds of HN-paragangliomas express vascular endothelial growth factor (VEGF), specifically in the chief cells.[49] VEGF is induced by hypoxia, and its up-regulation in HN-paragangliomas may explain their hypervascularity.

The exciting corollary of this hypothesis is that mitochondrial complex II is involved in oxygen sensing, for which some experimental evidence is in fact beginning to emerge (reviewed in Ref. 50). In response to hypoxia, mitochondria increase their levels of reactive oxygen species, which apparently act as second messengers in a variety of cell types. Moreover, some of the signaling cascades thus elicited appear to participate in the control of cell death pathways (apoptosis). It is thus possible that the carotid body hypertrophy seen in individuals living at high altitudes, and the slow developmental pattern of carotid body tumors in SDHD carriers, is caused by a defect in this apoptotic pathway. Indeed, one study observed that the chief cells of most

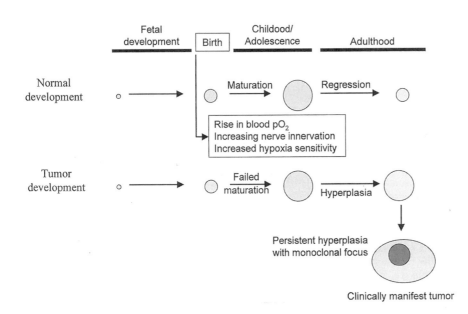

Figure 36-4 Model for the role of the mitochondrial complex II in the development of a carotid body tumor. Normal maturation of the type I carotid body cells, accompanied by a rise in hypoxia sensitivity, occurs simultaneously with the rise in partial pressure of oxygen in arterial blood around the time of birth. Failed maturation (caused by chronic hypoxia or a gene-defect in SDHB, -C, or -D) results in glomus cell hypertrophy. A persistent hyperplastic state increases the chance of acquiring further gene mutations and monoclonal tumor growth (in dark grey).

carotid body tumors express moderate to high levels of the antiapoptotic protein *bcl-2*.[51] Yet this hypothesis doesn't explain tumorigenesis in the paraganglia other than those at the carotid bifurcation, such as those in the jugular bulb and middle ear. It also remains to be seen whether noninherited sporadic HN-paragangliomas arise by a maturation defect in hypoxia sensing.

SDHD and the Inheritance Pattern of HN-Paragangliomas

The simplest model explaining the inheritance pattern of PGL1-linked HN-paragangliomas is one in which the maternally derived allele is not expressed. After the molecular nature of the gene-defect was discovered, this model predicted that SDHD would behave as a maternally imprinted gene. However, measurements of allele-specific mRNA expression patterns in fetal brain and kidney, and adult brain and blood lymphocytes, show that both alleles are expressed at equal levels.[40] The possibility remains that the allele-specific expression of SDHD is specific for the paraganglia cells in the head and neck region. Investigating this is hampered by the size of normal human paraganglia and the difficulty in obtaining these tissues postmortem. Nonetheless, several arguments speak against a classic genomic imprinting model for SDHD. First, the preferential loss of the normal maternal SDHD allele in tumors suggests that it is expressed in paraganglia cells and that its loss provides a selective growth advantage in the development of paraganglioma. By analogy, loss of the wild-type allele was also observed in two tumors caused by SDHC, and, indeed, this family showed no evidence for maternal imprinting.[44] Second, if all individuals would inherit an imprinted inactive maternal copy from their mother, Knudson's two-hit hypothesis would effectively be reduced to a one-hit variant, because only a single mutation event would be needed to inactivate the paternal allele and to initiate tumor growth. This is at odds with the rarity of HN-paragangliomas in the general population. Third, SDHD does not map to a chromosomal region known to harbor imprinted genes, or syntenic to mouse chromosome regions that are known to contain genes with parent-of-origin effects. It has been suggested that the SDHD gene is not completely imprinted in normal paraganglia or that secondary relaxation of imprinting occurs prior to tumor formation.[40] Even more complex models, invoking a linked, oppositely imprinted gene whose inactivation determines tumor progression, can be conjured up.

Can anything be gleaned from the fact that mitochondria play an essential role as energy suppliers for the cell, while having an exclusive maternal inheritance? Here, the available information is also puzzling. Genetic defects are now known in all subunits of complex II (Table 36-1). Mutations in SDHA are recessive, but are found in a small proportion of patients affected with the Leigh syndrome,[52,53] which is characterized by the presence of developmental delay and lactic acidosis and by a mean life expectancy of less than 5 years (MIM 256000). By contrast,

mutations in SDHB, SDHC and SDHD are dominant, causing tumor susceptibility in carriers, although the imprinting phenomenon is seen only for SDHD. Knowledge on the effect of these mutations on mitochondrial function is essentially still lacking, but all can apparently be maternally transmitted without reduction of fitness. If all these mutations simply "inactivate" complex II, then one would predict some Leigh syndrome patients to be compound heterozygote or homozygote for SDHB, SDHC or SDHD mutations. Conversely, heterozygote carriers of an SDHA mutation would be at risk for developing HN-paragangliomas. Neither has been found to date, suggesting that SDHA, -B, -C, and -D mutations have differential effects on mitochondrial function. Although we know little about the oxidative requirements of primary and haploid secondary oocytes, it is conceivable that those carrying an SDHD mutation are specifically capable of correcting the defect by an epigenetic mechanism affecting the expression of one or more other genes. This expression pattern might persist throughout adult life, effectively suppressing the development of paraganglioma.

Specific Genes Involved in Sporadic HN-Paragangliomas. As explained, the definition of sporadic HN-paragangliomas is somewhat problematic given their benign clinical behavior and typical inheritance pattern. In the Dutch population, inherited cases appear to comprise a much higher proportion than previously estimated.[8] Accordingly, the two SDHD founder mutations were found in the germ line of 20 of 55 (36 percent) Dutch patients who had previously been classified as "sporadic" on the basis of lack of an apparent family history.[42] Ten of the isolated patients had multiple paragangliomas, and in eight of these patients, SDHD germ-line mutations were found, indicating that multicentricity is a strong predictive factor for the hereditary nature of the disorder in isolated patients. Further work on SDHD mutation prevalence in patients from other ethnicities should discover whether or not such high proportions are a peculiarity of the founder effect in the Dutch population.

Regardless of the genetic origin of HN-paraganglioma, other genes are likely involved in the progression toward clinically manifest disease. The glomus jugulare tumor of one of two affected brothers was found to contain missense mutations in TP53 and CDKN2A,[54] but these may have been induced by radiotherapy. The clinical association between pheochromocytoma and HN-paragangliomas, although weak, might point to common genetic etiology. Pheochromocytomas occur in the context of a number of cancer syndromes, including multiple endocrine neoplasia (MEN1 and MEN2), von Hippel-Lindau disease (VHL), and neurofibromatosis type 1 (NF1). Genes underlying these syndromes are known, and thus form candidates for their involvement in HN-paragangliomas. The RET oncogene, causing MEN2, does not seem to play a role in HN-paraganglioma.[55] Another study found LOH at 3p21 in two of four informative cases, but not including the VHL locus at 3p25.[56]

Table 36-1 Inherited Defects in Mitochondrial Complex II Subunits

Subunit (chrom. location)	Syndrome	Inheritance pattern	Heterozygous carriers
SDHA (5p15)	Leigh syndrome	Recessive	Unaffected
SDHB (1p36)	Familial pheochromocytoma with or without paraganglioma	Dominant	Susceptible to PHEO (and PGL)
SDHC (1q21)	HN-paragangliomas	Dominant	Susceptible to PGL
SDHD (11q22.3)	HN-paragangliomas	Dominant with imprinting	Susceptible to PGL (and PHEO)

PGL = Head and neck paraganglioma; PHEO = adrenal pheochromocytoma.

IMPLICATIONS FOR DIAGNOSIS AND PREDICTIVE TESTING

Hereditary paragangliomas of the head and neck caused by SDHD mutations present a unique tumor syndrome that does not conform to mendelian rules of inheritance. This has considerable consequences for the genetic counseling of affected families.[8] The gene is nonpenetrant in carriers who derive it from their mother. Yet "imprinted" male carriers can transmit the disease risk to their children. Even though tumors develop later in adult life, are clinically indolent in their growth pattern and rarely metastasize, they can cause severe disabling symptoms and do require extensive surgery. Hereditary patients have a tendency to develop multicentric and bilateral lesions, which, at the base of the skull, carry a strong risk to invalidating bilateral cranial nerve palsy. For these patients accurate risk assessment is an important aid in planning clinical decisions. Surgery remains difficult, is not always radical,[57] and has a risk of complications and postoperative morbidity, such as cranial nerve palsy and decreased quality of life. Therefore radiation therapy is advocated even though there is no strong evidence that these tumors are radiosensitive. The choice for either treatment modality should be based on tumor characteristics relating to the dynamics of their growth pattern.[12,13] For extremely slow-growing tumors, a wait-and-see option probably serves the patients' interests best.

Histology, DNA flow cytometry, and immunohistochemistry are poor predictors of tumor behavior. Presymptomatic carrier detection of SDHD mutations in families with this disease will provide the opportunity to perform selective and efficient screening by MRI.[5] As a consequence, tumors can be detected at much earlier stages, and can be monitored to establish their growth dynamics. This allows the surgeon to adopt the wait-and-see policy and time the excision of the tumor in such a way that the chances of radical removal are optimal and those of associated morbidity are minimal.

Acknowledgments

The authors thank Drs. Peter Taschner, Jeroen Jansen, and Pancras Hogendoorn for critical reading of the manuscript.

REFERENCES

1. Gulya A: The glomus tumor and its biology. *Laryngoscope* **103(Suppl 60)**:7, 1993.
2. Blumenfeld J, Cohen N, Laragh J, Ruggiero D: Hypertension and catecholamine biosynthesis associated with a glomus jugulare tumor. *N Engl J Med* **327**:894, 1992.
3. Donnelly DF: Developmental aspects of oxygen sensing by the carotid body. *J Appl Physiol* **88**:2296, 2000.
4. Parry D, Li F, Strong L, Carney J, Schottenfeld D, Reimer R, Grufferman S: Carotid body tumors in humans: Genetics and epidemiology. *J Natl Cancer Inst* **68**:573, 1982.
5. Van Gils A, Van der Mey A, Hoogma R, Sandkuijl L, Maaswinkel-Mooy P, Falke T, Pauwels E: MRI screening of kindred at risk of developing paragangliomas: Support for genomic imprinting in hereditary glomus tumours. *Br J Cancer* **65**:903, 1992.
6. McCaffrey T, Meyer F, Michels V, Piepgras D, Marion M: Familial paragangliomas of the head and neck. *Arch Otolaryngol Head Neck Surg* **120**:1211, 1994.
7. Lack EE, Cubilla AL, Woodruff JM: Paragangliomas of the head and neck region. A pathologic study of tumors from 71 patients. *Hum Pathol* **10**:191, 1979.
8. Oosterwijk JC, Jansen JC, Van Schothorst EM, Oosterhof AW, Devilee P, Bakker E, Zoeteweij MW, et al: First experiences with genetic counseling based on predictive DNA diagnosis in hereditary glomus tumours (paragangliomas). *J Med Genet* **33**:379, 1996.
9. Van Baars F, Cremers C, Van den Broek P, Geerts S, Veldman J: Genetic aspects of nonchromaffin paraganglioma. *Hum Genet* **60**:305, 1982.
10. Van Baars F, Cremers C, Van den Broek P, Veldman J: Familiar non-chromaffin paragangliomas (glomus tumors). *Acta Otolaryngol* **91**:589, 1981.
11. Grufferman S, Gillman M, Pasternak L, Peterson C, Young W: Familial carotid body tumors: Case report and epidemiologic review. *Cancer* **46**:2116, 1980.
12. Van der Mey AGL, Frijns JH, Cornelisse CJ, Brons EN, van Dulken H, Terpstra HL, Schmidt PH: Does intervention improve the natural course of glomus tumors? A series of 108 patients seen in a 32-year period. *Ann Otol Rhinol Laryngol* **101**:635, 1992.
13. Jansen JC, Van den Berg R, Kuiper A, Van der Mey AGL, Zwinderman AH, Cornelisse CJ: Estimation of growth rate in patients with head and neck paragangliomas influences the treatment proposal. *Cancer* **88**:2811, 2000.
14. Gonzalez C, Almaraz L, Obeso A, Rigual R: Carotid body chemoreceptors: from natural stimuli to sensory discharges. *Physiol Rev* **74**:829, 1994.
15. Solcia E, Kloppel G, Sobin LH: Histological typing of endocrine tumors, in Sobin LH (ed): *WHO International Histological Classification of Tumors*, 2nd ed. Berlin, Springer Verlag, 2000.
16. Zak FG, Lawson W. *The Paraganglionic Chemoreceptor System*. New York, Springer Verlag, 1982.
17. Guild SR: The glomus jugulare, a non-chromaffin paraganglion in man. *Ann Otol Rhinol Laryngol* **62**:1045, 1953.
18. Hurst G, Heath D, Smith P: Histological changes associated with ageing of the human carotid body. *J Pathol* **147**:181, 1985.
19. Heath D: The human carotid body in health and disease. *J Pathol* **164**:1, 1991.
20. Smith P, Jago R, Heath D: Anatomical variation and quantitative histology of the normal and enlarged carotid body. *J Pathol* **137**:287, 1982.
21. Van der Mey A, Maaswinkel-Mooy P, Cornelisse C, Schmidt P, Van de Kamp J: Genomic imprinting in hereditary glomus tumours: evidence for new genetic theory. *Lancet* **2**:1291, 1989.
22. Baysal BE, Farr JE, Rubinstein WS, Galus RA, Johnson KA, Aston CE, Myers EN, et al: Fine mapping of an imprinted gene for familial nonchromaffin paragangliomas, on chromosome 11q23. *Am J Hum Genet* **60**:121, 1997.
23. Milunsky J, Destefano AL, Huang XL, Baldwin CT, Michels VV, Jako G, Milunsky A: Familial paragangliomas: Linkage to chromosome 11q23 and clinical implications. *Am J Med Genet* **72**:66, 1997.
24. Kennedy D, Nager G: Glomus tumor and multiple endocrine neoplasia. *Otolaryngol Head Neck Surg* **94**:644, 1986.
25. DeAngelis L, Kelleher B, Post K, Fetell M: Multiple paragangliomas in neurofibromatosis: A new neuroendocrine neoplasia. *Neurology* **37**:129, 1987.
26. Schimke RN, Collins DL, Rothberg PG: Functioning carotid paraganglioma in the von Hippel-Lindau syndrome. *Am J Med Genet* **80**:533, 1998.
27. Sato T, Saito H, Yoshinga K, Shibota Y, Sasano N: Concurrence of carotid body tumor and pheochromocytoma. *Cancer* **34**:1787, 1974.
28. Bogdasarian R, Lotz P, Arbor M: Multiple simultaneous paragangliomas of the head and neck in association with multiple retroperitoneal pheochromocytomas. *Otolaryngol Head Neck Surg* **87**:648, 1979.
29. Heutink P, Van der Mey A, Sandkuijl L, Van Gils A, Bardoel A, Breedveld G, Van Vliet M et al: A gene subject to genomic imprinting and responsible for hereditary paragangliomas maps to chromosome 11q23-qter. *Hum Mol Genet* **1**:7, 1992.
30. Mariman E, Van Beersum S, Cremers C, Van Baars F, Ropers H: Analysis of a second family with hereditary non-chromaffin paragangliomas locates the underlying gene at the proximal region of chromosome 11q. *Hum Genet* **91**:357, 1993.
31. Mariman E, Van Beersum S, Cremers C, Struycken P, Ropers H: Fine mapping of a putatively imprinted gene for familial non-chromaffin paragangliomas to chromosome 11q13.1: Evidence for genetic heterogeneity. *Hum Genet* **95**:56, 1995.
32. Struycken PM, Cremers CW, Mariman EC, Joosten FB, Bleker RJ: Glomus tumours and genomic imprinting: Influence of inheritance along the paternal or maternal line. *Clin Otolaryngol* **22**:71, 1997.
33. Niemann S, Steinberger D, Muller U: PGL3, a third, not maternally imprinted locus in autosomal dominant paraganglioma. *Neurogenetics* **2**:167, 1999.
34. Van Schothorst EM, Jansen JC, Grooters E, Prins DEM, Wiersinga LJ, Van der Mey AGL, Van Ommen G-JB et al: Founder effect at PGL1 in hereditary head and neck paraganglioma families from The Netherlands. *Am J Hum Genet* **63**:468, 1998.
35. Baysal BE, Van Schothorst EM, Farr JE, Grashof P, Myssiorek D, Rubinstein WS, Taschner P et al: Repositioning the hereditary paraganglioma critical region on chromosome band 11q23. *Hum Genet* **104**:219, 1999.

36. Van der Mey A, Cornelisse C, Hermans J, Terpstra J, Schmidt P, Fleuren G: DNA flow cytometry of hereditary and sporadic paragangliomas (glomus tumours). *Br J Cancer* **63**:298, 1991.

37. Devilee P, Van Schothorst E, Bardoel A, Bonsing B, Kuipers-Dijkshoorn N, James M, Van der Mey A et al: Allelotype of head and neck paragangliomas: allelic imbalance is confined to the long arm of chromosome 11, the site of the predisposing locus PGL. *Genes Chromosomes Cancer* **11**:71, 1994.

38. Dannenberg H, De Krijger RR, Zhao J, Speel EJ, Saremaslani P, Dinjens WN, Mooi WJ et al: Differential loss of chromosome 11q in familial and sporadic parasympathetic paragangliomas detected by comparative genomic hybridization. *Am J Pathol* **158**:1937, 2001.

39. Van Schothorst EM, Beekman M, Torremans P, Kuipers-Dijkshoorn NJ, Wessels HW, Bardoel AFJ, Van der Mey AGL et al: Para-gangliomas of the head and neck region show complete loss of heterozygosity at 11q22-q23 in chief cells and the flow-sorted DNA aneuploid fraction. *Hum Pathol* **29**:1045, 1998.

40. Baysal BE, Ferrell RE, Willett-Brozick JE, Lawrence EC, Myssiorek D, Bosch A, Van der Mey AGL et al: Mutations in SDHD, a mitochondrial complex II gene, in hereditary paraganglioma. *Science* **287**:848, 2000.

41. Hirawake H, Taniwaki M, Tamura A, Amino H, Tomitsuka E, Kita K: Characterization of the human SDHD gene encoding the small subunit of cytochrome b (cybS) in mitochondrial succinate-ubiquinone oxidoreductase. *Biochim Biophys Acta* **1412**:295, 1999.

42. Taschner PEM, Jansen JC, Bosch A, Rosenberg EH, Van der Mey AGL, Van Ommen G-JB, Cornelisse CJ et al: Nearly all hereditary paragangliomas in the Netherlands are caused by two founder mutations in the SDHD gene. *Genes Chromosomes Cancer* **31**:274, 2001.

43. Gimm O, Armanios M, Dziema H, Neumann HP, Eng C: Somatic and occult germ-line mutations in SDHD, a mitochondrial complex II gene, in nonfamilial pheochromocytoma. *Cancer Res* **60**:6822, 2000.

44. Niemann S, Muller U: Mutations in SDHC cause autosomal dominant paraganglioma, type 3. *Nat Genet* **26**:268, 2000.

45. Astuti D, Latif F, Dallol A, Dahia PL, Douglas F, George E, Skoldberg F et al.: Gene mutations in the succinate dehydrogenase subunit SDHB cause susceptibility to familial pheochromocytoma and to familial paraganglioma. *Am J Hum Genet* **69**:49, 2001.

46. Nurse CA, Vollmer C: Role of basic FGF and oxygen in control of proliferation, survival, and neuronal differentiation in carotid body chromaffin cells. *Dev Biol* **184**:197, 1997.

47. Lack EE: Hyperplasia of vagal and carotid body paraganglia in patients with chronic hypoxemia. *Am J Pathol* **91**:497, 1978.

48. Saldana MJ, Salem LE, Travezan R: High altitude hypoxia and chemodectomas. *Hum Pathol* **4**:251, 1973.

49. Jyung RW, LeClair EE, Bernat RA, Kang TS, Ung F, McKenna MJ, Tuan RS: Expression of angiogenic growth factors in paragangliomas. *Laryngoscope* **110**:161, 2000.

50. Chandel NS, Schumacker PT: Cellular oxygen sensing by mitochondria: Old questions, new insight. *J Appl Physiol* **88**:1880, 2000.

51. Wang DG, Barros AAB, Johnston CF, Buchanan KD: Oncogene expression in carotid body tumors. *Cancer* **77**:2581, 1996.

52. Bourgeron T, Rustin P, Chretien D, Birch-Machin M, Bourgeois M, Viegas-Pequignot E, Munnich A, et al: Mutation of a nuclear succinate dehydrogenase gene results in mitochondrial respiratory chain deficiency. *Nat Genet* **11**:144, 1995.

53. Parfait B, Chretien D, Rotig A, Marsac C, Munnich A, Rustin P: Compound heterozygous mutations in the flavoprotein gene of the respiratory chain complex II in a patient with Leigh syndrome. *Hum Genet* **106**:236, 2000.

54. Guran S, Tali ET: p53 and p16INK4A mutations during the progression of glomus tumor. *Pathol Oncol Res* **5**:41, 1999.

55. De Krijger RR, Van der Harst E, Muletta-Feurer S, Bruining HA, Lamberts SW, Dinjens WN, Roth J et al: RET is expressed but not mutated in extra-adrenal paragangliomas. *J Pathol* **191**:264, 2000.

56. Vargas MP, Zhuang Z, Wang C, Vortmeyer A, Linehan WM, Merino MJ: Loss of heterozygosity on the short arm of chromosomes 1 and 3 in sporadic pheochromocytoma and extra-adrenal paraganglioma. *Hum Pathol* **28**:411, 1997.

57. Gstoettner W, Matula C, Hamzavi J, Kornfehl J, Czerny C: Long-term results of different treatment modalities in 37 patients with glomus jugulare tumors. *Eur Arch Otorhinolaryngol* **256**:351, 1999.

58. Badenhop RF, Cherian S, Lord RS, Baysal BE, Taschner PEM, Schofield PR: Novel mutations in the SDHD gene in pedigrees with familial carotid body paraganglioma and sensorineural hearing loss: *Genes Chrom Cancer* **31**:225, 2001.

59. Astuti D, Douglas F, Lennard TWJ, Aligianis IA, Woodward ER, Evans DGR, Eng C et al.: Germline SDHD mutation in familial phaeochromocytoma. *Lancet* **357**:1181, 2001.

60. Milunsky JM, Maher TA, Michels VV, Milunsky A: Novel mutations and the emergence of a common mutation in the SDHD gene causing familial paraganglioma. *Am J Med Genet* **100**:311, 2001.

Familial Cylindromatosis

Michael R. Stratton ▪ *Graham R. Bignell*

1. Cylindromas are benign neoplasms of the skin that originate from skin appendage structures. Sporadic cylindromas are usually small, solitary tumors with few complications. Familial cylindromatosis is a rare, autosomal dominant genetic predisposition to the development of multiple cylindromas. This can be a severely disfiguring condition associated with considerable morbidity.

2. There is a single familial cylindromatosis susceptibility gene (*CYLD*) located on chromosome 16q12. Loss of heterozygosity on chromosome 16q in both familial and sporadic cylindromas indicates that *CYLD* is a tumor-suppressor gene/recessive oncogene. Germ line mutations of *CYLD* are found in cylindromatosis families and somatic mutations in sporadic and familial cylindromas. However, no somatic mutations have been found in other types of neoplasm. All currently identified mutations are predicted to cause truncation or absence of the encoded protein.

3. *CYLD* encodes a 956-amino acid protein. It includes three Cytoskeletal-Associated Protein-Glycine conserved (CAP-GLY) domains that are found in proteins coordinating the attachment of organelles to microtubules. It also has sequence homology to the catalytic domain of ubiquitin C-terminal hydrolases, a family of enzymes that act to deubiquitinate proteins. However, the critical biological activities that are subverted by the *CYLD* mutations that result in cylindromatosis have yet to be elucidated.

Cylindromas are neoplasms derived from skin appendage structures. To inform understanding of the pathogenesis and phenotype of these tumors, we review briefly the anatomy and function of appendageal skin structures. The skin is composed of the epidermis, the dermis, and a set of epidermal appendageal structures that serve a wide range of functions. The latter include hair follicles, eccrine glands, apocrine glands, and sebaceous glands. Figure 37-1 shows a representation of the skin appendages and their anatomic interrelationship. During development, the progenitors of skin appendages are believed to originate from the embryologic basal cell layer (stratum germinativum) of the epidermis.

Hair follicles are found in most areas of the skin, excluding the palms of the hands and soles of the feet, and are present at highest density in the scalp and pubic regions. Most of the five million hair follicles that are present in adult humans are formed by the fifth month of gestation, and new follicles probably do not form after birth. Sebaceous glands are closely associated with hair follicles and are similarly distributed on all skin surfaces with the exception of the palms and soles. They secrete sebum, an oily substance that functions as a lubricant, prevents excess evaporation from the skin surface, and protects the hair from becoming brittle. After birth, sebaceous glands are relatively inactive, but are activated by the increased circulating concentration of sex hormones at puberty. Eccrine glands are also widely distributed over the skin except for a few areas such as the margins of the lips, nail beds of the fingers and toes, and eardrums. In contrast to hair follicles and sebaceous

glands they are most abundant in the skin of the palms and soles. They produce sweat for temperature control. Apocrine glands initially develop over the whole body. However, most are subsequently lost during fetal development and in the adult are restricted to the axillae and pubic regions. At puberty, apocrine glands begin to secrete a complex mixture of substances that become odorous through bacterial metabolism. In many animals, these secretions are pheromonal signals important in courtship and territorial behavior. However, their role in modern humans is less certain, and they may be predominantly vestigial.

CLINICAL ASPECTS OF CYLINDROMAS AND CYLINDROMATOSIS

Pathology and Histogenesis

Cylindromas are benign tumors of the skin. They belong to the highly diverse and complex group of skin neoplasms that are derived from and/or show differentiation toward elements of the skin appendages.[1] They are well-demarcated lesions, situated in the dermis or subcutis and are composed of islands of small, epithelial cells, each island surrounded by a narrow band of homogeneous, hyaline, eosinophilic, basement membrane-like material (Fig. 37-2). The tumor cells are often arranged in palisades around the periphery of the island and occasionally form tubules. Cylindromas acquired their unusual name because of the characteristic microscopic architecture, which resembles tightly packed cylinders of cells cut in cross-section.

The histogenesis and/or major direction of differentiation of cylindromas is controversial. The debate usually centers on whether the neoplastic cells show eccrine or apocrine features, with morphologic, histochemical, and ultrastructural studies invoked to support both hypotheses. However, the distribution of cylindromas predominantly on the scalp (see below) and absence from the palms, soles, and axilla argues against a close association with either eccrine or apocrine glands. Indeed, the distribution of cylindromas tends to mirror most closely that of hair follicles, although the tumors are rarely found in the beard area. The associations of cylindromatosis with trichoepitheliomas (adnexal skin tumors that show features of pilosebaceous differentiation) and eccrine spiradenomas similarly provide inconclusive evidence of histogenesis. Together, these arguments do not convincingly support a very close association with or similarity to any adult skin appendage structure. Instead, they suggest that cylindromas arise from relatively undifferentiated progenitor cells (possibly associated with a subset of hair follicles) that may show incipient differentiation toward several adnexal structures once transformed into neoplastic clones.

Sporadic Cylindromas

Cylindromas arising in individuals without a family history of the disease are relatively common, solitary skin nodules, usually measuring less than 1 cm in diameter. They arise mainly on the scalp or face of middle-aged or elderly individuals. They are rarely associated with any mortality or morbidity. Surgical removal, if required, is almost always for cosmetic reasons. Malignant

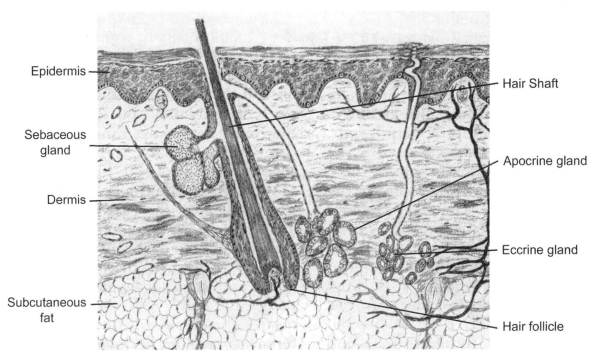

Fig. 37-1 Representation of the skin and its appendageal (adnexal) structures.

cylindromas are extremely rare, with only 30 case reports in the literature. Many of these occur on the background of familial cylindromatosis.

Familial Cylindromatosis

Familial cylindromatosis (MIM 132700) is a rare, autosomal dominant predisposition to multiple cylindromas that was first reported in 1842 by Ancell. In such families, the cylindromas arise predominantly in hairy areas of the body, with approximately 90 percent on the head and neck[2] (Fig. 37-3). The development and coalescence of many tumors on the scalp sometimes leads to the formation of a confluent mass, from which the designation *turban tumor syndrome* derives. Cylindromas have occasionally been reported in the parotid gland and lung of individuals with the disease. Malignant change with distant metastasis in familial cylindromatosis is well recognized,[3] but is unusual despite the profusion of benign lesions. Other tumors of skin appendages,

such as trichoepitheliomas (which show hair follicle differentiation) and eccrine spiradenomas (which show features of sweat glands) have been reported in cylindromatosis. However, no other neoplasms or developmental abnormalities are known to be associated with the disease.

In familial cylindromatosis, the cylindromas usually begin to appear in the second or third decades, accumulating in number and increasing slowly in size throughout adult life. Several reports suggest that women are more frequently and severely affected than men. Overall, however, the expression and penetrance of the disease are highly variable. Carriers of *CYLD* gene mutations may show few (if any) lesions, even at an advanced age. Indeed, within a single family some carriers may be affected by very severe disease, while others remain unaffected or bear a few, inconspicuous tumors. Although this variation in expression within a single family could conceivably be a result of environmental factors, it is much more suggestive of the influence of modifying

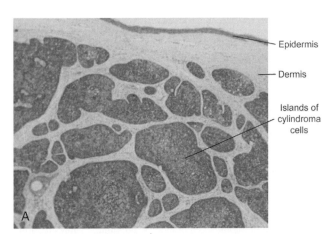

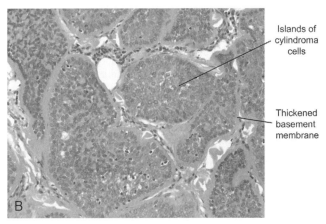

Fig. 37-2 Microscopical appearances of cylindromas. *A*, H&E stained section ×40 magnification of a familial cylindroma, showing surface epidermis, dermis, and islands of neoplastic tissue. *B*,

H&E stained section ×400 magnification of a familial cylindroma showing islands of cylindroma cells surrounded by thickened basement membrane.

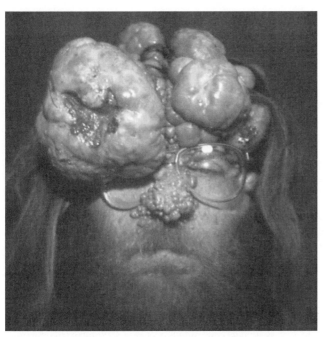

Fig. 37-3 A severely affected individual with familial cylindromatosis showing multiple cylindromas on the scalp and face.

genes that modulate the phenotypic expression of germline mutations in *CYLD*.

Familial cylindromatosis has a low mortality, but can be associated with substantial morbidity. In severely affected individuals, lesions frequently ulcerate and become infected, causing severe discomfort. One affected individual in our series reported that she could only obtain pain relief by pouring a kettle of boiling water onto her head. Rarely, cylindromas may cause deafness or interfere with vision. Unsurprisingly, the severe disfigurement sometimes associated with the disease can have attendant psychological problems. Recurrent surgical intervention to remove troublesome nodules is common and, in severe cases, removal of the scalp with reconstruction using skin grafts is required.

GENETIC LOCI

By genetic linkage analysis of two extended pedigrees with familial cylindromatosis, the location of a predisposition gene (designated *CYLD*) on chromosome 16q12-13 was established in 1995.[4] Subsequently, 14 additional informative families have been reported, all of which have exhibited evidence of linkage to this locus.[5–7] The latter included families with trichoepitheliomas and eccrine spiradenomas (in addition to cylindromas) indicating that the presence of other skin adnexal tumors does not reflect the existence of additional susceptibility loci. Indeed, data from genetic linkage analyses, analyses of loss of heterozygosity in familial cylindromas, and mutational analyses of the gene itself strongly suggest that there is no heterogeneity in genetic predisposition to familial cylindromatosis, and that *CYLD* is the only susceptibility gene.

Approximately 70 percent of cylindromas from individuals with familial cylindromatosis exhibit loss of heterozygosity (LOH) on chromosome 16q in the vicinity of *CYLD*. Indeed, analysis of the remainder of the genome has revealed that chromosome 16 is the only region that shows LOH in familial cylindromas.[8] In all tumors examined, the lost allele has been the wild-type allele inherited from the non–mutation-carrying parent.[4,6,7] Loss of heterozygosity on chromosome 16q is also present in the majority of sporadic cylindromas.[8] These patterns of allele loss in familial and sporadic tumors are characteristic of a tumor suppressor

gene/recessive oncogene, and indicate that, like most cancer susceptibility genes, *CYLD* falls into this category.

SPECIFIC GENES

The *CYLD* Gene

By fine-mapping of meiotic recombinants in cylindromatosis families and use of positional cloning techniques, the *CYLD* gene was identified in 2000.[9] *CYLD* is composed of 20 exons (the smallest being 9 bp) and extends over approximately 56 kb of genomic DNA. The first three exons are untranslated; exon 3 (in the 5' untranslated region) and the 9 bp exon 7 (which is coding) both show alternative splicing. Overlapping exon 1 is a GC-rich region, within which there are numerous CpG dinucleotides, and which has the properties of a CpG island.

Germ line *CYLD* mutations have been found in 21 of 24 cylindromatosis families studied. Because the remaining families show evidence of linkage to the *CYLD* locus on chromosome 16q, it is likely that these are also due to cryptic mutations in this gene. Only two pairs of families had identical mutations, while the remaining mutations were unique. One of these pairs of families also shared a polymorphic marker haplotype in the vicinity of the gene, suggesting that they derived from a common founder mutation and were distant branches of each other. The other pair of families with an identical mutation did not share a polymorphic marker haplotype, indicating that this mutation (2272C > T which is at a CpG dinucleotide) arose independently. Indeed, this mutation was also found as a somatic mutation in a familial cylindroma (see below), indicating that this is likely to be a mutation hotspot.

In addition to germ line mutations, a small number of somatic *CYLD* mutations have been reported. Four of 23 familial cylindromas without chromosome 16q LOH carried intragenic *CYLD* somatic mutations and 1 contained a somatic deletion of approximately 300 kb that removes *CYLD* completely. One of three sporadic cylindromas had a somatic *CYLD* mutation. However, a screen of more than 100 primary cancers, including breast, colorectal, ovary, sarcoma, prostate, and a further 150 cancer cell lines, failed to reveal any additional somatic *CYLD* mutations (unpublished observations).

As expected of a tumor-suppressor gene/recessive oncogene, all mutant alleles of *CYLD* reported thus far are predicted to abolish function of the protein. This is achieved by deletion of the entire gene, by reduction in messenger ribonucleic acid (mRNA) levels through nonsense-mediated RNA decay or by protein truncation. Of the 25 independent intragenic *CYLD* mutations reported, 9 cause translational frameshifts as a result of small insertions or deletions, 12 are base substitutions that directly generate translational termination codons, and 4 are base substitutions in splice sites.

The known truncating mutations in *CYLD* are all located in the 3' two-thirds of the coding sequence. This clustering may be a consequence of the presence of a domain in the N-terminal part of CYLD that mediates a dominant negative effect of the truncated protein. Under this model, mutations that truncate CYLD N-terminal to this domain would abolish the dominant negative effect, would be associated with lower disease penetrance, and would not be ascertained as classical cylindromatosis pedigrees. Alternatively, there may be a second start codon from which a smaller CYLD product would be translated. If this smaller protein has tumor suppressor activity it would rescue the effect of truncating mutations located 5' to the alternative initiation site. However, *in vitro* transcription/translation of full-length *CYLD* cDNA yielded a single protein consistent in size with the full translation.

FUNCTION OF CYLD

Full-length CYLD is predicted to be a protein of 956 amino acids, with the exon − 7 splice variant encoding 953 amino acids

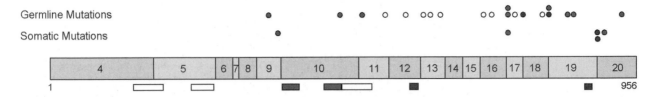

Fig. 37-4. Representation of the *CYLD* gene. The complete coding sequence (CDS) from codon 1 to 956 is represented with the exons numbered. The positions of germ line and somatic mutations are shown as dots above the CDS (nonsense mutations in red, frameshift mutations in yellow, and splice site mutations in blue). The relative positions of the known motifs are shown as rectangles below the CDS (CAP-GLY domains in yellow, putative SH3 binding domain in red and the UCH domains in blue).

(Fig. 37-4). Likely orthologues, identified by regions of extensive amino acid identity, are present in *Drosophila melanogaster* and *Caenorhabditis elegans*. Although the predicted protein does not show extensive sequence similarity to other known human proteins, a number of previously defined motifs are present (Fig. 37-4).

There are three CAP-GLY domains.[10] Two of these domains (approximately from amino acids 127 to 203 and amino acids 472 to 540) show strong similarity to previously described CAP-GLY domains, while the third (from amino acids 232 to 285) exhibits weaker similarity. The third CAP-GLY domain is present in the *D. melanogaster* CYLD orthologue.

Comparison of the CYLD sequence against itself reveals a short repeated segment of approximately 25 amino acids (between amino acids 388 to 413 and 446 to 471) that is rich in proline residues. This proline-rich region may constitute an SH3 binding domain that mediates protein-protein interactions in signal transduction or vesicle transport pathways.[11]

There are two short regions that exhibit homology to the two halves of a split ubiquitin C-terminal hydrolase (UCH) catalytic domain (reference 12 and http://www.expasy.ch/cgi-bin/get-prodoc-entry?PDOC00127; http://www.expasy.ch/cgi-bin/get-prodoc-entry?PDOC00750) amino acids 871 to 889 showing homology to a UCH2-2 domain and amino acids 593 to 610 showing weaker homology to a UCH2-1 domain. These domains are highly conserved in both *D. melanogaster* and *C. elegans* orthologues.

There are four Cys-X-X-Cys pairs (between amino acids 788 and 856) that may represent finger-like metal-binding domains. Three of the four Cys-X-X-Cys pairs are conserved in *D. melanogaster* and *C. elegans,* despite relative lack of conservation of the surrounding amino acids.

CAP-GLY domains were originally identified in CLIP170/Restin, a protein that acts as a linker between endocytic vesicles and microtubules.[13,14] Subsequently, CAP-GLY domains have been identified in a number of proteins that are believed to coordinate the attachment of cellular organelles, such as vesicles or chromosomes, to microtubules and thus assist their movements within the cell.[11] The CAP-GLY domains themselves are responsible for microtubule binding.[15] Included among this group of proteins are p150Glued which forms part of the dynactin complex[16] (necessary for the docking of cargoes to the minus end directed microtubule associated motor, dynein) and BIK1 (mutations of which cause disorders of mitotic segregation in yeast).[17,18] CLIP170 and a number of other proteins have two CAP-GLY domains, while the majority of CAP-GLY proteins contain a single copy. CYLD is the first protein, to our knowledge, that has three CAP-GLY motifs (although one of these is quite divergent from the consensus sequence). All truncating *CYLD* mutations are predicted to leave intact the N-terminal two CAP-GLY domains. Similar to CYLD, several other proteins with CAP-GLY domains have C-terminal metal-binding finger-like domains.[11]

The mechanism by which inactivation of a protein containing CAP-GLY domains might contribute to neoplastic transformation is not clear. Several CAP-GLY proteins are implicated in the attachment of the mitotic spindle to chromosomes.[19–21] It is, therefore, plausible that CYLD is required for appropriate segregation of chromosomes during mitosis and that abnormalities of CYLD result in gains or losses of chromosomes. However, examination of 25 familial cylindromas for LOH on almost all chromosomal arms failed to reveal any evidence of allele loss other than on chromosome 16q.[8] Similarly, comparative genomic hybridization (CGH) performed on 10 familial cylindromas showed very few copy number changes (Shipley and Stratton, unpublished data). These results therefore provide no evidence in favor of a phenotype of chromosomal instability in familial cylindromas carrying *CYLD* mutations.

Another major clue to the function of CYLD is the presence of two regions that could form a putative UCH Type 2 catalytic domain toward the C-terminus of the protein (http://www.expasy.ch/cgi-bin/get-prodoc-entry?PDOC00127; http://www.expasy.ch/cgi-bin/get-prodoc-entry?PDOC00750). UCH catalyzes the hydrolysis of ubiquitin resulting in deubiquitination, reducing degradation of target proteins by the proteasome.[12] Therefore, inactivation of CYLD could conceivably contribute to oncogenesis by enhancing the degradation of proteins that, for example, suppress cell proliferation or promote apoptosis.[22]

Germ line mutations in the *CYLD* gene are remarkable for their tumor-type specificity. With the exceptions of trichoepitheliomas and eccrine spiradenomas (both of which also show features of skin adnexal structures), there is no evidence for predisposition to other types of neoplasm, either in the skin or other organs. Similarly, somatic *CYLD* mutations appear restricted to cylindromas and are not found in other tumors. Nevertheless, *CYLD* is highly expressed in fetal brain, testis, and skeletal muscle, and at a lower level in adult brain, leukocytes, liver, heart, kidney, spleen, ovary, and lung. It therefore seems unlikely that the propensity of *CYLD* mutations to cause neoplastic transformation in skin appendageal tissues is attributable simply to the tissue or cell-type specific expression pattern of the gene.

The biological activities of CYLD predicted on the basis of amino acid sequence require direct experimental confirmation. However, the presence of functional motifs that have not previously been found in proteins implicated in oncogenesis promises new insights into mechanisms of neoplastic transformation.

IMPLICATIONS FOR DIAGNOSIS

Identification of *CYLD* will, of course, enable presymptomatic carrier testing of at-risk individuals. The main utility of such testing is to implement, at an early stage, strategies that might prevent the development of tumors. Currently, no such treatment modalities exist and it therefore seems unlikely that there will be substantial uptake of *CYLD* carrier diagnosis. However, experience of other, similar heritable conditions suggests that, for a variety of reasons (for example "simply wanting to know") there will be a low level of uptake. It would also not be surprising if, in severely affected families, there might be requests for antenatal diagnosis upon which early gestation termination might be based.

REFERENCES

1. Abenoza P, Ackerman AB: *Neoplasms with Eccrine Differentiation.* Philadelphia, Lea and Febiger, 1990.
2. van Balkom ID, Hennekam RC: Dermal eccrine cylindromatosis. *J Med Genet* **31**:321, 1994.
3. Gerretsen AL, Beemer FA, Deenstra W, et al: Familial cutaneous cylindromas: Investigations in five generations of a family. *J Am Acad Dermatol* **33**:199, 1995.
4. Biggs PJ, Wooster R, Ford D, et al: Familial cylindromatosis (turban tumour syndrome) gene localised to chromosome 16q12–q13: Evidence for its role as a tumour suppressor gene. *Nat Genet* **11**:441, 1995.
5. Verhoef S, Schrander-Stumpel CT, Vuzevski VD, et al: Familial cylindromatosis mimicking tuberous sclerosis complex and confirmation of the cylindromatosis locus, CYLD1, in a large family. *J Med Genet* **35**:841, 1998.
6. Thomson SA, Rasmussen SA, Zhang J, et al: A new hereditary cylindromatosis family associated with CYLD1 on chromosome 16. *Hum Genet* **105**:171, 1999.
7. Takahashi M, Rapley E, Biggs PJ, et al: Linkage and LOH studies in 19 cylindromatosis families show no evidence of genetic heterogeneity and refine the *CYLD* locus on chromosome 16q12–q13. *Hum Genet* **106**:58, 2000.
8. Biggs PJ, Chapman P, Lakhani SR, et al: The cylindromatosis gene (CYLD) on chromosome 16q may be the only tumour suppressor gene involved in the development of cylindromas. *Oncogene* **12**:375, 1996.
9. Bignell GR, Warren W, Seal S, et al: Identification of the familial cylindromatosis tumor-suppressor gene. *Nat Genet* **25**:160, 2000.
10. Riehemann K, Sorg C: Sequence homologies between four cytoskeleton-associated proteins. *Trends Biochem Sci* **18**:82, 1993.
11. Feng S, Chen JK, Yu H, et al: Two binding orientations for peptides to the Src SH3 domain: Development of a general model for SH3-ligand interactions. *Science* **266**:1241, 1994.
12. D'Andrea A, Pellman D: Deubiquitinating enzymes: A new class of biological regulators. *Crit Rev Biochem Mol Biol* **33**:337, 1998.
13. Pierre P, Scheel J, Rickard JE: CLIP-170 links endocytic vesicles to microtubules. *Cell* **70**:887, 1992.
14. Bilbe G, Delabie J, Bruggen J, et al: Restin: A novel intermediate filament-associated protein highly expressed in the Reed-Sternberg cells of Hodgkin's disease. *EMBO J* **11**:2103, 1992.
15. Pierre P, Pepperkok R, Kreis TE: Molecular characterization of two functional domains of CLIP-170 in vivo. *J Cell Sci* **107**:1909, 1994.
16. Waterman-Storer CM, Holzbaur EL: The product of the *Drosophila* gene, Glued, is the functional homologue of the p150Glued component of the vertebrate dynactin complex. *J Biol Chem* **271**:1153, 1996.
17. Berlin V, Styles CA, Fink GR: BIK1, a protein required for microtubule function during mating and mitosis in *Saccharomyces cerevisiae*, colocalizes with tubulin. *J Cell Biol* **111**:2573, 1990.
18. Pellman D, Bagget M, Tu YH, et al: Two microtubule-associated proteins required for anaphase spindle movement in *Saccharomyces cerevisiae*. *J Cell Biol* **130**:1373, 1995.
19. Karki S, Holzbaur EL: Cytoplasmic dynein and dynactin in cell division and intracellular transport. *Curr Opin Cell Biol* **11**:45, 1999.
20. Dujardin D, Wacker UI, Moreau A, et al: Evidence for a role of CLIP-170 in the establishment of metaphase chromosome alignment. *J Cell Biol* **141**:849, 1998.
21. Kahana JA, Schlenstedt G, Evanchuk DM, et al: The yeast dynactin complex is involved in partitioning the mitotic spindle between mother and daughter cells during anaphase B. *Mol Biol Cell* **9**:1741, 1998.
22. Hershko A: Roles of ubiquitin-mediated proteolysis in cell cycle control. *Curr Opin Cell Biol* **9**:788, 1997.

Familial Cardiac Myxomas and Carney Complex

Mark Veugelers ▪ *Carl J. Vaughan* ▪ *Craig T. Basson*

1. **Cardiac myxomas are neoplasms that occur in at least 7 per 10,000 individuals. They are the most common primary cardiac tumor in adults.[1] The typical cardiac myxoma is a sporadic, benign, nonrecurring left atrial tumor. These neoplasms are thought to arise from primitive, subendocardial, pluripotent, mesenchymal cells.[2] Morbidity and mortality from cardiac myxomas is the result of embolic stroke, heart failure, and/or constitutional symptoms. Prompt surgical resection of cardiac myxomas is recommended.**

2. **A significant portion of cardiac myxomas is related to Carney complex,[3] a familial autosomal dominant syndrome. Familial cardiac myxomas are associated with spotty pigmentation of the skin; endocrine dysfunction; extracardiac (most often cutaneous) myxomas; schwannomas; pituitary adenomas; thyroid tumors; testis tumors; ovarian tumors; and breast tumors. Not all patients with Carney complex develop cardiac myxomas, but affected individuals usually have at least two components of the complex, or one component as well as a significant family history.**

3. **Clinical evaluation and genetic linkage analyses[4,5] of families affected by Carney complex have suggested two chromosomal loci: chromosome 2p16 and chromosome 17q24. Linkage to the chromosome 17q24 locus was initially observed in 4 families affected by Carney complex.[4] Positional cloning studies have determined that familial cardiac myxomas and Carney complex, linked to chromosome 17q24, are caused by mutations in the *PRKAR1α* gene that encodes the R1α regulatory subunit of cyclic adenosine monophosphate (cAMP)-dependent protein kinase A (PKA). Haploinsufficiency of *PRKAR1α* in Carney complex patients predicts a tumor-suppressor function for this gene.[6,7] Although some tumors of Carney complex patients with mutations of *PRKAR1α* show loss-of-heterozygosity (LOH) at chromosome 17q24, this is not a universal finding and is apparently not required for tumorigenesis.[6,7] Thus, Carney complex is a multiple neoplasia syndrome which, like Peutz-Jeghers syndrome, is associated with dermatologic abnormalities and is caused by gene mutations that modify the activity of a protein kinase.**

Carney complex is a familial multiple neoplasia syndrome characterized by cardiac myxomas in the setting of spotty skin pigmentation and endocrinopathy.[8] First described in 1973 by Rees et al.,[9] the disorder was initially referred to by the acronyms NAME (Nevi, Atrial myxoma, Myxoid neurofibromata, Ephelides)[10] or LAMB (Lentigines, Atrial myxoma, Mucocutaneous myxoma, Blue nevi).[11] Others have called this disease "Syndrome Myxoma"[12] and Swiss-syndrome.[13] Several detailed clinicopathologic analyses of familial and sporadic cardiac myxoma cohorts have led to the commonly used eponym Carney

complex.[3] Although cardiac myxomas are usually benign nonmetastatic lesions that are readily amenable to surgical resection, individuals with Carney complex account for an unusual subset of cardiac myxoma patients with an aggressive recurrent autosomal dominant tumor syndrome. Recent molecular analyses have demonstrated that the genetic etiologies of Carney complex are heterogeneous but that the major cause of Carney complex are mutations in the *PRKAR1α* gene encoding the R1α subunit of cAMP-dependent protein kinase A.

CLINICAL ASPECTS

Cardiac Myxoma

Although primary tumors of the heart are rare, their incidence at autopsy is variably reported as between 0.0017 percent and 0.19 percent, and myxomas account for nearly half of all such primary cardiac neoplasms. Typically, these are benign solitary tumors that arise in middle-aged women at the *fossa ovalis* on the left atrial side of the interatrial septum.[14,15] These tumors do not metastasize. Cardiac myxomas can present with a variety of constitutional symptoms, heart failure, and embolic stroke, and diagnosis of a cardiac myxoma is typically made by echocardiography. Prompt surgical resection is recommended to avoid embolic events, and surgical resection is usually curative without tumor recurrence. Several hematologic, immunologic, and rheumatologic disorders (e.g., anemia, polycythemia, fever, rheumatoid arthritis, vasculitis, lupus-like syndrome, and Raynaud phenomenon) have all been associated with the presence of myxomas. These systemic abnormalities have been reported to result from myxoma secretion of interleukin-6, and they can resolve with tumor resection.[16] Histologically, cardiac myxomas are comprised of small stellate cells against a bland proteoglycan myxoid background (Fig. 38-1).[2] The tumors are thought to arise from a subendothelial pluripotent stem cell, sometimes referred to as a "reserve" cell.[17] Accordingly, a number of organized structures, including acinar elements, regions of extramedullary hematopoiesis, and blood vessels, are occasionally noted within these tumors consistent with differentiation along a variety of lineages such as epithelial, hematopoietic, endothelial, muscular, and osteogenic.

Approximately 7 percent of individuals with cardiac myxomas are affected by the familial disorder Carney complex and have associated noncardiac findings.[12,18] More than two-thirds of Carney complex patients have developed one or more cardiac myxomas.[3,12,15,18] Although cardiac myxomas in Carney complex are histologically indistinguishable from the more common sporadic cardiac myxomas (Fig. 38-1),[2] their clinical presentation and course can be quite distinct (Table 38-1).[12,15,18,19] Consistent with Carney complex's transmission as an autosomal dominant trait, cardiac myxomas in this complex exhibit no age or gender preference. Although they most often arise, like their sporadic counterparts, in the left atrium, they can occur in any of the four cardiac chambers and may present with multiple lesions in the

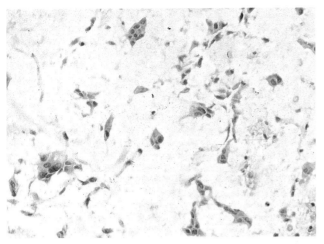

Figure 38-1 Histopathology of a cardiac myxoma. Cardiac myxomas are comprised of small stellate cells against a myxoid proteoglycan background. Shown is a cardiac myxoma from a patient with Carney complex.

Table 38-1 Differences in Clinical Features Between Nonfamilial and Familial Cardiac Myxomas

Clinical Feature	Sporadic	Familial
Female gender preference	Yes	No
Typical age of presentation	Middle age	Postpuberty
Left atrial predominance	Yes	Yes
Ventricular and right atrial tumors	Rare	Common
Multicentric tumors	Rare	Common
Other noncardiac tumors	Rare	Common
Spotty pigmentation of the skin	No	Yes
Endocrinopathy	Rare	Common

same or different chambers. Furthermore, despite adequate resection, Carney complex cardiac myxomas can recur at sites distant from the initial surgery within even a single year or many years later. Patients have experienced multiple recurrences and have required more than three cardiac surgeries in their lifetime.[12,15,18,19] Because of the high risk of tumor recurrence, patients with Carney complex, unlike patients with sporadic cardiac myxomas, should undergo annual surveillance echocardiography throughout their lifetime (Fig. 38-2C).

Skin Pigmentation

Spotty skin pigmentation, usually lentigines, is present in almost all patients with Carney complex (≥95 percent).[3–5] Lentigines are skin lesions characterized by basal cell layer hyperpigmentation associated with melanocytic hyperplasia.[20] Small (pinpoint to 6 mm), round, irregularly shaped brown-to-black macules characteristically occur in the center of the face and vermilion border of the lips (Fig. 38-2A). Spotty pigmented lesions of the conjunctiva, eyelids, and external ears are also frequently observed.[21] Other affected areas include genitalia, trunk and, less commonly, oral and perianal mucosae. In about 20 percent of Carney complex patients, spotty skin pigmentation may include the common blue nevus and/or the exceptionally rare epithelioid blue nevus, which has only been reported in Carney complex patients.[22,23] Blue nevi are nonmalignant blue to black, domed,

small (< 1 cm) lesions, occurring on the face, head, neck, trunk, and extremities. These nonmalignant lesions do not recur at the initial site after excision.

Skin and Other Extracardiac Myxomas

Cutaneous myxomas are usually present as small (less than 1 cm), multicentric, recurring lesions, which occur in about 75 percent of Carney complex patients.[3–5,21,24] The eyelid and external ear are preferentially involved, but these tumors also occur on the face, head, neck, trunk, and limbs with rare involvement of the hands and feet.[25,26] There are no unusual histologic features to these cutaneous myxomas. Similar benign myxomas have also been observed in visceral organs including the liver (Fig. 38-2B) and spleen.[4]

Endocrinopathy and Primary Pigmented Nodular Adrenocortical Disease

Carney complex patients may present with several forms of adrenal, pituitary, and thyroid dysfunction (Fig. 38-2B). Although generally associated with endocrine overactivity, Carney complex may also involve endocrine underactivity, such as hypothyroidism.[27] Endocrine dysfunction may occur in the absence of glandular neoplasms, which are also independently associated with Carney complex. Most commonly, Carney complex patients present with Cushing syndrome due to primary pigmented nodular adrenocortical disease (PPNAD), a bilateral adrenal disorder leading to hypercortisolism.[3–5] In this disorder, which occurs in about 20 percent of Carney complex patients, multiple, small, black-brown pigmented, autonomously functioning nodules are present in an atrophic adrenal cortex.[28] Symptoms of Cushing syndrome are generally treated by bilateral adrenalectomy. Pharmacologic adrenalectomy is occasionally used with unusual durable results.[17]

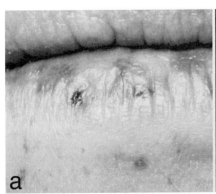

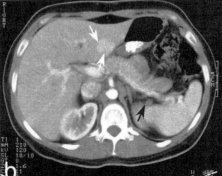

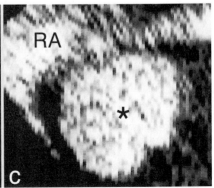

Figure 38-2 Clinical features of Carney complex. Examples of cutaneous, endocrinologic, and cardiac manifestations in a family affected by Carney complex. *A*, Multiple lentigines: irregularly shaped brown-to-black macules are present on the face and vermilion border of the lips. *B*, Abdominal CAT scan imaging showing liver myxoma (white arrow) and adrenal hypertrophy (black arrow). *C*, Echocardiogram showing a large myxoma (*) arising from the wall of the right atrium (RA). Individuals in this family are affected by a ΔFST163 mutation in the *PRKAR1α* gene.[6]

Nonmyxomatous Tumors

Psammomatous Melanotic Schwannoma. The psammomatous melanotic schwannoma is a very rare tumor associated with Carney complex in approximately half of occurrences.[29] The presence of melanin, psammoma bodies, and fat in the tumor cells is unusual and differentiates this neoplasm from a common schwannoma. The tumor can involve the spinal nerve roots and vertebrae, and can also can affect the skin, stomach, or esophagus. Although psammomatous melanotic schwannoma is usually benign, metastasis has been documented in 10 percent of cases.[29]

Pituitary Tumors. Growth hormone-producing pituitary adenomas, resulting in gigantism and/or acromegaly, have been observed in approximately 10 percent of Carney complex patients.[4,5] Prolactin-secreting adenomas have also been noted.[30,31] Upon resection by transsphenoidal hypophysectomy, most Carney-complex pituitary tumors have been found to be macroadenomas.[32]

Thyroid Tumors. Thyroid tumors are infrequently observed in Carney complex. Benign thyroid nodules and cysts, Hürthle-cell adenoma, and thyroid papillary and follicular carcinoma, have all been reported.[33]

Breast Tumors. Mammary gland lesions occur in both females and males and have been estimated to occur in about one-fourth of Carney complex patients. They are usually asymptomatic and generally are of two histologic types: ductal adenoma with tubular features and myxoid fibroadenoma.[34,35] Both neoplasms may be bilateral and tend to be multicentric within a single breast.

Ovarian Tumors. In a prospective study of female Carney complex patients, 60 percent had ovarian cysts. In two patients, the cysts progressed to cystadenomas and required surgery. Cystic teratoma, endometrioid carcinoma, and metastatic adenocarcinoma (but not stromal tumors) have all been observed.[36]

Testicular Tumors. Large-cell, calcifying, Sertoli cell tumors[37] are one of the rarest forms of testicular neoplasms. However, they occur in 30 percent of male Carney complex patients.[3] While these tumors may be asymptomatic, they may produce estrogens and cause sexual precocity and/or gynecomastia. All identified cases showed multicentric foci within each testis and usually exhibited bilateral involvement. One Carney complex patient has died with metastasis of his testicular tumor.[38] In addition to Sertoli cell tumors, other testicular lesions, including Leydig cell tumors and adrenocortical rest tumors, have been observed in Carney complex patients.[5]

Miscellaneous

Other neoplasms that have been reported in Carney complex patients include osteochondromyxoma; gastric carcinoma; Barrett metaplasia of the esophagus; colonic polyps/colorectal cancer; myxoid uterine leiomyoma; trichofolliculoma; pancreatic adenocarcinoma; pheochromocytoma; angiomyxoma; fibrolamellar hepatoma; lung granuloma; spermatocele; and cerebellopontine angle tumor.[3,5,39,40] The significance of these lesions' association with Carney complex remains unknown.

A definitive clinical diagnosis of Carney complex is possible when at least two of the following major manifestations are present: cardiac myxomas, characteristic spotty pigmentation of the skin, or PPNAD. Any one of those major findings coupled with a family history of Carney complex is also sufficient to establish the diagnosis. The presence of a noncardiac myxoma, a psammomatous melanotic schwannoma or a Sertoli cell tumor along with any major manifestation is also highly suggestive of Carney complex. The role of other tumors or endocrinopathies in establishing a clinical diagnosis of Carney complex are less clear given the propensity of those disorders to occur in other settings as well.

PARTIAL PHENOCOPY SYNDROMES

Several related syndromes share some manifestations with Carney complex. Careful analysis of subtle clinical features of patient presentations usually permits their differentiation from Carney complex.

Peutz-Jeghers Syndrome

Peutz-Jeghers syndrome is an autosomal dominant lentiginosis and multiple neoplasia syndrome that shares several cutaneous and oncologic features with Carney complex. The syndrome is characterized by skin and mucosal lentigines, gastrointestinal polyps, and breast, thyroid, ovarian, and testicular tumors.[41] The skin and mucosal lentigines in Peutz-Jeghers syndrome are clinically similar to those observed in Carney complex patients. The extremely rare large-cell, calcifying, Sertoli cell tumor of the testis is almost exclusively seen in familial cases of Peutz-Jeghers syndrome and Carney complex. All Peutz-Jeghers-associated tumors, except the gastrointestinal lesions, are observed in Carney complex, although some Carney complex patients have developed intestinal polyposis and gastrointestinal tumors.[5,39] Thus, making clinical differentiation between the two syndromes may be difficult.[5,42] The presence of cardiac or cutaneous myxomas, which do not occur in Peutz-Jeghers syndrome, within a family suggests a diagnosis of Carney complex. At least one pedigree in which individuals had been assigned a diagnosis of Peutz-Jeghers syndrome, proved to be affected by Carney complex after development of cardiac myxoma in the proband.[42] Peutz-Jeghers syndrome is genetically heterogeneous with one locus at chromosome 19p13. Loss-of-function mutations at this locus in the *STK11/LKB-1* gene, coding for a serine/threonine kinase, have been identified in several Peutz-Jeghers pedigrees.[43,44]

LEOPARD Syndrome

LEOPARD syndrome is an autosomal dominant lentiginosis syndrome. The acronym describes the association of lentigines, electrocardiographic abnormalities, ocular hypertelorism, pulmonary stenosis, abnormalities of the genitalia, retardation, and deafness. The syndrome shows variable expression within the same family and has also been referred to as cardiocutaneous syndrome. A hallmark of LEOPARD syndrome is hypertrophic cardiomyopathy, which is not a feature of Carney complex. Some families have initially been diagnosed with LEOPARD syndrome, but their diagnoses were reassigned as Carney complex after the development of cardiac myxomas in probands from the pedigrees.[45,46]

MOLECULAR GENETIC ASPECTS OF CARNEY COMPLEX

Carney complex is transmitted in families in an autosomal dominant fashion (Fig. 38-3).[3–5,38] Despite highly variable expressivity, the penetrance is nearly complete, with all affected patients exhibiting at least one of the stigmata before 30 years of age. The disease occurs in all races, and to date, more than 50 different familial cases have been reported.[4,5,47] In addition, about 200 sporadic cases have been described. Cytogenetic rearrangements involving chromosomes 2p, 17p, and 12p were initially described in sporadic atrial myxomas.[48–50] These observations suggested that genes involved in Carney complex tumorigenesis might map to these locations.[48] Linkage and positional cloning studies[4,5] have now described two loci for Carney complex: chromosome 2p16 and chromosome 17q24.

Genetic Mapping of the 2p Locus

Initial linkage analysis[5] of 11 Carney complex families suggested a locus on chromosome 2p16 with an aggregate LOD score of 5.97. However, no single family exhibited a statistically significant LOD score >3.6. In subsequent experiments, several of the families from this study proved to be linked to another locus at chromosome 17q24 (Refs. 4, 7, and 47, and see below). To date,

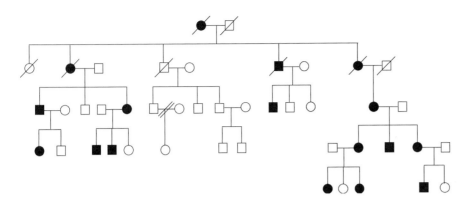

Figure 38-3. Pedigree of Carney complex family YA. Family YA is a typical large family affected by Carney complex.[4] Squares denote male family members; circles denote female family members. Affected and unaffected individuals are represented by closed and open symbols, respectively. Carney complex is transmitted in an autosomal dominant fashion and is linked in this family to chromosome 17q24. Further mutational analysis[6] demonstrated that Carney complex in family YA is caused by *PRKAR1α* haploinsufficiency, which is a result of a ΔFSG208 mutation.

the existence of a Carney complex locus at chromosome 2p16 remains uncertain.[47] Several small families of limited statistical power failed to show evidence of linkage to 17q24, but did exhibit haplotype sharing over an approximately 2 Mb interval between D2S391 and D2S153.[5,47,51] However, further genetic heterogeneity of the disorder is likely; there are several families, which exhibit significant discordance at both chromosomes 17q24 and 2p16 (Ref. 47 and unpublished data).

Genetic Mapping of the 17q24 Locus

Linkage analysis of a large family (Fig. 38-3; YA) definitively excluded linkage to the 2p16 locus[52] and demonstrated highly statistically significant (LOD score = 5.9) linkage of Carney complex to chromosome 17q24.[4] Meiotic fine mapping in this and other families[4,26] indicated that the disease gene was located in the 17-cM interval between D17S807 and D17S785. This interval was subsequently further refined by haplotype analysis of several other 17q24 linked families to a minimal genetic interval of ≈12 cM between D17S1882 and D17S929.[6]

Identification of *PRKAR1α* Mutations

The *PRKAR1α* gene, encoding the R1α-regulatory subunit of cAMP-dependent protein kinase A, had previously been mapped as *TSE1* (*Tissue-Specific Extinguisher* locus) to chromosome 17q23-q24 by somatic cell hybrid analysis.[53,54] PKA activity variably regulates proliferation rates and differentiation of a number of transformed and nontransformed cell types, and antagonism of R1α via several molecular strategies has been

attempted as a chemotherapeutic strategy in several malignancies.[55] Given the ubiquitous expression pattern of the *PRKAR1α* gene along with its chromosomal location and PKA participation in cell growth, differentiation, and cancer, *PRKAR1α* was an attractive candidate disease gene for Carney complex.

To analyze the *PRKAR1α* gene for mutations, the genomic structure of the gene was determined by comparison of the cDNA sequence with genomic sequence from chromosome 17q23-q24 elaborated by the Human Genome Project. Interestingly, although the *PRKAR1α* gene had previously been suggested[56] to be comprised of 11 exons (with two alternatively spliced exons—1a and 1b—containing 5′ untranslated sequence and 9 exons containing coding sequence), we noted that there were in fact 12 exons and that 1146 bp of coding sequence were divided amongst 10 exons (Fig. 38-4); the exon previously referred[56] to as exon 4 was actually divided into 2 exons. Elucidation of the *PRKAR1α* genomic structure permitted establishment of oligonucleotide primers that could be used first to polymerase chain reaction (PCR) amplify each of these 10 exons (Table 38-2) for Carney complex patient genomic DNA samples and then to sequence each exon to identify sequence variants.

Such sequence analysis of the coding sequence of the *PRKAR1α* gene demonstrated heterozygous sequence variants that were coinherited with Carney complex in several unrelated families.[6] These variants all introduced frameshift (deletions/ insertions) or nonsense mutations into the *PRKAR1α* gene, and were not present in panels of unrelated unaffected individuals.[6] Therefore, we concluded that mutation of the *PRKAR1α* gene is a

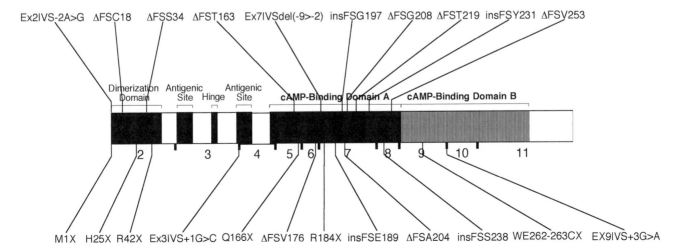

Figure 38-4. Schematic of the *PRKAR1α* cDNA and Carney complex-causing mutations. Exons encoding protein are denoted and numbered 2 to 11. cDNA regions that encode specific R1α protein functional domains are noted. *PRKAR1α* mutations known to cause Carney complex are shown. (Adapted from references 6, 7, 17, and 47, and from our unpublished data (manuscript in preparation).)

Table 38-2 PCR Primers for the Amplification of *PRKAR1α* Coding Exons

Exon	Forward primer	Reverse Primer
2	AAATCCCTGTGAATCAGT TGTC	CAACTGTCACAATCACCTCATC
3	GAAT TGGTGT T T TCCTCT TAACT T	TATGAT TCAT TCATCAAAGGAGAC
4	GT TGTAGTGAAACACTACAAAG	GACTGTCATCTGGTGAACAAT TACT
5	GACAGTCTGGGGTCT T TAAT TCTA	TCAAAGAGGAAAACAAACT TCAAT
6	T T TCT T TAAT T TGGAATATGCT TC	ATCTGACATACAAGGGATGTAATG
7	T T T T TAAAACAAAGT TCAGGAT TG	CTAAATCACACTCTCAAACACCAT
8	AT TAT TCCATAGCAT TATGTGGTG	AGTCACAGAGGAAATAACTGTGAA
9	GGCTAT T TGGT TGAATCTCT T TAT	TGAGT TCT T TACCTCTAAAAT TCAA
10	T TGT T TAGCT T T T TGGTGAT T T TA	GGAGAAGACAAAAT TATGGAAGAC
11	TAT TGTCT TCT T TCTCAGAAGTGC	GTGCAATAAAAGCAACT T TCAATA

major cause of Carney complex. Kirschner et al.[7] similarly identified *PRKAR1α* mutations in the same gene in Carney complex patients. To date, multiple frameshift, nonsense, and splicing mutations have been identified (Fig. 38-4) but no missense mutations in both Carney complex kindreds[6,7,47] and in sporadic Carney complex patients.[7,17,47] One major mutation hotspot has been identified (in eight unrelated kindreds; see references 6, 7, 17, and 47) that is located in a repetitive region of sequence, TGTG, in exon 5, and therefore may be related to polymerase slippage. Otherwise, mutations fail to demonstrate a predilection for any particular exon.

Despite the variable manifestations of the disease between families, no *PRKAR1α* genotype-phenotype correlations have been observed amongst Carney complex kindreds.[6,7,17,47] All mutations thus far identified lead to *PRKAR1α* haploinsufficiency. Mutant mRNAs or truncated proteins have not been detected in tissue samples from affected patients, and mutant mRNAs are likely degraded by nonsense-mediated mRNA decay.[6,7,47] Expression of mutant RNAs is enhanced in lymphocytes by pharmacologic inhibition of protein synthesis, which is required for nonsense-mediated decay.[47] Western blot analyses[6] show that lymphocytes from individuals with Carney complex contain 40 percent of the R1α protein that is contained in normal lymphocytes; these data are consistent with *PRKAR1α* haploinsufficiency in Carney complex. In several series,[6,7,17,47] mutations in the *PRKAR1α* gene were detected in approximately half of unrelated Carney complex patients. The remaining portion of patients may include patients with mutations that are refractory to currently employed technologies,[57] but given the disorder's heterogeneity, at least some of these individuals are likely to have mutations in genes other than *PRKAR1α*.

PRKAR1α in Carney Complex Tumorigenesis

Carney complex tumors exhibit considerable genomic instability. Initial microsatellite analyses and cytogenetic studies of Carney complex tumors and cardiac myxomas demonstrated that several chromosomal regions including 2p, 17p, 12p, and Y, as well as a number of other chromosomes, can exhibit rearrangements, deletions, and duplications.[48–50,58] Notably, these studies reported no significant loss of heterozygosity at chromosome 17q. More recently, coupled with identification of constitutional *PRKAR1α* mutations in Carney complex, studies that focused on chromosome 17q24 microsatellites revealed that Carney complex tumors can show loss of heterozygosity at the *PRKAR1α* locus.[7] However, other Carney complex tumors, including some cardiac myxomas, show no instability at this locus and retain the wild-type *PRKAR1α* allele.[6,7] In fact, the conclusion that loss of *PRKAR1α* heterozygosity is not absolutely required for Carney complex tumorigenesis is further supported by detection of full-length R1α protein in cardiac myxoma cells[6] and pituitary tumor cells[7] from Carney complex patients. Nonetheless, it is likely that somatic mutation(s) of *PRKAR1α* or as yet unidentified tumor-suppressor

gene(s) are required for tumorigenesis in Carney complex. In fact, loss of heterozygosity, gain of heterozygosity, and deletions are observed in a significant portion (44 to 73 percent) of Carney complex tumors at loci other than chromosome 17q24 including chromosomes 6, 11, 22, 10, and 19.[58]

Protein Kinase A Activity and Carney Complex

We[6] and others[7] have hypothesized that the mutations in *PRKAR1α* affect Carney complex patients via alteration in protein kinase A activity. The PKA holoenzyme is a tetramer comprised of two catalytic (C) subunits and two regulatory (R) subunits. Genes for four regulatory subunits—R1α, R1β, R2α, and R2β—have been identified, and the subunits differ in size, cAMP-affinity, and regional expression patterns.[59] The two classes of R subunits R1 and R2 define two types of PKA holoenzymes: type 1 and type 2. In its tetrameric form, protein kinase A is inactive. Upon binding of two molecules of cAMP to each regulatory subunit, the regulatory subunits undergo a conformational change and dissociate from the catalytic subunits, releasing two enzymatically active catalytic subunits (Fig. 38-5). The active catalytic subunit phosphorylates serine and threonine residues on specific substrate proteins. cAMP-dependent protein kinase A activity can either inhibit or stimulate cell proliferation depending on the cell type.[60]

PKA activity in any given cell type may be altered not only by the concentration of free catalytic subunit but also by the concentration ratio of R1:R2 regulatory subunits.[60] Regulatory subunit levels are modulated not only at the level of each gene's expression but also at the protein level by a wide array of different cell type-specific binding proteins for the regulatory subunits (so-called A Kinase Anchoring Proteins or AKAPs),[61] which may sequester regulatory subunits at intracellular sites. Importantly, the ratios of R1:R2 can change dramatically during development, differentiation, and transformation, and alterations in one regulatory subunit concentration may be incompletely compensated by changes in another. For instance, knockout of *prkar1β* or *prkar2β* in mouse leads to a partial increase in *prkar1α*.[62,63] The net result is an increased level of basal PKA activity with a decreased level of cAMP stimulated activity.

In some Carney complex tumors, cAMP-stimulated PKA activity is increased.[7] Such increased cAMP responsiveness may be due to overexpression of other PKA regulatory subunits in the setting of R1α deficiency. We have observed an excess of R1α as compared with R2β in both normal and Carney complex lymphocytes.[6] However, in cardiac myxomas from Carney complex patients, we have observed a reversal of this ratio with an excess of R2β as compared to R1α.[6] This altered regulatory subunit ratio may contribute not only to tumor growth in Carney complex but also to nontumor Carney complex phenotypes. For instance, lipomatous hypertrophy of the interatrial septum, a common finding in healthy elderly individuals, is observed in young individuals affected by Carney complex.[6] Interestingly, the

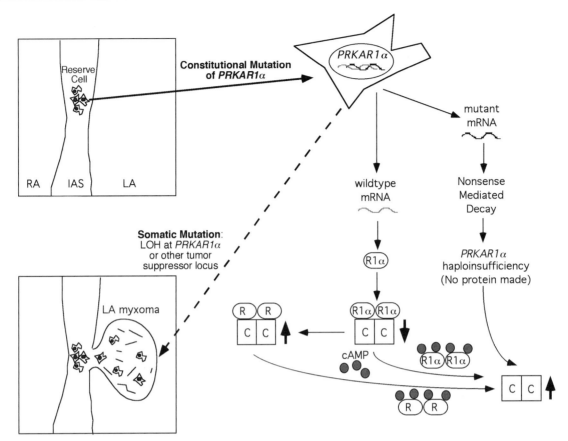

Figure 38-5 *PRKAR1α* haploinsufficiency and somatic mutation leading to myxoma formation in the heart. Constitutional *PRKAR1α* mutation in Carney complex patients results in *PRKAR1α* haploinsufficiency, because of nonsense-mediated mRNA decay of mutant PRKAR1α RNA. The result is decreased levels of R1α to associate with catalytic subunits (C) to form R1α type 1 PKA holoenzyme and a relative increase in the proportion of PKA holoenzymes containing other regulatory (R) subunits, i.e., R2α, R1β, R2β. A consequent increase in PKA activity after cAMP-dependent release of catalytic subunit is hypothesized. Subsequent somatic mutation or loss of heterozygosity at the *PRKAR1α* or other tumor-suppressor gene loci results in tumorigenesis and myxoma formation from reserve cells in the subendocardium. These tumors often arise from the interatrial septum (IAS) and most commonly extend into the left atrium (LA), but can involve the right atrium (RA), as well as the ventricles.

prkar2β null mice with a compensatory augmentation in *prkar1α* expression exhibit a lean phenotype caused by a marked increase in lipolysis.[64] Conversely, lipomatous hypertrophy of the interatrial septum in Carney complex patients may relate to decreased lipolysis in the setting of diminished *PRKAR1α* expression and compensatory increase in *PRKAR2β* expression.

Hyperendocrine states, benign endocrine neoplasms (e.g., pituitary and thyroid adenomas) and cutaneous spotty pigmentation in Carney complex are all likely also to result from increased PKA activity secondary to *PRKAR1α* haploinsufficiency. Elevated PKA activity is well known to be associated with endocrine cell growth and function. Constitutive activation of cAMP-dependent protein kinase activity results in unregulated growth of autonomous hyperfunctioning human thymocytes[65] and mutations in Gsα, and a consequent increase in cAMP levels and PKA activity cause growth hormone-secreting pituitary adenomas and thyroid adenomas in McCune-Albright syndrome.[66] Thus, loss of the R1α regulatory subunit in Carney complex may result in increased PKA activity and endocrine tumors. Similarly, PKA activity is required for tyrosine hydroxylase (TH) activity that contributes to catecholamine synthesis and biosynthesis of melanin skin pigmentation.[67] It has been hypothesized that somatic mutation of the STK11 protein kinase in addition to constitutional *STK11* mutations in autosomal dominant Peutz-Jeghers syndrome is required to result in lentiginosis,[43] but this is as yet unproven. Similarly, it remains unknown whether loss of a single *PRKAR1α* allele is sufficient to result in nonneoplastic endocrine hyperactivity or lentiginosis, or whether additional somatic mutation of

the *PRKAR1α* wild-type allele or of other genes is required for development of these phenotypes.

IMPLICATIONS FOR DIAGNOSIS

Because approximately half of Carney complex probands have detectable mutations in the *PRKAR1α* gene, and because, thus far, all Carney complex families large enough to generate a statistically significant (P < 0.05) LOD score exhibit linkage to chromosome 17q24, both mutational analysis of the *PRKAR1α* gene and linkage analysis with chromosome 17q24 polymorphisms can be potent tools in the diagnosis of Carney complex. As noted above, clinical differentiation between Carney complex and other multiple neoplasia disorders with associated dermatologic findings, such as Peutz-Jeghers syndrome, can sometimes be difficult. DNA-based diagnosis may, then, provide definitive answers.[17] We previously demonstrated that haplotype analysis can be sufficient to establish a Carney complex diagnosis in individuals who are members of a family that is of sufficient size that it can be shown to be linked to *PRKAR1α* with a LOD score >1.3.[26] Several intragenic microsatellites and single nucleotide polymorphisms associated with the *PRKAR1α* gene have been described,[6,7] and these can all be used to generate such haplotypes. In the case of single probands or small families, mutational analysis of the *PRKAR1α* gene can be performed.[17] If the disease haplotype is detected in an individual from a family linked to chromosome 17q24 or if a *PRKAR1α* mutation is detected, a Carney complex diagnosis can be unambiguously assigned, and appropriate surveillance evaluations should be initiated to detect cardiac and other tumors prior to clinical presentation.

However, it is critical to recognize that failure to detect a *PRKAR1α* mutation, or to establish significant evidence of nonlinkage (i.e., LOD score < −2.0) to chromosome 17q24 does not exclude a diagnosis of Carney complex. Such failures may be results of inability to detect refractory mutations in *PRKAR1α*[57] or of the disorder's genetic heterogeneity. Thus, in these individuals, clinical judgment still needs to be assiduously applied to determine the need for surveillance evaluations, such as annual echocardiography. In the future, improved methods of mutational analysis[57] and further definition of additional genes mutated in Carney complex will likely minimize these issues. In addition, improved understanding of the biochemical mechanisms by which *PRKAR1α* mutations result in tumorigenesis may suggest novel genetic and pharmacologic strategies that may be useful as adjunctive, or even as primary, nonsurgical therapies for these tumors.

REFERENCES

1. Roberts WC: Primary and secondary neoplasms of the heart. *Am J Cardiol* **80**:671, 1997.
2. Burke AP, Virmani R: Cardiac myxomas: a clinicopathologic study. *Am J Clin Pathol* **100**:671, 1993.
3. Carney JA, Gordon H, Carpenter PC, et al: The complex of myxomas, spotty pigmentation, and endocrine overactivity. *Medicine* **64**:270, 1985.
4. Casey M, Mah C, Merliss AD, et al: Identification of a novel genetic locus for familial cardiac myxomas and Carney complex. *Circulation* **98**:2560, 1998.
5. Stratakis CA, Carney JA, Lin JP, et al: Carney complex, a familial multiple neoplasia and lentiginosis syndrome: Analysis of 11 kindreds and linkage to the short arm of chromosome 2. *J Clin Invest* **97**:699, 1996.
6. Casey M, Vaughan CJ, He J, et al: Mutations in the protein kinase A R1alpha regulatory subunit cause familial cardiac myxomas and Carney complex. *J Clin Invest* **106**:R31, 2000.
7. Kirschner LS, Carney JA, Pack SD, et al: Mutations of the gene encoding the protein kinase A type I-alpha regulatory subunit in patients with the carney complex. *Nat Genet* **26**:89, 2000.
8. Carney JA: Familial multiple endocrine neoplasia syndromes:- Components, classification, and nomenclature. *J Intern Med* **243**:425, 1998.
9. Rees JR, Ross FG, Keen G: Lentiginosis and left atrial myxoma. *Br Heart J* **35**:874, 1973.
10. Atherton DJ, Pitcher DW, Wells RS, et al: A syndrome of various cutaneous pigmented lesions, myxoid neurofibromata and atrial myxoma: The NAME syndrome. *Br J Dermatol* **103**:421, 1980.
11. Rhodes AR, Silverman RA, Harris TJ, et al: Mucocutaneous lentigines, cardiomucocutaneous myxomas, and multiple blue nevi: The "LAMB" syndrome. *J Am Acad Dermatol* **10**:72, 1984.
12. Vidaillet HJ Jr, Seward JB, Fyke FE 3d, et al: "Syndrome myxoma": A subset of patients with cardiac myxoma associated with pigmented skin lesions and peripheral and endocrine neoplasms. *Br Heart J* **57**:247, 1987.
13. Meyer BJ, Weber R, Jenzer HR, et al: Rapid growth and recurrence of atrial myxomas in two patients with Swiss syndrome. *Am Heart J* **120**:220, 1990.
14. Reynen K: Cardiac myxomas. *N Engl J Med* **333**:1610, 1995.
15. Carney JA: Differences between nonfamilial and familial cardiac myxoma. *Am J Surg Pathol* **9**:53, 1985.
16. Seino Y, Ikeda U, Shimada K: Increased expression of interleukin 6 mRNA in cardiac myxomas. *Br Heart J* **69**:565, 1993.
17. Basson CT, Aretz HT: A 27-year-old woman with previous endocrinopathy and now with TIAs and two intracardiac masses. *N Engl J Med* In press, 2001.
18. McCarthy PM, Piehler JM, Schaff HV, et al: The significance of multiple, recurrent, and "complex" cardiac myxomas. *J Thorac Cardiovasc Surg* **91**:389, 1986.
19. Vatterott PJ, Seward JB, Vidaillet HJ, et al: Syndrome cardiac myxoma: More than just a sporadic event. *Am Heart J* **114**:886, 1987.
20. Lucky AW: Pigmentary abnormalities in genetic disorders. *Dermatol Clin* **6**:193, 1988.
21. Kennedy RH, Waller RR, Carney, JA: Ocular pigmented spots and eyelid myxomas. *Am J Ophthalmol* **104**:533, 1987.
22. Carney JA, Ferreiro JA: The epithelioid blue nevus. A multicentric familial tumor with important associations, including cardiac myxoma and psammomatous melanotic schwannoma. *Am J Surg Pathol* **20**:259, 1996.
23. Carney JA, Stratakis CA: Epithelioid blue nevus and psammomatous melanotic schwannoma: The unusual pigmented skin tumors of the Carney complex. *Semin Diagn Pathol* **15**:216, 1998.
24. Carney JA, Headington JT, Su WP: Cutaneous myxomas. A major component of the complex of myxomas, spotty pigmentation, andendocrine overactivity. *Arch Dermatol* **122**:790, 1986.
25. Ferreiro JA, Carney JA: Myxomas of the external ear and their significance. *Am J Surg Pathol* **18**:274, 1994.
26. Goldstein MM, Casey M, Carney JA, et al: Molecular genetic diagnosis of the familial myxoma syndrome (Carney complex). *Am J Med Genet* **86**:62, 1999.
27. Takasu N, Ohara N, Yamada T, et al: Development of autoimmune thyroid dysfunction after bilateral adrenalectomy in a patient with Carney's complex and after removal of ACTH-producing pituitary adenoma in a patient with Cushing's disease. *J Endocrinol Invest* **16**:697, 1993.
28. Shenoy BV, Carpenter PC, Carney JA: Bilateral primary pigmented nodular adrenocortical disease. Rare cause of the Cushing syndrome. *Am J Surg Pathol* **8**:335, 1984.
29. Carney JA: Psammomatous melanotic schwannoma. A distinctive, heritable tumor with special associations, including cardiac myxoma and the Cushing syndrome. *Am J Surg Pathol* **14**:206, 1990.
30. Handley J, Carson D, Sloan J, et al: Multiple lentigines, myxoid tumours and endocrine overactivity; four cases of Carney's complex. *Br J Dermatol* **126**:367, 1992.
31. Raff SB, Carney JA, Krugman D, et al: Prolactin secretion abnormalities in patients with the "syndrome of spotty skin pigmentation, myxomas, endocrine overactivity and schwannomas" (Carney complex). *J Pediatr Endocrinol Metab* **13**:373, 2000.
32. Watson JC, Stratakis CA, Bryant-Greenwood PK, et al: Neurosurgical implications of Carney complex. *J Neurosurg* **92**:413, 2000.
33. Stratakis CA, Courcoutsakis NA, Abati A, et al: Thyroid gland abnormalities in patients with the syndrome of spotty skin pigmentation, myxomas, endocrine overactivity, and schwannomas. *J Clin Endocrinol Metab* **82**:2037, 1997.
34. Carney JA, Toorkey BC: Myxoid fibroadenoma and allied conditions (myxomatosis) of the breast. A heritable disorder with special associations including cardiac and cutaneous myxomas. *Am J Surg Pathol* **15**:713, 1991.
35. Carney JA, Toorkey BC: Ductal adenoma of the breast with tubular features. A probable component of the complex of myxomas, spotty pigmentation, endocrine overactivity, and schwannomas. *Am J Surg Pathol* **15**:722, 1991.
36. Stratakis CA, Papageorgiou T, Premkumar A, et al: Ovarian lesions in Carney complex: Clinical genetics and possible predisposition to malignancy. *J Clin Endocrinol Metab* **85**:4359, 2000.
37. Proppe KH, Scully RE: Large-cell calcifying Sertoli cell tumor of the testis. *Am J Clin Pathol* **74**:607, 1980.
38. Koopman RJ, Happle R: Autosomal dominant transmission of the NAME syndrome (nevi, atrial myxoma, mucinosis of the skin and endocrine overactivity). *Hum Genet* **86**:300, 1991.
39. Nwokoro NA, Korytkowski MT, Rose S, et al: Spectrum of malignancy and premalignancy in Carney syndrome. *Am J Med Genet* **73**:369, 1997.
40. Carney JA, Boccon-Gibod L, Jarka DE, et al: Osteochondromyxoma of bone: A congenital tumor associated with lentigines and other unusual disorders. *Am J Surg Pathol* **25**:164, 2001.
41. Hemminki A: The molecular basis and clinical aspects of Peutz-Jeghers syndrome. *Cell Mol Life Sci* **55**:735, 1999.
42. Stratakis CA, Kirschner LS, Taymans SE, et al: Carney complex, Peutz-Jeghers syndrome, Cowden disease, and Bannayan-Zonana syndrome share cutaneous and endocrine manifestations, but not genetic loci. *J Clin Endocrinol Metab* **83**:2972, 1998.
43. Jenne DE, Reimann H, Nezu J, et al: Peutz-Jeghers syndrome is caused by mutations in a novel serine threonine kinase. *Nat Genet* **18**:38, 1998.
44. Hemminki A, Markie D, Tomlinson I, et al: A serine/threonine kinase gene defective in Peutz-Jeghers syndrome. *Nature* **391**:184, 1998.
45. Jozwiak S, Schwartz RA, Janniger CK, et al: Familial occurrence of the LEOPARD syndrome. *Int J Dermatol* **37**:48, 1998.

46. Coppin BD, Temple IK: Multiple lentigines syndrome (LEOPARD syndrome or progressive cardiomyopathic lentiginosis). *J Med Genet* **34**:582, 1997.

47. Kirschner LS, Sandrini F, Monbo J, et al: Genetic heterogeneity and spectrum of mutations of the *PRKAR1A* gene in patients with the Carney complex. *Hum Mol Genet* **9**:3037, 2000.

48. Richkind KE, Wason D, Vidaillet HJ: Cardiac myxoma characterized by clonal telomeric association. *Genes Chromosomes Cancer* **9**:68, 1994.

49. Dewald GW, Dahl RJ, Spurbeck JL, et al: Chromosomally abnormal clones and nonrandom telomeric translocations in cardiac myxomas. *Mayo Clin Proc* **62**:558, 1987.

50. Dijkuizen T, van den Berg E, Molenaar WM, et al: Cytogenetics of a case of cardiac myxoma. *Cancer Genet Cytogenet* **63**:73, 1992.

51. Taymans SE, Kirschner LS, Giatzakis C, et al: Radiation hybrid mapping of chromosomal region 2p15-p16: Integration of expressed and polymorphic sequences maps at the Carney complex (CNC) and Doyne honeycomb retinal dystrophy (DHRD) loci. *Genomics* **56**:344, 1999.

52. Basson CT, MacRae CA, Korf B, et al: Genetic heterogeneity of familial atrial myxoma syndromes (Carney complex). *Am J Cardiol* **79**:994, 1997.

53. Boshart M, Weih F, Nichols M, et al: The tissue-specific extinguisher locus TSE1 encodes a regulatory subunit of cAMP-dependent protein kinase. *Cell* **66**:849, 1991.

54. Jones KW, Shapero MH, Chevrette M, et al: Subtractive hybridization cloning of a tissue-specific extinguisher: TSE1 encodes a regulatory subunit of protein kinase A. *Cell* **66**:861, 1991.

55. Cho-Chung YS: Role of cyclic AMP receptor proteins in growth, differentiation, and suppression of malignancy: New approaches to therapy. *Cancer Res* **50**:7093, 1990.

56. Solberg R, Sandberg M, Natarajan V, et al: The human gene for the regulatory subunit R1α of cyclic adenosine 3′,5′-monophosphate-dependent protein kinase: Two distinct promoters provide differential regulation of alternatively spliced messenger ribonucleic acids. *Endocrinology* **138**:169, 1997.

57. Yan H, Kinzler KW, Vogelstein B: Genetic testing—present and future. *Science* **289**:1890, 2000.

58. Stratakis CA, Jenkins RB, Pras E, et al: Cytogenetic and microsatellite alterations in tumors from patients with the syndrome of myxomas, potty skin pigmentation, and endocrine overactivity (Carney complex). *J Clin Endocrinol Metab* **81**:3607, 1996.

59. Taylor SS, Buechler JA, Yonemoto W: cAMP-dependent protein kinase: Framework for a diverse family of regulatory enzymes. *Annu Rev Biochem* **59**:971, 1990.

60. Beebe SJ: The cAMP-dependent protein kinases and cAMP signal transduction. *Semin Cancer Biol* **5**:285, 1994.

61. Skalhegg BS, Tasken K: Specificity in the cAMP/PKA signaling pathway. Differential expression, regulation, and subcellular localization of subunits of PKA. *Front Biosc* **5**:D678, 2000.

62. Amieux PS, Cummings DE, Motamed K, et al: Compensatory regulation of RIα protein levels in protein kinase A mutant mice. *J Bio Chem* **272**:3993, 1997.

63. Planas JV, Cummings DE, Idzerda RL, et al: Mutation of the RIIbeta subunit of protein kinase A differentially affects lipolysis but not gene induction in white adipose tissue. *J Biol Chem* **274**:36281, 1999.

64. Cummings DE, Brandon EP, Planas JV, et al: Genetically lean mice result from targeted disruption of the RII beta subunit of protein kinase A. *Nature* **382**:622, 1996.

65. Parma J, Duprez L, Van Sande J, et al: Somatic mutations in the thyrotropin receptor gene cause hyperfunctioning thyroid adenomas. *Nature* **365**:649, 1993.

66. Weinstein LS, Shenker A, Gejman PV, et al: Activating mutations of the stimulatory G protein in the McCune-Albright syndrome. *N Engl J Med* **325**:1688, 1991.

67. Kim KS, Park DH, Wessel TC, et al: A dual role for the cAMP-dependent protein kinase in tyrosine hydroxylase gene expression. *Proc Natl Acad Sci U S A* **90**:3471, 1993.

Genetic Testing for Familial Cancer

Gloria M. Petersen ■ *Ann-Marie Codori*

1. Cancer gene discoveries have led to important changes in the clinical practice of cancer risk assessment. Genetic tests, in conjunction with family history information, can be used to a) clarify the diagnosis of inherited cancer syndromes in patients with tumors and b) provide information about cancer susceptibility to asymptomatic persons in high-risk families. The promise of cancer gene testing is reduced cancer incidence and mortality through directed prevention and screening.

2. In addition to the medical and health benefits of cancer gene testing, the power to identify high-risk persons has led to considerable discussion of the implications from consumer, epidemiologic, technologic, ethical, legal, policy, psychological, and genetic counseling perspectives.

3. Cancer gene testing can include a variety of modalities, including linkage, direct detection when the mutation is known, and mutation analysis, such as protein truncation test or sequencing. In addition, tests for microsatellite instability in colon tumors and gene expression assays may provide indirect evidence supporting a diagnosis of hereditary nonpolyposis colorectal cancer.

4. Commercial availability of germline cancer gene tests (i.e., BRCA1, BRCA2, APC, hMSH2, hMLH1, p16, NF2) has outpaced the awareness among health professionals of the need for careful implementation of testing algorithms and patient education on the issues.

5. Surveys of persons at varying risks for cancer show that most persons are interested in having a gene test. The actual uptake of cancer gene testing has been more modest; the decision to undergo gene testing is influenced by psychosocial factors, including perception of cancer risk, perceived ability to cope with gene test results, depression, and fear of insurance discrimination. Among persons who are tested, there appears to be no significant short-term (1–3 months) psychological distress following disclosure of results.

6. Cancer genetic risk assessment is a multistep process and incorporates medical, psychological, genetic, and counseling dimensions. Clinical indications and a model algorithm for cancer risk assessment and gene testing are provided. For persons who are at risk for cancer, gene test interpretation will depend upon whether the specific germline cancer gene mutation is known for the family. Careful evaluation of the pedigree for characteristic aggregation of tumor types among affected individuals and availability of affected persons for testing are important issues in implementing genetic testing.

7. Health professionals will need to be aware of the variety of issues that contribute to the process of helping patients to understand their risk, make informed decisions, and appreciate the implications for cancer prevention and risks for other family members. Genetic counseling is an essential component of cancer genetic risk assessment services.

The translation of cancer gene discoveries into the clinical setting by the introduction of genetic testing has undergone a remarkable evolution in a few short years. Cancer genetic testing has become a significant focus from a variety of perspectives because it represents a potentially powerful means to identify high-risk individuals. From a medical and public health perspective, cancer genetic testing provides a more precise way to intervene with measures that may detect cancer at an earlier stage or to prevent cancer altogether. From a patient or consumer perspective, cancer genetic testing offers a new way to learn about individual and family cancer risk but also raises concern about job and insurance discrimination. From an epidemiologic perspective, cancer genetic testing provides a means to better understand the etiology of cancer through the interaction of genetic and environmental factors and to better characterize cancer risk. From the technologic perspective, cancer genetic testing represents an application that mandates development of faster and more cost-effective assays that are clinically valid. From the ethical, legal, and policy perspective, cancer genetic testing reinforces and recasts the basic premise that genetic information is different and requires special protection. Finally, from the psychological and counseling perspective, cancer genetic testing is part of a challenging multidimensional process that involves communication with patients about different types of risk information and requires that patients understand the implications, benefits, and risks.

The confluence of these perspectives and the intensity with which their proponents have addressed genetic testing are due to several factors: the inherent appeal of perceived benefit from cancer genetic knowledge, the potential impact on a broad segment of the population, and the concern that the public and health professional communities are unprepared for this new technology. In this nascent period of gene testing for cancer risk, few of the issues are fully resolved and many continue to arise. This chapter reviews cancer genetic testing from different perspectives and provides an overview of the current status of clinical cancer risk assessment and genetic testing.

PERSPECTIVES ON CANCER GENETIC TESTING

Medical and Public Health Perspective

The identification of genes that are responsible for hereditary forms of cancer has resulted in efforts to apply this knowledge clinically, primarily in the form of gene tests. There is no doubt that information derived from genetic testing will lead in many instances to an improvement in cancer risk assessment and clinical management of cancer patients and their families.[1,2]

Table 39-1 Hereditary syndromes with increased cancer risk and identified susceptibility genes and chromosomal localizations

Syndrome	Predominate Tumor Types	Chromosome	Gene	Reference
Ataxia telangiectasia	Breast cancer, chromosome breakage/rearrangement syndrome	11q22.3	ATM	154
Cowden disease	Multiple hamartomas of skin and mucous membranes, breast cancer, thyroid cancer, renal cell adenocarcinoma, dysplastic cerebellar gangliocytoma	10q23	PTEN	155, 156
Familial adenomatous polyposis	Multiple colorectal adenomas	5q21	APC	157, 158
Familial gastric cancer	Gastric cancer	16q22.1	CDH1	159
Familial melanoma	Melanoma, glioblastoma, lung cancer	9p21	CDKN^2(p16)	160
Gorlin syndrome	Nevoid basal cell carcinoma of skin	9q	NBCCS	161–163
Hereditary breast-ovarian cancer syndrome	Breast, ovarian, prostate carcinoma; increased risk of other tumors	17q21 13q12–q13	BRCA1 BRCA2	150, 151
Hereditary nonpolyposis colorectal cancer	Colon, endometrial, ovarian, stomach, small bowel, ureteral carcinomas	2p16 3p21 2q31–q33 7q11.2 2p16	hMsh2 hMLH1 hPMS1 hPMS2 hMSH6	81, 83 164
Hereditary prostate cancer	Prostate carcinoma	1q24–25 Xq27–28	HPC1 HPCX	165, 166
Li-Fraumeni syndrome	Leukemia, soft-tissue sarcoma, osteosarcoma, brain tumor, breast and adrenal cortical carcinoma	17p13	TP53	167
Multiple endocrine neoplasia type 1	Parathyroid, endocrine pancreas, and pituitary tumors	11q	MEN–1	168
Multiple endocrine neoplasia type 2a	Medullary thyroid carcinoma, pheochromocytoma	10q11.2	RET	169
Multiple endocrine neoplasia type 2b	Familial medullary thyroid carcinoma	10q11.2	RET	170, 171
Neurofibromatosis type 1	Multiple peripheral neurofibromas, optic glioma, neurofibrosarcoma	17q11.2	NF1	172–176
Neurofibromatosis type 2	Central schwannomas and meningiomas, acoustic neuromas	22q11.2	NF2	177
Peutz-Jeghers syndrome	Multiple gastrointestinal tract polyps hamartomatous and adenomatus cancer of intestinal tract, pancreas, ovary, testis, breast, uterus	19p13.3	STK11	178, 179
Retinoblastoma	Retinoblastomas, osteosarcomas	13q14	RB	180, 181
von Hippel–Lindau syndrome	Renal cell carcinoma, pheochromocytoma, hemangioblastoma	3p25–p26	VHL	182

In conjunction with family history information, gene tests can be used to clarify the diagnosis of inherited cancer syndromes in patients with tumors and to provide information about cancer susceptibility to asymptomatic persons in high-risk families. Table 39-1 summarizes some hereditary cancer syndromes, detailed elsewhere in this volume, for which genetic testing can potentially improve cancer risk management of patients and their families.

Genetic testing for cancer holds the promise of reducing cancer mortality through timely screening and early intervention in those with predisposing mutations. The anticipated health benefits of testing rest on the assumption that persons at increased risk for cancer will be given options for preventive screening regimens or other interventions (such as prophylactic surgery or chemoprevention). Several decision analysis studies have evaluated the theoretical health and cost benefits of cancer gene testing for retinoblastoma[3] and familial adenomatous polyposis (FAP),[4,5] and those of management decisions (surveillance and prophylactic surgery) for hereditary breast cancer,[6,7] and hereditary colorectal cancer[8] and have generally found that the use of genetic test information or targeted interventions in cancer gene mutation carriers can be an improvement over conventional methods of cancer prevention. The parameters and construction of these decision analysis models vary, and some may only approximate the actual clinical situation, but they do appear to support the concept that genetic testing has a valid medical rationale.

It is becoming apparent that gene tests can and will change the way in which cancer risk assessment will be performed.[1,2,9–13] Indeed, certain gene tests (APC, RET, RB1, VHL) may now be considered part of the standard management of the respective hereditary cancer syndrome families, while the medical benefit of other gene tests (hMSH2, hMLH1, hMSH6, hPMS1, hPMS2, BRCA1, BRCA2, and p53) is presumed but not established.[14] The gene test outcome for an individual patient or at-risk family member can lead to more informed and directed recommendations for preventive interventions. As a general example, Fig. 39-1 illustrates the way in which colon cancer risk assessment has been conventionally performed. That is, health professionals often evaluate family histories of persons at risk for colon cancer who seek to learn their cancer risk but less often assess family histories of patients with colon cancer. Conventional risk assessment is based almost exclusively on evaluation of the family history, after which cancer screening recommendations can be made, tailored according to whether an inherited syndrome can be diagnosed. Fig. 39-2 illustrates a potential scenario in which colon cancer

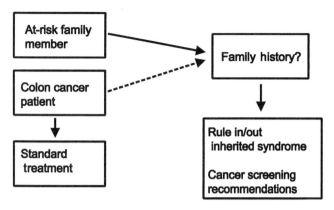

Fig. 39-1 Current view of conventional colon cancer risk assessment.

gene tests will alter this process. When gene tests are offered in conjunction with family history evaluation, not only will the two sources of information help make a firmer diagnosis, but clinical management of colon cancer patients may be influenced by this diagnosis. Likewise, more refined follow-up recommendations may be given to at-risk persons, whether they test positive or negative for a colon cancer gene. Genetic testing for cancer risk carries psychosocial implications that should be communicated through careful genetic counseling to persons considering cancer gene tests, both patients and family members. On one hand, genetic counseling will entail directive counseling toward cancer prevention where indicated, but on the other, it will entail communication about complex issues related to heredity, genetic test performance, probabilities, and uncertainty of outcome.

From the public health perspective, cancer gene discoveries may potentially be translated into genetic screening programs to identify high-risk groups to whom interventions (lifestyle modification, chemoprevention, or early detection) can be more effectively applied. There is agreement that much research is required prior to implementing any kind of public health program that involves genetic screening for cancer.[15-18] There is a need for more research into the issues surrounding technical and policy implications when applied to large-scale screening.[19] There is also a need to understand the frequency and attributable risks of cancer susceptibility genes and the efficacy and effectiveness of interventions in susceptible individuals, including examination of the premise that health prevention behaviors would be enhanced by knowledge of one's genetic susceptibility status. The difficulties are underscored by a recent study using decision analysis to investigate the role of genetic screening in cancer prevention. Grann and coworkers found that the theoretical cost-benefit ratio and survival rate would make screening all Ashkenazi Jewish women for specific BRCA1 and BRCA2 mutations cost-

effective only if prophylactic surgery were performed on mutation carriers.[20]

Patient/Consumer Perspective

A variety of studies have found that there is great interest in cancer genetic testing across all risk groups, whether for breast, ovarian, prostate, or colon cancers.[21-29] Studies among first-degree relatives of cancer patients have found that when presented with the hypothetical possibility of cancer genetic testing, the majority of respondents probably or definitely want genetic testing. Cancer risk perception is increased among those with a positive family history, and these individuals may be more likely to choose genetic testing to learn more about their cancer risk.[25-31] Generally, those with a family history of a given disorder are more likely to engage in disease prevention behaviors for that disorder,[32-34] and most persons tend to overestimate their personal risk of cancer[25] or probability of carrying a cancer gene mutation.[35] Adherence to screening recommendations after genetic testing is likely to be associated with pre-genetic testing screening behavior[32-34,36] and with previous symptoms suggestive of cancer.[37]

In clinical and research experience, the reasons patients give for wanting cancer genetic testing are cancer worry and/or desire to know if more screening tests are needed (personal cancer risk concern), childbearing concerns or need to learn if one's children are at risk (concern for relatives), and wanting to take better care of oneself (general health concern).[30,31,38-41] As will be discussed later, there are a number of psychosocial factors that influence the actual decision to have a cancer gene test. Among those that can damp interest are perceived inability to cope with the gene test result and worry about insurance discrimination.

Epidemiologic Perspective

The epidemiologic challenges offered by genetic testing are threefold. First, it is necessary to understand the frequency, attributable risk, and heterogeneity of cancer-associated gene mutations. In general, the mutations in genes that are known to be associated with hereditary forms of cancer (e.g., breast cancer[42]) are not common, and obtaining estimates is complicated by the logistic difficulties of conducting population-based genetic testing, and by ethnic variation. For example, certain types of BRCA1, BRCA2, and APC mutations are more common in the Ashkenazi Jewish population,[43-45] and certain hMLH1 mutations are more common in the Finnish population, due to a founder effect.[46,47] In addition, it is recognized from a number of studies that not all hereditary forms of cancer are accounted for by the currently known genes.[48,49]

Second, the opportunity to understand genetic and nongenetic contributions to cancer causation is enhanced by the existence of persons, either with or without clinical manifestations of malignancy, who are known to carry cancer gene mutations. The respective roles of genes and environment may be more efficiently addressed in such defined risk groups. Although studying more common polymorphisms of genes associated with metabolism of carcinogens has been one strategy to investigate this relationship, it may be increasingly possible to study high-penetrance cancer gene mutations. For example, Brunet and coworkers examined the relationship of smoking to breast cancer risk using only BRCA1 or BRCA2 mutation carriers and found a protective effect of smoking.[50] While this result contradicts our widespread understanding of the more typical harmful effect of smoking, this study design yielded an example of the type of knowledge that can be obtained from samples of gene-tested patients.

Third, the necessity to more carefully characterize and communicate cancer risk has been reinforced by cancer genetic testing.[51,52] In particular, there are two main ways in which risk associated with cancer gene mutations is usually given to patients: (1) *The probability that a person will carry a cancer gene mutation*, given information such as age, gender, ethnicity, and family history. A number of studies have investigated ways to estimate these risks and have obtained varying results, depending

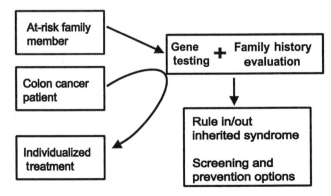

Fig. 39-2 Future view of colon cancer risk assessment.

upon the subjects studied and the factors employed in computing risks.[53–56] Predictive models have been developed for hereditary breast and ovarian cancer[57–59] and for hereditary nonpolyposis colorectal cancer (HNPCC).[60] (2) *The probability that a mutation carrier is going to develop cancer* (also termed *lifetime risk* or *penetrance* of a gene mutation). These studies are more difficult to perform, but estimates have been made, using both high-risk samples and larger population studies.[44,61–63] As the volume of gene-tested persons increases, the current methods for computing risks will be refined to more accurately inform the risk assessment process.

Technology Perspective

Two of the most consistent patterns to emerge from genetic studies of inherited cancer syndromes are that there are many causal mutations in associated loci and that many families have unique mutations. Thus, testing laboratories will have to develop a variety of different strategies for detecting mutations in patients or diagnosing at-risk individuals in cancer-carrying families.[64–66] These tests range from linkage analysis[67–69] and single-stranded conformational polymorphism analysis[70] to protein truncation tests[71,72] and direct end-to-end DNA sequencing and allele specific oligonucleotide assays.[64] The relative merits and drawbacks of mutation detection approaches have been reviewed elsewhere,[64–66,73,74] and different laboratories vary in their strategies for gene testing. Potential new strategies include DNA chip technology,[64] conversion of diploidy to haploidy,[75] and mass spectrometry,[76] but it is unlikely that there will ever be tests that meet the ideal criteria for DNA-based genetic tests, as set forth by Eng and Vijg:[64] 100% sensitivity, 100% specificity, cost-effectiveness (< $100 per gene or combination of genes), throughput and speed of testing that fit into clinical laboratory routine, and being user friendly.

Because of the relatively high sophistication of current mutation analysis technology, it is not necessarily a simple process for the clinician to understand and interpret the potential implications of gene test results. The Task Force on Genetic Testing of the National Institutes of Health–Department of Energy Working Group on the Ethical, Legal, and Social Implications of Human Genome Research has set forth general principles on gene testing relative to gene test validation and testing laboratory quality control[77] and has proposed revisions to policies regulating laboratories that perform gene tests, which notably mandate the inclusion of clinical validation of tests.[78] This group argues that gene tests are different from other clinical tests because of the complexities in assessment and interpretation and that they require more intake information. In addition, it says health care providers must describe the features of the genetic test, including potential consequences, prior to testing. When a clearcut test result is obtained, either because a disease-predisposing mutation is detected (positive gene test) or because a mutation is not detected in an at-risk person from a family where a known mutation is segregating (true negative gene test), the subsequent counseling and management options are more apparent. Inconclusive or uninformative negative gene tests will occur when no mutation is detected in a cancer family but, because of the limitations of the testing method, a mutation in the tested locus (or elsewhere) cannot be ruled out. At-risk members in these families should not reduce their vigilance in cancer screening.

Tissue sources for clinical gene testing. The most common tissue source for gene testing is leukocyte DNA; a simple blood sample is often all that is required to perform a gene test. DNA obtained from paraffin-embedded tissue blocks obtained at surgery is also an option, if an affected relative is deceased or obtaining a blood sample is not feasible.

Specific tumor DNA studies may also yield information to aid in the diagnosis of inherited susceptibility to cancer. In the case of HNPCC, a special tumor analysis to identify microsatellite instability (MSI, also known as replication error [RER]) can be performed.[79,80] In this analysis, DNA from both normal tissue and tumor tissue is analyzed by highly polymorphic microsatellite DNA markers and their banding patterns compared. Allele alterations (band shifts) seen between tumor and normal DNA suggest that the patient may have an impaired ability to repair DNA, which is an indirect assessment of forms of HNPCC that are due to mutations in mismatch repair genes (hMSH2, hMLH1, hPMS1, and hPMS2).[79–83] Because MSI analysis is less time consuming and expensive than gene tests based on mutation analysis, it offers a useful first screening test for HNPCC.[55]

The utility of gene expression assays in tumors as an adjunct to germline mutation detection in a genetically heterogeneous syndrome has also been evaluated. For example, in the case of a suspected HNPCC mutation carrier whose tumor is MSI-positive, immunohistochemistry expression assays of hMSH2 and hMLH1 may help to identify which gene to sequence.[84,85] RNA expression assays of BRCA1 have been investigated as a means of screening for germline mutations.[86]

Commercial availability of testing. With the discovery of specific genes responsible for inherited cancer syndromes, commercial laboratories have been quick to invest in the development of marketable gene tests. Among the cancers that may affect a larger segment of the population, hereditary breast and ovarian cancer (*BRCA1, BRCA2*), HNPCC (*hMSH2, hMLH1*), FAP and its variants (*APC*), hereditary melanoma (*p16*), and neurofibromatosis type 2 (*NF2*) now have commercially available gene tests.[14,87–89]

The widening commercial availability of germline cancer gene tests has outpaced the awareness among health professionals of the need for careful implementation of testing algorithms and patient education on the issues.[88,89] There have been calls for caution in moving genetic tests out of the research labs and into the commercial labs[87,90–94] until their impact and the effectiveness of cancer prevention strategies can be studied. Specifically, some professional organizations advise that genetic testing and counseling for cancer risk may be safely integrated into clinical practice only after there have been studies of gene frequencies and associated cancer risks, test sensitivity and specificity, the efficacy of interventions for decreasing cancer morbidity and mortality, counseling methods, and genetic discrimination among those found to be at high risk.[92–94]

Ethical, Legal, and Policy Perspective

The ethical, legal, and policy issues in genetic testing have been discussed in numerous reviews and position statements,[92–103] and certain themes are emerging. Perhaps the most important overarching theme is that genetic information is different from other types of information (whether medical, demographic, or social), because of implications for future risk of disease and because of implications for other relatives. As a result, genetic testing that reveals intrinsic genetic status mandates special consideration.

As with all ethical dilemmas, there are no absolute right or wrong answers to many of the questions raised by cancer genetic testing. Inherent in medical and genetic service is the principle of beneficence. Discussions and decisions related to genetic testing can further be guided by the relevant principles of bioethics identified by the Committee on Assessing Genetic Risks of the National Academy of Sciences and Institute of Medicine,[91] including: respect for autonomy, privacy, confidentiality, and equity. These have implications for shaping how clinicians should approach and manage cancer patients and their families. Some common ethical issues for clinicians to consider are the right to know/not to know, sharing of genetic information, coercion by family members to participate in genetic testing, privacy of medical and genetic information, reproductive decision-making, and testing of minors.

The legal and social ramifications of genetic susceptibility testing for cancer are also taking shape. Some issues that may have

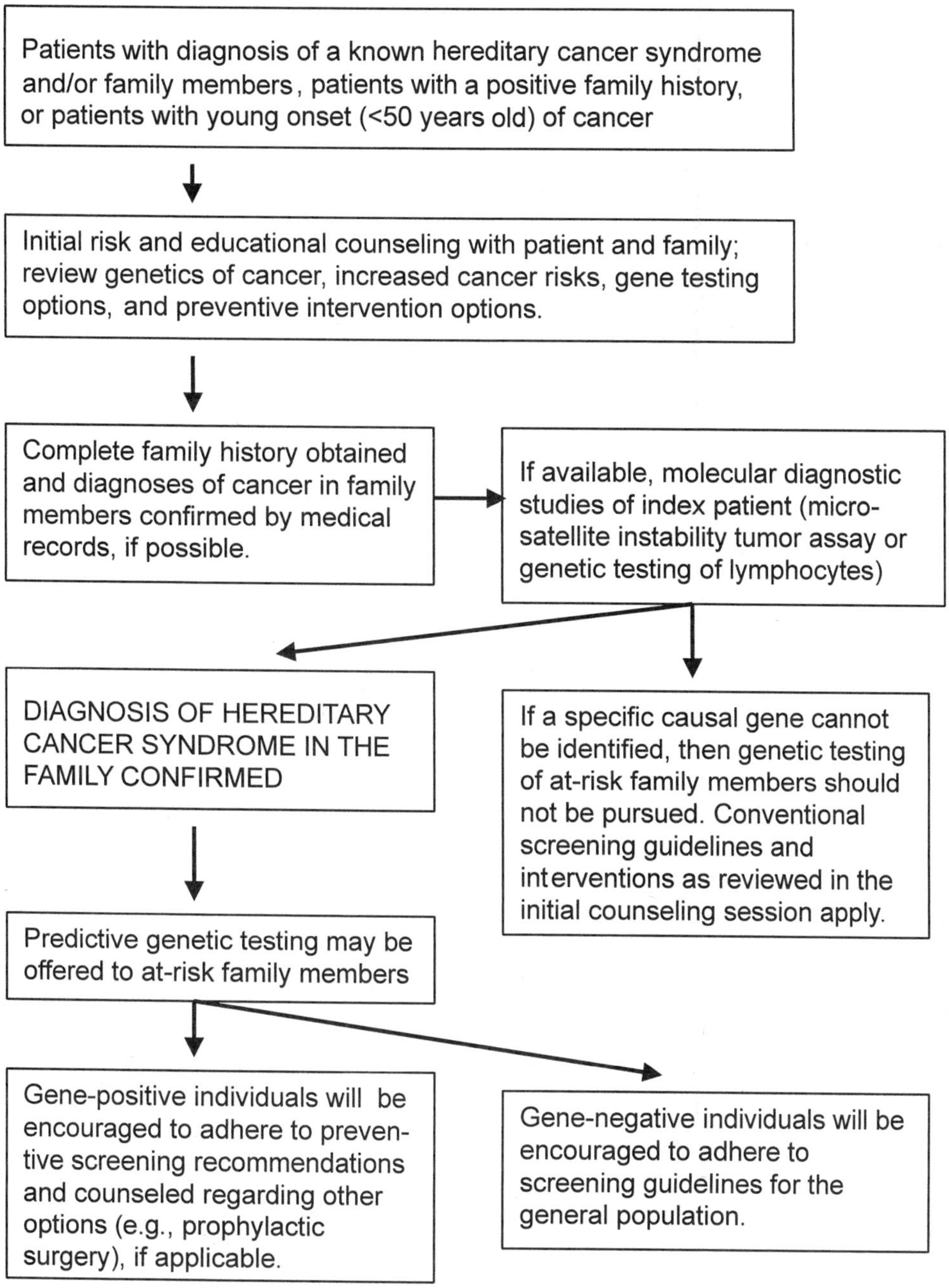

Patients with diagnosis of a known hereditary cancer syndrome and/or family members, patients with a positive family history, or patients with young onset (<50 years old) of cancer

↓

Initial risk and educational counseling with patient and family; review genetics of cancer, increased cancer risks, gene testing options, and preventive intervention options.

↓

Complete family history obtained and diagnoses of cancer in family members confirmed by medical records, if possible.

→

If available, molecular diagnostic studies of index patient (microsatellite instability tumor assay or genetic testing of lymphocytes)

DIAGNOSIS OF HEREDITARY CANCER SYNDROME IN THE FAMILY CONFIRMED

If a specific causal gene cannot be identified, then genetic testing of at-risk family members should not be pursued. Conventional screening guidelines and interventions as reviewed in the initial counseling session apply.

↓

Predictive genetic testing may be offered to at-risk family members

Gene-positive individuals will be encouraged to adhere to preventive screening recommendations and counseled regarding other options (e.g., prophylactic surgery), if applicable.

Gene-negative individuals will be encouraged to adhere to screening guidelines for the general population.

Fig. 39-3 Basic algorithm for cancer risk assessment that employs gene testing.

legal implications for clinicians are disclosing benefits, risks, and limitations of cancer genetic testing; following up and recontacting patients and family members when new information emerges; maintaining confidentiality of genetic information; and warning of inherited cancer risk ("genetic transferability") to others.

Privacy of genetic information. Genetic information should be considered confidential, and it is incumbent upon health professionals and laboratories to exercise all means of preventing unauthorized disclosure of gene test results to third parties. In practice, it is recommended that results should be released only to those individuals to whom the patient has consented or requested in writing to have them released, and care should be taken to minimize the likelihood that results will become available to unauthorized persons or organizations.[77] Garber and Patenaude point out, however, that physicians may breach confidentiality unintentionally by placing information in medical charts that may be reviewed by insurers or other third parties.[96] The dilemma is

that omitting this information compromises the patient's future medical care, yet including the information would compromise the ability of the patient or family members to obtain health, life, or disability insurance (and therefore coverage for preventive screening tests or procedures).

Another crucial issue is the revelation of gene test results to family members. As shown in Fig. 39-3, the optimal algorithm for gene testing of at-risk persons is to first test a family member who is affected with cancer; this patient must be willing to have the resulting genetic information shared with relatives. It is an important principle of gene testing that health care providers have an obligation to the person being tested not to inform other family members without the permission of the person tested.[77,91] There are also circumstances in which certain individuals may not want their test results known, yet by virtue of the pedigree structure this information will become known (e.g., an identical twin of a gene-positive patient); or family members may refuse to have their gene test results shared. The resolution of these issues may not always be easy, but it will call for careful planning and thorough genetic counseling with the family members involved, well before gene test results are made available.[103–105]

Risk of genetic discrimination. Persons at risk for cancer face other risks in the form of genetic discrimination (insurance, employment, educational, or other opportunities). Insurance companies may use genetic information, much as they use any other medical information, to underwrite an insurance policy. In these cases, insurance companies may deny insurance to those whom they consider to be at too great a risk for an illness or to those with pre-existing conditions.[106,107] Such denials are predicted to become more commonplace as new predisposition tests are developed.[108,109] Billings et al.[108] and Lapham et al.[107] have identified cases in which insurance or employment discrimination has occurred. They found discrimination against the "asymptomatic ill" — those with a genetic predisposition who remain healthy — who usually lost their insurance after undertaking preventive care. Overall, the problems encountered included difficulty obtaining coverage, finding or retaining employment, and being given permission for adoptions. Insurance problems often arose when people tried to alter existing policies because of relocations or job changes. Information provided by physicians often had little or no influence on the adverse outcomes. Many people dealt with this by giving incomplete or dishonest information.[107,108]

With respect to discrimination in the workplace, there may be risk of loss of employability if gene status or genetic risk of cancer is known or required by employers.[110] Recent attempts to remedy this include laws to protect access to health insurance, including the Health Insurance Portability and Accountability Act, which took effect in July 1997; protection of access to employment by an interpretation of the Americans with Disabilities Act of 1990 to include genetic information, and state laws to prevent genetic information from being used in employment considerations.

Psychological and Genetic Counseling Perspective.

The areas of psychological importance in cancer genetic testing include interest in and uptake of testing, impact of both positive and negative gene test results on cancer prevention behaviors and interventions (e.g., prophylactic surgery), and genetic testing of children.[111]

Uptake of cancer genetic testing. It has been observed in a number of studies that while interest in a hypothetical cancer gene test may be high, the actual uptake rates are more modest, even when persons are offered the gene test at no monetary cost. A person's decision to have a gene test is affected by a number of factors, including demographic, psychological, social, and personality.[38–41,112,113] Indeed, research suggests that psychological rather than medical factors appear to predominate in decisions about genetic testing. For example, Codori and coworkers[38] found that strength of cancer family history did not predict a patient's decision to be tested for HNPCC. Instead, tested persons had greater perceived confidence in their ability to cope with a positive test, thought more frequently about cancer, and had greater perceived risk for developing colorectal cancer. Of some concern was the fact that gene test decliners also were less likely to have had a colonoscopy, leading the authors to posit that those who choose not to take cancer gene tests may also be those who are unlikely to undertake the surveillance interventions. Bowen et al. suggest that while clinicians may think of the benefit of genetic testing as a medical decision, the predominance of emotion and self-perception of risk may lead to difficulties in patient-provider communication.[114] To overcome this barrier, some at-risk persons may need more psychological support and counseling to increase perceived ability to handle unfavorable medical information. One lesson from the research thus far is that recognition of psychologically vulnerable persons may require different

or tailored genetic counseling to prompt appropriate screening behaviors in those persons who might otherwise avoid screening.

Psychological consequences of positive gene tests. A favorable balance of health benefits versus costs depends on determining whether the medical benefits will outweigh any psychological "side effects." For at-risk persons, cancer gene testing is not without potential side effects, as it may pose risks to psychological well-being and to the very cancer prevention practices it is meant to promote. These risks derive from several factors, including the predictable stress reaction that can follow the delivery of unfavorable medical information.

Surveys of persons at risk for cancer have shown that they expect significant distress in the face of a positive cancer gene test. Eighty percent of 121 female first-degree relatives of ovarian cancer patients reported that they would become depressed if they tested positive for a breast cancer mutation; 77 percent reported that they would become anxious.[30] Similarly, 60 percent of male and female first-degree relatives of colon cancer patients reportedly expected to become depressed and 52 percent anxious upon receiving a positive gene test.[31] It is possible that distress caused by a positive gene test may interfere with subsequent preventive health behavior. This has been shown in other situations: Of women notified of an abnormal mammogram, those who experienced high levels of psychological distress after notification were less likely to perform subsequent breast self-exam than those with moderate levels of distress;[115] persons psychologically distressed after having been notified of their risk for hypertension adhered less to their medication regimens;[116] and distressed persons delay seeking medical attention for possible cancer symptoms[117]

There is concern that persons distressed by their cancer risk will make irrevocable decisions to have unproven prophylactic surgeries.[118] This prediction has some support from a study of first-degree relatives of breast cancer patients. Those who subsequently chose prophylactic mastectomy were more anxious and had higher levels of cancer worry than women who later chose continued screening or a chemoprevention trial.[119] The finding suggests that women undertake prophylactic surgery to more fully eliminate their cancer risk. However, prophylactic mastectomy, while effective,[120] does not eliminate breast cancer risk,[121,122] and some of the women studied may never develop cancer. Moreover, basing decisions on probabilistic genetic information means that short-term relief from cancer worry could be followed by regret if later, more definitive information reveals that the surgery was unnecessary.

A positive genetic test can have favorable psychological consequences, including removal of uncertainty and being better able to prepare for future events, as has been seen in Huntington disease[123,124] and FAP.[10] Surveys of persons at risk for cancer suggest that they anticipate benefits from "bad news." For example, 68 percent of first-degree relatives of ovarian cancer patients reported that they would feel more "in control" of their lives even if they tested positive.[125] Several studies that measured psychological parameters at baseline and 1 to 3 months following gene testing have found no adverse reactions in persons who received positive test results: Lerman et al. studied 279 male and female members of BRCA1-linked hereditary breast and ovarian cancer families and found no short-term increased depression or functional impairment in those who tested gene positive.[112] Croyle and coworkers found that distress declines after gene testing but that women who are mutation positive for BRCA1 experience more distress than noncarriers in followup.[126] In a study of 42 children at risk for FAP and their parents, Codori et al. also did not observe any significant increase in distress or behavioral problems in the gene-positive children.[127] The response to genetic testing is likely complex,[128] and research to examine these observations in the context of longer-term impact are ongoing.

Psychological Consequences of Negative Gene Tests. Those whose receive negative gene tests often experience relief at removal of uncertainty and doubt.[10,112,127] These persons are likely to be spared anxiety-provoking,[10,129] costly, and sometimes invasive screening procedures and to be relieved to know that their children's and their own personal risk for cancer is no greater than in the general population.

It is possible that some proportion of those who learn that they do not carry the cancer gene mutation in their family are at risk for psychological distress. In Huntington disease, "survivor guilt" was reported in 25 percent of people who tested negative,[130] and individual cases of depression and marital disruption have been reported.[130,131] Twenty-five percent of persons at risk for colon cancer predict feeling guilty, and 50 percent expect to continue worrying about cancer even after learning that they are noncarriers.[31] Similar rates were reported by women at risk for breast and ovarian cancer.[125]

Genetic Testing of Children. There has been debate on the appropriateness of genetic testing of minors, particularly for cancers that have their onset later in adulthood or for which there is no intervention to change the outcome. The medical and legal ramifications need to be explored and the interests of the children and their parents weighed.[91,132] Issues to consider include assessment of the significance of the potential benefits and harms of the gene test, determination of the decision-making capacity of the child, and advocacy on behalf of the child.[132,133] Certainly, the medical benefit to the child should be the primary justification for gene testing of children.

Certain hereditary cancer syndromes (e.g., multiple endocrine neoplasia type 2, FAP, retinoblastoma) involve onset of tumors in childhood and warrant genetic testing of children[10,12,134,135] because interventions are feasible.[91] Genetic testing of children requires special counseling adjusted to their age level, taking into consideration their awareness of cancer risk and perceptions of family attitudes toward cancer.[10] While screening and prophylactic surgery for gene-positive persons are currently available modalities, there is potential for chemoprevention or other interventions for which initiation in childhood would be most effective.[136] This would reopen the issue of performing gene tests in childhood for cancer syndromes that have their onset in adulthood.[9]

In summary, the available data suggest that interest in cancer gene testing may be high but that actual uptake may be more modest, being affected by psychological factors. The data also suggest that there may be psychological risks from cancer genetic testing, including emotional distress from positive and negative test results, unintended and inappropriate decreases in cancer screening behavior, irrevocable decisions made in a state of anxiety, false reassurances about cancer risk, distressing and unwanted genetic knowledge, and insurance and employment discrimination. These issues warrant carefully planned implementation of testing protocols. These factors, in large measure, call for sensitive, thorough preparation and follow-up, including education and psychological evaluation and support.

CURRENT STATUS OF CANCER RISK ASSESSMENT AND GENETIC TESTING

Cancer Risk Assessment Clinical Services

Within the last several years, there have been numerous clinical initiatives to provide cancer genetic risk assessment and genetic testing services.[137-140] Many are located in major medical university or comprehensive cancer center settings, but an increasing number of health professionals in health maintenance organization and private practice settings have begun to offer cancer genetic testing. While clinical geneticists and genetic counselors can provide this service, it is more often the case that the medical specialties that are generally associated with treatment of cancer have begun to recognize the importance of providing this component of a comprehensive service to their patients. In particular, professional societies of clinical oncologists, surgeons, and oncology nurses have initiated educational programs to keep their members current.[141-144]

The cancer risk assessment service is interdisciplinary (medicine, genetics, genetic counseling) and at a minimum should include a physician (oncologist or clinical geneticist), and genetic counselor, or nurse/nurse practitioner with cancer genetics experience. The service should have access to resource support personnel, including social workers, psychologists, specialists in cancer treatment and management, and ethicists, and to genetic testing laboratories certified under Clinical Laboratory Improvement Act (CLIA) regulations.

Indications for Cancer Risk Assessment

The increased understanding of the relationship of clinical features, epidemiology, and aggregation of cancers in families has allowed the compilation of guidelines to clues for clinicians that would warrant further evaluation for familial or hereditary cancer:[1,13,137]

- A cancer occurring at an unusually young age compared with the usual presentation of that type of cancer
- Multifocal development of cancer in a single organ or bilateral development of cancer in paired organs
- Development of more than one primary tumor of any type in a single individual
- Family history of cancer of the same type in a close relative(s)
- High rate of cancer within a family
- Occurrence of cancer in an individual or a family exhibiting congenital anomalies or birth defects
- Ashkenazi Jewish heritage
- Family known to segregate a hereditary gene mutation

More recently, resources for clinical cancer genetics have become available, in the form of both textbooks[1,13] and handbooks.[137] Internet-based resources and government-sponsored programs, such as the National Cancer Institute's Cancer Genetics Network, Cancer Information Service, and the Physician Data Query (PDQ) database, are other emerging new resources (Table 39-2).

Indications for Cancer Gene Tests

At this time, cancer gene tests have two primary clinical applications. When affected individuals are tested, gene tests may be used to molecularly diagnose an inherited cancer syndrome. When asymptomatic persons are tested, gene tests may be used to identify whether or not they are at increased risk because they carry a known predisposing mutation. The appropriate use of gene tests, particularly in determining who should be tested, is relatively straightforward in clearcut hereditary cancer syndrome families. However, this distinction is rapidly becoming blurred as further characterization of cancer gene loci appears to indicate that gene tests may be used for familial cancers due to mutations associated with lower penetrance in families that do not fit known criteria for hereditary syndromes, or for screening specific populations in which cancer susceptibility genes occur at high frequency.

Testing Affected Individuals to Clarify the Diagnosis. A patient with cancer might be offered gene testing to rule in or out a suspected inherited syndrome. In this case, there may be indications from family history or from clustering of specific tumors in family members suggestive of a hereditary syndrome (such as leukemia, soft-tissue sarcoma, brain tumors, or breast cancer in Li-Fraumeni syndrome[145]). Table 39-1 lists some of the tumor types that are associated with known cancer syndromes. Gene tests may also be offered to patients with apparently sporadic cancer if the cancer occurs at an unusually young age or if the patient has other stigmata suggestive of a hereditary syndrome. For

Table 39-2 Internet-Based Cancer Genetics Resources

Resource	Internet (Web Page) Address	Description
Alliance of Genetic Support Group	http://www.geneticalliance.org/index.html	Nonprofit organization that addresses the concerns of people with, and at risk for, genetic conditions.
American Cancer Society	http://www.cancer.org/	Nationally recognized non profit organization site contains a variety of information on cancer.
Association of Cancer Online Resources – Breast Cancer Information Clearinghouse	http://www.acor.org/	Established in 1994, this contains a directory of organizations that provide information and support for breast cancer patients and their families and access to online discussion groups.
Avon Breast Cancer Awareness Crusade	http://www.avoncrusade.com/	Avon's Internet crusade to provide more women, particularly low-income, minority, and older women, with access to breast cancer education and early detection screening services.
Cancer and Genetics	http://www.cancergenetics.org/	The Robert H. Lurie Comprehensive Cancer Center of Northwestern University site contains information for the general public, primary care physician, nurse practitioners, and other health care professionals.
Cancer Genetics Network	http://www.-dccps.ims.nci.nih.gov/CGN/	Newly established network sponsored by the National Cancer Institute.
Cancer Information Network	http://www.cancernetwork.com/	Containing separate sections for professional and patients, this site is a good source of facts and news on various cancers.
Cancer information Service	http://cis.nci.nih.gov/	Sponsored by the National Cancer Institute, this site is the home of the national information and education network, available at 1-800-4-CANCER, that provides the most up-to-date and accurate information on cancer.
CancerNet	http://cancernet.nci.nih.gov/	Sponsored by the National Cancer Institute, this site provides access to several NCI databases, including the PDQ (Physician Data Query) and Cancerlit.
Clinical Genetics: Information for Genetic Professionals	http://www.kumc.edu/gec/geneinfo.html	University of Kansas Medical Center site contains clinical, research, and educational resources for genetics professionals.
Division of Cancer Epidemiology and Genetics	http://www-dceg.ims.nci.nih.gov/index.html	Part of the National Cancer Institute, this site contains information on population-based research on environmental and genetic determinants of cancer.
ELSI	http://www.nhgri.nih.gov/ELSI/	The Ethical, Legal, and Social Implications program is a branch of the National Human Genome Research Institute, established in 1990 to address issues related to human gene mapping research.
Healthfinder	http://www.healthfinder.gov/	Developed by the U.S. Department of Health and Human Services, this site contains links to over 1400 health-related sites.
Human Genome Project	http://www.nhgri.nih.gov/HGP/	Home of the international effort to determine the DNA sequence of the entire human genome.
InteliHealth	http://www.intelihealth.com/IH/ihtIH	Developed by Aetna U.S. Healthcare and the Johns Hopkins University Hospital and Health System, this comprehensive site contains information for both consumers and professional.
International Collaborative Group on Hereditary Non-polyposis Colorectal Cancer	http://www.nfdht.nl/	Mainly for physicians and researchers, this site contains a mutation database and a set of clinical guidelines.
Johns Hopkins Breast Center	http://www.med.jhu.edu/breastcenter/	This site is the Internet link to the Breast Center, part of the Johns Hopkins Oncology Center, a National Cancer institute–designated Comprehensive Cancer Center.
Johns Hopkins Colon Cancer Center	http://www.hopkins-coloncancer.org/	This site is the Internet link to the Johns Hopkins Colon Cancer Center, part of the Johns Hopkins Oncology Center, a National Cancer Institute–designated Comprehensive Cancer Center
Medscape Oncology	http://oncology.medscape.com/Home/Topics//oncology.html	A commercial, comprehensive web service for both clinicians and consumers.
National Cancer Institute	http://cancer.gov/	The U.S. goverment's primary agency for cancer research and training.
National Institutes of Health	http://www.nih.gov/	One of eight agencies that make up the Public Health Service in the Department of Health and Human Services.
Office of Genetics and Disease Prevention	http://www.cdc.gov/genetics/	Maintained by the Centers for Disease Control and Prevention, this site contains information on the impact of human genetic research and the Human Genome Project on public health and disease prevention, including HuGE Net.

Table 39-2 (Continued).

Resource	Internet (Web page) Address	Description
OncoLink: Genetics and Cancer	http://Oncolink.upenn.edu/causeprevent/ genetics/	Part of the University of Pennsylvania Cancer Center OncoLink site.
Principles and Recommendation: Task Force on Genetic Testing	http://www.med.jhu.edu/tfgtelsi/promoting/	Final report of the Task Force on Genetic Testing, a working group of the National Institutes of Health and Department of Energy human genome programs.
The Susan G. Komen Foundation	http://www.komen.org	For both patients and professionals, this site contains information on breast cancer detection and coping as well as grant and funding opportunities.
US TOO International, Inc.	http://www..ustoo.com/	Home to the largest prostate cancer support group in the world, this site provides access to information on prostate cancer and to counseling and educational meetings.

example, FAP might be suspected in a patient who has multiple colonic adenomas, congenital hypertrophy of the retinal pigment epithelium, and desmoid tumor[146] but no family history of colon polyps or cancer. *APC* gene testing is an indicated diagnostic test, as such a patient could have a *de novo* mutation in the *APC* gene.[147] If the *APC* gene test is positive, the patient can be presumed to have FAP and his or her children to be at 50 percent risk for inheriting the mutation.

Because genetic heterogeneity is seen in some hereditary cancer phenotypes, gene tests may be used help to identify the specific locus that is involved. For example, Turcot syndrome, a rare colon polyposis/cancer syndrome associated with central nervous system malignancies, has been shown to be genetically heterogeneous, with at least three loci (*APC, hMLH1,* and *hPMS2*) that independently produce a similar clinical picture.[148] Patients from suspected hereditary breast cancer families may need to be tested for at least two genes, *BRCA1* and *BRCA2*, because both genes may produce similar family histories.[149–151]

Testing At-risk Individuals for Inherited Susceptibility to Cancer. Asymptomatic at-risk persons from known hereditary cancer syndrome families may benefit from gene testing. In particular, when a mutation in a cancer gene is known to be segregating in the family, at-risk persons who test negative for the mutation may be relieved of years of surveillance, while persons who test positive for the mutation may approach the screening regimen with greater willingness to adhere to the recommendations.

When a mutation is not known to segregate in a cancer family, or if the diagnosis of a cancer syndrome is less clearcut, gene testing of at-risk persons in these families is more problematic. Often there is not a living family member with cancer who can undergo gene testing to identify the mutation. In such instances a negative gene test result in an at-risk person is not a "true" negative result that places him or her at the general population's risk for that cancer. Rather, this person has an "inconclusive" or "uninformative" negative test result that does not rule out other cancer gene loci, or even other mutations in the tested locus that the gene test was not able to detect. A person receiving an inconclusive test result should continue to maintain a cancer surveillance regimen as though no gene test was ever done.

Cancer Genetic Risk Assessment Process

The risk assessment process has multiple steps and incorporates multiple dimensions: medicine, psychology, genetics, and counseling. Health professionals trained in cancer genetics will need to have an awareness of the variety of issues that contribute to the process of helping patients to understand their risk, make informed decisions, and appreciate the implications for cancer prevention and risks for other family members.

Algorithm for genetic testing. With due consideration given to the issues surrounding cancer gene testing, a basic algorithm for integrating gene tests in cancer risk assessment can be constructed (Fig. 39-3). In this algorithm, eligible persons might include patients with a diagnosis of a known hereditary cancer syndrome and/or family members, patients with a positive family history, and patients with young onset of cancer (generally before age 50). Such patients should receive initial face-to-face counseling about cancer risk, with an educational component that includes a review of the genetics of the specific cancer(s) relevant to the patient, factors influencing increased cancer risk, and preventive intervention options, all adjusted to each patient's level of understanding. If it has not already been done, a detailed family history should be elicited and follow-up confirmation of cancer diagnoses in family members obtained, if possible.

The novel aspect of cancer risk assessment is genetic testing. The gene test may consist of mutation analysis or of tumor analysis for microsatellite instability (in the case of colorectal cancer). Following initial counseling, a careful explanation of the risks and benefits of the gene test should be given to the patient, with ample opportunity to check understanding and to answer questions or concerns. Genetic testing may not necessarily be the best option for some patients or families and should be entered into voluntarily, after careful deliberation on the implications.

If a specific causal gene mutation cannot be identified, then genetic testing of at-risk family members should not be pursued. Conventional screening guidelines and interventions as reviewed in the initial counseling session apply. If a specific causal gene mutation is identified, then the diagnosis of the corresponding hereditary cancer syndrome can be confirmed. In this instance, genetic counseling and predictive gene testing may be offered to at-risk family members who may wish to have this test done.

If an at-risk person tests positive for the gene, then he or she will be encouraged to adhere to preventive screening recommendations specific to the hereditary syndrome and counseled regarding other options, such as prophylactic surgery or chemoprevention, if applicable. In the case of FAP, hereditary breast and ovarian cancer, and HNPCC, recommendations have been developed, mostly based on expert opinion.[1,122,147,152]

If an at-risk person from a family in which the mutation in the cancer gene is known to segregate tests negative for the mutation, then he or she will be encouraged to adhere to cancer screening guidelines for the general population.

Genetic counseling in cancer gene testing. *Genetic counseling must accompany genetic testing, because of the implications for family members and for reproductive decision-making.* While a conventional, non genetic diagnostic test pertains primarily to the health of the person who has been tested, a genetic test often has implications for the health of other relatives, such as offspring, parents, and siblings. For example, a person who learns that he or she has a gene for an autosomal dominant form of cancer immediately knows that all of his or her offspring have a 50 percent risk of having inherited the mutation and his or her grandchildren a 25 percent risk. When an affected person tests positive, without prior evidence that the cancer was hereditary, the entire family may be suddenly suspected to be at increased risk for cancer. An identical twin cannot be tested without automatically revealing the co-twin's status, whether or not she or he wants the information. Similarly, a person at 25 percent risk for cancer (i.e., with an affected grandparent and healthy at-risk parent) who tests positive for the mutation automatically reveals a genetic diagnosis to the at-risk parent. Thus, genetic information may have serious implications for many persons who were not even tested.

Pre-test Counseling. *Genetic counseling accompanying gene tests for inherited cancer risk should include*:

a) Educating the family about the clinical and management aspects of hereditary cancer, the risks of cancer within the syndrome, and the consequences of receiving gene-positive or gene-negative test results, including the recommended screening guidelines for each possible test outcome.

b) Exploration of the issues related to the family history and experiences with cancer. These experiences can be multigenerational and include quite personal involvement with relatives who have died from cancer and/or who had oncologic or surgical interventions. Family relationships can be profoundly marked by issues such as guilt and blame, and personal and familial identity may be strongly linked with cancer status. Other issues include the denial of disease risk or stigmatization of cancer within the family and the acceptability, convenience, and affordability of screening regimens. Thus, genetic testing is imbued with meaning for certain patients far beyond its function as a simple determiner of genetic status. The at-risk patient may have pre-formed, well-entrenched conceptions of what having cancer entails, and family relationships and identity may be strongly linked with disease or gene status. Understanding of the patient's perspective is crucial so that it can be taken into account in assisting her or him to adjust to genetic test results.

c) Exploration of the perception of risk and its meaning and anticipated meaning of any test results. With parents of at-risk minor children, time should also be devoted to discussing how and when the test results and risk will be communicated to the children. In certain countries, employability or loss of insurability (life or health) is a risk, although the magnitude of this risk is at present unknown.

Informed Consent for Gene Testing. The decision to move forward with the gene test should be freely made by the at-risk person after carefully considering the consequences of genetic testing. It is strongly recommended that a consent form that outlines the meaning of test results and the consequences of the gene test be utilized.[14,77,91,153] If patients are to make fully informed decisions about gene testing, the informed consent process must include discussions of several complex issues, listed below. This is a time-consuming process and can require at least an hour of counseling time. The genetic counseling process that accompanies gene testing should incorporate the basic elements of informed consent, including:[14,153]

- Information on the specific test being performed
- Implications of a positive and a negative result
- Possibility that the test will not be informative
- Options for risk estimation without genetic testing
- Risk of passing a mutation to children
- Technical accuracy of the test
- Fees involved in testing and counseling
- Risks of psychological distress
- Risks of insurance or employer discrimination
- Confidentiality issues

- Options for and limitations of medical surveillance and screening following testing

Disclosure and Post-disclosure Counseling. Disclosure of gene test results, which can occur 2 weeks to 2 months later, depending upon the laboratory, provides another opportunity to meet again with the at-risk family member, explore the meaning of the test, and discuss in a more substantial way the likely follow-up regimen and cancer risks to future offspring.

For persons who test positive for the tested cancer gene, we recommend a third, follow-up session (either by telephone or in person), in which the patient is allowed a second opportunity, free from the initial emotional reaction to the test result, to ask questions about clinical management and the clinician can determine if referral to a mental health professional for additional support is indicated.

SUMMARY

In summary, new research developments in the molecular genetics of cancer have led to the feasibility of cancer genetic testing for many patients and family members. Gene tests have the potential to identify high-risk persons, and gene tests results will have clinical implications for cancer risk management: Conventional preventive recommendations can be modified in light of gene test results such that those at higher risk for cancer (gene positive) will be identified for increased cancer surveillance, while those at lower risk (true gene negative) may be reassured. There is a very real potential for misinterpretation of inconclusive gene test results. The new genetic technology also has psychosocial consequences for patients and families and ethical, legal, and policy implications for health care providers. Genetic counseling is an important added component in cancer risk assessment and management, particularly in helping those at risk to understand the variety of implications gene test results have in the context of their experience with cancer and intervention options.

REFERENCES

1. Offit K: *Clinical Cancer Genetics: Risk Counseling and Management.* New York, Wiley-Liss, 1998.
2. Ponder B: Genetic testing for cancer risk. *Science* **278**:1050, 1997.
3. Noorani HZ, Khan HN, Gallie BL, Detsky AS: Cost comparison of molecular versus conventional screening of relatives at risk for retinoblastoma. *Am J Hum Genet* **59**:301, 1996.
4. Cromwell DM, Moore RD, Brensinger JD, Petersen GM, Bass EB, Giardiello FM: Cost analysis of alternative approaches to colorectal screening in familial adenomatous polyposis. *Gastroenterology* **114**:893, 1998.
5. Bapat B, Noorani H, Cohen Z, Berk T, Mitri A, Gallie B, Pritzker K, et al: Cost comparison of predictive genetic testing versus conventional screening for familial adenomatous polyposis. *Gut* **44**:698, 1999.
6. Schrag D, Kuntz KM, Garber JE, Weeks JC: Decision analysis — effects of prophylactic mastectomy and oophorectomy on life expectancy among women with BRCA1 or BRCA2 mutations. *N Engl J Med* **336**:1465, 1997.
7. Grann VR, Panageas KS, Whang W, Antman KH, Neugut AI: Decision analysis of prophylactic mastectomy and oophorectomy in BRCA1-positive or BRCA2-positive patients. *J Clin Oncol* **16**:979, 1998.
8. Syngal S, Weeks JC, Schrag D, Garber JE, Kuntz KM: Benefits of colonoscopic surveillance and prophylactic colectomy in patients with hereditary nonpolyposis colorectal cancer mutations. *Ann Intern Med* **129**:787, 1998.
9. Knudson AG: Hereditary cancers: from discovery to intervention. *J Natl Inst Cancer Monogr* **17**:5, 1995.
10. Petersen GM, Boyd PA: Gene tests and counseling for colorectal cancer risk: Lessons from familial polyposis. *J Natl Inst Cancer Monogr* **17**:67, 1995.
11. Li FP, Garber JE, Friend SH, Strong LC, Patenaude AF, Juengst ET, Reilly PR, et al: Recommendations on predictive testing for germ line p53 mutations among cancer-prone individuals. *J Natl Cancer Inst* **84**:1156, 1992.
12. Neumann HPH, Eng C, Mulligan LM, Glavac D, Zäuner I, Ponder BAJ, Crossey PA, et al: Consequences of direct genetic testing for

germline mutations in the clinical management of families with multiple endocrine neoplasia, type II. *JAMA* **274**:1149, 1995.

13. Hodgson SV, Maher ER: *A Practical Guide to Human Cancer Genetics.* Cambridge, Cambridge University Press, 1993.

14. Statement of the American Society of Clinical Oncology: Genetic testing for cancer susceptibility. *J Clin Oncol* **14**:1730, 1996.

15. Li FP: Cancer control in susceptible groups: Opportunities and challenges. *J Clin Oncol* **17**:719, 1999.

16. Khoury MJ: Genetic epidemiology and the future of disease prevention and public health. *Epidemiol Rev* **19**:175, 1997.

17. Perera FP: Environment and cancer: Who are susceptible? *Science* **278**:1068, 1997.

18. Kelloff GJ, Boone CW, Crowell JA, Nayfield SG, Hawk E, Malone WF, Steele VE, et al: Risk biomarkers and current strategies for cancer chemoprevention. *J Cell Biochem Suppl* **25**:1, 1996.

19. Holtzman NA: Scale-up technology: Moving predictive tests for inherited breast, ovarian, and colon cancers from the bench to the bedside and beyond. *J Natl Cancer Inst Monogr* **17**:95, 1995.

20. Grann VR, Whang W, Jacobson JS, Heitjan DF, Antman KH, Neugut AI: Benefits and costs of screening Ashkenazi Jewish women for BRCA1 and BRCA2. *J Clin Oncol* **17**:494, 1999.

21. Tambor ES, Rimer BK, Strigo TS: Genetic testing for breast cancer susceptibility: Awareness and interest among women in the general population. *Am J Med Genet* **68**:43, 1997.

22. Andrykowski MA, Munn RK, Studts JL: Interest in learning of personal genetic risk for cancer: A general population survey. *Prev Med* **25**:527, 1996.

23. Lerman C, Seay J, Balshem A, Audrain J: Interest in genetic testing among first-degree relatives of breast cancer patients. *Am J Med Genet* **57**:385, 1995.

24. Graham ID, Logan DM, Hughes-Benzie R, Evans WK, Perras H, McAuley LM, Laupacis A, Stern H: How interested is the public in genetic testing for colon cancer susceptibility? Report of a cross-sectional population survey. *Cancer Prev Control* **2**:167, 1998.

25. Petersen GM, Larkin E, Codori A-M, Wang C-Y, Booker SV, Bacon J, Giardiello FM, Boyd PA: Attitudes toward colon cancer gene testing: Survey of relatives of colon cancer patients. *Cancer Epidemiol Biomark Prev* **8**:337, 1999.

26. Glanz K, Grove J, Lerman C, Gotay C, Le Marchand L: Correlates of intentions to obtain genetic counseling and colorectal cancer gene testing among at-risk relatives from three ethnic groups. *Cancer Epidemiol Biomark Prev* **8**:329, 1999.

27. Smith KR, Croyle RT: Attitudes toward genetic testing for colon cancer risk. *Am J Public Health* **85**:1435, 1995.

28. Struewing JP, Lerman C, Kase RG, Giambarresi TR, Tucker MA: Anticipated uptake and impact of genetic testing in hereditary breast and ovarian cancer families. *Cancer Epidemiol Biomark Prev* **4**:169, 1995.

29. Bratt O, Kristoffersson U, Lundgren R, Olsson H: Sons of men with prostate cancer: Their attitudes regarding possible inheritance of prostate cancer, screening, and genetic testing. *Urology* **50**:360, 1997.

30. Lerman C, Daly M, Masny A, Balshem A: Attitudes about genetic testing for breast-ovarian cancer susceptibility. *J Clin Oncol* **12**:843, 1994.

31. Lerman C, Marshall J, Audrain J, Gómez-Caminero A: Genetic testing for colon cancer susceptibility: Anticipated reactions of patients and challenges to providers. *Int J Cancer* **69**:58, 1996.

32. Rodríguez C, Plasencia A, Schroeder DG: Predictive factors of enrollment and adherence in a breast cancer screening program in Barcelona. *Soc Sci Med* **40**:1155, 1995.

33. Kelly RB, Shank JC: Adherence to screening flexible sigmoidoscopy in asymptomatic patients. *Med Care* **30**:1029, 1992.

34. Kendall C, Hailey BJ: The relative effectiveness of three reminder letters on making and keeping mammogram appointments. *Behav Med* **19**:29, 1993.

35. Bluman LG, Rimer BK, Berry DA, Borstelmann N, Iglehart JD, Regan K, Schildkraut J, Winer EP: Attitudes, knowledge, and risk perceptions of women with breast and ovarian cancer considering testing for BRCA1 and BRCA2. *J Clin Oncol* **17**:1040, 1999.

36. Kash KM, Holland JC, Halper MS, Miller DG: Psychological distress and surveillance behaviors of women with a family history of breast cancer. *J Natl Cancer Inst* **84**:24, 1992.

37. Champion VL: Compliance with guidelines for mammography screening. *Cancer Detect Prev* **16**:253, 1992.

38. Codori A-M, Petersen GM, Miglioretti DL, Larkin EK, Bushey MT, Young C, Brensinger JD, et al: Attitudes toward colon cancer gene

testing: Factors predicting test uptake. *Cancer Epidemiol Biomark Prev* **8**:345, 1999.

39. Jacobsen PB, Valdimarsdottir HB, Brown KL, Offit K: Decision-making about genetic testing among women at familial risk for breast cancer. *Psychosomat Med* **59**:459, 1997.

40. Lynch HT, Watson P, Tinley S, Snyder C, Durham C, Lynch J, Kirnarsky Y, et al: An update on DNA-based BRCA1/BRCA2 genetic counseling in hereditary breast cancer. *Cancer Genet Cytogenet* **109**:91, 1999.

41. Evans DG, Maher ER, Macleod R, Davies DR, Craufurd D: Uptake of genetic testing for cancer predisposition. *J Med Genet* **34**:746, 1997.

42. Newman B, Mu H, Butler LM, Millikan RC, Moorman PG, King M-C: Frequency of breast cancer attributable to BRCA1 in a population-based series of American women. *JAMA* **279**:915, 1995.

43. Struewing JP, Beliovich D, Peretz T, Avishai N, Kaback MM, Collins FS, Brody LC: The carrier frequency of the BRCA1 185delAG mutation is approximately 1 percent in Ashkenazi Jewish individuals. *Nature Genet* **11**:198, 1995.

44. Struewing JP, Hartge P, Wacholder S, Baker SM, Berlin M, McAdams M, Timmerman MM, et al: The risk of cancer associated with specific mutations of BRCA1 and BRCA2 among Ashkenazi Jews. *N Engl J Med* **336**:1401, 1997.

45. Laken SJ, Petersen GM, Gruber SB, Oddoux C, Ostrer H, Giardiello FM, Hamilton SR, et al: Familial colorectal cancer in Ashkenazim due to a hypermutable tract in APC. *Nat Genet* **17**:79, 1997.

46. Nyström-Lahti M, Kristo P, Nicolaides NC, Chang SY, Aaltonen LA, Moisio AL, Järvinen HJ, et al: Founding mutations and Alu-mediated recombination in hereditary colon cancer. *Nat Med* **1**:1203, 1995.

47. Moisio AL, Sistonen P, Weissenbach J, de la Chapelle A, Peltomaki P: Age and origin of two common MLH1 mutations predisposing to hereditary colon cancer. *Am J Hum Genet* **59**:1243, 1996.

48. Serova OM, Mazoyer S, Puget N, Dubois V, Tonin P, Shugart YY, Goldgar D, et al: Mutations in BRCA1 and BRCA2 in breast cancer families: Are there more breast cancer-susceptibility genes? *Am J Hum Genet* **60**:486, 1997.

49. Liu B, Parsons R, Papadopoulos N, Nicolaides NC, Lynch HT, Watson P, Jass JR, et al: Analysis of mismatch repair genes in hereditary non-polyposis colorectal cancer patients. *Nature Med* **2**:169, 1996.

50. Brunet JS, Ghadirian P, Rebbeck TR, Lerman C, Garber JE, Tonin PN, Abrahamson J, et al: Effect of smoking on breast cancer in carriers of mutant BRCA1 or BRCA2 genes. *J Natl Cancer Inst* **90**:761, 1998.

51. Bottorff JL, Ratner PA, Johnson JL, Lovato CY, Joab SA: Communicating cancer risk information: The challenges of uncertainty. *Patient Educ Counseling* **33**:67, 1998.

52. Welch HG, Burke W: Uncertainties in genetic testing for chronic disease. *JAMA* **280**:1525, 1998.

53. Cornelis RS, Vasen HFA, Meijers-Heijboer H, Ford D, van Vliet M, van Tilborg AAG, Cleton FJ, et al: Age at diagnosis as an indicator of eligibility for BRCA1 DNA testing in familial breast cancer. *Hum Genet* **95**:539, 1995.

54. Rubin SC, Blackwood MA, Bandera C, Behbakht K, Benjamin I, Rebbeck TR, Boyd J: BRCA1, BRCA2, and hereditary nonpolyposis colorectal cancer gene mutations in an unselected ovarian cancer population—relationship to family history and implications for genetic testing. *Am J Obstet Gynecol* **178**:670, 1998.

55. Aaltonen LA, Salovaara R, Kristo P, Canzian F, Hemminki A, Peltomaki P, Chadwick RB, et al: Incidence of hereditary nonpolyposis colorectal cancer and the feasibility of molecular screening for the disease. *N Engl J Med* **338**:1481, 1998.

56. Shattuck-Eidens D, Oliphant A, McClure M, McBride C, Gupte J, Rubano T, Pruss D, et al: BRCA1 sequence analysis in women at high risk for susceptibility mutations. *JAMA* **278**:1242, 1997.

57. Couch FJ, DeShano ML, Blackwood MA, Calzone K, Stopfer J, Campeau L, Ganguly A, et al: BRCA1 mutations in women attending clinics that evaluate the risk of breast cancer. *N Engl J Med* **336**:1409, 1997.

58. Berry DA, Parmigiani G, Sánchez J, Winder E: Probability of carrying a mutation of breast ovarian cancer gene BRCA1 based on family history. *J Natl Cancer Inst* **89**:227, 1997.

59. Parmigiani G, Berry D, Aguilar O: Determining carrier probabilities for breast cancer-susceptibility genes BRCA1 and BRCA2. *Am J Hum Genet* **62**:145, 1998.

60. Wijnen JT, Vasen HFA, Khan PM, Zwinderman AH, Vanderklift H, Mulder A, Tops C, et al: Clinical findings with implications for genetic

testing in families with clustering of colorectal cancer. *N Engl J Med* **339**:511, 1998.

61. Ford D, Easton DF, Bishop DT, Narod SA, Goldgar DE, Breast Cancer Linkage Consortium: Risks of cancer in BRCA1 mutation carriers. *Lancet* **343**:692, 1994.

62. Aarnio M, Mecklin JP, Aaltonen LA, Nyström-Lahti M, Järvinen HJ: Life-time risk of different cancers in hereditary non-polyposis colorectal cancer (HNPCC) syndrome. *Int J Cancer* **64**:430, 1995.

63. Aarnio M, Sankila R, Pukkala E, Salovaara R, Aaltonen LA, de la Chapelle A, Peltomäki P, et al: Cancer risk in mutation carriers of DNA-mismatch-repair genes. *Int J Cancer* **81**:214, 1999.

64. Hawkins JR: *Finding Mutations.* New York, Oxford University Press, 1997.

65. Cotton RGH: *Mutation Detection.* Oxford, Oxford University Press, 1997.

66. Eng C, Vijg J: Genetic testing: The problems and the promise. *Nature Biotechnol* **15**:422, 1997.

67. Petersen GM, Slack J, Nakamura Y: Screening guidelines and premorbid diagnosis of familial adenomatous polyposis using linkage. *Gastroenterology* **100**:1658, 1991.

68. Maher ER, Bentley E, Payne SJ, Latif F, Richards FM, Chiano M, Hosoe S, et al.: Presymptomatic diagnosis of von Hippel-Lindau disease with flanking DNA markers. *J Med Genet* **29**:902, 1992.

69. Shimotake T, Iwai N, Yanagihara J, Tokiwa K, Tanaka N, Yamamoto M, Takai S: Prediction of affected MEN2A gene carriers by DNA linkage analysis for early total thyroidectomy: A progress in clinical screening program for children with hereditary cancer syndrome. *J Pediatr Surg* **27**:444, 1992.

70. Gayther SA, Sud R, Wells D, Tsioupra K, Delhanty JD: Rapid detection of rare variants and common polymorphisms in the APC gene by PCR-SSCP for presymptomatic diagnosis and showing allele loss. *J Med Genet* **32**:568, 1995.

71. Powell SM, Petersen GM, Krush AJ, Booker S, Jen J, Giardiello FM, Hamilton SR, et al: Molecular diagnosis of familial adenomatous polyposis. *N Engl J Med* **329**:1982, 1993.

72. Luce MC, Marra G, Chauhan DP, Laghi L, Carethers JM, Cherian SP, Hawn M, et al: In vitro transcription/translation assay for the screening of hMLH1 and hMSH2 mutations in familial colon cancer. *Gastroenterology* **109**:1368, 1995.

73. Forrest S, Cotton R, Landegren U, Southern E: How to find all those mutations. *Nature Genet* **10**:375, 1996.

74. Cotton RGH: Detection of unknown mutations in DNA: A catch-22. *Am J Hum Genet* **59**:289, 1996.

75. Yan H, Papadopoulos N, Marra G, Perrera C, Jiricny J, Boland CR, Lynch HT, et al: Conversion of diploidy to haploidy. *Nature* **403**:723, 2000.

76. Laken SJ, Jackson PE, Kinzler KW, Vogelstein B, Strickland PT, Groopman JD, Friesen MD: Genotyping by mass spectrometric analysis of short DNA fragments. *Nat Biotechnol* **16**:1352, 1998.

77. Holtzman NA, Watson MS (eds): *Promoting Safe and Effective Genetic Testing in the United States. Final Report of the Task Force on Genetic Testing.* Baltimore, Johns Hopkins University Press, 1998.

78. Holtzman NA, Murphy PD, Watson MS, Barr PA: Predictive genetic testing: From basic research to clinical practice. *Science* **278**:602, 1997.

79. Rodríguez-Bigas MA, Boland CR, Hamilton SR, Henson DE, Jass JR, Khan PM, Lynch H, et al: A National Cancer Institute workshop on hereditary nonpolyposis colorectal cancer syndrome: Meeting highlights and Bethesda Guidelines. *J Natl Cancer Inst* **89**:1758, 1997.

80. Boland CR, Thibodeau SN, Hamilton SR, Sidransky D, Eshleman JR, Burt RW, Meltzer SJ, et al: A National Cancer Institute workshop on microsatellite instability for cancer detection and familial predisposition: Development of international criteria for the determination of microsatellite instability in colorectal cancer. *Cancer Res* **58**:5248, 1998.

81. Leach FS, Nicolaides N, Papadopoulos N, Liu B, Jen J, Parsons R, Peltomäki P, et al: Mutations of a MutS homolog in hereditary non-polyposis colorectal cancer. *Cell* **75**:1215, 1993.

82. Papadopoulos N, Nicolaides NC, Wei Y-F, Ruben SM, Carter KC, Rosen CA, Haseltine WA, et al: Mutation of a mutL homolog in hereditary colon cancer. *Science* **263**:1625, 1994.

83. Nicolaides NC, Papadopoulos N, Liu B, Wei Y-F, Carter KC, Ruben SM, Rosen CA, et al: Mutations of two PMS homologues in hereditary nonpolyposis colon cancer. *Nature* **371**:75, 1994.

84. Thibodeau SN, French AJ, Cunningham JM, Tester D, Burgart LJ, Roche PC, McDonnell SK, et al: Microsatellite instability in colorectal

cancer: Different mutator phenotypes and the principal involvement of hMLH1. *Cancer Res* **58**:1713, 1998.

85. Cunningham JM, Kim CY, Tester DJ, Christensen ER, Parc Y, Halling K, Burgart LJ, et al: The frequency and mechanism of defective DNA mismatch repair in unselected colorectal carcinomas. *Am Assn Cancer Res Proc* **40**:243, 1999.

86. Kainu T, Kononen J, Johansson O, Olsson H, Borg A, Isola J: Detection of germline BRCA1 mutations in breast cancer patients by quantitative messenger RNA in situ hybridization. *Cancer Res* **56**:2912, 1996.

87. Hubbard R, Lewontin RC: Pitfalls of genetic testing. *N Engl J Med* **334**:1192, 1996.

88. Giardiello FM, Brensinger JD, Petersen GM, Luce MC, Hylind LM, Bacon JA, Booker SV, et al: The use and interpretation of commercial APC gene testing for familial adenomatous polyposis. *N Engl J Med* **336**:823, 1997.

89. Cho MK, Sankar P, Wolpe PR, Godmilow L: Commercialization of BRCA1/2 testing: Practitioner awareness and use of a new genetic test. *Am J Med Genet* **83**:157, 1999.

90. Nelson NJ: Caution guides genetic testing for hereditary cancer genes. *J Natl Cancer Inst* **88**:70, 1996.

91. Andrews LB, Fullarton JE, Holtzman NA (eds): *Assessing Genetic Risks: Implications for Health and Social Policy.* Washington, DC: National Academy Press, 1994.

92. National Advisory Council for Human Genome Research: Statement on use of DNA testing for presymptomatic detection of cancer risk. *JAMA* **271**:785, 1994.

93. Statement of the American Society of Human Genetics on genetic testing for breast and ovarian cancer predisposition. *Am J Hum Genet* **55**:i, 1994.

94. National Action Plan on Breast Cancer: Position paper: Hereditary susceptibility testing for breast cancer. *J Clin Oncol* **14**:1738, 1996.

95. Rothstein MA: Genetic testing: employability, insurability, and health reform. *Monogr Natl Cancer Inst* **17**:87, 1995.

96. Garber JE, Patenaude AF: Ethical, social and counseling issues in hereditary cancer susceptibility. *Cancer Surv* **25**:381, 1995.

97. Kash KM: Psychosocial and ethical implications of defining genetic risk for cancers. *Ann NY Acad Sci* **768**:41, 1995.

98. Patenaude AF: The genetic testing of children for cancer susceptibility: Ethical, legal and social issues. *Behav Sci Law* **14**:393, 1996.

99. Wilfond BS, Rothenberg KH, Thomson EJ, Lerman C: Cancer genetic susceptibility testing—ethical and policy implications for future research and clinical practice. *J Law Med Ethics* **25**:243, 1997.

100. Jeffords JH, Daschle T: Political issues in the genome era. *Science* **291**:1249, 2001.

101. Grady C: Ethics and genetic testing. *Adv Intern Med* **44**:389, 1999.

102. Ad Hoc Committee on Genetic Testing/Insurance Issues: Genetic testing and insurance. *Am J Hum Genet* **56**:327, 1995.

103. American Society of Human Genetics Social Issues Subcommittee on Familial Disclosure: Professional disclosure of familial genetic information. *Am J Hum Genet* **62**:474, 1998.

104. Lerman C, Peshkin BN, Hughes C, Isaacs C: Family disclosure in genetic testing for cancer susceptibility: Determinants and consequences. *J Health Care Law Policy* **1**:353, 1998.

105. Clayton EW: What should the law say about disclosure of genetic information to relatives? *J Health Care Law Policy* **1**:373, 1998.

106. ASHG Background Statement: Genetic testing and insurance. *Am J Hum Genet* **56**:327, 1995.

107. Lapham EV, Kozma C, Weiss JO: Genetic discrimination: Perspectives of consumers. *Science* **274**:621, 1996.

108. Billings PR, Kohn MA, de Cuevas M, Beckwith J, Alper JS, Natowicz MR: Discrimination as a consequence of genetic testing. *Am J Hum Genet* **50**:476, 1992.

109. Natowicz MR, Alper JK, Alper JS: Genetic discrimination and the law. *Am J Hum Genet* **50**:465, 1992.

110. Billings PR, Beckwith J: Genetic testing in the workplace: A view from the USA. *Trends Genet* **8**:198, 1992.

111. Hopwood P: Psychological issues in cancer genetics: Current research and future priorities. *Patient Educ Counseling* **32**:19, 1997.

112. Lerman C, Narod S, Schulman K, Hughes C, Gómez-Caminero A, Bonney G, Gold K, et al: BRCA1 testing in families with hereditary breast-ovarian cancer. A prospective study of patient decision making and outcomes. *JAMA* **275**:1885, 1996.

113. Lerman C, Hughes C, Trock BJ, Myers RE, Main D, Bonney A, Abbaszadegan MR, et al: Genetic testing in families with hereditary nonpolyposis colon cancer. *JAMA* **281**:1618, 1999.

114. Bowen DJ, Patenaude AF, Vernon SW: Psychosocial issues in cancer genetics: From the laboratory to the public. *Cancer Epidemiol Biomark Prev* **8**:326, 1999.

115. Lerman C, Trock B, Rimer BK, Jepson C, Brody D, Boyce A: Psychological side effects of breast cancer screening. *Health Psychol* **10**:259, 1991.

116. Macdonald LA, Sackett DL, Haynes RB, Taylor DW: Labelling in hypertension: A review of the behavioural and psychological consequences. *J Chron Dis* **37**:933, 1984.

117. Greenwald HP, Becker SW, Nevitt MC: Delay and noncompliance in cancer detection: A behavioral perspective for health planners. *Milbank Mem Fund Quart* **56**:212, 1978.

118. Biesecker BB, Boehnke M, Calzone K, Markel DS, Garber JE, Collins FS, Weber BL: Genetic counseling for families with inherited susceptibility to breast and ovarian cancer. *JAMA* **269**:1970, 1993.

119. Stefanek ME, Helzlsouer KJ, Wilcox PM, Houn F: Predictors of and satisfaction with bilateral prophylactic mastectomy. *Prev Med* **24**:412, 1995.

120. Hartmann LC, Schaid DJ, Woods JE, Crotty TP, Myers JL, Arnold PG, Petty PM, et al: Efficacy of bilateral prophylactic mastectomy in women with a family history of breast cancer. *N Engl J Med* **340**:77, 1999.

121. King M-C, Rowell S, Love SM: Inherited breast and ovarian cancer. What are the risks? What are the choices? *JAMA* **269**:1975, 1993.

122. Burke W, Daly M, Garber J, Botkin J, Kahn MJE, Lynch P, McTiernan A, et al: Recommendations for follow-up care of individuals with an inherited predisposition to cancer. II. *BRCA1* and *BRCA2*. *JAMA* **277**:997, 1997.

123. Codori AM, Brandt J: Psychological costs and benefits of predictive testing for Huntington's disease. *Am J Med Genet* **54**:174, 1994.

124. Wiggins S, Whyte P, Huggins M, Adam S, Theilmann J, Bloch M, Sheps SB, et al: The psychological consequences of predictive testing for Huntington's disease. *N Engl J Med* **327**:1401, 1992.

125. Lerman C, Daly M, Masney A, Balshem A: Attitudes about genetic testing for breast-ovarian cancer susceptibility. *J Clin Oncol* **12**:843, 1994.

126. Croyle RT, Smith KR, Botkin JR, Baty B, Nash J: Psychological responses to BRCA1 mutation testing: Preliminary findings. *Health Psychol* **16**:63, 1997.

127. Codori A-M, Petersen GM, Corazzini K, Bacon J, Loth DM, Boyd PA, Brandt J, et al: Genetic testing for cancer in children: Short-term psychological impact. *Arch Pediatr Adolesc Med* **150**:1131, 1996.

128. Dudok deWit AC, Tibben A, Duivenvoorden HJ, Niermeijer MF, Passchier J: Predicting adaptation to presymptomatic DNA testing for late onset disorders: Who will experience distress? Rotterdam Leiden Genetics Workgroup. *J Med Genet* **35**:745, 1998.

129. Lerman C, Rimer BK: Psychosocial impact of cancer screening. *Oncology* **7**:67, 1993.

130. Codori AM, Brandt J: Psychological costs and benefits of predictive testing for Huntington's disease. *Am J Med Genet* **54**:174, 1994.

131. Huggins M, Bloch M, Wiggins S, Adam S, Suchowersky O, Trew M, Klimek M, et al: Predictive testing for Huntington disease in Canada: Adverse effects and unexpected results in those receiving a decreased risk. *Am J Med Genet* **42**:508, 1992.

132. The American Society of Human Genetics Board of Directors and the American College of Medical Genetics Board of Directors: ASHG/ACMG Report. Points to consider: Ethical, legal, and psychosocial implications of genetic testing in children and adolescents. *Am J Hum Genet* **57**:1233, 1995.

133. Grosfeld FJM, Lips CJM, Beemer FA, van Spijker HG, Brouwers-Smalbraak GJ, ten Kroode HFJ: Psychological risks of genetically testing children for a hereditary cancer syndrome. *Patient Educ Counseling* **32**:63, 1997.

134. Learoyd DL, Marsh DJ, Richardson AL, Twigg SM, Delbridge L, Robinson BG: Genetic testing for familial cancer. Consequences of RET proto-oncogene mutation analysis in mutiple endocrine neoplasia, type 2. *Arch Surg* **132**:1022, 1997.

135. Gallie BL, Dunn JM, Chan HSL, Hamel PA, Phillips RA: The genetics of retinoblastoma: Relevance to the patient. *Pediatr Clin North Am* **38**:299, 1991.

136. Giardiello FM, Hamilton SR, Krush AJ, Piantadosi S, Hylind LM, Celano P, Booker SV, et al: Treatment of colonic and rectal adenomas with Sulindac in familial adenomatous polyposis. *N Engl J Med* **328**:1313, 1993.

137. Lindor NM, Greene MH, Mayo Familial Cancer Program: The concise handbook of family cancer syndromes. *J Natl Canc Inst* **90**:1039, 1998.

138. Lynch HT, Fitzsimmons ML, Lynch J, Watson P: A hereditary cancer consultation clinic. *Nebr Med J* **74**:351, 1989.

139. McKinnon WC, Guttmacher AE, Greenblatt MS, Compas BE, May S, Cutler RE, Yandell DW: The familial cancer program of the Vermont cancer center: Development of a cancer genetics program in a rural area. *J Genet Counseling* **6**:131, 1997.

140. Stadler MP, Mulvihill JJ: Cancer risk assessment and genetic counseling in an academic medical center: Consultants' satisfaction, knowledge, and behavior in the first year. *J Genet Counseling* **7**:279, 1998.

141. American Society of Clinical Oncology: Resource document for curriculum development in cancer genetics education. *J Clin Oncol* **15**:2157, 1997.

142. Niederhuber JE: Genetic testings for cancer: The surgeon's critical role. *J Am Coll Surg* **188**:74, 1999.

143. Webb MJ: Genetic testing and management of the cancer patient and cancer families. *Obstet Gynecol Symposium* **187**:449, 1998.

144. Engelking C: Genetics in cancer care: Confronting a Pandora's box of dilemmas. *Oncol Nurs Forum* **22**:27, 1995.

145. Li FP, Fraumeni JF Jr, Mulvihill JJ, Blattner WA, Dreyfus MG, Tucker MA, Miller RW: A cancer family syndrome in twenty-four kindreds. *Cancer Res* **48**:5358, 1988.

146. Herrera L (ed.): *Familial Adenomatous Polyposis*. New York, Liss, 1990.

147. Petersen GM, Brensinger J: Gene tests and genetic counseling in familial adenomatous polyposis. *Oncology* **10**:89, 1996.

148. Hamilton SR, Liu B, Parsons RE, Papadopoulos N, Jen J, Powell SM, Krush AJ, et al: The molecular basis of Turcot's syndrome. *N Engl J Med* **332**:839, 1995.

149. Ford D, Easton DF: The genetics of breast and ovarian cancer. *Br J Cancer* **72**:805, 1995.

150. Futreal PA, Liu Q, Shattuck-Eidens D, Cochran C, Harshman K, Tavtigian S, Bennett LM, et al: BRCA1 mutations in primary breast and ovarian carcinomas. *Science* **266**:120, 1994.

151. Tavtigian SV, Simard J, Rommens J, Couch F, Shattuck-Eidens D, Neuhausen S, Merajver S, et al: The complete BRCA2 gene and mutations in chromosome 13q-linked kindreds. *Nature Genet* **12**:333, 1996.

152. Burke W, Petersen G, Lynch P, Botkin J, Daly M, Garber J, Kahn MJE, et al: Recommendations for follow-up care of individuals with HNPCC-associated mutations. *JAMA* **277**:915, 1997.

153. Geller G, Botkin JR, Green MJ, Press N, Biesecker BB, Wilfond B, Grana G, et al: Genetic testing for susceptibility to adult-onset cancer. The process and content of informed consent. *JAMA* **277**:1467, 1997.

154. Savitsky K, Bar-Shira A, Gilad S, Rotman G, Ziv Y, Vanagaite L, Tagle DA, et al: A single ataxia telangiectasia gene with a product similar to PI-3 kinase. *Science* **268**:1749, 1995.

155. Li J, Yen C, Liaw D, Podsypanina K, Bose S, Wang SI, Puc J, et al: PTEN, a putative protein tyrosine phosphatase gene mutated in human brain, breast, and prostate cancer. *Science* **275**:1943, 1997.

156. Liaw D, Marsh DJ, Li J, Dahia PL, Wang SI, Zheng Z, Bose S, et al: Germline mutations of the PTEN gene in Cowden disease, an inherited breast and thyroid cancer syndrome. *Nature Genet* **16**:64, 1997.

157. Kinzler KW, Nilbert MC, Su L-K, Vogelstein B, Bryan TM, Levy DB, Smith KJ, et al: Identification of FAP locus genes from chromosome 5q21. *Science* **253**:661, 1991.

158. Groden J, Thliveris A, Samowitz W, Carlson M, Gelbert L, Albertsen H, Joslyn G, et al: Identification and characterization of the familial adenomatous polyposis coli gene. *Cell* **66**:589, 1991.

159. Guilford P, Hopkins J, Harraway J, McLeod M, McLeod N, Harawira P, Taite H, et al: E-cadherin germline mutations in familial gastric cancer. *Nature* **392**:402, 1998.

160. Kamb A, Shattuck-Eidens D, Eeles R, Liu Q, Gruis NA, Ding W, Hussey C, et al: Analysis of the p16 gene (CDKN2) as a candidate for the chromosome 9p melanoma susceptibility locus. *Nat Genet* **8**:23, 1994.

161. Farndon PA, Del Mastro RG, Evans DGR, Kilpatrick MW: Location of the gene for Gorlin syndrome. *Lancet* **339**:581, 1992.

162. Reis A, Kuster W, Linss G, Gebel E, Fuhrmann W, Groth W, Kuklik M, et al: Localisation of gene for the nevoid basal cell carcinoma syndrome. *Lancet* **339**:617, 1992.

163. Gailani MR, Bale SJ, Leffell DJ, DiGiovanna JJ, Peck GL, Poliak S, Drum MA, et al: Developmental defects in Gorlin syndrome related to a putative tumor suppressor gene on chromosome 9. *Cell* **69**:111, 1992.

164. Miyaki M, Konishi M, Tanaka K, Kikuchi-Yanoshita R, Muraoka M, Yasuno M, et al: Germline mutation of MSH6 as the cause of

hereditary nonpolyposis colorectal cancer. *Nat Genet* **17**:271, 1997.

165. Smith JR, Freije D, Carpten JD, Grönberg H, Xu J, Isaacs SD, Brownstein MJ, et al: Major susceptibility locus for prostate cancer on chromosome 1 suggested by a genome-wide search. *Science* **274**:1301, 1996.

166. Xu J, Meyers D, Freije D, Isaacs S, Wiley K, Nusskern D, Ewing C, et al: Evidence for a prostate cancer susceptibility locus on the X chromosome. *Nature Genet* **20**:175, 1998.

167. Malkin D, Li FP, Strong LC, Fraumeni JF Jr., Nelson CE, Kim DH, Kassel J, et al: Germ line p53 mutations in a familial syndrome of breast cancer, sarcomas, and other neoplasms. *Science* **250**:1233, 1990.

168. Larsson C, Skogseid B, Oberg K, Nakamura Y, Nordenskjold M: Multiple endocrine neoplasia type 1 gene maps to chromosome 11 and is lost in insulinoma. *Nature* **332**:85, 1988.

169. Mulligan LM, Kwok JBJ, Healey CS, Elsdon MJ, Eng C, Gardner E, Love DR, et al: Germ-line mutations of the RET proto-oncogene in multiple endocrine neoplasia type 2A. *Nature* **363**:458, 1993.

170. Hofstra RM, Landsvater RM, Ceccherini I, Stulp RP, Stelwagen T, Luo Y, Pasini B, et al: A mutation in the RET proto-oncogene associated with multiple endocrine neoplasia type 2B and sporadic medullary thyroid carcinoma. *Nature* **367**:375, 1994.

171. Carlson KM, Dou S, Chi D, Scavarda N, Toshima K, Jackson CE, Wells SA Jr., et al: Single missense mutation in the tyrosine kinase catalytic domain of the RET protooncogene is associated with multiple endocrine neoplasia type 2B. *Proc Natl Acad Sci USA* **91**:1579, 1994.

172. Rouleau GA, Wertelecki W, Haines JL, Hobbs WJ, Trofatter JA, Seizinger BR, Martuza RL, et al: Genetic linkage of bilateral acoustic neurofibromatosis to a DNA marker on chromosome 22. *Nature* **329**:246, 1987.

173. Barker D, Wright E, Nguyen K, Cannon L, Fain P, Goldgar D, Bishop DT, et al: Gene for von Recklinghausen neurofibromatosis is in the pericentromeric region of chromosome 17. *Science* **236**:1100, 1987.

174. Seizinger BR, Rouleau GA, Ozelius LJ, Lane AH, Faryniarz AG, Chao MV, Huson S, et al: Genetic linkage of von Recklinghausen neurofibromatosis to the nerve growth factor receptor gene. *Cell* **49**:589, 1987.

175. Wallace MR, Marchuk DA, Andersen LB, Letcher R, Odeh HM, Saulino AM, Fountain JW, et al: Type 1 neurofibromatosis gene: Identification of a large transcript disrupted in three NF1 patients. *Science* **249**:181, 1990.

176. Cawthon RM, Weiss R, Xu GF, Viskochil D, Culver M, Stevens J, Robertson M, et al: A major segment of the neurofibromatosis type 1 gene: cDNA sequence, genomic structure, and point mutations. *Cell* **62**:193, 1990.

177. Trofatter JA, MacCollin MM, Rutter JL, Murrell JR, Duyao MP, Parry DM, et al.: A novel moesin-, ezrin-, radixin-like gene is a candidate for the neurofibromatosis 2 tumor suppressor. *Cell* **75**:826, 1993.

178. Hemminki A, Markie D, Tomlinson I, Avizienyte E, Roth S, Loukola A, Bignell G, et al: A serine/threonine kinase gene defective in Peutz-Jeghers syndrome. *Nature* **391**:184, 1998.

179. Jenne DE, Reimann H, Nezu J-I, Friedel W, Loff S, Jeschke R, Müller O, et al: Peutz-Jeghers syndrome is caused by mutations in a novel serine threonine kinase. *Nature Genet* **18**:38, 1998.

180. Cavenee WK, Hansen MF, Nordenskjold M, Kock E, Maumenee I, Squire JA, Phillips RA, et al: Genetic origin of mutations predisposing to retinoblastoma. *Science* **228**:501, 1985.

181. Lee W-H, Bookstein R, Hong F, Young L-J, Shew J-Y, Lee EYP: Human retinoblastoma susceptibility gene: Cloning, identification, and sequence. *Science* **235**:1394, 1987.

182. Latif F, Tory K, Gnarra J, Yao M, Duh F-M, Orcutt ML, Stackhous T, et al: Identification of the von Hippel-Lindau disease tumor suppressor gene. *Science* **260**:1317, 1993.

CANCER BY SITE

Pancreatic Cancer

Ralph H. Hruban ■ *Charles J. Yeo* *Scott E. Kern*

1. Pancreatic ductal adenocarcinoma is the fifth leading cause of cancer death in the United States. It is estimated that approximately 28,000 Americans were diagnosed with pancreatic cancer in 2000. It is a nearly uniformly fatal disease, and the mortality rate closely follows that of the incidence. Pancreatic cancer presents clinically with pain, with symptoms related to obstruction of the biliary or pancreatic ducts, or with protean symptoms such as weight loss and cachexia.

2. Although most carcinomas of the pancreas appear to be sporadic, a number of anecdotal case reports and case-control studies suggest that as many as 10 percent of all cases of pancreatic carcinoma are hereditary. The gene or genes responsible for the familial aggregation of pancreatic cancer largely are unknown, but germ-line mutations in the *BRCA2*, *STK11/LKB11*, *PRSS1* and *p16* genes, have been shown to predispose to pancreatic cancer, although with incomplete penetrance.

3. The profile of genetic mutations in pancreatic cancer is distinct from other neoplasms. The K-*ras* oncogene is commonly activated by somatic mutations in pancreatic cancer, whereas three tumor-suppressor genes are commonly inactivated. Ninety percent or more of pancreatic cancers harbor activating point mutations in codon 12 of K-*ras*. The *p16* tumor-suppressor gene is inactivated in 90 to 100 percent of pancreatic cancers, *p53* in 50 to 75 percent, and *DPC4* in 55 percent. In addition, occasional somatic mutations of the *RB1*, *MKK4*, *STK11/LKB1*, *ALK4* and *TGFβ* receptor genes also have been reported. Various gene amplifications affect a minority of carcinomas.

4. Inactivation of the *DPC4* gene may be rather specific for pancreatic neoplasia. *DPC4* is inactivated in as few as 15 percent of colorectal cancers and in less than 10 percent of other major cancer types. Dpc4 belongs to a class of proteins that mediate signals of the TGFβ superfamily.

5. Microsatellite instability (RER+) is seen in a small minority (~4 percent) of pancreatic cancers. These RER+ cancers have a characteristic histologic appearance and frequently have wild-type K-*ras* genes.

6. Pancreatic cancer is likely to harbor changes in additional yet uncharacterized genes. Chromosome arms with unexplained losses of heterozygosity at frequencies of greater than 40 percent in pancreatic cancer include 1p, 6p, 8p, 12q, 13q, 21q, and 22q.

7. A large number of pancreatic cancers have been karyotyped. Double minute chromosomes, possibly representing gene amplification, were identified in 8 percent of pancreatic cancers in one study. These karyotyping studies also provide an understanding of the structural basis for genetic losses identified at the molecular level. Sites having loss of heterozygosity tend to correspond to sites of karyotypic abnormalities in individual tumors.

8. The diagnosis of pancreatic cancer is suspected based on clinical findings and often can be confirmed with radiologic and endoscopic techniques. Effective screening tests are not available yet.

Adenocarcinoma of the pancreas is one of the most aggressive of human malignancies. It typically presents late in the course of the disease, with nonspecific symptoms. As a result, patients with pancreatic cancer have an extremely poor prognosis, with an overall 5-year survival rate of less than 5 percent.[1] However, those patients with early, surgically resectable carcinomas have a substantially improved prognosis. Clearly, early detection of the carcinoma, before it has spread beyond the pancreas, is the key to the successful treatment of patients with pancreatic carcinoma. A better understanding of the molecular genetic alterations in pancreatic cancer may lead to the development of new tests to detect this cancer earlier.

Until recently, our understanding of the genetics of pancreatic cancer was very incomplete. In large part, this was because of difficulties presented by the carcinomas themselves. Pancreatic cancers induce a prominent nonneoplastic reaction. As a result, the neoplastic cells constitute only a small minority of the cells in the tumor. This problem of low neoplastic cellularity has hampered the molecular analyses of pancreatic cancer. Recent efforts, however, have overcome this obstacle by selectively enriching for neoplastic cells by propagating the cancers in tissue culture or in immunodeficient mice. Once a mutation is identified in these enriched populations, it can be confirmed by a sensitive assay of the original primary tumor. Indeed, these techniques are a major advance in our ability to analyze pancreatic cancers, and pancreatic cancer now boasts an extensive molecular description.[2] Whereas much of what is known about pancreatic cancer has been learned by the study of sporadic pancreatic cancers, some genes that have been identified in sporadic carcinomas also have been found to play a role in the development of inherited forms of pancreatic cancer.

In this chapter we will focus on the advances in our understanding of the molecular genetic alterations in human ductal adenocarcinoma of the pancreas, since this tumor type accounts for the majority of pancreatic neoplasms.

CLINICAL ASPECTS OF ADENOCARCINOMA OF THE PANCREAS

Incidence

Adenocarcinoma of the pancreas is the fifth leading cause of cancer death in the United States.[1] In 2000, approximately 28,000 new cases of pancreas cancer were diagnosed in the United States, and nearly the same number died from it.[1] These patients are mostly elderly.[3] The incidence of pancreatic cancer increases steadily with age, and approximately 80 percent of the cancers

---

A list of standard abbreviations is located immediately preceding the index. Nonstandard abbreviations used in this chapter include: HNPCC = hereditary nonpolyposis colorectal carcinoma; FAMMM = familial atypical multiple-mole melanoma; LOH = loss of heterozygosity; RDA = representational difference analysis; PanIN = pancreatic intraepithelial neoplasia.

occur in the seventh and eight decades of life.[4] Pancreatic cancer is extremely uncommon before the age of 40, although cases have been reported in children.[5] Pancreatic cancer appears to occur slightly more commonly in men than in women and, in the United States, in African-Americans more frequently than in whites.[3,4] The incidence of pancreatic cancer is higher among Jews than among non-Jews, and it is higher in Western industrialized countries than it is in the third world.[6,7] Among white males, the incidence and mortality rates from pancreatic cancer have been decreasing slowly since the 1970s, but during this same period of time, the mortality rates among African-American women have increased slightly.[1]

A number of environmental factors have been studied as possible etiologic agents in the development of pancreatic cancer, and cigarette smoking has the highest association with pancreatic cancer.[3,8–11] For example, smoking during college has been associated with a 2.6-fold risk of developing pancreatic cancer.[12] In addition, the risk of developing pancreatic cancer increases in relation to the duration of smoking and the number of cigarettes smoked.[4,13]

Diets high in meat and fat and low in fiber also may predispose to the development of pancreatic cancer, but the role of alcohol consumption is less clear.[4,13–17] Based on an early well-publicized study, coffee was once thought to be a possible risk factor for the development of pancreatic cancer. This study, however, had serious methodologic flaws, and coffee is now not felt to be a significant risk factor.[15,16] Thus age and cigarette smoking remain the greatest risk factors for developing pancreatic cancer.

Familial Patterns of Pancreatic Cancer

Almost all cancers show a tendency to aggregate in families, but the fraction of cancer that is hereditary varies substantially among different cancer types.[18] There have been a number of case reports in the literature that suggest that there is a familial form of pancreatic cancer.[19–34] For example, Lynch et al. described 47 individuals with pancreatic cancer in 18 families in which multiple family members had pancreatic cancer.[20] The age of onset (median 70 years), histologic types, and survival times of these 47 patients were comparable with published data on unselected patients with pancreatic cancer, and there appeared to be an autosomal dominant mode of transmission in several of the families.[20,34] Based on these family studies, it has been suggested that as many as 10 percent of the cases of pancreatic cancer are hereditary.[24] Similarly, Ghadirian et al. interviewed 179 patients with pancreatic cancer and 179 controls matched for gender and age, and they reported that 7.8 percent of the patients with pancreatic cancer had a family history of pancreatic cancer, compared with only 0.6 percent of control patients without pancreatic cancer ($p < 0.01$).[35] Fernandez et al. also studied the relationship of family history to the development of pancreatic cancer.[36] They conducted a case-control study in northern Italy of 362 patients with histologically confirmed pancreatic cancer and 1408 controls admitted to the hospital for acute, nonneoplastic, non-digestive tract disorders.[36] Significantly more of the patients with pancreatic cancer had a family history of pancreatic cancer than did the controls ($RR = 3.0$). From their data they estimated that 3 percent of newly diagnosed pancreatic cancers were familial.[36] Similarly, we recently analyzed 212 kindreds enrolled in the National Familial Pancreas Tumor Registry (NFPTR).[*] *Familial* pancreatic kindreds were defined as those families in which there had been at least two first-degree relatives diagnosed with pancreatic cancer, and we found that second-degree relatives of patients with familial pancreatic cancer are at increased risk for developing pancreatic cancer.[37]

Thus anecdotal reports and several case-control studies suggest that between 3 and 10 percent of pancreatic cancers are caused by

inherited factors, and even second-degree relatives of patients with pancreatic cancer are at increased risk for developing the disease.

Diagnosing Pancreatic Cancer

Although the pancreas is located deep in the retroperitoneal space, it can be visualized with sophisticated imaging techniques.[38] Spiral (or helical) computed tomography (CT) is the best of these techniques, and other commonly used techniques include real-time ultrasonography, magnetic resonance imaging (MRI), angiography, endoscopic retrograde cholangiopancreatography, and endoscopic ultrasonography. Despite the introduction of these new techniques, the death rate for pancreatic carcinoma has not changed significantly. This is not surprising, since the biggest determinant of patient outcome is stage at diagnosis, and these tools do not currently influence the timing of patient presentation.[38] The survival rate for pancreatic cancer will not improve significantly until new tests are developed to screen for the disease before patients become symptomatic.

Although all the imaging techniques may reveal a suspicious mass in the pancreas, the "gold standard" for diagnosing pancreatic cancer remains histopathology. Tissue for microscopic examination can be obtained either by fine-needle aspiration, by tissue needle core biopsy, or by excisional biopsy at the time of laparotomy.[38,39] Again, as was true for imaging, the need for biopsy is likely to be apparent only after the disease has advanced.[40]

Pathology of Pancreatic Cancer

The most common type of exocrine pancreatic cancer is the duct cell adenocarcinoma.[41–43] The majority of these cancers arise in the head of the pancreas (60 percent) and the remainder in the body (13 percent), tail (5 percent) or infiltrate diffusely throughout the gland (21 percent).[42] By light microscopy, adenocarcinomas of the pancreas are composed of neoplastic glands infiltrating a dense nonneoplastic stroma (Fig. 40-1). Numerous inflammatory cells, including lymphocytes, also are frequently admixed with the tumor cells. This nonneoplastic host response is characteristic of pancreatic cancers, and it must be considered when conducting molecular analyses of allelic loss, since DNA isolated from most pancreatic cancers contains predominantly normal DNA. Perineural (Fig. 40-2) and vascular invasion is seen frequently in pancreatic cancers, as is infiltration of adjacent structures and metastases to regional lymph nodes (Fig 40-3).

Infiltrating adenocarcinoma of the pancreas frequently is associated with dramatic histologic changes in the pancreatic ducts and ductules. The normal pancreatic ducts and ductules are lined by a single layer of cuboidal to columnar epithelial cells, but in most pancreata with cancer this epithelium is regionally replaced by a proliferative epithelium with varying degrees of cytologic and architectural atypia.[44] A new international nomenclature has recently been adopted for these duct lesions.[43–46,46A] The term *pancreatic intraepithelial neoplasia-1A (PanIN-1A)* refers to a uniform increase in the mucin content of the epithelial cells *PanIN-1B* to the presence of papillae lined by columnar cells without atypia and *PanIN-2* to papillary lesions with moderate nuclear enlargement and a moderate increase in nuclear-to-cytoplasmic ratio. Finally, *PanIN-3* is used to designate duct lesions with significant nuclear enlargement, a significantly increased nuclear-to-cytoplasmic ratio, loss of cellular polarity, and significant nuclear pleomorphism.[46A] It is hoped that this new nomenclature will help standardize the classification of these lesions and therefore facilitate their molecular analysis. The histology of selected duct lesions is illustrated in Fig. 40-4.

These various duct lesions are more common in pancreata with cancer than they are in pancreata without cancer.[45–48] For example, Cubilla and Fitzgerald compared the duct changes in 227 pancreata with pancreatic cancer with the duct changes in 100 age- and sex-matched controls without pancreatic cancer.[45] They

---

*The National Familial Pancreas Tumor Registry, The Johns Hopkins Hospital, Department of Pathology, Weinberg 2242, 401 N. Broadway, Baltimore, MD 21231 (410) 955-9132; (410) 955-0115 (fax); e-mail: *rhruban@jhmi.edu*.

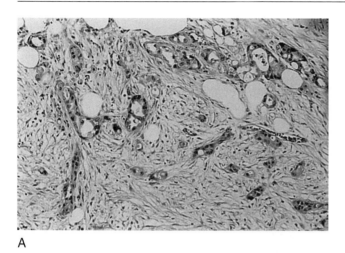

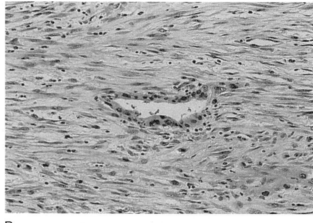

A   B

Fig. 40-1 Infiltrating adenocarcinoma of the pancreas. Note the haphazard arrangement of markedly atypical glands (**A**) and the intense nonneoplastic inflammatory and fibroblastic response elicited by the carcinoma (**B**). (**A,B** both hematoxylin and eosin).

found that papillary lesions were three times more common in the pancreata obtained from patients with pancreatic cancer than they were in pancreata obtained from patients without pancreatic cancer and that atypical papillary lesions were seen only in pancreata with pancreas cancer.[45] These findings have been confirmed by Kozuka et al. and Pour et al.[47,48] More recently Furukawa et al., using three-dimensional mapping techniques, have demonstrated a stepwise progression from mild dysplasia to severe dysplasia in pancreatic duct lesions.[46] These results suggest that infiltrating cancers of the pancreas arise from precursors in the pancreatic ducts—that there is a progression in the pancreas from PanIN-1A (Fig. 40-4A), to PanIN-1B (Figs. 40-4A–C), to PanIN-2 (Fig. 40-4D), to PanIN-3, to infiltrating adenocarcinoma[41,43,49] (see Figs. 40-1 and 40-2). This hypothesis, however, is based on observations of fixed static specimens. Serial samples taken over time would be needed to demonstrate that, in fact, these lesions in pancreatic ducts can progress to infiltrating cancer.[49] Brat et al. have recently done just that, in a series of patients followed after partial pancreatectomy. Brat et al. reported three patients in whom PanIN-3 was documented 17 months, 9 years, and 10 years before the development of an infiltrating cancer of the pancreas.[43,49] These morphologic observations therefore strongly suggest that just as there is a progression from adenoma to infiltrating cancer in the colorectum, so too is there a progression from PanINs to infiltrating cancer in the pancreas.[49] Furthermore, these results suggest that these lesions in the pancreatic ducts are

not in actuality hyperplasias but instead represent part of the neoplastic process—hence the new PanIN nomenclature.

GENETIC LOCI

Genetic Loci Involved in Hereditary Pancreatic Cancer

It has proven difficult to perform classic linkage studies in families with pancreatic cancer because of the small size of most kindreds and the short life expectancy of patients with carcinoma of the pancreas. Nonetheless, analyses of families in which there is an aggregation of pancreatic cancer may provide clues as to which genes are involved in hereditary pancreatic cancer.

Families with an aggregation of pancreatic cancer can be divided into three general groups: (1) those associated with known syndromes, (2) those in which there is an aggregation of pancreatic cancers but not part of a known syndrome, and (3) those in which there is an association of pancreatic with nonpancreatic cancers.

Syndromes Associated with Pancreatic Cancer. Several well-characterized genetic syndromes have been shown to predispose affected family members to the development of pancreatic cancer.[33,37] These include hereditary pancreatitis, hereditary nonpolyposis colorectal carcinoma (HNPCC, Lynch syndrome), a subset of the familial atypical multiple-mole melanoma

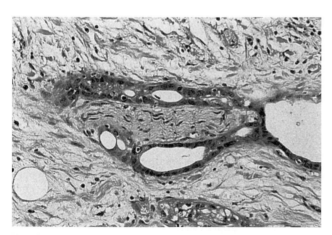

Fig. 40-2 Infiltrating adenocarcinoma of the pancreas growing along a nerve. Pain is a common symptom of pancreatic cancer (hematoxylin and eosin).

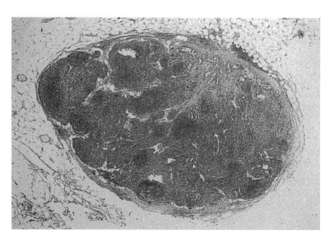

Fig. 40-3 Metastatic adenocarcinoma of the pancreas in a lymph node. The carcinoma has metastasized to the upper right-hand corner of this node (hematolylin and eosin).

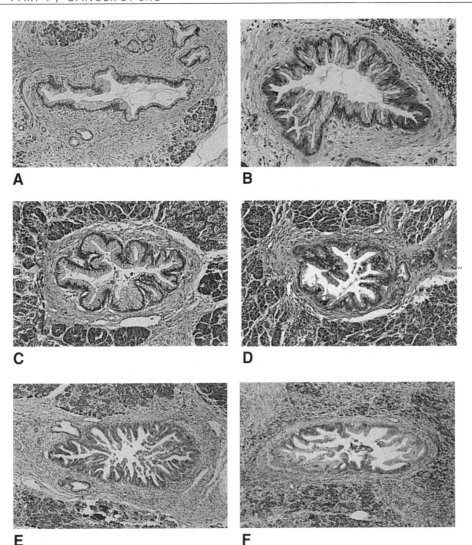

A

B

C

D

E

F

Fig. 40-4 PanINs, from pancreata with cancer. Note the progression from PanIN-1A (*A*), to PanIN-1B (*B, C*), to PanIN-2 (*D*), to PanIN-3 (*E, F,* carcinoma *in situ*) (all hematoxylin and eosin).

(FAMMM) syndrome, the Peutz-Jeghers syndrome, familial breast cancer (*BRCA2*), and ataxia telangiectasia[33,34] (Table 40-1).

Hereditary Pancreatitis. Hereditary pancreatitis is an autosomal dominant disorder with incomplete penetrance characterized by recurrent episodes of severe pancreatitis in blood-related family members over two generations.[50–53] There is often an early age of

onset of the pancreatitis, and the patients frequently develop chronic pancreatitis. Men are affected at the same rate as women.[34] Familial pancreatitis recently has been shown by Whitcomb et al. to be caused by mutations in the *cationic trypsinogen* gene on 7q35.[53,54] These authors constructed a 500-member pedigree from a U.S. kindred centered in eastern Kentucky and Western Virginia, and using microsatellite markers

Table 40-1 Hereditary Syndromes Associated with Pancreatic Cancer

Syndrome	Mode of Inheritance	Gene	Chromosome Locus	Manifestation
Hereditary pancreatitis	AD	*cationic trypsinogen*	7q35	Recurrent episodes of severe pancreatitis occurring at an early age
HNPCC	AD	*MSH2*	2p	Colonic, endometrial, and stomach cancers; mutator penotype
		MLH1	3p	
		PMS2	7p	
		PMS1	2q	
FAMMM	AD	*p16*	9p	Multiple nevi, atypical nevi, melanomas
Peutz-Jeghers	AD	*LKB1*	19p	Hamartomatous polyps of the gastrointestinal tract, mucocutaneous melanin macules
Familial breast cancer 2	AD	*BRCA2*	13q	Breast, ovarian, and pancreatic cancer
Ataxia telangiectasia	AR	*ATM*	11q22–23	Cerebellar ataxia, oculocutaneous telangiectasia, thymic hypoplasia

NOTE: HNPCC = hereditary nonpolyposis colorectal cancer; FAMMM = familial atypical mole–multiple melanoma; AD = autosomal dominant; AR = autosomal recessive.

and linkage analysis, they were able to establish cosegregation between the familial pancreatitis phenotype and the 7q35 locus.[53] The *cationic trypsinogen* gene resides at 7q35, and Whitcomb et al. demonstrated that an Arg-His substitution at residue 117 of this gene segregates with the hereditary pancreatitis in some families.[54] Mutations at this site block the inactivation of trypsin, resulting in autodigestion of the pancreas. The mechanism by which pancreatitis leads to the development of pancreatic cancer is not clear; however, some have suggested that the increased risk of pancreatic cancer observed in patients with chronic pancreatitis is secondary to chronic injury and regeneration from the pancreatitis itself.[33,55,56]

HNPCC. Hereditary nonpolyposis colorectal cancer is another syndrome that predisposes affected individuals to pancreatic cancers.[19,34] This syndrome is characterized by the autosomal dominant transmission of a predisposition to colonic cancer in association with other cancers, including endometrial, stomach, and pancreatic cancer.[23,57–59] HNPCC is caused by germ-line mutations in one of the DNA mismatch repair genes.[60–65] These genes include *hMSH2, hMSH1, hPMS2, hPMS1, hMSH6/GTBP,* and *hMSH3,* and they code for proteins that repair single-base-pair changes and small insertions/deletions that occur during DNA replication.[61,62,66–69] When one of these genes is inactivated in a neoplasm, the neoplastic cells accumulate mutations in small noncoding regions of the genome called *microsatellite repeats,* resulting in changes in length of these repeats, a phenotype called *microsatellite instability.* Of note, replication errors, such as those found in HNPCC, are found in approximately 4 percent of pancreatic cancers,[67,70,71,71A] and as noted previously, pancreatic cancer has been reported in some HNPCC kindreds.[23,57–59]

Peutz-Jeghers. The Peutz-Jeghers syndrome is a hereditary disease with an autosomal dominant pattern of inheritance characterized by hamartomatous polyps of the gastrointestinal tract and mucocutaneous melanocytic macules.[72] Forty-eight percent of 31 patients with Peutz-Jeghers syndrome followed by Giardiello et al. developed cancer, and 4 of these cancers were pancreatic cancer.[73] This represents a 100-fold excess of pancreatic cancer compared with that expected.[73A] The Peutz-Jeghers syndrome recently has been shown to be caused by germ-line mutations in the *LKB1/STK11* gene on 19p.[74,75] *LKB1* has strong homology to a cytoplasmic *Xenopus* serine threonine protein kinase, *XEEK1.* Peutz-Jeghers is therefore the first cancer-susceptibility syndrome to be identified that is attributable to inactivating mutations in a protein kinase.[74,75] Su et al. recently have demonstrated loss of the wild-type *LKB1* allele in a pancreatic cancer from a patient with a germ-line *LKB1* mutation and the Peutz-Jeghers syndrome.[76]

FAMMM. A subset of patients with the FAMMM syndrome appear to be at increased risk for developing pancreatic cancer.[21,33,34] The FAMMM syndrome is inherited in an autosomal dominant fashion and is characterized by multiple nevi, multiple atypical nevi, and multiple cutaneous malignant melanomas.[21,77,78] Germ-line mutations in *p16* have been shown to segregate with the increased risks of pancreatic cancer in some kindreds with the FAMMM syndrome.[77,78] Of interest, although the risk of pancreatic cancer is increased in these kindreds, it is not a highly penetrant trait. In these families there may be a tendency for mutations at the C-terminal end of the *p16* gene to be associated with a higher penetrance for pancreatic cancer.[79]

Ataxia Telangectasia. Although the association is not as well established as it is for the other syndromes, patients with ataxia telangiectasia also may be at increased risk for developing pancreatic cancer.[33,34] Ataxia telangiectasia is characterized by progressive cerebellar ataxia with degeneration of Purkinje cells, telangiectasias (primarily conjuctival), thymic hypoplasia with cellular and humoral immunodeficiencies, and oculomotor apraxia. Ataxia telangiectasia is inherited in an autosomal recessive pattern, and the gene responsible for this syndrome has been cloned recently. The *ATM* gene resides on chromosome 11q22-23, and it encodes for a protein that is similar to several yeast and mammalian phosphatidylinositol 3' kinases involved in mitogenic signal transduction, meiotic recombination, and cell cycle control.[80] Patients with ataxia telangiectasia are at increased risk for developing a number of neoplasms, including ovarian cancer, biliary cancer, gastric cancer, leukemia, lymphoma, and possibly pancreatic cancer.[33,34,80]

Families with an Aggregation of Pancreatic Cancer. Although a number of well-characterized syndromes have been associated with an increased risk of pancreatic cancer, the majority of pancreatic cancers cannot be explained in this way. In many families, pancreatic cancer occurs independent of a known syndrome. For example, Henry Lynch at Creighton University has reported over 30 extended families with multiple cases of pancreatic carcinoma.[19–25,34] He identified a suspected autosomal dominant mode of transmission in some of his pedigrees and estimated that between 5 and 10 percent of all pancreatic cancers have a hereditary origin.[24,34] Lynch notes, however, that the clustering of a cancer in a family does not necessarily mean that the cancer is hereditary. Environmental exposures need to be considered. For example, it is possible that several members of a family developed cancer because they each had smoked cigarettes.[33] Nonetheless, these families provide a unique opportunity to study efficiently the clinical patterns and genetics of pancreatic cancer.

We therefore established the National Familial Pancreas Tumor Registry (NFPTR) at Johns Hopkins in 1994 . This is now one of the largest registries of families in which more than one family member is affected with pancreatic cancer.[*] Two-hundred fifty-five families with two or more first-degree relatives having cancer of the pancreas have enrolled in this registry as of January 2001. The average age at diagnosis for patients with pancreatic cancer in these families (65.5 years) does not appear to differ from the age of onset of pancreatic carcinomas that are apparently sporadic.[37] Approximately 20 percent of the patients with pancreatic cancer enrolled in this registry developed a second non-pancreatic cancer.[37] These cancers included breast cancer, colon cancer, melanoma, bladder cancer, lung cancer, and prostate cancer.[37] As discussed previously, analyses of the kindred enrolled in this registry have demonstrated that second-degree relatives of patients from kindreds with familial pancreatic cancer are at increased risk for developing pancreatic cancer compared with second-degree relatives of patients from families in which only one first-degree relative developed pancreatic cancer (3.7 percent versus 0.6 percent, $p < 0.0001$).[37] Nonpancreatic cancers also were increased in second-degree relatives of the familial pancreatic cancer cases (27.2 percent versus 12.1 percent, $p < 0.0001$). The other types of cancer that developed in these patients included breast cancer, lung cancer, and colon cancer.[37] More recently, Tersmette et al. followed the first 241 kindreds enrolled in the NFPTR to estimate the prospective risk of pancreatic cancer among first-degree relatives of pancreatic cancer patients in familial pancreatic cancer kindreds.[80A] Risk was estimated by comparing observed new cases of pancreatic cancer to expected numbers based on United States population-based Surveillance, Epidemiology, and End Results (SEER) program data. Remarkably, there was a significantly increased 18-fold risk (95% CI=4.7–44.5) of pancreatic cancer among first-degree relatives in the familial pancreatic cancer kindreds (Table 40-2).[80A] This risk rose to 57-fold if there were three or more affected family members at the time of enrollment.

Members of these registries, as well as those of registries created for other cancer types, are an important resource that can

---

*The National Familial Pancreas Tumor Registry, The Johns Hopkins Hospital, Department of Pathology, Weinberg 2242, 401 N. Broadway, Baltimore, MD 21231 (410) 955-9132; (410) 955-0115 (fax); e-mail: *rhruban@jhmi.edu.*

Table 40-2 Prospective Risk and Incidence of Pancreatic Cancer (PC) Among At-Risk First-Degree Relatives in the National Familial Pancreatic Tumor Registry (NFPTR).

Number of PC in Kindred at Time of Registry in NFPTR	Number of At-Risk First-Degree Relatives Followed	Age Group (years)	Person-years at Risk	Number of Incident Pancreatic Cancers				Incidence (per 10^5/year)
				Observed	Expected	O/E	95% C.I.	
1*		0–29	167	0	0	1.00	–	0
		30–59	971	1	0.04	25.2	0.63–139	20.6
		60–84	493	1	0.27	3.8	0.09–20.6	40.6
	642	Total	1631	2	0.31	6.5	0.78–23.3	24.5
2 or more**		0–29	81	0	0	1.00	–	0
		30–59	612	1	0.03	39.3	0.84–186	32.7
		60–84	359	3	0.19	15.5	3.3–46.1	167.0
	598	Total	1052	4	0.23	18.3	4.74–44.50	76.0
		0–29	16	0	0	1.00	–	0
		30–59	93	0	0	1.00	–	0
		60–84	91	3	0.05	61.09	12.4–175.0	660.8
3 or more**	105	Total	199	3	0.05	56.6	12.4–175.0	301.4

* Sporadic PC kindreds. These kindreds did not have a pair of first-degree relatives with pancreatic cancer, but may have contained family members with PC who were more distantly related to the index case.
** Familial PC kindreds. Kindreds containing at least a pair of first-degree relatives with PC. Kindreds with 3 or more are a subset of kindreds with 2 or more.
SOURCE: Reproduced with permission from American Association for Cancer Research, Inc., Tersmette AC et al: *Clin Cancer Res*, 7:738, 2001.

be used to determine the contribution of environmental risk factors, the patterns of inheritance of pancreatic cancer, and the types and prevalence of other tumor types (such as melanoma, breast cancer, and ovarian cancer) in familial pancreatic cancer.[81,82] The results of these analyses should provide a basis for counseling families with a familial aggregation of pancreatic cancer.

Families in Which There Is an Association of Pancreatic with Nonpancreatic Cancers. Several other cancers, including those of the breast and ovary, have been associated with pancreatic cancer in some families.[34] Tulinius et al. analyzed the cancer risk for family members of 947 randomly selected female breast cancer patients in the Icelandic Cancer Registry.[83] They found more cases of pancreatic cancer than expected in male first-degree relatives of the breast cancer patients ($RR = 1.66$).[83] Kerber and Slattery, in a case-control study of the Utah Population Database, found that a family history of pancreatic cancer is significantly associated with an increased risk of ovarian cancer.[84] From this Kerber and Slattery estimate that a family history of pancreatic cancer accounted for 4.8 percent of the cases of ovarian cancer.[84] Similarly, genetically defined subsets of families with familial melanoma and with familial breast cancer have been found to have an increased incidence of pancreatic cancer.[77,78,85–88]

Currently, a minority of the cases in which there is an aggregation of pancreatic cancer can be accounted for by known syndromes or by an association of nonpancreatic with pancreatic cancers. Each form of familial pancreatic cancer has, however, provided insights and fresh opportunities to study the genetics of pancreatic cancer. In turn, the results of these analyses will provide insight into the etiology of pancreatic cancers that are apparently sporadic.

Genetic Loci Involved in Sporadic Pancreatic Cancer

Three general approaches have been taken in the search for the genetic loci involved in the development of pancreatic cancer. The identity of specific chromosomes lost or gained by the pancreatic cancer can be determined by the karyotypes of metaphase spreads obtained from fresh cancers. These cytogenetic studies provide structural information about the mechanisms responsible for the loss or gain of genetic material, but the resolution of this technique

is limited. More detailed information can be obtained by looking for loss of heterozygosity (LOH) using a panel of molecular probes specific for each chromosome arm. Such allelotypes were used in the identification of the novel *DPC4* tumor-suppressor gene in a panel of pancreatic cancers and in defining the roles of the *p16* and *p53* genes. Finally, the relatively new technique of representational difference analysis (RDA) has been applied to pancreatic cancer. RDA is a method for isolating DNA fragments that are present in only one of two nearly identical complex genomes. It uses subtraction hybridization methods and has been shown to enrich for difference products over 1 million-fold. RDA is a particularly attractive technique for isolating new tumor-suppressor genes because it can strongly favor the enrichment of homozygously deleted regions. Homozygous deletions are smaller than most heterozygous losses, and so this technique promises to focus attention on smaller regions of the genome to serve as candidate loci for new tumor-suppressor genes.

Karyotype of Sporadic Pancreatic Cancer. A number of recurrent chromosome abnormalities have been identified in sporadic pancreatic cancers, providing clues to the specific genes involved in the pathogenesis of pancreatic cancer.[89–92] Griffin et al. have karyotyped 62 primary pancreatic cancers resected at The Johns Hopkins Hospital and found clonally abnormal karyotypes in 44 of the cancers.[91,92] The karyotypes generally were complex and included both numerical and structural changes. Losses were more frequent than gains and included a high prevalence of losses of chromosomes 18, 13, 12, 17, and 6. The losses of chromosome 6q were confirmed by fluorescent *in situ* hybridization using a biotin-labeled microdissection probe from 6q24-ter. The most frequent whole-chromosome gains were of chromosomes 20 and 7. Recurrent structural abnormalities most frequently involved 1p, 3p, 11p, 17p, 1q, 6q, and 19q.[91,92] In addition, double-minute chromatin bodies suggestive of gene amplification were identified in six of the cancers. These karyotype studies, when combined with smaller reports by Johansson et al., suggest that chromosomes 1p, 3p, 6q, and 11p may harbor yet unidentified tumor-suppressor genes.[89,91,92] More recently Höglund et al. have combined karyotyping with fluorescence *in situ* hybridization to demonstrate that chromosome 19 aberrations are common in pancreatic cancer.[93]

Allelotype of Sporadic Pancreatic Cancer. Hahn et al. and Seymour et al. have allelotyped two series of pancreatic cancers.[70,94] High frequencies (60 percent) of allelic loss were found at 1p, 9p, 17p, and 18q, whereas moderate frequencies (40–60 percent) of allelic loss were seen at 3p, 6p, 8p, 10q, 12q, 13q, 18p, 21q, and 22q.[70,94] These patterns of allelic loss suggest regions of the genome as harboring candidate tumor-suppressor loci. For example, the *p53* gene is located on 17p, and 17p was lost in 100 percent of the cancers allelotyped by Hahn et al.[70] Similarly, the *DPC4* gene on 18q and the *p16* gene on 9p each suffered LOH in nearly 90 percent of the tumors.[70] In these studies, chromosome 1p had the highest frequency of allelic loss (67 percent) not accounted for by a known tumor-suppressor gene.

Allelotype and karyotype studies produce different kinds of information, and a comparison of these results provides new insight into the structural basis of the molecular genetic alterations. Brat et al. compared the chromosomal abnormalities of primary pancreatic adenocarcinomas, as determined by classic cytogenetics, with the molecular changes, as determined by the studies of LOH, in the same cancers.[95] In the 14 cancers with abnormal karyotypes, 65 percent (123 of 188) of the chromosomal arms with molecular LOH were associated with karyotypic structural abnormalities. Karyotypic changes accounting for these losses included 83 whole-chromosomal losses, 18 partial deletions, 9 isochromosomes, 8 additions, and 5 translocations. The greatest degree of correlation between the cytogenetic and molecular studies was found at sites of known tumor-suppressor genes such as *p53*, *DPC4*, *p16*, and *BRCA2*. These results generally validate both techniques and indicate that, in pancreatic cancer, large structural abnormalities can account for two-thirds of the LOH. Of note, there were 13 chromosomes that had extensive regions of LOH yet appeared normal on karyotypic analysis. This finding suggests that chromosome loss with reduplication of the remaining chromosome occurs in pancreatic cancer.[95] Finally, homozygous deletions tended to be small and were not detected in the karyotype analyses.

RDA Applied to Sporadic Pancreas Cancer. As discussed previously, RDA is a powerful technique that can be used to isolate small regions of homozygous deletion in a cancer. Schutte et al. applied RDA to a sporadic pancreatic cancer and identified a homozygous deletion that mapped to a 180-kb region on chromosome 13q.[96] This deletion mapped to the area of the *BRCA2* locus, and the map of this deletion provided the first published partial sequences of the *BRCA2* gene, including exon 2 and intron 24.[96] The mapping of this deletion, a critical advance aiding in the discovery of the *BRCA2* gene by Stratton et al. and by Myriad Genetics, provided the first clue that the *BRCA2* was a tumor-suppressor gene as opposed to a proto-oncogene and showed that *BRCA2* served such a role in the pancreas.[97,98]

SPECIFIC GENES

Specific Genes Involved in Hereditary Pancreatic Cancer

The short life expectancy of patients with pancreatic carcinoma has made it difficult to perform classic linkage studies on families with pancreatic cancer. Simply put, it is extremely unusual to find more than one patient alive with disease at a time in any family. Because of these difficulties, most studies of familial pancreatic cancer have relied on the candidate gene approach. In this approach, a tumor-suppressor gene that is known to be inactivated in sporadic pancreatic cancers is selected as the candidate gene, and then germ-line tissues from affected individuals from families in which there is an aggregation of pancreatic cancer can be tested for mutations in this candidate gene. This approach is possible because, at the molecular level, familial and sporadic forms of cancer often involve the same genes.[99] For example, familial adenomatous polyposis (FAP) has been shown to be caused by

inherited mutations in the *APC* gene, and inactivation of *APC* is a common and early event in sporadic adenocarcinomas of the colon.[100,101] Similarly, missense germ-line mutations in the *RET* proto-oncogene are responsible for the multiple endocrine neoplasia type 2 (MEN2) syndrome, and these same mutations have been identified in sporadic medullary carcinomas of the thyroid.[102,103]

The candidate gene approach has been applied to familial pancreatic cancer, and in a few of the families, the pancreatic cancers appear to be caused by germ-line mutations in the *p16*, *LKB1*, or *BRCA2* gene.[104,105] In contrast, a number of these families have been examined for germ-line mutations in *DPC4*, but to date, none have been found.[79]

Germ-Line *p16* Mutations in Pancreatic Cancer Families. The *p16* (*MTS1/p16/CDKN2*) gene is genetically inactivated in approximately 80 percent of sporadic adenocarcinomas of the pancreas.[71] In 40 percent of these cancers, these inactivations are caused by somatic homozygous deletions of the gene and in another 40 percent by somatic intragenic mutations in one allele coupled with loss of the second allele. *p16* therefore would appear to be a good candidate to examine in patients with familial pancreatic cancers. Moskaluk et al. analyzed 21 kindreds with familial pancreatic carcinoma for germ-line mutations in *p16* and in the related *CDK4* gene.[104] Kindreds known to have the FAMMM syndrome were excluded. Germ-line *CDK4* mutations were not seen, and germ-line *p16* mutation were identified in only one family. The mutation was found in two individuals affected with pancreatic cancer in this family, and the alteration destroyed the donor splice site of intron 2, causing premature termination after the addition of two new codons at the 3′ end of exon 2.[104] Of interest, one of the two carriers in this kindred also had a melanoma, suggesting that this kindred, in fact, had the FAMMM syndrome. All other patients in this series were found to be wild type for both *p16* and for *CDK4*.[104] Thus germ-line *p16* mutations could account for the pancreatic cancers in only 1 (5 percent) of the 21 kindreds studied with familial pancreatic cancer, and they were seen in a patient who also had melanoma. Germ-line mutations in *p16* therefore should be suspected when there is an aggregation of both melanoma and pancreatic cancer in a family.[77,78]

Germ-Line *BRCA2* Mutations in Pancreatic Cancer Families. The *BRCA2* gene was another logical choice for the candidate gene approach. *BRCA2* may play a role in the development of sporadic pancreatic cancer. Twenty-five to 35 percent of sporadic pancreatic cancers show LOH at the *BRCA2* locus on 13q, and karyotypic losses of chromosome 13 are common in pancreatic cancer.[70,89,91,92,94] Furthermore, a critical advance in the discovery of *BRCA2* was the identification of a homozygous deletion of the *BRCA2* locus in a pancreatic cancer.[96,97] Finally, as noted previously, there have been some reports suggesting that the risk of pancreatic cancer is increased in families of breast cancer patients and in carriers of *BRCA2* mutations.[83,85–88] Goggins et al. therefore screened a panel of 41 adenocarcinomas of the pancreas for *BRCA2* mutations.[105] Four of the 41 cancers had both a loss of one allele of *BRCA2* and a mutation in the second allele. Three of these four mutations were present in the germ-line. The three germ-line mutations identified included two germ-line 6174 delT at codon 1982 and a germ-line 2481 insT mutation.[105] Because of these findings, the utility of a cross-sectional population screen was evaluated. Normal tissues from 245 consecutive surgical patients with adenocarcinoma of the pancreas were screened near the 6174 nucleotide. Sequence analysis of this limited region of the *BRCA2* gene revealed two additional germ-line mutations, a 6174 delT mutation and a second nearby 6158 insT mutation. Thus a total of 5 germ-line mutations in *BRCA2* were identified. Remarkably, only 1 of the 5 patients with germ-line mutations had a relative with breast cancer, and 1 had a relative with prostate cancer. None had a family history of pancreatic cancer.[105] Ozcelik et al. confirmed these findings by Goggins and estimated that 10

Table 40-3 Genetic Alterations in Apparently Sporadic Pancreatic Carcinomas

Genes	Chromosome Locus	Mechanism of Alteration	Frequency (%)
Oncogenes			
K-*ras*	12	Point mutations codons 12, 13	80–100
Tumor-suppressor genes			
p16	9p	Homozygous deletion, LOH and IM, hypermethylation	95
p53	17p	LOH and IM	50–75
DPC4	18q	Homozygous deletion, LOH and IM	55
BRCA2	13q	Germ-line IM and acquired LOH	4–7
MKK4	17p	Homozygous deletion, LOH and IM	4
LKB1	19p	Homozygous deletion, LOH and IM	5
ALK4	12q	LOH and IM	2
RB	13q	Mutation/small deletion	0–7
Genome maintenance genes			
hMSH2, hMLH1, hPMS1, hPMS2, hMSHG/GTBP, hMSH3	Multiple	Often undetermined; gives phenotype of microsatellite instability	4

NOTE: LOH = loss of heterozygosity; IM = intragenic mutation.

percent of pancreatic cancers in Ashkenazi Jews are caused by germ-line *BRCA2* 6174 delT mutations and suggested that carriers of the 6174 delT mutation have a 10-fold increased risk of developing pancreatic cancer.[106]

Germ-line mutations in *BRCA2* therefore represent the most common inherited predisposition to pancreatic carcinoma identified to date, and the results of screening for *BRCA2* mutations suggest that the classic definition of a familial case of pancreatic cancer is too stringent. Clearly, some cases of pancreatic cancer that appear sporadic are, in fact, caused by inherited mutations in *BRCA2.*

LKB1. As noted previously, the Peutz-Jeghers syndrome is associated with an increased risk of pancreatic cancer,[73,73A] and Su et al. have demonstrated recently loss of the wild-type *LKB1* allele in a pancreatic cancer obtained from a patient with the Peutz-Jeghers syndrome and a germ-line *LKB1* mutation.[76]

Absence of Germ-Line *DPC4*, K-*ras* and *p53* Mutations in Pancreatic Cancer Families. The *DPC4* (*Smad4*) gene was an attractive candidate gene to study in families with pancreatic cancer.[107] *DPC4* was identified in a locus of consensus homozygous deletions in sporadic pancreatic carcinomas. It is biallelically inactivated in almost 50 percent of pancreatic carcinomas.[107] Moskaluk et al. therefore sequenced the complete *DPC4* coding sequence of 25 individuals from 11 separate kindreds with a familial aggregation of pancreatic carcinoma, but no mutations were found.[79] Similarly, the K-*ras* oncogene frequently is activated and the *p53* tumor suppressor frequently is inactivated in pancreatic carcinomas, but to date, germ-line mutations have not been identified in either of these two genes in patients with familial or sporadic cancer.[107,108]

In summary, the gene or genes responsible for the majority of cases of familial pancreatic cancer have not yet been identified. A small minority of these cases may be caused by germ-line mutations in *p16*, particularly in patients in whom there is a family history of melanoma. Germ-line mutations in *BRCA2* also predispose to the development of pancreatic cancer, and because of their low penetrance, these mutations appear responsible for some cases of pancreatic cancer that appear to be sporadic.

Specific Genes Involved in Sporadic Pancreatic Cancer (Table 40-3)

The development of an adenocarcinoma of the pancreas is complex and involves the accumulation of mutations in the K-*ras* oncogene and in numerous tumor-suppressor genes. K-*ras* appears to be activated in the vast majority of pancreatic cancers, whereas the tumor-suppressor genes *p53*, *p16*, *DPC4*, and *BRCA2* frequently are inactivated.[108] These mutations dysregulate the cell cycle and lead to inappropriate cell proliferation. Of interest, a high concordance of *DPC4* and *p16* inactivation ($p < 0.007$) has been reported in pancreatic cancer, suggesting that inactivation of the *p16/RB* pathway might increase the selective pressure for subsequent mutations of *DPC4* in this tumor type.[2] This section will begin with a discussion of K-*ras*, the most frequently altered gene in pancreatic cancer, and it will then be followed by a discussion of the tumor-suppressor genes that are most frequently inactivated in pancreatic cancer. It will conclude with a discussion of microsatellite instability in pancreatic cancer.

Activation of K-*ras*. Oncogenes encode for proteins that, when overexpressed or activated by a mutation, possess transforming properties. In normal cells, K-*ras* is a proto-oncogene that encodes for a G protein involved in signal transduction.[109] Point mutations in codons 12, 13, or 61 of K-*ras* activate the gene product.[110] These mutations impair the intrinsic GTPase activity of this protein and cause it to be constitutively active in signal transduction.[109] K-*ras* is the most frequently mutated gene in pancreatic cancer, with reported mutation rates ranging 71 to 100 percent.[108,111–124] This is the highest reported prevalence of K-*ras* mutations in any tumor type. The vast majority of these mutations occur in codon 12 of K-*ras*.[108] These mutations appear to be early events in the development of pancreatic neoplasia. This has been demonstrated by studies of the noninvasive duct lesions that are found in the pancreata with and without cancer.[125] In humans and in the Syrian golden hamster animal model of pancreatic neoplasia, these duct lesions have been shown to harbor activating point mutations in K-*ras*.[125–133] For example, several investigators have microdissected the pancreatic duct lesions from pancreata obtained from patients without cancer, and they have shown that these noninvasive duct lesions can harbor activating clonal mutations in K-ras.[125,128,129] Thus activation of the K-ras oncogene appears to be a fairly early event in the development of adenocarcinoma of the pancreas. Furthermore, as will be discussed later, the high prevalence of K-ras mutations in invasive cancers, their presence early in the neoplastic process, and the limitation of these mutations largely to a pair of codons all make K-ras a promising marker for a molecular-based test to detect early pancreatic carcinomas.

Amplification of Oncogenes

The most common amplicon in pancreatic cancer (10 percent of the cases) also was the first to be identified. Originally found as the amplification of the PD-1 gene, the leading current candidate to explain the amplification on chromosome 19q is the AKT2 gene.[134,135] Other sites of amplification exist, however, at much lower frequencies.[136]

Tumor-Suppressor Genes. Tumor-suppressor genes differ from oncogenes in that tumor-suppressor genes normally function to restrict the expansion of cell populations. Their loss, by deletion or mutation, leads to dysregulated cell growth.

p53 Inactivation. The p53 tumor-suppressor gene is inactivated in more than half of all pancreatic carcinomas.[2,117,137–143] In almost all these cancers this inactivation occurs by loss of one allele coupled with an intragenic mutation of the other. Evidence for the loss of one allele comes from allelotyping and karyotyping studies that have identified 17p as a site of frequent loss in pancreatic cancers.[70,91,92,94] When sequenced, the second allele of p53 is mutated in about 50 to 75 percent of the cancers.[2,121,140] The majority of mutations reported have been transitions (pyrimidine-to-pyrimidine or purine-to-purine) in the conserved regions of the gene. Redston et al. and Rozenblum et al. also noted a high prevalence of small frameshift mutations in the p53 gene in pancreatic cancers.[2,140] p53 is a nuclear DNA-binding protein that acts as a G1/S checkpoint, and it also plays a role in the induction of apoptosis.[144–148] Inactivation of p53 in pancreatic cancers therefore results in the loss of two important controls of cell number, the initiation of replication and the induction of cell death.

p16 Inactivation. p16 is a tumor-suppressor gene that is inactivated in a variety of tumors.[149] p16 resides on chromosome 9p, and as noted earlier, 9p was found to be a frequent site of allelic loss in allelotypes of pancreatic cancer.[70,94] Caldas et al. demonstrated loss of one allele of p16 accompanied by sequence changes in p16 in the second allele in 38 percent of tumors.[70,71,94,150–154] Furthermore, Caldas et al. demonstrated homozygous deletions of p16 in nearly 40 percent of the tumors. Therefore, p16 is genetically inactivated in nearly 80 percent of pancreatic cancers. In addition, Schutte et al. demonstrated that p16 is inactivated by hypermethylation of its promoter in most of the remaining cancers.[155,156] p16 inhibits the promotion of the cell cycle by competing with cyclin D in binding to CDK4, preventing CDK4 from phosphorylating the RB protein. Hypophosphorylated RB protein binds and may sequester transcription factors that otherwise promote the G1/S transition, whereas hyperphosphorylation of RB releases these factors.[157] Therefore, the inactivation of p16 in approximately 95 percent of pancreatic cancers dysregulates another important cell cycle checkpoint.

DPC4. One of the most frequently lost chromosome arms in both the allelotypes and karyotypes of pancreatic cancer is 18q.[91,92,94,158] Based on this observation, Hahn et al. performed detailed genome scanning of 18q on a panel of pancreatic carcinomas.[107] These analyses not only confirmed the high frequency of LOH on 18q but also revealed a consensus locus of homozygous deletions. These homozygous deletions did not include the DCC locus. Further positional cloning of the locus lead to the discovery of the DPC4 gene. This tumor-suppressor

gene, also known as SMAD4, is biallelically inactivated in almost 55 percent of pancreatic carcinomas.[107] In 35 percent, this inactivation is by homozygous deletion, and in 20 percent, by loss of one allele coupled with an intragenic mutation of the other.[107]

Recently, Wilentz et al. have demonstrated that immunohistochemical labeling for the DPC4 gene product directly mirrors gene status, providing a simple test for DPC4 inactivation in tissue.[158A] Remarkably, although DPC4 appears to be a common target of inactivation in pancreatic cancer, it is only infrequently inactivated in other neoplasms.[159] The specificity of DPC4 inactivation for pancreatic cancer suggests that the DPC4 status may be useful in determining if a particular metastatic carcinoma in a patient had arisen in the pancreas.

DPC4 has homology to the Smad family of proteins, and the Smad proteins play a role in signal transduction from transforming growth factor beta (TGFβ) superfamily cell surface receptors.[160–163] Normally, TGFβ provides a growth-inhibitory signal to epithelial cells.[164] When TGFβ binds to the TGFβ receptor, it promotes the dimerization of the TGFβ receptors type I and type II, which in turn activate the kinase activity of the TGFβ type I receptor.[164] The signal is transferred to Smad proteins by phosphorylation. These proteins then complex with DPC4, and relocalization to the nucleus occurs.[165]

The importance of DPC4 in TGFβ signaling was proven conclusively by Zhou et al.[166] They homozygously deleted the DPC4 gene of cultured human colonic cancer cells using homologous recombination and demonstrated that this deletion abrogated signaling from TGFβ, as well as from the TGFβ family member activin.[166] Takaku et al. demonstrated the importance of DPC4 (Smad4) inactivation in tumorigenesis.[167] They made mice that were compound heterozygotes to mutant APC and DPC4 alleles. Because these genes lie close on the same chromosome in mice, an LOH event results in a tumor lacking functional copies of both genes.[167] The intestinal neoplasms that developed in these mice were unusually invasive and had a greater stromal response than did neoplasms that developed in simple APC mutant mice.[167] Therefore, by extension, the inactivation of DPC4 in pancreatic cancer may lead to the loss of an important pathway in TGFβ-related signaling, and it may play a significant role in the malignant progression of these tumors.

Mutations in Multiple Genes in Pancreatic Cancer. Rozenblum et al. have determined the status of K-ras, p53, p16, DPC4, and BRCA2 in a series of 42 pancreatic carcinomas.[2] This extensive molecular analysis of a series of cancers provides a unique opportunity to determine if there are any relationships among the mutations in these various genes. All 42 carcinomas harbored a mutation in codon 12 of K-ras, and inactivation of all three tumor-suppressor genes occurred in 37 percent of the cancers.[2] A high concordance was found between DPC4 and p16 inactivation ($p < 0.007$), suggesting that inactivation of the p16/RB pathway increased the selective pressure for subsequent mutations of DPC4. Of note, one carcinoma carried a germ-line mutation in BRCA2 and eight additional selected genetic events, highlighting the complexity of the molecular genetic events responsible for the development of pancreatic cancer. Furthermore, small homozygous deletions appear to be a common mechanism for inactivating tumor-suppressor genes in pancreatic cancer. One or more homozygous deletions were found in 64 percent of the cancers.[71,107,159,168]

Other Tumor-Suppressor Genes. A number of other tumor-suppressor genes appear to be inactivated in only a small minority of pancreatic carcinomas. For example, the MKK4 gene on 17p encodes for the mitogen-activated protein kinase 4 (MKK4) protein. MKK4 is an important component of a stress- and cytokine-induced signal transduction pathway involving the mitogen-activated protein kinase (MAPK) proteins.[169] Su et al. recently have confirmed the findings of Teng et al. that MKK4 is inactivated in about 4 percent of pancreatic carcinomas.[169] Two percent of the carcinomas harbored an intragenic mutation coupled with LOH, and in 2 percent *MKK4* was inactivated by homozygous deletion.[169] Some of the allelic loss patterns did not extend to the *p53* locus on 17p, and inactivation of *MKK4* may therefore explain some of the LOH seen on 17p in pancreatic adenocarcinomas.

Chromosome 19p is also frequently lost in pancreatic cancer, and as discussed earlier, the gene responsible for the Peutz-Jeghers syndrome, *LKB1*, has been identified recently at 19p13.3.[74,75,93] Höglund et al. karyotyped a series of pancreatic cancers and reported that structural arrangements of chromosome 19 resulting in loss of 19p were common.[93] Su et al. extended these studies and demonstrated, at the molecular level, that *LKB1* is indeed inactivated in 5 percent of apparently sporadic pancreatic carcinomas.[76] In 1 to 2 percent of the cancers this was by homozygous deletion and in 3 to 4 percent by LOH coupled with an intragenic mutation. The inactivation of *LKB1* in both familial (Peutz-Jeghers syndrome) and sporadic pancreatic cancers confirms the hypothesis that the same genes are frequently responsible for the development of both sporadic and familial forms of cancer.[99]

Although one report suggested that *APC* might be inactivated in pancreatic cancers, more detailed studies, which examined large numbers of pancreatic cancers, demonstrated that inactivation of *APC* or its pathway partner *β-catenin* is rare in pancreatic cancers.[94,170–172] These genes are almost universally mutated in colorectal neoplasia, and the rarity of *APC* pathway alterations in pancreatic cancer demonstrates further that the mutation spectrum of pancreatic ductal carcinoma is distinct from that seen in other gastrointestinal neoplasms. Of interest, Abraham et al. have recently shown that the *β-catenin/APC* pathway is frequently targeted in some non-ductal pancreatic neoplasms, including solid and pseudopapillary tumors, pancreaticoblastomas, and acinar cell carcinomas (personal communication).

There have been conflicting reports on the expression levels of the *DCC* gene product in pancreatic carcinomas, but only rare homozygous deletions have been reported to date for *DCC* in pancreatic cancer.[70,107,173]

Mutations of *RB* are reported in pancreatic cancer, but at a very low rate. Huang et al. found that immunohistologic staining for RB expression was lost in 3 of 30 pancreatic cancers. In one of these three cases a truncating mutation was found, and in a second a missense mutation was verified by DNA sequencing.[94,173–175]

Recently, Su et al. examined 96 pancreatic adenocarcinomas and demonstrated biallelic inactivation of the *ACVR1B (ALK4)* gene in two of these cancers.[175A] In one of these cancers, the gene was inactivated by loss of one allele coupled with an intragenic mutation in the second allele. In the second cancer the gene was inactivated by a 5 base pair frame-shift deletion.[175A] *ACVR1B* codes for a type 1 activin receptor.

Microsatellite Instability. Goggins et al. screened 82 xenografted sporadic adenocarcinomas of the pancreas for DNA replication errors (RER+) using polymerase chain reaction amplification of microsatellite markers.[67] Three (3.7 percent) of the 82 carcinomas were RER+ and contained associated mutations in the *TGFBRII* gene. In contrast to typical gland-forming adenocarcinomas of the pancreas, all these RER+ carcinomas were poorly differentiated and had expanding borders and a prominent syncytial growth pattern[67] (Fig. 40-5). Furthermore, all the RER+ carcinomas were K-*ras* wild type, and the one case that was karyotyped showed a near diploid pattern.[71A] These data by Goggins et al. suggest that DNA replication errors occur in approximately 4 percent of pancreatic carcinomas and that wild-type K-*ras* gene status coupled with the histologic findings of poor differentiation, a syncytial growth pattern, and pushing borders should suggest the possibility of DNA replication errors in carcinomas of the pancreas. Wilentz et al. recently extended the studies of Goggins et al. and demonstrated that patients with medullary carcinomas of

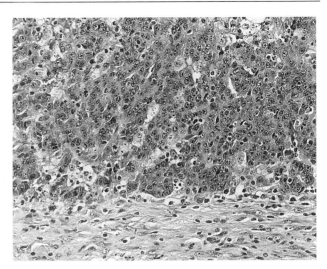

Fig. 40-5 Pancreatic carcinoma with DNA replication errors (RER+). RER+ carcinomas of the pancreas are associated with wild-type K-*ras* and poor differentiation, a syncytial growth pattern, and pushing borders.

the pancreas are more likely to have a family history of cancer than are patients with conventional ductal adenocarcinomas.[71A]

DNA Hypermethylation. Recently Ueki et al. have demonstrated that multiple genes are hypermethylated in pancreatic adenocarcinomas.[175B,175C] Using methylation-specifc PCR (MSP) they demonstrated aberrant methylation of at least one locus in 60 percent of pancreatic carcinomas. The loci methylated included *RARβ* (methylated in 20 percent), *p16* (18 percent), *CACNA1G* (16 percent), *TIMP-3* (11 percent), *E-cad* (7 percent), *THBS1* (7 percent), *hMLH1* (4 percent) and *DAP kinase* (2 percent).[175B] Simultaneous methylation of at least four loci was observed in ~15 percent of the carcinomas—a subgroup the authors classified as "CpG island–methylator-phenotype positive (CIMP+)." Thus, many pancreatic carcinomas hypermethylate a small percentage of genes, and a small subset displays a CIMP+ phenotype.

IMPLICATIONS FOR DIAGNOSIS

There are no molecular tests currently being used to screen for pancreatic carcinomas. However, the recent advances in our understanding of how molecular biology can be used to screen for cancer, coupled with an improved understanding of the molecular genetics of this tumor, provide several avenues for developing such a test.[176] Probably the best example is the K-*ras* oncogene. K-*ras* is a particularly attractive target for a molecular screening test for pancreatic cancer for three reasons. First, the vast majority of pancreatic carcinomas harbor mutations in K-*ras*, suggesting that K-*ras* will be a sensitive genetic marker.[108,111–124] Second, mutations in this oncogene essentially are limited to two codons, and so a limited number of probes can be employed to detect these mutations, greatly simplifying the analyses.[108] Finally, as discussed earlier, these mutations appear to be early events in the development of pancreatic neoplasia, suggesting that K-*ras* could be used to detect early and therefore curable cancers.[125–129,137] Indeed, K-*ras* mutations have been used to identify cells shed from pancreatic cancers in pancreatic juice samples, in cytologic preparations, and in stool and blood specimens.[122,129,130,177–183] For example, Caldas et al. screened stool specimens obtained from patients with chronic pancreatitis, cholangiocarcinoma, and pancreatic cancer.[129] They found K-*ras* mutations in stool specimens from nine patients. Six of these nine patients had pancreatic cancer, and in five of the six cases the mutation found in the patients' invasive pancreatic cancer was the same as the one identified in the stool. In the remaining four patients, mutations identified in the stool were identical to those present in duct lesions (PanINs) found in the patients' resected pancreatic specimens.[129] This study established that screening for genetic alterations can be used to detect rare cells shed from pancreatic cancers. It also demonstrated that an improved understanding of the genetic alterations in PanINs and in early invasive pancreatic cancers will be essential for the development of genetic-based screening tests. A significant investigative effort has therefore been focused on defining the genetic alterations in PanINs in the pancreas. The majority of PanINs examined to date have been found to harbor activating point mutations with codon 12 of the K-*ras* oncogene,[125,126,128–133,177,184] and some PanINs with cytologic and architectural atypia have been shown to accumulate the *p53* gene product to immunohistologically detectable levels, suggesting that those PanINs harbor *p53* mutations.[137,185] More recently, Moskaluk et al. examined PanINs adjacent to infiltrating pancreatic cancers known to harbor inactivating *p16* mutations, and one-third of these PanINs harbored *p16* alterations.[132] Wilentz et al. have confirmed that *p16* and *DPC4* are inactivated in PanINs using immuno-histochemical stains.[186,186A] Importantly, these genetic alterations in K-ras, p53, DPC4 and p16 occur while the neoplasm is still *in situ,* before it has spread beyond the pancreatic duct system.

Recent studies of gene expression patterns in pancreatic cancer using serial analysis of gene expression (SAGE) and expression arrays have identified a number of potential new markers of pancreatic cancer including tissue inhibitor of metalloproteinase type 1 (Timp-1), prostate stem cell antigen (PSCA) and mesothelin.[187–189]

In addition to leading to the development of new screening tests for early pancreatic neoplasms, an improved understanding of the genetics of pancreatic cancer will lead to the discovery of additional germ-line mutations in cancer-causing genes that predispose to pancreatic cancer, and geneticists will be able to screen at-risk individuals for these germ-line mutations. Carriers of germ-line mutations can then be clinically screened more thoroughly and may even choose prophylactic surgery, while those found not to carry germ-line mutations will have their anxiety relieved and can be spared unnecessary screening tests.

Clearly, we need to advance our understanding of the molecular genetics of pancreatic cancer so that new tests can be developed that are both sensitive and specific for early stages of this disease.

ACKNOWLEDGMENTS

We would like to thank Jennifer Galford for her assistance, energy, and enthusiasm in preparing this manuscript and Kieran Brune for her tireless dedication to the National Familial Pancreas Tumor Registry. For the latest on pancreatic cancer, visit our Web site (*http://pathology.jhu.edu/pancreas*).

REFERENCES

1. Parker SL, Tong T, Bolden S, Wingo PA: Cancer statistics, 1997. *CA Cancer J Clin* **47**:5, 1997.
2. Rozenblum E, Schutte M, Goggins M, et al: Tumor-suppressive pathways in pancreatic carcinoma. *Cancer Res* **57**:1731, 1997.
3. Gold EB, Goldin SB: Epidemiology of and risk factors for pancreatic cancer. *Surg Oncol Clin North Am* **7**:67, 1998.
4. Gold EB: Epidemiology of and risk factors for pancreatic cancer. *Surg Clin North Am* **75**:819, 1995.
5. Taxy JB: Adenocarcinoma of the pancreas in childhood: Report of a case and a review of the English language literature. *Cancer* **37**:1508, 1976.
6. Newill VA: Distribution of cancer mortality among ethnic subgroups of the white population in New York City, 1953-1958. *J Natl Cancer Inst* **26**:405, 1961.
7. Seidman H: Cancer death rates by site and sex for religions and socioeconomic groups in New York City. *Environ Res* **3**:234, 1970.
8. Durbec JP, Chevillotte C, Bidart JM, Berthezene P, Sarles H: Diet, alcohol, tobacco, and risk of cancer of the pancreas: A case-control study. *Br J Cancer* **47**:463, 1983.
9. Ghadirian P, Simard A, Baillargeon J: Tobacco, alcohol, and coffee and cancer of the pancreas: A population-based, case-control study in Quebec, Canada. *Cancer* **67**:2664, 1991.
10. Doll R, Peto R: Mortality in relation to smoking: Twenty years observation on male British doctors. *Br Med J* **2**:1525, 1976.
11. Kahn HA: The Dorn study of smoking and mortality among U.S. Veterans: Report on eight and one-half years of observation. *Natl Cancer Inst Monogr* **19**:1, 1966.
12. Whittemore AS, Paffenbarger RS Jr, Anderson D, Lee JE: Early precursors of pancreatic cancer in college men. *J Chron Dis* **36**:251, 1983.
13. Howe GR, Ghadirian P, DeMesquita HB, et al: A collaborative case-control study of nutrient intake and pancreatic cancer within the search programme. *Int J Cancer* **51**:365, 1992.
14. Hirayama T: Epidemiology of pancreatic cancer in Japan. *Jpn J Clin Oncol* **19**:208, 1989.
15. Gold EB, Gordis L, Diener MD, Seltser R, Boitnott JK, Bynum TE, Hutcheon DF: Diet and other risk factors for cancer of the pancreas. *Cancer* **55**:460, 1985.
16. LaVecchia C, Liati P, Decarlie A, Negri E, Franceschi S: Coffee consumption and risk of pancreatic cancer. *Int J Cancer* **40**:309, 1987.
17. Velema JP, Walker AM, Gold EB: Alcohol and pancreatic cancer: Insufficient epidemiiologic evidence for a causal relationship. *Epidemiol Rev* **8**:28, 1986.
18. Li FP: Molecular epidemiology studies of cancer in families. *Br J Cancer* **68**:217, 1993.
19. Lynch HT, Voorhees GJ, Lanspa S, McGreevy PS, Lynch J: Pancreatic carcinoma and hereditary nonpolyposis colorectal cancer: A family study. *Br J Cancer* **52**:271, 1985.
20. Lynch HT, Fitzsimmons ML, Smyrk TC, Lanspa SJ, Watson P, McClellan J, Lynch JF: Familial pancreatic cancer: Clinicopathologic study of 18 nuclear families. *Am J Gastroenterol* **85**:54, 1990.
21. Lynch HT, Fusaro RM: Pancreatic cancer and the familial atypical multiple mole melanoma (FAMMM) syndrome. *Pancreas* **6**:127, 1991.
22. Lynch HT, Fusaro L, Lynch JF: Familial pancreatic cancer: A family study. *Pancreas* **7**:511, 1992.
23. Lynch HT, Smyrk TC, Watson P, et al: Genetics, natural history, tumor spectrum, and pathology of hereditary nonpolyposis colorectal cancer: An updated review. *Gastroenterology* **104**:1535, 1993.
24. Lynch HT: Genetics and pancreatic cancer. *Arch Surg* **129**:266,1994.
25. Lynch HT, Fusaro L, Smyrk T, Watson P, Lanspa S, Lynch J: Medical genetic study of eight pancreatic cancer-prone families. *Cancer Invest* **13**:141, 1995.
26. Bergman W, Watson P, de Jong J, Lynch HT, Fusaro RM: Systemic cancer and the FAMMM syndrome. *Br J Cancer* **61**:932, 1990.
27. Dat N, Sontag S: Pancreatic carcinoma in brothers. *Ann Intern Med* **97**:282, 1982.
28. Ehrenthal D, Haeger L, Griffin T, Compton C: Familial pancreatic adenocarcinoma in three generations. *Cancer* **59**:1661, 1987.
29. Grajower MM: Familial pancreatic cancer. *Ann Intern Med* **98**:111, 1983.
30. Katkhouda N, Mouiel J: Pancreatic cancer in mother and daughter. *Lancet* **2**:747, 1986.
31. MacDermott RP, Kramer P: Adencarcinoma of the pancreas in four siblings. *Gastroenterology* **65**:137, 1973.
32. Reimer R, Fraumeni JF Jr, Ozols R, Bender R: Pancreatic cancer in father and son. *Lancet* **1**:911, 1977.
33. Lumadue JA, Griffin CA, Osman M, Hruban RH: Familial pancreatic cancer and the genetics of pancreatic cancer. *Surg Clin North Am* **75**:845, 1995.
34. Lynch HT, Smyrk T, Kern SE, et al: Familial pancreatic cancer: a review. *Semin Oncol* **23**:251, 1996.
35. Ghadirian P, Boyle P, Simard A, Baillargeon J, Maisonneuve P, Perret C: Reported family aggregation of pancreatic cancer within a population-based case-control study in the Francophone community in Montreal, Canada. *Int J Pancreatol* **10**:183, 1991.
36. Fernandez E, La Vecchia C, D'Avanzo B, Negri E, Franceschi S: Family history and the risk of liver, gallbladder, and pancreatic cancer. *Cancer Epidemiol Biomark Prev* **3**:209, 1994.
37. Hruban RH, Petersen GM, Ha PK, Kern SE: Genetics of pancreatic cancer: From genes to families. *Surg Oncol Clin North Am* **7**:1, 1998.
38. Moossa AR, Gamagami RA: Diagnosis and staging of pancreatic neoplams. *Surg Clin North Am* **75**:871, 1995.
39. Christoffersen P, Poll P: Preoperative pancreas aspiration biopsies. *Acta Pathol Microbiol Immunol Scand (Suppl)* **212**:28, 1970.
40. American Cancer Society: *Cancer Facts and Figures 1996.* New York, 1996 (abstract).

41. DiGiuseppe JA, Yeo CJ, Hruban RH: Molecular biology and the diagnosis and treatment of adenocarcinoma of the pancreas. *Adv Anat Pathol* **3**:139, 1996.

42. Solcia E, Capella C, Klöppel G: *Tumors of the Pancreas*. 3rd Series, Armed Forces Institute of Pathology, Washington, DC, 1997.

43. Wilentz RE, Hruban RH: Pathology of cancer of the pancreas. *Surg Oncol Clin North Am* **7**:43, 1998.

44. Wilentz RE, Slebos RJC, Hruban RH: Screening for pancreatic cancer using techniques to detect altered gene products, in Reber HA (ed): *Advances in Pancreatic Cancer*. 1997.

45. Cubilla AL, Fitzgerald PJ: Morphological lesions associated with human primary invasive nonendocrine pancreas cancer. *Cancer Res* **36**:2690, 1976.

46. Furukawa T, Chiba R, Kobari M, Matsuno S, Nagura H, Takahashi T: Varying grades of epithelial atypia in the pancreatic ducts of humans: Classification based on morphometry and multilvariate analysis and correlated with positive reactions of carcinoembryonic antigen. *Arch Pathol Lab Med* **118**:227, 1994.

46A. Hruban RH, Adsay NV, Albores-Saavedra J, Compton C, Garrett E, Goodman SN, Kern SE, Klimstra DS, Klöppel G, Longnecker DS, Lüttges J, Offerhaus GJA: Pancreatic intraepithelial neoplasia (PanIN): A new nomenclature and classification system for pancreatic duct lesions. *Am J Surg Pathol* **25**:579, 2001.

47. Kozuka S, Sassa R, Taki T, et al: Relation of pancreatic duct hyperplasia to carcinoma. *Cancer* **43**:1418, 1979.

48. Pour PM, Sayed S, Sayed G: Hyperplastic, preneoplastic and neoplastic lesions found in 83 human pancreases. *Am J Clin Pathol* **77**:137, 1982.

49. Brat DJ, Lillemoe KD, Yeo CJ, Warfield PB, Hruban RH: Progression of pancreatic intraductal neoplasias to infiltrating adenocarcinoma of the pancreas. *Am J Surg Pathol* **22**:163, 1998.

50. de la Garza M, Hill ID, Lebenthal E: Hereditary pancreatitis, in Go VLW, DiMango EP, Gardner JD, et al (eds): *The Pancreas: Biology, Pathobiology, and Disease*, vol 2. New York, Raven Press, 1993, p 1095.

51. Davidson P, Costanza D, Swieconek JA, Harris JB: Hereditary pancreatitis: A kindred without gross aminoaciduria. *Ann Intern Med* **68**:88, 1968.

52. Comfort MW, Steinberg AG: Pedigree of a family with hereditary chronic relapsing pancreatitis. *Gastroenterology* **21**:54, 1952.

53. Whitcomb DC, Preston RA, Aston CE, et al: A gene for hereditary pancreatitis maps to chromosome 7q35. *Gastroenterology* **110**:1975, 1996.

54. Whitcomb DC, Gorry MC, Preston RA, et al: Hereditary pancreatitis is caused by a mutation in the cationic trypsinogen gene. *Nature Genet* **14**:141, 1996.

55. Ekbom A, McLaughlin JK, Karlsson B-M, Nyren O, Gridley G, Adami H-O, Fraumeni JF J: Pancreatitis and pancreatic cancer: A population-based study. *J Natl Cancer Inst* **86**:625, 1994.

56. Lowenfels AB, Maisonneuve P, Cavallini G, et al: Pancreatitis and the risk of pancreatic cancer. *New Engl J Med* **328**:1433, 1993.

57. Lynch HT, Krush AJ: Heredity and adenocarcinoma of the colon. *Gastroenterology* **53**:517, 1967.

58. Lynch HT, Krush AJ, Guirgis H: Genetic factors in families with combined gastrointestinal and breast cancer. *Am J Gastroenterol* **59**:31, 1973.

59. Lynch HT, Schuelke GS, Kimberling WJ, et al: Hereditary non-polyposis colorectal cancer (Lynch syndromes I and II): II. Biomarker studies. *Cancer* **56**:939, 1985.

60. Liu B, Parsons R, Papadopoulos N, et al: Analysis of mismatch repair genes in hereditary non-polyposis colorectal cancer patients. *Nature Med* **2**:169, 1996.

61. Leach FS, Nicolaides NC, Papadopoulos N, et al: Mutations of a *mutS* homolog in hereditary nonpolyposis colorectal cancer. *Cell* **75**:1215, 1993.

62. Fishel R, Lescoe MK, Rao MRS, et al: The human mutator gene homolog *MSH2* and its association with hereditary nonpolyposis colon cancer. *Cell* **75**:1027, 1993.

63. Aaltonen LA, Peltomaki P, Mecklin J-P, et al: Replication errors in benign and malignant tumors from hereditary nonpolyposis color-ectal cancer patients. *Cancer Res* **54**:1645, 1994.

64. Thibodeau SN, Bren G, Schaid D: Microsatellite instability in cancer of the proximal colon. *Science* **260**:816, 1993.

65. Ionov Y, Peinado MA, Malkhosyan S, Shibata D, Perucho M: Ubiquitous somatic mutations in simple repeated sequences reveal a new mecanism for colonic carcinogenesis. *Nature* **363**:558, 1993.

66. Strand M, Prolla TA, Liskay RM, Petes TD: Destabilization of tracts of simple repetitive DNA in yeast by mutations affecting DNA mismatch repair. *Nature* **365**:274, 1993.

67. Goggins M, Offerhaus GJA, Hilgers W, et al: Pancreatic adenocar-cinomas with DNA replication errors (RER+) are associated with wild-type k-*ras* and characteristic histopathology: poor differentiation, a syncytial growth pattern, and pushing borders suggest RER+. *Am J Pathol* **152**:1501, 1998.

68. Parsons R, Li G-M, Longley MJ, et al: Hypermutability and mismatch repair deficiency in RER+ tumor cells. *Cell* **75**:1227, 1993.

69. Kunkel TA: Slippery DNA and diseases. *Nature* **365**:207, 1993.

70. Hahn SA, Seymour AB, Hoque ATMS, et al: Allelotype of pancreatic adenocarcinoma using xenograft enrichment. *Cancer Res* **55**:4670, 1995.

71. Caldas C, Hahn SA, da Costa LT, et al: Frequent somatic mutations and homozygous deletions of the *p16* (*MTS1*) gene in pancreatic adenocarcinoma. *Nature Genet* **8**:27, 1994.

71A. Wilentz RE, Goggins M, Redston M, Marcus VA, Adsay NV, Sohn TA, Kadkol SS, Yeo CJ, Choti M, Zahurak M, Johnson K, Tascilar M, Offerhaus GJA, Hruban RH, Kern SE: Genetic, immunohisto-chemical, and clinical features of medullary carcinoma of the pancreas: A newly described and characterized entity. *Am J Pathol* **156**:1641, 2000.

72. Bowlby LS: Pancreatic adenocarcinoma in an adolescent male with Peutz-Jeghers syndrome. *Hum Pathol* **17**:97, 1986.

73. Giardiello FM, Welsh SB, Hamilton SR, et al: Increased risk of cancer in the peutz-jeghers syndrome. *New Engl J Med* **316**:1511, 1987.

73A. Giardiello FM, Bresinger JD, Tersmette AC, Goodman SN, Petersen GM, Booker SV, Cruz-Correa M, Offerhaus JA: Very high risk of cancer in familial Peutz-Jeghers syndrome. *Gastroenterology* **119**(6):1447, 2000.

74. Jenne DE, Reimann H, Nezu J, et al: Peutz-Jeghers syndrome is caused by mutations in a novel serine threonine kinase. *Nature Genet* **18**:38, 1998.

75. Hemminki A, Markie D, Tomlinson I, et al: A serine/threonine kinase gene defective in Peutz Jeghers syndrome. *Nature* **391**:184, 1998.

76. Su GH, Hruban RH, Bansal RK, et al: Germline and somatic mutations of the *STK11/LKB1* Peutz-Jeghers gene in pancreatic and biliary cancers. *Am J Pathol* **154**:1835, 1999.

77. Whelan AJ, Bartsch D, Goodfellow PJ: Brief report: a familial syndrome of pancreatic cancer and melanoma with a mutation in the *CDKN2* tumor-suppressor gene. *New Engl J Med* **333**:975, 1995.

78. Goldstein AM, Fraser MC, Struewing JP, et al: Increased risk of cancer in melanoma-prone kindreds with p16 *INK4* mutations. *New Engl J Med* **333**:970, 1995.

79. Moskaluk CA, Hruban RH, Schutte M, et al: Polymerase chain reaction and cycle sequencing of DPC4 in the analysis of familial pancreatic carcinoma. *Diagn Mol Pathol* **6**:85, 1997.

80. Savitsky K, Bar-Shira A, Gilad S, et al: A single ataxia telangiectasia gene with a product similar to P1-3 kinase. *Science* **268**:1749, 1995.

80A. Tersmette AC, Petersen GM, Offerhaus GJA, Falatko FC, Brune K, Goggins M, Rozenblum E, Wilentz RE, Yeo CJ, Camerson JL, Kern SE, Hruban RH: Increased risk of incident pancreatic cancer among first-degree relatives of patients with familial pancreatic cancer. *Clin Cancer Res*, **7**:738, 2001.

81. Aston CE, Banke MG, McNamara PJ, et al: Segregation analysis of pancreatic cancer (abstract). *Am J Hum Genet* **61**:A194, 1997.

82. Crowley KE, Aston CE, MacNamara PJ, et al: Familial aggregation of other cancers in families with pancreatic cancer (abstract). *Am J Hum Genet* **61**:A196, 1997.

83. Tulinius H, Olafsdottir GH, Sigvaldason H, Tryggvadottir L, Bjarnadottir K: Neoplastic diseases in families of breat cancer patients. *J Med Genet* **31**:618, 1994.

84. Kerber RA, Slattery ML: The impact of family history on ovarian cancer risk. *Arch Intern Med* **155**:905, 1995.

85. Thorlacius S, Olafsdottir G, Tryggvadottir L, et al: A single BRCA2 mutation in male and female breast cancer families from Iceland with varied cancer phenotypes. *Nature Genet* **13**:117, 1996.

86. Phelan CM, Lancaster J, Tonin P, et al: Mutation analysis of the BRCA2 gene in 49 site-specific breast cancer families. *Nature Genet* **13**:120, 1996.

87. Couch FJ, Farid LM, DeShano ML, et al: *BRCA2* germline mutations in male breast cancer cases and breast cancer families. *Nature Genet* **13**:123, 1996.

88. Berman DB, Costalas J, Schultz DC, Grana G, Daly M, Godwin AK: A common mutation in BRCA2 that predisposes to a variety of cancers is found in both Jewish Ashkenazi and non-Jewish individuals. *Cancer Res* **56**:3409, 1996.

89. Johansson B, Bardi G, Heim S, et al: Nonrandom chromosomal rearrangements in pancreatic carcinomas. *Cancer* **69**:1674, 1992.

90. Johansson B, Mandahl N, Heim S, Mertens F, Andrén-Sandberg Å, Mitelman F: Chromosome abnormalities in a pancreatic adenocarcinoma. *Cancer Genet Cytogenet* **37**:209, 1989.

91. Griffin CA, Hruban RH, Long PP, Morsberger LA, Douna-Issa F, Yeo CJ: Chromosome abnormalities in pancreatic adenocarcinoma. *Genes Chromosom Cancer* **9**:93, 1994.

92. Griffin CA, Hruban RH, Morsberger L, et al: Consistent chromosome abnormalities in adenocarcinoma of the pancreas. *Cancer Res* **55**:2394, 1995.

93. Höglund M, Gorunova L, Andrén-Sandberg Å, Dawiskiba S, Mitelman F, Johansson B: Cytogenetic and fluorescence in situ hybridization analyses of chromosome 19 aberrations in pancreatic carcinomas: Frequent loss of 19p13.3 and gain of 19q13.1-13.2. *Genes Chromosom Cancer* **21**:8, 1998.

94. Seymour A, Hruban RH, Redston MS, et al: Allelotype of pancreatic adenocarcinoma. *Cancer Res* **54**:2761, 1994.

95. Brat DJ, Hahn SA, Griffin CA, Yeo CJ, Kern SE, Hruban RH: The structural basis of molecular genetic deletions: An integration of classical cytogenetic and molecular analyses in pancreatic adenocarcinoma. *Am J Pathol* **150**:383, 1997.

96. Schutte M, daCosta LT, Hahn SA, et al: Identification by representational difference analysis of a homozygous deletion in pancreatic carcinoma that lies within the *BRCA2* region. *Proc Natl Acad Sci USA* **92**:5950, 1995.

97. Wooster R, Bignell G, Lancaster J, et al: Identification of the breast cancer susceptibility gene *BRCA2*. *Nature* **378**:789, 1995.

98. Tavtigian SV, Simard J, Rommens J, et al: The complete *BRCA2* gene and mutations in chromosome 13q linked kindreds. *Nature Genet* **12**:335, 1996.

99. Knudson AG: Mutation and cancer: Statistical study of retinoblastoma. *Proc Natl Acad Sci USA* **68**:820, 1971.

100. Powell SM, Petersen GM, Krush AJ, et al: Molecular diagnosis of familial adenomatous polyposis. *New Engl J Med* **329**:1982, 1993.

101. Powell SM, Zilz N, Beazer-Barclay Y, et al: *APC* mutations occur early during colorectal tumorigenesis. *Nature* **359**:235, 1992.

102. Mulligan L, Kwok JBJ, Healey CS, et al: Germ-line mutations of the *RET* proto-oncogene in multiple endocrine neoplasia type 2A. *Nature* **363**:458, 1993.

103. Blaugrund JE, Johns MM Jr, Eby YJ, Ball DW, Baylin SB, Hruban RH, Sidransky D: *RET* proto-oncogene mutations in inherited and sporadic medullary thyroid cancer. *Hum Mol Genet* **3**:1895, 1994.

104. Moskaluk CA, Hruban RH, Lietman A, et al: Low prevalence of p16^INK4a and CDK4 mutations in familial pancreatic carcinoma. *Hum Mutat* **12**:70, 1998.

105. Goggins M, Schutte M, Lu J, et al: Germline *BRCA2* gene mutations in patients with apparently sporadic pancreatic carcinomas. *Cancer Res* **56**:5360, 1996.

106. Ozcelik H, Schmocker B, DiNicola N, et al: Germline BRCA2 6174delT mutations in Ashkenazi Jewish pancreatic cancer patients. *Nature Genet* **16**:17, 1997.

107. Hahn SA, Schutte M, Hoque ATMS, et al: *DPC4*, a candidate tumor suppressor gene at human chromosome 18q21.1. *Science* **271**:350, 1996.

108. Hruban RH, van Mansfeld ADM, Offerhaus GJA, et al: K-*ras* oncogene activation in adenocarcinoma of the human pancreas: A study of 82 carcinomas using a combination of mutant-enriched polymerase chain reaction analysis and allele-specific oligonucleotide hybridization. *Am J Pathol* **143**:545, 1993.

109. Barbacid M: *Ras* genes. *Annu Rev Biochem* **56**:779, 1987.

110. Scheffzek K, Ahmadian MR, Kabsch W, Wiesmuller L, Lautwein A, Schmitz F, Wittinghofer A: The Ras-RasGAP complex: Structural basis for GTPase activation and its loss in oncogenic *ras* mutants. *Science* **277**:333, 1997.

111. Almoguera C, Shibata D, Forrester K, Martin J, Arnheim N, Perucho M: Most human carcinomas of the exocrine pancreas contain mutant c-K-*ras* genes. *Cell* **53**:549, 1988.

112. Smit VTHBM, Boot AJM, Smits AMM, Fleuren GJ, Cornelisse CJ, Bos JL: K-*ras* codon 12 mutations occur very frequently in pancreatic adenocarcinomas. *Nucleic Acids Res* **16**:7773, 1988.

113. Mariyama M, Kishi K, Nakamura K, Obata H, Nishimura S: Frequency and types of point mutation at the 12th codon of the c-Ki-*ras* gene found in pancreatic cancers from Japanese patients. *Jpn J Cancer Res* **80**:622, 1989.

114. Grünewald K, Lyons J, Frolich A, et al: High frequency of Ki-*ras* codon 12 mutations in pancreatic adenocarcinomas. *Int J Cancer* **43**:1037, 1989.

115. Nagata Y, Abe M, Motoshima K, Nakayama E, Shiku H: Frequent glycine-to-aspartic acid mutations at codon 12 of c-Ki-*ras* gene in human pancreatic cancer in Japanese. *Jpn J Cancer Res* **81**:135, 1990.

116. Tada M, Yokosuka O, Omata M, Ohto M, Isono K: Analysis of ras gene mutations in biliary and pancreatic tumors by polymerase chain reaction and direct sequencing. *Cancer* **66**:930, 1990.

117. Berrozpe G, Schaeffer J, Peinado MA, Real FX, Perucho M: Comparative analysis of mutations in the *p53* and K-*ras* genes in pancreatic cancer. *Int J Cancer* **58**:185, 1994.

118. Motojima K, Urano T, Nagata Y, Shiku H, Tsunoda T, Kanematsu T: Mutations in the Kirsten-*ras* oncogene are common but lack correlation with prognosis and tumor stage in human pancreatic carcinoma. *Am J Gastroenterol* **86**:1784, 1991.

119. Motojima K, Urano T, Nagata Y, Shiku H, Tsurifune T, Kanematsu T: Detection of point mutations in the Kirsten-*ras* oncogene provides evidence for the multicentricity of pancreatic carcinoma. *Ann Surg* **217**:138, 1993.

120. Pellegata NS, Losekoot M, Fodde R, et al: Detection of K-*ras* mutations by denaturing gradient gel electrophoresis (DGGE): A study on pancreatic cancer. *Anticancer Res* **12**:1731, 1992.

121. Pellegata NS, Sessa F, Renault B, Bonato MS, Leone BE, Solcia E, Ranzani GN: K-*ras* and p53 gene mutations in pancreatic cancer: ductal and nonductal tumors progress through different genetic lesions. *Cancer Res* **54**:1556, 1994.

122. Suzuki H, Yoshida S, Ichikawa Y, et al: Ki-ras mutations in pancreatic secretions and aspirates from two patients without pancreatic cancer. *J Natl Cancer Inst* **86**:1547, 1994.

123. Tabata T, Fujimori T, Maeda S, Yamamoto M, Saitoh Y: The role of *ras* mutation in pancreatic cancer, precancerous lesions, and chronic pancreatitis. *Int J Pancreatol* **14**:237, 1993.

124. Yashiro T, Fulton N, Hara H, et al: Comparison of mutations of ras oncogen in human pancreatic exocrine and endocrine tumors. *Surgery* **114**:758, 1993.

125. DiGiuseppe JA, Hruban RH, Offerhaus GJA, Clement MJ, van den Berg FM, Cameron JL, van Mansfeld ADM: Detection of K-*ras* mutations in mucinous pancreatic duct hyperplasia from a patient with a family history of pancreatic carcinoma. *Am J Pathol* **144**:889, 1994.

126. Cerny WL, Mangold KA, Scarpelli DG: K-*ras* mutation is an early event in pancreatic duct carcinogenesis in the syrian golden hamster. *Cancer Res* **52**:4507, 1992.

127. Tada M, Omata M, Ohto M: *Ras* gene mutations in intraductal papillary neoplasms of the pancreas: Analysis in five cases. *Cancer* **67**:634, 1991.

128. Yanagisawa A, Ohtake K, Ohashi K, Hori M, Kitagawa T, Sugano H, Kato Y: Frequent c-Ki-*ras* oncogene activation in mucous cell hyperplasias of pancreas suffering from chronic inflammation. *Cancer Res* **53**:953, 1993.

129. Caldas C, Hahn SA, Hruban RH, Redston MS, Yeo CJ, Kern SE: Detection of K-*ras* mutations in the stool of patients with pancreatic adenocarcinoma and pancreatic ductal hyperplasia. *Cancer Res* **54**:3568, 1994.

130. Berthélemy P, Bouisson M, Escourrou J, Vaysse N, Rumeau JL, Pradayrol L: Identification of K-*ras* mutations in pancreatic juice in the early diagnosis of pancreatic cancer. *Ann Intern Med* **123**:188, 1995.

131. Sugio K, Molberg K, Albores-Saavedra J, Virmani AK, Koshimoto Y, Gazdar AF: K-*ras* mutations and allelic loss at 5q and 18q in the development of human pancreatic cancers. *Int J Pancreatol* **21**:205, 1997.

132. Moskaluk CA, Hruban RH, Kern SE: *p16* and K-*ras* gene mutations in the intraductal precursors of human pancreatic adenocarcinoma. *Cancer Res* **57**:2140, 1997.

133. Tada M, Ohashi M, Shiratori Y, et al: Analysis of K-*ras* gene mutation in hyperplastic duct cells of the pancreas without pancreatic disease. *Gastroenterology* **110**:227, 1996.

134. Cheng JQ, Ruggeri B, Klein WM, Sonoda G, Altomare DA, Watson DK, Testa JR: Amplification of *AKT2* in human pancreatic cells and inhibition of *AKT2* expression and tumorgenicity by antisense RNA. *Proc Natl Acad Sci* **93**:3636, 1996.

135. Batra SK, Metzgar RS, Hollingsworth MA: Isolation and characterization of a complementary DNA (PD-1) differentially expressed by human pancreatic ductal cell tumors. *Cell Growth Differ* **2**:385, 1991.

136. Wallrapp C, Müeller-Pillasch F, Solinas-Toldo S, et al: Characterization of a high copy number amplification at 6q24 in pancreatic cancer identifies *c-myb* as a candidate oncogene. *Cancer Res* **57**:3135, 1997.

137. DiGiuseppe JA, Hruban RH, Goodman SN, et al: Overexpression of p53 protein in adenocarcinoma of the pancreas. *Am J Clin Pathol* **101**:684, 1994.

138. Casey G, Yamanaka Y, Friess H, et al: *p53* mutations are common in pancreatic cancer and are absent in chronic pancreatitis. *Cancer Lett* **69**:151, 1993.

139. Nakamori S, Yashima K, Murakami Y, et al: Association of *p53* gene mutations with short survival in pancreatic adenocarcinoma. *Jpn J Cancer Res* **86**:174, 1998.

140. Redston MS, Caldas C, Seymour AB, Hruban RH, da Costa L, Yeo CJ, Kern SE: *p53* mutations in pancreatic carcinoma and evidence of common involvement of homocopolymer tracts in DNA microdeletions. *Cancer Res* **54**:3025, 1994.

141. Scarpa A, Capelli P, Mukai K, Zamboni G, Oda T, Iacono C, Hirohashi S: Pancreatic adenocarcinomas frequently show *p53* gene mutations. *Am J Pathol* **142**:1534, 1993.

142. Suwa H, Yoshimura T, Yamaguchi N, et al: K-*ras* and *p53* alterations in genomic DNA and transcripts of human pancreatic adenocarcinoma cell lines. *Jpn J Cancer Res* **85**:1005, 1994.

143. Weyrer K, Feichtinger H, Haun M, et al: *p53, Ki-ras,* and DNA ploidy in human pancreatic ductal adenocarcinomas. *Lab Invest* **74**:279, 1996.

144. Yonish-Rouach E, Resnitzky D, Lotem J, Sach L, Kimchi A, Oren M: Wildtype p53 induces apoptosis of myeloid leukemic cells that is inhibited by interleukin-6. *Nature* **352**:345, 1991.

145. Bates S, Vousden KH: p53 in signaling checkpoint arrest or apoptosis. *Curr Opin Genet Dev* **6**:12, 1996.

146. Kern SE, Pietenpol JA, Thiagalingam S, Seymour A, Kinzler KW, Vogelstein B: Oncogenic forms of p53 inhibit p53-regulated gene expression. *Science* **256**:827, 1992.

147. Kern SE, Kinzler KW, Bruskin A, Jarosz D, Friedman P, Prives C, Vogelstein B: Identification of p53 as a sequence-specific DNA-binding protein. *Science* **252**:1708, 1991.

148. Yin Y, Tainsky MA, Bischoff FZ, Strong LC, Wahl GM: Wild-type p53 restores cell cycle control and inhibits gene amplification in cells with mutant *p53* alleles. *Cell* **70**:937, 1992.

149. Kamb A, Gruis NA, Weaver-Feldhaus J, et al: A cell cycle regulator potentially involved in genesis of many tumor types. *Science* **264**:436, 1994.

150. Hu YX, Watanabe H, Ohtsubo K, Yamaguchi Y, Ha A, Okai T, Sawabu N: Frequent loss of p16 expression and its correlation with clinicopathological parameters in pancreatic carcinoma. *Clin Cancer Res* **3**:1473, 1997.

151. Huang L, Goodrow TL, Zhang S, Klein-Szanto AJP, Chang H, Ruggeri BA: Deletion and mutation analyses of the *P16/MTS-1* tumor-suppressor gene in human ductal pancreatic cancer reveals a higher frequency of abnormalities in tumor-derived cell lines than in primary ductal adenocarcinomas. *Cancer Res* **56**:1137, 1996.

152. Bartsch D, Shevlin DW, Callery MP, Norton JA, Wells SA, Goodfellow PJ: Reduced survival in patients with ductal pancreatic adenocarcinoma associated with *CDKN2* mutation. *J Natl Cancer Inst* **88**:680, 1996.

153. Naumann M, Savitskaia N, Eilert C, Schramm A, Kalthoff H, Schmiegel W: Frequent codeletion of *p16/MTS1* and *p15/MTS2* and genetic alterations in *p16/MTS1* in pancreatic tumors. *Gastroenterology* **110**:1215, 1996.

154. Bartsch D, Shevlin DW, Tung WS, Kisker O, Wells SA, Goodfellow PJ: Frequent mutations of *CDKN2* in primary pancreatic adenocarcinomas. *Genes Chromosom Cancer* **14**:189, 1995.

155. Herman JG, Merlo A, Mao L, et al: Inactivation of the *CDKN2/p16/MTS1* gene is frequently associated with aberrant DNA methylation in all common human cancer. *Cancer Res* **55**:4525, 1995.

156. Schutte M, Hruban RH, Geradts J, et al: Abrogation of the *Rb/p16* tumor-suppressive pathway in virtually all pancreatic carcinomas. *Cancer Res* **57**:3126, 1997.

157. Whyte P: The retinoblastoma protein and its relatives. *Semin Cancer Biol* **6**:83, 1995.

158. Longnecker DS: The quest for preneoplastic lesions in the pancreas. *Arch Pathol Lab Med* **118**:226, 1994.

158A. Wilentz RE, Su GH, Dai JL, Sparks AB, Argani P, Sohn TA, Yeo CJ, Kern SE, Hruban RH: Immunohistochemical labeling for Dpc4 mirrors genetic status in pancreatic adenocarcinomas: A new marker of *DPC4* inactivation. *Am J Pathol* **156**:37, 2000.

159. Schutte M, Hruban RH, Hedrick L, et al: *DPC4* gene in various tumor types. *Cancer Res* **56**:2527, 1996.

160. Niehrs C: Mad connection to the nucleus. *Nature* **381**:561, 1996.

161. Derynck R, Gelbart WM, Harland RM, et al: Nomenclature: Vertebrate mediators of TGFβ family signals. *Cell* **87**:173, 1996.

162. Riggins GJ, Thiagalingam S, Rozenblum E, et al: Mad-related genes in the human. *Nature Genet* **13(3)**:347, 1996.

163. Grau AM, Zhang L, Wang W, et al: Induction of p21^waf1 expression and growth inhibition by transforming growth factor *β* involve the tumor suppressor gene *DPC4* in human pancreatic adenocarcinoma cells. *Cancer Res* **57**:3929, 1997.

164. Polyak K: Negative regulation of cell growth by TGFβ. *Biochim Biophys Acta* **1242**:185, 1996.

165. White RL: Tumor suppressing pathways. *Cell* **92**:591, 1998.

166. Zhou S, Buckhaults P, Zawel L, et al: Targeted deletion of Smad4 shows it is required for transforming growth factor *β* and activin signaling in colorectal cancer cells. *Proc Natl Acad Sci USA* **95**:2412, 1998.

167. Takaku K, Oshima M, Miyoshi H, Matsui M, Seldin MF, Taketo MM: Intestinal tumorigenesis in compound mutant mice of both *Dpc4(Smad4)* and *Apc* genes. *Cell* **92**:645, 1998.

168. Hahn SA, Hoque ATMS, Moskaluk CA, et al: Homozygous deletion map at 18q21.1 in pancreatic cancer. *Cancer Res* **56**:490, 1996.

169. Su GH, Hilgers W, Shekher M, Tang D, Yeo CJ, Hruban RH, Kern SE: Alterations in pancreatic, biliary, and breast carcinomas support *MKK4* as a genetically targeted tumor-suppressor gene. *Cancer Res* **58**:2339, 1998.

170. Horii A, Nakatsuru S, Miyoshi Y, et al: Frequent somatic mutations of the *APC* gene in human pancreatic cancer. *Cancer Res* **52**:6696, 1992.

171. Yashima K, Nakamori S, Murakami Y, et al: Mutations of the adenomatous polyposis coli gene in the mutation cluster region: Comparison of human pancreatic and colorectal cancers. *Int J Cancer* **59**:43, 1994.

172. McKie AB, Filipe MI, Lemoine NR: Abnormalities affecting the *APC* and *MCC* tumour suppressor gene loci on chromosome 5q occur frequently in gastric cancer but not in pancreatic cancer. *Int J Cancer* **55**:598, 1993.

173. Barton CM, McKie AB, Hogg A, et al: Abnormalities of the *RB1* and *DCC* tumor suppressor genes: uncommon in human pancreatic adenocarcinoma. *Mol Carcinog* **13**:61, 1995.

174. Ruggeri B, Zhang S-Y, Caamano J, DiRado M, Flynn SD, Klein-Szanto AJP: Human pancreatic carcinomas and cell lines reveal frequent and multiple alterations in the *p53* and *Rb-1* tumor-suppressor genes. *Oncogene* **7**:1503, 1992.

175. Huang L, Lang D, Geradts J, Obara T, Klein-Szanto AJP, Lynch HT, Ruggeri BA: Molecular and immunochemical analyses of RB1 and cyclin D1 in human ductal pancreatic carcinomas and cell lines. *Mol Carcinog* **15**:85, 1996.

175A. Su GH, Bansal R, Murphy KM, Montgomery E, Yeo CJ, Hruban RH, Kern SE. *ACVR1B* (*ALK4*, activin receptor type 1B) Gene mutation in pancreatic carcinoma. *Proc Natl Acad Sci USA* **98**: 3254, 2001.

175B. Ueki T, Toyata M, Sohn T, Yeo CJ, Issa J-P J, Hruban RH, Goggins M: Hypermethylation of multiple genes in pancreatic adenocarcinoma. *Cancer Res* **60**:1835, 2000.

175C. Ueki T, Toyota M, Skinner H, Walter KM, Yeo CJ, Issa J-P J, Hruban RH, Goggins M: Identification and characterization of differentially methylated CpG islands in pancreatic carcinoma. *Cancer Res* **61**:8540, 2001.

176. Hruban RH, van der Riet P, Erozan Y, Sidransky D: Molecular biology and the early detection of carcinoma of the bladder: The case of Hubert H. Humphrey. *New Engl J Med* **330**:1276, 1994.

177. Tada M, Omata M, Kawai S, Saisho H, Ohto M, Saiki RK, Sninsky JJ: Detection of *ras* gene mutations in pancreatic juice and peripheral blood of patients with pancreatic adenocarcinoma. *Cancer Res* **53**:2472, 1993.

178. Apple SK, Hecht JR, Novak JM, Nieberg RK, Rosenthal DL, Grody WW: Polymerase chain reaction-based K-*ras* mutation detection of

pancreatic adenocarcinoma in routine cytology smears. *Am J Clin Pathol* **105**:321, 1996.

179. Brentnall TA, Chen R, Kimmey MB, et al: *Ras* mutations and microsatellite instability detected in ERCP-derived pancreatic juice from patients with pancreatic cancer (abstract). *Gastroenterology* **108**:A452, 1995.

180. Iguchi H, Sugano K, Fukayama N, et al: Analysis of Ki-*ras* codon 12 mutations in the duodenal juice of patients with pancreatic cancer. *Gastroenterology* **110**:221, 1996.

181. Kondo H, Sugano K, Fukayama N, et al: Detection of point mutations in the K-*ras* oncogene at codon 12 in pure pancreatic juice for diagnosis of pancreatic carcinoma. *Cancer* **73**:1589, 1994.

182. Uehara H, Nakaizumi A, Baba M, et al: Diagnosis of pancreatic cancer by K-*ras* point mutation and cytology of pancreatic juice. *Am J Gastroenterol* **91**:1616, 1996.

183. Wilentz RE, Chung CH, Sturm PDJ, et al: Detection of K-*ras* mutations in duodenal fluid-derived DNA from patients with pancreatic cancer. *Cancer* **82**:96, 1998.

184. Hruban RH, Yeo CJ, Kern SE: Screening for pancreatic cancer, in Kramer B, Provok P, Gohagan J (eds): *Screening Theory and Practice*. New York, Marcel Dekker 1998.

185. Hameed M, Marrero AM, Conlon KC, et al: Expression of p53 nucleophosphoprotein in *in situ* pancreatic ductal adenocarcinoma: An immunohistochemical analysis of 100 cases (abstract). *Lab Invest* **70**:132A, 1994.

186. Wilentz RE, Geradts J, Maynard R, et al: Inactivation of the *p16 (INK4A)* tumor-suppressor gene in pancreatic duct lesions: loss of intranuclear expression. *Cancer Res.* **58**:4740, 1998.

186A. Wilentz RE, Geradts J, Maynard R, Offerhaus GJA, Kang M, Goggins M, Yeo CJ, Kern E, Hruban RH. Inactivation of the p16 (INK4A) tumor-suppressor gene in pancreatic duct lesions: Loss of intranuclear expression. *Cancer Res* **58**(20):4740, 1998.

187. Zhou W, Sokoll LJ, Bruzek DJ, Zhang L, Velculescu VE, Goldin SB, Hruban RH, Kern SE, Hamilton SR, Chan DW, Vogelstein B, Kinzler KW: Identifying markers for pancreatic cancer by gene expression analysis. *Cancer Epidemiol Biomarkers Prev* **7**: 109, 1998.

188. Argani P, Rosty C, Reiter RE, Wilentz RE, Murugesan SR, Leach SD, Ryu B, Skinner HG, Goggins M, Jaffee EM, Yeo CJ, Cameron JL, Kern SE, Hruban RH: Discovery of new markers of cancer through serial analysis of gene expression (SAGE): Prostate stem cell antigen (PSCA) is overexpressed in pancreatic adeno-carcinoma. *Cancer Res* **61**:4320, 2001.

189. Argani P, Iacobuzio-Donahue CA, Ryu B, Rosty C, Goggins M, Wilentz RE, Murugesan SR, Kaushal M, Leach SD, Jaffee E, Yeo CJ, Cameron JL, Kern SE, Hruban RH: Mesothelin is over-expressed in the vast majority of adenoccarcinomas of the pancreas: Identification of a new pancreatic cancer marker by serial analysis of gene expression (SAGE). *Clin Cancer Res*, 2001. (In press.)

Ovarian Cancer

Louis Dubeau

1. Ovarian carcinomas are the fifth leading cause of death from cancer among women. These tumors are morphologically similar to those arising from Müllerian-derived gynecologic organs despite the ovary itself not being embryologically derived from Müllerian ducts.
2. That ovarian carcinomas rarely spread outside the pelvic and abdominal cavities should facilitate usage of molecular genetic tests to document the presence or absence of residual tumor cells in treated patients.
3. Ovarian carcinomas are thought to arise from the mesothelial layer lining the ovarian surface. This theory does not account for the Müllerian-like appearance of these tumors and remains unproven.
4. The development of a suitable animal model for ovarian carcinomas is complicated by the low frequencies of these tumors in lower mammals. That such tumors are associated with frequent ovulation in birds supports theories linking incessant ovulation to risk of ovarian cancer in humans.
5. *In vitro* cultures of cells regarded as possible candidates for the origin of ovarian carcinomas, as well as of benign ovarian tumors, are available. Such cultures provide experimental systems to clarify the association between these different cell types and ovarian tumorigenesis.
6. Ovarian epithelial tumors are a good model to study tumor development because they are subdivided into benign, low malignant potential, and different grades of malignant subgroups which can each be regarded as representing varying degress of neoplastic transformation.
7. Although most ovarian carcinomas occur sporadically, a significant proportion arise in individuals with familial predisposition to this disease. The best-characterized genetic determinants of such predisposition are inherited mutations in either the *BRCA1* gene (familial breast/ovarian cancer syndrome) or in genes coding for mismatch repair enzymes (Lynch II syndrome).
8. Molecular genetic changes distinguishing ovarian cystadenomas, LMP tumors, and different grades of carcinomas from each other have been described. A gene that possibly escapes X chromosome inactivation may control the development of tumors of low malignant potential. Abnormalities in the same gene may be associated with increased biological aggressiveness in carcinomas.
9. Molecular genetic studies suggest that benign and malignant ovarian epithelial tumors are usually not part of a disease continuum. Benign tumors that progress to malignancy are probably those that are predisposed to such progression from their onset because of the presence of molecular genetic abnormalities associated with malignancy.
10. A genetic model for ovarian epithelial tumor development can be formulated based on known molecular genetic differences between benign, low malignant potential, and malignant tumors.

CLINICOPATHOLOGIC FEATURES OF OVARIAN CARCINOMAS

Ovarian carcinoma is the fifth leading cause of death from cancer among women in the United States. This heterogeneous group of tumors includes several histopathologic subtypes, such as serous, mucinous, endometrioid, clear cell, as well as other less common forms.[1] One of the most intriguing features of these different subtypes is their striking resemblance to carcinomas arising from other organs of the female genital tract. For example, serous ovarian carcinomas are morphologically similar to epithelial tumors arising in the fallopian tubes. Mucinous carcinomas resemble those arising in endocervix. Endometrioid ovarian carcinomas are similar to carcinomas of the endometrium. Clear-cell tumors are likewise similar to a variant of endometrial carcinomas. These morphologic similarities are difficult to reconcile with there being no fallopian, endocervical, or endometrial-like epithelia present in normal ovaries. In addition, whereas the above organs are derived embryologically from the Müllerian ducts, the ovary is thought to be of mesonephric origin. The histogenesis of ovarian epithelial tumors is, therefore, still unclear, greatly complicating the development screening protocols for precursor lesions or early disease.

Ovarian carcinomas usually remain confined to the pelvic and abdominal cavities even at advanced disease stages. Thus, these tumors should be suitable for molecular genetic tests aimed at documenting the presence of residual disease following completion of adjuvant chemotherapy protocols. Recent studies[2] suggest that the presence of measurable levels of the enzyme telomerase in abdominal washings of patients may be a useful indicator of active disease for that purpose.

CURRENT THEORIES ABOUT THE CELL OF ORIGIN OF OVARIAN EPITHELIAL TUMORS

According to the currently favored theory, ovarian epithelial tumors arise in the mesothelial layer lining the ovarian surface (surface epithelium).[1] This cell layer may invaginate to create small cysts, which eventually lose their connection to the ovarian surface and may give rise to ovarian tumors. That ovarian epithelial tumors resemble tumors of Müllerian origin is often explained by the suggestion that the ovarian surface epithelium is not the direct precursor of ovarian epithelial neoplasms; instead, it must first undergo metaplasia to become Müllerian-like. If this hypothesis is correct, knowledge of the factors responsible for such metaplastic changes could lead to effective approaches for the prevention of ovarian cancer. Indeed, if metaplasia of the ovarian surface epithelium is a necessary step preceding tumor development, controlling this step would put us one step ahead of the cancer. However, the above theory is largely based on morphologic observations and remains unproved.[3] Recently, an argument was made that the components of the secondary Müllerian system, which include rete ovarii, paraovarian Müllerian rests, and endosalpingiosis, as well as pathologic conditions

A list of standard abbreviations is located immediately preceding the index. Additional abbreviations used in this chapter include: LMP = low malignant potential such as endometriosis, may be the site of origin of ovarian carcinomas.[3]

ANIMAL MODELS

Development of a suitable animal model for spontaneous ovarian carcinoma is complicated by these tumors being rare in most animals, including lower mammals. Knowledge of the reasons for the relatively low incidence of spontaneous ovarian epithelial tumors in lower mammals as compared to humans could provide important clues about the origin and risk factors of the human tumors. That tumors resembling human ovarian carcinomas are frequently present in the domestic hen[2] may prove particularly relevant. The high frequency of ovarian tumors in those animals has been linked to the activity of incessant egg production.[4] Wild hens or other wild birds, in which continuous egg production is not artificially induced, do not develop ovarian tumors. These observations are intriguing in light of the extensive epidemiologic data suggesting an association between incessant ovulation and risk of ovarian cancer in humans.[5] Such studies indicate that interruption of chronic menstrual cycling by either pregnancy or anovulatory drugs has an important protective effect against this disease.[5] Recent findings that the *BRCA1* gene, which is important for familial predisposition to breast and ovarian cancer, is strongly expressed in cells responding to pituitary gonadotropin hormones,[6] and that ovaries from patients with familial predisposition to the above cancers show various changes related to ovulatory activity,[7] provide additional support for a link between ovulatory activity and ovarian cancer development. These observations raise the possibility that ovarian carcinomas result from an artifact of civilization, that of incessant ovulation, as chronic menstrual cycling was unlikely in early humans due to more frequent pregnancies and longer lactation periods.

In Vitro MODELS

Several authors succeeded in culturing mesothelial cells lining the surface of ovaries of either adult humans or experimental animals, and were able to keep the cells in culture over several passages.[8–10] Cultures of epithelial cells derived from rete ovarii were also reported.[11] Godwin *et al.*[12] reported a high transformation rate in cultured ovarian surface mesothelial cells, suggesting that they may indeed be prone to malignant development. Support for the hypothesis that such cells may be prone to undergo metaplastic changes comes from the demonstration that steroid hormone responsiveness, a characteristic of Müllerian-derived epithelia, was induced by v-*ras* transformation in cultured ovarian surface epithelial cells.[13]

Several strains of ovarian cystadenomas, which are benign tumors of the same cell lineage as carcinomas, were recently developed and characterized.[14] Given the divergent differentiation pathways of ovarian epithelial tumors and ovarian surface mesothelium, and because definitive evidence that the former originates in the latter is still missing, these strains may constitute attractive models to investigate the molecular mechanisms of ovarian tumor progression in *in vitro* environments.

OVARIAN EPITHELIAL TUMORS AS A MODEL FOR TUMOR DEVELOPMENT

In addition to being an important clinical entity, ovarian epithelial tumors are attractive for studying tumor development because they can be subdivided into well-defined and phenotypically stable categories that may be regarded as representing varying degrees of neoplastic transformation (Fig. 41-1). Cystadenomas are made up of the same cell type as carcinomas, but are readily distinguished from the latter based on their total absence of invasive or metastatic abilities. Ovarian tumors of low malignant potential (LMP) are histologically more complex than cystadenomas and show some histopathologic features that are normally associated

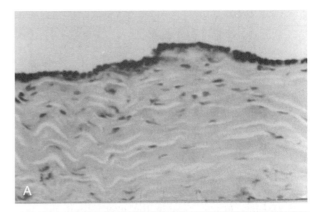
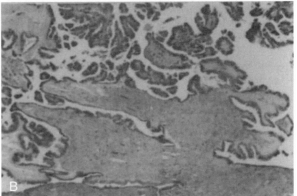
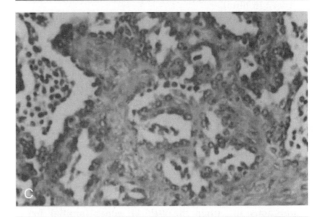
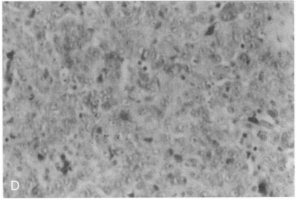

Fig. 41-1 Components of the ovarian epithelial tumor model. *A.* Cystadenoma: Incessant but ordered cell proliferation. *B.* Low malignant potential: Disorganized cell proliferation resulting in complex histologic architectures. *C.* Low grade carcinoma: Invasive and metastatic; incessant but ordered cell proliferation allowing maintenance of glandular or other specialized structures. *D.* High grade carcinoma: Invasive and metastatic; disorganized cell proliferation resulting in solid and amorphous tumor blocks.

with carcinomas, but have absent (or greatly reduced) invasive abilities.[1,15] The further subdivision of ovarian carcinomas into low and high histologic grades allows further dissection of their phenotypic features. Low-grade carcinomas form organized structures, such as glandular acini, whereas high-grade lesions form solid, poorly organized cell masses according to the criteria used in Fig. 41-1, which were adopted in the author's laboratory because of their simplicity and reproducibility.

FAMILIAL PREDISPOSITION TO OVARIAN CARCINOMA

Although this review focuses primarily on sporadic ovarian epithelial tumors, it is estimated that up to 10 percent of ovarian carcinomas occur in individuals with familial predisposition to this disease. Most familial ovarian cancers appear to fall into one of two major syndromes. The first syndrome is the familial breast and ovarian cancer syndrome that is associated with inherited mutations in the *BRCA1* and *BRCA2* genes. Tumors belonging to this group may show different clinicopathologic characteristics than sporadic ovarian tumors show,[16] and it has been suggested that their spectrum of somatic molecular genetic abnormalities may also be different.[17] Some features, however, are similar to those seen in sporadic ovarian cancers. For example, incessant ovulatory activity, which is an important risk factor for sporadic cancers, also increases disease risk in patients with germ-line mutations in either of these two genes. The second group of familial ovarian cancers is that associated with Lynch II syndrome, which is characterized by predisposition to cancers of the colon, endometrium, and ovary, and which is associated with inherited abnormalities in genes coding for mismatch repair enzymes. Both syndromes are described more fully in other chapters and are not discussed further here.

MOLECULAR CHANGES DISTINGUISHING DIFFERENT SUBTYPES OF OVARIAN EPITHELIAL TUMORS

A number of abnormalities involving cellular proto-oncogenes, including HER-2/*neu*,[18] AKT2,[19] c-*fms*,[20] Bcl-2,[21] FGF-3,[22] and *met*,[23] were described in ovarian carcinomas. Abnormalities involving tumor-suppressor genes such as *p53*,[24–27] *SPARC*,[28] and *nm23*,[29] were also reported. Novel genes were isolated based on their down-regulation in ovarian tumors, and may function as tumor suppressors,[30–32] although their exact roles in ovarian tumorigenesis are still unclear. Data on frequencies of losses of heterozygosity on various chromosomes are extensive, including several complete allelotypes.[33–35] In addition, comprehensive cytogenetic analyses of ovarian tumors have been reported.[36–39] Specific molecular abnormalities were shown to be associated with disease prognosis[21,22,40,41] and specific genes, such as HER-2/*neu*[42–44] and *p53*,[45] have been evaluated as potential targets for gene therapy. A comprehensive review of these data are beyond the scope of this chapter, which focuses on molecular genetic studies presented in the context of the ovarian epithelial tumor model described in Fig. 41-2. The intent of this chapter is to provide insights into the molecular genetic changes controlling the different tumor subtypes shown in Fig. 41-1, in order to develop a molecular genetic model for ovarian tumorigenesis similar to what was first achieved with colorectal cancer.[46]

The complexity of molecular genetic changes present in ovarian carcinomas clearly increases with increasing tumor histologic grades.[35,37,47,48] This observation is in agreement with classical tumor progression theories.[49] Grades of ovarian carcinomas, however, are not only a function of the mere number of molecular genetic abnormalities present in a given tumor genome as specific molecular abnormalities appear strongly associated with high histologic grades.[35,37,47,48,50,51] Thus, whereas losses of heterozygosity affecting certain chromosomes, such as 6q, 17p, and 17q, appear frequently in ovarian tumors of all histologic grades,[35] losses in chromosome 13 are frequent only in those of high histologic grades.[50,51] It may be that the gene(s) targeted by losses of heterozygosity in chromosome 13 control(s) a different cellular pathway associated perhaps with differentiation or other determinants of tumor grade, but not with cell-cycle regulation. Proof of this hypothesis awaits identification and characterization of the gene(s) targeted by these losses of heterozygosity.

Recent data[35,37] also provide insights into the molecular genetic differences distinguishing ovarian carcinomas from the noninvasive and nonmetastatic ovarian epithelial tumors (Fig. 41-2). Examination of the distribution and frequencies of losses of heterozygosity in these various tumor subtypes showed that such losses, which are frequent in ovarian carcinomas, are rare in the biologically less aggressive ovarian epithelial tumors (with the exception of losses affecting the X chromosome in LMP tumors discussed below).[35] Thus, the underlying defects responsible for loss of heterozygosity usually result in malignancy, implying that tumor-suppressor gene inactivation, which is an important consequence of such losses, is not a feature of cystadenoma or LMP tumor development.[35] Other published molecular genetic differences between the different subtypes of ovarian tumors mentioned in Fig. 41-2 include the presence of p53 mutations,[27,52] which is strongly associated with malignant tumors, and changes in DNA methylation,[53] which are associated with both LMP tumors and carcinomas, but not with cystadenomas. Telomerase, an enzyme necessary for unlimited cell growth, is usually not detected in cystadenomas, whereas it is expressed in most LMP tumors and carcinomas.[54]

The only exception to the rarity of losses of heterozygosity in LMP tumors are losses affecting the X chromosome, which are present in about 50 percent of cases.[35] The target(s) of the allelic losses involving this chromosome in LMP tumors is not known, although the candidate chromosomal region was recently narrowed down considerably.[55] That the reduced allele invariably affects the inactive copy of this chromosome suggests that the targeted gene(s) escapes X inactivation. This suggestion is attractive because individuals born with a single X chromosome (Turner syndrome)[56] show abnormal ovarian development (gonadal dysgenesis). Thus, the presence of the inactive X chromosome is necessary for normal ovarian development and it is conceivable that abnormalities in the same gene during adult life may lead to tumorigenesis. The X chromosome is also thought to be important for the establishment of *in vitro* immortality,[57,58] and was recently implicated in the development of prostate cancer.[59]

ARE OVARIAN CYSTADENOMAS, LMP TUMORS, AND CARCINOMAS PART OF A DISEASE CONTINUUM?

Whether ovarian cystadenomas, LMP tumors, and carcinomas represent distinct disease processes or are part of a disease continuum is important to our understanding of ovarian tumor development and is relevant to the clinical management of cystadenomas and LMP tumors. Arguments in favor of a disease continuum come from morphologic observations that areas that are histologically indistinguishable from typical ovarian cystadenomas are sometimes found contiguous to carcinomas.[60] The most straightforward interpretation for these lesions, which are sometimes called cystadenocarcinomas, is that the histologically malignant areas arose from the preexisting morphologically benign areas. This interpretation implies that any molecular genetic change associated with carcinomas, but that are normally not present in solitary cystadenomas, should be confined to the histologically malignant portions of cystadenocarcinomas. However, losses of heterozygosity and *p53* mutations, which are frequent in carcinomas and absent, or at least very rare, in solitary cystadenomas, are usually concordant in all portions of ovarian cystadenocarcinomas, including the morphologically benign areas.[27,61] Concordance for aneuploidy was likewise shown in different regions of cystadenocarcinomas using interphase

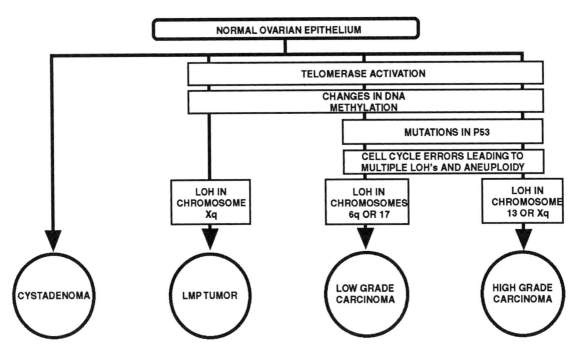

Fig. 41-2 A genetic model for sporadic (nonfamilial) ovarian epithelial tumor development.

cytogenetic approaches.[62] It seems clear based on these observations that histologically benign portions of cystadenocarcinomas are genetically different from typical (solitary) cystadenomas.[27,61] This conclusion supports the idea that cystadenomas do not generally progress to malignancy unless they carry a genetic predisposition to such progression, such as a mutation in the *p53* gene.[27]

A GENETIC MODEL FOR NONFAMILIAL OVARIAN EPITHELIAL TUMOR DEVELOPMENT

The genetic model in Fig. 41-2 is a working hypothesis based on information reviewed in the last section. Little is known about the genetic determinants of ovarian cystadenomas. These tumors appear to share few features with their malignant counterparts and may arise from a different mechanism. In contrast, some molecular changes, such as telomerase expression[54] and global changes in DNA methylation,[53] appear to be shared both by LMP tumors and carcinomas. These observations emphasize the merit of subdividing the biologically less aggressive ovarian tumors into cystadenomas and LMP tumors, in spite of the apparent clinically benign nature of the latter.[63] LMP tumors also show frequent losses of heterozygosity targeting a specific region of the inactive copy of the X chromosome. These changes, by themselves, are not sufficient to induce invasive and metastatic behavior because they occur in LMP tumors. However, if losses affecting the X chromosome occur in tumors where the malignant phenotype is already present, these may result in increased biological aggressiveness. This last conclusion accounts for the observation that losses affecting the X chromosome, although rare in low-grade carcinomas, are frequent in high-grade tumors.[35] Mutations in *p53*, as well as multiple losses of heterozygosity, the latter presumably resulting from cell-cycle errors that may be facilitated by the former, lead to the development of carcinomas. Specific losses of heterozygosity (such as in chromosome 13 or Xq) may be associated with specific features of the malignant phenotype, such as cellular differentiation, and may lead to higher tumor histologic grades. In contrast, losses in chromosomes 6q or 17 may be more directly associated with the malignant phenotype *per se* and are compatible with all histologic grades.

The nature of the specific genes targeted by the allelic deletions mentioned in the above model, as well as the exact consequences of other molecular genetic changes, such as in DNA methylation, are still largely unknown. These questions are the focus of current research efforts and significant progress is likely in the near future. These advances will result in a more comprehensive understanding of the mechanisms of ovarian epithelial tumors at the molecular level, and should also provide a basis for novel screening, diagnostic, and therapeutic approaches that are likely to improve the clinical management of these important tumors of women.

REFERENCES

1. Scully RE: Ovarian tumors. *Am J Pathol* **87:**686, 1977.
2. Duggan B, Wan M, Yu M, Roman L, Muderspach L, Delgadillo E, Li W-Z, Martin S, Dubeau L: Detection of ovarian cancer cells: Comparison of a telomerase assay and cytologic examination. *J Natl Cancer Inst* **90:**238, 1998.
3. Dubeau L: The cell of origin of ovarian epithelial tumors and the ovarian surface epithelium dogma: Does the emperor have no clothes? *Gynecol Oncol* **72:**437, 1999.
4. Fredrickson TN: Ovarian tumors of the hen. *Environ Health Perspect* **73:**35, 1987.
5. Whittemore AS, Harris R, Intyre J, Group CC: Characteristics relating to ovarian cancer risk: Collaborative analysis of 12 U.S. case-control studies. *Am J Epidemiol* **136:**1184, 1992.
6. Wan M, Sangiorgi F, Felix JC, Dubeau L: Association of BRCA1 with gonadotropin-responsive cells. *Lancet* **348:**192, 1996.
7. Salazar H, Godwin AK, Daly MB, Laub PB, Hogan WM, Rosenblum N, Boente MP, Lynch HT, Hamilton TC: Microscopic benign and invasive neoplasms and a cancer-prone phenotype in prophylactic oophorectomies. *J Natl Cancer Inst* **88:**1810, 1996.
8. Nicosia SV, Johnson JH, Streibel EJ: Growth characteristics of rabbit ovarian mesothelial (surface epithelial) cells. *Int J Gynecol Pathol* **4:**58, 1985.
9. Siemens CH, Auersperg N: Serial propagation of human ovarian surface epithelium in tissue culture. *J Cell Physiol* **134:**347, 1988.
10. Tsao SW, Mok SC, Fey EG, Fletcher JA, Wan TS, Chew EC, Muto MG, Knapp RC, Berkowitz RS: Characterization of human ovarian surface epithelial cells immortalized by human papilloma viral oncogenes (HPV-E6E7 ORFs). *Exp Cell Res* **218:**499, 1995.
11. Dubeau L, Velicescu M, Sherrod AE, Schreiber G, Holt G: Culture of human fetal ovarian epithelium in a chemically defined, serum-free medium: A model for ovarian carcinogenesis. *Anticancer Res* **10:**1233, 1990.
12. Godwin AK, Testa JR, Handel LM, Liu Z, Vanderveer LA, Tracey PA, Hamilton TC: Spontaneous transformation of rat ovarian surface

epithelial cells: Association with cytogenetic changes and implications of repeated ovulation in the etiology of ovarian cancer. *J Natl Cancer Inst* **84:**592, 1992.

13. Pan J, Roskelley CD, Luu The V, Rojiani M, Auersperg N: Reversal of divergent differentiation by ras oncogene-mediated transformation. *Cancer Res* **52:**4269, 1992.

14. Luo MP, Gomperts B, Imren S, DeClerck YA, Ito M, Velicescu M, Felix JC, Dubeau L: Establishment of long-term *in vitro* cultures of human ovarian cystadenomas and LMP tumors and examination of their spectrum of expression of matrix-degrading proteinases. *Gynecol Oncol* **67:**277, 1997.

15. Bell DA: Ovarian surface epithelial-stromal tumors. *Hum Pathol* **22:**750, 1991.

16. Johannsson OT, Idvall I, Anderson C, Borg A, Barkardottir RB, Egilsson V, Olsson H: Tumour biological features of BRCA1-induced breast and ovarian cancer. *Eur J Cancer* **33:**362, 1997.

17. Rhei E, Bogomolniy F, Federici MG, Maresco DL, Offit K, Robson ME, Saigo PE, Boyd J: Molecular genetic characterization of BRCA1- and BRCA2-linked hereditary ovarian cancers. *Cancer Res* **58:**3193, 1998.

18. Press MF, Jones LA, Godolphin W, Edwards CL, Slamon DJ: HER-2/ neu oncogene amplification and expression in breast and ovarian cancers. *Prog Clin Biol Res* **354A:**209, 1990.

19. Bellacosa A, DeFeo D, Godwin AK, Bell DW, Cheng JQ, Altomare DA, Wan M, Dubeau L, Scambia V, Masciullo V, Ferrandina G, Panici PB, Mancuso S, Neri G, Testa JR: Molecular alterations of the AKT2 oncogene in ovarian and breast carcinomas. *Int J Cancer* **64:**280, 1995.

20. Chambers SK, Wang Y, Gertz RE, Kacinski BM: Macrophage colony-stimulating factor mediates invasion of ovarian cancer cells through urokinase. *Cancer Res* **55:**1578, 1995.

21. Herod JJ, Eliopoulos AG, Warwick J, Niedobitek G, Young LS, Kerr DG: The prognostic significance of Bcl-2 and p53 expression in ovarian carcinoma. *Cancer Res* **56:**2178, 1996.

22. Rosen A, Sevelda P, Klein M, Dobianer K, Hruza C, Czerwenka K, Hanak H, Vavra N, Salzer H, Leodolter S, Medl M, Spona J: First experience with FGF-3 (INT-2) amplification in women with epithelial ovarian cancer. *Br J Cancer* **67:**1122, 1993.

23. Di-Renzo MF, Olivero M, Katsaros D, Crepaldi T, Gaglia P, Zola P, Sismondi P, Comoglio PM: Overexpression of the Met/HGF receptor in ovarian cancer. *Int J Cancer* **58:**658, 1994.

24. Teneriello MG, Ebina M, Linnoila RI, Henry M, Nash JD, Park RC, Birrer MJ: p53 and Ki-ras gene mutations in epithelial ovarian neoplasms. *Cancer Res* **53:**3103, 1993.

25. Mazars R, Pujol P, Maudelonde T, Jeanteur P, Theillet C: p53 mutations in ovarian cancer: A late event? *Oncogene* **6:**1685, 1991.

26. Kohler MF, Marks JR, Wiseman RW, Jacobs IJ, Davidoff AM, Clarke-Pearson DL, Soper JT, Bast RC, Berchuck A: Spectrum of mutation and frequency of allelic deletion of the p53 gene in ovarian cancer. *J Natl Cancer Inst* **85:**1513, 1993.

27. Zheng J, Benedict WF, Xu H-J, Hu S-X, Kim TM, Velicescu M, Wan M, Cofer KF, Dubeau L: Genetic disparity between morphologically benign cysts contiguous to ovarian carcinomas and solitary cystadenomas. *J Natl Cancer Inst* **87:**1146, 1995.

28. Mok SC, Chan WY, Wong KK, Muto MG, Berkowitz RS: SPARC, an extracellular matrix protein with tumor-suppressing activity in human ovarian epithelial cells. *Oncogene* **12:**1895, 1996.

29. Mandai M, Konishi I, Koshiyama M, Mori T, Arao S, Tashiro H, Okamura H, Nomura H, Hiai H, Fukumoto M: Expression of metastasis-related nm23-H1 and nm23-H2 genes in ovarian carcinomas: Correlation with clinicopathology, EGFR, c-erbB-2, and c-erbB-3 genes, and sex steroid receptor expression. *Cancer Res* **54:**1825, 1994.

30. Mok SC, Chan WY, Wong KK, Cheung KK, Lau CC, Ng SW, Baldini A, Colitti CV, Rock CO, Berkowitz RS: DOC-2, a candidate tumor suppressor gene in human epithelial ovarian cancer. *Oncogene* **16:**2381, 1998.

31. Schultz DC, Vanderveer L, Berman BD, Hamilton TC, Wong AJ, Godwin AK: Identification of 2 candidate tumor suppressor genes on chromosome 17.p13.3. *Cancer Res* **56:**1997, 1996.

32. Abdollahi A, Godwin AK, Miller PD, Getts LA, Schultz DC, Taguchi T, Testa JR, Hamilton TC: Identification of a gene containing zinc-finger motifs based on lost expression in malignantly transformed rat ovarian surface epithelial cells. *Cancer Res* **57:**2029, 1997.

33. Sato T, Saito H, Morita R, Koi S, Lee JH, Nakamura Y: Allelotype of human ovarian cancer. *Cancer Res* **51:**5118, 1991.

34. Cliby W, Ritland S, Hartmann L, Dodson M, Halling KC, Keeney G, Podratz KC, Jenkins RB: Human epithelial ovarian cancer allelotype. *Cancer Res* **53:**2393, 1993.

35. Cheng PC, Gosewehr JA, Kim TM, Velicescu M, Wan M, Zheng J, Felix JC, Cofer KF, Luo P, Biela BH, Godorov G, Dubeau L: Potential role of the inactivated X chromosome in ovarian epithelial tumor development. *J Natl Cancer Inst* **88:**510, 1996.

36. Pejovic T: Genetic changes in ovarian cancer. *Ann Med* **27:**73, 1995.

37. Iwabuchi H, Sakamoto M, Sakunaga H, Ma YY, Carcangiu ML, Pinkel D, Yang Feng TL, Gray JW: Genetic analysis of benign, low-grade, and high-grade ovarian tumors. *Cancer Res* **55:**6172, 1995.

38. Thompson FH, Emerson J, Alberts D, Liu Y, Guan XY, Burgess A, Fox S, Taetle R, Weinstein R, Makar R, Powell D, Trent J: Clonal chromosome abnormalities in 54 cases of ovarian carcinoma. *Cancer Genet Cytogenet* **73:**33, 1994.

39. Persons DL, Hartmann LC, Herath JF, Borell TJ, Cliby WA, Keeney GL, Jenkins RB: Interphase molecular cytogenetic analysis of epithelial ovarian carcinomas. *Am J Pathol* **142:**733, 1993.

40. Henriksen R, Wilander E, Oberg K: Expression and prognostic significance of Bcl-2 in ovarian tumors. *Br J Cancer* **72:**1324, 1995.

41. Berchuck A, Kamel A, Whitaker R, Kerns B, Olt G, Kinney R, Soper JT, Dodge R, Clarke Pearson DL, Marks P, McKenzie S, Yin S, Bast RC: Overexpression of HER-2/neu is associated with poor survival in advanced epithelial ovarian cancer. *Cancer Res* **50:**4087, 1990.

42. Yu D, Matin A, Xia W, Sorgi F, Huang L, Hung MC: Liposome-mediated in vivo E1A gene transfer suppressed dissemination of ovarian cancer cells that overexpress HER-2/neu. *Oncogene* **11:**1383, 1995.

43. Hung MC, Matin A, Zhang Y, Xing X, Sorgi F, Huang L, Yu D: HER-2/ neu-targeting gene therapy — a review. *Gene* **159:**65, 1995.

44. Pietras RJ, Fendly BM, Chazin VR, Pegram MD, Howell SB, Slamon DJ: Antibody to HER-2/neu receptor blocks DNA repair after cisplatin in human breast and ovarian cancer cells. *Oncogene* **9:**1829, 1994.

45. Mujoo K, Maneval DC, Anderson SC, Gutterman JU: Adenoviral-mediated p53 tumor suppressor gene therapy of human ovarian carcinoma. *Oncogene* **12:**1617, 1996.

46. Fearon ER, Vogelstein B: A genetic model for colorectal tumorigenesis. *Cell* **61:**759, 1990.

47. Zheng JP, Robinson WR, Ehlen T, Yu MC, Dubeau L: Distinction of low grade from high grade human ovarian carcinomas on the basis of losses of heterozygosity on chromosomes 3, 6, and 11 and HER-2/neu gene amplification. *Cancer Res* **51:**4045, 1991.

48. Dodson MK, Hartmann LC, Cliby WA, DeLacey KA, Keeney GL, Ritland SR, Su JQ, Podratz KC, Jenkins RB: Comparison of loss of heterozygosity patterns in invasive low-grade and high-grade epithelial ovarian carcinomas. *Cancer Res* **53:**4456, 1993.

49. Nowell PC: The clonal evolution of tumor cell populations. *Science* **194:**23, 1976.

50. Kim TM, Benedict WF, Xu H-J, Hu S-X, Gosewehr J, Velicescu M, Yin E, Zheng J, D'Ablaing G, Dubeau L: Loss of heterozygosity on chromosome 13 is common only in the biologically more aggressive subtypes of ovarian epithelial tumors and is associated with normal retinoblastoma gene expression. *Cancer Res* **54:**605, 1994.

51. Dodson MK, Cliby WA, Xu H-J, DeLacey KA, Hu S-X, Keeney GL, Li J, Podratz KC, Jenkins RB, Benedict WF: Evidence of functional RB protein in epithelial ovarian carcinomas despite loss of heterozygosity at the RB locus. *Cancer Res* **54:**610, 1994.

52. Wertheim I, Muto MG, Welch WR, Bell DA, Berkowitz RS, Mok SC: P53 gene mutation in human borderline epithelial ovarian tumors. *J Natl Cancer Inst* **86:**1549, 1994.

53. Cheng PC, Schmutte C, Cofer KF, Felix JC, Yu MC, Dubeau L: Alterations in DNA methylation are early, but not initial events in ovarian tumorigenesis. *Br J Cancer* **75:**396, 1997.

54. Wan M, Li W-Z, Duggan B, Felix J, Zhao Y, Dubeau L: Telomerase activity in benign and malignant epithelial ovarian tumors. *J Natl Cancer Inst* **89:**437, 1997.

55. Edelson MI, Lau CC, Colitti CV, Welch WR, Bell DA: A one-centimorgan deletion unit on chromosome Xq12 is commonly lost in borderline and invasive epithelial ovarian tumors. *Oncogene* **16:**197, 1998.

56. Turner HH: A syndrome of infantilism, congenital webbed neck, and cubitus valgus. *Endocrinol* **23:**566, 1938.

57. Klein CB, Conway K, Wang XW, Bhamra RK, Lin XH, Cohen MD, Annab L, Barrett JC, Costa M: Senescence of nickel-transformed cells by an X chromosome: Possible epigenetic control. *Science* **251:**796, 1991.

58. Wang XW, Lin X, Klein CB, Bhamra RK, Lee YW, Costa M: A conserved region in human and Chinese hamster X chromosomes can induce cellular senescence of nickel-transformed Chinese hamster cell lines. *Carcinogenesis* **13:**555, 1992.

59. Monroe KA, Yu MC, Kolonel LN, Coetzee GA, Wilkens LR, Ross RK, Henderson BE: Evidence of an X-linked or recessive genetic component to prostate cancer risk. *Nat Med* **1:**827, 1995.

60. Puls LE, Powell DE, DePriest PD, Gallion HH, Hunter JE, Kryscio RJ, van Nagell JR: Transition from benign to malignant epithelium in mucinous and serous ovarian cystadenocarcinoma. *Gynecol Oncol* **47:**53, 1992.

61. Zheng J, Wan M, Zweizig S, Velicescu M, Yu MC, Dubeau L: Histologically benign or low-grade malignant tumors adjacent to high-grade ovarian carcinomas contain molecular characteristics of high-grade carcinomas. *Cancer Res* **53:**4138, 1993.

62. Wolf NG, Abdul-Karim FW, Schork NJ, Schwartz S: Origins of heterogeneous ovarian carcinomas. A molecular cytogenetic analysis of histologically benign, low malignant potential, and fully malignant components. *Am J Pathol* **149:**511, 1996.

63. Kurman RJ, Trimble CL: The behavior of serous tumors of low malignant potential: Are they ever malignant? *Int J Gynecol Pathol* **12:**120, 1993.

Endometrial Cancer

Lora Hedrick Ellenson

1. Endometrial carcinoma is the most common malignancy of the female genital tract in the United States. In 2000 there were approximately 36,100 newly diagnosed cases of endometrial carcinoma and 6500 deaths as a result of this cancer.
2. Endometrial carcinoma is the most common noncolorectal carcinoma in women belonging to hereditary nonpolyposis colorectal carcinoma (HNPCC) families. Thus, mutations in the DNA mismatch repair genes (*hMSH2, hMLH1, hPMS1,* and *hPMS2*) that cause HNPCC are also thought to cause endometrial carcinoma in this setting.
3. Endometrial carcinoma encompasses two broad categories of malignant epithelial tumors that arise from endometrial epithelium. Epidemiologic and clinical features can distinguish them. Recently, it has been recognized that there are distinct histologic features of endometrial carcinomas that correlate, for the most part, with the two categories. The histologic types are called endometrioid carcinoma and uterine serous carcinoma. Recent molecular studies suggest that there may be differences in the molecular profiles of the two categories of endometrial carcinoma. Furthermore, it is suggested that these molecular differences may contribute to the differences in the clinical behavior of the tumor types.
4. Approximately 20 percent of sporadic endometrial carcinomas demonstrate microsatellite instability, yet only a fraction of these tumors have mutations in one of the four known DNA mismatch repair genes that cause HNPCC. Microsatellite instability has not been identified in uterine serous carcinomas, and may represent a molecular phenotype confined to endometrioid carcinomas.
5. The most common molecular abnormalities identified, to date, in endometrial carcinoma are *PTEN* mutations, microsatellite instability, K-*ras* mutations, and p53 gene mutations. *PTEN* is a recently identified tumor-suppressor gene on chromosome 10q23. Mutations in *PTEN* are the most common molecular alteration yet identified in endometrial cancer with 40–50 percent harboring such mutations. It appears that mutations in *PTEN* may be important early in the development of endometrioid carcinoma, as they are found in 20 percent of hyperplastic precursor lesions. K-*ras* mutations are thought to occur in 10–30 percent of endometrial carcinomas, and may also represent a relatively early alteration in endometrioid carcinoma, as mutations are present in atypical hyperplastic lesions.
6. p53 mutations are found in 10–30 percent of endometrial carcinomas. Recent data suggest that the majority occur in uterine serous carcinoma and in high-grade and high-stage endometrioid carcinomas. p53 mutations are very common in endometrial intraepithelial carcinoma, the precursor of

uterine serous carcinoma, and may, therefore, occur early in the pathogenesis of this aggressive type of endometrial carcinoma. Statistical analyses of p53 overexpression by immunohistochemistry have found that it is an independent indicator of poor prognosis.
7. The molecular genetics of endometrial carcinoma are just beginning to be elucidated. To date, only p53 overexpression offers promise as a useful molecular diagnostic tool.

CLINICAL ASPECTS

Incidence

Endometrial cancer is the fifth leading cause of cancer in women worldwide, with approximately 150,000 cases diagnosed each year. In the United States, it is the most common malignancy of the female genital tract, with 36,100 newly diagnosed cases and roughly 6500 deaths estimated in 2000.[1] It should be noted that the term *endometrial cancer* encompasses both malignant epithelial tumors (carcinomas) and malignant mesenchymal tumors (sarcomas). Because more than 95 percent of endometrial cancers are carcinomas, the terms *endometrial cancer* and *endometrial carcinoma* are often used synonymously in the literature.

Most cases of endometrial carcinoma are thought to be sporadic; however, some clearly have a hereditary basis. Mothers and sisters of women with endometrial carcinoma have 2.7 times the risk of developing endometrial carcinoma when compared to controls.[2] The vast majority of endometrial carcinomas recognized as inherited occur in affected women belonging to hereditary nonpolyposis colorectal cancer (HNPCC) families. HNPCC is an autosomal dominantly inherited disease, and members of HNPCC families have an increased risk of developing a number of different types of cancer, especially colorectal cancer.[3] Notably, endometrial carcinoma is the most common extracolonic cancer in HNPCC families.[4] Women who are gene carriers of HNPCC have a tenfold increased risk, compared to the general population, of developing endometrial carcinoma; however, the percentage of endometrial cancers due to HNPCC is not well defined.[5] A small amount of literature has suggested the possibility of a site-specific form of inherited endometrial carcinoma, but there are insufficient data to conclusively prove its existence as a clinical genetic entity.[6]

Clinical Behavior and Histology

The endometrium forms the lining of the uterine cavity and is a complex tissue composed of both glandular epithelial and stromal components. Endometrial carcinoma arises from the epithelial component, with most tumors displaying glandular differentiation. It most commonly arises in perimenopausal and postmenopausal women. In most cases, women with endometrial carcinoma seek medical attention for abnormal vaginal bleeding, and endometrial tissue is obtained by biopsy or curettage for a definitive microscopic diagnosis.

Although endometrial carcinoma is classically thought of as a single disease, there is substantial evidence to support that it consists of two broad categories of malignant epithelial tumors.

A list of standard abbreviations is located immediately preceding the index. Nonstandard abbreviations used in this chapter include: HNPCC = hereditary nonpolyposis colorectal carcinoma; LOH = loss of heterozygosity.

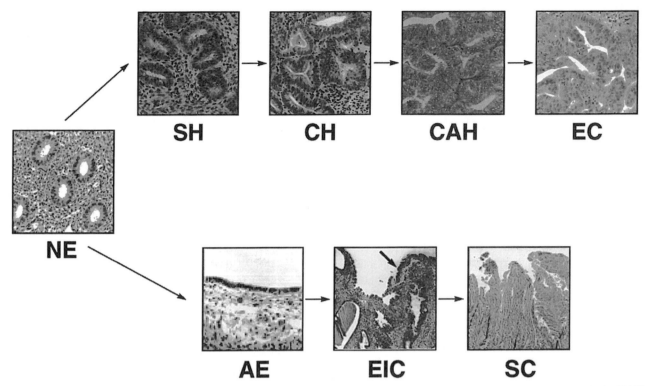

Fig. 42-1 Progression model of the two types of endometrial carcinoma. The development of endometrioid carcinoma (EC) from normal epithelium (NE) arises over time through a series of hyperplastic lesions that increase in both architectural complexity and cytologic atypia from simple hyperplasia (SH) to complex hyperplasia (CH) and finally complex atypical hyperplasia (CAH). Uterine serous carcinoma (SC) develops in the setting of atrophic endometrium (AE) from a precursor lesion called endometrial intraepithelial carcinoma (EIC).

The initial data suggesting the existence of two distinct types of endometrial carcinoma came from epidemiologic and clinical studies.[7] Recently it became apparent that these clinically defined categories of tumors correlate, for the most part, with specific light microscopic features.

Briefly, the initial clinical studies recognized that one group of women with endometrial carcinoma often have a history of exposure to estrogen, are slightly younger (mean age of 59) than the overall mean for the disease, and have tumors that usually behave in a relatively indolent manner. This group has been designated Type I endometrial carcinoma, and is often referred to as "estrogen-related."[8] Histologically, the majority of Type I tumors tend to have architectural features that resemble the appearance of normal endometrial glands, and are called endometrioid carcinomas to denote this resemblance. They are generally low-grade (i.e., well differentiated), low-stage (confined to the uterus), and have a good prognosis. Both epidemiologic and light microscopic studies have suggested that this type of carcinoma develops from normal epithelium, under the influence of estrogen stimulation, through a continuum of histopathologically recognizable lesions called hyperplasias (Fig. 42-1). Hyperplasia is defined as a proliferation of abnormal shaped and sized endometrial glands that leads to an imbalance in the normal glandular/stromal ratio of the endometrium. This proliferative process can, over time, undergo an increase in architectural complexity and cytologic atypia until it is difficult to distinguish from carcinoma, with the notable exception that there is a lack of detectable stromal invasion.[9] Hyperplasia, at any stage, can cause abnormal vaginal bleeding. As a result, many cases come to clinical attention and are treated prior to the development of frankly invasive carcinoma.

Type II carcinoma, in contrast to Type I, is unrelated to estrogenic stimulation (non-estrogen-related), occurs in older women (mean age of 68), and demonstrates aggressive behavior. Virtually all Type II carcinomas are composed of cuboidal cells showing marked cytologic atypia and nuclear pleomorphism that grow in either a glandular or papillary architecture.[10] These features are strikingly similar to those of the more common serous carcinoma of the ovary, giving rise to the name uterine serous carcinoma to distinguish them from primary serous ovarian tumors. By definition, serous carcinomas of the endometrium are all high-grade, frequently have extrauterine spread by the time of diagnosis, and carry a poor prognosis, behaving much like ovarian serous carcinomas.[11] Serous tumors of the endometrium generally arise in the setting of an atrophic, not a hyperplastic, endometrium. Recently, a putative precursor of uterine serous carcinoma has been described and termed endometrial intraepithelial carcinoma (Fig. 42-1).[12] It is characterized by a replacement of the preexisting endometrial epithelium with markedly atypical cells that are virtually indistinguishable from the cells found in invasive uterine serous carcinoma. Endometrial intraepithelial carcinoma, even in the absence of definitive invasion in the uterus, can be associated with intra-abdominal carcinoma illustrating the aggressive nature of this neoplastic endometrial process.

It is important to recognize that the histology of endometrial carcinoma is more complicated than presented above. For example, there are several other minor histologic variants of endometrial carcinoma (e.g., mucinous, villoglandular, and clear cell). The appropriate category in which these histologic variants belong is not well established. These histologic variants are rare and poorly understood, and are not considered further in this chapter.

That the two major types of endometrial carcinoma are distinct has been further supported by recent molecular studies, as is discussed in detail below. Until recently, many of the molecular genetic studies of endometrial carcinoma have failed to adequately recognize and separately study the two major types of tumors, creating a body of literature that is often difficult to interpret, as becomes evident later in this chapter.

HEREDITARY ENDOMETRIAL CARCINOMA

The only well-established form of inherited endometrial carcinoma is associated with HNPCC. Over the past several years, the genes responsible for the majority of families that meet the clinical criteria for HNPCC have been identified and cloned. Furthermore, the HNPCC families in which linkage studies have been informative demonstrate linkage to loci subsequently found to harbor one of the known genes. For these reasons, the discussion of the genetic loci and the specific genes involved in inherited endometrial carcinoma are combined.

HNPCC is discussed in great detail in Chap. 18. Therefore, it is presented only briefly here, with an emphasis on endometrial carcinoma. HNPCC is the most common hereditary family cancer syndrome and is transmitted as an autosomal dominant trait. It is clinically defined by these criteria: (a) at least three relatives with colorectal cancer with one a first-degree relative of the other two; (b) the presence of tumors in at least two successive generations; and (c) one family member affected by colorectal cancer before the age of 50.[13] Endometrial carcinoma is not a required criterion for the clinical definition of HNPCC. However, the International Collaborative Group on HNPCC has recognized that if these criteria are strictly followed, families with a high incidence of endometrial carcinoma, as well as colorectal carcinoma, would be excluded. Although the actual percentage of all endometrial carcinoma due to HNPCC is not known, it has been shown that the cumulative incidence of endometrial carcinoma in women belonging to HNPCC kindreds is 20 percent by age 70, in contrast to 3 percent in the general population.[5]

Genetic Loci and Specific Genes

As previously stated, endometrial carcinoma is the most common extracolonic tumor that occurs in HNPCC families. Linkage analysis of several large HNPCC kindreds identified susceptibility loci on the short arms of chromosomes 2 and 3.[14,15] Informative linkage studies have determined linkage to either of these two chromosomal arms in the majority of HNPCC families. However, in a small number of families linkage to either of these regions is lacking.

Over the past several years four genes have been identified that cause HNPCC in most of the kindreds meeting the clinical criteria of this inherited family cancer syndrome. The cloning of these genes resulted from the propitious coincidence of several different lines of scientific investigation, including studies aimed at identifying genes that play a role in human tumors, and others aimed at understanding fundamental molecular processes in microbial organisms.

Investigators were analyzing microsatellites (small repetitive sequences) in DNA isolated from tumors arising in HNPCC family members and found alterations in the length of microsatellite DNA sequences when compared to germ-line DNA from the same patients.[16] Other investigators reported a similar molecular phenotype in approximately 20 percent of sporadic colorectal tumors.[17,18] This molecular phenotype was referred to as microsatellite instability or replication errors. Microsatellite instability and its role, if any, in the neoplastic process was unclear. Shortly after the discovery of microsatellite instability in both sporadic and HNPCC-associated colorectal carcinomas, a study was published demonstrating that mutations in DNA mismatch repair genes led to a 100- to 700-fold increase in the instability of simple dinucleotide repeat sequences in the simple eukaryote *S. cerevisiae*.[19] This observation, along with previous work in both *E. coli* and *S. cerevisiae*, provided a crucial connection between microsatellite instability and mutations in DNA mismatch repair genes. This connection led to the ultimate

identification of human DNA mismatch repair genes and opened a new avenue of cancer research.

In a very short time, four human homologues of microbial DNA mismatch repair genes were cloned. At a somewhat later date a fifth gene involved in DNA mismatch repair, *GTPB*, was cloned, but it will not be discussed here.[20,21] The four human DNA mismatch repair genes known to cause HNPCC are named *hMSH2*, *hMLH1*, *hPMS1*, and *hPMS2*, in keeping with their microbial homologues, and are located on chromosomes 2p, 3p, 2q, and 7q, respectively.[22–26] The physical maps of *hMSH2* and *hMLH1* have shown that their locations correlate with chromosomal loci determined to have genetic linkage to HNPCC. The linkage and physical mapping data provided additional information suggesting that DNA mismatch repair genes play a role in the pathogenesis of neoplasms arising in HNPCC kindreds. Subsequent studies documented germ-line mutations in one of these four human mismatch repair genes in affected members of most HNPCC kindreds, with the *hMSH2* and *hMLH1* genes accounting for the vast majority. At present, there is not a reported difference in the frequency of endometrial carcinoma among the HNPCC kindreds that carry mutations in the different genes.

The contribution of how microsatellite instability and defects in the DNA mismatch repair system contributed to tumorigenesis remained unproved. In microorganisms, the DNA mismatch repair system was known to detect and repair mispaired bases introduced during replication of the cellular genome. Furthermore, microbial organisms lacking a functional DNA mismatch repair system have a marked increase in the rate at which mutations accumulate. In mammalian cells, the DNA mismatch repair system has been much less well characterized, but it is thought to have a similar function to its microbial counterpart. Microsatellite DNA sequences in both humans and microorganisms are prone to undergo alterations in their length (explaining their highly polymorphic nature) during DNA replication. Therefore, it follows that microsatellite DNA sequences might demonstrate numerous alterations in the absence of an intact DNA mismatch repair system. This suggests that microsatellite instability may simply serve as a marker of an increased rate of mutation caused by an underlying defect in the DNA mismatch repair system. This led directly to the notion that lack of a functional mismatch repair system would result in an increased rate of mutations in oncogenes and tumor-suppressor genes, thus predisposing cells to the accumulation of mutations now thought to be a cornerstone of the neoplastic process. In support of this idea, studies have demonstrated an increase in the rate of point mutations in an expressed gene (HPRT) in a mismatch repair-deficient mammalian cell line. The identification of mutations in DNA mismatch repair genes in human tumors created a new class of cancer-causing genes called mutator genes.

The high frequency of endometrial carcinoma in HNPCC families indicates that the genes responsible for HNPCC are involved in the pathogenesis of endometrial carcinoma in this setting. A review of the literature does not provide a straightforward analysis of mutations in women with endometrial carcinoma belonging to HNPCC families. Clearly, further studies of HNPCC-associated endometrial carcinomas are needed.

Sporadic Endometrial Carcinoma

As alluded to earlier, the identification and characterization of the genetic loci and specific genes involved in endometrial tumorigenesis have been hampered by the inadequate recognition of the distinct types of endometrial carcinomas. Much of the problem is related to the classification scheme, described earlier, being initially described in 1983 and only recently gaining widespread acceptance. In addition, uterine serous (Type II) carcinomas are relatively rare, comprising approximately 10 percent of all sporadic endometrial carcinomas. Consequently, and understandably, many of the studies have not clearly stated the type (or types) of endometrial carcinomas that were included. Additionally, many studies that have classified the tumors lack significant numbers to enable the results of the different tumor types to be assessed independently. When possible, this chapter discusses the molecular genetics of sporadic endometrial carcinoma in the context of these two tumor types.

Genetic Loci

Over the past several years a number of loss of heterozygosity (LOH) studies have attempted to locate regions of the genome that may harbor tumor-suppressor genes that play a role in endometrial tumorigenesis. In combining the results of the major studies, LOH has been detected on these chromosomes: 1, 3, 6, 8p, 9p, 9q, 10q, 11, 13, 14q, 15, 16q, 17p, 18p, 18q, 20, 21, and 22q.[28-32] A review of the literature reveals substantial variation in the regions that have been found to undergo LOH in endometrial carcinoma, and there are only several regions from this long list that have shown significant LOH in more than one study. These include loci on chromosomes 3p, 10q, 17p, and 18q. The 3p LOH is striking, as several candidate tumor-suppressor genes and the *hMLH1* gene map to this chromosome. The target(s) of 3p LOH have not yet been determined in endometrial carcinoma. Two separate groups of investigators have reported between 35 and 40 percent LOH of a region of 10q, and one group has suggested that there may be two discrete regions of 10q that undergo LOH.[29,31] A range of 9 to 35 percent of endometrial carcinomas has been reported to show 17p LOH. A recent study of uterine serous carcinoma detected LOH of 17p, specifically 17p13.1, in 100 percent of informative cases.[33] Because most of the LOH studies did not specify the tumor type, it will be of interest in the future to determine the percentage of each type that have 17p LOH. LOH of chromosome 18q has been found in three studies, all of which included tumors from Japanese women, with the highest reported frequency of 33 percent.[28,30,32] Other studies have failed to detect 18q LOH, including two studies confined to the analysis of tumors from American women, as well as one exclusively of Japanese women. Although 14q LOH has been identified in only one study, the association of 14q LOH with a poor prognosis led the authors to suggest that 14q LOH may indicate aggressive tumor behavior.[30] Interestingly, the authors note that several of the tumors with 14q LOH were uterine serous carcinomas. Further studies are necessary to confirm the possible association of 14q LOH and aggressive behavior of endometrial carcinoma.

As is easily imaginable, the variability among the LOH studies has hindered the identification of novel regions of the genome that may be important in the development of endometrial carcinoma. The reason(s) for the variability between studies are uncertain, but there are many possible explanations. For example, the polymorphic markers used in the various studies are not identical, and if relatively small deletions are responsible for LOH in endometrial carcinoma, the critical regions may only be detected with very specific markers. Furthermore, many of the studies have failed to carefully report the histologic types of the tumors analyzed. If the histologic types, which reflect the distinct categories of endometrial carcinoma, have different underlying molecular genetic alterations, the results of such studies may depend heavily on the types of tumors studied. This point is of further interest, as many studies have included tumors from Japanese and American patients and there is some evidence suggesting differences in the molecular basis of endometrial carcinomas in these two populations.

Specific Genes

The discussion of the specific genes is divided into three sections according to the general classification of genes currently recognized as cancer-causing genes: (a) mutator genes, (b) oncogenes, and (c) tumor-suppressor genes.

Mutator Genes. Due to the association of endometrial carcinoma and HNPCC, presumably sporadic cases of endometrial carcinoma were analyzed for instability of microsatellite DNA sequences. In several studies, microsatellite instability was detected in approximately 20 percent of endometrial tumors.[34-36] Given the association of microsatellite instability and mutations in human DNA mismatch repair genes, it seemed likely that mutations in these genes may be involved in the development of sporadic endometrial carcinomas that displayed microsatellite instability. A mutational analysis of four of the known DNA mismatch repair genes (*hMSH2, hMLH1, hPMS1,* and *hPMS2*) found that only a small number of sporadic endometrial carcinomas with microsatellite instability had mutations in one of these four genes.[37] In addition, mutations of *hMSH2* and *hMLH1* have been found in two endometrial carcinoma cell lines (HEC59 and AN$_{3CA}$) that demonstrate microsatellite instability.[38] These findings are similar to those seen in cases of microsatellite instability-positive sporadic colorectal cancers. The recent literature has found that the vast majority of microsatellite instability-positive sporadic endometrial carcinomas demonstrate hypermethylation of the *hMLH1* promoter. This, in turn, is thought to be related to lack of expression of hMLH1 and the disruption of DNA mismatch repair.[38a,38b]

Finally, a recent study found that 34 cases of uterine serous carcinoma failed to demonstrate microsatellite instability.[39] The observed difference in the frequency between endometrial and uterine serous carcinoma is statistically significant and provides support for differences in the molecular pathogenesis of the two most common types of endometrial carcinoma.

Oncogenes. A number of oncogenes have been studied over the years, yet there are very few that have been found to be altered in a substantial number of endometrial carcinomas. The proto-oncogene recognized as mutated most commonly in endometrial carcinoma is K-*ras*. It has been shown, in a number of independent studies, to be mutated in 10 to 30 percent of endometrial carcinomas.[40-45] K-*ras* is a member of the *ras* gene family that consists of three closely related genes (H-*ras*, K-*ras*, and N-*ras*). The H-*ras* gene was discovered due to its ability to transform an immortalized rodent cell line, and its identification led to the cloning of the two other family members. Each of the *ras* genes encodes a 21-kDa guanine nucleotide-binding protein (p21) that transduces signals from activated transmembrane receptors to protein kinases that regulate cell growth and differentiation. The oncogenic mutations occur most commonly at codons 12, 13, and 61 and result in a gain-of-function. The mutant *ras* proteins have a decreased ability to interact with the GTPase-activating protein called *ras*-GAP, reducing their ability to interact with the GTPase-activating protein *ras*-GAP, and reducing their ability to hydrolyze guanosine triphosphate (GTP) to guanosine diphosphate (GDP). Hence, the mutant *ras* protein remains in the GTP-bound or activated state. In endometrial carcinoma, most mutations are found in codon 12. A recent study of American patients, that separated the two types of endometrial carcinoma, found that 11.6 percent of endometrioid carcinomas contained codon 12 mutations, whereas uterine serous carcinomas were all negative for codon 12 mutations.[46] The numbers were not statistically significant; however, it suggests that K-*ras* mutations may be differentially mutated in the different types of endometrial carcinoma. K-*ras* mutations have also been found in complex atypical hyperplasia (the precursor of endometrioid carcinoma) leading investigators to suggest that K-*ras* mutations may be a relatively early event in endometrial tumorigenesis.[43-45] Investigators have analyzed the association of K-*ras* mutations with prognosis, but the results have been conflicting.

There are a small number of studies showing alterations in the expression and/or amplification of the *HER-2/neu* gene in endometrial carcinoma. *HER-2/neu* is a member of the epidermal growth factor receptor gene family. It encodes a transmembrane tyrosine kinase receptor and is overexpressed in a subset of breast and ovarian cancers. The data on this gene in endometrial carcinoma are limited, but several studies have shown that it is overexpressed in 11 to 59 percent of tumors, and amplified in 14 to 21 percent of tumors.[47,48] One study revealed that overexpression and amplification of *HER-2/neu* were associated with a poor prognosis, and a multivariate analysis indicated that overexpres-

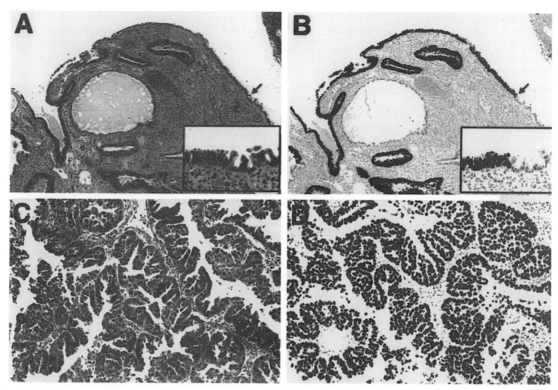

Fig. 42-2 Immunohistochemistry of p53 in uterine serous carcinoma and its precursor endometrial intraepithelial carcinoma. Endometrial intraepithelial carcinoma (EIC) arises abruptly from atrophic endometrium (*A*) and shows intense positive staining (*B*). A typical uterine serous carcinoma (*C*) also shows intense, diffuse staining for p53 protein (*D*). (Reprinted with permission from Tashiro H, et al.[33])

sion was an independent prognostic factor.[49,50] Independent studies have suggested that overexpression may be more common in uterine serous carcinomas.[51]

Recently, there have been several studies looking at expression of the *bcl-2* gene in endometrial carcinoma and hyperplasia. The *bcl-2* gene product prevents cells from undergoing apoptosis and is overexpressed in a number of different types of human tumors. The results of the studies in endometrial carcinoma are contradictory, with some demonstrating increased expression in endometrial carcinomas and others finding it decreased.[52,53] However, the results of several studies have found expression in normal proliferative endometrium and an absence of expression in normal secretory endometrium. These results suggest that *bcl-2* may play a role in the normal endometrial cycle. Hence, further studies on endometrial carcinoma seem needed to determine if *bcl-2* has a role in endometrial tumorigenesis.

Tumor-Suppressor Genes. As is true in many tumors, the *p53* gene has been the most extensively studied gene in endometrial carcinoma. *p53* is the prototype tumor-suppressor gene and it is the most frequently mutated gene in human cancers. It encodes a nuclear phosphoprotein with an apparent molecular weight of 53 kDa. For obvious reasons, this gene has been under intensive investigation for many years. Recent studies have begun to elucidate the mechanisms by which *p53* controls cell growth (reviewed in reference 54). Briefly, it has been found that p53 expression increases, posttranscriptionally, in response to DNA damage, resulting in a G1/S cell-cycle arrest. It is thought that this arrest gives cells the opportunity to repair the damaged DNA such that mutations are not fixed in the genomic template and, in turn, passed to daughter cells after cell division is complete. It has also been found that elevations in *p53* gene expression can lead to apoptosis. Recent data suggest that transcriptional activation of p21^{WAF1} by p53 is important in the G1/S arrest, but is not essential for apoptosis. Evidently, given its ubiquitous involvement in human tumorigenesis, mutations that inactivate the *p53* gene

provide a significant growth-promoting affect on many cell types.

Evaluation of p53 in endometrial carcinoma has largely been by immunohistochemistry, and overexpression of the protein has been reported in anywhere from 11 to 45 percent of endometrial carcinomas.[55–57] Evaluation of the data is troublesome due to a lack of description of the staining patterns (intensity and percent of cells staining) and the types of tumors analyzed. The staining pattern may be of utmost importance, as it is thought that detection of p53 by immunohistochemistry reflects the presence of mutations in the gene. Many studies have shown that there is considerable variability in staining and that only intense, diffuse staining may accurately predict the presence of mutations. One large study demonstrated that positive staining was more common in high-grade (41.7 percent) than in low-grade (12 percent) tumors, and another study revealed it more frequently in high-stage (41 percent) than in low-stage (9 percent) tumors.[56,58] Furthermore, when the tumor types have been separated, a higher frequency of staining is noted in uterine serous carcinomas (66 to 86 percent) as compared to the endometrioid type (Fig. 42-2).[33,59] Several studies have shown that overexpression of p53 by immunohistochemistry is an independent prognostic variable, predicting a poor prognosis.[57,60]

Analyses have also shown a wide range (9.5 to 23 percent) in the frequency of p53 mutations in endometrial carcinoma.[59,61] Again, these differences may be due to the types, grades, and stages of tumors analyzed. Many of the mutational studies have consistently shown that mutations are more common in high-grade tumors, and a recent study analyzing only uterine serous carcinomas detected mutations in 90 percent of tumors.[33] The strong association of p53 mutations and uterine serous carcinoma may offer an explanation for the prognostic significance of p53 overexpression and its association with a poor outcome.

Many of the p53 studies have focused on the clinical utility of the results. Recent studies suggest that they may also provide meaningful information about the molecular pathogenesis of endometrial carcinoma. As mentioned earlier, a putative precursor of uterine serous carcinoma has been described and p53 immunohistochemical studies revealed positivity in a very high percentage of endometrial intraepithelial carcinoma (Fig. 42-2).[62] This finding is in contrast to the very infrequent staining of atypical hyperplasia, the precursor of endometrioid carcinoma. Mutational analyses have shown that mutations in exons 5 to 8 of the *p53* gene are present in a majority of endometrial intraepithelial carcinomas (78 percent), suggesting, along with the high frequency of p53 mutations in uterine serous carcinoma, that *p53* mutations occur early in the pathogenesis of this tumor type.[33] It is reasonable to speculate that early mutation of the *p53* gene may be an important determinant of the aggressive biological behavior of uterine serous carcinoma, resulting in the poor outcome of patients with this tumor type.

Several recent studies have shown that mutations in *PTEN*, a tumor-suppressor gene located on chromosome 10q23.3, are common in endometrial carcinoma.[63,64,65] Approximately 40 to 50 percent of endometrioid carcinomas contain *PTEN* mutations, making it the most frequently mutated gene yet identified in this tumor type. The small number of uterine serous carcinomas analyzed for *PTEN* mutations are negative; however, before mutations in this tumor type are excluded more cases of serous carcinoma should be analyzed. Interestingly, *PTEN* mutations are more frequent in microsatellite instability-positive tumors than in those that lack instability.[63,64] Although the biological basis of this association is not yet understood it may represent an important finding with regards to the molecular pathogenesis of endometrioid carcinoma. Furthermore, *PTEN* mutations have been identified in approximately 20 percent of complex hyperplasias, with and without atypia, suggesting that *PTEN* mutations occur early in the pathogenesis of at least some endometrial carcinomas.[66,67] The predicted amino acid sequence of *PTEN* reveals significant homology to both tensin, a protein located in focal cell adhesions, and tyrosine phosphatases.[68] Biochemical studies have shown that PTEN is a dual-specificity protein and lipid phosphatase.[69,70] Notably, studies have shown that the lipid second messenger, phosphatidylinositol 3,4,5-triphosphate (PIP3), which controls the phosphorylation of AKT is a PTEN substrate.[70] AKT is a central regulator of a number of downstream effector molecules involved in cell proliferation and apoptosis. In addition, studies have also shown a role for PTEN in the regulation of cell migration and formation of focal cell adhesions.[71] In sum, the high frequency of *PTEN* mutations in endometrial carcinoma and their presence in hyperplastic lesions imply that inactivation of *PTEN* plays a significant role in its development. Clearly, the role of *PTEN* in endometrial tumorigenesis will be actively pursued in the near future.

Finally, a recent study found mutations in the β-catenin gene in 13 percent of endometrial carcinomas, and an accumulation of β-catenin protein in 38 percent of endometrial carcinomas.[53a] This finding is of considerable interest as it suggests a role for the *Wnt* signaling pathway, a pathway commonly involved in colorectal tumorigenesis, in the development of endometrial carcinoma. Additional studies are needed to determine the significance of this pathway in endometrial tumorigenesis.

IMPLICATIONS FOR DIAGNOSIS

As endometrial carcinoma remains poorly understood at the molecular level, there are very few molecular markers that are currently helpful in its diagnosis. The only gene, at present, with potential usefulness as a diagnostic tool is *p53*. It is very possible that *p53* immunohistochemistry may aid in the recognition of uterine serous carcinoma and its precursor lesion, endometrial intraepithelial carcinoma. The ability to consistently recognize this tumor, particularly in its early stages, may lead to better treatment approaches for this very aggressive tumor type. However, future studies are needed to better define the quality and quantity of *p53* immunostaining that accurately identify this type of tumor in the

endometrium. In addition, *p53* staining may help identify the more aggressive subset of endometrioid tumors that should perhaps be treated more rigorously than those subsets that lack positive staining.

SUMMARY

The role of steroid hormones and their receptors in the development of endometrial carcinoma is excluded from this chapter. This is not an oversight, but little is known at the genetic level about how they contribute to the neoplastic phenotype in the endometrium. It is an area that deserves attention in the future. Finally, there is much to be learned about the molecular basis of endometrial carcinoma. Hopefully, future investigations will more vigilantly include a record of the distinct histologic types of endometrial carcinoma and their specific molecular genetic alterations so that we can come to understand the distinct genetic differences, and similarities, of the two major types of endometrial carcinoma. If the molecular underpinnings of these two types of carcinoma can be determined, perhaps new tools can be developed for more effective diagnosis and treatment of this common malignancy of women.

REFERENCES

1. Greenlee RT, Murray T, Bolden S, Wingo PA: Cancer statistics. *Cancer J Clin* **50**:7, 2000.
2. Schildkraut JM, Risch N, Thompson WD: Evaluating genetic association among ovarian, breast, and endometrial cancer: Evidence for a breast/ovarian cancer relationship. *Am J Hum Genet* **45**:521, 1989.
3. Watson P, Lynch HT: The tumor spectrum in HNPCC. *Anticancer Res* **14**:1635, 1994.
4. Watson P, Lynch HT: Extracolonic cancer in hereditary nonpolyposis colorectal cancer. *Cancer* **71**:679, 1993.
5. Watson P, Vasen HFA, Mecklin JP, Jarvinen H, Lynch HT: The risk of endometrial cancer in hereditary nonpolyposis colorectal cancer. *Am J Med* **96**:516, 1994.
6. Sandles LG, Shulman LP, Elias S, Photopulos GJ, Smiley LM, Posten WM, Simpson JL: Endometrial adenocarcinoma: Genetic analysis suggesting heritable site-specific uterine cancer. *Gynecol Oncol* **47**:167, 1992.
7. Bokhman JV: Two pathogenetic types of endometrial carcinoma. *Gynecol Oncol* **15**:10, 1983.
8. Kurman RJ: *Blaustein's Pathology of the Female Genital Tract.* New York: Springer-Verlag, 1994.
9. Kurman RJ, Kaminski PF, Norris HJ: The behavior of endometrial hyperplasia: A long-term study of "untreated" hyperplasia in 170 patients. *Cancer* **56**:403, 1985.
10. Sherman ME, Bitterman P, Rosenheim NB, Delgado G, Kurman RJ: Uterine serous carcinoma. A morphologically diverse neoplasm with unifying clinicopathologic features. *Am J Surg Pathol* **16**:600, 1992.
11. Hendrickson M, Ross J, Eifel P, Martinez A, Kempson R: Uterine papillary serous carcinoma a highly malignant form of endometrial adenocarcinoma. *Am J Surg Pathol* **6**:93, 1982.
12. Ambros RA, Sherman ME, Zahn CM, Bitterman P, Kurman RJ: Endometrial intraepithelial carcinoma: A distinctive lesion specifically associated with tumors displaying serous differentiation. *Hum Pathol* **26**:1260, 1995.
13. Vasen HFA, Mecklin JP, Meera Khan P, Lynch HT: Hereditary non-polyposis colorectal cancer. *Lancet* **338**:877, 1991.
14. Lindblom A, Tannergard P, Werelius B, Nordenskjold M: Genetic mapping of a second locus predisposing to hereditary non-polyposis colon cancer. *Nat Genet* **5**:279, 1993.
15. Peltomäki P, Aaltonen LA, Sistonen P, Pylkkänen L, Mecklin J-P, Jarvinen H, Green JS, JR, J, Weber JL, Leach FS, Petersen GM, Hamilton SR, de la Chapelle A, Vogelstein B: Genetic mapping of a locus predisposing to human colorectal cancer. *Science* **260**:810, 1993.
16. Aaltonen LA, Peltomäki P, Leach FS, Sistonen P, Pylkkänen L, Mecklin JP, Jarvinen H, Powell SM, Jen J, Hamilton SR, Petersen GM, Kinzler KW, Vogelstein B, de la Chapelle A: Clues to the pathogenesis of familial colorectal cancer. *Science* **260**:812, 1993.
17. Thibodeau SN, Bren G, Schaid D: Microsatellite instability in cancer of the proximal colon [see comments]. *Science* **260**:816, 1993.

18. Ionov Y, Peinado MA, Malkhosyan S, Shibata D, Perucho M: Ubiquitous somatic mutations in simple repeated sequences reveal a new mechanism for colonic carcinogenesis. *Nature* **363**:558, 1993.

19. Strand M, Prolla TA, Liskay RM, Petes TD: Destabilization of tracts of simple repetitive DNA in yeast by mutations affecting DNA mismatch repair. *Nature* **365**:274, 1993.

20. Palombo F, Gallinari P, Iaccarino I, Lettieri T, Hughes M, D'Arrigo A, Truong O, Hsuan JJ, Jiricny J: GTBP, a 160-kilodalton protein essential for mismatch-binding activity in human cells. *Science* **268**:1912, 1995.

21. Papadopoulos N, Nicolaides NC, Liu B, Parsons R, Lengauer C, Palombo F, D'Arrigo A, Markowitz S, Willson JK, Kinzler KW, Jirichy J, Vogelstein B: Mutations of GTBP in genetically unstable cells [see comments]. *Science* **268**:1915, 1995.

22. Papadopoulos N, Nicolaides NC, Wei YF, Ruben SM, Carter KC, Rosen CA, Haseltine WA, Fleischmann RD, Fraser CM, Adams MD, Venter JC, Hamilton SR, Peterson GM, Watson P, Lynch HT, Peltomaki P, Mecklin J, de la Chapelle A, Kinzler KW, Vogelstein B: Mutation of a mutL homolog in hereditary colon cancer [see comments]. *Science* **263**:1625, 1994.

23. Nicolaides NC, Papadopoulos N, Liu B, Wei YF, Carter KC, Ruben SM, Rosen CA, Haseltine WA, Fleischmann RD, Fraser CM, Adams MD, Venter JC, Dunlop MG, Hamilton SR, Petersen GM, de la Chapelle A, Vogelstein B, Kinzler KW: Mutations of two PMS homologues in hereditary nonpolyposis colon cancer. *Nature* **371**:75, 1994.

24. Bronner CE, Baker SM, Morrison PT, Warren G, Smith LG, Lescoe MK, Kane M, Earabino C, Lipford J, Lindblom A, Tannergard P, Bollag RJ, Godwin AR, Ward DC, Nordenskjold M, Fishel R, Kolodner R, Liskay RM: Mutation in the DNA mismatch repair gene homologue hMLH1 is associated with hereditary non-polyposis colon cancer. *Nature* **368**:258, 1994.

25. Fishel R, Lescoe MK, Rao MR, Copeland NG, Jenkins NA, Garber J, Kane M, Kolodner R: The human mutator gene homolog MSH2 its association with hereditary nonpolyposis colon cancer. *Cell* **75**:1027, 1993.

26. Leach FS, Nicolaides NC, Papadopoulos N, Liu B, Jen J, Parsons R, Peltomaki P, Sistonen P, Aaltonen LA, Nystrom LM, Guan JZ, Meltzer PS, Yu J, Kao F, Chen DJ, Cerosaletti KM, Fournier REK, Todd S, Lewis T, Leach RJ, Naylor SL, Weissenbach J, Mecklin J, Jarvinen H, Petersen GM, Hamilton SR, Green J, Jass J, Watson P, Lynch HT, Trent JM, de la Chapelle A, Kinzler KW, Vogelstein B: Mutations of a mutS homolog in hereditary nonpolyposis colorectal cancer. *Cell* **75**:1215, 1993.

27. Eshleman JR, Markowitz SD, Donover S, Lang EZ, Lutterbaugh JD, Li G, Longley M, Modrich P, Veigl ML, Sedwick WD: Diverse hypermutability of multiple expressed sequence motifs present in a cancer with microsatellite instability. *Oncogene* **12**:1425, 1996.

28. Imamura T, Arima T, Kato H, Miyamoto S, Sasazuki T, Wake N: Chromosomal deletions and K-ras gene mutations in human endometrial carcinomas. *Int J Cancer* **51**:47, 1992.

29. Jones MH, Koi S, Fujimoto I, Hasumi K, Kato K, Nakamura Y: Allelotype of uterine cancer by analysis of RFLP and microsatellite polymorphisms: Frequent loss of heterozygosity on chromosome arms 3p, 9q, 10q, 17p. *Genes Chromosomes Cancer* **9**:119, 1994.

30. Fujino T, Risinger JI, Collins NK, Liu F-S, Nishii H, Takahashi H, Westphal E- M, Barrett JC, Sasaki H, Kohler MF, Berchuck A, Boyd J: Allelotype of endometrial carcinoma. *Cancer Res* **54**:4294, 1994.

31. Peiffer SL, Herzog TJ, Tribune DJ, Mutch DG, Gersell DJ, Goodfellow PJ: Allelic loss of sequences from the long arm of chromosome 10 and replication errors in endometrial cancers. *Cancer Res* **55**:1922, 1995.

32. Okamoto A, Sameshima Y, Yamada Y, Teshima S-I, Terashima Y, Terada M, Yokota J: Allelic loss on chromosome 17p and p53 mutations in human endometrial carcinoma of the uterus. *Cancer Res* **51**:5632, 1991.

33. Tashiro H, Isacson C, Levine R, Kurman RJ, Cho KR, Hedrick L: p53 gene mutations are common in uterine serous carcinoma and occur early in their pathogenesis. *Am J Pathol* **150**:177, 1997.

34. Burks RT, Kessis TD, Cho KR, Hedrick L: Microsatellite instability in endometrial carcinoma. *Oncogene* **9**:1163, 1994.

35. Duggan BD, Felix JC, Muderspach LI, Tourgeman D, Zheng J, Shibata D: Microsatellite instability in sporadic endometrial carcinoma. *J Natl Cancer Inst* **86**:1216, 1994.

36. Risinger JI, Berchuck A, Kohler MF, Watson P, Lynch HT, Boyd J: Genetic instability of microsatellites in endometrial carcinoma. *Cancer Res* **53**:5100, 1993.

37. Katabuchi H, van Rees B, Lambers AR, Ronnett BM, Blazes MS, Leach FS, Cho KR, Hedrick L: Mutations in DNA mismatch repair genes are not responsible for microsatellite instability in most sporadic endometrial carcinomas. *Cancer Res* **55**:5556, 1995.

38. Boyer JC, Umar A, Risinger JI, Lipford JR, Kane M, Yin S, Barrett JC, Kolodner RD, Kunkel TA: Microsatellite instability, mismatch repair deficiency, and genetic defects in human cancer cell lines. *Cancer Res* **55**:6063, 1995.

38a. Esteller M, Levine R, Baylin SB, Ellenson LH, Herman JG: MLH1 promoter hypermethylation is associated with the microsatellite instability phenotype in sporadic endometrial carcinomas. *Oncogene* **17**:2413, 1998.

38b. Simpkins SB, Bocker T, Swisher EM, Mutch DG, Gersell DJ, Kovatich AJ, Palazzo JP, Fishel R, Goodfellow PJ: MLH1 promoter methylation and gene silencing is the primary cause of microsatellite instability in sporadic endometrial cancers. *Hum Mol Genet* **8**:661, 1999.

39. Tashiro H, Lax SF, Gaudin PB, Isacson C, Cho KR, Hedrick L: Microsatellite instability is uncommon in uterine serous carcinoma. *Am J Pathol* **150**:75, 1997.

40. Mizuuchi H, Nasim S, Kudo R, Silverberg SG, Greenhouse S, Garrett CT: Clinical implications of k-ras mutations in malignant epithelial tumors of the endometrium. *Cancer Res* **52**:2777, 1992.

41. Ignar-Trowbridge D, Risinger JI, Dent GA, Kohler M, Berchuck A, McLachlan JA, Boyd J: Mutations of the Ki-ras oncogene in endometrial carcinoma. *Am J Obstet Gynecol* **167**:227, 1992.

42. Fujimoto I, Shimizu Y, Hirai Y, Chen J-I, Teshima H, Hasumi K, Masubuchi K, Takahashi M: Studies on ras oncogene activation in endometrial carcinoma. *Gynecol Oncol* **48**:196, 1993.

43. Duggan BD, Felix JC, Muderspach LI, Tsao J-L, Shibata DK: Early mutational activation of the c-Ki-ras oncogene in endometrial carcinoma. *Cancer Res* **54**:1604, 1994.

44. Enomoto T, Fujita M, Inoue M, Rice JM, Nakajima R, Tanizawa O, Nomura T: Alterations of the p53 tumor suppressor gene and its association with activation of the c-K-ras-2 proto-oncogene in premalignant and malignant lesions of the human uterine endometrium. *Cancer Res* **53**:1883, 1993.

45. Sasaki H, Nishii H, Takahashi H, Tada A, Furusato M, Terashima Y, Siegal GP, Parker SL, Kohler MF, Berchuck A, Boyd J: Mutations of the ki-ras proto-oncogene in human endometrial hyperplasia and carcinoma. *Cancer Res* **53**:1906, 1993.

46. Caduff RF, Johnston CM, Frank TS: Mutations of the Ki-ras oncogene in carcinoma of the endometrium. *Am J Pathol* **146**:182, 1995.

47. Esteller M, Garcia A, Martinez I Palones JM, Cabero A, Reventos J: Detection of c-erbB-2/neu and fibroblast growth factor-3/INT-2 but not epidermal growth factor receptor gene amplification in endometrial cancer by differential polymerase chain reaction. *Cancer* **75**:2139, 1995.

48. Czerwenka K, Lu Y, Heuss F: Amplification and expression of the c-erbB-2 oncogene in normal, hyperplastic, and malignant endometria. *Int J Gynecol Pathol* **14**:98, 1995.

49. Pisani AL, Barbuto DA, Chen D, Ramos L, Lagasse LD, Karlan BY: Her-2/neu, p53, and DNA analyses as prognosticators for survival in endometrial carcinoma. *Obstet Gynecol* **85**:729, 1995.

50. Saffari Jones LA, El-Naggar A, Felix JC, George J, Press MF: Amplification and overexpression of HER2/neu (c-erbB2) in endometrial cancers: Correlation with overall survival. *Cancer Res* **55**:5693, 1995.

51. Khalifa MA, Mannel RS, Haraway SD, Walker J, Min K-W: Expression of EGFR, HER-2/neu, p53, and PCNA in endometrioid, serous papillary, and clear cell endometrial adenocarcinomas. *Gynecol Oncol* **53**:84, 1994.

52. Yamauchi N, Sakamoto A, Uozaki H, Iihara K, Machinami R: Immunohistochemical analysis of endometrial adenocarcinoma for bcl-2 and p53 in relation to expression of sex steroid receptor and proliferative activity. *Int J Gynecol Pathol* **15**:202, 1996.

53. Henderson GS, Brown KA, Perkins SL, Abbott TM, Clayton F: bcl-2 is down-regulated in atypical endometrial hyperplasia and adenocarcinoma. *Mod Pathol* **9**:430, 1996.

53a. Fukuchi T, Sakamoto M, Tsuda H, Maruyama K, Nozawa S, Hirohashi S. β-Catenin mutation in carcinoma of the uterine endometrium. *Cancer Res* **58**:3526, 1998.

54. Kastan MB, Canman CE, Leonard CJ: p53, cell cycle control and apoptosis: Implications for cancer. *Cancer Metastasis Rev* **14**:3, 1995.

55. Inoue M, Okayama A, Fujita M, Enomoto T, Sakata M, Tanizawa O, Ueshima H: Clinicopathological characteristics of p53 overexpression in endometrial cancers. *Int J Cancer* **58**:14, 1994.

56. Kohler MF, Berchuck A, Davidoff AM, Humphrey PA, Dodge RK, Iglehart JD, Soper JT, Clarke-Pearson DL, Bast RC, Marks JR: Overexpression and mutation of p53 in endometrial carcinoma. *Cancer Res* **52**:1622, 1992.

57. Ito K, Watanabe K, Nasim S, Sasano H, Sato S, Yajima A, Silverberg SG, Garrett CT: Prognostic significance of p53 overexpression in endometrial cancer. *Cancer Res* **54**:4667, 1994.

58. Jiko K, Sasano H, Ito K, Ozawa N, Sato S, Yajima A: Immunohistochemical and in situ hybridization analysis of p53 in human endometrial carcinoma of the uterus. *Anticancer Res* **13**:305, 1993.

59. Kihana T, Hamada K, Inoue Y, Yano N, Iketani H, Murao S-I, Ukita M, Matsuura S: Mutation and allelic loss of the p53 gene in endometrial carcinoma. *Cancer* **76**:72, 1995.

60. Geisler JP, Wiemann MC, Zhou Z, Miller GA, Geisler HE: p53 as a prognostic indicator in endometrial cancer. *Gynecol Oncol* **61**:245, 1996.

61. Honda T, Kato H, Imamura T, Gima T, Nishida J, Sasaki M, Hosi K, Sato A, Wake N: Involvement of p53 gene mutations in human endometrial carcinomas. *Int J Cancer* **53**:963, 1993.

62. Sherman ME, Bur ME, Kurman RJ: p53 in endometrial cancer and its putative precursors: Evidence for diverse pathways of tumorigenesis. *Hum Pathol* **26**:1268, 1995.

63. Tashiro H, Blazes MS, Wu R, Cho KR, Bose S, Wang SI, Li J, Parsons R, Hedrick Ellenson L: Mutations in PTEN are frequent in endometrial carcinoma but rare in other common gynecologic malignancies. *Cancer Res* **57**:3935, 1997.

64. Kong D, Suzuki A, Zou T, Sakurada A, Kemp LW, Wakatsuki S, Yokoyama T, Yamakawa H, Furukawa T, Sato M, Ohuchi N, Sato S, Yin J, Wang S, Abraham JM, Souza RF, Smolinski KM, Meltzer SJ, Horii A: PTEN is frequently mutated in primary endometrial carcinomas. *Nat Genet* **17**:143, 1997.

65. Risinger JI, Hayes K, Berchuck A, Barrett JC: PTEN/MMAC1 mutations in endometrial cancers. *Cancer Res* **57**:4736, 1997.

66. Levine RL, Cargile CB, Blazes MS, van Rees B, Kurman RJ, Hedrick Ellenson L: PTEN mutations and microsatellite instability in complex atypical hyperplasia, a precursor lesion to uterine endometrioid carcinoma. *Cancer Res* **58**:3254, 1998.

67. Maxwell GL, Risinger JI, Gumbs C, Shaw H, Bentley RC, Barrett JC, Berchuck A, Futreal PA: Mutation of the PTEN tumor suppressor gene in endometrial hyperplasia. *Cancer Res* **58**:2500, 1998.

68. Li J, Yen C, Liaw D, Podsypanina K, Bose S, Wang SI, Puc J, Miliaresis C, Rodgers L, McCombie R, Bigner SH, Giovanella BC, Ittmann M, Tycko B, Hibshoosh H, Wigler MH, Parsons R: PTEN, a putative protein tyrosine phosphatase gene mutated in human brain, breast, and prostate cancer. *Science* **275**:1943, 1997.

69. Meyers MP, Stolarov JP, Eng C, Li J, Wang S, Wigler MH, Parsons R, Tonks NK: P-TEN, the tumor suppressor from human chromosome 10q23, is a dual-specificity phosphatase. *Proc Natl Acad Sci U S A* **94**:9052, 1997.

70. Maehama T, Dixon JE: The tumor suppressor, PTEN/MMAC1, dephosphorylates the lipid second messenger, phosphatidylinositol 3,4,5-triphosphate. *J Biol Chem* **273**:13375, 1998.

71. Tamura M, Gu J, Matsumoto K, Aota S, Parsons R, Yamada KM: Inhibition of cell migration, spreading, and focal adhesions by tumor suppressor PTEN. *Science* **280**:1614, 1998.

Cervical Cancer

Kathleen R. Cho

1. Based on available worldwide statistics, cervical cancer is the second most common cause of cancer-related mortality in women. Cervical cancers are curable when detected early, and the implementation of effective screening programs has reduced the incidence of and mortality from cervical cancer in industrialized countries substantially.

2. Neoplastic processes are undoubtedly complex, and cervical tumorigenesis is no exception. Like other adult solid tumors, cervical cancer appears to develop and progress largely as a consequence of activating mutation of oncogenes coupled with inactivation of tumor-suppressor genes. Alterations of such genes have profound effects on the exquisite control of cell growth and differentiation present in normal cells. Based on currently available information, it appears that inherited factors do not play a major role in cervical tumorigenesis.

3. Cervical cancer is different from most other common malignancies in that it is strongly associated with an infectious agent (human papillomavirus, HPV). This strong association has been used to great advantage in the research laboratory because the HPVs provide powerful tools with which to examine the molecular mechanisms underlying cervical tumor development and progression.

4. Most studies have focused on the E6 and E7 transforming proteins of the oncogenic HPV types. E6 and E7 interfere with function of the cellular tumor-suppressor proteins p53 and pRB via protein-protein interactions. By interfering with cell cycle control and DNA repair mechanisms, oncogenic HPVs appear to contribute indirectly to cervical tumorigenesis by promoting genetic instability and the accumulation of mutations in HPV-infected cells.

5. Relatively few specific genes have been identified that are often altered in cervical carcinomas, although frequent amplification of *c-myc* and *HER2-neu* has been reported. However, other cytogenetic and molecular genetic studies suggest that genes on chromosomes 1, 3, 5, 11, and others are likely to play important roles in cervical tumorigenesis. Intensive efforts are currently underway to identify specific genes targeted by alterations of these chromosomes.

6. Animal models of papillomavirus-associated tumorigenesis have been developed, including several species-specific systems. More recently, production of transgenic animals expressing HPV transforming proteins have provided new insights into the mechanisms by which HPVs contribute to cervical cancer.

7. Cervical cancers are particularly attractive targets for preventive and antitumor vaccines because they virtually always contain tumor-specific antigens (HPV proteins).

A list of standard abbreviations is located immediately preceding the index. Nonstandard abbreviations used in this chapter include: SILs = squamous intraepithelial lesions; LSILs = low-grade squamous intraepithelial lesions; HSILs = high-grade squamous intraepithelial lesions; HPV = human papillomavirus.

CLINICAL ASPECTS

Incidence

Of cancers affecting women worldwide, cervical cancer is second only to breast cancer in both incidence and mortality.[1] Nearly 500,000 women are diagnosed with cervical cancer each year, and many die of the disease. The majority of cervical cancer patients are socioeconomically disadvantaged and thus without access to routine gynecologic care and screening for precancerous lesions. As a result, cervical cancer is particularly prevalent in many developing nations.

Notably, carcinomas of the cervix usually are curable if detected early. In the United States, the incidence and death rate from cervical cancer have decreased markedly over the last few decades, largely because of early detection and effective treatment of noninvasive precursor lesions and minimally invasive carcinomas. In the United States during 1997, there were approximately 14,500 new cervical cancer cases and 4800 cervical cancer deaths.[2] Estimates of the prevalence of precursor lesions, collectively referred to as *squamous intraepithelial lesions* (SILs), range from 0.5 to 6.5 percent of the American female population and include at least 50,000 new cases of carcinoma *in situ* each year.

Histopathology

The cervix includes both vaginal (ectocervical) and internal (endocervical) portions. The ectocervix is covered by stratified squamous epithelium, whereas the endocervix is lined by mucin-producing columnar epithelium that invaginates into the underlying stroma to form gland-like structures. Most cervical cancers are of squamous-type differentiation and arise within a specific region of the cervix referred to as the *transformation zone*. The transformation zone is an area in which, via a process called *squamous metaplasia,* the columnar epithelium located at the junction between the ectocervix and endocervix is replaced by squamous epithelium. Less commonly, cervical carcinomas arise from the endocervical columnar/glandular epithelium (adenocarcinomas).

During the development of squamous carcinomas, metaplastic squamous cells within the transformation zone undergo distinctive morphologic changes reflecting a progression from normal epithelium to carcinoma (Fig. 43-1). Lesions confined to the epithelium can be categorized as low-grade squamous intraepithelial lesions (LSILs) or high-grade squamous intraepithelial lesions (HSILs) depending on their specific morphologic features. Histopathologically, the intraepithelial lesions are characterized by changes reflecting abnormal cellular proliferation and differentiation. LSILs (previously called *mild* or *low-grade dysplasias*) show mild expansion of the proliferative zone in the basal and parabasal portions of the epithelium. Cells toward the surface are arranged haphazardly and often contain enlarged, pleomorphic, and hyperchromatic nuclei surrounded by clear halos. Collectively, these changes are referred to as *koilocytotic atypia*. The HSILs show even greater expansion of the proliferative zone, with mitotic figures often identified in the middle and upper portions of the epithelium. Koilocytotic atypia usually is less prominent than in LSILs, but the cells are more crowded and disorganized, have

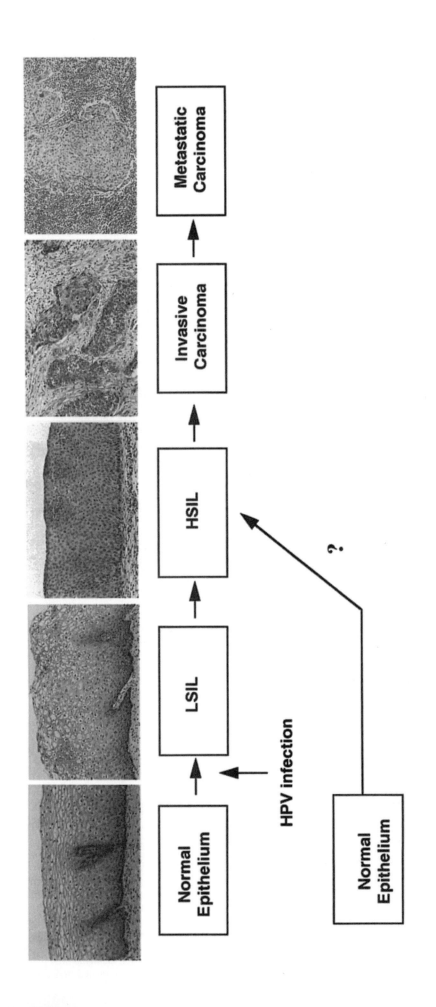

Fig. 43-1 Cervical tumorigenesis is associated with distinctive morphologic changes that reflect a progression from normal epithelium to carcinoma. HPV infection is an early, if not initiating, event in this process. Although all high-grade squamous intraepithelial lesions (HSILs) may not arise from low-grade lesions (LSILs), invasive carcinomas are almost always found in association with their HSIL precursors.

higher nuclear to cytoplasmic ratios, and show loss of polarity. The HSIL category includes lesions previously characterized as moderate and high-grade dysplasias as well as *in situ* carcinomas. Although HSILs may not always arise from preexisting LSILs, virtually all invasive squamous carcinomas arise from untreated HSILs.[3]

Biologic Behavior

If left untreated, SILs can either regress spontaneously, persist, or progress to a more advanced lesion. Based on several previous studies, it appears that the likelihood an LSIL will regress is about 60 percent, whereas the likelihood of progression to invasive carcinoma is only 1 percent.[4] In contrast, the highest grade of intraepithelial lesions regress only 33 percent of the time, and progression to invasive carcinoma occurs in greater than 12 percent of patients. Clearly, high-grade lesions are much more likely to progress to frank malignancy than those of low grade, but not all HSILs will progress to carcinoma, even if left untreated. Presently, lesions that will progress cannot be distinguished from those which will regress based on morphologic features alone.

Women with preinvasive and even early invasive cervical lesions usually are asymptomatic. Hence, without a strategy for early detection, those who develop cervical cancer would be more likely to be diagnosed with late-stage and often incurable disease. Fortunately, exfoliated cervical cells can be collected easily and examined microscopically, following staining, with the method originally described by Papanicolau. Detection of abnormal cells on these "Pap smears" is followed by diagnostic biopsy. Although some clinicians elect to closely follow patients with LSILs, some low-grade and virtually all high-grade lesions are treated by excisional biopsy or other ablative modalities such as laser therapy, cryotherapy, or electrocautery.

Even invasive cancers, when detected early, usually are cured by surgery alone. The 5-year survival of patients with tumors showing less than 3.0 mm of stromal invasion and maximum width of less than 7.0 mm (FIGO stage IA1) is nearly 100 percent.[5] Unfortunately, a substantial number of women in the United States fail to obtain even routine gynecologic care. As a consequence, nearly 50 percent of U.S. women with cervical cancer are diagnosed when the disease is stage II or higher.[6] Women with clinically visible cancers almost always report abnormal vaginal bleeding. Patients with high-stage disease usually are treated with surgery or radiation.

Cervical Cancer as an Infectious Disease

Essentially all human tumors are thought to arise because of mutations in oncogenes, tumor-suppressor genes, and genes encoding proteins involved in DNA damage recognition and repair. These mutations may be acquired somatically or inherited in the germ line. Based on the information available to date, it appears that inherited factors do not play a major role in cervical tumorigenesis, although some investigators have noted an association between the incidence of cervical cancer and particular major histocompatibility complex (MHC) alleles (HLA-DQ3 and, to a lesser extent, HLA-DR6).[7,8] Recently, Banks and colleagues reported a sevenfold increased risk of cervical cancer in individuals homozygous for the Arg allele at the polymorphic codon 72 of the *p53* tumor-suppressor gene.[9] Interestingly, the Arg allele was found to be more susceptible to human papillomavirus (HPV) E6-mediated degradation than the Pro allele (see discussion of E6 function below). Thus increased cervical cancer risk associated with the Arg/Arg genotype is plausible based on what is known about the mechanisms by which HPVs contribute to cervical tumorigenesis. Unfortunately, several larger case-control studies in a variety of populations could not find evidence to support this association.[9a–9e]

Although the contribution of inherited factors to cervical cancer risk remains uncertain, there is no doubt that cervical cancer is strongly associated with an infectious agent. The past few years have seen a remarkable convergence of several lines of investigation convincingly implicating involvement of certain types of HPVs in the development of cervical carcinoma. More recent molecular studies also have provided insight into probable mechanisms by which oncogenic HPVs contribute to cervical neoplasia.

Despite the fact that cervical cancer may, in many respects, be thought of as an infectious disease, it is important to recognize that of the millions of women infected by HPVs, only a small subset actually develops cervical cancer. This observation suggests that in the majority of patients, host immune surveillance may play an important role in limiting the growth and/or promoting regression of HPV-induced lesions. Humoral immunity does not appear to be a critical factor in controlling viral infection, particularly once the virus has entered the cell. Rather, HPV infection is more likely limited in most patients by the cell-mediated immune response.[10]

THE ROLE OF HPV INFECTION IN CERVICAL TUMORIGENESIS

Over 90 percent of invasive cervical carcinomas have been shown to contain DNA sequences from particular HPV types.[11] Papillomaviruses are small DNA viruses composed of an approximately 8-kb double-stranded circular genome enclosed by a 55-nm viral capsid. Over 100 different HPV types have been characterized on the basis of differences in DNA sequence, and a single host may be infected by multiple different HPVs. Based on extensive examination of the association of different HPV types with exophytic condylomas (genital warts), SILs, and cervical cancers, genital HPVs can be broadly classified into two groups: those associated with benign lesions (primarily HPVs 6 and 11) and those associated with invasive carcinomas (primarily HPVs 16 and 18). This classification into low-risk (non-cancer-associated) and high-risk (cancer-associated) types is reflected by *in vitro* evidence that cloned DNA of high-risk, but not low-risk, HPVs can efficiently immortalize primary human keratinocytes.[12–14] Moreover, only the E6 and E7 open reading frames of the high-risk HPV genome are required for this immortalization function.[15]

Nearly all invasive cervical cancers contain high-risk HPV sequences, providing compelling evidence for HPV infection as a causative factor. However, several lines of evidence suggest that HPV infection alone is insufficient to generate the fully malignant phenotype. First, while the HPV *E6* and *E7* genes from high-risk viruses can cooperate to efficiently immortalize primary cells in culture, a fully transformed phenotype is only seen after many *in vitro* cell doublings. Second, although infection with high-risk HPV types is very common, only a small percentage of infected women develop invasive cervical cancer. Third, those who develop cancer generally do so long after initial infection with HPV (many years in most cases). These observations suggest that in addition to infection with a high-risk HPV type, other events are required for the development of cervical cancer. Presumably, these events include alterations of oncogenes and tumor-suppressor genes in cervical cells harboring the HPV genome.

Functional Consequences of HPV Oncoprotein Expression

Given that infection with high-risk HPVs contributes to the pathogenesis of cervical cancer, studies over the past decade have sought to investigate the molecular mechanisms underlying HPV-associated tumor development. The HPV E6 and E7 oncoproteins have been shown to interact directly with tumor-suppressor gene products. Specifically, the E6 oncoprotein of high-risk HPV types 16 and 18 binds the tumor-suppressor protein p53 with much higher affinity than E6 of low-risk HPV types 6 and 11, and this binding appears to promote p53 degradation via the ubiquitin pathway.[16,17] The interaction between high-risk HPV E6 and p53 is mediated by a third protein, called *E6-AP*, that functions as a ubiquitin ligase in the ubiquitination of p53.[18–20] The HPV16 E7 protein has been shown to bind the retinoblastoma tumor-suppressor protein p105-RB (and other members of the RB family) with much greater affinity than its low-risk counterpart, presumably inactivating pRB's tumor-suppressor function.[21–23] Comparable to the p53-E6 interaction, studies by Boyer *et al.* provide evidence for E7-induced enhanced degradation of Rb protein via the ubiquitin-proteasome pathway.[23a]

Since high-risk HPV infection provides a means with which to inactivate these tumor suppressors through protein-protein interactions, it is not surprising that most HPV-positive cervical carcinomas and carcinoma-derived cell lines lack *p53* and *pRB* mutations.[24,25] However, a few HPV-positive tumors have been shown to contain *p53* gene mutations, suggesting that in at least some cases the gene mutation confers an additional growth advantage to the HPV-infected cell.[26–28] Other studies support the notion that *p53* gene mutation may play a role in the progression of at least some cervical tumors, since *p53* point mutations have been identified more frequently in metastases arising from HPV-positive cervical carcinomas than in primary tumors.[29]

The functional consequences of *p53* and *pRB* inactivation by HPV oncoproteins have been addressed by several studies. Cells damaged by irradiation or DNA strand-breaking drugs arrest in the late G1 portion of the cell cycle, presumably allowing the cells to repair DNA damage and avoid accumulation of genetic lesions.[30–32] This cell cycle arrest is temporally associated with accumulation of wild-type p53 protein and is not seen in cells lacking p53 or in those expressing mutant *p53* genes. When the HPV16 E6 protein is expressed in cells exhibiting a normal DNA damage response, baseline p53 protein levels are reduced dramatically, and the cell cycle arrest following DNA damage is abolished.[33,34] Hence high-risk HPVs may indirectly contribute to cervical tumorigenesis by promoting genomic instability and the accumulation of mutations in HPV-infected cells. HPV16 E7 also has been shown to effectively abrogate the p53-dependent growth arrest in response to DNA damage.[35–37] Several studies suggest that this may be explained by a role for pRB downstream of p53 in the growth-arrest pathway (Fig. 43-2). Abrogation of this important cellular response by the HPV transforming proteins suggests a plausible mechanism for the accelerated accumulation of genetic alterations necessary for cervical tumor progression that occurs in the setting of high-risk HPV infection.

There are several types of genetic alterations that may arise as a consequence of *p53* and *pRB* inactivation and the resulting abrogation of the growth arrest in response to DNA damage. When high-risk (HPV16) E6 is introduced into human fibroblasts, the cells show a marked increase in their ability to amplify drug-resistance genes in response to drug treatment.[38] In contrast, low-risk (HPV6) E6 has no effect. The idea that high-risk HPV infection may enhance gene amplification is particularly interest-ing because frequent amplification of *c-myc, HER2-neu,* and as yet unidentified gene(s) on the long arm of chromosome 3 (3q) has been reported in cervical cancers.[39–42] At least one study suggests that *c-myc* amplification may be a useful marker of poor prognosis, since patients whose tumors had *c-myc* amplification suffered early relapse more frequently than those whose tumors lacked the alteration.[40] The gains of chromosome 3q sequences also are particularly interesting because they appear to occur at the transition from severe dysplasia (HSIL) to invasive squamous carcinoma.[42] Specifically, over-representation of chromosome 3q sequences was observed in 90 percent of carcinomas but in less than 10 percent of HSILs, suggesting that the 3q gains may confer the potential for stromal invasion to affected cells.

Another genetic alteration that occurs frequently at the transition from HSIL to invasive carcinoma is integration of the viral genome into the host DNA. In condylomas and most SILs, the HPV genome is maintained as an episome (a free circular molecule replicating independently of the cellular genome). Regardless of HPV type, the production of progeny virions in these lesions is tightly linked to squamous epithelial differentia-tion.[43] In contrast, the majority of invasive carcinomas contain high-risk HPV DNA integrated into human chromosomal DNA as one or multiple tandem copies.[44,45] During the process of integration, substantial portions of the HPV genome may be deleted, but the *E6* and *E7* open reading frames virtually always are retained. Although several studies have failed to find a common site in the host genome where the virus integrates, viral integration almost invariably disrupts elements of the HPV genome (i.e., *E1* and/or *E2*) that regulate expression of the *E6* and *E7* transforming genes.[46] Not surprisingly, integration of HPV16 DNA into the genome of cervical epithelial cells was found to correlate with a selective growth advantage *in vitro,* providing further support for the notion that viral integration is an important step for *in vivo* tumor progression.[47] High-risk HPVs may themselves contribute to integration of HPV DNA into the host genome. Indeed, studies have shown that the frequency of foreign DNA integration is enhanced in cells expressing high-risk but not low-risk HPV E6 and E7.[48]

In other studies, inactivation of *p53* by the HPV16 E6 protein was found to increase the rate of spontaneous mutagenesis (particularly point mutations and small insertions or deletions) in human cells.[49] Interestingly, HPV16 E7 expression had no effect on the rate of mutagenesis, suggesting that the type of genetic alteration detected by this assay is enhanced by *p53* but not by *pRB* inactivation. A plausible explanation for this finding may be provided by the observation that p53's role in suppressing tumorigenesis is not likely to be restricted to its participation in

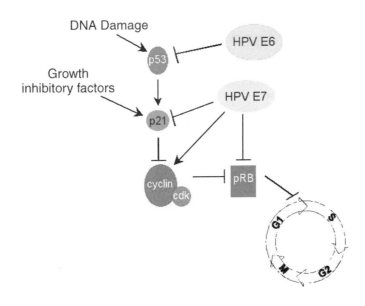

Fig. 43-2 A representation of the DNA damage-induced cell cycle checkpoint pathway in mammalian cells. DNA damage results in accumulation of the p53 protein. Accumulation of wtp53 increases levels of p21$^{waf1/cip1}$, which in turn inhibits activation of cyclin-cdk complexes. pRB therefore remains in the unphosphorylated (active) state, and pRB-associated E2F transcription factors are unable to activate transcription of genes required for progression from G1 into S phase. Consequently, cells arrest in late G1. High-risk HPVs can disrupt the pathway at multiple points: through interaction of E6 with p53 and, further downstream, through the effects of E7 on pRB, p21, and the G1 cyclins. (*Modified with permission from Alani and Münger K: Human papillomaviruses and associated malignancies. J Clin Oncol 16:330–337, 1998.*)

the DNA damage-response pathway. p53 is thought to play a more direct role in DNA repair also, because it has been found to be associated with other proteins involved in DNA repair such as the DNA helicases ERCC3/XPB and RPA.[49]

Clearly, we are beginning to develop an understanding of the molecular mechanisms underlying the difference in oncogenic potential between the high- and low-risk HPVs. The E6 and E7 proteins encoded by the low-risk HPVs appear to have substantially less impact on p53 and pRB function than their high-risk counterparts. However, it remains possible, if not likely, that the oncogenic potential of the various HPV types is owing to additional factors beyond their ability to directly interfere with p53 and pRB function. For example, in addition to its interaction with E6-AP, HPV E6 has been shown to bind to a putative calcium-binding protein called *ERC-55,* and the transforming ability of *E6* mutants was found to correlate with ERC-55 binding activity.[50] E6 proteins encoded by high-risk HPVs are also able to bind to the PDZ domain of HDLG, the mammalian homologue of the *Drosophila* disks large tumor-suppressor protein, which in turn has been shown to interact with the *APC* (adenomatous polyposis coli) tumor-suppressor gene product.[51,52] These findings raise the intriguing possibility that the interaction of HPV E6 with hDLG may represent a mechanism with which to inactivate APC function that bypasses the need for *APC* gene mutation. Additional studies are needed to further explore this possibility. The E6 transforming protein of bovine papillomavirus 1 (BPV1) has been shown to interact with the focal adhesion protein paxillin.[53,54] Paxillin is thought to participate in the transduction of signals from the plasma membrane to focal adhesions and the actin cytoskeleton. Hence E6-mediated disruption of the actin fiber network could alter important signal transduction pathways that regulate cell cycle control and cellular differentiation programs. HPV E7 has been shown to interact with a number of nuclear and cytoplasmic proteins, suggesting that the interaction of E7 with pRB is one of several protein-protein interactions relevant for cellular transformation.[54a] For example, E7 can bind and inactivate the cyclin-dependent kinase inhibitors p21 and p27, and expression of E7 leads to increased expression of the G1 cyclins A and E.[55-58] G1 cyclin-cdk complexes are important in regulating the phosphorylation status of pRB, which in turn regulates cell growth mediated by the E2F family of transcription factors.[59-61] In other studies, expression of HPV16 E6/E7 was shown to lead to increased cellular levels of cyclin B and p34[cdc2], suggesting that the HPV oncoproteins may affect other portions of the cell cycle in addition to the G1S checkpoint.[62]

The role of other HPV proteins in cellular transformation is also being actively investigated. E5 has been shown to act as a mitogen, presumably through growth factor receptor signal transduction pathways, and to induce anchorage-independent growth of immortalized fibroblasts in an epidermal growth factor (EGF)-dependent fashion.[63]

OTHER GENETIC LOCI IMPLICATED IN CERVICAL TUMORIGENESIS

Both cytogenetic and molecular genetic analyses have been used in an attempt to identify additional loci frequently altered during cervical tumorigenesis. In general, cytogenetic studies have failed to identify consistent specific chromosomal rearrangements or other karyotypic abnormalities in cervical cancer cells. Structural and numerical abnormalities of chromosome 1 have been reported most frequently.[64,65]

Other investigators have performed allelotype analyses of cervical carcinomas in an attempt to localize tumor-suppressor loci. In one study of 35 uterine cancers (including both endometrial and cervical carcinomas), high frequencies of allelic loss (i.e., > 35 percent) were found at loci on chromosomes 3p, 9q, 10q, and 17p.[66] In another study of 53 primary cervical carcinomas, more than 25 percent of informative tumors had allelic losses involving chromosomes 1q, 3p, 3q, 4q, 5p, 5q, 6p,

10q, 11p, 18p, and Xq.[67] Frequent deletions on 3p and 11p have been confirmed by other studies.[68-70] Deletion mapping of chromosome 3p has localized common regions of deletion to 3p13-14.3 and 3p13-p21.1.[68,69] The 3p losses are particularly interesting in part because deletions of this region are common not only in cervical carcinomas but also in several other tumor types, including clear cell renal carcinomas, lung carcinomas, and nasopharyngeal carcinomas. Recently, a candidate tumor-suppressor gene, *FHIT* at 3p14.2, was cloned.[71] Aberrant *FHIT* transcripts have been identified in several different tumor types, including esophageal, stomach, breast, and colon carcinomas.[71,72] The gene spans a fragile site called *FRA3B* that was found independently to contain a spontaneous HPV16 integration site.[73] Altered *FHIT* transcripts and markedly reduced or absent Fhit protein expression have been demonstrated in roughly 70 percent of primary cervical carcinomas but not in normal cervix, suggesting that *FHIT* inactivation may be important in cervical cancer pathogenesis.[74]

Functional studies have provided yet additional evidence suggesting involvement of tumor-suppressor genes in the development and/or progression of cervical cancer. For example, transfer of chromosome 11 into HeLa cells (derived from an HPV18-positive cervical carcinoma) and SiHa cells (derived from an HPV16-positive cervical carcinoma) resulted in complete suppression of tumorigenicity.[75,76] Similarly, expression of the *DCC* gene in keratinocytes transformed by HPV18 and nitrosomethylurea resulted in suppression of tumorigenicity, and tumorigenic reversion was associated with loss or rearrangement of transfected *DCC* sequences.[77]

ANIMAL MODELS

A better understanding of the role of HPV infection in the pathogenesis of cervical cancer undoubtedly will enhance our ability to effectively manage patients with this disease. Although *in vitro* systems are very powerful, they are often limited in their ability to provide insights into the processes driving neoplastic progression. Thus a long-standing goal of HPV and cervical cancer researchers has been to develop effective animal models of HPV-induced tumors. Such models, in addition to leading to improved preventive, diagnostic, and therapeutic strategies, also may facilitate identification of genetic and environmental cofactors that may profoundly influence both tumor development and progression.

The strong association of HPV infection with cervical tumorigenesis led to great optimism that useful animal models of cervical cancer could be developed easily. In general, animal models of viral diseases require a source of infectious virus and a susceptible host. Unfortunately, both have been problematic with respect to HPVs. These viruses are notoriously difficult to culture, largely because HPV virions are only produced in highly differentiated keratinocytes. Successful culture of HPV was not achieved until 1992.[78] To further complicate matters, infection with the various types of papillomaviruses is species-specific, and HPVs do not infect nonhuman species. Thus several models of papillomavirus-associated oncogenesis have been developed in species-specific systems, including those in rabbits, rodents, cattle, dogs, and non-human primates.[79,80] Fortunately, many researchers have successfully circumvented the species specificity of papillomaviruses by expressing viral genes in transgenic animals. Several groups have produced transgenic mice expressing high-risk HPV transforming genes.[79,80] Increased propensity to develop tumors has been observed in all transgenic lineages, with the specific location and type of tumor determined largely by the nature of the promoter used to express the transgenes. Transgenic mice expressing the *E6* and *E7* oncogenes of HPV16 under control of the β-actin promoter or α-A-crystallin promoter develop neuroepithelial carcinomas and lens tumors, respectively.[81,82] In one study, mice expressing the same genes under the control of the mouse mammary tumor virus promoter developed large testicular seminomas, whereas another group reported the development of salivary gland carcinomas, lymphomas, and cutaneous histiocyto-mas.[83,84] In the latter study, 77 percent of the female transgenic mice also developed dysplastic and/or hyperplastic changes in the cervix and vagina, although no anogenital tumors were observed. Probably the most illustrative transgenic model system is that recently described by Arbeit and colleagues.[85] These investigators generated transgenic mice expressing the early region of the HPV16 genome under the control of the human keratin-14 promoter. The mice developed squamous carcinomas exclusively in the vagina and cervix when treated chronically with 17β-estra-diol. Although the mechanisms for the synergism between chronic estrogen exposure and expression of HPV oncoproteins in squamous carcinogenesis remain to be determined, this animal model system is likely to prove invaluable in future studies.

IMPLICATIONS FOR DIAGNOSIS AND TREATMENT

HPV proteins provide tumor-specific antigens in the great majority of cervical carcinomas, and hence it should be feasible to develop prophylactic or antitumor vaccines to effectively prevent or treat cervical cancer.[86] The development of such vaccines has been hindered, at least in part, by the difficulty in propagating HPVs in culture and by only relatively recent availability of good animal model systems. Nonetheless, substantial progress has been made in the last few years. For example, several investigators are working to develop prophylactic vaccines based on the use of genetically engineered papillomavirus-like particles to elicit neutralizing anti-HPV antibodies or cell-mediated immune response.[87,88] Preliminary studies in animals have been encour-aging. Alternative approaches also have been employed. Non-capsid papillomavirus antigens (those consistently present in cervical cancer cells) are preferentially routed for MHC class I presentation, which typically is deficient in cervical cancer cells.[10] Thus a reasonable approach for an antitumor vaccine is one that attempts to route such antigens into the MHC class II processing and presentation pathway via the endosomal and lysosomal cellular compartments. In a recent study, Wu and colleagues fused a target tumor antigen (HPV16 E7) to a sequence of the lysosomal protein LAMP-1 in order to direct the antigen into the endosomal and lysosomal compartments and enhance MHC class II presentation of E7 peptides.[89] Expression of the fusion protein in appropriate recipient cells resulted in enhanced presentation to CD4+ cells in vitro. Moreover, in vivo immunization experiments using recombinant vaccinia viruses in mice demonstrated that immunization with the chimeric protein resulted in increased E7-specific lymphoproliferative activity, antibody titers, and cytotoxic T-lymphocyte activity compared with immunization with wild-type E7. In more recent studies, these investigators were able to use the same recombinant viral vaccines to cure mice with small established tumors.[90] Clinical trials of this type of vaccine in cervical cancer patients are likely to follow in the near future.

Certainly, another major goal of cervical cancer researchers in the future will be to identify specific genes involved in the progression of premalignant lesions. The identification of such genes is critical for developing potential screening protocols to augment those currently based on cytopathologic screening of Papanicolau smears alone. The knowledge gained also may prove useful for designing novel and more sensible therapeutic strategies as well as more reliable methods that can be used to predict which intraepithelial lesions may be more likely to progress to invasive disease.

REFERENCES

1. Beral V, Hermon C, Muñoz N, Devesa SS: Cervical cancer. *Cancer Surv* **19-20**:265, 1994.
2. Parker SL, Tong T, Bolden S, Wingo PA: Cancer statistics, 1997. *CA* **47**:5, 1997.
3. Kiviat NB, Critchlow CW, Kurman RJ: Reassessment of the morphological continuum of cervical intraepithelial lesions: Does it reflect different stages in the progression to cervical carcinoma? in

Muñoz N, Bosch FX, Shah KV, Meheus A (eds): *The Epidemiology of Cervical Cancer and Human Papillomavirus*. Lyon: International Agency for Research on Cancer, 1992, pp 59-66.
4. Östör AG: Natural history of cervical intraepithelial neoplasia: A critical review. *Int J Gynecol Pathol* **12**:186, 1993.
5. Benedet JL, Anderson GH: Stage IA carcinoma of the cervix revisited. *Obstet Gynecol* **87**:1052, 1996.
6. Jessup JM, McGinnis LS, Winchester DP, Eyre H, Fremgen A, Murphy GP, Menck HR: Clinical highlights from the National Cancer Data Base: 1996. *CA* **46**:185, 1996.
7. Wank R, Thomssen C: High risk of squamous cell carcinoma of the cervix for women with HLA-DQw3. *Nature* **352**:723, 1991.
8. Helland A, Borresen AL, Kaern J, Ronningen KS, Thorsby E: HLA antigens and cervical carcinoma (letter, comment). *Nature* **356**:23, 1992.
9. Storey A, Thomas M, Kalita A, Harwood C, Gardiol D, Mantovani F, Breuer J, [JKM4]et al: Role of a p53 polymorphism in the development of human papillomavirus-associated cancer. *Nature* **393**:229, 1998.
9a. Helland A, Langerod A, Johnsen H, Olsen AO, Skovlund E, Borresen-Dale AL: p53 polymorphism and risk of cervical cancer. *Nature* **396**: 530, 1998.
9b. Hildesheim A, Schiffman M, Brinton LA, Fraumeni JF Jr, Herrero R, Bratti MC, Schwartz P, Mortel R, Barnes W, Greenberg M, McGowan L, Scott DR, Martin M, Herrera JE, Carrington M: p53 polymorphism and risk of cervical cancer. *Nature* **396**: 531, 1998.
9c. Josefsson AM, Magnusson PK, Ylitalo N, Quarforth-Tubbin P, Ponten J, Adami HO, Gyllensten UB: p53 polymorphism and risk of cervical cancer. *Nature* **396**: 531, 1998.
9d. Klaes R, Ridder R, Schaefer U, Benner A, von Knebel Doeberitz M: No evidence of p53 allele-specific predisposition in human papillomavirus-associated cervical cancer. *J Mol Med* **77**: 299, 1999.
9e. Minaguchi T, Kanamori Y, Matsushima M, Yoshikawa H, Taketani Y, Nakamura Y: No evidence of correlation between polymorphism at codon 72 of p53 and risk of cervical cancer in Japanese patients with human papillomavirus 16/18 infection. *Cancer Res* **58**: 4584, 1998.
10. Altmann A, Jochmus I, Rösl F: Intra- and extracellular control mechanisms of human papillomavirus infection. *Intervirology* **37**:180, 1994.
11. Bosch FX, Manos MM, Muñoz N, Sherman ME, Jansen AM, Peto J, Schiffman MH, Moreno V, Kurman R, Shah KV: Prevalence of human papillomavirus in cervical cancer: A worldwide perspective. International Biological Study on Cervical Cancer (IBSCC) study Group. *J Natl Cancer Inst* **87**:796, 1995.
12. Pirisi L, Yasumoto S, Feller M, Doniger J, DiPaolo JA: Transformation of human fibroblasts and keratinocytes with human papillomavirus type 16 DNA. *J Virol* **61**:1061, 1987.
13. Pecoraro G, Morgan D, Defendi V: Differential effects of human papillomavirus type 6, 16, and 18 DNAs on immortalization and transformation of human cervical epithelial cells. *Proc Natl Acad Sci USA* **86**:563, 1989.
14. Woodworth CD, Doniger J, DiPaolo JA: Immortalization of human foreskin keratinocytes by various human papillomavirus DNAs corresponds to their association with cervical carcinoma. *J Virol* **63**:159, 1989.
15. Hawley-Nelson P, Vousden KH, Hubbert NL, Lowy DR, Schiller JT: HPV16 E6 and E7 proteins cooperate to immortalize human foreskin keratinocytes. *EMBO J* **8**:3905, 1989.
16. Werness BA, Levine AJ, Howley PM: Association of human papillomavirus types 16 and 18 E6 proteins with p53. *Science* **248**:76, 1990.
17. Scheffner M, Werness BA, Huibregtse JM, Levine AJ, Howley PM: The E6 oncoprotein encoded by human papillomavirus types 16 and 18 promotes the degradation of p53. *Cell* **63**:1129, 1990.
18. Huibregtse JM, Scheffner M, Howley PM: A cellular protein mediates association of p53 with the E6 oncoprotein of human papillomavirus types 16 or 18. *EMBO J* **10**:4129, 1991.
19. Huibregtse JM, Scheffner M, Howley PM: Cloning and expression of the cDNA for E6-AP, a protein that mediates the interaction of the human papillomavirus E6 oncoprotein with p53. *Mol Cell Biol* **13**:775, 1993.
20. Scheffner M, Huibregtse JM, Vierstra RD, Howley PM: The HPV-16 E6 and E6-AP complex functions as a ubiquitin-protein ligase in the ubiquitination of p53. *Cell* **75**:495, 1993.
21. Dyson N, Howley PM, Münger K, Harlow E: The human papillomavirus 16 E7 oncoprotein is able to bind to the retinoblastoma gene product. *Science* **243**:934, 1989.

22. Dyson N, Guida P, Münger K, Harlow E: Homologous sequences in adenovirus E1A and human papillomavirus E7 proteins mediate interaction with the same set of cellular proteins. *J Virol* **66**:6893, 1992.

23. Davies RC, Hicks R, Crook T, Morris JDH, Vousden K: Human papillomavirus type 16 E7 associates with a histone H1 kinase and with p107 through sequences necessary for transformation. *J Virol* **67**:2521, 1993.

23a. Boyer SN, Wazer DE, Band V: E7 protein of human papilloma virus-16 induces degradation of retinoblastoma protein through the ubiquitin-proteasome pathway. *Cancer Res* **56**:4620, 1996.

24. Scheffner M, Münger K, Byrne JC, Howley PM: The state of the *p53* and *retinoblastoma* genes in human cervical carcinoma cell lines. *Proc Natl Acad Sci USA* **88**:5523, 1991.

25. Crook T, Wrede D, Vousden KH: *p53* point mutation in HPV negative human cervical carcinoma cell lines. *Oncogene* **6**:873, 1991.

26. Helland A, Holm R, Kristensen G, Kaern J, Karlsen F, Trope C, Nesland JM, Borresen AL: Genetic alterations of the *tp53* gene, p53 protein expression, and HPV infection in primary cervical cancers. *J Pathol* **171**:105, 1993.

27. Fujita M, Inoue M, Tanizawa O, Iwamoto S, Enomoto T: Alterations of the *p53* gene in human primary cervical carcinoma with and without human papillomavirus infection. *Cancer Res* **52**:5323, 1992.

28. Kessis TD, Slebos RJC, Han S, Shah KV, Bosch FX, Muñoz N, Hedrick L, Cho KR: *p53* gene mutations and *mdm2* amplification are uncommon in primary carcinomas of the uterine cervix. *Am J Pathol* **143**:1398, 1993.

29. Crook T, Vousden KH: Properties of *p53* mutations detected in primary and secondary cervical cancers suggest mechanisms of metastasis and involvement of environmental carcinogens. *EMBO J* **11**:3935, 1992.

30. Kastan MB, Onyekwere O, Sidransky D, Vogelstein B, Craig RW: Participation of p53 protein in the cellular response to DNA damage. *Cancer Res* **51**:6304, 1991.

31. Kuerbitz SJ, Plunkett BS, Walsh WV, Kastan MB: Wild-type p53 is a cell cycle checkpoint determinant following irradiation. *Proc Natl Acad Sci USA* **89**:7491, 1992.

32. Kastan MB, Zhan Q, El-Deiry WS, Carrier F, Jacks T, Walsh W, Plunkett B, Vogelstein B, Fornace AJ Jr: A mammalian cell cycle checkpoint pathway utilizing p53 and GADD45 is defective in ataxia-telangiectasia. *Cell* **71**:587, 1992.

33. Kessis TD, Slebos RJC, Nelson WG, Kastan MB, Plunkett BS, Han SM, Lorincz AT, Hedrick L, Cho KR: Human papillomavirus 16 E6 expression disrupts the p53-mediated cellular response to DNA damage. *Proc Natl Acad Sci USA* **90**:3988, 1993.

34. Foster SA, Demers GW, Etscheid BG, Galloway DA: The ability of human papillomavirus E6 proteins to target p53 for degradation in vivo correlates with their ability to abrogate actinomycin D-induced growth arrest. *J Virol* **68**:5698, 1994.

35. Hickman ES, Picksley SM, Vousden KH: Cells expressing HPV16 E7 continue cell cycle progression following DNA damage induced p53 activation. *Oncogene* **9**:2177, 1994.

36. Demers GW, Foster SA, Halbert CL, Galloway DA: Growth arrest by induction of p53 in DNA damaged keratinocytes is bypassed by human papillomavirus 16 E7. *Proc Natl Acad Sci USA* **91**:4382, 1994.

37. Slebos RJ, Lee MH, Plunkett BS, Kessis TD, Williams BO, Jacks T, Hedrick L, Kastan MB, Cho KR: p53-dependent G1 arrest involves pRB-related proteins and is disrupted by the human papillomavirus 16 E7 oncoprotein. *Proc Natl Acad Sci USA* **91**:5320, 1994.

38. White AE, Livanos EM, Tlsty TD: Differential disruption of genomic integrity and cell cycle regulation in normal human fibroblasts by the HPV oncoproteins. *Genes Dev* **8**:666, 1994.

39. Baker VV, Hatch KD, Shingleton HM: Amplification of the *c-myc* proto-oncogene in cervical carcinoma. *J Surg Oncol* **39**:225, 1988.

40. Ocadiz R, Sauceda R, Cruz M, Graef AM, Gariglio P: High correlation between molecular alterations of the *c-myc* oncogene and carcinoma of the uterine cervix. *Cancer Res* **47**:4173, 1987.

41. Mitra AB, Murty VVVS, Pratap M, Sodhani P, Chaganti RSK: *ERBB2* (*HER2/neu*) oncogene is frequently amplified in squamous cell carcinoma of the uterine cervix. *Cancer Res* **54**:637, 1994.

42. Heselmeyer K, Schrock E, du Manoir S, Blegen H, Shah K, Steinbeck R, Auer G, Ried T: Gain of chromosome 3q defines the transition from severe dysplasia to invasive carcinoma of the uterine cervix. *Proc Natl Acad Sci USA* **93**:479, 1996.

43. Chow LT, Broker TR: Papillomavirus DNA replication. *Intervirology* **37**:150, 1994.

44. Dürst M, Kleinheinz A, Hotz M, Gissman L: The physical state of human papillomavirus type 16 DNA in benign and malignant genital tumours. *J Gen Virol* **66**:1515, 1985.

45. Cullen AP, Reid R, Champion M, Lorincz AT: Analysis of the physical state of different human papillomavirus DNAs in intraepithelial and invasive cervical neoplasia. *J Virol* **65**:606, 1991.

46. Choo KB, Pan CC, Han SH: Integration of human papillomavirus type 16 into cellular DNA of cervical carcinoma: Preferential deletion of the *E2* gene and invariable retention of the long control region and the *E6/E7* open reading frames. *Virology* **161**:259, 1987.

47. Jeon S, Allen-Hoffmann BL, Lambert PF: Integration of human papillomavirus type 16 into the human genome correlates with a selective growth advantage of cells. *J Virol* **69**:2989, 1995.

48. Kessis TD, Connolly DC, Hedrick L, Cho KR: Expression of HPV16 E6 or E7 increases integration of foreign DNA. *Oncogene* **13**:427, 1996.

49. Havre PA, Yuan JL, Hedrick L, Cho KR, Glazer PM: p53 inactivation by HPV16 E6 results in increased mutagenesis in human cells. *Cancer Res* **55**:4420, 1995.

50. Chen JJ, Reid CE, Band V, Androphy EJ: Interaction of papillomavirus E6 oncoproteins with a putative calcium-binding protein. *Science* **269**:529, 1995.

51. Kiyono T, Hiraiwa A, Fujita M, Hayashi Y, Akiyama T, Ishibashi M: Binding of high-risk human papillomavirus E6 oncoproteins to the human homologue of the *Drosophila* discs large tumor suppressor protein. *Proc Natl Acad Sci USA* **94**:11612, 1997.

52. Matsumine A, Ogai A, Senda T, Okumura N, Satoh K, Baeg GH, Kawahara T, [JKM13]et al: Binding of *APC* to the human homologue of the *Drosophila* discs large tumor suppressor protein. *Science* **272**:1020, 1996.

53. Tong X, Howley PM: The bovine papillomavirus E6 oncoprotein interacts with paxillin and disrupts the actin cytoskeleton. *Proc Natl Acad Sci USA* **94**:4412, 1997.

54. Tong X, Salgia R, Li JL, Griffin JD, Howley PM: The bovine papillomavirus E6 protein binds to the LD motif repeats of paxillin and blocks its interaction with vinculin and the focal adhesion kinase. *J Biol Chem* **272**:33373, 1997.

54a. Zwerschke W, Jansen-Durr P: Cell transformation by the E7 oncoprotein of human papillomavirus type 16: Interactions with nuclear and cytoplasmic target proteins. *Adv Cancer Res* **78**:1, 2000.

55. Zerfass-Thome K, Zwerschke W, Mannhardt B, Tindle R, Botz JW, Jansen-Durr P: Inactivation of the cdk inhibitor p27 (kip1) by the human papillomavirus type 16 E7 oncoprotein. *Oncogene* **13**:2323, 1996.

56. Jones DL, Alani RM, Münger K: The human papillomavirus E7 oncoprotein can uncouple cellular differentiation and proliferation in human keratinocytes by abrogating p21^Cip1-mediated inhibition of cdk2. *Genes Dev* **11**:2101, 1998.

57. Funk JO, Waga S, Harry JB, Espling E, Stillman B, Galloway DA: Inhibition of CDK activity and PCNA-dependent DNA replication by p21 is blocked by interaction with the HPV-16 E7 oncoprotein. *Genes Dev* **11**:2090, 1997.

58. Zerfass K, Schulze A, Spitkovsky D, Friedman V, Henglein B, Jansen-Durr P: Sequential activation of cyclin E and cyclin A gene expression by human papillomavirus type 16 E7 through sequences necessary for transformation. *J Virol* **69**:6389, 1995.

59. Ewen ME, Sluss HK, Sherr CJ, Matsushime H, Kato J, Livingston DM: Functional interactions of the retinoblastoma protein with mammalian D-type cyclins. *Cell* **73**:487, 1993.

60. Kato J, Matsushime H, Hiebert SW, Ewen ME, Sherr CJ: Direct binding of cyclin D to the retinoblastoma gene product (pRb) and pRb phosphorylation by the cyclin D-dependent kinase CDK4. *Genes Dev* **7**:331, 1993.

61. Hinds PW, Mittnacht S, Dulic V, Arnold A, Reed SI, Weinberg RA: Regulation of retinoblastoma protein functions by ectopic expression of human cyclins. *Cell* **70**:993, 1992.

62. Steinmann KE, Pei XF, Stoppler H, Schlegel R: Elevated expression and activity of mitotic regulatory proteins in human papillomavirus-immortalized keratinocytes. *Oncogene* **9**:387, 1994.

63. Straight SW, Hinkle PM, Jewers RJ, McCance DJ: The E5 oncoprotein of human papillomavirus type 16 transforms fibroblasts and effects the downregulation of the epidermal growth factor receptor in keratinocytes. *J Virol* **67**:4521, 1993.

64. Atkin NB, Baker MC: Chromosome 1 in 26 carcinomas of the cervix uteri: Structural and numerical changes. *Cancer* **44**:604, 1979.

65. Sreekantaiah C, De Braekeleer M, Haas O: Cytogenetic findings in cervical carcinoma: A statistical approach. *Cancer Genet Cytogenet* **53**:75, 1991.

66. Jones MH, Koi S, Fujimoto I, Hasumi K, Kato K, Nakamura Y: Allelotype of uterine cancer by analysis of RFLP and microsatellite

polymorphisms: Frequent loss of heterozygosity on chromosome arms 3p, 9q, 10q, and 17p. *Genes Chromosom Cancer* **9**:119, 1994.

67. Mitra AB, Murty VVVS, Li RG, Pratap M, Luthra UK, Chaganti RSK: Allelotype analysis of cervical carcinoma. *Cancer Res* **54**:4481, 1994.

68. Jones MH, Nakamura Y: Deletion mapping of chromosome 3p in female genital tract malignancies using microsatellite polymorphisms. *Oncogene* **7**:1631, 1992.

69. Kohno T, Takayama H, Hamaguchi M, Takano H, Yamaguchi N, Tsuda H, Hirohashi S, [JKM14]et al: Deletion mapping of chromosome-3p in human uterine cervical cancer. *Oncogene* **8**:1825, 1993.

70. Srivatsan ES, Misra BC, Venugopalan M, Wilczynski SP: Loss of heterozygosity for alleles on chromosome 11 in cervical carcinoma. *Am J Hum Genet* **49**:868, 1991.

71. Ohta M, Inoue H, Cotticelli MG, Kastury K, Baffa R, Palazzo J, Siprashvili Z, [JKM15]et al: The *FHIT* gene, spanning the chromosome 3p14.2 fragile site acid renal carcinoma-associated t(3-8) breakpoint, is abnormal in digestive tract cancers. *Cell* **84**:587, 1996.

72. Negrini M, Monaco C, Vorechovsky I, Ohta M, Druck T, Baffa R, Huebner K, Croce CM: The *FHIT* gene at 3p14.2 is abnormal in breast carcinomas. *Cancer Res* **56**:3173, 1996.

73. Wilke CM, Hall BK, Hoge A, Paradee W, Smith DI, Glover TW: FRA3B extends over a broad region and contains a spontaneous HPV16 integration site: Direct evidence for the coincidence of viral integration sites and fragile sites. *Hum Genet* **5**:187, 1996.

74. Greenspan DL, Connolly DC, Wu R, Lei RY, Vogelstein JTC, Kim Y, Mok JE, [JKM17]et al: Loss of *FHIT* expression in cervical carcinoma cell lines and primary tumors. *Cancer Res* **57**:4692, 1997.

75. Oshimura M, Kugoh H, Koi M, Shimizu M, Yamada H, Satoh H, Barrett JC: Transfer of a normal human chromosome 11 suppresses tumorigenicity of some but not all tumor cell lines. *J Cell Biochem* **42**:135, 1990.

76. Saxon PJ, Srivatsan ES, Stanbridge EJ: Introduction of human chromosome 11 via microcell transfer controls tumorigenic expression of HeLa cells. *EMBO J* **5**:3461, 1986.

77. Klingelhutz AJ, Hedrick L, Cho KR, McDougall JK: The *DCC* gene suppresses the malignant phenotype of transformed human epithelial cells. *Oncogene* **10**:1581, 1995.

78. Meyers C, Frattini MG, Hudson JB, Laimins LA: Biosynthesis of human papillomvirus from a continuous cell line upon epithelial differentiation. *Science* **257**:971, 1992.

79. Brandsma JL: Animal models of human-papillomavirus-associated oncogenesis. *Intervirology* **37**:189, 1994.

80. Griep AE, Lambert PF: Role of papillomavirus oncogenes in human cervical cancer: Transgenic animal studies. *Proc Soc Exp Biol Med* **206**:24, 1994.

81. Arbeit JM, Münger K, Howley PM, Hanahan D: Neuroepithelial carcinomas in mice transgenic with human papillomavirus type 16 E6/E7 ORFs. *Am J Pathol* **142**:1187, 1993.

82. Griep AE, Herber R, Jeon S, Lohse JK, Dubielzig RR, Lambert PF: Tumorigenicity by human papillomavirus type 16 E6 and E7 in transgenic mice correlates with alterations in epithelial cell growth and differentiation. *J Virol* **67**:1373, 1993.

83. Kondoh G, Murata Y, Aozasa K, Yutsudo M, Hakura A: Very high incidence of germ cell tumorigenesis (seminomagenesis) in human papillomavirus type 16 transgenic mice. *J Virol* **65**:3335, 1991.

84. Sasagawa T, Kondoh G, Inoue M, Yutsudo M, Hakura A: Cervical/vaginal dysplasias of transgenic mice harbouring human papillomavirus type 16 *E6-E7* genes. *J Gen Virol* **75**:3057, 1994.

85. Arbeit JM, Howley PM, Hanahan D: Chronic estrogen-induced cervical and vaginal squamous carcinogenesis in human papillomavirus type 16 transgenic mice. *Proc Natl Acad Sci USA* **93**:2930, 1996.

86. Galloway DA: Human papillomavirus vaccines: A warty problem. *Infect Agents Dis* **3**:187, 1994.

87. Greenstone HL, Nieland JD, de Visser KE, De Bruijn ML, Kirnbauer R, Roden RB, Lowy DR, Kast WM, Schiller JT: Chimeric papillomavirus virus-like particles elicit antitumor immunity against the E7 oncoprotein in an HPV16 tumor model. *Proc Natl Acad Sci USA* **95**:1800, 1998.

88. Balmelli C, Roden R, Potts A, Schiller J, De Grandi P, Nardelli-Haefliger D: Nasal immunization of mice with human papillomavirus type 16 virus-like particles elicits neutralizing antibodies in mucosal secretions. *J Virol* **72**:8220, 1998.

89. Wu TC, Guarnieri FG, Stavely-O'Carroll KF, Viscidi RP, Levitsky HI, Hedrick L, Cho KR, August JT, Pardoll DM: Engineering an intracellular pathway for major histocompatibility complex class II presentation of antigens. *Proc Natl Acad Sci USA* **92**:11671, 1995.

90. Lin KY, Guarnieri FG, Staveley-O'Carroll KF, Levitsky HI, August JT, Pardoll DM, Wu T-C: Treatment of established tumors with a novel vaccine that enhances major histocompatibility class II presentation of tumor antigen. *Cancer Res* **56**:21, 1996.

Bladder Cancer

Paul Cairns ■ *David Sidransky*

1. Bladder cancer is the fifth most common male cancer among Americans. Almost all bladder cancer in the United States is composed of transitional cell carcinoma. Familial cases are rare and usually part of the Lynch syndrome. Smoking is perhaps the greatest risk factor for sporadic disease.

2. Cytogenetic studies have identified a number of chromosomal changes in bladder cancer. Low-grade noninvasive tumors are usually diploid, whereas high-grade invasive tumors often contain gross aneuploidy. Monosomy of chromosome 9 is the most common abnormality seen in this disease.

3. Few proto-oncogene mutations or amplifications have been described in bladder cancer. However, chromosomal deletions are very common on chromosomes 9p, 17p, and 13q. Candidate genes inactivated at these loci include *p16, p53,* and *Rb,* respectively. Moreover, *p53* and *Rb* mutations usually are seen in flat (carcinoma *in situ*) or invasive lesions and are correlated with a poor prognosis.

4. Many bladder cancers appear as multifocal disease at presentation. Molecular studies have shown that multiple tumors in the same patient arise from the uncontrolled spread of a single progenitor cell. These tumors then proceed through variable genetic events during progression. A preliminary molecular progression model for bladder cancer suggests that chromosome 9p is an early loss event in most tumors. Conversely, loss of chromosomes 17p and 14q is more often associated with flat lesions and invasive tumors.

5. Genetic alterations can be detected in the urine sediment of patients with bladder cancer. Microsatellite analysis allows detection of loss of heterozygosity (LOH) or genomic instability in primary tumor and urine DNA. Pilot studies suggest that most bladder tumors can be detected by DNA analysis. Moreover, these approaches are amenable to automated techniques suitable for the clinical setting.

CLINICAL ASPECTS

Bladder cancer is the fifth most common male cancer among Americans.[1] There are over 50,000 new cases diagnosed yearly, with a male/female ratio of almost 3:1. There is no pathognomonic sign or symptom for bladder cancer, but most patients present with microscopic hematuria. Occasionally, gross hematuria and pain also can lead to the diagnosis. This year alone over 11,000 patients will die from advanced and/or metastatic disease.[1]

There are few reports of familial bladder cancer.[2] Clinical cases of bladder cancer owing to hereditary predisposition probably represent 1 percent or less of all tumors. The estimated relative risk of developing the disease, even with an affected family member under the age of 45, is only 1.45 per person.[3] The greatest risk for inherited urothelial cancer probably occurs as part of the Lynch

syndrome (hereditary nonpolyposis colorectal cancer, HNPCC).[4] In this syndrome, there is a high risk of bladder cancer, but it is often overshadowed by the high risk of other neoplasms, including colon cancer and uterine cancer.

Almost all bladder cancers in the United States are composed of transitional cell carcinoma (TCC). Bladder irritation or infections such as schistosomiasis can predispose to specific types of bladder cancer. In areas such as Egypt where these infection rates are high, squamous carcinoma is very common.[5] Exposure to certain chemical compounds including analgesics also may predispose to an increased risk of urothelial cancer.[6,7]

In the United States, cigarette smoking is perhaps the single greatest risk factor for bladder cancer. Compared with nonsmokers, smokers have been estimated to have a twofold increased risk of developing the disease. It is also clear that this risk may be dose-related, and in a similar fashion to lung cancer, patients who stop smoking develop an intermediate risk that begins to subside with increasing age.[8–10]

PATHOLOGY

The vast majority of bladder cancer originates in the urothelium, the characteristic transitional cell urothelial lining in the urinary tract.[11] Moreover, many tumors are already multifocal at presentation. A major and overwhelming distinction between superficial and invasive disease involves penetration into the lamina propria. The prognosis for invasive disease is much worse and depends on grade and stage. Although 85 to 95 percent of bladder cancers are TCCs, mixed tumors occasionally with squamous cell or adenocarcinoma elements are also found. Despite its low frequency in the United States, squamous cell carcinoma, for the reasons mentioned earlier, may be the most common malignancy in Egypt. Adenocarcinoma, thought to arise from the trigone of the bladder, occurs in less than 2 percent of all bladder cancers. A particular subset of adenocarcinomas also may arise from the urachus remnant located over the dome of the bladder.

There are two separate and clearly defined entities of superficial bladder cancer presentation.[12,13] The treatment for these two distinct clinical entities of bladder cancer is quite unique, since the outcome and prognosis of each are quite different.

Primary flat lesions with carcinoma *in situ* are notorious for their high likelihood of recurrence and progression.[14,15] A large retrospective study demonstrated that 40 percent of the patients with carcinoma *in situ* developed invasive disease within 5 years.[13] Papillary tumors have a strong propensity to recur, and over 70 percent of patients have a second primary lesion, usually within 2 years.[16,17] However, these lesions have no more than a 20 percent lifetime risk of progression to invasive tumors. Molecular studies have already shed some light as to the different genetic changes that may determine the morphologic appearance and progression of these two very different clinical and pathologic presentations of superficial bladder cancer.[18–20]

CHROMOSOMAL ABNORMALITIES

Neoplastic cells of the transitional cell epithelium contain many structural and numerical chromosomal changes that appear with some consistency.[21,22] These chromosomal changes in tumor cells

---

A list of standard abbreviations is located immediately preceding the index. Nonstandard abbreviations used in this chapter include: CGH = comparative genomic hybridization; ECFR = epidermal growth factor receptors; HNPCC = hereditary nonpolyposis colorectal cancer; LOH = loss of heterozygosity; TCC = transitional cell carcinoma.

include the underrepresentation or abnormally high numbers of chromosomes (aneuploidy) and the presence of easily identifiable structurally abnormal chromosomes that are stably inherited from one cell to another (markers). In general, it has been found that low-grade noninvasive tumors are associated with a normal (diploid) number of 46 chromosomes or with numerical deviations of only a few chromosomes. High-grade invasive tumors, on the other hand, are usually associated with gross aneuploidy and often contain marker chromosomes. The presence of marker chromosomes in low-grade noninvasive tumors has been associated with a strong tendency for recurrence and progression.[22]

Cytogenetic reports on bladder cancer have demonstrated the consistent gain or loss of specific chromosomes or chromosomal regions in most tumors.[22] Cytogenetic studies have identified loss of chromosome 9 as a very frequent change in bladder tumors.[23–25] These studies often described monosomy of chromosome 9 as the most common karyotypic change.[23] Loss of chromosome 10 or deletions of only a portion of 10q also have been described as the only karyotypic abnormality.[24,25] Another specific chromosomal abnormality in bladder cancer was first reported as an isochromosome of chromosome 5p. This appears cytogenetically as a symmetric duplication of the short arm of chromosome 5, specific for a subset of bladder cancers. Deletions and translocations of chromosome 5 are also frequently reported.[24,26]

In addition to traditional cytogenetics, novel methods now allow easier identification of genomic amplifications. A method called *comparative genomic hybridization* (CGH) allows fluorescent identification of amplified genomic regions in human cancers.[27,28] Recent CGH analysis of bladder cancer identified several areas of amplification and confirmed other areas of deletions.[29] Amplifications not previously seen by cytogenetics or molecular studies were identified on chromosomes 3p, 10p, 12q, 17q, 18p, and 22q. Thus, in many ways, CGH has become complementary to traditional cytogenetic and molecular studies.

GENETIC LOCI

As mentioned previously, there have been very few reported cases of inherited bladder cancer. Families have been described without any evidence of cytogenetic abnormalities.[2] Recently, a family was identified with a translocation of 20q and 5p.[30] In addition to bladder cancer, this family also demonstrated metastatic melanoma. In this family, however, a putative oncogene or tumor-suppressor gene has not been identified.

Sporadic Loci

Proto-oncogenes. Despite the initial discovery of a *ras* mutation in a bladder carcinoma cell line, very few *ras* gene mutations have been detected in primary TCC of the bladder.[31] It now appears that less than 10 percent of primary bladder tumors contain *ras* gene mutations.[32,33] Some investigators have observed increased expression of ras protein, but this result remains unproven because of questions about the specificity of the antibodies used.[34]

Growth factors are a class of proteins that bind to specific cell surface receptors, inducing a variety of responses including mitoses in susceptible target cells. Several laboratories have independently studied the expression of urothelial epidermal growth factor receptors (EGFR) using either immunohistochemistry to detect message with antibodies to various portions of the EGFR or autoradiography with isotope-labeled ligand.[18] Most groups have found a higher density of receptors on malignant cells compared with normal epithelium.[18,35] Moreover, epidermal growth factors are excreted in high concentrations in human urine, allowing incubation continually with normal premalignant and malignant urothelial cells. EGFRs are normally found only on the basal cell layer of the bladder epithelium. They also can be richly expressed on the superficial layers of malignant tissue. This abnormal distribution of receptors presumably allows greater access of malignant transitional cells to urinary epidermal growth

factor (EGF) and has led investigators to suspect that EGF plays a role in the development and growth of bladder cancer.[18] Others have reported that the *EGFR* gene is expressed mostly in high-grade invasive tumors, and increased staining has been correlated with increased stage and death from disease in patients with Ta or T1 lesions.[36,37] However, other investigators have found no gross abnormalities at the DNA level; thus overexpression may be owing to an increase in mRNA transcription alone.[38] The *c-erbB1* proto-oncogene that maps to chromosome 7 encodes the *EGFR* gene. Interestingly, trisomy of chromosome 7 is a frequent genetic observation in bladder tumors and could lead to an increase in EGFR expression in tumor cells.[21,22] Another gene on chromosome 7, *MET*, is a candidate proto-oncogene in bladder cancer because mutations of *MET* have been found in hereditary and sporadic papillary renal tumors with trisomy 7.[39] We have sequenced 48 primary bladder tumors and found no mutation of the critical exons of the tyrosine kinase domain.

DNA amplification and increased levels of expression of *c-erbB2* have been reported as well as alterations of *c-myc* and *c-src*.[40–43] However, gross alterations or amplifications of these genes have been described rarely in primary bladder tumors. Although many proto-oncogenes have been identified in human tumors, very few have been found to be consistently altered in bladder cancer. In contrast, chromosomal loss and inactivation of tumor-suppressor genes have been found to play a significant role in progression of bladder tumors.

Chromosomal Deletions and Tumor-Suppressor Genes. Southern analysis with RFLP markers followed by the recent availability of highly polymorphic small repeat sequences known as *microsatellites* has allowed genome-wide assessment of chromosomal loss in bladder cancer.[44–48] The most common loss is the genetic event identified as loss of chromosome 9.[49] Deletion of chromosome 9 appears to be just as common in superficial tumors and invasive tumors. Inactivation of a putative tumor-suppressor gene on chromosome 9 is therefore a key candidate for the initiating event in bladder carcinoma. Careful mapping of chromosome 9 with microsatellite markers has revealed that there are at least two distinct regions of loss: one on chromosome 9p21 and the second on chromosome 9q.[50–52] Southern blot analysis, comparative multiplex PCR, and FISH analysis have revealed the presence of small homozygous deletions of 9p21 in primary bladder tumors.[53,54] These deletions also have been seen in cell lines and have been implicated in the genesis of a variety of tumor types.[55,56]

Another common area of allelic loss is on chromosome 17p. Losses of 17p have correlated with mutations of *p53* and occur predominantly in invasive bladder tumors.[57,58] However, a subset of superficial tumors, especially flat lesions, has been found to contain a higher rate of 17p loss.[19,59]

Southern blot analysis of primary bladder tumors with polymorphic markers has revealed frequent loss of chromosome 13q at the *Rb* locus.[45] Loss of 13q also has been associated with tumors of high stage, and immunohistochemical studies recently have confirmed that *Rb* is the major target of 13q deletions in bladder tumors.[60]

A number of other areas of allelic loss have been identified in bladder cancer. Chromosome 11p loss originally was described by Southern blot analysis and has been confirmed by microsatellite analysis.[44,47,48] Although both Wilms' tumor loci are candidate targets for the deletion of 11p observed in bladder cancer, bladder tumors are not seen in the spectrum of urogenital abnormalities or as second primary malignancies in Wilms' tumors.[61]

Losses of 3p, 4, 5q, 8, 14q, and 18q also have been reported.[19,47,48,62] Two distinct regions of loss have been identified on chromosome 4, one on 4p and one on 4q.[63,64] There also has been a report of two distinct regions of loss on chromosome 14, one on proximal and one on distal 14q. These losses of chromosome 14q correlated closely with increasing grade and stage.[65]

The Clonal Origin of Bladder Cancer

Many bladder tumors present as multifocal disease at diagnosis. The concept of field cancerization was described originally by Slaughter to explain the occurrence of multiple skip lesions and second primary tumors in patients with aerodigestive tract tumors.[66] This hypothesis also was extended to bladder tumorigenesis to describe the possible presence of a field defect secondary to continued exposure of exogenous and endogenous compounds excreted in urine.[11]

We have examined the hypothesis of field cancerization in bladder cancer using molecular genetic techniques.[67] We tested tumors from four female patients with a method that analyzes X chromosome inactivation, which can determine whether tumors were derived from the same precursor cell. This technique was complimented by analysis of allelic loss on various chromosomes, as described previously. In each patient examined, all tumors had the same X chromosome inactivation, whereas normal bladder retained the same polyclonal X chromosome inactivation pattern as expected. Moreover, each of the evaluable tumors from a given patient had lost the same chromosome 9 allele, commonly found early in progression. Later events in progression, such as 17p and 18q loss, were not shared by different tumors from the same patient, implying that multiple tumors in the same patient arose from the uncontrolled early spread of a single transformed cell. These tumors then proceeded through independent and variable genetic events during progression. If a field defect existed, one would expect multiple independent transforming events in each tumor, implying a multiclonal origin for these lesions.

Since this study, other investigators have confirmed the hypothesis that most multiple tumors in the bladder arise from a single progenitor cell. In another study, multiple tumors from 28 of 30 patients were found to contain the same X chromosome inactivation pattern, implying evolution from the same progenitor cell.[68] This understanding about bladder cancer genesis has implications for our understanding of tumor progression and may be useful for cancer diagnosis (see below). It also has allowed the designation of a preliminary progression model for bladder cancer.

Molecular Progression Model

As mentioned previously, careful characterization of genetic alterations within histopathologic lesions at various stages of progression allows the delineation of a molecular progression model. We have previously defined a simple progression model for bladder cancer.[18] In this model, critical allelic losses have been placed in various steps of progression, but oncogenes are not demonstrated because they are involved, so far, in only a minority of primary bladder tumors at the genetic level. Critical steps in this model include initiation of bladder cancer owing to the inactivation of a putative tumor-suppressor gene on chromosome 9, loss of p53 function from the preinvasive to invasive state, and a variety of other genetic alterations associated with invasion and metastasis.

One interesting aspect of this progression model is the distinct differences between the progression of flat and papillary superficial lesions. Both these lesions share a high frequency of chromosome 9 loss that remains almost unchanged during the progression to invasive tumors. However, loss of chromosome 17p is far more frequent in flat lesions and has been associated with inactivation of the p53 gene.[19,59,69] This is intriguing because inactivation of p53 may lead to accumulation of further genetic changes and the propensity of these lesions to acquire a more invasive phenotype. Another distinct change is loss of chromosome 14q. 14q deletion is almost exclusively seen in flat lesions or invasive tumors and virtually absent in papillary lesions.[69] Interestingly, the frequency of 14q loss is even higher in flat lesions than in invasive tumors, suggesting that not all invasive tumors arise from flat lesions. 14q loss thus may lead to the initiation of flat lesions, from which only a fraction may continue to progress to invasive tumors. In this way, invasive tumors may be the final progression pathway for some papillary lesions and many flat lesions. Further characterization of the critical gene on chromosome 14q may lead to a better understanding of the events that lead to the development of flat lesions and their propensity for invasion.[65]

Specific Genes

Germ-Line Mutations. Although there is no common or defined syndrome for familial bladder cancer, familial uroepithelial tumors have been reported. Often these cases appear as a manifestation of the cancer family syndrome, known as *Lynch syndrome* (HNPCC).[4] Of the many neoplasms that occur in these families, TCC is the fourth most common, affecting individuals who manifest TCC alone, TCC and colon cancer, or TCC and other carcinomas.[70,71] Interestingly, in Lynch syndrome, TCC is predominant in the upper tract in contrast to sporadic TCC.

Mutations of mismatch repair genes, including *MSH2, MLH1, PMS1,* and *PMS2,* have been found to be responsible for the majority of cases.[72–75] These genes are involved in DNA mismatch repair and belong to a highly conserved group of repair proteins. As in other sporadic tumors from this syndrome, bladder tumors display characteristic genetic instability manifested by shifts or changes in the repeat size of microsatellite markers.[76] These shifts are actually expansions and contractions of small DNA repeat elements. Approximately 2 percent of all sporadic bladder tumors display characteristic microsatellite instability associated with Lynch syndrome and mismatch repair.[76]

Somatic Mutations. A candidate gene on chromosome 9p21, *p16* (*CDKN2/MTS-1*), is the most common inactivated gene in bladder cancer.[56,77] This gene has been found to be mutated in familial melanoma and pancreatic cancer.[78,79] Although a few point mutations are observed in bladder cancer cell lines, the vast majority of primary tumors with loss of heterozygosity (LOH) of 9p21 do not contain obvious mutations of *p16*.[80,81] This finding pointed to alternative mechanisms for gene inactivation or, potentially, that a second tumor-suppressor gene resided nearby. Recently, we have shown that homozygous deletions of chromosome 9p21 stretching into the *p16* locus are quite common in primary bladder tumors.[54] Much of the controversy surrounding this locus stems from difficulty in identifying homozygous deletions in primary tumors because of contaminating nonneoplastic cells. However, using the strategy of fine microsatellite mapping, homozygous deletions can be identified by the apparent retention of one or two closely spaced markers among a large region demonstrating LOH.[54] These results were confirmed in a number of cases by Southern blot and FISH analyses demonstrating the specificity of the technique. It is now clear that at least 50 percent of all bladder tumors contain a homozygous deletion that includes *p16*. Moreover, we have demonstrated other alternative mechanisms of inactivation including methylation of the *p16* promoter leading to transcriptional block and inactivation of *p16*.[82] Although methylation is common in many other tumor types, inactivation of *p16* by methylation is still uncommon in bladder cancer. The *p16* locus is quite complex and codes for a second transcript called *ARF*. This distinct protein appears to be involved in a separate p53 pathway. Although its exact role in tumor progression is not clear, deletion of the *p16* locus may inactivate genes involved in two critical tumor-suppressor gene pathways, *Rb* and *p53*.[83] Further analysis of a putative second tumor-suppressor locus on chromosome 9 is hampered in bladder cancer by the wide occurrence of monosomy, perhaps indicating inactivation of a gene on chromosome 9q. Although the *patched* gene, inactivated in Gorlin's syndrome and sporadic basal cell carcinoma, has been found on chromosome 9q, an important role in bladder cancer has not been defined.[84,85,85a,85b] Mutations of *p53* are ubiquitous in human cancer, and bladder cancer is no exception.[86] Losses of 17p have correlated well with sequence analysis of *p53* mutations and occur predominantly in invasive bladder tumors.[57] However, a subset of superficial tumors, especially flat lesions, has been found to contain these mutations. Importantly, a large study based on immunohistochemical analysis of *p53* demonstrated a significant decrease in overall survival for *p53* positive patients versus those with tumors that were *p53* negative.[87] It was implied that mutation of *p53* was an independently poor prognostic factor regardless of stage or therapy. Inactivation of *p53* is critical in many tumor types.[86] It has been postulated that *p53* is a critical regulator of response to DNA damage.[88] The appropriate presence of wild-type *p53* leads to growth arrest in the presence of damage and perhaps to apoptosis with excessive damage. Cells that lack p53 protein are unable to undergo a normal G1/S arrest and perhaps propagate further accumulated genetic damage.

A number of lines of evidence also point to a role for the *Rb* gene in bladder carcinogenesis. Immunohistochemical studies have confirmed that *Rb* is the target of 13q deletions in most bladder cancers.[60] A substantially worse prognosis for those tumors with negative standing also has been reported.[89,90] Moreover, reintroduction of the *Rb* gene leads to slowing of cell growth and tumorigenicity in bladder carcinoma cells.[91] The regulatory function of the Rb protein appears to be controlled by phosphorylation during the G1S phase of the cell cycle.[92] p16, one of a number of CDK inhibitors, is also critical for this pathway. In many ways, inactivation of both *p16* and *Rb* may be redundant, and in fact, tumors have demonstrated inactivation of one or the other of these genes but generally not both.[88] Analysis of *Rb* and *p16* status directly in bladder cancer has not been done on the same tumors. It is tempting to speculate, however, that the cyclin D1/p16/Rb pathway is vital in bladder cancer as in many other tumor types.

Bladder tumors are occasionally seen in patients with Cowden syndrome,[93] which arises from mutation of the *PTEN/MMAC1* tumor-suppressor gene located at chromosome 10q23.[94] Point mutations and homozygous deletions of *PTEN/MMAC1* have been found in a subset of bladder tumors with chromosome 10q LOH and are associated with advanced disease.[95]

IN VITRO SYSTEMS

In vitro models have been essential for much of the molecular work done on bladder cancers. Transformation of bladder epithelial cell lines that harbor allelic losses similar to those seen in primary human tumors have helped in the cloning of critical tumor-suppressor genes.[96,97] Transfection of human cell lines followed by reintroduction into animal bladders or renal capsules also have been important models.[98] Transfection of indolent transitional cell carcinoma with proto-oncogenes will not only increase expression of epidermal growth factor receptors but also can increase proliferate responses to epidermal growth factor as well.[99] Moreover, transfection of tumor-suppressor genes leads to diminished growth in these models. Furthermore, these models may be useful to test therapeutic efficacy before clinical trials.[100]

IMPLICATIONS FOR DIAGNOSIS

Microsatellite DNA markers are not only used for mapping primary tumors but also can be used for tumor detection. Microsatellite markers allow detection of LOH or genomic instability in primary tumors.[101] In a blinded study, urine samples from 25 patients with suspicious bladder lesions were analyzed by microsatellite analysis and compared with normal DNA from the same patients. Microsatellite changes matching those in the tumor were detected in the urine sediment in 19 of the 20 patients (95 percent) who were diagnosed with bladder cancer. Urine cytology detected cancer cells in only 50 percent of these same samples.[101]

The most common microsatellite abnormality detected in urine was LOH at critical chromosomal loci.[101] As mentioned earlier in the molecular progression model, early changes including loss of chromosome 9p and 14q were instrumental in the diagnosis of these patients. Moreover, although widespread microsatellite

instability is only associated with Lynch syndrome, occasional microsatellite alterations are not uncommon. These microsatellite expansions or deletions are rare in small repeats but are more common in larger repeats, including tri- and tetranucleotides repeat sequences.[102] It appears that certain repeats are more susceptible to alterations and can be found with a relatively high frequency in many sporadic tumors including bladder cancers. At least 15 percent of the patients in this study were diagnosed by microsatellite alterations that would not have been diagnosed by LOH.[101]

In the study, tumors of all grades and stages were detected, including the difficult to diagnose low-grade papillary tumors.[101] In many cases that were considered atypical but not diagnostic for cancer by cytology, the correct diagnosis was established by molecular analysis. Importantly, control patients without cancer did not demonstrate any of the abnormalities. In a second pilot study where patients were monitored for bladder cancer recurrence, molecular analysis was sensitive, identifying 10 of 11 recurrences. Moreover, at least 2 patients had a positive molecular analysis several months before a recurrence was definitively identified by cystoscopy.[103] The ability to automate this technique with fluorescent labeling and microcapillary electrophoresis may make this a rapidly useful clinical test.[104] The final implementation awaits the completion of large prospective clinical trials to assess overall efficacy.

The recent explosion in our understanding of the genetic events that underlie the progression of human cancer has allowed us to consider novel approaches for diagnosis and treatment. For bladder cancer, a preliminary progression model already suggests specific genetic differences between papillary and flat lesions that may be critical for the treatment of these patients. These models also have led to the development of molecular markers that promise exquisite specificity and sensitivity for the early detection of cancer and for diagnosis of recurrent cases. The fact that most recurrent disease is owing to the expansion of a single progenitor cell may allow us to develop rational therapeutic targets. Critical changes such as *p53* that may lead to a poor outcome also may yield novel, specific therapeutic strategies. It is certain that the future promises to bring exciting new discoveries that will bring molecular biology closer to the forefront of clinical medicine.

REFERENCES

1. Parker SL, Tong T, Bolden S, Wingo PA: Cancer statistics, 1996. *CA* **5**:27, 1996.
2. Schulte PA: The role of genetic factors in bladder cancer. *Cancer Detect Prev* **11**(3-6):379, 1988.
3. Kantor AF, Hartge P, Hoover RN, Fraumeni JF Jr: et al: Familial and environmental interaction in bladder cancer. *Int J Cancer* **35**:703, 1985.
4. Lynch HT: Genetics, natural history, tumor spectrum, and pathology of hereditary nonpolyposis colorectal cancer: An updated review. *Gastroenterology* **104**(5):1535, 1993.
5. Tawfik HN: Carcinoma of the urinary bladder associated with schistosomaisis in Egypt: The possible causal relationship. *Int Symp Princes Takamatsu Cancer Res Fund* **18**:197, 1987.
6. McCredie M, Stewart JH, Ford JM, MacLennan RA, et al: Phenacetin analgesics and cancer of the bladder or renal pelvis in women. *Br J Urol* **55**:220, 1983.
7. Piper JM, Tonocia J, Matanoski GM: Heavy phenacetin use and bladder cancer in women aged 20 to 49 years. *N Engl J Med* **313**:292, 1985.
8. Silverman DT, Hartge P, Morrison AS, Devesa SS, et al: Epidemiology of bladder cancer. *Hematol Oncol Clin North Am* **6**:1, 1992.
9. Augustine A, Hebert JR, Kabat GC, Wynder EL, et al: Bladder cancer in relation to cigarette smoking. *Cancer Res* **48**:4405, 1988.
10. Burch JD, Rohan TE, Howe GR, Risch HA, Hill GB, Steele R, Miller AB, et al: Risk of bladder cancer by source and type of tobacco exposure: A case study. *Int J Cancer* **44**:622, 1989.
11. Fair WR, Fuks ZY, Scher HI: Cancer of the bladder, in Devita VT, Hellman S, Rosenberg SA (eds): *Cancer: Principles and Practices of Oncology.* Philadelphia, Lippincott, 1993, pp 1052–1072.
12. Friedell GH, Soloway MS, Hilgar AG, Farrow GM, et al: Summary of workshop on carcinoma in situ of the bladder. *J Urol* **136**:1047, 1986.

13. Tannenbaum M, Romas NA, Droller MJ: The pathobiology of early urothelial cancer, in Skinner DG, Leiskovsky G (eds): *Genitourinary Cancer*. Philadelphia, Saunders, 1988.

14. Althausen AF, Prout GR Jr, Daly JJ: Noninvasive papillary carcinoma of the bladder associated with carcinoma *in situ*. *J Urol* **116**:575, 1976.

15. Farrow GM, Utz DC, Rife CC, Greene LF, et al: Clinical observation of sixty cases of *in situ* carcinoma of the urinary bladder. *Cancer Res* **37**:2794, 1977.

16. Heney NM, Ahmed S, Flanagan MJ: Superficial bladder cancer: Progression and recurrence. *J Urol* **130**:1083, 1983.

17. Fitzpatrick JM, West AB, Butler MR: Superficial bladder tumors (stage pTa, grade 1 and 2): The importance of recurrence pattern following initial resection *J Urol* **135**:920, 1986.

18. Sidransky D, Messing E: Molecular genetics and biochemical mechanisms in bladder cancer: Oncogenes, tumor suppressor genes, and growth factors. *Urol Clin North Am* **19**(4):629, 1992.

19. Dalbagni S, Presti JC, Reuter VE, Fair WR, Cordon-Cardo C: Genetic alterations in bladder cancer. *Lancet* **342**:469, 1993.

20. Spruck CH, Ohneseit PF, Gonzalez M, Esrig D, Miyao N, Tsai YC, Lerner SP, Schmütte C, Yang AS, Cote R, Dubeau L, Nichlos PW, Hermann GG, Steven K, Horn T, Skinner DG, Jones PA: Two molecular pathways to transition cell carcinoma of the bladder. *Cancer Res* **54**:784, 1994.

21. Sandberg AA: *The Chromosomes in Human Cancer and Leukemia*, 2d ed. New York, Elsevier Science, 1990.

22. Sandberg AA: Chromosome changes in bladder cancer: Clinical and other correlations. *Cancer Genet Cytogenet* **19**(1-2):163, 1986.

23. Smeets W, Pauwels R, Laarakkers L, Debruyne F, Geraedts J: Chromosomal analysis of bladder cancer: III. Nonrandom alterations. *Cancer Genet Cytogenet* **29**(1):29, 1987.

24. Berger CS, Sandberg AA, Todd IAD, Pennington RD, Haddad FS, Hecht BK, Hecht F: Chromosomes in kidney, ureter, and bladder cancer. *Cancer Genet Cytogenet* **23**:1, 1986.

25. Gibas Z, Prout GJ, Connolly JG, Prontes JE, Sandberg AA: Nonrandom chromosomal changes in transitional cell carcinoma of the bladder. *Cancer Res* **44**(3):1257, 1984.

26. Gibas Z, Prout GR, Pontes JE, Connolly JG, Sandberg AA: A possible specific chromosome change in transitional cell carcinoma of the bladder. *Cancer Genet Cytogenet* **19**(3):229, 1986.

27. Kallioniemi A, Kallioniemi OP, Sudar D, Rutovitz D, Gray JW, Waldman F, Pinkel D: Comparative genomic hybridization for molecular cytogenetic analysis of solid tumors. *Science* **258**(5083):818, 1992.

28. du Manoir S, Speicher MR, Joos S, Schrock E, Popp S, Dohner H, Kovacs G, Robert M, Lichter P, Cremer T: Detection of complete and partial chromosome gains and losses by comparative genomic *in situ* hybridization. *Hum Genet* **90**(6):590, 1993.

29. Voorter C, Joos S, Vallinga M, Poddighe P, Schalken J, du Manoir S, Ramaekers Lichter P, Hopman A: Detection of chromosomal imbalances in transitional cell carcinoma of the bladder by comparative genomic hybridization. *Am J Pathol* **146**(6):1341, 1995.

30. Schoenberg M, Kiemeney L, Walsh PC, Griffin CA, Sidransky D: Germline translocation t(5)(p15) and familial transitional cell carcinoma. *J Urol* **155**(3):1035, 1996.

31. Reddy EP, Reynolds RK, Santos E, Barbacid M: A point mutation is responsible for the acquisition of transforming properties by the T24 human bladder carcinoma oncogene. *Nature* **300**(5888):149, 1982.

32. Knowles MA, Williamson M: Mutation of Hras is infrequent in bladder cancer: Confirmation by single conformation polymorphism analysis, designed restriction fragment length polymorphisms, and direct sequencing. *Cancer Res* **53**:133, 1993.

33. Fujita J, Srivastava SK, Kraus MH, Rhim JS, Tronick SR, Aaronson SA: Frequency of molecular alterations affecting *ras* proto-oncogenes in human urinary tract tumors. *Proc Natl Acad Sci USA* **82**(11):3849, 1985.

34. Viola MV, Fromowitz F, Oravez S, Deb S, Schlom J: *ras* oncogene p21 expression is increased in premalignant lesions and high grade bladder carcinoma. *J Exp Med* **161**:1213, 1985.

35. Messing EM, Reznikoff CA: Normal and malignant urothelium: In effects of epidermal growth factor. *Cancer Res* **47**:2230, 1987.

36. Neal DE, Marsh C, Bennett MK, Abel PD, Hall RR, Sainsbury JR, Harris AL: Epidermal receptors in human bladder cancer: Comparison of invasive and superficial tumours. *Lancet* **1**(8425):366, 1985.

37. Neal DE, Sharples L, Smith K, Fennelly J, Hall RR, Harris AL: The epidermal growth factor receptor and the prognosis of bladder cancer. *Cancer* **65**:1619, 1990.

38. Berger MS, Greenfield C, Gullick WJ, Haley J, Downward J, Neal DE, Harris AL, Waterfieldm MD: Evaluation of epidermal growth factor receptors in bladder tumours. *Br J Cancer* **56**:533, 1987.

39. Schmidt L, Duh F-M, Chen F, Kishida T, Glenn G, Choyke P, Scherer SW, Zhuang Z, Lubensky Dean M, Allikmets R, Chidambaram, Bergerheim UR, Feltis JR, Casadevall C, Zamarron A, Bernues M, Richard S, Lips C, Walther MM, Tsui LC, Geil L, Orcutt ML, Stackhouse T, Lipan J, Slife L, Brauch H, Decker J, Niehans G, Hughson M, Moch H, Storkel S, Lerman MI, Linehan WM, Zbar B: Germline and somatic mutations in the tyrosine kinase domain of the *MET* proto-oncogene in papillary renal carcinomas. *Nature Genet* **16**:68, 1997.

40. Wright C, Mellon K, Neal DE, Johnston P, Corbett IP, Horne CH: Expression of c-erbB2 protein product in bladder cancer. *Br J Cancer* **62**:764, 1990.

41. Masters JR, Vesey SG, Munn CF, Evan GI, Watson JV: c-myc oncoprotein levels in bladder cancer. *Urol Res* **16**(5):341, 1988.

42. Del-Senno L, Maestri I, Piva R, Hanau S, Reggiani A, Romano A, Russo G: Differential hypomethylation of the *c-myc* proto in bladder cancers at different stages and grades. *J Urol* **142**:146, 1989.

43. Fanning P, Bulovas K, Saini KS: Elevated expression of pp60[c-src] in low grade bladder carcinomas. *Cancer Res* **52**:1457, 1992.

44. Fearon ER, Feinberg AP, Hamilton SH, Vogelstein B: Loss of genes on the short arm of chromosome 11 in bladder cancer. *Nature* **318**(6044):377, 1985.

45. Cairns P, Proctor AJ, Knowles MA: Loss of heterozygosity at the *Rb* locus is frequent and correlates with muscle invasion in bladder carcinoma. *Oncogene* **6**:2305, 1991.

46. Tsai YC, Nichols PW, Hiti AL, Williams Z, Skinner DG, Jones PA: Allelic losses of chromosomes 9, 11, and 17 in human bladder cancer. *Cancer Res* **50**:44, 1990.

47. Presti JC, Reuter VW, Galan T, Fair WR, Cordon C: Molecular genetic alterations in superficial and locally advanced human bladder cancer. *Cancer Res* **51**:5405, 1991.

48. Knowles MA, Elder PA, Williamson M, Cairns JP, Shaw ME, Law MG: Allelotype of human bladder cancer. *Cancer Res* **54**:531, 1994.

49. Cairns P, Shaw ME, Knowles MA: Initiation of bladder cancer may involve deletion of a tumor suppressor gene on chromosome 9. *Oncogene* **8**:1083, 1993.

50. Ruppert JM, Tokino K, Sidransky D: Evidence for two bladder cancer suppressor loci on human chromosome 9. *Cancer Res* **53**:5093-5095, 1993.

51. Cairns P, Shaw ME, Knowles MA: Preliminary mapping of the deleted region of chromosome 9 in bladder cancer. *Cancer Res* **53**:1230, 1993.

52. Linnenbach AJ, Pressler LB, Seng BA, Kimmel BS, Tomaszewski JE, Malkowicz SB: Characterization of chromosome 9 deletions in transitional cell carcinoma by microsatellite assay. *Hum Mol Genet* **2**(9):1407, 1993.

53. Cairns P, Tokino K, Eby Y, Sidransky D: Homozygous deletions of 9p21 in primary human bladder tumors detected by comparative multiplex PCR. *Cancer Res* **54**(6):1422, 1994.

54. Cairns P, Polascik TJ, Eby Y, Tokino K, Califano J, Merlo A, Mao L, Herath J, Jenkins R, Westra W, Rutter JL, Buckler A, Gabrielson E, Tockman M, Cho KR, Hedrick L, Bova GS, Isaacs W, Koch W, Schwab D, Sidransky D: Frequency of homozygous deletion at p16/CDKN2 in primary human tumors. *Nature Genet* **11**(2):210, 1995.

55. Olopade OI, Buchhagen DL, Malik K, Sherman J, Nobori T, Bader S, Nau MM, Gazdar AF, Minna J, Diaz MO: Homozygous loss of the interferon genes defines the critical region on 9p that is deleted in lung cancers. *Cancer Res* **53**:2410, 1993.

56. Kamb A, Gruis NA, Weaver-Feldhaus J, Liu Q, Harshmann K, Tavtigian SI, Stockert E, Day IIIRD, Johnson BE, Skolnick MH: A cell cycle regulator potentially involved in genesis of many tumor types. *Science* **264**:436, 1994.

57. Sidransky D, von Eschenbach A, Tsai YC, Jones P, Summerhayes I, Marshall F, Meera P, Green P, Hamilton SR, Frost P, Vogelstein E: Identification of *p53* gene mutations in bladder cancers and urine samples. *Science* **252**:706, 1991.

58. Habuchi T, Ogawa O, Kaheki Y, Sugiyama T, Yoshida O: Allelic loss of chromosome 17p in urothelial cancer: Strong association with invasive phenotype. *J Urol* **148**:1595, 1992.

59. Fujimoto K, Yamada Y, Okajima E: Frequent association of *p53* mutation in invasive bladder cancer. *Cancer Res* **52**:1393, 1992.

60. Xu HJ, Cairns P, Hu SX, Knowles MA, Benedict WF: Loss of Rb protein expression in primary bladder cancer correlates with loss of heterozygosity at the *Rb* locus and tumor progression. *Int J Cancer* **53**(5):781, 1993.

61. Hawkins MM, Draper GJ, Smith RA: Cancer among 1348 offspring of survivors of childhood cancer. *Int J Cancer* **43**(6):975, 1989.

62. Wu S, Storer BE, Bookland EA, Klingelhutz AJ, Gilchrsit KW, Meisner LF, Oyasu R, Reznikoff CA: Nonrandom chromosome losses in stepwise neoplastic transformation in vitro of human uroepithelial cells. *Cancer Res* **51**:3323, 1991.

63. Elder PA, Bell SM, Knowles MA: Deletion of two regions on chromosome 4 in bladder carcinoma: Definition of a critical 750-kb region at 4p16.3. *Oncogene* **9**(12):3433, 1994.

64. Polascik TJ, Cairns P, Chang WY, Schoenberg MP, Sidransky D: Distinct regions of allelic loss on human chromosome 4 in primary bladder carcinoma. *Cancer Res* **55**(22):5396, 1995.

65. Chang WY, Cairns P, Schoenberg MP, Polasick TJ, Sidransky D: Novel suppressor loci on chromosome 14q in primary bladder cancer. *Cancer Res* **55**(15):3246, 1995.

66. Slaughter DL, Southwick HW, Smejkal W: Field cancerization in oral stratified squamous epithelium: Clinical implications of multicentric origin. *Cancer* **6**:963, 1953.

67. Sidransky D, Frost P, Von Eschenbach A, Oyasu R, Preisinger AC, Vogelstein B: Clonal origin of bladder cancer. *N Engl J Med* **326**:737, 1992.

68. Miyao N, Tsai YC, Lerner SP, Olami AF, Spruck CH, Gonzalez-Zuleta M, Nichols PW, Skinner DG, Jones PA: Role of chromosome 9 in human bladder cancer. *Cancer Res* **53**(17):4066, 1993.

69. Rosin MP, Cairns P, Epstein JI, Schoenberg MP, Sidransky D: An allelotype of carcinoma *in situ* of the human bladder. *Cancer Res* **55**:5213, 1995.

70. Vasen HF, Offerhaus GJ, den Hartog Jager FC, Menko FH, Nagengast FM, Griffioen G, van Hogezand RB, Heintz : The tumour spectrum in hereditary non-polyposis colorectal cancer: A study of 24 kindreds in the netherlands. *Int J Cancer* **46**(1):31, 1990.

71. Lynch HT, Ens JA, Lynch JF: The Lynch syndrome II and urological malignancies. *J Urol* **143**:24, 1990.

72. Cleaver JE: It was a very good year for DNA repair. *Cell* **76**:1, 1994.

73. Bronner CE, Baker SM, Morrison PT, Warren G, Smith LG, Lescoe MK, Kane M, Earabino C, Lipford J, Lindbla Tannergard P, Bollag RJ, Godwin AR, Ward DC, Nordenskjold M, Fishel R, Kolodner R, Liskay RM: Mutation in the DNA mismatch repair gene homologue *hMLH1* is associated with hereditary non-polyposis colon cancer. *Nature* **368**:258, 1994.

74. Nicolaides NC, Popadopoulos N, Liu B, Wei YF, Carter KC, Ruben SM, Rosen CA, Haseltine WA, Fleischmann RD, Fraser CM, Adams MD, Venter JC, Dunlop M, Hamilton SR, Petersen GM, de la Chapelle A, Vogelstein B, Kinzler KW: Mutations of two PMS homologues in hereditary nonpolyposis colon cancer. *Nature* **371**:75, 1994.

75. Liu B, Parsons R, Papadopoulos N, Nicolaides NC, Lynch HT, Watson P, Jass JR, Dunlop M, Wyllie A, Peltomaki P, de la Chapelle Hamilton SR, Vogelstein B, Kinzler H: Analysis of mismatch repair genes in hereditary non-polyposis colorectal cancer patients. *Nature Med* **2**(2):169, 1996.

76. Gonzalez M, Ruppert JM, Tokino K, Tsai YC, Spruck CH III, Miyao N, Nichols PW, Hermann GG, Horn T, Steven K, Summerhayes IC, Sidransky D, Jones PA: Microsatellite instability in bladder cancer. *Cancer Res* **53**:5620, 1993.

77. Serrano M, Hannon GJ, Beach D: A new regulatory motif in cell control causing specific inhibition of cyclin D^{CDK4}. *Nature* **366**:704, 1993.

78. Hussussian CJ, Struewing JP, Goldstein AM, Higgins PAT, Ally DS, Sheahan M, Clark WH Jr, Tucker MA, Dracopoli NC: Germline *p16* mutations in familial melanoma. *Nature Genet* **8**:15, 1994.

79. Caldas C, Hahn SA, da Costa LT, Redston MS, Schutte M, Seymour AB, Weinstein CL, Hruban R, Yeo CJ, Kern SE: Frequent somatic mutations and homozygous deletions of the *p16* (*MTS1*) gene in pancreatic adenocarcinoma. *Nature Genet* **8**:27, 1994.

80. Cairns P, Mao L, Merlo A, Lee DJ, Schwab D, Eby Y, Tokino K, van der Riet P, Blaugrand JE, Sidransky D: Rates of *p16* (*MTS1*) mutations in primary tumors with 9p loss. *Science* **256**:415, 1994.

81. Spruck CH, Gonzalez-Zuleta M, Shibata A, Simoneau AR, Lin M-F, Gonzales F, Tsai Y, Jones PA: *p16* gene in uncultured tumors. *Nature* **370**:183, 1994.

82. Merlo A, Herman JG, Mao L, Lee DJ, Schwab D, Burger PC, Baylin SB, Sidransky D: 59 CpG island methylation is associated with transcriptional silencing of the tumour suppressor *p16/CDKN2/MTS1* in human cancers. *Nature Med* **7**(1):686, 1995.

83. Zhang Y, Xiong Y, Yarbrough WG: ARF promotes MDM2 degradation and stabilizes p53: ARF-INK4a locus deletion impairs both the *RB* and *p53* tumor suppression pathways. *Cell* **92**:725, 1998.

84. Johnson RL, Rothman AL, Xie J, Godrich LV, Bare JW, Bonifas JM, Quinn AG, Myers RM, Cox DR, Epstein EH, Scott MP: Human homologue of *patched*, a candidate gene for the basal cell nevus syndrome. *Science* **272**:1668, 1996.

85. Hahn H, Wicking C, Zaphiropoulos PG, Gailani MR, Shanley S, Chidambaram, Vorechovsky I, Holmberg E, Unden A, Gillies S, Negus K, Smyth I, Pressman C, Leffell DJ, Gerrard B, Goldstein AM, Dean M, Toftgard R, Chenevix-Trench G, Wainwright B, Bale AE: Mutations of the human homologue of *Drosophila patched* in the nevoid basel cell carcinoma syndrome. *Cell* **85**:841, 1996.

85a. McGarvey TW, Maruta Y, Tomaszewski JE, Linnenbach AJ, Malkowicz SB: PTCH gene mutations in invasive transitional cell carcinoma of the bladder. *Oncogene* **17**:1167, 1998.

85b. Simoneau AR, Spruck CH 3rd, Gonzalez-Zulueta M, Gonzalgo ML, Chan MF, Tasi YC, Dean M, Steven K, Horn T, Jones PA: Evidence for two tumor suppressor loci accosicated with proximal chromosome 9p to q and distal chromosome 9q in bladder cancer and the initial screening for GASI and PTC mutations. *Cancer Res* **56**:5039, 1996.

86. Hollstein M, Sidransky D, Vogelstein B, Harris C: *p53* mutations in human cancer. *Science* **253**:49, 1991.

87. Esrig D, Elmajian D, Groshen S, Freeman JA, Stein JP, Chen SC, Nicholls Skinner DG, Jones PA, Cote RJ: Accumulation of nuclear p53 and tumor progression in bladder cancer. *New Engl J Med* **331**(19):1259, 1994.

88. Hartwell LH, Kastan MB: Cell cycle control and cancer. *Science* **266**(5192):1821, 1994.

89. Cordon-Cardo C, Wartinger D, Petrylak D, Dalbagni G, Fair WR, Fuks Z, Renter VE: Altered expression of retinoblastoma gene product: Prognostic indicator in bladder cancer. *J Natl Cancer Inst* **84**:1251, 1992.

90. Logothetis CJ, Xu HJ, Ro JY, Hu SX, Sahin A, Ordonez N, Benedict WF: Altered expression of retinoblastoma protein and known prognostic variables in locally advanced bladder cancer. *J Natl Cancer Inst* **84**:1256, 1992.

91. Takahashi R, Hashimoto T, Hu HJ, Hu SX, Matsui T, Miki T, Bigo-Marshall H, Aaronson SA, Benedict WF: The retinoblastoma gene functions as a growth and tumor suppressor in human bladder carcinoma cells. *Proc Natl Acad Sci USA* **88**:5257, 1991.

92. Mihara K, Cao XR, Yen A, Chandler S, Driscoll B, Murphree AL, T'Ang A, Fung Y: Cell cycle regulation of phosphorylation of human Rb gene product. *Science* **246**:1300, 1989.

93. Starink TM, Van Der Veen JPW, Arwert F, De Waal LP, De Lange GG, Gille JJP, Eriksson AW: The Cowden syndrome: A clinical and genetic study in 21 patients. *Clin Genet* **29**:222, 1986.

94. Liaw D, Marsh DJ, Li J, Dahia PLM, Wang SI, Zheng Z, Bose S, Call KM, Tsou HC, Peacocke M, Eng C, Persons R: Germline mutations of the *PTEN* gene in Cowden disease, an inherited breast and thyroid cancer syndrome. *Nature Genet* **16**:64, 1997.

95. Cairns P, Evron E, Okami K, Halachmi N, Esteller M, Herman JG, Bose S, Wang SI, Persons R, Sidransky D: Point mutation and homozygous deletion of *PTEN/MMAC1* in primary bladder cancers. *Oncogene* **16**:3215, 1998.

96. Reznikoff CA, Kao C, Messing EM, Newton M, Swaminathan S: A molecular genetic model of human bladder carcinogenesis. *Semin Cancer Biol* **4**(3):143, 1993.

97. Kao C, Wu SQ, Bhatthacharya M, Meisner LF, Reznikoff CA: Losses of 3p, 11p, and 13q in EJ/ras simian virus 40 human uroepithelial cells. *Genes Chromosom Cancer* **4**(2):158, 1992.

98. Theodorescu D, Cornil I, Fernandez BJ, Kerbel RS: Over-expression of normal and mutated forms of *HRAS* induces orthotopic bladder invasion in a human transitional cell carcinoma. *Proc Natl Acad Sci USA* **87**(22):9047, 1990.

99. Theodorescu D, Cornil I, Sheehan C, Man MS, Kerbel RS: *Ha-ras* induction of the invasive phenotype results in up of epidermal growth factor receptors and altered responsiveness to epidermal growth factor in human papillary transitional cell carcinoma cells. *Cancer Res* **51**(16):4486, 1991.

100. Theodorescu D, Connors KM, Groce A, Hoffman RM, Kerbel RS: Lack of influence of c-ras expression on the drug sensitivity of human bladder cancer histocultured in three. *Anticancer Res* **13**(4):941, 1993.

101. Mao L, Schoenberg MP, Scicchitano M, Erozan YS, Merlo A, Schwab D, Sidransky D: Molecular detection of primary bladder cancer by microsatellite analysis. *Science* **271**:659, 1996.

102. Mao L, Lee DJ, Tockman MS, Erozan YS, Askin F, Sidransky D: Microsatellite alterations as clonal markers in the detection of human cancer. *Proc Natl Acad Sci USA* **91**:9871, 1994.

103. Steiner G, Schoenberg MP, Linn JF, Mao L, Sidransky D: Detection of bladder cancer recurrence by microsatellite analysis of urine. *Nature Med* **3**(6): 621, 1997.

104. Wang Y, Ju J, Carpenter BA, Atherton JM, Sensabaugh GF, Mathies RA: Rapid sizing of short tandem repeat alleles using capillary array electrophoresis and energy fluorescent primers. *Anal Chem* **67**(1):1197, 1995.

Stomach Cancer

Steven M. Powell

1. **Adenocarcinoma comprises the vast majority of malignant tumors arising from the stomach. Gastric carcinoma is a significant worldwide health burden, second only to lung tumors as a leading cause of cancer deaths. Significant geographic and temporal variances are observed in this cancer's incidence, predominantly of the intestinal type. Epidemiologic studies indicate a strong environmental component in the acquisition of this cancer. Developing countries that are noted to have a high prevalence of *Helicobacter pylori* infection early in life are distinctly prone to having high rates of gastric adenocarcinomas. Most gastric cancers are identified in advanced stages that present in the later decades of adult life, commonly resulting in a lethal outcome shortly thereafter.**

2. **Gastric cancers exhibit heterogeneity in clinical, biologic, and genetic aspects. Multiple pathologic classifications of gastric adenocarcinomas exist, including those with morphologic and histologic criteria. The TNM staging system is generally used as the basis for prognostication in this cancer, with depth of infiltration being an important parameter. Most cases of stomach cancer are sporadic in nature, with rare reports of inherited gastric cancer predisposition traits that can involve germ-line E-cadherin alterations or in conjunction with the hereditary nonpolyposis colon cancer disease entity.**

3. **Cytogenetic studies have been unsuccessful in identifying an obvious significant chromosomal aberration in gastric cancers. Loss of heterozygosity studies and comparative genomic hybridization analyses have identified several loci with significant allelic loss, thus indicating the possibility of harboring a tumor-suppressor gene important in gastric tumorigenesis. The exact target(s) of loss or gain in most of these chromosomal regions, including 4q, 5q, 9p, 17p, 18q, and 20q, remains to be clarified. Additionally, evidence of Epstein-Barr virus infection can be found in a minority of gastric cancer patients.**

4. **Multiple somatic alterations have been described in gastric carcinomas at the molecular level. The significance of these changes in gastric tumorigenesis remains to be established in most instances. The *p53* gene is consistently altered in a majority of gastric cancer cases. Microsatellite instability and associated alterations of the transforming growth factor βII receptor, *IGFRII*, *BAX*, *E2F-4*, *MSH3*, and *MSH6* genes are found in a subset of gastric carcinomas. Cell adhesion abnormalities such as E-cadherin or associated molecule alterations may play an important role in diffuse-type gastric cancer development. A detailed, clear working model of gastric tumorigenesis has yet to be formulated. Thus improved diagnostic, prognostic, therapeutic, and preventive strategies are eagerly awaited for gastric carcinomas. Critical molecular alterations that are** prevalent in these cancers, once fully characterized, ultimately may provide new avenues to combat this lethal disease.

CLINICAL ASPECTS

Gastric adenocarcinoma is the predominant cancer of the stomach, accounting for over 95 percent of cases. Lymphomas, leiomyosarcomas, and carcinoid lesions represent only a minority of stomach tumors. Once the leading cause of cancer deaths in the United States, the incidence of gastric cancer in developed countries has declined dramatically.[1] Adenocarcinomas of the gastroesophageal junction that commonly arise from Barrett's esophagus, on the other hand, appear to be on the rise most recently in several populations for unclear reasons.[2,3] Adenocarcinoma of the stomach remains a leading cause of cancer death worldwide and continues to be responsible for the majority of cancer deaths in developing countries.[4,5]

Most cases of gastric cancer appear to occur sporadically without an obvious inherited component. It is estimated that up to 10 percent of gastric cancer cases are related to a familial component. Familial clustering has been observed in 12 to 25 percent of cases.[6] Case-control studies suggest a small but consistent increased risk of gastric cancer in first-degree relatives of patients with gastric adenocarcinoma.[7–9]

A well-characterized inherited predisposition syndrome potentially involving gastric cancer development is hereditary nonpolyposis colon cancer (HNPCC), which includes potential tumor development in a variety of tissue types.[10] Germ-line genetic abnormalities of mismatch repair genes underlying this disease entity have been unveiled recently, as discussed in Chap. 18. The isolation of these genes should allow better definition of the fraction of gastric cancers that result from this inherited cancer predisposition trait. Interestingly, fewer gastric cancers have been noted to be associated with HNPCC, correlating with the recent general decline in incidence of gastric cancer in developed countries.

Rare kindreds exhibiting site-specific gastric cancer predilection have been reported, occasionally associated with other inherited abnormalities.[11–13] Notably, Napoleon Bonaparte's family was afflicted with this cancer. A few kindreds manifesting a diffuse, poorly differentiated gastric cancer predisposition trait have been shown recently to harbor E-cadherin alterations in their germ line that cosegregate with these cancers.[14] There has even been a report of gastric carcinoma in an extended Li-Fraumeni kindred.[15]

Epidemiology

Significant geographic variability in incidence both internationally and intranationally is observed. In the early 1990s, incidence rates varied from 60.1 per 100,000 in Costa Rica to 7.3 per 100,000 in the United States.[16] Epidemiologic studies that include migration and temporal analyses indicate that environmental factors, especially in the first decades of life, are important in the etiology of gastric cancers.[17,18] Notably, a consistent predominance of gastric cancers in males (approximately 2:1 ratio) is seen across worldwide populations.

A list of standard abbreviations is located immediately preceding the index. Nonstandard abbreviations used in this chapter include: HNPCC = hereditary nonpolyposis colon cancer; LOH = loss of heterozygosity.

Helicobacter pylori infection has been implicated recently as an etiologic factor in gastric cancer development, both adenocarcinoma and primary non-Hodgkin lymphoma.[19–21] Evidence continues to accumulate that this infection, especially when contracted early in life, as commonly occurs in developing countries, leads to chronic gastric inflammation with subsequent fivefold to sixfold risk of gastric cancer development.[22] This risk of cancer development in infected persons depends on as yet unidentified cofactors, and its pathophysiological mechanism remains to be elucidated. Similarly, chronic gastritis and resulting atrophy from pernicious anemia appear to be associated with an increased risk, albeit small, of gastric cancer development.[23]

Evidence of Epstein-Barr virus (EBV) infection has been demonstrated in a small proportion (approximately 10 percent) of gastric carcinomas by *in situ* hybridization with specific RNA probes.[24–27] The monoclonal nature of EBV genomes in virtually all neoplastic cells of these tumors along with significant prior antibody levels suggests that infection by this virus may not be so latent. The classic proteins associated with cell transformation of EBV infection, LMP1 and EBNA2, do not appear to be expressed in these gastric cancers; however, EBNA1 was shown to be expressed in most virus-associated tumor cells.[27,28] A significant lymphoid infiltration and tendency toward prolonged survival have been observed in gastric cancers harboring detectable EBV. Further studies are needed to determine the role of this infection in human gastric tumorgenesis.

Dietary irritants (i.e., salts or preservatives) and potential carcinogens (i.e., nitrates) have been suggested as etiologic factors of gastric cancer,[29] yet no specific agent has been indicted definitively. Additionally, several protective factors such as fruits, vegetables, ascorbic acid, α-tocopherol, onions, and gastric acidity have been indicated, yet the precise agents responsible for a specific action remain elusive. Molecular studies may help clarify these issues.

Pathology

Gastric adenocarcinomas display several distinct morphologic, histologic, and biologic characteristics. Thus multiple tumor classification systems have been created to characterize these lesions pathologically in attempts to confer their natural history. Lauren described histopathologic subtypes of gastric adenocarcinomas as intestinal type (expansive or gland-forming) or diffuse type (infiltrative or scattered neoplastic cells), and this classification is widely applied.[30] Evidence continues to accumulate suggesting that these two subtypes of gastric cancer arise in different settings and have distinctive biologic behavior.[31] Intestinal-type gastric adenocarcinomas tend to predominante in high-risk geographic regions, arise in association with precursor lesions (i.e., chronic atrophic gastritis or intestinal metaplasia), and occur more distally and later in life (usually after the sixth decade of life), whereas diffuse-type gastric cancers appear to have a relatively constant incidence, arise without identifiable precursor lesions, and present earlier in life and more diffusely in the stomach. Additionally, intestinal-type gastric cancers tend to spread hematogenously to the liver, whereas diffuse-type gastric cancers tend to spread more contiguously into the peritoneum. Moreover, although some molecular alterations are shared, distinct genetic abnormalities appear to occur with specific biologic phenotypes (see below).

Additional histologic classifications for gastric carcinoma have been developed (i.e., World Health Organization[32] and Ming[33]) that involve tissue architecture and differentiation criteria. The traditional classification of Borman is based on morphologic criteria.[34] Goeski has even developed criteria that examine mucin content and degree of cellular atypia as potentially distinctive prognostic features of gastric tumors.[35,36]

The TMN staging classification[37] is used primarily in staging cancers at diagnosis to assess resectability and prognoses. The primary tumor's depth is one of the most important parameters in this determination. The concept of early gastric adenocarcinomas[35] (tumors confined to the mucosa or submucosa) originated in Japan,[38] and patients are observed to have much better 5-year survival rates (over 90 percent) versus more advanced lesions (less than 20 percent for stage III or IV). Unfortunately, most cases of gastric cancer are diagnosed in more advanced stages, for which effective systemic therapy is limited and surgery reserved for palliation. Mass screening programs in high-risk regions such as Japan have helped in diagnosing some of these cancers at earlier stages, but significant improvements in diagnosis, prognostication, and therapy are eagerly awaited to make a substantial impact on this cancer's mortality.

ALTERED GENETIC LOCI

Large kindreds with an obvious highly penetrant inherited predisposition for the development of gastric cancer, having the potential power to link disease markers, are rare. Three Maroi kindreds with significant occurrence of diffuse gastric carcinomas were identified and found to have underlying germ-line E-cadherin mutations that cosegregated with disease.[14] HNPCC with underlying mismatch repair gene alterations is the only other well-defined inherited trait with germ-line mutations known to predispose to gastric cancer development. Of note, the blood group A phenotype was reported to be associated with gastric cancers[39,40] and the blood group O phenotype with gastric ulcers.[41] Interestingly, *H. pylori* was shown to adhere to the Lewis[b] blood group antigen and may be an important host factor that facilitates this chronic infection and subsequent risk of gastric cancer development.[42] Further studies are awaited to clarify this or any other host factor with genetic determinants that might predispose toward the development of gastric cancer.

Most molecular analyses of this cancer have involved studies of sporadic tumors for critical, acquired alterations. Cytogenetic studies of gastric adenocarcinomas are few in number and have failed to identify any consistent or noteworthy chromosomal abnormalities. A variable number of numerical or structural aberrations have been reported in gastric cancer cells, including those involving chromosomes 3 (rearrangements), 6 (deletion distal to 6q21), 8 (trisomy), 11 (11p13-p15 aberrations), and 13 (monosomy and translocations).[43–46] Alone, these findings are not compelling for a specific role in gastric tumorigenesis and may represent only nonspecific changes accompanying transformation.

Comparative genomic hybridization (CGH) analyses of xenografted and primary gastric and gastroesophageal junctional adenocarcinomas have revealed several regions of consensus change in DNA copy number.[47,48] Chromosomal arms 4q, 5q, 9p, 17p, and 18q showed frequent decreases in DNA copy number. On the other hand, chromosomes 7, 8, and 20q showed frequent increases in DNA copy number of cases analyzed in this fashion.

Loss of heterozygosity (LOH) analyses have identified several arms and regions of chromosomes that may contain tumor-suppressor genes important in gastric tumorigenesis. Genetic loci observed to be significantly lost in gastric tumors include those located on the following chromosomal arms: 17p (over 60 percent at the *p53* locus),[49] 18q (over 60 percent at the *DCC* locus),[50] and 5q (30 to 40 percent at or near the *APC* locus).[49,51,52] Less frequent but significant allelic losses have been reported on chromosome arms 1p, 1q, 7q, and 13q.[53] A 13-cM region between D1S201 and D1S197 on chromosome 1p commonly lost in gastric cancers has been delineated, but the critical target remains to be identified.[54] Moreover, a locus on 7q (D7S95) has been associated with peritoneal metastasis when lost.[55] Known, as well as candidate, tumor-suppressor genes have been isolated in some of these frequently lost regions, as described below, but the actual targets of genetic loss that provide gastric neoplastic cells with additional survival or growth advantages for clonal expansion remain to be clarified for many of these loci.

SPECIFIC MOLECULAR ALTERATIONS

The *p53* gene has been demonstrated consistently to be significantly altered in gastric adenocarcinomas. Allelic loss occurs in over 60 percent of patients, and mutations are identified in approximately 30 to 50 percent of patients depending on the mutational screening method employed [i.e., single-stranded conformational polymorphism (SSCP) assay or degenerative gradient gel electrophoresis assay] and sample sizes.[56] Some mutations of *p53* have even been identified in early dysplastic and apparent intestinal metaplasia gastric lesions. In general, however, alterations of this gene occur more frequently in the advanced stages of dysplasia in both histopathologic subtypes. The spectrum of mutations in this gene within gastric tumors appears similar to that which occurs in other cancers with a predominance of base transitions, especially at CpG dinucleotides. Inactivation of this important cell cycle regulator appears to confer a growth advantage and allow clonal expansion of transformed cells. Many studies have used immunohistochemical analysis of tumors in an effort to detect excessive expression of p53 as an indirect means to identify mutations of this gene, but this assay does not appear to have consistent prognostic value in patients with gastric cancers.[57,58]

Microsatellite instability has been found in a significant portion of sporadic gastric carcinomas.[59–61] Variability in classification of instability or histopathologic subtype and number of loci examined in studies account for some variation of this phenotype's frequency, with a trend toward more frequent occurrence in intestinal-type cancers at more advanced stages observed, although noted in early lesions as well (i.e., adenomas). The degree of genome-wide instability also varies, with more severe instability (e.g., >2 abnormal loci) associated with subcardial intestinal or atypical types. A negative association with p53 alterations also has been suggested, indicating different paths of alterations accumulating in individual gastric tumors. Studies have indicated less frequent lymph node or vessel invasion, prominent lymphoid infiltration, and better prognosis in those gastric cancers which displayed significant microsatellite instability.[59,62,63] However, it remains to be proven if this phenotype is a prognostic marker for improved survival, as suggested in colon cancers. The alterations responsible for producing this phenotype in a subset of sporadic gastric cancers remain to be elucidated.

At least one important target of the instability in those cancers displaying abnormally sized microsatellites appears to be the transforming growth factor beta (TGF-β) type II receptor. A study of gastric cancers displaying the microsatellite instability phenotype revealed that a majority (5 of 7) contained mutated TGF-β type II receptors at a polyadenine tract within its gene.[64] Moreover, altered TGF-β type II receptor genes could be found in gastric cancers not displaying microsatellite instability. Several gastric cancer cell lines resistant to the growth inhibitory and apoptotic effects of TGF-β were shown to have altered TGF-β type II genes (deletions and amplifications) and transcripts (truncated or absent).[65] Thus TGF-β type II receptor mutation appears to be a critical event in the development of at least a subset of gastric cancers, allowing escape from the growth control of TGF-β. Additional genes with simple tandom repeat sequences within their coding regions found to be altered in gastric cancers displaying microsatellite instability include *BAX, IGFRII, hMSH3, hMSH6,* and *E2F-4.*[66–68]

As mentioned earlier, E-cadherin germ-line mutations have been found in several large kindreds exhibiting a strong predisposition to diffuse gastric cancer development. Several sporadic gastric cancers also have displayed altered E-cadherin, mainly in diffuse cases. Reduced E-cadherin expression determined by immunohistochemical analysis was noted often (92 percent of 60 patients) in gastric carcinomas and observed to be significantly associated with diffuse-type cancers and more undifferentiated neoplastic cells (i.e., signet ring cells).[69] Genetic abnormalities of the E-cadherin gene (located on chromosome 16q22.1) and

transcripts also have been demonstrated in diffuse gastric cancers.[70] Half of 26 diffuse gastric carcinomas had abnormal E-cadherin transcripts detected by reverse transcription PCR (RT-PCR) analysis that were not seen in noncancerous tissue from the same patients. Moreover, a study of 10 gastric cancer cell lines displaying loose intercellular adhesion found absent E-cadherin transcripts in four lines and insertions or deletions in two other lines.[71] Splice-site alterations producing exon deletion and skipping, large deletions including allelic loss, and point mutations of the E-cadherin gene were all demonstrated in these diffuse-type cancers, some even exhibiting alterations in both alleles. In comparison of RT-PCR products from normal tissue and tumor tissue from patients, allelic expression imbalance of E-cadherin also has been shown in a porportion (42 percent of 35 informative cases) of gastric carcinomas.[72] E-cadherin is a transmembrane, calcium-ion-dependent adhesion molecule (important in epithelial cell homotypic interactions) that, when decreased in expression, is associated with invasive properties.[73] Additionally, α-catenin, which binds to the intracellular domain of E-cadherin and links it to actin-based cytoskeletal elements, was noted to have reduced immunohistochemical expression in 70 percent of 60 gastric carcinomas and correlated with infiltrated growth and poor differentiation.[74]

LOH studies suggest that chromosome 5q harbors at least one tumor-suppressor gene important in the development of gastric cancers.[49,51,52,75,76] The exact target(s), however, of this loss in gastric tumors is not fully clarified. Several somatic *APC* mutations, mostly missense in nature and of relatively low frequency, have been reported in Japanese patients with gastric adenocarcinomas and adenomas using ribonuclease protection or SSCP assays for partial screening.[77] On the other hand, several other reports including Japanese patients have not identified significant *APC* mutations in gastric carcinomas on similar partial screening analysis of the commonly mutated region and include direct nucleotide sequencing and the sensitive in vitro synthesis protein assay.[76,78–80] Interestingly, an increased risk of gastric cancer associated with familial adenomatous polyposis (patients with germ-line *APC* mutations) has been reported in high-risk regions such as Asia,[81,82] whereas no increased risk was exhibited in other populations.[83,84] Significant allelic loss (30 percent) at the *APC* locus suggests the existence of a tumor-suppressor gene important in gastric tumorigenesis nearby. Indeed, alternative loci have been mapped to commonly deleted regions in gastric cancers (the interferon regulatory factor 1 loci and D5S428)[75] and esophageal cancers (5q31.1).[85] Thus future studies should help define the important gene(s) on chromosome 5q, which is critically involved in gastric tumorigenesis.

The targets of loss on other chromosomes implicated to harbor important tumor-suppressor gene(s) in gastric cancer also remain to be defined. Significant allelic loss (60 percent) has been noted at the *DCC* locus on chromosome 18q in gastric cancers.[50] Only one of 35 gastric cancers contained an intragenic mutation of *Smad4* along with allelic loss, suggesting that this *MADD* homologue gene is infrequently altered in gastric tumorigenesis.[86]

Evidence of a tumor-suppressor loci on chromosome 3p has accumulated from a variety of studies, including allelic loss in primary gastric tumors (46 percent) and homozygous deletion in a gastric cancer cell line (KATO III).[87] A candidate tumor-suppressor gene, *FHIT*, recently isolated from the FRA3B site at 3p14.2, was reported to have abnormal transcripts of deleted exons in 5 of 9 gastric cancers in addition to transcript abnormalities noted in esophagus, colon, lung, and head and neck cancers as well.[88–90] One somatic missense mutation was identified in exon 6 of the *FHIT* gene during a coding region analysis of 40 gastric carcinomas.[91] Significant abnormalities of the *FHIT* gene were not observed in a study of 31 colorectal cancer patients.[92] Addtional studies should help clarify the role *FHIT* plays in gastric tumorigenesis.

The *c-met* gene encodes a tyrosine kinase receptor for the hepatocyte growth factor. Amplification of the *c-met* gene was reported to be associated with scirrhous-type gastric cancers.[93] Northern blot analyses of gastric cancer cell lines and resected primary carcinomas compared with paired nonneoplastic tissue showed overexpression of a 7.0-kb transcript of the *c-met* gene in 48 percent of 31 cancers, predominantly of the well-differentiated type.[94] Moreover, a 6.0-kb *c-met* transcript appeared to be preferentially expressed in scirrhous gastric tumor cells and correlated with latter stages of tumor development. Tumor and stromal cell interactions have been implicated with this growth factor and receptor signal system as well as involvement of multiple others, including epidermal growth factor (which is expressed in approximately one-quarter of gastric cancers), transforming growth factor alpha (TGF-α), interleukin-1a, criptor, amphiregulin, platelet-derived growth factor, K-sam, and others.[53,95] Telomerase activity has been detected by a PCR-based assay frequently in the late stages of gastric tumors (85 percent of 66 patients) and is associated with a poor prognosis.[96] The expression of telomerase, a ribonucleoprotein DNA polymerase, and stabilization of telomeres have been noted to be concomitant with immortalization in tumor cells.[97] Specific alterations and the true prevalence of significant changes in these genes or gene products in gastric tumors remain to be characterized.

Another potential marker of poor prognosis is overexpression of *c-erbB-2*, a transmembrane tyrosine kinase receptor proto-oncogene. Amplification of *c-erbB-2* has been demonstrated in a small subset of gastric cancers, approximately 10 percent.[98] Several reports have shown amplification or increased expression of erbB-2 immunohistochemically in gastric tumors to be associated with a worse prognosis.[99] Furthermore, enhanced expression of erbB-2 recently has been demonstrated to occur more frequently in gastric cancers displaying microsatellite instability.[100] The specific genetic or epigenetic alterations underlying these immunohistochemical findings remain to be characterized.

A number of other alterations have been reported in gastric carcinomas that remain to be defined, as well as the role they play in gastric tumorigenesis. Several splice variants of a transmembrane glycoprotein, CD44, seem to be preferentially expressed in gastric tumors cells.[101] Membrane-type matrix metalloproteinase was expressed preferentially in some gastric cancer cells with colocalization and activation of the zymogen proMMP-2.[102] Both loss and overexpression of Bc1-2 and nm23 have been reported in several gastric cancers, making their role unclear. Amplification of cyclin E and increased plasminogen activation have been reported as well in several gastric tumors.[103] A somatic mitochondrial deletion of 50 bp was even demonstrated in four gastric adenocarcinomas.[104]

Activation of the oncogene *K-ras* appears to be rare in gastric tumorigenesis.[79,105,106] Although allelic loss was noted in 18 percent gastric tumors at the locus for p16 on chromosome 9p, no inactivating somatic mutations were detected in over 70 patients screened by PCR-SSCP analysis.[107] No methylation abnormalities or genetic alterations of cycle regulators such as p16, p21, or p27 have as yet been reported.

IMPLICATIONS

Identification of important genetic alterations in gastric tumorigenesis has important practical as well as biologic implications. As evident from molecular genetic characterization of colorectal tumor development, genetic markers with potential clinical utility in diagnosis, prognosis, and therapeutic guidance can be discovered. A clear molecular working model of gastric tumorigenesis has yet to be delineated, but as genetic alterations are better characterized in these cancers, critical changes may emerge to provide new opportunities of earlier diagnosis, improved prognostication, and more rational design of therapeutic agents and preventive strategies. Since most gastric cancers are diagnosed in late stages of development with concomitant poor prognosis and little chance of cure, genetic changes occurring early and

frequently may enable identification of truly premalignant gastric lesions that would be beneficial to remove or warrant intervention in some manner. Directed screening efforts for this cancer are a pressing issue, and molecular markers may help address this important matter.

Characterization of somatic changes in these gastric tumors also may expose specific environmental factors (e.g., fingerprints[108]) and strongly indict agents for further mechanistic studies. Additionally, identification of a genetic predisposition marker for the development of gastric cancer may facilitate more effective preventive and screening programs. Identifying critical molecular alterations and defining the role played in gastric tumorigenesis also may provide unique opportunities for improved chemopreventive or chemotherapeutic agents to be developed and given at more opportune times.

Finally, since gastric cancer appears to be a rather heterogeneous disease biologically and genetically, characterization of the various pathways and events along the way should afford multiple opportunities to design more specific and therefore more effective therapies in the treatment of this tumor. For example, antibodies to the oncoprotein erbB-2 and epidermal growth factor receptor have shown promise in inhibiting growth of gastric cancer cell lines and xenografts.[95,109] Moreover, current systemic therapies are generally ineffective in controlling gastric cancer growth. Opportunities to explore whether a genetic marker's status such as p53 in these tumors will guide more effective therapy are welcomed. Improved prognostic markers are also eagerly awaited to help guide more aggressive surgical or systemic therapies (i.e., chemotherapy and/or radiotherapy) and ultimately may be derived from the molecular alterations indicated earlier or from as yet unidentified critical change in gastric cancer cells.

ACKNOWLEDGMENTS

This work was supported in part by NIH Grant CA67900-01 and a Foundation AGA Research Scholarship award.

REFERENCES

1. Correa P, Chen V: Gastric cancer. *Cancer Surv* **19/20**:55, 1994.
2. Blot WJ, Devesa SS, Kneller RW: Rising incidence of adenocarcinoma of the esophagus and gastric cardia. *JAMA* **265**:1287, 1991.
3. Locke RG, Talley NJ, Carpenter HA, Harmsen WS, Zinsmeister AR, Melton LJ: Changes in the site- and histology-specific incidence of gastric cancer during a 50-year period. *Gastroenterology* **109**:1750, 1995.
4. Parkin DM, Pisani P, Ferlay J: Estimates of the worldwide incidence of eighteen major cancers in 1985. *Int J Cancer* **54**:594, 1993.
5. Boffetta P, Parkin DM: Cancer in developing countries. *CA* **44**:81, 1994.
6. Goldgar DE, Easton DF, Cannon-Albright LA, Skolnock MH: Systematic population-based assessment of cancer risk in first-degree relatives of cancer probands. *J Natl Cancer Inst* **86**:1600, 1994.
7. La Vecchia C, Negri E, Franceschi S, Gentile A: Family history and the risk of stomach and colorectal cancer. *Cancer* **70**:50, 1992.
8. Zangheiri G, Di Gregorio C, Sacchetti R, et al: Familial occurrence of gastric cancer in the 2-year experience of a population-based registry. *Cancer* **66**:2047, 1990.
9. Graham S, Lilienfeld AM: Genetic studies of gastric cancer in humans: An appraisal. *Cancer* **11**:957, 1958.
10. Lynch HT, Smyrk TC, Watson P, Lanspa SJ, Lynch JF, Lynch PM, Cavalieri RJ, Boland CR: Genetics, natural history, tumor spectrum, and pathology of hereditary nonpolyposis colorectal cancer. *Gastroenterology* **104**:1535, 1993.
11. Maimon SN, Zinninger MM: An analysis of 5 stomach cancer families in the state of Utah. *Cancer* **14**:1005, 1953.
12. Woolf CM, Isaacson EA: An analysis of 5 stomach cancer families in the state of Utah. *Cancer* **1961**:1005, 1961.
13. Triantafillidis JK, Kosmidis P, Kottardis S: Genetic studies of gastric cancer in humans: An appraisal. *Cancer* **11**:957, 1958.
14. Guilford P, Hopkins J, Harraway J, McLeod M, McLeod N, Harawira P, Taite H: E-cadherin germline mutations in familial gastric cancer. *Nature* **392**:402–405, 1998.

15. Varley JM: An extended Li-Fraumeni kindred with gastric carcinoma and a codon 175 mutation of *TP53. J Med Genet* **32**:942–945, 1995.

16. Parker SL, Tong T, Bolden S, Wingo PA: Cancer statistics. *CA* **46**(1):5, 1996.

17. Haenszel W, Kurihara M, Segi M, Lee RK: Stomach cancer among Japanese in Hawaii. *J Natl Cancer Inst* **49**:969, 1972.

18. Correa P, Haenszel W: Epidemiology of gastric cancer, in Correa P, Haenszel W (eds): *Epidemiology of Cancer of the Digestive Tract*. The Hague, The Netherlands: Martinus Hijhoff, 1972, p 58.

19. Parsonnet J, Hansen S, Rodriguez L, Gelb AB, Warnke RA, Jellum E, Orentreich N, Vogelman JH, Friedman GD: *Helicobacter pylori* infection and gastric lymphoma. *New Engl J Med* **330**:1267, 1994.

20. Parsonnet J, Friedman GD, Vandersteen DP, Chang Y, Vogelman JH, Orenreich N, Sibley RK: *Helicobacter pylori* infection and the risk of gastric carcinoma. *N Engl J Med* **325**:1127, 1991.

21. Nomura A, Stemmerman GN, P-HC, Kato I, Perez-Perez GI, Blaser MJ: *Helicobacter pylori* infection and gastric carcinoma among Japanese Americans in Hawaii. *N Engl J Med* **325**:1132, 1991.

22. Blaser MJ, Chyou PH, Nomura A: Age at establishment of *Helicobacter pylori* infection and gastric carcinoma, gastric ulcer, and duodenal ulcer risk. *Cancer Res* **55**:562, 1995.

23. Elsborg L, Mosbech J: Pernicious anaemia as a risk factor in gastric cancer. *Acta Med Scand* **206**:315, 1979.

24. Rowlands DC, Ito M, Mangham DC, Reynolds G, Herlost H, Fielding JWL, Newbold KM, Jones EL, Young LS, Niedobitek G: Epstein-Barr virus and carcinomas: Rare association of the virus with gastric adenocarcinomas. *Br J Cancer* **68**:1014, 1993.

25. Shibata D, Weiss LM: Epstein-Barr virus-associated gastric adeno-carcinoma. *Am J Pathol* **140**:769, 1992.

26. Imai S, Koizumi S, Sugiura M, Toyunaga M, Uemura Y, Yanamoto N, Tanaka S, Sato E, Osato T: Gastric carcinoma: Monoclonal epithelial malignant cells expressing Epstein-Barr virus latent infection protein. *Proc Natl Acad Sci USA* **91**:9131, 1994.

27. Gulley ML, Pulitzer DR, Eagan PA, Schneider BG: Epstein-barr virus infection is an early event in gastric carcinogenesis and is independent of bcl-2 expression and p53 accumulation. *Hum Pathol* **27**(1):19, 1996.

28. Murray PG, Nieddobitek G, Kremmer E, Grasser F, Reynolds GM, Cruchley A, Williams DM, Muller-Lantzsh N, Young LS: *In situ* detection of the Epstein-Barr virus-encoded nuclear antigen 1 in oral hairy leukoplakia and virus-associated carcinomas. *J Pathol* **178**:44, 1996.

29. Fuchs CS, Mayer RJ: Gastric carcinoma. *N Engl J Med* **333**(1):32, 1995.

30. Lauren P: The two histological main types of gastric carcinoma: Diffuse and so-called intestinal-type carcinoma. *Acta Pathol Microbiol Scand* **64**:31, 1965.

31. Correa P, Shiao YH: Phenotypic and genotypic events in gastric carcinogenesis. *Cancer Res* **54**:1941, 1994.

32. Oota K, Sobin LH: Histological typing: Gastric and esophageal carcinogenesis, in *International Histological Classification of Tumors*. Geneva, World Health Organization, 1977.

33. Ming S-C: Gastric carcinoma: A pathobiological classification. *Cancer* **39**:2475, 1977.

34. Borrmann R: Gushwulste de magens and duodenums, in Henke F, Lubarsh O (eds): *Handbuch der Speziellen Pathologischen Anatomie und Histologie*. Berlin, Springer, 1926, p 865.

35. Dixon MF, Martin JG, Sue-Ling HM, Wyatt JI, Quirke P, Johnston D: Goseki grading in gastric cancer: Comparison with existing systems of grading and its reproducibility. *Histopathology* **25**:309, 1994.

36. Goseki N, Takizawa T, Koike M: Differences in the mode of extension of gastric cancer classified by histological type: New histological classification of gastric carcinoma. *Gut* **33**:606, 1992.

37. Sobin LH, Wittekind Ch (eds): *International Union Against Cancer (UICC): TNM Classification of Malignant Tumors* 5th ed. New York: John Wiley, 1997

38. Hirota T, Ming S-C, Itabashi M: *Pathology of early gastric cancer*, in *Gastric Cancer*, in Nishi M, Ichikawa, H, Nakajima T, Maruyama K, Tahara E (eds): Tokyo, New York, Springer-Verlag p. 66–86.

39. Aird I, Bentall H: A relationship between cancer of stomach and ABO groups. *Br J Med* **1**:799, 1953.

40. Haenszel W, Kurihara M, Locke F, Shimuzu K, Segi M: Stomach cancer in Japan. *J Natl Cancer Inst* **56**:265, 1976.

41. Clarke CA, Cowan WK, Edwards JW, Howel-Evans AW, McConnell RB, Woodrow JC, Sheppard PM: The relation of ABO bloodgroups to duodenal and gastric ulceration. *Br Med J* **4940**:643, 1955.

42. Boren T, Per F, Roth KA, Larson G, Normark S: Attachment of *Helicobacter pylori* to human gastric epithelium mediated by blood group antigens. *Science* **262**:1892, 1993.

43. Seruca R, Castedo S, Correia C, Gomes P, Carneiro F: Cytogenetic findings in eleven gastric carcinomas. *Cancer Genet Cytogenet* **68**:42–48, 1993.

44. Rodriguez E, Ladanyi M, Altorki N, Albino AP, Kelsen DP: 11p13-15 is a specific region of chromosomal rearrangement in gastric esophageal adenocarcinomas. *Cancer Res* **50**:6410–6416, 1990.

45. Ochi H, Douglass H, Sandberg AA: Cytogenetic studies in primary gastric cancer. *Cancer Genet Cytogenet* **22**:295, 1986.

46. Panani AD, Ferti A, Malliaros S, Raptis S: Cytogenetic study of 11 gastric adenocarcinomas. *Cancer Genet Cytogenet* **81**:169, 1995.

47. El-Rifai W, Harper JC, Cummings OW, Hyytinen E, Frierson HF, Knuutila S, Powell SM: Consistent genetic alterations in xenografts of proximal stomach and gastroesophageal junction adenocarcinomas. *Cancer Res* **58**:34, 1998.

48. Moskaluk CA, Hu J, Perlman EJ: Comparative genomic hybridization of esophageal and gastroesophageal adenocarcinomas reveals consensus areas of DNA gain and loss. *Genes Chromosom Cancer* **22**:305, 1998.

49. Sano T, Tsujino T, Yoshida K, Nakayama H, Haruma K, Ito H, Nakamura Y, Kajiyama G, Tahara E: Frequent loss of heterozygosity on chromosomes 1q, 5q and 17q in human gastric carcinomas. *Cancer Res* **51**:2926, 1991.

50. Uchino S, Hitoshi T, Masayuki N, Jun Y, Terada M, Saito T, Kobayashi M, Sugimura T, Hirohashi S: Frequent loss of heterozygosity at the *DCC* locus in gastric cancer. *Cancer Res* **52**:3099, 1992.

51. McKie AB, Filipe I, Lemoine NR: Abnormalities affecting the *APC* and *MCC* tumour suppressor gene loci on chromosome 5q occur frequently in gastric cancer but not in pancreatic cancer. *Int J Cancer* **55**:598, 1993.

52. Rhyu MG, Park WS, Jung YJ, Choi SW, Meltzer SJ: Allelic deletions of *MCC, APC* and *p53* are frequent late events in human gastric carcinogenesis. *Gastroenterology* **106**:1584, 1994.

53. Tahara E, Semba S, Tahara H: Molecular biological observations in gastric cancer. *Semin Oncol* **23**(3):307, 1996.

54. Ezaki T, Yanagisawa A, Ohta K, Aiso S, Watanabe M, Hibi T, Kato Y, Nakajima T, Ariyama T, Inzawa J, Nakamura Y, Horii A: Deletion mapping chromosome 1p in well-differentiated gastric cancer. *Br J Cancer* **73**:424, 1996.

55. Kuniyasu H, Yasui W, Yokosaki H: Frequent loss of heterozygosity of the long arm of chromosome 7 is often associated with progression of human gastric carcinoma. *Cancer* **59**:597, 1994.

56. Beroud C, Soussi T: *p53* and *APC* gene mutations: Software and databases. *Nucl Acids Res* **25**(1):138, 1997.

57. Gabber HE, Muller W, Schneiders A, Meier S, Hommel G: The relationship of p53 expression to the prognosis of 418 patients with gastric carcinoma. *Cancer* **76**(5):720, 1995.

58. Hurlimann J, Saraga EP: Expression of p53 protein in gastric carcinomas. *Am J Surg Pathol* **18**(12):1247, 1994.

59. Seruca R, Santos NR, David L, Constancia M, Barroca H, Carneiro F, Seixas M, Peltomaki R, Lothe R, Sobrinho-Simoes M: Sporadic gastric carcinomas with microsatellite instability display a particular clinicopathologic profile. *Int J Cancer* **64**(1):32–6, 1995.

60. Strickler JG, Zheng J, Shu Q, Burgart LJ, Alberts SR, Shibata D: *p53* mutations and microsatellite instability in sporadic gastric cancer: When guardians fail. *Cancer Res* **54**:4750, 1994.

61. Chong J-M, Fukayama M, Hayashi Y, Takizawa T, Koike M, Konishi M, Kikuchi-Yanoshita R, Miyaki M: Microsatellite instability in the progression of gastric carcinoma. *Cancer Res* **54**:4595, 1994.

62. Nakashima H, Hiroshi I, Mori M, Ueo H, Ikeda M, Akiyoshi T: Microsatellite instability in Japanese gastric cancer. *Cancer Suppl* **75**(6):1503, 1995.

63. Dos Santos NR, Seruca R, Constancia M, Seixas M, Sobrinho-Simoes M: Microsatellite instability at multiple loci in gastric carcinoma: Clinicopathologic implications and prognosis. *Gastroenterology* **110**:38, 1996.

64. Myeroff LL, Ramon P, Kim S-J, Hedrick L, Cho KR, Orth K, Mathis M, Kinzler K, Lutterbaugh J, Park K, Bang Y-J, Lee HY, Park J-G, Lynch H, Roberts AB, Vogelstein B, Markowitz SD: A transforming growth factor β receptor type II gene mutation common in colon and gastric but rare in endometrial cancers. *Cancer Res* **55**:5545, 1995.

65. Park K, Kim S-J, Bang Y-J, Park J-G, Kim NK, Roberts AB, Sporn MB: Genetic changes in the transforming growth fact beta (TGF-β) type II receptor gene in human gastric cancer cells: Correlation with sensitivity to growth inhibition by TGF-β. *Proc Natl Acad Sci USA* **91**:8772, 1994.

66. Yamamoto H, Sawai H, Perucho M: Frameshift somatic mutations in gastrointestinal cancer of the microsatellite mutator phenotype. *Cancer Res* **57**:4420, 1997.

67. Souza RF, Appel R, Jing Y, Wang S, Smolinski KN, Abraham JM, Zou T, Shi Y, Lei J, Cottrell J, Cymes K, Biden K, Simms L, Leggett B, Lynch PM, Frazier M, Powell SM, Harpaz N, Sugimura H, Young J, Meltzer SJ: Microsatellite instability in the insulin-like growth factor II receptor gene in gastrointestinal tumours. *Nature Genet* **14**:255, 1996.

68. Souza RF, Yin J, Smolinski KN, Zou TT, Wang S, Shi YQ, Ryu MG, Cottrell J, Abraham JM, Biden K, Simms L, Leggett B, Bova GS, Frank T, Powell SM, Sugimura H, Young J, Harpaz N, Shimizu K, Matsuvara N, Melzer SJ: Frequent mutations of the E2F-4 cell cycle gene in primary human gastrointestinal tumors. *Cancer Res* **57**:2350, 1997.

69. Mayer B, Johnson JP, Leitl F, Jauch KW, Heiss MM, Schildberg FW, Birchmeier W, Funke I: E-cadherin expression in primary and metastatic gastric cancer: Down-regulation correlates with cellular dedifferentiation and glandular disintegration. *Cancer Res* **53**:1690, 1993.

70. Becker KF, Atkinson MJ, Reich U, Becker I, Nekarda H, Siewart JR, Hofler H: E-cadherin gene mutations provide clues to diffuse type gastric carcinomas. *Cancer Res* **54**:3845, 1994.

71. Oda T, Kanai Y, Oyama T, Yoshiura K, Shimoyama Y, Birchmeier W, Sugimura T: E-cadherin gene mutations in human gastric carcinoma cell lines. *Proc Natl Acad Sci USA* **91**:1858, 1994.

72. Becker KF, Hofler H: Frequent somatic allelic inactivation of the E-cadherin gene in gastric carcinomas. *J Natl Cancer Inst* **87**(14):1082, 1995.

73. Birchmeier W, Behrens J: Cadherin expression in carcinomas: Role in the formation of cell junctions and the prevention of invasiveness. *Biochem Biophys Acta* **1198**:11, 1994.

74. Matsui S, Shiozaki H, Masatoshi I, Shigeyuke T, Doki Y, Kadowaki T, Iwazawa T, Shimaya K, Nagafuchi A, Tsukita S, Mori T: Immuno-histochemical evaluation of α-catenin expression in human gastric cancer. *Virchov Archov* **424**:375–381, 1997.

75. Tamura G, Ogasawara S, Nishizuka S, Sakata K, Maesawa C, Suzuki Y, Tershima N, Saito K, Satodate R: Two distinct regions of deletion on the long arm of chromosome 5 in differentiated adenocarcinomas of the stomach. *Cancer Res* **56**:612, 1996.

76. Powell SM, Cummings OW, Mullen JA, Asghar A, Fuga G, Piva P, Minacci C, Megha T, Piero T, Jackson CE: Characterization of the *APC* gene in sporadic gastric adenocarcinomas. *Oncogene* **12**:1953, 1996.

77. Nagase H, Nakamura Y: Mutation of the *APC* (adenomatous polyposis coli) gene. *Hum Mutat* **2**:425, 1993.

78. Ogaswarara S, Maesawa C, Tamura G, Satodate R: Lack of mutations of the adenomatous polyposis coli gene in oesophageal and gastric carcinomas. *Virchows Arch* **424**(6):607, 1994.

79. Maesawa C, Tamura G, Suzuki Y, Ogasawara S, Sakata K, Kashiwaba M, Satodate R: The sequential accumulation of genetic alterations characteristic of the colorectal adenoma-carcinoma sequence does not occur between gastric adenoma and adenocarcinoma. *J Pathol* **176**:249, 1995.

80. Sud R, Talbot IC, Delhanty JD: Infrequent alterations of the *APC* and *MCC* genes in gastric cancers from British patients. *Oncogene* **21**:1104, 1996.

81. Utsunomiya J: The concept of hereditary colorectal cancer and the implications of its study, in Utsunomiya J, Lynch HT (eds): *Hereditary Colorectal Cancer*. Tokyo, Springer-Verlag, 1990, p 3.

82. Park JG, Park KJ, Ahn YO, Song IS, Choi KW, Moon HY, Choo SY, Kim JP: Risk of gastric cancer among Korean familial adenomatous polyposis patients. *Dis Colon Rectum* **53**:996, 1992.

83. Offerhaus GJA, Giardello FM, Krush AJ, Booker SV, Tersmette AC, Kelley NC, Hamilton SR: The risk of upper gastrointestinal cancer in familial adenomatous polyposis. *Gastroenterology* **102**:1980, 1992.

84. Burt RW: Polyposis syndromes, in Yamada T, Alpers TH (eds): *Textbook of Gastroenterology*. New York, Lippincott, 1991.

85. Ogaswara S, Tamura G, Maesawa C, Suzuki Y, Iishida K, Satoh N, Uesugi N, Saito K, Satodate R: Common deleted region of the long arm of chromosome 5 in esophageal carcinoma. *Gastroenterology* **110**:52, 1996.

86. Powell SM, Harper J, Hamilton S, Robinson C, Cummings OW: Inactivation of *Smad4* in gastric carcinomas. *Cancer Res* **57**:4221, 1997.

87. Kastury K, Baffa R, Druck T, Cotticelli MG, Inoue H, Massimo N, Rugge M, Huang D, Croce CM, Palazzo J, Huebner K: Potential gastrointestinal tumor suppressor locus at the 3p14.2FRA3b site

identified by homozygous deletions in tumor cell lines. *Cancer Res* **56**:978, 1996.

88. Ohta M, Hiroshi I, Citticelli MG, Kastury K: The *FHIT* gene, spanning the chromosome 3p14.2 fragile site and renal carcinoma-associated t(3;8) breakpoint, is abnormal in digestive tract cancers. *Cell* **84**:587, 1996.

89. Sozzi G, Verosnese ML, Negrini M, Baffa R, Cotticelli MG, Enoue H, Tornielli S, Pilotti S, De Gregorio L, Pastorino U, Pierotti MA, Ohta M, Huebner K, Croce CM: The *FHIT* gene at 3p14.2 is abnormal in lung cancer. *Cell* **85**:17, 1996.

90. Virgilio L, Shuster M, Gollin SM, Veronese ML, Ohta M, Huebner K, Croce CM: *FHIT* gene alterations in head and neck squamous cell carcinomas. *Proc Natl Acad Sci USA* **93**:9770, 1996.

91. Gemma A, Hagiwara K, Ke Y, Burke LM, Khan MA, Nagashima M, Bennett WP, Harris CC: *FHIT* mutations in human primary gastric cancer. *Cancer Res* **57**:1435, 1997.

92. Thiagalingam S, Lisitsyn NA, Hamaguchi M, Wigler MH, Willson JKV, Markowitz SD, Leach FS, Kinzler KW, Vogelstein B: Evaluation of *FHIT* gene in colorectal cancers. *Cancer Res* **56**:2936, 1996.

93. Kuniyasu H, Yasui W, Kitadai Y, Yokosaki H, Ito H, Tahara E: Frequent amplification of the *c-met* gene in scirrhous type stomach cancer. *Biochem Biophys Res Commun* **189**:227, 1992.

94. Kuniyasu H, Yasui W, Kitadai Y, Tahar E: Aberrant expression of *c-met* mRNA in human gastric carcinomas. *Int J Cancer* **55**:72, 1993.

95. Tokunaga A, Onda M, Okuda T, Teramoto T, Fijita I, Mizutani T, Kiyama T, Yoshiyuki T, Nishi K, Matsukura N: Clinical significance of epidermal growth factor (EGF), EGF receptor, and c-erbB-2 in human gastric cancer. *Cancer* **75**:1418, 1995.

96. Hiyama E, Yokoyama T, Tatsumato N, Hiyama K, Imamura Y, Murakami Y: Telomerase activity in gastric cancer. *Cancer Res* **55**:3258–3262, 1995.

97. Kim JW, Piatyszek MA, Prowse MA, Harley KR, West CB, Peter LC, Ho GMC, Woodring EN, Weinrich SL, Shay JW: Specific association of human telomerase activity with immortal cells and cancer. *Science* **266**:2011, 1994.

98. Ooi A, Kobayashi M, Mai M, Nakanishi I: Amplification of *c-erbB2* in gastric cancer: Detection in formalin-fixed, paraffin-embedded tissue by fluorescence *in situ* hybridization. *Lab Invest* **78**(3):345, 1997.

99. Mizutani T, Onda M, Tokunaga A, Yamanaka N, Sugisaka Y: Relationship of c-erbB-2 protein expression and gene amplification to invasion and metastasis in human gastric cancer. *Cancer* **72**:2083, 1993.

100. Lin J-T, Wu MS, Shun C-T, Lee W-J, Wang T-H: Occurrence of microsatellite instability in gastric carcinoma is associated with enhanced expression of erbB-2 oncoprotein. *Cancer Res* **55**:1428, 1995.

101. Dammrich J, Vollmers HP, Heider K-H, Muller-Hermelink H-K: Importance of different CD44v6 expression in human gastric intestinal and diffuse type cancers for metastatic lymphogenic spreading. *J Mol Med* **73**:395, 1995.

102. Nomura H, Hiroshi S, Motoharu S, Masyoshi M, Yasunori O: Expression of membrane-type matrix metalloproteinase in human gastric cancer. *Cancer Res* **55**:3263, 1995.

103. Tahara E: Molecular mechanism of stomach carcinogenesis. *J Cancer Res Clin Oncol* **119**:265, 1993.

104. Burgart LJ, Zheng J, Shu Q, Strickler JG, Shibata D: A somatic mitochondrial mutation in gastric cancer. *Am J Pathol* **147**(4):1105, 1995.

105. Kihana T, Tsuda H, Teruyuki H, Shimosato Y, Hiromi S, Terada M, Hirohashi S: Point mutation of *c-Ki-ras* oncogene in gastric adenoma and adenocarcinoma with tubular differentiation. *Jpn J Cancer Res* **82**:308, 1991.

106. Koshiba M, Ogawaa O, Habuchi T, Hamazaki S, Thoshihide S: Infrequent *ras* mutation in human stomach cancers. *Jpn J Cancer Res* **84**:163–167, 1993.

107. Igaki H, Sasaki H, Tachimori Y, Watanabe H, Kimura T, Harada Y, Sugimura T, Tarada M: Mutation frequency of the *p16/CDKN2* gene in primary cancers in the upper digestive tract. *Cancer Res* **55**:3421, 1995.

108. Vogelstein B, Kinzler KW: Carcinogens leave finger prints. *Nature* **355**:209, 1992.

109. Kasprzyk PG, Song SU, Di Fiore PP, King CR: Therapy of an animal model of human gastric cancer using a combination of Anti-erbB-2 monoclonal antibodies. *Cancer Res* **52**:2771, 1992.

Prostate Cancer

William B. Isaacs ■ *G. Steven Bova*

1. **Prostate cancer is the most commonly diagnosed cancer in men. The incidence of this disease shows strong age, race, and geographic dependence, with African Americans and Asians being examples of high- and low-risk populations, respectively.**

2. **Although no hereditary prostate cancer genes have been cloned, familial clustering data and segregation analyses are consistent with the existence of dominant high-risk alleles for prostate cancer. Genome-wide scans for linkage in prostate cancer families have implicated loci on 1q and Xq as harboring prostate cancer-susceptibility genes.**

3. **Deletion of sequences from the short arm of chromosome 8 is perhaps the most frequent chromosomal alteration in prostate cancer, occurring at high frequency even in precursor lesions. Gain of sequences on chromosome 8q and loss of sequences on 13q are only slightly less common than 8p loss of heterozygosity (LOH). Gain and deletion of chromosome 7 sequences, along with deletions of chromosomes 5q, 6q, 10q, and 16q, are also frequent events in the prostate cancer cell genome. The genes driving the apparent selection of these abnormalities are largely unknown.**

4. **Methylation of a CpG island in the promoter of the *GSTP1* gene is the most common genomic alteration yet identified in prostate cancer, occurring in virtually every case. The common inactivation of this carcinogen-defense pathway suggests a potentially important role of environmental carcinogens during prostatic carcinogenesis.**

5. **Although mutations of *p53*, *PTEN*, *Rb*, *ras*, *CDKN2*, and other tumor-suppressors and oncogenes have been detected at varying frequencies in prostate cancer, no single gene has been identified as being mutated in the majority of prostate cancers.**

6. **The androgen receptor gene, when either mutated or amplified, may play a critical role in prostate tumorigenesis both at the early stages and during progression to androgen-insensitive disease. Polymorphic variants of the androgen receptor and other genes involved in androgen metabolism that differ in their biologic activity may modulate risk for prostate cancer or for the tendency to develop more aggressive forms of this disease.**

7. **Prostate cancers vary tremendously in their biologic aggressiveness. The ability of various genetic alterations to serve as much-needed molecular diagnostic and prognostic indicators is being evaluated.**

CLINICAL ASPECTS

Incidence

In 1990, prostate cancer became the most common form of cancer (other than skin cancer) diagnosed in the U.S. male. In 1997, over

200,000 new prostate cancer cases were diagnosed, accounting for over 35 percent of all cancers affecting men, and over 40,000 deaths resulted from this disease.[1] The number of prostate cancers diagnosed in the United States has been increasing since 1972 and in particularly dramatic fashion since 1988. This increase is due primarily to changes in methods used to detect the disease [e.g., the use of serum prostate-specific antigen (PSA)] as well as interest in detecting this disease (increased awareness and screening), coupled with what appears to be an actual but slight increase in the true incidence rate.[2]

The incidence of prostate cancer shows strong age, race, and geographic dependence. It is primarily a disease of older men, with the incidence rate for men over age 65 being 20-fold greater than that for men between 50 and 54 years of age. Less than 1 percent of cases are diagnosed under the age of 40, reaching a peak frequency of approximately 1 in 7 in the eighth and ninth decades of life.[3] This disease is uncommon in Asian populations and common in Scandinavian countries, and the highest incidence (and mortality) rates known are in African-American males, with the latter being twofold higher than for American white males.[4]

The *initiation* of prostate cancer, i.e., the formation of a histologically identifiable lesion, is a very frequent event, occurring in the nearly one-third of men over age 45.[5] Fortunately, the majority of such lesions do not progress to clinically detectable tumors. Interestingly, the rate of histologic cancer incidence is roughly the same worldwide,[6,7] suggesting an important role for environmental factors as potential promoting agents to explain the large regional differences observed in the incidence of clinically detectable disease.[8] In addition to environmental factors, studies of familial aggregation of this disease have suggested that between 5 and 10 percent of prostate cancers may be directly attributable to the inheritance of prostate cancer-susceptibility alleles (see below) that may act as genetic factors driving this progression independent of environmental exposure. Thus, as with numerous other cancers, there is evidence for both genetic and environmental factors in the etiology of prostate cancer, with the majority of disease most likely being a result of interaction of the two.[9]

Prostate cancer develops in two different regions of the gland, with most lesions (~80 percent) being found in the periphery, where more often than not the disease is multifocal. The remainder of cancers are found in a periurethral region, termed the *transition zone*.[10] Curiously, it is the latter region of the prostate in which the virtually ubiquitous process of benign prostatic hyperplasia (BPH) occurs.[11] Based primarily on this regional difference in the incidence of benign and malignant growth and on the fact that stromal cell proliferation is typically a major component of BPH, these benign lesions are not thought to be the precursors of invasive adenocarcinoma in the prostate. Instead, *prostatic intraepithelial neoplasia* (PIN) is the term given to characteristic foci of dysplastic ductal and acinar cells thought to be the precursor lesions of this disease.[12]

Diagnostic Criteria

Previously, the development of symptoms, either due to local disease resulting primarily in voiding dysfunction or due to disseminated disease commonly resulting in bone pain, has been the initial sign of prostatic malignancy, resulting in many men being diagnosed with advanced disease. This situation has changed

---

A list of standard abbreviations is located immediately preceding the index. Nonstandard abbreviations used in this chapter include: PSA = prostate-specific antigen; PIN = prostatic intraepithelial neoplasia; LOH = loss of heterozygosity.

dramatically with the use of PSA as a screening tool, which, when combined with digital rectal examination and transrectal ultrasound, results in a much greater ability to detect prostate cancer while it is still confined to the gland. The use of these latter methods is primarily responsible for the approximately threefold increase in incidence rates observed since 1988,[2] as well as the tremendous decline in the percentage of patients diagnosed annually with disseminated disease.

PSA is a serine protease with a chymotrpysin-like substrate specificity. It is normally secreted by the prostate in large amounts into the seminal plasma.[13] The PSA level in the bloodstream of men is normally below 4 ng/ml, although this varies with age.[14] With prostate pathology, this level can increase, in particularly dramatic fashion in the case of carcinoma. A current focus of intense research effort is on the ability to accurately interpret slightly elevated PSA levels that can be indicative of either benign or malignant disease.[15–17] Serum PSA detection after prostatectomy or other treatment for prostate cancer is a very reliable indication of disease progression.[18]

The histology of normal, cancerous, and benign hyperplastic prostate is illustrated in Fig. 46-1. Prostate cancer is graded based on tissue architectural patterns according to the system proposed by the Gleason.[19] Because of the common morphologic heterogeneity, two different grades are given for the first and second most prevalent patterns, and the sum of these two grades is added to give the Gleason score. Staging is categorized using the TNM (tumor, node, metastasis) classification.[20]

Unique Features of Prostate Carcinoma

Several features tend to distinguish adenocarcinoma of the prostate from other common cancers. The following list is not exhaustive but serves to highlight important questions in prostate cancer biology for which there is little understanding at the molecular level: (1) extreme age dependence of incidence—although the most common malignancy in men, this disease does not appear (at least in a clinically detectable form) at significant rates until the sixth decade of life (incidence of 1 in 2 million below the age of 40[3]); (2) slow growth rate-doubling times measured in years are not uncommon[21] (Does this slow growth rate simply explain the age-dependent incidence of prostate cancer?); (3) sensitivity to androgens—most prostate cancers respond to androgen ablation therapy, although virtually all become insensitive to this treatment; (4) multifocality—the prostate of a man diagnosed with prostate cancer contains an average of five apparently independent lesions[22] (these lesions are genetically heterogeneous, both inter- and intratumorally,[23–25] and this multifocality is independent of family history of prostate cancer[22]); and (5) lack of ability to establish cell lines in vitro from clinical specimens of prostate cancer (after hundreds of attempts by numerous investigators, only a handful of cell lines exist). Recent establishment of a series of useful human prostate cancer xenografts[26–30] has provided an important research alternative.

GENETIC LOCI

Hereditary Prostate Cancer

Although no prostate cancer-susceptibility genes have been cloned, there is substantial evidence that a hereditary form of this disease exists. A positive family history of prostate cancer is one of the strongest risk factors identified for this disease.[31–35] Segregation analyses of familial aggregation patterns suggest that these observations are most consistent with the existence of one or more hereditary prostate cancer genes that act in an autosomal dominant fashion to confer greatly increased risk of disease.[35–37] It is estimated that approximately 9 percent of all prostate cancer is attributable to such gene(s), although in the case of early-onset disease (i.e., diagnosis before age 55), a greater proportion (40 percent) may be due to an inherited susceptibility.[35,38]

Studies supporting the existence of hereditary forms of prostate cancer have led to the initiation of genome-wide searches for loci contributing to hereditary prostate cancer. The first such scan for linkage, reported by Smith et al.,[39] resulted in suggestive evidence for prostate cancer-susceptibility loci on several chromosomes, including 1q, 4q, 5p, 7p, 13q, and Xq. Statistically significant evidence was achieved for the locus 1q24-25 (*HPC1*). Families linked to *HPC1* tended to have an early mean age of diagnosis (under 65 years) and large number of affected members (> 4).[40] While three subsequent studies have corroborated linkage to *HPC1*,[40–42] three additional studies found no clear evidence for *HPC1*-predisposed disease within their study populations,[43–45] although evidence of linkage to a novel locus at 1q42.2-43 was observed in one report.[45] The disparity in these studies emphasizes the common set of obstacles for linkage detection in hereditary prostate cancer, most prominently, a high phenocopy rate and genetic locus heterogeneity.

A further confounding issue in prostate cancer linkage studies is the lack of a clear delineation of the mode(s) of inheritance. Although segregation analyses of familial prostate cancer have supported autosomal dominant inheritance, several population-based studies have reported a statistically significant excess risk of prostate cancer in men with affected brothers compared with those with affected fathers, consistent with the hypothesis of an X-linked, or recessive, model of inheritance.[46–50] Interestingly, in a follow-up study to the initial genome-wide search for prostate cancer linkage, Xu et al.[51] reported linkage to the X chromosome (q27-28) in a large collection of multiplex prostate cancers from North America and Europe. More precise information on inherited prostate cancer and its molecular mechanisms will have to await the cloning of the responsible genes.

As a result of various epidemiologic studies over the past four decades, a link between prostate and breast cancer etiology has been suspected.[52–56] More recent studies have demonstrated an association between *BRCA1* and *BRCA2* mutations and the incidence of prostate cancer in carriers.[57–60] The most direct evidence for a role of these genes in prostate cancer susceptibility comes from the study by Struewing et al.[60] of Ashkenazi men known to harbor *BRCA1* or *BRCA2* gene mutations. In this cohort, the rate of prostate cancer diagnosis by age 70 was 16 percent, compared with 3.8 percent for nonmutation carriers. Other studies examining a role for these genes in prostate cancer have been less supportive of a prominent effect. Lehrer et al.[61] reported an absence of *BRCA1* and *BRCA2* founder mutations in Ashkenazi prostate cancer cases, although only a limited number of these men reported a positive family history of the disease. Langston et al.[62] found a *BRCA1* 185delAG mutation in an affected member of a Jewish prostate cancer family, although no other family members were tested. A study of multiplex Ashkenazi Jewish prostate cancer families did not find elevated rates of common mutations in either *BRCA1* or *BRCA2*.[63] Overall, germ-line mutations in these genes are likely to account for only a small proportion of familial prostate cancer.

Sporadic Disease

Chromosomal Alterations in Sporadic Disease. Initial loss of heterozygosity (LOH) studies indicated that chromosomes 8p, 10q, and 16q may harbor prostate tumor-suppressor genes. These studies have been confirmed and extended to include chromosomes 7q and 13q as regions of frequent allelic loss.[64]

Chromosome 8. Of the regions analyzed, the short arm of chromosome 8 has received the most attention because it appears to be the most frequent site of LOH in prostate cancers, occurring in the majority of patients examined. Two or possibly three distinct region of LOH occur on this chromosomal arm, with the region 8p21-12 being deleted in the majority of prostate cancer precursor lesions (PIN), and more distally, 8p22 is deleted in most adenocarcinomas.[65–70] In this latter region, a homozygous deletion of approximately 1 megabase has been observed.[71]

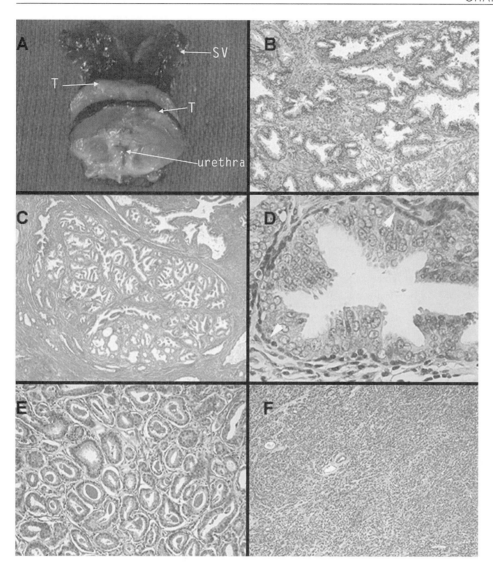

Fig. 46-1 Representative prostate histology. (*A*) Gross radical prostatectomy specimen. Serial section of the gland from apex to base. Bilateral tumor occurrence in the posterior portion (marked T). The position of the urethra is labeled. SV, seminal vesicles. (*B*) Normal. Histology of normal prostate. Open glands varying in size and form are separated by abundant stromal tissue (×20). (*C*) Benign prostatic hyperplasia (BPH). Well-defined nodule of crowded but non infiltrative, benign glands (×20). (*D*) Prostatic intraepithelial neoplasia (PIN). Cytologically malignant cells within a single architecturally benign gland. Note the presence of basal epithelial cell layer (*arroweads*) (×400). (*E*) Prostate adenocarcinoma. Low-grade (Gleason 2 + 2 = 4). Closely packed single, round glands, separated by scant stroma (×20). (*F*) Prostate adenocarcinoma. High grade (Gleason 5 + 5 = 10). Glandular differentiation is absent; sheets of anaplastic cells occasionally intermixed with smooth muscle fibers (×20). (*Photographs kindly provided by Joseph D. Kronz, M.D., and Jurgita Sauvageot.*)

The first reports of chromosome 8p abnormalities in prostate cancer were cytogenetic studies that suggested that loss of chromosome 8p material was correlated with loss of androgen responsiveness.[72] The finding of chromosome 8p LOH was first described by Bergerheim et al.[73] in a study of primary and metastatic deposits of prostate cancer. Since then, subregional deletion analysis of chromosome 8p in prostate cancer has been performed using a variety of molecular methods, all of which have confirmed a high frequency of loss in this region, especially but not exclusively within chromosome band 8p22.[24,65–68,73–80] The rate of 8p22 loss reported in these regions varies from 32 to 65 percent in primary tumors and 65 to 100 percent in DNA derived from metastases.

Separate discrete regions of loss in more proximal regions including 8p21[67,70] and 8p12[68,70] have been described. Frequent loss (63 percent) of portions of 8p21-p12 have been identified in PIN lesions,[69] suggesting that a gene in this area may become frequently inactivated at a relatively early stage in prostate tumorigenesis. Evidence of heterogeneity of 8p LOH among different PIN lesions within the same gland was observed.[69] A combined CGH, Southern, and microsatellite study has shown loss of chromosome 8p22-p12 in 80 percent of prostate cancer lymph node metastases,[81] and microcell transfer of human chromosome 8 into a rat prostate cancer cell line has been reported to suppress metastatic ability.[82] An association of chromosome 8p loss and higher stage has been reported.[68]

A candidate tumor-suppressor gene, termed *N33,* located in a homozygously deleted region of chromosome 8p22 has been

identified that is expressed in many normal tissues but not in some cancers, most notably those of the colon.[83] The contribution of this gene to prostatic carcinogenesis awaits further clarification.

The frequent loss of sequences on chromosome 8p provides a marker to determine the similarity or difference between primary prostate cancers and their metastases. This approach has been used to determine the concordance rates for 8p loss in a series of PIN, primary, and metastatic lesions obtained from the same patient.[24] Cases were observed in which there was a complete concordance in that all samples of cancer had retained or lost the same 8p marker, but there also were cases in which the PIN sample would show loss but not the primary tumor or the lymph node tumor samples. In addition, there were cases that showed differences among the multiple primary lesions within the prostate. These data and similar findings[23] demonstrate the complex genetic relationship that exists between primary and metastatic lesions and suggest that the primary prostate cancer that gives rise to a given metastatic deposit is not easily predicted on the basis of morphologic characteristics.

Concomitant with deletion of sequences from the short arm, chromosome 8 is frequently affected by gain of sequences on the long arm. First observed by Southern analysis,[65] a CGH study of lymph node metastases indicated that 85 percent of such tumors showed evidence of 8q gain, making this the most common numerical alteration observed in this study.[81] Van den Berg et al.[84] reported that gain of 8q sequences in prostate cancer was highly correlated with disease progression, and similarly, in the CGH study of Visakorpi et al.,[79] gain of 8q sequences was seen in 89 percent of tumor recurrences after hormonal therapy, whereas only 6 percent of primary tumors showed this alteration. An obvious candidate gene that may be the target of these amplification events in prostate cancer is the oncogene *c-myc* located at 8q24, although most of the amplification events on 8q are large, suggesting that many genes are affected. At present, the overall contribution of the *c-myc* gene to progression of prostate cancer is undefined.

Chromosome 7. Similar to chromosome 8, chromosome 7 also frequently undergoes both gain and loss events in prostate cancer. Trisomy 7 is common in both PIN[23] and cancer lesions,[85-89] and gain of chromosome 7 has been observed in 30 to 56 percent of cases in CGH studies.[70,80] The association of chromosome 7 aneusomy with advanced stage[88,90] and poor prognosis[89] indicates that gain of chromosome 7 material may play an important role in progression of some prostate cancers. Likewise, loss of discrete portions of chromosome 7q in prostate cancer,[91-94] with the most frequent region of deletion appearing at 7q31.1, suggests that this region also may harbor a gene important in tumor progression, since tumors deleting this region are usually of high grade and stage.

Chromosome 10. Cytogenetic analyses of prostate cancer have not revealed consistent chromosomal deletions (see refs. 87 and 95–97), which might provide information regarding the location of tumor-suppressor genes. However, an early study[98] employing direct preparations of prostate cancer cells, showed that four of four patients with late-stage prostate carcinomas exhibited chromosome 10q deletions and three of four exhibited chromosome 7q deletions. Since that time, alterations of the long arm of chromosome 10, while by no means ubiquitous, have been the most consistently observed karyotypic abnormality in prostate cancer. Initial studies examining chromosome 10 by RFLP analysis found losses solely on 10q[99] or on both arms of chromosome 10.[73] A number of reports since then using both RFLP and microsatellite analysis have found loss of chromosome 10 in 29 to 48 percent of informative cases, with a complex pattern of loss being observed, including monosomy and loss of 10p alone, loss of portions of 10p and 10q, and loss of sequences on 10q alone.[100-103] The most common region of deletion on the short and long arms has been mapped to 10p11.2 and 10q23.1, respectively (see *PTEN* below).

Chromosome 16q. Carter et al.[99] observed LOH of markers on chromosome 16q in approximately 30 percent of clinically localized tumors, whereas Bergerheim et al.[73] found a higher rate (56 percent) in a series of metastatic and localized tumors. Deletion mapping data presented in this latter study suggested that the critical region was located between D16S4 and 16qter. Employing a series of cosmid contigs in a FISH analysis, Cher et al.[104] suggested that the common region of loss was more distally located between 16q23.1 and 16qter.

Chromosome 17. Studies of loss of chromosome 17 sequences have focused primarily on two regions, one being in the vicinity of the *p53* gene at 17p13.1 and the other being in the area of the *BRCA1* gene on the proximal long arm. Allelic of loss the *p53* gene and distal markers is generally low in early-stage primary prostate cancer (< 20 percent), a finding consistent with the low frequency of *p53* gene mutations found in these tumors (see below). A study by Brooks et al.[105] demonstrates that there is a higher rate of 17p loss in higher-grade and later-stage prostate cancers but that this loss is not correlated with an increasing frequency of *p53* mutations, suggesting the presence of perhaps another tumor-suppressor gene that may contribute to the LOH events on this chromosomal arm.

Brothman et al.[106] and Williams et al.[107] used a variety of approaches to implicate a region on the proximal long arm of chromosome 17 in the vicinity of the *BRCA1* gene at 17q21 as harboring a gene important in prostate carcinogenesis. By using a

series of P1 clones in a FISH analysis, these workers were able to demonstrate that the common region of loss did not include *BRCA1* but was more distal, implicating a different gene in this region. These results are critical because it has been suggested repeatedly that the *BRCA1* gene may play an important role in prostate carcinogenesis, although little direct evidence of this has been reported.

Chromosome 18. Initial studies implicating chromosome 18 as harboring a prostate tumor-suppressor gene found LOH of markers in the vicinity of the *DCC* gene at band 21.2 on the long arm of this chromosome at rates of between 20 and 40 percent.[73,78,99] Latil et al.[74] found that one-third of clinically localized prostate cancers show loss of markers on 18q and suggest that the common region of deletion lies between the centromere and D18S19, located at 18q22.1, although a subsequent study narrowed this region, excluding *DCC*. Examinations of the *DPC4* gene at 18q21.1 in prostate cancer revealed an absence of inactivating mutations of this pancreatic tumor-suppressor gene.[108,109]

CGH Studies of Prostate Cancer. Visakorpi et al.[79] used comparative genomic hybridization (CGH) to survey the genome of a series of both untreated, localized prostate cancers and tumors from patients failing hormonal therapy. This study found chromosome 8p to be the most frequently deleted, followed by 13q, 6q, 16q, 18q, and 9p. In a series of nine advanced prostate cancers, there was a significant increase in deletions of chromosome 5q and gains of chromosomes 7p, 8q, and X when compared with untreated primary tumor samples. Similarly, Cher et al.[81] used CGH combined with Southern and microsatellite analyses to study a series of over 31 advanced prostate cancers (primarily lymph node deposits of prostate cancer). As expected, a high frequency of chromosome 8p loss was seen (71 percent). This study also revealed that portions of chromosome 13 were just as commonly deleted (65 percent), followed by chromosomes 17p (52 percent), 10q22.1-qter (42 percent), 2cen-q31 (42 percent), 16q (42 percent), 5cen-q23.3 (39 percent), and 6q14-q23.2 (39 percent). Increases in copy number of sequences on chromosome 8q were observed in 81 percent of samples, with gains of chromosomes 1q, 2p, 3p and q, 7p and q, and 11p being observed in over 40 percent of the samples. Although the CGH analysis was not able to detect a case containing a homozygous deletion on chromosome 8p22, in general, the concordance between the CGH data and that obtained by either Southern or microsatellite analysis was excellent, with agreement observed at 215 to 233 (92 percent) of informative loci. Thus these studies confirm previous studies of allelic loss in prostate cancer and at the same time greatly expand the chromosomal regions implicated as harboring "prostate cancer genes."

SPECIFIC GENES

Sporadic Disease

A number of genes have been found to be mutated in prostate cancer, including *p53*, *PTEN*, *Rb*, *RAS*, *CDKN2*, androgen receptor (*AR*), *MXI1*, and *POLB*, although the latter two, located on chromosomes 10q25 and 8p11.2, respectively, remain to be confirmed. *RAS* mutations are uncommon (< 5 percent of cases),[110-112] as are point mutations of *Rb*,[113] although loss of one copy of *Rb* readily occurs. To date, the most consistently observed site of point mutations is the *p53* gene, and these mutations are common only in advanced disease. Microsatellite instability is uncommon but detectable in prostate cancer,[114-117] and the *hPMS2* gene has been shown to be mutated in a prostate cancer cell line that exhibits this phenotype.[118]

p53. *p53* mutations are uncommon in localized disease but become quite frequent in deposits of metastatic prostate cancer, particularly those to bone.[119-125] Observed heterogeneity of *p53* mutations within different tumors in the same gland and within different regions of the same gland appears to be a unique feature of prostate cancer.[25] Furthermore, LOH and point mutation of *p53* do not appear to be tightly coupled in this disease.[105]

PTEN. A series of studies has examined prostate cancer specimens for alterations in the dual-function phosphatase gene *PTEN* and found that this gene is inactivated by a combination of mechanisms including hemi- and homozygous deletion,[126–129] point mutation,[126–128] and promoter methylation.[129] These changes are observed most commonly in advanced disease and may play a role in the acquisition of metastatic potential.

Rb. The importance of *Rb* gene inactivation in prostate cancer was suggested initially by the studies of Bookstein et al.,[130,131] who demonstrated the presence of inactivating mutations in the *Rb* gene in clinical specimens of prostate cancer, as well as the ability of reintroduction of a cloned copy of *Rb* to suppress the tumorigenicity of DU145 prostate cancer cells, which had been shown to produce a nonfunctional truncated Rb protein. Combined CGH and LOH studies reveal that one copy of *Rb* is lost in advanced prostate cancer at rates approaching 80 percent,[81] although limited sequencing studies suggest that point mutations are present in less than 20 percent of clinical samples.[113] Immunohistochemical studies of *Rb* expression demonstrate lack of expression in 10 to 22 percent of tumors, with a questionable correlation between tumor LOH of *Rb* and lack of expression.[132,133] These data, together with LOH events on 13q that do not include *Rb,* suggest the presence of an additional or alternative prostate tumor-suppressor gene near the *Rb* locus.[133]

CDKN2. Much attention has been focused on the *p16/CDKN2* gene, a negative regulator of cell cycle progression located at chromosome 9p21, since the finding of frequent homozygous deletions in a wide variety of cancer cell lines.[134] A relatively high frequency of homozygous (~20 percent)[135] and hemizygous losses of *CDKN2* have been observed in clinical specimens of prostate cancer.[136] In the latter case, loss events in the vicinity of the *CDKN2* gene are more common in metastatic deposits of prostate cancer (43 versus 20 percent in primary tumors), and in a small but detectable fraction of tumors (~15 percent), the *CDKN2* gene shows evidence of inactivation by promoter methylation.[136] Whether all the allelic loss events at 9p21 in prostate cancer are associated with *CDKN2* inactivation or whether they reflect inactivation of a neighboring gene, e.g., *p15*, has not been determined.

Androgen Receptor. The role of androgen in normal prostate physiology is unquestioned, since these hormones are strictly required for normal development and maintenance of prostate growth and function. However, the role of androgens and androgen receptors in prostate cancer is much less clear, and recent studies have generated a great deal of renewed interest in this pathway[137] and its role in the critical progression of prostate cancer to androgen independence. An initial hypothesis that loss of *AR* gene expression may be important in androgen-independent disease was not supported by several studies that showed continued or even elevated *AR* gene expression in androgen-independent tumors.[138,139] Newmark et al.[140] were the first to report a mutated androgen receptor in a clinical specimen of prostate cancer, found curiously in a localized cancer prior to any hormonal therapy. This and other findings of mutations prior to hormonal therapy[141] would suggest that mutant *AR* may provide a growth advantage even in the presence of normal androgen levels. Kelly et al.[142] and Sartor et al.[143] described a number of patients who underwent a paradoxical response to withdrawal of the antiandrogen flutamide in that a number of clinical parameters (e.g., PSA levels, bone pain) improved on cessation of drug treatment. One explanation proposed for this response is that such patients harbor *AR* gene mutations similar to that found in the prostate cancer cell line LNCaP (Thr to Ala change at codon 868) that alters the ligand specificity of the receptor such that both estrogens and antiandrogens, as well as androgens, can now act as agonists.[144,145] The frequency of such mutations in prostate cancer patients is unknown, but a study by Taplin et al.[146] found that 5 of 10 samples of hormone-refractory prostate cancer metastatic to bone had *AR* mutations and at least two of these mutations resulted in a shift in hormone specificity of the androgen receptor. Finally, Visakorpi et al.[147] demonstrated that up to 30 percent of prostate cancer specimens from men failing hormonal therapy are characterized by increases in copy number of X chromosomal region (q11-q13) containing the androgen receptor. These results suggest that instead of being insensitive to androgen, such tumors may become supersensitive to androgen by an as yet undetermined mechanism or perhaps sensitive to a different nonandrogen steroid hormone. Thus, whereas the precise role of androgen and the androgen receptor in this disease is not known, these studies imply a potential role of this pathway at a critical step in prostate cancer progression.

p27 (CDKN1B). A number of studies report that reduced levels of the cyclin kinase inhibitor p27 are associated with a more aggressive prostate cancer phenotype,[148–151] although the mechanism of this down-regulation is not clear. Interestingly, Kibel et al.[152] described a homozygous deletion of the *p27* gene in a lethal case of prostate cancer and a high frequency of LOH of *p27* in advanced prostate cancers in general. Thus it is possible that, in addition to increased ubiquitin-mediated p27 protein degradation that has been demonstrated in colon and other cancers, in prostate cancer, at least a subset of lesions may inactivate this gene via deletion.

Bcl-2: An Inhibitor of Apoptosis. The *bcl-2* gene, located on chromosome 18q21, is unique among oncogenes in that its expression does not enhance the rate of cell proliferation but instead decreases the rate of cell death.[153,154] The role of *bcl-2* in the development and progression of carcinoma of the prostate has been examined by McDonnell et al.[155] Using immunohistochemical techniques, *bcl-2* is not usually expressed in androgen-dependent prostatic cancer cells, whereas it was expressed in androgen-independent prostatic cancer cells.[155] This observation has been confirmed by Colombel et al.[156] These findings suggest that enhanced expression of bcl-2 protein in carcinomas of the prostate is associated with the transition to androgen independence, although Furuya et al.[157] demonstrated that there are bcl-2 independent pathways to this state as well.

E-cadherin and KAI-1. Genes whose down-regulation has been implicated in prostate cancer progression include the cell adhesion molecule genes *E-cadherin* and *KAI-1* located at chromosomes 16q22.1 (a frequent site of LOH) and 11p11.2, respectively.[158] E-cadherin protein levels are frequently reduced in high-grade prostate cancers, and this finding has prognostic significance.[159–161] *KAI-1* was identified by its ability to suppress metastasis in experimental animal studies.[162,163] Although the predominate mechanism for down-regulation of these genes has not been determined, in the case of *E-cadherin,* gene inactivation via promoter methylation has been found commonly in prostate cancer cell lines and at a low but detectable rate in clinical specimens of prostate cancer.

GSTπ. Similarly, the gene for the phase II detoxification enzyme glutathione *S*-transferase π also has been found to be extensively methylated in the promoter region, in a completely cancer-specific fashion, with concomitant absence of expression.[164–166] In fact, this methylation event, being found in over 90 percent of all prostate cancers, as well as in PIN lesions, is the most common genomic alteration yet observed in prostate cancer. The mechanism by which this region becomes specifically methylated in prostate cancer and the basis for its apparent selection in the carcinogenic pathway are unclear at present. Since this enzyme is a key part of an important cellular pathway to prevent damage from a wide range of carcinogens, its inactivation may result in increased susceptibility of prostate tissue to both tumor initiation and progression resulting from an increased rate of accumulated DNA damage. Indeed, reactivation of this or a similar cellular defense pathway, perhaps by dietary intervention, has been proposed as a treatment strategy aimed at blocking the progression of initiated prostate cancer foci.

Hereditary Cases

AR Gene. To date, no germ-line mutations have been identified that confer increased risk for prostate cancer, although multiple efforts are underway to identify such changes in prostate cancer families. Polymorphic variations in a variety of genes, however, have been suggested to modulate an individual's risk of prostate cancer development. A prime example of this is the *AR* gene, which has been implicated as a potentially important gene in modifying prostate cancer risk due to polymorphisms within the gene that result in variable androgen receptor activity. Specifically, there are two polymorphic triplet repeats in exon 1 that code for polyglutamine and polyglycine repeats of varying lengths of between 11 and 31 and 10 and 22 residues, respectively.[167–170] Although variations in the polyglycine repeat length are of unknown biologic consequence, it has been demonstrated that the polyglutamine repeat length is inversely related to the ability of the androgen receptor to stimulate androgen-specific transcriptional activity.[171–173] This is of particular interest because the population with the shortest average glutamine repeat length observed is the African-American population, which has the highest incidence and mortality rates reported for prostate cancer, whereas Asian individuals, who have low risk for prostate cancer, tend to have longer repeat lengths.[167,168] Hakimi et al.[137] have suggested that *AR* genes with shorter repeat lengths may increase the risk of developing more aggressive prostate cancer by virtue of conferring greater sensitivity to androgenic stimulation. Polymorphisms in other genes involved in androgen metabolism also have been implicated in determining one's risk for prostate cancer development (e.g., 5α-reductase, 3β-hydroxysteroid dehydrogenase).[174–177] Further study will be necessary to determine the overall role of these polymorphisms in determining or modifying prostate cancer risk.

Implications for Diagnosis

Whereas localized prostate cancer is readily curable by prostatectomy, there is presently no effective curative therapy for disseminated disease. Thus early detection is a critical aspect in prostate cancer diagnosis, although it is confounded by the presence of neoplastic lesions of limited clinical relevance in most aging men. Once the disease is detected, the ability to accurately determine the biologic aggressiveness of a given prostate cancer is a prime research goal. As mentioned earlier, certain molecular alterations such as gain and loss of sequences on chromosomes 7 and 8 have been shown to have prognostic significance, and loss of expression of the cell adhesion molecules, E-cadherin and possibly KAI-1, is strongly associated with more aggressive disease. In terms of diagnosis, PCR-based detection of methylation of the *GSTP1* promoter offers great potential as a highly sensitive and specific prostate cancer detection tool.[165,166]

New therapeutic approaches based on genetic alterations in prostate cancer cells have been limited, primarily due to lack of progress in the identification of genes that are mutated at high frequency in this disease. However, *p53* gene replacement and PSA (and other prostate-specific) promoter-based targeting of toxic gene expression to the prostate are examples of novel strategies that are under development.[178,179]

REFERENCES

1. Landis SH, Murray T, Bolden S, Wingo PA: Cancer statistics, 1998. *CA* **48**:6, 1998.
2. Brawley OW, Kramer BS: Epidemiology of prostate cancer, in Vogelsang NJ, Scardino PT, Shipley WU, Coffey DS (eds): *Comprehensive Textbook of Genitourinary Oncology.* Baltimore, Williams & Wilkins, 1996, pp 565-572.
3. National Cancer Institute: SEER Program, 1996.
4. Boring CC, Squires TS, Tong T: Cancer statistics, 1992 [published erratum appears in *CA* **42**(2):127,1992]. *CA* **42**:19, 1992.
5. Dhom G: Epidemiologic aspects of latent and clinically manifest carcinoma of the prostate. *J Cancer Res Clin Oncol* **106**:210, 1983.
6. Breslow N, Chan CW, Dhom G, Drury RA, Franks LM, Gellei B, Lee YS, Lundberg S, Sparke B, Sternby NH, Tulinius H: Latent carcinoma of prostate at autopsy in seven areas. *Int J Cancer* **20**:680, 1977.
7. Yatani R, Chigusa I, Akazaki K, Stemmermann GN, Welsh RA, Correa P: Geographic pathology of latent prostatic carcinoma. *Int J Cancer* **29**:611, 1982.
8. Carter BS, Carter HB, Isaacs JT: Epidemiologic evidence regarding predisposing factors to prostate cancer (review). *Prostate* **16**:187, 1990.
9. Taylor JA: Epidemiologic evidence of genetic susceptibility to cancer (review). *Birth Defects* **26**:113, 1990.
10. McNeal JE, Redwine EA, Freiha FS, Stamey TA: Zonal distribution of prostatic adenocarcinoma: Correlation with histologic pattern and direction of spread. *Am J Surg Pathol* **12**:897, 1988.
11. McNeal JE: Origin and evolution of benign prostatic enlargement. *Invest Urol* **15**:340, 1978.
12. Bostwick DG: Prostatic intraepithelial neoplasia (PIN). *Urology* **34**:16, 1989.
13. Lilja H, Abrahamsson PA: Three predominant proteins secreted by the human prostate gland. *Prostate* **12**:29, 1988.
14. Dalkin BL, Ahmann FR, Kopp JB: Prostate specific antigen levels in men older than 50 years without clinical evidence of prostatic carcinoma. *J Urol* **150**:1837, 1993.
15. Oesterling JE: Prostate specific antigen: A critical assessment of the most useful tumor marker for adenocarcinoma of the prostate (review). *J Urol* **145**:907, 1991.
16. Pannek J, Partin AW: The role of PSA and percent free PSA for staging and prognosis prediction in clinically localized prostate cancer. *Semin Urol Oncol* **16**(3):100, 1998.
17. Carter HB, Pearson JD: Prostate-specific antigen velocity and repeated measures of prostate-specific antigen. *Urol Clin North Am* **24**(2):333, 1997.
18. Oesterling JE, Chan DW, Epstein JI, Kimball AW Jr, Bruzek DJ, Rock RC, Brendler CB, Walsh PC: Prostate specific antigen in the preoperative and postoperative evaluation of localized prostatic cancer treated with radical prostatectomy. *J Urol* **139**:766, 1988.
19. Gleason DF: Histologic grading of prostate cancer: A perspective (review). *Hum Pathol* **23**:273, 1992.
20. Montie JE: 1992 staging system for prostate cancer (review). *Semin Urol* **11**:10, 1993.
21. Berges RR, Vukanovic J, Epstein JI, CarMichel M, Cisek L, Johnson DE, et al: Implication of cell kinetic changes during the progression of human prostatic cancer. *Clin Cancer Res* **1**:473, 1995.
22. Bastacky SI, Wojno KJ, Walsh PC, CarMichael MJ, Epstein JI: Pathologocal features of hereditary prostate cancer. *J Urol* **153**:987, 1995.
23. Qian JQ, Bostwick DG, Takahashi S, Borell TJ, Herath JF, Lieber MM, Jenkins RB: Chromosomal anomalies in prostatic intraepithelial neoplasia and carcinoma detected by fluorescence in situ hybridization. *Cancer Res* **55**:5408, 1995.
24. Sakr WA, Macoska JA, Benson P, Grignon DJ, Wolman SR, Pontes JE, Crissman JD: Allelic loss in locally metastatic, multisampled prostate cancer. *Cancer Res* **54**:3273, 1994.
25. Mirchandani D, Zheng J, Miller GJ, Ghosh AK, Shibata DK, Cote RJ, Roy-Burman P: Heterogeneity in intratumor distribution of *p53* mutations in human prostate cancer. *Am J Pathol* **147**:92, 1995.
26. Ellis WJ, Vessella RL, Buhler KR, Bladou F, True LD, Bigler SA, et al: Characterization of a novel androgen-sensitive, prostate-specific antigen-producing prostatic carcinoma xenograft: LuCaP 23. *Clin Cancer Res* **2**:1039, 1996.
27. Klein KA, Reiter RE, Redula J, Moradi H, Zhu XL, Brothman AR, et al: Progression of metastatic human prostate cancer to androgen independence in immunodeficient SCID mice. *Nature Med* **3**:402, 1997.
28. Nagabhushan M, Miller CM, Pretlow TP, Giaconia JM, Edgehouse NL, Schwartz S, et al: CWR22: The first human prostate cancer xenograft with strongly androgen-dependent and relapsed strains both in vivo and in soft agar. *Cancer Res* **56**:3042, 1996.

29. van Weerden WM, de Ridder CM, Verdaasdonk CL, Romijn JC, van der Kwast TH, Schroder FH, et al: Development of seven new human prostate tumor xenograft models and their histopathological characterization. *Am J Pathol* **149**:1055, 1996.

30. Stearns ME, Ware JL, Agus DB, Chang CJ, Fidler IJ, Fife RS, et al: Workgroup 2: Human xenograft models of prostate cancer. *Prostate* **36**:56, 1998.

31. Cannon L, Bishop DT, Skolnick M, Hunt S, Lyon JL, Smart CR: Genetic epidemiology of prostate cancer in the Utah Mormon genealogy. *Cancer Surv* **1**:47, 1982.

32. Meikle AW, Smith JA, West DW: Familial factors affecting prostatic cancer risk and plasma sex-steroid levels. *Prostate* **6**:121, 1985.

33. Spitz MR, Currier RD, Fueger JJ, Babaian RJ, Newell GR: Familial patterns of prostate cancer: a case-control analysis. *J Urol* **146**:1305, 1991.

34. Steinberg GD, Carter BS, Beaty TH, Childs B, Walsh PC: Family history and the risk of prostate cancer. *Prostate* **17**:337, 1990.

35. Carter BS, Beaty TH, Steinberg GD, Childs B, Walsh PC: Mendelian inheritance of familial prostate cancer. *Proc Natl Acad Sci USA* **89**:3367, 1992.

36. Gronberg H, Damber L, Damber JE, Iselius L: Segregation analysis of prostate cancer in Sweden: Support for dominant inheritance. *Am J Epidemiol* **146**:552, 1997.

37. Schaid DJ, McDonnell SK, Blute ML, Thibodeau SN: Evidence for autosomal dominant inheritance of prostate cancer. *Am J Hum Genet* **62**:1425, 1998.

38. Carter BS, Bova GS, Beaty TH, Steinberg GD, Childs B, Isaacs WB, Walsh PC: Hereditary prostate cancer: Epidemiologic and clinical features (review). *J Urol* **150**(3):797, 1993.

39. Smith JR, Freije D, Carpten JD, Gronberg H, Xu J, Isaacs SD, et al: Major susceptibility locus for prostate cancer on chromosome 1 suggested by a genome-wide search (see comments). *Science* **274**:1371, 1996.

40. Gronberg H, Xu J, Smith JR, Carpten JD, Isaacs SD, Freije D, et al: Early age at diagnosis in families providing evidence of linkage to the hereditary prostate cancer locus (*HPC1*) on chromosome 1 [published erratum appears in *Cancer Res* **15**:58(14):3191, 1998]. *Cancer Res* **57**:4707, 1997.

41. Cooney KA, McCarthy JD, Lange E, Huang L, Miesfeldt S, Montie JE, et al: Prostate cancer susceptibility locus on chromosome 1q: a confirmatory study (see comments). *J Natl Cancer Inst* **89**:955, 1997.

42. Guo Y, Sklar GN, Borkowski A, Kyprianou N: Loss of the cyclin-dependent kinase inhibitor p27(Kip1) protein in human prostate cancer correlates with tumor grade. *Clin Cancer Res* **3**:2269, 1997.

43. McIndoe RA, Stanford JL, Gibbs M, Jarvik GP, Brandzel S, Neal CL, et al: Linkage analysis of 49 high-risk families does not support a common familial prostate cancer-susceptibility gene at 1q24-25. *Am J Hum Genet* **61**:347, 1997.

44. Eeles RA, Durocher F, Edwards S, Teare D, Badzioch M, Hamoudi R, et al: Linkage analysis of chromosome 1q markers in 136 prostate cancer families. The Cancer Research Campaign/British Prostate Group U.K. Familial Prostate Cancer Study Collaborators. *Am J Hum Genet* **62**:653, 1998.

45. Berthon P, Valeri A, Cohen-Akenine A, Drelon E, Paiss T, Wohr G, et al: Predisposing gene for early-onset prostate cancer, localized on chromosome 1q42.2-43. *Am J Hum Genet* **62**:1416, 1998.

46. Woolf CM: An investigation of the fammilial aspects of carcinoma of the prostate. *Cancer* **13**:361, 1960.

47. Narod SA, Dupont A, Cusan L, Diamond P, Gomez JL, Suburu R, et al: The impact of family history on early detection of prostate cancer (letter). *Nature Med* **1**:99, 1995.

48. Monroe KR, Yu MC, Kolonel LN, Coetzee GA, Wilkens LR, Ross RK, et al: Evidence of an X-linked or recessive genetic component to prostate cancer risk (see comments). *Nature Med* **1**:827, 1995.

49. Whittemore AS, et al: Family history and prostate cancer risk in black, white, and Asian men in the United States and Canada. *Am J Epidemiol* **141**:732, 1997.

50. Hayes RB, Liff JM, Pottern LM, Greenberg RS, Schoenberg JB, Schwartz AG, et al: Prostate cancer risk in U.S. blacks and whites with a family history of cancer. *Int J Cancer* **60**:361, 1995.

51. Xu J, Meyers D, Freije D, Isaacs S, Wiley K, Nusskern D, et al: Evidence for a prostatecancer susceptibility locus on the X chromosome. *Nature Genet* **20**:175, 1998.

52. Macklin TM: The genetic basis of human mammary cancer, in *Proceedings of the Second National Cancer Conference,* vol 2. New York, 1954, pp 1074-1087.

53. Wynder EL, Hyams L, Shigematsu T: Correlations of international cancer death rates. An epidemiological exercise. *Cancer* **20**:113, 1967.

54. Thiessen EU: Concerning a familial association between breast cancer and both prostatic and uterine malignancies. *Cancer* **34**:1102, 1974.

55. McCahy PJ, Harris CA, Neal DE: Breast and prostate cancer in the relatives of men with prostate cancer. *Br J Urol* **78**:552, 1996.

56. Ekman P, Pan Y, Li C, Dich J: Environmental and genetic factors: A possible link with prostate cancer. *Br J Urol* **79**:35, 1997.

57. Ford D, Easton DF, Bishop DT, Narod SA, Goldgar DE: Risks of cancer in *BRCA1*-mutation carriers. Breast Cancer Linkage Consortium. *Lancet* **343**:692, 1994.

58. Easton DF, Steele L, Fields P, Ormiston W, Averill D, Daly PA, McManus R, Neuhausen SL, Ford D, Wooster R, Cannon-Albright LA, Stratton MR, Goldgar DE: Cancer risks in two large breast cancer families linked to *BRCA2* on chromosome 13q12-13. *Am J Hum Genet* **61**:120, 1997.

59. Sigurdsson S, Thorlacius S, Tomasson J, Tryggvadottir L, Benediktsdottir K, Eyfjord JE, Jonsson E: *BRCA2* mutation in Icelandic prostate cancer patients. *J Mol Med* **75**:758, 1997.

60. Struewing JP, Hartge P, Wacholder S, Baker SM, Berlin M, McAdams M, et al: The risk of cancer associated with specific mutations of *BRCA1* and *BRCA2* among Ashkenazi Jews. *New Engl J Med* **336**:1401, 1997.

61. Lehrer S, Fodor F, Stock RG, Stone NN, Eng C, Song HK, McGovern M: Absence of 185delAG mutation of the *BRCA1* gene and 6174delT mutation of the *BRCA2* gene in Ashkenazi Jewish men with prostate cancer. *Br J Cancer* **78**:771, 1998.

62. Langston AA, Stanford JL, Wicklund KG, Thompson JD, Blazej RG, Ostrander EA: Germ-line *BRCA1* mutations in selected men with prostate cancer (letter). *Am J Hum Genet* **58**:881, 1996.

63. Wilkens EP, Freije D, Xu J, Nusskern D, Suzuki H, Isaacs SD, Wiley K, Bujnovszky P, Walsh PC, Isaacs WB: No evidence for a role of *BRCA1* or *BRCA2* mutations in Ashkenazi Jewish families with hereditary prostate cancer. *Prostate* **39**:280, 1999.

64. Isaacs WB: Molecular genetics of prostate cancer, in Ponder BA, Cavenee WK, Solomon E (eds): *Genetics and Cancer: A Second Look.* Plainview, NY, Cold Spring Harbor Laboratory Press, 1995, pp 357–380.

65. Bova GS, Carter BS, Bussemakers MJ, Emi M, Fujiwara Y, Kyprianou N, Jacobs SC, Robinson JC, Epstein JI, Walsh PC, et al: Homozygous deletion and frequent allelic loss of chromosome 8p22 loci in human prostate cancer. *Cancer Res* **53**:3869, 1993.

66. MacGrogan D, Levy A, Bostwick D, Wagner M, Wells D, Bookstein R: Loss of chromosome arm 8p loci in prostate cancer: Mapping by quantitative allelic imbalance. *Genes Chromosom Cancer* **10**:151, 1994.

67. Trapman J, Sleddens HF, van der Weiden MM, Dinjens WN, Konig JJ, Schroder FH, Faber PW, Bosman FT: Loss of heterozygosity of chromosome 8 microsatellite loci implicates a candidate tumor suppressor gene between the loci D8S87 and D8S133 in human prostate cancer. *Cancer Res* **54**:6061, 1994.

68. Suzuki H, Emi M, Komiya A, Fujiwara Y, Yatani R, Nakamura Y, Shimazaki J: Localization of a tumor suppressor gene associated with progression of human prostate cancer within a 1.2 Mb region of 8p22-p21.3. *Genes Chromosom Cancer* **13**:168, 1995.

69. Emmert-Buck MR, Vocke CD, Pozzatti RO, Duray PH, Jennings SB, Florence CD, Zhuang Z, Bostwick DG, Liotta LA, Linehan WM: Allelic loss on chromosome 8p12-21 in microdissected prostatic intraepithelial neoplasia. *Cancer Res* **55**:2959, 1995.

70. Macoska JA, Trybus TM, Benson PD, Sakr WA, Grignon DJ, Wojno KD, Pietruk T, Powell IJ: Evidence for three tumor suppressor gene loci on chromosome 8p in human prostate cancer. *Cancer Res* **55**:5390, 1995.

71. Bova GS, MacGrogan D, Levy A, Pin SS, Bookstein R, Isaacs WB: Physical mapping of chromosome 8p22 markers and their homozygous deletion in a metastatic prostate cancer. *Genomics* **35**:46, 1996.

72. Konig JJ, Kamst E, Hagemeijer A, Romijn JC, Horoszewicz J, Schroder FH: Cytogenetic characterization of several androgen responsive and unresponsive sublines of the human prostatic carcinoma cell line LNCaP. *Urol Res* **17**:79, 1989.

73. Bergerheim US, Kunimi K, Collins VP, Ekman P: Deletion mapping of chromosomes 8, 10, and 16 in human prostatic carcinoma. *Genes Chromosom Cancer* **3**:215, 1991.

74. Latil A, Baron JC, Cussenot O, Fournier G, Soussi T, Boccon-Gibod L, Le Duc A, Rouesse J, Lidereau R: Genetic alterations in localized prostate cancer: Identification of a common region of deletion on chromosome arm 18q. *Genes Chromosom Cancer* **11**:119, 1994.

75. Macoska JA, Trybus TM, Sakr WA, Wolf MC, Benson PD, Powell IJ, Pontes JE: Fluorescence in situ hybridization analysis of 8p allelic loss and chromosome 8 instability in human prostate cancer. *Cancer Res* **54**:3824, 1994.

76. Cher ML, MacGrogan D, Bookstein R, Brown JA, Jenkins RB, Jensen RH: Comparative genomic hybridization, allelic imbalance, and fluorescence *in situ* hybridization on chromosome 8 in prostate cancer. *Genes Chromosom Cancer* **11**:153, 1994.

77. Matsuyama H, Pan Y, Skoog L, Tribukait B, Naito K, Ekman P, Lichter P, Bergerheim US: Deletion mapping of chromosome 8p in prostate cancer by fluorescence in situ hybridization. *Oncogene* **9**:3071, 1994.

78. Massenkeil G, Oberhuber H, Hailemariam S, Sulser T, Diener PA, Bannwart F, Schafer R, Schwarte-Waldhoff I: *P53* mutations and loss of heterozygosity on chromosomes 8p, 16q, 17p, and 18q are confined to advanced prostate cancer. *Anticancer Res* **14**:2785, 1994.

79. Visakorpi T, Kallioniemi A, Syvanen AC, Hyytinen ER, Karhu R, Tammela T, Isola JJ, Kallioniemi OP: Genetic changes in primary and recurrent prostate cancer by comparative genomic hybridization. *Cancer Res* **55**:342, 1995.

80. Joos S, Bergerheim USR, Pan Y, Matsuyama H, Bentz M, Dumanoir S, Lichter P: Mapping of chromosomal gains and losses in prostate cancer by comparative genomic hybridization. *Genes Chromosom Cancer* **14**:267, 1995.

81. Cher ML, Bova GS, Moore DH, Small EJ, Carroll PR, Pin SS, Epstein JI, Isaacs WB, Jensen RH: Genetic alterations in untreated prostate cancer metastases and androgen independent prostate cancer detected by comparative genomic hybridization and allelotyping. *Cancer Res* **56**:3091, 1996.

82. Ichikawa T, Nihei N, Suzuki H, Oshimura M, Emi M, Nakamura Y, Hayata I, Isaacs JT, Shimazaki J: Suppression of metastasis of rat prostatic cancer by introducing human chromosome 8. *Cancer Res* **54**:2299, 1994.

83. MacGrogan D, Levy A, Bova GS, Isaacs WB, Bookstein R: Structure and methylation-associated silencing of a gene within a homozygously deleted region of human chromosome band 8p22. *Genomics* **35**:55, 1996.

84. Van Den Berg C, Guan XY, Von Hoff D, Jenkins R, Bittner M, Griffin C, Kallioniemi O, Visakorpi T, McGill J, Herath J, Epstein J, Sarosdy M, Meltzer P, Trent J: DNA sequence amplification in human prostate cancer identified by chromosome microdissection: Potential prognostic implications. *Clin Cancer Res* **1**:11, 1995.

85. Macoska JA, Micale MA, Sakr WA, Benson PD, Wolman SR: Extensive genetic alterations in prostate cancer revealed by dual PCR and FISH analysis. *Genes Chromosom Cancer* **8**:88, 1993.

86. Micale MA, Sanford JS, Powell IJ, Sakr WA, Wolman SR: Defining the extent and nature of cytogenetic events in prostatic adenocarcinoma: Paraffin FISH vs metaphase analysis. *Cancer Genet Cytogenet* **69**(1):7, 1993.

87. Arps S, Rodewald A, Schmalenberger B, Carl P, Bressel M, Kastendieck H: Cytogenetic survey of 32 cancers of the prostate. *Cancer Genet Cytogenet* **66**(2):93, 1993.

88. Bandyk MG, Zhao L, Troncoso P, Pisters LL, Palmer JL, von Eschenbach AC, Chung LWK, Liang JC, Chung LW: Trisomy 7: A potential cytogenetic marker of human prostate cancer progression. *Genes Chromosom Cancer* **9**:19, 1994.

89. Alcaraz A, Takahashi S, Brown JA, Herath JF, Bergstralh EJ, Larson-Keller JJ, Lieber MM, Jenkins RB: Aneuploidy and aneusomy of chromosome 7 detected by fluorescence *in situ* hybridization are markers of poor prognosis in prostate cancer. *Cancer Res* **54**:3998, 1994.

90. Zitzelsberger H, Szucs S, Weier HU, Lehmann L, Braselmann H, Enders S, Schilling A, Breul J, Hofler H, Bauchinger M: Numerical abnormalities of chromosome 7 in human prostate cancer detected by fluorescence *in situ* hybridization (FISH) on paraffin-embedded tissue sections with centromere-specific DNA probes. *J Pathol* **172**:325, 1994.

91. Zenklusen JC, Thompson JC, Troncoso P, Kagan J, Conti CJ: Loss of heterozygosity in human primary prostate carcinomas: A possible tumor suppressor gene at 7q31.1. *Cancer Res* **54**(24):6370, 1994.

92. Takahashi S, Shan AL, Ritland SR, Delacey KA, Bostwick DG, Lieber MM, Thibodeau SN, Jenkins RB: Frequent loss of heterozygosity at 7q31.1 in primary prostate cancer is associated with tumor aggressiveness and progression. *Cancer Res* **55**(18):4114, 1995.

93. Watson DL, Mashal R, Krithivas K, Corless C, Kantoff P, Richie JP, Sklar J: Loss of heterozygosity at chromosomal locus 7q21-q31 in metastatic prostate cancer. *J Urol* **153**:271A, 1995.

94. Takahashi S, Qian J, Brown JA, Alcaraz A, Bostwick DG, Lieber MM, Jenkins RB: Potential markers of prostate cancer aggressiveness detected by fluorescence *in situ* hybridization in needle biopsies. *Cancer Res* **54**:3574, 1994.

95. Brothman AR, Peehl DM, Patel AM, McNeal JE: Frequency and pattern of karyotypic abnormalities in human prostate cancer. *Cancer Res* **50**:3795, 1990.

96. Lundgren R, Mandahl N, Heim S, Limon J, Henrikson H, Mitelman F: Cytogenetic analysis of 57 primary prostatic adenocarcinomas. *Genes Chromosom Cancer* **4**:16, 1992.

97. Micale MA, Mohamed A, Sakr W, Powell IJ, Wolman SR: Cytogenetics of primary prostatic adenocarcinoma: Clonality and chromosome instability. *Cancer Genet Cytogenet* **61**:165, 1992.

98. Atkin NB, Baker MC: Chromosome study of five cancers of the prostate. *Hum Genet* **70**:359, 1985.

99. Carter BS, Ewing CM, Ward WS, Treiger BF, Aalders TW, Schalken JA, Epstein JI, Isaacs WB: Allelic loss of chromosomes 16q and 10q in human prostate cancer. *Proc Natl Acad Sci USA* **87**:8751, 1990.

100. Ittmann M: Allelic loss on chromosome 10 in prostate adenocarcinoma. *Cancer Res* **56**:2143, 1996.

101. Gray IC, Phillips SMA, Lee SJ, Neoptolemos JP, Weissenbach J, Spurr NK: Loss of the chromosomal region 10q23-25 in prostate cancer. *Cancer Res* **55**:4800, 1995.

102. Eagle LR, Yin X, Brothman AR, Williams BJ, Atkin NB, Prochownik EV: Mutation of the *MXI1* gene in prostate cancer. *Nature Genet* **9**:249, 1995.

103. Trybus TM, Burgess AC, Wojno KJ, Glover TW, Macoska JA: Distinct areas of allelic loss on chromosomal regions 10p and 10q in human prostate cancer. *Cancer Res* **56**:2263, 1996.

104. Cher ML, Ito T, Weidner N, Carroll PR, Jensen RH: Mapping of regions of physical deletion on chromosome 16q in prostate cancer cells by fluorescence *in situ* hybridization (FISH). *J Urol* **153**(1):249, 1995.

105. Brooks JD, Bova GS, Ewing CM, Epstein JI, Carter BS, Piantadosi S, Robinson JC, Isaacs WB: An uncertain role for *p53* alterations in human prostate cancers. *Cancer Res* **56**:3814, 1996.

106. Brothman AR, Steele MR, Williams BJ, Jones E, Odelberg S, Albertsen HM, Jorde LB, Rohr LR, Stephenson RA: Loss of chromosome 17 loci in prostate cancer detected by polymerase chain reaction quantitation of allelic markers. *Genes Chromosom Cancer* **13**:278, 1995.

107. Williams BJ, Jones E, Zhu XL, Steele MR, Stephenson RA, Rohr LR, Brothman AR: Prostatic neoplasm, genes, tumor, *in situ* hybridization, chromosome deletion: Evidence for a tumor suppressor gene distal to *brca1* in prostate cancer. *J Urol* **155**:720, 1996.

108. Schutte M, Hruban RH, Hedrick L, Cho KR, Nadasdy GM, Weinstein CL, et al: *DPC4* gene in various tumor types. *Cancer Res* **56**:2527, 1996.

109. MacGrogan D, Pegram M, Slamon D, Bookstein R: Comparative mutational analysis of *DPC4* (*Smad4*) in prostatic and colorectal carcinomas. *Oncogene* **15**:1111, 1997.

110. Carter BS, Epstein JI, Isaacs WB: *ras* gene mutations in human prostate cancer. *Cancer Res* **50**:6830, 1990.

111. Gumerlock PH, Poonamallee UR, Meyers FJ, deVere White RW: Activated *ras* alleles in human carcinoma of the prostate are rare. *Cancer Res* **51**:1632, 1991.

112. Moul JW, Friedrichs PA, Lance RS, Theune SM, Chang EH: Infrequent *RAS* oncogene mutations in human prostate cancer. *Prostate* **20**:327, 1992.

113. Kubota Y, Fujinami K, Uemura H, Dobashi Y, Miyamoto H, Iwasaki Y, Kitamura H, Shuin T: Retinoblastoma gene mutations in primary human prostate cancer. *Prostate* **27**:314, 1995.

114. Egawa S, Uchida T, Suyama K, Wang C, Ohori M, Irie S, et al: Genomic instability of microsatellite repeats in prostate cancer: Relationship to clinicopathological variables. *Cancer Res* **55**:2418, 1995.

115. Watanabe M, Imai H, Shiraishi T, Shimazaki J, Kotake T, Yatani R: Microsatellite instability in human prostate cancer. *Br J Cancer* **72**:562, 1995.

116. Terrell RB, Wille AH, Cheville JC, Nystuen AM, Cohen MB, Sheffield VC: Microsatellite instability in adenocarcinoma of the prostate. *Am J Pathol* **147**:799, 1995.

117. Cunningham JM, Shan A, Wick MJ, McDonnell SK, Schaid DJ, Tester DJ, et al: Allelic imbalance and microsatellite instability in prostatic adenocarcinoma. *Cancer Res* **56**:4475, 1996.

118. Boyer JC, Umar A, Risinger JI, Lipford JR, Kane M, Yin S, Barrett JC, Kolodner RD, Kunkel TA: Microsatellite instability, mismatch repair

deficiency, and genetic defects in human cancer cell lines. *Cancer Res* **55**:6063, 1995.

119. Visakorpi T, Kallioniemi OP, Heikkinen A, Koivula T, Isola J: Small subgroup of aggressive, highly proliferative prostatic carcinomas defined by p53 accumulation. *J Natl Cancer Inst* **84**:883, 1992.

120. Bookstein R, MacGrogan D, Hilsenbeck SG, Sharkey F, Allred DC: *p53* is mutated in a subset of advanced-stage prostate cancers. *Cancer Res* **53**:3369, 1993.

121. Navone NM, Troncoso P, Pisters LL, Goodrow TL, Palmer JL, Nichols WW, von Eschenbach AC, Conti CJ: p53 protein accumulation and gene mutation in the progression of human prostate carcinoma. *J Natl Cancer Inst* **85**:1657, 1993.

122. Aprikian AG, Sarkis AS, Fair WR, Zhang ZF, Fuks Z, Cordon-Cardo C: Immunohistochemical determination of p53 protein nuclear accumulation in prostatic adenocarcinoma. *J Urol* **151**:1276, 1994.

123. Dinjens WN, van der Weiden MM, Schroeder FH, Bosman FT, Trapman J: Frequency and characterization of *p53* mutations in primary and metastatic human prostate cancer. *Int J Cancer* **56**:630, 1994.

124. Voeller HJ, Sugars LY, Pretlow T, Gelmann EP: *p53* oncogene mutations in human prostate cancer specimens. *J Urol* **151**:492, 1994.

125. Chi SG, deVere White RW, Meyers FJ, Siders DB, Lee F, Gumerlock PH: *p53* in prostate cancer: Frequently expressed transition mutations. *J Natl Cancer Inst* **86**:926, 1994.

126. Cairns P, Okami K, Halachmi S, Halachmi N, Esteller M, Herman JG, Jen J, Isaacs WB, Bova GS, Sidransky D: Frequent inactivation of *PTEN/MMAC1* in primary prostate cancer. *Cancer Res* **15**; **57**(22):4997, 1997.

127. Suzuki H, Freije D, Nusskern DR, Okami K, Cairns P, Sidransky D, Isaacs WB, Bova GS: Interfocal heterogeneity of *PTEN/MMAC1* gene alterations in multiple metastatic prostate cancer tissues. *Cancer Res* **15**; **58**(2):204, 1998.

128. Vlietstra RJ, van Alewijk DC, Hermans KG, van Steenbrugge GJ, Trapman J: Frequent inactivation of *PTEN* in prostate cancer cell lines and xenografts. *Cancer Res* **58**:2720, 1998.

129. Whang YE, Wu X, Suzuki H, Reiter RE, Tran C, Vessella RL, et al: Inactivation of the tumor suppressor *PTEN/MMAC1* in advanced human prostate cancer through loss of expression. *Proc Natl Acad Sci USA* **95**:5246, 1998.

130. Bookstein R, Shew JY, Chen PL, Scully P, Lee WH: Suppression of tumorigenicity of human prostate carcinoma cells by replacing a mutated *RB* gene. *Science* **247**:712, 1990.

131. Bookstein R, Rio P, Madreperla SA, Hong F, Allred C, Grizzle WE, Lee WH: Promoter deletion and loss of retinoblastoma gene expression in human prostate carcinoma. *Proc Natl Acad Sci USA* **87**:7762, 1990.

132. Ittmann MM, Wieczorek R: Alterations of the retinoblastoma gene in clinically localized, stage B prostate adenocarcinomas. *Hum Pathol* **27**:28, 1996.

133. Cooney KA, Wetzel JC, Merajver SD, Macoska JA, Singleton TP, Wojno KJ: Distinct regions of loss of 13q in prostate cancer. *Cancer Res* **56**:1142, 1996.

134. Kamb A, Gruis NA, Weaver-Feldhaus J, Liu Q, Harshman K, Tavtigian SV, Stockert E, Day RS, Johnson BE, Skolnick MH: A cell cycle regulator potentially involved in genesis of many tumor types (see comments). *Science* **264**:436, 1994.

135. Cairns P, Polascik TJ, Eby Y, Tokino K, Califano J, Merlo A, Mao L, Herath J, Jenkins R, Westra W, Bova GS, et al: Frequency of homozygous deletion at *p16/CDKN2* in primary human tumours. *Nature Genet* **11**:210, 1995.

136. Jarrard D, Bova GS, Ewing CM, Pin SS, Nguyen SH, Baylin SB, Cairns P, Sidransky D, Herman JG, Isaacs WB: Deletional, mutational, and methylation analyses of *CDKN2(p16/MTS1)* in primary and metastatic prostate cancer. *Genes Chromosom Cancer* **19**:90, 1997.

137. Hakimi JM, Rondinelli RH, Schoenberg MP, Barrack ER: Androgen-receptor gene structure and function in prostate cancer. *World J Urol* **14**:329, 1996.

138. Hobisch A, Culig Z, Radmayr C, Bartsch G, Klocker H, Hittmair A: Distant metastases from prostatic carcinoma express androgen receptor protein. *Cancer Res* **55**:3068, 1995.

139. Ruizeveld de Winter JA, Janssen PJ, Sleddens HM, Verleun-Mooijman MC, Trapman J, Brinkmann AO, Santerse AB, Schroder FH, van der Kwast TH: Androgen receptor status in localized and locally progressive hormone refractory human prostate cancer. *Am J Pathol* **144**:735, 1994.

140. Newmark JR, Hardy DO, Tonb DC, Carter BS, Epstein JI, Isaacs WB, Brown TR, Barrack ER: Androgen receptor gene mutations in human prostate cancer. *Proc Natl Acad Sci USA* **89**:6319, 1992.

141. Tilley WD, Buchanan G, Hickey TE, Bentel JM: Mutations in the androgen receptor gene are associated with progression of human prostate cancer to androgen independence. *Clin Cancer Res* **2**:277, 1996.

142. Kelly WK, Scher HI: Prostate specific antigen decline after antiandrogen withdrawal: The flutamide withdrawal syndrome. *J Urol* **149**:607, 1993.

143. Sartor O, Cooper M, Weinberger M, Headlee D, Thibault A, Tompkins A, Steinberg S, Figg WD, Linehan WM, Myers CE: Surprising activity of flutamide withdrawal, when combined with aminoglutethimide, in treatment of "hormone-refractory" prostate cancer [published erratum appears in *J Natl Cancer Inst* 16; **86**(6):463, 1994]. *J Natl Cancer Inst* **86**:222, 1994.

144. Harris SE, Rong Z, Harris MA, Lubahn DD: Androgen receptor in human prostate adenocarcinoma LNCaP/ADEP cells contains a mutation which alters the specificity of the steroid-dependent transcriptional activation region. *Endocrinology* **126**:93, 1990.

145. Veldscholte J, Berrevoets CA, Ris-Stalpers C, Kuiper GG, Jenster G, Trapman J, Brinkmann AO, Mulder E: The androgen receptor in LNCaP cells contains a mutation in the ligand binding domain which affects steroid binding characteristics and response to antiandrogens (review). *J Steroid Biochem Mol Biol* **41**:665, 1992.

146. Taplin ME, Bubley GJ, Shuster TD, Frantz ME, Spooner AE, Ogata GK, Keer HN, Balk SP: Mutation of the androgen-receptor gene in metastatic androgen-independent prostate cancer (see comments). *New Engl J Med* **332**:1393, 1995.

147. Visakorpi T, Hyytinen E, Koivisto P, Tanner M, Keinanen R, Palmberg C, Palotie A, Tammela T, Isola J, Kallioniemi OP: In vivo amplification of the androgen receptor gene and progression of human prostate cancer. *Nature Genet* **9**(4):401, 1995.

148. Guo Y, Sklar GN, Borkowski A, Kyprianou N: Loss of the cyclin-dependent kinase inhibitor p27(Kip1) protein in human prostate cancer correlates with tumor grade. *Clin Cancer Res* **3**:2269, 1997.

149. Yang RM, Naitoh J, Murphy M, Wang HJ, Phillipson J, deKernion JB, et al: Low p27 expression predicts poor disease-free survival in patients with prostate cancer. *J Urol* **159**:941, 1998.

150. Cote RJ, Shi Y, Groshen S, Feng AC, Cordon-Cardo C, Skinner D, et al: Association of p27Kip1 levels with recurrence and survival in patients with stage C prostate carcinoma. *J Natl Cancer Inst* **90**:916, 1998.

151. Cheville JC, Lloyd RV, Sebo TJ, Cheng L, Erickson L, Bostwick DG, et al: Expression of p27kip1 in prostatic adenocarcinoma. *Mod Pathol* **11**:324, 1998.

152. Kibel AS, Schutte M, Kern SE, Isaacs WB, Bova GS: Identification of 12p as a region of frequent deletion in advanced prostate cancer. *Cancer Res* **58**:5652, 1998.

153. Reed JC, Cuddy M, Slabiak T, Croce CM, Nowell PC: Oncogenic potential of *bcl-2* demonstrated by gene transfer. *Nature* **336**:259, 1988.

154. Hockenbery DM: The *bcl-2* oncogene and apoptosis (review). *Semin Immunol* **4**:413, 1992.

155. McDonnell TJ, Troncoso P, Brisbay SM, Logothetis C, Chung LW, Hsieh JT, Tu SM, Campbell ML: Expression of the protooncogene *bcl-2* in the prostate and its association with emergence of androgen-independent prostate cancer. *Cancer Res* **52**:6940, 1992.

156. Colombel M, Symmans F, Gil S, O'Toole KM, Chopin D, Benson M, Olsson CA, Korsmeyer S, Buttyan R: Detection of the apoptosis-suppressing oncoprotein *bcl-2* in hormone-refractory human prostate cancers. *Am J Pathol* **143**:390, 1993.

157. Furuya Y, Krajewski S, Epstein JI, Reed JC, Isaacs JT: Expression of *bcl2* in the progression of human and rodent prostatic cancers. *Clin Cancer Res* **2**:398, 1996.

158. Dong J-T, Suzuki H, Pin SS, Bova GS, Schalken JA, Isaacs WB, Barrett JC, Isaacs JT: Down-regulation of the *KAI1* metastasis suppressor gene during the progression of human prostatic cancer infrequently involves gene mutation and allelic loss. *Cancer Res* **56**:3091, 1996.

159. Umbas R, Isaacs WB, Bringuier PP, Schaafsma HE, Karthaus HF, Oosterhof GO, Debruyne FM, Schalken JA: Decreased E-cadherin expression is associated with poor prognosis in patients with prostate cancer. *Cancer Res* **54**:3929, 1994.

160. Umbas R, Schalken JA, Aalders TW, Carter BS, Karthaus HF, Schaafsma HE, Debruyne FM, Isaacs WB: Expression of the cellular adhesion molecule E-cadherin is reduced or absent in high-grade prostate cancer. *Cancer Res* **52**:5104, 1992.

161. Morton RA, Ewing CM, Nagafuchi A, Tsukita S, Isaacs WB: Reduction of E-cadherin levels and deletion of the alpha-catenin gene in human prostate cancer cells. *Cancer Res* **53**:3585, 1993.

162. Ichikawa T, Ichikawa Y, Dong J, Hawkins AL, Griffin CA, Isaacs WB, Oshimura M, Barrett JC, Isaacs JT: Localization of metastasis suppressor gene(s) for prostatic cancer to the short arm of human chromosome 11. *Cancer Res* **52**:3486, 1992.

163. Dong J-T, Lamb PW, Rinker-Schaeffer CW, Vukanovic J, Isaacs JT, Barrett JC. KAI-1: A metastasis suppressor gene for prostate cancer on human chromosome 11p11.2. *Science* **268**:884, 1995.

164. Lee WH, Morton RA, Epstein JI, Brooks JD, Campbell PA, Bova GS, Hsieh WS, Isaacs WB, Nelson WG: Cytidine methylation of regulatory sequences near the pi-class glutathione *S*-transferase gene accompanies human prostatic carcinogenesis. *Proc Natl Acad Sci USA* **91**(24):11733, 1994.

165. Lee WH, Isaacs WB, Bova GS, Nelson WG: CG island methylation changes near the *GSTP1* gene in prostatic carcinoma cells detected using the polymerase chain reaction: A new prostate cancer biomarker. *Cancer Epidemiol Biomark Prev* **6**:443, 1997.

166. Brooks JD, Weinstein M, Lin X, Sun Y, Pin SS, Bova GS, et al: CG island methylation changes near the *GSTP1* gene in prostatic intraepithelial neoplasia. *Cancer Epidemiol Biomark Prev* **7**:531, 1998.

167. Edwards A, Hammond HA, Jin L, Caskey CT, Chakraborty R: Genetic variation at five trimeric and tetrameric tandem repeat loci in four human population groups. *Genomics* **12**:241, 1992.

168. Irvine RA, Yu MC, Ross RK, Coetzee GA: The CAG and GGC microsatellites of the androgen receptor gene are in linkage disequilibrium in men with prostate cancer. *Cancer Res* **55**:1937, 1995.

169. Macke JP, Hu N, Hu S, Bailey M, King VL, Brown T, Hamer D, Nathans J: Sequence variation in the androgen receptor gene is not a common determinant of male sexual orientation. *Am J Hum Genet* **53**:844, 1993.

170. Sleddens HF, Oostra BA, Brinkmann AO, Trapman J: Trinucleotide (GGN) repeat polymorphism in the human androgen receptor (*AR*) gene. *Hum Mol Genet* **2**:493, 1993.

171. Chamberlain NL, Driver ED, Miesfeld RL: The length and location of CAG trinucleotide repeats in the androgen receptor N-terminal domain affect transactivation function. *Nucleic Acids Res* **22**:3181, 1994.

172. Kazemi-Esfarjani P, Trifiro MA, Pinsky L: Evidence for a repressive function of the long polyglutamine tract in the human androgen receptor: Possible pathogenetic relevance for the (CAG)n-expanded neuronopathies. *Hum Mol Genet* **4**:523, 1995.

173. Sobue G, Doyu M, Morishima T, Mukai E, Yasuda T, Kachi T, Mitsuma T: Aberrant androgen action and increased size of tandem CAG repeat in androgen receptor gene in X-linked recessive bulbospinal neuronopathy. *J Neurol Sci* **121**:167, 1994.

174. Reichardt JK, Makridakis N, Henderson BE, Yu MC, Pike MC, Ross RK: Genetic variability of the human *SRD5A2* gene: Implications for prostate cancer risk. *Cancer Res* **55**:3973, 1995.

175. Makridakis N, Ross RK, Pike MC, Chang L, Stanczyk FZ, Kolonel LN, et al: A prevalent missense substitution that modulates activity of prostatic steroid 5α-reductase. *Cancer Res* **57**:1020, 1997.

176. Devgan SA, Henderson BE, Yu MC, Shi CY, Pike MC, Ross RK, et al: Genetic variation of 3 beta-hydroxysteroid dehydrogenase type II in three racial/ethnic groups: Implications for prostate cancer risk. *Prostate* **33**:9, 1997.

177. Ross RK, Pike MC, Coetzee GA, Reichardt JK, Yu MC, Feigelson H, et al: Androgen metabolism and prostate cancer: Establishing a model of genetic susceptibility. *Cancer Res* **58**:4497, 1998.

178. Rodriguez R, Schuur ER, Lim HY, Henderson GA, Simons JW, Henderson DR: Prostate attenuated replication competent adenovirus (ARCA) CN706: A selective cytotoxic for prostate-specific antigen-positive prostate cancer cells. *Cancer Res* **57**:2559, 1997.

179. Simons JW, Marshall FF: The future of gene therapy in the treatment of urologic malignancies. *Urol Clin North Am* **25**:23, 1998.

Brain Tumors

Sandra H. Bigner ■ *Roger E. McLendon*
Naji Al-dosari ■ *Ahmed Rasheed*

1. **Glioblastoma multiforme, the most common malignant primary brain tumor of adults, is characterized by gains of chromosome 7 and losses of chromosome 10, which are seen in up to 80 to 90 percent of patients. Approximately 25 to 30 percent of patients with loss of chromosome 10 have mutations of the *PTEN/MMAC1* gene. More than half of these tumors also contain abnormalities of genes involved in cell cycle control. Specifically, about a third of patients have homozygous deletions of the *CDKN2A* gene, while some tumors with intact *CDKN2A* have loss of expression of the retinoblastoma gene or have amplification of the *CDK4* gene. In addition, approximately one-half of patients have amplification, often with rearrangement, of the epidermal growth factor receptor (*EGFR*) gene.**
2. **Low-grade astrocytomas, particularly anaplastic astrocytomas, as well as low-grade tumors that progress to glioblastomas, contain mutations of the *TP53* gene in up to 50 percent of patients in some series.**
3. **Oligodendrogliomas are frequently characterized by losses of 1p and 19q. The target genes for loss of these regions remain unknown.**
4. **A subset of ependymomas has loss of 22q. Mutation of the neurofibromatosis type 2 (*NF2*) gene has been described in a single patient with an ependymoma. Therefore, whether or not this gene is the target of the 22q loss in these tumors remains speculative.**
5. **The most consistent finding in medulloblastomas, the most common primary malignant brain tumor of children, is loss of 17p. Mapping of the deleted region to distal 17p and a low incidence of *TP53* gene mutations suggest that *TP53* is not the target of 17p loss in these tumors. Approximately 15 percent of patients have mutations of the *PTCH* gene, in association with loss of 9q. The incidence of gene amplification has variously been reported to be from less than 5 to 22 percent in medulloblastomas. The amplified gene is usually *c-myc*, with a few examples of *N-myc* gene amplification.**
6. **Approximately 60 percent of meningiomas and schwannomas have loss of 22q, which is usually associated with *NF2* gene mutations.**

ASTROCYTOMAS

The astrocyte, one form of glial cell that comprises much of the background substance of the brain and spinal cord, is believed to give rise to a large category of primary brain tumors, the astrocytomas. These neoplasms can occur in all areas of the brain and spinal cord in children and adults. Although the vast majority of astrocytic neoplasms occur sporadically, they can be seen in

---

A list of standard abbreviations is located immediately preceding the index. Nonstandard abbreviations used in this chapter include: LOH = loss of heterozygosity.

patients with the familial adenomatous polyposis syndrome, the Li-Fraumeni syndrome, and central neurofibromatosis (see Chaps. 23, 26 and 34). The incidence of astrocytomas is approximately 7.0 per 100,000,[1] which means that nearly 20,000 Americans will have an astrocytoma diagnosed each year. The World Health Organization (WHO) classification[2] recognizes four grades of astrocytoma (Fig. 47-1). Grade I astrocytomas are slow-growing, noninfiltrative neoplasms, occurring mainly in children and young adults, and include juvenile pilocytic astrocytomas and gangliogliomas. Grade II astrocytomas are mainly well-differentiated fibrillary astrocytomas, whereas grade III astrocytomas are a more aggressive neoplasm, the anaplastic astrocytoma.[3] The most malignant form of astrocytoma, the grade IV tumor, is the glioblastoma multiforme, which is the most common primary malignant brain tumor of adults. Although these tumors most commonly occur in the cerebral hemispheres of older individuals, they can be seen throughout the brain and spinal cord in patients of all ages.

Chromosomal Abnormalities in Astrocytomas (Table 47-1)

The most consistent chromosomal changes in glioblastomas are gains of chromosome 7, seen in about 80 percent of tumors with abnormal stem lines, losses of chromosome 10 in 60 percent of tumors, losses of 9p in about a third of tumors, and the presence of double minute chromosomes (Dmins) in up to 50 percent of tumors[4–9] (Figs. 47-2 and 47-3).

Genetic Alterations in Astrocytomas

Loss of heterozygosity (LOH) analyses have confirmed losses of all or part of chromosome 10 in more than 90 percent of tumors (Fig. 47-4) in some series and have narrowed the smallest region of overlapping deletion to 10q25.[10,11] Most series also have identified a second region on 10p, and a third site on proximal 10q also has been targeted by some observers.[12–14] Li *et al.*[15] and Steck *et al.*[16] have identified a gene located at 10q23 that was mutated or deleted in a subset of gliomas. This gene, called *PTEN* for phosphatase and tensin homologue deleted on chromosome 10 or *MMAC1* for mutated in multiple advanced cancers, is mutated in 24 to 60 percent of glioblastomas with LOH for 10q[17–21] and in approximately 40 percent of prostatic and endometrial cancers.[22,23] Germline mutations of the *PTEN/MMAC1* gene are seen in Cowden disease and the Bannayan-Zonana syndrome.[24,25] The product of this gene is a protein tyrosine phosphatase, transforming growth factor beta (TGF-β)-regulated and epithelial cell-enriched phosphatase, or TEP1.[26] Although mutations of the *PTEN/MMAC1* gene are common in high-grade astrocytomas (glioblastomas and anaplastic astrocytomas), they are rarely seen in low-grade astrocytomas.[27,28] In addition, among glioblastomas, mutations of this gene are seen more frequently in *de novo* rather than secondary tumors.[29]

Although the *PTEN/MMAC1* gene is clearly implicated in a subset of gliomas, the location of this gene is at 10q23, whereas the most frequent region of overlapping deletions in these tumors is at 10q25-6, and the observation that many astrocytomas with

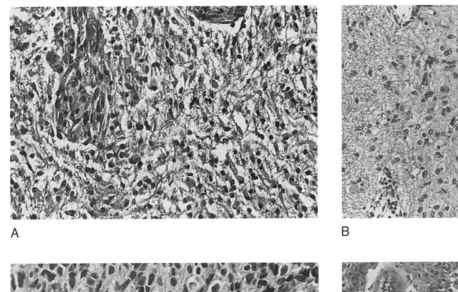

A

B

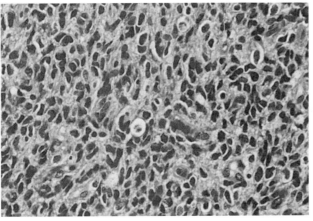

C

D

Fig. 47-1 Histology of astrocytomas. (*A*) WHO grade I astrocytomas are largely represented by pilocytic astrocytomas, which are moderately cellular neoplasms formed of bipolar astrocytes that occasionally produce Rosenthal fibers. (*B*) WHO grade II astrocytomas, also known as well-differentiated fibrillary astrocytomas, are composed of unipolar and stellate astrocytes with simplified processes that exhibit mild nuclear pleomorphism and a proliferation index of 1 percent or less. (*C*) Grade III astrocytomas, or anaplastic astrocytomas, are highly cellular neoplasms composed largely of unipolar astrocytes exhibiting nuclear pleomorphism and a brisk proliferation index but lacking in tumor necrosis and vascular proliferation. (*D*) Grade IV astrocytomas, or glioblastomas, form the most malignant end of the spectrum and are characterized by astrocytic neoplasms exhibiting nuclear pleomorphism, brisk proliferation index, vascular proliferation, and/or necrosis with pseudopalisading.

Table 47-1 Chromosomal and Genetic Alterations Characteristic of Specific Types of Brain Tumors

Tumor Type	Chromosomal or LOH Abnormality	Genetic Alteration
Glioblastoma	+7	Unknown
	−9p	CDKN2A, CDKN2B
	−10	PTEN/MMAC1 gene mutation, DMBT1 deletion?
	−17p	p53 gene mutation
	Dmins	EGFR gene amplification and rearrangement
Oligodendroglioma	−1p, −19q	Unknown
Ependymoma	−22	NF2 gene mutation?
Medulloblastoma	−17p	Unknown
	−9q	PTCH gene mutation
	Dmins	c-myc, N-myc gene amplification
Meningioma	−22	NF2 gene mutation
Schwannoma	−22	NF2 gene mutation

LOH for 10q lack mutations of this gene has raised the possibility that another chromosome 10 gene or genes may be involved in gliomas. Candidate genes in the 10q25 region include *MXI1* and *PAX-2*.[30–32] *DMBT1,* for deleted in malignant brain tumors, is located at 10q25.3-26.1. This gene, which shows homology to the scavenger receptor cysteine-rich superfamily, was shown to be homozygously deleted in 9 of 39 glioblastomas and 2 of 20 medulloblastomas by Mollenhauer et al.[33] Although this gene was not expressed in 4 of 5 brain tumor cell lines, the lack of demonstration of point mutations in these tumors raises the possibility that this gene may not be the target of the deletions.

LOH analyses of astrocytomas revealed that approximately one-third of these tumors have loss of all or part of 17p.[34–45] Unlike the chromosomal deviations described earlier, which are seen mainly in glioblastomas, LOH for 17p occurs in astrocytomas of all grades. Point mutations of the *p53* gene can be demonstrated in the majority of astrocytomas with 17p loss. The mutations are clustered in the same hot spots as are seen in colon, breast, and lung carcinomas. The incidence of *TP53* mutations, confirmed by sequence data, is about 25 percent (73 of 295) in glioblastomas, 34 percent (49 of 144) in anaplastic astrocytomas, and 30 percent (33 of 111) in astrocytomas.[38–40,45–54] Most of the *TP53* studies have concentrated on the conserved exons 5 through 8, but studies that included the entire coding sequence (exons 2–11) have uncovered

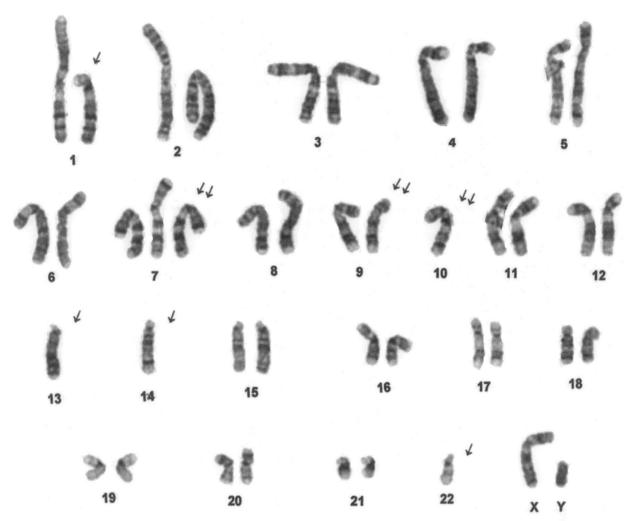

Fig. 47-2 Karyotype of glioblastoma. This Giemsa-trypsin–banded karyotype of glioblasoma xenograft D-643 MG shows gain of chromosome 7, a deletion of 9p, and loss of a chromosome 10 (double arrows). Additional, nonspecific changes are marked with single arrows.

only a handful of mutations outside of exons 5 through 8.[38,40,46,47,50] Similar to colon cancer, codons 175, 248, and 273 are frequently mutated in brain tumors, but the codon that is most frequently mutated in brain is codon 273, whereas in colon it is codon 175.[52] *TP53* mutations are associated with age of the patient. These alterations are rare among pediatric patients[43,45,50,52,55,56] but occur in nearly 50 percent of tumors in young adults, with a much lower incidence (< 20 percent) in patients over 50 years of age. Most of the *TP53* mutations identified in astrocytomas are G-to-C > A-to-T transitions located at CpG sites and resemble the pattern of mutations found in colon cancer, sarcomas, and lymphomas.

The cytogenetic observation of 9p loss in gliomas prompted evaluation of the α and β interferon genes, which are located at 9p22. Hemizygous or homozygous deletion of interferon genes

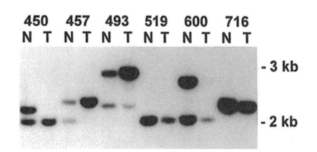

Fig. 47-3 FISH of glioblastoma. This interphase nucleus from a glioblastoma contains three chromosome 7 centromere signals (dark) and one centromere 10 signal (light).

Fig. 47-4 LOH of glioblastoma chromosome 10. A Southern blot of Taq I-digested DNA (5 μg) from blood (N) and glioblastoma tumor (T) was hybridized to the 10q marker D10S25. This marker showed LOH in tumors 450, 457, 493, and 600 and was uninformative in tumors 519 and 716. The size of the alleles ranged from 1.9 to 3 kb.

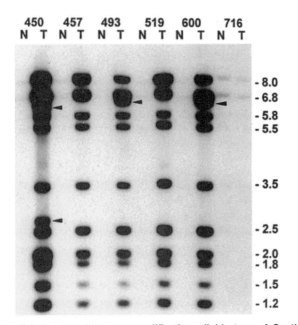

Fig. 47-5 Southern blot gene amplification, glioblastoma. A Southern blot of EcoRI-digested DNA (5 μg) from blood (N) and glioblastoma tumor (T) was hybridized with *EGFR* gene probe pE7. The hybridizing fragments, in samples with normal copy number of the gene (all blood and tumor 716), appear as faint bands, and their sizes (in kb) are indicated on the right. In tumors 457 and 519 the gene was amplified, and in 450, 493, and 600 the gene was amplified and rearranged. Arrows indicate variant bands resulting from gene rearrangement.

was reported in glioma cell lines and in biopsies of high-grade astrocytomas,[57,58] but it was not clear in these early studies whether the interferon genes were the target of 9p deletions in gliomas or were simply located near the region of the target gene. In 1994, the *CDKN2A* and *CDKN2B* genes, which are located at 9p21, were found to be homozygously deleted in various types of tumors including gliomas.[59] By combining data collected on tumor biopsies in several laboratories, the overall incidence of homozygous deletions is 33 percent (98 of 300) in glioblastomas and 24 percent in anaplastic astrocytomas (19 of 79) and for hemizygous deletion or LOH for 9p loci is 24 percent of glioblastomas and 18 percent of anaplastic astrocytomas. The incidence of homozygous deletions of both *CDKN2A* and *CDKN2B* is higher in xenografts, approaching 80 percent in some studies.[60] Among the 23 low-grade astrocytoma biopsies analyzed, none exhibited homozygous deletion, although 5 showed LOH, altogether there have been only 3 cases of mutations, all in glioblastomas.[61–70] The high frequency of homozygous deletions on chromosome 9 and the inclusion of *CDKN2A* and *CDKN2B* gene sequences in the deleted region in most cases has led observers to believe that *CDKN2A* and *CDKN2B* are the target suppressor genes for 9p loss in gliomas. Unlike the *p53* gene, which usually undergoes point mutation, the most common mechanism for *CDKN2A* gene inactivation in gliomas is homozygous deletion. However, alternative mechanisms such as transcriptional silencing by hypermethylation of CpG islands may be responsible for reduced expression in some gliomas with intact *CDKN2A/CDKN2B* genes.[71]

The majority of glioblastomas that possess Dmins contain amplification of the *EGFR* gene.[72] The *EGFR* gene has been shown to be amplified in one-third to one-half of glioblastomas but only in isolated cases of anaplastic astrocytomas and rarely in other lower-grade tumors. In many glioblastomas, the amplified *EGFR* gene is also rearranged[73,74] (Fig. 47-5). The most common class of mutants bears deletion of exons 2 through 7 of the gene, resulting in an in-frame deletion of 801 bp of coding sequence and

generation of a glycine residue at the fusion point. This variant receptor, designated EGFRvIII, has been reported in 17 to 62 percent of glioblastomas.[75–80] The tumor cell membrane fractions containing the mutant 140-kDa receptor show a significant elevation in tyrosine kinase activity without its ligand.[81] The mutant is still capable of binding with its ligand but at a significantly reduced affinity.[82]

Relationship Between Cell Cycle Regulators in Astrocytomas

In addition to deletions of the *CDKN2A* and *CDKN2B* genes as discussed earlier, alterations of other genes involved in cell cycle regulation have been described in subsets of astrocytomas. LOH for 13q or loss of expression of the retinoblastoma (*Rb*) gene product has been described in 20 to 40 percent of glioblastomas,[12,37,70,83–86] and amplification of the *CDK4* gene has been described in up to 15 percent of glioblastomas.[64,87] Furthermore, He et al.,[86] Biernat,[88] and Ueki et al.[70] have shown that most glioblastomas contain only one of these three alterations: (1) *CDKN2A/CDKN2B* deletion, (2) LOH for 13q or loss of *Rb* expression, or (3) *CDK4* gene amplification or increased expression.

Genetic Alterations in the Progression of Gliomas

It has long been recognized that there are two patterns for the development of glioblastomas. The majority of these tumors occur in patients over 50 years of age, in individuals with no previous indication of a brain tumor. A second group of patients involves younger people whose glioblastomas evolve out of lower-grade astrocytomas. Recent studies have provided molecular markers that in many cases distinguish between these two clinical patterns. The *de novo* pathway, occurring in older patients, includes tumors over 50 percent of which contain *EGFR* gene amplification and the majority of which lack *TP53* gene mutations.[42–44,88] Glioblastomas evolving through progression, in contrast, seldom have *EGFR* gene amplification, and more than 50 percent contain *TP53* gene mutations.[41,88–93]

Other molecular markers, including LOH for chromosome 10, *CDKN2A* and *CDKN2B* deletions, *Rb* and *CDK4* abnormalities, and amplification of other oncogenes do not appear to differ in tumors arising through these two pathways.

OLIGODENDROGLIOMAS

Oligodendrogliomas are a type of glioma that occur mainly in the cerebral hemispheres of adults and are derived from the oligodendrocyte. Well-differentiated oligodendrogliomas exhibiting benign cytologic features are considered grade II according to the WHO classification (Fig. 47-6), whereas anaplastic oligoden-

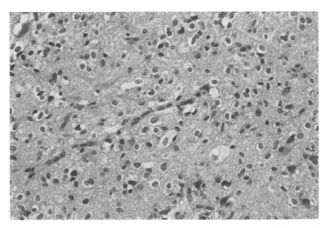

Fig. 47-6 Oligodendrogliomas are characterized by cells with round to oval nuclei surrounded by perinuclear cytoplasmic haloes and usually associated with a fine arcuating network of tubular vessels.

drogliomas exhibiting abundant mitotic activity, necrosis without pseudopalisading, and glomeruloid vascular proliferation are considered grade III tumors. According to data collected by the Survelliance, Epidemiology, and End Results (SEER) Project, the age-adjusted incidence of oligodendroglioma is 0.33 per 100,000.[1]

Chromosomal Abnormalities in Oligodendrogliomas

Although most cytogenetic analyses of oligodendrogliomas have failed to demonstrate consistent findings, LOH studies have shown that loss of 1p and 19q occurs in a substantial proportion of these tumors. Bello et al.[94] reported LOH for loci on 1p in up to 100 percent (6 of 6) oligodendrogliomas and in most (5 of 6) anaplastic oligodendrogliomas. Among other types of gliomas, only 2 of 11 glioblastomas exhibited 1p LOH, suggesting that 1p LOH is characteristic of tumors of oligodendroglial origin. A high incidence of 1p loss in tumors of oligodendroglial origin has been confirmed by Reifenberger et al.[95] using LOH techniques, and by in situ hybridization, Hashimoto et al.[96] found deletion of a 1p locus in 9 of 9 oligodendrogliomas.

Analysis with restriction fragment length polymorphism and microsatellite markers showed loss of markers on chromosome 19 in about 63 percent (17 of 27) of grade II oligodendrogliomas, 75 percent (18 of 24) of grade III or anaplastic oligodendrogliomas, and 48 percent (21 of 43) of mixed oligoastrocytomas.[95,97,98] This abnormality also has been reported in about 16 percent (4 of 25) of astrocytomas, 38 percent (13 of 34) of anaplastic astrocytomas, and 28 percent (37 of 130) of glioblastomas tested.[97,98] Loss of loci on 19q was more frequent among oligodendroglial tumors, whereas astrocytic tumors mostly lost 19p alleles.[98] The 19q minimal deletion region has been mapped to a 425-kb region on 19q13.3.[99,100]

EPENDYMOMAS

Ependymomas are a category of glioma derived from the ventricular lining that can occur at many locations within the brain and spinal cord of adults and children predominantly associated with the ventricular system. Favored sites include the posterior fossa (IVth ventricle) in children, the lateral ventricles in adults, and the cauda equina in patients of all ages. Most lesions are classified histologically as grade II (Fig. 47-7), whereas tumors with anaplastic features (anaplastic ependymomas, grade III) are sometimes seen. Central neurofibromatosis (NF type 2) is associated with ependymoma, most commonly of the spinal cord. SEER data indicate an age-adjusted incidence of 0.18 per 100,000.[1]

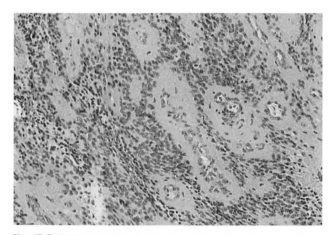

Fig. 47-7 Ependymomas often form perivascular pseudorosettes in which the tumor cells project slender fibrillar processes toward vessels while the nuclei appear excluded to a certain distance.

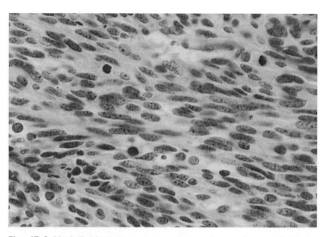

Fig. 47-8 Medulloblastomas are embryonal neoplasms that are markedly cellular, with tumor cells generally exhibiting minimal amounts of cytoplasm. Although the classic growth pattern is that of diffuse sheets of tumor cells, up to a third of cases will show a nodular growth pattern, of uncertain significance.

Chromosomal Abnormalities in Ependymomas

The most common cytogenetic abnormality in ependymomas is loss or structural alteration of chromosome 22, seen as an isolated finding in some patients and as part of a more complex picture in others. This alteration characterizes approximately 10 to 20 percent of patients with abnormal stem lines in most cytogenetic studies, and a similar incidence of chromosome 22 loss has been described in LOH studies.[101–112] Some observers, however, have noted this abnormality in a high proportion of patients by karyotype[103,106,110] or by LOH analysis.[113,114] Since the *NF2* gene is located on 22q, it has been considered as a possible target for loss of this chromosomal region in ependymomas. However, since only one somatic mutation of this gene has been reported among 25 ependymomas that were studied, the role of *NF2* mutations in ependymomas remains speculative.[115]

MEDULLOBLASTOMAS

Medulloblastoma, the most common malignant primary brain tumor of childhood, is a small cell neoplasm that arises in the cerebellum. Owing to the primitive morphology of the cells with lack of differentiation and their resemblance to some poorly differentiated supratentorial neoplasms, these tumors have been called "primitive neuroectodermal tumors (PNET)" by some observers. They are characterized by sheets of small cells with scant cytoplasm and a high mitotic rate (Fig. 47-8). Medulloblastomas are usually a sporadic tumor but can be seen in association with familial adenomatous polyposis (see Chap. 34). In the United Kingdom, the incidence of medulloblastoma has been estimated at 0.5 per 100,000 children less than 15 years old age,[116] with an overall age-adjusted incidence reported by the Central Brain Tumor Registry of the United States (CBTRUS) of 0.2 per 100,000.[117]

Chromosomal Abnormalities in Medulloblastomas

The most common specific chromosomal abnormality in medulloblastomas is loss of 17p, through formation of isochromosome 17q [i(17q)] or by unbalanced translocations[103,104,111,118–123] (Fig. 47-9). By karyotype as well as LOH studies, the incidence of this feature is approximately 30 to 40 percent.[113,124–129] Despite the location of the *TP53* gene on 17p, *TP53* gene mutations are uncommon in these tumors, seen in about 5 percent of cases.[126,128,130–135] This observation, along with mapping of the deleted region to 17p13.1-13.3, which is distal to the *p53* gene, suggests that another as yet undescribed gene is likely to be the target of 17p loss in these tumors.

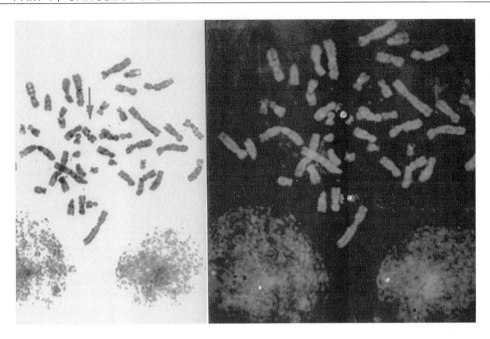

Fig. 47-9 Medulloblastoma with i(17q). The dark label that corresponds to a 17q probe stains the normal q arm of one chromosome 17 and both q arms of the i(17q). The light label marks the 17 centromere in both the normal chromosome 17 and i(17q).

Genetic Alterations in Medulloblastomas

Dmins are seen in about 5 percent of medulloblastoma biopsies but can be identified in almost all permanent cultured cell lines and xenografts derived from these.[118,136] In most samples with Dmins, amplification of the *c-myc* or, less often, the *N-myc* gene can be demonstrated[128,136–142] (Fig. 47-10). The true incidence of *myc* gene amplification is difficult to determine in these tumors because the observed incidence differs according to the method of analysis. However, a recent analysis by comparative genomic hybridization suggested that it may be as high as 18 percent.[143]

The gene for the nevoid basal cell carcinoma (Gorlin) syndrome was mapped to 9q22.3-q31 by linkage analysis. Since patients with this genetic defect are susceptible to developing medulloblastoma, this region was investigated by LOH studies in 3 medulloblastomas from patients with this syndrome and 17 sporadic medulloblastomas by Schofield *et al.*[144] They found loss of this region in both informative cases from Gorlin syndrome patients and in 3 of 17 (18 percent) sporadic tumors. All 3 sporadic tumors with loss were of the desmoplastic type. The Gorlin syndrome gene was identified as *PTCH,* the human homologue of the *Drosophila patched* gene, by Johnson *et al.*[145] and Hahn *et al.*[146] Raffel *et al.*[147] demonstrated mutations of *PTCH* in 3 of 5 sporadic medulloblastomas with 9q LOH. Reports from other laboratories have confirmed *PTCH* mutations in about 15 percent of sporadic medulloblastomas.[148–151] The majority of tumors containing the deletions have desmoplastic histology and exhibit LOH for 9q22. The *PTCH* gene product is a transmembrane receptor for the Sonic hedgehog protein. This observation has prompted investigators to evaluate other members of the *PTCH* gene pathway for alterations in medulloblastoma. Reifenberger *et al.*[152] have described one sporadic medulloblastoma with a mutation of the *SMOH* gene, the product of which is known to complex with *PTCH.*

Medulloblastomas are often seen in Turcot syndrome patients who carry germ-line mutations of the *APC* gene.[153] Although mutations of the *APC* gene have not been demonstrated in sporadic medulloblastomas, the β-catenin gene, the product of which

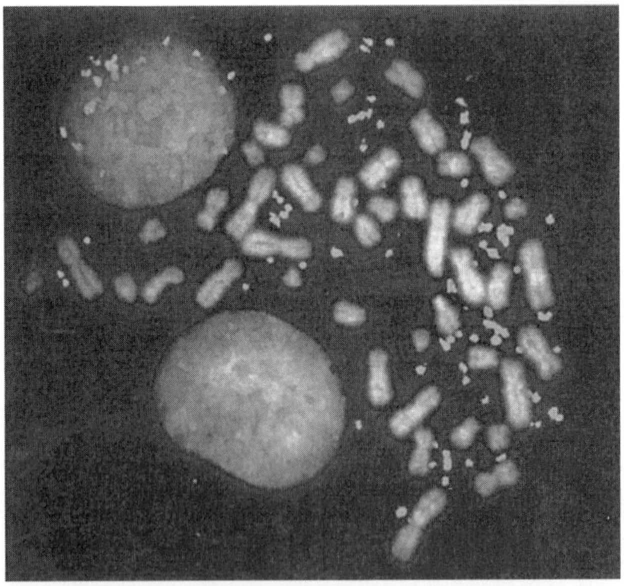

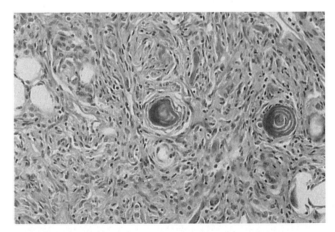

Fig. 47-10 Medulloblastoma with *c-myc* gene amplification. The *c-myc* probe, labeled darkly, is duplicated numerous times, as seen in the interphase nuclei and in the Dmins of a chromosomal spread.

Fig. 47-11 Meningiomas are dural-based neoplasms that grow as noninfiltrating masses, pushing brain away. These spindle cell tumors are often arranged in whorls and cords separated by collagen and occasionally are associated with eosinophilic psammoma bodies.

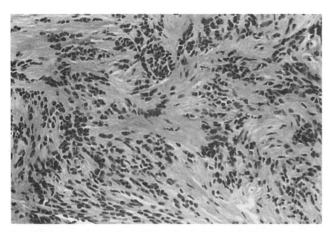

Fig. 47-12 Schwannomas also grow as solid, noninfiltrating tumors but are found along peripheral, and some cranial, nerves. The histologic hallmark of the schwannoma is the Verocay body, which is an anuclear zone formed by palisading tumor cell nuclei.

interacts with the *APC* gene product, has been shown to be mutated in 3 of 67 sporadic medulloblastomas.[154]

MENINGIOMA AND SCHWANNOMA

Meningiomas are slow-growing neoplasms derived from the meningothelial cell that forms the arachnoid membrane. These tumors are composed of swirling sheets of cells with oval nuclei, often forming whorls and psammoma bodies (Fig. 47-11). They are generally considered to be benign, because they often can be excised completely surgically, but occasional cases recur and can show aggressive clinical characteristics. SEER data indicate an age-adjusted incidence of 0.13 per 100,000, although data reported by CBTRUS support a much higher incidence of 2.5 per 100,000.[116,117]

Schwannomas are benign neoplasms, derived from the schwann cell that forms myelin in the peripheral nervous system. They are found attached to cranial or peripheral nerves, with favored sites being the acoustic and other sensory nerves. CBTRUS data report an overall incidence of nerve sheath tumors

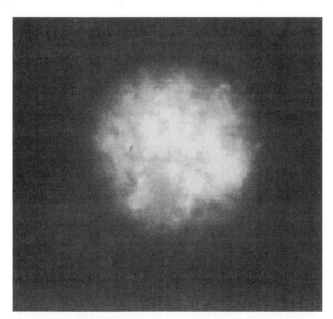

Fig. 47-13 FISH using a chromosome 22 probe in a meningioma. This interphase nucleus from a meningioma contains only one chromosome 22 signal.

of 0.7 per 100,000.[117] Histologically, they form masses of spindle-shaped cells and are usually benign (Fig. 47-12). Both schwannomas, particularly bilateral lesions involving the acoustic nerves, and meningiomas are components of central neurofibromatosis type 2, and peripheral schwannomas occur in peripheral neurofibromatosis or NF type 1 (see Chaps. 25 and 26).

Genetic Alterations in Meningiomas and Schwannomas

One of the first chromosomal abnormalities described in a solid human tumor was monosomy for a G-group chromosome.[155] With the implementation of banding techniques, the missing chromosome was identified as number 22 in the early 1970s.[156,157] Loss or deletion of chromosome 22 is the most consistent karyotypic abnormality seen in this tumor type, occurring in about 60 percent of cases[158] (Fig. 47-13). LOH studies confirmed loss of 22q in 40 to 60 percent of both meningiomas and schwannomas.[159–165] This observation, taken together with the occurrence of these tumors in NF2 and linkage studies that localized the NF2 locus to 22q, raised the possibility that the *NF2* gene was the target of chromosome 22 loss in these two tumor types. Isolation of the *NF2* gene and sequencing of this gene in these tumors confirmed that 40 to 60 percent of sporadic meningiomas and schwannomas contain *NF2* gene mutations.[166–172]

REFERENCES

1. Velema JP, Percy CL: Age curves of central nervous system tumor incidence in adults: Variation of shape by histologic type. *J Natl Cancer Inst* **79**:623, 1987.
2. Kleihues P, Burger PC, Scheithauer BW: *Histological Typing of Tumours of the Central Nervous System*, 2nd ed. New York, Springer-Verlag, 1993.
3. Burger PC, Scheithauer BW, Vogel FS: *Surgical Pathology of the Nervous System and Its Coverings*. New York, Churchill-Livingstone, 1991.
4. Rey JA, Bellow J, deCampos JM, Kusak EM, Ramos C, Benitez J: Chromosomal patterns in human malignant astrocytomas. *Cancer Genet Cytogenet* **29**:201, 1987.
5. Bigner SH, Mark J, Burger P, Mahaley MS Jr, Bullard DE, Muhlbaier LH, Bigner DD: Specific chromosomal abnormalities in malignant human gliomas. *Cancer Res* **48**:405, 1988.
6. Jenkins RJ, Kimmel DW, Moertel CA, Schultz CG, Schiethauer BW, Kelly PJ, Dewald GW: A cytogenetic study of 53 human gliomas. *Cancer Genet Cytogenet* **39**:253, 1989.
7. Thiel G, Losanowa T, Kintzel D, Nisch G, Martin H, Vorpahl K, Witkowski R: Karyotypes in 90 human gliomas. *Cancer Genet Cytogenet* **58**:109, 1992.
8. Hecht BK, Turc-Carel C, Chatel M, Grellier P, Gioanni J, Attias R, Gaudray P, Hecht F: Cytogenetics of malignant gliomas: 1. The autosomes with reference to rearrangements. *Cancer Genet Cytogenet* **84**:1, 1995.
9. Debiec-Rychter M, Alwasiak J, Liberski PP, Nedoszytko B, Babinska M, Mrózek K, Imielinski B, Borowska-Lehman J, Limon J: Accumulation of chromosomal changes in human glioma progression: A cytogenetic study of 50 cases. *Cancer Genet Cytogenet* **85**:61, 1995.
10. Fults D, Pedone C: Deletion mapping of the long arm of chromosome 10 in glioblastoma multiforme. *Genes Chromosom Cancer* **7**:173, 1993.
11. Rasheed BK, McLendon RE, Friedman HS, Friedman AH, Fuchs HE, Bigner DD, Bigner SH: Chromosome 10 deletion mapping in human gliomas: A common deletion region in 10q25. *Oncogene* **10**:2243, 1995.
12. Ransom DT, Ritland SR, Moertel CA, Dahl RJ, O'Fallon JR, Scheithauer BW, Kimmel DW, Kelly PJ, Olopade OI, Diaz MO, Jenkins RB: Correlation of cytogenetic analysis and loss of heterozygosity studies in human diffuse astrocytomas and mixed oligo-astrocytomas. *Genes Chromosom Cancer* **5**:357, 1992.
13. Karlbom AE, James CD, Boethius J, Cavenee WK, Collins VP, Nordenskjold M, Larsson C: Loss of heterozygosity in malignant gliomas involves at least three distinct regions on chromosome 10. *Hum Genet* **92**:169, 1993.
14. Kimmelman AC, Ross DA, Liang BC: Loss of heterozygosity of chromosome 10p in human gliomas. *Genomics* **34**:250, 1996.

15. Li J, Yen C, Liaw D, Podsypanina K, Bose S, Wang WI, Puc J, Millaresis C, Rodgers L, McCombie R, Bigner SH, Giovanelia BC, Ittmann M, Tycko B, Hibshoosh H, Wigler MH, Parsons R: *PTEN*, a putative protein tyrosine phosphatase gene mutated in human brain, breast, and prostate cancer. *Science* 273:1943, 1997.

16. Steck PA, Pershouse MA, Jasser SA, Yung WKA, Lin H, Ligon AH, Langford LA, Baumgard ML, Hattier T, Davis T, Frye C, Hu R, Swedland B, Teng DHF, Tavtigian SV: Identification of a candidate tumour suppressor gene, *MMAC1*, a chromosome 10q23.3 that is mutated in multiple advanced cancers. *Nature Genet* 15:356, 1997.

17. Wang SI, Pac J, Li J, Brace JN, Cairns P, Sidramsky D, Parsons R: Somatic mutations of *PTEN* in glioblastoma multiforme. *Cancer Res* 57:4183, 1997.

18. Liu W, James CD, Frederick L, Alderete BE, Jenkins RB: *PTEN/MAC1* mutations and *EGFR* amplification in glioblastomas. *Cancer Res* 57:5254, 1997.

19. Teng DHJ, Hu R, Lin H, Davis T, Ilev D, Frye C, Swedlund B, Hansen KL, Vinson VL, Gumpper KL, Ellis L, El-Naggar A, Frazier M, Jasser S, Langford LA, Lee J, Mills GB, Perhouse MA, Pollack RE, Tornos C, Troncoso P, Yung WKA, Fujii G, Berson A, Bookstein R, Boten JB, Tavtigian SV, Steck PA: *MMAC1/PTEN* mutations in primary tumor specimens and tumor cell lines. *Cancer Res* 57:5231, 1997.

20. Fults D, Pedone CA, Thompson GE, Uchiyama CM, Gumpper KL, Iliev D, Vinson VL, Tavtigian SV, Perry WL III: Microsatellite deletion mapping on chromosome 10q and mutation analysis of *MMAC1, FAS,* and *MX11* in human glioblastoma multiforme. *Int J Oncol* 12:905, 1998.

21. Boström J, Cobbers JMJL, Wolter M, Tabatabai G, Weber RG, Lichter P, Collins VP, Reifenberger G: Mutation of the *PTEN (MMAC1)* tumor suppressor gene in a subset of glioblastomas but not in meningiomas with loss of chromosome arm 10q. *Cancer Res* 51:29, 1998.

22. Cairns P, Okami K, Hatachmi S, Hatachmi N, Esteller M, Herman JG, Jen J, Isaacs WB, Bova GS, Sidransky D: Frequent inactivation of *PTEN/MMAC1* in primary prostate cancer. *Cancer Res* 57:4997, 1997.

23. Maxwell GL, Risinger JI, Gumbs C, Shaw H, Bentley RC, Barrett JC, Berchuck A, Futreal PA: Mutation of the *PTEN* tumor suppressor gene in endometrial hyperplasias. *Cancer Res* 58:2500, 1998.

24. Marsh DJ, Dahia PLM, Zheng Z, Liaw D, Parsons R, Gorlin RJ, Eng C: Germline mutations in *PTEN* are present in Bannayan-Zonana syndrome. *Nature Genet* 16:333, 1997.

25. Marsh DJ, Dahia PLM, Coulon V, Zheng Z, Dorion-Bonnet F, Call KM, Little R, Lin AY, Eles RA, Goldstein AM, Hodgson SV, Richardson A-L, Robinson BG, Weber HC Longy M, Eng C: Allelic imbalance, including deletion of *PTEN/MMAC1,* at the Cowden disease locus on 10q22-23, in hamartomas from patients with Cowden syndrome and germline *PTEN* mutation. *Genes Chromosom Cancer* 21:61, 1998.

26. Li DM, Sum H: *TEP1,* encoded by a candidate tumor suppressor locus is a novel protein tyrosine phosphatase regulated by transforming growth factor β1. *Cancer Res* 57:2124, 1997.

27. Rasheed BKA, Stenzel TT, McLendon RE, Parsons R, Friedman AH, Friedman HS, Bigner DD, Bigner SH: *PTEN* gene mutations are seen in high-grade but not in low-grade gliomas. *Cancer Res* 57:4187, 1997.

28. Duerr EM, Rollbrocker B, Hayashi Y, Peters N, Meyer-Puttlitz B, Louis DN, Schramm J, Wiestler OD, Parsons R, Eng C, von Deimling A: *PTEN* mutations in gliomas and glioneuronal tumors. *Oncogene* 16:2259, 1998.

29. Tohma Y, Gratas C, Biernat W, Peraud A, Foxuda M, Yonekawa Y, Kleihues P, Ohgaki H: *PTEN (MMAC1)* mutations are frequent in primary glioblastomas (de novo) but not in secondary glioblastomas. *J Neuropathol Exp Neurol* 57:684, 1998.

30. Eagle LR, Yin X, Brothman AR, Williams BJ, Atkin NB, Prochownik EV: Mutation of the *MX11* gene in prostate cancer. *Nature Genet* 9:249, 1995.

31. Stapleton P, Weith A, Urbanek P, Kozmik Z, Busslinger M: Chromosomal localization of seven *PAX* genes and cloning of a novel family member, *PAX-9. Nature Genet* 3:292, 1993.

32. Wechsler DS, Shelly CA, Petroff CA, Dang CV: *MX11,* a putative tumor suppressor gene, suppresses growth of human glioblastoma cells. *Cancer Res* 57:4905, 1997.

33. Mollenhauer J, Wiemann S, Scheurlen W, Korn B, Hayashi Y, Wilgenbus KK, von Diemling A, Poustka A: *DMBT1,* a new member of the SRCR superfamily, on chromosome 10q25.3-26.1 is deleted in malignant brain tumours. *Nature Genet* 17:32, 1997.

34. Eel-Azouzi M, Chung RY, Farmer GE, Martuza RL, Black PM, Rouleau GA, Hettlich C, Hedley-Whyte ET, Zervas NT, Panagopoulos K, Nakamura Y, Gusella JF, Seizinger BR: Loss of distinct regions on

35. Fults D, Tippets RH, Thomas RJ, Nakamura Y, White R: Loss of heterozygosity for loci on chromosome 17p in human malignant astrocytoma. *Cancer Res* 49:6572, 1989.

36. James CD, Carlbom E, Nordenskjold M, Collins VP, Cavenee WK: Mitotic recombination of chromosome 17 in astrocytomas. *Proc Natl Acad Sci USA* 86:2858, 1989.

37. Venter DJ, Bevan KL, Ludwig RL, Riley TEW, Jat PS, Thomas DGT, Noble MD: Retinoblastoma gene deletions in human glioblastomas. *Oncogene* 6:445, 1991.

38. Fults D, Brockmeyer D, Tullous MW, Pedone CA, Cawthon RM: *P53* mutation and loss of heterozygosity on chromosomes 17 and 10 during human astrocytoma progression. *Cancer Res* 52:674, 1992.

39. von Deimling A, Eibl RH, Ohgaki H, Louis DN, von Ammon K, Petersen I, Kleihues P, Chung RY, Wiestler OD, Seizinger BR: *p53* mutations are associated with 17p allelic loss in grade II and grade III astrocytoma. *Cancer Res* 52:2987, 1992.

40. Frankel RH, Bayona W, Koslow M, Newcomb EW: *p53* mutations in human malignant gliomas: Comparison of loss of heterozygosity with mutation frequency. *Cancer Res* 52:1427, 1992.

41. Lang FF, Miller DC, Koslow M, Newcomb EW: Pathways leading to glioblastoma multiforme: A molecular analysis of genetic alterations in 65 astrocytic tumors. *J Neurosurg* 81:427, 1994.

42. Leenstra S, Bijlsma EK, Troost D, Oosting J, Westerveld A, Bosch D, Huslebos TJM: Allele loss on chromosomes 10 and 17p and epidermal growth factor receptor amplification in human malignant astrocytoma related to prognosis. *Br J Cancer* 70:684, 1994.

43. Rasheed BK, McLendon RE, Herndon JE, Friedman HS, Friedman AH, Bigner DD, Bigner SH: Alterations of the *TP53* gene in human gliomas. *Cancer Res* 54:1324, 1994.

44. Tenan M, Colombo BM, Pollo B, Cajola L, Broggi G, Finocchiaro G: *P53* mutations and microsatellite analysis of loss of heterozygosity in malignant gliomas. *Cancer Genet Cytogenet* 74:139, 1994.

45. Hermanson M, Funa K, Koopmann J, Maintz D, Waha A, Westermark B, Heldin CH, Wiestler OD, Louis DN, von Deimling A, Nister M: Association of loss of heterozygosity on chromosome 17p with high platelet-derived growth factor alpha receptor expression in human malignant gliomas. *Cancer Res* 56:164, 1996.

46. Chung R, Whaley J, Kley N, Anderson K, Louis D, Menon A, Hettlich C, Freiman R, Hedley-Whyte ET, Martuza R, Jenkins R, Yandell D, Seizinger BR: *TP53* gene mutations and 17p deletions in human astrocytomas. *Genes Chromosom Cancer* 3:323, 1991.

47. Mashiyama S, Murakami Y, Yoshimoto T, Sekiya T, Hayashi K: Detection of *p53* gene mutations in human brain tumors by single-strand conformation polymorphism analysis of polymerase chain reaction products. *Oncogene* 6:1313, 1991.

48. Louis DN: The *p53* gene and protein in human brain tumors. *J Neuropathol Exp Neurol* 53:11, 1994.

49. Kraus JA, Bolln C, Wolf HK, Neumann J, Kindermann D, Fimmers R, Forster F, Baumann A, Schlegel U: *TP53* alterations and clinical outcome in low grade astrocytomas. *Genes Chromosom Cancer* 10:143, 1994.

50. Lang FF, Miller DC, Pisharody S, Koslow M, Newcomb E: High frequency of p53 protein accumulation without *p53* gene mutation in human juvenile pilocytic, low grade and anaplastic astrocytomas. *Oncogene* 9:949, 1994.

51. Alderson LM, Castleberg RL, Harsh GR, Louis DN, Henson JW: Human gliomas with wild-type p53 express bcl-2. *Cancer Res* 55:999, 1995.

52. Chen P, Iavarone A, Fick J, Edwards M, Prados M, Israel MA: Constitutional *p53* mutations associated with brain tumors in young adults. *Cancer Genet Cytogenet* 82:106, 1995.

53. Kyritsis AP, Xu R, Bondy ML, Levin V, Bruner JM: Correlation of p53 immunoreactivity and sequencing in patients with glioma. *Mol Carcinogen* 15:1, 1996.

54. Bogler O, Huang H-JS, Kleihues P, Cavenee WK: The *p53* gene and its role in human brain tumors. *Glia* 15:308, 1995.

55. Litofsky NS, Hinton D, Raffel C: The lack of a role for p53 in astrocytomas in pediatric patients. *Neurosurgery* 34:967, 1994.

56. Willert JR, Daneshvar L, Sheffield VC, Cogen PH: Deletion of chromosome arm 17p DNA sequences in pediatric high-grade and juvenile pilocytic astrocytomas. *Genes Chromosom Cancer* 12:165, 1995.

57. Miyakoshi J, Dobler KD, Allalunis-Turner J, McKean JD, Petruk K, Allen PBR, Aronyk KN, Weir B, Huyser-Wierenga D, Fulton D, Urtsun RC, Day RS III: Absence of *IFNA* and *IFNB* genes from human

malignant glioma cell lines and lack of correlation with cellular sensitivity to interferons. *Cancer Res* **50**:278, 1990.

58. Olopade OI, Jenkins RB, Ransom DT, Malik K, Pomykala H, Nobori T, Cowan JM, Rowley JD, Diaz MO: Molecular analysis of deletions of the short arm of chromosome 9 in human gliomas. *Cancer Res* **52**:2523, 1992.

59. Kamb A, Grui NA, Weaver-Feldhaus J, Liu Q, Harshman K, Tavtigian SV, Stockert E, Day RS, Johnson BE, Skolnick MH: A cell cycle regulator potentially involved in genes of many tumor types. *Science* **264**:436, 1994.

60. Jen J, Harper JW, Bigner SH, Bigner DD, Papadopoulos N, Markowitz S, Wilson JKV, Kinzler KW, Vogelstein B: Deletion of *p16* and *p15* genes in brain tumors. *Cancer Res* **54**:6353, 1994.

61. Ueki K, Rubio MP, Ramesh V, Correa KM, Rutter JL, von Deimling A, Buckler AJ, Gusella JF, Louis DN: *MTS1/CDKN2* gene mutations are rare in primary human astrocytomas with allelic loss of chromosome 9p. *Hum Mol Genet* **3**:1841, 1994.

62. Giani C, Finocchiaro G: Mutation rate of the *CDKN2* gene in malignant gliomas. *Cancer Res* **54**:6338, 1994.

63. He J, Allen JR, Collins VP, Allalunis-Turner MJ, Godbout R, Day RS, James CD: CDK4 amplifications is an alternative mechanism to *p16* gene homozygous deletion in glioma cell lines. *Cancer Res* **54**:5804, 1994.

64. Schmidt EE, Ichimura K, Reifenberger G, Collins VP: *CDKN2* (*p16/ MTS1*) gene deletion or CDK4 amplification occurs in the majority of glioblastomas. *Cancer Res* **54**:6321, 1994.

65. Moulton T, Samara G, Chung WY, Yuan L, Desai R, Sist, Bruce J, Tycko B: *MTS1/p16/CDKN2* lesions in primary glioblastoma multiforme. *Am J Pathol* **146**:613, 1995.

66. Nishikawa R, Furnari FB, Lin H, Arap W, Berger MS, Cavenee WK, Su Huang HJ: Loss of P16[INK4] expression is frequent in high grade gliomas. *Cancer Res* **55**:1941, 1995.

67. Walker DG, Duan W, Popovic EA, Kaye AH, Tomlinson FH, Lavin M: Homozygous deletions of the multiple tumor suppressor gene 1 in the progression of human astrocytomas. *Cancer Res* **55**:20, 1995.

68. Sonoda Y, Yoshimoto T, Sekiya T: Homozygous deletion of the *MTS1/ p16* and *MTS2/p15* genes and amplification of the *CDK4* gene in glioma. *Oncogene* **11**:2145, 1995.

69. Li YJ, Hoang-Xuan K, Delattre JY, Poisson M, Thomas G, Hamelin R: Frequent loss of heterozygosity on chromosome 9, and low incidence of mutations of cyclin-dependent kinase inhibitors *p15* (*MTS2*) and *p16* (*MTS1*) genes in gliomas. *Oncogene* **11**:597, 1995.

70. Ueki K, Ono Y, Henson JW, Efird JT, von Deimling A, Louis DN: *CDKN2/p16* or *RB* alterations occur in the majority of glioblastomas and are inversely correlated. *Cancer Res* **56**:150, 1996.

71. Herman JG, Merlo A, Mao L, Lapidus RG, Issa JPJ, Davidson NE, Sidransky D, Baylin SB: Inactivation of the *CDKN2/p16/MTS1* gene is frequently associated with aberrant DNA methylation in all common human cancers. *Cancer Res* **55**:4525, 1995.

72. Bigner SH, Wong AJ, Mark J, Muhlbaier LH, Kinzler KW, Vogelstein B, Bigner DD: Relationship between gene amplification and chromosomal deviations in malignant human gliomas. *Cancer Genet Cytogenet* **29**:165, 1987.

73. Wong AJ, Bigner SH, Bigner DD, Kinzler KW, Hamilton SR, Vogelstein B: Increased expression of the epidermal growth factor receptor gene in malignant gliomas is invariably associated with gene amplification. *Proc Natl Acad Sci USA* **84**:6899, 1993.

74. Bigner SH, Humphrey PA, Wong AJ, Vogelstein B, Mark J, Friedman HS, Bigner DD: Characterization of the epidermal growth factor receptor in human glioma cell lines and xenografts. *Cancer Res* **50**:8017, 1990.

75. Humphrey PA, Wong AJ, Vogelstein B, Zalutsky MR, Fuller GN, Archer GE, Friedman HS, Kwatra MM, Bigner SH, Bigner DD: Anti-synthetic peptide antibody reacting at the fusion junction of deletion-mutant epidermal growth factor receptors in human glioblastoma. *Proc Natl Acad Sci USA* **87**:4207, 1990.

76. Sugawa N, Ekstrand A, James CD, Collins VP: Identical splicing of aberrant epidermal growth factor receptor transcripts from amplified rearranged genes in human glioblastomas. *Proc Natl Acad Sci USA* **87**:8602, 1990.

77. Ekstrand AJ, James CD, Cavenee WK, Seliger B, Pettersson RF, Collins VP: Genes for epidermal growth factor receptor, transforming growth factor alpha, and epidermal growth factor and their expression in human gliomas in vivo. *Cancer Res* **51**:2164, 1991.

78. Ekstrand AJ, Sugawa N, James CD, Collins VP: Amplified and rearranged epidermal growth factor receptor genes in human glioblastomas reveal deletions of sequences encoding portions of the N- and/or C-terminal tails. *Proc Natl Acad Sci USA* **89**:4309, 1992.

79. Moscatello DK, Holgado-Madruga M, Godwin AK, Ramirez G, Gunn G, Zoltick PW, Biegel J, Hayes RL, Wong AJ: Frequent expression of a mutant epidermal growth factor receptor in multiple human tumors. *Cancer Res* **55**:5536, 1995.

80. Wikstrand CJ, Hale LP, Batra SK, Hill ML, Humphrey PA, Kurpad SN, McLendon RE, Moscatello D, Pegram CN, Reist CJ, Traweek T, Wong AJ, Zalutsky MR, Bigner DD: Monoclonal antibodies against EGFRvIII are tumor specific and react with breast and lung carcinomas and malignant gliomas. *Cancer Res* **55**:3140, 1995.

81. Yamazaki H, Fukui Y, Ueyama Y, Tamaoki N, Kawamoto T, Taniguchi S, Shibuya M: Amplification of the structurally and functionally altered epidermal growth factor receptor gene (*c-erbB*) in human brain tumors. *Mol Cell Biol* **8**:1816, 1988.

82. Batra SK, Castelino-Prabhu S, Wikstrand CJ, Zhu X, Humphrey PA, Friedman HS, Bigner DD: Epidermal growth factor ligand-independent, unregulated, cell-transforming potential of a naturally occurring human mutant *EGFRvIII* gene. *Cell Growth Diff* **6**:1251, 1995.

83. James CD, He J, Carlbom E, Dumanski JP, Hansen M, Nordenskjld M, Collins VP, Cavenee WK: Clonal genomic alterations in glioma malignancy stages. *Cancer Res* **48**:5546, 1988.

84. Fults D, Pedone CA, Thomas GA, White R: Allelotype of human malignant astrocytoma. *Cancer Res* **50**:5784, 1990.

85. Henson JW, Schnitker BL, Correa KM, von Deimling A, Fassbender F, Xu HJ, Benedict WF, Yandell DW, Louis DN: The retinoblastoma gene is involved in malignant progression of astrocytomas. *Ann Neurol* **3**:714, 1994.

86. He J, Olson JJ, James CD: Lack of p16[INK4] or retinoblastoma protein (pRb), or amplification-associated overexpression of cdk4 is observed in distinct subsets of malignant glial tumors and cell lines. *Cancer Res* **55**:4833, 1995.

87. Reifenberger G, Reifenberger J, Ichimura K, Meltzer PS, Collins VP: Amplification of multiple genes from chromosomal region 12q13-14 in human malignant gliomas: Preliminary mapping of the amplicons shows preferential involvement of *CDK4, SAS,* and *MDM2. Cancer Res* **54**:4299, 1994.

88. Biernat W, Yohma Y, Yonekawa Y, Kleihues P, Oligaki H: Alterations of cell cycle regulatory genes in primary (*de novo*) and secondary glioblastomas. *Acta Neuropathol* **94**:303, 1997.

89. von Deimling A, von Ammon K, Schoenfeld D, Wiestler OD, Seizinger BR, Louis DN: Subsets of glioblastoma multiforme defined by molecular genetic analysis. *Brain Pathol* **3**:19, 1993.

90. Ohgaki H, Schauble B, zur Hausen A, von Ammon K, Kleihues P: Genetic alterations associated with the evolution and progression of astrocytic brain tumours. *Virchows Arch* **427**:113, 1995.

91. Watanabe K, Tachibana O, Sato K, Yonekawa Y, Kleihues P, Ohgaki H: Overexpression of the EGF receptor and *p53* mutations are mutually exclusive in the evolution of primary and secondary glioblastomas. *Brain Pathol* **6**:217, 1996.

92. Louis DN: Clinicopathogenetic subsets of glioblastoma multiform: From both sides now. *Brain Pathol* **6**:223, 1996.

93. Kleihues P, Ohgaki H: Genetics of glioma progression and the definition of primary and secondary glioblastoma. *Brain Pathol* **7**:1131, 1997.

94. Bello MJ, Vaquero J, de Campos JM, Kusak ME, Sarasa JL, Szez-Castresana J, Pestana A, Rey JA: Molecular analysis of chromosome 1 abnormalities in human gliomas reveals frequent loss of 1p in oligodendroglial tumors. *Int J Cancer* **57**:172, 1994.

95. Reifenberger J, Reifenberger G, Liu L, James CD, Wechsler W, Collins VP: Molecular genetic analysis of oligodendroglial tumors shows preferential allelic deletions on 19q and 1p. *Am J Pathol* **145**:1175, 1994.

96. Hashimoto N, Ichikawa D, Arakawa Y, Date K, Ueda S, Nakagawa Y, Horil A, Nakamura Y, Abe T, Inazawa J: Frequent deletions of material from chromosome arm 1p in oligodendroglial tumors revealed by double-target fluorescence in situ hybridization and microsatellite analysis. *Genes Chromosom Cancer* **14**:295, 1995.

97. von Deimling A, Nagel J, Bender B, Lenartz D, Schramm J, Louis DN, Wiestler OD: Deletion mapping of chromosome 19 in human gliomas. *Int J Cancer* **57**:676, 1994.

98. Ritland SR, Ganju V, Jenkins RB: Region-specific loss of heterozygosity on chromosome 19 is related to the morphologic type of human glioma. *Genes Chromosom Cancer* **12**:277, 1995.

99. Rubio MP, Correa KM, Ueki K, Mohrenweiser HW, Gusella JF, von Deimling A, Louis DN: The putative glioma tumor suppressor gene on

chromosome 19q maps between *APOC2* and *HRC*. *Cancer Res* **54**:4760, 1994.

100. Yong WH, Chou D, Ueki K, Harsh GR IV, von Deimling A, Gusella JF, Mohrenweiser HW, Louis DN: Chromosome 19q deletions in human gliomas overlap telomeric to D19S219 and may target a 425 kb region centromeric to D19S112. *J Neuropathol Exp Neurol* **54**:622, 1995.

101. Brown NP, Pearson ADJ, Davison EV, Gardner-Medwin D, Crawford P, Perry RK: Multiple chromosome rearrangements in a childhood ependymoma. *Cancer Genet Cytogenet* **36**:25, 1988.

102. Stratton MR, Darling J, Lantos PL, Cooper CS, Reeves BR: Cytogenetic abnormalities in human ependymomas. *Int J Cancer* **44**:579, 1989.

103. Chadduck WM, Boop FA, Sawyer JR: Cytogenetic studies of pediatric brain and spinal cord tumors. *Pediatr Neurosurg* **17**:57, 1991.

104. Vagner-Capodano AM, Gentet JC, Gambarelli D, Pellissier JF, Gouzien M, Lena G, Genitori L, Choux M, Raybaud C: Cytogenetic studies in 45 pediatric brain tumors. *Pediatr Hematol Oncol* **9**:223, 1992.

105. Weremowicz S, Kupsky WJ, Morton CC, Fletcher JA: Cytogenetic evidence for a chromosome 22 tumor suppressor gene in ependymoma. *Cancer Genet Cytogenet* **61**:193, 1992.

106. Rogatto SR, Casartelli C, Rainho CA, Barbieri-Neto J: Chromosomes in the genes and progression of ependymomas. *Cancer Genet Cytogenet* **69**:146, 1993.

107. Neumann E, Kalousek DK, Norman MG, Stienbok P, Cochrane DD, Goddard K: Cytogenetic analysis of 109 pediatric central nervous system tumors. *Cancer Genet Cytogenet* **71**:40, 1993.

108. Sawyer JR, Sammartino G, Husain M, Boop FA, Chadduck WM: Chromosome aberrations in four ependymomas. *Cancer Genet Cytogenet* **74**:132, 1994.

109. Bijlsma EK, Voesten AMJ, Bijleveld EH, Troost D, Westerveld A, Mérel P, Thomas G, Huslebos TJM: Molecular analysis of genetic changes in ependymomas. *Genes Chromosom Cancer* **13**:272, 1995.

110. Wernicke C, Thiel G, Lozanova T, Vogel S, Kintzel D, Jünisch W, Lehmann K, Witkowski R: Involvement of chromosome 22 in ependymomas. *Cancer Genet Cytogenet* **79**:173, 1995.

111. Agamanolis DP, Malone JM: Chromosomal abnormalities in 47 pediatric brain tumors. *Cancer Genet Cytogenet* **81**:125, 1995.

112. Blaeker H, Rasheed BKA, McLendon RE, Friedman H, Batra SK, Fuchs HE, Bigner SH: Microsatellite analysis of childhood brain tumors. *Genes Chromosom Cancer* **15**:54, 1996.

113. James CD, He J, Carlbom E, Mikkelsen T, Ridderheim PA, Cavenee WK, Collins VP: Loss of genetic information in central nervous system tumors common to children and young adults. *Genes Chromosom Cancer* **2**:94, 1990.

114. Ransom DT, Ritland SR, Kimmel DW, Moertel CA, Dahl RJ, Scheithauer BW, Kelly PJ, Jenkins RB: Cytogenetic and loss of heterozygosity studies in ependymomas, pilocytic astrocytomas, and oligodendrogliomas. *Genes Chromosom Cancer* **5**:348, 1992.

115. Rubio M, Correa KM, Ramesh V, MacCollin MM, Jacoby .B, von Deimling A, Gusella JF, Louis DN: Analysis of the neurofibromatosis 2 gene in human ependymomas and astrocytomas. *Cancer Res* **54**:45, 1994.

116. Stevens MCG, Cameron AH, Muir KR, Parkes SE, Reid H, Whitwell H: Descriptive epidemiology of primary central nervous system tumours in children: A population-based study. *Clin Oncol* **3**:323, 1991.

117. Central Brain Tumor Registry of the United States: Annual Report. Chicago, 1995.

118. Bigner SH, Mark J, Friedman HS, Biegel JA, Bigner DD: Structural chromosomal abnormalities in human medulloblastomas. *Cancer Genet Cytogenet* **30**:91, 1988.

119. Griffin CA, Hawkins AL, Packer RJ, Rorke LB, Emanuel BS: Chromosome abnormalities in pediatric brain tumors. *Cancer Res* **48**:175, 1988.

120. Biegel JA, Rorke LB, Packer RJ, Sutton LN, Schut L, Bonner L, Emanuel S: Isochromosome 17q in primitive neuroectodermal tumors of the central nervous system. *Genes Chromosom Cancer* **1**:139, 1989.

121. Karnes PS, Tran TN, Cui MY, Raffel C, Gilles FH, Barranger JA, Ying KL: Cytogenetic analysis of 39 pediatric central nervous system tumors. *Cancer Genet Cytogenet* **59**:12, 1992.

122. Neumann E, Kalousek DK, Norman MG, Stienbok P, Cochrane DD, Goddard K: Cytogenetic analysis of 109 pediatric central nervous system tumors. *Cancer Genet Cytogenet* **71**:40, 1993.

123. Fuji Y, Hongo T, Hayashi Y: Chromosome analysis of brain tumors in childhood. *Genes Chromosom Cancer* **11**:205, 1994.

124. Thomas GA, Raffel C: Loss of heterozygosity on 6q, 16q and 17p in human central nervous system primitive neuroectodermal tumors. *Cancer Res* **51**:639, 1991.

125. Cogen P, Daneshvar L, Metzger AK, Edwards MSB: Deletion mapping of the medulloblastoma locus on chromosome 17p. *Genomics* **8**:279, 1990.

126. Biegel JA, Burk CD, Barr FG, Emanuel BS: Evidence for a 17p tumor related locus distinct from p53 in pediatric primitive neuroectodermal tumors. *Cancer Res* **52**:3391, 1992.

127. Albrecht S, von Deimling A, Pietsch T, Giangaspero F, Brandnert S, Kleiheust P, Wiestler OD: Microsatellite analysis of loss of heterozygosity on chromosomes 9q, 11p, and 17p in medulloblastoma. *Neuropathol Appl Neurobiol* **20**:74, 1994.

128. Batra SK, McLendon RE, Koo JS, Castelino-Prabhu S, Fuchs E, Krischer JP, Friedman HS, Bigner DD, Bigner SH: Prognostic implications of chromosome 17q deletions in human medulloblastomas. *J Neurooncol* **24**:39, 1995.

129. Scheurlen WG, Senf L: Analysis of the GAP-related domain of the neurofibromatosis type 1 (*NF1*) gene in childhood brain tumors. *Int J Cancer* **64**:234, 1995.

130. Ohgaki H, Eibl RH, Wiestler OD, Yasargil MG, Newcomb EW, Kleihues P: *P53* mutations in nonastrocytic human brain tumors. *Cancer Res* **51**:6202, 1991.

131. Saylors R, Sidransky D, Friedman HS, Bigner SH, Bigner DD, Vogelstein B, Brodeur GM: Infrequent *p53* gene mutations in medulloblastomas. *Cancer Res* **51**:4721, 1991.

132. Cogen PH, Daneshvar L, Metzgar AK, Geoffrey D, Edwards MSB, Sheffield VC: Involvement of multiple chromosome 17p loci in medulloblastoma tumorigenesis. *Am J Hum Genet* **50**:584, 1992.

133. Badiali M, Iolascon A, Loda M, Scheithauer B, Basso G, Trentini G, Giangaspero F: *p53* gene mutations in medulloblastoma, immunohistochemistry, gel shift analysis and sequencing. *Diagn Mol Pathol* **2**:23, 1993.

134. Raffel C, Thomas GA, Tishler DM, Lassof S, Allen JC: Absence of *p53* mutations in childhood central nervous system primitive neuroectodermal tumors. *Neurosurgery* **33**:301, 1993.

135. Adesina AM, Nalbantoglu J, Cavenee WK: *p53* gene mutation and *mdm2* gene amplification are uncommon in medulloblastoma. *Cancer Res* **54**:5649, 1994.

136. Bigner SH, Friedman HS, Vogelstein B, Oakes WJ, Bigner DD: Amplification of the *c-myc* gene in human medulloblastoma cell lines and xenografts. *Cancer Res* **50**:2347, 1990.

137. Raffel C, Gilles FE, Weinberg KI: Reduction to homozygosity and gene amplification in central nervous system primitive neuroectodermal tumors of childhood. *Cancer Res* **50**:587, 1990.

138. Badiali M, Pession A, Basso G, Andreini L, Rigobello L, Galassi E, Giangaspero F: *N-myc* and *c-myc* oncogenes amplification in medulloblastomas: Evidence of particularly aggressive behavior of a tumor with *c-myc* amplification. *Tumori* **77**:118, 1991.

139. Friedman HS, Burger PC, Bigner SH, Trojanowski JQ, Brodeur GM, He X, Wikstrand CJ, Kurtzberg J, Berens ME, Halperin EC, Bigner DD: Phenotypic and genotypic analysis of a human medulloblastoma cell line and transplantable xenograft (D341 Med) demonstrating amplification of *c-myc*. *Am J Pathol* **130**:472, 1988.

140. Wasson JC, Saylors RL, Zelter P, Friedman HS, Bigner SH, Burger PC, Bigner DD, Look AT, Douglass EC, Brodeur GM: Oncogene amplification in pediatric brain tumors. *Cancer Res* **50**:2987, 1990.

141. Batra SK, Rasheed A, Bigner SH, Bigner DD: Oncogenes and antioncogenes in human central nervous system tumors. *Lab Invest* **71**:621, 1994.

142. Pietsch T, Scharman T, Fonatsch CF, Schmidt D, Ockler R, Freihoff D, Albrecht S, Wiestler OW, Zeltzer P, Riehm H: Characterization of five new cell lines derived from human primitive neuroectodermal tumors of the central nervous system. *Cancer Res* **54**:3278, 1994.

143. Schütz BR, Scheurlen W, Krauss J, du Manoir S, Joos S, Bentz M, Lichter P: Mapping of chromosomal gains and losses in primitive neuroectodermal tumors by comparative genomic hybridization. *Genes Chromosom Cancer* **16**:196, 1996.

144. Schofield D, West DC, Anthony DC, Marshal R, Sklar J: Correlation of loss of heterozygosity at chromosome 9q with histological subtype in medulloblastomas. *Am J Pathol* **146**:472, 1995.

145. Johnson RL, Rothamn AL, Xie J, Goodrich LV, Bate JW, Bonifas JM, Quinn AC, Myers RM, Cox DR, Epstein EH Jr, Scott MP: Human homolog of patched, a candidate gene for the basal cell nevus syndrome. *Science* **272**:1668, 1996.

146. Hahn H, Wicking C, Zaphiropoulos C, Gailani MR, Stanley S, Chidanharam A, Vorechovsky J, Holmberg E, Unden AB, Giles S,

Negus K, Smyth I, Pressman C, Leffell DJ, Gerrard B, Goldstein AM, Dean M, Toftgard R, Chenevia-Trench G, Wainwright B, Bale AE: Mutations of the human homologue of *Drosophilia* patched in the nevoid basal cell carcinoma syndrome. *Cell* **85**:841, 1996.

147. Raffel C, Jenkins RB, Frederick L, Hebrink D, Alderete B, Fults DW, James CD: Sporadic medulloblastomas contain *PTCH* mutations. *Cancer Res* **57**:842, 1997.

148. Vorechovsky I, Tingby O, Hartman M, Strmberg B, Nister M, Collins VP, Toftgard R: Somatic mutations in the human homologue of *Drosophilia* patched in primitive neuroectodermal tumours. *Oncogene* **15**:361, 1997.

149. Pietsch T, Waha A, Koch A, Kraus J, Albrecht S, Tonn J, Srensen N, Berthold F, Henk B, Schmandt N, Wolf HK, von Diemling A, Wainwright B, Chenevix-Trench G, Wiestler OD, Wicking C: Medulloblastomas of the desmoplastic variant carry mutations of the human homologue of *Drosophilia* patched. *Cancer Res* **57**:2085, 1997.

150. Wolter M, Reifenberger J, Sommer C, Ruzicka T, Reifenberger G: Mutations in the human homologue of the *Drosophilia* segment polarity gene patched (*PTCH*) in sporadic basal cell carcinomas of the skin and primitive neuroectodermal tumors of the central nervous system. *Cancer Res* **57**:2581, 1997.

151. Xie J, Johnson RL, Zhang X, Bare JW, Waldman FM, Cogen PH, Menon AG, Warren RS, Chen L-C, Scott MP, Epstein EH Jr: Mutations of the *PATCHED* gene in several types of sporadic extracutaneous tumors. *Cancer Res* **57**:2369, 1997.

152. Reifenberger J, Wolter M, Weber RG, Megahed M, Ruzicka T, Lichter P, Reifenberger G: Missense mutations in *SMOH* in sporadic basal cell carcinomas of the skin and primitive neuroectodermal tumors of the central nervous system. *Cancer Res* **58**:1798, 1998.

153. Hamilton SR, Liu B, Parsons RE, Papdopoulos N, Jen J, Powell SM, Krush AJ, Berk T, Cohen Z, Titu B, Burger PC, Wood PA, Taqi F, Booker SV, Petersen GM, Offerhaus GJA, Tersmette AC, Giardiello FM, Vogelstein B, Kinzler KW: The molecular basis of Turcot's syndrome. *N Engl J Med* **392**:839, 1995.

154. Zurawell RH, Chiappa SA, Allen C, Raffel C: Sporadic medulloblastomas contain oncogenic β-catenin mutations. *Cancer Res* **58**:896, 1996.

155. Zang KD, Singer H: Chromosomal constitution of meningiomas. *Nature* **216**:84, 1967.

156. Mark J, Levan G, Mitelman F: Identification by fluorescence of the G chromosome lost in human meningiomas. *Hereditas* **71**:163, 1972.

157. Zankl H, Zang KD: Cytological and cytogenetical studies on brain tumors: IV. Identification of the missing G chromosome in human meningiomas as no. 22 by fluorescence technique. *Hum Genet* **14**:167, 1972.

158. Zang KD: Cytological and cytogenetical studies on human meningioma. *Cancer Genet Cytogenet* **6**:249, 1982.

159. Seizinger BR, De la Monte S, Atkins L, Gusella JF, Martuza RL: Molecular genetic approach to human meningioma: loss of genes on chromosome 22. *Proc Natl Acad Sci USA* **84**:5419, 1987.

160. Dumanski JP, Carlbom E, Collins VP, Nordenskjld M: Deletion mapping of a locus on human chromosome 22 involved in the oncogenesis of meningioma. *Proc Natl Acad Sci USA* **84**:9275, 1987.

161. Seizinger BR, Rouleau G, Ozelius LJ, Lane AH, St George-Hyslop P, Huson S, Gusella JF, Martuza RL: Common pathogenetic mechanism for three tumor types in bilateral acoustic neurofibromatosis. *Science* **236**:317, 1987.

162. Rouleau GA, Wertlecki W, Haines JL, Hobbs WJ, Trofatter JA, Seizinger BR, Martuza RL, Superneau DW, Conneally PM, Gusella JF: Genetic linkage of bilateral acoustic neurofibromatosis to a DNA marker on chromosome 22. *Nature* **329**:246, 1987.

163. Wertelecki W, Rouleau GA, Superneau DW, Forehand LW, Williams JP, Haines JL, Gusella JF: Neurofibromatosis 2: Clinical and DNA linkage studies of a large kindred. *N Engl J Med* **319**:278, 1988.

164. Dumanski JP, Rouleau GA, Nordenskjld M, Collin VP: Molecular genetic analysis of chromosome 22 in 81 cases of meningioma. *Cancer Res* **50**:5863, 1990.

165. Cogen PH, Daneshvar L, Bowcock AM, Metzger AK, Cavalli-Sforza LL: Loss of heterozygosity for chromosome 22 DNA sequences in human meningioma. *Cancer Genet Cytogenet* **53**:271, 1991.

166. Rouleau GA, Merel P, Lutchman M, Sanson M, Zucman J, Marineau C, Hoang-Xuan K, Demczuk S, Desmaze C, Plougastel B, Pulst SM, Lenoir G, Bijlsma E, Fashold R, Dumanski J, deJong P, Parry D, Eldrige R, Aurias A, Delattre O, Thomas G: Alteration in a new gene encoding a putative membrane-organizing protein causes neurofibromatosis type 2. *Nature* **363**:495, 1993.

167. Deprez RHL, Bianchi AB, Groen NA, Seizinger BR, Hagemeijer A, vanDrunen E, Bootsma D, Koper JW, Avezaat CJJ, Kley N, Zwarthoff EC: Frequent *NF2* gene transcript mutations in sporadic meningiomas and vestibular schwannomas. *Am J Hum Genet* **54**:1022, 1994.

168. Ruttledge MH, Xie Y-G, Han F-Y, Peyrard M, Collins V, Nordenskjld M, Dumanski JP: Deletions on chromosome 22 in sporadic meningioma. *Genes Chromosom Cancer* **10**:122, 1994.

169. Ruttledge MH, Sarrazin J, Rangaratnam S, Phelan CM, Twist E, Merel P, Delattre O, Thomas G, Nordenskjld M, Collins VP, Dumanski JP, Rouleau GA: Evidence of the complete inactivation of the *NF2* gene in the majority of sporadic meningiomas. *Nature Genet* **6**:180, 1994.

170. Jacoby LB, MacCollin M, Louis DN, Mohney T, Rubio M-P, Pulaski K, Trofatter JA, Kley N, Seizinger B, Ramesh V, Gusella JF: Exon scanning for mutations of the *NF2* gene in schwannomas. *Hum Mol Genet* **3**:413, 1994.

171. Irving RM, Moffat DA, Hardy DG, Barton DE, Xuereb JH, Raher ER: Somatic *NF2* gene mutations in familial and non-familial vestibular schwannoma. *Hum Mol Genet* **3**:347, 1994.

172. Bijlsma EK, Mérel P, Bosch DA, Westerveld A, Delattre O, Thomas G, Hulsebos TJM: Analysis of mutations in the *SCH* gene in schwannomas. *Genes Chromosom Cancer* **11**:7, 1994.

Lung Cancer

Barry D. Nelkin ∎ *Mack Mabry* ∎ *Stephen B. Baylin*

1. **Lung cancer is the leading cause of cancer-related death for both men and women in the United States and the solid tumor with the most defined relationship to a known environmental cause, cigarette smoking. The clinical and biologic aspects of this disease are complex in that four major histologic cancer types, all related to smoking, can arise from the bronchial epithelium, including large cell undifferentiated, squamous cell, adeno-, and small cell lung carcinomas. The first three types, collectively known as non-small cell lung cancer (NSCLC), metastasize later than the small cell tumors (SCLC) and can be cured by early surgery. SCLC is one of the most highly metastatic tumors in humans and has less than a 5 percent 5-year survival rate.**

2. **Hereditary aspects of lung cancer are probably less well understood than for any of the other common forms of solid tumors. There are no well-defined syndromes for inherited lung cancer. However, a growing body of evidence suggests that a complex Mendelian dominant inheritance pattern for genetic predisposition may play a significant role in determining which smokers eventually will get lung tumors. Animal models for carcinogen-induced lung cancers, particularly in mice, suggest a major locus for genetic predisposition to lung adenocarcinoma and may prove useful for defining a gene(s) important to the human disease. The specific gene(s) involved have not been defined, nor have the genetic loci involved been delineated.**

3. **In part because of the poorly defined hereditary aspects of lung cancer, little is known about the precise gene alterations that underly the earliest steps for lung carcinogenesis. However, multiple genetic alterations, in candidate gene regions (loss of heterozygosity at chromosomes 3p, 9p, 13q, and 17p) or in specific candidate genes (*p16, p53, K-ras, cyclin D1* genes), have been elucidated for established lung cancers. The most frequent of these changes, and those which occur earliest in disease progression, provide clues for genes involved in both the initial steps and the hereditary aspects of lung neoplasia.**

4. **Further definition of the genes mediating the evolution of lung cancers is essential to establish critically needed markers to facilitate risk assessment for and design of novel tests for early diagnosis of these neoplasms.**

CLINICAL AND BIOLOGIC ASPECTS

It is estimated that 169,500 new cases of lung cancer will be diagnosed, and 157,400 deaths from lung cancer will occur in the United States in 2001. Thus, lung cancer is the leading cause of cancer-related death in this country.[1] Ironically, considering the tremendous impact of this disease, lung cancer is arguably the most preventable solid tumor, since 90 percent of all patients with these malignancies develop their disease because of exposure to tobacco products and in virtually all instances through cigarette smoking.[2,3]

One of the difficulties in defining genetic predisposition for lung cancer, for making the diagnosis of this disease, and for treatment is that four major histologies of lung tumors evolve from the bronchial epithelium of smokers, and the precise cellular relationships between these tumor types still are not elucidated. From a clinical perspective, lung cancer can be divided into two treatment groups of four histologic types.[4] Squamous cell, adeno-, and large cell carcinomas are collectively referred to as non-small cell lung cancers (NSCLCs) and comprise approximately 75 percent of all lung tumors. These are different in their treatment approaches and responses from a fourth type, small cell lung cancer (SCLC), which constitutes the remaining 25 percent of lung neoplasms. Each of these major forms of lung cancer is intimately related to cigarette smoking. Of great interest for consideration of genetic predisposition to lung cancer and for studies of the genetic changes in these diseases is that only 10 percent of all smokers at risk develop lung carcinoma.[3] This is so despite the fact that virtually all these individuals have a degree of preneoplastic histologic change in their bronchial epithelium.[5] Also, the average age for diagnosis of lung cancer is approximately 60 years. All these data suggest that the evolution of lung cancer occurs over a protracted period of time and involves multiple genetic changes.

For all the lung cancer types, current therapeutic approaches are less than optimal, as reflected in the high death rate from these malignancies. The initial diagnosis for each tumor type almost always stems from clinical evaluation of a chronic cough, weight loss, dyspnea, hemoptysis, hoarseness, or chest pain in patients with a long history of smoking.[6] For the NSCLC group, successful therapies center on early surgery, since metastases occur later than for SCLC. For patients with the most limited stage of NSCLC at the time of initial diagnosis and surgery, 5-year cure rates are approximately 50 percent.[7,8] For patients with nonresectable initial NSCLC and those with recurrent disease, chemotherapy and irradiation are employed, but long-term response rates are only 35 percent, with a median survival time of only 25 weeks.[9,10]

The clinical course for SCLC is very different than that for NSCLC, as is the mode of and response pattern to treatment. This cancer is one of the most metastatic of all solid tumors and is extremely lethal.[11] Tumor spread occurs so early in the course of the disease that surgery is seldom used as a primary approach even for patients with no objective signs of metastasis at the time of initial diagnosis.[12,13] Treatment approaches rely primarily on combination chemotherapy, with thoracic irradiation added in patients with nonmetastatic disease.[14,15] Ironically, this highly lethal cancer has among the highest initial sensitivity among solid tumors to these approaches.[16] However, recurrent and resistant disease virtually always ensues, and the 5-year survival rate is only 5 percent, with an average survival time of 13 months, even for extensively treated patients presenting with detectable disease limited to the chest.[16]

The division of NSCLC and SCLC into two separate categories is useful for consideration of clinical behavior but is simplistic from a biologic standpoint and for considerations of inherited predisposition for these neoplasms. The heterogeneous histologic types of lung cancers may reflect different cells of origin for each tumor type within the bronchial epithelium.[17] For example, as discussed in a section that follows on animal models of lung carcinogenesis, the parent cell for bronchoalveolar carcinomas, a

A list of standard abbreviations is located immediately preceding the index. Nonstandard abbreviations used in this chapter include: NSCLC = non-small cell lung cancer; SCLC = small cell lung cancer; LOH = loss of heterozygosity.

subtype of adenocarcinomas, appears to be the type II pneumocyte within the bronchial epithelium. The cellular origins of SCLC are less certain, although they have been of particular interest because this tumor is characterized by having a neuroendocrine phenotype that most closely resembles that of a sparse population of normal neuroendocrine cells found throughout the bronchial epithelium.[18] The complex biology underlying lung cancer evolution is illustrated by the fact that it is not uncommon for individual lung cancers to manifest biochemical features of both SCLC and NSCLC, such as sharing of neuroendocrine features.[19,20] This fact suggests that lung cancers are capable of a transdifferentiation that reflects a common differentiation lineage in which they may arise.[20] This biology, as well as the discussed clinical aspects, must be taken into account in all studies to define the gene defects responsible for evolution of sporadic and inherited forms of these diseases. As will be discussed later, there are some patterns of genetic loci abnormalities and of altered function of tumor-suppressor genes and oncogenes that suggest segregation of specific genetic changes to NSCLC and SCLC.

GENETIC LOCI

Hereditary Cases: Linkage Analyses

The contribution of hereditary factors to the development of lung cancer is probably less well understood than for any of the common forms of solid tumors in humans. Unlike for breast, colon, renal, and other cancers, no distinct familial forms of the common types of lung cancer have been defined. Therefore, specific genetic loci responsible for predisposition to lung tumor development have not been elucidated. However, a building body of evidence indicates that there may be an exceedingly important role for genetic predisposition in determining risk of lung cancer development among smokers. This section briefly reviews the progress in this area and the prospects for defining the specific genetic loci responsible.

Proof that the familial occurrence of lung cancer has a genetic basis is complicated by the central role of cigarette smoking in causing these neoplasms. Smoking rates increased dramatically after World War I in American men, and this trend was followed by a later increase in the incidence of women who smoke.[21] Since there is a lag period of at least 20 years from the initiation of smoking until the development of lung cancer, smoking habits must be taken into account in analyzing multiple family generations.[22] This is especially important for the occurrence of lung cancer in women, since their incidence of smoking has increased dramatically over the past 40 years.[23,24] Finally, there is evidence that the likelihood of an individual choosing to smoke can be highly influenced on a familial basis, and this must be taken into account in all studies of familial lung cancer.[25]

Despite the problems, a growing number of studies over the past 30 years, using increasingly sophisticated statistical methods to factor in influence of smoking and other environmental factors, have demonstrated a twofold or more risk of lung cancer in relatives of patients with this disease.[25] However, the firm link to actual Mendelian inheritance of lung cancer itself still was difficult to establish. The most significant step in documenting this probability has come from the detailed investigations of Sellers and colleagues of a large number of families in southern Louisiana. Using sophisticated epidemiologic approaches that factor in pre- and post-World War I smoking histories of families and the effects of age, sex, and environment, these authors found validation for a Mendelian codominant inheritance pattern for lung cancer among smokers.[25-27] In fact, their data predict, in the population studied, that all smokers eventually develop lung cancer because they inherit a gene(s) that may have a high incidence in the general population.[25-27] As the authors are careful to point out, these results must be verified through studies of other families in other regions. However, the implications are enormous for considering approaches to the control of lung cancer and for

identifying specific genetic loci involved in predisposition to these neoplasms.

The cited evidence for the role of true inheritance in the development of lung cancer must be translated into formal searches for the involved genetic loci. The job will not be an easy one for multiple reasons. First, as discussed, the inheritance patterns for lung cancer even within a given family appear complex, and multiple loci may be involved. Second, although an earlier age of onset may be a result of inheriting lung cancer risk genes, particularly in women, disease onset still occurs primarily in older individuals.[25-27] These factors make standard linkage analysis of large kindreds with multiple generations very difficult. Early-age-onset lung cancer certainly occurs.[28-30] However, it remains to be determined whether patients with this phenotype develop their disease via the same mechanisms as do patients with typical late-age-onset lung cancer and whether familial patterns for this phenotype can be delineated to facilitate the search for lung cancer predisposition genes.

In addition, the complex array of lung cancer histologies dictates the need to decipher whether hereditary factors contribute to the occurrence of each major subtype. Recent studies indicate that adenocarcinoma of the lung may be the histologic type most linked to definite familial occurrence.[31,32] Interestingly, this is also the type that has been most associated with the few instances of early-age onset.[28-30,33,34]

Therefore, for all the reasons articulated, definition of the actual genetic loci involved for inherited forms of lung cancer will require acquisition of large numbers of families to facilitate nonclassical linkage analyses, such as segregation analyses and sib-pair linkage approaches. Consortium arrangements to conduct such studies are now being established and hopefully will yield at least chromosome assignment for lung cancer predisposition genes within the next several years.

Genetic Loci for Sporadic Forms of Lung Cancer

Cytogenetic Changes. The karyotypes of both SCLC and NSCLC exhibit extensive abnormalities. Whang-Peng et al. showed the first consistent cytogenetic abnormality in lung cancer, deletions on the short arm of chromosome 3, in virtually all SCLC cell lines examined.[35] As discussed in the following section, this observation has been confirmed and extended at the molecular level using polymorphic probes. Testa et al. have shown that in NSCLC primary tumors, an average of 31 clonal karyotypic abnormalities were evident.[36] Among the most common abnormalities were loss of chromosomes 9 and 13 (65 and 71 percent, respectively).

Loss of Heterozygosity. As suggested by the extensive cytogenetic abnormalities, loss of heterozygosity (LOH) is common in lung cancers, as in other solid tumors, and has been studied extensively. Most of these extensive studies,[37-43] summarized in Table 48-1, have relied on conventional RFLP or microsatellite methods. Most recently, whole genome allelotypes of lung cancer, based on high throughput PCR-based methods to detect DNA polymorphisms, have been reported.[43a,43b] Thus far these new studies have examined only a small number of pairs of tumor or tumor cell line DNA and their normal counterparts. Nevertheless, these studies are largely in agreement with the results of the earlier, lower resolution studies of LOH in lung cancer. In addition, these recent studies also suggest new regions of potential LOH in lung cancer, including areas of chromosomes 4p, 4q, 5q, 15q and X. Finally, these studies have begun to delineate further the extent of LOH in candidate tumor-suppressor gene regions. Definition of these loci will allow initiation of DNA sequence-based approaches to discover the tumor-suppressor genes in these regions; two such studies will be discussed below.

LOH areas commonly found in lung cancer are listed in Table 48-1, and those studied most extensively are discussed below. Although some LOH loci occur in all lung cancer types, several have distinct incidence differences between subtypes. For SCLC, there is a very high incidence (90-100 percent of specimens) of

LOH on chromosome 3p in the previously discussed area of frequent cytogenetic loss.[37,38] This last change also often occurs but is less frequent (50–80 percent) in NSCLC. There are at least three, and possibly as many as eight, distinct areas of LOH on chromosome 3p, indicating the presence of multiple tumor-suppressor genes on chromosome 3p[43c]. The individual regions of chromosome 3p that are lost differ somewhat among the histologic lung cancer subtypes. Chromosome areas within 3p21 are lost in NSCLC, whereas more distal regions, at 3p25-p26, and more proximal regions, at 3p12-p14, are more often lost in SCLC.[37,38] Studies of SCLC cell lines also have demonstrated areas of homozygous deletion within 3p21 and 3p12-14.[39,40] Importantly, this region is the site for the most common fragile site in the genome, FRA3B. As discussed below, delineation of these distinct and frequent chromosome 3 LOH areas in lung tumors has prompted intense efforts to identify associated tumor-suppressor genes.

LOH for chromosome region 17p also is extremely frequent in all types of lung cancer and especially in DNA from SCLC (90 percent).[41] The tumor-suppressor gene p53 is located at region 17p13.1 and, as discussed in a later section, is clearly a gene involved in the pathogenesis of established lung cancer.

13q also has a high frequency (75 percent) of LOH in SCLC but a low frequency (15 percent) in NSCLC.[41] As noted in a later section and in Table 48-1, this locus includes the site of the retinoblastoma susceptibility gene (Rb), which is almost always aberrantly expressed or mutated in SCLC.

As discussed previously, 9p is an area of frequent cytogenetic abnormality in NSCLC but not in SCLC. This site is the locus of two separate cyclin-dependent kinase inhibitors (CDKIs), *p15* and *p16*. These genes are described in more detail in a section that follows. Also, there is some evidence that a third tumor-suppressor gene may be located at 9p22-23, and a number of laboratories are attempting to identify genes in this region.[42]

LOH for chromosome 5q is observed in approximately half the SCLC cases studied and is most commonly localized to 5q13-21.[43] The region of loss has been intriguing because the tumor-suppressor gene *APC*, which plays a major role in colon cancer, is located within this region. However, analyses of lung cancers for inactivating mutations of *APC* using an RNAse protection screen have not identified any lesions despite the frequent LOH for this locus.[44]

Listed in Table 48-1 are additional, less well-characterized LOH loci that occur with significant frequency (30–50 percent) in lung cancer. These lesions presumably include loci for tumor-suppressor genes that may be of biologic importance, but more work is required to validate this assumption and to document the importance of these changes within the full spectrum of genetic alterations in lung tumors.

Timing of LOH during Lung Cancer Progression. Several studies have attempted to examine the stages in NSCLC tumor progression at which various genetic lesions accrue. Two groups have shown that 3p loss occurs early in NSCLC and is detectable in hyperplastic, precancerous bronchial lesions.[45,46] Similarly, 9p and 17p loss could be detected in preneoplastic hyperplasia.[47] Recently, it was shown that LOH at 3p, 9p, and 17p can often be detected even in the earliest stages of precancerous bronchial changes, in dysplastic or slightly abnormal foci.[47a] The small size of these clonal patches suggests that these chromosomal changes may be among the first molecular lesions in the development of lung cancer. In one study, K-*ras* mutations were found to occur later in NSCLC development than the preceding LOH changes and were not detectable until the later carcinoma *in situ* stage; another study suggested that the *ras* mutations may occur in earlier stages.[48,49] Allelic loss on chromosomes 2q, 18q, and 22q were relatively uncommon (20–33 percent) in primary NSCLC but were found often (63–83 percent) in brain metastases.[50] These results suggest that these latter genetic lesions provide growth advantages to NSCLC cells late in tumor development. The timing of genetic events in lung carcinogenesis needs much further study and will help to define genes for tumor initiation and clues to those involved in genetic predisposition.

Microsatellite Instability. In hereditary nonpolyposis colon cancer, defects in the mismatch repair pathway, which lead to instability changes in microsatellite repeat sequences, recently have been delineated (see Chap. 18). Instability in microsatellite markers also has been studied by several groups in lung cancers with diverse and occasionally conflicting results. Initial reports indicated that microsatellite markers were more likely to be altered in SCLC compared with NSCLC.[51–53] However, other investigators have found no significant differences. Most recently, it has been reported that microsatellite instability is not observed in SCLC but frequently observed in NSCLC and that the replication error phenotype was more likely in NSCLC metastases and in clinically advanced lung cancers.[52] Whether these conflicting results depend on the microsatellite markers selected for analyses, differences in the selection of cases for study, or technical factors in the assays remains to be determined.

SPECIFIC GENES

Genes Involved in Hereditary Lung Cancer

As mentioned previously, there are no distinct genetic syndromes for lung cancer to help identify gene mutations that specify absolute genetic predisposition to these malignancies. However, there are a few clues to genes for which inherited mutations or patterns of inherited polymorphisms could play a role.

Germ-Line Mutations in Genes Involved in Sporadic Lung Cancer. As noted in a section that follows, mutations in the Ha-*ras* gene occur with frequency in sporadic forms of NSCLC. A rare polymorphism in this gene, which involves differences in numbers of a tandemly arranged reiterated sequence, has been reported to occur with increased frequency in patients with lung cancer.[54] However, subsequent studies have provided conflicting results for the actual linkage of this *ras* polymorphism to lung cancer.[55] The majority of the most recent studies have failed to reveal a predictive relationship, and more work will be required to resolve this issue.

Genetic Syndromes for Other Types of Cancer and the Occurrence of Lung Cancer

There are at least three genetic syndromes that predominantly predispose to other forms of cancer in which lung cancer also may

Table 48-1 Commonly Altered Chromosomal Loci in Lung Cancer

Locus	Histologic Subtype	Gene	Frequency
A. Loci with defined or potential tumor suppressor gene			
3p12-p14	SCLC, NSCLC	FHIT	80†–100%,‡
3p21	NSCLC, SCLC	RASSFI ?	80†–100*,‡
9p21-p22	SCLC, NSCLC	p15, p16	60–70%
11q12-q24	NSCLC	PPP2R1B	65%†
13q14	SCLC, NSCLC	Rb	75–80%*
17p13.1	SCLC, NSCLC	p53	50†–95*
B. Loci without defined tumor suppressor gene			
3p25	SCLC, NSCLC		80†–100*,‡
5q21	SCLC, NSCLC		50%
22q	SCLC, NSCLC		55%
C. Other loci commonly (30–50%) altered in lung cancer			
1p, 1q, 2q, 3q, 6q, 7q, 8p, 9p, 11p, 12p, 17q, 18q, 19p, 21q			

*SCLC.
†NSCLC.
‡Combined frequency for LOH on 3p.

occur. Since these syndromes are so rare, it is not yet clear whether a specific histologic type of lung cancer is favored; moreover, the few reported cases have not yet reached the statistical significance to prove that there is increased incidence of lung cancer associated with these genetic disorders.

Lung cancer may occur with increased frequency in the Li-Fraumeni syndrome (LFS), caused by a germ-line mutation in the *p53* tumor-suppressor gene on chromosome 17p.[56] A substantial fraction of the lung cancers in LFS appear in nonsmokers and young (<45 years) patients, suggesting a biologic effect of LFS on lung cancer development. Similarly, transgenic mice expressing a mutant *p53* gene or lacking *p53* genes can develop lung adenocarcinomas.[57,58]

Patients harboring an inactivating mutation in the *Rb* tumor-suppressor gene on chromosome 13q commonly develop retinoblastoma and osteosarcoma.[59] Primary relatives of bilateral retinoblastoma patients, many of whom are carriers of the mutation, have been reported to develop a variety of secondary cancers, including lung cancer, at relatively high frequency.[60,61] In these studies, several of the lung cancers developed in relatively young (<55 years) patients. A recent study of long term survivors of hereditary retinoblastoma reported a sharply higher incidence of lung cancer in this population.[61a]

Bloom syndrome is an exceedingly rare recessive genetic disorder (165 patients reported) that is associated with defects in DNA repair (see Chap. 16). Leukemias and other cancers are quite common in this syndrome. One case of squamous cell carcinoma of the lung has been reported in a 38-year-old Bloom syndrome patient.[62]

Genetic Differences in Capacity to Metabolize Tobacco Carcinogens

Since cigarette smoking is so intimately involved in the development of lung cancer, it has been logical to search for specific lung cancer predisposition genes by investigating genetic differences between individuals in their capacity to metabolize the major carcinogens present in tobacco and in cigarette smoke. Clues to a role for such differences in determining lung cancer risk have emerged. Several enzymes associated with the cytochrome P450 system (CYP) are responsible for metabolizing tobacco carcinogens to forms that can be excreted readily from the body.[63] In so doing, however, functional groups can be altered on the parent molecules that result in enhancement of carcinogenicity through increased propensity to form bulky DNA adducts. Certain polymorphisms in the discussed enzymes are being associated with differing degrees of metabolic capacity between individuals and increased risk of developing lung cancer. For example, the ability to induce activity of the enzyme CYP2D6 by the antihypertensive drug debrisoquine has been associated with lung cancer risk.[63] The major tobacco carcinogen 4-(methylnitrosoamino)-1-(3-pyridyl)-1-butanone (NNK) is a substrate for CYP2D6.[64] High ability for induction of this enzyme now has been correlated with increased incidence of lung cancer (odds ratio of about 7.5 in one study) in several studies.[65,66] Poor ability to induce CYP2D6 was associated with mutations and polymorphisms in the gene.[67] Several studies have challenged the association between CYP2D6 activity and lung cancer risk.[68–70] Work to match allelotypes for these gene changes, using sensitive PCR based assays, with lung cancer incidence in larger populations should resolve these issues over the next several years.

Another cytochrome system enzyme, CYP1A1 (aromatic hydrocarbon hydroxylase, AHH), also demonstrates genetically determined differences between individuals for basal activity and inducibility by tobacco smoke.[63] This enzyme metabolically activates polyaromatic hydrocarbons (PAHs), and levels have been reported to be higher in patients with lung cancer than in control individuals without cancer.[71] Differences in activity of and association of polymorphisms for other CYP enzymes to lung cancer risk alone have been reported.[63] However, for all these enzymes, subsequent studies have yielded conflicting results with

regard to tightness of linkage to predisposition and occurrence of lung cancer, and future investigations will be required to resolve these issues.[63]

In addition to the described enzymes that may form carcinogenic metabolites from tobacco-related compounds, other enzymes can influence lung cancer risk by catalyzing detoxication reactions that enhance elimination of the described toxic products. Low or absent activity of one such enzyme, the M1 isoform of glutathione-*S*-transferase (GSTM1), which arises through autosomal recessive inheritance for homozygous deletion of the gene, has been linked to high lung cancer risk.[72] Again, this relationship has been challenged by some studies.[73] However, a recent report of PCR-detected deletion of the *GSTM1* gene showed an odds ratio of approximately 1.5 for linkage of the null phenotype with SCLC and adenocarcinoma of the lung.[72] Similarly, lung cancer patients have been reported to have a higher incidence of a specific *GSTP1* polymorphism associated with increased lung DNA adduct levels.[74] Future studies again will be necessary to establish the precise relationships between GSTM1 or *GSTP1* status and lung cancer risk.

In summary, there is a growing body of data for linking genetic differences in capacity to metabolize tobacco carcinogens with risk for developing lung cancer. The odds ratios being reported indicate that no one of the factors being studied has an overwhelming role in predisposition for an individual smoker to be at the highest risk for lung cancer susceptibility. However, a profile of each of the genetic differences in a given smoker might well define a truly significant indicator of risk status. It is clear, from the studies to date, that existing PCR assays for detecting genetic status of each important metabolizing enzyme require much additional refinement. As these improve, monitoring of inherited capacity for carcinogen metabolism may provide a significant way to assess predisposition to lung cancer in large populations.

Genes Involved in Sporadic Lung Cancer

Despite the large body of data for altered genetic loci in sporadic lung cancer, discussed earlier, few specific genes in these regions have been shown to have a role in lung tumorigenesis. However, as outlined below, alterations in both dominantly acting oncogenes and tumor-suppressor genes do occur in established lung tumors and provide clues to the progression steps for these cancers.

Oncogenes Involved in Sporadic Lung Cancer

Ras **Family Genes.** As for other solid tumors discussed in this book, mutations in *ras* family genes (see Chap. 11) occur frequently in lung cancer. In NSCLC tumors, *ras* mutations, primarily of K-*ras*, are observed at frequencies that may approach 50 percent of cases, as detected by sensitive PCR-based methods.[75] H-*ras* mutations are observed in NSCLC at a very low frequency, and mutations in N-*ras* are rare.[76–78] K-*ras* mutations are common in adenocarcinomas, less common in squamous cell lung cancers, extremely rare in bronchoalveolar carcinomas, and have not been described in SCLC.[79–84] In NSCLC, the presence of *ras* mutations has been reported to be a negative prognostic factor, especially in patients with adenocarcinomas.[75,82,86]

myc **Family Genes.** Members of the *myc* family of oncogenes, c-*myc*, N-*myc*, and L-*myc* (see Chap. 11), represent another dominant oncogene family that can be activated in lung cancer, usually by gene amplification. c-*myc* amplification in SCLC appears to be a negative prognostic factor; c-*myc* amplification is three times more common in cancers obtained from treated patients than in tumor specimens from untreated patients.[86–88] Amplification of c-*myc* also correlated with a twofold reduction in median patient survival.[88] A number of investigators have suggested that this poor prognosis occurs because increased c-*myc* protein modifies intrinsic drug resistance to certain treatment modalities.[89,90] Amplification or overexpression of L-*myc* and N-

myc are also found in SCLC and SCLC cell lines, but the prognostic implications of this overexpression are not certain.[91–93]

Cyclin D. Cyclin D is involved in traversing the G1 cell cycle checkpoint for entry into S phase, at least in part by inactivating the Rb tumor-suppressor protein (see Chap. 9). Thus cyclin D can act as an oncogene. Cyclin D1 is overexpressed in most cases of NSCLC[94,95]; in one recent study,[95] many of these instances of cyclin D1 overexpression were shown to be due to gene amplification. In NSCLC cases with cyclin D1 overexpression, normal Rb expression was seen. Cyclin D1 expression was not commonly seen in SCLC; presumably because the *Rb* gene is consistently altered in SCLC, a second abnormality in the same signal transduction pathway does not confer a further growth advantage.

Tumor-Suppressor Genes Involved in Sporadic Lung Cancer

As discussed in a previous section, there are many common sites of LOH, suggestive of alterations in tumor-suppressor loci in the major forms of lung cancer. However, only a few of the specific genes that may have altered function in these chromosome regions have been characterized. Several well-described tumor-suppressor genes (p53, p16, *Rb*) are altered in established lung cancers and almost certainly play a role in the evolution of these tumors, especially for progression stages of these cancers. Other genes including FHIT, PTEN/MMAC1, PP1, and PP2A have been found to be altered in some lung cancers.

p53 Gene. Perhaps the best defined tumor-suppressor gene change in lung cancer is mutation of the *p53* gene. This loss of gene function appears to be the major correlate to the previously discussed very frequent LOH that occurs for chromosome region 17p13.1 in all lung cancer types.[41] *p53* mutations are obviously one of the most common genetic changes in all types of human cancer, and these have been found in 50 percent of NSCLC and 90 percent of SCLC tumors.[96,97] The most frequently observed mutations in these tumors are G > T transversions, and these may reflect bulky DNA adducts resulting from carcinogens found in cigarette smoke.[96] Recently, it has been reported that the tobacco carcinogen benzo[a]pyrenediolepoxide (BPDE) binds directly to the hot spots for the mutations in the *p53* gene found in lung carcinomas.[98] Some studies suggest that lung cancers with *p53* mutations have a worse clinical prognosis, but this relationship remains to be clarified.[99,100]

p16 Gene. Alterations in the cyclin-dependent kinase inhibitor encoding gene *p16* occur frequently in lung cancers, as they do in most common forms of human cancer.[101–104] This gene is a strong tumor-suppressor candidate to account for the previously discussed frequent LOH and homozygous deletions that occur at chromosome region 9p21 in lung and other tumor types. As in many tumor types, point mutations in the *p16* gene are rare, and the homozygous deletions are most common in cell culture lines.[104–106] However, this latter change now has been documented in primary lung cancers as well.[105–107] In both cultures and primary tumors, loss of *p16* gene function also occurs frequently via transcriptional silencing associated with abnormal DNA methylation of the transcription start site region.[108] The methylation change occurs in the absence of *p16* gene coding region mutations.[108,109] Both the homozygous deletions of *p16* and the methylation changes occur almost always in NSCLC rather than in SCLC tumors.[108] This is thought to reflect the fact that the *p16* gene functions in the *cyclin D-Rb* gene pathway for control of cell proliferation. Tumor cells appear to require inactivation of only one gene in this pathway.[110–112] Since *Rb* gene mutations are very frequent, as noted below, in SCLC but are much less frequent in NSCLC, inactivation of the *cyclin D-Rb* pathway by loss of *p16* function may be advantageous primarily for NSCLC cells.[110–112]

The precise role for *p16* gene changes in the progression of NSCLC tumors has not been delineated yet. However, this loss of

gene function may play a very early role, since, as discussed earlier, LOH and homozygous deletions of chromosome 9p21 have been found in early lung cancer lesions. Further investigations of the role of the *p16* gene in lung carcinogenesis are critical and could be important for understanding of genetic susceptibility for lung cancer.

Rb Gene. The tumor-suppressor gene *Rb,* which plays a critical role in the cyclin D pathway for cell cycle control and is located in chromosome region 13q14, is altered in nearly all SCLC tumors and in 30 to 40 percent of NSCLC.[113–115] In NSCLC, aberrant *Rb* was more common in tumors of higher clinical stage.[115] As mentioned above, hereditary retinoblastoma patients, who have constitutional inactivation of one allele of the *Rb* gene, and their primary relatives, have increased incidence of lung cancer.

FHIT Gene. The frequent LOH observed on chromosome 3 in both SCLC and NSCLC has focused an intense search for tumor suppressor genes in this area. The *FHIT* gene, which is located in one of these areas of LOH, at chromosome 3p14.2, encompasses the fragile site FRA3B, at the breakpoint for a t(3;8) reciprocal translocation commonly seen in renal cancer (116, and references therein). Early studies showed abnormal *FHIT* mRNA transcripts in lung and other cancers. Subsequent studies have demonstrated loss of expression of FHIT protein, and deletion of the *FHIT* gene in lung cancer, including biallelic deletions in two lung cancer cell lines. Introduction of the *FHIT* gene into lung cancer cell lines has been shown to result in growth inhibition, induction of apoptosis, and inhibition of tumorigenicity. Together, these results suggest that *FHIT* may function as a tumor suppressor gene. FHIT has dinucleotide hydrolase activity, and it has been speculated that FHIT may function either by controlling intracellular levels of diadenosine polyphosphate, or that the FHIT-diadenosine polyphosphate complex may be active in signal transduction. Understanding the tumor suppressor mechanism of FHIT will require much further study.

PTEN/MMAC1 Gene. Two recent reports[117,118] document alterations in the *PTEN/MMAC1* gene in several SCLC cell lines and in primary SCLC tumors and, less commonly, in NSCLC. The *PTEN/MMAC1* gene is located in chromosome region 10q23.3, a region of frequent LOH in SCLC. PTEN/MMAC1 is a dual specificity phosphatase that is mutated in Cowden disease, which predisposes to several types of cancer, and in Bannayan-Zonana syndrome. However, several earlier reports[119–121] suggested that alterations of the *PTEN/MMAC1* gene in lung cancer are uncommon, and lung cancer is not associated with Cowden disease or Bannayan-Zonana syndrome. Further study, including larger numbers of lung cancers, will be necessary to resolve the role of *PTEN/MMAC1* in lung cancer.

PP2A. The locus 11q22-24 exhibits frequent LOH in lung cancer, and introduction of this chromosomal region can inhibit tumorigenicity in lung cancer cells. Wang and colleagues systematically screened this region for expressed sequences which might be candidate tumor suppressor genes.[121a] They found a subunit of the serine/threonine protein phosphatase PP2A, PPP2R1B, which was mutated in several primary lung tumors and lung cancer cell lines; in some of these samples, both alleles were affected. The critical demonstration that introduction of PPP2R1B can inhibit tumorigenicity in lung cancer cells has not yet been reported. Inhibition of protein phosphatases has been associated with several cellular functions leading to cell transformation, so PPP2R1B may be a strong candidate for a tumor suppressor gene.

PP1. PP1, like PP2A, is a serine/threonine protein phosphatase. One subunit of PP1, PPP1R3, has been shown to be mutated in a small number of lung cancers and lung cancer cell lines.[121b] The PPP1R3 gene is located at 7q31.1-31.2, which exhibits a moderate frequency of LOH in lung cancer.

With the completion of the human genome sequence, it will now be feasible to search for tumor suppressor genes by examination of the sequence of regions of LOH or interstitial chromosomal deletion. However, the potential difficulties in searching for tumor suppressor genes, based on LOH or chromosomal deletion, are evident in a recent report.[121c] The area of chromosome 3p21.3 has one of the highest frequencies of LOH in lung cancer. In addition, several cell lines have been shown to have homozygous deletions in this region. The entire region was sequenced and examined for potential genes. Twenty-five known or potential genes were identified, and examined for mutations or low expression in lung cancer cell lines. A low level of mutations was found in a few of these genes, but no robust candidate for a tumor suppressor gene was identified. It is possible that there are several tumor suppressor genes in this area. Alternatively, the predominant mechanism of inactivation of the tumor suppressor gene in this region may not be by mutation, but rather by haploinsufficiency or an epigenetic mechanism such as DNA methylation. In support of the latter possibility, it has recently been shown that one gene in the 3p21.3 region, RASSF1, can inhibit tumorigenicity in lung tumor cells, and is methylated in lung tumor DNA.[121d]

Animal Models for Defining Genetic Aspects of Lung Cancer

Animal models can prove invaluable for clarifying genetic determinants of human cancers, especially for tumors such as lung cancer where little is known about the initial molecular steps underlying tumorigenesis. Multiple animal types, including dogs, mice, and rats, are susceptible to development of either spontaneous lung cancers or lung neoplasms induced by exposure to carcinogens. The carcinogen models may be particularly valuable for determining genetic changes that contribute to predisposition to lung neoplasia and have been especially well studied in the mouse.[122] The most important features of the murine lung cancer models with regard to potential contribution to our understanding of human lung neoplasia will be discussed briefly below.

Controlled exposure of mice to tobacco-related carcinogens, such as NNK, and to various forms of irradiation consistently induce lung tumors. In the main, the lesions have a histology similar to human lung adenocarcinoma and appear to constitute an excellent model for this common form of tumor.[122-124] A particularly important feature of the tumor is that the lesions have been hypothesized to arise in a defined parent cell, the type II pneumocyte.[122,123] This postulation has been further strengthened by the finding that a distinct change, increase in DNA-methyl-transferase activity, occurs only in this cell type in the lung immediately after exposure of mice to NNK.[124] Also, following carcinogen exposure, the murine tumors evolve over a distinct course of progression from hyperplasia, to benign appearing adenomas, to frank carcinoma.[122-124] This cellular origin and the ability to examine defined stages of tumor progression offer an excellent opportunity to outline molecular steps responsible for multiple stages of lung tumor progression.

Importantly, susceptibility of mice to the described tumor induction is very strain-dependent, and this genetically determined response relates specifically to lung cancer.[122] This situation provides an opportunity to outline molecular events for predisposition to multiple stages of lung cancer evolution that may have great ramifications for defining genetic steps for human lung cancer. Several approaches to detecting genes responsible for strain susceptibility have been used already. For example, standard linkage analyses have been applied to study generations of mice bred from an initial cross between the A/J mouse, which is very sensitive to tumor induction with NNK exposure, and a resistant strain, the C3H mouse. A major susceptibility locus on distal chromosome 6, termed Pas1, has been identified and confirmed in subsequent studies including crosses between the sensitive strain and noninbred mice that are resistant to tumor induction.[122-125]

The gene(s) responsible for the contribution of the described Pas1 locus has not yet been identified but obviously will be of great interest for human lung cancer as well. One interesting candidate, the Kras2 gene, is near the locus and has been studied in detail. As noted in a previous section, this gene is mutated in a significant percentage of human lung adenocarcinomas and is mutated in an even higher proportion (70 to over 90 percent) of spontaneous and carcinogen-induced murine lung adenocarcinomas as well.[122,123] Furthermore, the alterations in the murine tumors occur very early in the hyperplasia and adenoma stages.[122,123] Intriguingly, in tumors induced in susceptible offspring from crosses between carcinogen-sensitive and -resistant mice, the Kras2 gene mutations are always in the allele inherited from the sensitive strain.[122] However, the Kras2 gene does not appear to fall within the tightest area of chromosome linkage on chromosome 6, and the presence of mutations in this gene is as high in tumors from the more resistant strains of mice as in those from sensitive strains.[122] Thus it is felt, at this time, that either the Kras2 gene mutations are an important step for early progression of the murine tumors but not for the initial steps influenced by inherited susceptibility, or the gene mutations are influenced in some way by a control locus that is contained within the nearby area of tight linkage on chromosome 6.[122]

Subsequent linkage studies to map quantitative trait loci (QTLs) that affect lung cancer incidence or development in mice have detected linkage on chromosomes 4, 6, 9, 10, 11, 12, 17, 18, and 19 (reviewed in ref. 126). Interestingly, the locus on chromosome 4 is near the $p16^{INK4a}$ gene. This locus may be of special importance because in a genome-wide search for LOH in murine lung tumors, the p16 region was the only region lost consistently, suggesting the presence of a tumor-suppressor gene.[122] Similarly, the frequency of p16 gene alterations in rat lung tumors is extremely high and consists of homozygous deletions and aberrant promoter region hypermethylation.[127] The relatively weak linkage for the chromosome 4 region to the strain differences in tumor susceptibility suggests that the p16 gene, or other genes in the LOH area, may, as for Kras2 mutations, play more of a role in progression than in tumor initiation. Direct studies of alterations in murine homologues of key tumor-suppressor genes for human neoplasia also have been used to search for molecular clues to strain differences in lung tumor susceptibility. No significant incidence for Rb or p53 gene mutations have been found in the murine tumors.[122]

In summary, animal models for lung carcinoma, especially those defined in mice, offer an important opportunity to help define genes that may be central to the development of and genetic predisposition to particularly human lung adenocarcinoma. The difficulty in acquiring large numbers of families with inherited human lung cancer that are suitable for standard linkage analyses emphasizes the importance of using animal models as adjuncts to the study of genetic predisposition to lung cancer in humans. The defined progression stages for the murine carcinogenesis-induced tumors and the differences in strain susceptibility both contribute to the inherent value of using these models to define genes for which human homologues can readily be identified. It will not be surprising if some of the genes discovered will have key roles for lung cancer evolution in both the murine and human settings.

IMPLICATIONS OF GENETIC CHANGES FOR THE DIAGNOSIS AND TREATMENT OF LUNG CANCER

The tremendous impact that lung cancer has on society and the distinct relationship to a known environmental cause for these tumors make this malignancy a prime target for defining genetic markers of risk and for use in early diagnosis. Hopefully, the evidence for an important role for genetic predisposition in determining which smokers develop lung cancer will be followed in the coming years by elucidation of the molecular events involved. In turn, these genetic changes may serve as the best markers for defining risk and marking the earliest stages of lung cancer.

As the best markers emerge, they can be incorporated into diagnostic strategies that are already providing proof of principle for use of genetic changes to provide for early diagnosis of lung cancer, such as the detection of *p53* and *ras* gene mutations in sputum DNA months to years before clinical signs of tumor have been reported.[122] These are retrospective studies in which the precise mutations that appeared in the eventual tumors were known, and prospective investigations will be needed to validate such approaches. However, the ability to use tissue samples obtained by such noninvasive procedures is most encouraging. In fact, other body fluids, including blood and urine, have now been used to detect genetic changes, such as microsatellite instability, that are present in established lung tumors of the patients studied.[128,129] Hopefully, germ-line DNA changes that reflect increased risk for the development of lung cancer also will come to play a role in population screening, since the rate of cigarette smoking remains high and is increasing, especially among young people and women, in many regions of the world.

Some of the genetic changes that already have been defined as frequent events in established lung cancers are being investigated as potential therapeutic targets for lung cancer. Recently, in an initial gene therapy study of patients with lung cancer, regression of tumors injected with a retrovirus for expression of the wild-type *p53* gene, has been reported.[120] Inhibitors of *ras* gene function hold promise for treatment of the many patients with lung cancers that harbor mutations in this family of genes.[131,132] Surely, as other gene alterations important for the various stages of lung cancer progression are discovered, these will present more potential molecular targets for new and novel therapeutic strategies for the current most lethal form of human neoplasia.

REFERENCES

1. Greenlee RT, Hill-Harmon MB, Murray T, Thun M: Cancer Statistics, 2001. *CA Cancer J Clin* **51**:15, 2001

2. Ferguson MK, Skosey C, Hoffman PL, Golomb HM: Sex differences in presentation and survival in patients with lung cancer. *J Clin Oncol* **8**:1402, 1990.

3. Mattson ME, Pollack ES, Cullen JW: What are the odds that smoking will kill you. *Am J Public Health* **77**:425, 1987.

4. Pass HI, Mitchell JB, Johnson DH, Turrisi AT: *Lung Cancer: Principles and Practice.* Philadelphia, Lippincott, 1996.

5. Fontana RS, Sanderson DR, Taylor WF: Early lung cancer detection: Results of the initial (prevalence) radiologic and cytologic screening in the Mayo Clinic study. *Am Rev Respir Dis* **130**:561, 1984.

6. Midthun DE, Jett JR: Clinical presentation of lung cancer, in Pass HI, Mitchell JB, Johnson DH, Turrisi AT (eds): *Lung Cancer: Principles and Practice.* Philadelphia, Lippincott, 1996, p 421.

7. Williams DE, Pairolero PC, Davis C, Bernatz PE, Payne WS, Taylor WF, Uhenhopp MA, Fontana RS: Survival of patients surgically treated for stage I lung cancer. *J Thorac Cardiovasc Surg* **82**:70, 1981.

8. Shimizu N, Ando A, Teramoto S, Moritani Y, Nishii K: Outcome of patients with lung cancer detected via mass screening as compared to those presenting with symptoms. *J Surg Oncol* **50**:7, 1992.

9. Einhorn LH, Loehrer PJ, Williams SD, Meyers S, Gabrys T, Nattan SR, Woodburn R, Drasga R, Songer J, Fisher W: Random prospective study of vindesine versus vindesine plus high cisplatin versus vindesine plus cisplatin plus mitomycin C in advanced non lung cancer. *J Clin Oncol* **4**:1037, 1986.

10. Bonomi P: Non small cell lung cancer chemotherapy, in Pass HI, Mitchell JB, Johnson DH, Turrisi AT (eds): *Lung Cancer: Principles and Practice.* Philadelphia, Lippincott, 1996, p 811.

11. Johnson DH, Greco FA: Small cell carcinoma of the lung. *Crit Rev Oncol Hematol* **4**:303, 1986.

12. Miller AB, Fox W, Tall R: Five year follow-up of the Medical Research Council comparative trial of surgery and radiotherapy for the primary treatment of small-celled or oat-celled carcinoma of the bronchus. *Lancet* **2**:501, 1969.

13. Johnson DH: Chemotherapy of small cell lung cancer, in Pass HI, Mitchell JB, Johnson DH, Turrisi AT (eds): *Lung Cancer: Principles and Practice.* Philadelphia, Lippincott, 1996, p 825.

14. Ihde DC: Chemotherapy of lung cancer. *N Engl J Med* **327**:1434, 1992.

15. Murray N, Coy P, Pater J, Hodson I, Arnold Z, Zee BC, Payne D, Kostashuk EC, Evans WK, Dixon P: Importance of timing for thoracic irradiation in the combined modality treatment of limited stage small cell lung cancer. *J Clin Oncol* **11**:336, 1993.

16. Arrigada R, Le Chevalier T, Pignon JP, Riviere A, Monnet I, Chomy P, Tuchais C, Tarayre M, Ruffie P: Initial chemotherapeutic doses and survival in patients with limited small cell lung cancer. *N Engl J Med* **329**:1848, 1993.

17. Gazdar AF, Carney DN, Guccion JG, Baylin SB: Small cell carcinoma of the lung: Cellular origin and relationship to other pulmonary tumors, in Greco FA, Oldham RK, Bunn PA (eds): *Small Cell Lung Cancer.* New York, Grune & Stratton, 1981, p 145.

18. Linnoila RI: in Kaliner MA, Barnes PJ, Kunkel GHH, Baraniuk JN (eds): *Neuropeptides in Respiratory Medicine.* N York, Marcel Dekker, 1994, p 197.

19. Linnoila RI, Mulshine JL, Steinberg SM, Funa K, Matthews MJ, Cotelingam JD, Gazdar AF: Neuroendocrine differentiation in endocrine and non lung carcinomas. *Am J Clin Pathol* **90**:641, 1988.

20. Mabry M, Nelkin BD, Falco JP, Barr LF, Baylin SB: Transitions between lung cancer phenotypes: implications for tumor progression. *Cancer Cell* **3**:53, 1991.

21. Giovino GA, Schooley MW, Zhu BP, Chrismon JH, Tomar SL, Peddicord JP, Merritt RK, Husten CG, Eriksen MP: Surveillance for selected tobacco behaviors: United States, 1900-1994. *MMWR CDC Surveill Summ* **43**:1, 1994.

22. Schottenfeld D: Epidemiology of lung cancer, in Pass HJ, Mitchell JB, Johnson DH, Turrisi AT (eds): *Lung Cancer: Principles and Practice.* Philadelphia, Lippincott, 1996, p 305.

23. Ernster VL: The epidemiology of lung cancer in women. *Ann Epidemiol* **4**:102, 1994.

24. Harris RE, Zang EA, Anderson JI, Wynder EL: Race and sex differences in lung cancer risk associated with cigarette smoking. *Int J Epidemiol* **22**:592, 1993.

25. Sellers TA: Familial predisposition to lung cancer, in Roth JA, Cox JP, Hong WK (eds): *Lung Cancer.* Boston, Blackwell, 1993, p 20.

26. Sellers TA, Bailey JE, Elston RC, Wilson AF, Elston GZ, Ooi WL, Rothschild H: Evidence for mendelian inheritance in the pathogenesis of lung cancer. *J Natl Cancer Inst* **82**:1272, 1990.

27. Sellers TA, Potter JD, Bailey JE, Rich SS, Rothschild H, Elston RC: Lung cancer detection and prevention for an interaction between smoking and predisposition. *Cancer Res* **52**:2694s, 1992.

28. Makimoto T, Tsuchiya S, Nakano H, Watanabe S, Takei Y, Nomoto T, Ishihara S, Saitoh R: Primary lung cancer in young patients. *Nippon Kyobu Shikkan Gakkai Zasshi* **33**:241, 1995.

29. Rocha MP, Fraire AE, Guntupalli KK, Greenberg SD: Lung cancer in the young. *Cancer Detect Prev* **18**:349, 1994.

30. Bourke W, Milstein D, Giura R, Donghi M, Luisetti M, Rubin AH, Smith LJ: Lung cancer in young adults. *Chest* **102**:1723, 1992.

31. Tsuji H, Hara S, Tagawa Y, Kawahara K, Ayabe H, Tomita M: Bilateral bronchiolalveolar carcinoma, showing familial aggregation of lung cancer. *Nippon Kyobu Geka Gakkai Zasshi* **42**:1061, 1994.

32. Ogawa H: Interaction between family history and smoking in lung cancer. *Gan No Rinsho* **33**:575, 1987.

33. Capewell S, Wathen CG, Sankaran R, Sudlow MF: Lung cancer in young patients. *Respir Med* **86**:499, 1992.

34. Larrieu AJ, Jamieson WR, Nelems JM, Fowler R, Yamamoto B, Leriche J, Murray N: Carcinoma of the lung in patients under 40 years of age. *Am J Surg* **149**:602, 1985.

35. Whang-Peng J, Knutsen T, Gazdar A, Steinberg SM, Oie H, Linnoila I, Mulshine J, Nau M, Minna JD: Nonrandom structural and numerical chromosome changes in non-small-cell lung cancer. *Genes Chromosom Cancer* **3**:168, 1991.

36. Testa JR, Siegfried JM, Liu Z, Hunt JD, Feder MM, Litwin S, Zhou J, Taguchi T, Keller SM: Cytogenetic analysis of 63 non cell lung carcinomas: Recurrent chromosome alterations amid frequent and widespread genomic upheaval. *Genes Chromosom Cancer* **11**:178, 1994.

37. Hibi K, Takahashi T, Yamakawa K, Ueda R, Sekido Y, Ariyoshi Y, Suyama M, Takagi H, Nakamura Y: Three distinct regions involved in 3p deletion in human lung cancer. *Oncogene* **7**:445, 1992.

38. Brauch H, Tory K, Kotler F, Gazdar AF, Pettengill OS, Johnson B, Graziano S, Winton T, Buys CH, Sorenson GD: Molecular mapping of deletion sites in the short arm of chromosome 3 in human lung cancer. *Genes Chromosom Cancer* **1**:240, 1990.

39. Rabbitts P, Bergh J, Douglas J, Collins F, Waters J: A submicroscopic homozygous deletion at the D3S3 locus in a cell line isolated from a small cell lung carcinoma. *Genes Chromosom Cancer* **2**:231, 1990.

40. Daly MC, Xiang RH, Buchhagen D, Hensel CH, Garcia DK, Killary AM, Minna JD, Naylor SL: A homozygous deletion on chromosome 3 in a small cell lung cancer cell line correlates with a region of tumor suppressor activity. *Oncogene* **8**:1721, 1993.

41. Yokota J, Wada M, Shimosato Y, Terada M, Sugimura T: Loss of heterozygosity of chromosomes 3, 13, and 17 in small cell carcinoma and on chromosome 3 in adenocarcinoma of the lung. *Proc Natl Acad Sci USA* **84**:9252, 1987.

42. Neville EM, Stewart M, Myskow M, Donnelly RJ, Field JK: Loss of heterozygosity at 9p23 defines a novel locus in non-small cell lung cancer. *Oncogene* **11**:581, 1995.

43. Hosoe S, Ueno K, Shigedo Y, Tachibana I, Osaki T, Kumagai T, Tanio Y, Kawase I, Nakamura Y, Kishimoto T: A frequent deletion of chromosome 5q21 in advanced small cell and non-small cell carcinoma of the lung. *Cancer Res* **54**:1787, 1994.

43a. Girard L, Zochbauer-Muller S, Virmani AK, Gazdar AF, Minna JD: Genome-wide allelotyping of lung cancer identifies new regions of allelic loss, differences between small cell lung cancer and non-small cell lung cancer, and loci clustering. *Cancer Res* **60**:4894, 2000.

43b. Lindblad-Toh K, Tanenbaum DM, Daly MJ, Winchester E, Lui WO, Villapakkam A, Stanton SE, Larsson C, Hudson TJ, Johnson BE, Lander ES, Meyerson M: Loss-of-heterozygosity analysis of small-cell lung carcinomas using single-nucleotide polymorphism arrays. *Nat Biotechnol* **18**:1001, 2000.

43c. Wistuba II, Behrens C, Virmani AK, Mele G, Milchgrub S, Girard L, Fondon JW, Garner HR, McKay B, Latif F, Lerman MI, Lam S, Gazdar AF, Minna JD: High resolution chromosome 3p allelotyping of human lung cancer and preneoplastic/preinvasive bronchial epithelium reveals multiple, discontinuous sites of 3p allele loss and three regions of frequent breakpoints. *Cancer Res* **60**:1949, 2000.

44. Horii A, Nakatsuru S, Miyoshi Y, Ichii S, Nagase H, Ando H, Yanagisawa A, Tsuchiya E, Kato Y, Nakamura Y: Frequent somatic mutations of *APC* gene in human pancreatic cancer. *Cancer Res* **52**:6696, 1992.

45. Sundaresan V, Ganly P, Haselton P, Rudd R, Sinha G, Bleehen NM, Rabbitts P: *p53* and chromosome 3 abnormalities, characteristic of malignant lung tumours, are detectable in preinvasive lesions of the bronchus. *Oncogene* **7**:1989, 1992.

46. Hung J, Kishimoto Y, Sugio K, Virmani A, McIntire DD, Minna JD, Gazdar AF: Allele-specific chromosome 3p deletions occur at an early stage in the pathogenesis of lung carcinoma. *JAMA* **273**:558, 1995.

47. Kishimoto Y, Sugio K, Hung JY, Virmani AK, McIntire DD, Minna JD, Gazdar AF: Allele loss in chromosome 9p loci in preneoplastic lesions accompanying non-small-cell lung cancers. *J Natl Cancer Inst* **87**:1224, 1995.

47a. Park IW, Wistuba II, Maitra A, Milchgrub S, Virmani AK, Minna JD, Gazdar AF: Multiple clonal abnormalities in the bronchial epithelium of patients with lung cancer. *J Natl Cancer Inst* **91**:1863, 1999.

48. Sugio K, Kishimoto Y, Virmani AK, Hung JY, Gazdar AF: *K-ras* mutations are a relatively late event in the pathogenesis of lung carcinomas. *Cancer Res* **54**:5811, 1994.

49. Westra WH, Slebos RJ, Offerhaus GJ, Goodman SN, Evers SG, Kensler TW, Askin FB, Rodenhuis S, Hruban RH: *K-ras* oncogene activation in lung adenocarcinomas from former smokers: Evidence that *K-ras* mutations are an early and irreversible event in the development of adenocarcinoma of the lung. *Cancer* **72**:432, 1993.

50. Shiseki M, Kohno T, Nishikawa R, Sameshima Y, Mizoguchi H, Yokota J: Frequent allelic losses on chromosome 2q, 18q, and 22q in advanced non-small cell lung carcinoma. *Cancer Res* **54**:5643, 1994.

51. Merlo A, Mabry M, Gabrielson E, Vollmer R, Baylin SB, Sidransky D: Frequent microsatellite instability in primary small cell lung cancer. *Cancer Res* **54**:2098, 1994.

52. Adachi J, Shiseki M, Okazaki T, Ishimaru G, Noguchi M, Hirohashi S, Yokota J: Microsatellite instability in primary and metastatic lung carcinomas. *Genes Chromosom Cancer* **14**:301, 1995.

53. Shridhar V, Siegfried J, Hunt J, del Mar Alonso M, Smith DI: Genetic instability of microsatellite sequences in many non-small cell lung carcinomas. *Cancer Res* **54**:2084, 1994.

54. Sugimura H, Caporaso NE, Modali RV, Hoover RN, Resau JH, Trump BF, Longeran JA, Krontiris TG, Mann DL, Weston A: Association of rare alleles of the Harvey ras protooncogene with lung cancer. *Cancer Res* **50**:1857, 1990.

55. Vineis P, Caporaso N: The analysis of restriction fragment length polymorphism in human cancer: A review from an epidemiologic perspective. *Int J Cancer* **47**:26, 1991.

56. Li FP, Fraumeni JF, Mulvihill JJ, Blattner WA, Dreyfus MG, Tucker MA, Miller RW: A cancer family syndrome in twenty kindreds. *Cancer Res* **48**:5358, 1988.

57. Lavigueur A, Bernstein A: *p53* transgenic mice: Accelerated erythroleukemia induction by Friend virus. *Oncogene* **6**:2197, 1991.

58. Donehower LA, Harvey M, Slagle BL, McArthur MJ, Montgomery CA, Butel JS, Bradley A: Mice deficient for p53 are developmentally normal but susceptible to spontaneous tumours. *Nature* **356**:215, 1992.

59. Goodrich DW, Lee W: The molecular genetics of retinoblastoma. *Cancer Surv* **9**:529, 1990.

60. Strong LC, Herson J, Haas C, Elder K, Chakraborty R, Weiss KM, Majumder P: Cancer mortality in relatives of retinoblastoma patients. *J Natl Cancer Inst* **73**:303, 1984.

61. Sanders BM, Jay M, Draper GJ, Roberts EM: Non-ocular cancer in relatives of retinoblastoma patients. *Br J Cancer* **60**:358, 1989.

61a. Kleinerman RA, Tarone RE, Abramson DH, Seddon JM, Li FP, Tucker MA: Hereditary retinoblastoma and risk of lung cancer. *J Natl Cancer Inst* **92**:2037, 2000.

62. German J: Bloom syndrome: A Mendelian prototype of somatic mutational disease. *Medicine* **72**:393, 1993.

63. Shields PG, Harris CC: Genetic predisposition to cancer, in Roth JA, Cox JD, Hong WK (eds): *Lung Cancer*. Boston, Blackwell, 1993, p 3.

64. Crespi CL, Penman BW, Gelboin HV, Gonzalez FJ: A tobacco smoke nitrosamine, 4(methylnitrosamino)(3) is activated by multiple cytochrome P450s including the polymorphic human cytchrome P450 2D6. *Carcinogenesis* **12**:1197, 1991.

65. Caporaso NE, Shields PG, Landi MT, Shaw GL, Tucker MA, Hoover R, Sugimura H, Weston A, Harris CC: The debrisoquine metabolic phenotype and DNA assays: Implications of misclassification for the association of lung cancer and the debrisoquine metabolic phenotype. *Environ Health Perspect* **98**:101, 1992.

66. Caporaso NE, Hayes RB, Dosemeci M, Hoover R, Ayesh R, Hetzel M, Idle J: Lung cancer risk, occupational exposure, and the debrisoquine metabolic phenotype. *Cancer Res* **49**:3675, 1989.

67. Gough AC, Miles JS, Spurr NK, Moss JE, Gaedigk A, Eichelbaum M, Wolf CR: Identification of the primary gene defect at the cytochrome P450 CYP2D locus. *Nature* **347**:773, 1990.

68. Shaw GL, Falk RT, Deslauriers J, Frame JN, Nesbitt JC, Pass HI, Issaq HJ, Hoover RN, Tucker MA: Debrisoquine metabolism and lung cancer risk. *Cancer Epidemiol Biomark Prev* **4**:41, 1995.

69. Shaw GL, Falk RT, Frame JN, Weiffenbach B, Nesbitt JC, Pass HI, Caporaso NE, Moir DT, Tucker MA: Genetic polymorphism of CYP2D6 and lung cancer risk. *Cancer Epidemiol Biomark Prev* **7**:215, 1998.

70. Legrand-Andreoletti M, Stucker I, Marez D, Galais P, Cosme J, Sabbagh N, Spire C, Cenee S, Lafitte JJ, Beaune P, Broly F: Cytochrome P450 CYP2D6 gene polymorphism and lung cancer susceptibility in Caucasians. *Pharmacogenetics* **8**:7, 1998.

71. Rudiger HW, Nowak D, Hartmann K, Cerutti PA: Enhanced formation of benzo(a) pyrene: DNA adducts in monocytes of patients with a presumed predisposition to lung cancer. *Cancer Res* **45**:5890, 1985.

72. To-Figueras J, Gene M, Gomez-Catalan J, Galan C, Firvida J, Fuentes M, Rodamilans M, Huguet E, Estape J, Corbella J: Glutathione *S*-transferase M1 and codon 72 p53 polymorphisms in a northwestern Mediterranean population and their relation to lung cancer susceptibility. *Cancer Epidemiol Biomark Prev* **5**:337, 1996.

73. London SJ, Daly AK, Cooper J, Navidi WC, Carpenter CL, Idle JR: Polymorphism of glutathione *S*-transferase M1 and lung cancer risk among African-Americans and Caucasians in Los Angeles County, California. *J Natl Cancer Inst* **87**:1246, 1995.

74. Ryberg D, Skaug V, Hewer A, Phillips DH, Harries LW, Wolf CR, Ogreid D, Ulvik A, Vu P, Haugen A: Genotypes of glutathione *S*-transferase M1 and P1 and their significance for lung DNA adduct levels and cancer risk. *Carcinogenesis* **18**:1285, 1997.

75. Clements NC, Nelson MA, Wymer JA, Savage C, Aquirre M, Garewal H: Analysis of *K-ras* gene mutations in malignant and nonmalignant endobronchial tissue obtained by fiberoptic bronchoscopy. *Am J Respir Crit Care Med* **152**:1374, 1995.

76. Rodenhuis S, Slebos R, Boot AJ, Evers SG, Mooi WJ, Wagenaar SS, van Bodegom PC, Bos JL: Incidence and possible clinical significance of *K-ras* oncogene activation in adenocarcinoma of the human lung. *Cancer Res* **48**:5738, 1988.

77. Mills NE, Fishman CL, Scholes J, Anderson SE, Rom WN, Jacobson DR: Detection of *K-ras* oncogene mutations in bronchoalveolar lavage fluid for lung cancer diagnosis. *J Natl Cancer Inst* **87**:1056, 1995.

78. Suzuki Y, Orita M, Shiraishi M, Hayashi K, Sekiya T: Detection of *ras* gene mutations in human lung cancers by single strand conformation polymorphism analysis of polymerase chain reaction products. *Oncogene* **5**:1037, 1990.

79. Slebos RJC, Evers SG, Wagenaar SS, Rodenhuis S: Cellular protooncogenes are infrequently amplified in untreated non-small cell lung cancer (NSCLC). *Br J Cancer* **59**:76, 1988.

80. Reynolds S, Anna CK, Brown KC, Wiest JS, Beattie EJ, Pero RW, Iglehart JD, Anderson MW: Activated oncogenes in human lung tumors from smokers. *Proc Natl Acad Sci USA* **88**:1085, 1991.

81. Li S, Rosell R, Urban A, Font A, Ariza A, Armengol P, Abad A, Navas JJ, Monzo M: *K-ras* gene point mutation: A stable tumor marker in non-small cell lung carcinoma. *Lung Cancer* **11**:19, 1994.

82. Rosell R, Li S, Skacel Z, Mate JL, Maestre J, Canela M, Tolosa E, Armengol P, Barnadas A, Ariza A: Prognostic impact of mutated *K-ras* gene in surgically resected non cell lung cancer patients. *Oncogene* **8**:2407, 1993.

83. Ohshima S, Shimizu Y, Takahama M: Detection of *c-Ki-ras* gene mutation in paraffin sections of adenocarcinoma and atypical bronchioloalveolar cell hyperplasia of human lung. *Virchows Arch* **424**:129, 1994.

84. Wagner SN, Muller R, Boehm J, Putz B, Wunsch PH, Hofler H: Neuroendocrine neoplasms of the lung are not associated with point mutations at codon 12 of the *Ki-ras* gene. *Virchows Arch [B]* **63**:325, 1993.

85. Rodenhuis S, Slebos RJ: Clinical significance of *ras* oncogene activation in human lung cancer. *Cancer Res* **52**:2665s, 1992.

86. Little CD, Nau MM, Carney DN, Gazdar AF, Minna JD: Amplification and expression of the *c-myc* oncogene in human lung cancer cell lines. *Nature* **306**:194, 1983.

87. Brennan J, O'Connor T, Makuch RW, Simmons AM, Russell E, Linnoila RI, Phelps RM, Gazdar AF, Ihde DC, Johnson BE: *Myc* family DNA amplification in 107 tumors and tumor cell lines from patients with small cell lung cancer treated with different combination chemotherapy regimens. *Cancer Res* **51**:1708, 1991.

88. Johnson BE, Ihde DC, Makuch RW, Gazdar AF, Carney DN, Oie H, Russell E, Nau MM, Minna JD: *c-myc* family oncogene amplification in tumor cell lines established from small cell lung cancer patients and its relationship to clinical status and course. *J Clin Invest* **79**:1629, 1987.

89. Sklar MD, Prochownik EV: Modulation of cis resistance in Friend erythroleukemia cells by *c-myc*. *Cancer Res* **51**:2118, 1991.

90. Niimi S, Nakagawa K, Yokota J, Tsunokawa Y, Nishio K, Terashima Y, Shibuya M, Terada M, Saijo N: Resistance to anticancer drugs in NIH3T3 cells transfected with *c-myc* and/or *c-H-ras* genes. *Br J Cancer* **63**:237, 1991.

91. Nau MM, Brooks BJ, Battey J, Sausville E, Gazdar AF, Kirsch IR, McBride OW, Bertness V, Hollis GF, Minna JD: *L-myc*, a new myc gene amplified and expressed in human small cell lung cancer. *Nature* **318**:69, 1985.

92. Nau MM, Brooks BJ, Carney DN, Gazdar AF, Battey JF, Sausville EA, Minna JD: Human small lung cancers show amplification and expression of the *N-myc* gene. *Proc Natl Acad Sci USA* **83**:1092, 1986.

93. Johnson BE: The role of MYC, JUN, and FOS oncogenes in human lung cancer, in Pass HI, Mitchell JB, Johnson DH, Turisi AT (eds): *Lung Cancer: Principles and Practice*. Philadelphia, Lippincott, 1996, p 83.

94. Schauer IE, Siriwardana S, Langan TA, Sclafani RA: Cyclin D1 overexpression vs retinoblastoma inactivation: Implications for growth control evasion in non-small cell and small cell lung cancer. *Proc Natl Acad Sci USA* **91**:7827, 1994.

95. Marchetti A, Doglioni C, Barbareschi M, Buttitta F, Pellegrini S, Gaeta P, La Rocca R, Merlo G, Chella A, Angeletti CA, Dalla Palma P, Bevilacqua G: Cyclin D1 and retinoblastoma susceptibility gene alterations in non-small cell lung cancer. *Int J Cancer* **75**:187, 1998.

96. Chiba I, Takashi T, Nau MM, D'Amico D, Curiel DT, Misudomi T, Buchhagen DL, Carbone D, Piantadosi S, Koga H: Mutations in the *p53* gene are frequent in primary, resected non-small cell lung cancer. *Oncogene* **5**:1603, 1990.

97. D'Amico D, Carbone D, Mitsudomi T, Nau M, Fedorko J, Russell E, Johnson B, Buchhagen D, Bodner S, Phelps R: High frequency of somatically acquired *p53* mutations in small cell lung cancer cell lines and tumors. *Oncogene* **7**:339, 1992.

98. Denissenko MF, Pao A, Tang M, Pfeifer GP: Preferential formation of benzo[a]pyrene adducts at lung cancer mutational hot spots in p53. *Science* **274**:430, 1996.

99. Quinlan DC, Davidson AG, Summers CL, Warden HE, Doshi HM: Accumulation of p53 protein correlates with a poor prognosis in human lung cancer. *Cancer Res* **52**:4828, 1992.

100. McLaren R, Kuzu I, Dunnill M, Harris A, Lane D, Gatter K: The relationship of p53 immunostaining to survival in carcinoma of the lung. *Br J Cancer* **66**:735, 1992.

101. Serrano M, Hannon GJ, Beach D: A new regulatory motif in cell control causing specific inhibition of cyclin D/CDK4. *Nature* **366**:704, 1993.

102. Sherr CJ: G1 phase progression: Cycling on cue. *Cell* **79**:551, 1994.

103. Larsen C: p16^{INK4}: A gene with a dual capacity to encode unrelated proteins that inhibit cell cycle progression. *Oncogene* **12**:2041, 1996.

104. Kamb A, Gruis NA, Weaver J, Liu Q, Harshman K, Tavtigian SV, Stockert E, Day RS, Johnson BE, Skolnick MH: A cell cycle regulator potentially involved in genesis of many tumor types. *Science* **264**:436, 1994.

105. Cairns P, Mao L, Merlo A, Lee DJ, Schwab D, Eby Y, Tokino K, van der Riet P, Blaugrund JE, Sidransky D: Rates of *p16* (*MTS1*) mutations in primary tumors with 9p loss. *Science* **265**:415, 1994.

106. Okamoto A, Hussain SP, Hagiwara K, Spillare EA, Rusin MR, Demetrick DJ, Serrano M, Hannon GJ, Shiseki M, Zariwala M, Xiong Y, Beach DH, Yokota J, Harris CC: Mutations in the *p16^{INK4}/MTS1/ CDKN2, p15^{INK4}/MTS2*, and *p18* genes in primary and metastatic lung cancer. *Cancer Res* **55**:1448, 1995.

107. Packenham JP, Taylor JA, White CM, Anna CH, Barrett JC, Devereux TR: Homozygous deletions at chromosome 9p21 and mutation analysis of p16 and p15 in microdissected primary non cell lung cancers. *Clin Cancer Res* **1**:687, 1995.

108. Merlo A, Herman JG, Mao L, Lee DJ, Gabrielson E, Burger PC, Baylin SB, Sidransky D: 59 CpG island methylation is associated with transcriptional silencing of the tumour suppressor *p16/CDKN2/ MTS1* in human cancers. *Nature Med* **1**:686, 1995.

109. Herman JG, Merlo A, Mao L, Lapidus RG, Issa J, Davidson NE, Sidransky D, Baylin SB: Inactivation of the *CDKN2/p16/MTS1* gene is frequently associated with aberrant DNA methylation in all common human cancers. *Cancer Res* **55**:4525, 1995.

110. Shapiro GI, Edwards CD, Kobzik L, Godleski J, Richards W, Sugarbaker DJ, Rollins BJ: Reciprocal *Rb* inactivation and *p16^{INK4}* expression in primary lung cancers and cell lines. *Cancer Res* **55**:505, 1995.

111. Otterson GA, Khleif SN, Chen W, Coxon AB, Kaye FJ: CDKN2 gene silencing in lung cancer by DNA hypermethylation and kinetics of *p16^{INK4}* protein induction by 5-aza 29deoxycytidine. *Oncogene* **11**:1211, 1995.

112. Otterson GA, Kratzke RA, Coxon A, Kim YW, Kaye FJ: Absence of *p16^{INK4}* protein is restricted to the subset of lung cancer lines that retains wildtype RB. *Oncogene* **9**:3375, 1994.

113. Sherr CJ: Mammalian G1 cyclins. *Cell* **73**:1059, 1993.

114. Hensel CH, Hsieh CL, Gazdar AF, Johnson BE, Sakaguchi AY, Naylor SL, Lee WH, Lee EY: Altered structure and expression of the retinoblastoma susceptibility gene in small cell lung cancer. *Cancer Res* **50**:3067, 1990.

115. Xu HJ, Hu SX, Cagle PT, Moore GE, Benedict WF: Absence of retinoblastoma protein expression in primary non-small cell lung carcinomas. *Cancer Res* **51**:2735, 1991.

116. Veronese, M-L, Sozzi G, Huebner K, Croce CM: The role of the *FHIT* gene in the pathogenesis of lung cancer, in Pass HI, Mitchell JB, Johnson DH, Turrisi AT, Minna JD: *Lung Cancer: Principles and Practice, Second Edition*. Philadelphia, Lippincott Williams and Wilkins, 2000, p. 156.

117. Kohno T, Takahashi M, Manda R, Yokota J: Inactivation of the *PTEN/MMAC1/TEP1* gene in human lung cancers. *Genes Chromosom Cancer* **22**:152, 1998.

118. Yokomizo A, Tindall DJ, Drabkin H, Gemmill R, Franklin W, Yang P, Sugio K, Smith DI, Liu W: *PTEN/MMAC1* mutations identified in small cell, but not in non-small cell lung cancers. *Oncogene* **17**:475, 1998.

119. Sakurada A, Suzuki A, Sato M, Yamakawa H, Orikasa K, Uyeno S, Ono T, Ohuchi N, Fujimura S, Horii A: Infrequent genetic alterations of the *PTEN/MMAC1* gene in Japanese patients with primary cancers of the breast, lung, pancreas, kidney, and ovary. *Jpn J Cancer Res* **88**:1025, 1997.

120. Kim SK, Su LK, Oh Y, Kemp BL, Hong WK, Mao L: Alterations of *PTEN/MMAC1*, a candidate tumor suppressor gene, and its homo-

logue, *PTH2,* in small cell lung cancer cell lines. *Oncogene* **16**:89, 1998.

121. Okami K, Wu L, Riggins G, Cairns P, Goggins M, Evron E, Halachmi N, Ahrendt SA, Reed AL, Hilgers W, Kern SE, Koch WM, Sidransky D, Jen J: Analysis of *PTEN/MMAC1* alterations in aerodigestive tract tumors. *Cancer Res* **58**:509, 1998.

121a. Wang SS, Esplin ED, Li JL, Huang L, Gazdar A, Minna J, Evans GA: Alterations of the PPP2R1B gene in human lung and colon cancer. *Science* **282**:284, 1998.

121b. Kohno T, Takakura S, Yamada T, Okamoto A, Tanaka T, Yokota J: Alterations of the PPP1R3 gene in human cancer. *Cancer Res* **59**:4170,1999.

121c. Lerman MI, Minna JD, for The International Lung Cancer Chromosome 3p21.3 Tumor Suppressor Gene Consortium: The 630-kb lung cancer homozygous deletion region on human chromosome 3p21.3: identification and evaluation of the resident candidate tumor suppressor genes. *Cancer Res* **60**:6116, 2000.

121d. Dammann R, Li C, Yoon JH, Chin PL, Bates S, Pfeifer GP: Epigenetic inactivation of an RAS association domain family protein from the lung tumour suppressor locus 3p21.3. *Nat Genet* **25**:315, 2000.

122. Dragani TA, Manenti G, Pierotti MA: Genetics of murine lung tumors. *Adv Cancer Res* **67**:83, 1995.

123. Belinsky SA, Devereux TR, Maronpot RR, Stoner GD, Anderson MW: Relationship between the formation of promutagenic adducts and the activation of *K-ras* protooncogene in lung tumors from A/J mice treated with nitrosamines. *Cancer Res* **49**:5305, 1989.

124. Belinsky SA, Nikula KJ, Baylin SB, Issa J: Increased cytosine DNA activity is target-cell-specific and an early event in lung cancer. *Proc Natl Acad Sci USA* **93**:4045, 1996.

125. Gariboldi M, Manenti G, Canzian F, Falvella FS, Radice MT, Pierotti MA, Della Porta G, Binelli G, Dragani TA: A major susceptibility locus to murine lung carcinogenesis maps on chromosome 6. *Nature Genet* **3**:132, 1993.

126. Herzog CR, Lubet RA, You M: Genetic alterations in mouse lung tumors: Implications for cancer chemoprevention. *J Cell Biochem Suppl* **28-29**:49, 1997.

127. Swafford DS, Middleton SK, Palmisano WA, Nikula KJ, Tesfaigzi J, Baylin SB, Herman JG, Belinsky SA: Frequent aberrant methylation of *p16^{INK4}* in primary rat lung tumors. *Mol Cell Biol* **17**:1366, 1997.

128. Mao L, Hruban RH, Boyle JO, Tockman M, Sidransky D: Detection of oncogene mutations in sputum precedes diagnosis of lung cancer. *Cancer Res* **54**:1634, 1994.

129. Chen XQ, Stroun M, Magnenat J, Nicod LP, Kurt A, Lyautey J, Lederrey C, Anker P: Microsatellite alterations in plasma DNA of small cell lung cancer patients. *Nature Med* **2**:1033, 1996.

130. Roth JA, Nguyen D, Lawrence DD, Kemp BL, Carrasco CH, Ferson DZ, Hong WK, Komaki R, Lee JJ, Nesbitt JC, Pisters KMW, Putnam JB, Schea R, Shin DM, Walsh GL, Dolormente MM, Han C, Martin FD, Yen N, Xu K: Retrovirus wild *p53* gene transfer to tumors of patients with lung cancer. *Nature Med* **2**:985, 1996.

131. Sun J, Qian Y, Hamilton AD, Sebti SM: *Ras* CAAX peptidomimetic FTI276 selectivity blocks tumor growth in nude mice of a human lung carcinoma with *K-ras* mutation and *p53* deletion. *Cancer Res* **55**:4243, 1995.

132. James GL, Goldstein JL, Brown MR, Rawson TE, Somers TC, McDowell RS, Crowley CW, Lucas BK, Levinson AD, Marsters JC: Benzodiazepine peptidomimetics: Potent inhibitors of *ras* farnesylation in animal cells. *Science* **260**:1937, 1993.

Hepatocellular Carcinoma

Lynne W. Elmore ■ *Curtis C. Harris*

1. Hepatocellular carcinoma (HCC) is an aggressive malignancy with a poor prognosis. The multifactorial and multistage pathogenesis of HCC has fascinated a wide spectrum of cancer researchers for decades. While a number of etiologic factors have been identified, the elucidation of their mechanistic roles in hepatocarcinogenesis has recently just begun. Clearly, in sub-Saharan Africa and Eastern Asia, viral and chemical carcinogenic components are involved, with the subsequent inactivation of the p53 tumor suppressor gene playing a central role. A better understanding of the molecular pathogenesis of HCC will provide clues for more effective preventive and therapeutic strategies.

2. HCC is the predominant cause of cancer mortality in Southern China and sub-Saharan Africa. Infection with hepatitis B virus (HBV) and food contamination with aflatoxin B_1 (AFB_1) are major and possible synergistic risk factors. A number of conditions associated with chronic hepatic inflammation and cirrhosis have also been identified as important etiologic factors worldwide.

3. HBV sequences randomly integrate into host chromosomal DNA, resulting in frequent rearrangements. HBV-induced chromosomal aberrations may in part explain the loss of heterozygosity reported on many chromosomes in HCCs. Allelic loss of the short arm of chromosome 17, which includes the p53 tumor suppressor gene, has commonly been found in human HCCs.

4. In specific geographic regions of Asia, Africa, and North America with high HCC risk, e.g., Qidong and Tongon, China, southern Africa, and Mexico, a G to T transversion at the third position of codon 249 of p53 has provided a molecular link between dietary AFB_1 exposure and liver cancer development. Data from laboratory studies indicate that this region of p53 is highly sensitive to AFB_1-induced DNA damage and that the resulting mutated protein provides a selective growth advantage in liver cells. Inactivation of p53 gene function may also result from its association with the HBV X protein (HBx). p53 and HBx physically associate, resulting in the inability of p53 to bind specific DNA sequences, transcriptionally transactivate p53-effector genes, associate with critical DNA repair proteins, and induce apoptosis. Abnormalities of the retinoblastoma tumor suppressor gene, typically in advanced lesions and associated with loss of p53, have also been reported in HCCs.

5. While mutation and amplification of protooncogenes, e.g., the ras family, are rarely detected in human HCCs, their overexpression is a common finding. *c-myc* and *c-fos* overexpression may result in part from HBV-encoded transcriptional transactivators, which are often expressed and functionally active in HCCs.

6. Insulin-like growth factor II (IGF-II) and insulin receptor substrate 1 (IRS-1) are frequently expressed at high levels in HCCs. The insulin growth factor signal transduction pathways may contribute to hepatocarcinogenesis by providing a strong proliferative stimulus, promoting tumor angiogenesis and/or preventing transforming growth factor-β_1(TGF-β_1)-induced apoptosis. Overexpression of transforming growth factor-α also is observed in many HCCs, particularly in those tumors associated with HBV infection.

7. A better understanding of the complex pathobiological process of hepatocarcinogenesis has resulted in more effective preventive measures, including the implementation of HBV vaccination programs. The possibility of *p53* as a target for HCC therapy is discussed.

Hepatocellular carcinoma is one of the most common malignancies worldwide, affecting 250,000 to 1,000,000 individuals annually (reviewed in[1,2]). HCC causes at least 200,000 deaths per year, and in some regions such as Qidong, China, this disease causes 10 percent of all deaths. Both epidemiologists and laboratory researchers have greatly contributed to the understanding of the multifactorial etiology and multistage pathogenesis of HCC[3,4] (Fig. 49-1).

EPIDEMIOLOGY AND ETIOLOGY

The geographic distribution of HCC is highly variable, with Eastern Asia and sub-Saharan Africa being the most prevalent regions (reviewed in[2,5]). Substantial epidemiologic evidence indicates that HBV is a major risk factor for the development of HCC (reviewed in[6]). HBV carriers with chronic active hepatitis have up to a 200-fold greater risk of developing HCC than age-matched noninfected controls.[7–12] Moreover, an estimated 80 percent of HCCs worldwide are in HBV-infected individuals. Aflatoxin B_1 (AFB_1) also is considered to be a significant etiologic agent in certain geographic areas (e.g., Asia, southern Africa, and Mexico) where food contaminated by this mycotoxin is consumed.[13–15] In the high-HCC incidence geographic area of China, exposure to dietary AFB_1 and chronic HBV infection are synergistic risk factors.[15–19] Other etiologic factors for hepatocarcinogenesis include conditions associated with chronic necroinflammatory liver disease and cirrhosis, such as hepatitis C virus (HCV) infection, chronic alcohol-induced liver disease, hemochromatosis, primary biliary cirrhosis, and alpha-1 antitrypsin deficiency.[2,6,20–25] Data from recent case series and case control studies indicate that synergistic interactions may also exist between HBV and HCV in the development of HCC.[26–29]

CHROMOSOMAL AND GENETIC ABNORMALITIES

Little is known regarding the specific alterations responsible for the development or progression of human HCC. Loss of heterozygosity (LOH) has been associated with inactivation of tumor suppressor genes.[30–36] In human HCCs, LOH has been reported on several chromosome arms, including 1p[37–39], 1q[39,40], 2q[39], 4q[38–42], 5q[43,44], 6q[39,45], 8p[39,40,46,47], 8q[38,40,44], 9p[44,48], 9q[39], 10q[40,49], 11p[44,50,51], 11q[44], 13q[39,40,44,51,52] and 17p[38,40,44,52,53]with some occurring irrespective of the presence of HBV infection.[49,54] It is noteworthy that four cases have been reported in which

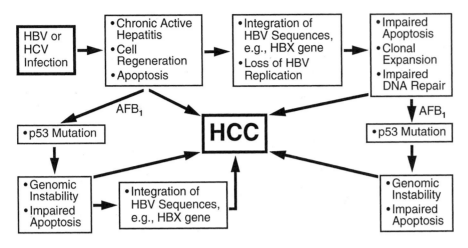

Fig. 49-1 Model of viral-chemical interactions in multistage hepatocellular carcinogenesis.

HBV-associated rearrangements have affected chromosome 17.[35,36,55,56] In two of these[35,36] the rearrangement mapped in the vicinity of the tumor suppressor gene p53, which is located on chromosome 17p13.1.[57] As described below ("Tumor Suppressor Genes"), p53 is the most common LOH site described in human HCCs,[58–62] and data are accumulating to strongly suggest that inactivation of this gene/protein may significantly contribute to the molecular pathogenesis of human HCC. A frequent LOH on 6q at the mannose-6-phosphate/insulin-like growth factor II receptor (M6P/IGF2r) locus in human hepatocellular carcinomas and adenomas has also been reported.[45,63,64] Since this receptor is necessary for both the activation of a growth inhibitor (transforming growth factor β_1 [TGF-β_1])[65] and the degradation of a potent mitogen (insulin growth factor II [IGF-II]),[66] its loss could facilitate liver cell growth.

Most HCCs in HBV carriers contain HBV DNA sequences integrated into the host chromosomal DNA.[6,67] Unlike woodchuck hepatitis virus DNA, which frequently integrates into the c-*myc* or N-*myc* protooncogenes, resulting in either their rearrangement or overexpression,[68,69] the sites of HBV integration in human HCC are highly variable and random.[70,71] Findings of amplification or a single base mutation of some oncogenes have been reported in human HCCs associated with HBV integration, but their incidence is very rare.[72,73] Instead, the sites of cellular DNA at which HBV integrates frequently undergo rearrangements,[74,75] resulting in translocations,[35,55] inverted duplications,[76] deletions,[50,55,77] and possibly recombinatorial events.[2,78] These HBV-induced chromosomal alterations may result in the loss of relevant cellular genes, such as tumor suppressor genes, important in cell cycle control and differentiation.

Tumor Suppressor Genes

The p53 tumor suppressor protein is involved in multiple cellular processes, including cell cycle control, senescence, DNA repair, genomic stability, and apoptosis (reviewed in[79,80]). p53 is functionally inactivated by either structural mutations, viral proteins, or endogenous cellular mechanisms in the majority of human cancers.[79,81–83] Certain domains of the p53 gene have been highly conserved, reflecting the functional importance and selection of this protein.[84] The majority of base substitutions fall within the highly conserved central portion of the gene,[85,86] which mediates sequence-specific DNA binding and transcriptional activation[81] (Fig. 49-2). An extensive analysis of p53 gene mutations indicates that the sites and features of DNA base changes differ among the various human tumor types.[82,85] In the case of HCC, a unique mutational spectrum has provided a strong molecular link between carcinogen exposure and cancer development. When primary HCCs in Qidong, China, were examined, we found that 8 of 16 had point mutations at the third position of codon 249, resulting in a G:C to T:A transversion.[88] This finding has been confirmed by others[89,90] and extended to HCCs from southern Africa and North

America and Tongon, China.[58,91–93] A dose-dependent relationship between dietary AFB$_1$ and codon 249^{ser} p53 mutations is observed in these geographic areas (Fig. 49-3). HCCs from geographic areas of low AFB$_1$ exposure have a different mutational spectrum,[58,94,95] further establishing a positive association between high dietary AFB$_1$ exposure and 249^{ser} mutations. An analysis of p53 mutations in several human HCC and hepatoblastoma cell lines indicates that this mutational hotspot is specific for liver tumors of hepatocellular origin and does not require the genomic integration of HBV.[96]

Using a highly sensitive genotypic mutation assay, Aguilar et al.[97] have demonstrated the relative abundance of the p53 249^{ser} mutant liver cells of nonmalignant specimens from Qidong when compared to specimens from Thailand and the United States. The biological basis for this frequently observed, early mutational event may be due to the high mutability of the third base at codon 249, as suggested by in vitro studies using human liver cells[98–100]. An alternate, but not mutually exclusive, explanation is that this mutation provides liver cells with a selective growth advantage. Supporting this hypothesis are the following observations: (1) p53-null human liver cancer cells exhibit an enhanced growth rate following transfection with the p53 249^{ser} mutant;[101] (2) introduction of a murine p53 mutation corresponding to human codon 249 into a murine hepatocyte cell line resulted in a selective growth advantage;[102] (3) the 249^{ser} mutant inhibits wild-type p53-mediated apoptosis, resulting in increased cell survival;[103] and (4) the 249^{ser} mutant is more effective than other p53 mutants in inhibiting wild-type p53 transactivation activity in human liver cells[103] (Fig. 49-4). One model concerning the generation of liver cancers with 249^{ser} mutation is that AFB$_1$ is metabolically activated to form the promutagenic N7dG adduct.[104,105] Enhanced cell proliferation due to chronic active hepatitis then allows both fixation of the G:C → T:A transversion in codon 249 of the p53 gene and selective clonal expansion of cells containing this mutated gene.

While the p53 249^{ser} mutant in HCCs correlates with high risk exposure to AFB$_1$, the absence of mutations in exons 5–8 of the p53 gene in 50 to 80 percent of HCCs[87,88,91,106,107] suggests that p53 inactivation may be achieved by another mechanism. The finding that p53 protein and HBx interact[108–110] prompted us to evaluate the functional consequences of this association. HBx strongly inhibits p53 sequence-specific binding[109] which is in contrast to the enhanced DNA binding specificity of the transcription factors CREB and AFT-2 when complexed to HBx, a non-DNA binding cotransactivator.[111,112] HBx also blocks p53-mediated transcriptional transactivation in vivo, as well as the in vitro association of p53 with either XPB (ERCC3)[109] or XPD,[113] transcriptional factors involved in nucleotide excision repair.[114–115] Moreover, HBx efficiently abrogates p53-mediated apoptosis[103] (Fig. 49-5). Recent data indicate that the same carboxyl-terminal domain of HBx (amino acids 111–154)

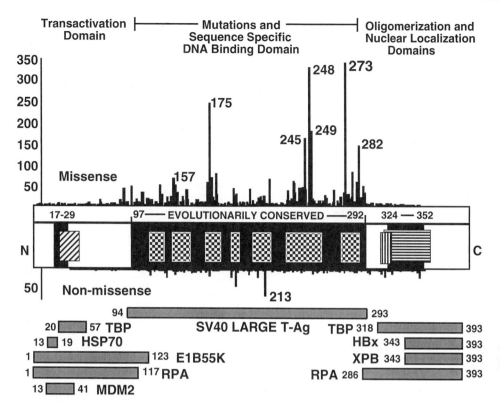

Fig. 49-2 Schematic representation of p53 molecule. The p53 protein consists of 393 amino acids with functional domains, evolutionarily conserved domains, and regions designated as mutational hotspots. Functional domains include the transactivation region (amino acids 20–42; diagonal striped block), sequence-specific DNA-binding region (amino acids 100–293), nuclear localization sequence (amino acids 316–325; vertical striped block), and oligomerization region (amino acids 319–360; horizontal striped block). Cellular or oncoviral proteins bind to specific areas of the p53 protein. Evolutionarily conserved domains (amino acids 17–29, 97–292, and 324–352; black areas) were determined using the MACAW program. Seven mutational hotspot regions within the large conserved domain are identified: amino acids 130–142, 151–164, 171–181, 193–200, 213–223, 234–258, and 270–286; checkered blocks). Functional domains and protein binding sites (gray bars underneath) were compiled from references. Vertical lines above the schematic, missense mutations; lines below schematic, nonmissense mutations.

necessary for binding to p53 (Fig. 49-6) is necessary for sequestering p53 in the cytoplasm and inhibiting p53-mediated apoptosis[116] (Fig. 49-7). The binding of HBx to the extreme carboxyl-terminal domain of p53 appears to inhibit the association of p53 with two putative downstream effectors of p53-mediated apoptosis, namely XPB and XPD[117]. Based on the above data we speculate that inactivation of p53-mediated transcriptional transactivation and apoptosis by HBx could lead to a disruption of normal cellular surveillance mechanisms for repairing and removing damaged cells, thus contributing to genomic instability.

In some cases of HCC, mutation of p53[106,118–121] or possibly inactivation of p53 by MDM-2[122] may be a late event in tumor progression. Tanaka et al.[123] have reported that p53 mutations are closely related to the progression of HCC and that in some cases, malignant cells which acquire the p53 mutations might develop into dedifferentiated subpopulations within a single HCC. Further suggesting an involvement of mutant p53 in the progression of liver cancer is the observation that some nodules consist of both p53 LOH and non-LOH, with the former being associated with cells of more severe cellular atypia.[118] It is noteworthy that abnormalities of the retinoblastoma tumor suppressor gene (Rb) have also been reported in advanced HCCs.[54,124,125,126] In one study, LOH at the Rb gene was detected in 6 of 7 (86 percent) HCCs with a p53 mutation, compared to none of 17 HCCs lacking mutation of p53.[124]

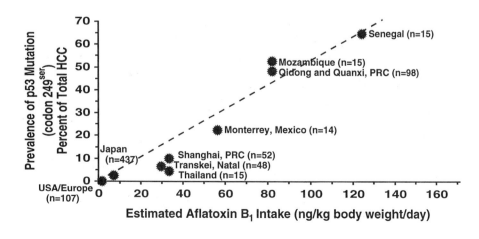

Fig. 49-3 Correlation of estimated aflatoxin B1 dietary exposure and frequency of codon 249ser p53 mutations in hepatocellular carcinoma.

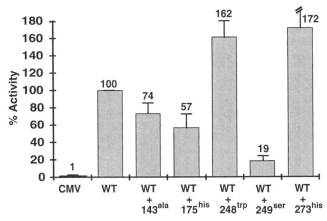

Fig. 49-4 Dominant negative effects of p53 mutants on the transcription of wild-type p53 in a p53-null human liver cancer cell line (Hep-3B).

ONCOGENES

Although activated protooncogenes are found in many spontaneous and experimentally induced HCCs in animal models,[127] no single oncogene has been shown to be preferentially activated in human HCCs.[128–130] By DNA transfection assay in NIH-3T3 cells, activated N-*ras* has been isolated from human HCC tissue; however, the gene was mutated in only a small fraction of the tumor cells.[103] Overexpression of N-*ras*, usually in the absence of a mutation, is often observed in human HCCs,[128,130] while mutations or overexpression of H- and K-*ras* are rare.[132] New oncogenes have been cloned from human HCC tissue,[5,133,134] but their role in hepatocarcinogenesis is unclear.

Mutations and amplification of c-*myc* are rarely detected in human HCCs, but overexpression of this protooncogene is a common finding.[125,130,135] Small studies have also demonstrated frequent overexpression of c-*fos* with an absence of mutations.[125,135,136] The HBV genome contains four open reading frames, two of which are potential transcriptional transactivators (reviewed in[137]). It is well established that HBx is a potent co-transactivator of many viral[138,139] and cellular[138,140–142] promoters including c-*myc*.[143,144] and c-*fos*.[144] The preS/S region of the HBV genome following 3′-truncation[145] also is able to co-transactivate these two protooncogenes.[146] In most cases of HCC, either or both transactivators are expressed and functionally active,[70,146–153] while the other HBV gene products are infrequently detected.[67,148,154] These data indicate that the transcriptional co-transactivation function of HBx and/or preS/S may significantly contribute to the development of HCC. However, considering the multiple functions of HBx, its role in hepatocarcinogenesis may not be limited to its ability to either inactivate p53 functions or transactivate cellular genes. In this regard, HBx can deregulate cell cycle checkpoints,[155] activate the ras-raf-mitogen-activated protein (MAP) kinase[156,157] and protein kinase C signaling cascades,[158,159] stimulate DNA synthesis[155] and cell cycle progression,[160] induce apoptosis,[161] bind to the DNA repair gene XAP-1/UV-DDB,[162,163] complex with cellular transcription

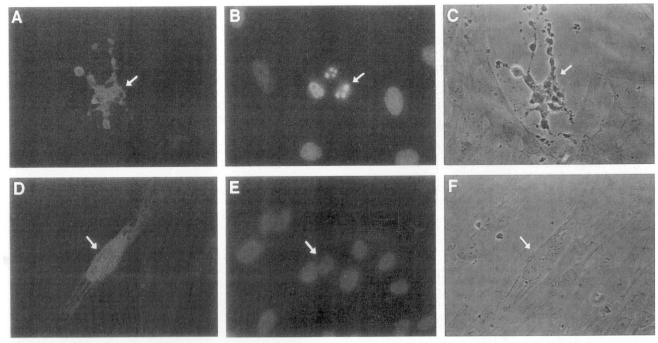

Fig. 49-5 Inhibition of p53-mediated apoptosis by the hepatitis B viral X gene. Induction of apoptosis in normal primary human fibroblasts was achieved by microinjection of a wild-type p53 expression vector. Cells were injected with the wild-type expression vector alone (A–C) or coinjected with wild-type p53 and HBx genes (D–F). Cells were processed and analyzed as described in ref. 103.

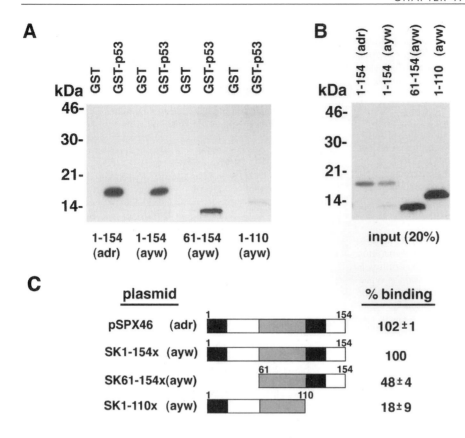

Fig. 49-6 The C-terminal domain of HBx is critical for in vitro association with GST-p53. (*A*) In vitro translated full-length HBx protein (lanes 1–4) and HBx deletion mutants (lanes 5–8) were incubated with glutathione-Sepharose beads loaded with either GST-p53 (lanes 2, 4, 6, 8) or GST (lanes 1, 3, 5, 7); (*B*) To reference input for binding, 20% of the volume of the various in vitro translated HBx proteins used for binding were immunoprecipitated by anti-HBx antibody;[116] (*C*) Schematic representation of full-length and truncated HBx as described in reference,[116] along with a summary of their binding to p53. Percent binding represents the mean ± SD from at least three independent binding assays with values made relative to SK1-154x.

factors,[112,164,165] inhibit hepatic serine proteases,[166–168] neoplastically transform rodent cells in vitro,[169,170] and, as a transgene, induce HCCs in mice.[171]

Growth Factors

The insulin growth factors, which include insulin and insulin-like growth factors I and II (IGF-I and -II, respectively), are potent hepatocellular mitogens.[172] IGF-II is overexpressed[66,172–177] and exhibits an allelic-expression imbalance[178–180] in many human HCCs. In some cases of HBV-associated HCCs, HBx may modulate the expression of IGF-II at the transcriptional level.[165,181] Insulin receptor substrate 1 (IRS-1), a main substrate for insulin and insulin-like growth factors I and II, is also highly expressed in many human HCC tumor tissues and cell lines.[178,182] IRS-1 exhibits transforming potential in NIH-3T3 cells, which is dependent in part on the presence of IGF-I.[183] As a transgene, IRS-1 overexpression leads to increased hepatocyte DNA synthesis.[182] Collectively, these data indicate that the insulin

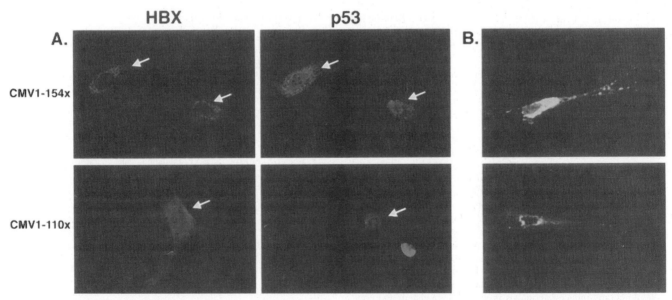

Fig. 49-7 HBx via its carboxyl terminal region sequesters p53 to the cytoplasm. (*A*) Normal human fibroblasts were microinjected with a p53 expression vector and either full-length HBx (CMV-1-154x) or a deletion mutant missing the last 44 amino acids (CMV-1-110x) followed by incubation for 24 hours. Immunostaining was performed as described in reference 116; (*B*) Confocal microscopic analysis of normal human fibroblasts coinjected with p53 and full-length HBx expression vectors. (*Upper*) Representative example of the degree of cytoplasmic sequestration typically observed in fibroblasts over-expressing p53 and HBx. (*Lower*) Fibroblast with all detectable p53 co-localizing with HBx in the cytoplasm.

growth factor signal transduction pathway may provide a critical proliferative stimulus during hepatocarcinogenesis. In addition, IGF-II may promote angiogenesis by upregulating the expression of vascular endothelial growth factor[184,185], a protein which may also play an importnt role in the invasion and metastasis of HCC[186]. Moreover, overexpression of at least one component of this pathway (i.e., IRS-1) may contribute to the development of HCC by preventing TGF-β1-induced apoptosis.[187]

Transforming growth factor-α (TGF-α), another potent hepatocellular mitogen, is present at elevated levels in human HCCs, with its detection often being closely linked to HBV infection.[175,188,189] Specifically, TGF-α was detected more frequently in patients whose adjacent nontumorous liver had detectable HBV surface antigen and/or HBV core antigen (91 percent) than in those whose liver lacked these viral protein products (61 percent).[189] It remains unclear, however, whether increased expression of this growth factor is mechanistically related to hepatocarcinogenesis or whether it results from liver regeneration in response to chronic HBV infection. The latter possibility is supported by the finding that elevated TGF-α expression is typically observed in the livers of patients with chronic hepatitis and without HCC.[175] As with IGF-II, TGF-α may promote tumor angiogenesis by upregulating vascular endothelial growth factor.[190]

IMPLICATIONS FOR TREATMENT AND PREVENTION

HCC is regarded as an aggressive malignancy with a poor prognosis.[1,191] Of the more than 250,000 cases diagnosed worldwide annually, less than 3 percent will survive 5 or more years. For some patients, surgical resection or orthotopic liver transplantation offers disease-free survival; however, most must rely on other modes of treatment, which are currently only palliative.[1,192]

Our better understanding of the complex pathobiologic processes during hepatocarcinogenesis has already resulted in more effective preventive measures. Vaccines for HBV are well developed, and vaccination programs are currently being implemented in 85 countries.[193] The Universal immunization program in Taiwan has resulted in a 10-fold reduction in the hepatitis B carrier rate and has significantly reduced the incidence of hepatocellular carcinoma in children.[194–196] Knowing that AFB$_1$ is a significant risk factor in the development of HCC, limiting the exposure to this mycotoxin by improving the storage of food grains would be another feasible strategy to decrease the incidence of HCC. The efficiency of this intervention could be monitored by measuring aflatoxin-albumin adducts in the blood of individuals consuming food grains.[197]

The frequent inactivation of p53 in HCCs makes this gene an attractive target for cancer therapy (reviewed in[79]). The development of drugs that would inhibit wild-type p53-HBx interactions may provide a means to rescue p53 tumor suppressor function. In those cases where p53 is mutated, agents that mimic wild-type p53 may be effective. Another possibility is p53 gene therapy. Laboratory studies have demonstrated the efficacy of p53 gene therapy in human cancer cells in vitro[198,199] and as a xenograph in athymic nude mice.[200–202] Based on this success, a phase I protocol for non-small cell lung cancer in humans is underway.[203] While the success of this approach is still speculative, it is encouraging that a p53 cDNA expression vector under the control of an α-fetoprotein promoter was successfully transferred into Hep-3B liver cells using a replication-defective retroviral vector, resulting in decreased cell growth and increased sensitivity to chemotherapy-induced apoptosis in vitro.[204] Vogelstein and coworkers[205] have devised a novel strategy of gene therapy, which may also be a future option for HCCs containing mutant p53. This approach relies on the ability of mutant p53 in tumor cells to selectively bind to exogenously introduced gene products resulting in the transcriptional activation of a toxic gene. As we continue to

better understand the molecular pathogenesis of human HCC, clues for additional, rational intervention and therapeutic strategies will likely follow.

ACKNOWLEDGMENTS

The editorial and graphic assistance of Dorothea Dudek and Amy Hancock is greatly appreciated.

REFERENCES

1. Haydon GH, Hayes PC: Hepatocellular carcinoma. *Br J Hosp Med* **53**:74–80, 1995.
2. Sherman M: Hepatocellular carcinoma. *Gastroenterologist* **3**:55–66, 1995.
3. Harris CC: Solving the viral-chemical puzzle of human liver carcinogenesis. *Cancer Epidemiol Biomarkers Prev* **3**:1–2, 1994.
4. Harris CC: The 1995 Walter Hubert Lecture: Molecular epidemiology of human cancer: insights from the mutational analysis of the p53 tumor suppressor gene. *Br J Cancer* **73**:261–269, 1996.
5. Okuda K: Hepatocellular carcinoma: recent progress. *Hepatology* **15**:948–963, 1992.
6. Robinson WS: Molecular events in the pathogenesis of hepadnavirus associated hepatocellular carcinoma. *Annu Rev Med* **45**:297–323, 1994.
7. Beasley RP, Hwang LY, Lin CC, Chien CS: Hepatocellular carcinoma and hepatitis B virus. A prospective study of 22707 men in Taiwan. *Lancet* **2**:1129–1133, 1981.
8. Yeh FS, Yu MC, Mo CC, Luo S, Tong MJ, Henderson BE: Hepatitis B virus, aflatoxins, and hepatocellular carcinoma in southern Guangxi, China. *Cancer Res* **49**:2506–2509, 1989.
9. Beasley RP: Hepatitis B virus. The major etiology of hepatocellular carcinoma. *Cancer* **61**:1942–1956, 1988.
10. McMahon BJ, Lanier AP, Wainwright RB, Kilkenny SJ: Hepatocellular carcinoma in Alaska Eskimos: epidemiology, clinical features, and early detection. *Prog Liver Dis* **9**:643–655, 1990.
11. Iijma T, Saitoh N, Nobutomo K, Nambu M, Sakuma K: A prospective cohort study of hepatitis B surface antigen carriers in a working population. *Gann* **75**:571–573, 1984.
12. Obata H, Hayashi N, Motoike Y, Hisamitsu T, Okuda H, Kobayashi S, Nishioka K: A prospective study on the development of hepatocellular carcinoma from liver cirrhosis with persistent hepatitis B virus infection. *Int J Cancer* **25**:741–747, 1980.
13. Wogan GN: Aflatoxins as risk factors for hepatocellular carcinoma in humans. *Cancer Res* **52**:2114s–2118s, 1992.
14. Harris CC: Hepatocellular carcinogenesis: recent advances and speculations. *Cancer Cells* **2**:146–148, 1990.
15. Ross RK, Yuan JM, Yu MC, Wogan GN, Qian GS, Tu JT, Groopman JD: Urinary aflatoxin biomarkers and risk of hepatocellular carcinoma. *Lancet* **339**:943–946, 1992.
16. Qian GS, Ross RK, Yu MC, Yuan JM, Gao YT, Henderson BE, Wogan GN, et al: A follow-up study of urinary markers of aflatoxin exposure and liver cancer risk in Shanghai, People's Republic of China. *Cancer Epidemiol Biomarkers Prev* **3**:3–10, 1994.
17. Hsia CC, Kleiner DE Jr, Axiotis CA, Di Bisceglie A, Nomura AM, Stemmermann GN, Tabor E: Mutations of p53 gene in hepatocellular carcinoma: role of hepatitis B virus and aflatoxin contamination in the diet. *J Natl Cancer Inst* **84**:1638–1641, 1992.
18. Chen CJ, Yu MW, Liaw YF: Epidemiological characteristics and risk factors of hepatocellular carcinoma. *J Gastroenterol Hepatol* **12**:S294–308, 1997.
19. Lunn RM, Zhang YJ, Wang LY, Chen CJ, Lee PH, Lee CS, Tsai WY et al: p53 mutations, chronic hepatitis B virus infection, and aflatoxin exposure in hepatocellular carcinoma in Taiwan. *Cancer Res* **57**:3471–3477, 1997.
20. Tsukuma H, Hiyama T, Tanaka S, Nakao M, Yabuuchi T, Kitamura T, Nakanishi K et al: Risk factors for hepatocellular carcinoma among patients with chronic liver disease. *N Engl J Med* **328**:1797–1801, 1993.
21. Robinson WS: The role of hepatitis B virus in development of primary hepatocellular carcinoma: Part II. *J Gastroenterol Hepatol* **8**:95–106, 1993.
22. Thompson SC, Lin A, Warren R, Giles G, Crofts N: Risk factors associaated with hepatocellular carcinoma notified to the Anti-Cancer Council of Victoria in 1991-1992. *Aust N Z J Public Health* **21**:626–630, 1997.

23. Caselmann WH, Alt M: Hepatitis C virus infection as a major risk factor for hepatocellular carcinoma. *J Hepatol* **24**: 61–66, 1996.

24. Izzo F, Cremona F, Ruffolo F, Palaia R, Parisi V, Curley SA: Outcome of 67 patients with hepatocellular cancer detected during screening of 1125 patients with chronic hepatitis. *Ann Surg* **227**:513–518, 1998.

25. Di Bisceglie AM: Hepatitis C and hepatocellular carcinoma. *Hepatology* **26**: 34S–38S, 1997.

26. Yu MW, Chen CJ: Hepatitis B and C viruses in the development of hepatocellular carcinoma. *Crit Rev Oncol Hematol* **17**:71–91, 1994.

27. Kubo S, Nishiguchi S, Tamori A, Hirohashi K, Kinoshita H, Kuroki T: Development of hepatocellular carcinoma in patients with HCV infection, with or without past HBV infection, and relationship to age at the time of transfusion. *Vox sang* **74**: 129, 1998.

28. Donato F, Boffetta P, Puoti M: A meta-analysis of epidemiological studies on the combined effect of hepatitis B and C virus infections in causing hepatocellular carcinoma. *Int J Cancer* **75**: 347–354, 1998.

29. Tsai JF, Jeng, JE, Ho MS, Chang WY, Hsieh MY, Lin ZY, Tsai JH: Effect of hepatitis C and B virus infection on risk of hepatocellular carcinoma: a prospective study. *Br J Cancer* **76**: 968–974, 1997.

30. Shiraishi M, Morinaga S, Noguchi M, Shimosato Y, Sekiya T: Loss of genes on the short arm of chromosome 11 in human lung carcinomas. *Jpn J Cancer Res* **78**:1302–1308, 1987.

31. Kovacs G, Erlandsson R, Boldog F, Ingvarsson S, Muller R, Klein G, Sumegi J: Consistent chromosome 3p deletion and loss of heterozygosity in renal cell carcinoma. *Proc Natl Acad Sci USA* **85**:1571–1575, 1988.

32. Bodmer WF, Bailey CJ, Bodmer J, Bussey HJ, Ellis A, Gorman P, Lucibello FC et al: Localization of the gene for familial adenomatous polyposis on chromosome 5. *Nature* **328**:614–616, 1987.

33. Solomon E, Voss R, Hall V, Bodmer WF, Jass JR, Jeffreys AJ, Lucibello FC et al: Chromosome 5 allele loss in human colorectal carcinomas. *Nature* **328**:616–619, 1987.

34. Johnson BE, Sakaguchi AY, Gazdar AF, Minna JD, Burch D, Marshall A, Naylor SL: Restriction fragment length polymorphism studies show consistent loss of chromosome 3p alleles in small cell lung cancer patients' tumors. *J Clin Invest* **82**:502–507, 1988.

35. Meyer M, Wiedorn KH, Hofschneider PH, Koshy R, Caselmann WH: A chromosome 17:7 translocation is associated with a hepatitis B virus DNA integration in human hepatocellular carcinoma DNA. *Hepatology* **15**:665–671, 1992.

36. Zhou YZ, Slagle BL, Donehower LA, vanTuinen P, Ledbetter DH, Butel JS: Structural analysis of a hepatitis B virus genome integrated into chromosome 17p of a human hepatocellular carcinoma. *J Virol* **62**:4224–4231, 1988.

37. Zhang W, Hirohashi S, Tsuda H, Shimosato Y, Yokota J, Terada M, Sugimura T: Frequent loss of heterozygosity on chromosomes 16 and 4 in human hepatocellular carcinoma. *Jpn J Cancer Res* **81**:108–111, 1990.

38. Kuroki T, Fujiwara Y, Tsuchiya E, Nakamori S, Imaoka S, Kanematsu T, Nakamura Y: Accumulation of genetic changes during development and progression of hepatocellular carcinoma: loss of heterozygosity of chromosome arm 1p occurs at an early stage of hepatocarcinogenesis. *Genes Chrom Cancer* **13**:163–166, 1995.

39. Nagai H, Pineau P, Tiollais P, Buendia MA, Dejean A: Comprehensive allelotyping of human hepatocellular carcinoma. *Oncogene* **14**: 2927–2933, 1997.

40. Piao Z, Park C, Park JH, Kim H: Allelotype analysis of hepatocellular carcinoma. *Int J Cancer* **75**: 29–33, 1998.

41. Sheu JC: Molecular mechanism of hepatocarcinogenesis. *J Gastroenterol Hepatol* **12**: S309–13, 1997.

42. Chou YH, Chung KC, Jeng LB, Chen TC, Liaw YF: Frequent allelic loss on chromosomes 4q and 16q associated with human hepatocellular carcinoma in Taiwan. *Cancer Lett* **123**:1–6, 1998.

43. Ding SF, Habib NA, Dooley J, Wood C, Bowles L, Delhanty JD: Loss of constitutional heterozygosity on chromosome 5q in hepatocellular carcinoma without cirrhosis. *Br J Cancer* **64**:1083–1087, 1991.

44. Hubbard AL, Harrison DJ, Moyes C, Wyllie AH, Cunningham C, Mannion E, Smith CA: N-acetyltransferase 2 genotype in colorectal cancer and selective gene retention in cancers with chromosome 8p deletions. *Gut* **41**:229–234, 1997.

45. De Souza AT, Hankins GR, Washington MK, Fine RL, Orton TC, Jirtle RL: Frequent loss of heterozygosity on 6q at the mannose 6-phosphate/insulin-like growth factor II receptor locus in human hepatocellular tumors. *Oncogene* **10**:1725–1729, 1995.

46. Emi M, Fujiwara Y, Nakajima T, Tsuchiya E, Tsuda H, Hirohashi S, Maeda Y et al: Frequent loss of heterozygosity for loci on chromosome 8p in hepatocellular carcinoma, colorectal cancer, and lung cancer. *Cancer Res* **52**:5368–5372, 1992.

47. Yuan BZ, Miller MJ, Keck CL, Zimonjic DB, Thorgerison SS, Popescu NC: Cloning, characterization, and chromosomal localizaation of a gene frequently deleted in human liver cancer (DLC-1) homologous to rat RhoGAP. *cancer Res* **58**:2196–2199, 1998.

48. Piao Z, Park C, Lee JS, Yang CH, Choi KY, Kim H: Homozygous delections of the CDKN2 gene and loss of heterozygosity of 9p in primary hepatocellular carcinoma. *Cancer Lett* **122**: 201-207, 1998.

49. Fujimori M, Tokino T, Hino O, Kitagawa T, Imamura T, Okamoto E, Mitsunobu M et al: Allelotype study of primary hepatocellular carcinoma. *Cancer Res* **51**:89–93, 1991.

50. Rogler CE, Sherman M, Su CY, Shafritz DA, Summers J, Shows TB, Henderson A et al: Deletion in chromosome 11p associated with a hepatitis B integration site in hepatocellular carcinoma. *Science* **230**:319–322, 1985.

51. Wang HP, Rogler CE: Deletions in human chromosome arms 11p and 13q in primary hepatocellular carcinomas. *Cytogenet Cell Genet* **48**: 72–78, 1988.

52. Nishida N, Fukuda Y, Kokuryu H, Sadamoto T, Isowa G, Honda K, Yamaoka Y et al: Accumulation of allelic loss on arms of chromosomes 13q, 16q and 17p in the advanced stages of human hepatocellular carcinoma. *Int J Cancer* **51**:862–868, 1992.

53. Nishida N, Fukuda Y, Kokuryu H, Toguchida J, Yandell DW, Ikenega M, Imura H et al: Role and mutational heterogeneity of the p53 gene in hepatocellular carcinoma. *Cancer Res* **53**:368–372, 1993.

54. Fujimoto Y, Hampton LL, Wirth PJ, Wang NJ, Xie JP, Thorgeirsson SS: Alterations of tumor suppressor genes and allelic losses in human hepatocellular carcinomas in China. *Cancer Res* **54**:281–285, 1994.

55. Hino O, Shows TB, Rogler CE: Hepatitis B virus integration site in hepatocellular carcinoma at chromosome 17;18 translocation. *Proc Natl Acad Sci USA* **83**:8338–8342, 1986.

56. Tokino T, Fukushige S, Nakamura T, Nagaya T, Murotsu T, Shiga K, Aoki N et al: Chromosomal translocation and inverted duplication associated with integrated hepatitis B virus in hepatocellular carcinomas. *J Virol* **61**:3848–3854, 1987.

57. McBride OW, Merry D, Givol D: The gene for human p53 cellular tumor antigen is located on chromosome 17 short arm (17p13). *Proc Natl Acad Sci USA* **83**:130–134, 1986.

58. Ozturk M: p53 mutation in hepatocellular carcinoma after aflatoxin exposure. *Lancet* **338**:1356–1359, 1991.

59. Oda T, Tsuda H, Scarpa A, Sakamoto M, Hirohashi S: Mutation pattern of the p53 gene as a diagnostic marker for multiple hepatocellular carcinoma. *Cancer Res* **52**:3674–3678, 1992.

60. Bressac B, Galvin KM, Liang TJ, Isselbacher KJ, Wands JR, Ozturk M: Abnormal structure and expression of p53 gene in human hepatocellular carcinoma. *Proc Natl Acad Sci USA* **87**:1973–1977, 1990.

61. Piao Z, Kim H, Jeon BK, Lee WJ, Park C: Relationship between loss of heterozygosity of tumor suppressor genes and histologic differentiation in hepatocellular carcinoma. *Cancer* **80**: 865–872, 1997.

62. Kishimoto Y, Shiota G, Kamisaki Y, Wada K, Nakamoto K, Yamawaki M, Kotani M, et al: Loss of the tumor suppressor p53 gene at the liver cirrhosis stage in Japanese patients with hepatocellular carcinoma. *Oncology* **54**: 304–310, 1997.

63. Yamada T, De Souza AT, Finkelstein S, Jirtle RL: Loss of the gene encoding mannose 6-phosphate/insulin-like growth factor II receptor is an early event in liver carcinogenesis. *Proc Natl Acad Sci U S A* **94**: 10351–10355, 1997.

64. Piao Z, Choi Y, Park C, Lee WJ, Park JH, Kim H: Deletion of the M6P/IGF2r gene in primary hepatocellular carcinoma. *Cancer Lett* **120**: 39–43, 1997.

65. Takiya S, Tagaya T, Takahashi K, Kawashima H, Kamiya M, Fukuzawa Y, Kobayashi S et al: Role of transforming growth factor beta 1 on hepatic regeneration and apoptosis in liver diseases. *J Clin Pathol* **48**:1093–1097, 1995.

66. Seo JH, Park BC: Expression of insulin-like growth factor II in chronic hepatitis B, liver cirrhosis, and hepatocellular carcinoma. *Gan To Kagaku Ryoho* **22**(**Suppl 3**):292–307, 1995.

67. Diamantis ID, McGandy CE, Chen TJ, Liaw YF, Gudat F, Bianchi L: Hepatitis B X-gene expression in hepatocellular carcinoma. *J Hepatol* **15**:400–403, 1992.

68. Fourel G, Trepo C, Bougueleret L, Henglein B, Ponzetto A, Tiollais P, Buendía MA: Frequent activation of N-myc genes by hepadnavirus insertion in woodchuck liver tumours. *Nature* **347**:294–298, 1990.

69. Hsu T, Moroy T, Etiemble J, Louise A, Trepo C, Tiollais P, Buendia MA: Activation of c-myc by woodchuck hepatitis virus insertion in hepatocellular carcinoma. *Cell* **55**:627–635, 1988.

70. Matsubara K, Tokino T: Integration of hepatitis B virus DNA and its implications to hepatocarcinogenesis. *Mol Biol Med* **7**:243–260, 1990.

71. Rogler CE, Chisari FV: Cellular and molecular mechanisms of hepatocarcinogenesis. *Semin Liver Dis* **12**:265–278, 1992.

72. de The H, Marchio A, Tiollais P, Dejean A: A novel steroid thyroid hormone receptor related gene inappropriately expressed in human hepatocellular carcinoma. *Nature* **330**:667–670, 1987.

73. Wang J, Chenivesse X, Henglein B, Brechot C: Hepatitis B virus integration in a cyclin A gene in a hepatocellular carcinoma. *Nature* **343**:555–557, 1990.

74. Ogata N, Tokino T, Kamimura T, Asakura H: A comparison of the molecular structure of integrated hepatitis B virus genomes in hepatocellular carcinoma cells and hepatocytes derived from the same patient. *Hepatology* **11**:1017–1023, 1990.

75. Hino O, Kajino K: Hepatitis virus related hepatocarcinogenesis. *Intervirology* **37**:133–135, 1994.

76. Hino O, Nomura K, Ohtake K, Kawaguchi T, Sugano H, Kitagawa T: Instability of integrated hepatitis B virus DNA with inverted repeat structure in a transgenic mouse. *Cancer Genet Cytogenet* **37**:273–278, 1989.

77. Nakamura T, Tokino T, Nagaya T, Matsubara K: Microdeletion associated with the integration process of hepatitis B virus DNA. *Nucleic Acids Res* **16**:4865–4873, 1988.

78. Hino O, Tabata S, Hotta Y: Evidence for increased in vitro recombination with insertion of human hepatitis B virus DNA. *Proc Natl Acad Sci USA* **88**:9248–9252, 1991.

79. Harris CC: Structure and function of the p53 tumor suppressor gene: clues for rational cancer therapeutic strategies. *J Natl Cancer Inst* **88**:1442–1455, 1996.

80. Ko LJ, Prives C: p53: puzzle and paradigm. *Genes Devel* **10**:1054–1072, 1996.

81. Levine AJ, Momand J, Finlay CA: The p53 tumour suppressor gene. *Nature* **351**:453–456, 1991.

82. Hollstein M, Sidransky D, Vogelstein B, Harris CC: p53 mutations in human cancers. *Science* **253**:49–53, 1991.

83. Greenblatt MS, Bennett WP, Hollstein M, Harris CC: Mutations in the p53 tumor suppressor gene: clues to cancer etiology and molecular pathogenesis. *Cancer Res* **54**:4855–4878, 1994.

84. Soussi T, Caron de Fromentel C, May P: Structural aspects of the p53 protein in relation to gene evolution. *Oncogene* **5**:945–952, 1990.

85. Hollstein M, Rice K, Greenblatt MS, Soussi T, Fuchs R, Sorlie T, Hovig E et al: Database of p53 gene somatic mutations in human tumors and cell lines. *Nucleic Acids Res* **22**:3547–3551, 1994.

86. Hollstein M, Shomer B, Greenblatt M, Soussi T, Hovig E, Montesano R, Harris CC: Somatic point mutations in the p53 gene of human tumors and cell lines: updated compilation. *Nucleic Acids Res* **24**:141–146, 1996.

87. Murakami Y, Hayashi K, Sekiya T: Detection of aberrations of the p53 alleles and the gene transcript in human tumor cell lines by single conformation polymorphism analysis. *Cancer Res* **51**:3356–3391, 1991.

88. Hsu IC, Metcalf RA, Sun T, Welsh JA, Wang NJ, Harris CC: Mutational hotspot in the p53 gene in human hepatocellular carcinomas. *Nature* **350**:427–428, 1991.

89. Scorsone KA, Zhou YZ, Butel JS, Slagle BL: p53 mutations cluster at codon 249 in hepatitis B virus-positive hepatocellular carcinomas from China. *Cancer Res* **52**:1635–1638, 1992.

90. Li D, Cao Y, He L, Wang NJ, Gu J: Aberrations of p53 gene in human hepatocellular carcinoma from China. *Carcinogenesis* **14**:169–173, 1993.

91. Bressac B, Kew M, Wands J, Ozturk M: Selective G to T mutations of p53 gene in hepatocellular carcinoma from southern Africa. *Nature* **350**:429–431, 1991.

92. Soini Y, Chia SC, Bennett WP, Groopman JD, Wang JS, DeBenedetti VM, Cawley H et al: An aflatoxin-associated mutational hotspot at codon 249 in the p53 tumor suppressor gene occurs in hepatocellular carcinomas from Mexico. *Carcinogenesis* **17**:1007–1012, 1996.

93. Yang M, Zhou H, Kong RY, Fong WF, Ren LQ, Liao XH, Wang Y et al: Mutations at codon 249 of p53 gene in human hepatocellular carcinomas from Tongan, China. *Mutat Res* **381**: 25–29, 1997.

94. Oda T, Tsuda H, Scarpa A, Sakamoto M, Hirohashi S: p53 gene mutation spectrum in hepatocellular carcinoma. *Cancer Res* **52**:6358–6364, 1992.

95. Kress S, Jahn UR, Buchmann A, Bannasch P, Schwarz M: p53 mutations in human hepatocellular carcinomas from Germany. *Cancer Res* **52**:3220–3223, 1992.

96. Hsu IC, Tokiwa T, Bennett W, Metcalf RA, Welsh JA, Sun T, Harris CC: p53 gene mutation and integrated hepatitis B viral DNA sequences in human liver cancer cell lines. *Carcinogenesis* **14**:987–992, 1993.

97. Aguilar F, Harris CC, Sun T, Hollstein M, Cerutti P: Geographic variation of p53 mutational profile in nonmalignant human liver. *Science* **264**:1317–1319, 1994.

98. Aguilar F, Hussain SP, Cerutti P: Aflatoxin B1 induces the transversion of $G \to T$ in codon 249 of the p53 tumor suppressor gene in human hepatocytes. *Proc Natl Acad Sci USA* **90**:8586–8590, 1993.

99. Cerutti P, Hussain P, Pourzand C, Aguilar F: Mutagenesis of the H-ras protooncogene and the p53 tumor suppressor gene. *Cancer Res* **54**:1934s–1938s, 1994.

100. Mace K, Aguilar F, wang JS, Vautravers P, Gomez-Lechon M, Gonzealea FJ, Groopman J et al: Aflatoxin B1 induced DNA adduct formation and p53 mutations in CYP450-expressing human liver cell lines. *Carcinogenesis* **18**: 1291–1297, 1997.

101. Ponchel F, Puisieux A, Tabone E, Michot JP, Froschl G, Morel AP, Frebourg T et al: Hepatocarcinoma mutant p53 induces mitotic activity but has no effect on transforming growth factor beta 1-mediated apoptosis. *Cancer Res* **54**:2064–2068, 1994.

102. Dumenco L, Oguey D, Wu J, Messier N, Fausto N: Introduction of a murine p53 mutation corresponding to human codon 249 into a murine hepatocyte cell line results in growth advantage, but not in transformation. *Hepatology* **22**:1279–1288, 1995.

103. Wang XW, Gibson MK, Vermeulen W, Yeh H, Forrester K, Sturzbecher HW, Hoeijmakers JHJ, et al: Abrogation of p53-induced apoptosis by the hepatitis B virus X gene. *Cancer Res* **55**:6012–6016, 1995.

104. Guengerich FP, Johnson WW, Ueng Y-F, Yamazaki H, Shimada T: Involvement of cytochrome P450, glutathione S-transferase, and epoxide hydrolase in the metabolism of aflatoxin B1 and relevance to risk of human liver cancer. *Environ Health Perspect* **104**:557–562, 1996.

105. Buss P, Caviezel M, Lutz WK: Linear dose-response relationship for DNA adducts in rat liver from chronic exposure to aflatoxin B1. *Carcinogenesis* **11**:2133–2135, 1990.

106. Hosono S, Chou MJ, Lee CS, Shih C: Infrequent mutation of p53 gene in hepatitis B virus positive primary hepatocellular carcinomas. *Oncogene* **8**:491–496, 1993.

107. Kung YK, Kim CJ, Kim WH, Kim HO, Kang GH, Kim YI: p53 mutation and overexpression in hepatocellular carcinoma and dysplastic nodules in the liver. *Virchows Arch* **432**: 27-32, 1998.

108. Feitelson MA, Zhu M, Duan LX, London WT: Hepatitis B x antigen and p53 are associated in vitro and in liver tissues from patients with primary hepatocellular carcinoma. *Oncogene* **8**:1109–1117, 1993.

109. Wang XW, Forrester K, Yeh H, Feitelson MA, Gu JR, Harris CC: Hepatitis B virus X protein inhibits p53 sequence-specific DNA binding, transcriptional activity, and association with transcription factor ERCC3. *Proc Natl Acad Sci USA* **91**:2230–2234, 1994.

110. Ueda H, Ullrich SJ, Gangemi JD, Kappel CA, Ngo L, Feitelson MA, Jay G: Functional inactivation but not structural mutation of p53 causes liver cancer. *Nat Genet* **9**:41–47, 1995.

111. Maguire HF, Hoeffler JP, Siddiqui A: HBV X protein alters the DNA binding specificity of CREB and ATF-2 by protein-protein interactions. *Science* **252**:842–844, 1991.

112. Williams JS, Andrisani OM: The hepatitis B virus X protein targets the basic region evcine zipper domain of CREB. *Proc Natl Acad Sci USA* **92**:3819–3823, 1995.

113. Jia L, Wang XW, Sun Z, Harris CC: Interactive effects of p53 tumor suppressor gene and hepatitis B virus in hepatocellular carcinogenesis. Tahara E (ed) *In Molecular Pathology of Gastroeuterological Cancer: Application to Clinical Practice*, Tahara E (ed), Tokyo, Springer-Verlag, 1997, pp. 209–218.

114. Schaeffer L, Roy R, Humbert S, Moncollin V, Vermeulen W, Hoeijmakers JH, Cambon P, et al.: DNA repair helicase: a component of BTF2 (TFIIH) basic transcription factor. *Science* **260**:58–63, 1993.

115. Weeda G, van Ham RC, Vermeulen W, Bootsma D, Van der Eb AJ, Hoeijmakers JH: A presumed DNA helicase encoded by ERCC3 is involved in the human repair disorders xeroderma pigmentosum and Cockayne's syndrome. *Cell* **62**:777–791, 1990.

116. Elmore LW, Hancock AR, Chang SF, Wang XW, Chang S, Callahan CP, Geller DA. et al.: Hepatitis B virus X protein and p53 tumor suppressor interactions in the modulation of apoptosis. *Proc Natl Acad Sci USA* **94**:14707–14712, 1997.

117. Wang XW, Yeh H, Schaeffer L, Roy R, Moncollin V, Egly JM, Wang Z, et al.: p53 modulation of TFIIH-associated nucleotide excision repair activity. *Nature Genet* **10**:188–195, 1995.

118. Teramoto T, Satonaka K, Kitazawa S, Fujimori T, Hayashi K, Maeda S: p53 gene abnormalities are closely related to hepatoviral infections and occur at a late stage of hepatocarcinogenesis. *Cancer Res* **54**:231–235, 1994.

119. Jaskiewicz K, Banach L, Izycka E: Hepatocellular carcinoma in young patients: histology, cellular differentiation, HBV infection and oncoprotein p53. *Anticancer Res* **15**:2723–2725, 1995.

120. Mise K, Tashiro S, Yogita S, Wada D, Harda M, Fukuda Y, Mikaye H. et al.: Assessment of the biological malignancy of hepatocellular carcinoma: relationship of clinicopathological facotrs and prognosis. *Clin Cancer Res* **4**:1475–1482, 1998.

121. Qin G, Su J, Ning Y, Duan X, Luo D, Lotlikar PD: p53 protein expression in patients with hepatocellular carcinoma from the high incidence area of Guangxi, Southern China. *Cancer Lett* **121**:203–210, 1997.

122. Qiu SJ, Ye SL, Wu ZQ, TangZY, Liu YK: The expression of the mdm2 gene may be related to the aberration of the p53 gene in human hepatocellular carcinoma. *J Cancer Res Clin Oncol* **124**:253–258, 1998.

123. Tanaka S, Toh Y, Adachi E, Matsumata T, Mori R, Sugimachi K: Tumor progression in hepatocellular carcinoma may be mediated by p53 mutation. *Cancer Res* **53**:2884–2887, 1993.

124. Murakami Y, Hayashi K, Hirohashi S, Sekiya T: Aberrations of the tumor suppressor p53 and retinoblastoma genes in human hepatocellular carcinomas. *Cancer Res* **51**:5520–5525, 1991.

125. Tabor E: Tumor suppressor genes, growth factor genes, and oncogenes in hepatitis B virus-associated hepatocellular carcinoma. *J Med Virol* **42**:357–365, 1994.

126. Ashida K, Kishimoto Y, Nakamoto K, Wada K, Shiota G, Hirooka Y, Kamisaki Y. et al.: Loss of heterozygosity of the retinoblastoma gene in liver cirrhosis accompanying hepatocellular carcinoma. *J Cancer Res Clin Oncol* **123**:489–495, 1997.

127. Pascale RM, Simile MM, Feo F: Genomic abnormalities in hepatocarcinogenesis. Implications for a chemopreventive strategy. *Anticancer Res* **13**:1341–1356, 1993.

128. Gu JR: Molecular aspects of human hepatic carcinogenesis. *Carcinogenesis* **9**:697–703, 1988.

129. Zhang XK, Huang DP, Chiu DK, Chiu JF: The expression of oncogenes in human developing liver and hepatomas. *Biochem Biophys Res Commun* **142**:932–938, 1987.

130. Gu JR, Hu LF, Cheng YC, Wan DF: Oncogenes in human primary hepatic cancer. *J Cell Physiol Suppl* **4**:13–20, 1986.

131. Takada S, Koike K: Activated N-ras gene was found in human hepatoma tissue but only in a small fraction of the tumor cells. *Oncogene* **4**:189–193, 1989.

132. Ogata N, Kamimura T, Asakura H: Point mutation, allelic loss and increased methylation of c-Ha-ras gene in human hepatocellular carcinoma. *Hepatology* **13**:31–37, 1991.

133. Yang SS, Modali R, Parks JB, Taub JV: Transforming DNA sequences of human hepatocellular carcinomas, their distribution and relationship with hepatitis B virus sequence in human hepatomas. *Leukemia* **2**:102S–113S, 1988.

134. Yuasa Y, Sudo K: Transforming genes in human hepatomas detected by a tumorigenicity assay. *Jpn J Cancer Res* **78**:1036–1040, 1987.

135. Arbuthnot P, Kew M, Fitschen W: c-fos and c-myc oncoprotein expression in human hepatocellular carcinomas. *Anticancer Res* **11**:921–924, 1991.

136. Farshid M, Tabor E: Expression of oncogenes and tumor suppressor genes in human hepatocellular carcinoma and hepatoblastoma cell lines. *J Med Virol* **38**:235–239, 1992.

137. Feitelson MA: Biology of hepatitis B virus variants. *Lab Invest* **71**:324–349, 1994.

138. Twu JS, Schloemer RH: Transcriptional trans-activating function of hepatitis B virus. *J Virol* **61**:3448–3453, 1987.

139. Spandau DF, Lee CH: Trans-activation of viral enhancers by the hepatitis B virus X protein. *J Virol* **62**:427–434, 1988.

140. Twu JS, Lai MY, Chen DS, Robinson WS: Activation of protooncogene c-jun by the X protein of hepatitis B virus. *Virology* **192**:346–350, 1993.

141. Aufiero B, Schneider RJ: The hepatitis B virus X-gene product transactivates both RNA polymerase II and III promoters. *EMBO J* **9**:497–504, 1990.

142. Natoli G, Avantaggiati ML, Chirillo P, Costanzo A, Artini M, Balsano C, Levrero M: Induction of the DNA-binding activity of c-jun/c-fos heterodimers by the hepatitis B virus transactivator pX. *Mol Cell Biol* **14**:989–998, 1994.

143. Balsano C, Avantaggiati ML, Natoli G, De Marzio E, Will H, Perricaudet M, Levrero M: Full-length and truncated versions of the hepatitis B virus (HBV) X protein (pX) transactivate the c-myc protooncogene at the transcriptional level. *Biochem Biophys Res Commun* **176**:985–992, 1991.

144. Levrero M, Balsano C, Avantaggiati ML, Natoli G, De Marzio E, Will H: Hepatitis B virus and hepatocellular carcinoma: a possible role for the viral transactivators. *Ital J Gastroenterol* **23**:576–583, 1991.

145. Caselmann WH, Meyer M, Kekulî AS, Lauer U, Hofschneider PH, Koshy R: A trans-activator function is generated by integration of hepatitis B virus preS2/S sequences in human hepatocellular carcinoma DNA. *Proc Natl Acad Sci USA* **87**:2970–2974, 1990.

146. Kekulî AS, Lauer U, Meyer M, Caselmann WH, Hofschneider PH, Koshy R: The preS2/S region of integrated hepatitis B virus DNA encodes a transcriptional transactivator. *Nature* **343**:457–461, 1990.

147. Unsal H, Yakicier C, Marcais C, Kew M, Volkmann M, Zentgraf H, Isselbacher KJ, et al.: Genetic heterogeneity of hepatocellular carcinoma. *Proc Natl Acad Sci USA* **91**:822–826, 1994.

148. Paterlini P, Poussin K, Kew M, Franco D, Brechot C: Selective accumulation of the X transcript of hepatitis B virus in patients negative for hepatitis B surface antigen with hepatocellular carcinoma. *Hepatology* **21**:313–321, 1995.

149. Caselmann WH: Transactivation of cellular gene expression by hepatitis B viral proteins: a possible molecular mechanism of hepatocarcinogenesis. *J Hepatol* **22**:34–37, 1995.

150. Wei Y, Etiemble J, Fourel G, Vitvitski-Trepo L, Buendía MA: Hepadnavirus integration generates virus-cell cotranscripts carrying 3′ truncated X genes in human and woodchuck liver tumors. *J Med Virol* **45**:82–90, 1995.

151. Su Q, Schroder CH, Hofmann WJ, Otto G, Pichlmayr R, Bannash P: Expression of hepatitis B virus X protein in HBV-infected human livers and hepatocellular carcinomas. *Hepatology* **27**:1109–1120, 1998.

152. Su TS, Hwang WL, Yauk YK: Characterization of hepatitis B virus integrant that results in chromosomal rearrangement. *DNA Cell Biol* **17**:415–425, 1998.

153. Kobayashi S, Saigoh Ki, Urashima T, Asano T, Isono K: Detection of hepatitis B virus x transcripts in human hepatocellular carcinoma tissues. *J Surg Res* **73**:97–100, 1997.

154. Laskus T, Radkowski M, Nowicki M, Wang LF, Vargas H, Rakela J: Association between hepatitis B virus core promoter rearrangements and hepatocellular carcinoma. *Biochem Biophys Res Commun* **244**:812–814, 1998.

155. Benn J, Schneider RJ: Hepatitis B virus HBx protein deregulates cell cycle checkpoint controls. *Proc Natl Acad Sci USA* **92**:11215–11219, 1995.

156. Benn J, Schneider RJ: Hepatitis B virus HBx protein activates Ras-GTP complex formation and establishes a Ras, Raf, MAP kinase signaling cascade. *Proc Natl Acad Sci USA* **91**:10350–10354, 1994.

157. Doria M, Klein N, Lucito R, Schneider RJ: The hepatitis B virus HBx protein is a dual specificity cytoplasmic activator of Ras and nuclear activator of transcription factors. *EMBO J* **14**:4747–4757, 1995.

158. Kekulî AS, Lauer U, Weiss L, Luber B, Hofschneider PH: Hepatitis B virus transactivator HBx uses a tumor promoter signalling pathway. *Nature* **361**:742–745, 1993.

159. Luber B, Lauer U, Weiss L, Hohne M, Hofschneider PH, Kekul AS: The hepatitis B virus transactivator HBx causes elevation of diacylglycerol and activation of protein kinase C. *Res Virol* **144**:311–321, 1993.

160. Koike K, Moriya K, Yotsuyanagi H, Iino S, Kurokawa K: Induction of cell cycle progression by hepatitis B virus HBx gene expression in quiescent mouse fibroblasts. *J Clin Invest* **94**:44–49, 1994.

161. Kim H, Lee H, Yum Y: X-gene product of hepatitis B virus induces apoptosis in liver cells. *J Biol Chem* **273**: 381-385, 1998.

162. Lee TH, Elledge SJ, Butel JS: Hepatitis B virus X protein interacts with a probable cellular DNA repair protein. *J Virol* **69**:1107–1114, 1995.

163. Becker SA, Lee TH, Butel JS, Slagle BL: Hepatitis B virus X protein interferes with cellular DNA repair. *J Virol* **72**: 266-272, 1998.

164. Lucito R, Schneider RJ: Hepatitis B virus X protein activates transcription factor NF-kappa B without a requirement for protein kinase C. *J Virol* **66**:983–991, 1992.

165. Lee YI, Lee Y, Bong YS, Hyun SW, Yoo YD, Kim SJ. et al.: The human hepatitis B virus transactivator X gene product regulates Sp1 mediated transcription of an insulin-like growth factor II promoter 4. *Oncogene* **16**: 2367-2380, 1997.

166. Fischer M, Runkel L, Schaller H: HBx protein of hepatitis B virus interacts with the C-terminal portion of a novel human proteasome alpha-subunit. *Virus Genes* **10**:99–102, 1995.

167. Takada S, Kido H, Fukutomi A, Mori T, Koike K: Interaction of hepatitis B virus X protein with a serine protease, tryptase TL2 as an inhibitor. *Oncogene* **9**:341–348, 1994.

168. Takada S, Tsuchida N, Kobayashi M, Koike K: Disruption of the function of tumor-suppressor gene p53 by the hepatitis B virus X protein and hepatocarcinogenesis. *J Cancer Res Clin Oncol* **121**:593–601, 1995.

169. Höhne M, Schaefer S, Seifer M, Feitelson MA, Paul D, Gerlich WH: Malignant transformation of immortalized transgenic hepatocytes after transfection with hepatitis B virus DNA. *EMBO J* **9**:1137–1145, 1990.

170. Shirakata Y, Kawada M, Fujiki Y, Sano H, Oda M, Yaginuma K, Kobayashi M, et al.: The X gene of hepatitis B virus induced growth stimulation and tumorigenic transformation of mouse NIH3T3 cells. *Jpn J Cancer Res* **80**:617–621, 1989.

171. Kim CM, Koike K, Saito I, Miyamura T, Jay G: HBx gene of hepatitis B virus induces liver cancer in transgenic mice. *Nature* **351**:317–320, 1991.

172. Macaulay VM: Insulin-like growth factors and cancer. *Br J Cancer* **65**:311–320, 1992.

173. Su Q, Liu YF, Zhang JF, Zhang SX, Li DF, Yang JJ: Expression of insulin-like growth factor II in hepatitis B, cirrhosis and hepatocellular carcinoma: its relationship with hepatitis B virus antigen expression. *Hepatology* **20**:788–799, 1994.

174. Cariani E, Lasserre C, Seurin D, Hamelin B, Kemeny F, Franco D, Czech MP, et al.: Differential expression of insulin-like growth factor II mRNA in human primary liver cancers, benign liver tumors, and liver cirrhosis. *Cancer Res* **48**:6844–6849, 1988.

175. Park BC, Huh MH, Seo JH: Differential expression of transforming growth factor alpha and insulin-like growth factor II in chronic active hepatitis B, cirrhosis and hepatocellular carcinoma. *J Hepatol* **22**:286–294, 1995.

176. Sohda T, Iwata K, Soejima H, Kamimura S, Shijo H, Yun K: In situ detection of insuline-like growth factor II (IGF2) and H19 gene expression in hepatocellular carcinoma. *J Hum Genet* **43**:49–53, 1998.

177. Sohda T, Kamimura S, Iwata K, Shijo H, Okumura M: Immunohistochemical evidence of insulin-like growth factor II in human small hepatocellular carcinoma with hepatitis C virus infection: relationship to fatty change in carcinoma cells. *J Gastroenterol Hepatol* **12**:224–228, 1997.

178. Takeda S, Kondo M, Kumada T, Koshikawa T, Ueda R, Nishio M, Osada H, et al.: Allelic-expression imbalance of the insulin-like growth factor 2 gene in hepatocellular carcinoma and underlying disease. *Oncogene* **12**:1589–1592, 1996.

179. Aihara T, Noguchi S, Miyoshi Y, Nakano H, Sasaki Y, Nakamura Y, Monden M. et al.: Allelic imbalance of insulin-like growth factor II gene expression in cancerous and precancerous lesions of the liver. *Hepatology* **28**:86–89, 1998.

180. Uchida K, Kondo M, Takeda S, Osada H, Takahashi T, Nakao A: Altered transcriptional regulation of the insulin-like growth factor 2 gene in human hepatocellular carcinoma. *Mol Carcinog* **18**:193–198, 1997.

181. Seo JH, Kim KW, Murakami S, Park BC: Lack of colocalization of HBx Ag and insulin like growth factor II in the livers of patients with chronic hepatitis B, cirrhosis and hepatocelular carcinoma. *J Korean Med Sci* **12**:523–531, 1997.

182. Tanaka S, Mohr L, Schmidt EV, Sugimachi K, Wands JR: Biological effects of human insulin receptor substrate-1 overexpression in hepatocytes. *Hepatology* **26**:598–604, 1997.

183. Ito T, Sasaki Y, Wands JR: Overexpression of human insulin receptor substrate 1 induces cellular transformation with activation of mitogen activated protein kinases. *Mol Cell Biol* **16**:943–951, 1996.

184. Kim KW, Bae SK, Lee OH, Bae MH, Lee MJ, Park BC: Insulin-like growth factor II induced by hypoxia may contribute to angiogenesis of human hepatocellular carcinoma. *Cancer Res* **58**:384–351, 1998.

185. Bae MH, Lee MJ, Bae SK, Lee YM, Park BC, Kim KW: Insulin-like growth factor II (IGF-II) secreted from HepG2 human hepatocellular carcinoma cells shows angiogenic activity. *Cancer Lett* **128**:41–46, 1998.

186. Li XM, Tang ZY, Zhou G, Lui YK, Ye SL: Significance of vascular endothelial growth factor mRNA expression in invasion and metastasis of helpatocellular carcinoma. *J Exp Clin Cancer Res* **17**:13–17, 1998.

187. Tanaka S, Wands JR: Insulin receptor substrate 1 overexpression in human hepatocellular carcinoma cells prevents transforming growth factor beta 1 apoptosis. *Cancer Res* **56**:3391–3394, 1996.

188. Nalesnik MA, Lee RG, Carr BI: Transforming growth factor alpha (TGFalpha) in hepatocellular carcinomas and adjacent hepatic parenchyma. *Hum Pathol* **29**:228–234, 1998.

189. Hsia CC, Axiotis CA, Di Bisceglie AM, Tabor E: Transforming growth factor-alpha in human hepatocellular carcinoma and coexpression with hepatitis B surface antigen in adjacent liver. *Cancer* **70**:1049–1056, 1992.

190. Yamaguchi R, Yano H, Iemura A, Ogasawara S, Haramaki M, Kojiro M: Expression of vascular endothelial growth factor in human hepatocellular carcinoma. *Hepatology* **28**: 68–77, 1998.

191. Di Bisceglie AM, Rustgi VK, Hoofnagle JH, Dusheiko GM, Lotze MT: NIH conference: Hepatocellular carcinoma. *Ann Intern Med* **108**:390–401, 1988.

192. Lin DY, Lin SM, Liaw YF: Non-surgical treatment of hepatocellular carcinoma. *J Gastroenterol Hepatol* **12**:S319–28, 1997.

193. Zuckerman AJ: Prevention of primary liver cancer by immunization. *N Engl J Med* **336**:1906–1907, 1997.

194. Lee CL, Ko YC: Hepatitis B vaccination and hepatocellular carcinoma in Taiwan. *Pediatrics* **99**:351–353, 1997.

195. Chang MH: Hepatitis B: long-term outcome and benefits from mass vaccination in children. *Acta Gastroenterol Belg* **61**:210–213, 1998.

196. Chang MH, Chen CJ, Lai MS, Hsu HM, Wu TC, Kong MS, Liang DC. et al.: Universal hepatitis B vaccination in Taiwan and the incidence of hepatocellular carcinoma in children. Taiwan Childhood Hepatoma Study Group. *N Engl J med* **336**:1855–1859, 1997.

197. Kew MC: Increasing evidence that hepatitis B virus X gene protein and p53 protein may interact in the pathogenesis of hepatocellular carcinoma. *Hepatology* **25**:1037–1038, 1997.

198. Harris CC: p53 Tumor suppressor gene: from the basic research laboratory to the clinic: An abridged historical perspective. *Carcinogenesis* **17**: 1181–1198.

199. Lee JM, Bernstein A: Apoptosis, cancer and the p53 tumor suppressor gene. *Cancer Metastasis Rev* **14**:149–161, 1995.

200. Mullen CA, Blaese RM: Gene therapy of cancer. *Cancer Chemother Biol Response Modif* **15**:176–189, 1994.

201. Clayman GL, el-Naggar AK, Roth JA, Zhang WW, Goepfert H, Taylor DL, Liu TJ: In vivo molecular therapy with p53 adenovirus for microscopic residual head and neck squamous carcinoma. *Cancer Res* **55**:1–6, 1995.

202. Liu TJ, el-Naggar AK, McDonnell TJ, Steck KD, Wang M, Taylor DL, Clayman GL: Apoptosis induction mediated by wild-type p53 adenoviral gene transfer in squamous cell carcinoma of the head and neck. *Cancer Res* **55**:3117–3122, 1995.

203. Roth JA, Nguyen D, Lawrence DD, Kemp BL, Carrasco CH, Ferson DZ, Hong WK. et al.: Retrovirus-mediated wild-type p53 gene transfer to tumors of patients with lung cancer. *Nat Med* **2**:985–991, 1996.

204. Xu GW, Sun ZT, Forrester K, Wang XW, Coursen J, Harris CC: Tissue-specific growth suppression and chemosensitivity promotion in human hepatocellular carcinoma cells by retroviral-mediated transfer of the wild-type p53 gene. *Hepatology* **24**:1264–1268 1996.

205. da Costa LT, Jen J, He TC, Chan TA, Kinzler KW, Vogelstein B: Converting cancer genes into killer genes. *Proc Natl Acad Sci USA* **93**:4192–4196, 1996.

Clinical and Biological Aspects of Neuroblastoma

Garrett M. Brodeur

- **Neuroblastoma, a tumor of the postganglionic sympathetic nervous system, is the most common extracranial solid tumor of childhood.**
- **No environmental exposures or agents have been associated with an increased risk of neuroblastoma. However, a subset has a genetic predisposition that follows an autosomal dominant pattern of inheritance.**
- **Primary tumors generally arise in the adrenal medulla (50 percent) or elsewhere in the abdomen or pelvis (30 percent). Only 20 percent arise in the chest.**
- **Metastases usually are found in the regional lymph nodes, bone, bone marrow, skin, or liver. Paraneoplastic syndromes characteristic of neuroblastomas are seen in a small percentage of patients.**
- **Tissue biopsy or characterization of cells in the bone marrow diagnoses neuroblastomas. Catecholamine metabolites are elevated in the urine in over 90 percent of cases.**
- **There is an international neuroblastoma staging system for categorizing the extent and resectability of the primary tumor and the presence or absence of metastases.**
- **A number of prognostic variables have been identified that allow better prediction of clinical behavior: MYCN amplification, allelic loss of 1p36, gain of 17q, expression of TrkA, tumor cell ploidy, and tumor pathology.**
- **Histologically, neuroblastic tumors can be immature (neuroblastoma), partially mature (ganglioneuroblastoma), or completely mature (ganglioneuroma). However, other features, such as the presence or absence of Schwannian stroma, mitoses, or karyorrhectic cells, may have more prognostic importance.**
- **Localized, resectable tumors can be cured by surgery alone. Unresectable tumors or metastatic disease in infants require mild to moderately intensive chemotherapy. Metastatic disease in older patients, and regional tumors with unfavorable biological features in any age, require intensive chemotherapy, frequently with bone marrow or stem cell rescue.**
- **Screening of infants for neuroblastoma by measuring urinary catecholamine metabolites has resulted in a doubling of the apparent incidence rate in infants with no decrease in advanced disease in older children.**

- **Future therapeutic approaches may be aimed at the induction of differentiation or programmed cell death through retinoid or neurotrophin receptor pathways. Alternate approaches may focus on the product of the MYCN gene, the 1p36 suppressor gene, other specific genetic changes, or antiangiogenesis.**

Few tumors have engendered as much fascination and frustration for clinical and laboratory investigators as neuroblastoma. This tumor of the postganglionic sympathetic nervous system is the most common solid tumor in childhood. Interestingly, some infants with metastatic disease can experience complete regression of their disease without therapy, and some older patients have complete maturation of their tumor into a benign ganglioneuroma. Unfortunately, the majority of patients have metastatic disease that grows relentlessly despite even the most intensive multimodality therapy. Indeed, despite dramatic improvements in the cure rate for other common pediatric neoplasms, such as acute lymphoblastic leukemia or Wilms tumor, the improvement in the overall survival rate of patients with neuroblastoma has been relatively modest.

Recent advances in understanding the biology of neuroblastoma, however, have provided considerable insight into the genetic and biochemical mechanisms underlying these seemingly disparate behaviors. Near triploidy with whole chromosome gains is a characteristic feature of favorable neuroblastoma in infants. High expression of the nerve growth factor receptor (called *TrkA*) is found in the majority of these tumors, and this may mediate either apoptosis or differentiation in these tumors. On the other hand, amplification of the *MYCN* oncogene is found in a substantial number of patients with advanced stages of disease and a poor prognosis. Finally, evidence for allelic loss at 1p, 11q, 14q, or other sites suggests the location of tumor-suppressor genes that may be important in the molecular pathogenesis of more aggressive neuroblastomas. These and other biological observations have given us tremendous insight into mechanisms of malignant transformation and progression, as well as spontaneous differentiation and regression.

The specific genetic changes that have been identified allow tumors to be classified into subsets with distinct biological features and clinical behavior. Indeed, certain genetic abnormalities are very powerful predictors of response to therapy and outcome, and as such, they have become essential components of tumor characterization at diagnosis. Thus, neuroblastoma serves as a model solid tumor in which the genetic and biological analysis of the tumor cells have become conventional determinants of optimal patient management. The challenge of the next decade is to translate this information into more effective and less toxic therapy for these patients.

In this chapter, the epidemiologic, genetic, and pathologic features of neuroblastomas are reviewed. In addition, the essential clinical features of tumor presentation and management are discussed, including several paraneoplastic syndromes that are associated with neuroblastomas. The cytogenetic and molecular

A list of standard abbreviations is located immediately preceding the index. Nonstandard abbreviations used in this chapter include: BMT = bone marrow transplantation; CCG = Children's Cancer Group; CGH = comparative genomic hybridization; DI = DNA index; Dmins = double-minute chromatin bodies; HSR = homogeneously staining region; HVA = homovanillic acid; INSS = International Neuroblastoma Staging System; LNTR = low-affinity neurotrophin receptor; LOH = loss of heterozygosity; MIBG = meta-iodobenzylguanidine; NGF = nerve growth factor; NSE = neuron-specific enolase; POG = Pediatric Oncology Group; VIP = vasoactive intestinal peptide; VMA = vanillylmandelic acid

genetic features of the tumor cells and their implications are reviewed. Current clinical management is discussed briefly. Finally, the current results of mass screening for neuroblastoma, and the implications for understanding the genetic heterogeneity of this disease, are presented.

EPIDEMIOLOGY

Incidence

Neuroblastomas account for 7 to 10 percent of all childhood cancers. The prevalence is about 1 case per 7500 live births, and there are about 600 new cases of neuroblastoma per year in the United States.[7] This corresponds to an incidence of 10.5 per million per year in Caucasian children and 8.8 per million per year in African-American children less than 15 years of age.[7,8] Evidence indicates that this incidence is fairly uniform throughout the world, at least for industrialized nations. The tumor is slightly more common in boys than in girls, with a male/female sex ratio of 1.2:1 in most large studies.

The median age at diagnosis of 1001 consecutive children with neuroblastoma seen at Pediatric Oncology Group (POG) institutions from 1981 to 1989 is 22 months.[1] Thus, 37 percent of patients are less than 1 year of age, 81 percent are less than 4 years of age, and 97 percent are diagnosed by 10 years of age (Fig. 50-1). Some studies have shown a bimodal age distribution, with an initial peak before 1 year of age and a second peak around 3 years of age.[8,9] This observation suggests that there may be at least two subpopulations of neuroblastoma, the first of which may represent a genetically predisposed subset, as seen in retinoblastoma. Alternatively, there may be two genetically distinct types of neuroblastoma with different ages of onset (see below). However, a bimodal age distribution is not always seen.

Embryology

In 1963, Beckwith and Perrin reported that microscopic neuroblastic nodules, resembling neuroblastoma *in situ*, were found frequently in infants less than 3 months of age who died of other causes.[10] This finding was interpreted initially to indicate that neuroblastomas develop up to 40 times more often than they are detected clinically, but that the tumor regresses spontaneously in the vast majority of cases. However, others subsequently demonstrated that these neuroblastic nodules occurred uniformly in all fetuses studied, peaked between 17 and 20 weeks of gestation, and gradually regressed by the time of birth or shortly after.[11,12] Thus, the microscopic neuroblastic nodules seen in the earlier study were likely remnants of fetal adrenal development. Nevertheless, these neuroblastic cell rests may be the cells from which neuroblastomas develop, at least in the adrenal medulla.

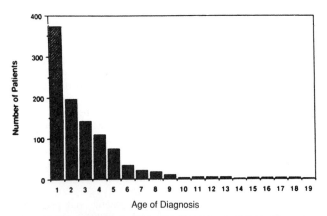

Fig. 50-1 Age at diagnosis in 1001 consecutive patients diagnosed with neuroblastoma in the Pediatric Oncology Group (POG) between 1981 and 1989. (*Reprinted from Brodeur*[1] *with permission of CV Mosby Year Book.*)

Although some controversy still exists concerning the initial observation of *in situ* neuroblastoma, the latter interpretation is generally accepted.

Microscopic neuroblastic nodules, as described above, would never be detected clinically, nor would they be detected by screening infants for neuroblastoma by measuring urinary catecholamine metabolites (see below). However, the concept of *in situ* neuroblastoma has been used to support the argument that many neuroblastomas arise and regress spontaneously. Indeed, there are a number of well-documented cases in infants with neuroblastoma that have had complete regression of their tumor.[13] The actual frequency of neuroblastomas that are detected clinically and subsequently regress without treatment more likely represents 5 to 10 percent of all neuroblastoma patients.[14-16] However, based on estimates from the mass screening studies, the frequency of true asymptomatic neuroblastomas that regress spontaneously is probably much higher, and may be equal to the number detected clinically (see below).

Environmental Studies

The etiology of neuroblastoma is unknown in most cases, but, based on current information, it appears unlikely that environmental exposures play a major role. There have been a few reports of neuroblastoma associated with the fetal hydantoin, phenobarbital, or alcohol syndromes,[17-19] suggesting that prenatal exposure to these substances may increase the risk of neuroblastoma. However, this association has not been confirmed with certainty. Two studies have reported a weak association between neuroblastoma and paternal occupational exposure to electromagnetic fields, but this was not confirmed in another study.[20-22] The latter group previously had shown an association between maternal use of hair-coloring products, but this also has not been confirmed.[23] Moreover, no prenatal or postnatal exposure to drugs, chemicals, or radiation has been either strongly or consistently associated with an increased incidence of neuroblastoma.

CONSTITUTIONAL GENETICS

Genetic Predisposition

A subset of patients with neuroblastoma exhibits a predisposition to develop this disease, and this predisposition follows an autosomal dominant pattern of inheritance. Knudson and Strong have estimated that as much as 22 percent of all neuroblastomas could be the result of a germinal mutation.[24] Regression analysis of these data from neuroblastoma fits the two-mutation hypothesis proposed by Knudson for the origin of childhood cancer.[25] According to this hypothesis, the nonhereditary form of neuroblastoma would result from two postzygotic (somatic) mutations in a single cell, causing malignant transformation of the cell that then develops into a single tumor. Hereditary tumors would arise in individuals in whom the first mutation is acquired as a prezygotic (germinal) event, so it is present in all cells. Only one additional mutation in any cell of the target tissue would be needed to induce malignant transformation, so these individuals would have a higher incidence of neuroblastoma with a peak incidence at an earlier age. In addition, they may develop tumors at multiple primary sites, either simultaneously or sequentially. If such persons survive, half of their offspring would be carriers of the germinal mutation, with an estimated 63 percent chance of developing neuroblastoma.[24,26]

There have been a number of reports of familial neuroblastoma, as well as bilateral or multifocal disease, consistent with hereditary predisposition, which were reviewed by Kushner and colleagues.[27] The median age at diagnosis of patients with familial neuroblastoma is 9 months, which contrasts with a median age of 22 months for neuroblastoma in the general population. At least 20 percent of patients with familial neuroblastoma have bilateral adrenal or multifocal primary tumors. The concordance for neuroblastoma in monozygotic siblings during infancy suggests that hereditary

Table 50-1 Constitutional Chromosome Abnormalities in Patients with Neuroblastoma

Chromosome Abnormality	Comments	Reference
del(21)(p11); inv(11)(q21q23)	One from each parent	31–33
t(4;7)(p?;q?)	Balanced; normal phenotype	34
t(11;16)(q?;q?)	Balanced; normal phenotype	34
Partial trisomy 2p and monosomy 16p	Congenital anomalies	35
Partial trisomy 3q and monosomy 8p	Congenital anomalies	35
Partial trisomy 15q and monosomy 13q	Congenital anomalies	36
Trisomy 18	Congenital anomalies	37
fra(1)(p13.1)	Hereditary fragile site	38
t(1;?)(p36;?)	Mosaic?	39
t(1;17)(p36;q12–21)	Balanced	40, 41
t(1;13)(q22;q12)	Balanced	42
t(8;11)(q22.1;q21)	Balanced	43
t(2;11)(p23;q22)	Balanced	43
t(2;6)(q32.2;q25.3)	Balanced	43
del(1)(p36.2–p36.3)	Dysmorphic, retarded	44
t(1;10)(p22;q21)	Balanced	45, 46

factors may be predominant, whereas the discordance in older twins suggests that random mutations or other factors may play a role.[28] A recent report examined the genetic linkage of neuroblastoma predisposition to several candidate loci in families segregating the disease, but linkage was not found.[29] Nevertheless, an international registry has been developed to identify familial neuroblastoma throughout the world.[29,30]

Constitutional Chromosome Abnormalities

A constitutional predisposition syndrome or associated congenital anomalies have not yet been identified in human neuroblastoma.[5] Several cases of constitutional chromosome abnormalities detected by banding have been reported in individuals with neuroblastoma, but no consistent pattern has emerged as yet (Table 50-1).[31–46] There have been three reports of constitutional abnormalities involving the short arm of chromosome 1, which frequently is deleted or rearranged in neuroblastoma cells. Laureys and colleagues described a patient with neuroblastoma who had a constitutional translocation between chromosomes 1 and 17, with the breakpoint on chromosome 1 in 1p36, the region frequently deleted in neuroblastoma cells.[40,41] A second interesting case, reported by Biegel, had a constitutional deletion of 1p36 and neuroblastoma, confirmed by both cytogenetic and molecular analysis.[44] A third case with a similar deletion was reported by White and colleagues.[47] Together with the frequent deletion of 1p36 in sporadic neuroblastomas, these cases suggested that constitutional deletions or rearrangements involving a gene on 1p36 may play a role in malignant transformation or predisposition to neuroblastoma in some cases. However, a recent report that familial neuroblastoma is not linked to 1p36 suggests that the predominant predisposition locus lies elsewhere.[29]

Two series reporting the routine constitutional karyotype analysis of a series of neuroblastoma patients have identified several cases with balanced translocations, suggesting that balanced translocations per se may be more common than in the general population (Table 50-1).[34,43] No consistent breakpoint has been identified, however, so routine karyotypic analysis is unlikely to be rewarding. Individuals with neuroblastoma who also have mental retardation, dysmorphic features, or other evidence of gross genetic abnormalities should be examined cytogenetically, because this may help identify the neuroblastoma predisposition locus (or loci).[44]

Other Genetic Syndromes

Neuroblastoma has been associated with neurofibromatosis type 1 (von Recklinghausen disease) suggesting that it might be part of a spectrum of syndromes involving maldevelopment of the neural crest.[48–50] However, an analysis of reported instances of the simultaneous occurrence of neuroblastoma and neurofibromatosis in the same patient suggests that these cases probably can be accounted for by chance alone.[51] Aganglionosis of the colon (Hirschsprung disease) is also a disorder of neural crest origin that has been associated with neuroblastoma, but linkage to genes associated with this disorder also has not been seen.[29] A variety of other congenital anomalies and genetic syndromes have been reported in association with neuroblastoma, but no specific abnormality has been identified with increased frequency.[52–54] Interestingly, there may be an increased prevalence of neuroblastoma in patients with Turner syndrome, and a decreased prevalence in patients with Down syndrome, but the reasons for this are unclear.[55–57]

GENETICS OF TUMOR CELLS

Oncogene Activation and Allelic Gain

Amplification of *MYCN* and Other Loci. Some neuroblastomas are characterized cytogenetically by double-minute chromatin bodies (dmins) and homogeneously staining regions (HSRs), which are cytogenetic manifestations of gene amplification (Fig. 50-2).[58–61] However, the gene or genetic region amplified was not known initially. Schwab and others identified a novel *c-myc*-related oncogene that was amplified in a series of neuroblastoma cell lines.[62,63] The amplified sequence, known as *MYCN,* is normally located on the distal short arm of chromosome 2, but maps to the dmins or HSRs in tumors with *MYCN* amplification.[63,64] Apparently a large region from 2p24 (including the *MYCN* locus) becomes amplified initially as extrachromosomal dmins, but may become linearly integrated into a chromosome as one or more HSR, particularly in established cell lines.[65,66]

Brodeur and colleagues have demonstrated that *MYCN* amplification occurs in about 25 percent of primary neuroblastomas from untreated patients (Figs. 50-3 and 50-4).[5,65,67,68] Amplification of *MYCN* is associated predominantly with advanced stages of disease and a poor outcome, but it is also associated with rapid tumor progression and a poor prognosis, even in infants and patients with lower stages of disease.[60,68–71] These studies have been extended to 3000 patients participating in cooperative group protocols in the United States. (Table 50-2).[3–5] *MYCN* amplification can be detected by Southern blot, fluorescence *in situ* hybridization, quantitative PCR, comparative genomic amplification, or other techniques.[66,72]

Interestingly, a consistent pattern was found of *MYCN* copy number (either amplified or unamplified) in different tumor

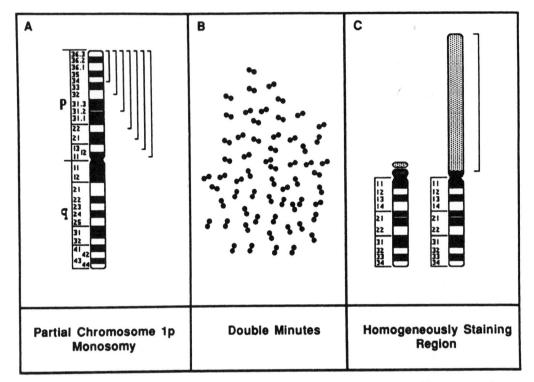

A	B	C
Partial Chromosome 1p Monosomy	Double Minutes	Homogeneously Staining Region

Fig. 50-2 Common cytogenetic abnormalities in human neuroblastomas. Shown are representations of three common cytogenetic abnormalities seen in human neuroblastomas. *A*, Deletions of the short arm of chromosome 1. The brackets indicate that the region deleted in different tumors is variable in terms of its proximal breakpoint, but the distal short arm appears to be deleted in all cases, resulting in partial 1p monosomy. *B*, Extrachromosomal double-minute chromatin bodies (dmins). Dmins are seen in about 30 percent of primary neuroblastomas and are a cytogenetic manifestation of gene amplification. *C*, Homogeneously staining region (HSR). A representative HSR on the short arm of chromosome 13 is shown in this example. HSRs are a cytogenetic manifestation of gene amplification in which the amplified sequences are chromosomally integrated. (*Reprinted from Brodeur[68] with permission of Brain Pathology.*)

samples taken from an individual patient, either simultaneously or consecutively.[73] These results suggest that *MYCN* amplification is an intrinsic biological property of a subset of aggressive neuroblastomas, and tumors without amplification at diagnosis rarely, if ever, develop this abnormality subsequently. Currently, neuroblastomas from patients on clinical trials in the United States, Europe, and Japan are routinely assessed for the presence of *MYCN* amplification, because it is a powerful predictor of a poor prognosis.

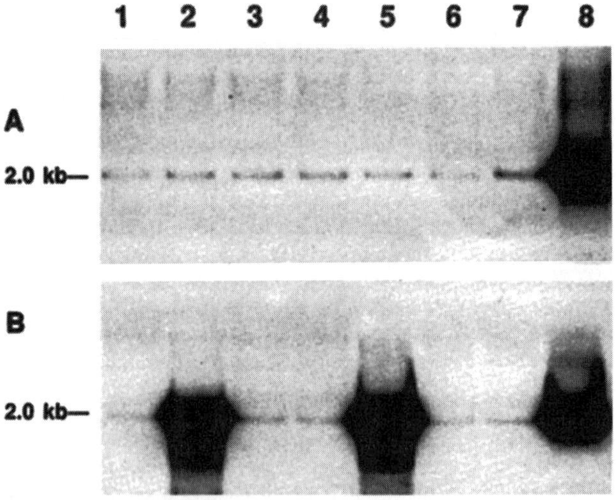

Our studies have also shown a strong correlation between *MYCN* amplification and 1p loss of heterozygosity (LOH).[74–76] Both *MYCN* amplification and deletion of 1p are strongly correlated with a poor outcome and with each other, but it is not yet clear if they are independent prognostic variables.[77–81] Nevertheless, they appear to characterize a genetically distinct subset of very aggressive neuroblastomas. Most cases with *MYCN* amplification also have 1p LOH, but not all cases with 1p LOH have amplification. This suggests that 1p deletion may precede the development of amplification. Indeed, it may be necessary to delete a gene that regulates *MYCN* expression, or one that mediates programmed cell death in the presence of high *MYCN* gene expression, for amplification to occur. Alternatively, there may be an underlying genetic abnormality that leads to genomic instability that predisposes to both 1p LOH and *MYCN* amplification.

About 25 percent of neuroblastomas have *MYCN* amplification, and virtually all of these cases have very high *MYCN* expression at the RNA and protein levels.[70] Indeed, there is heterogeneity in the level of expression of *MYCN* in single-copy tumors, but higher expression in nonamplified tumors does not consistently correlate with a worse outcome.[82–85] It is possible that the level of expression in nonamplified tumors seldom, if ever, exceeds a certain threshold level necessary to confer an unfavorable outcome, whereas almost all tumors with *MYCN* amplification exceed this threshold.[86] Furthermore, activation of *MYCN* by mechanisms other than amplification or overexpression may play an important role.[87] Finally, *DDX1*, a member of the DEAD box family of RNA helicases, is coamplified with *MYCN* in about half the cases.[88–91] However, the clinical significance of this finding is unclear.

Fig. 50-3 Southern blots showing *MYCN* amplification. In both rows, lane 1 represents DNA from a normal lymphoblastoid cell line as a single-copy control, and lane 8 represents DNA from the NGP cell line, with 150 copies of *MYCN* per haploid genome. (Row A). Lanes 2-7 represent 6 neuroblastomas with a single copy of *MYCN* per haploid genome. (Row B). Lanes 2 and 5 show examples of tumors with *MYCN* amplification, whereas the other tumors have the normal single-copy signal. (*Reprinted from Brodeur[68] with permission of Brain Pathology.*)

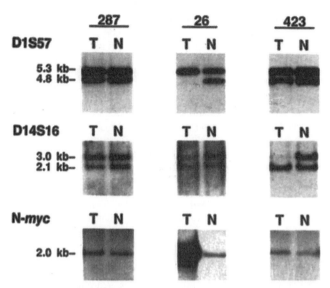

D1S57

5.3 kb—
4.8 kb—

D14S16

3.0 kb—
2.1 kb—

N-myc

2.0 kb—

Fig. 50-4 Patterns of genetic change in neuroblastomas. The first row shows assessment of LOH for the short arm of chromosome 1 (1p34) using the hypervariable probe D1S57 and the enzyme *Taq*I. The second row shows assessment of LOH for the long arm of chromosome 14 (14p32) using the probe D14S16 and the enzyme *Taq*I. The third row shows assessment of *MYCN* amplification using the pNB-1probe and *Eco*RI digestion of the DNAs. The first column (patient no. 287) shows no LOH for 1p or 14q, and normal *MYCN* copy number. The second column (patient no. 26) shows LOH for 1p and *MYCN* amplification, without allelic loss for 14q. The third column (patient no. 423) shows LOH for 14q, without LOH for 1p or *MYCN* amplification, which was the second most common pattern of genetic change. (T = tumor DNA; N = normal DNA from the same patient). (*Reprinted from Fong and colleagues[75] with permission of Cancer Research.*)

Amplification of Other Loci. We sought evidence for amplification of other oncogenes in a large series of neuroblastomas and tumor-derived cell lines, but none was found.[61] However, there are at least six examples of neuroblastoma cell lines or primary tumors that amplify regions that are remote from the *MYCN* locus at 2p24. These examples include amplification of genes from 2p22 and 2p13 in the IMR-32 cell line, as well as coamplification of *MYCN* and *MDM2* (from 12q13) in the NGP, TR-14, and LS cell lines.[92–95] Finally, there is one report of coamplification of *MYCN* and *MYCL* in a neuroblastoma cell line, which has been seen in at least one primary tumor as well.[4,5,66,96] These findings indicate that more than one locus can be amplified, but no neuroblastoma has been shown to amplify another gene that did not also amplify *MYCN*. Allelic gain of several other loci, such as 2p, 4q, 6p, 7q, 11q, and 18q, has been identified using comparative genomic hybridization (CGH) approaches.[97–102] However, the true prevalence, as well as the biological and clinical significance of these findings, is unclear at present.

Trisomy for 17q. To date, the only other specific karyotypic abnormality that has been detected with increased frequency is

Table 50-2 Correlation between MYCN Amplification and Stage in 3000 Neuroblastomas[2–6]

Stage at Diagnosis	*MYCN* Amplification	3-yr. Survival
Benign ganglioneuromas	0/64 (0%)	100%
Low stages (1, 2)	31/772 (4%)	90%
Stage 4-S	15/190 (8%)	80%
Advanced States (3, 4)	612/1974 (31%)	30%
TOTAL	658/3000 (22%)	50%

trisomy for the long arm of chromosome 17 (17q).[58,77,103] This finding was first noted by conventional cytogenetic studies and by FISH analysis, but its real frequency was not appreciated until recently. Allelotyping and CGH studies have suggested that gain of the long arm of chromosome 17 may occur in over half of all neuroblastomas.[97–101,104] Even accounting for near-triploid cases with gain of the entire chromosome, 17q trisomy may be the most prevalent genetic abnormality identified to date in neuroblastomas. Although gain of 17q can occur independently, it frequently occurs as part of an unbalanced translocation between chromosomes 1 and 17.[101,105–107] The 17q breakpoints vary, but a region has been defined from 17q22-qter that suggests a dosage effect rather than interruption of a gene.[108] Gain of 17q appears to be associated with a more aggressive subset of neuroblastomas, although its significance relative to other genetic and biological markers awaits a large prospective trial and multivariate analysis.

Tumor DNA Content: Near-Diploidy vs. Hyperdiploidy. Although the majority of tumors that have been karyotyped are in the diploid range, a substantial number of tumors from patients with lower stages of disease are hyperdiploid or near triploid. The modal karyotype number has been shown to have prognostic value.[109–111] Karyotypic analysis of tumor cells, however, is a tedious process that is generally successful in less than 25 percent of the cases attempted. Flow cytometric analysis of DNA content is a simple and semiautomated way of measuring total cell DNA, which correlates well with modal chromosome number. Recent studies by Look and others demonstrate that determination of the DNA index (DI) of neuroblastomas from infants provides important information that can be predictive of response to particular chemotherapeutic regimens as well as outcome.[112–115] Although this analysis cannot detect specific chromosome rearrangements, such as deletions, translocations, or gene amplification, it is a relatively simple test that correlates with biological behavior, at least in subsets of patients. Unfortunately, the DNA index loses its prognostic significance for patients over 2 years of age.[113] This is probably because hyperdiploid tumors from infants generally have whole chromosome gains without structural rearrangements, whereas hyperdiploid tumors in older patients usually have a number of structural rearrangements as well.

Tumor-Suppressor Genes and Allelic Loss

Chromosome Deletion or Allelic Loss at 1p. Deletion of the short arm of chromosome 1(1p) is a common abnormality that has been identified in 70 to 80 percent of the near-diploid tumors that have been karyotyped (Fig. 50-2).[59,61,103,116,117] However, using DNA polymorphism approaches that do not require tumor cells in mitosis, the actual prevalence is probably closer to 35 percent (Fig. 50-4).[74,76,78–80,118–121] Deletions of chromosome 1 are found more commonly in patients with advanced stages of disease, but the independent prognostic significance of 1p LOH is controversial.[77–81] Distal 1p36 appears to be deleted in almost all cases, including 1p36.2–.3, although the breakpoints are quite variable (Fig. 50-5). Indeed, another area of controversy is whether there is a single site of consistent deletion on distal 1p or two independent sites.[76,119–122] Finally, there is disagreement about whether distal 1p undergoes genomic imprinting, based on preferential parental allelic loss.[123,124] The resolution of these controversies must await additional studies, but it appears clear that at least one (and possibly more) tumor-suppressor gene resides at this locus.[4,5]

Unfortunately, no good candidate for the neuroblastoma tumor-suppressor gene on 1p36 has been identified, but several have been proposed (Fig. 50-5), including the tumor necrosis factor receptor 2 gene,[125] a zinc finger gene called *HKR3*,[126] a cell-cycle control gene called *CDC2L1*,[127] a tumor-suppressor gene in mice called *DAN*,[128] and a TP53 homolog called *TP73*.[129] Indeed, *TP73* is particularly interesting because of its homology to the prevalent tumor-suppressor gene *TP53*, but mutations have not been identified in neuroblastomas lacking one copy of the gene.[130]

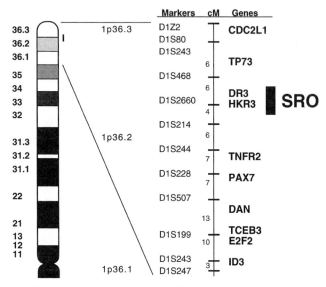

Fig. 50-5 Consistent region of 1p LOH in neuroblastomas. Diagrammatic representation of the short arm of chromosome 1 (1p), as well as the expanded genetic map of 1p36 and the approximate location of several candidates for the neuroblastoma tumor-suppressor gene (shown in bold). Also shown (SRO) is the region of consistent deletion of 1p36 in neuroblastomas (6 cM, 1 to 2 Mb), based on PCR-based polymorphisms. This map is described in more detail by White and colleagues.[47,76] *(Modified from Brodeur[5] with permission of Lippincott-Raven Press.)*

Moreover, with the exception of *HKR3*, these other candidate genes have been excluded from the region of consistent deletion, and careful analysis of *HKR3* has failed to identify any mutations.[47,76,126] Thus, further narrowing of the region of consistent deletion and analysis of candidate genes is required.

Chromosome Deletion or Allelic Loss at 11q, 14q, and Other Sites

Allelic Loss at 11q. Allelic loss of 11q has been detected by analysis of DNA polymorphisms and by CGH techniques.[75,98–101,131,132] In a recent study, 11q allelic loss occurs in 114 of 267 cases (43 percent), making it the most common deletion detected to date in neuroblastomas.[132] 11q deletion was associated with 14q deletion, but it was inversely correlated with 1p deletion and *MYCN* amplification. Interestingly, 11q LOH was associated with decreased event-free survival, but only in patients lacking *MYCN* amplification. Loss of 11q was not associated with other clinical or biological variables.

Allelic Loss at 14q. There is evidence that LOH for the long arm of chromosome 14 also occurs with increased frequency in neuroblastomas (Fig. 50-4).[75,131,133,134] The frequency of 14q allelic loss varies in different studies from 25 percent to 50 percent in several smaller studies, but it appears to be a consistent finding that probably represents loss of another suppressor gene. A more recent study found allelic loss in 64 of 280 cases (23 percent).[135] A consensus region of deletion was found in 14q23–32. There was a strong correlation with 11q allelic loss and an inverse relationship with 1p deletion and *MYCN* amplification. However, no correlation was found with other biological or clinical features or outcome.

Allelic Loss at Other Sites. Deletion or allelic loss has been demonstrated at a variety of other sites by genome-wide allelotyping or by CGH. The most consistent sites, in addition to those mentioned above, include 3p, 4p, 6q, 9p, 13q, and 18q.[98–102,104] However, none of these other sites have been studied in as much detail as the above sites, so their biological or clinical significance is unclear.

Other Tumor-Suppressor Genes

Involvement of TP53. The *TP53* gene, encoding the p53 protein, is one of the most commonly involved genes in human neoplasia. Several studies have examined neuroblastomas for mutation in the *TP53* gene, but mutations are rarely found.[136–140] Nevertheless, there is still controversy about the involvement of this gene in human neuroblastomas. Some reports have shown cytoplasmic sequestration in undifferentiated neuroblastomas, and this impairs the normal G1 checkpoint after DNA damage.[141,142] However, others have demonstrated that, although p53 is primarily located in the cytoplasm, ionizing radiation induces normal translocation to the nucleus of p53 that is capable of inducing G1 arrest.[143] At present this apparent discrepancy remains unresolved.

Involvement of CDK Inhibitors and the Neurofibromatosis 1 Gene. The *CDKN2A* (*INK4A*/p16) gene is deleted or mutated in many types of adult cancer, especially in established cell lines. Nevertheless, three studies have found no evidence of inactivation in neuroblastomas.[144–146] Indeed, two of these studies also examined the related genes *CDKN2B* (*KIP1*/p27) and *CDKN2C* (*INK4C*/p18) genes, but no deletions or rearrangements were found in these genes either.[145,146] One report, however, found frequent loss of 9p in neuroblastomas, and although only one tumor had a missense mutation, a number of others had absence of expression, suggesting inactivation in these cases.[147] Finally, two studies have found evidence of deletions or mutations in the neurofibromatosis 1 (*NF1*) gene in neuroblastoma cell lines, but it is unclear if this occurs commonly in primary tumors.[148,149]

ABNORMAL PATTERNS OF GENE EXPRESSION

Expression of Neurotrophin Receptors

Neuroblastoma cells are derived from sympathetic neuroblasts, and they frequently exhibit features of neuronal differentiation. Indeed, because neuroblastomas may show spontaneous or induced differentiation to ganglioneuroblastoma or ganglioneuroma, the malignant transformation of these cells may result in part from a failure to respond fully to the normal signals to undergo this maturation process. The factors responsible for regulating normal differentiation are not well understood at present, but they probably involve one or several neurotrophin-receptor pathways that signal the cell to differentiate. Recently, three tyrosine kinase receptors for a homologous family of neurotrophin factors were cloned. The main ligand for the *TrkA*, *TrkB*, and *TrkC* receptors is nerve growth factor (NGF), brain-derived neurotrophic factor (BDNF), and neurotrophin-3 (NT-3), respectively; neurotrophin-4/5 (NT-4) appears to function through *TrkB*.[150–159] Another transmembrane receptor binds all the neurotrophins with low affinity (LNTR), but its role in mediating responses to the presence or absence of these homologous ligands is controversial.[150,160,161]

To evaluate the clinical significance of *TrkA* expression in neuroblastomas, we studied the relationship between *TrkA* mRNA expression and patient survival in frozen tumors from 77 children with neuroblastomas and 5 children with ganglioneuromas.[162] High levels of *TrkA* expression (> 100 density units) were detected in 63 of the 77 neuroblastomas (82 percent). All tumors that had low-stage and no *MYCN* amplification showed a high level of *TrkA* expression. All but one tumor with *MYCN* amplification, however, had an extremely low or undetectable level of *TrkA* expression. The expression of *TrkA* correlated strongly with survival: the 5-year cumulative-survival rate of the group with a high level of *TrkA* expression was 86 percent, whereas that of the group with a low level of *TrkA* expression was 14 percent (p < 0.001). Indeed, the combination of *TrkA* expression and *MYCN* amplification had a strong influence on overall survival (see below). The group with high levels of *TrkA* expression and no *MYCN* amplification showed a cumulative 5-year survival of 87 percent. The patients whose tumors had a

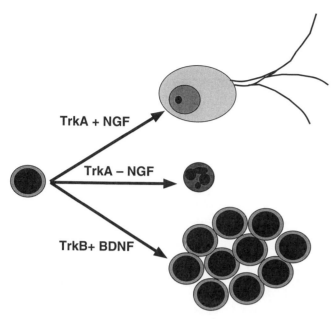

Fig. 50-6 Diagrammatic representation of the potential fates of neuroblastoma cells, depending on the pattern of expression of neurotrophin receptors and the availability of neurotrophins in their microenvironment. Favorable neuroblastoma cells expressing TrkA (with or without TrkC), if deprived of NGF, frequently undergo programmed cell death in vitro. These same cells will survive and differentiate if provided with adequate amounts of neurotrophins. In contrast, unfavorable neuroblastomas frequently express TrkB as well as its ligand BDNF. This autocrine loop apparently favors survival of these cells independent of exogenous neurotrophins. Furthermore, these cells generally do not express TrkA (or TrkC), and they do not respond to NGF by undergoing differentiation. (Modified from Brodeur[5] with permission of Lippincott-Raven Press.)

normal *MYCN* copy number and a low level of expression of *TrkA* had a 50 percent survival (p = 0.03), and all patients with *MYCN* amplification died within 2 years. Similar results have been obtained independently by others, supporting the strong correlation between high *TrkA* expression and a favorable outcome.[163–166]

The NGF/*TrkA* pathway may play an important role in the propensity of some neuroblastomas to regress or differentiate in selected patients. The association of *Trk* expression with tumors that have a favorable outcome suggests that it may play some role in the behavior of the tumors. Indeed, the expression of *TrkA* is required for biological responsiveness to NGF. In the presence of ligand, neuronal differentiation is induced and survival is promoted.[167] However, neurotrophic-factor deprivation may lead to programmed cell death (apoptosis) at this stage (Fig. 50-6).[168,169] Thus, the *in vivo* differentiation or regression that is seen either spontaneously or in response to treatment may be mediated by the NGF/*TrkA* pathway.[162]

Recently, we examined the expression and function of *TrkB* and *TrkC* in neuroblastomas. Both of these neurotrophin receptors can be expressed in a truncated form (lacking the tyrosine kinase) and a full-length form. Interestingly, expression of full-length *TrkB* was strongly associated with *MYCN*-amplified tumors.[170] Because these tumors also express the *TrkB* ligand (BDNF), this may represent an autocrine or paracrine loop providing some survival or growth advantage (Fig. 50-6).[171–173] Maturing tumors were more likely to express the truncated *TrkB*, whereas most immature, nonamplified tumors expressed neither.[170] In contrast, the expression of *TrkC* was found predominantly in lower stage tumors, and, like *TrkA*, was not expressed in *MYCN* amplified tumors.[174,175] This suggests that favorable tumors are characterized by the expression of *TrkA* with or without *TrkC*, but unfavorable tumors express full-length *TrkB* plus its ligand *BDNF*.

Expression of *HRAS* and Other Oncogenes

Although *NRAS* was first identified as the transforming gene of a human neuroblastoma cell line, subsequent studies of primary neuroblastomas by ourselves and others indicate that *RAS* activation by mutation of codons 12, 13, 59, or 61 is rare.[176–178] On the contrary, there is evidence that high expression of *HRAS* in neuroblastomas is associated with lower stage and better outcome.[179–181] The pattern of oncogene expression may be used to distinguish neuroblastomas from other histologically similar tumors, such as neuroepithelioma.[182] However, the ultimate clinical utility of the analysis of oncogene expression in neuroblastomas remains to be determined. Thus, in the subset of the patients lacking *MYCN* amplification, there is no consistent evidence to date for amplification or activation of any other oncogene.

Expression of the Multidrug Resistance Genes

Some tumor cells become resistant to a large number of chemotherapeutic agents simultaneously by overexpressing genes that confer this resistance, probably by enhanced efflux of the agents. The genes associated with this phenomenon are the multidrug resistance gene *MDR1* and the gene for multidrug resistance-related protein *MRP*. Most of the investigation of these genes and their encoded proteins has been performed *in vitro*, but their expression and potential clinical significance in neuroblastomas was addressed recently.[183–186] The data concerning the clinical significance of expression of *MDR1* in neuroblastomas are controversial, but the one study examining *MRP* expression shows a strong correlation with advanced clinical stages and a poor prognosis.[183–186] If this is confirmed by a larger independent study, analysis of *MRP* expression could become an important variable to examine to determine a patient's prognosis and to, in turn, influence the choice of agents or the intensity of treatment.

Telomerase Expression and Activity

Hiyama and colleagues[187] have studied 79 neuroblastomas from untreated patients for telomerase activity. They found that 16 had high telomerase activity, 60 had low activity, and 3 had no detectable activity. Interestingly, the three with no activity were among eight with stage 4S, a stage with a special pattern of limited dissemination found in infants whose tumors sometimes undergo spontaneous regression. None of these children died. In fact, only 2 of 60 patients with low activity died, whereas 12 of 16 with high activity died. Interestingly, all 11 with *MYCN* amplification had high activity, including the one patient with stage 4-S who died. These results show a correlation between telomerase activity and outcome of neuroblastoma patients, with a very good outcome seen in the few with no activity and a poor outcome in those with high activity (most with *MYCN* amplification). Thus, the extremes of telomerase activity (high or absent) may provide some useful information, but telomerase activity per se is correlated more with malignancy in general and not with specific types or behavior.[188] In further support of the potential clinical importance of telomerase expression, Reynolds and coworkers have shown a correlation of high expression of the RNA component with stage 4 disease and a poor outcome.[189]

Expression of Apoptosis Genes

Neuroblastoma has the highest rate of spontaneous regression observed in human cancers, and delayed activation of normal apoptotic pathways may play a role in this phenomenon.[190] Activation of programmed cell death can originate from a variety of stimuli, such as the presence or absence of exogenous ligand or from DNA damage. Indeed, NGF withdrawal is an important signal for apoptosis in the developing nervous system, and mediates the elimination of redundant cells. However, other cell surface proteins may be involved with initiation of apoptosis in neuronal cells and neuroblastomas (reviewed by Brodeur and Castle[191]). Members of the tumor necrosis factor receptor (TNFR) family, such as p75 (binds NGF with low affinity) and CD95/FasL (binds Fas ligand), as well as members of the retinoic acid receptor family, can mediate the induction of apoptosis in some neuroblastoma cell lines.[192,193] In addition, increased CD95 expression appears to be an essential component of chemotherapy induced apoptosis in neuroblastomas.[193]

Intracellular molecules responsible for relaying the apoptotic signal include the Bcl-2 family of proteins. *BCL-2* is highly expressed in most neuroblastoma cell lines and primary tumors and the level of expression is inversely related to the proportion of cells undergoing apoptosis and the degree of cellular differentiation.[190,194–198] There have been conflicting reports regarding the correlation between the level of expression of Bcl-2 in primary tumors and prognostic variables,[194,196,197,199,200] but taken together the evidence suggests that there is no significant correlation. However, the Bcl-2 family of proteins may play an important role in acquired resistance to chemotherapy.[201,202] Finally, caspases are the proteolytic enzymes responsible for the execution of the apoptotic signal, and there is evidence that increased expression of interleukin-1β-converting enzyme (ICE, caspase-1) and other caspases in primary neuroblastoma is associated with favorable biological features and improved disease outcome.[203] These observations are consistent with the hypothesis that neuroblastomas prone to undergoing apoptosis are more likely to spontaneously regress and/or respond well to cytotoxic agents.

GENETIC MODEL OF NEUROBLASTOMA DEVELOPMENT

In summary, there is increasing evidence for at least two genetic subsets of neuroblastomas that are highly predictive of clinical

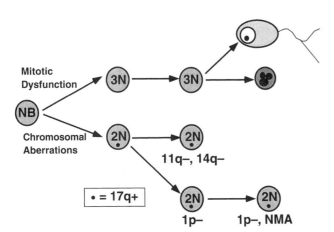

Fig. 50-7 Genetic model of neuroblastoma development. According to this model, all neuroblastomas have a common precursor (NB) and may have a common mutation (the one responsible for familial neuroblastoma). However, a commitment is made to develop into one of two major types. The first type is characterized by mitotic dysfunction leading to a hyperdiploid or near-triploid modal karyotype (3N) with whole chromosome gains, but few if any structural cytogenetic rearrangements. These tumors usually express high levels of TrkA, so they are prone to either differentiation or apoptosis, depending on the presence or absence of NGF in their microenvironment. The second type generally has a near-diploid (2N) or near-tetraploid karyotype but is characterized by gross chromosomal aberrations. No consistent abnormality has been identified to date, but 17q gain is very common. Within this type, two subsets can be distinguished. 11q deletion and/or 14q deletion characterize one subset, whereas the second subset is characterized by 1p LOH, with or without MYCN amplification (NMA). The latter tumors frequently express TrkB plus BDNF, probably representing an autocrine survival pathway. Thus, neuroblastoma represents fundamentally two major types and three subtypes, but they may all arise from a common precursor cell. (*Reprinted from Ambros and Brodeur*[347] *with permission from Lippincott-Raven Press.*)

Table 50-3 Biological/Clinical Types of Neuroblastoma[3–5,347]

Feature	Type 1	Type 2A	Type 2B
MYCN	Normal	Normal	Amplified
DNA Ploidy	Hyperdiploid	Near diploid	Near diploid
	Near triploid	Near tetraploid	Near tetraploid
17q gain	Rare	Common	Common
11q, 14q LOH	Rare	Common	Rare
1p LOH	Rare	Rare	Common
TrkA exp.	High	Low or absent	Low or absent
TrkB exp.	Truncated	Low or absent	High (full length)
TrkC exp.	High	Low or absent	Low or absent
Age	Usually <1 yr.	Usually >1 yr.	Usually 1–5 yr.
Stage	Usually 1, 2, 4S	Usually 3, 4	Usually 3, 4
3-yr. Survival	95%	25–50%	20%

behavior. One recently proposed classification takes into account abnormalities of 1p, *MYCN* copy number, and assessment of DNA content, and distinct genetic subsets of neuroblastomas can be identified (Fig. 50-7; Table 50-3).[2–6] The first is characterized by mitotic dysfunction leading to a hyperdiploid or near-triploid modal karyotype, with few if any cytogenetic rearrangements. These tumors lack specific genetic changes like *MYCN* amplification or 1p LOH. These patients are generally less than 1 year of age with localized disease and a very good prognosis. The second is characterized by gross chromosomal aberrations and they generally have a near-diploid karyotype. No consistent abnormality has been identified to date, but 17q gain is common. Within this type, two subsets can be distinguished. One subset is characterized by 11q deletion, 14q deletion, or other changes, but patients in this subset lack *MYCN* amplification and generally lack 1p LOH. Patients with these tumors are generally older with more advanced stages of disease that is slowly progressive and often fatal. The second subset has amplification of *MYCN*, usually with 1p36 LOH. These patients are generally between 1 and 5 years of age with advanced stages of disease that is rapidly progressive and frequently fatal. It is unknown if a tumor from one type ever converts to a less favorable type, but current evidence suggests that they are genetically distinct.[73,113]

Indeed, it is possible that all neuroblastomas have a single mutation in common. This is because one can see the spectrum from ganglioneuroma to metastatic neuroblastoma in a single family.[29,30] However, a commitment is made shortly after to develop into one of two major types: (a) a favorable type characterized by mitotic dysfunction and whole chromosome gains, leading to hyperdiploidy or near triploidy, or (b) an unfavorable type characterized by structural chromosomal rearrangements. The first type of tumors generally expresses high levels of *TrkA*, and these tumors are prone to differentiation or programmed cell death, depending on the presence or absence of NGF. The second type frequently has gain of 17q and expresses little, if any, *TrkA*. However, subsets can be distinguished by different patterns of genetic change (Fig. 50-7). A less aggressive subtype is characterized by deletion of 11q, 14q, or other rearrangements. The most aggressive subtype is characterized by *MYCN* amplification, frequently with 1p LOH, and these tumors frequently express *TrkB* plus *BDNF*, representing an autocrine survival pathway. Thus, neuroblastoma represents fundamentally two different types, but it can be seen as one or three diseases as well, depending on the perspective.

CLINICAL MANIFESTATIONS AND PATTERN OF SPREAD

Primary Tumors

About half of all neuroblastomas originate in the adrenal medulla; 30 percent occur in nonadrenal abdominal sites in the paravertebral ganglia, pelvic ganglia, or the organ of Zuckerkandl; and 20 percent occur in the paravertebral ganglia of the thorax.[1,2] Most primary tumors cause symptoms of abdominal mass or pain. However, because of the paraspinal location of many tumors, they may invade the spinal canal through neural foramina and cause compression of the spinal cord. In the thoracic or upper lumbar region, this usually leads to paraplegia, whereas lower lumbar invasion leads to a cauda equina syndrome with loss of bowel or bladder function. Midline tumors can displace or compress other structures such as the trachea or esophagus, and lead to obstructive symptoms. Finally, involvement of the superior cervical ganglion can produce Horner syndrome, which consists of unilateral ptosis, myosis, and anhydrosis.

Metastatic Disease

Most neuroblastomas are metastatic at the time of diagnosis. Frequent sites of metastasis are: regional or distant lymph nodes, cortical bone, bone marrow, liver, and skin. In infants (<1 year old), a characteristic pattern of small primary tumors with dissemination limited to liver and skin (with or without minimal marrow involvement) is associated with a favorable outcome. This special pattern is referred to as stage 4-S.[204–207] However, in older patients (>1 year old), the dissemination most frequently involves bone marrow and bone, particularly the bones of the skull and orbits. Rarely, disease may spread to lung and brain parenchyma, usually as a manifestation of relapsing or end-stage disease. The outlook for these older patients is very poor, even with intensive multimodality therapy. However, there has been recent progress in elucidating the genetic and biochemical basis of these very different patterns of behavior.

Paraneoplastic Syndromes

Several paraneoplastic syndromes have been associated with neuroblastoma, although each is seen in only 1 to 3 percent of patients. Intractable secretory diarrhea and abdominal distension, sometimes associated with hypokalemia and dehydration (Kerner-Morrison syndrome), is a manifestation of tumor secretion of vasoactive intestinal peptide (VIP).[208,209] VIP is a 28 amino acid polypeptide hormone that is related in structure to glucagon, secretin, and several other polypeptide hormones.[210] It is encoded by the third exon of a large, 6-exon gene that also encodes a closely related polypeptide hormone, PHM-27, in exon 4.[211] However, these two proteins are expressed differentially in some cells.[212] The biological functions of VIP are relaxation of smooth muscle, stimulation of intestinal water and electrolyte secretion, and stimulation of release of other polypeptide hormones.[210] The VIP syndrome usually is associated with ganglioneuroblastoma or ganglioneuroma, and these symptoms resolve after eradication of the tumor.[208,209]

Opsomyoclonus, sometimes called myoclonic encephalopathy, is a syndrome that consists of myoclonic jerking and random eye movement, sometimes associated with cerebellar ataxia. This syndrome has been observed in up to 4 percent of patients.[213–217] Other neuromuscular disorders have been seen in association with neuroblastoma as well, but they are less common. These symptoms may diminish or even disappear with eradication of the tumor, and these patients usually have a favorable outcome from the oncologic perspective.[215] It is, however, becoming increasingly apparent that many patients have residual neurologic abnormalities.[218–220] The symptoms may vary in severity, especially worsening in association with intercurrent illnesses. Recent evidence suggests that the opsoclonus syndrome may be caused by antineuronal autoantibodies.[221–223]

The third paraneoplastic syndrome is due to increased secretion of catecholamines, but this appears to occur in less than 1 percent of patients. The syndrome consists of episodes of tachycardia, palpitations, profuse sweating, and flushing, which is produced by secretion of norepinephrine.[224] Indeed, symptoms attributed to excess catecholamine secretion reportedly were seen in a mother who had a fetus with a neuroblastoma.[225] This syndrome is more common in patients with pheochromocytomas, because these tumors secrete epinephrine, which is a more potent inducer of these symptoms than norepinephrine.

METHODS OF DIAGNOSIS

Diagnostic Criteria

To confirm a diagnosis of neuroblastoma, some histologic evidence that demonstrates neural origin or differentiation by light microscopy, electron microscopy, or immunohistology is usually required. Alternatively, because the bone marrow is frequently involved, some patients are considered to have neuroblastoma based on the presence of "compatible" tumor cells involving the bone marrow, accompanied by increased urinary catecholamine metabolites. Differences in diagnostic criteria used by different groups or countries have led to some difficulties in comparing studies. However, proposals have been made to develop international criteria to confirm a diagnosis of neuroblastoma.[206,207]

Catecholamine Metabolism

When sensitive techniques are used, usually 90 to 95 percent of tumors produce sufficient catecholamines to result in increased urinary metabolites. This provides a great diagnostic advantage in confirming the diagnosis of neuroblastoma, as well as in following disease activity in those patients whose tumors are secretors.[226–228] Fig. 50-8 depicts catecholamine synthesis and metabolism. Although the major pathways and products of catecholamine catabolism are shown, the actual pathways of intracellular and extracellular catecholamine breakdown are more complex.

The precursor amino acids for catecholamine synthesis are phenylalanine and tyrosine. Phenylalanine is converted by phenylalanine hydroxylase to tyrosine (Fig. 50-8). Tyrosine is then converted by tyrosine hydroxylase to 3,4-dihydroxy-phenyl-alanine (DOPA), which is a catecholamine precursor. DOPA is converted by DOPA decarboxylase to the first catecholamine in the pathway, dopamine. Dopamine is converted by dopamine-β-hydroxylase to norepinephrine, which is then converted by phenylethanolamine-N-methyltransferase to epinephrine. Neuroblastoma cells lack this last enzyme, which is present in adrenal chromaffin cells and pheochromocytomas. The two enzymes primarily responsible for the catabolism of catecholamines are catechol-O-methyl transferase and monoamine oxidase. DOPA and dopamine are converted primarily to homovanillic acid (HVA), whereas norepinephrine and epinephrine are converted primarily to vanillylmandelic acid (VMA). Most laboratories involved in neuroblastoma diagnosis measure both urinary VMA and HVA.

Differential Diagnosis

Because of the many potential clinical presentations, neuroblastoma may be confused with a variety of other neoplasms as well as nonneoplastic conditions. This is particularly a problem in the 5 to 10 percent of tumors that do not produce catecholamines, as well as in the 1 percent or so of patients who do not have an obvious primary tumor.[213–217] Patients with the VIP syndrome can be confused with infectious or inflammatory bowel disease, and those with the opsoclonus-myoclonus and ataxia syndromes can resemble primary neurologic disease. Histologically, neuroblastoma tissue from primary or metastatic sites may be quite undifferentiated, and may be confused with other embryonal pediatric cancers such as rhabdomyosarcoma, Ewing sarcoma, neuroepithelioma, lymphoma, or leukemia (especially megakaryoblastic leukemia). Fortunately, a battery of monoclonal antibodies are being developed that should allow these various disease entities to be made with greater objectivity and confidence.[229–233]

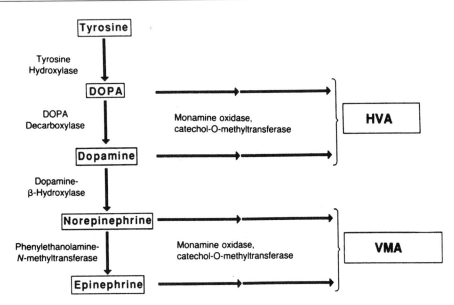

Fig. 50-8 Pathway of catecholamine metabolism. Shown is a simplified diagram of catecholamine synthesis and metabolism. HVA and VMA are the urinary catecholamine metabolites usually measured. (*Reprinted from Brodeur[1] with permission of Mosby–Year Book.*)

CLINICAL EVALUATION AND STAGING

Diagnostic Testing

A standard set of recommended tests to define the clinical stage or extent of disease has been established.[206,207] Certainly, the more tests that are done, the greater the likelihood of finding disseminated disease. This applies particularly to the number of bone marrow aspirates and biopsies that are done, and the manner in which marrow disease is detected.[234–236] For this purpose, a standard set of immunologic reagents to detect occult neuroblastoma are being developed.[207] This immunocytologic approach may obviate the need for multiple aspirates and biopsies in the future. Uniformity with respect to minimum testing should improve the comparability of studies, but the tests recommended should be available in most medical centers.

The conventional diagnostic imaging modalities include plain radiographs, bone scintigraphy,[237–239] ultrasound,[240] computerized tomography (CT scan),[241,242] and magnetic resonance imaging (MRI scan).[243,244] In addition, the potential specificity and sensitivity of meta-iodobenzylguanidine (MIBG) scintigraphy for evaluation of bone and soft tissue involvement by neuroblastoma is attractive.[245,246] MIBG is taken up by catecholaminergic cells, which includes most neuroblastomas. Radiolabeled MIBG scintigraphy thus has the potential to be a very specific and sensitive method of assessment of the primary tumor and focal metastatic disease. Unfortunately, MIBG scintigraphy is not readily available throughout the industrialized countries of the world.

Tumor Pathology

Neuroblastomas arise from primitive, pluripotential sympathetic nerve cells (sympathogonia), which are derived from the neural crest. These cells differentiate into the different normal tissues of the sympathetic nervous system, such as the spinal sympathetic ganglia, the supporting Schwannian cells, and adrenal chromaffin cells. The three classic histopathologic patterns of neuroblastoma, ganglioneuroblastoma, and ganglioneuroma reflect a spectrum of morphologic and biochemical differentiation. The typical neuroblastoma is composed of small, but uniformly sized, cells containing dense, hyperchromatic nuclei and scant cytoplasm. The presence of neuritic processes, or neuropil, is a pathognomonic feature of all but the most primitive neuroblastoma. The fully differentiated, and benign, counterpart of neuroblastoma is the ganglioneuroma. It is composed of mature ganglion cells, surrounded by a matrix of Schwannian cells and neuropil.

Ganglioneuroblastomas are a heterogeneous group of tumors with histopathologic features spanning the extremes of maturation represented by neuroblastoma and ganglioneuroma. Ganglioneuroblastomas may be either focal or diffuse, depending on the pattern seen, but diffuse ganglioneuroblastoma is associated with less aggressive behavior.[247]

Several pathologic classification systems of neuroblastoma have been proposed that have some value in predicting the behavior of the tumor. Some utilize features of neuronal differentiation, whereas others consider the amount of Schwannian stroma, mitotic figures, karyorrhexis, or tumor calcification.[247–249] At the current time the "Shimada" classification is the most popular and has the most clinical utility in predicting outcome.[247] However, in the future, an international neuroblastoma pathology classification based on the Shimada classification will be used.[250] The Schwannian stroma was presumed to arise from the clonal proliferation of malignant cells, because both Schwann cells and neuroblasts are of neural crest origin. Also, neuroblastoma cells in culture could have either a neuronal or a substrate-adherent phenotype.[251] Recent evidence from Ambros and colleagues has shown, however, that the Schwann cells appear to be normal diploid cells that are reactive and infiltrate the tumor.[252] In contrast, the neuroblasts and ganglion cells in such differentiating tumors are near triploid. Thus, the tumors with Schwannian stroma probably make a tropic factor that results in the infiltration and proliferation of these cells.

Staging

The distribution of patients by stage or extent of disease differs depending on the age at diagnosis. For instance, in a consecutive series of 1001 patients enrolled on POG protocols from 1981 to 1989 and staged by the POG staging system, only about 40 percent of patients less than 1 year of age had unresectable or metastatic disease, whereas almost 80 percent of older patients had advanced stages of disease.[1,2,206,207] These findings explain, in part, the generally better outcome of infants with neuroblastoma compared to their older counterparts, but biological differences of the tumors in the two age groups appear to be very important also.

Until recently there were several different staging systems used for neuroblastoma throughout the world.[204,253–257] In general, the various staging systems give comparable results in distinguishing low-stage, good-prognosis patients from high-stage, poor-prognosis patients. However, some of the differences between the staging systems are substantial, particularly as applied to patients with intermediate stages. Therefore, a group of individuals met in 1986 and again in 1991 to formulate an International Neuro-

Table 50-4 International Neuroblastoma Staging System[206,207]

STAGE 1	Localized tumor with complete gross excision, with or without microscopic residual disease; representative ipsilateral lymph nodes negative for tumor microscopically (nodes attached to and removed with the primary tumor may be positive).
STAGE 2A	Localized tumor with incomplete gross excision; representative ipsilateral nonadherent lymp nodes negative for tumor microscopically.
STAGE 2B	Localized tumor with or without complete gross excision, with ipsilateral nonadherent lymph nodes positive for tumor. Enlarged contralateral lymph nodes must be negative microscopically.
STAGE 3	Unresectable unilateral tumor infiltrating across the midline,* with or without regional lymph node involvement; *or* localized unilateral tumor with contralateral regional lymph node involvement; *or* midline tumor with bilateral extension by infiltration (unresectable); *or* by lymph node involvement.
STAGE 4	Any primary tumor with dissemination to distant lymph nodes, bone, bone marrow, liver, skin, and/or other organs (except as defined for Stage 4S).
STAGE 4S	Localized primary tumor (as defined for Stage 1, 2A, or 2B), with dissemination limited to skin, liver, and/or bone marrow† (limited to infants < 1 year of age)

Multifocal primary tumors (e.g., bilateral adrenal primary tumors) should be staged according to the greatest extent of disease, as defined above, followed by a subscript "M" (e.g., 3_M).
* The midline is defined as the vertebral column. Tumors originating on one side and "crossing the midline" must infiltrate to or beyond the opposite side of the vertebral column.
† Marrow involvement in stage 4S should be minimal, i.e., less than 10% of total nucleated cells identified as malignant on bone marrow biopsy or on marrow aspirate. More extensive marrow involvement would be considered to be Stage 4. The MIBG scan (if done) should be negative in the marrow.

blastoma Staging System that would lead to uniformity in staging of patients with neuroblastoma for clinical trials and biological studies around the world.

The International Neuroblastoma Staging System (INSS) is based on clinical, radiographic, and surgical evaluation of children with neuroblastoma.[206,207] This staging system (Table 50-4) utilizes the most important components of previous systems. To distinguish the INSS from previous systems, Arabic numbers are used rather than Roman numerals or letters of the alphabet. Recently, modifications have been proposed in this system to clarify definitions of stages, as well as criteria for diagnosis and response to treatment.[206,207] In addition, suggestions were made to develop biological risk groups that incorporate clinical and laboratory variables in determining prognosis.[207]

PROGNOSTIC CONSIDERATIONS — CLINICAL AND BIOLOGICAL FEATURES

Clinical Features

The most important clinical variables are the stage of disease, the age of the patient at diagnosis, and the site of the primary tumor.[114,258–266] The overall prognosis of patients with stages 1, 2, and 4-S is between 75 and 90 percent, whereas those with stages 3 and 4 have a two-year disease-free survival range of 30 to 40 percent. The outcome of infants less than 1 year of age is substantially better than older patients with the same stage of disease, particularly those with more advanced stages of disease. Patients with primary tumors in the adrenal gland appear to do

worse than patients with tumors originating at other sites, particularly the thorax, but this does not appear to add substantially to the prognosis once the variables of age and stage are considered.

Biological Features

A variety of biological variables (pathology, serum markers, genetic features) have been studied that appear to have predictive value as independent prognostic markers in patients with neuroblastoma. The serum markers include ferritin, neuron-specific enolase (NSE), a cell membrane ganglioside (G_{D2}), and lactate dehydrogenase (LDH). The genetic features of the tumor that have been proposed as prognostic markers include tumor-cell DNA index, *MYCN* oncogene copy number, deletion or LOH involving 1p, and unbalanced gain of 17q. Additional markers have been proposed, such as expression of the H-*ras* oncogene, the multidrug resistance gene, or the multidrug resistance-related protein, but the value of these markers is still unclear.[179,180,184–186,267–269] Moreover, no study to date has examined all variables in a large set of patients, so it is somewhat difficult to say which single variable or combination of variables are the most powerful predictors of outcome, in addition to the more conventional clinical features of patient age and stage.

Tumor Pathology

Differentiated histology, such as ganglioneuroblastoma, generally is associated with localized tumors,[248] but this type of histologic classification does not have prognostic value that adds substantially to age and stage. More detailed analysis of histology, such as the classifications by Shimada or Joshi, considers the amount of Schwannian stroma, mitotic figures, karyorrhexis, and calcification.[247,249] These classifications appear to be more powerful predictors of outcome. Soon there will be an international neuroblastoma pathology classification (INPC) that will supersede the abovementioned systems and become the international standard for histopathologic classification, particularly as a prognostic variable.[207,250] Expression of the cell surface glycoprotein CD44 has also been shown to have prognostic significance, with high expression associated with more differentiated tumors and a better outcome.[270–273]

Serum Markers

Ferritin. Analysis of serum from patients with neuroblastoma has determined that ferritin levels are increased in some patients with actively growing tumors.[274–277] Ferritin levels are rarely elevated in patients with low stages of disease, whereas up to half of patients with advanced stages have significant elevations and a much worse outcome. *In vitro* evidence suggests that the tumor cells may produce this ferritin. Increased ferritin levels may be simply a marker of rapid tumor growth and/or large tumor burden. On the other hand, ferritin or iron may be particularly important for growth of neuroblastoma cells. In this regard, it is interesting that some therapeutic approaches are targeting the increased levels of ferritin and iron in patients with advanced disease.

NSE. NSE is a cytoplasmic protein with enolase activity that is associated with neural cells. Analysis of serum NSE from patients with neuroblastoma has indicated that survival is substantially worse in advanced patients with high serum NSE levels.[278–281] Although marked increases in serum NSE were associated with neuroblastomas, mild to moderate elevations were seen with other pediatric tumors, also. Thus, NSE is not as specific as was once thought, but it may have prognostic value, and perhaps it may be useful to follow disease activity and response to treatment in individual patients.

Ganglioside G_{D2}. Several independently derived monoclonal antibodies against neuroblastoma cells recognize gangliosides, which are sialic acid-containing glycosphingolipids. The most characteristic ganglioside on human neuroblastoma cell membranes is called G_{D2}. Not only is the presence of this ganglioside useful for identifying neuroblastoma cells, but also increased levels have been found in the plasma of patients with neuroblastoma. Measurement of circulating G_{D2} may serve as another useful marker of disease activity or response to treatment.[282–285] Indeed, gangliosides shed by tumor cells may play a role in accelerating tumor progression, and antibodies against G_{D2} may be useful for therapy of neuroblastoma as well.[283,286]

LDH. Although it is not specific to neuroblastoma, serum LDH level has been proposed as a prognostic marker for neuroblastoma. Increased LDH levels may be a reflection of rapid cellular turnover or of large tumor burden. Increased levels are more common in patients with extensive or progressive disease, and levels of greater than 1500 μm/ml have been associated with a poor prognosis in infants with neuroblastoma.[287–289]

Genetic Markers

Tumor Cell DNA Index. Tumor cells with an increased DNA content (or "hyperdiploid" karyotype) have been associated with a favorable outcome in infants with neuroblastoma.[109–115,290–293] In addition, hyperdiploid tumors are more likely to have lower stages of disease and require little, if any, therapy, whereas those with a "diploid" DNA content are more likely to have advanced stages of disease and require more intensive therapy. However, this variable appears to be useful primarily for patients less than 1 year of age with advanced stages of disease.[113]

MYCN amplification. The presence of *MYCN* amplification in tumor cells is found predominantly in patients with advanced stages of disease.[67] However, *MYCN* amplification is associated with rapid tumor progression and a poor prognosis, regardless of the age of the patient or the stage of the disease.[60,67–71,113,290] Although not all patients with a poor outcome have *MYCN* amplification, most patients with amplification treated with conventional therapy have rapid progression and die (Fig. 50-9).[1,2]

Allelic Loss for 1p, 11q, or 14q. Finally, there appears to be a strong correlation between 1p deletion and poor event-free survival.[74,76–81,117,273] Because there is an association between *MYCN* amplification and 1p deletion, it remains controversial as to whether this finding has independent prognostic significance.[77–81] Although 11q LOH occurs with substantial frequency and correlates with event-free survival in some series, its overall clinical significance is unclear.[75,98–101,131,132] Finally, 14q LOH does not appear to have prognostic significance other than its association with advanced stages of disease in some studies.[75,131,133–135]

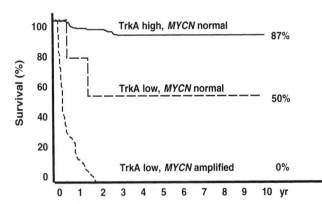

Fig. 50-9 MYCN Amplification, *TrkA* expression and survival in children with neuroblastoma. Survival according to *MYCN* copy number (amplified or not) and *TrkA* expression (high versus low or absent) in 82 children with neuroblastoma. (*Reprinted from Nakagawara*[162] *with permission from the New England Journal of Medicine.*)

Trk Gene Expression. Recent studies suggest that high levels of expression of the *TrkA* gene are associated with a favorable outcome in neuroblastoma patients.[86,162–166] Although prospective studies need to be done to confirm these observations, current evidence suggests that high *TrkA* gene expression may be a very powerful prognostic marker (Fig. 50-9). Indeed, it may predict the propensity of selected tumors to undergo either programmed cell death, leading to regression, or neuronal differentiation, leading to a benign ganglioneuroma. Similar results have been obtained by analysis of *TrkC*, which is also associated with a biologically favorable outcome, but they appear to be a subset of the *TrkA*-positive tumors, so *TrkC* expression does not have independent prognostic significance.[174,175] In contrast, *TrkB* expression is associated with advanced stage tumors with *MYCN* amplification.[170] Tumors expressing *TrkB*, along with its ligand *BDNF*, may have an autocrine survival pathway that provides them with a survival advantage.[170–173]

Biological/Clinical Subsets of Neuroblastoma. As described above, neuroblastomas can be separated into genetically distinct subsets, with characteristic clinical behavior and prognosis (Table 50-4; Fig. 50-7). They represent two fundamentally different types that are either biologically favorable or unfavorable. However, the latter type can be divided into subtypes, based on the pattern of genetic abnormalities, with distinct clinical behavior. This concept has been validated by several recent studies.[113,273,294] Thus, genetic analysis of neuroblastoma cells provides prognostic information that can direct more appropriate choice of treatment.

THERAPEUTIC APPROACHES

The treatment modalities traditionally employed in the management of neuroblastoma are surgery, chemotherapy, and radiotherapy. The role of each is determined by the natural history of individual cases considering stage, age, and biological features. With few exceptions (e.g., patients with localized primary tumors and many infants with 4-S disease), chemotherapy remains the backbone of the multimodality treatment plan. For this discussion, stage is defined by the INSS criteria (Table 50-3).[206,207]

Surgery

Surgery plays a pivotal role in the management of neuroblastoma. Depending on the timing, operative procedures can have diagnostic as well as therapeutic functions.[253,295–298] The goals of primary surgical procedures, performed prior to any other therapy, are to establish the diagnosis, to provide tissue for biological studies, to excise the tumor if feasible, and to stage the tumor surgically. In delayed primary or second-look surgery, the surgeon determines response to therapy and removes residual disease when possible. Surgery can also have palliative benefit for recurrent or progressive disease.

Chemotherapy

Chemotherapy is the predominant modality of management in neuroblastoma. Single-agent phase II trials conducted in patients with recurrent or advanced neuroblastoma have identified a number of effective drugs.[2] Cyclophosphamide, ifosfamide, cisplatin, carboplatin doxorubicin (Adriamycin), and the epipodophyllotoxins (teniposide, VM-26; and etoposide, VP-16) yield complete and partial response rates of 25 to 50 percent, and have become the cornerstone of multiagent regimens. Drug combinations have been developed that take advantage of drug synergism, mechanisms of cytotoxicity, and differences in side effects.[299,300] Treatment of children with advanced stage neuroblastoma using these combinations has resulted in improved response rates with minimal increase in toxicity.[2,301–305]

Radiation Therapy

Neuroblastoma is considered a radiosensitive tumor, and radiotherapy is very effective in achieving local control or palliation.

However, long-term control of neuroblastoma is seldom achieved with radiation therapy alone because of the propensity of this tumor to widespread metastases.[306,307] Historically, radiation has been used in the multimodality management of residual neuroblastoma, bulky unresectable tumors, and disseminated disease. More recently, the role of radiotherapy in neuroblastoma continues to be refined with the improvement in multiagent chemotherapy and the increasing trend toward developing risk-related treatment groups based upon age, stage, and biological features.

Bone Marrow and Stem Cell Transplantation

Attempts have been made to improve on the modest gains of intensive, combined-modality therapy to increase intensity of therapy. Dose-limiting marrow toxicity can be ameliorated to some extent by the use of colony-stimulating factors for the granulocyte or granulocyte-macrophage lineages, which increase the rate of marrow recovery. However, therapy that is more intensive can be administered if accompanied by bone marrow transplantation (BMT). Although allogeneic BMT is practiced by some centers, the most popular approach is autologous BMT, frequently with a purged marrow.[308–318] Marrow purging usually is accomplished by covalently attaching a cocktail of antineuroblastoma antibodies to magnetic beads and mixing beads with the marrow, followed by passing the marrow over powerful magnets.[309,310,319–322] A variation on this approach that is undergoing clinical trials currently is the use of peripheral blood-stem cells (with or without CD34-positive selection) as the source of cells for marrow rescue.[323,324] Although these approaches may increase the median survival of older patients with advanced stages of neuroblastoma, it is not clear that the long-term, disease-free survival has been affected appreciably.

Biologically Based Risk Groups

Most current studies for the treatment of neuroblastoma patients are based on risk groups that consider various biological features (*MYCN* copy number, histopathology, and tumor ploidy in infants) in addition to patient age and INSS stage. Preliminary data, adjusted for age and stage, indicate that analysis of DNA content in infants and *MYCN* copy number in all patients, allow more precise determination of risk.[68,112,113,325] Tumor histopathology by the Shimada classification also appears to be an important independent prognostic marker, at least for certain subsets of patients. It is likely that tumor histopathology as determined by the INPC classification will replace the Shimada classification in these risk assessments.[247] Judging the prognostic impact of other biological variables, such as 1p LOH, 11q LOH, unbalanced 17q gain, *TrkA* expression, or others, must await prospective therapeutic and biological studies.

Second Malignant Neoplasms

Other malignant diseases have been observed in individuals with neuroblastoma, such as pheochromocytoma, brain tumors, acute leukemia, and renal cell carcinoma.[326–330] However, none of these second cancers have occurred with sufficient frequency to indicate a specific relationship between neuroblastoma and any other neoplasm.[331] Furthermore, it is not clear if second malignant neoplasms are more common in survivors who had hereditary predisposition to develop neuroblastoma. Analysis of this question requires more precise methods to detect predisposed individuals, as well as improved patient survival. Thus, it currently appears that most second malignant neoplasms are either coincidental or related to the therapy, so future modifications of treatment aimed at eliminating potentially carcinogenic agents are warranted.

Future Treatment Strategies

The use of dose-intensified chemotherapy combinations, with or without autologous bone marrow transplantation, has produced better immediate disease control in neuroblastoma. Unfortunately, this has not translated into durable remissions in children with high-risk tumors. Future treatment strategies will address: (a) the

identification of new drugs and drug combinations; (b) the use of biological agents targeted at killing neuroblastoma cells, such as radiolabeled MIBG or antineuroblastoma antibodies; (c) agents that might induce differentiation, such as retinoic acid or NGF; and (d) antiangiogenesis therapy or other approaches.[332–337]

NEUROBLASTOMA SCREENING STUDIES

Another approach to improve the long-term outcome of patients with neuroblastoma is to identify patients with this disease earlier in the course of their disease. Because neuroblastomas frequently produce increased levels of catecholamines whose metabolites are detectable in the urine, mass urinary screening of infants for neuroblastoma has been undertaken in Japan for over 20 years.[338–341] The rationale of such a mass screening program assumes that patients with aggressive, biologically unfavorable disease and low likelihood of survival evolve over time from more localized, biologically favorable tumors. Alternatively, early detection of patients with biologically unfavorable disease may lead to an improved outcome. Similar efforts have been recently undertaken in North America (especially Quebec, Canada) and in Europe to answer questions concerning the feasibility and utility of screening for neuroblastoma.[342–346]

Studies of the clinical and cytogenetic features of tumors identified as a result of mass screening of infants for neuroblastomas in Japan suggest that the majority of patients identified have lower stages of disease, and virtually all of the tumors are in the hyperdiploid or near-triploid range.[109,291] Previous studies demonstrated that such findings generally are associated with a very favorable outcome.[109–115] Therefore, the results of the screening study have suggested at least two possibilities: either (a) all neuroblastomas begin as tumors with a more favorable genotype and phenotype, and some evolve into more aggressive tumors with adverse genetic features; or (b) there are at least two different subsets of neuroblastoma, and the more favorable group presents earlier, and therefore is the predominant group detected by screening. The accumulating body of genetic information, as discussed above (Table 50-4, Fig. 50-7), is more consistent with the latter explanation.[5,73,113,293,347–351]

In addition to the genetic data discussed above, the accumulating evidence suggests that the prevalence of neuroblastoma in screened populations is increased by 50 to 100 percent over that seen in unscreened populations, and the prevalence of neuroblastoma in patients over 1 year of age has not changed appreciably.[293,343,344,348,351] Taken together with the biological information, this suggests that screening is detecting tumors in a substantial number of patients who likely would never develop symptomatic disease because their tumors would have regressed or matured without therapy. Many of the tumors detected by screening at 6 months of age have favorable biological features and could be cured easily with relatively mild therapy. A few patients with unfavorable biological features have presented clinically during the first 6 to 12 months of age in the screened population, and some have had an unfavorable outcome. It remains to be determined if screening at a later time will permit early detection of tumors with intermediate or unfavorable biological features and thereby improve their prognosis.

FUTURE CONSIDERATIONS

In addition to the improvements and prospects for future therapy discussed herein, there are a variety of areas in which improvement in the management of patients with neuroblastoma may come, including: (a) the identification of individuals with a genetic predisposition to develop this disease; (b) general population screening approaches for early detection and treatment; (c) additional markers besides urinary catecholamine metabolites to follow tumor response to treatment; and (d) better biological characterization of tumors for classification and prognostication.

As improvements occur in the long-term outcome of patients with neuroblastoma, it becomes increasingly important to identify individuals who are predisposed to develop this tumor. Not only will this be useful for the siblings of neuroblastoma patients, but it will also provide useful information for genetic counseling of patients and their offspring. No predisposition locus has been identified as yet, although several loci have been excluded recently, including 1p36.[29] Thus, it appears that the familial neuroblastoma predisposition gene resides elsewhere, although there is the formal possibility that more than one predisposition locus exists. In any case, a genome-wide search is underway to identify the familial neuroblastoma predisposition gene.

The urinary VMA/HVA screening programs in Japan, North America, and Europe initially were very promising, leading to cautious optimism. However, characterization of the tumors identified by screening indicates that the majority of these tumors have favorable biological features, more like those seen in infants with lower stages of disease. Indeed, the screening may just be increasing the prevalence of neuroblastoma by detection of tumors that might regress spontaneously, without lowering the prevalence of more advanced stages of disease in patients over 1 year of age. Indeed, despite this "overdetection," there has been no decrease in the prevalence of neuroblastoma in older patients. Thus, it is not clear if mass screening at an older age will lead to detection of genetically unfavorable, aggressive tumors, or if this early detection will ultimately improve their outcome.

Following the levels of catecholamine metabolites in the urine of patients with neuroblastoma does not appear to be as sensitive as α-fetoprotein or β-human chorionic gonadotropin for following germ-cell tumors. Additional markers have been proposed, including serum ferritin, NSE, G_{D2}, chromogranin A, and others, but none has yet emerged as superior. As more is understood about the biology of neuroblastomas, additional candidates might emerge that could be used to follow response to treatment and to predict early relapse. Such markers might obviate the need for multiple diagnostic imaging studies and marrow sampling in patients in remission.

The biological characterization of neuroblastomas by such features as DNA index, *MYCN* amplification, 1p LOH, *TrkA* expression, and others, has provided powerful prognostic variables. It remains to be determined which will emerge as the most clinically useful prognostic variable when subjected to multivariate analysis. It is possible that these biological features will become more important than clinical distinctions such as age, stage, primary site, and tumor histology. The mandate for the future is to translate promising biological studies into clinical applications, and to continue to look for new insights into mechanisms of neuroblastoma transformation and progression that can be used to clinical advantage.

ACKNOWLEDGMENTS

Some of this material has been published previously.[1-6]

REFERENCES

1. Brodeur GM: Neuroblastoma and other peripheral neuroectodermal tumors, in Fernbach DJ, Vietti TJ (eds): *Clinical Pediatric Oncology*. St. Louis, Mosby–Year Book, 1991, p. 337.
2. Brodeur GM, Castleberry RP: Neuroblastoma, in Pizzo PA, Poplack DG (eds): *Principles and Practice of Pediatric Oncology*. Philadelphia, JB Lippincott, 1997, p. 761.
3. Brodeur GM, Nakagawara A: Molecular basis of clinical heterogeneity in neuroblastoma. *Am J Pediatr Hematol Oncol* **14**:111, 1992.
4. Brodeur GM: Molecular basis for heterogeneity in human neuroblastomas. *Eur J Cancer* **31A**:505, 1995.
5. Brodeur GM, Maris JM, Yamashiro DJ, Hogarty MD, White PS: Biology and genetics of human neuroblastomas. *J Pediatr Hematol Oncol* **19**:93, 1997.
6. Brodeur GM: Clinical and biological aspects of neuroblastomas, in Scriver CR, Beaudet AL, Sly WS, Valle D, Stanbury JB, Wyngaarden JB, Fredrickson DS, Vogelstein B (eds): *The Molecular and Metabolic Basis of Inherited Disease*. New York, McGraw-Hill, 1997, p. 691.
7. Miller RW, Young JLJ, Novakovic B: Childhood cancer. *Cancer* **75**:395, 1995.
8. Voute PA: Neuroblastoma, in Sutow WW, Fernbach DJ, Vietti TJ (eds): *Clinical Pediatric Oncology*. St. Louis, CV Mosby, 1984, p. 559.
9. Sawada T, Sugimoto T, Tanaka T, Kawakatsu H, Ishii T, Matsumura T, Horii Y: Number and cure rate of neuroblastoma cases detected by the mass screening program in Japan: Future aspects. *Med Pediatr Oncol* **15**:14, 1987.
10. Beckwith J, Perrin E: In situ neuroblastomas: A contribution to the natural history of neural crest tumors. *Am J Pathol* **43**:1089, 1963.
11. Turkel SB, Itabashi HH: The natural history of neuroblastic cells in the fetal adrenal gland. *Am J Pathol* **76**:225, 1975.
12. Ikeda Y, Lister J, Bouton JM, Buyukpamukcu M: Congenital neuroblastoma, neuroblastoma in situ, and the normal fetal development of the adrenal. *J Pediatr Surg* **16**:636, 1981.
13. Haas D, Ablin AR, Miller C, Zoger S, Matthay KK: Complete pathologic maturation and regression of stage IVS neuroblastoma without treatment. *Cancer* **62**:818, 1988.
14. Evans AE, Baum E, Chard R: Do infants with stage IV-S neuroblastoma need treatment? *Arch Dis Child* **56**:271, 1981.
15. McWilliams NB: Stage IV-S neuroblastoma: Treatment controversy revisited. *Med Pediatr Oncol* **14**:41, 1986.
16. Carlsen NLT: How frequent is spontaneous remission of neuroblastomas? Implications for screening. *Br J Cancer* **61**:441, 1990.
17. Allen RW, Ogden B, Bentley FL, Jung AL: Fetal hydantoin syndrome, neuroblastoma, and hemorrhagic disease in a neonate. *JAMA* **244**:1464, 1980.
18. Kinney H, Faix R, Brazy J: The fetal alcohol syndrome and neuroblastoma. *Pediatrics* **66**:130, 1980.
19. Seeler RA, Israel JN, Royal JE, Kaye CI, Rao S, Abulaban M: Ganglioneuroblastoma and fetal hydantoin-alcohol syndromes. *Pediatrics* **63**:524, 1979.
20. Spitz MR, Johnson CC: Neuroblastoma and paternal occupation. A case-control analysis. *Am J Epidemiol* **121**:924, 1985.
21. Wilkins JRI, Hundley VD: Paternal occupational exposure to electromagnetic fields and neuroblastoma in offspring. *Am J Epidemiol* **131**:995, 1990.
22. Bunin GR, Ward E, Kramer S, Rhee CA, Meadows AT: Neuroblastoma and parental occupation. *Am J Epidemiol* **131**:776, 1990.
23. Kramer S, Ward E, Meadows AT, Malone KE: Medical and drug risk factors associated with neuroblastoma: A case-control study. *J Natl Cancer Inst* **78**:797, 1987.
24. Knudson AGJ, Strong LC: Mutation and cancer: Neuroblastoma and pheochromocytoma. *Am J Hum Genet* **24**:514, 1972.
25. Knudson AG: Mutation and cancer: Statistical study of retinoblastoma. *Proc Natl Acad Sci U S A* **68**:8820, 1971.
26. Knudson AGJ, Meadows AT: Developmental genetics of neuroblastoma. *J Natl Cancer Inst* **57**:675, 1976.
27. Kushner BH, Gilbert F, Helson L: Familial neuroblastoma: Case reports, literature review, and etiologic considerations. *Cancer* **57**:1887, 1986.
28. Kushner BH, Helson L: Monozygotic siblings discordant for neuroblastoma: Etiologic implications. *J Pediatr* **107**:405, 1985.
29. Maris JM, Kyemba SM, Rebbeck TR, White PS, Sulman EP, Jensen SJ, Allen C, Biegel JA, Yanofsky RA, Feldman GL, Brodeur GM: Familial predisposition to neuroblastoma does not map to chromosome band 1p36. *Cancer Res* **56**:3421, 1996.
30. Maris JM, Chatten J, Meadows AT, Biegel J, Brodeur GM: Familial neuroblastoma: New affected members and a further association with Hirschsprung disease. *Med Pediatr Oncol* **28**:1, 1997.
31. Pegelow CH, Ebbin AJ, Powars D, Towner JW: Familial neuroblastoma. *J Pediatr* **87**:763, 1975.
32. Hecht F, Kaiser-McCaw B: Chromosomes in familial neuroblastoma [letter]. *J Pediatr* **98**:334, 1981.
33. Hecht F, Hecht BK, Northrup JC, Trachtenberg N, Wood ST, Cohen JT: Genetics of familial neuroblastoma: Long-range studies. *Cancer Genet Cytogenet* **7**:227, 1982.
34. Moorhead PS, Evans AE: Chromosomal findings in patients with neuroblastoma. *Prog Cancer Res Ther* **12**:109, 1980.
35. Nagano H, Kano Y, Kobuchi S, Kajitani T: A case of partial 2p trisomy with neuroblastoma. *Jpn J Hum Genet* **25**:39, 1980.
36. Sanger WG, Howe J, Fordyce R, Purtilo DT: Inherited partial trisomy #15 complicated by neuroblastoma. *Cancer Genet Cytogenet* **11**:153, 1984.

37. Robinson MG, McCorquodale MM: Trisomy 18 and neurogenic neoplasia. *J Pediatr* **99**:428, 1981.
38. Rudolph B, Harbott J, Lampert F: Fragile sites and neuroblastoma: Fragile site at 1p13.1 and other points on lymphocyte chromosomes from patients and family members. *Cancer Genet Cytogenet* **31**:83, 1988.
39. Lampert F, Rudolph B, Christiansen H, Franke F: Identical chromosome 1p breakpoint abnormality in both the tumor and the constitutional karyotype of a patient with neuroblastoma. *Cancer Genet Cytogenet* **34**:235, 1988.
40. Laureys G, Speleman F, Opdenakker G, Leroy J: Constitutional translocation t(1;17)(p36;q12-21) in a patient with neuroblastoma. *Genes Chromosomes Cancer* **2**:252, 1990.
41. Laureys G, Speleman F, Versteeg R, van der Drift P, Chan A, Leroy J, Francke U, Opdenakker G, van Roy N: Constitutional translocation t(1;17)(p36.31-p36.13;q11.2-q12.1) in a neuroblastoma patient. Establishment of somatic cell hybrids and identification of PND?A12M2 on chromosome 1 and NF1/SCYA7 on chromosome 17 as breakpoint flanking single copy markers. *Oncogene* **10**:1087, 1995.
42. Michalski AJ, Cotter FE, Cowell JK: Isolation of chromosome-specific DNA sequences from an Alu polymerase chain reaction library to define the breakpoint in a patient with a constitutional translocation t(1;13)(q22;q12) and ganglioneuroblastoma. *Oncogene* **7**:1595, 1992.
43. Bown NP, Pearson ADJ, Reid MM: High incidence of constitutional balanced translocations in neuroblastoma. *Cancer Genet Cytogenet* **69**:166, 1993.
44. Biegel JA, White PS, Marshall HN, Fujimori M, Zackai EH, Scher CD, Brodeur GM, Emanuel BS: Constitutional 1p36 deletion in a child with neuroblastoma. *Am J Hum Genet* **52**:176, 1993.
45. Mead RS, Cowell JK: Molecular characterization of a (1;10)(p22;q21) constitutional translocation from a patient with neuroblastoma. *Cancer Genet Cytogenet* **81**:151, 1995.
46. Roberts T, Chernova O, Cowell JK: Molecular characterization of the 1p22 breakpoint region spanning the constitutional translocation breakpoint in a neuroblastoma patient with a t(1;10)(p22;q21). *Cancer Genet Cytogenet* **100**:10, 1998.
47. White PS, Thompson PM, Jensen SJ, Sulman EP, Sulman EP, Guo C, Maris JM, Hogarty MD, Allen C, Biegel JA, Matise TC, Gregory SG, Reynolds CP, Brodeur GM: Detailed molecular analysis of 1p36 in neuroblastoma. *Eur J Cancer* (in press), 2000.
48. Knudson AGJ, Amromin GD: Neuroblastoma and ganglioneuroma in a child with multiple neurofibromatosis. Implications for the mutational origin of neuroblastoma. *Cancer* **19**:1032, 1966.
49. Bolande R, Towler WF: A possible relationship of neuroblastoma to von Recklinghausen's disease. *Cancer* **26**:162, 1970.
50. Bolande RP: The neurocristopathies: A unifying concept of disease arising in neural crest maldevelopment. *Hum Pathol* **5**:409, 1974.
51. Kushner BH, Hajdu SI, Helson L: Synchronous neuroblastoma and von Recklinghausen's disease: A review of the literature. *J Clin Oncol* **3**:117, 1985.
52. Miller RW, Fraumeni JFJ: Neuroblastoma: Epidemiologic approach to its origin. *Am J Dis Child* **115**:253, 1968.
53. Sy WM, Edmonson JH: The developmental defects associated with neuroblastoma—Etiologic implications. *Cancer* **22**:234, 1968.
54. Nakissa N, Constine LS, Rubin P, Strohl R: Birth defects in three common pediatric malignancies: Wilms' tumor, neuroblastoma and Ewing's sarcoma. *Oncology* **42**:358, 1985.
55. Blatt J, Olshan AF, Lee PA, Ross JL: Neuroblastoma and related tumors in Turner's syndrome. *J Pediatr* **131**:666, 1997.
56. Maris JM, Brodeur GM: Are certain children more likely to develop neuroblastoma? *J Pediatr* **131**:656, 1997.
57. Satge D, Sasco AJ, Carlsen NL, Stiller CA, Rubie H, Hero B, de Bernardi B, de Kraker J, Coze C, Kogner P, Langmark F, Hakvoort-Cammel FG, Beck D, von der Weid N, Parkes S, Hartmann O, Lippens RJ, Kamps WA, Sommelet D: A lack of neuroblastoma in Down syndrome: A study from 11 European countries. *Cancer Res* **58**:448, 1998.
58. Biedler JL, Ross RA, Shanske S, Spengler BA: Human neuroblastoma cytogenetics: Search for significance of homogeneously staining regions and double minute chromosomes. *Prog Cancer Res Ther* **12**:81, 1980.
59. Brodeur GM, Green AA, Hayes FA, Williams KJ, Williams DL, Tsiatis AA: Cytogenetic features of human neuroblastomas and cell lines. *Cancer Res* **41**:4678, 1981.
60. Brodeur GM, Seeger RC, Sather H, Dalton A, Siegel SE, Wong KY, Hammond D: Clinical implications of oncogene activation in human neuroblastomas. *Cancer* **58**:541, 1986.

61. Brodeur GM, Fong CT: Molecular biology and genetics of human neuroblastoma. *Cancer Genet Cytogenet* **41**:153, 1989.
62. Schwab M, Alitalo K, Klempnauer KH, Varmus HE, Bishop JM, Gilbert F, Brodeur G, Goldstein M, Trent JM: Amplified DNA with limited homology to myc cellular oncogene is shared by human neuroblastoma cell lines and a neuroblastoma tumour. *Nature* **305**:245, 1983.
63. Kohl NE, Kanda N, Schreck RR, Bruns G, Latt SA, Gilbert F, Alt FW: Transposition and amplification of oncogene-related sequences in human neuroblastomas. *Cell* **35**:359, 1983.
64. Schwab M, Ellison J, Busch M, Rosenau W, Varmus HE, Bishop JM: Enhanced expression of the human gene N-myc consequent to amplification of DNA may contribute to malignant progression of neuroblastoma. *Proc Natl Acad Sci U S A* **81**:4940, 1984.
65. Brodeur GM, Seeger RC: Gene amplification in human neuroblastomas: Basic mechanisms and clinical implications. *Cancer Genet Cytogenet* **19**:101, 1986.
66. Hogarty MH, Brodeur GM: Oncogene amplification, in Vogelstein B, Kinzler K (eds): *Genetic Basis of Human Cancer.* New York, McGraw Hill, 1998, p. 161–172
67. Brodeur GM, Seeger RC, Schwab M, Varmus HE, Bishop JM: Amplification of N-myc in untreated human neuroblastomas correlates with advanced disease stage. *Science* **224**:1121, 1984.
68. Brodeur GM: Neuroblastoma—Clinical applications of molecular parameters. *Brain Pathol* **1**:47, 1990.
69. Seeger RC, Brodeur GM, Sather H, Dalton A, Siegel SE, Wong KY, Hammond D: Association of multiple copies of the N-myc oncogene with rapid progression of neuroblastomas. *N Engl J Med* **313**:1111, 1985.
70. Seeger RC, Wada R, Brodeur GM, Moss TJ, Bjork RL, Sousa L, Slamon DJ: Expression of N-myc by neuroblastomas with one or multiple copies of the oncogene. *Prog Clin Biol Res* **271**:41, 1988.
71. Brodeur GM, Fong CT, Morita M, Griffith RC, Hayes FA, Seeger RC: Molecular analysis and clinical significance of N-myc amplification and chromosome 1 abnormalities in human neuroblastomas. *Prog Clin Biol Res* **271**:3, 1988.
72. Wasson JC, Brodeur GM: Molecular analysis of gene amplification in tumors, in Dracopoli NC, Haines JL, Korf BR, Moir DT, Morton CC, Seidman CE, Seidman JG, Smith DR (eds): *Current Protocols in Human Genetics.* New York, Greene Publishing and John Wiley & Sons, 1994, p. 10.5.1.
73. Brodeur GM, Hayes FA, Green AA, Casper JT, Wasson J, Wallach S, Seeger RC: Consistent N-myc copy number in simultaneous or consecutive neuroblastoma samples from sixty individual patients. *Cancer Res* **47**:4248, 1987.
74. Fong CT, Dracopoli NC, White PS, Merrill PT, Griffith RC, Housman DE, Brodeur GM: Loss of heterozygosity for the short arm of chromosome 1 in human neuroblastomas: Correlation with N-myc amplification. *Proc Natl Acad Sci U S A* **86**:3753, 1989.
75. Fong CT, White PS, Peterson K, Sapienza C, Cavenee WK, Kern S, Vogelstein B, Cantor AB, Look AT, Brodeur GM: Loss of heterozygosity for chromosome 1 or 14 defines subsets of advanced neuroblastomas. *Cancer Res* **52**:1780, 1992.
76. White PS, Maris JM, Beltinger C, Sulman E, Marshall HN, Fujimori M, Kaufman BA, Biegel JA, Allen C, Hilliard C, Valentine MB, Look AT, Enomoto H, Sakiyama S, Brodeur GM: A region of consistent deletion in neuroblastoma maps within 1p36.2-.3. *Proc Natl Acad Sci U S A* **92**:5520, 1995.
77. Caron H: Allelic loss of chromosome 1 and additional chromosome 17 material are both unfavourable prognostic markers in neuroblastoma. *Med Pediatr Oncol* **24**:215, 1995.
78. Maris JM, White PS, Beltinger CP, Sulman EP, Castleberry RP, Shuster JJ, Look AT, Brodeur GM: Significance of chromosome 1p loss of heterozygosity in neuroblastoma. *Cancer Res* **55**:4664, 1995.
79. Gehring M, Berthold F, Edler L, Schwab M, Amler LC: The 1p deletion is not a reliable marker for the prognosis of patients with neuroblastoma. *Cancer Res* **55**:5366, 1995.
80. Martinsson T, Shoberg P-M, Hedborg F, Kogner P: Deletion of chromosome 1p loci and microsatellite instability in neuroblastomas analyzed with short-tandem repeat polymorphisms. *Cancer Res* **55**:5681, 1995.
81. Caron H, van Sluis P, de Kraker J, Bokkerink J, Egeler M, Laureys G, Slater R, Westerveld A, Voute PA, Versteeg R: Allelic loss of chromosome 1p as a predictor of unfavorable outcome in patients with neuroblastoma. *N Engl J Med* **334**:225, 1996.
82. Nisen PD, Waber PG, Rich MA, Pierce S, Garvin JRJ, Gilbert F, Lanzkowsky P: N-myc oncogene RNA expression in neuroblastoma. *J Natl Cancer Inst* **80**:1633, 1988.

83. Slavc I, Ellenbogen R, Jung W-H, Vawter GF, Kretschmar C, Grier H, Korf BR: myc gene amplification and expression in primary human neuroblastoma. *Cancer Res* 50:1459, 1990.

84. Chan HSL, Gallie BL, DeBoer G, Haddad G, Ikegaki N, Dimitroulakos J, Yeger H, Ling V: MYCN protein expression as a predictor of neuroblastoma prognosis. *Clin Cancer Res* 3:1699, 1997.

85. Bordow SB, Norris MD, Haber PS, Marshall GM, Haber M: Prognostic significance of MYCN oncogene expression in childhood neuroblastoma. *J Clin Oncol* 16:3286, 1998.

86. Nakagawara A, Arima M, Azar CG, Scavarda NJ, Brodeur GM: Inverse relationship between trk expression and N-myc amplification in human neuroblastomas. *Cancer Res* 52:1364, 1992.

87. Cohn SL, Salwen H, Quasney MW, Ikegaki N, Cowan JM, Herst CV, Kennett RH, Rosen ST, DiGiuseppe JA, Brodeur GM: Prolonged N-myc protein half-life in a neuroblastoma cell line lacking N-myc amplification. *Oncogene* 5:1821, 1990.

88. Squire JA, Thorner PS, Weitzman S, Maggi JD, Dirks P, Doyle J, Hale M, Godbout R: Co-amplification of *MYCN* and a DEAD box gene (*DDX1*) in primary neuroblastoma. *Oncogene* 10:1417, 1995.

89. Manohar CF, Salwen HR, Brodeur GM, Cohn SL: Co-amplification and concomitant high levels of expression of a DEAD box gene with MYCN in human neuroblastoma. *Genes Chromosomes Cancer* 14:196, 1995.

90. George RE, Kenyon RM, McGuckin AG, Malcolm AJ, Pearson ADJ, Lunec J: Investigation of the coamplification of the candidate genes ornithine decarboxylase, ribonucleotide reductase, syndecan-1 and a DEAD box gene, DDX1, with N-myc in neuroblastoma. *Oncogene* 12:1583, 1996.

91. Amler LC, Shurmann J, Schwab M: The DDX1 gene maps within 400 kbp 5' to MYCN and is frequently coamplified in human neuroblastoma. *Genes Chromosomes Cancer* 15:134, 1996.

92. Shiloh Y, Shipley J, Brodeur GM, Bruns G, Korf B, Donlon T, Schreck RR, Seeger R, Sakai K, Latt SA: Differential amplification, assembly and relocation of multiple DNA sequences in human neuroblastomas and neuroblastoma cell lines. *Proc Natl Acad Sci U S A* 82:3761, 1985.

93. Corvi R, Savelyeva L, Amler L, Handgetinger R, Schwab M: Cytogenetic evolution of MYCN and MDM2 amplification in the neuroblastoma LS tumor and its cell line. *Eur J Cancer* 31A:520, 1995.

94. Corvi R, Savelyeva L, Breit S, Wenzel A, Handgretinger R, Barak J, Oren M, Amler L, Schwab M: Non-syntenic amplification of MDM2 and MYCN in human neuroblastoma. *Oncogene* 10:1081, 1995.

95. Van Roy N, Forus A, Myklebost O, Cheng NC, Versteeg R, Speleman F: Identification of two distinct chromosome 12-derived amplification units in neuroblastoma cell line NGP. *Cancer Genet Cytogenet* 82:151, 1995.

96. Jinbo T, Iwamura Y, Kaneko M, Sawaguchi S: Coamplification of the L-myc and N-myc oncogenes in a neuroblastoma cell line. *Jpn J Cancer Res* 80:299, 1989.

97. Meddeb M, Danglot G, Chudoba I, Venuat AM, Benard J, Avet-Loiseau H, Vasseur B, Le Paslier D, Terrier-Lacombe MJ, Hartmann O, Bernheim A: Additional copies of a 25 Mb chromosomal region originating from 17q23.1-17qter are present in 90% of high-grade neuroblastomas. *Genes Chromosomes Cancer* 17:156, 1996.

98. Brinkschmidt C, Christiansen H, Terpe HJ, Simon R, Boecker W, Lambert F, Stoerkel S: Comparative genomic hybridization (CGH) analysis of neuroblastomas — An important methodological approach in paediatric tumour pathology. *J Pathol* 181:394, 1997.

99. Plantaz D, Mohapatra G, Matthay KK, Pellarin M, Seeger RC, Feuerstein BG: Gain of chromosome 17 is the most frequent abnormality detected in neuroblastoma by comparative genomic hybridization. *Am J Pathol* 150:81, 1997.

100. Vandesompele J, Van Roy N, Van Gele M, Laureys G, Ambros P, Heimann P, Devalck C, Schuuring E, Brock P, Otten J, Gyselinck J, De Paepe A, Speleman F: Genetic heterogeneity of neuroblastoma studied by comparative genomic hybridization. *Genes Chromosomes Cancer* 23:141, 1998.

101. Lastowska M, Nacheva E, McGuckin A, Curtis A, Grace C, Pearson A, Bown N: Comparative genomic hybridization study of primary neuroblastoma tumors. United Kingdom Children's Cancer Study Group. *Genes Chromosomes Cancer* 18:162, 1997.

102. Altura RA, Maris JM, Li H, Boyett JM, Brodeur GM, Look AT: Novel regions of chromosomal loss in familial neuroblastoma by comparative genomic hybridization. *Genes Chromosomes Cancer* 19:176, 1997.

103. Gilbert F, Feder M, Balaban G, Brangman D, Lurie DK, Podolsky R, Rinaldt V, Vinikoor N, Weisband J: Human neuroblastomas and abnormalities of chromosome 1 and 17. *Cancer Res* 44:5444, 1984.

104. Takita J, Hayashi Y, Kohno T, Shiseki M, Yamaguchi N, Hanada R, Yamamoto K, Yokota J: Allelotype of neuroblastoma. *Oncogene* 11:1829, 1995.

105. Van Roy N, Laureys G, Cheng NC, Willem P, Opdenakker G, Versteeg R, Speleman F: 1;17 translocations and other chromosome 17 rearrangements in human primary neuroblastoma tumors and cell lines. *Genes Chromosomes Cancer* 10:103, 1994.

106. Savelyeva L, Corvi R, Schwab M: Translocation involving 1p and 17q is a recurrent genetic alteration of human neuroblastoma cells. *Am J Hum Genet* 55:334, 1994.

107. Caron H, van Sluis P, van Roy N, de Kraker J, Speleman F, Voute PA, Westerveld A, Slater R, Versteeg R: Recurrent 1;17 translocations in human neuroblastoma reveal nonhomologous mitotic recombination during the S/G2 phase as a novel mechanism for loss of heterozygosity. *Am J Hum Genet* 55:341, 1994.

108. Lastowska M, Van Roy N, Bown N, Speleman F, Lunec J, Strachan T, Pearson ADJ, Jackson MS: Molecular cytogenetic delineation of 17q translocation breakpoints in neuroblastoma cell lines. *Genes Chromosomes Cancer* 23:116, 1998.

109. Hayashi Y, Hanada R, Yamamoto K, Bessho F: Chromosome findings and prognosis in neuroblastoma. *Cancer Genet Cytogenet* 29:175, 1986.

110. Kaneko Y, Kanda N, Maseki N, Sakurai M, Tsuchida Y, Takeda T, Okabe I, Sakurai M: Different karyotypic patterns in early and advanced stage neuroblastomas. *Cancer Res* 47:311, 1987.

111. Christiansen H, Lampert F: Tumour karyotype discriminates between good and bad prognostic outcome in neuroblastoma. *Br J Cancer* 57:121, 1988.

112. Look AT, Hayes FA, Nitschke R, McWilliams NB, Green AA: Cellular DNA content as a predictor of response to chemotherapy in infants with unresectable neuroblastoma. *N Engl J Med* 311:231, 1984.

113. Look AT, Hayes FA, Shuster JJ, Douglass EC, Castleberry RP, Brodeur GM: Clinical relevance of tumor cell ploidy and N-myc gene amplification in childhood neuroblastoma. A Pediatric Oncology Group Study. *J Clin Oncol* 9:581, 1991.

114. Oppedal BR, Storm-Mathisen I, Lie SO, Brandtzaeg P: Prognostic factors in neuroblastoma. Clinical, histopathologic, immunohisto-chemical features, and DNA ploidy in relation to prognosis. *Cancer* 72:772, 1988.

115. Taylor SR, Blatt J, Constantino JP, Roederer M, Murphy RF: Flow cytometric DNA analysis of neuroblastoma and ganglioneuroma. A 10-year retrospective study. *Cancer* 62:749, 1988.

116. Brodeur GM, Sekhon GS, Goldstein MN: Chromosomal aberrations in human neuroblastomas. *Cancer* 40:2256, 1977.

117. Hayashi Y, Kanda N, Inaba T, Hanada R, Nagahara N, Muchi H, Yamamoto K: Cytogenetic findings and prognosis in neuroblastoma with emphasis on marker chromosome 1. *Cancer* 63:126, 1989.

118. Weith A, Martinsson T, Cziepluch C, Bruderlein S, Amler LC, Berthold F: Neuroblastoma consensus deletion maps to 1p36.1-2. *Genes Chromosomes Cancer* 1:159, 1989.

119. Takeda O, Homma C, Maseki N, Sakurai M, Kanda N, Schwab M, Nakamura Y, Kaneko Y: There may be two tumor suppressor genes on chromosome arm 1p closely associated with biologically distinct subtypes of neuroblastoma. *Genes Chromosomes Cancer* 10:30, 1994.

120. Schleiermacher G, Peter M, Michon J, Hugot J-P, Viehl P, Zucker J-M, Magdelénat H, Thomas G, Delattre O: Two distinct deleted regions on the short arm of chromosome 1 in neuroblastoma. *Genes Chromosomes Cancer* 10:275, 1994.

121. Caron H, Peter M, van Sluis P, Speleman F, de Kraker J, Laureys G, Michon J, Brugieres L, Voute PA, Westerveld A, Slater R, Delattre O, Versteeg R: Evidence for two tumour suppressor loci on chromosomal bands 1p35-36 involved in neuroblastoma: One probably imprinted, another associated with N-myc amplification. *Hum Mol Genet* 4:535, 1995.

122. Cheng NC, Van Roy N, Chan A, Beitsma M, Westerveld A, Speleman F, Versteeg R: Deletion mapping in neuroblastoma cell lines suggests two distinct tumor suppressor genes in the 1p35-35 region, only one of which is associated with N-myc amplification. *Oncogene* 10:291, 1995.

123. Caron H, van Sluis P, van Hoeve M, de Kraker J, Bras J, Slater R, Mannens M, Voute PA, Westerveld A, Versteeg R: Allelic loss of chromosome 1p36 in neuroblastoma is of preferential maternal origin and correlates with N-myc amplification. *Nat Genet* 4:187, 1993.

124. Cheng JM, Hiemstra JL, Schneider SS, Naumova A, Cheung N-KV, Cohn SL, Diller L, Sapienza C, Brodeur GM: Preferential amplification of the paternal allele of the N-myc gene in human neuroblastomas. *Nat Genet* 4:191, 1993.

125. Beltinger CP, White PS, Maris JM, Sulman EP, Jensen SJ, LePaslier D, Stallard BJ, Goeddel DV, deSauvage FJ, Brodeur GM: Physical mapping and genomic structure of the human TNFR2 gene. *Genomics* **35**:94, 1996.

126. Maris JM, Jensen SJ, Sulman EP, Beltinger CP, Gates K, Allen C, Biegel JA, Brodeur GM, White PS: Cloning, chromosomal localization, and physical mapping and genomic characterization of HKR3. *Genomics* **35**:289, 1996.

127. Lahti JM, Valentine M, Xiang J, Jones B, Amann J, Grenet J, Richmond G, Look AT, Kidd VJ: Alterations in the PITSLRE protein kinase gene complex on chromosome 1p36 in childhood neuroblastoma. *Nat Genet* **7**:370, 1994.

128. Enomoto H, Ozaki T, Takahashi E-i, Nomura N, Tabata S, Takahashi H, Ohnuma N, Tanabe M, Iwai J, Yoshida H, Matsunaga T, Sakiyama S: Identification of human *DAN* gene, mapping to the putative neuroblastoma tumor suppressor locus. *Oncogene* **9**:2785, 1994.

129. Kaghad M, Bonnet H, Yang A, Creancier L, Biscan J, Valent A, Minty A, Chalon P, Lelias J, Dumont X, Ferrara P, McKeon F, Caput D: Monoallelically expressed gene related to p53 at 1p36, a region frequently deleted in neuroblastoma and other human cancers. *Cell* **90**:809, 1997.

130. Ichimiya S, Nimura Y, Sunahara M, Shishikura T, Kageyama H, Nakamura Y, Sakiyama S, Seki N, Ohira M, Kaneko Y, McKeon F, Caput D, Nakagawara A: Genetic analysis of p73 localized at chromosome 1p36.3 in primary neuroblastomas. *Eur J Cancer* (in press), 2000.

131. Srivatsan ES, Ying KL, Seeger RC: Deletion of chromosome 11 and of 14q sequences in neuroblastoma. *Genes Chromosomes Cancer* **7**:32, 1993.

132. Maris JM, Guo C, White PS, Hogarty MD, Thompson PM, Stram DO, Matthay K, K., Seeger RS, Brodeur GM: Chromosome 11q22 allelic deletion is common in neuroblastomas. *Eur J Cancer* (in press), 2000.

133. Suzuki T, Yokota J, Mugishima H, Okabe I, Ookuni M, Sugimura T, Terada M: Frequent loss of heterozygosity on chromosome 14q in neuroblastoma. *Cancer Res* **49**:1095, 1989.

134. Takayama H, Suzuki T, Mugishima H, Fujisawa T, Ookuni M, Schwab M, Gehring M, Nakamura Y, Sugimura T, Terada M, Yokota J: Deletion mapping of chromosomes 14q and 1p in human neuroblastoma. *Oncogene* **7**:1185, 1992.

135. Thompson PM, Kyemba SK, Jensen SJ, Guo C, Maris JM, Brodeur GM, Stram DO, Matthay KK, Seeger RC, White PS: Loss of heterozygosity (LOH) for chromosome 14q in neuroblastoma. *Eur J Cancer* (in press), 2000.

136. Imamura J, Bartram CR, Berthold F, Harms D, Nakamura H, Koeffler HP: Mutation of the p53 gene in neuroblastoma and its relationship with N-myc amplification. *Cancer Res* **53**:4053, 1993.

137. Vogan K, Bernstein M, Brisson L, Leclerc J-M, Brossard J, Brodeur GM, Pelletier J, Gros P: Absence of p53 gene mutations in primary neuroblastomas. *Cancer Res* **53**:5269, 1993.

138. Komuro H, Hayashi Y, Kawamura M, Hayashi K, Kaneko Y, Kamoshita S, Hanada R, Yamamoto K, Hongo T, Yamada M, Tsuchida Y: Mutations of the p53 gene are involved in Ewing's sarcomas but not in neuroblastomas. *Cancer Res* **53**:5284, 1993.

139. Hosoi G, Hara J, Okamura T, Osugi Y, Ishihara S, Fukuzawa M, Okada A, Okada S, Tawa A: Low frequency of the p53 gene mutations in neuroblastoma. *Cancer* **73**:3087, 1994.

140. Castresana JS, Bello MJ, Rey JA, Nebreda P, Queizan A, Garcia-Miguel P, Pestana A: No TP53 mutations in neuroblastomas detected by PCR-SSCP analysis. *Genes Chromosomes Cancer* **10**:136, 1994.

141. Moll UM, LaQuaglia M, Benard J, Riou G: Wild-type p53 protein undergoes cytoplasmic sequestration in undifferentiated neuroblastomas but not in differentiated tumors. *Proc Ntnl Acad Sci U S A* **92**:4407, 1995.

142. Moll UM, Ostermeyer AG, Haladay R, Winkfield B, Frazier M, Zambetti G: Cytoplasmic sequestration of wild-type p53 protein impairs the G1 checkpoint after DNA damage. *Mol Cell Biol* **16**:1126, 1996.

143. Goldman SC, Chen CY, Lansing TJ, Gilmer TM, Kastan MB: The p53 signal transduction pathway is intact in human neuroblastoma despite cytoplasmic localization. *Am J Pathol* **148**:1381, 1996.

144. Beltinger CP, White PS, Sulman EP, Maris JM, Brodeur GM: No CDKN2 mutations in neuroblastomas. *Cancer Res* **55**:2053, 1995.

145. Kawamata N, Seriu T, Koeffler HP, Bartram CR: Molecular analysis of the cyclin-dependent kinase inhibitor family: p16(CDKN2/MTS1/INK4A), p18 (INK4C) and p27 (Kip1) genes in neuroblastomas. *Cancer* **77**:570, 1996.

146. Iolascon A, Giordani L, Moretti A, Tonini GP, Lo Cunsolo C, Mastropietro S, Borriello A, Ragione FD: Structural and functional analysis of cyclin-dependent kinase inhibitor genes (CDKN2A, CDKN2B, and CDKN2C) in neuroblastoma. *Pediatr Res* **43**:139, 1998.

147. Takita J, Hayashi Y, Kohno T, Yamaguchi N, Hanada R, Yamamoto K, Yokota J: Deletion map of chromosome 9 and p16 (CDKN2A) gene alterations in neuroblastoma. *Cancer Res* **57**:907, 1997.

148. The I, Murthy AE, Hannigan GE, Jacoby LB, Menon AG, Gusella JF, Bernards A: Neurofibromatosis type 1 gene mutations in neuroblastoma. *Nat Genet* **3**:62, 1993.

149. Johnson MR, Look AT, DeClue JE, Valentine MB, Lowy DR: Inactivation of the NF1 gene in human melanoma and neuroblastoma cell lines without impaired regulation of GTP-ras. *Proc Ntnl Acad Sci U S A* **90**:5539, 1993.

150. Hempstead BL, Martin-Zanca D, Kaplan DR, Parada LF, Chao MV: High-affinity NGF binding requires coexpression of the trk proto-oncogene and the low-affinity NGF receptor. *Nature* **350**:678, 1991.

151. Kaplan DR, Martin-Zanca D, Parada LF: Tyrosine phosphorylation and tyrosine kinase activity of the trk proto-oncogene product induced by NGF. *Nature* **350**:158, 1991.

152. Kaplan DR, Hempstead BL, Martin-Zanca D, Chao MV, Parada LF: The trk proto-oncogene product: A signal transducing receptor for nerve growth factor. *Science* **252**:554, 1991.

153. Klein R, Jing S, Nanduri V, O'Rourke E, Barbacid M: The trk proto-oncogene encodes a receptor for nerve growth factor. *Cell* **65**:189, 1991.

154. Klein R, Nanduri V, Jing S, Lamballe F, Tapley P, Bryant S, Cordon-Cardo C, Jones KR, Reichardt LF, Barbacid M: The trkB tyrosine protein kinase is a receptor for brain-derived neurotrophic factor and neurotrophin-3. *Cell* **66**:395, 1991.

155. Lamballe F, Klein R, Barbacid M: trkC, a new member of the trk family of tyrosine protein kinases, is a receptor for neurotrophin-3. *Cell* **66**:967, 1991.

156. Squinto SP, Stitt TN, Aldrich TH, Davis S, Bianco SM, Radziejewski C, Glass DJ, Masiakowski P, Furth ME, Valenzuela DM, DiStefano PS, Yancopoulos GD: trkB encodes a functional receptor for brain-derived neurotrophic factor and neurotrophin-3 but not nerve growth factor. *Cell* **65**:885, 1991.

157. Ip NY, Ibanez CF, Nye SH, McClain J, Jones PF, Gies DR, Belluscio L, Le Beau MM, Espinsosa III R, Squinto SP, Persson H, Yancopoulos GD: Mammalian neurotrophin-4: Structure, chromosomal localization, tissue distribution, and receptor specificity. *Proc Natl Acad Sci U S A* **89**:3060, 1992.

158. Berkemeier LR, Winslow JW, Kaplan DR, Nikolics K, Goeddel DV, Rosenthal A: Neurotrophin-5: A novel neurotrophic factor that activates trk and trkB. *Neuron* **7**:857, 1991.

159. Soppet D, Escandon E, Maragos J, Middlemas DS, Reid SW, Blair J, Burton LE, Stanton BR, Kaplan DR, Hunter T, Nikolics K, Parada LF: The neurotrophic factors brain-derived neurotrophic factor and neurotrophin-3 are ligands for the trkB tyrosine kinase receptor. *Cell* **65**:895, 1991.

160. Chao MV, Bothwell MA, Ross AH, Koprowski H, Lanahan AA, Buch CR, Sehgal A: Gene transfer and molecular cloning of the human NGF receptor. *Science* **232**:518, 1986.

161. Hempstead BL, Patil N, Olson K, Chao MV: Molecular analysis of the nerve growth factor receptor. *Cold Spring Harb Symp Quant Biol* **53**:477, 1988.

162. Nakagawara A, Arima-Nakagawara M, Scavarda NJ, Azar CG, Cantor AB, Brodeur GM: Association between high levels of expression of the TRK gene and favorable outcome in human neuroblastoma. *N Engl J Med* **328**:847, 1993.

163. Suzuki T, Bogenmann E, Shimada H, Stram D, Seeger RC: Lack of high-affinity nerve growth factor receptors in aggressive neuroblastomas. *J Natl Cancer Inst* **85**:377, 1993.

164. Kogner P, Barbany G, Dominici C, Castello MA, Raschella G, Persson H: Coexpression of messenger RNA for TRK protooncogene and low affinity nerve growth factor receptor in neuroblastoma with favorable prognosis. *Cancer Res* **53**:2044, 1993.

165. Borrello MG, Bongarzone I, Pierotti MA, Luksch R, Gasparini M, Collini P, Pilotti S, Rizzetti MG, Mondellini P, DeBernardi B, DiMartino D, Garaventa A, Brisgotti M, Tonini GP: TRK and RET protooncogene expression in human neuroblastoma specimens: High-frequency of trk expression in non-advanced stages. *Int J Cancer* **54**:540, 1993.

166. Tanaka T, Hiyama E, Sugimoto T, Sawada T, Tanabe M, Ida N: trkA gene expression in neuroblastoma. *Cancer* **76**:1086, 1995.

167. Levi-Montalcini R: The nerve growth factor 35 years later. *Science* **237**:1154, 1987.

168. Martin DP, Schmidt RE, DiStefano PS, Lowry OH, Carter JG, Johnson EMJ: Inhibitors of protein synthesis and RNA synthesis prevent neuronal death caused by nerve growth factor deprivation. *J Cell Biol* **106**:829, 1988.

169. Koike T, Tanaka S: Evidence that nerve growth factor dependence of sympathetic neurons for survival in vitro may be determined by levels of cytoplasmic free Ca^{2+}. *Proc Natl Acad Sci U S A* **88**:3892, 1991.

170. Nakagawara A, Azar CG, Scavarda NJ, Brodeur GM: Expression and function of TRK-B and BDNF in human neuroblastomas. *Mol Cell Biol* **14**:759, 1994.

171. Kaplan DR, Matsumoto K, Lucarelli E, Thiele CJ: Induction of TrkB by retinoic acid mediates biologic responsiveness to BDNF and differentiation of human neuroblastoma cells. *Neuron* **11**:321, 1993.

172. Acheson A, Conover JC, Fandi JP, DeChiara TM, Russell M, Thadani A, Squinto SP, Yancopoulos GD, Lindsay RM: A BDNF autocrine loop in adult sensory neurons prevents cell death. *Nature* **374**:450, 1995.

173. Matsumoto K, Wada RK, Yamashiro JM, Kaplan DR, Thiele CJ: Expression of brain-derived neurotrophic factor and p145^{TrkB} affects survival, differentiation, and invasiveness of human neuroblastoma cells. *Cancer Res* **55**:1798, 1995.

174. Yamashiro DJ, Nakagawara A, Ikegaki N, Liu X-G, Brodeur GM: Expression of TrkC in favorable human neuroblastomas. *Oncogene* **12**:37, 1996.

175. Ryden M, Sehgal R, Dominici C, Schilling FH, Ibanez CF, Kogner P: Expression of mRNA for the neurotrophin receptor trkC in neuroblastomas with favourable tumour stage and good prognosis. *Br J Cancer* **74**:773, 1996.

176. Ballas K, Lyons J, Jannsen JWG, Bartram CR: Incidence of ras gene mutations in neuroblastoma. *Eur J Pediatr* **147**:313, 1988.

177. Ireland CM: Activated N-ras oncogenes in human neuroblastoma. *Cancer Res* **49**:5530, 1989.

178. Moley JF, Brother MB, Wells SA, Spengler BA, Biedler JL, Brodeur GM: Low frequency of ras gene mutations in neuroblastomas, pheochromocytomas and medullary thyroid cancers. *Cancer Res* **51**:1596, 1991.

179. Tanaka T, Slamon DJ, Shimoda H, Waki C, Kawaguchi Y, Tanaka Y, Ida N: Expression of Ha-ras oncogene products in human neuroblastomas and the significant correlation with a patient's prognosis. *Cancer Res* **48**:1030, 1988.

180. Tanaka T, Slamon DJ, Shimada H, Shimoda H, Fujisawa T, Ida N, Seeger RC: A significant association of Ha-ras p21 in neuroblastoma cells with patient prognosis. *Cancer* **68**:1296, 1991.

181. Tanaka T, Sugimoto T, Sawada T: Prognostic discrimination among neuroblastomas according to Ha-ras/Trk A gene expression. *Cancer* **83**:1626, 1998.

182. Thiele CJ, McKeon C, Triche TJ, Ross RA, Reynolds CP, Israel MA: Differential protooncogene expression characterizes histopathologically indistinguishable tumors of the peripheral nervous system. *J Clin Invest* **80**:804, 1987.

183. Goldstein LJ, Galski H, Fojo A, Willingham M, Lai SL, Gazdar A, Pirker R, Green A, Crist W, Brodeur GM, Grant C, Lieger M, Cossman J, Gottesman MM, Pastan I: Expression of a multidrug resistance gene in human tumors. *J Natl Cancer Inst* **81**:116, 1989.

184. Goldstein LJ, Fojo AT, Ueda K, Crist W, Green A, Brodeur G, Pastan I, Gottesman MM: Expression of the multidrug resistance, MDR1, gene in neuroblastomas. *J Clin Oncol* **8**:128, 1990.

185. Chan HSL, Haddad G, Thorner PS, DeBoer G, Lin YP, Ondrusek N, Yeger H, Ling V: P-glycoprotein expression as a predictor of the outcome of therapy for neuroblastoma. *N Engl J Med* **325**:1608, 1991.

186. Norris MD, Bordow SB, Marshall GM, Haber PS, Haber M: Association between high levels of expression of the multidrug resistance-associated protein (MRP) gene and poor outcome in primary human neuroblastoma. *N Engl J Med* **334**:231, 1996.

187. Hiyama E, Hiyama K, Yokoyama T, Matsuura Y, Piatyszek MA, Shay JW: Correlating telomerase activity levels with human neuroblastoma outcomes. *Nat Med* **1**:249, 1995.

188. Brodeur GM: Do the ends justify the means? *Nat Med* **1**:203, 1995.

189. Reynolds CP, Zuo JJ, Kim NW, Wang H, Lukens JN, Matthay KK, Seeger RC: Telomerase expression in primary neuroblastomas. *Eur J Cancer* **33**:1929, 1997.

190. Oue T, Fukuzawa M, Kusafuka T, Kohmoto Y, Imura K, Nagahara S, Okada A: In situ detection of DNA fragmentation and expression of bcl-2 in human neuroblastoma: Relation to apoptosis and spontaneous regression. *J Pediatr Surg* **31**:251, 1996.

191. Brodeur GM, Castle VP: The role of apoptosis in human neuroblastomas, in Hideman JA, Oive C (eds): *Apoptosis in Cancer Chemotherapy*. Totowa, NJ, Human Press Inc, p. 305.

192. Bunone G, Mariotti A, Compagni A, Morandi E, Della Valle G: Induction of apoptosis by p75 neurotrophin receptor in human neuroblastoma cells. *Oncogene* **14**:1463, 1997.

193. Fulda S, Sieverts H, Friesen C, Herr I, Debatin KM: The CD95 (APO-1/Fas) system mediates drug-induced apoptosis in neuroblastoma cells. *Cancer Res* **57**:3823, 1997.

194. Castle VP, Heidelberger KP, Bromberg J, Ou X, Dole M, Nunez G: Expression of the apoptosis-suppressing protein bcl-2, in neuroblastoma is associated with unfavorable histology and N-myc amplification. *Am J Pathol* **143**:1543, 1993.

195. Hanada M, Krajewski S, Tanaka S, Cazals-Hatem D, Spengler BA, Ross RA, Biedler JL, Reed JC: Regulation of Bcl-2 oncoprotein levels with differentiation of human neuroblastoma cells. *Cancer Res* **53**:4978, 1993.

196. Ramani P, Lu QL: Expression of bcl-2 gene product in neuroblastoma. *J Pathol* **172**:273, 1994.

197. Ikegaki N, Katsumata M, Tsujimoto Y, Nakagawara A, Brodeur GM: Relationship between bcl-2 and myc gene expression in human neuroblastoma. *Cancer Lett* **91**:161, 1995.

198. Hoehner JC, Gestblom C, Olsen L, Pahlman S: Spatial association of apoptosis-related gene expression and cellular death in clinical neuroblastoma. *Br J Cancer* **75**:1185, 1997.

199. Mejia MC, Navarro S, Pellin A, Castel V, Llombart-Bosch A: Study of bcl-2 protein expression and the apoptosis phenomenon in neuroblastoma. *Anticancer Res* **18**:801, 1998.

200. Tonini GP, Mazzocco K, di Vinci A, Geido E, de Bernardi B, Giaretti W: Evidence of apoptosis in neuroblastoma at onset and relapse. An analysis of a large series of tumors. *J Neurooncol* **31**:209, 1997.

201. Dole M, Nunez G, Merchant AK, Maybaum J, Rode CK, Bloch CA, Castle VP: Bcl-2 inhibits chemotherapy-induced apoptosis in neuroblastoma. *Cancer Res* **54**:3253, 1994.

202. Dole MG, Jasty R, Cooper MJ, Thompson CB, Nunez G, Castle VP: Bcl-xL is expressed in neuroblastoma cells and modulates chemotherapy-induced apoptosis. *Cancer Res* **55**:2576, 1995.

203. Nakagawara A, Nakamura Y, Ikeda H, Hiwasa T, Kuida K, Su MS, Zhao H, Cnaan A, Sakiyama S: High levels of expression and nuclear localization of interleukin-1-beta-converting enzyme (ICE) and CPP-32 in human neuroblastomas. *Cancer Res* **57**:4578, 1997.

204. Evans AE, D'Angio GJ, Randolph JA: A proposed staging for children with neuroblastoma. Children's Cancer Study Group A. *Cancer* **27**:374, 1971.

205. D'Angio GJ, Evans AE, Koop CE: Special pattern of widespread neuroblastoma with a favorable prognosis. *Lancet* **1**:1046, 1971.

206. Brodeur GM, Seeger RC: International criteria for diagnosis, staging and response to treatment in patients with neuroblastoma. *J Clin Oncol* **6**:1874, 1988.

207. Brodeur GM, Pritchard J, Berthold F, Carlsen NLT, Castel V, Castleberry RP, De Bernardi B, Evans AE, Favrot M, Hedborg F, Kaneko M, Kemshead J, Lampert F, Lee REJ, Look AT, Pearson ADJ, Philip T, Roald B, Sawada T, Seeger RC, Tsuchida Y, Voute PA: Revisions of the international criteria for neuroblastoma diagnosis, staging and response to treatment. *J Clin Oncol* **11**:1466, 1993.

208. Kaplan S, Holbrook C, McDaniel H, Buntain W, Crist W: Vasoactive intestinal peptide secreting tumors of childhood. *Am J Dis Child* **134**:21, 1980.

209. El Shafie M, Samuel D, Klippel CH, Robinson MG, Cullen BJ: Intractable diarrhea in children with VIP-secreting ganglioneuroblastomas. *J Pediatr Surg* **18**:34, 1983.

210. Said SI: Vasoactive intestinal peptide (VIP): Current status. *Peptides* **5**:143, 1984.

211. Bodmer M, Fridkin M, Gozes I: Coding sequences for vasoactive intestinal peptide and PHM-27 peptide are located on two adjacent exons in the human genome. *Proc Natl Acad Sci U S A* **82**:3548, 1985.

212. Beinfeld MC, Brick PL, Howlett AC, Holt IL, Pruss RM, Moskal JR, Eiden LE: The regulation of vasoactive intestinal peptide synthesis in neuroblastoma and chromaffin cells. *Ann N Y Acad Sci* **527**:68, 1988.

213. Robinson MJ, Howard RN: Neuroblastoma, presenting as myasthenia gravis in a child aged 3 years. *Pediatrics* **43**:111, 1969.

214. Roberts KB, Freeman JM: Cerebellar ataxia and "occult neuroblastoma" without opsoclonus. *Pediatrics* **56**:464, 1975.

215. Altman AJ, Baehner RL: Favorable prognosis for survival in children with coincident opsomyoclonus and neuroblastoma. *Cancer* **37**:846, 1976.

216. Nickerson BG, Hutter JJ: Opsoclonus and neuroblastoma. Response to ACTH. *Clin Pediatr* **18**:446, 1979.

217. Kinast M, Levin HS, Rothner AD, Erenberg G, Wacksman J, Judge J: Cerebellar ataxia, opsoclonus, and occult neural crest tumor. Abdominal computerized tomography in diagnosis. *Am J Dis Child* **134**:1057, 1980.

218. Telander RL, Smithson WA, Groover RV: Clinical outcome in children with acute cerebellar encephalopathy and neuroblastoma. *J Pediatr Surg* **24**:11, 1989.

219. Mitchell WG, Snodgrass SR: Opsoclonus-ataxia due to childhood neural crest tumors: A chronic neurologic syndrome. *J Child Neurol* **5**:153, 1990.

220. Koh PS, Raffensperger JG, Berry S, Larsen MB, Johnstone HS, Chou P, Luck SR, Hammer M, Cohn SL: Long-term outcome in children with opsoclonus-myoclonus and ataxia and coincident neuroblastoma. *J Pediatr* **125**:712, 1994.

221. Noetzel MJ, Cawley LP, James VL, Minard BJ, Agrawal HC: Anti-neurofilament protein antibodies in opsoclonus-myoclonus. *J Neuroimmunol* **15**:137, 1987.

222. Budde-Steffen C, Anderson NE, Rosenblum MK, Graus F, Ford D, Synek BJ, Wray SH, Posner JB: An antineuronal autoantibody in paraneoplastic opsoclonus. *Ann Neurol* **23**:528, 1988.

223. Pranzatelli MR: The neurobiology of the opsoclonus-myoclonus syndrome. *Clin Neuropharmacol* **3**:186, 1992.

224. Kedar A, Glassman M, Voorhess ML, Fisher J, Allen J, Jenis E, Freeman AI: Severe hypertension in a child with ganglioneuroblastoma. *Cancer* **47**:2077, 1981.

225. Mason GA, Hart-Mercer J, Miller EJ, Strang LB, Wynne NA: Adrenaline-secreting neuroblastoma in an infant. *Lancet* **2**:322, 1957.

226. Laug WE, Siegel SE, Shaw KNF, Landing B, Baptista J, Gutenstein M: Initial urinary catecholamine metabolite concentrations and prognosis in neuroblastoma. *Pediatrics* **62**:77, 1978.

227. LaBrosse EH, Com-Nougue C, Zucker JM, Comoy E, Bohuon C, Lemerle J, Schweisguth O: Urinary excretion of 3-methoxy-4-hydroxymandelic acid and 3-methoxy-4-hydroxyphenylacetic acid by 288 patients with neuroblastoma and related neural crest tumors. *Cancer Res* **40**:1995, 1980.

228. Graham-Pole J, Salmi T, Anton AH, Abramowsky C, Gross S: Tumor and urine catecholamines (CATS) in neurogenic tumors. Correlations with other prognostic factors and survival. *Cancer* **51**:834, 1983.

229. Triche TJ, Askin FB, Kissane JM: Neuroblastoma, Ewing's sarcoma, and the differential diagnosis of small-, round-, blue-cell tumors, in Finegold M (eds): *Pathology of Neoplasia in Children and Adolescents.* Philadelphia, WB Saunders, 1986, p. 145.

230. Kemshead JT, Goldman A, Fritschy J, Malpas JS, Pritchard J: Use of panels of monoclonal antibodies in the differential diagnosis of neuroblastoma and lymphoblastic disorders. *Lancet* **1**:12, 1983.

231. Donner K, Triche TJ, Israel MA, Seeger RC, Reynolds CP: A panel of monoclonal antibodies which discriminate neuroblastoma from Ewing's sarcoma, rhabdomyosarcoma, neuroepithelioma, and hematopoietic malignancies. *Prog Clin Biol Res* **175**:367, 1985.

232. Sugimoto T, Sawada T, Arakawa S, Matsumura T, Dakamoto I, Takeuchi Y, Reynolds CP, Kemshead JT, Helson L: Possible differential diagnosis of neuroblastoma from rhabdomyosarcoma and Ewing's sarcoma by using a panel of monoclonal antibodies. *Jpn J Cancer Res* **76**:301, 1985.

233. Moss TJ, Seeger RC, Kindler-Rohrborn A, Marangos PJ, Rajewsky MF, Reynolds CP: Immunohistologic detection and phenotyping of neuroblastoma cells in bone marrow using cytoplasmic neuron specific enolase and cell surface antigens. *Prog Clin Biol Res* **175**:367, 1985.

234. Bostrom B, Nesbit ME, Brunning RD: The value of bone marrow trephine biopsy in the diagnosis of metastatic neuroblastoma. *Am J Pediatr Hematol Oncol* **7**:303, 1985.

235. Franklin IM, Pritchard J: Detection of bone marrow invasion by neuroblastoma is improved by sampling at two sites with both aspirates and trephine biopsies. *J Clin Pathol* **36**:1215, 1983.

236. Moss TJ, Reynolds CP, Sather HN, Romansky SG, Hammond GD, Seeger RC: Prognostic value of immunocytologic detection of bone marrow metastases in neuroblastoma. *N Engl J Med* **324**:219, 1991.

237. Daubenton JD, Fisher RM, Karabus CD, Mann MD: The relationship between prognosis and scintigraphic evidence of bone metastases in neuroblastoma. *Cancer* **59**:1586, 1987.

238. Heisel MA, Miller JH, Reid BS, Siegel SE: Radionuclide bone scan in neuroblastoma. *Pediatrics* **71**:206, 1983.

239. Podrasky AE, Stark DD, Hattner RS, Gooding CA, Moss AA: Radionuclide bone scanning in neuroblastoma: Skeletal metastases and primary tumor localization of 99mTc-MDP. *AJR Am J Roentgenol* **141**:469, 1983.

240. White SJ, Stuck KJ, Blane CE, Silver TM: Sonography of neuroblastoma. *AJR Am J Roentgenol* **141**:465, 1983.

241. Couanet D, Hartmann O, Piekarski JD, Vanel D, Masselot J: The use of computed tomography in the staging of neuroblastomas in childhood. *Arch Pediatr* **38**:315, 1981.

242. Golding SJ, McElwain TJ, Husband JE: The role of computed tomography in the management of children with advanced neuroblastoma. *Br J Radiol* **57**:661, 1984.

243. Fletcher BD, Kopiwoda SY, Strandjord SE, Nelson AD, Pickering SP: Abdominal neuroblastoma: Magnetic resonance imaging and tissue characterization. *Radiology* **155**:699, 1985.

244. Smith FW, Cherryman GR, Redpath TW, Crosher G: The nuclear magnetic resonance appearances of neuroblastoma. *Pediatr Radiol* **15**:329, 1985.

245. Geatti O, Shapiro B, Sisson JC, Hutchinson RJ, Mallette S, Eyre P, Beierwaltes WH: Iodine-131 metaiodobenzylguanidine (131-I-MIBG) scintigraphy for the location of neuroblastoma: Preliminary experience in ten cases. *J Nucl Med* **26**:736, 1985.

246. Voute PA, Hoefnagel CA, Marcuse HR, de Kraker J: Detection of neuroblastoma with ^{131}I-meta-iodobenzylguanidine. *Prog Clin Biol Res* **175**:389, 1985.

247. Shimada H, Chatten J, Newton WA, Jr., Sachs N, Hamoudi AB, Chiba T, Marsden HB, Misugi K: Histopathologic prognostic factors in neuroblastic tumors: Definition of subtypes of ganglioneuroblastoma and an age-linked classification of neuroblastomas. *J Natl Cancer Inst* **73**:405, 1984.

248. Hughes M, Marsden HB, Palmer MK: Histologic patterns of neuroblastoma related to prognosis and clinical staging. *Cancer* **34**:1706, 1974.

249. Joshi V, Cantor A, Altshuler G, Larkin E, Neill J, Shuster J, Holbrook T, Hayes A, Castleberry R: Prognostic significance of histopathologic features of neuroblastoma: A grading system based on the review of 211 cases from the Pediatric Oncology Group [Abstract]. *Proc Am Soc Clin Oncol* **10**:311, 1991.

250. Castleberry RP, Pritchard J, Ambros P, Berthold F, Brodeur GM, Castel V, Cohn SL, De Bernardi B, Dicks-Mireaux C, Frappaz D, Haase GM, Haber M, Jones DR, Joshi VV, Kaneko M, Kemshead JT, Kogner P, Lee REJ, Matthay KK, Michon JM, Monclair R, Roald BR, Seeger RC, Shaw PJ, Shimada H, Shuster JJ: The International Neuroblastoma Risk Groups (INRG): A preliminary report. *Eur J Cancer* **33**:2113, 1997.

251. Ciccarone V, Spengler BA, Meyers MB, Biedler JL, Ross RA: Phenotypic diversification in human neuroblastoma cells: Expression of distinct neural crest lineages. *Cancer Res* **49**:219, 1989.

252. Ambros IM, Zellner A, Roald B, Amann G, Ladenstein R, Printz D, Gadner H, Ambros PF: Role of chromosome 1p and Schwann cells in the maturation of neuroblastoma. *N Engl J Med* **334**:1505, 1996.

253. Nitschke R, Smith EI, Shochat S, Altshuler G, Travers H, Shuster JJ, Hayes FA, Patterson R, McWilliams N: Localized neuroblastoma treated by surgery — A Pediatric Oncology Group Study. *J Clin Oncol* **6**:1271, 1988.

254. Hayes FA, Green AA, Hustu HO, Kumar M: Surgicopathologic staging of neuroblastoma: Prognostic significance of regional lymph node metastases. *J Pediatr* **102**:59, 1983.

255. De Bernardi B, Rogers D, Carli M, Madon E, de Laurentis T, Bagnulo S, di Tullio MT, Paolucci G, Pastore G: Localized neuroblastoma. Surgical and pathological staging. *Cancer* **60**:1066, 1987.

256. Nagahara N, Ohkawa H, Suzuki H, Tsuchida Y, Nakajou T: Staging of neuroblastoma. *J Clin Oncol* **8**:179, 1990.

257. Nakagawara A, Morita K, Okabe I, Uchino J, Ohi R, Iwafuchi M, Matsuyama S, Nagashima K, Takahashi H, Nakajo T, Hirai Y, Tshchida Y, Saeki M, Yokoyama J, Nishi T, Okamoto E, Suita S: Proposal and assessment of Japanese Tumor Node Metastasis postsurgical histopathological staging system for neuroblastoma based on an analysis of 495 cases. *Jpn J Clin Oncol* **21**:1, 1990.

258. Altman AJ, Schwartz AD: Tumors of the sympathetic nervous system, in Altman AJ, Schwartz AD (eds): *Malignant Diseases of Infancy, Childhood and Adolescence.* Philadelphia, WB Saunders, 1983, p. 368.

259. Carlsen NLT, Christensen IJ, Schroeder H, Bro P, Erichsen G, Hambort-Pedersen B, Jensen KB, Nielsen OH: Prognostic factors in neuroblastomas treated in Denmark from 1943 to 1980. A statistical estimate of prognosis based on 253 cases. *Cancer* **58**:2726, 1986.

260. Coldman AJ, Fryer CJH, Elwood JM, Sonley MJ: Neuroblastoma: Influence of age at diagnosis, stage, tumor site, and sex on prognosis. *Cancer* **46**:1896, 1980.

261. Evans AE, D'Angio GJ, Propert K, Anderson J, Hann H-WL: Prognostic factors in neuroblastoma. *Cancer* **59**:1853, 1987.

262. Grosfeld JL, Schatzlein M, Ballantine TVN, Weetman RM, Baehner RL: Metastatic neuroblastoma: Factors influencing survival. *J Pediatr Surg* **13**:59, 1978.

263. Grosfeld JL: Neuroblastoma in infancy and childhood, in Hays DM (ed): *Pediatric Surgical Oncology*. New York, Grune & Stratton, 1986, p. 63.

264. Jaffe N: Neuroblastoma: Review of the literature and an examination of factors contributing to its enigmatic character. *Cancer Treat Rev* **3**:61, 1976.

265. Jereb B, Bretsky SS, Vogel R, Helson L: Age and prognosis in neuroblastoma. Review of 112 patients younger than 2 years. *Am J Pediatr Hem Oncol* **6**:233, 1984.

266. Kinnier-Wilson LM, Draper GJ: Neuroblastoma, its natural history and prognosis: A study of 487 cases. *BMJ* **3**:301, 1974.

267. Bourhis J, Benard J, Hartmann O, Boccon-Gibod L, Lemerle J, Riou G: Correlation of MDR1 gene expression with chemotherapy in neuroblastoma. *J Natl Cancer Inst* **81**:1401, 1989.

268. Nakagawara A, Kadomatsu K, Sato S-I, Kohno K, Takano H, Akazawa K, Nose Y, Kuwano M: Inverse correlation between expression of multidrug resistance gene and N-myc oncogene in human neuroblastomas. *Cancer Res* **50**:3043, 1990.

269. Corrias MV, Cornaglia-Ferraris P, Di Martino D, Stenger AM, Lanino E, Boni L, Tonini GP: Expression of multidrug resistance gene, MDR1, and N-myc oncogene in an Italian population of human neuroblastoma patients. *Anticancer Res* **10**:897, 1990.

270. Gross N, Beck D, Beretta C, Jackson D, Perruisseau G: CD44 expression and modulation on human neuroblastoma tumours and cell lines. *Eur J Cancer* **31A**:471, 1995.

271. Combaret V, Gross N, Lasset C, Frappaz D, Beretta-Brognara C, Philip T, Beck D, Favrot MC: Clinical relevance of CD44 cell surface expression and MYCN gene amplification in neuroblastoma. *Eur J Cancer* **33**:2101, 1997.

272. Kramer K, Cheung NK, Gerald WL, LaQuaglia M, Kushner BH, LeClerc JM, LeSauter L, Saragovi HU: Correlation of MYCN amplification, Trk-A and CD44 expression with clinical stage in 250 patients with neuroblastoma. *Eur J Cancer* **33**:2098, 1997.

273. Christiansen H, Sahin K, Berthold F, Hero B, Terpe H-J, Lampert F: Comparison of DNA aneuploidy, chromosome 1 abnormalities, MYCN amplification and CD44 expression as prognostic factors in neuroblastoma. *Eur J Cancer* **31A**:541, 1995.

274. Hann HW, Evans AE, Cohen IJ, Leitmeyer JE: Biologic differences between neuroblastoma stage IV-S and IV. Measurement of serum ferritin and E-rosette inhibition in 30 children. *N Engl J Med* **305**:425, 1981.

275. Hann HWL, Evans AE, Siegel SE, Wong KY, Sather H, Dalton A, Hammond D, Seeger RC: Prognostic importance of serum ferritin in patients with stages III and IV neuroblastoma. The Children's Cancer Study Group Experience. *Cancer Res* **45**:2843, 1985.

276. Hann HWL, Stahlhut MW, Evans AE: Basic and acidic isoferritins in the sera of patients with neuroblastoma. *Cancer* **62**:1179, 1988.

277. Silber JH, Evans AE, Fridman M: Models to predict outcome from childhood neuroblastoma: The role of serum ferritin and tumor histology. *Cancer Res* **51**:1426, 1991.

278. Marangos P: Clinical studies with neuron specific enolase. *Prog Clin Biol Res* **175**:285, 1985.

279. Tsuchida Y, Honna T, Iwanaka T, Saeki M, Taguchi N, Kaneko T, Koide R, Tsunematsu Y, Shimizu KI, Makino SI, Hashizume K, Nakajo T: Serial determination of serum neuron-specific enolase in patients with neuroblastoma and other pediatric tumors. *J Pediatr Surg* **22**:419, 1987.

280. Zeltzer PM, Parma AM, Dalton A, Siegel SE, Marangos PJ, Sather H, Hammond D, Seeger RC: Raised neuron-specific enolase in serum of children with metastatic neuroblastoma. *Lancet* **2**:361, 1983.

281. Zeltzer PM, Marangos PJ, Evans AE, Schneider SL: Serum neuron-specific enolase in children with neuroblastoma. Relationship to stage and disease course. *Cancer* **57**:1230, 1986.

282. Ladisch S, Wu ZL: Detection of a tumour-associated ganglioside in plasma of patients with neuroblastoma. *Lancet* **1**:136, 1985.

283. Ladisch S, Kitada S, Hays EF: Gangliosides shed by tumor cells enhance tumor formation in mice. *J Clin Invest* **79**:1879, 1987.

284. Schulz G, Cheresh DA, Varki NM, Yu A, Staffileno LK, Reisfeld RA: Detection of ganglioside GD2 in tumor tissues and sera of neuroblastoma patients. *Cancer Res* **44**:5914, 1984.

285. Schengrund CL, Repman MA, Shochat SJ: Ganglioside composition of human neuroblastomas—Correlation with prognosis. A Pediatric Oncology Group Study. *Cancer* **56**:2640, 1985.

286. Valentino L, Moss T, Olson E, Wang H-J, Elshoff R, Ladisch S: Shed tumor gangliosides and progression of human neuroblastoma. *Blood* **75**:1564, 1990.

287. Quinn JJ, Altman AJ, Frantz CN: Serum lactic dehydrogenase, an indicator of tumor activity in neuroblastoma. *J Pediatr* **97**:89, 1980.

288. Woods WG: The use and significance of biologic markers in the evaluation and staging of a child with cancer. *Cancer* **58**:442, 1986.

289. McWilliams NB, Hayes FA, Shuster JJ, Smith EI, Green A, Castleberry R: Prognostic indicators in babies less than 1 with stage D neuroblastoma [Abstract]. *Pediatr Res* **23**:344A, 1988.

290. Cohn SL, Rademaker AW, Salwen HR, Franklin WA, Gonzales-Crussi F, Rosen ST, Bauer KD: Analysis of DNA ploidy and proliferative activity in relation to histology and N-myc amplification in neuroblastoma. *Am J Pathol* **136**:1043, 1990.

291. Hayashi Y, Habu Y, Fujii Y, Hanada R, Yamamoto K: Chromosome abnormalities in neuroblastomas found by VMA mass screening. *Cancer Genet Cytogenet* **22**:363, 1986.

292. Hayashi Y, Inabada T, Hanada R, Yamamoto K: Chromosome findings and prognosis in 15 patients with neuroblastoma found by VMA mass screening. *J Pediatr* **112**:67, 1988.

293. Kaneko Y, Kanda N, Maseki N, Nakachi K, Okabe I, Sakuri M: Current urinary mass screening or catecholamine metabolites at 6 months of age may be detecting only a small portion of high-risk neuroblastomas: A chromosome and N-myc amplification study. *J Clin Oncol* **8**:2005, 1990.

294. Bourhis J, De Vathaire F, Wilson GD, Hartmann O, Terrier-Lascombe MJ, Boccon-Gibod L, McNally NJ, Lemerle J, Riou G, Bernard J: Combined analysis of DNA ploidy index and N-myc genomic content in neuroblastoma. *Cancer Res* **51**:33, 1991.

295. Kiely EM: The surgical challenge of neuroblastoma. *J Pediatr Surg* **29**:128, 1994.

296. La Quaglia MP, Kushner BH, Heller G, Bonilla MA, Lindsley KL, Cheung NK: Stage 4 neuroblastoma diagnosed at more than 1 year of age: Gross total resection and clinical outcome. *J Pediatr Surg* **29**:1162, 1994.

297. Morris JA, Shochat SJ, Smith EI, Look AT, Brodeur GM, Cantor AB, Castleberry RP: Biological variables in thoracic neuroblastoma: A Pediatric Oncology Group Study. *J Pediatr Surg* **30**:296, 1995.

298. Smith EI, Castleberry RP: Neuroblastoma, in Wells SA Jr. (ed): *Current Problems in Pediatric Surgery*. St. Louis, CV Mosby, 1990, p. 577.

299. Green AA, Hustu HO, Kumar M: Sequential cyclophosphamide and doxorubicin for induction of complete remission in children with disseminated neuroblastoma. *Cancer* **48**:2310, 1981.

300. Hayes FA, Green AA, Casper J, Cornet J, Evans WE: Clinical evaluation of sequentially scheduled cisplatin and VM26 in neuroblastoma; response and toxicity. *Cancer* **48**:1715, 1981.

301. Castleberry RP: Biology and treatment of neuroblastoma. *Pediatr Clin North Am* **44**:919, 1997.

302. Cheung NKV, Heller G: Chemotherapy dose intensity correlates strongly with response, median survival and median progression-free survival in metastatic neuroblastoma. *J Clin Oncol* **9**:1050, 1991.

303. Kushner BH, LaQuaglia MP, Bonilla MA, Lindsley K, Rosenfield N, Yeh S, Eddy J, Gerald WL, Heller G, Cheung NKV: Highly effective induction therapy for stage 4 neuroblastoma in children over 1 year of age. *J Clin Oncol* **12**:2607, 1994.

304. Matthay KK: Neuroblastoma: Biology and therapy. *Oncology* **11**:1857, 1997.

305. Matthay KK, Perez C, Seeger RC, Brodeur GM, Shimada H, Atkinson JB, Black CT, Gerbing R, Haase GM, Stram DO, Swift P, Lukens JN: Successful treatment of stage III neuroblastoma based on prospective biologic staging: A Children's Cancer Group study. *J Clin Oncol* **16**:1256, 1998.

306. Halperin E: Neuroblastoma, in Halperin E, Kun L, Constine L, Tarbell N (eds): *Pediatric Radiation Oncology*. New York, Raven Press, 1989, p. 134.

307. Castleberry RP, Kun L, Shuster JJ, Altshuler G, Smith EI, Nitschke R, Wharam M, McWilliams N, Joshi V, Hayes FA: Radiotherapy improves the outlook for children older than one year with POG stage C neuroblastoma. *J Clin Oncol* **9**:789, 1991.

308. August CS, Serota FT, Koch PA, Burkey E, Schlesinger H, Elkins WL, Evans AE, D'Angio GJ: Treatment of advanced neuroblastoma with supralethal chemotherapy, radiation and allogeneic or autologous marrow reconstitution. *J Clin Oncol* **2**:609, 1984.

309. Gee AP, Graham Pole J: Use of bone marrow purging and bone marrow transplantation for neuroblastoma, in Pochedly C (ed): *Neuroblastoma: Tumor Biology and Therapy*. Boca Raton, FL, CRC Press, 1990, p. 317.

310. Graham-Pole J, Casper J, Elfenbein G, Gee A, Gross S, Janssen W, Koch P, Marcus R, Pick T, Shuster J, Spruce W, Thomas P, Yeager A: High-dose chemoradiotherapy supported by marrow infusions for advanced neuroblastoma: A Pediatric Oncology Group study. *J Clin Oncol* **9**:152, 1991.

311. Hartmann O, Kalifa C, Benhamou E, Patte C, Flamank F, Jullien C, Beaujean F, Lemerle J: Treatment of advanced neuroblastoma with high-dose melphalan and autologous bone marrow transplantation. *Cancer Chemother Pharmacol* **16**:165, 1986.

312. Hartmann O, Benhamou E, Beaujean F, Kalifa C, Lejars O, Patte C, Behard C, Flamant F, Thyss A, Deville A, Vannier JP, Pautard-Muchemble E, Lemerle J: Repeated high-dose chemotherapy followed by purged autologous bone marrow transplantation as consolidation therapy in metastatic neuroblastoma. *J Clin Oncol* **5**:1205, 1987.

313. Philip T, Bernard JL, Zucker JM, Pinkerton R, Lutz P, Bordigoni P, Plouvier E, Robert A, Carton R, Philippe N, Philip I, Chauvin F, Favrot M: High-dose chemoradiotherapy with bone marrow transplantation as consolidation treatment in neuroblastoma: An unselected group of stage IV patients over 1 year of age. *J Clin Oncol* **5**:266, 1987.

314. Philip T, Zucker JM, Bernard JL, et al: Bone marrow transplantation in an unselected group of 65 patients with stage IV neuroblastoma, in Dicke KA, Spitzer G, Jagannath S (eds): *Autologous Bone Marrow Transplantation III.* Houston, TX, University of Texas, 1987, p. 407.

315. Pinkerton CR, Philip T, Biron P, Frapaz D, Philippe N, Zucker JM, Bernard JL, Philip I, Kemshead J, Favrot M: High-dose melphalan, vincristine and total-body irradiation with autologous bone marrow transplantation in children with relapsed neuroblastoma: A phase II study. *Med Pediatr Oncol* **15**:236, 1987.

316. Pritchard J, McElwain TJ, Graham-Pole J: High dose melphalan with autologous marrow for treatment of advanced neuroblastoma. *Br J Cancer* **45**:86, 1982.

317. Seeger R, Moss TJ, Feig SA, Lenarsky C, Selch M, Ramsay N, Harris R, Wells J, Sather W, Reynolds CP: Bone marrow transplantation for poor prognosis neuroblastoma. *Prog Clin Biol Res* **271**:203, 1988.

318. Treleaven JG, Gibson FM, Ugelstad J, Rembaum A, Philip T, Caine GD, Kemshead JT: Monoclonal antibodies and magnetic microspheres for the removal of tumor cells from bone marrow. *Lancet* **1**:70, 1984.

319. Matthay KK, Seeger RC, Reynolds CP, al e: Allogeneic versus autologous purged bone marrow transplantation for neuroblastoma: A report from the Childrens' Cancer Group. *J Clin Oncol* **12**:2382, 1994.

320. Seeger RC, Matthay KK, Villablanca JG, Harris R, Feig SA, Selch M, Stram D, Reynolds CP: Intensive chemoradiotherapy and autologous bone marrow transplantation (ABMT) for high risk neuroblastoma [abstract]. *Proc Am Soc Clin Oncol* **10**:310, 1991.

321. Stram DO, Matthay KK, O'Leary M, Reynolds CP, Haase GM, Atkinson JB, Brodeur GM, Seeger RC: Consolidation chemoradiotherapy and autologous bone marrow transplantation versus continued chemotherapy for metastatic neuroblastoma: A report of two concurrent Children's Cancer Group studies. *J Clin Oncol* **14**:2417, 1996.

322. Zucker JM, Bernard JL, Philip T, Gentet JC, Michon J, Bouffet E: High dose chemotherapy with BMT as consolidation treatment in neuroblastoma — The LMCE 1 unselected group of patients revisited with a median follow up of 55 months after BMT [abstract]. *Proc Am Soc Clin Oncol* **9**:294, 1990.

323. Philip T, Ladenstein R, Lasset C, Hartmann O, Zucker JM, Pinkerton R, Pearson AD, Klingebiel T, Garaventa A, Kremens B, Bernard JL, Rosti G, Chauvin F: 1070 myeloablative megatherapy procedures followed by stem cell rescue for neuroblastoma: 17 years of European experience and conclusions. European Group for Blood and Marrow Transplant Registry Solid Tumour Working Party. *Eur J Cancer* **33**:2130, 1997.

324. Ladenstein R, Philip T, Lasset C, Hartmann O, Garaventa A, Pinkerton R, Michon J, Pritchard J, Klingebiel T, Kremens B, Pearson A, Coze C, Paolucci P, Frappaz D, Gadner H, Chauvin F: Multivariate analysis of risk factors in stage 4 neuroblastoma patients over the age of one year treated with megatherapy and stem-cell transplantation: A report from the European Bone Marrow Transplantation Solid Tumor Registry. *J Clin Oncol* **16**:953, 1997.

325. Bowman LC, Castleberry RP, Altshuler G, Smith EI, Cantor A, Shuster J, Yu A, Look AT, Hayes FA: Therapy based on DNA index (DI) for infants with unresectable and disseminated neuroblastoma (NB): Preliminary results of the Pediatric Oncology Group "Better Risk" study [abstract]. *Med Pediatr Oncol* **18**:364, 1990.

326. Fairchild RS, Kyner JL, Hermreck A, Schimke RN: Neuroblastoma, pheochromocytoma and renal cell carcinoma. Occurrence in a single patient. *JAMA* **242**:2210, 1979.

327. Secker-Walker LM, Stewart EL, Todd A: Acute lymphoblastic leukaemia with t(4;11) follows neuroblastoma: A late effect of treatment? *Med Pediatr Oncol* **13**:48, 1985.

328. Shah NR, Miller DR, Steinherz PG, Garbes A, Farber P: Acute monoblastic leukemia as a second malignant neoplasm in metastatic neuroblastoma. *Am J Pediatr Hem Oncol* **7**:309, 1983.

329. Weh HJ, Kabisch H, Landbeck G, Hossfeld DK: Translocation (9;11)(p21;q23) in a child with acute monoblastic leukemia following 21/2 years after successful chemotherapy for neuroblastoma. *J Clin Oncol* **4**:1518, 1986.

330. Ben-Arush MW, Doron Y, Braun J, Mendelson E, Dar H, Robinson E: Brain tumor as a second malignant neoplasm following neuroblastoma stage IV-S. *Med Pediatr Oncol* **18**:240, 1990.

331. Meadows AT, Baum E, Fossati-Bellani F, Green D, Jenkin RDT, Marsden B, Nesbit M, Newton W, Oberlin O, Sallan SG, Siegel S, Strong LC, Voute PA: Second malignant neoplasms in children: An update from the Late Effects Study Group. *J Clin Oncol* **3**:532, 1985.

332. Cheung NK, Kushner BH, Yeh SDJ, Larson SM: 3F8 monoclonal antibody treatment of patients with stage 4 neuroblastoma: A phase II study. *Int J Cancer* **12**:1299, 1998.

333. Frost JD, Hank JA, Reaman GH, Frierdich S, Seeger RC, Gan J, Anderson PM, Ettinger LJ, Cairo MS, Blazar BR, Krailo MD, Matthay KK, Reisfeld RA, Sondel PM: A phase I/IB trial of murine monoclonal anti-GD2 antibody 14.G2a plus interleukin-2 in children with refractory neuroblastoma: A report of the Children's Cancer Group. *Cancer* **80**:317, 1997.

334. Matthay KK, DeSantes K, Hasegawa B, Huberty J, Hattner RS, Ablin A, Reynolds CP, Seeger RC, Weinberg VK, Price D: Phase I dose escalation of 131I-metaiodobenzylguanidine with autologous bone marrow support in refractory neuroblastoma. *J Clin Oncol* **16**:229, 1998.

335. Meitar D, Crawford SE, Rademaker AW, Cohn SL: Tumor angiogenesis correlates with metastatic disease, N-myc amplification, and poor outcome in human neuroblastoma. *J Clin Oncol* **14**:405, 1996.

336. Villablanca JG, Khan AA, Avramis VI, Seeger RC, Matthay KK, Ramsay NK, Reynolds CP: Phase I trial of 13-cis-retinoic acid in children with neuroblastoma following bone marrow transplantation. *J Clin Oncol* **13**:894, 1995.

337. Wassberg E, Christofferson R: Angiostatic treatment of neuroblastoma. *Eur J Cancer* **33**:2020, 1997.

338. Sawada T, Hirayama M, Nakata T, Takeda T, Takasugi N, Mori T, Maeda K, Koide R, Hanawa Y, Tsunoda A, Shimizu K, Nagahara N, Yamamoto K: Mass screening for neuroblastoma in infants in Japan. *Lancet* **2**:271, 1984.

339. Nishi M, Miyake H, Takeda T, Shimada M, Takasugi N, Sato Y, Hanai J: Effects of the mass screening of neuroblastoma in Sapporo City. *Cancer* **60**:433, 1987.

340. Sawada T, Kidowaki T, Sakamoto I, Hashida T, Matsumura T, Nakagawara M, Kusunoki T: Neuroblastoma. Mass screening for early detection and its prognosis. *Cancer* **53**:2731, 1984.

341. Takeda T, Hatae Y, Nakadate H, Nishi M, Hanai J, Sato Y, Takasugi N: Japanese experience of screening. *Med Pediatr Oncol* **17**:368, 1989.

342. Woods WG, Tuchman M, Bernstein ML, Leclerc J-M, Brisson L, Look T, Brodeur GM, Shimada H, Hann HL, Robison LL, Shuster JJ, Lemieux B: Screening for neuroblastoma in North America. Two-year results from the Quebec project. *Am J Pediatr Hem Oncol* **14**:312, 1992.

343. Woods WG, Lemieux B, Leclerc JM, Bernstein ML, Brisson L, Broussard J, Brodeur GM, Look AT, Robison LL, Schuster JJ, Weitzman S, Tuchman M: Screening for neuroblastoma (NB) in North America: The Quebec Project, in Evans AE, Brodeur GM, Biedler JL, D'Angio GJ, Nakagawara N (eds): *Advances in Neuroblastoma Research.* New York, Wiley Liss, 1994, p. 377.

344. Woods WG, Tuchman M, Robison LL, Bernstein M, Leclerc J-M, Brisson L, Brossard J, Hill G, Shuster J, Luepker R, Weitzman S, Bunin G, Lemieux B: A population-based study of the usefulness of screening for neuroblastoma. *Lancet* **348**:1682, 1996.

345. Schilling FH, Erttmann R, Ambros PF, Strehl S, Christiansen H, Kovar H, Kabisch H, Treuner J: Screening for neuroblastoma. *Lancet* **344**:1157, 1994.

346. Kerbl R, Urban CHE, Ladenstein R, Ambros IM, Spuller E, Mutz I, Amann G, Kovar H, Gadner H, Ambros PF: Neuroblastoma screening

in infants postponed after the sixth month of age: A trial to reduce "overdiagnosis" and to detect cases with "unfavorable" biologic features. *Med Pediatr Oncol* **29**:1, 1997.

347. Ambross PF, Brodeur GM: The concept of tumorigenesis in neuroblastoma, in Brodeur GM, Sawada T, Tsuchida Y, Voute PA (eds): *Neuroblastoma*. Amsterdam: Elsevier Science, 2000(in press).

348. Bessho F, Hashizume K, Nakajo T, Kamoshita S: Mass screening in Japan increased the detection of infants with neuroblastoma without a decrease in cases in older children. *J Pediatr* **119**:237, 1991.

349. Hachitanda Y, Ishimoto K, Hata J-i, Shimada H: One hundred neuroblastomas detected through a mass screening system in Japan. *Cancer* **74**:3223, 1994.

350. Hayashi Y, Hanada R, Yamamoto K: Biology of neuroblastomas in Japan found by screening. *Am J Pediatr Hem Oncol* **14**:342, 1992.

351. Hayashi Y, Ohi R, Yaoita S, Nakamura M, Kikuchi Y, Konno T, Tsuchiya S, Shiraishi H: Problems of neuroblastoma screen for 6 month olds, and results of second screening for 18 month olds. *J Pediatr Surg* **30**:467, 1995.

Cancers of the Oral Cavity and Pharynx

Saman Warnakulasuriya

1. Oral and pharyngeal cancer is the sixth most common malignancy reported worldwide. About 62 percent arise in developing countries. Oral neoplasms are uncommon in Western countries, but in the past decade rising trends have been reported among young males. Malignancies of this site are a serious public health problem in Asia.

2. Major risk factors, tobacco and excess alcohol consumption, are well established. The primary cause of high incidence in Asians is the widespread habit of chewing betel quid. Antioxidant micronutrients such as β carotene and vitamin C are protective. Some viruses, such as HPV (types 16 & 18), are also implicated.

3. Most mouth cancers are asymptomatic at early stages. Many present at a late stage, approximately 70 percent with nodal metastases. There is also a high incidence of second primary tumors in the upper aerodigestive tract following an oral or pharyngeal, squamous cell carcinomous (SCC). In most Western countries, the reported 5-year survival is around 50 percent.

4. Several potentially malignant lesions and conditions that arise on the oral mucosa are known. This makes oral cancer a candidate site for screening. Knowledge of molecular markers may assist in the detection of high-risk individuals.

5. Multiple chromosome losses and gains are described with substantial variations in loss of heterozygosity in individual tumors. Clustering of fragile sites is demonstrated in 3p and 9p, and by gene amplification at 11q13.

6. While ras mutations are rare in white caucosoid populations, they are frequently seen in tobacco/areca-chewing Asian subjects with oral SCC. When mutated or amplified, ras may cooperate with cyclin D1 in altering G0/G1 transition.

7. p53 mutations and overexpression of the protein may be demonstrated in at least half of oral SCC. Mutations are predominant in exon 8, but may occur in exon 5 as well. Codons 176, 245-8, 273, and 296-8 appear to harbor a high proportion of the mutations described so far. The profiles of these results, so far, are discordant against other tobacco-induced cancers. p53 mutations are uncommon in the preinvasive stage but appear to occur in the transition from preinvasive to the invasive stage. p53 therefore does not serve as a potential biomarker to detect which precancers may progress with time. p53 overexpression is an independent prognostic marker in advanced tumors.

8. Other cell-cycle regulatory proteins, namely, p21, p27, and pRb, have been investigated. Some tumors appear to have independent pathways of expression, or inactivation of these molecules that is unrelated to p53 status. P16 inactivation may occur in nearly half of oral cancers causing dysregulation of growth arrest.

9. p53 and CYFRA 21-1 may serve as tumor markers but are not universally present. Immunogenicity of p53 needs further study. Saliva may also serve as a useful biological fluid in tumor marker assessments.

10. Although multiple genetic hits are observed in individual tumors, their temporal sequence is yet to be elucidated.

Oral and pharyngeal cancer is the sixth most common neoplasm encountered globally and contributes to a large proportion of upper aerodigestive tract (UADT) and head and neck cancers seen in any specialist unit. This specific site includes cancers of the lip, tongue, mouth, and pharynx. Nasopharynx is excluded from the discussion because it has specific characteristics different from other pharyngeal subsites. Over the last few years, we have begun to understand the molecular basis of the malignant phenotype and some key genes involved in the complex, multistep process of carcinogenesis of the lining squamous epithelium of UADT. While the majority of the studies of interest have specifically involved oral or pharyngeal sites, some publications have used tumor samples from various sites of the head and neck, which carry some biological diversity. Data derived from several of these heterogeneous sites are included in this chapter for comparisons. The molecular variations in oral cancer may reflect the diverse etiology related to ethnic origins and these issues are discussed in the later sections of this chapter.

EPIDEMIOLOGY

Oral and pharyngeal cancers have striking geographic and ethnic variations around the globe. Worldwide, an estimated 306,000 new cases were reported in 1990,[1] about two-thirds of them arising in developing countries. Highest rates are reported in most south Asian countries. In these countries, such as India and Sri Lanka, up to 40 percent of all reported cancers may occur in mouth or pharynx. Outside Asia, the highest rates for oral and pharyngeal cancer are reported for France and Brazil.

In the United States, an estimated 30,200 new cases (20,000 in men and 10,000 in women) of oral cavity and pharyngeal cancers were diagnosed in the year 2000.[2] In terms of frequency of cancer incidence, oral and oropharyngeal sites together rank seventh among black American and twelfth among white Americans. Among blacks, pharyngeal cancer is more common as compared to other oral sites. In the United States, an estimated 7800 (5100 men and 2700 women) died in the year 2000 from cancer at these two sites. For all stages combined, the 5-year survival rate is 53 percent and the 10-year survival rate is 43 percent. Overall the death rates from oral cancer have been decreasing since the early 1980s, but this is confined to white males (probably a reflection of reduction in tobacco smoking) as has been shown for all male cancer deaths in the United States.[3] Rising trends however, are reported among blacks, particularly for pharyngeal cancer, and among all Americans of younger ages (probably linked to increased smokeless tobacco use).[4] Poor survival in black Americans, with an excess mortality of 30 to 40 percent for oropharyngeal cancer has been attributed to lower socioeconomic status, more advanced stage, and differences in treatment, which accounted for 86 percent of excess hazard of death.[5] A comparison of registrations and deaths from UADT cancers from neighboring Canada with data taken from Ontario Cancer Registry against the Surveillance, Epidemiology, and End Results (SEER) Registry of the United States shows a higher incidence in the United States and differences in 5-year survival. These are attributable to much higher incidence of cancer at this site among African Americans.[6]

In the United Kingdom (U.K.), around 3500 people are newly diagnosed with oral and pharyngeal (excluding nasopharynx) cancer each year.[7] The male-to-female ratio is around 2:1 and annual death-to-registration ratio is 0.5. There are marked regional variations within Britain, with high rates reported from Scotland and northern regions of England. Since 1970, several studies have reported rising trends, particularly for tongue cancer, among young adults.[8] These trends are also apparent in many parts of continental Europe[9] and are linked to increased per capita consumption of alcohol in several European countries, including the U.K. Asian ethnic minority communities resident in the U.K. are reported to have a higher incidence of oral cancer as compared to the native population.[10] Oral cancer incidence and mortality is also higher in lower socioeconomic groups.[11]

The Indian subcontinent, its neighboring countries, France, and Brazil are widely recognized as high incidence countries for oral cancer. In most of these populations, the incidence rates approximate 40 per 100,000 per annum. For a long time it was thought that the incidence of oral cancer was decreasing in India, but new evidence suggests oral cancer is now approaching epidemic proportions because of a sharp rise in oral submucous fibrosis in the younger population, a potentially malignant condition attributable to use of manufactured areca products.[12] Special risk factors operate in these individual populations in high-risk countries. The urban/rural and socioeconomic differences in incidence of cancers at this site, as well as the sex and racial variations, are consistent with patterns of recognized risk factors within the community.[13]

Risk Factors

Tobacco and Alcohol. Tobacco consumption and excess alcohol use are the major risk factors for cancers of the oral cavity and pharynx. The risk from these two agents are synergistic and heavy smokers (+40 cigarettes/d) and heavy drinkers (+30 drinks per week) have 38 times the risk of oral cancer that abstainers from both products have.[14] In the United States, the mouth and pharynx attributable fraction for these two factors amounts to approximately 80 percent.[15] For other countries, the attributable ratio is variable. For example, in France alcohol drinking appears to be the major factor and a case series of oral cancer patients in Paris reported drinking on average 80 to 100 drinks per week.[16] While all types of alcohol are implicated, in Brittany, France, apple brandies, and in Brazil, cachaca, distilled from sugarcane,[17] and mate drinking appear to be linked to oral and pharyngeal cancer.

Smokeless Tobacco. Worldwide oral use of smokeless tobacco (ST) takes many forms. In the West, ST is available as oral snuff or in moist pouches. ST is a well-recognized risk factor for oral cancers in the United States [with a relative risk (RR) approaching 50], and "snuff dipper's cancer" is particularly prevalent in the southern states.[18] There is controversy as to the carcinogenicity of Swedish snuff as claimed by Axell[19] based on the low incidence of mouth cancer in Swedish snuff dippers. The most written about is ST use among Asians who use it with betel /areca quid.[20] Addition of ST to the areca quid raises the relative risk of the product by nearly 15 times.[21] Areca nut contributes to the development of a potentially malignant condition known as submucous fibrosis, which is linked to the high copper content in areca.[22] Other ST products that carry significant mutagenicity are toombak in the

Sudan; shamma in the Jizan province of Saudi Arabia; khaini, a mixture of ST and lime, in India; and boiled/sweetened ST, which is called zarda, that is mostly used by people from Bangladesh.[23]

Diet and Nutrition. Protective effect of fruits and fresh vegetables was shown for U.S. populations;[24] serum levels of β carotene was lower in men who later developed oral cancer;[25] and vitamin C is associated with decreased risks.[26] A recent study shows extension of these protective effects of antioxidant micronutrients among Japanese against the development of oral leukoplakia[27] and chemoprevention with β-carotene is reported to result in sustained remissions of oral leukoplakia.[28]

Clinical Aspects

In most case series, the average age at presentation is around 60 years. Most oral cancers are asymptomatic in their earlier stages. As the malignancy progresses, symptoms vary according to the intraoral site. The large majority of symptoms clinically present as exophytic growths and/or as deeply invasive indurated ulcers with everted margins. On occasions, they appear as white or red plaques, clinically indistinguishable from precancer. In practice, a large majority of oral cancers still present very late in their natural history as large lesions, and metastasis to the regional nodes is not uncommon. Blood-borne metastasis is, however, rare. TNM classification is used for staging; the criteria are the same for both Union Internationale Contre le Cancer (UICC) and American Joint Committe on Cancer (AJCC) systems.[29,30] Significant changes in the N criteria have been made in these last editions. Assessment of patients to establish whether neck nodes are positive may need general anaesthesia. Occult metastatic disease can be found in nearly 30 percent of elective N0 neck dissections.[31] Based on the TNM scores, the tumors can be assigned to a stage grouping 0 to IV.

The occurrence of synchronous and metachronous multiple primaries in the UADT can be observed. A second primary tumor (SPT) of the UADT (mouth, pharynx, larynx, upper esophagus), tracheobronchial tree and lung arises, probably as a result of chronic exposure to carcinogens common to these sites particularly tobacco and alcohol. The incidence of SPT in other UADT sites following a primary tumor in the oral, cavity or pharynx is up to 20 percent[32-38] (Table 51-1). In one study between 1985 and 1994, the occurrence of SPT increased from 7 percent to 17 percent for the oral cavity.[38] Panendoscopy for at least 4 years of followup is recommended to detect a SPT,[36] but this remains controversial.[35] Supplementation with β-carotene reduces SPTs.[39]

Despite advances in reconstructive surgery, prognosis has not improved over the past three decades in most of Western Europe,[40] except in very specialized treatment centers. Factors of independent prognostic value include the size of the primary tumor, its estimated depth, and its anterior location within the oral cavity.[41]

Several oral precancerous lesions (leukoplakia and erythroplakia) and conditions (e.g., submucous fibrosis) are recognized; however, their transformation rates vary (1 to 28 percent; average of 4 percent overall) and are not guaranteed to eventually to transform to cancer.[42] However, many oral cancers reported from India and Sri Lanka have a premalignant phase (Fig. 51-1); the proportion of oral cancers preceded by a potentially malignant lesion in Western populations is not well established, and one recent Dutch study[43] suggests as much as 50 percent may arise from a preceeding oral lesion. Detection of any alterations in gatekeeper genes or genomic instability in oral precancers might aid the recognition of those lesions with the highest risk of transformation.

Tumor detection is aided by the use of suitable agents such as toluidine blue (Oratest), particularly in high-risk subjects.[44] Some areas with dysplasia that may be missed by the naked eye are reported to be picked up by the dye and confirmed by biopsy to be dysplasia or frank carcinoma.[44,45] Additional aids to assist diagnosis include computer-assisted screening of mucosal brush biopsies, recently described from a large-scale multicenter study.[46]

Table 51-1 Reported Studies on Second Primary Tumor (SPT) in UADT Following a Primary-Tumor, in Lip, Oral Cavity, or Pharynx

Author	Country	Year	Primary	Cases	Follow up (years)	Any SPT*
Winn & Blot	U.S.	1935–82	Oral	8000	3.4	11%
Soderholm	Finland	1953–89	Lip + Oral	9092		12%
Cianfriglia	Italy	1989–92	Oral	200	3.2	14%
Jovanovic	Netherlands	1971–91	Oral	727	3.9	13%
Van der Tol	Netherlands	1971–91	Lip	56	5.5	17.8%
Ogawa	Japan	1995–98	Oral	25	3	20%
Popella	Germany	1985–94	Oral + OP	467	9	7–20%

*Including all UADT or lung; OP, oropharynx

The sensitivity and specificity of these aids need critical evaluation in various settings.

PATHOLOGY

Cancers of the upper aerodigestive tract arise from the covering or lining mucosa, and in oral and oropharyngeal sites, more than 85 percent are squamous cell carcinomas. Among tobacco chewers however, verrucous carcinomas are increasingly encountered, particularly on the labial mucosa of lips, oral commisures, and vestibular sulci, where the tobacco quid is retained. Verrucous carcinomas show minimal or lack of invasion and spread laterally. Other histologic variants to conventional squamous cell carcino-

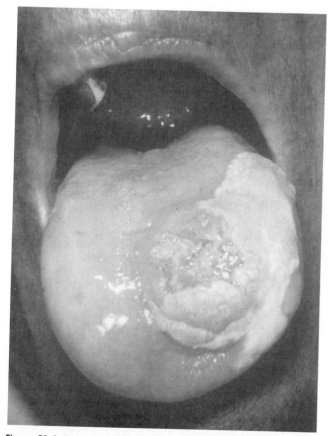

Figure 51-1 Oral carcinoma arising from an extensive white patch on the dorsum of tongue. This white patch (leukoplakia) preceded the development of the tumor and is a component in the natural history of the disease in many Asian subjects. Development of genetic markers will allow these precancer lesions to be screened to assess which may progress and which may not.

mas include spindle cell carcinoma, basaloid squamous cell carcinoma, and papillary squamous carcinoma. Cytokeratins are potentially good tumor markers and assist in the diagnosis of these rare histologic variants, particularly when all other histologic features may be lost in the change to the malignant phenotype.[47–48] Detailed descriptions on histologic patterns are beyond the scope of this chapter and can be found in some excellent texts on oral pathology.[49–50]

Over several decades, grading systems of oral malignant tumors have been devised and improved. Initially reported by Broders,[51] the system that has been in use in routine pathology diagnosis is based on the proportion of differentiated keratinocytes to undifferentiated or anaplastic cells. This allows grading of tumors into well, moderate, and poorly differentiated categories or to distinguish anaplastic SCC. The state of tissue differentiation may also be further examined by the selected use of cytokeratin markers.[48] An evaluation of the down-regulation of K13 and K20, coupled with anomalous expression of simple epithelial keratins K8, K18, and K19, may be useful research tools. The currently favored system for grading oral SCC in investigational pathology was devised by Bryne and colleagues,[52] and this gives a better prognostic indication than the Broders' system. The following five histologic parameters are scored at the worst advancing front, each on a 0 to 4 scale: degree of keratinization, nuclear polymorphism, number of mitosis per high-power field, pattern of invasion, and lymphocytic infiltration within the stroma. A score of 10 or more is considered by Bryne's group as a poor prognostic indicator. The practical difficulties encountered are the heterogeneous cell populations in SCC biopsies and the subjectivity involved in selecting the worst invasive front for scoring. Additional factors to be considered for research evaluations are the depth of invasion or tumor thickness[53] and the measure of angiogenesis.[54] Studies on mode and depth of invasion may be facilitated by examining laminin expression at the basement membrane region of invading tumor fronts,[55] and can be quantified as continuous/linear and for focal loss.[56]

The status of surgical resection margins when reported as clear, close, and uninvolved is useful to determine the need for postoperative radiotherapy.[57] The presence and extent of extracapsular spread of the tumor in desected nodes is prognostic[58] and are recommended for pathologic N staging.[59]

At an experimental level, focal or extensive loss of E-cadherin[60] α_6 and β_4 integrin subunits[61] and the de novo expression of $\alpha v \beta_6$ integrin has been shown to promote the epithelial cell migration associated with tumorigenesis.[62] Dysregulation of CD44 (variant 6)—a cell-surface glycoprotein—occurs, in metastatic cells of oral cancer,[63] but its significance to disease progression at this site is yet to be established.

Familial and Genetic Susceptibility

Despite the clearly defined evidence of the role of environmental risk factors in the development of squamous cell carcinomas of head and neck (SCCHN), there is also a possibility that inherited susceptibility may be operational in some cases. Oral and oropharyngeal cancers rarely feature in rare familial cancer syndromes such as Bloom syndrome and Fanconi anemia. A condition in which oral cancer could develop in children includes dyskeratosis congenita, a rare syndrome in which it has been shown that p53 activation might play a part.[64] Cancer families with a cluster of several affected individuals with oral cancer have been reported.[65,66] Five case-control studies indicate that in four of the studies, a family history of SCCHN is a significant risk factor. Excluding the U.S. study,[67] which reported slightly or nonsignificantly raised ORs, the relative risk of SCCHN in relatives of SCCHN cases in the other studies ranged from 3.4 to 4.3.[68–71] Among subgroups studied, the siblings had the highest risk (RR=14 in one study) and pharyngeal tumors also had a higher risk as compared to other AUDT sites. In cancer families, oral cancer that occurs at a young age and with multiple primary tumors is common. We await the results of a prospective collaborative study on familial SCCHN currently being undertaken in southern England.[72]

Association of oral SCC susceptibility with various genotypic polymorphisms such as cytochrome P450 (CYP1A1) and glutathione-S-transferase (GSTM1), indicating a loss in detoxification of carcinogens and reactive oxygen species, has been reported by several Japanese workers. Katoh and colleagues[73] examined genetic polymorphisms in 92 Japanese subjects with oral SCC and 147 unrelated noncancer controls. The frequency of GSTM1 null genotype was significantly higher in cancers (58.7 percent) as compared with controls (46.3 percent). They concluded that GSTM1 null genotype has a weak correlation with oral cavity cancer but other polymorphisms examined by them had no correlation with oral cancer. Two further studies[74,75] confirmed that those individuals with polymorphisms in GSTM1, as well as CYP1A1, have a genetically high risk of oral cancer, even cigarette smoking frequency was quite low.

Other genetic susceptibilities reported among Japanese subjects included polymorphism of N-acetyltransferase 1 and a finding that NAT1*10 allele had a significantly high relative risk of 5.9 for nonsmokers and 3.1 for smokers.[76]

In a comparative study of African American and white American patients with oral cancer in the United States, GSTM1 null genotype was found to carry a significantly high oral cancer risk among African Americans but not among whites.[77] The lack of significant associations between GSTM genotype and oral cancer risk in whites was further confirmed by a study on GSTM1, GSTM3, GSTT1, and CYP1A1 in 100 British oral cancer subjects matched to 467 control individuals.[78] These authors remarked on a possible mutant allele on CYP2D6 in oral cancer cases, but the significance of this finding is not yet clear as the carcinogen this may detoxify is yet not known.

Genetic polymorphisms of aldehyde dehydrogenase-2, which eliminates acetaldehyde generated during alcohol metabolism, was examined in 901 Japanese male alcoholics,[79] of whom 33 had SCC of AUDT. Seventeen of 33 (51.5 percent) who had SCC of AUDT had the mutant ALDH2*2 allele, and the blood concentration of acetaldehyde in the affected 17 subjects was 6 times greater than in the homozygotes, and in this subset, significantly more multiple primary tumors were found. Inactive ALDH2 is a risk factor for multiple carcinomas of AUDT in Japanese. This is of significance as only about 10 percent of Japanese alcoholics have the ALDH2*2 allele.[80]

Chromosomal Losses and Gains

Allelic imbalance or loss of heterozygosity (LOH) studies by cytogenetic methods, restriction fragment length polymorphism (RFLP), and molecular studies with highly polymorphic microsatellite markers have been used to identify regions on chromosomes that may contain putative tumor suppressor genes in oral, oropharyngeal, and other head and neck cancers. Cytogenetic studies also suggest chromosomal gains, but losses are more common than gains at specific sites.[81] Contrasting findings, that gains of genetic material dominate as compared with losses, were put forward by Wolff and colleagues.[82]

3p. The significance of frequent deletions in the long-arm of chromosome 3 in oral cancer was first highlighted by Partridge and colleagues[83] by using RFLP analysis. LOH in 3p is now recognized as a very common event in oral carcinomas, occurring in approximately 70 percent of all SCC.[84] Moreover, allelic imbalance or LOH in 3p was shown in oral dysplastic mucosa, but not in histologically normal oral mucosa, suggesting this is an early event in the carcinogenesis process.[85] In the precancers deletions of 3p at 3p21.3-22.1 and 3p12.1-13 were most frequent, and increased in frequency when dysplasias recurred, or when SCC developed. 3p deletions thus might serve as a marker to identify lesions that may recur or progress to cancer. The overall results from many investigations is fairly compatible with recent evidence that there are three discrete regions—3p21, 3p24-26, and 3p13-14—recognized as fragile sites showing frequent allelic losses.[86–88] Some of the likely genes residing in these chromosome loci are hMLH1, one of the DNA repair genes; VHL, though the syndrome is not clinically implicated in oral cancer; T β R-II; and FHIT-1. FHIT gene may have a significant involvement in oral SCC. Furthermore, introducing an intact human chromosome 3 into different oral tumorigenic cell lines completely suppressed the tumorigenicity of each cell line, with significant decreases in in vitro growth rate and morphologic changes.[87]

9p. Frequent loss of loci in chromosome 9p in head and neck cancers was reported by a Dutch group.[89] Loss of 9p21-22 is associated with homozygous deletion at p16/CDKN2, observed at a high frequency in many other types of sporadic human tumors.[90] Inactivation of p16/CDKN2 was recently described as a near-universal step in the development of oral and oropharyngeal SCC, and the homozygous deletion of this gene locus is the most common mechanism of its inactivation.[91] By using 24 highly polymorphic markers mapped to chromosome 9, more than half of the informative cases were found to have LOH at 9p21-22.[92] In addition to p15/p16 genes, several other TSG may exist at this focus.

11q. 11q13 amplification provides a selective advantage to many carcinomas and the region amplified is 2.5 to 5 Mb in size. In a meta-analysis of 890 cancers reported from the Netherlands in the head and neck and upper aerodigestive tract sites, amplification of the chromosomal region 11q13 was found in 36 percent of the cases.[93] A slightly lower frequency of 20 percent gene amplification affecting the 11q13 band was reported from France,[94] with some differences in frequency of amplification in the subsites of UADT. In most oral SCC with an 11q13 amplification, cyclin D1—involved in cell-cycle regulation[95]—is overexpressed. Although early studies suggested that amplification was found in less than 15 percent of SCCHN,[96] subsequent work on large panels of SCCHN show that 30 to 50 percent of the tumors may overexpress cyclin D1.[97,98] Amplification of this gene product appears to be associated with poor prognosis.[99] Gene transfer of cyclin D1 to keratinocyte cell lines result in in vitro morphologic transformation.

Assuming that the responsible genes will be overexpressed because of DNA amplification, Schuuring and colleagues,[100] used cDNA-cloning procedures to show another candidate gene, EMS1, which fulfills this criterion in carcinomas with 11q13 amplification. Both cyclin-D1 and EMS1 were coamplified in carcinomas with 11q13 amplification.[101] The EMS1 gene encodes the human cortactin protein, which might mediate the increased metastatic potential of tumors showing 11q13 amplification.

Int-2 gene localized to the chromosomal band 11q13, has also been shown to be amplified up to ~3-fold in SCCHN,[102] and particularly in hypopharyngeal cancers (ninefold amplification shown by Southern blots quantitatively analyzed by densitometry). The hypopharynx has the worst prognosis among head and neck tumors.

While loss of LOH at 3p and 9p correspond to several tumor-suppressor genes and chromosomal gains at 11q13 are striking, a review of literature reveals substantial variations in LOH in other fragile sites, including 1p36 (p58, FRAP,TNF-RII), 8p12 and 8p23, 4q25, 5q21-22 (APS region), 18q, and 21q.[103–110] Some of these loci hint at known putative tumor-suppressor genes (shown in parenthesis) and at others that have not yet been precisely mapped.[103] On the other hand, for the recently described putative tumor-suppressor genes such as DOC-1 mapped to chromosome 12q24,[111] corresponding LOH at this site has not been reported. From presently available evidence, it appears that complex patterns of allelic imbalance occur in primary oral SCC. Frequent loss at 3p21 and 9p21 shown by both early and advanced lesions suggest important critical roles for these losses in the development and progression of SCC at this specific cancer site.[104] In general, these findings point to the existence of multiple tumor-suppressor genes within several of these chromosomal regions.

Specific Genes

ras. Members of the *ras* protooncogene family—*H-ras* (Harvey), *K ras* (Kirsten), and N ras encoding p21 protein with GTPase activity—are frequently activated in a wide range of human malignancies, including adenocarcinoma of pancreas, colon, and lung. Patterson and colleagues[112] reviewed the interesting population (ethnic) differences that have been described with respect to the incidence of ras mutations in oral and head and neck cancer (Table 51-2). Although *ras* mutations in oral and oropharyngeal cancer are rare (< 5 percent in the Western and Japanese populations,[113–121]) among Indian subjects with chewing tobacco-associated oral cancer *ras* mutations are reported to be frequent (35 percent).[122] A subsequent study from Indian samples reported 20 percent to be mutated, with a novel codon 59 mutation of *Ha-ras*.[123] In nontobacco-chewing Taiwanese subjects, 18 percent of oral cancers harbored *Ki ras* mutations linked to areca chewing.[124] These ethnic/cultural differences in the frequency of *ras* mutations is striking, with different environmental factors resulting in a high or low pattern of point mutations in the family of *ras* genes.

p53. Alterations in p53 tumor-suppressor gene constitute one of the most common genetic aberrations in a broad spectrum of human tumors.[125,126] Indeed there is a plethora of publications on p53 alterations in various sites of the head and neck. Reports on p53 mutations in oral and oropharyngeal and other head and neck cancers from various populations in the United States, United Kingdom, France, the Netherlands, Nordic countries, Japan, Taiwan, India, and Sri Lanka indicate a frequency ranging from 39 to 80 percent. Because some studies examine exons 5 to 8 only,[127,128] the spectrum of mutations reported is limited. By using data from the International Agency for Research on Cancer's p53 mutation database (R1), the distribution and nature of p53 mutations in 793 head and neck cancers described in the literature were analyzed. An examination of entries from studies reported on oral, oropharyngeal, and other head and neck cancers does not display distinct mutation patterns for various sites examined (Fig. 51-2). Predominantly, mutations are in exon 8 involving codons 288, 296, and 298,[129] but some studies suggest the presence of hot spots in exon 5 as well.[130] The most frequently reported p53 mutations in oral cancer so far lie in codons 176, 245 to 248, 273, and 296 to 298; some of these correspond to sites reported in lung cancer, but a detailed comparison of mutations of oral and oropharyngeal sites suggest that the pattern of mutations is more complex and different from classical tobacco-associated cancers such as lung, larynx, and the bladder. It would be interesting to further examine whether oral cancers from smokers or alcohol abusers show a distinct, unique, p53 mutation spectrum that is not observed in areca-chewing oral cancer subjects from Asia or nonhabitues.

Base changes observed in oral and oropharyngeal cancer (Table 51-3) are not predominantly the G-T substitutions that are noted, for example, in lung cancer.[131] This observation suggests

Table 51-2 Reported Frequency of Point Mutations in *ras* Oncogenes in Oral, Paraoral, and Head and Neck Malignancies

Reference	Cases (n)	Ha	N	Ki	Remarks
ORAL					
1. Chang et al.	22	—	—	2	Neither associated with 1° oral SCC
2. Warnakulasuriya et al.	48	1	—	—	Tongue SCC (in a nonresident)
3. Howell et al.	11	—	—	1	Ca gingiva
4. Yeudall et al.	06	1	—	—	Ca floor of mouth
	07*	1	—	—	
5. Clark et al.	67	—	—	—	None reported
6. Saranath et al.	57	20	—	—	All 1° oral SCC
7. Munirajan et al.	46	9	—		Novel codon 59 *Ha-ras*
8. Kuo et al.	33	—	—	6	SCC: 5 buccal, 1 tongue
7. Xu et al.	34	—	—	—	No mutations detected
8. Matsuda	20	—	—	1	No p53/p16 alterations in this case of SCC
HEAD & NECK					
9. Rumsby et al.	37	2	—	—	Lip SCC
	8*				Received prior irradiation
10. Kiaris et al.	120	—	—	2	14/26 tumors Overexpressed *Ha-ras*
11. Tadokoro et al.	4*	2	—	—	established from nodal metastases
12. Sheng et al.	54*	2	—	—	1°SCC and nodes

*Cell lines
Studies 6,7, land 8 were in populations from India and Taiwan
Reported *ras* mutations: In Western populations 10/331=3%; India and Taiwan 35/136=26%

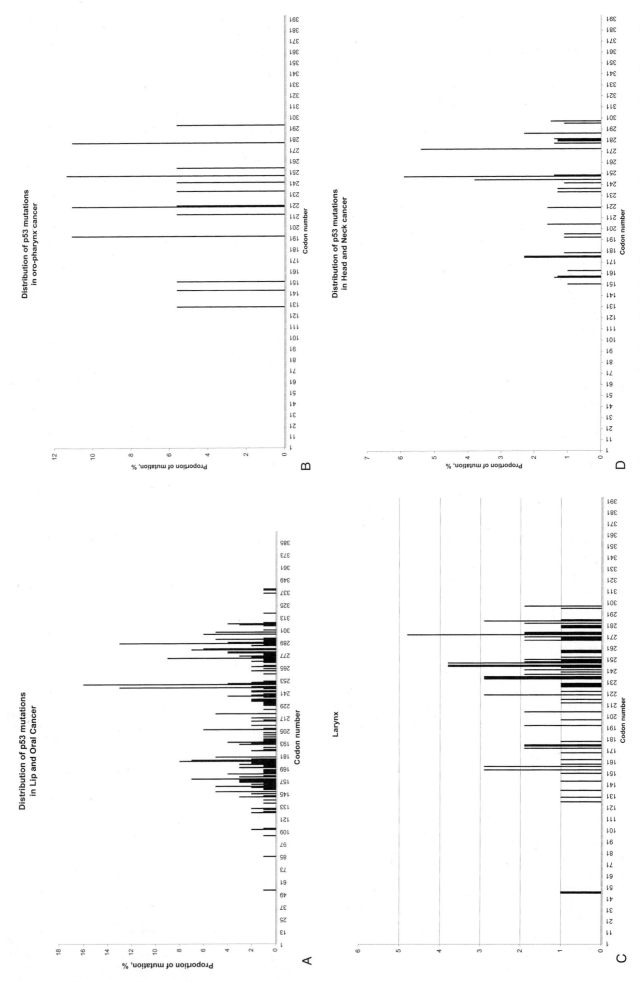

Figure 51-2 Hotspot codons for p53 mutations in oral, oropharyngeal, larynx, and head and neck cancer. For head and neck cancers (n=793) only sites that contain more than 1 percent of a specific mutation are shown.

that the mutagenesis of p53 by metabolism of benzo(a)pyrene occurs in a tissue-specific manner.

p53 mutations can give rise to conformationally related, functionally defective proteins that have a longer half-life than their wild-type form and therefore are detectable by immunohistochemistry. Overexpression of p53 has been found in 40 to 80 percent of head and neck cancers. The overexpression of p53 protein generally reflects a missense mutation (greater than 70 percent in most publications), but lack of concordance between genetic analysis and protein expression has been reported in many studies of oral carcinoma.[130,132] The many reasons for such discrepancies are discussed by Partridge et al.[133] and the explanation based on p53-MDM2 interaction is gaining popularity.[134] It has been apparent since the early 1990s that p53 overexpression is demonstrable in a large proportion of oral carcinomas and in a minority of oral potentially malignant lesions, but we concluded at the onset of these studies that p53 aberration was neither sufficient nor necessary for the development of malignancy.[135]

Most studies demonstrating p53 overexpression of oral cancer have not found a correlation with a diverse range of patient or tumor factors.[137] The exception being Field's group,[137] which reported a correlation between p53 expression and heavy smoking, mutations related to advanced stage and high-grade tongue tumors.[138] Several detailed investigations, including a recent study from our laboratory[139] and others, suggest that p53 overexpression may correlate with poor survival.[140,141] Oral carcinomas have a significantly increased cell proliferation and several key molecules, including p53, may contribute to this altered homeostasis.[142]

p53 overexpression in oral precancers, particularly leukoplakia has been reported with a wide variation and a meta-analysis suggests that p53 can be detected in at least half of these potentially malignant lesions.[143,144] This has lead many authors in the early writings to erroneously conclude that p53 overexpression is an early event in the pathogenesis of oral carcinoma,[145,146] or to suggest a potential use of p53 as a biomarker to assess the risk status of leukoplakia to identify those lesions with an increased risk of converting to the malignant phenotype.[132,140,147] Although overexpression is commonly reported, p53 mutations are uncommon in preinvasive lesions.[148] The exception appears to be erythroplakia lesions,[149] with 46 percent of the cases harboring a p53 mutation, a frequency significantly higher than that reported for leukoplakia. Proliferative verrucous leukoplakia, with a high risk of malignancy that approaches 100 percent, also demonstrated universal presence of p53 protein in all sequential biopsies taken from 10 subjects who all developed carcinoma.[150] Three studies examining sequential biopsies taken over several years with adequate followup information on which precancers transformed or not, report that p53 involvement apparently occurs in the transition from preinvasive to the invasive state,[151–152] and that the presence or absence of p53 staining could not predict the outcome.[153] Based on these observations, p53 cannot be considered a potential biomarker to detect which oral precancers may progress to cancer over time.[154]

Other Cell-Cycle Regulatory Proteins

Dysregulation of several cell-cycle regulatory proteins is apparent in oral SCC. Available evidence on some related cell-cycle proteins—p21, p27, p16, pRb, and cyclins—is reviewed here. At present, available information on MDM2, p130, and p19ARF is meager.

p21. Among many proteins that wild-type p53 may activate,[155] p21 (WAF1/Cip1) protein is thought to be the main downstream effector of p53 that mediates growth arrest following DNA damage.[156] However, several studies point to positive or increased p21 protein expression in oral and head and neck SCC.[157–163] P21 expression in these studies was found in both p53+ and p53− tumors. p21 overexpression has been detected even when the carcinoma revealed a nonsense mutation by molecular analysis.[158]

In a study reported from our laboratory, 14 of 24 oral SCC showed loss of p21 expression, but among these 14 tumors (p21-negative), 8 SCC did not overexpress p53, indicating other mechanisms are involved in switching off this gene. These independent observations taken together suggest that p53-independent pathways of p21 induction. Overexpression of p21 alone appeared to be insufficient to suppress tumor progression in oral SCC.

p27. Reduced p27Kip1 expression is associated with an increase in cell proliferation. p27 protein (with 42 percent homology with p21) is able to inhibit cdk activity, mediating cell-cycle arrest. Data concerning the occurrence of down-regulation of p27 in oral SCC leading to cell-cycle alterations was presented in three reported studies.[160,162,164] The study by Jordan and colleagues[164] demonstrated a reduction in p27Kip1 levels (a score decreasing from 49.6 in normal to a low 28.7 in carcinomas) associated with an increased cell proliferation (a score rising from 16.3 in normal to 51.8 in carcinoma) in oral SCC. Data so far indicate p27 is down-regulated in oral SCC providing an alternative p53-independent mechanism to mediate growth arrest.

p16. Multiple tumor-suppressor gene 1-MTS1 (also called p16, p16INK4, and CDKN) mapped to the region of 9p21 has been found mutated or deleted in a variety of malignancies, including melanomas.[165] In head and neck cancers, p16 is commonly inactivated by homozygous deletions and promoter methylation,[166] and rarely by point mutation. That a minor proportion of oral SCC has p16 gene mutation leading to its inactivation has been shown.[167] Three subsequent studies used Western blotting and immunolocalization and showed an absence of p16 in 63 to 89 percent of the primary oral SCC malignancies.[166,168,169] p16 gene alteration and lack of protein expression is more common in oral SCC cell lines[168,170] than in primary SCC. Data from several laboratories indicate that p16 pathway is a critical target for G1-S checkpoint in oral malignancies.

p16 exhibits its functions of cell-cycle regulation through inhibition of CDK 4-mediated phosphorylation of retinoblastoma protein (pRb110). Phosphorylation of pRb during G1 phase of the cell cycle allows for transcription of G1 to S phase, and thus plays an important role in G1-S check point. Absence of retinoblastoma gene product in oral SCC was first described by Pavelic and colleagues,[171,172] but contradictory results were reported recently.[162] Two studies have examined the interrelationship of p16/pRb in oral carcinoma.[168,169] One study has confirmed that pRb is expressed in about half of oral SCC and that its expression is inversely correlated with p16/MTS1 expression.[168] An association between absence of p16 (89 percent) and detectable pRb (94 percent) proteins has been reported independently.[166]

Cyclins. An increase in dysregulation of cell proliferation plays a role in oral carcinogenesis. The progression of cells through the cell cycle is governed by CDKs, which are activated by binding to cyclin proteins. Passage through G1 to S phase is regulated by the activities of cyclin D and cyclin A. On the other hand, B-type cyclins regulate G2/M transition. Overexpression of cyclin D1 (in conjunction with amplification of the chromosomal region 11q 13) has been shown in at least one-third to nearly one-half of oral and head and neck SCCs,[97,98,166] and in the presence of aberrant expression of cyclin A,[173] this is crucial in the regulation of the G1 to S phase transition. Furthermore, cyclin B1 is also cooperative to cell-cycle dysregulation, particularly in poorly differentiated tumors leading to aberrant cell-cycle progression at the G2/M checkpoint in oral SCC.[173]

Genetic Progression Models in Head and Neck and Oral Cancer

Taking clues from the Feron and Vogelstein model[174] of genetic progression for colon neoplasia, tumors that have a definable natural history progressing from precancer to carcinoma to nodal metastasis can be examined to identify whether the genetic events

Table 51-3 p53 Mutation Types in Oral Cancer and Other AUDT Sites

Type	Lip + Oral	Other pharynx	Nasopharynx	Larynx	Head and neck
AT:CG	5.1	0	0	1.0	1
AT:GC	11.5	10.2	2.63	16.35	16.35
AT:TA	5.4	10.2	5.26	11.54	11.54
GC:AT	**21**	**28.6**	5.26	11.54	11.54
GC:AT at CpG	13.7	14.3	**52.63**	7.69	7.69
GC:CG	8	4	18.42	6.73	6.73
GC:TA	16.6	14.3	0	**25.96**	**25.96**
INS/DEL Complex	18.2	18.4	15.79	18.27	18.27
Other tandem	0.3		0	1	1

occurring during tumorigenesis can be described in a set sequence. To enable such modeling, data from serial biopsies should be obtained following multiple marker studies. In Western countries, the samples available for study from progressing and nonprogressing oral premalignant lesions are rare, particularly because the recognizable high-risk lesions are selectively excised at detection. By using limited molecular information available on head and neck cancers, Califano[104] and Field[175] attempted to illustrate the order of genetic progression at this site. Califano's group[175] restricted their model to loss of chromosomal material, taking into account 9p loss as the earliest detectable genetic event. An essential step in progression from precancer to cancer is described as loss of LOH at 3p and/or at 9p.[176] Several overlapping genetic events are found during initiation and progression in the model presented by Field.[175] It is clear that the sequence of genetic events is still poorly understood and incapable of providing clues to molecular fingerprinting during tumorigenesis at this site. The concept of a gatekeeper gene (see Chap. 13) has yet to be applied to this specific site, although a network of gatekeeper tumor suppressor genes can be speculated. A detailed knowledge of the processes involved and the genetic sequences in malignant transformation, particularly the genes involved in the early stages, will better define the biomarker screening tools for evaluation of oral precancers and high-risk subjects. Knowledge of the complete spectrum of alterations involved in individual tumors and their precursors may be required to provide this clinical information.

Studies that have examined clonal relationships in oral carcinoma by using genetic markers have contradictory results.[177–179] Some studies indicate that multiple lesions arise because of the transfer of the progeny of clonally related altered cells, while other studies point to independent origins of multiple foci that are diverse.[175,180–182] Most studies of head and neck use p53 as the clonal marker, but one cannot exclude the possibility that a tumor may change its p53 mutational profile during progression by acquiring new mutations or by losing mutations originally present.[182]

Serologic Markers

p53 antibodies are found predominantly in human cancer patients with a specificity of 96 percent and a sensitivity of about 30 percent.[183] Few studies have demonstrated p53 in sera of head and neck patients (309/1063=29 percent)[184–186] and recently in sera,[187–188] and in saliva[189,190] of oral carcinoma cases. The clinical significance of p53 as a serum tumor marker remains to be explored, and it is of interest to note that few heavy smokers (4/63) without oral lesions have been detected by enzyme-linked immunosorbent assay (ELISA) to be p53 antibody-positive.[188] Followup studies on the utility of p53 as a serum or saliva marker at this site are awaited.

CYFRA 21-1, a measure of the serum-soluble fragments of cytokeratin 19, is reported to be significantly higher in patients with SCCHN as compared to healthy controls.[191] At a cut-off value of 2.2 ng/mL, this marker has a 95 percent specificity and the sensitivity in 378 UADT SCCs examined was 60 percent, but smaller and earlier stages of SCC showed significantly lower CYFRA levels, reducing its potential diagnostic use.

Viruses and Oral Cancer

Viral infections of the oral epithelium may promote oral carcinogenesis by deactivating tumor-suppressor genes and their products, e.g., p53, up-regulating oncogenes, and increasing the population of cells with genomic damage beyond a certain threshold. Human papillomavirus (HPV 16 and 18) has been studied extensively in oral carcinoma with contradictory results; prevalence of HPV varying from 0 to 100 percent has been reported.[192,193] It is possible that the low copy number of HPV-infected cells desires highly sensitive detection methods and to answer this application of nested PCR using two sets of HPV consensus primers yielded a prevalence of 50 percent.[194] Multicentric studies are in progress to account for population differences and for interlaboratory variations in HPV detection. Another virus that has received attention is Epstein-Barr virus (EBV), again found in healthy oral mucosa.[195] The oral lesion referred to as hairy leukoplakia ascribed to EBV infection commonly found in HIV seropositive subjects is not known to transform to malignancy.

SUMMARY

Exogenous mutagens, such as smoked or chewed tobacco, alcohol, and some viral oncogenes, play a major role in the pathogenesis of multiple genetic changes in the lining epithelium of the UADT. Variations in activity of metabolizing enzymes and DNA repair competence among individuals can contribute to susceptibility. Over the past decade, the key genetic abnormalities in oral and pharyngeal SCC and some of their precursors have been mapped. Some genomic sites seemingly are nonrandomly involved in the genesis of cancers in these specific sites. With potential precursor lesions as targets, this basic and translational research should provide ways for early detection and to monitor treatment. Despite progress from numerous studies of p53 protein expression and p53 gene mutations, and the downstream molecules that control cell proliferation and cell death, much remains unknown about the early events in the natural history. This is likely a result of independent and mutually exclusive genetic pathways that cascade the multistep process of carcinogenesis that trigger the involution of tumor cells.

ACKNOWLEDGMENTS

I wish to acknowledge my colleagues C. Trevedy, M. Tavassoli, N. Johnson, and M. Partridge for the many years of collaborative research and academic activity from which I have gained enormous benefits, and which have enriched this review. I wish to thank Magali Oliver at the p53 database IARC, Lyon, France, for allowing me access to their user-friendly databases.

REFERENCES

1. Parkin DM, Pisani P, Ferlay J: Estimates of the worldwide incidence of twenty-five major cancers in 1990. *Int J Cancer* **80**:827, 1999.
2. American Cancer Society: Oral cavity and oropharyngeal resource Center. http://www3cancer.org. 2000
3. Greenlee RT, Murray T, Bolden S, Wingo PA: Cancer statistics, 2000. *CA Cancer J Clin* **50**:7, 2000.
4. Davies S, Severson RK: Increasing incidence of cancer of the tongue in the United States among young adults. *Lancet* **2**:910, 1987.
5. Arbes SJ Jr, Olshan AF, Caplan DJ, Schoenbach VJ, Slade GD, Symons MJ: Factors contributing to the poorer survival of black Americans diagnosed with oral cancer (United States). *Cancer Causes Control* **10**:513, 1999.

6. Skarsgard DP, Groome PA, Mackillop WJ, Zhou S, Rothwell D, Dixon PF, O'Sullivan B, Hall SF, Holwaty EJ: Cancers of the upper aerodigestive tract in Ontario, Canada, and the United States. *Cancer* **88**:1728, 2000.

7. Cancer Research Campaign. Oral Cancer in UK. *Factsheet* **14**, 2000

8. Johnson NW, Warnakulasuriya KAAS: Epidemiology and etiology of oral cancer in the United Kingdom. *Comm Dent Health* **10(Suppl 1)**:13, 1993.

9. La Vecchia C, Tavani A, Franceschi S, Levi F, Corrao G, Negri E: Epidemiology and prevention of oral cancer. *Eur J Cancer (Oral Oncology)* **33**:302, 1997.

10. Warnakulasuriya KAAS, Johnson NW, Linklater KM, Bell J: Cancer of mouth, pharynx and nasopharynx in Asian and Chinese immigrant residents in Thames regions. *Eur J Cancer* **35B**:471, 1999.

11. Edwards D, Johnson NW: Treatment of upper aerodigestive tract cancers in England and its effects on survival. *Br J Cancer* **81**:323, 1999.

12. Gupta PC: Mouth cancer in India: A new epidemic? *J Indian Med Assoc* **97**:370, 1999.

13. Blot WJ, McLaughlin JK, Devesa SS, Fraumeni JF. Cancer of the oral cavity and pharynx, in Schottenfeld D, Fraumeni JF Jr (eds): *Cancer Epidemiology and Prevention.* Oxford, England, Oxford University Press, 1996 p. 666.

14. Blot WJ: Alcohol and cancer. *Cancer Res (Suppl)* **52**:2119, 1992.

15. Thomas DB: Alcohol as a cause of cancer. *Environ Health Perspect* **103(Suppl 8)**:153, 1995.

16. Brugere LA, Guenel P, Leclerc A et al: Differential effects of tobacco and alcohol in cancer of the larynx, pharynx and the mouth. *Cancer* **57**:391, 1986.

17. Franco EL, Kowalski LP, Oliveira BV et al: Risk factors for oral cancer in Brazil: A case-control study. *Int J Cancer* **43**:992, 1989.

18. Winn DM, Blot WJ, Fraumeni JF Jr: Snuff dipping and oral cancer. *N Engl J Med* **305**:230, 1981.

19. Axell T: Oral mucosal changes related to smokeless tobacco usage: Research findings in Scandinavia. *Eur J Cancer* **29B**:299, 1993.

20. Zain RB, Ikeda N, Gupta PC, Warnakulasuriya S, van Wyk CW, Shrestha P, Axell T: Oral mucosal lesions associated with betel quid, areca nut and tobacco chewing habits: Consensus from a workshop held in Kuala Lumpur, Malaysia, November 25–27, 1996. *J Oral Med Pathol* **28**:1, 1999.

21. Warnakulasuriya S: Analytical studies of the evaluation of the role of betel-quid in oral carcinogenesis, in Bedi R (ed): *Betel Quid and Tobacco Chewing: Usage and Health Issues,* London, Transcultural Health, 1994, p.61

22. Trivedy C, Baldwin D, Warnakulasuriya S, Johnson NW, Peters T: Copper content in Areca catechu (betel nut) products in oral submucous fibrosis. *Lancet* **349**:1447, 1997.

23. International Agency Research on Cancer: *Evaluation of the Carcinogenic Risk of Chemicals to Humans,* Monograph vol 37. Lyon, France, IARC, 1985.

24. McLauughlin JK, Gridley G, Block G et al: Dietary factors in oral and pharyngeal cancer. *J Natl Cancer Inst* **80**:1237, 1988.

25. Zheng W, Blot WJ, Diamond EL: Serum micronutrients and subsequent risk of oral and pharyngeal cancer. *Cancer Res* **53**:795, 1993.

26. Rossing MA, Vaughan TL, McKnight B: Diet and pharyngeal cancer. *Int J Cancer* **44**:593, 1989.

27. Nagao T, Ikeda N, Warnakulasuriya S: Serum antioxident micronutrients and the risk of oral leukoplakia. *Eur J Cancer* **368**:466, 2000.

28. Garewal HS, Katz RV, Meyskens F, Pitcock J, Morse D, Friedman S, Peng Y, Pendrys DG, Mayne S, Alberts D, Kiersch T, Graver E: Beta-carotene produces sustained remissions in patients with oral leukoplakia: Results of a multicenter prospective trial. *Arch Otolaryngeal Head Neck Surg* **125**:1305, 1999.

29. Sobin LH, Wittekind C (eds): *UICC TNM Classification of Malignant Tumours.* New York, John Wiley, 1997.

30. *American Joint Committee on Cancer. Manual for Staging of Cancer.* Philadelphia, Lippincott, 1997.

31. O'Brien CJ, Traynor SJ, McNeil E, McMahon JD, Chaplin JM: The use of clinical criteria alone in the management of the clinically negative neck among patients with squamous cell carcinoma of the oral cavity and oropharynx. *Arch Otolaryngol Head Neck Surg* **126**:360, 2000.

32. Winn DM, Blot WJ: Second cancer following cancers of the buccal cavity and pharynx in Connecticut, 1935–81. *Natl Cancer Inst Monogr* **68**:23, 1985.

33. Cianfriglia F, Di Gregoria DA, Manieri A: Multiple primary tumours in patients with oral SCC. *Oral Oncol* **35**:157, 1999.

34. Soderholm AL, Pukkala E, Lindqvist C, Teppo L: Risk of new primary cancer in patients with oropharyngeal cancer. *Br J Cancer* **69**:784, 1994.

35. Jovanovic A, van der Tol IGH, Schulten EAJM, Kostense PJ, de Vries N, Snow GB, van der Wall I: Risk of multiple primary tumours following oral squamous cell carcinoma. *Int J Cancer* **56**:320, 1994.

36. Ogawa T, Matsuura K, Hashimoto S, Nakano H, Sasaki H, Suzaki T, Kondo Y, Tateda M, Hozawa K, Takasaka T: Multiple primary cancers of oral cavity and pharynx. *Nippon Jibiinkoka Gakki Kaiho* **102**:1198, 1999.

37. Van der Tol IG, de Visscher JG, Jovanovic A, van der Waal I: Risk of second primary cancer following treatment of squamous cell carcinoma of the lower lip. *Eur J Cancer* **35B**:571, 1999.

38. Popella C, Bodeker R, Glanz H, Kohl S: Multiple carcinomas in the upper aerodigestive tract. 1. Oral cavity and oropharynx. *Laryngorhinootologie* **78**:671, 1999.

39. Hong WK, Lippman SM, Itri L: Prevention of second primary tumors with isotretinoin in squamous cell carcinoma of the head and neck. *N Engl J Med* **323**:795, 1990.

40. Berrino F, Sant M, Verdecchia R, Capocaccia R, Hakulimen T, Esteve J: Survival of oral cancer patients in Europe: The EUROCARE study. *IARC Sci Publ* **132**, 1995.

41. DOSAK. Prognoses of Oral Cavity Carcinomas. Munchen, Hanser 1986. p. 70.

42. Van der Wall I, Schepman KP, Meij van der EH, Smeele LE: Oral leukoplakia: A clinicopathological review. *Eur J Cancer* **33B**:291, 1997.

43. Schepman KP, van der Meij EH, Smeele LE, van der Wall I. Malignant transformation of oral leukoplakia: A follow-up study of a hospital-based population of 166 patients with oral leukoplakia from the Netherlands. *Eur J Cancer* **34B**:270, 1999.

44. Warnakulasuriya KAAS, Johnson NW: Sensitivity and specificity of OraScan toluidine blue mouthrinse in the detection of oral cancer and precancer. *J Oral Pathol Med* **25**:97, 1996.

45. Vacher C, Legens M, Rueff B, Lezy JP: Screening of cancerous and precancerous lesions of the oral mucosa in an at-risk population. *Rev Stomatol Chir Maxillofac* **100**:180, 1999.

46. Sciubba JJ. Improving detection of precancerous and cancerous oral lesions. Computer-assisted analysis of the oral brush biopsy. *J Am Dental Assoc* **130**:1445, 1999.

47. Morgan PR, Leigh Im, Purkis PE, Gardner ID, vanMuijen GNP, Lane EB: Site variation of keratin expression in human oral epithelia; an immunohistochemical study of individual keratins. *Epithelia* **1**:31, 1987.

48. Ogden GR: Cytokeratins as tumour markers. *Oral Dis* **6**:57, 2000.

49. Odell EW, Morgan PR: *Biopsy Pathology of the Oral Tissues.* London, Chapman and Hall, p. 214.

50. Cawson RA, Binnie, Speight PM, Barrett AW, Wright JM: *Lucas's Pathology of Tumours of the Oral Tissues.* London, Churchill Livingstone, 1998.

51. Broders AC: The microscopic grading of cancer. *Surg Clin North Am* **21**:947, 1941.

52. Bryne M, Koopang HS, Lilleng R, Stene T, Bang G, Dabelsteen E: New malignancy grading is a better prognostic indicator than Broders' grading in oral squamous cell carcinomas. *J Oral Pathol Med* **18**:432, 1989.

53. Onercl M, Yilmaz T, Gedikoglu G: Tumour thickness as a predictor of cervical lymph node metastasis in squamous cell carcinoma of the lower lip. *Otolaryngol Head Neck Surg* **122**:139, 2000.

54. Zatterstrom UK: Angiogenesis in squamous cell carcinoma of head and neck. *Oral Dis* **6**:61, 2000.

55. Haas M, Berndt A, Hyckel P, Stiller KJ, Kosmehl H: Laminin-5 in diseases of the oral cavity. *Mund Kiefer Gesichtschir* **4**:25, 2000.

56. Noguchi M, Kohama G, Hiratsuka H, Sekiguchi T: Clinical significance of laminin deposition and T-cell infiltration in oral cancer. *Head Neck* **15**:125, 1993.

57. Woolgar JA, Rogers S, West CR, Errington RD, Brown JS, Vaughan ED: Survival and patterns of recurrence in 200 oral cancer patients treated by radical surgery and neck dissection. *Eur J Cancer* **35B**:257, 1999.

58. Woolgar JA, Scott J, Vaughan ED, Brown JS, West CR, Rogers S: Survival, metastasis and recurrence of oral cancer in relation to pathological features. *Ann R Coll Surg Engl* **77**:325, 1995.

59. Helliwell TR, Woolgar JA: Minimum dataset for head and neck carcinoma histopathology reports. *The R Coll Pathol* Nov 1998, London, RCP.

60. Downer CS, Speight PM: E-cadherin expression in normal, hyperplastic and malignant oral epithelium. *Eur J Cancer* **29B**:303, 1993.

61. Downer CS, Watt FM, Speight PM: Loss of α6 and β4 integrin subunits coincides with loss of basement membrane components in oral squamous cell carcinoma. *J Pathol* **171**:183, 1993.

62. Speight PM, Poomsawat S, Thomas GJ: The role and regulation of integrins in oral cancer. *Oral Dis* **6**:59, 2000.

63. Bahar R, Kunishi M, Kayada K, Yoshiga K: CD 44 variant 6 (CD44v6) expression as a progression marker in benign, premalignant and malignant oral epithelial tissues. *Int J Oral Maxillofac Surg* **26**:443, 1997.

64. Ogden GR: Dyskeratosis congenita: report of a case and review of literature. *Oral Surg Oral Med Oral Pathol Oral Radio Endod* **65**:586, 1988.

65. Hara H, Ozeki S, Shiratsuchi Y, et al: Familial occurance of oral cancer: Reported cases. *J Oral Maxillofac Surg* **46**:1098, 1988

66. Ankanthil R, Mathew A, Joseph F: Is oral cancer susceptibility inherited? *Eur J Cancer* **32B**:63, 1996.

67. Goldstein A, Blot W, Greenberg R: Familial risk in oral and pharyngeal cancer. *Eur J Cancer* **30B**:319, 1994.

68. Cooper M, Jovanic A, Nauta J: Role of genetic factors in the aetiology of squamous cell carcinoma of the head and neck. *Arch Otolaryngol Head Neck Surg* **121**:157, 1995.

69. Foulkes WD, Brunet J-S, Kowalski LP: Family history is a risk factor for squamous cell carcinoma of the head and neck in Brazil: A case-control study. *Int J Cancer* **63**:769, 1995.

70. Foulkes WD, Brunet J-S, Sieh W, Black MJ, Shenouda G, Narod SA: Familial risk of squamous cell carcinoma a retrospective case-control study. *BMJ* **313**:716, 1996.

71. Mork J, Moller B, Glattre E: Familial risk in head and neck squamous cell carcinoma diagnosed before the age of 45: A population-based study. *Eur J Cancer* **35B**:360, 1999.

72. Jefferies S, Eeles R, Goldgar D, A'Hern RA, Henk JM, Gore M: The role of genetic factors in predisposition to squamous cell cancer of the head and neck. *Br J Cancer* **79**:865, 1999.

73. Katoh T, Kaneko S, Kohshi K, Munaka M, Kitagawa K, Kunugita N, Ikemura K, Kawamoto T: Genetic polymorphisms of tobacco-and alcohol-related metabolizing enzymes and oral cavity cancer. *Int J Cancer* **26**:83, 1999.

74. Sato M, Sato T, Izumo T, Amagasa T: Genetic polymorphism of drug-metabolizing enzymes and susceptibility to oral cancer. *Carcinogenesis* **20**:1927, 1999.

75. Tanimoto K, Hayashi S, Yoshiga K, Ichikawa T: Polymorphisms of CYP1A1 and GSTM1 gene involved in oral squamous cell carcinoma in association with cigarette dosage. *Eur J Cancer* **35B**:191, 1999.

76. Katoh T, Kaneko S, Boissy R, Watson M, Ikemura K, Bell DA: A pilot study testing the association between *N*-acetyltransferases 1 and 2 and risk of oral squamous cell carcinoma in Japanese people. *Carcinogenesis* **19**:10, 1998.

77. Park LY, Muscat JE, Kaur T, Schantz SP, Stern JC, Richie JP Jr, Lazarus P: Comparison of GSTM polymorphisms and risk for oral cancer between African-Americans and Caucasians. *Pharmacogenetics* **10**:123, 2000.

78. Worrall SF, Corrigan M, High A, Starr D, Matthias C, Wolf CR, Jones PW, Hand P, Gilford J, Farrell WE, Hoben P, Fryer AA, Strane RC: Susceptibility and outcome in oral cancer: Preliminary data showing an association with polymorphism in cytochrome P450 CYP2D6. *Pharmacogenetics* **8**:433, 1998.

79. Yokoyama A, Muramatsu T, Ohmori T, Makuuchi H, Higuchi S, Matsushita S, Yohino K, Maruyama K, Nakano M, Ishii H: Multiple primary esophageal and concurrent upper aerodigestive tract cancer and the aldehyde dehydrogenase-2 genotype of Japanese alcoholics. *Cancer* **77**:1986, 1996.

80. Higuchi S, Matsushita S, Imazeki H, Kinoshita T, Takagi S, Kono H: Aldehyde dehydrogenase genotypes in Japanese alcoholics. *Lancet* **343**:741, 1994.

81. Wennerberg J, Mertens F, Jin Y, Akervall J: Chromosomal abnormalities in squamous cell carcinoma of the head and neck. *Oral Dis* **6**:51, 2000.

82. Wolff E, Girod S, Liehr T, Vorderwulbecke U, Ries J, Steininger H, Gebhart E: Oral squamous cell carcinomas are characterised by a rather uniform pattern of genomic imbalances detected by comparative genomic hybridisation. *Eur J Cancer* **34B**:186, 1998.

83. Partridge M, Kiguwa S, Langdon JD: Frequent deletion of chromosome 3p in oral squamous cell carcinoma. *Eur J Cancer* **30B**:248, 1994.

84. Partridge M, Warnakulasuriya S: The biology of cancer, in Ward Booth P, Schendel SA, Hausamen J-E (eds)*Maxillofacial Surgery*. Edinburgh, Churchill Livingstone, 1999, p. 309.

85. Emilion G, Langdon JD, Speight P, Partridge M: Frequent gene deletions in potentially malignant oral lesions. *Br J Cancer* **73**:809, 1996.

86. Wu Cl, Sloan P, Read AP, Harris RH, Thakker NS: Deletion mapping on the short arm of chromosome 3 in oral squamous cell carcinoma of the oral cavity. *Cancer Res* **54**:6484, 1994.

87. Uzawa N, Yoshida MA, Hosoe S, Hosimura M, Amagasa T, Ikeuchi T: Functional evidence for involvement of multiple putative tumour suppressor genes on the short arm of chromosome 3 in the human oral squamous cell carcinogenesis. *Cancer Genet Cytogenet* **107**:125, 1998.

88. Partridge M, Emilion G, Lalworth M, A'Hern R, Phillips E, Pateromichelakis S, Langdon J: Patient-specific mutation databases for oral cancer. *Int J Cancer* **84**:284, 1999.

89. Reit van der P, Nawroz H, Hruban RH, et al: Frequent loss of chromosome 9p21-22 in head and cancer progression. *Cancer Res* **54**:1156, 1994.

90. Cairns P, Polascik T, Eby Y, et al: Frequency of homozygous deletion at p16/CDKN2 in primary human tumours. *Nat Genet* **11**:210, 1995.

91. Wu CL, Roz L, McKown S, Sloan P, Read AP, Holland S, Porter S, Scully C, Paterson I, Tavassoli M, Thakker N: DNA studies underestimate the major role of CDKN2A inactivation in oral and orophyngeal squamous cell carcinomas. *Genes Chromosomes Cancer* **25**:16, 1999.

92. Nakanishi H, Wang XL, Imai FL, Kato J, Shiiba M, Miya T, Imai Y, Tanzawa H: Localization of a novel tumor suppressor gene loci on chromosome 9p21-22 in oral cancer. *Anticancer Res* **19**:29, 1999.

93. Schuuring E: The involvement of the chromosome 11q 13 region in human malignancies: *cyclin D1* and *EMS1* are two new candidate oncogenes—review. *Gene* **59**:83, 1995.

94. Fortin A, Guerry M, Guerry R, Talbot M, Parise O, Schwaab G, Bosq J, Bourhis J, Salvatori P, Janot F, Busson P: Chromosome 11q13 gene amplifications in oral and oropharyngeal carcinomas: no correlation with subclinical lymph node invasion and disease recurrence. *Clin Cancer Res* **3**:1609, 1997.

95. Hall M, Peters G: Genetic alterations of cyclins, cyclin-dependent kinases, and Cdk inhibitors in human cancer. *Adv Cancer Res* **68**:67, 1996.

96. Akervall J, Jin Y-S, Zatterstrom U, et al: Chromosome abnormalities involving 11q13 are associated with poor prognosis in squamous cell carcinoma of the head and neck. *Cancer* **76**:853, 1995.

97. Bartkova J, Lukas J, Muller H, Strauss, Gusterson B, Bartek J: Abnormal patterns of D-type cyclin expression and G1 regulation in human head and neck cancer. *Cancer Res* **55**:949, 1995.

98. Michalides RJAM, van Vee NMJ, Kristel PMP, Hart AAM, Loftus BM, Hilgers FJM, Balm AJM: Overexpression of cyclin D1 indicates a poor prognosis in squamous cell carcinoma of the head and neck. *Arch Otolaryngeal Head Neck Surg* **123**:497, 1997.

99. Akervall JA, Michalides RJAM, Mineta H, et al: Amplification of *cyclin D1* in squamous cell carcinoma of the head and neck and the prognostic value of chromosomal abnormalities and cyclin D1 expression. *Cancer* **79**:380, 1997.

100. Schuuring E, Verhoeven E, Mooi WJ: Identification and cloning of two overexpressed genes, *U21B31/PRAD1* and *EMS1*, within the amplified chromosome 11q13 region in human carcinomas. *Cancer Res* **52**:5229, 1992.

101. Van Rossum A, van Damme, Scurring-Scholtes W, de Graaf J, Brok H, van Buuren V, Vaandrager JW, Verheijen M, Takes R, Baatenburg-de Jong R, van Krieken J, Kluin PM, Schuuring E: The role of amplified chromosome 11q13 gene, *EMS1/Cortactin*, in head and neck carcinomas. *Oral Dis* **6**:52, 2000.

102. Somers KD, Cartwright SL, Schechter GL: Amplification of the *int-2* gene in human head and neck squamous cell carcinomas. *Oncogene* **5**:915, 1990.

103. Grafti FR, Sirchia SM, Garagiola I, Sironi E, Galioto S, Rossella F, Serafini P, Dulcetti F, Bozzetti A, Brusati R, Simoni G: Losses of heterozygosity in oral and oropharyngeal epithelial carcinomas. *Cancer Genet Cytogenet* **118**:57, 2000.

104. Califano J, van der Riet P, Westra W, Nawroz H, Clayman G, Piantadosi S, Corio R, Lee D, Greenberg B, Koch W, Sidransky D: Genetic progression model for head and neck cancer: Implications for field cancerization. *Cancer Res* **56**:2488, 1996.

105. Kimura T: Studies on deletion of 1p36 in oral squamous cell carcinoma. *Nippon Jibiinkoka Gakkai Kaiho* **101**:1430, 1998.

106. Ishward CS, Shuster M, Bockmuhl U, Thakker N, Shah P, Toomes C, D Re, Gollin SM: Frequent allelic loss and homozygous deletion in chromosome 8p in oral cancer. *Int J Cancer* **80**:25, 1999.

107. Sunwoo JB, Sun PC, Gupta VK, Schmidt AP, El-Mofty S, Schlnick SB: Localization of a putative tumor suppressor gene in the sub-telomeric region of chromosome 8p. *Oncogene* **18**:2651, 1999.

108. Wang XL, Uzawa K, Imai FL, Tazawa H: Localization of a novel tumour suppressor gene associated with cancer on chromosome 4q25. *Oncogene* **18**:823, 1999.

109. Mao EJ, Schwartz SM, Daling JR, Beckmann AM: Loss of heterozygosity at 5q21-22 (adenomatous polyposis coli gene region) in oral squamous cell carcinoma is common and correlated with advanced disease. *J Oral Pathol Med* **27**:297, 1998.

110. Yamamoto N, Uzawa K, Miya T, Watanabe T, Yokoe H, Shibahara T, Noma H, Tanzawa H: Frequent allelic loss/imbalance on the long arm of chromosome 21 in oral cancer: Evidence for three discrete tumour suppressor gene loci. *Oncol Rep* **6**:1223, 1999.

111. Tsuji T, Duh FM, Latif F, Popescu NC, Zimonjic DB, McBride J, Matsuo K, Ohyama H, Todd R, Nagata E, Terakado N, Sasaki A, Matsumura T, Lerman MI, Wong DT: Cloning, mapping, expression, function, and maturation analyses of the human ortholog of the hamster putative tumor suppressor gene DOC-1. *J Biol Chem* **273**:6704, 1998.

112. Paterson IC, Eveson JW, Prime SS: Molecular changes in oral cancer may reflect aetiology and ethnic origin. *Eur J Cancer* **32B**:150, 1996.

113. Rumsby G, Carter RL, Gusterson BA: Low incidence of *ras* oncogene activation in human squamous cell carcinomas. *Br J Cancer* **61**:365, 1990.

114. Howell RE, Wong FSH, Fenwick RG: Activated *Kirsten ras* oncogene in an oral squamous cell carcinoma. *J Oral Pathol Med* **19**:301, 1990.

115. Chang SE, Bhatia P, Johnson NW, Morgan P, McCormick F, Young B, Hiorns L: *Ras* mutations in United Kingdom examples of oral malignancies are infrequent. *Int J Cancer* **48**:409, 1991.

116. Warnakulasuriya KAAS, Chang SE, Johnson NW: Point mutations in the *Ha-ras* oncogene are detectable in formalin-fixed tissues of oral squamous cell carcinomas, but are infrequent in British cases. *J Oral Pathol Med* **21**:225, 1992.

117. Yeudall WA, Torrance LK, Elsegood KA, Speight P, Scully C, Prime SS: *Ras* gene point mutation is a rare event in premalignant and malignant cells and tissues from oral mucosal lesions. *Eur J Cancer* **29B**:63, 1993.

118. Clark LJ, Edington K, Swan IR, Mclay KA, Newlands WJ, Wills LC, Young HA, Johnston PW, Mitchell R, Robertson G: The absence of Harvey *ras* mutations during development and progression of squamous cell carcinomas of the head and neck. *Br J Cancer* **68**:617, 1993.

119. Kiaris H, Spandidos DA, Jones AS, Vaughan ED, Field JK: Mutations, expression and genomic instability of the H-ras proto-oncogene in squamous cell carcinomas of the head and neck. *Br J Cancer* **72**:123, 1995.

120. Xu J, Gimenez-Conti IB, Cunningham JE, Collet AM, Luna MA, Lanfranchi HE, Spitz MR, Conti CJ: Alterations of p53, cyclin D1, Rb and H-ras in human oral carcinomas related to tobacco use. *Cancer* **83**:204, 1998.

121. Matsuda H, Konishi N, Hiasa Y, Hayashi I, Tsuzuki T, Tao M, Kitahori Y, Yoshioka N, Kirita T, Sugimura M: Alterations of p16/CDKN2, p53 and ras genes in oral squamous cell carcinomas and premalignant lesions. *J Oral Pathol Med* **25**:232, 1996.

122. Saranath D, Chang SE, Bhotie LT, Panchal RG, Kerr IB, Mehta AR, Johnson NW, Deo MG: High frequency mutation in codons 12 and 61 of H-ras oncogene in chewing tobacco-related human oral carcinoma in India. *Br J Cancer* **63**:573, 1991.

123. Munirajan AK, Mohanprasad BK, Shanmugam G, Tsuchida N: Detection of a rare point mutation at codon 59 and relatively high incidence of H-ras mutation in Indian oral cancer. *Int J Oncol* **13**:971, 1998.

124. Kuo MYP, Jeng FH, Chiang CP, Hahn LJ: Mutations of Ki-ras oncogene codon 12 in betel quid chewing-related human oral squamous cell carcinoma in Taiwan. *J Oral Pathol Med* **23**:70, 1994.

125. Harris CC: The 1995 Walter Hubert Lecture—molecular epidemiology of human cancer: Insight from mutational analysis of the p53 tumour-suppressor gene. *Br J Cancer* **73**:261, 1996.

126. Hussain SP, Harris CC: Molecular epidemiology of human cancer: Contributions of mutational spectra studies of tumor suppressor genes. *Cancer Res* **58**:4023, 1998.

127. Ranasinghe AW, Macgeoch C, Dyer S, Spurr N, Johnson NW: Some carcinomas from Sri Lankan betel/tobacco chewers overexpress p53 oncoprotein but lack mutations in exons 5-9. *Anticancer Res* **13**:2065, 1993.

128. Kuo MY, Huang JS, Hsu HC, Chiang CP, Kok SH, Kuo YS, Hong CY: Infrequent p53 mutations in patients with areca quid chewing-associated oral squamous cell carcinomas in Taiwan. *J Oral Pathol Med* **28**:221, 1999.

129. El-Naggar AD, Lai S, Luna MA, Zhou X-D, Weber RS, Goepfert H, Batsakis JG: Sequential p53 mutation analysis of preinvasive and invasive head and neck squamous cell carcinoma. *Int J Cancer* **64**:196, 1995.

130. Penhallow J, Steingrimsdottir H, Elamin F, Warnakulasuriya S, Farzaneh F, Johnson NW, Tavassoli M: p53 alterations and HPV infections are common in oral SCC: p53 gene mutations correlate with the absence of HP16-E6 DNA. *Int J Oncol* **12**:59, 1998.

131. Hainaut P, Hollstein M: p53 and human cancer: The first ten thousand mutations. *Adv Cancer Res* **77**:81, 2000.

132. Saranath D, Tandle AT, Teni TR, Dedhia PM, Borges AM, Parikh D, Sanghavi V, Mehta AR: p53 inactivation in chewing tobacco-induced oral cancers and leukoplakias from India. *Eur J Cancer* **35B**:242, 1999.

133. Partridge M, Kiguwa S, Emilion G, Pateromichelakis S, A'Hern R, Langdon JD: New insights into p53 protein stabilization in oral squamous cell carcinoma. *Eur J Cancer* **35B**:45, 1999.

134. Lane DP, Hall PA: MDM2-arbiter of p53's destruction. *Trends Biochem Sci* **22**:372, 1997.

135. Warnakulasuriya KAAS, Johnson NW: Expression of p53 mutant nuclear phosphoprotein in oral carcinoma and potentially malignant oral lesions. *J Oral Pathol Med* **21**:404, 1992.

136. Raybaud-Diogene H, Tetu B, Morency R, Fortin A, Monteil RA: p53 overexpression in head and neck squamous cell carcinoma: review of the literature. *Eur J Cancer* **32B**:143, 1996.

137. Field JK, Spandidos DA, Maliri A, Yiagnisis M, Gosney JR, Stell PM: Elevated p53 expression correlates with a history of heavy smoking in squamous cell carcinoma of the head and neck. *Br J Cancer* **64**:573, 1991.

138. Atula S, Kurvinen K, Grenman R, Syrjanen S: SSCP pattern indicative for p53 mutation is related to advanced stage and high grade of tongue cancer. *Eur J Cancer* **32B**:222, 1996.

139. Warnakulasuriya S, Jia C, Johnson NW, Houghton J: p53 and p glycoprotein expression are significant prognostic markers in advanced head and neck cancer treated with chemo/radiotherapy. *J Pathol* **191**:33, 2000.

140. Kaur J, Srivastava A, Ralhan R: Prognostic significance of p53 protein overexpression in betel and tobacco related oral oncogenesis. *Int J Cancer* **79**:370, 1998.

141. Girod SC, Pfeiffer P, Ries J, Pape HD: Proliferative activity and loss of function of tumour suppressor genes as "biomarkers" in diagnosis and prognosis of benign and preneoplastic oral lesions and oral squamous cell carcinoma. *Br J Oral Maxillofac Surg* **36**:252, 1998.

142. Warnakulasuriya KAAS, Johnson NW: Association of overexpression of p53 oncoprotein with the state of cell proliferation in oral carcinoma. *J Oral Pathol Med* **23**:246, 1994.

143. Warnakulasuriya S: p53 and oral precancer—a review, in Varma AK (ed): *Oral Oncology, vol VI. Proceedings of the Sixth International Congress on Oral Cancer*, New Delhi, Macmillan, 1998, p. 93.

144. Warnakulasuriya S: p53 as an early marker in the natural history of oral carcinoma. *Oral Dis* **6**:56, 2000.

145. Yan JJ, Tzeng CC, Jin YT: Overexpression of p53 protein in squamous cell carcinoma of buccal mucosa and tongue in Taiwan: An immunohistochemical and clinicopathological study. *J Oral Pathol Med* **25**:55, 1996.

146. Slootweg PJ, Koole R, Hordijk GJ: The presence of p53 protein in relation to Ki-67 cellular proliferation marker in head and neck squamous cell carcinoma and adjacent dysplastic mucosa. *Eur J Cancer* **30B**:138, 1994.

147. Saranath D, Tandle AT, Deo MG, Mehta AR, Sanghivi V: Loss of p53 gene as a biomarker of high risk oral leukoplakia. *Indian J Biochem Biophys* **34**:266, 1997.

148. Boyle JO, Hakim J, Koch W et al: The incidence of p53 mutations increases with progression of head and neck cancer. *Cancer Res* **53**:4477, 1993.

149. Qin GZ, Park JY, Chen SY, Lazarus P: A high prevalence of p53 mutations in pre-malignant oral erythroplakia. *Int J Cancer* **80**:345, 1999.

150. Warnakulasuriya S, Speight PM, Tavassoli M, Elamin F, Penhallow J, Johnson NW: Association between proliferative verrucous leukoplakia, p53 protein and HPV infection. *Oral Dis* **3(Suppl 2)**:S28, 1997.

151. Murti PR, Warnakulasuriya KAAS, Johnson NW, Bhonsle RB, Gupta PC, Daftary DK, Mehta FS: p53 expression in oral precancer as a marker for malignant potential. *J Oral Pathol Med* **27**:191, 1998.

152. Shahnavaz SA, Regezi JA, Bradley G, Dube ID, Jordan RC: p53 gene mutations in sequential oral epithelial dysplasias and squamous cell carcinomas. *J Pathol* **190**:417, 2000.

153. Rich AM, Kerdpon D, Reade PC: p53 expression in oral precancer and cancer. *Aust Dent J* **44**:103, 1999.

154. Warnakulasuriya S: Lack of molecular markers to predict malignant potential of precancer. [editorial]. *J Pathol* **190**:407, 2000.

155. Hall PA, Meek D, Lane DP: p53-integrating the complexity. *J Pathol* **180**:1, 1996.

156. Harper JW, Adami GR, Wei N, Keyomarsi K, Elledge SJ: The p21 cdk-inhteracting protein Cip1 is a potent inhibitor of G1 cyclin-dependent kinases. *Cell* **75**:805, 1993.

157. Erber R, Klein W, Andl T, Enders C, Born AI, Conradt C, Bartek J, Bosch FX: Aberrant p21 (CIPI/WAF1) protein accumulation in head and neck cancer. *Int J Cancer* **74**:383, 1997.

158. Yook JI, Kim J: Expression of p21WAF1/CIP1 is unrelated to p53 tumour suppressor gene status in oral squamous cell carcinomas. *Eur J Cancer* **34B**:198, 1998.

159. Agarwal S, Mathur M, Shukla NK, Ralhan R: Expression of cyclin-dependent kinase inhibitor p21waf1/cip1 in premalignant and malignant oral lesions: Relationship with p53 status. *Eur J Cancer* **34B**:353, 1998.

160. Warnakulasuriya KAAS, Tavassoli M, Johnson NW: Relationship of p53 overexpression to other cell-cycle regulatory proteins in oral squamous cell carcinoma. *J Oral Pathol* **27**:376, 1998.

161. Regezi JA, Dekker NP, McMillan A, Ramirez-Amador V, Meneses-Garcia A, Ruiz-Godoy Rivera LM, Chysomali E, Ng IOL: p53, p21, Rb, and MDM2 proteins in tongue carcinoma from patients < 35 versus > 75 years. *Eur J Cancer* **35B**:379, 1999.

162. Schoelch M, Regezi JA, Dekker NP, Ng IOL, McMillan A, Ziober BL, Thu Le Q, Silverman S, Fu KK: Cell-cycle proteins and the development of oral squamous cell carcinoma. *Eur J Cancer* **35B**:333, 1999.

163. Ng IOL, Lam KY, Ng M, Regezi JA: Expression of p21/waf1 in oral squamous cell carcinomas—correlation with p53 and mdm2 and cellular proliferation index. *Eur J Cancer* **35B**:63, 1999.

164. Jordan RCK, Bradley G, Slingerland J: Reduced levels of the cell-cycle inhibitor p27^{Kip1} in epithelial dysplasia and carcinoma of the oral cavity. *Am J Pathol* **152**:585, 1998.

165. Fountain JW, Karayiorgou M, Ernstoff MS, Kirkwood JM, Vlock DR, Ernstoff TL, Bouchard B, Vijayasaradhi S, Houghton AN, Lahti J, Kidd VJ, Housman DE, Dracopoli NC: Homozygous deletion within human chromosome band 9p21 in melanoma. *Proc Natl Acad Sci U S A* **89**:10557, 1992.

166. El-Naggar AK, Lai S, Clayman GL, Zhou JH, Tucker SA, Meyers J, Luna MA, Benedict WF: Expression of p16, Rb, and cyclin D1 gene products in oral and laryngeal squamous carcinoma: biological and clinical implications. *Hum Pathol* **30**:1013, 1999.

167. Dawson CD, Chang K-W, Solt DB: MTS1 gene mutations in archival oral squamous cell carcinomas. *J Oral Pathol Med* **25**:541, 1996.

168. Sartor M, Steingrimsdottir H, Elamin F, Gaken J, Warnakulasuriya S, Partridge M, Thakker N, Johnson NW, Tavassoli M: Role of p16/MTS1, cyclin D1 and RB in primary oral cancer and oral cancer cell lines. *Br J Cancer* **80**:79, 1999.

169. Pande P, Mathur M, Shukla NK, Ralhan R: pRb and p16 protein alterations in human oral tumorigenesis. *Eur J Cancer* **34B**:396, 1998.

170. Zhang SY, Klein Szanto AJ, Sauter ER, Shaffarenko M, Mitsunga S, Nobori T, Carson DA, Ridge JA, Goodrow TL: Higher frequency of alterations in the p16/CDKN2 gene in squamous cell lines than in primary tumours of the head and neck. *Cancer Res* **54**:5050, 1994.

171. Pavelic ZP, Lasmar M, Pavelic LJ et al: Absence of retinoblastoma gene product in human primary oral cavity carcinomas. *Eur J Cancer* **32B**:347, 1996.

172. Pavelic ZP, Lasmar M, Pavelic LJ, et al: Altered expression of retinoblastoma gene in human oral cavity squamous cell carcinoma. *Proc Am Assoc Cancer Res* **36**:639, 1995.

173. Kushner J, Bradley G, Young B, Jordan RCK: Aberrant expression of cyclin A and cyclin B1 proteins in oral carcinoma. *J Oral Pathol Med* **28**:77, 1999.

174. Fearon ER, Vogelstein B: A genetic model for colorectal tumorigenesis. *Cell* **61**:759, 1990.

175. Field JK: The role of oncogenes and tumour-suppressor genes in the aetiology of oral, head and neck squamous cell carcinoma. *J Roy Soc Med* **88**:35, 1995.

176. Rosin MP, Cheng X, Poh C, Lam WL, Huang Y, Lovas J, Berean K, Epstein JP, Priddy R, Le ND, Zhang L: Use of allelic deletions to predict malignant risk for low-grade oral epithelial dyaplasia. *Clin Cancer Res* **6**:357, 2000.

177. Tjebbes GWA, Leppers vd Straat FGJ, Tilanus MGJ, Hordijk GJ, Slootweg PJ: p53 tumour suppressor gene as a clonal marker in head and neck squamous cell carcinoma: p53 mutations in primary tumour and matched lymp node metastases. *Eur J Cancer* **35B**:384, 1999.

178. Zariwala M, Schmid S, Pfaltz M, Ohgaki H, Kleihues P, Schafer R: p53 gene mutations in oropharyngeal carcinoma: A comparison of solitary and multiple primary tumours and lymph node metastases. *Int J Cancer* **56**:807, 1994

179. Bongers V, Snow GB, van der Wall I, Braakhuis BJM: Value of p53 expression in oral cancer and adjacent normal mucosa in relation to the occurrence of multiple primary carcinomas. *Eur J Cancer* **31B**:392, 1995.

180. Ogden GR, Hall PA: Field change, clonality, and early epithelial cancer: Possible lessons from p53. *J Pathol* **181**:127, 1997.

181. Partridge M, Emilion, Pateromichelakis S, Phillips E, Langdon J: Field cancerisation of the oral cavity: Comparison of the spectrum of molecular alterations in cases presenting with both dysplastic and malignant lesions. *Eur J Cancer* **33B**:332, 1997.

182. Slootweg PJ, van Oijen MGCT, Tjebbes GWA, Leppers vd Straat FGJ, Hordijk GJ, Koole R, Tilanus MGJ: p53 as a clonal marker in head and neck cancer. *Oral Dis* **6**:55, 2000.

183. Soussi T: p53 antibodies in sera of patients with various types of cancer: A review. *Cancer Res* **60**:1777, 2000.

184. Cough MJ, Koch M, Brenan JA, Sidransky D: The humoral response to oncoprotein p53 in head and neck cancer. *Head Neck* **16**:495, 1994.

185. Maass JD, Gottschlich S, Niemann AM, Goeroegh T, Lippert BM, Werner JA: Serum p53 antibodies in head and neck cancer, in Werner JA, Lippert BM, Lippert HH (eds): *Head and Neck Cancer: Advances in Basic Research.* London, Elsevier, 1996, p 351.

186. Bourhis J, Lubin R, Roche B, Koscielny S, Bosq J, Dubois I, Talbot M, Marandas P, Schwaab G, Wibault P, Luboinski B, Eschwege F, Soussi T: Analysis of p53 serum antibodies in patients with head and neck squamous cell carcinoma. *J Natl Cancer Inst* **88**:1228, 1996.

187. Friedrich RE, Barttel Friedrich S, Plambeck K, Bahlo M, Klapdor R: p53 auto-antibodies in the sera of patients with oral squamous cell carcinoma. *Anti cancer Res* **17**:3183, 1997.

188. Ralhan R, Nath N, Agarwal S, Wasylyk B, Shukla NK: Circulating p53 antibodies as early markers of oral cancer: Correlation with p53 alterations. *Clin Cancer Res* **4**:2147, 1998.

189. Tavassoli M, Brunel N, Maher R, Johnson NW, Soussi T: p53 antibodies in the saliva of patients with squamous cell carcinoma of the oral cavity. *Int J Cancer* **78**:390, 1998.

190. Warnakulasuriya S, Soussi T, Maher R, Johnson NW, Tavassoli M: Expression of p53 in oral squamous cell carcinoma is associated with the presence of IgG and IgA p53 autoantibodies in sera and saliva of the patients. *J Pathol* **192**:52, 2000.

191. Niemann AM, Paulsen JI, Lippert BM, Henze E, Goeroegh T, Gottschlich S, Werner JA: CYFRA 21-1 in patients with head and neck cancer. In Werner JA, Lippert BM, Rudert HH (eds): *Head and Neck Cancer: Advances in Basic Research.* London, Elsevier, 1996, p 529.

192. Ogura H, Watanabe S, Fukushima K, Masuda Y, Fujiwara T, Yebe Y: Human papillomavirus DNA in squamous cell carcinomas of the respiratory tract and upper digestive tracts. *Jpn J Clin Oncol* **23**:221, 1993.

193. Yeudall WA, Paterson IC, Patel V, Prime SS: Presence of human papillomavirus sequence in tumour-derived human oral keratinocytes expressing mutant p53. *Eur J Cancer* **2**:136, 1995.

194. Elamin F, Steingrimsdottir H, Warnakulasuriya S, Johnson N, Tavassoli M: Prevalence of human papillomavirus infection in premalignant and malignant lesions of the oral cavity in UK subjects: A novel method of detection. *Eur J Cancer* **34B**:191, 1998.

195. Mao EJ, Smith CJ: Detection of Epstein-Barr virus (EBV) DNA by polymerase chain reaction (PCR) in oral smears from healthy individuals and patients with squamous cell carcinoma. *J Oral Pathol Med* **22**:12, 1993.

Genetic Abnormalities in Lymphoid Malignancies

Dan L. Longo

1. Lymphoid neoplasms accounted for about 90,000 new cases of cancer in 2001 (fourth most-common cancer). Lymphoid malignances include acute and chronic forms of leukemia, entities that manifest as solid tumors generally classed as either Hodgkin disease or non-Hodgkin lymphomas, and plasma cell tumors. They have been increasing in incidence at an approximate rate of 5 percent per year since the 1950s. The etiologies are largely unknown.

2. More than 90 percent of lymphoid neoplasms are derived from B lymphocytes (all plasma cell tumors, 99 percent of Hodgkin disease, 85 percent of non-Hodgkin lymphomas, 95 percent of chronic lymphoid leukemias, and 80 percent of acute lymphoid leukemias). The World Health Organization Classification of Tumors of Lymphoid Tissues defines discrete clinicopathologic entities based on histology, cell surface phenotype, genetic abnormalities and clinical features. While there are 43 named entities in this classification, the 10 most common diseases account for about 90 percent of the cases.

3. Acute lymphoid leukemias are associated with several common chromosomal translocations. Chronic lymphoid leukemia is associated with trisomy 12 (20 percent) and deletions of chromosome 13q14 (up to 50 percent). Hodgkin disease is characterized by aneuploidy, but no consistent clonal genetic abnormality has been detected. Non-Hodgkin lymphomas of B-cell origin frequently have characteristic chromosomal translocations that involve the immunoglobulin genes (for example, t(14;18)(q32;q21) in follicular lymphoma, t(11;14)(q13;q32) in mantle cell lymphoma, and t(8;14)(q24;q32) in Burkitt lymphoma), and those of T-cell origin often have translocations involving the T-cell receptor loci on chromosomes 7 and 14 attached to a variety of partners. Plasma cell tumors have been difficult to study but often show evidence of errors occurring during heavy-chain switch recombination, and contain gains and losses of multiple chromosomal segments. Lymphoid tumors tend to accumulate genetic damage over time. The lymphoid follicle is the site of somatic mutation to generate antibody diversity, and tumors derived from the lymphoid follicle are characterized by ongoing mutation in immunoglobulin and nonimmunoglobulin genes.

4. At least three human viruses are lymphomagenic: Epstein-Barr virus, human T-cell lymphotropic virus (HTLV) I, and human herpesvirus (HHV)-8. Many individuals are infected with Epstein-Barr virus worldwide, yet the incidence of Epstein-Barr virus-related lymphoma is low. Similarly, of the many people in endemic areas infected with HTLV I, few develop lymphoid malignancy. Less is known about the epidemiology of HHV-8. A fourth virus, human hepatitis C virus, is associated with lymphoplasmacytic lymphoma, but the relationship is complex and viral products are not found in the tumor cells.

5. Lymphomas of mucosa-associated lymphatic tissue (MALT) appear to be initiated by chronic antigenic stimulation, and they retain dependence on the initial stimulating antigen even after evidence of a clonal malignancy develops. The most common MALT lymphoma occurs in the stomach as a consequence of *Helicobacter pylori* infection. More than half of these gastric MALT lymphomas are cured by eradication of the bacterium even though the tumor cells contain clonal immunoglobulin gene rearrangements. In those not responding to *H. pylori* eradication, many tumors contain a characteristic chromosome translocation, t(11;18)(q21;q21).

6. A search of the MIM database for lymphoid malignancy turns up more than 70 entries. However, none of these familial syndromes has led to the elucidation of one or more genes involved in lymphomagenesis. Many are associated with secondary lymphomagenesis by Epstein-Barr virus because the germ line mutation produces a serious immune deficiency that destroys host control of the viral replication.

THE MAGNITUDE OF THE PROBLEM

Nearly 90,000 people in the United States were diagnosed with a lymphoid malignancy in 2001.[1] The cancers derived from lymphoid cells are diverse in clinical features, natural history, cell of origin, genetic abnormalities, and response to therapy. Clinicians have approached lymphoid malignancies as a set of diseases grouped largely by their dominant clinical manifestations and natural history (Table 52-1). Acute lymphoid leukemias (ALL) include pre-B-cell ALL, pre-T-cell ALL, and B-cell ALL (also known as Burkitt leukemia/lymphoma) and account for 3500 new cases per year. Chronic lymphoid leukemia (CLL) is the most common leukemia in the United States and accounts for 8100 new cases per year. Hodgkin disease incidence is declining slowly and accounted for 7400 new cases in 2001. The lymphoid neoplasms that grow as solid tumors are called non-Hodgkin lymphomas and have been increasing in incidence about 5 percent per year since the 1950s;[2] 56,200 cases were diagnosed in 2001. Plasma cell disorders include multiple myeloma, plasmacytoma, immunoglobulin deposition diseases, and heavy-chain disease; 14,400 cases were diagnosed in 2001. Figure 52-1 displays the distribution of lymphoid neoplasms.

Until recently, each of the named disease entities had a distinct classification system. However, it was recognized that despite diverse clinical features, the lymphoid malignancies shared derivation from lymphocytes and their precursors. Therefore, the World Health Organization undertook the creation of a new unifying classification for lymphoid neoplasms.[3] The classification for lymphoid tumors is given in Table 52-2. It is a listing of diseases based on the lymphocyte lineage, B cell or T cell, and the degree of differentiation of the cell of origin (either precursor, failing to express mature antigen receptors, or mature, expressing mature antigen receptors).

Table 52-1 Clinical Schema of Lymphoid Malignancies

Acute lymphoid leukemia
Chronic lymphoid leukemia
Hodgkin disease
Non-Hodgkin lymphomas
  Indolent lymphomas
  Aggressive lymphomas
Plasma cell disorders

The classification is clinically useful in that the diagnostic criteria for each named entity are clearly defined, were arrived at by international consensus, and include several features of disease including histologic appearance, immunologic phenotype, clinical features, and genetic abnormalities. Old schemes relied heavily on the interpretation of the appearance of the tumor on light microscopy, often ignoring relevant clinical, immunologic and genetic features. As our capacity to perform genetic analysis has become more sophisticated, new disease entities have emerged that were formerly grouped with other similar-appearing diseases.

The drawbacks of the new system are several. It groups the diseases based upon lymphocyte lineage, which is not useful. Dividing a large collection of diseases into two groups in which one group contains 90 percent of the diseases and the other less than 10 percent of the diseases seems to ignore the purpose of a classification system. The distinction between precursor and mature entities is also without clear meaning. It does not identify diseases that behave more aggressively — precursor leukemias are not more aggressive than B-cell ALL (Burkitt leukemia). Furthermore, here again, the mature category includes more than 90 percent of the diseases. In addition, the high frequency of translocations in lymphomas associated with the recombination events that create the antigen receptors suggest that genetic lesions develop at the precursor stage that then transform the cells at the mature stage. Therefore, precursor versus mature does not provide any pathogenetic insight. Thus, the basis for listing the diseases in this way is not well considered.

In addition, the list of named entities is enormous and is very difficult to teach without added simplifications. One could also quibble with holding Hodgkin disease in a separate group from the other B-cell diseases, but I won't do that here. The WHO Classification requires further revision as current disease categories that are obviously heterogeneous give rise to distinct subsets. This is already happening. In diffuse large B-cell lymphoma, cDNA microarray analysis is defining molecular subsets that may have distinct natural histories and responses to treatment.[4] In CLL, two subsets of roughly equal size have been noted, one with mutated immunoglobulin genes and one with germ line immunoglobulin genes.[5,6] Nevertheless, the WHO Classification will be the basis for lymphoma taxonomy for years to come.

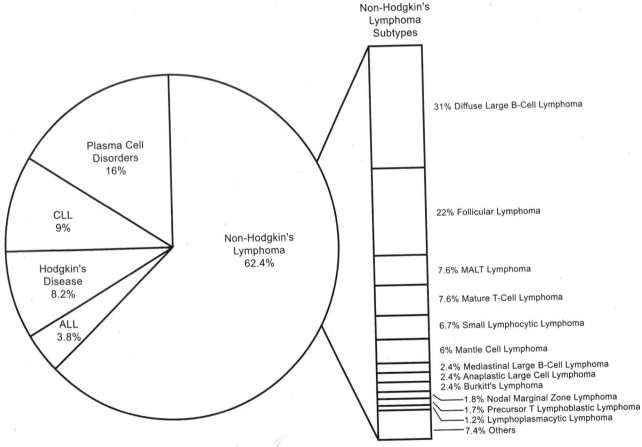

Figure 52-1. Distribution of diagnoses among the 90,000 cases of lymphoid malignancy diagnosed in 2001. There were 3500 cases of acute lymphoid leukemia (ALL), 8100 cases of chronic lymphoid leukemia (CLL), 7400 cases of Hodgkin disease, 14,400 cases of plasma cell disorders, chiefly multiple myeloma, and 56,200 cases of non-Hodgkin lymphoma. Among non-Hodgkin lymphomas, the distribution of diagnoses within that heterogeneous group is provided in the bar graph. These data are derived from an international study, A clinical evaluation of the International Lymphoma Study Group classification of non-Hodgkin lymphoma. The non-Hodgkin lymphoma classification project. *Blood* 89:3909, 1997. In the United States, diffuse large B-cell lymphoma accounts for about 40 percent of cases and follicular lymphoma about 33 percent; thus, these two diagnoses account for nearly 3 of 4 patients in the United States.

Table 52-2 World Health Organization Classification of Lymphoid Tumors

B-Cell Neoplasms
 Precursor B-cell neoplasm
  Precursor B lymphoblastic leukemia/lymphoma
 Mature B-cell neoplasms
  Chronic lymphocytic leukemia/small lymphocytic lymphoma
  B-cell prolymphocytic leukemia
  Lymphoplasmacytic lymphoma
  Splenic marginal zone lymphoma
  Hairy cell leukemia
  Plasma cell myeloma
  Solitary plasmacytoma of bone
  Extraosseous plasmacytoma
  Extranodal marginal zone B-cell lymphoma
   of mucosa-associated lymphoid tissue (MALT lymphoma)
  Nodal marginal zone B-cell lymphoma
  Follicular lymphoma
  Mantle cell lymphoma
  Diffuse large B-cell lymphoma
  Mediastinal (thymic) large B-cell lymphoma
  Intravascular large B-cell lymphoma
  Primary effusion lymphoma
  Burkitt lymphoma/leukemia
 B-cell proliferations of uncertain malignant potential
  Lymphomatoid granulomatosis
  Posttransplant lymphoproliferative disorder, polymorphic
T-Cell and NK-Cell Neoplasms
 Precursor T-cell neoplasms
  Precursor T lymphoblastic leukemia/lymphoma
  Blastic NK cell lymphoma
 Mature T-cell and NK-cell neoplasms
  T-cell prolymphocytic leukemia
  T-cell large granular lymphocytic leukemia
  Aggressive NK cell leukemia
  Adult T-cell leukemia/lymphoma
  Extranodal NK/T cell lymphoma, nasal type
  Enteropathy-type T-cell lymphoma
  Hepatosplenic T-cell lymphoma
  Subcutaneous panniculitis-like T-cell lymphoma
  Mycosis fungoides
  Sezary syndrome
  Primary cutaneous anaplastic large cell lymphoma
  Peripheral T-cell lymphoma, unspecified
  Angioimmunoblastic T-cell lymphoma
  Anaplastic large cell lymphoma
 T-cell proliferation of uncertain malignant potential
  Lymphomatoid papulosis
Hodgkin Lymphoma
 Nodular lymphocyte predominant Hodgkin lymphoma
 Classical Hodgkin lymphoma
  Nodular sclerosis classical Hodgkin lymphoma
  Lymphocyte-rich classical Hodgkin lymphoma
  Mixed cellularity classical Hodgkin lymphoma
  Lymphocyte-depleted classical Hodgkin lymphoma

This chapter reviews what is known about lymphocyte ontogeny and then discusses what is known about the genetic abnormalities that contribute to lymphomagenesis in the most common disease entities. I then discuss what is known about viral lymphomagenesis and close the chapter with a brief discussion of familial clustering of lymphoid malignancies.

LYMPHOCYTE DEVELOPMENT

All the molecular events involved in the step-wise progression of lymphocyte development have not yet been elucidated. Much of what we know of lymphocyte development has emerged from the careful study of immunodeficient patients and mice in which particular genes are knocked out. From all appearances, the development of the immune system has been largely conserved from mouse to man. Thus, I freely extrapolate between species, while recognizing that some details may later prove to be incorrect. In both species, the progression of lymphocyte maturation occurs as a consequence of the action of particular combinations of transcription factors that are often induced by specific growth and differentiation factors expressed in the anatomic niche.

Although some debate continues, most evidence supports the notion that a common lymphocyte progenitor cell emerges from a pluripotent hematopoietic stem cell at least in part through the induction of expression of the zinc finger transcription factor *Ikaros*. If *Ikaros* is deleted in the mouse, lymphocytes do not develop.[7] Similarly, *Pu.1* is an ets winged helix transcription factor that is also essential to lymphoid cell development.[8] It is not known whether these transcription factors are induced by some extracellular signal or are a part of the cell's natural developmental program of differentiation. The common lymphoid progenitor expresses CD34, CD117 (c-kit), and IL-7 receptors.

T cells and B cells then go their separate paths while retaining the common feature of using recombinase activating genes-1 and -2 (*Rag-1, -2*) to form unique clonally expressed antigen receptors by recombining distinct genes.

B-Cell Development

Figure 52-2 depicts the schema of normal B-cell development and maturation, and the putative normal counterparts for certain common B-cell lymphomas.

The first cell type recognized as committed to the B cell lineage is the pro-B-cell. This cell depends on the expression of at least four transcription factors: E2A[9] (both gene products E12 and E47 generated through alternative splicing[10]), a helix-loop-helix (bHLH) transcription factor; EBF[11] (early B-cell factor, also a bHLH family member); PAX-5[12] (B-cell-specific activator protein, BSAP), an IL-7-regulated gene necessary to synthesize a rearranged transcript; and SOX-4.[13] PAX-5 seems to prevent the cell from switching to the myeloid or other lineages.[14] This pro-B-cell expresses CD34, CD38, and CD10 on its surface and the VpreB surrogate light chain that is later expressed on the surface as the pre-B-cell receptor. The immunoglobulin genes remain in germ line configuration in the pro-B-cell.

The pro-B-cell becomes a pre-B-cell stage I when it expresses CD19 on the surface in addition to CD34 and CD10, loses surface CD38 expression, and expresses the RAG genes and terminal deoxynucleotide transferase (TdT). This cell makes the first heavy-chain gene recombination, the D-J rearrangement. CD79a and b are detectable intracellularly but no cytoplasmic μ heavy chain is present.

The pre-B-cell stage II comes in two varieties. The large one is the less mature of the two; it loses surface CD34 expression, loses c-kit (CD117) expression, completes V-D-J rearrangement, contains cytoplasmic heavy chains, and expresses the pre-B-cell receptor on its surface consisting of CD79a and b and an immunoglobulin-like molecule with the distinctive rearranged μ heavy chain together with the nonpolymorphic VpreB plus $\lambda5$ as light-chain counterparts. Signals through this receptor are essential for continued development.[15] The gene rearrangement occurs through the action of the RAG genes mediating recombination at specific signal sequences.[16] The small pre-B-cell stage II loses TdT and VpreB, stops expressing the pre-B-cell receptor, and begins V-J rearrangement of its light chain genes. After the immunoglobulin genes are rearranged, the heterodimeric transcription factor comprised by Oct-2 and Bob-1 is required for transcription of the rearranged gene.[17]

The next stage of development is the immature B cell, which expresses IgM and CD20 on its surface and loses CD10 expression. Cytoplasmic heavy chains are no longer detected. The cell becomes a mature B cell when it further rearranges the heavy

		B Cells	Heavy Chain Genes	Light Chain Genes	Intracellular Proteins	Surface Proteins	Neoplasms	Translocations
BONE MARROW / **ANTIGEN INDEPENDENT**		Stem Cell	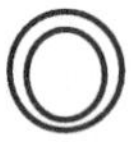 germline	germline		CD34 CD45 IL7R		
		Pro-B Cell	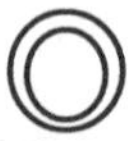 germline	germline	TdT λ5, VpreB RAG-1, RAG2	CD34, CD38 CD45, c-kit CD10	precursor B cell tumors	see table 3
		Pre-B I Cell	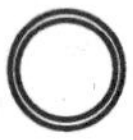 D-J rearrangement	germline	TdT λ5, VpreB CD79 a,b	CD34, CD10 CD19, c-kit	precursor B cell tumors	see table 3
		Pre-B II Large Cell	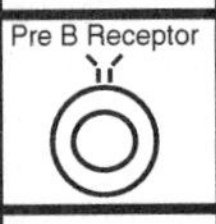 V-DJ rearrangement	germline	TdT RAG-1, RAG2 μ heavy chain λ5, VpreB CD79 a,b	CD10, CD19 CD20, CD40		
		Pre-B II Small Cell	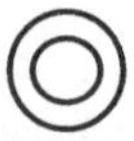 VDJ rearranged	V-J rearrangement	μ CD79 a,b	CD19, CD20 CD40, CD10		
		Immature B	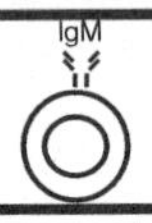 VDJ rearranged	VJ rearranged	RAG-1, RAG-2 for receptor editing	IgM CD19, CD20 CD40		
		Mature B	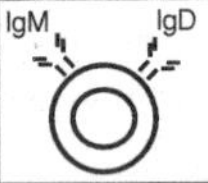 VDJ switch rearrangement	VJ rearranged		IgM, IgD CD19, CD20 CD21, CD40		
PERIPHERY / **ANTIGEN DRIVEN**					**Lymph node regions**			
		Centro-Blast	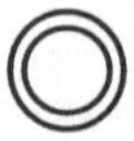 Somatic Hypermutation	Somatic Hypermutation	Follicle Dark Zone		Diffuse Large B Cell	3q27
		Centro-Cyte	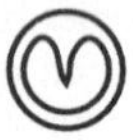 Antigen Selection	Antigen Selection	Follicle Light Zone	CD10, CD20	Follicular Lymphoma	t(14;18)
		Post-Germinal Center	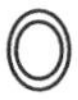 VDJ Rearranged Switched and Mutated	VJ Rearranged and Mutated	Interfollicular Area		Burkitt's Lymphoma	t(8;14)
			VDJ Rearranged Switched and Mutated	VJ Rearranged and Mutated			Hodgkin's Disease	none
			VDJ Rearranged Switched and Mutated	VJ Rearranged and Mutated	Marginal Zone		MALT Lymphoma	t(11;18)
			VDJ Rearranged Switched and Mutated	VJ Rearranged and Mutated			Lymphoplasma-cytoid Lymphoma	t(9;14)
			VDJ Rearranged Switched and Mutated	VJ Rearranged and Mutated	Bone Marrow	CD38	Myeloma	various 14q32
			" "	" "		?CD38⁻ sIgMdim ?CD38⁺ CD5	CLL	trisomy 12
			unmutated	unmutated				
			unmutated	unmutated	Mantle Zone	CD5	Mantle Cell	t(11;14)

Figure 52-2. Schema of normal B-cell development and maturation, and the putative normal counterparts for certain common B-cell lymphomas.

chain gene to generate a δ heavy chain, and expresses both IgM and IgD on its surface. It is then ready to migrate to peripheral lymph node sites. A number of B cells die in the bone marrow at the immature stage of development (surface IgM only) presumably because the expressed immunoglobulin is capable of binding to an autoantigen; this is B-cell negative selection.[18] Some cells expressing forbidden receptors can survive by undergoing further immunoglobulin gene rearrangements and by expressing a new receptor; this is called receptor editing.[19] A subset of mature B cells will express CD5 on their surface, and traffic to lymph node mantle zones and to the peritoneal and pleural cavities. It is not entirely clear whether this subset develops as a branch point in normal B-cell differentiation or whether these cells are derived from cells with features of the monocyte lineage.[20]

Up to this point, maturation has proceeded in an antigen-independent fashion mainly in the bone marrow. Subsequent maturation steps occur after exposure to antigen. Antigen exposure occurs in peripheral lymphoid organs, the spleen, the lymph nodes, and the mucosa-associated lymphatic tissue of the gut and other organs. Short-lived self-tolerant naive B cells emerge from the bone marrow and either enter or fail to enter lymphoid follicles. B cells not entering lymphoid follicles die in a few days. Figure 52-3 is a schematic view of the lymph node.

B cells generally encounter antigen first in the T-cell-rich paracortical zone of the lymphoid tissue. They interact there with T cells that are specific for the same antigen and that have the antigen presented to them by dendritic cells.[21] The T-cell/B-cell interaction fosters the proliferation of the cells (which is influenced by CD40 stimulation), the switching of the immuno-globulin isotype (the particular isotype being influenced by the cytokines secreted by the T cell), and the production of antibody.

A small proportion of the B cells become plasma cells and a larger proportion migrate to the dark zone of the lymphoid follicle where they undergo proliferation and somatic hypermutation of the variable regions of their immunoglobulin genes.[22] The small number of clones that enter the follicle then give rise to many progeny in the dark zone that then migrate to the light zone as they stop proliferating. In the light zone, cells with the highest affinity for antigen are positively selected through tight and long-lived interactions with specialized follicular dendritic cells that present the antigen to the B cells. Those B cells not interacting with the follicular dendritic cells undergo apoptosis. Positively selected B cells expand further, undergo additional isotype switching, and either become memory B cells or plasma cells.

The B cells occupying the follicular mantle zone do not depend on interactions with T cells that recognize the same antigen. They produce IgM and IgG antibody almost exclusively, and usually express CD5 on their surface. They recognize antigens with a repeating subunit structure such as polysaccharides. Their immunoglobulin genes tend to have few or no changes from the germ line sequence, and they do not pass through germinal centers during their maturation.[23]

The anatomic specialization in peripheral lymphoid tissues is important for antigen-induced maturation process of B cells. Most of what we know about the formation of lymph nodes and lymphoid tissue is derived from effects observed in knockout mice. Such studies have documented important roles for tumor necrosis factor (TNF), lymphotoxin-α, and a variety of transcription factors, chemokines, and cell surface proteins in the processes (reviewed in Ref. 24). Another important molecule in germinal center formation and the regulation of lymphoid cell function is BCL-6 or LAZ3, a transcriptional repressor that when knocked out

Schematic representation of a germinal center

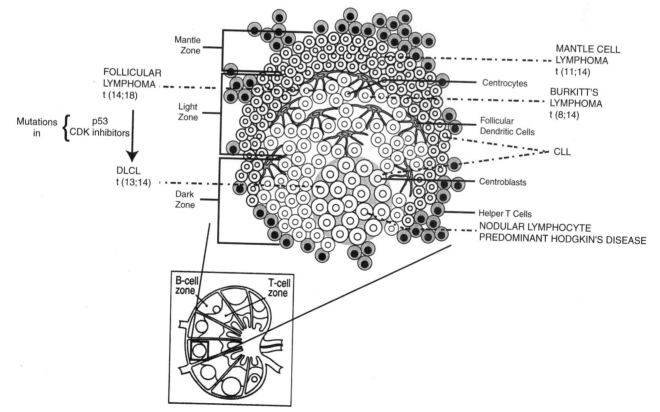

Figure 52-3. Schematic depiction of the events that occur in lymph nodes and the lymphomas derived from particular nodal segments.

leads to widespread inflammation and the absence of germinal centers.[25]

Using the expression of certain cell surface markers and the presence or absence of mutations in the immunoglobulin genes, it is possible to assign particular B-cell neoplasms to corresponding stages of normal B-cell development. For example, a lymphoma that expresses CD5 on its surface and has immunoglobulin genes of germ line sequence corresponds to a mantle zone lymphocyte. A lymphoma that contains mutated immunoglobulin genes is felt to be a postgerminal center tumor. A lymphoma that contains mutated immunoglobulin genes and shows evidence of continued intraclonal variation through accumulation of additional mutations in different cells within the tumor is felt to be of follicular center origin. This exercise is not of particular clinical importance nor has it led to special insights about lymphomagenesis as yet. However, with further elucidation of the molecular steps that mediate the maturation of B cells, it may become possible to better understand what goes wrong to produce a lymphoma of a particular type. It is anticipated that most of the discrete lymphoma entities will have their own distinctive pathogenetic pathways.

T-Cell Development

Figure 52-4 depicts the schema of normal T-cell development and maturation and the putative normal counterparts for T-cell lymphomas.

The commitment of the common lymphoid cell progenitor to the T-cell lineage is mediated by expression of at least two transcription factors, GATA-3,[26] a zinc finger protein, and Notch-1,[27] a transmembrane receptor containing epidermal growth factor

repeats in its ectodomain and ankyrin repeats and a transcription factor dimerization site called RAM23 in the cytoplasmic domain. The Notch-1 receptor encounters its ligand, Jagged, on the surface of a bone marrow stromal cell, which leads to cleavage of the Notch-1 receptor at the transmembrane domain. The intracellular portion of Notch-1 then activates two pathways. It translocates to the nucleus and heterodimerizes with a helix-loop-helix transcription factor called recombination signal binding protein or RBP-Jκ converting the RBP-Jκ from a transcriptional repressor to a transcriptional activator of T-cell lineage-specific genes. Another portion of the intracellular Notch-1 receptor is a molecule called Deltex, which prevents the phosphorylation and activation of the B-cell specific transcription factor, E2A. Thus, Notch-1 signaling leads to T-lineage commitment and B-lineage inhibition.[28] Notch-1 signaling is also involved in the commitment to express either $\alpha\beta$ or $\gamma\delta$ T-cell receptors and in the decision to become either CD4+ or CD8+ (see below).

The first T-lineage-committed cell is a pro-T cell that is CD34, CD38, and CD44 positive, but which does not express CD3, CD4, or CD8. It migrates to the thymus where it enters the cortex, expresses CD2, and proceeds through steps of maturation while migrating toward the medulla. The pro-T cell is tripotential. It can generate T cells expressing $\gamma\delta$ T-cell receptors, T cells expressing $\alpha\beta$ T-cell receptors, or it can generate NK cells, which do not rearrange the T-cell receptor genes. The commitment to NK cell lineage appears to depend in part on the expression of helix-loop-helix transcription factors in the Id family, which interfere with receptor gene rearrangement.[29] During fetal development, two waves of $\gamma\delta$ T cells are produced and are the first T cells. However, after birth, the production of $\alpha\beta$ T cells predominates,

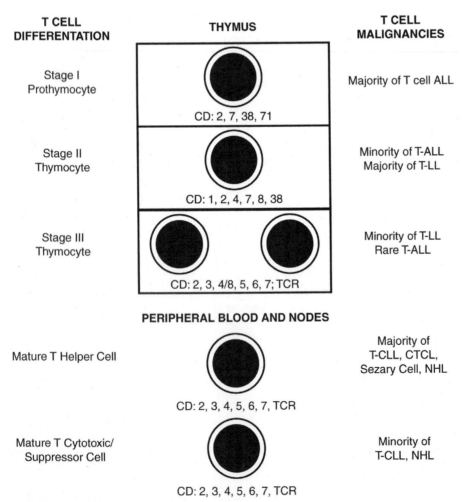

Figure 52-4. Schema of normal T-cell development and maturation and the putative normal counterparts for T-cell lymphomas.

perhaps under the influence of Notch-1. The $\gamma\delta$ T cell subset differs from $\alpha\beta$ T cells in their antigen specificity, in pattern of CD4 and CD8 expression, and in anatomic distribution. $\gamma\delta$ T cells are often found in the gastrointestinal tract, liver, and reproductive tract, rather than in peripheral lymphoid organs.

Because they do not express either CD4 or CD8, the most immature cells in the thymus are called double-negative thymocytes. They are CD44 positive and CD25 negative at their most immature stage; then they express CD25. When CD25 comes on, CD44 levels decline, and at this stage, the T-cell receptor β-chain genes begin to rearrange. After β chain protein is made, it pairs with a surrogate α chain called pre-T-cell α and is expressed on the cell surface. Expression of this pre-T-cell receptor arrests further rearrangement of the β genes and leads to expression of both CD4 and CD8, the double-positive thymocyte. This is the largest population in the thymus.

Subsequently, the α chain genes rearrange and permit the cell to express a mature $\alpha\beta$ T-cell receptor. The small double-positive cells express relatively low levels of T cell receptors and 95 percent of these cells are destined to die in the thymus. Those double-positive cells that recognize self major histocompatibility complex (MHC) antigens are permitted to mature, to express high levels of T-cell receptors, and to stop expressing either CD4 or CD8 to become single positive thymocytes. These cells undergo negative selection to eliminate autoreactive cells, and by this time, the cells have reached the medulla where they express a mature phenotype and are then exported to the periphery.[30]

It remains unclear why T cell malignancies are so much less frequent than B cell malignancies. The T cell does not undergo somatic mutation of its receptor in the periphery like B cells do and it is possible that this protects T cells from promiscuous mutations directed inadvertently at nonreceptor genes. Alternatively, DNA repair mechanisms may be more efficient in T cells, or

turnover mechanisms may be more efficient at recognizing and eliminating damaged T cells than damaged B cells. No evidence speaks to these notions. Nevertheless, T-cell malignancies account for less than 10 percent of lymphoid neoplasms and the reasons for this imbalance seem likely to be important.

LYMPHOID MALIGNANCIES: THE USUAL SUSPECTS

Despite the extensive information elucidating various steps in lymphoid cell ontogeny and functional maturation, little is known of the stepwise genetic changes that lead to lymphomagenesis. Lymphocytes are distinctive in having directed gene recombination events as crucial elements of their normal development. It is also clear that a large number of errors in these recombination events have been documented in lymphomas and the resulting chromosomal translocations have been implicated in the neoplastic transformation. Table 52-3 lists translocations associated with particular types of lymphoid malignancy. In most cases, however, the precise linkage between the chromosomal translocation and the transformation of the translocation-bearing cell remains hypothetical. For example, the t(14;18) translocation is characteristic of follicular lymphomas (see below). This translocation activates expression of *bcl-2* in follicular center B cells that normally do not express it. However, the overexpression of *bcl-2* in follicular center B cells does not lead to uncontrolled growth[31], the translocation has been found in normal people without lymphoma[32], and some lymphomas that bear the characteristic translocation do not even express bcl-2 protein[33]. Thus, if the translocation is involved in the neoplastic transformation at all, it is certainly not necessary to maintain the transformed phenotype in vivo. The translocation may be only one step of a multistep process that for most tumors is not understood.

Table 52-3 **Chromosomal Translocations Associated with Lymphoid Malignancies**

Disease	Translocation	Genes Involved	Mechanism	Effects
Precursor B-cell	t(9;22)(q34;q11.2)	Abl 9q34; Bcr 22q11.2	Oncogene fusion	Tyrosine kinase activation
	t(v;11)(v;q23)	Various partners; MLL 11q23	Oncogene fusion	Drosophila trithorax transcription
	t(12;21)(p13;q22)	TEL 12p13; CBFA2 21q22	Oncogene fusion	Ets-related transcription with core binding factor
	t(1;19)(q23;p13.3)	PBX 1q23; E2A 19p13.3	Oncogene fusion	Homeodomain plus bHLH transcription factor
Precursor T-cell	See Table 52-4			
Follicular lymphoma	t(14;18)(q32;q21)	IgH 14q32; bcl2 18q21 Rare bcl 2 association with light-chain genes	Transcriptional deregulation	Prevention of apoptosis
Diffuse large B-cell	t(3;v)(q27;v)	bcl6 3q27 with various partners	Transcriptional deregulation	Interferes with transcriptional repression of bcl 6
Burkitt lymphoma	t(8;14)(q24;q32)	IgH 14q32; Myc 8q24 Also associates with light-chain genes	Transcriptional deregulation	Promotes cell proliferation
MALT lymphoma	t(11;18)(q21;q21)	API1 11q21; MLT 18q21	Fusion protein	Inhibits apoptosis
	t(1;14)(p22;q32)	bcl-10 1p22; IgH 14q32	Transcriptional deregulation	Inhibits apoptosis
Mantle cell lymphoma	t(11;14)(q13;q32)	bcl-1 11q13; IgH 14q32	Transcriptional deregulation	Overexpression of cyclin D1
Lymphoplasmacytoid	t(9;14)(p13;q32)	Pax5 9p13; IgH 14q32	Transcriptional deregulation	Expression of B cell transcription factor
Anaplastic large cell	t(2;5)(p23;q35)	ALK 2p23; NPM 5q35	Fusion protein	Tyrosine kinase activation
T-prolymphocytic leukemia	t(7;14)(q34;q32.1)	TCRβ 7q34; TCL1 14q32.1	Transcriptional deregulation	β Barrel protein transcription
	t(14;14)(q11;q32.1)	TCRα/δ 14q11; TCL1 14q32.1	Transcriptional deregulation	β Barrel protein transcription
	t(X;14)(q28;q11)	MTCP1 Xq28; TCRα/δ 14q11	Transcriptional deregulation	β Barrel protein transcription

Chromosome translocations can result in altered cell biology in at least two major ways: (a) a novel chimeric gene product can be created that has new biologic activities; or (b) a normally unexpressed or tightly regulated gene can be placed under the control of an expressed gene promoter (in lymphomas, usually the antigen receptor gene) resulting in abnormal or unregulated expression of the normally unexpressed or regulated gene. While distinctive chromosomal translocations are the dominant genetic abnormalities in most types of lymphoid malignancy, activating mutations in dominant oncogenes, inactivating mutations in tumor-suppressor genes, and viral gene expression also contribute to lymphoid neoplasia. The more common entities with defined genetic lesions are discussed.

Non-Hodgkin Lymphomas

Diffuse Large B-Cell Lymphoma. Diffuse large B-cell lymphoma (DLBCL) is the most common lymphoma, accounting for about 40 percent of cases in the United States, and is the lymphoma whose incidence is increasing at the fastest rate. This tumor is composed of diffuse infiltrates that are large neoplastic B cells, which can be diverse cytologically. Attempts to subclassify these heterogeneous tumors by microscopic features have been unsuccessful and no constellation of immunophenotypic markers identifies distinct subsets. Patients present with a dominant rapidly growing mass, either in lymph nodes or in extranodal sites (40 percent of cases) such as the gastrointestinal tract, central nervous system, skin, testis, bone. The cause is unknown. About half of patients are curable with combination chemotherapy. Clinical poor prognostic factors include age >60 years, high lactic acid dehydrogenase (LDH), poor performance status, advanced stage disease, and 2 or more extranodal sites of involvement.

The tumor cells express clonal immunoglobulin gene rearrangements and the V regions are mutated suggesting that DLBCL is a tumor of germinal center or postgerminal center B-cell origin.

About 30 to 35 percent of tumors contain a balanced translocation between chromosome 3q27 and one of the immunoglobulin genes, the heavy-chain genes on 14q32, κ chain genes on 2p11, and λ chain genes on 22q11.[34] Other partner genes have been identified on chromosomes 1q21, 2q23, 5q13, 5q31, 9p13, 11q13, 12p11, 12q11, and 12q23 in other tumors, and in some cases, a der(3) is identified without identification of the reciprocal partner. The gene on 3q27 involved in these cases is *bcl6*, which encodes a zinc finger transcriptional repressor important in the formation of germinal centers. Normally, bcl6 protein is detectable in germinal center B cells, but it is not normally expressed in pre- or postgerminal center cells.[35] It remains unclear why the aberrant expression of a transcriptional repressor contributes to the neoplasia. The translocations involving 3q27 usually truncate *bcl6* in its 5′ flanking region or within the first exon or intron and the coding sequence is usually intact; thus, the gene is translocated under the influence of a heterologous promoter, a mechanism called promoter substitution. Translocations involving this gene are generally not found in other lymphomas. The gene can also be altered by the somatic mutation that introduces alterations in the V gene sequences in the germinal center. Other more indolent B-cell lymphomas can evolve to DLBCL. Nearly all follicular lymphomas at some time in their course ultimately acquire mutations in p53 and become more aggressive in pattern of growth and natural history.[36] This progression from follicular lymphoma may explain why about 20 percent of patients with DLBCL have tumors containing the t(14;18) (see below). Chronic lymphoid leukemia converts to DLBCL in about 5 percent of cases. MALT lymphomas can undergo histologic progression to DLBCL. When DLBCL contains a translocation typical of another type of lymphoma, it often signals that the DLBCL evolved from additional genetic damage in a more indolent lymphoma.

The application of cDNA microarray technology to DLBCL has led to the definition of at least two subsets of disease with differences in their gene expression profiles. One group of patients (about 40 percent of the total) have tumors that express genes suggesting that the cells are of germinal center origin and the other group has tumors with a pattern of gene expression that resembles mitogen-activated peripheral blood B cells.[37] Interestingly, these molecular profiles seem to reflect distinct prognoses; the 5-year survival of patients with germinal center-like DLBCL was 75 percent as compared to < 25 percent for the activated B-cell-like DLBCL group. Thus, gene expression profiling is likely to provide additional insight into the cell biology of lymphomas and may provide information that can be exploited clinically in their management.

Follicular Lymphoma. Follicular lymphoma is the second most common lymphoma accounting for about one-third of cases in the United States. It is characterized by a follicular pattern of growth of two morphologically distinct cell types: small cells with cleaved nuclear contour and large cells that are similar to DLBCL cells. In most cases, the fraction of the tumor consisting of large cells is 5 percent or less. As the fraction of large cells increases, the clinical aggressiveness of the tumor appears to increase and the natural history of follicular large cell lymphoma resembles DLBCL. The disease is predominantly lymph node-based, but a large fraction of patients have disease spread to the bone marrow. Few patients have involvement of other extranodal sites. The clinical prognostic factors that have been noted in DLBCL also apply to follicular lymphoma, but fewer patients have poor prognostic factors. Median survival for patients with follicular lymphoma is about 12 years. Many types of therapy cause temporary regression of the disease, but it often recurs. More aggressive therapy appears to be achieving longer remissions, but in contrast to the curable DLBCL, it is not yet clear that permanent remission can be achieved in follicular lymphoma. At autopsy, over 90 percent of patients with follicular lymphoma have sites of disease that contain DLBCL.

The tumor cells contain clonal immunoglobulin gene rearrangements and the V segments are heavily mutated. There is also evidence of ongoing V gene mutation and the accumulation of mutations in other genes as well.[36] Thus, this tumor is thought to be derived from germinal center B cells.

Virtually all cases show cytogenetic abnormalities. The most common change (85 percent) is the t(14;18)(q32;q21) translocation that places the *bcl2* gene on chromosome 18 under the influence of the immunoglobulin heavy-chain gene promoter, usually joining to the J_H region.[38] Rare translocations juxtapose *bcl2* with the κ or λ genes. The bcl2 protein is involved in the inhibition of programmed cell death or apoptosis.[39] Bcl2 is not normally expressed in the germinal center. Its overexpression might permit a cell to survive that was destined to die because it contains nonadaptive mutations that do not result in high affinity binding to antigen being presented by the follicular dendritic cells. However, the protein does not promote growth or block maturation. The translocation apparently occurs early in B-cell development at the time of the initial immunoglobulin gene rearrangements, yet it permits maturation to surface IgM and IgD expressing follicular center B cells.

The effects of bcl2 on cell death may not be its primary effect in lymphoma cells. In addition to its capacity to heterodimerize with death promoters such as Bax and Bad, bcl2 may also interfere with the activation of transcription factors, thus altering gene expression.[40] In mice overexpressing bcl2, generalized polyclonal expansion of B cells is detected, but tumors do not occur unless another genetic lesion is introduced.[41] It may play a role at a critical time in lymphomagenesis, and then no longer be needed to maintain the transformed state, as tumors in which *bcl2* has been silenced have been detected.

Bcl6 can be rearranged in 15 percent of cases or mutated in up to 40 percent of cases; trisomy 7 and trisomy 18 may be seen in 20 percent of cases; none of these appear to influence the natural history of disease. However, 6q23-26 lesions and 17p (p53) mutations alter the natural history and the prognosis.[42] *p16*

(INK4a) inactivation by deletion, mutation or methylation has been noted in histologic transformation to DLBCL.[43]

MALT Lymphoma. Extranodal marginal zone B-cell lymphoma of mucosa-associated lymphoid tissue (MALT lymphoma) occurs in extranodal sites and is comprised by small lymphocytes and monocytoid B-cells that infiltrate the marginal zone of reactive B-cell follicles and extend into the interfollicular region. In epithelial tissues, the infiltrate can replace the mucosa and extend deeper into the tissue. These lesions are usually (50 percent) gastric in origin, but lesions involving the thyroid (4 percent), salivary (14 percent) and lacrimal glands (12 percent), skin (11 percent), bronchial epithelium (10 percent), and small intestine (mainly in the Middle East) also occur. The underlying pathogenesis of the disease appears to be chronic infection or autoimmunity. In gastric lesions, *Helicobacter pylori* is detected in over 90 percent of cases.[44] Sjögren syndrome precedes salivary MALT lymphoma,[45] Hashimoto thyroiditis precedes thyroid MALT lymphoma,[46] *Borrelia* infection is associated with skin MALT lymphoma,[47] and intestinal parasites appear to predispose to small intestinal MALT (formerly called α heavy-chain disease or IPSID, immunoproliferative small intestinal disease).[48] The tumors may show plasmacytic differentiation, but the presence of a serum paraprotein is unusual except in the case of IPSID. Patients present with either an extranodal mass of an involved organ, or with stomach symptoms, in the case of gastric MALT. The tumors are usually not disseminated and a high proportion of patients is curable. The differential diagnosis is usually not difficult for an experienced hematopathologist. The tumors are monoclonal B cells that express CD20, CD79a, and CD21. They are distinguished from small lymphocytic lymphoma through the absence of CD5 and from mantle cell lymphoma through the absence of cyclin D1 expression and from follicular lymphoma through the absence of CD10 expression.

The clonal immunoglobulin gene rearrangements in MALT lymphoma typically show mutated V regions and the cell of origin in felt to be a postgerminal center marginal zone B cell.

Most genetic data have been obtained in gastric MALT lymphoma. In about half the patients, the lesions regress completely when *H. pylori* is eradicated with antibiotics and these tumors often do not have detectable genetic lesions. Of those tumors that do not regress, nearly all contain genetic lesions. Trisomy 3 is noted in 50 to 60 percent of cases,[49] and t(11;18)(q21;q21) is noted in 20 to 25 percent of cases.[50] The translocation involves a gene called *API2*, apoptosis inhibitor-2, a member of the inhibitor of apoptosis protein (IAP) family on 11q21 being brought together with a gene called *MLT* (translocated in MALT lymphoma) on chromosome 18q21.[51] The resulting fusion protein is thought to inhibit apoptosis, but its precise role in the biology of the lymphoma is not well understood. *MLT* appears to encode a protein that contains immunoglobulin-like domains and has some homology to caspases. The molecular anatomy of the fusion frequently involves several sites within exon 7 of *API2* and various exons of *MLT*. The chromosomes do not appear to have immunoglobulin gene-signal sequences. The fusion appears to suggest nonhomologous end joining following multiple double-strand breaks. However, aside from this translocation, the cells are genetically stable. Tumors bearing t(11;18) do not appear to progress to DLBCL, even though they are resistant to *H. pylori* eradication.[52] By contrast, MALT lymphoma of the stomach or other organs can progress to DLBCL, and when that occurs, the tumors have heterogeneous genetic lesions including amplification of *rel* or *myc*, deletions of 13q, gains on chromosome 3, 7, 9, 12, and 18, but they do not have t(11;18).[53] Histologic progression is often associated with mutations in p53 and bcl6.[54]

In a few cases of MALT lymphoma, a t(1;14)(p22;q32) has been noted that results in the juxtaposition of *bcl-10* with the immunoglobulin heavy-chain gene.[55] Bcl-10 is capable of activating NF-κB and is thought to be involved in apoptosis as it contains a caspase recruitment domain (CARD). The translocation generates a truncated version of the molecule that is overexpressed, but it ceases functioning as a pro-apoptotic molecule and therefore, may favor cell survival. In some cases, bcl-10 seems to retain the capacity to activate NF-κB and in some cases this activity is lost. Like most of the genetic lesions observed in lymphoma, its role in the disease remains speculative.

Mantle Cell Lymphoma. Mantle cell lymphoma is a diffusely growing neoplasm composed of small to medium-sized lymphoid cells with slightly irregular nuclei. The infiltrates can appear vaguely nodular but they do not have the structure of follicles in follicular lymphoma. In most cases, nodal involvement is dominant but when extranodal sites are involved, most commonly the gastrointestinal tract is affected. Multiple lymphomatous polyposis can be an extreme manifestation of mantle cell lymphoma involvement of the gastrointestinal tract. The median survival is 3 to 5 years and the disease is relatively refractory to standard treatment approaches. A blastic variant has been described with more rapid tumor growth and a considerably shorter survival (6 months).[56]

The malignant cell is a CD5-positive B cell with unmutated immunoglobulin genes. It is thought to be derived from mantle zone lymphocytes.

The typical genetic abnormality is t(11;14)(q13;q32), which activates the transcription of the cyclin D1 gene on chromosome 11. The overexpression of cyclin D1 is a reliable diagnostic marker for this disease. Cyclin D1 normally regulates the activity of cyclin-dependent kinase 4/6, which promotes phosphorylation of the retinoblastoma protein. This leads to the release of E2F transcription factors and cell cycle progression. The relationship between the overexpression of cyclin D1 and the tumor progression is unclear. All the tumor cells express cyclin D1, but not all of the cells are in cycle. Thus, the laboratory studies suggesting that overexpression of cyclin D1 in rat fibroblasts can lead to abnormalities in growth and cell cycle control bear an unclear relationship to the generation of lymphoma.[57] Overexpression of cyclin D1 in lymphoid cells does not lead to transformation.[58] Therefore, the translocation appears to remove the G1 cell cycle checkpoint as a component of the transformation process, but the other steps that drive proliferation have not been defined. A minority of cases demonstrate other genetic lesions associated with the G1 checkpoint, including mutations in p53, inactivation of the cyclin-dependent kinase inhibitors p16 and p18, and deletion of RB. Mutation in p53 is often seen in the blastic variant.

Burkitt Lymphoma/Leukemia. Burkitt lymphoma is a highly aggressive, rapidly growing malignancy with a growth fraction of nearly 100 percent. The histologic picture is a diffuse monotonous infiltrate of medium-sized cells. It exists in three clinical forms: endemic Burkitt lymphoma occurs in Africa, affecting children aged 4 to 7 years; sporadic Burkitt lymphoma occurs throughout the world in children (accounting for about 50 percent of lymphoma in children) and young adults (adult median age 30 years); and immunodeficiency-associated Burkitt lymphoma is associated with HIV infection and may be a presenting sign of AIDS or may occur years after the AIDS diagnosis.[3] Extranodal sites are commonly involved: the jaw in endemic, the abdomen (masses often start in the ileocecal region) in sporadic, the central nervous system (CNS) in AIDS-associated Burkitt lymphoma. CNS spread is a risk for any of the forms. Sporadic Burkitt lymphoma can involve the lymph nodes or organs such as breasts, kidneys, and ovaries. Nodal presentations are more common in adults. When the bone marrow is involved, the malignant cells may circulate; Burkitt leukemia (FAB L3) is also known as B-cell ALL, and is the most aggressive form of acute lymphoid leukemia (see below).

Because of the high growth rate, tumors may reach massive proportions before diagnosis and treatment. The tumor cells are readily killed by chemotherapy, resulting in rapid tumor lysis syndrome, as the burden of nucleic acids places metabolic stress on the host (hyperkalemia, hyperuricemia, hyperphosphatemia, hypocalcemia, arrhythmia, renal failure).

The tumor cells express monoclonal surface IgM, CD19, CD20, CD79a, bcl6, and CD10, and are negative for CD5, CD23, terminal deoxynucleotide transferase, and bcl2. The immunoglobulin molecules contain mutations in the variable regions and the tumor is thought to be derived from a germinal center B cell.

All cases have translocations that activate the expression of the *myc* oncogene on chromosome 8q24.[59] In 80 percent of cases, the translocation is to the heavy-chain gene complex on 14q32; in 15 percent of cases, the partner is the κ chain genes on chromosome 2; in 5 percent of cases, rearrangement involves the λ chain genes on chromosome 22. The chromosome 8 breakpoints are 5' of *c-myc* when they rearrange to chromosome 14 and 3' when they partner with 2 and 22. Heterogeneity in breakpoints is also noted in different forms of Burkitt lymphoma. In endemic Burkitt, the chromosome 8 breakpoint is more than 1000 kilobases 5' of *c-myc* and the chromosome 14 breakpoint is within the JH region. In sporadic Burkitt, the chromosome 8 breakpoint is within 3 kilobases 5' of *c-myc* and the chromosome 14 breakpoint is in the switch region.[60] These translocations result in the continuous unregulated expression of c-myc by at least two mechanisms, promotion from the immunoglobulin gene expression mechanism, and disruption of the negative regulatory site that would normally control c-myc expression. The c-myc exon 1-intron 1 border, a site containing regulatory sequences for gene expression, is routinely mutated in translocated genes. Furthermore, mutations are also noted in c-myc exon 2 that interfere with the ability of the RB-related regulatory protein p107 to suppress the transactivation domain of c-myc.[61] Unlike so many other translocated genes in lymphoma, *c-myc* is an authentic transforming gene that induces telomerase expression, promotes growth, and is directly responsible for the neoplasia.

In addition to c-myc expression in all cases of Burkitt lymphoma, p53 is mutated and 6q is deleted in about 30 percent of both sporadic and endemic cases.[62] The role of the Epstein-Barr virus in the disease is unclear. Nearly 100 percent of endemic Burkitt lymphoma and about 30 percent of sporadic cases contain clonal episomes of the Epstein-Barr virus genome. In endemic and AIDS-related Burkitt lymphoma, the virus is latent in the cells, and only EBNA-1 and the two small RNAs, EBER-1 and EBER-2, are expressed. The form of latency in sporadic Burkitt lymphoma is type II, in which LMPs are also expressed. It remains unclear how Epstein-Barr virus contributes to the lymphomagenesis in Burkitt lymphoma.[63]

Mature T-Cell Lymphomas. As shown in Table 52-2, a number of entities are considered under the heading of mature T-cell lymphomas. In general, lymphomas of mature T-cell origin are not associated with signature chromosomal translocations. T-cell lymphomas are more rare and have been less well studied. Like B-cell lymphomas, they are identifiable as monoclonal through the expression of clonal T-cell receptor gene rearrangements. Cell surface markers shared by mature peripheral T cells are often noted, such as CD2, CD3, CD5, and CD7. In many cases, one of these will be undetected, usually CD7, and this is a clue to the malignant nature of the infiltrate.[64] The tumors often possess bizarre karyotypes with multiple abnormalities often involving the T-cell receptor gene loci on chromosomes 7q35 (β chain genes) and 14q11 (α and δ chain genes). The chromosomes most often altered in structure are 1, 6, 2, 4, 11, 14, and 17. Breakpoints at 6q23 are common. Aneuploidy typically involves trisomies of 3 or 5 and an extra X chromosome.[65] The diversity of these findings has not allowed the construction of a consistent model of molecular pathogenesis.

Two entities are exceptions to this conclusion: anaplastic large cell lymphoma (see below) and T-cell prolymphocytic leukemia (T-PLL). T-PLL is rare, accounting for < 2 percent of cases of small lymphocytic leukemia. The disease always involves the bone marrow and peripheral blood, and frequently produces hepato-

splenomegaly, adenopathy, and skin infiltrations. In 80 percent of patients, the tumor cells bear a t(14;14)(q11;q32.1), a reciprocal tandem translocation that joins the T-cell receptor α genes to a region containing a pair of oncogenes called *TCL1* and *TCL1b*.[66] Alternative ways of activating *TCL1* include chromosomal inversion inv(14)(q11q32.1) and translocating it to the β-chain genes on chromosome 7 [t(7;14)(q35;q32.1)]. The Tcl1 protein is an 8-stranded β barrel protein. A structural homolog of Tcl1 called Mtcp1 maps to the X chromosome and is also involved in translocations to chromosome 14 in some cases of T-PLL [t(X;14)(q28;q11)].[67] The function of β barrel proteins is not defined, but expression of both gene products in transgenic mice leads to a T-cell leukemia at the age of 15 months.[68,69]

Abnormalities of chromosome 8 [deletions, trisomy 8q, t(8;8)p11-12;q12)] are also seen in 70 to 80 percent of cases of T-PLL.[70] Deletions and mutations at the *ATM* gene (mutated in ataxia telangiectasia) at 11q23 are also common,[71,72] implying a role for abnormal DNA repair in the pathogenesis of the disease.

Anaplastic Large-Cell Lymphoma. Anaplastic large-cell lymphoma (ALCL) is derived from peripheral T cells that are pleomorphic, large, and have horseshoe-shaped nuclei. The majority of patients (70 percent) have advanced stage disease with extensive peripheral and abdominal adenopathy, often with involvement of bone marrow and other extranodal disease sites such as skin, soft tissue, and lung. High fever is often seen. The tumor cells often express CD30, a member of the tumor necrosis factor receptor family that is a signal transduction molecule expressed on activated T cells. The major differential diagnosis is with Hodgkin disease, but Hodgkin disease often expresses CD15 and B-cell markers that ALCL cells lack, and ALCL cells express EMA and granzyme B that Hodgkin cells lack.

Ninety percent of ALCLs show clonal rearrangement of the T-cell receptor genes and in the remainder both immunoglobulin and T-cell receptor genes are in the germline configuration.[73] The most frequent genetic abnormality (found in 70 to 80 percent) in ALCL is t(2;5)(p23;q35), a translocation in which the *NPM* gene for nucleophosmin on 5q35 is fused to *ALK*, a gene called anaplastic lymphoma kinase on 2p23.[74] *ALK* encodes a tyrosine kinase receptor belonging to the insulin receptor family and is not normally expressed in lymphoid cells. Nucleophosmin is normally expressed in the nucleus and nucleolus. The fusion truncates the N-terminal nuclear localization signal of nucleophosmin and it is thought that the fusion protein NPM-ALK (p80) localizes to the nucleus through dimerization with wild-type nucleophosmin. The ALK component of the fusion protein consists mainly of the intracellular catalytic domain of the kinase. The NPM-ALK fusion proteins also homodimerize, which activates the kinase. The precise substrates for the chimeric gene product are not well defined. However, retroviral introduction of a chimeric gene into mice causes T-cell lymphomas.[75]

A number of other *ALK*-activating translocations have been detected in the 20 percent or so of ALCL patients lacking t(2;5). These include rearrangement to the tropomyosin 3 gene on chromosome 1, a TRK-fusion gene on chromosome 3, the ATIC (5-aminoimidazole-4-carboxamide-ribonucleotide transformylase-inosine monophosphate cyclohydrolase) gene on chromosome 2, the clathrin heavy-chain gene on chromosome 17, and an unidentified partner on chromosome 19.[76] ALK negative ALCL is unusual and has not been carefully studied.

Mediastinal Large B-Cell Lymphoma. Mediastinal or thymic large B-cell lymphoma arises in the mediastinum and consists of sheets of large pleomorphic tumor cells with abundant pale cytoplasm associated with dense fibrotic strands that compartmentalize the tumor. The disease is often localized to the chest and affects young women disproportionately. The tumor cells express CD19 and CD20 and their immunoglobulin genes are clonally rearranged; however, no immunoglobulin molecules are expressed.[77] The tumor cells are often hyperdiploid with gains in chromosome 9p and amplification of *REL*.[78] In addition, the tumor cells appear to overexpress a gene called *MAL* that encodes a proteolipid normally found in association with glycosphingolipids in myelin and in T cells.[79] It is unclear how *MAL* expression relates to the biology of the tumor.

Lymphoplasmacytic Lymphoma. Lymphoplasmacytic lymphoma produces the clinical syndrome known as Waldenstrom macroglobulinemia. It is a tumor of small lymphocytes, some with features of plasma cell differentiation, that affects the lymph nodes, bone marrow, and spleen. The median age of patients is 63 years with men and women roughly equally affected. The clinical features are dominated by the IgM paraprotein secreted by the tumor. Symptoms are related to hyperviscosity; neuropathy, if the specificity of the secreted antibody is for a myelin sheath antigen; coagulopathy, if the antibody interferes with clotting factors, platelets, or fibrin; and cryoglobulinemia. A proportion of patients are infected with hepatitis C, but it is not clear whether the virus is promoting lymphoid cell growth or the immune system is responding to the viral infection or a particular viral protein. A disproportionate number of the tumors appear to use the VH 1-69 gene in the tumor immunoglobulin and it has been shown that antibodies to hepatitis C E2 protein also frequently use this gene.[80] The possibility that a viral antigen is driving the tumor is intriguing.

The immunoglobulin gene V regions contain somatic mutations suggesting the cell is of postgerminal center origin. However, the cell has not undergone successful class switching. About 50 percent of cases have a characteristic translocation t(9;14) (p13;q32) bringing the *PAX5* gene on 9 under the influence of the immunoglobulin heavy-chain gene promoter.[81] The *PAX5* gene product is B-cell-specific activation protein, BSAP, the transcription factor cited above as important for specification of the B-lineage during B-cell development. How the expression of BSAP leads to the tumor is unknown. No other recurrent genetic lesions have been identified in this tumor.

Hodgkin Disease

Hodgkin disease is now divided into two disease entities: nodular lymphocyte predominant Hodgkin disease (NLPHD) comprises about 5 percent of all cases, and classical Hodgkin disease (CHD) comprises the other 95 percent (with nodular sclerosis and mixed cellularity accounting for 90 percent). For many years, the fundamental nature of Hodgkin disease eluded study because in all subtypes of this disease, the malignant cell is a rare cell within a mass of normal polyclonal reactive inflammatory and immune cells. However, the ability to microdissect tumor tissue and harvest and analyze gene expression in individual tumor cells has markedly advanced our understanding.

NLPHD is a monoclonal B-cell tumor characterized by a nodular pattern of growth and scattered expansion of neoplastic cells with nuclear contours that resemble popcorn kernels called L&H cells (for lymphocytic and histiocytic Reed-Sternberg cell variants). A network of follicular dendritic cells establishes the background and these cells are associated with small B cells and numerous CD57+ T cells. The disease tends to cause localized adenopathy usually in the neck and it has a slow natural history. Local radiation therapy often cures the disease but in the small subset who relapse, subsequent therapy is usually effective at inducing subsequent remissions such that very few patients die from the disease.

L&H cells typically express CD20, CD79a, Bcl-6, CD45, and usually express J (joining) chain of immunoglobulin M and CD75. They are usually CD30- and CD15-negative, distinguishing them from Reed-Sternberg cells in CHD. The cells usually express both the Oct2 and Bob.1 chains of the transcription factor that assures immunoglobulin gene transcription. This, too, is distinct from Reed-Sternberg cells that are always missing one (20 percent) or both (80 percent) factors.[82] The immunoglobulin genes are clonally rearranged and carry a heavy load of somatic mutations with evidence of intraclonal variations that document ongoing

mutation.[83,84] The inference from these data is that the L&H cell is derived from the dark zone of the germinal center where the somatic mutation cell machinery is active. Progression to DLBCL is seen in about 3 percent of cases and the lymphoma is clonally related to the NLPHD.[85]

CHD is characterized by malignant cells called Reed-Sternberg cells that are multinucleated and reside in a cellular infiltrate composed of nonneoplastic lymphocytes, eosinophils, neutrophils, macrophages, plasma cells, fibroblasts, and fibrosis. The disease commonly originates in cervical lymph nodes and spreads contiguously to adjacent lymph node groups. The disease commonly involves the mediastinum, and about one-third of patients have spleen involvement, which implies hematogenous spread because the spleen has no afferent lymphatics. The marrow is involved in less than 5 percent of cases. About 90 percent of patients with CHD are curable with therapies widely available today.

Reed-Sternberg cells are nearly always CD30- and CD15-positive, and are usually negative for CD45, the J chain, and CD75. CD20 is present on some tumor cells in about 40 percent of cases. The cells are readily distinguishable from CD30-positive ALCL because they express BSAP, a B-cell-restricted protein, and do not express ALK. Reed-Sternberg cells express a wide range of cytokines and chemokines. In about 98 percent of cases, the Reed-Sternberg cells contain clonally rearranged immunoglobulin genes, and the genes contain somatic mutations, but no immunoglobulin transcription takes place and no intraclonal variation is noted suggesting that mutations are not ongoing.[86] A small number of cases appear to have clonal T-cell receptor rearrangements.[87]

Genetic studies of Reed-Sternberg cells have documented hypertetraploidy consistent with the multinucleated nature of the cells, but no recurrent specific chromosomal changes have been documented in CHD.[88] Comparative genomic hybridization demonstrates recurrent gains on chromosomes 2p, 9p, and 12q, and amplifications on 4p16, 4q23-24, and 9p23-24.[89] Appropriate models to approach the problem of lymphomagenesis in Hodgkin disease are lacking. However, one reasonable inference from the presence of functional immunoglobulin gene rearrangements that do not lead to gene transcription is that there is a problem with the apoptosis pathway. Normal B cells that fail to express surface immunoglobulin die. Convincing evidence of an apoptotic defect in Reed-Sternberg cells is unavailable. It is also unclear what role, if any, Epstein-Barr virus plays in CHD. About 50 percent of patients with mixed cellularity CHD have clonal Epstein-Barr virus episomes detected and the association is stronger in developing countries. When Epstein-Barr virus is present, the tumor cells appear to express only LMP-1 and EBNA-1 (see below). Additional studies are necessary to clarify the relationship between Epstein-Barr virus and CHD.

Chronic Lymphoid Leukemia

CLL is the most common leukemia in the West. It comprises 90 percent of chronic leukemias of lymphoid origin. Typically, the bone marrow contains infiltrates of small lymphoid cells and the peripheral lymphocyte count is >10,000/mm^3. The morphology of the circulating cells is similar to normal small lymphocytes. When the peripheral lymphocyte count is not elevated but lymphadenopathy and/or splenomegaly are present, the patient is said to have small lymphocytic lymphoma. The main difference between CLL and small lymphocytic lymphoma is the pattern of disease involvement. The difference is most likely related to the expression of an adhesion molecule or a chemokine receptor that permits the neoplastic cells to home to lymph nodes.

CLL kills people by replacing the marrow thereby inhibiting normal hematopoiesis. About 50 percent of patients with CLL die from infection. About 25 percent of patients with CLL develop autoimmune hemolytic anemia or thrombocytopenia that can mimic marrow failure, but when the cytopenias are due to an autoimmune mechanism, they are readily controlled with glucocorticoids and do not exert an adverse influence on survival. The autoantibody is usually not the tumor immunoglobulin.

CLL is not a homogeneous disease, despite the appearance of the neoplastic cells. About 50 percent of cases contain cells bearing mutated immunoglobulin suggesting a follicular center origin, and about 50 percent of cases contain cells bearing unmutated immunoglobulin suggesting a mantle zone origin.[5,6] The presence of unmutated immunoglobulin genes predicts for a shorter natural history and more resistance to treatment. The cells in both types of CLL express CD5, low levels of surface IgM, and CD23. Controversy surrounds the issue of the role of CD38. Without question CD38 expression has an adverse influence on survival in CLL.[90] However, it is not completely clear whether CD38 expression predicts for unmutated immunoglobulin genes. One can usually distinguish CLL from mantle cell lymphoma (another CD5-bearing malignancy) by the presence of cyclin D 1 in mantle cell lymphoma, but not in CLL.

Trisomy 12 has been noted in about 20 to 25 percent of cases of CLL,[91] and tends to identify cases with more aggressive natural history, but the correlation with unmutated immunoglobulin genes has not yet been assessed. About 50 percent of cases show deletions at 13q14;[92] it is thought that such deletions involve tumor suppressor gene(s) that may be important in the pathogenesis of CLL. Several groups are attempting to identify such gene(s) (for example, Ref. 93). In 5 percent of cases, CLL or small lymphocytic lymphoma may become DLBCL, a change that signals a more aggressive natural history and is usually heralded by mutations in p53.[94] About 10 percent of CLL patients have tumors with p53 mutations and no progression to DLBCL. A small number of CLL patients have mutations in *ATM*. Deletions in 6q are seen in patients with somewhat more aggressive B-cell prolymphocytic leukemia.[95]

Acute Lymphoid Leukemia

ALL occurs mainly (75 percent) in children under age 6 years; 80 to 85 percent are of precursor B-cell origin and 15 to 20 percent are of precursor T-cell origin. These precursor lymphoid cell neoplasms usually present with fatigue and weakness from anemia. The vast majority of cases show greater than 25 percent of the marrow cells replaced by the malignant cells with tumor cells present in the peripheral blood. A small fraction of patients will present with mass lesions and less than 25 percent marrow involvement; these cases are called lymphoblastic lymphoma. Lymphoblastic lymphoma is more commonly of T-cell than B-cell origin. T-cell lymphoblastic lymphoma can produce a large mediastinal mass as it originates from the thymus. The lineage is relatively unimportant clinically. All the leukemias derived from precursor B or T cells are of the FAB L1 or L2 type morphologically. FAB L3 is Burkitt leukemia or B-cell ALL, so-called because it is derived from a mature peripheral surface immunoglobulin-expressing B cell. Acute leukemias of both lineages can spread to the central nervous system and require intensive chemotherapy for treatment together with maintenance therapy and CNS prophylaxis.

Despite clinical similarities, precursor B-cell tumors differ from precursor T-cell tumors in immunophenotype and genetic abnormalities. Precursor B-cell tumors of the earliest stage are HLA-DR-positive and express CD19, cytoplasmic CD22, and cytoplasmic CD79a. Intermediate stage or common ALL is characterized by CD10 expression. In the most mature pre-B-cell stage, blasts express cytoplasmic μ heavy chains. Six genetic lesions are commonly associated with precursor B-cell neoplasms: hyperdiploidy (51 to 65 chromosomes) is noted in about 20 to 25 percent of cases and t(12;21)(p13;q22), the *TEL/CBFA2(AML1)* translocation, is associated with 16 to 29 percent of cases, and both of these genetic lesions are associated with a good prognosis.[96] The four other genetic lesions are associated with a poor prognosis and each is noted in 3 to 6 percent of all cases: hypodiploidy, t(9;22)(q34; q11.2), the *BCR/ABL* translocation; t(4;11)(q21;q23), the *AF4/MLL* translocation; and t(1;19)(q23;p13.3), the *PBX/E2A* translocation.

The *TEL* gene is a promiscuous partner in leukemias. When translocated to the *PDGFRb* gene on chromosome 5, the disease

that develops is chronic myelomonocytic leukemia.[97] When translocated to the *ABL* gene on chromosome 9, the disease that develops is acute myeloid leukemia.[98] When *TEL* translocates to the core binding-factor component gene *CBFA2* (also sometimes called *AML1*), pre-B-cell ALL develops. *TEL* (also known as *ETV6*) is member of the ETS family of transcription factors that contain a conserved 90-amino acid winged helix-turn-helix DNA binding domain. *CBFA2* is a component of core binding factor. It contains a runt domain (so called because of homology to Drosophila runt protein) that serves as its DNA binding site, recognizing an enhancer motif associated with a number of important genes in hematopoiesis.[99] The runt domain also facilitates heterodimerization. The C-terminus of CBFA2 contains a transactivating domain that binds with p300, a transcriptional activator involved in acetylation of histone proteins and chromatin remodeling.[100] Unlike other fusions with *CBFA2*, the fusion with *TEL* retains essentially the full length *CBFA2* including the runt domain and the transactivation domain. It has been proposed that the chimeric TEL/CBFA2 protein acts as a dominant negative to interfere with CBFA2 function.[101] The wild-type *TEL* allele is nearly always deleted in cells bearing the translocation.[102] How these changes lead to leukemia and why they occur in pre-B cells is unclear. ALL with t(12;21) shows high levels of expression of CD10 and HLA-DR and no CD20.

The *MLL* gene on chromosome 11q23 is also a promiscuous partner in acute leukemia fusing with over 30 other genes and leading to AML, ALL, and mixed lineage leukemias. In ALL, the *MLL* translocation to *AF4* occurs as a primary event. However, *MLL* translocation can also occur secondary to the use of topoisomerase inhibitors to treat other forms of cancer.[103] Nearly all the translocations involving *MLL* disrupt the gene between exons 5 and 11 joining the amino-terminal half of MLL to the partner gene. The transcribed chimeric fusion protein always contains the amino-terminal portion of MLL and the C-terminal portion of the translocated partner.[104] Yet little is known how the *AF4* gene fused to *MLL* functions. *MLL* gene rearrangements are seen in about 80 percent of infant ALL cases, and in about 50 percent of infant acute myeloid leukemia.[105] ALL associated with *MLL* translocations are usually CD10- and CD24-negative and CD15-positive.[106]

The ALL cells associated with the t(1;19) translocation contain cytoplasmic μ heavy chains. In this translocation, the E2A transcription factor important for B-lineage commitment on chromosome 19 is fused to a homeobox gene called *PBX* on chromosome 1 that is normally not expressed in B cells. The fusion severs the C-terminal basic helix-loop-helix DNA binding domain but leaves the amino-terminal transactivating domains of E2A. *PBX1* has no transactivating capability on its own, but its portion of the fusion protein dictates the interaction of E2A with other homeobox factors and allows for DNA binding and activation of genes controlled by PBX1-HOX complexes.[107] A small number of cases of ALL bear a t(17;19)(q22;p13), in which the hepatic leukemia factor (HLF), a basic leucine zipper transcription factor, moves to the *E2A* site.[108] HLF bears homology with the proapoptotic protein of *C. elegans* called CES-2. However, the HLF-E2A fusion appears to have strong antiapoptotic effects that may contribute to leukemogenesis.[109]

The features of the t(9;22) translocation gene product that are important in producing chronic myeloid leukemia are well defined and include the activities of the SH2 domain, the tyrosine kinase domain, and the F-actin binding domain.[110] However, it is unclear how this translocation leads to ALL. About 50 percent of adult ALLs with this translocation generate a fusion protein called p210; the other half generate an alternative form of the protein that is p190. In children with ALL, the p190 form predominates. The differences between the diseases promoted by p210 and p190 are also not clear.

The lymphoblasts in T-cell ALL are terminal transferase positive, and variably express CD1a, CD2, CD4, CD8, CD7, and cytoplasmic CD3. Myeloid antigens such as CD13 and CD33 may

Table 52-4 Chromosomal Rearrangements in Precursor T-Cell Neoplasms

Gene-Activation Rearrangement	Rearranged Gene at Breakpoint	Activated Gene Near Breakpoint	Encoded Protein Domain
t(8;14)(q24;q11)	TCRα (14q11)	c-MYC (8q24)	bHLH
t(1;14)(p33;q11)	TCRδ (14q11)	SCL-TAL/TCL5 (1p33)	bHLH
t(1;7)(p33;q35)	TCRβ (7q35)	SCL/TAL/TCL5 (1p33)	bHLH
t(1;3)(p33;q21)	TCTA (3p21)	SCL/TAL/TCL5 (1p33)	bHLH
t(7;9)(q35;q34)	TCRβ (7q35)	TAL2 (9q34)	bHLH
t(7;19)(q35;q13)	TCRβ (7q35)	LYL1 (19p13)	bHLH
t(11;14)(p15;q11)	TCRδ (14q11)	RBTN1/TTG1 (11p15)	LIM
t(11;14)(p13;q11)	TCRα/δ (14q11)	RBTN2/TTG1 (11p13)	LIM
t(7;11)(q35;p13)	TCRβ (7q35)	RBTN2/TTG1 (11p13)	LIM
t(10;14)(q24;q11)	TCRα (14q11)	HOX11 (10q24)	Homeobox
t(7;10)(q35;q13)	TCRβ (7q35)	HOX11	Homeobox
t(7;9)(q34;q34)	TCRβ	TAN1 (9q34.3)	Notch
t(1;7)(p34;q34)	TCRβ (7q34)	LCK (1p34)	Receptor tyrosine kinase

Gene Fusion Rearrangement	Fusion Gene	Genes Involved in Fusion	Encoded Protein Domains
t(11;19)(p23;p13.3)	ALL1/ENL	ALL1/MLL/HRX (11q23)	Trithorax
		ENL (19p13.3)	Zinc finger
t(X;11)(q13;q23)	ALL1/AFX	ALL1/MLL/HRX (11q23)	Trithorax
		AFX (Xq13)	Zinc finger

bHLH, basic helix-loop-helix

be expressed. In about one-third of T-cell ALL, translocations may be present bringing a number of different genes under the transcriptional influence of the T-cell antigen receptor genes, the α and δ loci on 14q11.2, the β locus at 7q35, or the γ locus at 7p14-15 (see Table 52-4). Partner genes include the transcription factors MYC (8q24); TAL1 (1p32); TAL2 (9q34); RBTN1 or LMO1 (11p15); RBTN2 or LMO2 (11p13); LYL1 or ENL (19p13); and HOX11 (10q24); as well as the src family kinase LCK (1p34.3-35).[111] In about 25 percent of cases, deletions in the 5′ regulatory sequence of TAL1 promote its expression without translocation. In both B-cell and T-cell ALL, deletions interfere with the expression of the cyclin-dependent kinase inhibitors p15 and p16; these may be detected in up to 60 percent of T-cell ALL and 25 percent of B-cell ALL.[112]

Despite all this descriptive biology, we do not fully understand the number of genetic lesions necessary to develop ALL, nor the order in which the lesions appear. The development of an effective treatment that interferes with the kinase activity of the BCR-ABL fusion protein (Gleevec) raises some hope that targeting a gene fusion translocation can have therapeutic efficacy.[113] However, in the instance of BCR-ABL, strong evidence was available in animal models that the kinase activity was necessary and sufficient to develop the neoplasm. Most of the translocations in ALL involve gene-activating rearrangements, and it is not clear how such gene products would be selectively targeted. In addition, complete dependence of the tumor on the translocation product may be involved in Burkitt lymphoma/leukemia, but little supportive data have been developed for most of the other genetic lesions.

Plasma Cell Disorders

Plasma cell disorders include multiple myeloma; extramedullary plasmacytoma; solitary plasmacytoma of bone; immunoglobulin deposition diseases such as amyloidosis, osteosclerotic myeloma [associated with the POEMS syndrome: polyneuropathy (sensorimotor demyelination), organomegaly (hepatosplenomegaly), endocrinopathy (diabetes, gynecomastia, testicular atrophy, impotence), monoclonal gammopathy, and skin changes (hyperpigmentation, hypertrichosis)]; and the heavy-chain diseases (γμα). Myeloma is by far the most common of these disorders.

Myeloma is a multifocal bone marrow disease characterized by a monoclonal immunoglobulin in the serum (a tumor product); decreased synthesis and an increased catabolism of other normal immunoglobulins; destructive osteolytic bony lesions without an osteoblastic component; pathologic fractures; bone pain; hypercalcemia; renal failure (from hypercalcemia, recurrent infections and damage from the tumor immunoglobulin); and anemia. The most important differential diagnosis is with monoclonal gammopathy of uncertain significance (MGUS), which affects about 6 percent of people over age 70 years. MGUS typically has lower levels of serum paraprotein, less than 10 percent plasma cells in the bone marrow, and absence of lytic lesions. The risk of MGUS evolving to myeloma is about 1 percent per year.

The malignant cells in myeloma are plasma cells that contain clonally rearranged and usually class-switched immunoglobulin, and the variable region genes are mutated consistent with derivation from a postgerminal center B cell.[114] The cells have lost bcl6 expression, but have cytoplasmic immunoglobulin, and are CD38- and CD138 (syndecan)-positive. In some patients, light chains alone are secreted; tumor cells sometimes delete their heavy chain genes or portions of them.

About 40 percent of patients with myeloma contain activating mutations of N- or K-ras,[115] and 25 percent have deletions in p53.[116] Both of these genetic lesions are associated with a more rapid course of disease. Heavy-chain gene translocations appear to occur in most myelomas, generally associated with errors during switch recombination; a wide range of chromosomal partners and oncogenes are involved but the three most common involve the FGFR3 (MMSET) gene on 4p16.3, the cyclin D1 gene on 11q13, and the c-maf gene on 16q23, each occurring in 10 to 20 percent of cases.[117] The application of new cytogenetics techniques is identifying a large number of structural errors in myeloma cells including gains in chromosomes 3, 5, 7, 9, 11, 15, and 19, and losses on 8, 13, 14, 17, and X.[118] Given that plasma cells have undergone three processes involving double-strand DNA breaks (VDJ rearrangement, somatic hypermutation, and switch rearrangement), it may not be surprising that so many structural errors are detected and the errors seem to increase in patients over time.[119] What is surprising is the paucity of information on the role of the genetic instability in the behavior of the disease.

VIRAL LYMPHOMAGENESIS

The viruses that can cause lymphoma tend to be widespread but are inefficient at inducing neoplasia, and they nearly never induce neoplasia in patients with normal levels of immune function.

Epstein-Barr Virus

Epstein-Barr virus contributes to the development of endemic Burkitt lymphoma; acquired immune deficiency syndrome (AIDS)-related lymphoma; posttransplantation lymphoproliferative disease; Hodgkin disease; some lymphomas associated with primary immune deficiencies; nasopharyngeal cancer (particularly in China); and nasal NK/T cell lymphoma. The virus infects about 90 percent of people gaining access through oral and respiratory system contact.[120] The virus infects cells bearing CD21, including B cells and oropharyngeal epithelium, and can produce infectious progeny. Under the influence of the host immune system, viral replication generally ceases and the virus becomes latent in infected cells. Latent infection is characterized by a circularized viral genome that replicates episomally in low copy number. Of the approximately 100 viral genes, only a small fraction are expressed in the latent state.

Three forms of latency exist. In type I latency, EBNA-1 and two nontranslated small RNAs, EBER-1 and -2, are expressed. This type of latency is characteristic of endemic Burkitt lymphoma. Although EBNA-1 can exert some influence on lymphoid cell proliferation, its main role is to bind to viral DNA and to protect it within the cell. EBNA-1 is insufficient to cause neoplastic transformation. Essentially all tumors expressing type I latency Epstein-Barr virus are likely to be independent of the viral effects. Burkitt lymphoma in both endemic and AIDS-associated forms expresses type I latency and relies on activation of the *myc* oncogene. Type II latency involves the additional expression of the latent membrane proteins (LMP-1, -2A, -2B) in addition to EBNA-1. LMP-1 is the true oncogene of Epstein-Barr virus.[121] It binds to and activates the signaling pathway of CD40, an important costimulatory molecule in B cells.[122] The tumor necrosis factor receptor-associated factor (TRAF) is bound and activated leading to activation of NF-κB, c-jun, cytokine production, and B-cell proliferation. Evidence of signal transduction is present in all forms of lymphoproliferative disease stimulated by Epstein-Barr virus in the presence of LMP-1, as in type II latency. A number of lymphoid tumors associated with the virus have type III latency in which the same genes expressed in type II are expressed plus the other latent proteins.

Additional study is required to be certain that LMP-1 plays a critical role in the non-B-cell malignancies with which Epstein-Barr virus is associated. However, at the moment, LMP-1 appears to be a critical target for removing the effects of the virus on associated tumors.

Human T-Cell Lymphotropic Virus I

Human T-cell lymphotropic virus I (HTLV-I) is a retrovirus that infects many people in the regions of the world where it is endemic (southwestern Japan, Caribbean, Central Africa, South America, Southeast Asia), and in a small fraction of infected people, the virus can cause adult T-cell leukemia/lymphoma, a mature peripheral T-cell neoplasm, or tropical spastic paraparesis. The virus replicates poorly in vivo; it is generally transmitted vertically through infected lymphocytes in the mother's milk, and to a lesser degree horizontally through sex and blood transfusion. The lifetime risk of developing lymphoma in an infected person is 3 to 5 percent.

Adult T-cell leukemia/lymphoma is usually a rapidly progressive disease affecting CD4-positive peripheral T cells. Clinical manifestations of disease include opportunistic infections from an underlying immune deficiency; high peripheral blood counts with large lymphocytes containing flower-shaped nuclei; hypercalcemia; lytic bone lesions; adenopathy; skin lesions; and pulmonary infiltrates.[123] Most patients survive less than 1 year from diagnosis.

HTLV-I does not have a transforming oncogene.[124] Where a transforming oncogene would be in its genome it has a 1.6-kb segment called the pX region, which codes for several proteins (including Tax, Rex, p21X-III, p12 and others) by altering the reading frame and by alternate splicing of the gene. However, in HTLV-I associated lymphomas, the only viral gene product that is universally detected is Tax, a 40-kDa protein that is mainly present in the nucleus. Tax seems highly likely to be the major HTLV-I gene involved in the pathogenesis of the HTLV-I-associated diseases, but unlike chronic myeloid leukemia and some other diseases in which expression of the causative gene product in transgenic mice elicits a disease similar to that seen in people, transgenic mice carrying the tax gene develop mesenchymal tumors.[125]

The initial function described for Tax was as a transactivator of viral gene expression. However, subsequent study has revealed pleiotropic effects of tax expression. Although a wide range of biological effects can be controlled by Tax, it remains a mystery as to which particular functions lead to neoplasia or to neurologic disease and why those manifestations occur so rarely and in the particular individuals in whom they occur. Four sets of biological activities have been identified for tax: transcriptional activation, transcriptional repression, inhibition of tumor-suppressor proteins, and possibly the promotion of DNA instability. Tax can bind to cyclic AMP response element-binding protein (CREB), NF-κB, and serum response factor (SRF), promoting viral replication, production of cytokines, cell proliferation, and prevention of cell death. Tax can also interfere with transcription; target genes for this effect include the cyclin-dependent kinase inhibitor p18, p53, Bax, a proapoptotic protein, and DNA polymerase β, an enzyme involved in DNA repair. Tax can also directly bind to and inhibit cyclin-dependent kinase inhibitors such as p15 and p16, which are considered tumor-suppressor genes because of their blocking effects on cell cycle progression.

Thus, Tax has a myriad of effects on the cell. It remains unclear which of its many effects are critical to cell transformation. It is also unclear whether some of these effects are more important than others and what keeps them from happening all the time in Tax-carrying cells. The implication is that Tax alone is insufficient to initiate the full cascade of its biological functions. Host factors may also play a role, but what they are is not yet defined.

Human Herpesvirus-8

Also known as Kaposi sarcoma-associated herpes virus, human herpesvirus-8 (HHV-8) is a γ2-herpesvirus of the *Rhadinovirus* family and the first member of that family known to infect people.[126] It has been linked causally to all forms of Kaposi sarcoma, AIDS-associated primary effusion lymphoma, and multicentric Castleman disease. HHV8 is necessary but probably insufficient to cause any of these conditions by itself; in addition to immune deficiency, other cofactors are probably necessary but they have not been defined.[127]

HHV-8 is related to Epstein-Barr virus. It is a double-stranded DNA virus that encodes 80 to 90 genes. Many of its genes are homologues of cellular genes involved in inflammation (cytokines and chemokines and their receptors), cell-cycle regulation and angiogenesis. A viral version of cyclin D is seen in primary effusion lymphoma and in Kaposi sarcoma tumors.[128] The virus seems to be equipped to avoid the apoptosis of the host cell and to foster the generation of new blood vessels. It has a number of mechanisms for avoiding the host response and for interfering with attempts to eliminate the infected cell. A viral open reading frame represses p53 transcriptional activity and apoptosis.[129] The biology of the virus remains at the descriptive stage. Much excitement has been generated over what the virus can do.[130] Not enough work has been focused on what it actually does and must do to induce neoplasia.

FAMILIAL DISEASES ASSOCIATED WITH LYMPHOMA

Many of the familial disorders associated with lymphoma are primary immune deficiency diseases. The lymphomas that occur in this setting are heterogeneous. Those associated with profound defects in T-cell function, such as X-linked lymphoproliferative disease or Duncan syndrome and DiGeorge syndrome (thymic aplasia), are usually caused by a failure of immune surveillance to control Epstein-Barr virus.[131] Those associated with defects in DNA repair mechanisms, such as ataxia telangiectasia and Bloom syndrome, develop lymphomas with multiple chromosomal abnormalities and deletions.[132] Autoimmune lymphoproliferative syndrome (ALPS) or Canale-Smith syndrome is an immune defect characterized by defective apoptosis, usually as a consequence of Fas mutations; 10 people among 130 members of 8 families were described to develop B- (including Hodgkin disease) and T-cell lymphomas that were not Epstein-Barr virus related.[133] Thus, inability of lymphocytes to undergo apoptosis is also a risk factor for lymphoma. The individual pathophysiology of the inherited condition must be considered to understand the associated risk. Not all inherited immune diseases lead to Epstein-Barr virus-caused cancers.

Other familial syndromes are associated with an increased risk of lymphoid tumors. A search of Mendelian Inheritance in Man (MIM), available through PubMed, reveals 291 matches when lymphoma diagnoses are searched. Familial forms of the major disease categories have been known for many years. Epidemiologic studies have found that a history of lymphoma in the family increases the risk of lymphoma about threefold.[134–137] However, systematic investigation of familial clusters of lymphoid malignancies has not yielded insights about the pathogenesis of lymphoid tumors. No new lymphoma genes have been found. Unlike other cancers, little insight into the nature of lymphomagenesis has yet to emerge from family studies.

Many readers may find useful a special issue of *Nature Genetics,* published in April 1997, in which Mitelman, Mertens, and Johansson compiled a breakpoint map of recurrent chromosomal rearrangements in human neoplasia (vol 15, pages 417–474).

REFERENCES

1. Greenlee RT, Hill-Harmon MB, Murray T, Thun M: Cancer statistics, 2001. *CA Cancer J Clin* **51**:15, 2001.
2. Devesa SS, Fears T: Non-Hodgkin's lymphoma time trends: United States and international data. *Cancer Res* **52**:5432s, 1992.
3. Jaffe ES, Harris NL, Stein H, Vardiman JW (eds): , *World Health Organization Classification of Tumours. Pathology and Genetics of Tumours of Haematopoietic and Lymphoid Tissues.* Lyon, France, IARC Press, 2001.
4. Alizadeh AA, Eisen MB, Davis RE, et al: Distinct types of diffuse large B-cell lymphoma identified by gene expression profiling. *Nature* **403**:503, 2000.
5. Damle RN, Wasil T, Fais F, et al: IgV gene mutation status and CD38 expression as novel prognostic indicators in chronic lymphocytic leukemia. *Blood* **94**:1840, 1999.
6. Hamblin TJ, Davis Z, Gardiner A, Oscier DG, Stevenson FK: Unmutated IgV(H) genes are associated with a more aggressive form of chronic lymphocytic leukemia. *Blood* **94**:1848, 1999.
7. Wang JH, Nichogiannopoulou A, Wu L, et al: Selective defects in the development of the fetal and adult lymphoid system in mice with an Ikaros null mutation. *Immunity* **5**:537, 1996.
8. Scott EW, Simon MC, Anastasi J, Singh H: Requirement of transcription factor PU.1 in the development of multiple hematopoietic lineages. *Science* **258**:1573, 1994.
9. Zuang Y, Soriano P, Weintraub H: The helix-loop-helix gene E2A is required for B cell formation. *Cell* **79**:885, 1994.
10. Bain G, Robanus Maandag EC, te Reile AJ, et al: Both E12 and E47 all commitment to the B cell lineage. *Immunity* **6**:145, 1997.
11. Lin H, Grosshedl R: Failure of B-cell differentiation in mice lacking the transcription factor EBF. *Nature* **376**:263, 1995.
12. Urbanek P, Wang ZQ, Fetka I, Wagner EF, Busslinger M: Complete block in early B cell differentiation and altered patterning of the posterior midbrain in mice lacking Pax5/BSAP. *Cell* **79**:901, 1994.
13. Schilham MW, Oosterwegel MA, Moerer P, et al: Defects in cardiac outflow tract formation and pro-B-lymphocyte expansion in mice lacking Sox-4. *Nature* **380**:711, 1996.
14. Chiang MY, Monroe JG: BSAP/Pax5a expression blocks survival and expansion of early myeloid cells implicating its involvement in maintaining commitment to the B-lymphocyte lineage. *Blood* **94**:3621, 1999.
15. Minegishi Y, Coustan-Smith E, Wang YH, Cooper MD, Campana D, Conley ME: Mutations in the human lambda 5/14.1 gene result in B-cell deficiency and agammaglobulinemia. *J Exp Med* **187**:71, 1998.
16. Fugmann SD, Lee AI, Shockett PE, Villey IJ, Schatz DG: The RAG proteins and V(D)J recombination: Complexes, ends, and transposition. *Annu Rev Immunol* **18**:495, 2000.
17. Ernst P, Smale ST: Combinatorial regulation of transcription II. The immunoglobulin mu heavy chain gene. *Immunity* **2**:427, 1995.
18. Goodnow CC, Crosbie J, Adelstein S, et al: Altered immunoglobulin expression and functional silencing of self-reactive B lymphocytes in transgenic mice. *Nature* **334**:676, 1988.
19. Chen C, Nagy Z, Prak EL, Weigert M: Immunoglobulin heavy chain gene replacement Ba mechanism of receptor editing. *Immunity* **3**:747, 1995.
20. Borrello MA, Palis J, Phipps RP: The relationship of CD5+ B lymphocytes to macrophages: Insights from normal biphenotypic B/macrophage cells. *Int Rev Immunol* **20**:137, 2001.
21. Cyster JG: Signaling thresholds and interclonal competition in preimmune B-cell selection. *Immunol Rev* **156**:87, 1997.
22. Liu Y-J, Arpin C: Germinal center development. *Immunol Rev* **156**:111, 1997.
23. Hardy RR, Hayakawa K: B-cell development pathways. *Annu Rev Immunol* **19**:595, 2001.
24. Kosco-Vilbois MH, Bonnefoy J-Y, Chvatchko Y: The physiology of murine germinal center reactions. *Immunol Rev* **156**:127, 1997.
25. Dent AL, Shaffer AL, Yu X, et al: Control of inflammation, cytokine expression, and germinal center formation by BCL-6. *Science* **276**:589, 1997.
26. Ting CN, Olson MC, Barton KP, Leiden, JM: Transcription factor GATA-3 is required for the development of the T-cell lineage. *Nature* **384**:474, 1996.
27. Radtke F, Wilson A, Stark M, et al: Deficient T cell fate specification in mice with an induced inactivation of Notch1. *Immunity* **10**:547, 1999.
28. MacDonald HR, Wilson A, Radtke F: Notch1 and T-cell development: Insights from conditional knockout mice. *Trends Immunol* **22**:155, 2001.
29. Heemskerk MH, Blom B, Nolan G, et al: Inhibition of T cell and promotion of natural killer cell development by the dominant negative helix-loop-helix factor Id3. *J Exp Med* **186**:1597, 1997.
30. VonBoehmer H: The developmental biology of T lymphocytes. *Annu Rev Immunol* **6**:309, 1993.
31. Nunez G, Seto M, Seremetis S, et al: Growth- and tumor-promoting effects of deregulated Bcl2 in human B-lymphoblastoid cells. *Proc Natl Acad Sci U S A* **86**:4589, 1989.
32. Liu Y, Hernandez AM, Shibata D, Cortopassi GA: Bcl2 translocation frequency rises with age in humans. *Proc Natl Acad Sci U S A* **91**:8910, 1994.
33. Wang J, Raffeld M, Medeiros LJ, et al: Follicular center cell lymphoma with the t(14;18) translocation in which the Bcl2 gene is silent. *Leukemia* **7**:1834, 1993.
34. Baron BW, Nucifora G, McNabe N, et al: Identification of the gene associated with the recurring chromosomal translocations t(3;14) (q27;q32) and t (3;22)(q27;q11) in B-cell lymphomas. *Proc Natl Acad Sci U S A* **90**:5262, 1993.
35. Cattoretti G, Chang C, Cechova K, et al: Bcl-6 protein is expressed in germinal center B cells. *Blood* **86**:45, 1995.
36. Sander CA, Yano T, Clark HM, et al: p53 mutation is associated with progression in follicular lymphoma. *Blood* **82**:1994, 1993.
37. Alizadeh AA, Eisen MB, Davis RE, et al: Identification of molecularly and clinically distinct types of diffuse large B-cell lymphoma by gene expression profiling. *Nature* **403**:503, 2000.
38. Bakhshi A, Jensen JP, Goldman P, et al: Cloning the chromosomal breakpoint of t(14;18) of human lymphomas: Clustering around *JH* on chromosome 14 and near a transcriptional unit on 18. *Cell* **41**:889, 1985.
39. Chao DT, Korsmeyer SJ: Bcl-2 family: regulators of cell death. *Annu Rev Immunol* **16**:395, 1998.

40. Srivastava RK, Sasaki CY, Hardwick JM, Longo DL: Bcl-2-mediated drug resistance: Inhibition of apoptosis by blocking nuclear factor of activated T-lymphocytes (NFAT)-induced Fas ligand transcription. *J Exp Med* **190**:253, 1999.

41. McDonnel TJ, Korsmeyer SJ: Progression from lymphoid hyperplasia to high-grade malignant lymphoma in mice transgenic for the t(14;18). *Nature* **349**:254, 1991.

42. Tilly H, Rossi A, Stamatoulias A, et al: Prognostic value of chromosomal abnormalities in follicular lymphoma. *Blood* **84**:1043, 1994.

43. Pinyol M, Cobo F, Bea S, et al: p16(INK4a) gene inactivation by deletions, mutations, and hypermethylation is associated with transformed and aggressive variants of non-Hodgkin's lymphomas. *Blood* **91**:2977, 1998.

44. Wotherspoon AC, Ortiz-Hidalgo C, Falzon MR, Isaacson PG: *Helicobacter pylori*-associated gastritis and primary B-cell gastric lymphoma. *Lancet* **338**:1175, 1991.

45. Kassan SS, Thomas TL, Moutsopoulos HM, et al: Increased risk of lymphoma in sicca syndrome. *Ann Intern Med* **89**:888, 1978.

46. Kato I, Tajima K, Suchi T, et al: Chronic thyroiditis as a risk factor for B-cell lymphoma of the thyroid gland. *Jpn J Cancer Res* **76**:1085, 1985.

47. Cerroni L, Zochling N, Putz B, Kerl H: Infection by *Borrelia burgdorferi* and cutaneous B-cell lymphoma. *J Cutan Pathol* **24**:457, 1997.

48. Price SK: Immunoproliferative small intestinal disease: A study of 13 cases with alpha heavy chain disease. *Histopathology* **17**:7, 1990.

49. Wotherspoon AC, Finn TM, Isaacson PG: Trisomy 3 in low-grade B-cell lymphomas of mucosa-associated lymphoid tissue. *Blood* **85**:2000, 1995.

50. Ott G, Katzenberger T, Greiner A, et al: The t(11;18)(q21;q21) chromosome translocation is a frequent and specific aberration in low-grade but not high-grade malignant non-Hodgkin's lymphoma of the mucosa-associated lymphoid tissue (MALT)-type. *Cancer Res* **57**:3944, 1997.

51. Dierlamm J, Baens M, Wlodarska I, et al: The apoptosis inhibitor gene API2 and a novel 18q gene, MLT, are recurrently rearranged in the t(11;18)(q21;q21) associated with mucosa-associated lymphoid tissue lymphoma. *Blood* **93**:3601, 1999.

52. Liu H, Ruskon-Fourmestraux A, Lavergne-Slove A, et al: Resistance of t(11;18) positive gastric mucosal-associated lymphoid tissue lymphoma to *Helicobacter pylori* eradication therapy. *Lancet* **357**:39, 2001.

53. Barth TFE, Bentz M, Dohner H, Moller P: Molecular aspects of B-cell lymphomas of the gastrointestinal tract. *Clin Lymphoma* **2**:57, 2001.

54. Gaidano G, Volpe G, Pastore C, et al: Detection of bcl6 rearrangements and p53 mutations in MALT lymphomas. *Am J Hematol* **56**:206, 1997.

55. Willis TG, Jadayel DM, Du MQ, et al: Bcl10 is involved in t(1;14)(p22;q32) of MALT B cell lymphoma and mutated in multiple tumor types. *Cell* **96**:35, 1999.

56. Bookman MA, Lardelli P, Jaffe ES, Duffey PL, Longo DL: Lymphocytic lymphoma of intermediate differentiation: Morphologic, immunophenotypic and prognostic factors. *J Natl Cancer Inst* **82**:742, 1990.

57. Jiang W, Kahn SM, Zhou P, et al: Overexpression of cyclin D1 in rat fibroblasts causes abnormalities in growth control, cell cycle progression and gene expression. *Oncogene* **8**:3447, 1993.

58. Bodrug S, Warner B, Bath M, et al: Cyclin D1 transgene impedes lymphocyte maturation and collaborates with the myc gene. *EMBO J* **13**:2124, 1994.

59. Dalla-Favera R, Martinotti S, Gallo RC, Erikson J, Croce CM: Translocation and rearrangements of the c-myc oncogene in human undifferentiated B-cell lymphomas. *Science* **219**:963, 1982.

60. Pelicci PG, Knowles DK, Magrath I, Dalla-Favera R: Chromosomal breakpoints and structural alterations of the c-myc locus differ in sporadic and endemic forms of Burkitt's lymphoma. *Proc Natl Acad Sci U S A* **83**:2984, 1986.

61. Gu W, Bhatia K, Magrath IT, Dang CV, Dalla-Favera R: Binding and suppression of the c-Myc transcriptional activation domain by p107. *Science* **264**:251, 1994.

62. Gaidano G, Hauptschein RS, Parsa NZ, et al: Deletions involving two distinct regions of 6q in B-cell non-Hodgkin's lymphoma. *Blood* **80**:1781, 1992.

63. Komano J, Maruo S, Kuozumi K, Oda T, Takada K: Oncogenic role of Epstein-Barr virus-encoded RNAs in Burkitt's lymphoma cell line Akata. *J Virol* **73**:9827, 1999.

64. Pinkus GS, O'Hara CJ, Said JW, et al: Peripheral/post-thymic T-cell lymphomas: A spectrum of disease. Clinical, pathologic, and immunologic features of 78 cases. *Cancer* **65**:971, 1990.

65. Lepretre S, Buchonnet G, Stamatoulias A, et al: Chromosome abnormalities in peripheral T-cell lymphoma. *Cancer Genet Cytogenet* **117**:71, 2000.

66. Russo G, Isobe M, Gatti R, et al: Molecular analysis of a t(14;14) translocation in leukemic T-cells of an ataxia telangiectasia patient. *Proc Natl Acad Sci U S A* **86**:602, 1989.

67. Stern MH, Soulier J, Rosenzwajg M, et al: MTCP-1: A novel gene on human chromosome Xq28 translocated to the T cell receptor alpha/delta locus in mature T cell proliferations. *Oncogene* **8**:2475, 1993.

68. Virgilio L, Lazzeri C, Bichi B, et al: Deregulated expression of TCL1 causes T cell leukemia in mice. *Proc Natl Acad Sci U S A* **95**:3885, 1998.

69. Griti C, Dastot H, Soulier J, et al: Transgenic mice for MTCP1 develop T-cell prolymphocytic leukemia. *Blood* **92**:368, 1998.

70. Sorour A, Brito-Babapulle V, Smedley D, Yuille M, Catovsky D: Unusual breakpoint distribution of 8p abnormalities in T-prolymphocytic leukemia: A study with YACS mapping to 8p11-12. *Cancer Genet Cytogenet* **121**:128, 2000.

71. Stilgenbauer S, Schaffner C, Litterst A, et al: Biallelic mutations in the ATM gene in T-prolymphocytic leukemia. *Nat Med* **3**:1155, 1997.

72. Vorechovsky I, Luo L, Dyer MJ, et al: Clustering of missense mutations in the ataxia-telangiectasia gene in a sporadic T-cell leukemia. *Nat Genet* **17**:96, 1997.

73. Foss HD, Anagnostopoulos I, Araujo I, et al: Anaplastic large-cell lymphomas of T-cell and null-cell phenotype express cytotoxic molecules. *Blood* **88**:4005, 1996.

74. Morris SW, Kirstein MN, Valentine MB, et al: Fusion of a kinase gene, ALK, to a nucleolar protein gene, NPM, in non-Hodgkin's lymphoma. *Science* **263**:1281, 1994.

75. Kuefer MU, Look AT, Pulford K: Retrovirus-mediated gene transfer of NPM/ALK causes lymphoid malignancy in mice. *Blood* **90**:2901, 1997.

76. Touriol C, Greenland C, Lamant L, et al: Further demonstration of the diversity of chromosomal changes involving 2p23 in ALK-positive lymphoma: 2 cases expressing ALK kinase fused to CLTCL (clathrin chain polypeptide-like). *Blood* **95**:3204, 2000.

77. Kanavaros P, Gaulard P, Charlotte F, et al: Discordant expression of immunoglobulin and its associated molecule mb-1/CD79a is frequently found in mediastinal large B cell lymphomas. *Am J Pathol* **146**:735, 1995.

78. Joos S, Otano-Joos MI, Ziegler S, et al: Primary mediastinal (thymic) B-cell lymphoma is characterized by gains of chromosomal material including 9p and amplification of the *REL* gene. *Blood* **87**:1571, 1996.

79. Copie-Bergman C, Gaulard P, Maouche-Chretein L, et al: The *MAL* gene is expressed in primary mediastinal large B-cell lymphoma. *Blood* **94**:3567, 1999.

80. Chan CH, Hadlock KG, Foung SK, Levy S: V(H)1-69 gene is preferentially used by hepatitis C virus-associated B cell lymphomas and by normal B cells responding to the E2 viral antigen. *Blood* **97**:1023, 2001.

81. Iida S, Rao PH, Mallasivam P, et al: The t(9;14)(p13;q32) chromosomal translocation associated with lymphoplasmacytoid lymphoma involves the PAX-5 gene. *Blood* **88**:4110, 1996.

82. Stein H, Marafioti T, Foss HD, et al: Down-regulation of BOB.1/OBF.1 and Oct-2 in classical Hodgkin disease but not in lymphocyte predominant Hodgkin disease correlates with immunoglobulin transcription. *Blood* **97**:496, 2001.

83. Braeuninger A, Kuppers R, Strickler JG, et al: Hodgkin and Reed-Sternberg cells in lymphocyte predominant Hodgkin disease represent clonal populations of germinal center derived tumor B cells. *Proc Natl Acad Sci U S A* **94**:9337, 1997.

84. Marafioti T, Hummel M, Anagnostopoulos I, et al: Origin of nodular lymphocyte-predominant Hodgkin's disease from a clonal expansion of highly mutated germinal center B cells. *N Engl J Med* **337**:453, 1997.

85. Wickert RS, Weisenburger DD, Tierens A, Greiner TC, Chan WC: Clonal relationship between lymphocyte predominance Hodgkin's disease and concurrent or subsequent large-cell lymphoma of B lineage. *Blood* **86**:2312, 1995.

86. Marafioti T, Hummel M, Foss HD, et al: Hodgkin and Reed-Sternberg cells represent an expansion of a single clone originating from a germinal center B-cell with functional immunoglobulin gene rearrangements but defective immunoglobulin transcription. *Blood* **95**:1443, 2000.

87. Seitz V, Hummel M, Marafioti T, et al: Detection of clonal T-cell receptor gamma-chain gene rearrangements in Reed-Sternberg cells of classic Hodgkin disease. *Blood* **95**:3020, 2000.

88. Schlegelberger B, Weber-Matthiesen K, Himmler A, et al: Cytogenetic findings and results of combined immunophenotyping and karyotyping in Hodgkin's disease. *Leukemia* **8**:72, 1994.

89. Joos S, Kupper M, Ohl S, et al: Genomic imbalances including amplification of the tyrosine kinase gene, JAK2 in CD30+ Hodgkin cells. *Cancer Res* **60**:549, 2000.

90. Ibrahim S, Keating M, Do KA, et al: CD38 expression as an important prognostic factor in B-cell chronic lymphocytic leukemia. *Blood* **98**:181, 2001.

91. Juliusson G, Oscier DG, Fitchett M, et al: Prognostic subgroups in B-cell chronic lymphocytic leukemia defined by specific chromosomal abnormalities. *N Engl J Med* **323**:720, 1990.

92. Brown AG, Ross FM, Dunne EM, Steel CM, Weir-Thompson EM: Evidence for a new tumor suppressor locus (DBM) in human B-cell neoplasia telomeric to the retinoblastoma gene. *Nat Genet* **3**:67, 1993.

93. Mabuchi H, Fujii H, Calin G, et al: Cloning and characterization of CLLD6, CLLD7, and CLLD8, novel candidate genes for leukemogenesis at chromosome 13q14, a region commonly deleted in B-cell chronic lymphocytic leukemia. *Cancer Res* **61**:2870, 2001.

94. Gaidano G, Ballerini P, Gong JZ, et al: p53 mutations in human lymphoid malignancies: Association with Burkitt lymphoma and chronic lymphocytic leukemia. *Proc Natl Acad Sci U S A* **88**:5413, 1991.

95. Offit K, Louie DC, Parsa NZ, et al: Clinical and morphologic features of B-cell small lymphocytic lymphoma with del(6)(q21q23). *Blood* **83**:2611, 1994.

96. Rubnitz JE, Pui CH, Downing JR: The role of TEK fusion genes in pediatric leukemias. *Leukemia* **13**:6, 1999.

97. Golub TR, Barker GF, Lovett M, Gilliland DG: Fusion of PDGF receptor beta to a novel ets-like gene, tel, in chronic myelomonocytic leukemia with t(5;12) chromosomal translocation. *Cell* **77**:307, 1994.

98. Papadopoulos P, Ridge SA, Boucher CA, Stocking C, Wiedemann LM: The novel activation of ABL by fusion to an ets-related gene, TEL. *Cancer Res* **55**:34, 1995.

99. Downing JR: The AML1-ETO chimaeric transcription factor in acute myeloid leukaemia: Biology and clinical significance. *Br J Haematol* **106**:296, 1999.

100. Kitabayashi I, Yokoyama A, Simizu K, Ohki M: Interaction and functional cooperation of the leukemia-associated factors AML1 and p300 in myeloid cell differentiation. *EMBO J* **17**:2994, 1998.

101. Hiebert SW, Sun W, Davis JN, et al: The t(12;21) translocation converts AML-1B from an activator to a repressor of transcription. *Mol Cell Biol* **16**:1349, 1996.

102. Raynaud S, Cave H, Baens M, et al: The 12;21 translocation involving TEL and deletion of the other TEL allele: Two frequently associated alterations found in childhood acute lymphoblastic leukemia. *Blood* **87**:2891, 1996.

103. Hunger SP, Tkachuk DC, Amylon MD, et al: HRX involvement in de novo and secondary leukemias with diverse chromosome 11q23 abnormalities. *Blood* **81**:3197, 1993.

104. Rowley JD: The der(11) chromosome contains the critical breakpoint junction in the 4;11, 9;11, and 11;19 translocations in acute leukemia. *Genes Chromosomes Cancer* **5**:264, 1992.

105. Greaves MF: Infant leukaemia: Biology, aetiology and treatment. *Leukemia* **10**:372, 1996.

106. Parkin JL, Arthur DC, Abramson CS, et al: Acute leukemia associated with the t(4;11) chromosome rearrangement: Ultrastructural and immunologic characteristics. *Blood* **60**:1321, 1982.

107. Van Dijk MA, Voorhoeve PM, Murre C: Pbx1 is converted into a transcriptional activator upon acquiring the N-terminal region of E1A in pre-B-cell acute lymphoblastoid leukemia. *Proc Natl Acad Sci U S A* **90**:6061, 1993.

108. Hunger SP, Ohyashiki K, Toyama K, Cleary ML: Hlf, a novel hepatic bZIP protein, shows altered DNA-binding properties following fusion to E2A in t(17;19) acute lymphoblastic leukemia. *Genes Dev* **6**:1608, 1992.

109. Inukai T, Inaba T, Ikushima S, Look AT: The AD1 and AD2 transactivation domains of E2A are essential for the antiapoptotic activity of the chimeric oncoprotein E2A-HLF. *Mol Cell Biol* **18**:6035, 1998.

110. Sawyers CL: Chronic myeloid leukemia. *N Engl J Med* **340**:1330, 1999.

111. Okuda T, Fisher R, Downing JR: Molecular diagnostics in pediatric acute lymphoblastic leukemia. *Mol Diagn* **1**:139, 1996.

112. Drexler HG: Review of alterations of the cyclin-dependent kinase inhibitor INK4 family genes p15, p16, p18 and p19 in human leukemia-lymphoma cells. *Leukemia* **12**:845, 1998.

113. Druker BJ, Sawyers CL, Kantarjian H, et al: Activity of a specific inhibitor of the BCR-ABL tyrosine kinase in the blast crisis of chronic myeloid leukemia and acute lymphoblastic leukemia with the Philadelphia chromosome. *N Engl J Med* **344**:1038, 2001.

114. Bakkus MH, Heirman C, Van R, et al: Evidence that multiple myeloma Ig heavy chain VDJ genes contain somatic mutations but show no intraclonal variation. *Blood* **80**:2326, 1992.

115. Liu P, Leong T, Quam L, et al: Activating mutations of N- and K-ras in multiple myeloma show different clinical associations: Analysis of the Eastern Oncology Group Phase III Trial. *Blood* **88**:2699, 1996.

116. Konigsberg R, Zojer N, Ackermann J, et al: Predictive role of interphase cytogenetics for survival of patients with multiple myeloma. *J Clin Oncol* **18**:804, 2000.

117. Bergsagel PL, Chesi MC, Nardini E, Brents LA, Kirby SL, Kuehl WM: Promiscuous translocations into immunoglobulin heavy chain switch regions in multiple myeloma. *Proc Natl Acad Sci U S A* **93**:13931, 1996.

118. Sawyer JR, Lukacs JL, Munshi N, et al: Identification of new nonrandom translocations in multiple myeloma with multicolor spectral karyotyping. *Blood* **92**:4269, 1998.

119. Lai JL, Zandecki M, Mary JY, et al: Improved cytogenetics in multiple myeloma: A study of 151 patients including 117 patients at diagnosis. *Blood* **85**:2490, 1995.

120. Cohen JI: Epstein-Barr virus infection. *N Engl J Med* **343**:3309, 2000.

121. Wang D, Liebowitz D, Kieff E: An EBV membrane protein expressed in immortalized lymphocytes transforms established rodent cells. *Cell* **43**:831, 1985.

122. Liebowitz D: Epstein-Barr virus and a cellular signaling pathway in lymphomas from immunosuppressed patients. *N Engl J Med* **338**:1413, 1998.

123. Blayney DW, Jaffe ES, Blattner WA, et al: The human T-cell leukemia/lymphoma virus associated with American adult T-cell leukemia/lymphoma. *Blood* **62**:401, 1983.

124. Yoshida M: Multiple viral strategies of HTLV-1 for dysregulation of cell growth control. *Annu Rev Immunol* **19**:475, 2001.

125. Nerenberg M, Hinrichs SH, Reynolds RK, Khoury G, Jay G: The tax gene of human T-lymphotropic virus type I induces mesenchymal tumors in transgenic mice. *Science* **237**:1324, 1987.

126. Cannon M, Cesarman E: Kaposi's sarcoma-associated herpes virus and acquired immunodeficiency syndrome-related malignancy. *Semin Oncol* **27**:409, 2000.

127. Kedes DH, Operskalski E, Busch M, et al: The seroepidemiology of human herpesvirus 8 (Kaposi's sarcoma-associated herpesvirus): distribution of infection in KS risk groups and evidence for sexual transmission. *Nat Med* **2**:918, 1996.

128. Cesarman E, Nador RG, Bai F, et al: Kaposi's sarcoma-associated herpesvirus contains G-protein-coupled receptor and cyclin D homologs which are expressed in Kaposi's sarcoma and malignant lymphoma. *J Virol* **70**:8218, 1996.

129. Gwack Y, Hwang S, Byun H, et al: Kaposi's sarcoma-associated herpesvirus open reading frame 50 represses p53-induced transcriptional activity and apoptosis. *J Virol* **75**:6245, 2001.

130. Boshoff C, Weiss RA: Epidemiology and pathogenesis of Kaposi's sarcoma-associated herpesvirus. *Phil Trans R Soc Lond B* **356**:517, 2001.

131. Purtilo DT, Strobach RS, Okano M, Davis JR: Epstein-Barr-virus-associated lymphoproliferative disorders. *Lab Invest* **67**:5, 1992.

132. Elenitoba-Johnson KS, Jaffe ES: Lymphoproliferative disorders associated with congenital immunodeficiencies. *Semin Diagn Pathol* **14**:35, 1997.

133. Straus SE, Jaffe ES, Puck JM, et al: The development of lymphomas in families with autoimmune lymphoproliferative syndrome with germ-line Fas mutations and defective lymphocyte apoptosis. *Blood* **98**:194, 2001.

134. Shpilberg O, Modan M, Modan B, Chetrit A, Fuchs Z, Ramot B: Familial aggregation of haematological neoplasms: A controlled study. *Br J Haematol* **87**:75, 1994.

135. Zhu K, Levine RS, Gu Y, et al: Non-Hodgkin's lymphoma and family history of malignant tumors in a case-control study (United States). *Cancer Causes Control* **9**:77, 1998.

136. Brown LM, Linet MS, Greenberg RS, et al: Multiple myeloma and family history of cancer among blacks and whites in the US. *Cancer* **85**:2385, 1999.

137. Paltiel O, Schmit T, Adler B, et al: The incidence of lymphoma in first-degree relatives of patients with Hodgkin disease and non-Hodgkin lymphoma: results and limitations of a registry-linked study. *Cancer* **88**:2357, 2000.

Page numbers followed by an "f" indicate figures; numbers followed by a "t" indicate tables.